Whittington Health

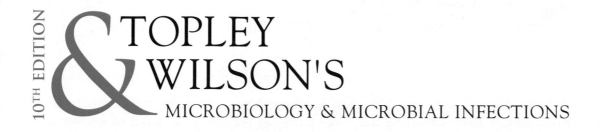

10TH EDITION

&TOPLEY &WILSON'S
MICROBIOLOGY & MICROBIAL INFECTIONS

VIROLOGY
VOLUME 2

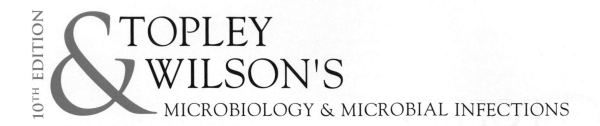

10ᵀᴴ EDITION

&TOPLEY WILSON'S

MICROBIOLOGY & MICROBIAL INFECTIONS

Topley & Wilson's Microbiology and Microbial Infections has grown from one to eight volumes since first published in 1929, reflecting the ever-increasing breadth and depth of knowledge in each of the areas covered. This tenth edition continues the tradition of providing the most comprehensive reference to microorganisms and the resulting infectious diseases currently available. It forms a unique resource, with each volume including examples of the best writing and research in the fields of virology, bacteriology, medical mycology, parasitology, and immunology from around the globe.

www.topleyandwilson.com

VIROLOGY Volumes 1 and 2

Edited by Brian W.J. Mahy and Volker ter Meulen
Volume 1 ISBN 0 340 88561 0; Volume 2 ISBN 0 340 88562 9; 2 volume set ISBN 0 340 88563 7

BACTERIOLOGY Volumes 1 and 2

Edited by S. Peter Borriello, Patrick R. Murray, and Guido Funke
Volume 1 ISBN 0 340 88564 5; Volume 2 ISBN 0 340 88565 3; 2 volume set ISBN 0 340 88566 1

MEDICAL MYCOLOGY

Edited by William G. Merz and Roderick J. Hay
ISBN 0 340 88567 X

PARASITOLOGY

Edited by F.E.G. Cox, Derek Wakelin, Stephen H. Gillespie, and Dickson D. Despommier
ISBN 0 340 88568 8

IMMUNOLOGY

Edited by Stephan H.E. Kaufmann and Michael W. Steward
ISBN 0 340 88569 6

Cumulative index

ISBN 0 340 88570 X

8 volume set plus CD-ROM

ISBN 0 340 80912 4

CD-ROM only

ISBN 0 340 88560 2

For a full list of contents, please see the *Complete table of contents* on page 1759

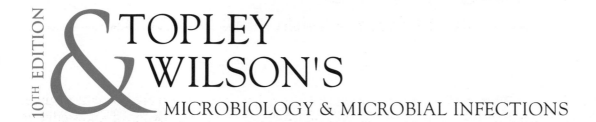

VIROLOGY

VOLUME 2

EDITED BY

Brian W.J. Mahy MA PhD ScD DSc
Senior Scientific Research Advisor, National Center for Infectious Diseases
Centers for Disease Control and Prevention, Atlanta, GA, USA

Volker ter Meulen MD
Professor Emeritus of Clinical Virology and Immunology
Former Chairman of the Institute for Virology and Immunobiology
University of Würzburg, Würzburg, Germany

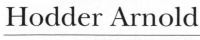

Hodder Arnold
A MEMBER OF THE HODDER HEADLINE GROUP

ASM
PRESS

First published in Great Britain in 1929
Second edition 1936; Third edition 1946
Fourth edition 1955; Fifth edition 1964; Sixth edition 1975
Seventh edition 1983 and 1984; Eighth edition 1990
Ninth edition 1998.
This tenth edition published in 2005 by
Hodder Arnold, an imprint of Hodder Education and a member of the Hodder Headline Group,
338 Euston Road, London NW1 3BH

http://www.hoddereducation.com

Distributed in the United States of America by ASM Press, the book publishing division of the American Society for Microbiology, 1752 N Street, N.W. Washington, D.C. 20036, USA

Hodder Headline's policy is to use papers that are natural, renewable and recyclable products and made from wood grown in sustainable forests. The logging and manufacturing processes are expected to conform to the environmental regulations of the country of origin.

Whilst the advice and information in this book are believed to be true and accurate at the date of going to press, neither the author[s] nor the publisher can accept any legal responsibility or liability for any errors or omissions that may be made. In particular (but without limiting the generality of the preceding disclaimer) every effort has been made to check drug dosages; however it is still possible that errors have been missed. Furthermore, dosage schedules are constantly being revised and new side-effects recognized. For these reasons the reader is strongly urged to consult the drug companies' printed instructions before administering any of the drugs recommended in this book.

British Library Cataloguing in Publication Data
A catalogue record for this book is available from the British Library

Library of Congress Cataloging-in-Publication Data
A catalog record for this book is available from the Library of Congress

Volume 1 ISBN-10   0 340 885 610   ISBN-13 978 0 340 88561 1
Volume 2 ISBN-10   0 340 885 629   ISBN-13 978 0 340 88562 8
Two volume set ISBN-10 0 340 885 637   ISBN-13 978 0 340 88563 5
Complete set and CD-ROM ISBN-10   0340 80912 4   ISBN-13   978 0 340 80912 9
Indian edtion ISBN-10   0 340 88559 9   ISBN-13   978 0 340 88559 8

1 2 3 4 5 6 7 8 9 10

Commissioning Editor: Serena Bureau / Joanna Koster
Development Editor: Layla Vandenberg
Project Editor: Zelah Pengilley
Production Controller: Deborah Smith
Cover Designer: Sarah Rees
Cover image: Herpes simplex virus, TEM. Dr. Linda Stannard, UCT / Science Photo Library

Typeset in 9/11 Times New Roman by Lucid Digital, Salisbury, UK
Printed and bound in Italy

What do you think about this book? Or any other Hodder Arnold title? Please send your comments to www.hoddereducation.com

Contents

Please note: Chapter names shown in gray can be found in Virology Volume 1

Contributors

Adriano Aguzzi MD PHD hcFRCP FRCPATH
Institute of Neuropathology
University Hospital of Zürich
Zürich, Switzerland

Antonio Alcami PHD
Department of Medicine
University of Cambridge
Addenbrooke's Hospital, Cambridge, UK; and
Centro Nacional de Biotecnologia (CSIC)
Campus Universidad Autónoma
Madrid, Spain

L. Andrew Ball DPHIL
Professor of Microbiology
University of Alabama at Birmingham
Birmingham, AL, USA

Jangu E. Banatvala CBE MA MD FRCP FRCPATH
FMEDSCI
Emeritus Professor of Clinical Virology
Guy's, King's and St Thomas' Medical
and Dental School
London, UK

Bettina Bankamp PHD
Measles, Mumps, Rubella and Herpes Team
Respiratory and Enteric Viruses Branch
Division of Viral and Rickettsial Diseases
National Center for Infectious Diseases
Centers for Disease Control and Prevention
Atlanta, GA, USA

Alan D.T. Barrett PHD
Department of Pathology
University of Texas Medical Branch
Galveston, TX, USA

Thomas Barrett PHD
Institue for Animal Health
Pirbright Laboratory
Pirbright, UK

William J. Bellini PHD
Chief, Measles, Mumps, Rubella and
Herpesviruses Team
Respiratory and Enteric Viruses Branch
Division of Viral and Rickettsial Diseases
National Center for Infectious Diseases
Centers for Disease Control and Prevention
Atlanta, GA, USA

Mauro Bendinelli MD PHD
Professor of Microbiology; and
Director of Virology and Retrovirus Center
Department of Experimental Pathology
Virology Section, University of Pisa
Pisa, Italy

Kenneth I. Berns MD PHD
Director, UF Genetics Institute; and
Professor, Molecular Genetics and Microbiology
College of Medicine
University of Florida
Gainesville, FL, USA

Jennifer M. Best PHD FRCPATH
Reader in Virology,
Department of Infectious Diseases
King's College London,
London, UK

Roumiana S. Boneva MD PHD
Medical Epidemiologist
National Center for Infectious Diseases
Centers for Disease Control and Prevention
Atlanta, GA, USA

Thomas Briese PHD
Jerome L. and Dawn Greene
Infectious Disease Laboratory
Mailman School of Public Health
Columbia University
New York, NY, USA

William J. Britt MD
Department of Pediatrics
University of Alabama at Birmingham
Birmingham, AL, USA

Jo Ellen Brunner PHD
Instructional Support Group
School of Biological Sciences
University of California
Irvine, CA, USA

Michael J. Carter BA PHD
School of Biomedical and Molecular Sciences
University of Surrey
Guildford, UK

Pierre-Emmanuel Ceccaldi PHD
Senior Scientist
Unit 'Epidémiologie et Physiopathologie
des Virus Oncogènes'
Institut Pasteur
Paris, France

Ian N. Clarke BSC PHD
Professor of Virology
Division of Infection, Inflammation and Repair
School of Medicine
University of Southampton
Southampton, UK

J. Barklie Clements FRSE FMEDSCI
Professor of Virology
Division of Virology
Institute of Biological and Life Sciences
University of Glasgow
Glasgow, UK

Leslie Collier MD DSC FRCP FRCPATH
Professor Emeritus of Virology
The London Hospital and Medical College, London;
Formerly Director, Vaccines and Sera Laboratories
The Lister Institute of Preventive Medicine
Elstree, Hertfordshire, UK

Richard C. Condit PHD
Department of Molecular Genetics and Microbiology
University of Florida College of Medicine
Gainesville, FL, USA

James F. Conway BSC PHD
Group Leader
Laboratoire de Microscopie Electronique Structurale
Institut de Biologie Structurale
Grenoble, France

Samantha Cooray MBIOCHEM PHD
Department of Virology
Wright Fleming Institute
Imperial College Faculty of Medicine
London, UK

Susan F. Cotmore PHD
Senior Research Scientist
Department of Laboratory Medicine
Yale University School of Medicine
New Haven, CT, USA

Nancy J. Cox PHD
Chief, Influenza Branch
Division of Viral and Rickettsial Diseases
Centers for Disease Control and Prevention
Atlanta, GA, USA

Dorothy H. Crawford MBBS PHD MD FRCP
DSC FRSE
Professor of Medical Microbiology
School of Biomedical & Clinical Laboratory Sciences
University of Edinburgh
Edinburgh, UK

Andrew J. Davison MA PHD
MRC Virology Unit
Institute of Virology
University of Glasgow
Glasgow, UK

Terence S. Dermody MD
Professor of Pediatrics and Microbiology
and Immunology
Elizabeth B. Lamb Center for Pediatric Research
Vanderbilt University School of Medicine
Nashville, TN, USA

Ulrich Desselberger MD FRCPATH FRCP
Clinical Microbiology and Public Health Laboratory
Addenbrooke's Hospital
Cambridge, UK (until July 2002)

Charlene S. Dezzutti PHD
HIV and Retrovirology Branch
Division of AIDS, STD, and TB Laboratory Research
National Center for HIV, STD, and TB Prevention
Centers for Disease Control and Prevention
Atlanta, GA, USA

Esteban Domingo PHD
Professor CSIC
Centro de Biología Molecular "Severo Ochoa"
CSIC-UAM, Universidad Autónoma de Madrid
Cantoblanco, Madrid, Spain

Ruben O. Donis DVM PHD
Chief, Molecular Genetics Section
Influenza Branch
Division of Viral and Rickettsial Diseases
National Centers for Infectious Diseases
Centers for Disease Control and Prevention
Atlanta, GA, USA

Bernadette M. Dutia BSC PHD
Senior Research Fellow
Laboratory for Clinical and Molecular Virology
Division of Veterinary Biomedical Sciences
University of Edinburgh
Edinburgh, UK

Andrew J. Easton BSC PHD
Professor of Virology
Department of Biological Sciences
University of Warwick
Coventry, UK

Richard M. Elliott BSC DPHIL FRSE
Professor of Molecular Virology
Division of Virology
Institute of Biomedical and Life Sciences
University of Glasgow
Glasgow, UK

Gisela Enders MD
Professor of Virology
Head of the Institute of Virology
Infectiology and Epidemiology; and
Chief, Laboratory Prof. G. Enders and Partners
Stuttgart, Germany

M. Anthony Epstein MA MD DSC PHD FRS
Nuffield Department of Clinical Medicine
University of Oxford, John Radcliffe Hospital
Oxford, UK

Dean D. Erdman Dr PH
Team Leader
Respiratory Virus Diagnostics Section
Division of Viral and Rickettsial Diseases
National Center for Infectious Diseases
Centers for Disease Control and Prevention
Atlanta, GA, USA

Mary K. Estes PHD
Professor, Department of Molecular Virology
and Microbiology
Baylor College of Medicine
Houston, TX, USA

Heinz Feldmann MD
Chief, Special Pathogens Program
National Microbiology Laboratory

Public Health Agency of Canada; and
Associate Professor
Department of Medical Microbiology
University of Manitoba
Winnipeg, MB, Canada

Hugh J. Field SCD FRCPATH
Reader in Comparative Virology
Centre for Veterinary Science
University of Cambridge
Cambridge, UK

Bernhard Fleckenstein MD
Professor and Chairman
Institute for Clinical and Molecular Virology
University of Erlangen-Nürnberg
Erlangen, Germany

Thomas M. Folks PHD
HIV and Retrovirology Branch
Division of AIDS, STD, and
TB Laboratory Research
National Center for HIV, STD, and TB Prevention
Centers for Disease Control and Prevention
Atlanta, GA, USA

Ilya V. Frolov PHD
Department of Microbiology and Immunology
University of Texas Medical Branch
Galveston, TX, USA

Yves Gaudin PHD
Director
Laboratoire de Virologie Moléculaire et Structurale
UMR-CNRS 2472; UMR-INRA 1157 CNRS
Gif-sur-Yvette, Cedex, France

Wolfram H. Gerlich PHD
Professor and Director
Institute of Medical Virology
Justus Liebig University Giessen
Giessen, Germany

Alexander E. Gorbalenya PHD DSCI
Associate Professor
Department of Medical Microbiology
Leiden University Medical Center
Leiden, The Netherlands

Jim Gray FIBMS PHD FRCPATH
Head, Enteric Virus Unit
Virus Reference Department
Health Protection Agency, Centre for Infections
London, UK

Duane J. Gubler ScD
Director of Asia-Pacific Institute for Tropical Medicine
and Infectious Diseases; and
Chair, Department of Medicine and
Medical Microbiology
John A. Burns School of Medicine
Honolulu, HI, USA

Stephen C. Hadler MD
Senior Advisor for Strengthening Childhood
Immunization, Global Immunization Division
National Immunization Program
Centers for Disease Control and Prevention
Atlanta, GA, USA

Walid Heneine PHD
HIV and Retrovirology Branch,
Division of AIDS, STD, and TB Laboratory Research
National Center for HIV, STD, and TB Prevention
Centers for Disease Control and Prevention
Atlanta, GA, USA

John J. Holland PHD
Emeritus Professor
Division of Biology and Institute of
Molecular Genetics, University of California
San Diego, La Jolla, CA, USA

Mady Hornig MA MD
Director of Translational Research
Jerome L. and Dawn Greene Infectious Disease
Laboratory; and
Associate Professor of Epidemiology
Mailman School of Public Health
Columbia University
New York, NY, USA

Li Jin MD PHD MRCPATH
Clinical Scientist, Enteric Virus Reference
Department, Health Protection Agency
Centre for Infections, London, UK

Michael Kann MD
Professor of Virology
Justus Liebig University Giessen
Giessen, Germany

Yoshihiro Kawaoka DVM PHD
Professor and Director
International Research Center for Infectious Diseases;
and Division of Virology
Department of Microbiology and Immunology
Institute of Medical Science
University of Tokyo, Tokyo, Japan; and
Professor, Department of Pathobiological Sciences
School of Veterinary Medicine

University of Wisconsin-Madison
Madison, WI, USA

Kamel Khalili PHD
Professor and Director
Center for Neurovirology and Cancer Biology
Temple University
Philadelphia, PA USA

Michael P. Kiley † PHD
Formerly USDA, Agricultural Research Service
Animal Production, Product Value
Beltsville, MD, USA

Hans-Dieter Klenk MD
Institute of Virology Medical School
Philipps-University
Marburg, Germany

Wendy A. Knowles BSC PHD MIBIOL
Clinical Scientist, Enteric, Respiratory and
Neurological Virus Laboratory
Specialist and Reference Microbiology Division
Health Protection Agency, Centre for Infections
London, UK

Myriam S. Künzi PHD
Postdoctoral Fellow, John Hopkins Oncology Center
Baltimore, MD, USA

Paul R. Lambden BSC PHD
Senior Research Fellow, Molecular Microbiology
University Medical School
Southampton General Hospital
Southampton, UK

R. Michael Linden PHD
Associate Professor
Department of Gene and Cell Medicine, and
Department of Microbiology
Mount Sinai School of Medicine
New York, NY, USA

W. Ian Lipkin MD
Jerome L. and Dawn Greene Infectious
Disease Laboratory
Mailman School of Public Health
Columbia University
New York, NY, USA

Graham Lloyd BSC MSC PHD FIBMS
Head, Special Pathogens Reference Unit
Health Protection Agency
Centre for Emergency, Preparedness and Response
Porton Down, Salisbury, UK

Fabrizio Maggi MD PhD
Assistant, Clinical Virology
Department of Experimental Pathology
Virology Section, University of Pisa
Pisa, Italy

Brian W.J. Mahy MA PhD ScD DSc
Senior Scientific Research Advisor
National Center for Infectious Diseases
Centers for Disease Control and Prevention
Atlanta, GA, USA

Myra McClure PhD DSc FRCPATH
Professor of Retrovirolgy and
Honorary Consultant in GU Medicine
Head of Section of Infectious Diseases
Jefferiss Research Trust Laboratories
Wright-Fleming Institute, Faculty of Medicine
Imperial College London
London, UK

Philip Minor BA PhD
National Institute for Biological Standards and
Control (NIBSC), Division of Virology
South Mimms, Potters Bar
Herts, UK

Anthony C. Minson BSc PhD
Professor of Virology, Virology Division
Department of Pathology, University of Cambridge
Cambridge, UK

Arnold S. Monto MD
Professor of Epidemiology, Director
The University of Michigan Bioterrorism
Preparedness Initiative
University of Michigan School of Public Health
Ann Arbor, MI, USA

Anne Moscona MD
Professor, Pediatrics and Microbiology/Immunology
Vice Chair of Pediatrics for Research
Weill Medical College
Cornell University
New York, NY, USA

Richard W. Moyer PhD
Senior Associate Dean for Research
Development; and
Professor, Department of Molecular Genetics
and Microbiology
University of Florida College of Medicine
Gainesville, FL, USA

Frederick A. Murphy DVM PhD
School of Veterinary Medicine
University of California Davis
Davis, CA, USA

David Mutimer MBBS MD FRACP FRCP
Reader in Hepatology, University of Birmingham; and
Consultant Hepatologist, Liver and Hepatobiliary Unit
Queen Elizabeth Hospital
Birmingham, UK

Anthony A. Nash PhD FRSE
Laboratory for Clinical and Molecular Virology
Centre for Infectious Diseases
University of Edinburgh
Edinburgh, UK

Neal Nathanson MD
Associate Dean, Global Health Programs
University of Pennsylvania School of Medicine
Philadelphia, PA, USA

James C. Neil BSc PhD FRSE
Professor of Virology and Molecular Oncology
Institute of Comparative Medicine
University of Glasgow Veterinary School
Glasgow, UK

Frank Neipel MD
Institute for Clinical and Molecular Virology
University of Erlangen-Nürnberg
Erlangen, Germany

Gabriele Neumann PhD
Department of Pathobiological Sciences
School of Veterinary Medicine
University of Wisconsin-Madison
Madison, WI, USA

Jessica Otte BS
Center for Neurovirology and Cancer Biology
Temple University
Philadelphia, PA, USA

Richard W. Peluso PhD
Vice President Process Sciences and
Manufacturing, Targeted Genetics
Seattle, WA, USA

Mark Pett MA PhD
Postdoctoral Research Associate
MRC Cancer Cell Unit
Hutchinson MRC Research Centre
Cambridge, UK

Paula M. Pitha MS PhD
Sidney Kimmel Comprehensive Cancer Centre
Johns Hopkins School of Medicine
Baltimore, MD, USA

Craig R. Pringle BSc PhD
Emeritus Professor, Biological Sciences Department
University of Warwick
Coventry, UK

Axel Rethwilm MD
Institut für Virologie und Immunbiologie
Universität Würzburg
Würzburg, Germany

Betty Robertson PhD
Division of Viral Hepatitis
Centers for Disease Control and Prevention
Division of Viral Hepatitis
Atlanta, GA, USA

Juan D. Rodas DVM MSc PhD
Assistant Professor
Facultad de Ciencias Agrarias y
Laboratorio de Immunovirologia
Universidad de Antioquia
Medellin, Columbia

John T. Roehrig PhD
Chief, Arbovirus Diseases Branch
Division of Vector-Borne Infectious Diseases
National Center for Infectious Diseases
Centers for Disease Control
and Prevention Public Health Service
Fort Collins, CO, USA

Paul A. Rota PhD
Measles, Mumps, Rubella and Herpesvirus Team
Respiratory and Enteric Viruses Branch
Division of Viral and Rickettsial Diseases
Centers for Disease Control and Prevention
Atlanta, GA, USA

David J. Rowlands PhD
School of Biochemistry and Microbiology
University of Leeds
Leeds, UK

Rob W.H. Ruigrok PhD
Laboratoire de Virologie Moléculaire et Structurale
FRE 2854 CNRS-Université Joseph Fourier
Grenoble, France

Willie Russell BSc PhD FRSE
Emeritus Research Professor
School of Biology
University of St Andrews
Fife, UK

Mahmut Safak PhD
Head, Laboratory of Molecular Virology
Center for Neurovirology and Cancer Biology
Temple University
Philadelphia, PA USA

Maria S. Salvato PhD
Professor, Institute of Human Virology
University of Maryland Biotechnology Institute
Baltimore, MD, USA

Jürgen Schneider-Schaulies PhD
Professor of Virology
Institute for Virology and Immunobiology
University of Würzburg, Würzburg, Germany

Sibylle Schneider-Schaulies PhD
Professor of Virology
Institute for Virology and Immunobiology
University of Würzburg
Würzburg, Germany

Guy Schoehn PhD
Laboratoire de Virologie Moléculaire et Structurale
FRE 2854 CNRS-Université Joseph Fourier
Grenoble, France

Ulrich Schubert PhD
Institute for Clinical and Molecular Virology
University of Erlangen-Nürnberg
Erlangen, Germany

Bert L. Semler PhD
Professor and Chair
Department of Microbiology and Molecular Genetics
University of California
Irvine, CA, USA

Jane F. Seward MBBS MPH
Chief, Viral Vaccine Preventable Diseases Branch
Epidemiology and Surveillance Division
National Immunization Program
Centers for Disease Control and Prevention
Atlanta, GA, USA

Robert E. Shope MD†
Formerly John S. Dunn Distinguished
Chair in Biodefense
Department of Pathology
University of Texas Medical Branch
Galveston, TX, USA

Stuart G. Siddell BSc PhD
Professor of Virology
Department of Pathology and Microbiology
University of Bristol
Bristol, UK

Peter Simmonds BM PhD MRCPATH
Centre for Infectious Diseases
University of Edinburgh
Edinburgh, UK

Anthony Simmons MA MB BCHIR PhD
Professor, Pediatrics, Pathology, Microbiology
and Immunology, 2.330 Children's Hospital
University of Texas Medical Branch at Galveston
Galveston, TX, USA

Geoffrey L. Smith PhD FRS
Professor of Virology; and
Wellcome Trust Research Fellow
Department of Virology
Faculty of Medicine
Imperial College London
London, UK

Eric J. Snijder PhD
Associate Professor,
Department of Medical Microbiology
Leiden University Medical Center
Leiden, The Netherlands

Steven Specter PhD
Professor, Medical Microbiology and Immunology and
Associate Dean for Admissions and Student Affairs
University of South Florida College of Medicine
Tampa, FL, USA

Margaret Stanley PhD
Professor of Epithelial Biology
Department of Pathology
University of Cambridge, UK

Peter Tattersall PhD
Professor, Departments of Laboratory
Medicine and Genetics
Yale University School of Medicine
New Haven, CT, USA

John M. Taylor PhD
Senior Member
Fox Chase Cancer Center
Philadelphia, PA, USA

Volker ter Meulen MD
Professor Emeritus of Clinical Virology
and Immunology
Former Chairman of the Institute for Virology
and Immunbiology
University of Würzburg
Würzburg, Germany

Noël Tordo PhD
Chief of Laboratory; and
Head, Unit 'Stratégies Antivirales'
Virology Department, Institut Pasteur
Paris, France

Ralph A. Tripp PhD
Professor and GRA Chair, University of Georgia,
College of Veterinary Medicine
Department of Infectious Diseases
Athens, GA, USA

Kenneth L. Tyler MD
Reuler-Lewin Family Professor of Neurology and
Professor of Medicine
Microbiology and Immunology
University of Colorado Health Sciences
Center and Chief, Neurology Service
Denver Veterans Affairs Medical Center
Denver, CO, USA

Marc H.V. Van Regenmortel PhD
Emeritus Research Director, CNRS
Biotechnology School of the University of Strasbourg
Illkirch, France

Alex I. Wandeler PhD
Canadian Food Inspection Agency
Ontario Laboratory Fallowfield
Nepean, Ontario, Canada

Scott C. Weaver PhD
Director for Tropical and Emerging Infectious Diseases
UTMB Center for Biodefense and
Emerging Infectious Disease; and
Professor, Departments of Pathology
Microbiology & Immunology
University of Texas Medical Branch
Galveston, TX, USA

Sandra K. Weller PhD
Professor and Chair
Molecular, Microbial and Structural Biology
University of Connecticut Health Center
Farmington, CT, USA

Richard J. Whitley MD
Professor of Pediatrics, Microbiology,
Medicine and Neurosurgery
University of Alabama at Birmingham
Children's Hospital
Birmingham, AL, USA

Margaret M. Willcocks BSc PhD
School of Biomedical and Molecular Sciences
University of Surrey
Guildford, UK

John A. Wyke MA, VetMB, PhD, MRCVS, FRSE
Senior Research Fellow
Institute of Comparative Medicine

University of Glasgow Veterinary School
Glasgow, UK

John Ziebuhr MD
Associate Professor, Institute of Virology
and Immunology, University of Würzburg
Würzburg, Germany

Preface

The remarkable progress of research in virology has led to the expansion from 47 chapters in the 9th edition to 70 in this 10th edition. Since the preparation of the 9th edition we have seen the emergence of several hitherto unknown human viruses as well as some remarkable examples of viruses of animals or birds crossing the species barrier and infecting humans. So far as the latter phenomenon is concerned, two incidents occurred involving avian influenza viruses. In 1997, avian influenza subtype H5N1 was recovered for the first time from humans, when it caused 18 cases of severe influenza with six deaths in children and adults in Hong Kong. The slaughter of more than a million chickens in early 1998 ended this disease outbreak, but in 1999 another avian influenza subtype, H9N2, was recovered from two young children in Hong Kong. The H5N1 virus has continued to infect poultry and other birds in South East Asia, and to cause further morbidity and mortality in humans in 2005. In both these incidents the viruses which affected humans were found to have all gene segments derived from the avian virus, a situation never previously encountered in influenza virology.

A second example of crossing the species barrier occurred in 1999 and involved a newly recognized paramyxovirus, Nipah virus, which caused disease outbreaks with severe mortality in Malaysia and Singapore. The causative virus was acquired from infected pigs, and disease control measures included the slaughter of more than a million pigs in Malaysia. Nipah virus appears to have a wide host range including dogs and cats as well as pigs and humans, and will be an important new area for investigation over the next several years. The virus is now causing human disease outbreaks in Bangladesh, apparently without the involvement of pigs as an intermediate host.

New human viruses that have recently emerged include TT virus, originally thought to be associated with transfusion-acquired hepatitis in Japan, but now not thought to be a cause of hepatitis. TT virus has a small circular, single-stranded DNA genome, and appears to have a global distribution. There is evidence that infection is acquired at an early age in some parts of the world, but its disease significance remains unknown. TT virus thus joins GB virus C/Hepatitis G virus as a newly recognized human virus infection of unknown disease significance.

In 2003, a new disease was recognized in Asia which became known as severe acute respiratory syndrome (SARS). Unexpectedly, the causative agent of this disease was identified as a hitherto unknown coronavirus. A remarkable international collaboration led to rapid determination of the complete genome sequence of the SARS human coronavirus which showed that this virus had not previously been seen. The precise origin of this virus remains unknown. As outlined in the preface to the 9th edition, it is likely that the identification of new viruses by gene sequencing or other technologies will continue to raise questions for virologists, who need to investigate their relevance.

The chapters in this 10th edition are grouped into four parts.

Several new chapters are now included in Part I (General Characteristics of Viruses).

The changes in virus classification and nomenclature that were approved by the International Committee on Taxonomy of Viruses (ICTV) in August 1999 are outlined in Chapters 3 and 4. During this period three new Orders were established, and the characteristics of those infecting vertebrates are described in two new chapters on Mononegavirales and Nidovirales (Chapters 19 and 20). We have also included three new chapters on replication of negative strand RNA viruses, positive-strand RNA viruses, and DNA viruses (Chapters 8-10), and a new chapter on Viral evasion of the immune response (Chapter 16), an increasingly recognized component of viral pathogenesis.

In Part II, the number of chapters on specific viruses and viral infection has increased from 26 to 40 in this 10th edition. There are new chapters on Borna disease virus (Chapter 52), an increasingly studied member of the Mononegavirales that may be a cause of some human psychiatric disorders, and on TT virus and other members of the *Anellovirus* genus (Chapter 57).

Other new chapters deal with polyoma viruses (Chapter 24), human herpes virus 8 (Chapter 28), poxvirus replication (Chapter 31) paramyxoviruses (Chapters 34-38), rotaviruses (Chapter 44), foamy viruses (Chapter 59), human immunodeficiency virus

(Chapter 65), and viral vectors for gene therapy (Chapter 68).

Chapters from the 9th edition that have undergone substantial revision include those on Human enteric RNA viruses (Chapters 41 and 42); Retroviruses and associated diseases in humans (Chapter 58); Bunyaviruses (Chapter 48); Betaherpesviruses (Chapter 27); Orthomyxoviruses (Chapter 32); Prions of human and animals (Chapter 61); Coronaviruses, Toroviruses, and Arteriviruses (Chapter 39); Reoviruses (Chapter 43); Hepatitis C (Chapter 54); Parvoviruses (Chapter 21); Immunoprophylaxis of viral diseases (Chapter 67); and Antiviral Chemotherapy (Chapter 69).

We are extremely indebted to all the authors for their excellent contributions to this text, which now provides a realistic representation of the state of the art in understanding human viral infections. As in previous editions, little prominence has been given to infections of nonhuman species, except where they bear upon human infections as zoonoses, models of pathogenesis, or economic importance.

We wish to thank Penny Mahy for her excellent editorial work.

During the preparation of this text, we deeply regret that two of our authors passed away. Michael Kiley (Chapter 65), a world expert on biosafety, died on 24th January 2004 (Johnson 2004) and Robert Shope (Chapter 48), the world's most distinguished arbovirologist, died on 19th January 2004 (Murphy and Calisher 2004). Their obituaries can be found in Archives of Virology (see below), but we hope that this text will serve as a continuing tribute to their memory.

References

Johnson, K.M., 2004. In Memoriam Michael Patrick Kiley (1942–2004). *Arch Virol* **149**, 1467–8.

Murphy, F.A., Calisher, C.H. et al. 2004. In Memoriam Robert Ellis Shope (1929–2004). *Arch Virol* **149**, 1061–6.

Brian W.J. Mahy and Volker ter Meulen
Atlanta and Würzburg
May 2005

Abbreviations

aa	amino acid
AB	antibody
AAFP	American Academy of Family Physicians
A+T	adenine and thymine
AAP	American Academy of Pediatrics
AAV	adeno-associated virus
ABLV	Australian bat lyssavirus
ABSV	Absettarov virus
ACE2	angiotensin-converting enzyme 2
ACIP	Advisory Committee on Immunization Practices (USA)
ACMHV-2	avian carcinoma virus Mill Hill virus 2
ACOG	American College of Obstetricians and Gynecologists
ACTG	acquired immunodeficiency syndrome clinical trial group
ACV	aciclovir; or acyclovir
ACV-MP	acyclovir monophosphate
ACV-TP	acyclovir triphosphate
AD	autodisable
ADC	acquired immunodeficiency syndrome dementia complex
ADCC	antibody-dependent cell-mediated cytotoxicity
ADE	antibody-dependent enhancement
Ad pol	adenovirus polymerase
ADRP	adenosine diphosphate-ribose1′-phosphatase
Ad35	adenovirus type 35
AFP	α-fetoprotein
AGMK	African green monkey kidney
AGUS	atypical glandular cells of undetermined significance
AHC	acute hemorrhagic conjunctivitis
AHSV	African horse sickness virus
AIDS	acquired immunodeficiency syndrome
ALFV	Alfuy virus
ALT	alanine amino transferase
ALV	avian leukosis virus
ALV-E	avian leukosis virus subgoup E
AM	'aseptic' meningitis
AMDV	Aleutian mink disease virus
AMP-RT	amplified reverse transcriptase
AMV	avian myeloblastosis virus
ANP	acyclic nucleoside phosphonate
ANV	avian nephritis virus
APC	antigen presenting cell
APD	average pore diameter
APOBEC3G	apolipoprotein B mRNA editing enzyme
APOIV	Apoi virus
APV	avian pneumovirus
Ara-A	adenine arabinoside
Ara-C	1-β-D-arabinofuranosylcytosine
Ara-MP	adenine arabinoside-monophosphate
Ara-TP	adenine arabinoside-triphosphate
ARDS	acute respiratory distress syndrome
ARIMA	autoregressive integrated moving average
AROAV	Aroa virus
ART	antiretroviral therapy
ARV	Adelaide river virus
ASCUS	atypical squamous cells of undetermined significance
ASFV	African swine fever virus
AST	alkaline phosphatase
As$_2$O$_3$	arsenic trioxide
ATCC	American Type Culture Collection
α-TIF	α-*trans*-inducing factor
ATL	acute T-cell leukemia; or adult T-cell leukemia
AZT	azidothymidine; or 3′-azido-3′-deoxythymidine
AZT-DP	azidothymidine diphosphate
AZT-TP	azidothymidine triphosphate
BaEV	baboon endogenous virus
BAGV	Bagaza virus
BAL	bronchoalveolar lavage
BANV	Banzi virus
BAstV	bovine astrovirus
BBB	blood–brain barrier
BBV	Bukalasa bat virus
BCC	basal cell carcinoma
BCoV	bovine coronavirus
BCR	B-cell receptor
BCRF	B-cell regulatory factor
BCV	Batu Cave virus
BD	borna disease
bDNA	branched DNA; or branched-chain DNA
BDPV	Barbarie duck parvovirus
BDV	Border disease virus; or borna disease virus
BEFV	bovine ephemeral fever virus
BFDV	beak and feather disease virus
BFPyV	budgerigar fledgling polyomavirus
BFU-E	burst-forming units erythroid

BFV	Barmah Forest virus; or bovine foamy virus
Bgp1	biliary glycoprotein 1
BH	black-hooded
BHK	baby hamster kidney
BIV	bovine immunodeficiency virus
BKPyV	BK polyomavirus
BKV	BK virus
BKVN	BKV-associated nephropathy
BL	Burkitt's lymphoma
BLV	bovine leukemia virus
BMI	body mass index
B19	human parvovirus B19
BOUV	Boul800ui virus
BPL	β-propiolactone
BPV	bovine parvovirus; or bovine papillomavirus
BPV-1	bovine papillomavirus type 1
BPyV	bovine polyomavirus
BSE	bovine spongiform encephalopathy
BSL	biosafety level
BSQV	Bussuquara virus
BToV	bovine torovirus
BTV 10	bluetongue virus type 10
BVaraU	bromovinylarabinosyl-uracil
BVDU	bromovinyl deoxyuridine
BVDU-DP	bromovinyl deoxyuridine-diphosphate
BVDU-MP	bromovinyl deoxyuridine-monophosphate
BVDV	bovine viral diarrhea virus
BVU	bromovinylarabinosyl-uracil
C	cytosine
CA	capsid
CAdV	canine adenovirus
CAH	chronic active hepatitis
CAM	cell adhesion molecule; or chorioallantoic membrane
CAR	coxsackie adenovirus receptor
CART	combined antiretroviral therapy
CAT	chloramphenicol acetyl transferase
CAV	chicken anemia virus
CCA	chimpanzee coryza agent
cccDNA	covalently closed circular DNA
CCE	cornified cell envelope
CCHFV	Crimean–Congo hemorrhagic fever virus
CCPP	contagious caprine pleuropneumonia
CCoV	canine enteric coronavirus
CCV	channel catfish virus
CD	circular dichroism
CDC	Centers for Disease Control and Prevention (USA)
CDI	conformation-dependent immunoassay
CDKI	cyclin-dependent kinase inhibitor
CDV	canine distemper virus
CEA	carcinoembryonic antigen
CEE	central European encephalitis
CEV	cell-associated enveloped virus
CF	complement fixation; or cystic fibrosis
CFU-E	colony-forming units erythroid

CHIKV	Chikungunya virus
CHO	Chinese hamster ovary
CI	complementation index
CIC	circulating immune complex
CID	cytomegalic inclusion disease
CIEBOV	Côte d'Ivoire ebola virus
CIN	cervical intraepithelial neoplasia
CIV	Carey island virus
CJD	Creutzfeldt–Jakob disease
CK II	casein kinase II
CLP	core-like particle
CMI	cell-mediated immunity
CMV	cytomegalovirus
CnMV	canine minute virus
CNS	central nervous system
COPV	canine oral papillomavirus
cp	cytopathic
CPCV	Cacipacore virus
CPD	cyclic phosphodiesterase
CPE	cytopathic effect
CPH	chronic persistent hepatitis
CPMV	cowpea mosaic virus
CPSF	cleavage and polyadenylation specificity factor
CPT	cycling probe technology
CPV	canine parvovirus
CPXV	cowpox virus
CRE	*cis*-acting replication element
CREB	cyclic AMP-responsive element-binding protein
CRF	circulating recombinant forms
CRM	chromosome region maintenance
CrmA	cytokine response modifier A
CRPV	cottontail rabbit papillomavirus
CRS	congenital rubella syndrome
CRV	Cowbone Ridge virus
cryo-EM	cryo-electron microscopy
CsA	cyclosporin A
CSD	Cambridge Structural Database (UK)
CSE	conserved sequence element
CSF	cerebrospinal fluid; or colony stimulating factor
CSFV	classical swine fever virus
CT	computer tomography
CTE	constitutive RNA transport element
CTFV	Colorado tick fever virus
CTL	cytotoxic T-lymphocyte
CVB3	coxsackie virus B3
cVDPV	circulating vaccine-derived poliovirus
CVS	challenge virus standard; or chorionic villi sampling; or congenital varicella syndrome
CWD	chronic wasting disease
CypA	cyclophilin A
D	aspartate
DA	dopamine
DAF	decay accelerating factor
DANA	2,3-didehydro-2-deoxy-N-acetylneuraminic acid
DBP	DNA-binding protein
DBS	dried blood spots

DBV	Dakar bat virus
DC	dendritic cell
DD	death domains
DDA-TP	dideoxyadenosine 5′ triphosphate
DDC	dideoxycytidine
DDI	2′,3′-dideoxyinosine
DDI-MP	2′,3′-dideoxyinosine monophosphate
DED	death effector domain
DEET	diethylmethylbenzamide; or diethyltoluamide
DENV	dengue virus
D4T	2′,3′-didehydro-2′-deoxythymidine; or didehydrodeoxyuridine
D4T-DP	D4T diphosphate
D4T-TP	D4T triphosphate
DHBV	duck hepatitis B virus
DHF	dengue hemorrhagic fever
DHF/DDS	Dengue hemorrhagic fever/dengue shock syndrome
DI	defective interfering
DIC	disseminated intravascular coagulation
DMSO	dimethyl sulfoxide
DMV	dolphin morbillivirus; or double membrane vesicle
DNApol	DNA polymerase
DNCB	dinitrochlorobenzene
DR	direct repeat
DRADA	double-stranded RNA adenosine deaminase activity
DRM	detergent-resistant membrane
dsRNA	double-stranded RNA
DSS	dengue shock syndrome
DTaP	diphtheria and tetanus toxoids and acellular pertussis vaccine
DY	drowsy
E	glutamate
EA	early antigen
EAE	experimental allergic encephalomyelitis
EAV	equine arteritis virus; or endogenous avian virus
EBER	Epstein–Barr virus-encoded small RNA
EBHSV	European brown hare syndrome virus
EBLV	European bat lyssavirus
EBNA	Epstein–Barr virus nuclear antigen
EBOV	Ebola virus
EBV	Epstein–Barr virus
EC50	effective concentration
ECTV	ectromelia virus
EDTA	ethylenediaminetetraacetic acid
EEEV	eastern equine encephalomyelitis virus
EEV	extracellular enveloped virus
EF-1α	elongation factor 1 alpha
EFV	equine foamy virus
EGF	epidermal growth factor
EHDV	epizootic hemorrhagic disease virus
EHV	Edge hill virus
EHV-2	equine herpesvirus 2
EI	erythema infectiosum
EIA	enzyme immunoassay
EIAV	equine infectious anemia virus
eIF-2α	eukaryotic translation initiation factor 2α
eIF3	eukaryotic translation initiation factor 3
EIPV	enhanced potency inactivated poliovirus vaccine
ELISA	enzyme linked immunosorbent assay
ELVIS	enzyme-linked virus-inducible system
EM	electron microscopy
EMCV	encephalomyocarditis virus
ENTV	Entebbe bat virus
EP	early palindrome
EPI	expanded program on immunization
EPO	erythropoietin
ER	endoplasmic reticulum
ERGIC	endoplasmic reticulum–Golgi intermediate compartment
ES	embryonic stem
EToV	equine torovirus
EV	epidermodysplasia verruciformis
F	fusion; or phenylalanine
FADD	Fas-associated death domain
FasL	Fas ligand
FAstV	feline astrovirus
FAT	fluorescent antibody test
FCoV	feline coronavirus
FcR	Fc receptor
FCV	famciclovir; or feline calicivirus
FDA	Food and Drug Administration (USA)
FDC	follicular dendritic cell
FeLV	feline leukemia virus
FFI	fatal familial insomnia
ffu	focus-forming unit
FFV	feline foamy virus
4-GuDANA	4-guanidino-Neu5Ac2en
FI-RSV	formalin-inactivated respiratory syncytial virus
FIPV	feline infectious peritonitis virus
FIV	feline immunodeficiency virus
5HT	serotonin
FMDV	foot-and-mouth disease virus
FPV	feline panleukopenia virus; or fowlpox virus
FRET	fluorescence resonance energy transfer
FrMLV	Friend murine leukemia virus
FSE	feline spongiform encephalopathy
FTIR	Fourier-transformed infrared
FV	foamy virus
GABA	γ-amino butyric acid
GAG	glycosaminoglycans
GalC	galactosylceramide
G+C	guanosine and cytosine
GAPDH	glyceraldehyde-3-phosphate dehydrogenase
GAV	gill-associated virus
GAVI	Global Alliance for Vaccines and Immunization
gB	glycoprotein B
GBV-A	GB virus A
GBV-B	GB virus B

GBV-C	GB virus C
GCV	ganciclovir
GCV-MP	ganciclovir monophosphate
GCV-TP	ganciclovir triphosphate
GDD	glycine–aspartic acid–aspartic acid
GETV	Getah virus
gG	glycoprotein G
GGTP	γ-glutamyl transpeptidase
GGYV	Gadget's gully virus
GM	growth medium
GM-CSF	granulocyte/macrophage colony stimulation factor
GmDNV	*Galleria mellonella* densovirus
GP	glycoprotein
GPCR	G-protein-coupled receptor
GPI	glycophosphatidylinositol
GPV	Goose parvovirus
GR	glycine–arginine-rich
GRE	glucocorticoid-responsive element
GREP	Global Rinderpest Eradication Programme
GSHV	ground squirrel hepatitis virus
GSS	Gerstmann–Sträussler–Scheinker
H	hemagglutinin; or histidine
HA	hemagglutination; or hemagglutinin
HAA	human T-cell leukemia virus-associated arthropathy
HAART	highly active antiretroviral therapy
HAD	human immunodeficiency virus-associated dementia
HAI	hemagglutination inhibition
HAM	human T-cell leukemia virus-associated myelopathy
HAM/TSP	human T-cell leukemia virus-1-associated myelopathy/tropical spastic paraparesis
HANV	Hanzalova virus
HaPyV	hamster polyomavirus
HAstV	human astrovirus
HAV	hepatitis A virus
Hb	hemoglobin
HBeAg	hepatitis B e antigen
HBIG	hepatitis B immunoglobulin
HBcAg	hepatitis B virus core antigen
HBsAg	hepatitis B surface antigen
HBSP	hepatitis B spliced protein
HBSS	Hank's balanced salt solution
HBV	hepatitis B virus
HCC	hepatocellular carcinoma
hCG	human chorionic gonadotropin
HCMV	human cytomegalovirus
HCoV	human coronavirus OC43, 229E, or NL63
HCV	hepatitis C virus; or hog cholera virus
HD	helper dependent; or Hodgkin's disease
HDCS	human diploid cell strain
HDV	hepatitis delta virus
HE	hemagglutinin–esterase; or hematoxylin and eosin
HECoV	human enteric coronavirus
HEF	hemagglutinin–esterase fusion
HEK	human embryonic kidney
HEPA	high efficiency particulate air
HERV	human endogenous retroviruses
HEV	hepatitis E virus
HF	host factor; or hydrops fetalis
HFMD	hand-foot-and-mouth disease
HFRS	hemorrhagic fever with renal syndrome
HFV	human foamy virus
HGH	human grown hormone
HGSIL	high-grade squamous intraepithelial lesion
HGV	hepatitis G virus
HHBV	heron hepatitis B virus
HHV-1	human herpesvirus 1
HHV-6	human herpesvirus 6
HHV-7	human herpesvirus 7
HHV-8	human herpesvirus 8
HI	hemagglutination inhibition
Hib	*Haemophilus influenzae* type b
HIV	human immunodeficiency virus
HIV-1	human immunodeficiency virus type 1
HIV-2	human immunodeficiency virus type 2
HL	hemolysis
HMO	health maintenance organization
hMPV	human metapneumovirus
HN	hemagglutinin-neuraminidase
HNF	hepatonuclear factor
HNIG	human normal immunoglobulin
hnRNP	heterogeneous nuclear ribonucleoprotein
Hoc	highly antigenic outer capsid
HPIV-3	human parainfluenza virus type 3
HPLC	high performance liquid chromatography
HPMPC	hydroxyphosphonylmethoxycytosine
HPV	human papilloma virus
HR	heptad repeat
HR-HPV	high-risk human papillomavirus
HRIG	human anti-rabies immunoglobulin
HRSV	human respiratory syncytial virus
HRV	human rhinovirus
HS	heparan sulfate
Hsc	heat-shock cognate
HSC	hematopoietic stem cell
HSK	herpes simplex virus-induced keratitis
HSV	herpes simplex virus; or herpesvirus saimiri
HSV-1	herpes simplex virus type 1
HSV-2	herpes simplex virus type 2
HTLV	human T-cell leukemia virus
HTLV-1	human T-cell leukemia virus-1
HTLV-2	human T-cell leukemia virus-2
HToV	human torovirus
HU	human T-cell leukemia virus-associated uveitis
Hu	human
huIgG	unspecific pooled human immunoglobulin
HuR	human RNA-binding protein
HVEM	herpesvirus entry mediator

HVR	hypervariable region
HVS	herpesvirus saimiri
HY	hyper
HYPRV	Hypr virus
I	isoleucine
IAA	infection-associated antigen
IAP	inhibitor of apoptosis protein
IATA	International Air Transport Association
IBV	infectious bronchitis virus
ICA	islet cell antibody
ICAM	intracellular adhesion molecule
ICAM-1	intercellular adhesion molecule 1
ICAO	International Civil Aviation Organization
ICE	interleukin-1β-converting enzyme
iCJD	iatrogenic Creutzfeldt–Jakob disease
ICNV	International Committee on Nomenclature of Viruses
ICTV	International Committee on Taxonomy of Viruses
ICTVdB	International Committee on Taxonomy of Viruses database
ID	immunodiffusion; or infective dermatitis
IDDM	insulin-dependent diabetes mellitus
IDU	idoxuridine; or injecting drug user
IDU-TP	idoxuridine triphosphate
IE	immediate–early
IEF	isoelectric focusing
IEM	immunoelectron microscopy
IEV	intracellular enveloped virus
IF	immunofluorescence; or intermediate filament
IFA	immunofluorescence assay
IFAT	indirect fluorescent antibody test
IFN	interferon
IFN-α	interferon-alpha
IFN-γ	interferon-gamma
IFT	immunofluorescence testing
Ig	immunoglobulin
IgA	immunoglobulin A
IgG	immunoglobulin G
IgM	immunoglobulin M
IHA	indirect hemagglutination
IL	interleukin
IL-6	interleukin-6
ILHV	Ilhéus virus
IM	infectious mononucleosis
IMP	inflammation modulatory protein
IMV	intracellular mature virus
IN	integrase
iNOS	inducible nitric oxide synthetase
Int	integrase
IOM	Institute of Medicine (USA)
IP	inflammatory protein; or internal promoter
IPA	immunoperoxidase assay
IPV	inactivated poliovirus vaccine
IR	inverted repeat
IRES	internal ribosomal entry site

IRF	interferon regulatory factor
IRF-3	interferon regulatory factor 3
IRF-7	interferon regulatory factor 7
ISAV	infectious salmon anemia virus
ISDR	interferon-sensitivity determining region
ISG	interferon-stimulated gene
ISRE	interferon-specific response element
ISVP	infectious subvirion particle
ITAM	immunoreceptor tyrosine-based activation motif
ITIM	immunoreceptor tyrosine-based inhibitory motif
ITR	inverted terminal repeat
ITV	Israel turkey meningo-encephalitis virus
IU	international unit
IUMS	International Union of Microbiological Societies
IV	immature virion
IVDU	intravenous drug user
IVF	in vitro fertilization
IVIG	intravenous immunoglobulin
IVN	nucleoid-containing IV
JAK	Janus kinase
JAM1	junctional adhesion molecule 1
JCPyV	JC polyoma virus
JCV	Jamestown Canyon virus
JEV	Japanese encephalitis virus
JLP	juvenile laryngeal papillomatosis
JSRV	jaagsiekte sheep retrovirus
JUGV	Jugra virus
JUTV	Jutiapa virus
JV	Jena virus
K	lysine
KADV	Kadam virus
KEDV	Kedougou virus
KFDV	Kyasanur Forest disease virus
KIR	killer cell immunoglobulin-like receptor; or killer inhibitory receptor
KOKV	Kokobera virus
KOUV	Koutango virus
KRV	Kilham rat virus
KS	Kaposi's sarcoma
KSHV	Kaposi's sarcoma herpesvirus
KSIV	Karshi virus
KUMV	Kumlinge virus
KUNV	Kunjin virus
L	large; or late; or leucine
LA	latex agglutination
LAIV	live-attenuated influenza vaccine
LAK	L-associated kinase
LAP	leukemia-associated protein
LAT	latency-associated transcript
LCL	lymphoblastoid cell line
LCMV	lymphocytic choriomeningitis virus
LCR	ligase chain reaction
LDL	low density lipoprotein

LDLR	low density lipoprotein-related		**MK**	monkey kidney
LDV	lactate dehydrogenase-elevating virus		**MLV**	murine leukemia virus
LGSIL	low-grade squamous intraepithelial lesion		**MM**	maintenance medium
LGTV	Langat virus		**MMLV**	Montana myotis leukoencephalitis virus
LIP	lymphoid interstitial pneumonitis		**MMP**	matrix metalloproteinase
LIV	Louping ill virus		**MMR**	measles, mumps, and rubella
LMP	last menstrual period; or latent membrane protein; or low-molecular-weight protein		**MMTV**	mouse mammary tumor virus
			MMV	mice minute virus
LMP1	latent membrane protein 1		**Mo**	mouse
LNYV	lettuce necrotic yellows virus		**MOCV**	molluscum contagiosum virus
LOD	logarithm of odds		**MODV**	Modoc virus
LP	leader protein		**MOI**	multiplicity of infection
LPD	lymphoproliferative disease		**MoMLV**	Moloney murine leukemia virus
LPMV	La-Piedad Michoacan-Mexico virus		**MPGN**	membranoproliferative glomerulonephritis
LPS	lipopolysaccharide		**MPMV**	Mason–Pfizer monkey virus
LPV	lymphotropic papovavirus		**MPV**	murine pneumonia virus
LR-HPV	low-risk human papillomavirus		**MPyV**	murine polyomavirus
LRSV	lychnis ringspot virus		**MRA**	microbiological risk assessment
LT	lymphotoxin		**MRI**	magnetic resonance imaging
LT-βR	LT-β receptor		**mRNA**	messenger RNA
LT-βR-IgFcγ	LT-βR-immunoglobulin fusion protein		**MS**	multiple sclerosis
LTR	long terminal repeat		**MSM**	men who have sex with men
			MST	mean survival time
M	matrix; or methionine		**MT**	methyltransferase
MA	matrix; or membrane antigen		**MuLV**	murine leukemia virus
mAb	monoclonal antibody		**MuV**	mumps virus
MADT	morphological alteration and disintegration test		**MV**	measles virus
MALT	mucosal-associated lymphoid system		**MVA**	modified virus Ankara
MAP	mitogen-activated protein		**MVB**	multivesicular body
MAR	monoclonal antibody-resistant		**MVEV**	Murray valley encephalitis virus
MARV	Marburg virus		**MVM**	minute virus of mice
MAYV	Mayaro virus		**MYXV**	myxoma virus
MBL	mannose-binding lectin			
MBM	meat and bone-meal		**N**	asparagine; or nucleocapsid; or nucleoprotein
MBP	myelin basic protein		**NA**	neuraminidase
MCA	middle cerebral artery		**nAChR**	nicotinic acetylcholine receptor
MCD	multifocal Castleman disease		**NACI**	National Advisory Committee on Immunization (Canada)
M cells	membranous epithelial cell		**NANB**	non-A, non-B
MCMV	murine cytomegalovirus		**NANBH**	non-A, non-B hepatitis
MCP	membrane co-factor protein		**NaPTA**	sodium phosphotungstate
MCV	molluscum contagiosum virus		**NAS**	nuclear addressing signal
MDBK	Madin–Darby bovine kidney		**NASBA**	nucleic acid sequence-based amplification
MDCK	Madin–Darby canine kidney		**NAT**	nucleic acid amplification technique
MDPV	muscovy duck parvovirus		**NC**	nucleocapsid
ME	myalgic encephalomyelitis		**NCAM**	neuronal cell adhesion molecule
MEAV	Meaban virus		**NCCLS**	National Committee for Clinical Laboratory Standards (USA)
MEK	MAPK/ERK kinase		**NCR**	noncoding region
MeV	measles virus		**NDUV**	Ndumu virus
MEV	Meaban virus		**NDV**	Newcastle disease virus
MGF	myxoma growth factor		**NE**	norepinephrine
MHC	major histocompatibility complex		**NEGV**	Negishi virus
MHV	murine hepatitis virus; or mouse hepatitis virus		**NEP**	nuclear export protein
MHV-68	murine gammaherpesvirus 68		**NES**	nuclear export signal
MHVR	mouse hepatitis virus receptor		**NFAT**	nuclear factor activated T cell
MIBE	measles inclusion body encephalitis		**NF-κB**	nuclear factor-κB
MIDV	Middelburg virus			
MIP	macrophage inflammatory protein			

NF1	nuclear factor I		**Pap**	papanicolaou
NFT	neurofibrillary tangles		**PAS**	periodic acid–Schiff
NGF	nerve growth factor		**PAstV**	porcine astrovirus
NHEJ	nonhomologous end joining		**PBL**	peripheral blood lymphocyte
NHP	nonhuman primate		**PBMC**	peripheral blood mononuclear cell
NID	national immunization days		**PBS**	phosphate-buffered saline; or primer binding site
NIH	National Institutes of Health (USA)		**PCBP**	poly(rC) binding protein
NIV	Nipah virus		**PCBP1**	poly(rC) binding protein 1
NJLV	Naranjal virus		**PCBP2**	poly(rC) binding protein 2
NK	natural killer		**PcG**	polycomb group
NLS	nuclear localization signal		**PCNA**	proliferating cell nuclear antigen
NLV	Norwalk-like viruses		**PCoV**	puffinosis coronavirus
NMSC	nonmelanoma skin cancer		**PCR**	polymerase chain reaction
NNRTI	nonnucleoside reverse transcriptase inhibitor		**PCV**	porcine circovirus; or penciclovir
NNS	nonsegmented negative-strand		**PCV-MP**	penciclovir-monophosphate
NO	nitric oxide		**PCV-TP**	penciclovir-triphosphate
noncp	noncytopathic		**PD**	prenatal diagnosis
NP	nucleocapsid-associated protein; or nucleo-protein		**PDB**	protein database
			PDGF	platelet derived growth factor
NPC	nasopharyngeal carcinoma; or nuclear pore complex		**PDR**	Physicians' Desk Reference (USA)
			PDV	phocine distemper virus
n-PCR	nested polymerase chain reaction		**PEDV**	porcine epidemic diarrhea virus
NPS	nasopharyngeal secretion		**PEG**	polyethylene glycol
NRE	negative regulatory element		**PEL**	primary effusion lymphoma
NRTI	nucleoside reverse transcriptase inhibitor		**PEMS**	poult enteritis mortality syndrome
nRT-PCR	nested reverse transcription-polymerase chain reaction		**PEP**	postexposure prophylaxis
			PFA	phosphonoformic acid
NS	nonstructural		**pfu**	plaque forming unit
NSP	nonstructural protein		**PFV**	prototype foamy virus
nt	nucleotide		**PHC**	primary hepatocellular carcinoma
NT	virus-neutralizing		**PHCoV**	pheasant coronavirus
NTAV	Ntaya virus		**PHEV**	porcine haemagglutinating encephalomyelitis virus
NTR	non-translated region; or noncoding region; or non-translated RNA			
			PHLS	Public Health Laboratory Service (UK)
NtRTI	nucleotide reverse transcriptase inhibitor		**PI**	protease inhibitor
NV	Nipah virus; or nonvirion		**PIC**	preintegration complex
nvCJD	new variant Creutzfeldt–Jakob disease		**PIE**	postinfectious encephalitis
			PIF	parvoviral initiation factor
OAE	otoacoustic emission		**PIV2**	parainfluenza virus 2
OAS	2′,5′-oligoadenylate synthetase		**PKCε**	protein kinase Cε
OAstV	ovine astrovirus		**PKR**	protein kinase dsRNA
OHFV	Omsk hemorrhagic fever virus		**PLpro**	papainlike cysteine proteinase
OIE	World Organization for Animal Health		**PMEA**	9-(2-phosphonylmethoxyethyl) adenine
ONNV	O'nyong-nyong virus		**PMKC**	primary cynomolgus or rhesus monkey kidney cell
OPV	oral poliovirus vaccine			
ORF	open reading frame		**PML**	progressive multifocal leukoencephalopathy
ORI	origin of replication		**PMLP**	promyelocyte leukemia protein
ORS	oral rehydration solution		**PMPA**	R-9-(2-phosphonylmethoxypropyl) adenine
			PMTV	potato mop-top virus
P	phosphoprotein; or pneumonia; or proline		**PMV**	porpoise morbillivirus
PA	platelet-aggregating		**PoEV**	porcine endogenous retrovirus
PABP	poly(A) binding protein		**poly(A)**	polyadenylate
PABPII	poly(A) binding protein II		**POTV**	Potiskum virus
PAGE	polyacrylamide gel electrophoresis		**POWV**	Powassan virus
PAHO	Pan American Health Organization		**PPBV**	Phnom Penh bat virus
PAMP	pathogen-associated molecular pattern		**PPD**	purified protein derivative
P&I	pneumonia and influenza		**PPlase**	peptidyl-prolyl isomerase

PPRV	peste des petits ruminants virus
PPS	postpolio syndrome
PPV	porcine parvovirus
PR	protease
PRCoV	porcine respiratory coronavirus
PRE	post-transcriptional regulatory element
PRN	plaque reduction neutralization
PRNT	plaque reduction neutralization test
PRR	pattern recognition receptor
PRRSV	porcine reproductive and respiratory syndrome virus
PR-RT/RN	protease-reverse transcriptase/RNase H
PSG	peripheral sensory ganglia
PSLV	poa semilatent virus
PSV	peak systolic velocity
PT/SAP	Pro–Thr/Ser–Ala–Pro
PTA	phosphotungstate
PTB	polypyrimidine tract binding
PTK	protein tyrosine kinase
PTLD	post-transplant lymphoproliferative disease
PToV	porcine torovirus
pTP	precursor of the terminal protein
PV	papillomavirus; or polyomavirus
PVC	polvinylchloride
PVR	poliovirus receptor
PYV	polyomavirus
Q	glutamine
R	arginine; or direct repeat
RABV	rabies virus
RANTES	regulated upon activation of normal T cell expressed and secreted
RBC	red blood cell
RBS	rep binding site
RBV	Rio Bravo virus; or ribavirin
rc	relaxed circular
RD	rhabdomyosarcoma cells
RdRp	RNA-dependent RNA polymerase
REA	restriction enzyme analysis
REBOV	Reston ebola virus
RER	rough endoplasmic reticulum
RF	recombination frequency; or replicative form; or retroperitoneal fibromatosis; or rheumatoid factors
RF-C	replication factor C
RFLP	restriction fragment length polymorphism
RFV	Royal Farm virus
RHDV	rabbit hemorrhagic disease virus
RHR	rolling hairpin replication
RI	replicative intermediate
RIA	radioimmunoassay
RID	receptor internalization and degradation
RKV	rabbit kidney vacuolating virus
RML	Rocky Mountain Laboratory
RNAi	RNA interference
RNP	ribonucleocapsid particle; or ribonucleoprotein

ROCV	Rocio virus
RPA	replication protein A
RPC	replication protein C
RPV	rinderpest virus; or rabbitpox virus
RPXV	rabbitpox virus
RR	ribonucleotide reductase
RRE	rev responsive element
RREID	rapid rabies enzyme immunodiagnosis
rRNA	ribosomal RNA
RRP	recurrent respiratory papillomatosis
RRV	rhesus monkey rhadinovirus; or Ross river virus
RSP	recombinant subviral particle
RSSE	Russian spring–summer encephalitis
RSV	respiratory syncytial virus
RT	reverse transcriptase
RTA	replication and transcription activator
RTC	reverse transcription complex
RtCoV	rat coronavirus
RT-PCR	reverse transcriptase polymerase chain reaction
RUBV	rubella virus
RV	rabies virus
RVV	rhesus–human reassortant rotavirus
S	serine
SA	sialic acid; or splice acceptor
SA12	simian agent 12
SABV	Saboya virus
SAC	Staphylococcus aureus Cowan strain I
SAF	scrapie-associated fibril
SAg	superantigen
SaHV-1	herpes saimiri
SAR	secondary attack rate; or structure–activity relationship
SARS	severe acute respiratory syndrome
SARS-CoV	severe acute respiratory syndrome coronavirus
SCBV-IM	sugarcane bacilliform virus-Ireng Maleng
SCC	squamous cell carcinoma
SCID	severe combined immunodeficiency
sCJD	sporadic Creutzfeldt–Jakob disease
SCR	short consensus repeat
SD	splice donor
SDA	strand displacement amplification
SDAV	sialodacryoadenitis virus
SDD	serine–aspartic acid–aspartic acid
SDS-PAGE	sodium dodecyl sulfate polyacrylamide gel electrophoresis
SEBOV	Sudan ebola virus
SELP	simian virus 40 early leader protein
SEPV	Sepik virus
SFA	sanglifehrin A
SFFV	spleen focus-forming virus
SFGF	Shope fibroma growth factor
SFV	Semliki Forest virus; or simian foamy virus
sg	subgenomic
SH	small hydrophobic
SHa	Syrian hamster
SHa/Mo	Syrian hamster/mouse

SHFV	simian haemorrhagic fever virus		**3D**	three-dimensional
SIL	squamous intraepithelial lesion		**TF**	transcription factor
SIN	self-inactivating		**TfR**	transferrin receptor
SINV	Sindbis virus		**TFT**	trifluridine; or trifluorothymidine
SIV	simian immunodeficiency virus		**Tg**	transgenic
SL	stem-loop		**TGEV**	transmissible gastroenteritis virus
SLAM	signaling lymphocyte activation molecule		**TGF-β**	transforming growth factor β
SLEV	St. Louis encephalitis virus		**TGF-β1**	tumor growth factor β1
SLV	Sapporo-like viruses		**Th**	T helper
SN	serum neutralization		**Th1**	T-helper-1
SNHL	sensorineural hearing loss		**Th2**	T-helper-2
SNS	segmented negative-stranded		**TH**	tyrosine hydroxylase
Soc	small outer capsid		**TIBO**	thiobenzimidazolone
SOKV	Sokoluk virus		**TIR**	terminal inverted sequence region; or Toll/inter-leukin-1 receptor
SP	structural protein			
SPDV	salmon pancreas disease virus		**TK**	thymidine kinase
SPIEM	solid-phase immunoelectron microscopy		**TLMV**	TTV-like minivirus
SPOV	Spondweni virus		**TLR**	Toll-like receptor
SPV	San Perlita virus		**TLR2**	Toll-like receptor 2
SREV	Saumarez Reef virus		**TM**	transmembrane
SRF	serum-response factor		**TMA**	transcription-mediated amplification
SRH	single radial hemolysis		**TMEV**	Theiler's murine encephalomyelitis virus
SRP	signal recognition particle		**TMUV**	Tembusu virus
SRSV	small round structured virus		**TMV**	tobacco mosaic virus
SRV	Saumarez Reef virus; or simian type D virus; or small round virus		**TNF**	tumor necrosis factor
			TNF-α	tumor necrosis factor α
ssDNA	single-stranded DNA		**TNFR**	tumor necrosis factor receptor
SSPE	subacute sclerosing panencephalitis		**T1L**	type 1 Lang (virus)
ssRNA	single-stranded RNA		**TOP**	termination of pregnancy
SST	sodium silicotungstate		**topo I**	topoisomerase I
STAT	signal transducers and activators of transcription		**TORCH**	toxoplasma gondii, other diseases, rubellavirus, cytomegalovirus, herpes simplex virus
STD	sexually transmitted disease			
STE	surface tubule element		**TORCHES-CLAP**	toxoplasma gondii, other diseases, rubellavirus, cytomegalovirus, herpes simplex virus, entero-virus, syphilis, chickenpox virus, Lyme disease, AIDs, parvovirus B19
STIKO	German Vaccinee Commission			
STLV	simian T-lymphotropic virus			
STMV	stump-tailed macaque virus			
STORCH	syphilis, toxoplasma, other diseases, rubella, cytomegalovirus, herpes simplex virus			
			TP	terminal protein
STRV	Stratford virus		**TPA**	tetradecanoylphorbol acetate
SU	surface		**TR**	terminal repeat
SV	subvirion		**TRAF**	tumor necrosis factor receptor activating factor
SV-5	simian virus 5		**TRBP**	tat region binding protein
SV40	simian vacuolating virus 40; or simian virus 40		**TRE-1**	tax response element 1
SVDV	swine vesicular disease virus		**TR-FIA**	time-resolved fluoroimmunoassay
SVP	subviral particle		**TRIS**	tris(hydroxymethyl)amino-methane
SVV	Sal Vieja virus		**tRNA**	transfer RNA
			TROCV	Trocara virus
			TRS	terminal resolution sequence; or transcription-regulating sequence
T	thymine			
TABV	Tamana bat virus		**ts**	temperature-sensitive
TAP	transporter associated with antigen processing		**TS**	thymidylate synthase
TAstV	turkey astrovirus		**TSE**	transmissible spongiform encephalopathy
TBEV	tick-borne encephalitis virus		**TSG**	tumor suppressor gene
TBP	TATA-binding protein		**TSP**	tropical spastic paraparesis
3CLp	3C-like protease; or 3C-like proteinase		**TSP/HAM**	tropical spastic paraparesis/human T-cell leukemia virus-I associated myelopathy
TCoV	turkey coronavirus			
TCR	T-cell receptor		**3TC**	2'-deoxy-3'-thiacytidine
2D	two-dimensional		**T3D**	type 3 Dearing (virus)

T2J	type 2 Jones (virus)	**VLP**	virus-like particle
TTMV	torque-teno-minivirus	**VLTF**	viral late transcription factor
TTP	thymidine triphosphate	**VMK**	vervet monkey kidney
TTV	torque-teno-virus	**VN**	virus neutralization
TUT	terminal uridylate transferase	**VNA**	virus-neutralizing antibody
TYUV	Tyuleniy virus	**Vpr**	viral protein R
		Vpu	viral protein U
UEV	ubiquitin E2 variant	**VSIV**	vesicular stomatitis Indiana virus
UGSV	Uganda S virus	**VSV**	vesicular stomatitis virus
ULBP	UL16 binding protein	**VTF**	viral termination factor
UNICEF	United Nations International Children's Emergency Fund	**VTM**	viral transport medium
		VZIG	varicella-zoster immune globulin
UPS	ubiquitin proteasome system	**VZV**	varicella zoster virus
UPU	Universal Postal Union		
URR	upstream regulatory region	**W**	Tryptophan
USUV	Usutu virus	**WB**	western blot
UTR	untranslated region	**WEEV**	western equine encephalomyelitis virus
UV	ultraviolet	**WESSV**	Wesselsbron virus
		WG	week of gestation
V	valine	**WHO**	World Health Organization
VA	virus-associated	**WHV**	woodchuck hepatitis virus
VACV	vaccinia virus; or valaciclovir	**WNV**	West Nile virus
VAERS	vaccine adverse events reporting system		
VAP	virus attachment protein	**X-SCID**	X-linked severe combined immunodeficiency
VAPP	vaccine-associated paralytic poliomyelitis	**XLA**	X-linked agammaglobulinemia
vCJD	variant Creutzfeldt–Jakob disease	**XLPS**	X-linked lymphoproliferative syndrome
vCKBP	viral chemokine binding protein		
vCKR	viral chemokine receptor	**Y**	tyrosine
VCP	viral complement control protein	**YAOV**	Yaounde virus
VEEV	Venezuelan equine encephalitis virus	**YFV**	yellow fever virus
VEGF	vascular endothelial growth factor	**YHV**	yellow head virus
VETF	viral early transcription factor	**YLDV**	yaba-like disease virus
vFLIP	viral FLICE inhibitory protein	**YMTV**	yaba monkey tumor virus
VHSV	viral hemorrhagic septicemia virus	**YOKV**	yokose virus
Vif	virus infectivity factor		
VIG	vaccinia immunoglobulin	**ZDV**	zidovudine
vIL-18BP	viral interleukin-18 binding protein	**ZEBOV**	Zaire ebola virus
vIL-1βR	viral interleukin-1β receptor	**ZF**	zinc-finger
VITF	viral intermediate transcription factor	**ZIG**	zoster immunoglobulin
VL	viral load	**ZIKV**	Zika virus
VLBW	very low birth weight		

PART II

SPECIFIC VIRUSES AND
VIRAL INFECTION (CONTINUED)

Picornaviruses

PHILIP MINOR

The picornaviruses cause a number of diseases of animals and humans of varying degrees of severity. The earliest record of a human disease believed to be caused by a virus is an Egyptian funerary stela of about 1 300 BC depicting a priest with the typical withered limb and dropped foot deformity of poli omyelitis, caused by *Poliovirus*, a picornavirus of the *Enterovirus* genus. In 1909, the virus was transmitted from the spinal cord of a fatal case to monkeys by Landsteiner and Popper. Enders et al. (1949) showed that poliovirus could be grown in primate cells of non-neural origin, and the isolation of other enteroviruses followed. Coxsackie virus was isolated from two children with paralytic disease from the town of Coxsackie in New York State in 1948 by the inoculation of newborn mice with fecal extracts (Dalldorf and Sickles 1948). Robbins and co-workers isolated echoviruses (enterocytopathic human orphan viruses) from healthy children in 1951. The echo-, polio- and coxsackie viruses, with more recently discovered viruses identified by number, are classified as enteroviruses, as shown in Table 40.1. The classification of the picornaviruses has been extensively reviewed and modified over the last few years and now relies mainly on molecular approaches.

The *Rhinovirus* genus of the picornavirus family is one of the causative agents of the common cold. Kruse (1914) first demonstrated that a cold could be transmitted by bacteria-free filtrates. The Common Cold Research Unit at Salisbury (UK) was established in 1946 and investigation of transmission of the common cold to human volunteers eventually led to the cultivation of the virus in vitro. In the USA, two cytopathogenic agents, JH and 2060, were described (Price et al. 1959) and were originally classified as echovirus 28, later being reclassified as *human rhinovirus A*, the type species of the genus (Kapikian et al. 1967). In 1960, Tyrrell and Parsons found that other viruses that caused common colds could be propagated in cultures of human embryonic kidney cells rolled at 33°C in medium with low pH (Tyrrell and Parsons 1960). This observation and the introduction of semicontinuous strains of diploid human embryonic lung fibroblasts (Hayflick and Moorhead 1961) led to a rapid increase in the number of

Table 40.1 Enterovirus *serotypes*

Group[a]	Major disease
Polioviruses 1–3	Paralytic poliomyelitis Aseptic meningitis
Coxsackie viruses A1–22, 24	Aseptic meningitis Herpangina Conjunctivitis (A24)
Coxsackie viruses B1–6	Aseptic meningitis Fatal neonatal disease Pleurodynia Myo- or pericarditis
Echoviruses 1–9, 11–21, 24–27, 29–34	Aseptic meningitis Rashes Febrile illness
Enteroviruses 68–71	Conjunctivitis (enterovirus 70) Polio-like illness (enterovirus 71)

Echovirus 9 = coxsackie virus A23; echovirus 10 = reovirus; echovirus 28 = rhinovirus; echovirus 34 = coxsackie virus A24.
a) In the current report of the International Committee on Taxonomy of Viruses these viruses are prefixed 'human' to distinguish them from animal viruses where relevant.

viruses isolated. Rhinoviruses were also isolated from horses (Plummer 1963) and cattle (Bögel and Böhm 1962).

The Rhinovirus Collaborative Programme of the World Health Organization authenticated 100 serotypes of rhinovirus over the next 20 years (Hamparian et al. 1987).

Foot-and-mouth disease virus (FMDV) was the first non-plant virus to be discovered (Loeffler and Frosch 1898).

PROPERTIES OF THE VIRUSES

The picornaviruses are small RNA-containing viruses. The complete sequences of the genomic RNA of many strains of picornaviruses have been determined, the first being that of the type 1 poliovirus strain Mahoney (Kitamura et al. 1981), and the atomic structures of representative viruses of each of the various genera have been resolved by X-ray crystallography (Hogle et al. 1985; Rossmann et al. 1985; Ming et al. 1987; Acharya et al. 1989). The discussion of the detailed molecular virology that follows refers to poliovirus except where stated otherwise.

Classification

The six genera that make up the *Picornaviridae* are:

- the enteroviruses (Table 40.1)
- the rhinoviruses
- the aphthoviruses, which cause foot-and-mouth disease of cattle
- the cardioviruses of mice, which include mengo virus and *Encephalomyocarditis virus* (EMCV) as well as Theiler's virus
- the hepatoviruses, which include hepatitis A viruses (described in Chapter 53, Hepatitis A and E)
- the parechoviruses, which encompass the viruses previously designated echovirus 22 and echovirus 23.

Comparisons of the sequences of the virus genomes play an essential role in the classification scheme. In particular, Theiler's virus and *Hepatitis A virus* were moved from the enteroviruses mainly because of the nature of their genomic organization and sequence, although they also have particular pathogenic features, whereas echovirus 22 and echovirus 23 appear to be typical enteroviruses in all except their sequences, which are very different.

Molecular classification of the picornaviruses

Theiler's virus of mice is an acid-stable picornavirus which produces symptoms analogous to those of poliomyelitis in humans, and for many years it was classified as an *Enterovirus*. Determination of the sequence and later the structure of the virus showed that it was much more closely related to the cardioviruses of mice such as EMCV, and it was reassigned on this basis. Likewise, *Hepatitis A virus* was categorized as an *Enterovirus*, largely on the basis of its acid stability and its occurrence in the stool of infected individuals, but its pathogenesis is strikingly different from that of other enteroviruses and its sequence is uniquely placed among those of the other picornaviruses. It was also therefore reclassified.

Sequence comparisons made it clear that the rhinoviruses were very similar to the enteroviruses and a re-evaluation of the whole basis of the classification took place, which has revealed the relationships between picornaviruses and enabled subclassifications to be made. The increasing use of molecular methods in clinical virology makes this a valuable and logical development.

Complete sequences of many picornaviruses are known and viruses can be classified into the appropriate genus on the basis of comparison of the amino acid sequences of any part of the coding region of the genome, including those encoding the structural proteins, P1, or the polymerase 3D (King et al. 2000). Dendrograms showing the relationships between the different picornavirus genera based on the P1 region are shown in Figure 40.1. Variation between genera is typically greater than 70 percent in terms of sequence, and the rhinoviruses and the enteroviruses are surprisingly closely related. If the nucleic acid sequence of the 5′ noncoding region is considered, however, only two clusters are evident.

Subclusters can be identified within a genus giving rise to the concept of the species. Members of a species are defined as sharing greater than 70 percent amino acid identity within P1, greater than 70 percent amino acid identity within the nonstructural proteins 2C and 3D combined, sharing a limited range of host cell receptors and natural host range, and having a degree of compatibility in certain aspects of virus multiplication. Species within the *Enterovirus* genus are shown in Figure 40.2. *Poliovirus* is currently classified in a different subspecies to the other group C species. There is reason to believe that the members of a species are able to exchange segments of their genomes by recombination more or less freely. Thus within the B species the P1 region is sufficient to identify a virus as a coxsackie virus B1 distinct from a coxsackie virus B3, for example, while comparisons of the nonstructural protein 3D are believed to be only able to identify a virus as a B species. Similarly within the C species it is not currently possible to distinguish a coxsackie virus A21 strain from a poliovirus by examination of the nonstructural proteins. This finding, if confirmed, implies that viruses within a species infect the same cell types and show a great deal of compatibility between their genomes, while

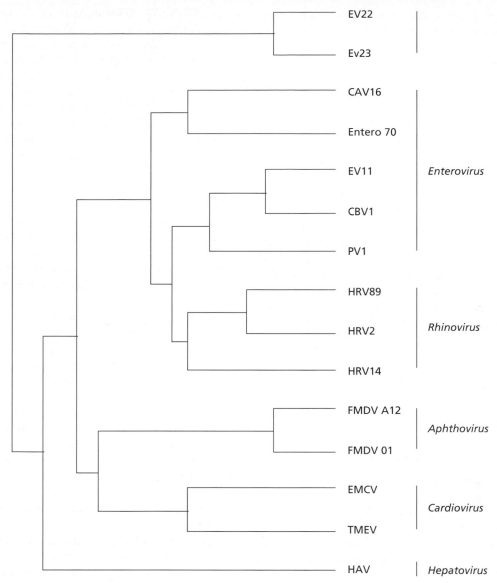

Figure 40.1 *Clustering of the picornavirus genera on the basis of comparison of the complete sequences of the genome. The viruses designated EV22 and EV23 (enterovirus 22 and enterovirus 23) are now classified as parechovirus 1 and parechovirus 2, respectively, on the basis of their highly distinct genomic sequences.*

those of different species are either unable to infect the same cell type naturally or have genomes which are incompatible with each other when segments are exchanged. Polioviruses which are recombinants between the vaccine strains and unknown species C enteroviruses have been isolated on several occasions, as discussed below (Kew et al. 2002).

Physical properties of picornaviruses of different genera

The viruses of the picornavirus genera share a number of characteristics (Palmenberg 1987), including size, icosahedral morphology, lack of a lipid envelope, a positive-sense RNA genome and the general arrangement of

their structural proteins. The sedimentation coefficient is ca. 155–160S. The enteroviruses, cardioviruses, hepatoviruses, and parechsoviruses have a buoyant density in cesium chloride of 1.34 g/cm^3, the rhinoviruses of 1.40 g/cm^3, and the aphthoviruses of 1.43 g/cm^3. The enteroviruses and parechoviruses, unlike rhinoviruses or aphthoviruses, are totally stable at pH 4 and resistant at pH 2, and this property formed the basis of early classification schemes for the picornaviruses.

The genomes of both the aphtho- and the cardioviruses include a tract of cytidine residues not found in the other genera, and share a similar genomic structure distinct from that of the enteroviruses and rhinoviruses, as described below. The properties of the picornavirus genera are summarized in Table 40.2, p. 861.

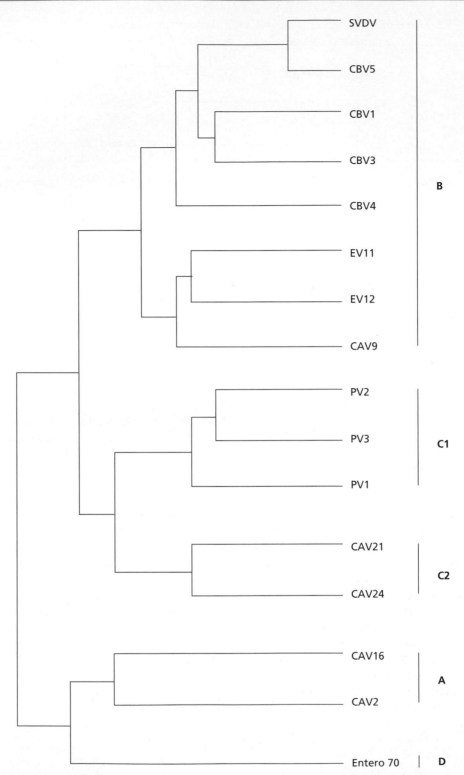

Figure 40.2 *Clustering of the human enteroviruses based on comparisons of the sequences of the structural proteins P1, showing the occurrence of species (clusters) A, B, C, and D.*

Biological and antigenic properties of subgroups

The enteroviruses are divided into various biological subgroups, which in general reflect the sequence classifications imperfectly. However, some are apparently related both serologically and by the sequence of the P1 region. For example, poliovirus 1 and poliovirus 2 share common antigens. Cross-relationships also exist between coxsackie viruses A3 and A8, A11 and A15, A13 and A18, echoviruses 1 and 8, 6 and 30, and 12 and 29.

Table 40.2 *Properties of the picornavirus genera*

Property	Enterovirus	Hepatovirus	Rhinovirus	Cardiovirus	Aphthovirus	Parechovirus[a]
Particle size	27 nm	27 nm	27 nm	27 nm	27 nm	27 nm
Sense or virion RNA	Messenger	Messenger	Messenger	Messenger	Messenger	Messenger
Sedimentation coefficient (S) of virion	156	156	149	156	142–146	156
RNA in virion (%)	31	31	31	34	38	31
Size of virion proteins (kDa)						
VP1	35	35	35	34	29	30.5
VP2	30	30	30	30	30	38
VP3	24	24	23	23	22	30
VP4	7	?[b]	7	7	8	…
Poly(A) tract	+	+	+	+	+	+
Size of genome						
kb	7 445	7 450	7 155	7 832	8 400	7 340
kDa	2 200	2 200	2 200	2 300	2 500	2 200
Buoyant density in CsCl (g/cm³)	1.34	1.34	1.41	1.34	1.43	1.36
Acid stability	+	+	−	+	−	+
Poly(C) tract	−	−	−	+	+	−
Base composition						
A (%)	30	29	32	26	26	32
U (%)	24	33	28	25	21	29
C (%)	23	16	20	26	28	19
G (%)	23	22	20	23	25	20

a) Echoviruses 22 and 23.
b) It is not clear whether hepatoviruses contain VP4.

In general, the echoviruses may be biologically distinguished from the coxsackie viruses by their failure to cause pathological changes in newborn mice. However, most strains of echovirus 9 can produce flaccid paralysis in newborn mice, a finding that led to its early classification as coxsackie virus A23. Some strains of enterovirus 71 grow better in newborn mice than in cultures of primate cells. Conversely, coxsackie virus A9 is not pathogenic for mice unless passaged in cell culture, in which it grows readily, thus resembling the echoviruses.

The neutralization of rhinovirus infectivity by antisera is largely type specific, and is the basis of the numbering system by which rhinoviruses are classified into 100 serotypes (Hamparian et al. 1987). Minor serological variations may exist within a serotype. Within type 1 there are two subtypes, A and B: the low degree of cross-reaction between these subtypes may be reciprocal or one-way (Monto and Johnson 1966). 'Prime' strains of rhinovirus 22 that are antigenically broader than the prototype strain have been isolated (Schieble et al. 1970; Hamparian et al. 1987).

Resemblances to other viruses

A number of other viruses seem to be superficially similar to the picornaviruses. Astroviruses, which contain RNA and lack a lipid bilayer, are of similar size to picornaviruses, although with distinct morphology in electron micrographs. The caliciviruses are similar, but significantly larger, with a particle diameter of 30 nm, a characteristic morphology, and a capsid consisting of a single protein species. Other small round viruses are found in the intestinal tract and may be confused with the true enteroviruses; their relationship, if any, with the enteric picornaviruses is not clear (see Chapter 41, Human enteric RNA viruses: Astroviruses).

However, the picornaviruses are similar in many ways, including particle structure and genomic organization to the spherical plant viruses such as cowpea mosaic virus and to insect viruses such as cricket paralysis virus. Similarly, the picornaviruses and togaviruses share some features of genomic strategy and organization. These relationships, which have been revealed by detailed molecular biological characterization of the viruses, suggest intriguing possibilities for the evolutionary origin of picornaviruses (see, for example, Rossmann 1987).

Morphology and structure

Picornaviruses usually appear in electron micrographs as roughly spherical particles not penetrated by negative

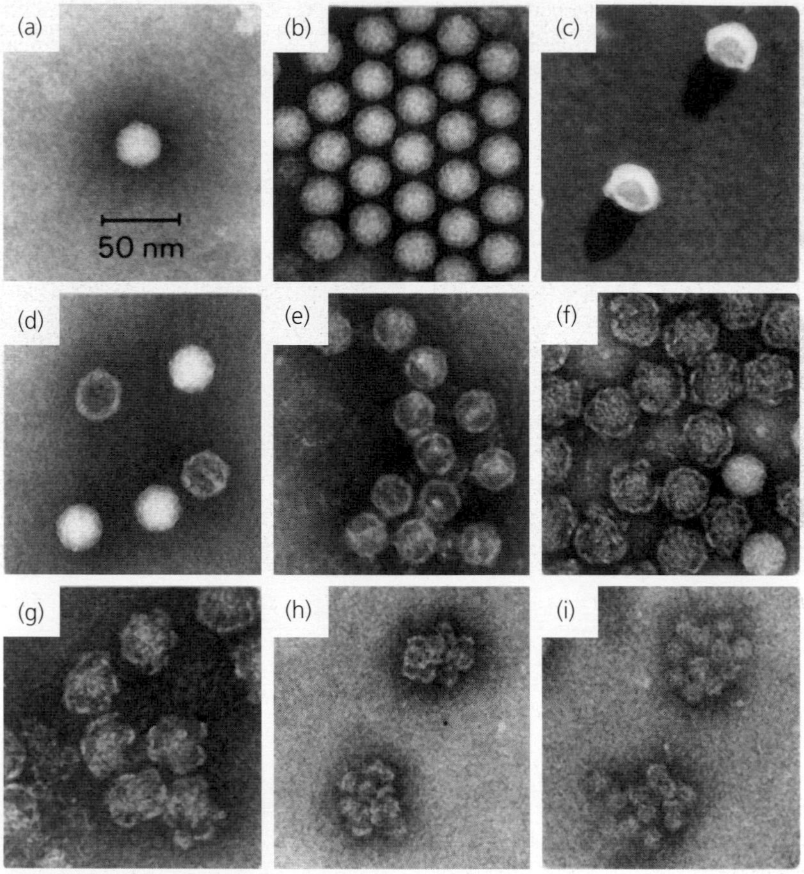

Figure 40.3 *Electron micrographs of poliovirus; all specimens (except c) stained with 4 percent sodium silicotungstate and all magnified ×200 000. (a) Whole virus particle (D antigen) ca. 30 nm in diameter and displaying a hexagonal profile. (b) High concentration of virus in hexagonal array. (c) Freeze-dried virus with low angle platinum shadowing (print reversed to give black shadows); virus particles produce either pointed or blunt-ended shadows, which are consistent with an icosahedral particle. (d) Penetration of stain into empty particles reveals outer capsid. (e) Empty particles (C antigen) showing small central unstained portions representing incomplete contents. (f) Flattened particles showing complete contents and outer capsid. (g) Flattened particles showing breakdown of capsid into angular or crescentlike portions. (h and i) Particles heated at 56°C for 2 min produce aggregates of ca. 12 crescentlike or circular structures.*

staining methods. Figure 40.3 demonstrates some of the features of poliovirus, but similar results would be obtained with all picornaviruses. The viruses are 25–30 nm in diameter (Figure 40.3a), and can occasionally present a hexagonal appearance (Figure 40.3a) or form hexagonal arrays (Figure 40.3b). Similarly, shadowed preparations can produce blunt-ended or pointed shadows, consistent with an icosahedral structure (Figure 40.3c). In preparations positively stained after drying of the virus from ethanol where the RNA is extruded, the capsid may remain negatively stained and so the thickness of the virion wall can be seen to be ca. 2.5 nm. A similar thickness has been determined for the empty capsids, which are in general penetrated by negative stain (Figure 40.3d), although frequently there are regions from which the stain is excluded (Figure 40.3e). When the particle is distorted during drying, it may expand and break into circular or crescent-like portions (Figure 40.3g). Similarly, heating (Figure 40.3h, i) can give rise to 12 crescentic or circular structures, which are believed to correspond to the pentamers of the icosahedron.

Understanding of picornaviruses was extended immensely by the determination of the atomic structures of rhinovirus 14 (Rossmann et al. 1985), the type 1 poliovirus strain Mahoney (Hogle et al. 1985), the cardiovirus mengo virus (Ming et al. 1987) and FMDV (Acharya et al. 1989). The structure of the type 1 poliovirus strain Mahoney is shown in Figure 40.4. Although all picornavirus structures solved to date are strikingly similar to each other, and to the spherical plant viruses such as southern bean mosaic virus and tomato bushy stunt virus, there are also clear differences between them.

The capsid of poliovirus is composed of 60 protomers, each being made up of one molecule of each of the four virion proteins VP1, VP2, VP3, and VP4. The protomers are arranged with icosahedral symmetry. Each of the 20 faces of the icosahedron is made up of three protomers, orientated so that the 12 apices of the icosahedron are occupied by five copies of VP1 while the center of each face is occupied by three copies each of VP2 and VP3, alternating around the threefold axis of symmetry. The overall thickness of the shell is about 3 nm, extending

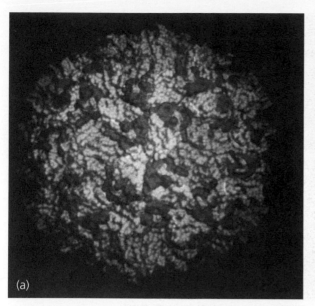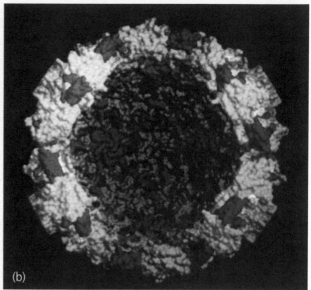

Figure 40.4 *Structure of the Mahoney strain of type 1 poliovirus showing* **(a)** *the complete capsid, and* **(b)** *the capsid with one pentamer removed to reveal the inside of the virion.*

11–14 nm from the particle center. However, the apices of the icosahedron and the face at the threefold axis of symmetry form two elevated features separated by a cleft or 'canyon' that circles the apex, which, for the enteroviruses and rhinoviruses, is believed to be the site by which the virus attaches to the specific receptor site on the cell.

The structural organization of the individual proteins that make up the virion is similar, (Figure 40.5). Each protein has a wedge-shaped core structure composed of eight strands of protein, shown as broad arrows in Figure 40.5, arranged in an antiparallel β-sheet array, the eight strands collectively forming a barrel (termed the β barrel). The core structure of polioviruses, rhinoviruses, and other spherical viruses, including plant viruses, are very similar in this respect. The features that are unique to the individual virus, including antigenic sites, arise from the loops that join the different β strands and the sequences at the N and C termini.

The narrow end of the β barrel of VP1 is located near the icosahedral apex of the virus while the corresponding regions of VP2 and VP3 alternate around the threefold axis of symmetry. VP4 forms a lattice around the inside of the pentameric apex. Interactions between adjacent pentamers include regions of secondary structure in the form of β sheets between the β barrels of VP2 and VP1.

In addition to the protein components of the virus shell, the N terminus of each VP4 protein is covalently bound to a myristic acid residue (Chow et al. 1987). The myristate sequences penetrate the pentameric apex, possibly forming a framework for assembly.

The structures of poliovirus and rhinovirus are very similar but differ from that of the cardioviruses, typified by mengo virus (Ming et al. 1987), where the pentameric apex is surrounded by five distinct pores rather than

a canyon. The 15 C-terminal residues of VP1 are disordered but exposed on the virus surface, whereas all C-terminal residues of VP1 are ordered in the poliovirus and rhinovirus.

The particle shell of FMDV is relatively smooth because of the truncation of certain loops, and there is no canyon or series of pits around the pentameric apex (Acharya et al. 1989). One loop in VP1 forms a disordered surface structure known to be a major antigenic site. The C terminus of VP1 is also a disordered surface feature lying in the region of the disordered loop. A residue in VP2 is covalently linked by a disulfide bridge to a residue in the disordered VP1 loop, and is therefore itself faint in the structure. It is believed that the highly exposed, disordered loop forms the site on the virus by which it attaches to the host cell, in contrast to the other picornaviruses which attach to the cell via the canyon or pit regions.

Genome structure and function

Sequences of the genomes of many picornaviruses representing strains from each genus have been determined. The genomic RNA, constituting about 33 percent of the mass of the virion, varies in size from about 7 200 nt for rhinovirus to 8 500 nt for FMDV (mol. mass 2 000–3 000 kDa). Virion RNA is of messenger sense and therefore infectious for cells, although less so than intact virus. The layout of the genome of poliovirus is presented in Figure 40.6. The 5′ terminus of the RNA is covalently linked to a small protein (VPg) of 22 amino acids via the phenolic hydroxyl group of the tyrosine at residue 3 from the N terminus, a residue conserved in all picornaviral sequences of VPg to date. The following 740 nucleotides of the RNA constitute the 5′ noncoding region preceding the coding region of the genome,

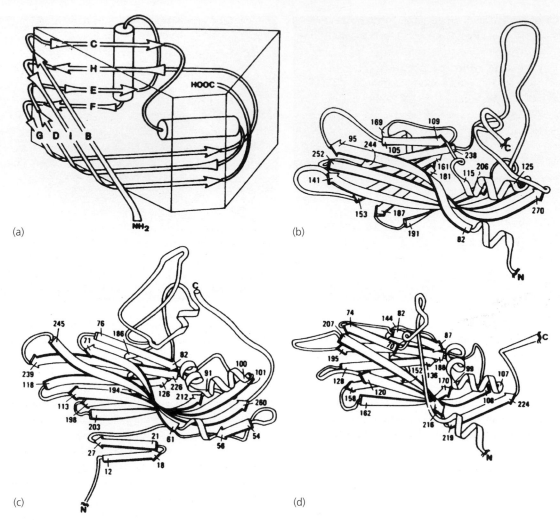

Figure 40.5 *Structure of the proteins making up the poliovirus capsid:* **(a)** *schematic diagram of β-barrel structure (arrow) and connecting α helices (cylinders);* **(b)** *VP1;* **(c)** *VP2;* **(d)** *VP3.*

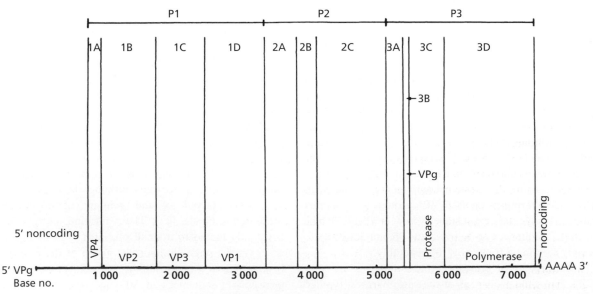

Figure 40.6 *Organization of the genome of enteroviruses showing the 5′ and 3′ noncoding regions and the location of the regions coding for the various proteins. Nomenclature is according to Rueckert and Wimmer (1984) and the common name where appropriate.*

which is translated as a single large protein cleaved by virus-encoded proteases as it is translated and post-translation. The genome terminates in a short untranslated 3′ noncoding region of about 70 nt, to which a sequence of 40–100 adenosine residues is attached, comparable to that found on many eukaryotic mRNAs. Sequence analysis of viral proteins has defined the genomic location and proteolytic cleavage sites used in processing. The structural proteins are encoded in the order VP4, VP2, VP3, and VP1, or 1A, 1B, 1C, 1D in the formal nomenclature (Rueckert and Wimmer 1984), from the 5′ end, making up the P1 region of the polyprotein which is excised as a single unit during replication. The nonstructural proteins P2, consisting of proteins 2A, 2B, and 2C, and P3, consisting of proteins 3A, 3B, 3C, and 3D, are also considered to be single units. The rhinoviruses closely resemble the enteroviruses except that the 5′ noncoding region lacks the poorly conserved 100 nt region immediately preceding the open reading frame.

The genomic organization of the cardioviruses and aphthoviruses differs from this general structure in that they encode a leader protein (L) before the P1 region and contain a polycytidylate tract in the 5′ noncoding region. In addition, protein 2A of FMDV is very small, and the genome includes three distinct copies of the protein VPg, any of which may be covalently linked to virus-derived RNA.

Complete cDNA copies of the picornavirus genome can be generated and used either to recover infectious virus directly from the DNA (Racaniello and Baltimore 1981) or, after linking to transcription systems such as SP6 or T7, to generate infectious RNA. It is thus possible to study the effect of defined genetic manipulations on the phenotype of the virus. For technical reasons, complete infectious copies of aphthovirus or cardiovirus genomes are more difficult to produce than those of the other genera.

Antigens

Most studies of the antigenic properties of enteroviruses, and of poliovirus in particular, have been concerned with humoral immunity to structural proteins, which is believed to be the major factor in protection from disease, although some work has concerned sites involved in recognition by T cells (Mahon et al. 1995). In infection by FMDV, however, a major immune response is directed against the infection-associated antigen (IAA) which has been shown to correspond to the nonstructural RNA polymerase protein 3D.

Antigenic differences may occur between different isolates; for example, isolates of type 3 polioviruses in Finland during 1984/85 differed from classic type 3 strains (Huovilainen et al. 1987) and UK strains of coxsackie virus B5 from 1973 were very different from the coxsackie virus Faulkner strain isolated in 1952.

The infectious virus particles of polioviruses and other picornaviruses differ antigenically from the empty capsids. Mayer et al. (1957) resolved poliovirus preparations into distinct fractions by centrifugation on a sucrose step gradient; most of the infectious material appeared in the fourth layer (D) and reacted preferentially with convalescent sera, but viral antigens could also be detected in the lighter third layer (C) which reacted preferentially with acute phase sera. D antigenic material corresponds to infectious particles, and C to empty capsids. Others showed that the natural virus expressed one antigenic determinant (termed N antigen), whereas material heated at 56°C for 30 minutes expressed another (H antigen) (Hummeler and Tumilowicz 1960); in general, N and D antigens are equated, as are C and H antigens. Relatively mild treatments have a pronounced effect on antigenicity (Le Bouvier 1955). Rhinoviruses also exhibit D and C antigen characteristics (Butterworth et al. 1976).

Monoclonal antibodies derived from mice immunized with poliovirus can bind to the D or to the C antigenic forms of the virus (Rombaut et al. 1983), or to both (Ferguson et al. 1984). In addition, some D-specific antibodies bind to subunits that are precursors to virions in the assembly pathway, whereas others bind only to mature virus. The particular sites recognized by antibodies were identified by generating antigenic mutants resistant to neutralization by monoclonal antibodies (Minor et al. 1986a; Page et al. 1988).

The specific amino acid substitutions found in antigenic mutants of poliovirus selected with murine antibodies are largely located in the loops decorating the β barrels and clustered into several non-overlapping sites on the surface of the virion. The regions in which mutations have been identified are shown in Table 40.3, and each site is complex and conformational in nature. For poliovirus of both type 2 and type 3, site 1 seems to be the major target of the murine immune response, whereas antibodies against the corresponding region of type 1 have not been induced by immunization with native virus.

Antibodies directed against site 3 of poliovirus serotypes 1 and 3 tend to be highly strain specific, even to the extent that antigenic drift can be demonstrated during the period of excretion by vaccinees.

Neutralizing antibody is difficult to induce with isolated viral proteins or with short peptides based on sequences found within them except where, as in FMDV, the immunogenic sequence is disordered in the structure (Bittle et al. 1982). The difference is attributable to the highly integrated and conformational nature of the antigenic sites. Even where viruses have been constructed in which entire sites have been exchanged between different serotypes (Burke et al. 1988; Murray et al. 1988) and can have antigenic and immunogenic properties of both parents, the inserted site is imperfectly expressed (Minor et al. 1990, 1991). The viruses usually grow poorly.

Table 40.3 *Antigenic sites for the neutralization of poliovirus and Rhinovirus by monoclonal antibodies*

Poliovirus			Rhinovirus 14		
Site	Amino acids involved		Site	Amino acids involved	
1	VP1	89–100	Nim 1a	VP1	91, 95
	VP1	142	Nim 1b	VP1	83, 85, 138, 139
	VP1	166	. . .	. . .	. . .
	VP1	253	. . .	. . .	. . .
2	VP1	220–222	Nim II	VP1	210
	VP2	164–170	. . .	VP2	158, 159, 161, 162
	VP2	273	. . .	. . .	. . .
3	VP1	286–290	Nim III	VP1	287
	VP3	58–60	. . .	VP3	72, 73, 75, 78, 203
	VP3	70–72	. . .	. . .	. . .
4	VP3	77–80	. . .	. . .	. . .
	VP2	72	. . .	. . .	. . .

Similar antigenic studies have been performed for rhinovirus 14. Sherry and colleagues (1986) identified four antigenic sites recognized by monoclonal antibodies (Table 40.3). All are surface features and in general the antigenic structures identified in all picornaviruses correspond to all of the prominent surface features in the structure, which are usually loops between strands of β barrels (Minor 1990). In contrast to poliovirus, no sites are strongly immunodominant or recessive.

When virus infection is initiated, the capsid undergoes a major rearrangement with the extrusion of the N terminus of VP1, which is normally internal. Antibodies to this region have been described in post-infection human sera and are believed to have neutralizing capacity.

Replication

ENTRY INTO HOST CELLS

Viral RNA from poliovirus is able to induce a single round of replication in rabbit kidney cells, which are not normally susceptible to infection (Holland et al. 1959), indicating that the blockage is at the level of virus entry. Saturable receptors have been demonstrated (Lonberg-Holm et al. 1976) and competition experiments showed that the three serotypes of poliovirus attach to the same site, distinct from that used by other enteroviruses. Monoclonal antibodies directed against cellular components have been raised that specifically block the binding of poliovirus (Minor et al. 1984), coxsackie viruses (Campbell and Cords 1983), and rhinovirus 14.

The gene coding for the poliovirus receptor was identified by Mendelsohn et al. (1986, 1989). It is a three-domain protein of the immunoglobulin superfamily with an unglycosylated molecular mass of 42 kDa. The cellular receptor for most rhinoviruses is the cell adhesion protein ICAM-1, a five-domain protein of the same superfamily (Greve et al. 1989; Staunton et al. 1989).

Other picornavirus receptors identified include decay accelerating factor (DAF), implicated in the complement pathway as the receptor for echovirus 7, among others (Ward et al. 1994) and integrin VLA2 for echovirus 1 (Bergelson et al. 1992). The possible need for additional molecules in attachment or penetration is suggested by the failure of mouse cells transfected with the genes for either ICAM-1 or DAF to support the growth of rhinovirus 14 or echovirus 7. Moreover, whereas mouse cells transfected with the poliovirus receptor are highly susceptible to poliovirus (Pipkin et al. 1993), it has been suggested that CD44 may also play a role (Shepley and Racaniello 1994). The poliovirus receptor and susceptibility to coxsackie virus B3 and echovirus 11 have been shown to be encoded on human chromosome 19 (Medrano and Green 1973; Miller et al. 1974). Transgenic mice carrying the gene for the human poliovirus receptor are susceptible to poliovirus infection by a variety of routes, developing paralysis similar to that seen in primates (Ren and Racaniello 1992) and such animals have been extensively used in pathogenesis studies in place of primates. A summary of the receptor sites used by some picornaviruses is given in Table 40.4, but the situation is complex except for polio in that the receptor sites listed alone do not in general confer susceptibility when transfected into nonsusceptible cells alone (Rieder and Wimmer 2002).

UNCOATING

When virus is allowed to bind to cells at room temperature and the cultures are then incubated at 37°C, up to 90 percent of the virus may be released into the medium. The released virus (A particles) has lost VP4, and has converted from D (N) antigenicity to C (H) antigenicity, although it retains the virion RNA (Joklik and Darnell 1961). Similar particles can be identified in the cells, and their production can be catalyzed by soluble receptor in the case of poliovirus.

PROTEIN SYNTHESIS

The genomic RNA is infectious and translated into virion proteins directly. The 5' terminus of many

Table 40.4 *Receptors and accessory factors used by picornavirus genera and species*

Genus	Species	Receptor	Accessory factors
Enterovirus	**B**		β_2–m
	Coxsackie virus A9	$\alpha_v\beta_3$; alternative receptor likely	MAP-70
	Coxsackie virus B1–6	HCAR	. . .
	Coxsackie viruses B1, 3, 5	DAF (= CD55)	$\alpha_v\beta_6$
	Echoviruses 1, 8	VLA-2 (= $\alpha_2\beta_1$)	. . .
	Echoviruses 3, 6, 7, 11, 12, 13, 19, 21, 24, 25, 29, 30, 33	DAF	β_2–m, CD59
	Echovirus 6	Heparin sulfate?	. . .
	Echovirus 69	ND	. . .
	C		
	Polioviruses 1–3	CD155 (Pvr)	. . .
	Coxsackie viruses A13, 17, 18, 20, 21, 24	ICAM-1	. . .
	Coxsackie virus A21	DAF	62
	Coxsackie virus 24v	ICAM-1, second receptor?	. . .
	D		
	Enterovirus 70 (68)	DAF	. . .
	E		
	Bovine enterovirus types 1 and 2	ND	. . .
Parechovirus	Human echovirus types 22 and 23	$\alpha_v\beta_3$	. . .
Rhinovirus	Major receptor group rhinovirus (>90 serotypes)	ICAM-1	. . .
	Minor receptor group rhinovirus (>10 serotypes)	LDL receptor related	. . .
Hepatovirus	Hepatitis A virus	HAVcr-1	. . .
Aphthovirus	FMDV	$\alpha_v\beta_3$, $\alpha_v\beta_6$	. . .
	A12 strains of foot-and-mouth disease virus 0_1	Heparan sulfate	. . .
Cardiovirus	Encephalomyocarditis virus, mengo virus	VCAM-1, sialylated glycophorin	. . .
	Theiler's murine encephalomyocarditis virus	ND	. . .
	Vilyuisk virus	ND	. . .

eukaryotic mRNA species is blocked by a 'cap' or 7-methylguanosine residue linked in the reverse orientation to the 5′ terminal residue by phosphate groups. Ribosomes bind close to the free capped 5′ end of the RNA and then 'scan' the sequence for the first suitable initiation codon (defined in part by the nucleotides that flank it) at which protein synthesis commences. Picornavirus RNAs are translated by another mechanism in which the 5′ noncoding region acts as an internal initiation site for translation not requiring a free terminus (Pelletier and Sonenberg 1988). Following the initiation of viral protein synthesis, host protein synthesis is rapidly shut off by mechanisms that are not fully understood but include the proteolytic cleavage of initiation factors required for the cap-dependent protein synthesis of the host cell by a mechanism involving virus-coded protease 2A.

POST-TRANSLATION PROCESSING

The proteases of polioviruses and other enteroviruses are extremely specific and have been proposed as possible targets for chemotherapeutic agents. In the case of poliovirus, the P1 protein comprising all the structural proteins is excised as a single unit by protease 2A, which cleaves between a tyrosine–glycine pair. This has the effect of removing the structural from the nonstructural proteins before they are processed any further. The corresponding protease in coxsackie virus B3 is believed to cleave between a threonine–isoleucine pair. Later processing is carried out by protease 3C or the precursor molecule 3CD. It may be difficult to identify the active moiety, which may be an intermediate or a final product of the cleavage pathway. The processing protease in poliovirus cleaves between glutamine–glycine pairs, including those found in the P1 region between VP2 and VP3, and VP3 and VP1. The exposure and possibly the amino acid sequence surrounding the dipeptide govern whether cleavage occurs, as many such pairs are not cleaved. A similar sequence specificity seems to function in coxsackie virus B viruses, but the situation is less clear in viruses such as hepatitis A virus, or other picornaviruses, such as EMC, in which cleavage does not seem to involve a specific dipeptide (Palmenberg 1987).

Two further proteolytic cleavages take place in the viral growth cycle. One occurs in protein 3D, at a tyrosine–glycine pair, and is thus probably performed by protein 2A. This may have the effect of reducing the amount of active polymerase in the cell, but the advantage of this is not understood, especially as at least the Sabin type 3 vaccine strain of poliovirus and viruses related to it do not carry out this step, although they grow to high titer in vivo and in vitro. The final cleavage involves the formation of VP2 and VP4 from the precursor VP0, which occurs as the last stage of maturation.

REPLICATION OF RNA

The synthesis of RNA requires an RNA template that is read from the 3′ to 5′ direction, whereas protein synthesis requires an RNA template read in the opposite direction. The two processes are therefore mutually exclusive, and the factors influencing the fate of a particular RNA molecule are not known.

The replication of poliovirus RNA requires the synthesis of both negative and positive strands of RNA (Kuhn and Wimmer 1987; Paul 2002). Messenger-sense (positive-strand) RNA is synthesized in a great excess over the complementary-sense RNA. Infected cells contain complete double-stranded copies of one positive and one negative strand of viral RNA, termed replicative forms (RF) and partial double-stranded structures termed replicative intermediates (RI). All nascent strands of polio RNA of either sense are covalently linked to VPg at the 5′ terminus. This protein is absent from RNA associated with ribosomes. The association of VPg with nascent RNA presumably accounts for the fact that inhibitors of protein synthesis, such as puromycin, rapidly inhibit RNA synthesis.

All of the nonstructural proteins are involved in RNA replication in some way. Viral protein 3D is present in replication complexes isolated from infected cells (Lundquist et al. 1974) and is able to synthesize poly(U) from a poly(A) template if primed with oligo(U) (Flanegan and Baltimore 1977). Protein 3B (VPg) is associated with nascent RNA strands. Guanidine inhibits poliovirus RNA synthesis, and mutants that are either resistant to it or dependent on its presence for growth possess base changes in protein 2C, which is therefore also implicated in synthesis in some way. This protein may influence host range in polioviruses and in rhinoviruses. It is therefore likely that some host factor is involved, although this could, for example, involve structural factors contributed by the host, such as cell membranes.

The detailed mechanism of viral RNA synthesis is controversial, although it is accepted that it occurs in particulate or membranous regions of the infected cell. Replication of virus in vitro has been reported in protein translation systems primed with polioviral RNA. Protein 3D is the main component of replicative complexes which may be prepared from infected cells by mild detergents. Such complexes synthesize both virion (+) and complementary (−) sense RNAs in vitro. Three models for RNA synthesis have been put forward.

1 Dasgupta et al. (1980) reported the presence of a 67 kDa protein able to initiate viral RNA synthesis in the absence of oligo(U). The protein has kinase activity, and the implication of host proteins in viral nucleic acid synthesis in other systems is well documented. However, this factor [host factor (HF)] leaves no clear role for VPg.

2 Flanegan and co-workers (Young et al. 1985) have reported a host enzyme-terminal uridylate transferase (TUT) – which is able to add uridine residues to the 3′ termini of viral nucleic acid. Uridine bases added to the 3′ end of the virion RNA that carries a poly(A) tail would form a tail that could loop back and anneal to the poly(A) sequence as a primer for 3D. The 3′ terminus of the complementary RNA is UUUUAA, so there is a short sequence for such a hairpin structure to form and prime RNA synthesis on the negative-sense RNA. An analogous mechanism has been suggested in the replication of parvoviruses. The hairpin structure would be cleaved by VPg or a precursor, in the course of which VPg would be transferred to the 5′ end of the nascent strand.

3 There is a proposal that uridine residues are added to VPg to make VPg pUpU, which then functions as a primer. Such an intermediate has been reported.

Combinations of these models have been proposed and the reader is referred to Paul (2002) for further details and discussions of the experimental evidence available.

ASSEMBLY OF CAPSIDS

The structural proteins are synthesized and processed as a unit and assemble to form pentamers of VP0, VP1, and VP3 (Putnak and Phillips 1981). Isolated pentamers (or 14S particles) are able to assemble into procapsids, which are complete but empty viral shells, sedimenting at 75S. It is possible to prepare soluble fractions from infected cells containing 14S subunits able to assemble to give 75S empty shells. If the pH is allowed to fall, however, the 75S units become altered, adopting the C antigenic form, and are no longer dissociable.

The last step in the maturation of the infectious virion is the cleavage of VP0 to give VP2 and VP4. It has been proposed that this occurs autocatalytically by insertion of the nucleic acid as a proton donor in the presence of a serine residue at position 10 of VP2 close to the cleavage point (Rossmann et al. 1985). However, specific mutagenesis of residue 10 does not prevent cleavage of VP0. A possible model for virion assembly is that the empty 75S capsids act as a dissociable reservoir of structural proteins. As the units reassociate around the genomic RNA, the cleavage of VP0 to VP2 and VP4 occurs, making assembly essentially irreversible under the conditions pertaining in the infected cell. This scheme remains speculative but plausible.

Effects on host cells

Replication of enteroviruses is normally accompanied by apoptosis of the host cell. The viruses almost certainly encode proteins that affect this process, but this remains a subject of study. Non-lytic persistent virus infections have been reported for poliovirus (Sarnow et al. 1986), hepatitis A virus, echovirus 6, and the coxsackie virus B viruses (Matteucci et al. 1985) in appropriate cells. There is evidence for the persistent enterovirus infection in vivo of humans and rats (Bowles et al. 1986; Schnurr and Schmidt 1988; Yousef et al. 1988).

Resistance to physical and chemical agents

Enteroviruses can remain viable for years at −20°C and −70°C, and for weeks at 4°C, but lose infectivity slowly at room temperature and with increasing rapidity as the temperature is raised. Their inactivation at all environmental temperatures is inhibited by molar magnesium chloride; this property has led to the widespread use of magnesium chloride as a stabilizer of oral poliovaccine.

In the absence of organic matter, enteroviruses are rapidly inactivated by ultraviolet light and usually by drying.

Enteroviruses are insensitive to alcoholic and phenolic disinfectants, ether, chloroform, and deoxycholate. Treatment with formaldehyde (0.3 percent), 0.1 M HCl, or free residual chlorine (0.3–0.5 p.p.m.) causes rapid inactivation. The activity of chlorine is diminished by a high pH, low temperature, and the presence of organic matter, and it may therefore be less effective when used under field conditions.

CLINICAL AND PATHOLOGICAL ASPECTS

Enteroviruses

The alimentary tract is the predominant site of replication of enteroviruses. Although infection is usually asymptomatic, enteroviruses are recognized causes of paralytic poliomylitis, encephalitis, aseptic meningitis, myocarditis, conjunctivitis, and numerous other syndromes associated with target organs outside the alimentary tract. The serotypes comprising each group and the main disease caused by them are listed in Table 40.1.

HOST RANGE

The only natural host of polioviruses are humans, although most strains will infect Old World monkeys and chimpanzees. However, cotton rats, mice and hamsters, and fertile hens' eggs may be infected by strains adapted in the laboratory. Other enteroviruses, notably the coxsackie viruses, will infect mice under laboratory conditions. Swine vesicular disease virus (SVDV) is closely related to coxsackie virus B5.

PATHOGENESIS

Enteroviruses infect via the mouth or oropharynx. The incubation period is usually 7–14 days, with extremes of 2–35 days. Virus infects the mucosal tissues of the pharynx, gut or both, finally entering the bloodstream and gaining access to cells of the reticuloendothelial system and specific target organs such as the meninges, myocardium, and skin. Enteroviruses can generally be recovered from the pharynx during the first week of illness and from the feces for 1–4 weeks after onset of illness; they have been isolated from cerebrospinal fluid (CSF), spinal cord, brain, heart, conjunctivae, and skin lesions.

Two or more enteroviruses may propagate simultaneously in the alimentary tract but usually multiplication of one virus interferes with the growth of the heterologous type.

Poliomyelitis

Poliomyelitis is the most serious disease caused by any of the enteroviruses. According to one view (Bodian 1955), the virus first multiplies in the tonsils and Peyer's patches of the small intestine before spreading to the more distant lymph nodes and thence by a viremia to other sites, including the spinal cord. According to another view (Sabin 1955), the virus multiplies at mucosal surfaces and accumulates in the draining lymph nodes where some, but not all, strains may replicate. From there virus seeds peripheral sites, including peripheral nerves, and the virus generated at the distant sites is the source of the detectable viremia. Antibodies appear early and are protective even when given as passive immunoglobulin (Hammon et al. 1953).

Virus may pass to the spinal cord along nerves under certain conditions; for example, in children with inapparent infection either at the time of tonsillectomy or at the time of injection with material causing local inflammation.

The anterior horn cells of the spinal cord are most readily infected by poliovirus, but in severe cases the intermediate gray ganglia and even the posterior horn and dorsal root ganglia may also be involved. In the brain, the reticular formation, the vestibular nuclei, the cerebellar vermis, and the deep cerebellar nuclei are most often affected.

Other enteroviruses

The pathogenesis of nonpolio enteroviruses is similar to that of poliovirus in the initial stages but the target organs vary. For example, echoviruses 6 and 9 may infect the CNS, causing meningitis. Coxsackie virus A7 and enterovirus 71 can cause paralysis, and others, such as coxsackie virus B viruses, may infect the heart or muscle.

Coxsackie virus A24 and enterovirus 70 resemble rhinoviruses, being spread by fomites and direct inoculation of the conjunctiva by contaminated fingers. The incubation period is very short (12–48 hours); recovery is usually complete within 1–2 weeks.

HOST FACTORS

Age is an important determinant of the severity of enterovirus disease, the incidence of some syndromes being greatest in neonates (e.g. myo- or pericarditis).

Malnutrition may worsen disease. When marasmus was induced in normally resistant postweaning mice, challenge with coxsackie virus B3 gave more severe disease.

Physical exertion while incubating poliovirus infection is associated with a higher incidence or greater extent of paralysis. The severity of paralysis is increased in monkeys infected experimentally with poliovirus and made to swim until exhausted. Similarly, exercising mice infected with coxsackie virus A9 or coxsackie virus B3 results in increased virus titers in their myocardium, in higher mortality rates, or both.

Pregnancy and parturition may be associated with a greater risk of paralysis with poliovirus infection or a greater risk of myocarditis with coxsackie virus B infection. Hypo- or agammaglobulinemic individuals with impaired or absent B-cell function but normal T-cell function clear enterovirus infections more slowly than those with a normal immune system. This provides further evidence for the importance of humoral immunity in the control of enteroviral infection. Maternal antibody may not protect from infection but will prevent disease.

CLINICAL SYNDROMES

The description of clinical syndromes below is not exhaustive. Further details concerning enteroviral diseases may be found in reviews by Moore and Morens (1984); Melnick (1990), and Bendinelli and Friedman (1988).

Most enterovirus infections produce clinically inapparent or minor illness. The consequences of infection, when they do occur, range from specific clinical syndromes, such as fatal paralytic or cardiac illness, to minor undifferentiated febrile illnesses. Asymptomatic infection rates are reported as 90–95 percent for the polioviruses, 76 percent for the coxsackie viruses and 43 percent for the echoviruses.

Poliomyelitis

Exposure to poliovirus may have the following consequences:

- **inapparent infection** (90–95 percent)
- **'abortive'** or **'minor' illness** (4–8 percent) with symptoms of upper respiratory tract infection, gastrointestinal upset, or influenza-like illness. The patient recovers within a few days
- **non-paralytic poliomyelitis** (1–2 percent), an illness of about 2–10 days similar to 'aseptic' meningitis, often accompanied by back pain and muscle spasm. Recovery usually is rapid and complete
- **paralytic poliomyelitis** (0.1–2 percent). The major illness, paralysis, usually follows a prodromal illness similar to the minor illness described above, especially in children. Thereafter the predominant feature is flaccid paralysis resulting from lower motor neuron damage. Paralytic poliomyelitis is termed **spinal** if the lower spine is involved or **bulbar** (from 'bulb' or medulla oblongata) if the upper spine and brainstem are involved. Bulbar poliomyelitis is the more serious because it affects the respiratory system.

A paralysed patient may recover completely or have varying degrees of residual deficit. A review of 203 cases between 1969 and 1981 in the USA (Moore et al. 1982) showed that residual paralysis was minor in 11 percent and significant or severe in 79 percent; 10 percent of the cases were fatal.

Post-polio syndrome has been described in which individuals who have survived an initial attack suffer a degeneration of function many years later. This may be anatomic in origin as advancing age results in the loss of nerve cells from an already damaged pathway. Sequences of enterovirus-related nucleic acid have been reported in the CSF of such cases, however, and some workers believe that the virus may persist.

'Aseptic' meningitis

Nonbacterial 'aseptic' meningitis (AM) is a common manifestation of enterovirus infection. Pleocytosis of the CSF is characteristically lymphocytic but may show transient predominance of polymorphonuclear leukocytes when cell counts are high in the early stage of illness, temporarily mimicking bacterial meningitis. Recovery is usually complete within a few weeks, although irritability and fatigue may persist for some weeks and there is a small risk of serious neurological damage in the first year of life (Wilfert et al. 1981). Second attacks of AM may occur from infection with other serotypes.

Paralytic disease

Polioviruses have been the dominant viral cause of paralysis in most of the world but are approaching eradication as described later. Sporadic cases of paralysis associated with coxsackie virus A7 continue to be reported (Gear 1984).

Paralysis has also been reported in association with coxsackie viruses B2–6 and echovirus types 3 (transverse myelitis), 4, 6, 9, 11, and 19.

Enterovirus 71 is capable of causing severe CNS disease with persisting flaccid paralysis, although it can also cause meningitis, encephalitis, and hand-foot-and-mouth disease (HFMD), depending on the outbreak (Melnick 1984).

Enterovirus 70, an agent of acute hemorrhagic conjunctivitis (AHC), has caused poliomyelitis-like illness (Kono et al. 1977).

Encephalitis

The dominant enterovirus associated with outbreaks of encephalitis is enterovirus 71, although poliovirus, coxsackie viruses A9, B3, B5, and B6 and echoviruses 6, 9, 17, and 19 have all been isolated from CSF or brain tissues.

Myalgic encephalomyelitis (postviral fatigue syndrome)

Multiple symptoms are associated with this illness (Behan 1980), but always include extreme muscle fatigue following slight physical effort, muscle pain, and psychological upset. The lack of objective physical signs, pronounced emotional lability, and neuroticism and the unknown nature of the disorder have made it easy for some physicians to dismiss the illness as hysterical. Myalgic encephalomyelitis (ME) is not a fatal disease but recovery may take months or years; relapses during periods of physical or mental stress are common. Chronic infection with enteroviruses has been reported (Yousef et al. 1988).

Pleurodynia (Bornholm disease)

The group B coxsackie viruses are the main identified causes of pleurodynia, also known as Bornholm disease, epidemic myalgia, or the devil's grippe. The chest pain is spasmodic, intensified by movement and may be severe. Abdominal pain resulting from involvement of the diaphragm occurs in approximately half the cases; in children this may be the chief complaint. The illness lasts for 2–14 days and is self-limited; recovery is complete although short relapses are common.

Sporadic cases of pleurodynia have also been associated with coxsackie viruses A4, A6, and A10; coxsackie virus A9 has been implicated in this syndrome and also in chronic diseases of the muscle and joints.

Congenital and neonatal infection

Prematurity, low birth weight, onset of illness within the first few days of life, occurrence during the 'enterovirus season' and recent antepartum or postpartum febrile illness in the mother are risk factors for the most severe, generalized and fatal neonatal enteroviral disease, most commonly associated with the coxsackie virus B, particularly coxsackie virus B2, and coxsackie virus B4. Neonatal illness has seldom been attributed to coxsackie virus A viruses but echoviruses (e.g. echoviruses 4, 9, 11, 17–20, 22, and 31) have been incriminated in both nursery outbreaks and sporadic infections. Fatal cases of echovirus infection generally present with progressive severe hepatitis and CNS involvement, whereas fulminant coxsackie virus B infections can be distinguished by the presence of severe myocarditis.

Cardiac disease

Severe myocarditis is usually a prominent feature of disseminated enterovirus infections of neonates; less severe myocarditis or pericarditis may follow infection of older children and adults. It has been estimated that ca. 5 percent of all symptomatic coxsackie virus infections induce heart disease.

Nucleic acid hybridization has been used to detect enterovirus RNA in myocardial biopsies. Replicating enterovirus RNA was found in 19 of 81 patients with suspected myocarditis (Kandolf 1988) but in none of the controls. Endomyocardial biopsies from >100 patients with heart muscle disease were investigated by Archard et al. (1988). Enterovirus genomic RNA was detected in 60 percent with active myocarditis and 47 percent with healing myocarditis; tissue from cases of other specific heart muscle diseases was consistently negative. All patients who made a coxsackie virus B-specific IgM response also had detectable enterovirus RNA in biopsy tissue. Enterovirus-infected myocardial cells have also been detected by hybridization in situ in dilated myocardiomyopathy (Kandolf 1988). Persistence of enteroviral genomes may therefore be implicated in chronic heart disease.

Mucocutaneous syndromes

Herpangina Herpangina is characterized by fever and a vesicular exanthem that typically involves the fauces and soft palate. It is chiefly associated with coxsackie virus A types 1–10, 16, and 22, and less commonly with coxsackie viruses B1–5 and some echoviruses. The disease occurs during the summer season and generally involves clusters of patients. Herpangina mainly affects young children but occasionally is seen in young adults. The illness is self-limited, with recovery in a few days.

Hand-foot-and-mouth disease (HFMD) HFMD is predominantly a childhood illness, usually associated with infection by coxsackie virus A16 or enterovirus 71. Occasionally, cases due to coxsackie viruses A5, A7, A9, A10, B2, and B5 have been reported. Typical cases of HFMD have vesicles and ulcers mainly in the front of the mouth, most frequently on the tongue, and a vesicular exanthem, mostly localized on the palms and soles;

virus can be isolated readily from these sites. During outbreaks, ca. 60–70 percent of cases show the complete clinical picture of HFMD. Recovery from HFMD is usually complete within 1–2 weeks.

Swine vesicular disease (SVD) in humans   Swine vesicular disease virus (SVDV) is a porcine enterovirus that is closely related to coxsackie virus B5 (Zhang et al. 1993). The disease in pigs was first recognized in Italy in 1966. Since then SVD has been seen throughout Europe as well as in Hong Kong and Japan. The lesions in pigs resemble those caused by foot-and-mouth disease and other vesicular diseases of pigs. No vesicles have been seen in workers with pigs affected with SVD although, in laboratories, inapparent human infection has occurred and antibodies have been detected. There are on record four human cases with presumptive evidence of infection with SVDV. One patient had a severe illness with fever, myalgia, weakness, and abdominal pain, in two the disease was mild and the fourth had meningitis. In three of these patients infection occurred after exposure to pigs; the other was exposed to the virus in the laboratory.

Exanthems   Usually transient and erythematous (rubelliform, maculopapular, rarely morbilliform, or vesicular) exanthems have been reported in infections by enteroviruses, notably during outbreaks of infection with coxsackie viruses A9, A16, and B5 or echoviruses 4, 9, and 16. Rash is seldom the sole clinical feature in symptomatic enterovirus infections. Fever, malaise, cervical lymphadenopathy, and aseptic meningitis may also occur in patients with rash. Rashes associated with coxsackie virus A9 and echovirus 9 can mimic rubella virus infection so closely as to merit diagnostic differentiation, particularly in pregnant women. Congenital abnormalities following maternal enterovirus infection have only rarely been reported.

Acute epidemic hemorrhagic conjunctivitis   In 1970 there was a large epidemic of acute epidemic hemorrhagic conjunctivitis (AHC) in Singapore with more than 60 000 reported cases. The causal agent was identified as a variant of coxsackie virus A24. After an incubation period of 18–48 hours, mild to severe conjunctivitis developed, with subconjunctival hemorrhage in a minority of cases; recovery was usually complete within 1–2 weeks. Epidemics of AHC recurred in southeast Asia in 1975 and again in 1985 and in the Americas.

Enterovirus 70 first emerged in an epidemic of AHC in Ghana in 1969, spread through the coastal areas of Africa, eventually reaching India, southeast Asia, and Japan by 1970, ultimately involving hundreds of millions of people. Serological surveys in Ghana, Indonesia, and Japan confirmed that the virus was not prevalent before the pandemic. The illness had a short incubation period (24 hours), acute subconjunctival hemorrhage being the most characteristic sign; corneal involvement was usually

transient and the prognosis good. The first outbreak in the western hemisphere was in Brazil in 1981 from where it then spread north, reaching Florida.

Rare cases of neurological complications accompanying or following enterovirus 70 conjunctivitis have been reported.

Respiratory disease

Respiratory illness caused by enteroviruses cannot be distinguished clinically from that caused by viruses such as rhinoviruses, parainfluenza viruses, respiratory syncytial virus, and adenoviruses. However, these viruses predominate in the winter months, whereas respiratory infection by enteroviruses typically occurs during the summer and autumn.

Diabetes

A possible association of insulin-dependent diabetes mellitus (IDDM) with coxsackie virus B infection was first suggested by Gamble in 1969. Reviews by Gamble (1980); Barrett-Connor (1985) and Toniolo et al. (1988) provide comprehensive interpretations of the available data.

A long euglycogenic period, characterized by the presence of islet cell antibodies (ICA) and T-lymphocyte responses, precedes the appearance of hyperglycemia following the near total disappearance of the β cells of the islets of Langerhans. There is some correlation of HLA haplotype (DR3 mainly in males, DR4 mainly in females) with this illness, suggesting that an autoimmune process is responsible for the chronic and irreversible loss of β cells. What triggers pancreatic autoimmunity in individuals is unknown.

Strains of coxsackie virus B4 and coxsackie virus B5 shown to be diabetogenic in mice have been isolated from people developing diabetes (Toniolo et al. 1988). It has now been shown that most of the group B coxsackie viruses are potentially able to infect and damage pancreatic endocrine cells, causing hyperglycemia. Serological studies have demonstrated that about one-third of the cases of IDDM in children are probably preceded by coxsackie virus B infection, although this may be a precipitating rather than causative factor.

Gastroenteritis

Although enteroviruses readily replicate within the gut, they are seldom the cause of gastroenteritis when this is the predominant feature.

Hepatitis

Hepatitis can accompany generalized coxsackie virus B and echovirus infections in neonates or occasionally in older children as well as following infection with hepatitis A virus (Chapter 53, Hepatitis A and E).

Rhinoviruses

Rhinoviruses are the major cause of common colds. In the US National Health Interview Survey for 1985, colds were associated with 161 million days of restricted activity and accounted for 26 million days of school absenteeism, 23 million days lost from work and 27 million visits to physicians. More than 800 oral cold remedies are available and the annual expenditure on such treatments exceeds $2 billion in the USA.

CLINICAL MANIFESTATIONS

About 30 percent of human volunteers inoculated intranasally with nasal secretions or tissue culture fluid containing rhinoviruses develop colds, whereas less than 5 percent of volunteers given uninfected material have symptoms (Tyrrell 1965). When virus is given to adults without antibody, up to 100 percent develop colds (D'Allessio et al. 1976). At least 15 different serotypes have been given to volunteers, with essentially the same results.

In studies of university students (Gwaltney and Jordan 1966; Hamre et al. 1966; Phillips et al. 1968), industrial workers (Hamparian et al. 1964; Gwaltney et al. 1966), military personnel (Bloom et al. 1963), and civilian families (Elveback et al. 1966; Higgins et al. 1966; Hendley et al. 1969; Monto and Cavallaro 1972; Fox et al. 1975, 1985), rhinoviruses were isolated from 7–40 percent of people (including children) with upper respiratory illness but from less than 2 percent of healthy people. These findings probably underestimate the importance of rhinoviruses, because virus can be isolated from only half of known infections. The same epidemiologic studies also indicate that between 10 percent and 40 percent of rhinovirus infections are subclinical, with substantial differences in pathogenicity between serotypes.

Rhinovirus infections are more common and severe in young children than in adults (Fox et al. 1975). Rhinoviruses are also associated with lower respiratory disease in children or those with a history of chronic respiratory disease. However, in controlled studies, rhinoviruses were found in 3–8 percent of children in hospital either with lower respiratory illness or without respiratory symptoms (Chanock and Parrott 1965; Holzel et al. 1965; Stott and Walker 1967; Mufson et al. 1970). Hence, the precise role of rhinoviruses in acute respiratory disease of children is unclear (Cherry 1973). In children with a history of wheezy bronchitis or asthma, rhinoviruses are associated with up to 33 percent of acute attacks, and virus was found more often in sputum than in the nose or throat, suggesting that virus multiplies in the lower respiratory tract (Horn et al. 1979).

Rhinoviruses can cause lower respiratory tract illness in adult volunteers infected with virus in a fine particle aerosol (Cate et al. 1965). Transient abnormal pulmonary function has also been found in a small proportion of healthy volunteers after intranasal instillation of rhinovirus and in a minority of natural infections. Although rhinoviruses have been isolated postmortem from the lungs of adults who died of pneumonia, they are not implicated as a significant cause of adult pneumonia. However, in people with chronic bronchitis, rhinovirus infections have been associated with 12–43 percent of exacerbations and virus frequently seems to invade the lower respiratory tract (Stott et al. 1968). Although Buscho and colleagues (1978) found that rhinoviruses could infect patients without exacerbating their chronic bronchitis, such patients are more susceptible to rhinovirus infection than are otherwise healthy people. Furthermore, Horn and Gregg (1973) found lower respiratory tract signs in 85–90 percent of rhinovirus infections in adults with a previous history of asthma or bronchitis but in only 5 percent of such infections in otherwise healthy adults.

Bovine rhinovirus types 1 and 3 have been isolated from cattle with respiratory disease but there is little evidence to show that they are clinically important (Stott et al. 1980; Yamashita et al. 1985). There is one reported isolation of bovine type 2 virus (Reed et al. 1971). Similarly, although infection with equine rhinoviruses is widespread in horses, their precise contribution to the problem of respiratory disease is not yet clear (Powell et al. 1978).

PATHOGENESIS

Hand contact rather than aerosol is the prime mode of transmission of rhinoviruses (Gwaltney et al. 1978). Virus has not been recovered from air in rooms occupied by infected people and it is not possible to transmit rhinovirus colds between volunteers separated by a double wire mesh allowing free flow of air but no direct contact. Under the same conditions, coxsackie virus A21 was readily transmitted. Aerosols produced by talking, coughing, and sneezing derive primarily from the saliva, which has a low titer of virus, and not from the nasal secretions in which titers are highest.

By contrast, rhinovirus can readily be isolated from the hands of people during the acute stage of a cold. Furthermore, the hand contacts the eye or nose, on average, once every 3 hours. Thus, in a comparison of routes of rhinovirus transmission, 11 or 15 hand-contact exposures initiated infection but only 1 of 22 aerosol exposures was successful. Epidemiologic findings indicate that colds spread poorly in workplaces where many people share the same air space but direct contact is minimal. By contrast, transmission occurs readily within families where direct contact is frequent.

Rhinoviruses replicate in and destroy the ciliated epithelium of both nasal and tracheal mucosae, but grow to highest titer in nasal epithelium (Hoorn and Tyrrell

1965). Ciliated cells are extruded from the epithelium, leaving a generally smooth surface (Reed and Boyde 1972). Mycoplasma replication is enhanced in such virus-damaged tissue (Reed 1972), which is also probably more susceptible to secondary invasion by bacteria and mycoplasmas. Although the target cell in the lower respiratory tract is not known, type II pneumocytes may be infected by rhinoviruses in vitro (Tyrrell et al. 1979). Rhinoviruses are rarely found outside the respiratory tract, partly because their growth is restricted by temperatures above 37°C.

Host responses to infection may cause the vascular engorgement, increased vascular permeability with transudation of serum proteins and increased mucus production that are characteristic of colds. Host responses include release of inflammatory mediators, such as kinins; influxes of inflammatory cells, including polymorphonuclear leukocytes; interferon; and probably neuroreflexes and associated cholinergic stimulation and neuropeptide release (Naclerio et al. 1988). Further evidence for the role of kinins is provided by the finding that intranasal instillation of bradykinin causes some of the symptoms and alterations in nasal mucus seen in rhinovirus colds.

IMMUNE RESPONSES

Rhinovirus infection stimulates an antibody response in 47–77 percent of cases (Fox et al. 1975). The response is greater in adults than in children. Severe lower respiratory infection induces higher antibody titers than mild upper respiratory infection. Furthermore, certain serotypes are more effective antigens than others. Specific antibody in the circulation is related to protection against reinfection of volunteers. In families in which exposure to known serotypes occurred, pre-existing serum antibody was 52–69 percent effective in preventing infection. Rhinovirus infections also stimulate local IgA production. Whether secretory IgA in the mucus of the upper respiratory tract or circulating antibody in the serum is the more important in protection remains contentious (Perkins et al. 1969; Douglas and Couch 1972).

Foot-and-mouth disease

Foot-and-mouth disease is a highly infectious disease of ungulates. There are a few reports of infection in humans and experimental infections of laboratory animals are readily initiated. Seven serotypes of FMDV are recognized – O, A, C, SAT1, SAT2, SAT3, and Asia 1 – and existing vaccines are based on inactivated preparations of the appropriate serotype.

The first signs of disease in cattle are dullness, anorexia, and rising temperature, followed by nasal discharge and the appearance of vesicles in the mouth and on the feet. Initially, the vesicles in the mouth are present on the tongue, hard palate and dental pad, lips and muzzle,

and on the feet in the interdigital space or along the coronary band, giving rise to lameness. The incubation period varies from 1 to 14 days.

The main routes of infection are inhalation, ingestion, or penetration of the epithelium. Virus may persist in the pharyngeal area for prolonged periods.

EPIDEMIOLOGY

Epidemiology is discussed in two sections: enteroviruses and rhinoviruses.

Enteroviruses

MODE OF TRANSMISSION

Humans are the only known reservoir for members of the human enterovirus group. Virus is generally shed for longer periods in feces (1 month or more) than from the oropharynx, and fecal contamination is the usual source of infection although enterovirus 70, the agent of acute hemorrhagic conjunctivitis, has been found almost exclusively in conjunctival and throat specimens.

INFLUENCE OF CLIMATE

In temperate climates enteroviruses are more prevalent in the summer and autumn (i.e. when warmth and humidity are at their peak). In tropical climates they tend to circulate all the year round or are associated with the rainy season.

SPREAD WITHIN FAMILIES

Young children are the usual reservoir of enterovirus infection. The secondary attack rates in susceptible family members are reported as 92 percent for polioviruses, 76 percent for coxsackie viruses and 43 percent for echoviruses. The greater spread of polioviruses and coxsackie viruses may be related to their longer periods of excretion. Secondary coxsackie virus infections were more common in mothers (78 percent) than in fathers (47 percent). Coxsackie viruses spread to 75 percent of exposed susceptibles but to only 25 percent of exposed people who already had antibody to the infecting type; echoviruses infected 43 percent of susceptibles and only one person with homotypic antibody.

EPIDEMIOLOGICAL SURVEILLANCE
International data

In 1963 the World Health Organization established a system for the collection and dissemination of information on viral infections. Although the level of reporting may be low and variable, the data are of interest in identifying viruses implicated in clinical syndromes. Examples from 1975 to 1983 are shown in Tables 40.5 and 40.6.

The commonest coxsackie virus reported was coxsackie virus A9, the serotype most readily detectable in

Table 40.5 *Reports of coxsackie virus infections by main clinical features, 1975–83*

Systems affected	Coxsackie virus A infections		Coxsackie virus B infections	
	Number	Predominant serotypes	Number	Predominant aerotypes
Central nervous system				
Total	1 627	A9	4 364	B5, 4
Paralytic	68	A9, 1	112	B4, 5
Cardiac	57	A9	596	B4, 2
Muscle/joint	35	A9	302	B4
Skin/mucosa	1 262	A16	360	B5, 4
Respiratory	741	A9	2 880	B4, 2
Gastrointestinal	996	A9	2 921	B4
Ophthalmic	30	A24	33	B4
Others	644	...	2 169	...
No illness/data	395	...	1 309	...
Totals	5 787	...	14 934	...

Data from the Global Surveillance Programme, World Health Organization, Geneva.

cell cultures. Coxsackie virus A16 is the main cause of HFMD. Over all, coxsackie virus B4 was the serotype associated with the widest range of syndromes; coxsackie virus B5 was the predominant serotype linked with nonparalytic CNS infections and rashes.

Almost half the reported echovirus infections were associated with CNS disease, especially aseptic meningitis (Table 40.6). Echoviruses 6, 9, 11, 19, and 30 are regularly encountered during outbreaks of aseptic meningitis, sometimes accompanied by a rash in echovirus 6 and 9 infections. Parechovirus 1, echovirus 22 is usually associated with a 'failure to thrive' syndrome in infants less than 1 year old and is seldom associated with CNS infection. The apparent role of coxsackie viruses A and B and, to a lesser extent, the echoviruses in paralytic disease should be interpreted with caution because most reports are based on virus isolation from feces alone.

Table 40.6 *Reports of echovirus infection by main clinical features, 1975–83*

Systems affected	Echovirus infections	
	Number	Predominant serotypes
Central nervous system		
Total	16 668	E30, 11, 19, 9, 6
Paralytic	178	E11, 9
Cardiac	266	E11, 6, 22
Muscle/joint	223	E11, 6
Skin/mucosa	976	E9, 11
Respiratory	4 620	E11, 22
Gastrointestinal	7 763	E11, 22
Ophthalmic	72	E11
Others	4 106	...
No illness/data	3 497	...
Total	38 191	...

Data from the Global Surveillance Programme, World Health Organization, Geneva.

Infections due to enterovirus serotypes 68–71 reported to WHO during 1975–83 and the associated illnesses are listed in Table 40.7.

Illness due to enteroviruses 68 and 69 is uncommon. Although the figures clearly show the association of enterovirus 70 with eye infections, they fail to reveal the pandemic nature of this virus in acute hemorrhagic conjunctivitis; enterovirus 70 is difficult to isolate in cell culture and this alone might explain the discrepancy. Enterovirus 71 is more readily isolated from clinical specimens, and its associations with CNS infections and HFMD (or both concurrently) are apparent from Table 40.7.

Peak virus activity was seen in July in the northern hemisphere, and during December to January in the southern hemisphere.

As shown in Table 40.8, enterovirus infections were more common in children, especially in those aged 1–4 years.

Rhinoviruses

Rhinovirus infections are seen throughout the year but are most prevalent in the spring and autumn when sudden changes in temperature are common. It has been suggested that rapid temperature changes are closely associated with the incidence of colds (Hope-Simpson 1958). Rhinoviruses are distributed throughout the world, and antibodies to them have been detected even in the remote communities of Alaskan Eskimos, Pacific Micronesians, and Kalahari Hottentots.

The multiplicity of rhinovirus serotypes is a major factor in their epidemiology. Several serotypes circulate simultaneously within a community, and an individual may be infected with two serotypes at the same time (Cooney and Kenny 1977). Some serotypes persist continuously in a population for several years whereas others may appear transiently. The distribution of sero-

Table 40.7 *Reports of enterovirus 68–71 infections in 217 cases by main clinical features, 1975–83*

Systems affected	Number of infections			
	Ev 68	Ev 69	Ev 70	Ev 71
Central nervous system				
Total	1	0	1	93
Paralytic	0	0	1	3
Cardiac	0	0	0	0
Muscle/joint	0	0	0	0
Skin/mucosa	0	0	0	41
Respiratory	1	1	0	9
Gastrointestinal	0	4	0	10
Ophthalmic	0	0	33	0
Others	0	0	0	10
No illness/data	1	2	0	10
Totals	3	7	34	173

Data from the Global Surveillance Programme, World Health Organization, Geneva.

types has changed over the years. Before 1967 most isolates belonged to the first 55 serotypes; in 1968 and 1969 fewer than half the isolates were serotypes 1–55 and an increasing number were types 56–89. Between 1970 and 1975, 50 percent of rhinoviruses isolated did not belong to the first 89 types (Fox 1976). However, more recent publications indicate that over 90 percent of rhinoviruses isolated can now be identified as known serotypes (Fox et al. 1985; Hamparian et al. 1987). Some serotypes, such as 1B, 12, 15 and 38, are isolated more often than others, possibly because they spread more effectively. Certainly, the more frequently isolated serotypes cause a higher secondary attack rate in family surveys (Fox et al. 1975). However, it must be remembered that frequency of isolation may just reflect the sensitivity of the cell cultures used rather than the distribution of viruses in a population.

LABORATORY DIAGNOSIS

Enteroviruses

Detailed descriptions of the principles and procedures for the diagnosis of enterovirus infections are published elsewhere (Grist et al. 1979).

COLLECTION OF SPECIMENS

The usual specimens for virus isolation are feces (or rectal swabs) and throat swabs. **Fecal** excretion of virus commences within a few days of infection and may continue for weeks in children with poliovirus and coxsackie virus infections, although it rarely exceeds 1 month with the echoviruses; in adults it is usually of shorter duration (1–2 weeks). Excretion in the feces is often intermittent, so, ideally, more than one sample should be collected at least 1–2 days apart. Isolation of virus from pharyngeal secretions is possible up to 1 week after onset of symptoms. Culture of virus from the CSF is an essential part of the routine laboratory diagnosis of patients with aseptic meningitis.

VIRUS ISOLATION IN CELL CULTURES

Polioviruses, the coxsackie B group viruses, and the echoviruses have been readily isolated in kidney cell cultures prepared from rhesus or cynomolgus monkeys or baboons which may not be readily available nowadays. Other susceptible cultures can be obtained from human amnion, diploid cells of human embryo lung, and the RD cell line derived from a human rhabdomyosarcoma. Polioviruses can be isolated in HEp-2c cells or the L20B line (Pipkin et al. 1993).

IDENTIFICATION OF SEROTYPES

Serotypes may be identified by reference antisera. These LBM pools (devised by Lim, Benyesh, and Melnick) are issued in freeze-dried form to reference centers after formal requests to WHO, Geneva. There are eight pools of antisera (A–H) against 42 enteroviruses that grow readily in cell culture and a further seven pools (J–P) of antisera against 19 coxsackie virus A serotypes that grow readily only in newborn mice (Table 40.9) (Melnick and Wimberly 1985).

ANTIGENIC VARIATION

Antigenic variation in the enteroviruses can give rise to prime strains that may not be neutralized by sera to the prototype strain, but can induce antibodies that neutralize the homologous and prototype strains equally well. Intratypic variants have also been described for coxsackie viruses A24, B1–4, B6, echoviruses 4, 9, and

Table 40.8 *Global surveillance of enteroviral infections by age, 1975–83*

Viruses (no. of infections)	Percentage in each age group					
	<1 year	1–4 years	5–14 years	15–24 years	25+ years	Unknown
Coxsackie virus A (5 787)	18	41	20	5	11	5
Coxsackie virus B (14 934)	25	34	18	5	14	4
Echovirus (38 191)	28	26	24	7	11	4
Enteroviruses 68–71[a] (217)	25	32	22	3	14	3

Data from the Global Surveillance Programme, World Health Organization, Geneva.
a) Details available from only 217 of total of 864 infections reported to WHO.

Table 40.9 *Type-specific antisera included in each of eight 'intersecting' LBM pools A–H*

Pool			Enteroviruses represented in each pool	
A	A7	B1, 4	E1, 4, 5, 7, 15, 29, 33	None
B	A7, 9	B2	E2, 3, 9, 19, 21, 26	P2
C	None	B1, 3, 5	E2, 6, 12, 24, 29, 30	P1
D	None	B2	E6, 13, 14, 16, 25, 26, 32, 33	P3
E	None	B4, 5	E5, 11, 13, 17, 18, 22, 30, 32	P2
F	None	B6	E7, 9, 14, 18–20, 26, 27, 29	P1
G	A9	B3	E4, 5, 16, 17, 20, 23, 30, 31	None
H	A16	B6	E1, 3, 9, 12, 22, 23, 32	P3

Antisera against 19 additional coxsackie A viruses are contained in pools J–P. Data from Melnick and Wimberly (1985).

33 and enterovirus 70. Unlike prime strains, intratypic variants have a narrower antigenic spectrum than their corresponding prototype strains.

Aggregation of virions may also cause problems in the neutralization test. The Pesascek strain of echovirus 4 is poorly neutralized by homologous antisera, whereas the Du Toit strain is readily neutralizable. Virus in non-neutralizable aggregates was found to constitute up to 30 percent of untreated Pesascek stock virus preparations but only 0.1 percent of Du Toit stocks. Methods used to disaggregate enteroviruses include filtration or treatment with chloroform.

VIRUS ISOLATION IN NEWBORN MICE

Coxsackie virus A is not readily detected in cell cultures (Table 40.10). Isolation requires that specimens should be injected into litters of newborn mice (24–48 hours old) by intracerebral, intraperitoneal, and subcutaneous routes. The group A viruses induce general myositis of striated muscle, causing flaccid paralysis and death. The B group cause spastic paralysis and degenerative changes in the brain and necrosis of the brown fat.

TEST FOR ANTIBODIES

A few diseases – notably pleurodynia, HFMD, and acute hemorrhagic conjunctivitis – are so regularly associated with particular serotypes (viz. coxsackie viruses B1–5, coxsackie virus A16, and enterovirus 70, respectively) that their serological diagnosis is often feasible; in other situations virus isolation is the best approach. Antibody

titers are compared in paired sera, the first sample being collected in the acute phase and the second 1–14 days later. Enzyme-linked immunosorbent assay (ELISA) or radioimmunoassay may be used as well as neutralization or, in some cases, hemagglutination inhibitor. Such methods can be used to assay for IgM specifically, and thus identify acute infections.

MOLECULAR BIOLOGICAL METHODS

Polymerase chain reaction (PCR) is increasingly applied to clinical specimens and isolates, particularly using primers able to amplify a wide range of enterovirus sequences, which can then be studied further. The use of PCR obviates the need for specific sera if regions of the genome encoding structural proteins are amplified (see above under Classification). Isolation may also be unnecessary, and this may change the spectrum of enteroviruses detected, specifically where they are difficult to grow in culture as for the coxsackie A viruses. Viral sequences have been commonly reported from samples of CSF and serum which is usually a poor source for virus isolation. The advantage of isolation is that it provides permanent specimens for later study. It is likely to become less common except in specialized centers in the future.

Rhinoviruses

Rhinovirus infections are normally diagnosed by isolation of virus from respiratory secretions. As for the

Table 40.10 *Comparative sensitivity of enterovirus isolation systems*

Virus group	Primary monkey[a]/ baboon	Primary human amnion	Human embryo lung (semi-continuous)	RD[b]	Newborn mice
Poliovirus	++	+	+	++	−
Coxsackie virus A	±[c]	±	±[d]	+	++
Coxsackie virus B	++	±	±	−	+
Echovirus	++	+	+	++	±
Enteroviruses	+	Variable	+	Variable	±

a) Rhesus or cynomolgus.
b) RD, human rhabdomyosarcoma continuous cell line.
c) Coxsackie virus A7, A9, A10, A16.
d) Coxsackie virus A21: −, nil; ±, poor; +, good; ++, very good.

enteroviruses, serological techniques have only limited value because of the large number of serotypes and the absence of a specific rhinovirus group antigen.

Rhinoviruses are most often isolated from nasal washings but throat or nasal swabs and sputa are suitable alternative samples. Virus is rarely isolated from blood.

Specimens should be transported to the laboratory in a buffered medium containing about 1 mg of protein (e.g. bovine plasma albumin) per milliliter and inoculated into cell cultures as soon as possible. Most rhinoviruses are strictly species-specific. Therefore, apart from the few strains that grow in monkey kidney cells, human rhinoviruses will grow only in cells of human origin. Semicontinuous cell strains from human embryonic lung are the most widely used for virus isolation, although certain virus strains are isolated more readily in diploid cells from human embryonic kidney or tonsils. Semicontinuous cell strains from different human embryos vary considerably in their sensitivity to rhinoviruses and these differences are not always revealed by titration of laboratory passaged viruses (Stott and Walker 1967; Fox et al. 1975). A continuous line of HeLa cells, sensitive to rhinoviruses, may also be used for primary isolation (Cooney and Kenny 1977). Bovine rhinoviruses are usually isolated in secondary calf kidney cells. All cell cultures inoculated with rhinoviruses should be rolled at 33°C in medium with pH below 7.6. Virus-infected cultures develop small areas of refractile cells, usually within 7 days. Such cytopathic agents are tentatively identified as rhinoviruses by demonstrating that they resist chloroform or ether, pass through a 50 nm filter, grow in the presence of bromodeoxyuridine (a DNA inhibitor) and are destroyed at pH 5. Final identification of a rhinovirus serotype requires neutralization by specific antiserum but this procedure can be simplified by combining antisera into a scheme of pools (Kenny et al. 1970).

Organ cultures of human embryonic trachea or nasal epithelium support the growth of some rhinoviruses that cannot be isolated in cell cultures. Although most of these viruses can subsequently be passaged in cell culture, some apparently replicate only in organ cultures.

When the infecting serotype is known, as in volunteer trials, virus antigen can be detected in nasal washings by ELISA, using specific polyclonal or monoclonal antibodies.

Molecular methods can also be applied. Deoxyoligonucleotides complementary to conserved sequence of the 5′ noncoding region hybridize to the RNAs of all 57 rhinovirus serotypes so far tested and also detect virus in nasal washings specifically and efficiently (Bruce et al. 1988). This approach has the further advantage that cDNA to this region of viral RNA may be specifically amplified by PCR, increasing the sensitivity of the technique.

Serological diagnosis of rhinovirus infection by demonstrating rising antibody titers is practicable only when the serotype of the infecting virus is known. The microneutralization test has been widely used for the detection of rhinovirus antibodies. The hemagglutination inhibition test is particularly useful for the rapid screening of volunteers for antibodies before inoculation (Reed and Hall 1973) but can, of course, be used only for serotypes that hemagglutinate. This restriction does not apply to ELISA or complement fixation tests.

CONTROL OF ENTEROVIRAL INFECTIONS

There are no established antiviral agents for the prevention or treatment of enteroviral diseases although a number of experimental drugs have been used in clinical trials. Pleconaril, an agent which inserts into the viral capsid and prevents the virus binding to the cell and subsequently uncoating, has been used in trials to attempt to interrupt chronic enterovirus infections of hypogammaglobulinemic patients. Quarantine of patients, or contacts, is of little use because most infections are inapparent and spread among close contacts is rapid. A degree of control can be achieved in special baby-care units (where enterovirus infections can often prove fatal), by 'barrier nursing,' an increase in general hygiene of the staff, and exclusion of staff and parents with even 'minor' illnesses. Similar precautions in eye clinics may help when acute hemorrhagic conjunctivitis is present in the community.

Use of immunoglobulin

Commercially prepared γ-globulin may be useful in preventing enteroviral disease, especially in nurseries threatened by serious outbreaks of group B coxsackie viruses. Its use halted an outbreak of echovirus 11 in a premature baby unit in England in 1983.

Prophylaxis: rhinoviruses

The use of formalin-inactivated rhinovirus 1A vaccine to induce antibody was first described in 1963 (Doggett et al. 1963; Mufson et al. 1963). Subsequently, similar inactivated vaccines made from rhinoviruses 2 and 13 have been administered by subcutaneous, intramuscular, or intranasal routes and have protected volunteers against live virus challenge. The problem of numerous serotypes with little or no cross-protection remains.

SPECIFIC THERAPY

In a review of chemotherapy for rhinovirus infections, Sperber and Hayden (1988) have pointed out that treatment may be aimed at either the virus or the symptoms it induces.

Many compounds specifically inhibit rhinoviruses in vivo but few have beneficial effects against infection in vivo, although some are used in symptom relief. Interferon, zinc salts, synthetic antiviral agents, and monoclonal antibodies have been tested against rhinovirus colds in placebo-controlled trials.

Natural and recombinant human interferons have been tested clinically. Recombinant interferon-$\alpha 2$, administered intranasally, protects against natural and experimental rhinovirus infections. However, no therapeutic benefit is observed even if treatment is started within 30 hours of virus challenge.

A number of compounds are now available that specifically bind to rhinovirus capsids and block uncoating. The Sterling–Winthrop compound disoxaril and its derivatives have powerful antiviral effects both in vitro and in animals inhibiting viral uncoating. It has been established by X-ray crystallography that this drug acts within the VP1 β barrel of the capsid. Two other compounds, dichloroflavan and R61837, also inhibit rhinovirus uncoating, and probably bind to a similar region of the capsid. In clinical trials, dichloroflavan was ineffective but R61837 had significant benefit when given intranasally before an experimental rhinovirus challenge. Enviroxime, a benzimidazole derivative, seems to inhibit the formation of the viral RNA polymerase replication complex. When given orally and intranasally before the challenge, enviroxime significantly reduced production of nasal mucus. However, no therapeutic benefit has yet been demonstrated.

Murine monoclonal antibodies directed against the major group cell receptor compete with rhinoviruses in vitro and displace previously bound virions from cells, thus inhibiting infection. One of these monoclonal antibodies, administered intransally and prophylactically to humans, modified experimental rhinovirus infection both clinically and virologically.

A major pharmacokinetic obstacle to effective therapy is the maintenance of an adequate concentration of drug in respiratory mucosae where rhinoviruses replicate. Furthermore, successful therapies must work rapidly and be free of any side effects.

Prophylaxis: the eradication of poliomyelitis

Polioviruses are believed to have been established throughout most of the population of the world from ancient times, surviving in an endemic form by infection of susceptible infants. Because of the universal presence of antibody to all three serotypes in women of childbearing age, and the protective effect of maternal antibody on disease but not gut infection, most infants would be infected while still protected. Improvements in standards of hygiene in the late nineteenth century led to a delay in the exposure of infants to an age when maternal antibody had declined to non-protective levels. Patterns of disease then changed from the relatively uncommon and endemic kind to the occurrence of large epidemics, and poliomyelitis also became known as infantile paralysis. Safe and effective polio vaccines were developed and used in the 1950s and had an immediate and impressive effect in developed countries. The incidence of poliomyelitis in the USA between 1951 and 1979 is shown in Figure 40.7.

INACTIVATED POLIO VACCINE

The first of the currently used vaccines to be developed was the formalin-inactivated preparation of Salk (1960). Virus was treated with low concentrations of formalin under carefully controlled conditions to ensure that infectivity but not immunogenicity was lost. The resulting inactivated polio vaccine (IPV) is administered

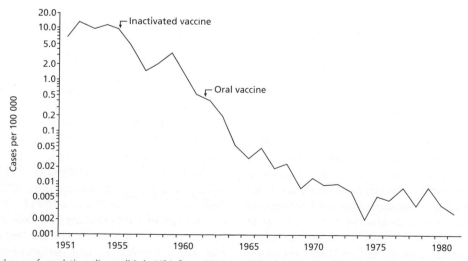

Figure 40.7 *Incidence of paralytic poliomyelitis in USA from 1951 to 1979, showing the effect of vaccination*

by injection; in the early days there were significant problems of production, particularly of the type 1 component which is the least immunogenic of the serotypes in IPV. Immediately after the licensure of the vaccine, batches were used that contained imperfectly inactivated virus, resulting in paralysis in recipients. This was the Cutter incident (Nathanson and Langmuir 1963), and is attributed to the presence of aggregates in which the virus at the center of a clump was protected from inactivation. Production was revised at once to introduce filter steps before and after treatment to remove aggregates, and no case of poliomyelitis attributable to IPV has been reported since. However, filtration removed viral antigen, making the supply problems more intense, and it was not until the 1980s with the development of improved high-density cell culture systems that high-potency IPV [enhanced potency IPV (EIPV)] became available. Its use in developed countries is increasing at the expense of the live attenuated vaccine.

LIVE POLIO VACCINE

The relative merits of inactivated polio vaccine and live attenuated vaccines were and remain a matter of heated debate. Both are highly effective and safe, but it is argued that the live, oral polio vaccine OPV developed by Sabin (Sabin and Boulger 1973), which imitates natural gut infection, also stimulates gut immunity effectively, preventing reinfection and thus interrupting transmission. Whilst it can be shown that even recent OPV vaccinees can be reinfected by wild-type strains, OPV is effective in breaking transmission in epidemics. This may be due to gut immunity or to simple competition. OPV is known to spread from person to person to some extent, which can be an advantage if not all susceptible individuals are immunized directly. Where countries have used IPV alone, unimmunized subpopulations can suffer outbreaks. For example, a religious group in Holland experienced outbreaks of type 1 in 1976 and type 3 in 1993.

The Sabin vaccine strains were developed by passage in vivo or in vitro and selected for reduced neurotropism by tests in primates. The molecular basis of this attenuation for primates was studied intensively in the 1980s and 1990s (Minor 1992).

The type 3 strain was studied in particular because it failed the primate safety test more often than types 1 and 2. Complete sequences of the genomes of the virulent precursor strain (Leon), the vaccine strain (Leon 12$_{a1b}$), and a virulent revertant isolated from a fatal case of vaccine-associated poliomyelitis were determined and compared to identify features common to the virulent strains that distinguished them from the vaccine strain. Recombinant viruses were made in which portions of the attenuated vaccine strain genome were exchanged for the equivalent region of the Leon genome to identify

changes that would attenuate. Finally, a deattenuated version of the Sabin type 3 vaccine strain was made in which all bases thought to have an attenuating effect were reverted to the virulent form. The conclusion from these studies was that only two mutations were responsible for the great majority of the attenuation of the Sabin type 3 vaccine strain. They were a base change at residue 472 in the 5' noncoding region, and a coding change leading to a substitution of a phenylalanine residue for a serine residue at position 91 of the capsid protein VP3. The 5' noncoding change leads to a loss of efficiency in the initiation of protein synthesis in in vitro translation systems (Svitkin et al. 1985), and the change in VP3 affects capsid assembly and is responsible in large part for the fact that growth of the Sabin vaccine strain is greatly inhibited at high temperatures. Other changes may make some contribution to the attenuated phenotype, but these two cause the only effects readily detectable in the standard virulence tests.

Comparable recombinants were made between the type 1 Sabin and the virulent type 1 Mahoney strains. The relatively large number of differences between the strains made detailed analysis more difficult, but it was concluded that a major attenuating mutation was to be found at base 480 in the 5' noncoding region, comparable to that found in type 3, and that other mutations were scattered through the genome, most if not all in the structural proteins. For type 2, there is evidence for a mutation in a similar location in the 5' noncoding region at residue 481, and in structural protein VP1 at residue 143. There is evidence from examination of the rare cases of vaccine-associated poliomyelitis that occur that the mutations identified in the animal model systems also attenuate the vaccine for humans.

THE ERADICATION OF WILD POLIOMYELITIS

In 1988 the World Health Organization declared the goal of eradicating all wild-type poliovirus and thus the cases of poliomyelitis that they caused by the year 2000. While this target date has passed, there is every possibility that the goal will be achieved in the near future. The reader is referred to the website for current information (www.polioeradication.org). Both live and killed vaccines have been shown to be highly effective but the live attenuated vaccine has been the most widely used because of ease of administration and cost; it is also proven to be able to interrupt epidemics of disease, although initially it was widely considered that it was not effective in developing countries. Various reasons were given to explain this, including possible interference with vaccine take by intercurrent intestinal infections, but the main reasons are probably twofold. First, the infrastructure in tropical countries is usually less well developed than in the temperate climates where the vaccine was shown to work, so that the quality of the vaccine could be very poor by the time it was used. Second, infection with poliovirus in temperate climates is markedly seasonal, with transmissions occurring only in the warmer summer months. Thus, when following the usual practice of immunizing children at a set age, the pool of susceptible individuals could be reduced greatly during the winter, when no virus transmission occurred, so that transmission was more difficult in the summer when the virus returned. By contrast, in tropical climates infection is year round, although there may be an element of seasonality. It is therefore a matter of chance whether an individual encounters the vaccine or the wild-type virus first, and there is no period of respite when immunization can make sufficient inroads on the susceptible population to affect person-to-person spread.

The solution to the problems was first to develop systems (cold chains) by which the quality of vaccines could be maintained by keeping them cold from the point of manufacture to the point of use. Second, the vaccine was used in a way that mimics an epidemic, namely by immunizing very large numbers of susceptibles within a very short period. This has taken the form of National Immunization Days (NID), which may involve the vaccination of 120 million children in a single country in a single day. As all susceptible intestines are occupied by vaccine, or are immune because of the vaccine, transmission of the wild-type virus is interrupted and in practice the wild-type virus can be eradicated in a particular limited region by a few well-conducted NIDs. Problems of access to regions of conflict or areas of particularly poor infrastructure arise, but the effect of the strategy has been to reduce the number of countries in which the virus is endemic to ten or less as of late 2002, with most concern arising from India and Nigeria. The Americas were certified free of polio in 1991, the Western Pacific Region of WHO including China in 1994, and the European Region in 2002. Even areas such as the Democratic Republic of Congo where savage wars are in progress and numbers of vaccine workers have been killed in the course of immunization programs are credibly free of poliomyelitis caused by the wild-type virus. Whilst wild-type poliovirus is still present in a few parts of the world, and in 2002 there were setbacks in both India and Africa in terms of numbers of cases identified, it is likely that the last wild-type 2 virus in the world was isolated in 1999, and that sooner rather than later the other two serotypes will also be eliminated.

One of the important factors in monitoring the progress of this exercise was the demonstration that virus transmission in a particular region had been interrupted. This depended on the specific identification of virus strains, accomplished by sequencing a relatively small part of the genome encoding the region around the *VP1-2A* gene (Rico-Hesse et al. 1987) or the region encoding the whole of VP1. Such sequences can be used to construct dendrograms of relatedness, and it has been possible to identify 'genotypes' of the different sero-types, defined as strains differing by 15 percent or less in sequence. The genotypes were found to be geographically clustered; thus an isolate from the Middle East would closely resemble other isolates from the Middle East, including those made some time ago. It was therefore possible to identify a particular virus as indigenous to the country of origin or imported, and if so, from where. For example, in 1984 a small outbreak of type 3 poliomyelitis occurred in Finland in which there were nine paralytic cases and one case of aseptic meningitis. Circulation of the strain was widespread despite the use of IPV in Finland, and there was some evidence that the strain was antigenically unusual. Genomic analysis revealed that the strain originated from the Middle East, possibly imported by soldiers serving with the UN.

CESSATION OF VACCINATION

One of the anticipated benefits of eradication is the cessation of vaccination, with consequent savings. It is also likely to be difficult and possibly unethical to maintain vaccination programs after the disease is eradicated. Stopping vaccinating is easier said than safely done, however. The molecular basis of the attenuation of the live vaccine strains of poliovirus developed by Sabin established in the 1980s and 1990s (Minor 1992) shows that for each of the strains there were relatively few mutations involved, two for each of the type 2 and 3 strains and a few more for the type 1 strain. In each case a mutation in the 5′ noncoding region had an effect with one or more mutations in the structural proteins and so far as can be seen there are no attenuating mutations in the nonstructural proteins.

The vaccines are extremely safe and effective but they all derive from original circulating natural isolates; the type 3 strain came from a fatal case. Moreover, it has been conclusively demonstrated that in rare instances, estimated at about one per 750 000 first-time vaccinees or one in 2 million overall, the vaccine can itself cause poliomyelitis in recipients or their contacts. In view of the small number of attenuating mutations, this is not surprising.

However, even when normal healthy vaccinees were examined it was found that the virus was capable of extraordinarily rapid and accurate adaptation and mutation (Minor et al. 1986b). For type 3, the mutation in the 5′ noncoding region, which is one of two that attenuate, the virus was lost at the latest within 6 days and usually within 3. The other mutation in the structural proteins is usually suppressed by changes at other positions rather than back mutation at about 11 days after vaccination; the suppressor mutations may affect other steps in the assembly of the virus than that affected by the attenuating mutation, and therefore compensate for its effects indirectly.

In addition, it was found that recombination between the viruses in the vaccine was extremely common. In fact it has been found to be the rule that a child excreting type 3 poliovirus more than 11 days after vaccination will be producing a recombinant virus in which the structural proteins derive from type 3 and the nonstructural proteins from types 1 or 2. Complex recombinants of all three serotypes are common.

The fact that the vaccine strains were derived from transmissible paralytic circulating strains of virus, that they can, albeit rarely, cause paralysis in recipients and in their contacts, coupled with the rapid evolution of the virus in vaccine recipients, suggests that it should be possible to select an epidemic, transmissible paralytic strain of poliovirus from the vaccine given the right conditions. Current observations confirm this possibility and give cause for concern.

PERSISTENCE AND CIRCULATION OF VACCINE-DERIVED VIRUS

One strategy for the cessation of vaccination would be simply to stop when it was certain that wild-type virus had been eradicated. The assumption on which this is based is that the vaccine virus does not circulate readily, and that it will therefore die out before sufficient susceptible individuals accumulate to maintain it in circulation. It is possible that this strategy would be successful. In certain countries vaccine is given at one set time. In Cuba, vaccine is only given twice at the beginning of the year and virus cannot be isolated from sewage specimens 6 months later. It has been shown that on average a vaccinee excretes poliovirus for about 5 or 6 weeks, with only one percent continuing for 10 weeks. It is believed that immunocompetent individuals never excrete the virus for longer than 6 months. Moreover, early studies showed that in the population studied which was in Louisiana, USA, the virus died out after three person-to-person transmissions. Thus virus excretion in the main is of limited duration and transmission is not very effective.

However, there have been several separate incidents in which small outbreaks of poliomyelitis have occurred after the eradication of the wild-type and where the causative virus is clearly related to the vaccine strain (Figure 40.8). They include type 2 strains isolated in Egypt between 1988 and 1993, strains responsible for an outbreak on the island of Hispaniola in Haiti and the Dominican Republic, which caused more than 20 cases in 2000–01 (Kew et al. 2002), a very small outbreak in the Philippines in 2001, and in Madagascar in 2002. The strains had some features in common. It is possible to date the origin of the strain by examining the sequence of the viral genome. During epidemics, the sequence drifts at a remarkably constant rate of about 3 percent for the silent mutations that do not cause amino acid changes, or about 1 percent if all mutations are considered (Martin et al. 2000a, 2000b). The rate seems to be independent of the type or the specific outbreak, and based on this molecular clock the strains in the incidents listed above had been circulating undetected

for 1–2 years. When they were examined in more detail, it was found that all were recombinant viruses between the vaccine strains and an unknown virus, which was not any of the vaccine strains. As poliovirus was either rare or eradicated in each of the countries concerned, it is assumed that the partner virus was a nonpolio group C enterovirus. As described above, the sequence data available suggest that recombination between members of this group occurs readily. In Hispaniola and in Madagascar there were several distinct recombinant viruses, indicating that multiple recombination events had taken place. The reason why all so far have been recombinants is not known, nor is there any understanding of what makes the viruses readily transmissible when the parent vaccine strain is not. The level of virus excreted is very similar in the outbreak cases and in normal vaccinees; it is tempting to speculate that the recombinant nature of the viruses plays a part, but it may be fortuitous. As stated above, all the vaccine strains originated from circulating strains of some sort and in principle it should be possible for them to regain transmissibility, particularly in the light of the rapid adaptation of the viruses in vaccine recipients. The origin of the strains is also speculative, but plausible. When poliomyelitis is eradicated from a region, the motivation for continuing vaccination dwindles and other health issues get attention. In Haiti, vaccine uptake was about 50 percent; in the other regions it was higher, typically about 80 percent overall. Thus while some of the susceptible children were given live vaccine, which they excreted, others were not, a situation that persisted for several years. This scenario is ideal for the selection of transmissible viruses and it seems almost inevitable that they would arise wherever vaccine programs gradually fade away. The solution could be to immunize the population to high coverage and then stop vaccinating altogether. This would at least reduce the time available for selecting transmissible strains.

CHRONIC EXCRETION OF POLIOVIRUS

A second hazard to the cessation of vaccination arises from the existence of hypogammaglobulinemic patients who may excrete virus for very long periods. So far as is known, such patients are relatively rare; at the time of writing the total number is fewer than 20. Moreover, there is no documented case of any of them acting as a source of infection for others. Some excrete virus for a prolonged period of 1 or 2 years and then stop spontaneously for known or unknown reasons; in one case excretion of virus stopped 3 years after a *Shigella* infection but usually there is no identifiable cause. However, there are instances where virus excretion had persisted for 10 years or more before it was detected, based on the sequence of the viruses, where the molecular clock seems to operate at the same rate as in an epidemic. Most patients have been identified because they develop poliomyelitis; exceptions include

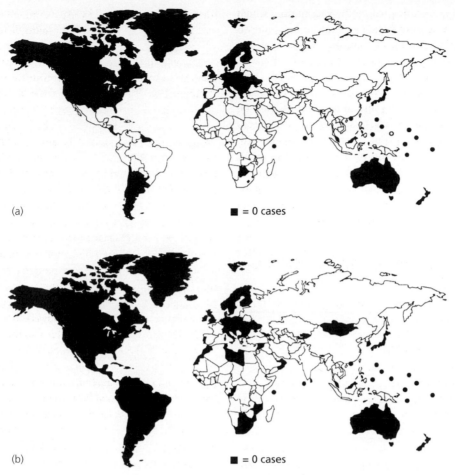

Figure 40.8 *Global distribution of poliomyelitis in* **(a)** *1988 and* **(b)** *1994. Shaded areas indicate countries with no reports of poliomyelitis due to wild-type virus.*

two patients who were deliberately given vaccine in the 1960s to investigate residual responses and protect them from wild-type poliovirus which was epidemic in the UK at the time. Some patients have been discovered by accident in the course of other investigations. Probably the best documented case is an individual who is currently known to have been excreting poliovirus in 1995 and was still doing so in 2002. Based on the sequence data, the patient is likely to have been excreting virus for 20 years. The virus is excreted at high levels in the stool and is highly virulent in animal models; it has also lost all molecular markers of attenuation. It seems likely that such individuals could act as origins of the virus in a post-eradication setting. They are rare, but nonetheless they occur. As hypogammaglobulinemia is mainly a disease of Caucasians, it may be that the hazard they pose is less by virtue of the high living standards and level of public hygiene than if they occurred in poorer parts of the world. The possible effect of AIDS has been raised; so far as is known, it does not increase the risk of long-term excretion of poliovirus, which is associated with a defect in humoral immunity. Extensive studies have not been carried out, however.

POSSIBLE SOLUTIONS

At the time of writing, the solution to the persistence of poliovirus from whatever source is not clear. Many developed countries have switched to the use of inactivated polio vaccine which at worst will maintain immunity while the significance of the issues raised can be evaluated. It has been proposed that vaccination should continue indefinitely, or that it should cease abruptly, which is likely to make the occurrence of the circulating strains found in Hispaniola and the other instances cited above less likely. New vaccines based on stabilized strains or nonreplicating vaccines have also been suggested. The possibility of bioterrorism or the escape of wild-type poliovirus from laboratory or other sources, or even the re-evolution of the virus from one of the other group C enteroviruses means that some reserve vaccine stock will be required. The form it will take and the strategies for its use remain to be established.

FUTURE PROSPECTS

Poliomyelitis due to wild-type virus is very likely to be eliminated in the near future. At that point the only way of contracting poliomyelitis will be by vaccination, which will therefore presumably stop. The strategy for doing so has not yet been elaborated, but the risk is that the vaccine strains will occupy the niche occupied by wild poliovirus, and, in view of their ability to adapt, that they will become virulent. It will therefore be necessary to protect individuals for some time until it can be shown that the vaccine-derived strains are not circulating freely but have died out. It is likely that this will be done by changing to the use of IPV rather than OPV, accompanied by suitable environmental monitoring. In Finland after the 1984/85 outbreak, OPV was used extensively but was only detectable in sewage for a period of a few months. It is therefore possible that circulation will not be prolonged, and that poliomyelitis will become the second disease to be eliminated, after smallpox.

REFERENCES

Acharya, R., Fry, E., et al. 1989. The three-dimensional structure of foot-and-mouth disease virus at 2.9 Å resolution. *Nature (Lond)*, **337**, 709–16.

Archard, L.C., Banner, M., et al. 1988. Persistence of enterovirus RNA in dilated myocardiopathy. A progression from myocarditis. In: Schultheib, H.-P. (ed.), *New concepts in viral heart disease*. New York: Springer-Verlag, 349–62.

Barrett-Connor, E. 1985. Is insulin-dependent diabetes mellitus caused by coxsackievirus B infection? A review of the epidemiologic evidence. *Rev Infect Dis*, **7**, 207–15.

Behan, P.O. 1980. Epidemic myalgic encephalomyelitis. *Practitioner*, **224**, 805–7.

Bendinelli, M. and Friedman, H. 1988. *Coxsackieviruses: a general update*. New York/London: Plenum Press.

Bergelson, J.M., Shepley, M.P., et al. 1992. Identification of the integrin VLA-2 as a receptor for echovirus 1. *Science*, **255**, 1718–20.

Bittle, J.L., Houghten, R.A., et al. 1982. Protection against foot-and-mouth disease by immunization with a chemically synthesized peptide predicted from the viral nucleotide sequence. *Nature (Lond)*, **298**, 30–3.

Bloom, H.H., Forsyth, B.R., et al. 1963. Relationship of rhinovirus infection to mild upper respiratory disease. 1. Results of a survey in young adults and children. *JAMA*, **186**, 38–45.

Bodian, D. 1955. Emerging concept of poliomyelitis infection. *Science*, **122**, 105–8.

Bögel, K. and Böhm, H. 1962. Ein rhinovirus des Rindes. *Zentralbl Bakteriol Orig Abt 1*, **187**, 2–14.

Bowles, N.E., Richardson, P.J., et al. 1986. Detection of Coxsackie-B-virus-specific RNA sequences in myocardial biopsy samples from patients with myocarditis and dilated cardiomyopathy. *Lancet*, **1**, 1120–3.

Bruce, C.B., Al-Nakib, W., et al. 1988. Synthetic oligonucleotides as diagnostic probes for rhinoviruses. *Lancet*, **2**, 53, [letter].

Burke, K.L., Dunn, G., et al. 1988. Antigen chimaeras of poliovirus as potential new vaccines. *Nature (Lond)*, **332**, 81–2.

Buscho, R.O., Saxtan, D., et al. 1978. Infections with viruses and *Mycoplasma pneumoniae* during exacerbations of chronic bronchitis. *J Infect Dis*, **137**, 377–83.

Butterworth, B.E., Grunert, R.R., et al. 1976. Replication of rhinoviruses. *Arch Virol*, **51**, 169–89.

Campbell, B.A. and Cords, C.E. 1983. Monoclonal antibodies that inhibit attachment of group B coxsackieviruses. *J Virol*, **48**, 561–4.

Cate, T.R., Couch, R.B., et al. 1965. Production of tracheobronchitis in volunteers with rhinovirus in a small particle aerosol. *Am J Epidemiol*, **81**, 95–105.

Chanock, R.M. and Parrott, R.H. 1965. Acute respiratory disease in infancy and childhood: present understanding and prospects for prevention. *Pediatrics*, **36**, 21–39.

Cherry, J.D. 1973. Newer respiratory viruses: their role in respiratory illness of children. *Adv Pediatr*, **20**, 225–90.

Chow, M., Newman, J.F.E., et al. 1987. Myristylation of picornavirus capsid protein VP4 and its structural significance. *Nature (Lond)*, **327**, 482–4.

Cooney, M.K. and Kenny, G.E. 1977. Demonstration of dual rhinovirus infection in humans by isolation of different serotypes in human heteroploid (HeLa) and human diploid fibroblast cell cultures. *J Clin Microbiol*, **5**, 202–7.

D'Allessio, D.J., Peterson, J.A., et al. 1976. Transmission of experimental rhinovirus colds in volunteer married couples. *J Infect Dis*, **133**, 28–36.

Dalldorf, G. and Sickles, G.M. 1948. An unidentified, filtrable agent isolated from the faeces of children with paralysis. *Science*, **108**, 61–3.

Dasgupta, A., Zabel, P. and Baltimore, D. 1980. Dependence of the activity of the poliovirus replicase on the host cell protein. *Cell*, **19**, 423–9.

Doggett, J.E., Bynoe, M.L., et al. 1963. Some attempts to produce an experimental vaccine with rhinoviruses. *Br Med J*, **1**, 34–6.

Douglas, R.G. Jr and Couch, R.B. 1972. Parenteral inactivated rhinovirus vaccine: minimal protective effect. *Proc Soc Exp Biol Med*, **139**, 899–902.

Elveback, L.R., Fox, J.P., et al. 1966. The virus watch program: a continuing surveillance of viral infections in metropolitan New York families. 3. Preliminary report on association of infections with disease. *Am J Epidemiol*, **83**, 436–54.

Enders, J.F., Weller, T.H. and Robbins, F.C. 1949. Cultivation of the Lansing strain of poliomyelitis virus in cultures of various human embryonic tissues. *Science*, **109**, 85–7.

Ferguson, M., Minor, P.D., et al. 1984. Neutralization epitopes on poliovirus type 3 particles: an analysis using monoclonal antibodies. *J Gen Virol*, **65**, 197–201.

Flanegan, J.B. and Baltimore, D. 1977. Poliovirus specific primer dependent RNA polymerase able to copy poly(A). *Proc Natl Acad Sci U S A*, **74**, 3677–80.

Fox, J.P. 1976. Is a rhinovirus vaccine possible? *Am J Epidemiol*, **103**, 345–54.

Fox, J.P., Cooney, M.K. and Hall, C.E. 1975. The Seattle virus watch. V. Epidemiologic observations of rhinovirus infections, 1965–1969, in families with young children. *Am J Epidemiol*, **101**, 122–43.

Fox, J.P., Cooney, M.K., et al. 1985. Rhinoviruses in Seattle families, 1975–1979. *Am J Epidemiol*, **122**, 830–46.

Gamble, D.R. 1980. The epidemiology of insulin dependent diabetes with particular reference to the relationship of virus infection to its etiology. *Epidemiol Rev*, **2**, 49–70.

Gear, J.H.S. 1984. Nonpolio causes of polio-like paralytic syndromes. *Rev Infect Dis*, **6**, Suppl 2, S379–84.

Greve, J., Davis, G., et al. 1989. The major human rhinovirus receptor is ICAM-1. *Cell*, **56**, 839–47.

Grist, N.R., Bell, E.J., et al. 1979. *Diagnostic methods in clinical virology*, 3rd edn. Oxford: Blackwell Scientific, 129–45.

Gwaltney, J.M. and Jordan, W.S. 1966. Rhinoviruses and respiratory illnesses in university students. *Am Rev Respir Dis*, **93**, 362–71.

Gwaltney, J.M., Hendley, J.O., et al. 1966. Rhinovirus infections in an industrial population. 1. The occurrence of illness. *N Engl J Med*, **275**, 1261–8.

Gwaltney, J.M., Moskalski, P.B. and Hendley, J.O. 1978. Hand-to-hand transmission of rhinovirus colds. *Ann Intern Med*, **88**, 463–7.

Hammon, W.M., Coriell, L.L., et al. 1953. Evaluation of Red Cross gamma globulin as prophylactic agent for poliomyelitis; final report of results based on clinical diagnosis. *JAMA*, **151**, 1272–85.

Hamparian, V.V., Leagus, M.B., et al. 1964. Epidemiologic investigations of rhinovirus infections. *Proc Soc Exp Biol Med*, **117**, 469–76.

Hamparian, V.V., Colonno, R.J., et al. 1987. A collaborative report: rhinoviruses – extension of the numbering system from 89 to 100. *Virology*, **159**, 191–2.

Hamre, D., Connelly, A.P. Jr and Procknow, J.J. 1966. Virologic studies of acute respiratory disease in young adults. IV. Virus isolations during four years of surveillance. *Am J Epidemiol*, **83**, 238–49.

Hayflick, L. and Moorhead, P.S. 1961. The serial cultivation of human diploid cell strains. *Exp Cell Res*, **25**, 585–621.

Hendley, J.O., Gwaltney, J.M. Jr and Jordan, W.S. Jr 1969. Rhinovirus infections in an industrial population. IV. Infections within families of employees during two fall peaks of respiratory illness. *Am J Epidemiol*, **89**, 184–96.

Higgins, P.G., Ellis, E.M. and Boston, D.G. 1966. The isolation of viruses from acute respiratory infections. 3. Some factors influencing the isolation of viruses from cases studied during 1962–64. *Mon Bull Minist Health Public Health Lab Serv*, **25**, 5–17.

Hogle, J.M., Chow, M. and Filman, D.J. 1985. Three dimensional structure of poliovirus at 2.9 Å resolution. *Science*, **229**, 1358–65.

Holland, J.J., McLaren, L.C., et al. 1959. The mammalian cell virus relationship. IV. Infection of naturally insusceptible cells with enterovirus ribonucleic acid. *J Exp Med*, **110**, 65–80.

Holzel, A., Parker, L., et al. 1965. Virus isolations from throats of children admitted to hospital with respiratory and other diseases, Manchester 1962–4. *Br Med J*, **1**, 614–19.

Hoorn, B. and Tyrrell, D.A.J. 1965. On the growth of certain 'newer' respiratory viruses in organ cultures. *Br J Exp Pathol*, **46**, 109–18.

Hope-Simpson, R.E. 1958. Discussion on the common cold. *Proc R Soc Med*, **51**, 267–74.

Horn, M.E. and Gregg, I. 1973. Role of viral infection and host factors in acute episodes of asthma and chronic bronchitis. *Chest*, **63**, Suppl, 44S–8.

Horn, M.E., Reed, S.E. and Taylor, P. 1979. Role of viruses and bacteria in acute wheezy bronchitis in childhood: a study of sputum. *Arch Dis Child*, **54**, 587–92.

Hummeler, K. and Tumilowicz, J.S. 1960. Studies on the complement fixing antigens of poliomyelitis. II. Preparation of the type-specific anti-N and anti-H indicator sera. *J Immunol*, **84**, 630–4.

Huovilainen, A., Hovi, T., et al. 1987. Evolution of poliovirus during an outbreak: sequential type 3 poliovirus isolates from several persons show shifts of neutralization determinants. *J Gen Virol*, **68**, 1373–8.

Joklik, W.L. and Darnell, J.E. 1961. The adsorption and early fate of purified poliovirus in HeLa cells. *Virology*, **13**, 439–47.

Kandolf, R. 1988. The impact of recombinant DNA techniques on the study of enterovirus heart disease. In: Bendinelli, M. and Friedman, H. (eds), *Coxsackieviruses: a general update*. New York/London: Plenum Press, 293–318.

Kapikian, A.Z., Conant, R.M., et al. 1967. Rhinoviruses: a numbering system. *Nature (Lond)*, **213**, 761–2.

Kenny, G.E., Cooney, M.K. and Thompson, D.J. 1970. Analysis of serum pooling schemes for identification of large numbers of viruses. *Am J Epidemiol*, **91**, 439–45.

Kew, O.M., Morris-Glasgow, V., et al. 2002. Outbreak of poliomyelitis in Hispaniola associated with circulating type vaccine derived poliovirus. *Science*, **296**, 356–9.

King, A.M.Q., Brown, F. et al. 2000. Picornaviridae. In van Regenmortel, M.H.V., Fauquet, C.M. et al. (eds), *Virus taxonomy. Seventh report of the International Committee on the Taxonomy of Viruses*. New York: Academic Press.

Kitamura, N., Semler, B.L., et al. 1981. Primary structure, gene organization and polypeptide expression of poliovirus RNA. *Nature (Lond)*, **291**, 547–53.

Kono, R., Miyamura, K., et al. 1977. Virological and serological studies of neurological complications of acute hemorrhagic conjunctivitis in Thailand. *J Infect Dis*, **135**, 706–13.

Kruse, W.V. 1914. Die Erreger von Husten und Schnupfen. *Münch Med Wochenschr*, **61**, 1547.

Kuhn, R.J. and Wimmer, E. 1987. The replication of picornaviruses. In Rowlands, D.J., Mayo, M.A. and Mahy, B.W.J. (eds), *The molecular biology of the positive strand RNA viruses*. FEMS Symposium No 32. London: Academic Press, 17–52.

Le Bouvier, G.L. 1955. The modification of poliovirus antigens by heat and ultraviolet light. *Lancet*, **2**, 1013–16.

Loeffler, F. and Frosch, P. 1898. Berichte der Kommission zur Erforschung der Maul- und Klauenseuche bei dem Institut für Infektionskrankheiten in Berlin. *Zentralbl Baktreriol Parsitenkd Infectionskr Hyg Abt 1 Orig*, **23**, 371–91.

Lonberg-Holm, K., Crowell, R.L. and Philipson, L. 1976. Unrelated animal viruses share receptors. *Nature (Lond)*, **259**, 679–81.

Lundquist, R.E., Ehrenfeld, E. and Maizel, J.V. Jr 1974. Isolation of a viral polypeptide associated with poliovirus RNA polymerase. *Proc Natl Acad Sci U S A*, **71**, 4773–7.

Luo, M., Vriend, G., et al. 1987. The atomic structure of Mengo virus at 3.0 Å resolution. *Science*, **235**, 182–91.

Mahon, B.P., Katrak, K., et al. 1995. Poliovirus-specific CD4+ Th1 clones with both cytotoxic and helper activity mediate protective humoral immunity against a lethal poliovirus infection in transgenic mic expressing the human poliovirus receptor. *J Exp Med*, **181**, 1285–92.

Martin, J., Dunn, G., et al. 2000a. Evolution of the Sabin strain of type 3 poliovirus in an immunodeficit patient during the entire 637-day period of virus excretion. *J Virol*, **74**, 3001–10.

Martin, J., Ferguson, G., et al. 2000b. The vaccine origin of the 1968 epidemic of type 3 poliomyelitis in Poland. *Virology*, **278**, 42–9.

Matteucci, D., Paglianti, M., et al. 1985. Group B coxsackieviruses readily establish persistent infections in human lymphoid cell lines. *J Virol*, **56**, 651–4.

Mayer, M.M., Rapp, H.J., et al. 1957. The purification of poliomyelitis virus as studied by complement fixation. *J Imunol*, **78**, 435–55.

Medrano, L. and Green, H. 1973. Picornavirus receptors and picornavirus multiplication in human-mouse hybrid cell lines. *Virology*, **54**, 515–24.

Melnick, J.L. 1984. Enterovirus type 71 infections: a varied clinical pattern sometimes mimicking paralytic poliomyelitis. *Rev Infect Dis*, **6**, S387–90.

Melnick, J.L. 1990. Enteroviruses: polioviruses, coxsackieviruses, echoviruses and newer enteroviruses. In: Fields, B.N. and Knipe, D.M. (eds), *Fields virology*, 2nd edn. New York: Raven Press, 549–605.

Melnick, J.L. and Wimberly, I.L. 1985. Lyophilized combination pools of enterovirus equine antisera: new LBM pools prepared from reserves of antisera stored frozen for two decades. *Bull W H O*, **63**, 543–50.

Mendelsohn, C., Johnson, B., et al. 1986. Transformation of a human poliovirus receptor gene into mouse cells. *Proc Natl Acad Sci U S A*, **83**, 7845–9.

Mendelsohn, C., Wimmer, E., et al. 1989. Cellular receptor for poliovirus: molecular cloning, nucleotide sequence, and expression of a new member of the immunoglobulin superfamily. *Cell*, **56**, 855–65.

Miller, D.A., Miller, O.J., et al. 1974. Human chromosome 19 carries a poliovirus receptor gene. *Cell*, **1**, 167–73.

Minor, P.D. 1990. Antigenic structure of picornaviruses. *Curr Top Microbiol Immunol*, **161**, 121–54.

Minor, P.D. 1992. The molecular biology of poliovaccines. *J Gen Virol*, **73**, 3065–77.

Minor, P.D., Pipkin, P.A., et al. 1984. Monoclonal antibodies which block cellular receptors of poliovirus. *Virus Res*, **1**, 203–12.

Minor, P.D., Ferguson, M., et al. 1986a. Antigenic structure of polioviruses of serotypes 1, 2 and 3. *J Gen Virol*, **67**, 1283–91.

Minor, P.D., John, A., et al. 1986b. Antigenic and molecular evolution of the vaccine strain of type 3 poliovirus during the period of excretion by a primary vaccinee. *J Gen Virol*, **67**, 693–706.

Minor, P.D., Ferguson, M., et al. 1990. Antigenic structure of chimeras of type 1 and type 3 poliovirus involving antigenic site 1. *J Gen Virol*, **71**, 2543–51.

Minor, P.D., Ferguson, M., et al. 1991. Antigenic structure of chimeras of type 1 and type 3 polioviruses involving antigenic sites 2, 3 and 4. *J Gen Virol*, **72**, 2475–81.

Monto, A.S. and Cavallaro, J.J. 1972. The Tecumseh study of respiratory illness. IV. Prevalence of rhinovirus serotypes, 1966–1969. *Am J Epidemiol*, **86**, 352–60.

Monto, A.S. and Johnson, K.M. 1966. Serologic relationships of the B632 and ECHO-28 rhinovirus strains. *Proc Soc Exp Biol Med*, **121**, 615–19.

Moore, M. and Morens, D.M. 1984. Enteroviruses, including polioviruses. In: Belshe, R.B. (ed.), *Textbook of human virology*. Littleton, MA: PSG Publishing, 407–84.

Moore, M., Katona, P., et al. 1982. Poliomyelitis in the United States, 1969–1981. *J Infect Dis*, **146**, 558–63.

Mufson, M.A., Ludwig, W.M., et al. 1963. Effect of neutralizing antibody on experimental rhinovirus infection. *JAMA*, **186**, 578–84.

Mufson, M.A., Krause, H.E., et al. 1970. The role of viruses, mycoplasmas and bacteria in acute pneumonia in civilian adults. *Am J Epidemiol*, **86**, 526–44.

Murray, M.G., Kuhn, R.J., et al. 1988. Poliovirus type 1/type 3 antigenic hybrid virus constructed in vitro elicits type 1 and type 3 neutralizing antibodies in rabbits and monkeys. *Proc Natl Acad Sci U S A*, **85**, 3203–7.

Naclerio, R.M., Proud, D., et al. 1988. Kinins are generated during experimental rhinovirus colds. *J Infect Dis*, **157**, 133–42.

Nathanson, N. and Langmuir, A.D. 1963. The Cutter Incident. Poliomyelitis following formaldehyde inactivated poliovirus vaccination in the United Stantes during the spring of 1955. *Am J Hyg*, **78**, 16–18.

Page, G.S., Mosser, A.G., et al. 1988. Three-dimensional structure of poliovirus serotype 1 neutralizing determinants. *J Virol*, **62**, 1781–94.

Palmenberg, A. 1987. Genome organisation, translation and processing in picornaviruses. In Rowlands, D.J., Mayo, M.A. and Mahy, B.W.J. (eds), *The molecular biology of the positive strand RNA viruses*. FEMS Symposium No 32. London: Academic Press, 1–16.

Paul, A.V. 2002. Possible unifying mechanism of picornavirus genome replication. In: Semler, B.L. and Wimmer, E. (eds), *Molecular biology of picornaviruses*. Washington, DC: ASM Press, 227–46.

Pelletier, J. and Sonenberg, N. 1988. Internal initiation of translation of eukaryotic mRNA directed by a sequence derived from poliovirus RNA. *Nature (Lond)*, **334**, 320–5.

Perkins, J.C., Tucker, D.N., et al. 1969. Evidence for protective effect of an inactivated rhinovirus vaccine administered by the nasal route. *Am J Epidemiol*, **90**, 319–26.

Phillips, C.A., Melnick, J.L., et al. 1968. Rhinovirus infections in a student population: isolation of five new serotypes. *Am J Epidemiol*, **87**, 447–56.

Pipkin, P.A., Wood, D.J., et al. 1993. Characterisation of L cells expressing the human poliovirus receptor for the specific detection of polioviruses in vitro. *J Virol Methods*, **41**, 333–40.

Plummer, G. 1963. An equine respiratory enterovirus. Some biological and physical properties. *Arch Ges Virusforsch*, **12**, 694–700.

Powell, D.G., Burrows, R., et al. 1978. A study of the infectious respiratory diseases among horses in Great Britain, 1971–1976. In: Bryans, J.T. and Gerber, H. (eds), *Equine infectious diseases IV*. Princeton: Veterinary Publications, 451–9.

Price, W.H., Emerson, H., et al. 1959. Studies of the JH and 2060 viruses and their relationship to mild upper respiratory disease in humans. *Am J Hyg*, **69**, 224–49.

Putnak, J.R. and Phillips, B.A. 1981. Picornaviral structure and assembly. *Microbiol Rev*, **45**, 287–315.

Racaniello, V.R. and Baltimore, D. 1981. Cloned poliovirus complementary DNA is infectious in mammalian cells. *Science*, **214**, 916–19.

Reed, S.E. 1972. Viral enhancement of mycoplasma growth in tracheal organ cultures. *J Comp Pathol*, **82**, 267–78.

Reed, S.E. and Boyde, A. 1972. Organ cultures of respiratory epithelium infected with rhinovirus or parainfluenza virus studied in a scanning electron microscope. *Infect Immun*, **6**, 68–76.

Reed, S.E. and Hall, T.S. 1973. Hemagglutination-inhibition test in rhinovirus infections of volunteers. *Infect Immun*, **8**, 1–3.

Reed, S.E., Tyrell, D.A., et al. 1971. Studies on a rhinovirus (EC11) derived from a calf. I. Isolation in calf tracheal organ cultures and characterization of the virus. *J Comp Pathol*, **81**, 33–40.

Ren, R. and Racaniello, V.R. 1992. Poliovirus spreads from muscle to the central nervous system by neural pathways. *J Infect Dis*, **166**, 747–52.

Rico-Hesse, R., Pallansch, M.A., et al. 1987. Geographic distribution of wild poliovirus type 1 genotypes. *Virology*, **160**, 311–22.

Rieder, E. and Wimmer, E. 2002. Cellular receptors of picornaviruses: an overview. In: Semler, B.L. (ed.), *Molecular biology of picornaviruses*. Washington, DC: ASM Press, 61–9.

Rombaut, B., Vrijsen, R. and Boeye, A. 1983. Epitope evolution in poliovirus maturation. *Arch Virol*, **76**, 289–98.

Rossmann, M.G. 1987. The evolution of RNA viruses. *BioEssays*, **7**, 99–103.

Rossmann, M.G., Arnold, E., et al. 1985. Structure of a human common cold virus and functional relationship to other picornaviruses. *Nature (Lond)*, **317**, 145–53.

Rueckert, R.R. and Wimmer, E. 1984. Systematic nomenclature of picornavirus proteins. *J Virol*, **50**, 957–9.

Sabin, A.B. 1955. Pathogenesis of poliomyelitis: reappraisal in the light of new data. *Science*, **123**, 1151–7.

Sabin, A.B. and Boulger, L.R. 1973. History of Sabin attenuated poliovirus oral live vaccine strains. *J Biol Standard*, **1**, 115–18.

Salk, J.E. 1960. Persistence of immunity after administration of formalin-treated poliovirus vaccine. *Lancet*, **2**, 715–23.

Sarnow, P., Bernstein, H.D. and Baltimore, D. 1986. A poliovirus temperature-sensitive RNA synthesis mutant located in a noncoding region of the genome. *Proc Natl Acad Sci U S A*, **83**, 571–5.

Schieble, J.H., Lennette, E.H. and Fox, V.L. 1970. Antigenic variation of rhinovirus type 22. *Proc Soc Exp Biol Med*, **133**, 329–33.

Schnurr, D.P. and Schmidt, N.J. 1988. Persistent infections. In: Bendinelli, M. and Friedman, H. (eds), *Coxsackieviruses: a general update*. New York/London: Plenum Press, 181–201.

Shepley, M.P. and Racaniello, V.R. 1994. A monoclonal antibody that blocks poliovirus attachment recognizes the lymphocyte homing receptor CD44. *J Virol*, **68**, 1301–8.

Sherry, B., Mosser, A.G., et al. 1986. Use of monoclonal antibodies to identify four neutralization immunogens on a common cold picornavirus, human rhinovirus 14. *J Virol*, **57**, 246–57.

Sperber, S.J. and Hayden, F.G. 1988. Chemotherapy of rhinovirus colds. *Antimicrob Agents Chemother*, **32**, 409–19.

Staunton, D.E., Merluzzi, V.J., et al. 1989. A cell adhesion molecule, ICAM-1, is the major surface receptor for rhinoviruses. *Cell*, **56**, 849–53.

Stott, E.J. and Walker, M. 1967. Human embryo kidney fibroblasts for the isolation and growth of rhinoviruses. *Br J Exp Pathol*, **48**, 544–51.

Stott, E.J., Grist, N.R. and Eadie, M.B. 1968. Rhinovirus infections in chronic bronchitis: isolation of eight possibly new rhinovirus serotypes. *J Med Microbiol*, **1**, 109–17.

Stott, E.J., Thomas, L.H., et al. 1980. A survey of virus infections of the respiratory tract of cattle and their association with disease. *J Hyg*, **85**, 257–70.

Svitkin, Y.V., Maslova, S.V. and Agol, V.I. 1985. The genomes of attenuated and virulent poliovirus strains differ in their in vitro translation efficiencies. *Virology*, **147**, 243–52.

Toniolo, A., Federico, G., et al. 1988. Diabetes mellitus. In: Bendinelli, M. and Friedman, H. (eds), *Coxsackieviruses: a general update*. New York/London: Plenum Press, 351–82.

Tyrrell, D.A.J. 1965. *Common colds and related diseases*. London: Edward Arnold, 197.

Tyrrell, D.A.J. and Parsons, R. 1960. Some virus isolates from common colds. III cytopathic effects in tissue cultures. *Lancet*, **1**, 239–42.

Tyrrell, D.A., Mika-Johnson, M., et al. 1979. Infection of cultured human type II pneumonocytes with certain respiratory viruses. *Infect Immun*, **26**, 621–9.

Ward, T., Pipkin, P.A., et al. 1994. Decay-accelerating factor CD55 is identified as the receptor for echovirus 7 using CELICS, a rapid immuno-focal cloning method. *EMBO J*, **13**, 5070–4.

Wilfert, C.M., Thompson, R.J. Jr, et al. 1981. Longitudinal assessment of children with enteroviral meningitis during the first three months of life. *Pediatrics*, **67**, 811–15.

Yamashita, H., Akashi, H. and Inaba, Y. 1985. Isolation of a new serotype of bovine rhinovirus from cattle. Brief report. *Arch Virol*, **83**, 113–16.

Young, D.C., Tuschall, D.M. and Flanegan, J.B. 1985. Poliovirus RNA-dependent RNA polymerase and host cell protein synthesize product RNA twice the size of poliovirion RNA in vitro. *J Virol*, **54**, 256–64.

Yousef, G.E., Bell, E.J., et al. 1988. Chronic enterovirus infection in patients with postviral fatigue syndrome. *Lancet*, **1**, 146–50.

Zhang, G., Wilsden, G., et al. 1993. Complete nucleotide sequence of a coxsackie B5 virus and its relationship to swine vesicular disease virus. *J Gen Virol*, **74**, 845–53.

Human enteric RNA viruses: astroviruses

MICHAEL J. CARTER AND MARGARET M. WILLCOCKS

Astroviruses are a relatively newly classified family of nonenveloped small RNA viruses. They appear to be widespread in nature and the list of family members and their known host species is increasing steadily. Most members are enteric and are an important cause of diarrhea and vomiting in the young of both humans and animals. In common with most agents of this type, the viruses seem to be highly resilient and survive well in the environment.

Human astroviruses (HAstV) were the first to be identified and were observed during electron microscopic examination of diarrheal stools from infants (Appleton and Higgins 1975; Madeley and Cosgrove 1975a). Their distinctive and unique appearance under negative stain (Figure 41.1) immediately suggested a novel type of virus. The particles were rounded in shape, 28 nm in diameter with a smooth margin, and, most distinctively, approximately 10 percent of them displayed a five- or six-pointed star motif on their surface. The term 'astrovirus' (Greek: astron – star) was coined to refer to this feature (Madeley and Cosgrove 1975b). Viruses showing this characteristic appearance have since been found in the stools of a variety of mammals including cattle (Woode and Bridger 1978), sheep (Snodgrass and Gray 1977), pigs (Bridger 1980), cats (Hoshino et al. 1981; Harbour et al. 1987), dogs (Williams 1980), mink (Englund et al. 2002), and mice (Kjeldsberg and Hem 1985). All were associated with mild diarrhea, generally in the young of the species.

Astroviruses have also been found to infect birds including turkeys (McNulty et al. 1980), chickens (Yamaguchi et al. 1979), and ducks (Gough et al. 1984), but in avian species the symptoms may vary. The duck

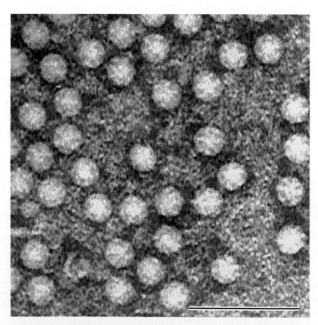

Figure 41.1 *Human fecal astroviruses negatively stained with phosphotungstic acid and viewed under the EM. Star-like motifs are visible on the surface of some particles, those showing both five- and six-pointed stars are visible. Bar 100 nm*

astrovirus DHV II causes a necrotic hepatitis, turkey astroviruses (TAstV) are associated with immunosuppressive disease or diarrhea, and the chicken virus causes nephritis. Astroviruses are a significant cause of mortality in all these species.

As is the case with other viruses infecting the gut, astroviruses are also observed in stools from symptom-free individuals and are also found in association with other enteric viruses. These features complicate attempts to assess the significance of astroviruses in human disease. Electron microscopy (EM)-based studies showed relatively few diarrheas were astrovirus-associated even though infection was known to be widespread. This in turn suggested that infections must usually be relatively mild or inapparent. Although this remains probable, recent evidence suggests that the 'typical' astrovirus structure described above may not have been a reliable feature for identification and studies using alternative technologies indicate a more significant virus association with symptomatic illness.

Initial attempts to culture these viruses failed and so the first investigations were carried out using ovine astrovirus (OAstV) since this could be obtained relatively easily from experimentally infected lambs (Herring et al. 1981). A major landmark in astrovirus research occurred with the adaptation of HAstV to cell culture; Lee and Kurtz (1981), working in Oxford, UK, repeatedly passaged virus from an adult volunteer through primary human embryo kidney cells in the presence of trypsin. Although the virus did not cause cytopathic effect in these cells, its presence could be demonstrated by immunofluorescence. After six passages it was able to infect a continuous monkey kidney cell line (LLC-MK2 cells), again requiring the addition of trypsin and without the production of cytopathic effect. This cultivation method enabled the production of antigens and subsequently both polyclonal (Lee and Kurtz 1982) and monoclonal (Herrmann et al. 1988) antibodies to HAstV were produced. These led to the recognition of antigenic variation between viruses and five serotypes were identified (Kurtz and Lee 1984). This list has now reached eight serotypes of HAstV. There are thought to be at least two serotypes of bovine astrovirus (BAstV) but apart from this, serotypic variation amongst animal strains is unknown. Enzyme-linked immunoassays were also developed (Herrmann et al. 1990), and these are now available commercially superseding to a large extent diagnosis by EM.

The Oxford adapted astrovirus strains continue to form the basis for much astrovirus research and although these represent each of the five serotypes initially identified, the procedure required to produce more isolates is relatively cumbersome and the number of characterized clinical isolates remained small. This bottleneck was overcome with the finding that a continuous human gut cell line (CaCo-2) was able to support the growth of HAstV directly from stool specimens without the need for prior adaptation; most clinical samples could now be isolated routinely by conventional laboratory procedures (Willcocks et al. 1990).

Subsequently, molecular cloning techniques were applied to both the Oxford strains and isolates from elsewhere, leading to the complete sequence determination of several virus genomes. The information derived from this has in turn led to the development of more sensitive detection systems using the reverse transcription-polymerase chain reaction (RT-PCR). All these advances have in turn fed an increase in our understanding of astrovirus genomic structure and replication strategy that ultimately led to the recognition of the unique identity of these agents and to the definition of a new family of viruses – the *Astroviridae* (Monroe et al. 1995).

CLASSIFICATION

In the 1970s, the application of EM to human stools revealed a number of small round viruses. These were originally classified according to their morphology and in 1982, Caul and Appleton proposed an interim classification scheme dividing them into 'featureless' and 'structured' particles. The featureless viruses included the enteroviruses, parvoviruses, and parvovirus-like particles, whilst the 'small round structured viruses' included the astroviruses, human caliciviruses (now termed sapoviruses) and the Norwalk-like viruses (now termed noroviruses). The 'structured' group was further divided into smooth-edged particles (the astroviruses) and those whose particles had a ragged outline (the sapo- and noroviruses). Since this time, increased knowledge of the protein composition and replication strategies of these viruses has permitted their more detailed and definitive classification. Astroviruses and human caliciviruses were soon recognized as distinct entities and the term small round structured virus (SRSV) was then used simply to refer to noroviruses.

Historically, astroviruses were identified as such simply from their morphology. Virus particles were nonenveloped and were thought to contain a single-stranded, presumptive positive-sense RNA genome but little more was known about them. These features are shared by two other families of animal viruses (the *Picornaviridae* and the *Caliciviridae*). Astroviruses were better defined when the growing database of their properties enabled their ready differentiation from other virus families. Features of polypeptide composition and genome structure were used to distinguish astroviruses from those other families above and thus permit their formal classification as a distinct virus family, the *Astroviridae* (Monroe et al. 1995). In common with modern trends in virus taxonomy, astroviruses are increasingly defined and grouped according to their genomic sequences; indeed, avian nephritis virus (ANV) was first isolated in 1976 but it was not until 2000 that molecular

Table 41.1 *Human and animal astroviruses*

Genus	Species	Serotypes	Host	Disease	Abbreviation
Mamastrovirus	*Human astrovirus*	8	Humans	Gastroenteritis	HAstV
	Bovine astrovirus	2	Cattle	None	BAstV
	Ovine astrovirus	1	Sheep	Gastroenteritis	OAstV
	Porcine astrovirus	1	Pigs	Gastroenteritis	PAstV
	Feline astrovirus	1	Cats	Gastroenteritis	FAstV
	Canine astrovirus[a]	1	Dogs	Mild enteritis	CAstV
	Murine astrovirus[a]	1	Mice and other rodents	Diarrhea	MAstV
Avastrovirus	*Duck astrovirus*	1	Ducks	Hepatitis	DAstV
	Turkey astrovirus type 1	1	Turkeys and chickens	Gastroenteritis	TAstV-1
	Turkey astrovirus type 2	. . .	Turkeys	Poultry enteritis mortality syndrome	TAstV-2
	Avian nephritis virus	1	Chickens	Acute nephritis	ANV

a) Tentative member of the *Astroviridae* awaiting molecular characterization.

cloning and sequence determination of the virus genome indicated that it should be classified within the *Astroviridae* (Imada et al. 2000). At first only one genus (*Astrovirus*) was recognized within the family. As sequence data accumulated, it became clear that the astroviruses obtained from mammals resembled each other more closely than those newly characterized viruses isolated from birds. The avian viruses likewise appear to be more closely related to each other than to astroviruses of mammals. Thus the *Astroviridae* have now been divided into two genera, *Mamastrovirus* (mammalian viruses) and *Avastrovirus* (avian astroviruses). The members currently assigned to each genus are listed in Table 41.1. Sequence comparisons such as these have the potential to illuminate much of the history of this virus family and this matter is discussed again under sequence phylogeny (see below).

BIOPHYSICAL PROPERTIES

Astrovirus particles are nonenveloped and have a buoyant density of between 1.34 and 1.40 g/ml in cesium chloride. HAstV particles have been reported with densities of 1.35–1.37 g/ml (Caul and Appleton 1982; Kurtz and Lee 1987; Willcocks et al. 1990; Matsui et al. 1993). Porcine astrovirus (PAstV) has been reported to have a buoyant density of 1.34–1.35 g/ml (Shimizu et al. 1990) and ovine of 1.38–1.40 g/ml. Aggregates of OAstV produced two peaks on cesium chloride density sedimentation: 1.365 and 1.39 g/ml (Herring et al. 1981). Similarly two distinct bands of 1.32 and 1.34 g/ml (Willcocks et al. 1990) and 1.33 and 1.37 g/ml (Matsui et al. 1993) were obtained using HAstV grown in vitro. Since the polypeptide composition of each band appeared identical in both cases, it had been speculated that the material of lower density consisted of empty virions. This was confirmed when Matsui and colleagues analyzed both peaks by hybridization analysis and

showed that the lower density material contained no viral RNA (Matsui et al. 1993).

In common with other nonenveloped viruses, astroviruses show the expected resistance to lipid solvents such as chloroform and are able to resist a variety of detergents (non-ionic, anionic, and zwitterionic). They are relatively resistant to inactivation by chlorine, titer is not reduced at levels below 30 p.p.m. of free chlorine. The virus can withstand heating to 60°C for 5 but not for 10 minutes (Kurtz and Lee 1987). As enteric viruses, they also display resistance to inactivation at acid pH, although stability is actually quite broad and the viruses withstand a range of pHs from 2 to 11 (Kurtz and Lee 1987). Amongst the enteric viruses their general stability appears second only to hepatitis A virus (Carter and Adams 2000) and they persist well in the environment. These properties have an important influence on the potential routes for transmission of the virus and this is discussed below.

MORPHOLOGY

Electron microscopy

HAstV particles of 'typical' morphology were originally reported as approximately 28 nm in diameter with a clearly defined margin and a characteristic star-like motif in their center. However, the characteristic star-like motif is visible only on some 10 percent of the virions (Figure 41.1) – or fewer in some preparations (Madeley 1979). The stellate structures are five- or six-pointed, but neither of their centers is penetrated by stain. Consequently both stars have a characteristic solid white center in electron microscopy (EM). This contrasts with the six-pointed 'star of David' feature visible on the surface of caliciviruses when viewed along their threefold axis of symmetry. The surface features of caliciviruses are ring-like hollows in which stain can accumulate. Calicivirus stars thus have a dark center surrounded by darker patches (Carter and Madeley 1987). It is not clear how the astrovirus star motifs are produced but insight may come from recent analyses of frozen particles using the technique of cryoelectron microscopy.

Astrovirus particles are usually attributed a smooth margin; however, in many micrographs there are indications of spike-like protrusions. Furthermore, particles are often present in very large numbers in stool samples and can sometimes be seen in paracrystalline arrays. Even when packed closely together, the edges of the particles seem not to make contact and it has been suggested that this even spacing between the virions could imply the existence of surface projections beyond the resolution of the electron microscope (Risco et al. 1995).

Particle size differs depending on the virus; OAstV has been reported to have a diameter of 29 nm (Gray et al. 1980), BAstV had an average diameter of 30 nm (but varied between 27 and 35 nm) (Woode et al. 1984). Interestingly, cell culture grown virus particles appear to be slightly larger, bovine astrovirus serotype 2 propagated in primary bovine kidney cells was 34 nm in diameter (varied between 30 and 37 nm) (Aroonprasert et al. 1989). This difference in diameter found between viruses propagated in cell culture and those derived from the natural host is also seen in HAstV and in general, HAstV particles grown in vitro and released from cell cultures appear less distinct and more ragged-edged than those observed in stool preparations. In fact, their average diameter has been reported to be as large as 34 nm for particles derived during the first five passages in CaCo-2 cells and such particles exhibited a remarkable similarity to caliciviruses in appearance (Willcocks et al. 1990; Risco et al. 1995). Viruses of more classical appearance were observed in later micrographs. Risco and colleagues (1995) similarly described virus released from LLC-MK2 cells and visualized in the electron microscope by negative staining as having a yet larger particle diameter (41 nm) and exhibiting a clear layer of surface spikes as suggested above.

Studies by Risco and colleagues (1995) also shed some light on this variability in appearance. These workers found that the larger particles shed from cell culture could be induced to display star-like motifs after a brief exposure to alkali (pH 10 for 10 minutes). Exposure like this is not likely under conditions of natural infection or sample collection, and most EM stains are acidic, but nonetheless local alkaline concentrations might conceivably occur during sample preparation and grid drying. The atypical larger particles were also infectious and it was proposed that these larger particles with the surface projections may represent the true native form of the virus, and the so-called 'typical' particles bearing surface stars might result from artifacts during preparation.

However, it should be borne in mind that the gut is a complex environment; although astroviruses can be grown in CaCo-2 and LLC-MK2 cells, it is likely that neither mimics exactly the true host cell, the enterocyte. Similarly, production of infectious virus requires supplementation with a protease (trypsin) and capsid protein processing appears to proceed both inside and outside the cell and may involve several stages (see below). Perhaps other extracellular factors are needed to allow released virions to 'mature' fully, although present in the intestinal lumen these would be absent in cell cultures. Consequently, it is not clear at present whether the star-bearing astroviruses represent an artifactually rearranged ragged-edged particle, or whether the ragged particles might represent partially matured forms of those showing surface stars. However, it is clear that both types are infectious and that this variation may well have affected some of the EM-based studies of virus prevalence.

Cryo-electron microscopy

Cryo-electron microscopy uses computer analysis of digitized images of hydrated virus particles to generate an electron density map and eventually a three-dimensional reconstruction of the particle. The technique is powerful and recent data have been obtained using Oxford adapted virus grown in LLC-MK2 cells. The final reconstructions (Figure 41.2) show that astrovirus particles consist of a smooth but rippled icosahedral capsid some 33 nm in diameter. The ripples do give a faint indication of star-like patterning on the capsid surface but this is not a prominent feature in these images. Thirty dimeric spikes arise from this capsid and are situated at the twofold axes of symmetry. These extend some 5 nm from the particle surface to give an overall diameter around 41–43 nm. Little detail was obtained concerning the structure of the RNA within the particle but it appeared to adopt a partially icosahedral confirmation.

THE VIRION-ASSOCIATED PROTEINS

The polypeptide composition has been determined for several serotypes of HAstV as well as the ovine and porcine viruses. The results have shown heterogeneity both in the number and the size of the structural proteins. Initial studies on OAstV found two polypeptides of about 33 kDa (Herring et al. 1981), Shimizu and colleagues (1990) purified PAstV grown in cell culture in the presence of trypsin and identified five polypeptides (of 39, 36, 31, 30, and 13 kDa).

The protein composition of various serotypes of HAstV has been investigated. All were analyzed following propagation in the presence of trypsin. Kurtz and Lee (1987) identified proteins of 36.5, 34, 33, and 32 kDa in an HAstV-4 isolate and later Kurtz (1989) found proteins of 34, 33, 26.5, and 5.2 kDa in HAstV-1.

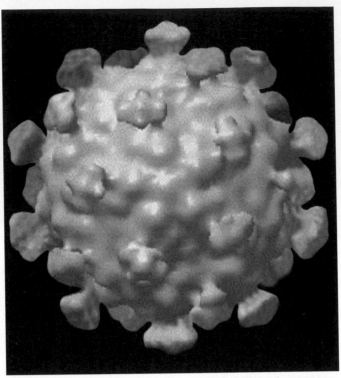

Figure 41.2 *Cryo-electron microscopic reconstruction of cell-culture-grown human astrovirus (resolution 2.4 nm). Structural predictions are derived by mathematical amalgamation of digitized images of frozen hydrated particles observed under the EM. The reconstruction shows surface projections rising from a smoothly rippled capsid surface. A five-pointed star-like feature is visible as a raised area in the center of the capsid surface. Image reproduced (with permission) from Matsui et al. 2001. We thank Dr S. Matsui and Dr M. Yeager for provision of this illustration.*

The small protein has never been confirmed but this may be due to variation between isolates or to differences in the polyacrylamide gel analysis system used. Willcocks and colleagues (1990) examined a serotype 1 astrovirus propagated in CaCo-2 cells and found proteins of 33.5, 31.5, and 24 kDa. Monroe and colleagues examined an HAstV-2 isolate adapted to growth in LLC-MK2 cells and found a similar pattern with proteins of 31, 29, and 20 kDa when the virus was propagated in the presence of trypsin (10 µg/ml). When trypsin was absent, virions contained a single protein of 90 kDa. Treatment of these virions with trypsin restored the normal pattern of polypeptides, confirming that the 90 kDa protein was an immature precursor to the normal forms (Monroe et al. 1991b). These reports have been combined to suggest a consensus protein composition for HAstV, although the actual sizes seem to vary with strain (Willcocks et al. 1992; Monroe et al. 1995). HAstV were thought to contain at least three structural proteins. Together the sum of their molecular masses suggested that they would account for almost all of the structural protein precursor. Two of these proteins formed a doublet on polyacrylamide gel analysis around 33 kDa, whilst the third was smaller and variable in size between isolates. This protein was not always detected, and was shown to be stripped from the virion by detergent treatment, which suggested that it may be loosely associated on the surface of the particle and thus be easily lost (Willcocks et al. 1990). Recently, Belliot and colleagues compared structural protein sizes in HAstV 1–5 and reconfirmed the basic pattern above; the largest two proteins varied very little between serotype and were always seen as a doublet of about 33 kDa. The third protein was consistently observed and varied between 25 and 28 kDa. This protein was largest in HAstV-2 and HAstV-4 and most variable in size amongst HAstV-5 isolates (Belliot et al. 1997a). The origin of these proteins is discussed below.

GENOME ORGANIZATION

The astrovirus genome consists of a single strand of positive-sense RNA of approximately 6 800 nucleotides, the 3′ terminus is polyadenylated (Jiang et al. 1993; Lewis et al. 1994; Willcocks et al. 1994b). The structure of the 5′ terminus is not known but it is anticipated that it is covalently linked to a small virus-encoded protein (VPg) as has been found in the calici- and picornaviruses.

The complete nucleotide sequences were first determined for HAstV serotypes 1 [Oxford reference strain adapted to growth in LLC-MK2 cells (Lewis et al. 1994) and Newcastle strain isolated in CaCo-2 cells (Willcocks et al., 1994b)] and 2 (Oxford reference strain; Jiang et al. 1993). All astrovirus genomes sequenced to date (including those of animal strains) show the same basic organization. The RNA contains three sequential open reading frames (ORF) termed 1a, 1b, and 2 (Figure 41.3) and has a short nontranslated region at each end of the genome (approx. 85 bases at the 5′ end and 83 at the 3′ end). The sizes of these ORFs for representative types of astrovirus are given in Table 41.2. The nonstructural proteins are encoded in the 5′ section of the genome in ORFs 1a and 1b; the structural proteins are specified by ORF 2. However, whilst both ORF 1a and ORF 2 possess 5′ initiation codons in a good context for activity (Kozak 1989), and whilst ORF 1a closes at a termination codon, there is no obvious start codon for ORF 1b and no separate mRNA for this region has ever been observed. ORF 1b is encoded in the −1 frame relative to ORF 1a, and examination of the 71 nt region of overlap (Figure 41.4) revealed features resembling the translational frameshifting elements seen in other virus families (e.g. the retroviruses (Jacks et al. 1988), coronaviruses, and arteriviruses (Bredenbeek et al. 1990)). These features comprised a 7 nt AU-rich sequence typical of 'slippery' sequences at which translating ribosomes could move back one base into ORF 1b. Slippery sequences alone have little effect and all are combined with features of strong secondary structure. In the astroviruses this is a stem–loop rather than a pseudoknot (Jiang et al. 1993; Lewis et al. 1994; Willcocks et al. 1994b). These features are conserved in all sequences determined to date. Mapping studies have supported the existence of the predicted secondary structures (Marczinke et al. 1994). Testing of this region of the RNA by translation in vitro has confirmed that it does direct −1 ribosome translation frameshifting at the ORF 1a/1b junction with an efficiency of approximately 5 percent in

vitro (Marczinke et al. 1994). This efficiency is about the same as that seen in retroviruses, but experiments in which the same signals were introduced into living cells indicated that frameshifting may be rather more efficient (25–28 percent) when translation takes place inside the cell (Lewis and Matsui 1996). Frameshifting ribosomes avoid the termination codon that closes ORF 1a and progress instead into ORF 1b. The product is an ORF 1a/1b fusion protein. Since not all ribosomes slip, this mechanism results in the manufacture of rather more ORF 1a products than those of ORF 1b. This latter frame encodes the virus RNA-dependent RNA polymerase which may be required in smaller amount. Thus the frameshifting events may be viewed as a refinement in the replication process, minimizing production of unnecessary RNA polymerase without requirement for a separate mRNA.

Replication of the virus

Replication of astrovirus is relatively poorly understood although the derivation of infectious clones of HAstV-1 (Geigenmuller et al. 1997) and ANV (Imada et al. 2000) should enable further analysis of the astrovirus life cycle and determination of structural features essential for replication and encapsidation.

The cell-surface receptor for astroviruses has not been identified; experiments with polarized gut epithelial cells (CaCo-2) have suggested that the receptor may be located on the basolateral rather than the apical membranes in this case (Willcocks et al. 1992). This appears unusual at first sight, but other enterically infecting viruses such as murine reovirus also show such

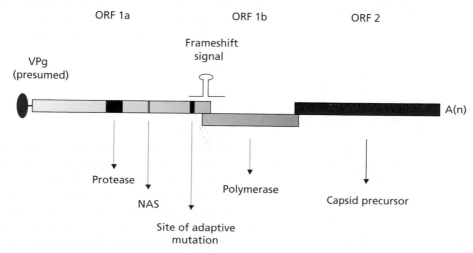

Figure 41.3 *Genome organization of human astrovirus. The basic three-open reading frame structure of HAstV-1 is illustrated (not to scale). A presumptive VPg is indicated at the 5′ terminus but its presence has not been formally demonstrated and the poly(A) tail is indicated at the 3′ terminus. The slippery sequence/stem–loop structure driving the frameshifting expression of ORF 1b is indicated at the overlap of ORFs 1a and 1b. These ORFs encode the virus nonstructural proteins and are both expressed from the genome. ORF 2 specifies precursors to virion structural proteins and is expressed from a subgenomic mRNA. The relative positions of functional motifs and other features of interest are indicated. Protease, site of virus serine protease; NAS, location of the bipartite nuclear addressing sequence; Site of adaptive mutation, location of repetitive sequences apparently deleted between strains and that may assist growth in some cell types.*

Table 41.2 *Genome and open reading frame sizes for characterized* Astroviridae

Astrovirus	Genome size (if complete)	ORF 1a amino acids	ORF 1b amino acids	ORF 2 amino acids	Accession number
HAstV-1 (Newcastle)	6 813	924	512	786	NC_001943
HAstV-1 (Oxford)	6 771	920	519	787	L23513
HAstV-2	6 797	920	519	796	L06802
HAstV-3	6 815	927	515	794	AF141381
HAstV-4	. . .	. . .	. . .	771	AB025801–AB025812
	. . .	. . .	. . .	771	Z33883
HAstV-5	. . .	. . .	. . .	783	AB037274–AB037273
HAstV-6	. . .	. . .	. . .	778	Z66541
	. . .	. . .	. . .	. . .	AB031030–AB031031
	. . .	. . .	. . .	. . .	AB013618
HAstV-7	. . .	. . .	. . .	791	AF248738
	. . .	. . .	. . .	791	Y08632
HAstV-8	6 759	921	518	842[a]	AF260508
	. . .	. . .	. . .	782	Z66541
TAstV-1	7 003	1 099	512	671	NC_002470
	. . .	. . .	. . .	. . .	Y15936
TAstV-2	7 355	1 125	527	724	AF206663
ANV	6 927	1 029	483	683	NC_003790
FAstV	. . .	. . .	. . .	816	AF056197
PAstV	. . .	. . .	. . .	783	Y15938
	. . .	. . .	. . .	776	AB037272
OAstV	6 440	844	523	762	NC_002496
	. . .	. . .	. . .	. . .	Y15937

a) Sequence reveals 60 additional residues at the N terminus preceding the usual start sequence MASK. . . . It is not known if these are present in the astrovirus mRNA and consequently whether they are translated to protein. Similar sequences present in some strains of HAstV-1 are not transcribed into subgenomic mRNA.

a distribution of receptors. In that case it is believed that virus is taken up whole through the M cells overlying the Peyer's patches, and released on the other side, so gaining access to the basolateral cell surfaces. In this regard it may be significant that BAstV has an affinity for M cells (see below). Cell penetration proceeds via absorptive receptor-mediated endocytosis. Virus entry to the cytoplasm is presumably triggered by pH decrease in the endosome since procedures that elevate intra-endosomal pH have been shown to reduce virus infection (Donelli et al. 1992). The astrovirus genome is infectious if transfected into susceptible cells so it is assumed that translation of the incoming genome is sufficient to initiate the replication process. Full-length transcripts of a cDNA clone of the virus are also infectious on transfection but a synthetic cap structure must be added. This result is reminiscent of that obtained for the caliciviruses (Sosnovtsev and Green 1995) and suggests that some structure at the 5′ terminus (presumably a VPg) is required to initiate translation and that the role of this structure can be substituted by a cap. Proteins are generated from the genome by direct translation to express ORF 1a and via a −1 ribosomal frameshifting event to express ORF 1b. Processing of the polyproteins thus produced is described below.

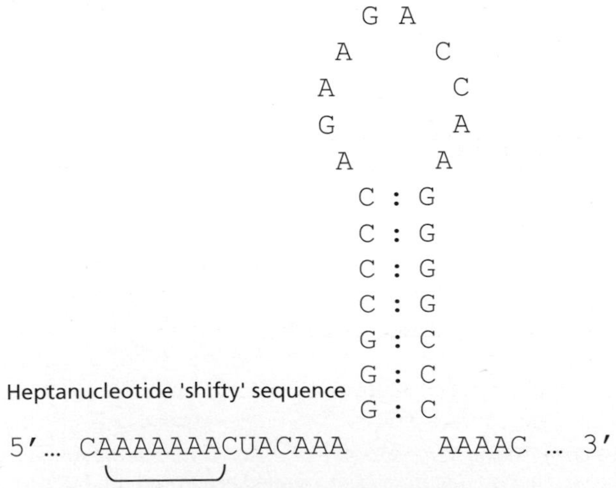

There have been reports of a nuclear involvement in both BAstV and HAstV replication. Aroonprasert and colleagues (1989) studied BAstV infection in vitro using immunofluorescent antibodies and found fluorescence initially in the cytoplasm of infected cells, followed shortly by brilliantly fluorescing intranuclear granules, suggesting nucleolar involvement. Similarly, experiments

Figure 41.4 *Frameshift signal derived from HAstV-1. The sequence illustrated shows the A-rich heptanucelotide slippery or shifty sequence preceding the stable stem–loop structure. The stem is highly stable and GC-rich; sequence of the stem and the loop appear less important than the overall stability of the structure (Marczinke et al. 1994).*

RNA transcripts

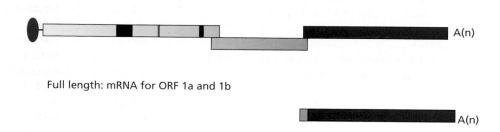

Full length: mRNA for ORF 1a and 1b

A(n)

Subgenomic transcript: mRNA for ORF 2

Figure 41.5 *Astrovirus-induced intracellular RNA. Full-length genome is present and acts as mRNA for ORFs 1a and 1b. A subgenomic mRNA is also synthesized to express the virus ORF 2 proteins. This is co-terminal with the virus genomic 3′ end and extends partially into ORF1b sequences. However, these precede the initiation codon and are not translated. In some viruses, ORF 2 in the genome is potentially longer than the subgenomic mRNA. In these cases any potential initiation codon (s) opening ORF 2 in the genomic RNA are usually in a poor context for activity and are not transcribed into the subgenomic mRNA. The subgenomic mRNA thus presents the ORF 2 initiation codon in the best context for activity as the first such codon in the message. Translation commences with the sequence 'M A S K ---' in almost all cases.*

studying HAstV replication in LLC-MK2 cells showed fluorescence in the nucleus at relatively late times in infection (W.D. Cubitt, personal communication). This fluorescence could suggest movement of structural protein to the nucleus since it has been detected with sera raised to the capsid protein. However, early cloning experiments used such sera to select clones expressing virus antigen (Matsui et al. 1993) and this approach led to the identification of regions specifying the so-called immunoreactive epitopes. Although one of these was derived from the capsid protein as expected, another was surprisingly located in the nonstructural genes close to the nuclear locating signal. When sera were raised to this part of the nonstructural protein, they also reacted with infected cell nuclei (Willcocks et al. 1999). The role of the nucleolus or nucleus in astrovirus infection is not known but replication is not affected by actinomycin D and thus DNA-directed information flow is presumably not required.

A second viral mRNA is also found during astrovirus replication (Monroe et al. 1991b); this subgenomic RNA is approximately 2 800 bases long and is also polyadenylated. It has been found by hybridization and sequence analysis to be co-terminal with the 3′ end of the genome (Matsui et al. 1993; Willcocks and Carter 1993) and is also believed to bear a VPg at its 5′ end (Figure 41.5). The subgenomic RNA has been found only in infected cells and does not become packaged into virus particles. During infection it is synthesized in five- to tenfold molar excess over the genomic RNA, presumably to allow synthesis of structural proteins in larger quantities than the nonstructural (Monroe et al. 1993). Since this RNA is not present in the virus, it must

be generated from the incoming full-length genomic RNA; however, little is known of RNA synthesis by this virus. Promoters have not been characterized and it is not known whether the subgenomic mRNA is subsequently replicated independently via its own separate negative-strand template, or produced only from the full-length antigenome. The 5′ terminus of the subgenomic RNA has been mapped (Monroe et al. 1993) and primer extension analysis reveals the bulk of the product to commence at position 4 359 in the sequence (coordinates refer to HAstV-1). Although the bulk of the molecule does indeed extend in a 3′ direction from this position, a small fraction of the product is slightly longer by 12 or 16 bases (Willcocks and Carter 1993).

Early in infection, capsid antigen is detected in the cytoplasm as a diffuse fluorescence in the perinuclear area. As infection proceeds this becomes more granular, and EM shows dense deposits of virus capsids in these areas (Aroonprasert et al. 1989). Cytopathic effect is not well observed because the trypsin required to allow the particles to mature causes detachment of the cells such that cytopathic effect is not visible. The exception to this has been in some CaCo-2 cell cultures where a shriveling and rounding of the cells can be seen. In this case cytopathic effect is usually limited to the margins of the cell sheet (Willcocks et al. 1990). This is presumably because receptors are located on the basolateral membranes of the cells and the virus has ready access to these only at the edges of the monolayer. Most others are presumably shielded below the tight junctions that bind the cells together. Virus is presumed to be released by cell lysis.

PROTEIN CODING AND EXPRESSION

ORFs 1a and 1b specify the virus nonstructural proteins; the arrangement of the sequences for which a potential role has been identified is given in Figure 41.3. ORF 1a has the potential to specify a 101 kDa protein that, in common with other positive-strand RNA viruses, is subsequently cleaved to release functional processed molecules. Both the polyprotein and a number of cleavage products have been identified inside cells, although function has not been allocated to all of them. Sequence analysis has revealed the presence of a chymotrypsin (3C)-like serine protease (Jiang et al. 1993); this is in contrast to the picorna- and caliciviruses which have a cysteine residue at the active site of their 3C protease. However, no sequence motifs indicative of RNA helicase, methyltransferases, or papain-like proteases have been detected in astroviruses. It is possible that small RNA viruses of this type do not require a helicase for efficient replication (Koonin 1991b; Jiang et al. 1993). It has been suggested that astrovirus may encode a VPg, based on the absence of a methyltransferase and the similarity of the polymerase to those of other VPg-containing viruses. Sequence analysis has indicated that it might be encoded upstream of the protease but VPg has not been observed experimentally (Matsui and Greenberg 1996). Towards its C-terminus, ORF 1a contains a bipartite nuclear localization signal (Willcocks et al. 1992; Jiang et al. 1993). Antisera raised to this region of the polyprotein have shown that nonstructural proteins do enter the cell nucleus during infection (Willcocks et al. 1999), but the purpose of this movement is not clear. This region of ORF 1a is also the site of a mutation that seems to accompany adaptation of HAstV to growth in continuous cell lines of nongut origin (e.g. LLC-MK2 cells). The Oxford adapted viruses were obtained by serial passage in primary human embryo kidney. During this process the host cell range of the virus became altered. Comparison with samples of the same virus that had been passaged in volunteers rather than human embryo kidney, cells showed that the cell-adapted virus contained a deletion of 45 nt. This removes a partially repetitive 15 amino acid sequence. Isolates made directly in gut cell lines (e.g. CaCo-2 cells) did not contain this deletion (Willcocks et al. 1994a). It has been suggested that this deletion might improve 'fit' between a virus protein and a cellular protein with which it must interact, thus extending host cell range. However, other features of this region also seem variable between strains and so the extent to which this modification represents adaptation to a particular host cell type rather than a coincidental or strain-related variation is not fully understood.

ORF 1b encodes a 59 kDa polypeptide whose amino acid sequence is that of an RNA-dependent RNA polymerase; it contains all the motifs typical of a polymerase belonging to supergroup I (Jiang et al. 1993). This group includes polymerases of the picorna- and caliciviruses, as well as some plant viruses (such as the bymoviruses and potyviruses), although the similarities between astroviruses and the plant viruses in this region do not necessarily indicate a common origin for the viruses (Koonin 1991a).

ORF 2 encodes the virion structural proteins and is expressed from a subgenomic mRNA that is 3′ co-linear with the genome (Monroe et al. 1993; Willcocks and Carter 1993). The structural proteins are produced as a precursor (90 kDa), which is then proteolytically cleaved. This protein has a well-conserved N terminus which is highly basic, and contains a serine/arginine repeat motif (Jonassen et al. 2001). This is similar to the basic region found in some coronaviruses (those related to transmissible gastroenteritis virus), and is also reminiscent of some plant viruses where such a sequence is involved in RNA binding (Carter 1994). By contrast, the 3′ end of ORF 2 specifies a highly acidic region. The function of these two areas is not known, but it is likely that these regions of strong charge localization do play a role in protein–protein interactions or protein–RNA interactions.

A highly conserved 35 nt stem–loop structure is located near the ORF 2 stop codon in all the astrovirus sequences examined to date (except that of TAstV-2). This feature straddles the termination codon and is formed from both translated and nontranslated sequences. The function of this structure is not known, but it is likely to be vital to the virus. Any change in one nucleotide of the stem structure is always accompanied by a compensatory mutation in the other strand of the stem such that base pairing and thus secondary structure is maintained (Jonassen et al. 1998).

Processing of nonstructural proteins

The nonstructural proteins are generated from two polyproteins corresponding to ORF 1a (101 kDa) or the ORF 1a/1b fusion resulting from ribosomal frameshifting during translation (160 kDa). The processing of these proteins remains to be fully elucidated but several workers have now examined processing either in infected CaCo-2 cells, transfected baby hamster kidney (BHK) cells or in vitro. A synthesis of the resultant data is presented in Figure 41.6.

Processing has been examined during productive infections of CaCo-2 cells using sera raised to specific sections of the nonstructural protein ORFs. Sera recognizing the C-terminal third of ORF 1a (residues 643–920 in HAstV-1) detected multiple cleavage products; the complete ORF 1a product was not observed, the largest protein being only 75 kDa. This indicated that some 26 kDa had been rapidly cleaved from the N terminus of ORF 1a and could not be detected using this serum. The 75 kDa protein appeared to be further cleaved,

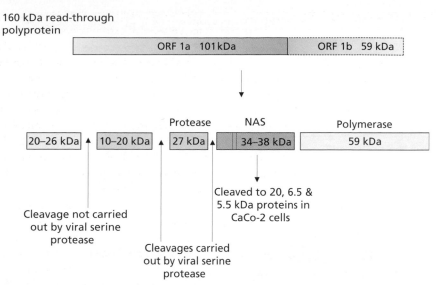

Figure 41.6 *Processing of astrovirus nonstructural proteins. Here the processing of the ORF1a/1b fusion generated by read-through translation of both ORFs is illustrated; 20–26 kDa is cleaved from the N terminus by a nonviral protease soon after translation (whilst other cleavages are performed by the virus-encoded enzyme). This releases the 27 kDa protease molecule and a presumptive second protein that has not been directly observed. The third section released from ORF 1a (34–38 kDa) includes the bipartite nuclear addressing signal (NAS) and is further cleaved to at least three products 20, 6.5, and 5.5 kDa in size. The ORF 1b product (polymerase) is believed to be cleaved at or near the frameshift position and is not markedly cleaved subsequently.*

producing a 34 kDa C-terminal product that could be detected by the serum used. Any other product(s) that derived from the N terminus of the molecule were not detectable by this method. The 34 kDa molecule appeared to be unstable and did not accumulate to high levels in the cell; instead it appeared to be processed to cleavage products of 20, 6.5, and 5.5 kDa that were observed to accumulate. The proteins that would be recognized by this serum would include any that contain the nuclear localization signal, and these were identified in the cell nucleus (Willcocks et al. 1999).

ORF 1a sequences have also been expressed in BHK cells transfected with expression constructs containing ORF 1a (Geigenmuller et al. 2002a). These workers also observed a cleavage near the N terminus, removing in this instance a 19 kDa section. This cleavage also took place if the virus protease was inactivated, thus confirming that it is not mediated by this enzyme and is probably a host-cell-specified event. Further processing was dependent on a functional viral protease and led to a product of 27 kDa that spanned the serine protease motifs. This corresponds to the 27 kDa protein identified in astrovirus-infected CaCo-2 cells and which can now be identified as the virus protease itself.

Gibson and colleagues (1998) reported the in vitro expression of both the full-length ORF 1a polyprotein and that of the combined ORF 1a/1b but presented no information on processing. A second study examined processing in vitro using antisera raised to synthetic peptides; a single autocatalytic event was observed in the ORF 1a polyprotein. This yielded an N-terminal 64 kDa and a C-terminal 38 kDa product. This cleavage was accomplished by the virus-specified serine protease

since mutation of the serine at the active site obviated this event (Kiang and Matsui 2002). The 38 kDa protein is probably analogous to the 34 kDa protein identified in CaCo-2 cells and their nuclei. The removal of 26 kDa from the N terminal was not observed, indicating again that this may be a host-cell-dependent cleavage.

Willcocks and colleagues (1999) also detected synthesis of the polymerase (ORF 1b product) in CaCo-2 cells using sera raised to the expressed ORF 1b protein. A single product of 59 kDa was detected. This is approximately the size expected for the whole of ORF 1b (786 aa). This suggests that little if any internal cleavage takes place in the polymerase and similarly that most or all of ORF 1a is effectively removed when the fusion protein is processed.

Processing of structural proteins

The astrovirus structural protein is translated from ORF 2 as a 90 kDa precursor protein and it has long been recognized that trypsin plays a vital role in cleavage of this precursor (Monroe et al. 1991b). Willcocks and colleagues (1990) showed that particles released in the absence of trypsin were non-infectious. Bass and Qui (2000) confirmed this finding and showed that such particles contained only minimally processed capsid precursor protein; 71 amino acids were cleaved from the N terminus intracellularly to generate a 79 kDa capsid precursor from which particles were formed. Treatment of these particles with trypsin after release led to the formation of three structural proteins and increased infectivity by 50 000–100 000-fold. Other workers have

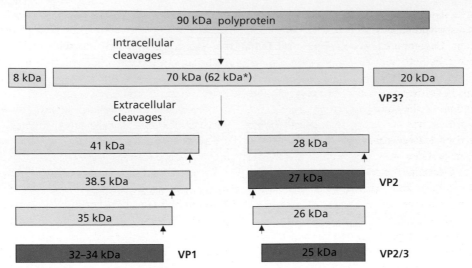

Figure 41.7 *Processing of astrovirus structural proteins. The illustration attempts to bring together data from a variety of sources, not all of which are compatible. Consequently the actual processing pathways used by any one virus may vary depending on either serotype of virus and/or host cell. In the model presented, primary translation generates a molecule of 90 kDa (VP90) that is subsequently processed. One report states that 8 kDa may be cleaved from the N terminus rapidly after translation (indicated by '*') but this does not appear to be general and does not occur in other systems where it has been sought. VP20 is cleaved from the C terminus and at least one report finds that this occurs intracellularly. In this case VP20 was not subsequently present in the virion (Mendez et al. 2002) and particles were formed exclusively from VP70. Other reports indicate that particles form from VP90 (and thus must include residues derived from VP20) (Geigenmuller et al. 2002b). Thus the backbone of the virion may indeed be formed from sequences contained within VP70 but the C-terminal residues contained within VP20 may be superficially located. Once cleaved (intracellularly or extracellularly), they may readily dissociate from the particles. Maturation of VP70 (or VP90 where particles are constructed from this protein) occurs extracellularly and is mediated by trypsin. Several sequential cuts are made and the efficiency of each may vary with both the strain of virus (and the accessibility of the scissile bond) and the activity of trypsin supplied in the growth medium. As a result, particle compositions may appear complex but VP32–34, and the overlapping proteins VP25 and VP27 may predominate (indicated in deeper color). Differences in the extent of maturational cleavage could also explain the lack of stoichiometric relationship observed in some preparations where levels of VP27 appear far lower than those of VP25. Past attempts to use a conventional nomenclature in which virus proteins are numbered VP1–3 are complicated. This nomenclature is best avoided since the proteins could be potentially assigned different names depending on the degree of cleavage and/or VP20 dissociation in any one preparation (indicated above).*

not observed this trimming of the N terminus and report structural proteins in the virion that extend completely to the N terminus of the protein. (Geigenmuller et al. 2002b; Mendez et al. 2002).

Determination of the cleavage sites and the manner of processing of virion proteins has been complicated by uncertainty as to the protein composition of the virions (see above). In a study of the Oxford HAstV-2 strain, Sanchez-Fauquier and colleagues (1994) found that the capsid precursor was cleaved to three polypeptides (34, 29, and 26 kDa) in the presence of trypsin. These sizes would account for almost all the structural protein precursor. However, N-terminal sequencing revealed surprising features. VP29 and VP26 were not distinct molecules. Instead, these moieties overlapped substantially; they shared a common C terminus and were both derived from the center of the precursor protein. The residues extending from the N terminus of the precursor to the N terminus of VP29 could form the 34 kDa protein (although this was not confirmed), but this analysis left the fate of some 27 kDa from the C terminal of the precursor protein unexplained. A further study of structural protein processing in HAstV-8 offered a possible explanation for these findings

(Figure 41.7). Mendez and colleagues (2002) found that 20 kDa was cleaved from the C terminus of the capsid precursor intracellularly. This molecule was not detected in virions and its fate has not been determined. The remaining 70 kDa molecule was processed extracellularly and only to completion when high levels of trypsin (>100 μg/ml) were present. The 70 kDa polyprotein was cleaved firstly to 41 and 28 kDa products and subsequently the size of each was further reduced through a series of trimming cuts. Three products were prominent in preparations of virions; VP34 and two forms derived from VP28: VP25 and VP27. The relationship between these two molecules agrees with the findings of Sanchez-Fauquier et al. (1994). The variability in the detection of the third virion protein could then result simply from differing efficiencies of trypsin cleavage and this might also explain some of the earlier reports of multiple protein components in the virion.

However, this explanation also fails to provide a role for the C-terminal 20 kDa removed intracellularly from the precursor in these experiments. This section of the protein is highly variable in sequence between serotypes. This suggests exposure to host antibody selection pressure and thus implies a structural (or at least extracellular) role. Furthermore, its presence on the same mRNA as the structural proteins would suggest that it is manufactured in similar amount. Geigenmuller and colleagues (2002b) infected CaCo-2 cells with mutant virus bearing a tag sequence at either the N or C terminus of the capsid protein. They also observed the removal of up to 20 kDa from the C terminus of the capsid precursor protein, but in this case the process was inefficient; the majority of the protein remained uncleaved regardless of the position of the tag. However, particles were observed in these cells, suggesting that C-terminal cleavage is not essential for particle formation and consequently C-terminal sequences can be incorporated at least into immature forms of the capsid inside the cell. Although these facts are suggestive of a structural role, this region has not been demonstrated in mature, extracellular virions by N-terminal sequence determination, indicating that it may be lost during particle maturation or sample preparation in the laboratory.

SEROLOGY

In the 1980s, Kurtz and Lee identified five serotypes of HAstV (HAstV-1–5) by immunofluorescence and immunosorbent electron microscopy (Lee and Kurtz 1982; Kurtz and Lee 1984). Each of these reference strains had been adapted to growth in LLC-MK2 cells (Lee and Kurtz 1981). Since then, three more serotypes have been recognized (HAstV-6–8); all were originally isolated in the UK (Lee and Kurtz 1994; Kurtz, unpublished data). However, they have remained uncommon in the UK. The HAstV are antigenically distinct from the animal viruses (Kurtz and Lee 1984); however, feline astrovirus (FAstV) is detected efficiently by enzyme-linked immunosorbent assay (ELISA) kits engineered using sera and monoclonal antibodies raised to HAstV.

In many viruses, genogroup analysis based on sequence phylogeny is superseding conventional classification by serotyping. Although genogroup analysis can be performed on any part (or the whole) virus sequence, serotyping by definition depends only on the structural proteins. For the most part, genogroupings are based on nonstructural sequences since these are well conserved and thus relatively easily accessed by PCR for sequence determination. In general, this type of analysis does give similar, if not identical, patterns regardless of the section of the genome used for analysis, but even so the potential for recombination events that might combine structural genes from one serotype with nonstructural genes from another should not be ignored. These problems can be largely overcome in the case of the astroviruses provided that the structural protein is used for genotyping. Noel and colleagues (1995) examined a short PCR product derived from ORF 2 of each serotype and showed that genotyping in this instance led to the same result as serotyping. Since then, additional capsid precursor sequences have become available, but the

coincidence of the two types of grouping has been maintained. Wang and colleagues (2001) compared capsid precursor sequences of 46 strains of HAstV and found that the genogroups obtained corresponded exactly to the serotypes. Comparisons have shown that within any given serotype, where more than one ORF 2 complete sequence is available, the strains are more than 94 percent identical. By contrast, the highest identity level seen between serotypes was 75 percent between types 5 and 6 (Mendez-Toss et al. 2000).

Jonassen and colleagues (2001) examined variation within the capsid sequence and also found that the N-terminal half was well conserved, while the C-terminal portion was hypervariable with large inserts or deletions. Neutralizing monoclonal antibodies prepared to the astrovirus capsid have all been found to be specific to the VP29 protein encoded in the midsection of the capsid polyprotein (Bass and Upadhyayula 1997).

The largest protein, on the other hand, is more conserved, and a common epitope has been predicted from sequence analysis (Mendez et al. 2002). All the serotypes of HAstV are recognized by a single non-neutralizing monoclonal antibody produced by Herrmann and colleagues (1988). The monoclonal antibody is directed at the capsid protein (Lewis et al. 1994), but the site it recognizes has not been fully defined. Current data suggest that the antibody binds to two discontinuous regions of the capsid protein, both located in the largest protein VP34 between residues 82–115 and 215–260 (residue numbers given for HAstV-1 strain A2/88 Newcastle) (M.M. Willcocks et al., unpublished data). This monoclonal antibody has been used to develop a commercial ELISA for astrovirus and also reacts with FAstV.

SEQUENCE PHYLOGENY

Genome nucleotide sequences

The complete nucleotide sequences have now been determined for four serotypes of HAstV:

1 HAstV-1 both Oxford (Lewis et al. 1994) and Newcastle (Willcocks et al. 1994b) strains
2 the Oxford strain of HAstV-2 (Jiang et al. 1993)
3 HAstV-3 from Germany (Oh and Schreier 2001)
4 HAstV-8 from Mexico (Mendez-Toss et al. 2000).

Three of the avian astroviruses have been sequenced, two from the turkey [TAstV-1; (Jonassen et al. 1998) and TAstV-2 (Koci et al. 2000a)] and one from the chicken (ANV; Imada et al. 2000). One other mammalian virus, that of the sheep, has also been sequenced – OAstV (Jonassen et al. 2001). The sequence of the structural gene *ORF2* has been obtained for the remaining serotypes of HAstV: HAstV-4 (Willcocks et al. 1995), HAstV-5 (Wang et al. 2001; S.S. Monroe et al., unpublished data), HAstV-6 (M.M. Willcocks et al.,

I. Oishi et al., both unpublished data), and for HAstV-7 (Jonassen et al. 2001; Walter et al. 2001b). Structural gene sequences are also available for the feline (M.M. Willcocks et al., unpublished data) and porcine astroviruses (Jonassen et al. 2001; Wang et al. 2001).

An analysis of the nine complete sequences available showed that they could be divided into two groups (Figure 41.8), with one containing the mammalian astroviruses (OAstV being an outlier) and the second containing the avian astrovirus sequences. The same two groups were also derived using either ORF 1a or 1b alone for the comparison (Lukashov and Gouldsmit 2002). Comparison, by these authors, of all the available ORF 2 sequences groups all the HAstV serotypes together with the feline virus being most closely related to them, followed by the porcine, and with the ovine capsid sequence showing considerable variation from the other mammalian capsid nucleotide sequences. Again the avian astroviruses formed a separate cluster. The authors speculate that the topology of the phylogenetic trees suggests that cross-species transmission may have occurred during astrovirus evolution with a PAstV-like virus being passed to cats and then to humans. This sort of cross-species transfer occurring during virus speciation and over evolutionary time must be clearly distinguished from zoonotic infections whereby animal viruses may infect humans, although this may also occur (see below). Grouping of the structural proteins on the basis of their more conserved sections should indicate underlying relatedness between viruses and strip out the effects of antigenic variation driven independently by immune responses in different host species. When performed this way, FAstV was even more closely grouped with the human strains, again indicating an evolutionary relationship (Wang et al. 2001). A comparison based on ORF 2 amino acid sequences reached similar conclusions (Jonassen et al. 2001).

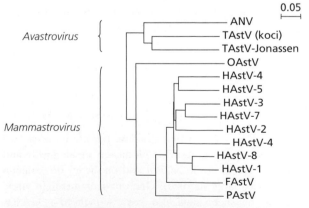

Figure 41.8 *Phylogenetic analysis of representative astrovirus capsid sequences. Sequences fall into two clear genogroups that have now been recognized as separate genera: Mamastrovirus containing sequences from mammalian viruses and Avastrovirus containing sequences from avian isolates. FAstV groups closest to human strains whilst OAstV is an outlier from the Mamastrovirus group.*

Analysis of virus sequences can always be complicated by the potential for recombination between genomes. The two phylogenetic groups identified above are not affected by these concerns, but recombination between human astroviruses can almost certainly take place. Four isolates of HAstV-5 from Houston, TX and Mexico City were analyzed at the junction of ORF 1b to ORF 2. These new isolates were closely related to serotype 3 in ORF 1b but closest to serotype 5 in ORF 2. These data, combined with the strong sequence conservation in this region seen in all HAstV serotypes, indicated a possible recombination site at the ORF 1b/ORF 2 junction (Walter et al. 2001a). Recombination events like this could exchange capsid protein genes between viruses in the case identified between serotypes of human virus, but presumably this could also exchange genes between an animal and a human virus under appropriate circumstances.

TRANSMISSION

Person to person

The virus is transmitted by the fecal–oral route and therefore spreads readily among babies and small children where infection is most common. There have been many reports of outbreaks in childcare facilities and schools (Lew et al. 1991; Mitchell et al. 1993, 1999b). Prevention or control of astrovirus infection in such settings is generally best achieved by careful attention to hygiene (hand washing, cleaning, or disposal of potentially contaminated items). It has been suggested (Abad et al. 2001) that astroviruses are able to survive on inert surfaces long enough for fomites to play a role in transmission of astrovirus diarrhea, and disinfection of any potentially contaminated surfaces, door handles, etc., is also required. The virus has been shown to be relatively resistant to disinfection by ethanol or isopropanol (Kurtz et al. 1980). It is also relatively resistant to inactivation by heat, acidification, detergent treatment, and treatment with phenolic, quaternary ammonium chloride, or benzalconium chloride-based products (Kurtz and Lee 1987). However, 70 percent methanol was found to decrease infectivity by 3 $\log_{10}$ and 90 percent decreased it to less than 10 infective units/ml and proprietary virucidal surface cleaners are effective. Since the virus is relatively temperature stable, attention should be paid to the operating temperature of bedpan washers. Infected individuals should be separated from those not infected and particular care should be taken to ensure that those who handle food do not continue to work while infected.

Foodborne

Foodborne transmission is not generally assumed to be significant in the case of astrovirus infection. This arises since the bulk of astrovirus infections occur in the young, an age group where direct fecal–oral person-to-person transmission is more likely. However, foodborne transmission between adults is likely to be more significant, and although most individuals are likely to have had prior experience of astrovirus types 1 and 2 (with resulting protective or ameliorating antibody memory), many would not have encountered the rarer serotypes which could therefore induce symptomatic illness. Astrovirus outbreaks have been associated with the consumption of shellfish contaminated with sewage (Kurtz and Lee 1987). A recent study in France found that 17 percent of oysters sampled were contaminated with the virus; and that, when sampling was carried out in an area routinely impacted by human sewage, 50 percent of mussels examined contained detectable levels of viral RNA (Le Guyader et al. 2000). Mussels and cockles are generally cooked before consumption and regulations brought in to control hepatitis A virus contamination will also control astroviruses. Astroviruses have been associated with single-exposure outbreaks similar to those more usually associated with Norwalk viruses, but these seem relatively uncommon. These have been well studied in Japan where Oishi and colleagues (1994) reported data from a multi-school outbreak in Osaka; and Utagawa and colleagues (1994) reported three outbreaks associated with restaurants and schools. In each case, astroviruses were the organisms most frequently identified although other agents were also present in some samples from the outbreak. Consequently, the contribution of individual viruses to the overall pattern of these events is not completely clear. Nevertheless, the potential for widespread and significant astrovirus-induced foodborne illness must be acknowledged.

Astroviruses survive well in water (see below) and transmission from contaminated streams has been reported (Cubitt 1991). They are also relatively difficult to inactivate with chlorine (the normal method of rendering water potable) being considerably more resistant than poliovirus (Abad et al. 1997). If the virus survives chlorination, then further inactivation could be quite slow, astroviruses can persist for a long time in dechlorinated tapwater: after 60 days the infectivity was reduced by 3.6 logs when the water was maintained at 20°C and only 2 logs at 4°C (Bosch et al. 1997). Astrovirus has been detected in water samples from an area where a concurrent astrovirus-induced gastroenteritis outbreak had occurred (Pinto et al. 1996).

Environmental transmission

Until recently relatively little was known of the circulation of astroviruses through the environment and particularly through surface waters and water treatment systems. A recent survey of seawater bathers in the UK implied that astrovirus survived well enough to pose a risk of infection in coastal waters and the presence of virus in shellfish (above) is also indicative. Higher levels of gastroenteritis were reported by surfers compared to age-matched controls who did not sea-bathe. Of the surfers surveyed, 93 percent showed serological evidence of exposure to HAstV-4 compared to 39 percent of controls (Myint et al. 1994). Molecular methods have detected astroviruses in 21 percent of river water samples and 3 percent of Dam water samples in South Africa (D. Steele, personal communication). Virus was found in samples where all usual microbiological indicators of fecal pollution were absent or within acceptable limits implying that astrovirus may present a risk in samples that could be assessed as 'safe' by usual methods (Taylor et al. 2001). The stability of the virus means that particles survive well and are detectable in waters flowing both into and out of water treatment works, indicating that viruses survive at least some forms of water processing. A quantitative assessment of astrovirus in such waters found that titers of 4×10^5– 1.4×10^7 particles per 100 ml in the water flowing into treatment plants and levels of 6×10^2–9×10^4 per 100 ml in the treated water flowing out (P. LeCann, personal communication). Astrovirus (and enteroviruses) has also been detected in sludge (Chapron et al. 2000). Consequently, it is hard to avoid the conclusion that astroviruses represent a hitherto underestimated environmental contaminant. Given recent data from Koopmans and colleagues (1998) that exposure to one serotype carries little protective effect against infection by other serotypes, then adults will continue to be at risk from the higher serotypes to which they are only rarely exposed.

PREVALENCE

Even from the first small-scale studies it was apparent that HAstV infections are very common, exposure occurs early in life (at least to the more common serotypes), and seropositivity rises steeply in early childhood. A survey in the UK found that 64 percent of children had antibodies to HAstV-1 by 4 years of age and this figure rose to 87 percent by age 10 (Kurtz and Lee 1978). A more recent age-stratified assessment of seroconversion to types 1 and 6 in London showed that children rapidly seroconverted to type 1 as maternal immunity waned. Infections commenced around 5–6 months of age and by age 5 nearly 90 percent of samples were positive for type 1 antibody. Seroconversion to type 6 was seen to commence slightly later (7–11 months) and to rise more slowly, reaching only some 20 percent even by adulthood (Kriston et al. 1996). A similar study addressing seroconversion in the USA found again that seroconversion to type 1 occurred rapidly after loss of maternal antibody, reaching 94 percent by age 6–9 years. In this case infections by HAstV-3 were also studied and a similar pattern observed. Infections occurred during the same time frames as those by HAstV-1 but were less frequent, with 55 percent of 6–9-year-olds remaining seronegative (Mitchell et al. 1999a). Midthun and colleagues (1993) found 45 percent of adults were seropositive for type 5 virus, 55 percent having presumably not contracted the virus. A seroprevalence survey in the Netherlands reached similar conclusions (Koopmans et al. 1998), finding antibodies to HAstV-1 in 91 percent; HAstV-2 in 31 percent; to HAstV-3 in 69 percent; to HAstV-4 in 50 percent and to HAstV-5 in 36 percent of persons sampled.

Several surveys have examined the incidence of astrovirus in diarrheal stools. In general, these fall into two classes: those using predominantly EM as the means of diagnosis, and those using alternative techniques (RT-PCR or ELISA). The former class generally report astroviruses at a frequency of 1–5 percent in diarrheal stools, whilst the latter find an increased prevalence and report values in the region of 5–15 percent. The second type of survey generally suggests that astrovirus is second only to rotavirus as a cause of enteric illness in children. A potential explanation of this discrepancy is addressed under diagnostic methods. Despite their differences, these surveys do reveal some underlying patterns, as follows.

First, where seasonality was detected, astrovirus incidence mirrored that of rotavirus. A peak of infection was observed in the winter months in Europe and the developed world (Guix et al. 2002; Lew et al. 1990; Maldonado 1996; Monroe et al. 1991a; Mustafa et al. 2000; Rodriguez-Baez et al. 2002; Sakamoto et al. 2000). Infection peaks in the rainy seasons elsewhere, e.g. Guatemala (Cruz et al. 1992) and rural Mexico (Maldonado et al. 1998). Infections in Japan showed a peak between March and April (Utagawa et al. 1994). The explanation of seasonality is not clear for any enteric virus, although it possibly involves contributions from a variety of factors. These may include: an increased efficiency of person-to-person transmission in colder weather (due to increased virus survival in the environment and more crowding in public places); the possibility of watercourse contamination (due to increased rainfall and blockage of drains, etc., by leaves); and even an increase in the levels of virus in filter-feeding shellfish consumed in the colder months.

Second, whilst co-circulation of different serotypes, and also of distinct genetic variants within a serotype, is often seen (McIver et al. 2000; Traore et al. 2000), serotype 1 is usually the most common virus detected, a finding expected from the seroprevalence studies above. Kurtz and Lee (1984) determined the serotypes of astroviruses acquired in the community in Oxford (UK) and found serotype 1 accounted for 77 percent of virus identifications in clinical samples. Serotypes 2–5 each accounted for 5–7 percent of the isolates. This was, however, a relatively small survey, but a more recent repeat (covering the period 1976–92) yielded similar data (Lee and Kurtz 1994). Serotype 1 was again the

most common (65 percent), with all the other serotypes having much lower incidence (HAstV-2 and HAstV-4 both 11 percent; HAstV-3 9 percent; HAstV-5 2 percent; and HAstV-6 and HAstV-7 both less than 1 percent). These findings are repeated across the world, serotype 1 being the most common serotype found in surveys carried out in a variety of geographical regions (Australia – Palombo and Bishop 1996; Chile – Gaggero et al. 1998; Mexico – Mendez-Toss et al. 2000; Korea – Kang et al. 2002; and Spain – Guix et al. 2002).

Third, this relative prevalence of serotype 1 is not universally true. Some fluctuation in relative prevalence of the individual serotypes is observed. In the UK survey described above, serotype 1 was the most common throughout the period surveyed except in 1991 when serotype 2 was the most prevalent (Lee and Kurtz 1994). Analysis of the age-stratified seroprevalence studies in London also indicates that infection by serotype 1 viruses may have increased in the years since 1990–91 and a sharp decrease in the seroprevalence rates (from 90 to 50 percent) is observed in children above the age of 6 years. This suggests that infection was less common when these individuals were aged <12 months, the peak age period for acquisition of the virus. Evidence from seroconversion of seawater bathers (Myint et al. 1994) and from serotyping studies in Oxford (Willcocks et al. 1995) indicate that serotype 4 increased in prevalence in the UK in 1993. Similarly, HAstV-2 was found as the most common serotype in Mexico City in two reports (Guerrero et al. 1998; Walter et al. 2001b), and in Malawi, HAstV-1 and HAstV-2 were found in approximately equal incidence (Cunliffe et al. 2002).

In common with rotavirus and the noroviruses, astrovirus is frequently acquired nosocomially. Two surveys in California found astrovirus and rotavirus at a similar frequency in the hospital setting. In both surveys, about half the astrovirus infections were thought to have been nosocomially acquired (Shastri et al. 1998; Rodriguez-Baez et al. 2002). The later survey (conducted 1998–2000) reported that 21 percent of hospitalized children (<6 years) had symptoms of gastroenteritis during their stay. Astrovirus was detected in 5.2 percent of the samples and 75 percent of these infections were symptomatic. Rotavirus accounted for only marginally more positive samples at 6.8 percent, suggesting that astrovirus has a similar incidence to rotavirus in this context. Rotavirus infections were, however, more severe and more likely to lead to dehydration (Rodriguez-Baez et al. 2002). Dennehy and colleagues (2001) obtained similar results in Australia; rotavirus was found to be the major cause of nosocomially acquired infection with astrovirus accounting for 16 percent. Community-acquired astrovirus was observed at a rate of 6.8 percent of samples. Once more rotavirus infection was clinically more severe. A survey in France examined the incidence of norovirus and astrovirus in hospitalized patients.

Infections were assigned as community or nosocomially acquired, depending on the delay between admission and development of illness. Where this period exceeded typical incubation times, infection had presumably been acquired in hospital. Approximately half the astrovirus infections identified and a third of the norovirus infections were found to be nosocomial (Traore et al. 2000). Foley and colleagues (2000) also found an approximately equal incidence of astrovirus and norovirus in presumed nosocomial infections in Ireland. Thus the majority of reports find that infection by all three agents can occur at about the same frequency in the hospital setting.

A further question to be considered is to what extent if any, animal strains of astrovirus might regularly cross-infect between species to reach humans. Sequence relatedness between feline and human astroviruses does suggest an evolutionary relationship, but this neither implies nor excludes more frequent traffic of viruses between these species. Certainly a recent large-scale survey of infectious intestinal disease in England and Wales found that recent contact with pets (cats and dogs) with diarrhea (but not with healthy animals) did carry an increased risk of developing intestinal disease. However, these cases tended to be associated with failure to detect a causative organism which was surprising (Food Standards Agency 2000). This in turn suggests that any zoonotically infecting agent might not be detected by the usual diagnostic methods used. Recent experimental data have shown that FAstV can infect human cells (CaCo-2) in culture, inducing cytopathic effect and leading to the release of progeny particles. These could not, however, be passaged further even when trypsin treated. This suggests that humans might be infectable with FAstV. Recombinant FAstV antigen was then used to modify an enzyme immunoassay (EIA) already developed for the type-specific detection of antibody to human astroviruses (Mitchell et al. 1999a). This test was then used to examine a panel of human sera previously characterized for antibody to HAstV types 1 and 6 (Kriston et al. 1996). The FAstV antigen was found to react with a panreactive non-neutralizing monoclonal antibody (Herrmann et al. 1988) but had no reactivity with rabbit sera raised to individual serotypes 1–7 of human astrovirus. This survey found that 7/262 (2.6 percent) of sera showed a specific reaction towards the feline virus antigen that did not correlate with cross-reacting seroconversion to any of the HAstV strains tested. Furthermore, samples from two different infants were negative for all seven human astroviruses tested, yet were positive for antibody recognizing the feline virus (W. D. Cubitt, unpublished observations). These data suggest that feline virus can infect humans, inducing seroconversion. However, it is not clear whether this is associated with any illness or if the infection is 'dead-end' and cannot be spread further between humans.

CLINICAL MANIFESTATIONS

Human and mammalian astroviruses

Human astroviruses are generally associated with fairly mild, self-limiting gastroenteritis in infants and young children. To some extent this view is likely to be an oversimplification (reviewed by Glass et al. 1996) Recent studies report that astrovirus is the second most common viral agent (after rotavirus) found in young children with diarrhea (Herrmann et al. 1991). However, astroviruses are also frequently identified in symptom-free individuals and it is clear that infection does not always result in clinical signs. The highest reported incidence was observed in rural Mayan infants. In this study 61 percent of a 3-year birth cohort showed astrovirus infection. Astrovirus was associated with 26 percent of all diarrheas observed and 17 percent of astrovirus positives were associated with diarrhea and a further 8 percent with other symptoms. In this study, astrovirus was found to be the major pathogen in that community, outstripping even rotavirus in incidence (Maldonado et al. 1998). However, findings from other surveys have revealed infection rates and symptom associations that were somewhat lower, e.g. 4.9 percent in Barcelona (Guix et al. 2002) and varied between 1.4 and 4.4 percent from 1995 to 1998 in Melbourne, Australia (Mustafa et al. 2000). However, it does not necessarily follow that illness is mild and astroviruses do result in hospitalization for severe diarrhea. In a study of such admissions in South Africa, rotavirus was found to be the most common viral cause at just under 30 percent but astroviruses were a highly significant second at 7.4 percent (D. Steele, personal communication). Even in the USA it has been estimated that astroviruses account for some 5 percent of all hospital admissions due to diarrhea (CDC 1990). There is currently no vaccine for astrovirus infection but an active program has targeted rotavirus for many years. Should such a vaccine enter general use, the relative significance of astrovirus-induced disease would rise.

The virus has an incubation period of 3–4 days that is followed by the appearance of diarrhea (typically two to six motions/day). This is the predominant clinical symptom of infection by these viruses and is accompanied by shedding of virus, which generally lasts for 2–3 days but may persist for up to 14 days (Kurtz and Lee 1987). Other reported symptoms include nausea and vomiting, headache, fever, and abdominal discomfort. A survey in London, UK found that 82 percent of children infected with astrovirus experienced diarrhea, 64 percent vomiting, 25 percent abdominal discomfort, and 18 percent mild dehydration (Nazer et al. 1982). A larger scale survey of infectious intestinal disease in the UK has analyzed symptoms reported by those infected with astroviruses: all those affected reported diarrhea as the major symptom with 60 percent% of infected children described as incapacitated by the infection (Food Standards Agency 2000).

Further astrovirus-induced illness is not always mild in adults. An outbreak of severe gastroenteritis amongst French military recruits was associated with HAstV-3 (Belliot et al. 1997c) whilst the Food Standards Agency (2000) study in England and Wales found diarrhea as the major symptom in astrovirus-infected adults attending their GP surgeries; 65 percent described it as 'severe' and nearly 90 percent were 'incapacitated' by the illness. Abdominal pain and loss of appetite were also common in both children and adults but febrile effects (temperature, muscle ache, etc.) seemed more frequent in adults than in children and vomiting was more frequent in children (75 percent) than in adults (29 percent). It may well be that many adults remain at risk of symptomatic infection by higher serotypes of astrovirus to which cross-protective immunity resulting from infection with serotype 1 is poor (Koopmans et al. 1998).

Symptom severity has been investigated by means of volunteer studies: bacteria-free filtrates of astrovirus-containing stools have been introduced orally to adult volunteers; in general these have shown that the virus has low pathogenicity in healthy adults. Kurtz and colleagues (1979) inoculated eight volunteers with HAstV-1 and found that only one developed diarrheal illness (and shed large numbers of astrovirus particles) and a second volunteer reported mild symptoms (accompanied by a lower level of virus shedding). However, most of this panel would have been exposed previously to this virus serotype. A second study in the USA exposed 19 volunteers to serotype 5 virus; 47 percent of these persons had undetectable titers of astrovirus-specific serum antibodies when inoculated. One volunteer developed mild illness and nine had a serological response to the virus but did not report symptoms (Midthun et al. 1993). The conclusion from these studies is that astrovirus infection is usually relatively mild in otherwise healthy adults whilst the clinical pattern tells us that this cannot be universally true.

Astrovirus infections may be especially significant in vulnerable groups; outbreaks have also been reported in residential communities of elderly people (Gray et al. 1987; Lewis et al. 1989). In Marin County, California (Oshiro et al. 1981), 51 percent of the residents of a convalescent hospital (and 12 percent of the staff) developed symptoms. Most experienced minor illness lasting about 3 days and consisting only of diarrhea, although 13 percent of the patients also experienced fever. In the immunocompromised, virus shedding has been reported for several months following infection (Noel and Cubitt 1994) and the gastroenteritis caused may be severe (Coppo et al. 2000). Infections of hospitalized children undergoing immunosuppressive regimens may be prolonged and can prove difficult to eradicate from the unit (Cubitt et al. 1999). Prolonged infections may also

be occurring in Bangladesh where a study found astrovirus was more frequently present in children <5 years who suffered from persistent diarrhea (15 percent) than in those with acute and short-lived illness (4 percent) (Unicomb et al. 1998). This suggests that in Bangladesh astrovirus may be an important contributor to the prolonged illness (defined as >14 days' duration) observed in 7 percent of diarrheal patients. In this setting, prolonged diarrhea is a serious condition and frequently results in death. However, it was not determined whether astrovirus was actually the cause of this persistent condition or simply secondary to it, nor was astrovirus linked to clinical severity. There have been few reports of any long-term consequences of astrovirus infection; however, short-term lactose intolerance and occasionally cows' milk intolerance lasting several months have been reported (Nazer et al. 1982; Kurtz and Lee 1987).

In other mammals, it is also generally the young of the species that show symptomatic infection and again diarrhea is the predominant symptom. These include lambs (Snodgrass and Gray 1977), calves (Woode and Bridger 1978; Woode et al. 1984), pigs (Shirai et al. 1985; Shimizu et al. 1990), mink (Englund et al. 2002), and cats (Hoshino et al. 1981; Harbour et al. 1987). The virus is clearly responsible for illness in the sheep and in cats it was severe enough to require hospitalization. However, in pigs and calves it appears relatively mild and the bulk of any symptoms observed may be due to coinfection by other agents.

Avian astroviruses

In birds, the range of symptoms produced by astrovirus is more diverse and generally more severe than in mammals. Astrovirus infection (DHV II) causes a rapidly fatal hepatitis in ducklings (Gough et al. 1984). Mortality rates can exceed 25 percent and have been reported up to 70 percent. Symptoms usually appear in 3–6-week-old birds. Examination revealed that the ducklings died of acute hepatitis with hepatocellular necrosis and generally, hyperplasia of the bile duct. Astrovirus-like particles were found by EM in the liver and feces and experimental transmission of the virus resulted in hepatitis and death within 2–4 days in five of 20 ducklings inoculated. Thus far the UK is the only reported country in which DHV II has struck and the origin of the virus remains unknown but is believed to result from contact with wild birds. The virus caused no symptoms in mature ducks, suggesting that adult birds might harbor the infection.

An avian astrovirus was first reported as a cause of gastroenteritis and mortality in turkey poults (6–11 days of age) in 1980 (McNulty et al. 1980). Since then there have been other reports of astrovirus outbreaks in turkeys resulting in enteritis and stunting of growth (Reynolds and Saif 1986). These features have been linked to a temporary reduction in maltase activity in the small intestine, resulting in disaccharide maldigestion (Thouvenelle et al. 1995). More recently TAstV has been implicated as the causative agent of poult enteritis mortality syndrome (PEMS) in turkeys. This emerging disease is characterized by enteritis, growth depression, lymphoid atrophy, and, interestingly, immunosuppression (Koci et al. 2000a). The virus can be detected in the intestines, thymus, and bursa of infected birds. The virus can reduce macrophage viability and phagocytosis in vitro, thus leading to increased susceptibility of infected turkeys to secondary bacterial infections (Qureshi et al. 2001).

ANV infection of young chickens results in growth retardation of the birds by causing acute interstitial nephritis (Imada et al. 1979). The virus has been shown to be widely distributed in chickens, and turkeys may also be susceptible (Imada et al. 1980). Field strains of the virus show vastly different degrees of pathogenicity ranging from subclinical infections to death (Frazier et al. 1990; Shirai et al. 1991).

PATHOGENESIS

HAstV pathogenesis has not been extensively studied; duodenal biopsy taken during infection showed that the virus had infected the epithelial cells of the lower part of the intestinal villi (Phillips et al. 1982). In lambs experimentally infected with OAstV, lesions were seen throughout the small intestine, especially in the midgut and ileum (Snodgrass et al. 1979). The virus was found to replicate in the mature columnar epithelial cells situated in the apical two-thirds of the villi (virus was detected in the cytoplasm of these cells by EM). The damaged cells were replaced by immature crypt cells – resulting in villus atrophy and malabsorption typical of virus-induced enteric illness (Gray et al. 1980). By contrast, BAstV infection was confined to the specialized M cells that overlay Peyer's patches in the jejunum and ileum of the calves; these infected cells were then shed and replaced by immature crypt cells (Woode et al. 1984). It has been suggested that the limited number of susceptible cells in the bovine gut compared to that in the sheep could explain the lack of symptoms in experimentally infected calves (Kurtz and Lee 1987).

Little is known of immunity to astroviruses. Certainly antibody is developed early in life but Koopmans and colleagues (1998) suggest that little heterotypic protection may result and cross-neutralization activity was not detected in those serotypes where it was sought. HLA-restricted CD4$^+$ T cells specific for astrovirus have been identified in the duodenal mucosa of eight of eight normal (asymptomatic) individuals and these were thought to be of the Th1 phenotype. The fact that astrovirus-specific T cells can be isolated from normal small intestinal biopsies strongly suggests that the precursor frequency of virus-specific T cells in the mucosa is likely to be higher than in peripheral blood. This could suggest that the gut immune system frequently encounters these viruses, regularly reactivating any T cells to proliferate. The presence of these cells might then promote immunity to reinfection (Molberg et al. 1998). All the T-cell clones tested recognized a recombinant HAstV-1 capsid protein, demonstrating that the T-cell epitopes concerned must reside in that protein. The extent to which this cellular immunity is heterotypic has not been determined (O. Molberg, personal communication).

DETECTION AND DIAGNOSIS

Electron microscopy

Astroviruses were originally detected, and for many years could only be diagnosed by EM. This has almost certainly resulted in a reduced efficiency of diagnosis since the technique relies on specimens that contain high levels of virus particles exhibiting good morphological preservation. Astroviruses may be shed in large numbers during infection (up to 10^{10} particles/g feces; Kurtz and Lee 1987), but this is by no means always the case; particles may be hard to find and their preservation may not be good. It has been found that the virions are unstable if pelleted from cesium chloride gradients and are better purified using potassium tartrate (Ashley and Caul 1982). Astrovirus morphology may itself be inherently variable (see section on Morphology, above). Although a typical astrovirus can be safely identified as such, specimens lacking these features cannot readily be discounted. If stars are not visible, a featureless particle would be observed and these can easily be mistaken for parvovirus-like agents. Reanalysis by culture and blotting of a panel of EM-identified parvoviruses revealed the majority to be astrovirus (Willcocks et al. 1991).

Oliver and Phillips (1988) carried out retrospective analyses of samples that had originally been classified on the basis of their appearance in the electron microscope and showed that several samples (14 of 53 re-examined) originally identified as 'small round' or 'parvovirus-like' viruses were in fact astroviruses. This particular confusion is significant since some laboratories have reported the small round virus (parvovirus-like) agents as the second most frequently identified virus (Lew et al. 1990). Alternatively, particles may be larger than expected, (possibly coated in antibody) and the margins of the particle might not be smooth. Indeed, Marin County virus was initially identified as a calicivirus due to these affects (Oshiro et al. 1981). These variations in structural parameters have undoubtedly clouded attempts to assess the significance of astroviruses in disease. The recent large-scale survey of infectious intestinal disease in the UK has identified astroviruses by EM, using ELISA methods only to confirm those found as positive by this means. Presumptive 'parvoviruses' have not been further examined. This is likely to underestimate the occurrence of astrovirus and this survey has yielded incidence figures similar to other EM-based surveys rather than the higher values usually associated with ELISA methods. One major advantage of EM, however, is that it is a 'catch-all' diagnostic tool, allowing any other potential pathogens in the specimen to also be detected. A survey in London, UK found that of 28 infants infected with astrovirus 16 were also infected with another enteric pathogen (Nazer et al. 1982). In patients shedding fewer particles, immune electron microscopy has proved a valuable tool (Berthiaume et al. 1981).

Cell culture

It was initially difficult to establish cell culture methods for astroviruses, and to date only the porcine and human strains can be cultured in vitro. Both were originally propagated in renal cells of the host species (Lee and Kurtz 1981; Shimizu et al. 1990). The viruses were only able to grow with the addition of trypsin (at 5–10 μg/ml) to the culture medium. In the absence of trypsin, infection could occur but did not give rise to infectious progeny (Lee and Kurtz 1981). This trypsin level caused disruption of the cell monolayer and no cytopathic effect was apparent. However, Hudson and colleagues (1989) did succeed in developing both a plaque assay for three of the serotypes (again with the addition of trypsin to the overlay), and a virus neutralization assay. PAstV required the addition of 0.5 μg trypsin to grow and limited cytopathic effect was visible in the porcine embryonic kidney cells (Shimizu et al. 1990).

Since these experiments, three human cell lines have been identified that are able to support the replication of HAstV directly from clinical samples. Two of these (CaCo-2 and T84) are gut-cell lines and one (PLC/PRF/5) is derived from a hepatoma.

Willcocks and colleagues (1990) found that a human colonic carcinoma cell line (CaCo-2 cells) could be infected with HAstV. Trypsin was required (at 5 μg/ml) for productive growth and at this concentration these cell monolayers remained relatively intact. Cytopathic effect became apparent from 2 days post-infection. These cells also supported the partial replication of FAstV in that infections could be established using viruses from feline diarrheal feces; mRNA and protein synthesis occurred and progeny particles were released. However these were found to be non-infectious and infectivity could not be rescued by addition of trypsin.

Taylor and colleagues (1997) found that a human hepatoma cell line (PLC/PRF/5) was also able to support the replication of human astroviruses directly from clinical samples. Trypsin was required (10 μg/ml) and the disruption caused by this to the cell monolayers did not permit detection of any cytopathic effect. Virus growth was monitored by EM or indirect immunofluorescence. In addition to these cells, the Oxford adapted astrovirus strains have a wider host cell range (Brinker et al. 2000).

Although cell culture is essential for isolating viruses from clinical samples, it is not generally the method of choice for diagnostic purposes because it is labor intensive, slow, expensive, and less sensitive than immunologically based or PCR-based assays. It has, however, been used successfully to enhance the detection level of RT-PCR for samples where virus particles should be highly dilute, e.g. drinking water. Concentrated samples were propagated in CaCo-2 cells before analysis by RT-PCR (Abad et al. 1997). A similar approach has been used in environmental water samples (where propagation in PLC/PRF/5 cells was employed; Marx et al. 1995) or in sludge biosolids (where integrated cell culture/RT-PCR was coupled with nested PCR; Chapron et al. 2000).

Enzyme immunoassays

Herrmann and co-workers (1988) developed an enzyme immunoassay (EIA) for astrovirus, using a monoclonal antibody to the group antigen to capture virus; this detected all astroviruses grown in cell culture. These workers later modified the test to detect astroviruses in stool samples (Herrmann et al. 1990). Compared with immune electron microscopy, this assay has as high a sensitivity (91 percent) and specificity (98 percent). Moe and colleagues (1991) developed a modified version of the assay using a biotinylated detector antibody. These assays have been particularly useful in epidemiologic studies, where large numbers of samples need to be assayed (Herrmann et al. 1991; Lew et al. 1991; Moe et al. 1991; Cruz et al. 1992; Walter et al. 2001b). A latex agglutination test specific for HAstV-1 has also been reported for this application (Kohno et al. 2000).

Modifications to these tests using recombinant antigen have also allowed the development of ELISA or immune fluorescence-based methods to detect serum antibody and thus determine the prevalence of antibodies to astroviruses in various communities. When used in this way, baculovirus-expressed antigen reacts in a serotype-specific manner, allowing antibody to each serotype to be assessed independently (Kriston et al. 1996; Mitchell et al. 1999a).

Molecular methods

A dot-blot hybridization procedure for detecting astroviruses in fecal samples has been described (Willcocks et al. 1991) but has only been used in a small-scale study (Silcock et al. 1993). A liquid hybridization assay was successfully tested on 26 wild strains of the virus (Belliot et al. 2001). As sequence data has accumulated a number of RT-PCR tests have been developed (Monroe et al. 1993; Jonassen et al. 1995; Noel et al. 1995; Yue and Ushijima 1996; Sakamoto et al. 2000; Traore et al. 2000). These have facilitated the rapid diagnosis of human astrovirus outbreaks (Cubitt et al. 1999). Oligo-nucleotide primers designed to match conserved sequences can detect all serotypes. Primer pairs have been reported targeting the 3′ end of the genome (Monroe et al. 1993; Jonassen et al. 1995), the RNA-dependent RNA polymerase gene (Belliot et al. 1997b) and from the 5′ end of the capsid gene (Sakon et al. 2000). RT-PCR has also been used for genotyping of human astroviruses by sequencing of a 348-bp amplimer from the capsid gene (Noel et al. 1995). However, this method has epidemiologic rather than diagnostic applic-ability. An RT-PCR has also been reported for the detection of TAstV in PEMS-affected commercial turkey flocks (Koci et al. 2000b).

The technique has also been useful in confirming results with specimens that gave ambiguous results in other tests (Grohmann et al. 1993) and has been able to provide more detail on outbreaks. Mitchell and colleagues (1995) used EIA and RT-PCR to screen fecal specimens in an outbreak of gastroenteritis in a child-care center. EIA found that stools from 75 percent of the infants, 50 percent of the toddlers, and 20 percent of the children were positive, whilst using RT-PCR increased the numbers to 100, 79, and 90 percent, respectively. This changed the interpretation of the outbreak; the virus had not selectively infected some of the children but had in fact infected almost all of them. The number of days of virus shedding was also found to be longer using this more sensitive method and increased from 1 to 9 days (as detected by EIA) to up to 35 days (as detected by PCR).

CONCLUSIONS

Astroviruses are becoming increasingly appreciated as agents of human disease to which we are regularly exposed from each other and the environment, and possibly from animals. Infections within institutional settings, often affecting those at particular risk, pose a particular problem. The significance of these agents as the second most frequent cause of gastroenteritis in chil-dren worldwide, and their possible association with prolonged illness in the third world, demands attention. Rotavirus remains the single most significant cause of childhood diarrhea and rightly receives the attention required to develop vaccines. However, control of rota-virus infection does not control gastroenteritis; vaccinees would remain susceptible to astrovirus infection and this could lead to a perceived lack of vaccine efficacy that could restrict vaccine uptake.

REFERENCES

Abad, F.X., Pinto, R.M., et al. 1997. Astrovirus survival in drinking water. *Appl Environ Microbiol*, **63**, 3119–22.

Abad, F.X., Villena, C., et al. 2001. Potential role of fomites in the vehicular transmission of human astroviruses. *Appl Environ Microbiol*, **67**, 3904–7.

Appleton, H. and Higgins, P.G. 1975. Viruses and gastroenteritis in infants. *Lancet*, **1**, 1297.

Aroonprasert, D., Fagerland, J.A., et al. 1989. Cultivation and particle characterisation of bovine astrovirus. *Vet Microbiol*, **19**, 113–25.

Ashley, C.R. and Caul, E.O. 1982. Potassium tartrate-glycerol as a density gradient substrate for separation of small, round viruses from human feces. *J Clin Microbiol*, **16**, 377–81.

Bass, D.M. and Qui, S. 2000. Proteolytic processing of the astrovirus capsid. *J Virol*, **74**, 1810–14.

Bass, D.M. and Upadhyayula, U. 1997. Characterization of human astrovirus serotype 1 astrovirus-neutralizing epitopes. *J Virol*, **71**, 8666–71.

Belliot, G., Laveran, H. and Monroe, S.S. 1997a. Capsid protein composition of reference strains and wild isolates of human astroviruses. *Virus Res*, **49**, 49–57.

Belliot, G., Laveran, H. and Monroe, S.S. 1997b. Detection and genetic differentiation of human astroviruses: phylogenetic grouping varies by coding region. *Arch Virol*, **142**, 1323–4.

Belliot, G., Laveran, H. and Monroe, S.S. 1997c. Outbreak of gastroenteritis in military recruits associated with serotype 3 astrovirus infection. *J Med Virol*, **51**, 101–6.

Belliot, G.M., Fankhauser, R.L. and Monroe, S.S. 2001. Characterization of 'Norwalk-like viruses' and astroviruses by liquid hybridization. *J Virol Methods*, **91**, 119–30.

Berthiaume, L., Alain, R., et al. 1981. Rapid detection of human viruses in faeces by a simple and routine immune electron microscopy technique. *J Gen Virol*, **55**, 223–7.

Bosch, A., Pinto, R.M., et al. 1997. Persistence of human astrovirus in fresh and marine water. *Water Sci Technol*, **35**, 243–7.

Bredenbeek, P.J., Pachuk, C.J., et al. 1990. The primary structure and expression of the second open reading frame of the polymerase gene of the coronavirus MHV-A59; a highly conserved polymerase is expressed by an efficient ribosomal frameshifting mechanism. *Nucleic Acids Res*, **18**, 1825–32.

Bridger, J.C. 1980. Detection by electron microscope of caliciviruses, astroviruses and rotavirus-like particles in the faeces of piglets with diarrhoea. *Vet Rec*, **107**, 532–3.

Brinker, J.P., Blacklow, N.R. and Herrmann, J.E. 2000. Human astrovirus isolation and propagation in multiple cell lines. *Arch Virol*, **145**, 1847–56.

Carter, M.J. 1994. Genomic organisation and expression of astroviruses and caliciviruses. *Arch Virol*, **9**, Suppl, 429–39.

Carter, M.J. and Adams, M.R. 2000. Microbiological hazards and their control: viruses. In: Adams, M.R. and Nout, M.J.R. (eds), *Fermentation and food safety*. Gaithersburg, MD: Aspen Publishers, 159–74.

Carter, M.J. and Madeley, C.R. 1987. Caliciviruses. In: Nermut, M.V. and Steven, A.C. (eds), *Virus structure*. London: Academic Press, 121–8.

Caul, E.O. and Appleton, H. 1982. The electron microscopical and physical characteristics of small round human fecal viruses: an interim scheme for classification. *J Med Virol*, **9**, 257–65.

CDC. 1990. Viral agents of gastroenteritis. Public health importance and outbreak management. *Morbid Mortal Wkly Rev* **39**, 1–24.

Chapron, C.D., Ballester, N.A. and Margolin, A.B. 2000. The detection of astrovirus in sludge biosolids using an integrated cell culture nested PCR technique. *J Appl Microbiol*, **89**, 11–15.

Coppo, P., Scieux, C., et al. 2000. Astrovirus enteritis in a chronic lymphocytic leukemia patient treated with fludarabine monophosphate. *Ann Hematol*, **79**, 43–5.

Cruz, J.R., Bartlett, A.V., et al. 1992. Astrovirus-associated diarrhea among Guatemalan ambulatory rural children. *J Clin Microbiol*, **30**, 11140–4.

Cubitt, W.D. 1991. A review of the epidemiology and diagnosis of water-borne viral infections. *Water Sci Technol*, **24**, 193–203.

Cubitt, W.D., Mitchell, D.K., et al. 1999. Application of electron microscopy, enzyme immunoassay and RT-PCR to monitor an outbreak of astrovirus type 1 in a pediatric bone marrow transplant unit. *J Med Virol*, **57**, 313–21.

Cunliffe, N.A., Dove, W., et al. 2002. Detection and characterisation of human astroviruses in children with acute gastroenteritis in Blantyre, Malawi. *J Med Virol*, **67**, 563–6.

Dennehy, P.H., Nelson, S.M., et al. 2001. A prospective case-control study of the role of astrovirus in acute diarrhoea among hospitalized young children. *J Infect Dis*, **184**, 10–15.

Donelli, G., Superti, F., et al. 1992. Mechanism of astrovirus entry into Graham 293 cells. *J Med Virol*, **38**, 271–7.

Englund, L., Chriel, M., et al. 2002. Astrovirus epidemiologically linked to pre-weaning diarrhea in mink. *Vet Microbiol*, **85**, 1–11.

Foley, B., O'Mahony, J., et al. 2000. Detection of sporadic cases of Norwalk-like virus (NLV) and astrovirus infection in a single Irish hospital from 1996 to 1998. *J Clin Virol*, **17**, 109–17.

Food Standards Agency. 2000. *A report of the study of infectious intestinal disease in England*. London: The Stationery Office.

Frazier, J.A., Howes, K., et al. 1990. Isolation of noncytopathic viruses implicated in the aetiology of nephritis and baby chick nephropathy and serologically related to avian nephritis virus. *Avian Pathol*, **19**, 139–60.

Gaggero, A., O'Ryan, M., et al. 1998. Prevalence of astrovirus infection among Chilean children with acute gastroenteritis. *J Clin Microbiol*, **36**, 3691–3.

Geigenmuller, U., Ginzton, N.H. and Matsui, S.M. 1997. Construction of a genome-length cDNA clone for human astrovirus serotype 1 and synthesis of infectious RNA transcripts. *J Virol*, **71**, 1713–17.

Geigenmuller, U., Chew, T., et al. 2002a. Processing of nonstructural proteins 1a of human astrovirus. *J Virol*, **76**, 2003–8.

Geigenmuller, U., Ginzton, N.H. and Matsui, S.M. 2002b. Studies on intracellular processing of the capsid protein of human astrovirus serotype 1 in infected cells. *J Gen Virol*, **83**, 1691–5.

Gibson, C.A., Chen, J., et al. 1998. Expression and processing of non structural proteins of human astroviruses. *Adv Exp Med Biol*, **440**, 387–91.

Glass, R.I., Noel, J., et al. 1996. The changing epidemiology of astrovirus-associated gastroenteritis: a review. *Arch Virol*, **12**, Suppl, 287–300.

Gough, R.E., Collins, M.S., et al. 1984. Astrovirus-like particles associated with hepatitis in ducklings. *Vet Rec*, **114**, 279.

Gray, E.W., Angus, K.W. and Snodgrass, D.R. 1980. Ultrastructure of the small intestine in astrovirus infected lambs. *J Gen Virol*, **49**, 71–82.

Gray, J.J., Wreghitt, T.G., et al. 1987. An outbreak of gastroenteritis in a home for the elderly associated with astrovirus type 1 and human calicivirus. *J Med Virol*, **23**, 377–81.

Grohmann, G.S., Glass, R.I., et al. 1993. Enteric viruses and diarrhea in HIV-infected patients. *N Engl J Med*, **329**, 14–20.

Guerrero, M.L., Noel, J.S., et al. 1998. A prospective study of astrovirus diarrhea of infancy in Mexico City. *Pediatr Infect Dis J*, **17**, 723–7.

Guix, S., Caballero, S., et al. 2002. Molecular epidemiology of astrovirus infection in Barcelona, Spain. *J Clin Microbiol*, **40**, 133–9.

Harbour, D.A., Ashley, C.R., et al. 1987. Natural and experimental astrovirus infection of cats. *Vet Rec*, **120**, 555–7.

Herring, A.J., Gray, E.W. and Snodgrass, D.R. 1981. Purification and characterization of ovine astrovirus. *J Gen Virol*, **53**, 47–55.

Herrmann, J.E., Hudson, R.W., et al. 1988. Antigenic characterization of cell cultivated astrovirus serotypes and development of astrovirus-specific monoclonal antibodies. *J Infect Dis*, **158**, 182–5.

Herrmann, J.E., Nowak, N.A., et al. 1990. Diagnosis of astrovirus gastroenteritis by antigen detection with monoclonal antibodies. *J Infect Dis*, **161**, 226–9.

Herrmann, J.E., Taylor, D.N., et al. 1991. Astroviruses as a cause of gastroenteritis in children. *N Engl J Med*, **324**, 1757–60.

Hoshino, Y., Zimmer, J.F., et al. 1981. Detection of astrovirus in faeces of a cat with diarrhoea. *Arch Virol*, **70**, 373–6.

Hudson, R.W., Herrmann, J.E. and Blacklow, N.R. 1989. Plaque quantitation and virus neutralization assays for human astrovirus. *Arch Virol*, **108**, 33–8.

Imada, T., Yamaguchi, S. and Kawamura, H. 1979. Pathogenicity for baby chicks of the G-4260 strain of the picornavirus 'avian nephritis virus'. *Avian Dis*, **23**, 582–8.

Imada, T., Yamaguchi, S., et al. 1980. Antibody survey against avian nephritis virus among chickens in Japan. *Natl Inst Anim Health Q (Tokyo)*, **20**, 79–80.

Imada, T., Yamaguchi, S., et al. 2000. Avian nephritis virus (ANV) as a new member of the family *Astroviridae* and construction of infectious ANV cDNA. *J Virol*, **74**, 8487–93.

Jacks, T., Power, M.D., et al. 1988. Characterization of ribosomal frameshifting in HIV-1 *gag-pol* expression. *Nature (Lond)*, **331**, 280–3.

Jiang, B., Monroe, S.S., et al. 1993. RNA sequence of astrovirus: distinctive genomic organization and a putative retrovirus-like ribosome frameshifting signal that directs the viral replicase synthesis. *Proc Natl Acad Sci U S A*, **90**, 10539–43.

Jonassen, C.M., Jonassen, T.O. and Grinde, B. 1998. A common RNA motif in the 3′ end of the genomes of astroviruses, avian infectious bronchitis and an equine rhinovirus. *J Gen Virol*, **79**, 715–18.

Jonassen, C.M., Jonassen, T.O., et al. 2001. Comparison of capsid sequences from human and animal astroviruses. *J Gen Virol*, **82**, 1061–7.

Jonassen, T.O., Monceyron, C., et al. 1995. Detection of all serotypes of human astrovirus by the polymerase chain reaction. *J Virol Methods*, **52**, 327–34.

Kang, Y.H., Park, Y.K., et al. 2002. Identification of human astrovirus infections from stool samples with diarrhea in Korea. *Arch Virol*, **147**, 1821–7.

Kiang, D. and Matsui, S.M. 2002. Proteolytic processing of a human astrovirus nonstructural protein. *J Gen Virol*, **83**, 25–34.

Kjeldsberg, E. and Hem, A. 1985. Detection of astrovirus in gut contents of nude and normal mice. *Arch Virol*, **84**, 135–40.

Koci, M.D., Seal, B.S. and Schultz-Cherry, S. 2000a. Molecular characterization of an avian astrovirus. *J Virol*, **74**, 6173–7.

Koci, M.D., Seal, B.S. and Schultz-Cherry, S. 2000b. Development of an RT-PCR diagnostic test for an avian astrovirus. *J Virol Methods*, **90**, 79–83.

Kohno, H., Watanabe, K., et al. 2000. Development of a simple latex agglutination test for detection of astrovirus serotype 1. *Rinsho Biseibutsu Jinsoku Shindan Kenkyukai Shi*, **11**, 87–91.

Koonin, E.V. 1991a. The phylogeny of RNA-dependent RNA polymerases of positive strand viruses. *J Gen Virol*, **72**, 2197–206.

Koonin, E.V. 1991b. Similarities in RNA helicases. *Nature (Lond)*, **352**, 290.

Koopmans, M.P., Bijen, M.H., et al. 1998. Age-stratified seroprevalence of neutralizing antibodies to astrovirus types 1 to 7 in humans in The Netherlands. *Clin Diagn Lab Immunol*, **5**, 33–7.

Kozak, M. 1989. The scanning model for translation: an update. *J Cell Biol*, **108**, 229–41.

Kriston, S., Willcocks, M.M., et al. 1996. Seroprevalence of astrovirus types 1 and 6 in London, determined using recombinant virus antigen. *Epidemiol Infect*, **117**, 159–64.

Kurtz, J.B. 1989. Astroviruses. In: Farthing, M.J.G. (ed.), *Viruses and the gut. Proceedings of the Ninth BSG SK & F International Workshop*. Welwyn Garden City, Herts: Smith Kline & French Laboratories Ltd, 84–7.

Kurtz, J.B. and Lee, T.W. 1978. Astrovirus gastroenteritis, age distribution of antibody. *Med Microbiol Immunol*, **166**, 227–30.

Kurtz, J.B. and Lee, T.W. 1984. Human astrovirus serotypes. *Lancet*, **2**, 1405.

Kurtz, J.B. and Lee, T.W. 1987. Astroviruses: human and animal. In Bock, G. and Whelan, J. (eds), *Novel diarrhoea viruses*. Ciba Foundation Symposium 128. Chichester: Wiley, 92–107.

Kurtz, J.B., Lee, T.W., et al. 1979. Astrovirus infection in volunteers. *J Med Virol*, **3**, 221–30.

Kurtz, J.B., Lee, T.W. and Parsons, A.J. 1980. The action of alcohols on rotavirus, astrovirus and enterovirus. *J Hosp Infect*, **1**, 321–5.

Lee, T.W. and Kurtz, J.B. 1981. Serial propagation of astrovirus in tissue culture with the aid of trypsin. *J Gen Virol*, **57**, 421–4.

Lee, T.W. and Kurtz, J.B. 1982. Human astrovirus serotypes. *J Hyg (Camb)*, **89**, 539–40.

Lee, T.W. and Kurtz, J.B. 1994. Prevalence of human astrovirus serotypes in the Oxford region 1976–92, with evidence for two new serotypes. *Epidemiol Infect*, **112**, 187–93.

Le Guyader, F., Haugarreau, L., et al. 2000. Three-year study to assess human enteric viruses in shellfish. *Appl Environ Microbiol*, **66**, 3241–8.

Lew, J.F., Glass, R.I., et al. 1990. Six year retrospective surveillance of gastroenteritis viruses identified at ten electron microscopy centers in the United States and Canada. *Pediatr Infect Dis*, **9**, 709–14.

Lew, J.F., Moe, C.L., et al. 1991. Astrovirus and adenovirus associated with diarrhea in children in day care settings. *J Infect Dis*, **164**, 673–8.

Lewis, D.C., Lightfoot, N.F., et al. 1989. Outbreaks of astrovirus type 1 and rotavirus gastroenteritis in a geriatric in-patient population. *J Hosp Infect*, **14**, 9–14.

Lewis, T.L. and Matsui, S.M. 1996. Astrovirus ribosomal frameshifting in an infection-transfection transient expression system. *J Virol*, **70**, 2869–75.

Lewis, T.L., Greenberg, H.B., et al. 1994. Analysis of astrovirus serotype 1 RNA, identification of the viral RNA-dependent RNA polymerase motif, and expression of a viral structural protein. *J Virol*, **68**, 77–83.

Lukashov, V.V. and Goudsmit, J. 2002. Evolutionary relationships among *Astroviridae*. *J Gen Virol*, **83**, 1397–405.

Madeley, C.R. 1979. Comparison of the features of astroviruses and caliciviruses seen in samples of faeces by electron microscopy. *J Infect Dis*, **139**, 519–23.

Madeley, C.R. and Cosgrove, B.P. 1975a. Viruses in infantile gastroenteritis. *Lancet*, **2**, 124.

Madeley, C.R. and Cosgrove, B.P. 1975b. 28 nm particles in faeces in infantile gastroenteritis. *Lancet*, **2**, 451–2.

Maldonado, Y.A. 1996. Astrovirus infections in children. *Rep Pediatr Infect Dis*, **6**, 39–40.

Maldonado, Y.A., Cantwell, M., et al. 1998. Population-based prevalence of symptomatic and asymptomatic astrovirus infection in rural Mayan infants. *J Infect Dis*, **178**, 334–9.

Marczinke, B., Bloys, A.J., et al. 1994. The human astrovirus RNA-dependent RNA polymerase coding region is expressed by ribosomal frameshifting. *J Virol*, **68**, 5588–95.

Marx, F.E., Taylor, M.B. and Grabow, W.O.K. 1995. Optimization of a PCR method for the detection of astrovirus type 1 in environmental samples. *Water Sci Technol*, **31**, 359–62.

Matsui, S.M. and Greenberg, H.B. 1996. Astroviruses. In: Fields, B.N., Knipe, D.M., et al. (eds), *Fields virology*, 3rd edn. Philadelphia: Lippincott-Raven, 811–24.

Matsui, S.M., Kim, J.P., et al. 1993. Cloning and characterization of human astrovirus immunoreactive epitopes. *J Virol*, **67**, 1712–15.

Matsui, S.M., Kiang, D., et al. 2001. Molecular biology of astroviruses: selected highlights. *Novartis Found Symp*, **238**, 219–33.

McIver, C.J., Palombo, E.A., et al. 2000. Detection of astrovirus gastroenteritis in children. *J Virol Methods*, **84**, 99–105.

McNulty, M.S., Curran, W.L. and McFerran, J.B. 1980. Detection of astroviruses in turkey faeces by direct electron microscopy. *Vet Rec*, **106**, 561.

Mendez, E., Fernandez-Luna, T., et al. 2002. Proteolytic processing of a serotype 8 human astrovirus ORF 2 polyprotein. *J Virol*, **76**, 7996–8002.

Mendez-Toss, M., Romero-Guido, P., et al. 2000. Molecular analysis of a serotype 8 human astrovirus genome. *J Gen Virol*, **81**, 2891–7.

Midthun, K., Greenberg, H.B., et al. 1993. Characterization and seroepidemiology of a type 5 astrovirus associated with an outbreak of gastroenteritis in Marin County, California. *J Clin Microbiol*, **31**, 955–62.

Mitchell, D.K., Van, R., et al. 1993. Outbreaks of astrovirus gastroenteritis in day care centers. *J Pediatr*, **123**, 725–32.

Mitchell, D.K., Monroe, S.S., et al. 1995. Virologic features of an astrovirus diarrhea outbreak in a day care center revealed by reverse transcription-polymerase chain reaction. *J Infect Dis*, **172**, 1437–44.

Mitchell, D.K., Matson, D.O., et al. 1999a. Prevalence of antibodies to astrovirus types 1 and 3 in children and adolescents in Norfolk, Virginia. *Pediatr Infect Dis J*, **18**, 249–54.

Mitchell, D.K., Matson, D.O., et al. 1999b. Molecular epidemiology of childhood astrovirus infection in child care centers. *J Infect Dis*, **180**, 514–17.

Moe, C.L., Allen, J.R., et al. 1991. Detection of astrovirus in pediatric stool samples by immunoassay and RNA probe. *J Clin Microbiol*, **29**, 2390–5.

Molberg, O., Nilsen, E.M., et al. 1998. CD4+ T-cells with specific reactivity against astrovirus isolated from normal human small intestine. *Gastroenterology*, **114**, 115–22.

Monroe, S.S., Glass, R.I., et al. 1991a. Electronmicroscopic reporting of gastrointestinal viruses in the United Kingdom, 1985–87. *J Med Virol*, **33**, 193–8.

Monroe, S.S., Stine, S.E., et al. 1991b. Temporal synthesis of proteins and RNAs during human astrovirus infection of cultured cells. *J Virol*, **65**, 641–8.

Monroe, S.S., Jiang, B., et al. 1993. Subgenomic RNA sequence of human astrovirus supports classification of *Astroviridae* as a new family of RNA viruses. *J Virol*, **67**, 3611–14.

Monroe, S.S., Carter, M.J., et al. 1995. *Astroviridae*. In: Murphy, F.A., Fauquet, C.M., et al. (eds), *Virus taxomony. 6th Report of the International Committee on the Taxonomy of Viruses*. Wien: Springer-Verlag, 364–7, *Archives of Virology* **Suppl. 10**.

Mustafa, H., Palombo, E.A. and Bishop, R.F. 2000. Epidemiology of astrovirus infection in young children hospitalized with acute gastroenteritis in Melbourne, Australia, over a period of four consecutive years, 1995 to 1998. *J Clin Microbiol*, **38**, 1058–62.

Myint, S., Manley, R. and Cubitt, W.D. 1994. Viruses in bathing water. *Lancet*, **343**, 1640–1.

Nazer, H., Rice, S. and Walker-Smith, J.A. 1982. Clinical associations of astrovirus in childhood. *J Pediatr Gastroenterol Nutr*, **1**, 555–8.

Noel, J. and Cubitt, W.D. 1994. Identification of astrovirus serotypes from children treated at the Hospital for Sick Children, London 1981–93. *Epidemiol Infect*, **113**, 153–9.

Noel, J.S., Lee, T.W., et al. 1995. Typing of human astroviruses from clinical isolates by enzyme immunoassay and nucleotide sequencing. *J Clin Microbiol*, **33**, 797–801.

Oh, D. and Schreier, E. 2001. Molecular characterization of human astroviruses in Germany. *Arch Virol*, **146**, 433–55.

Oishi, I., Yamazaki, K., et al. 1994. A large outbreak of acute gastroenteritis associated with astrovirus among students and teachers in Osaka, Japan. *J Infect Dis*, **170**, 439–43.

Oliver, A.R. and Phillips, A.D. 1988. An electron microscopical investigation of faecal small round viruses. *J Med Virol*, **24**, 211–18.

Oshiro, L.S., Haley, C.E., et al. 1981. A 27 nm virus isolated during an outbreak of acute infectious non-bacterial gastroenteritis in a convalescent hospital: a possible new serotype. *J Infect Dis*, **143**, 791–5.

Palombo, E.A. and Bishop, R.F. 1996. Annual incidence, serotype distribution and genetic diversity of human astrovirus isolates from hospitalized children in Melbourne, Australia. *J Clin Microbiol*, **34**, 1750–3.

Phillips, A.D., Rice, S.J. and Walker-Smith, J.A. 1982. Astrovirus within human small intestinal mucosa. *Gut*, **23**, A923–924.

Pinto, R.M., Abad, F.X., et al. 1996. Detection of infectious astroviruses in water. *Appl Environ Microbiol*, **62**, 1811–13.

Qureshi, M.A., Saif, Y.M., et al. 2001. Induction of functional defects in macrophages by a poult enteritis and mortality syndrome-associated turkey astrovirus. *Avian Dis*, **45**, 853–61.

Reynolds, D.L. and Saif, Y.M. 1986. Astrovirus: a cause of an enteric disease in turkey poults. *Avian Dis*, **30**, 728–35.

Risco, C., Carrascosa, J.L., et al. 1995. Ultrastructure of human astrovirus serotype 2. *J Gen Virol*, **76**, 2075–80.

Rodriguez-Baez, N., O'Brien, R., et al. 2002. Astrovirus, adenovirus, and rotavirus in hospitalized children: prevalence and association with gastroenteritis. *J Pediatr Gastroenterol Nutr*, **35**, 64–8.

Sakamoto, T., Negishi, H., et al. 2000. Molecular epidemiology of astroviruses in Japan from 1995 to 1998 by reverse transcription-polymerase chain reaction with serotype-specific primers. *J Med Virol*, **61**, 326–31.

Sakon, N., Yamazaki, K., et al. 2000. Genomic characterization of human astrovirus type 6 Katano virus and the establishment of a rapid and effective reverse transcription-polymerase chain reaction to detect all serotypes of human astrovirus. *J Med Virol*, **61**, 125–31.

Sanchez-Fauquier, A., Carrascosa, A.L., et al. 1994. Characterization of a human astrovirus serotype 2 structural protein (VP26) that contains an epitope involved in virus neutralization. *Virology*, **201**, 312–20.

Shastri, S., Doane, A.M., et al. 1998. Prevalence of astroviruses in a children's hospital. *J Clin Microbiol*, **36**, 2571–4.

Shimizu, M., Shirai, J., et al. 1990. Cytopathic astrovirus isolated from porcine acute gastroenteritis in an established cell line derived from porcine embryonic kidney. *J Clin Microbiol*, **28**, 201–6.

Shirai, J., Shimizu, M. and Fukusyo, A. 1985. Coronavirus-, calicivirus-, and astrovirus-like particles associated with acute porcine gastroenteritis. *Jpn J Vet Sci*, **47**, 1023–6.

Shirai, J., Nakamura, K., et al. 1991. Pathogenicity and antigenicity of avian nephritis isolates. *Avian Dis*, **35**, 49–54.

Silcock, J.G., Willcocks, M.M., et al. 1993. Virus involvement in community acquired diarrhoea examined by stool dot-blot hybridisation and electron microscopy. *Eur J Gastroenterol Hepatol*, **5**, 601–6.

Snodgrass, D.R. and Gray, E.W. 1977. Detection and transmission of 30 nm virus particles (astroviruses) in faeces of lambs with diarrhoea. *Arch Virol*, **55**, 287–91.

Snodgrass, D.R., Angus, K.W., et al. 1979. Pathogenesis of diarrhoea caused by astrovirus infections in lambs. *Arch Virol*, **60**, 217–26.

Sosnovtsev, S. and Green, K.Y. 1995. RNA transcripts derived from a cloned full-length copy of the feline calicivirus genome do not require VPg for infectivity. *Virology*, **210**, 383–90.

Taylor, M.B., Grabow, W.O.K. and Cubitt, W.D. 1997. Propagation of human astrovirus in the PLC/PRF/5 hepatoma cell line. *J Virol Methods*, **67**, 13–18.

Taylor, M.B., Cox, N., et al. 2001. The occurrence of hepatitis A and astrovirus in selected river and dam waters in South Africa. *Water Res*, **35**, 2653–60.

Thouvenelle, M.L., Haynes, J.S., et al. 1995. Astrovirus infection in hatchling turkeys: alterations in intestinal maltase activity. *Avian Dis*, **39**, 343–8.

Traore, O., Belliot, G., et al. 2000. RT-PCRT identification and typing of astrovirus and Norwalk-like viruses in hospitalized patients with gastroenteritis: evidence of nosocomial infections. *J Clin Virol*, **17**, 151–8.

Unicomb, L.E., Banu, N.N., et al. 1998. Astrovirus infection in association with acute, persistent and nosocomial diarrhea in Bangladesh. *Pediatr Infect Dis J*, **17**, 611–14.

Utagawa, E.T., Nishizawa, S., et al. 1994. Astrovirus as a cause of gastroenteritis in Japan. *J Clin Microbiol*, **32**, 1841–5.

Walter, J.E., Briggs, J., et al. 2001a. Molecular characterization of a novel recombinant strain of human astrovirus associated with gastroenteritis in children. *Arch Virol*, **146**, 2357–67.

Walter, J.E., Mitchell, D.K., et al. 2001b. Molecular epidemiology of human astrovirus diarrhea among children from a periurban community of Mexico City. *J Infect Dis*, **183**, 681–6.

Wang, Q.H., Kakizawa, J., et al. 2001. Genetic analysis of the capsid region of astroviruses. *J Med Virol*, **64**, 245–55.

Willcocks, M.M. and Carter, M.J. 1993. Identification and sequence determination of the capsid protein gene of human astrovirus serotype 1. *FEMS Microbiol Lett*, **114**, 1–8.

Willcocks, M.M., Carter, M.J., et al. 1990. Growth and characterisation of human faecal astrovirus in a continuous cell line. *Arch Virol*, **113**, 73–82.

Willcocks, M.M., Carter, M.J., et al. 1991. A dot-blot hybridisation procedure for the detection of astrovirus in stool samples. *Epidemiol Infect*, **107**, 405–10.

Willcocks, M.M., Carter, M.J. and Madeley, C.R. 1992. Astroviruses. *Rev Med Virol*, **2**, 97–106.

Willcocks, M.M., Aston, N., et al. 1994a. Cell culture adaptation of astrovirus involves a deletion. *J Virol*, **68**, 6057–8.

Willcocks, M.M., Brown, T.D.K., et al. 1994b. The complete sequence of a human astrovirus. *J Gen Virol*, **75**, 1785–8.

Willcocks, M.M., Kurtz, J.B., et al. 1995. Prevalence of human astrovirus serotype 4: Capsid protein sequence and comparison with other strains. *Epidemiol Infect*, **114**, 385–91.

Willcocks, M.M., Boxall, A.S. and Carter, M.J. 1999. Processing and intracellular location of human astrovirus non-structural proteins. *J Gen Virol*, **80**, 2607–11.

Williams, F.P. Jr 1980. Astrovirus-like, coronavirus-like and parvovirus-like particles detected in the diarrhoeal stools of beagle pups. *Arch Virol*, **66**, 216–26.

Woode, G.N. and Bridger, J.C. 1978. Isolation of small viruses resembling astroviruses and caliciviruses from acute enteritis of calves. *J Med Microbiol*, **11**, 441–52.

Woode, G.N., Pohlenz, J.F., et al. 1984. Astrovirus and Breda virus infections of dome cell epithelium of bovine ileum. *J Clin Microbiol*, **19**, 623–30.

Yamaguchi, S., Imada, T. and Kawamura, H. 1979. Characterization of a picornavirus isolated from broiler chicks. *Avian Dis*, **23**, 571–81.

Yue, H.J. and Ushijima, H. 1996. Detection and genotyping of astroviruses by RT-PCR and sequencing. *J Jpn Assoc Infect Dis*, **70**, 1220–6.

42

Human enteric RNA viruses: Noroviruses and Sapoviruses

IAN N. CLARKE AND PAUL R. LAMBDEN

HISTORICAL PERSPECTIVES

Diarrheal disease in humans, clinically distinct from bacterial gastroenteritis, was first reported in the southern USA. It was originally described as 'hyperemesis hiemis' or winter vomiting disease (Zahorsky 1929), a term that reflects its seasonality. The illness occurred in widespread epidemics with a high secondary attack rate, and was documented as a short, self-limiting episode of vomiting with some diarrhea. Later, this syndrome was also recognized by clinicians in the UK (Bradley 1943; Gray 1939; Miller and Raven 1936). Its distinction from bacterial gastroenteritis was confirmed by investigations of institutional outbreaks in which stool cultures were consistently negative for pathogenic bacteria.

Between the 1940s and the early 1970s, a variety of synonymous terms were used for this syndrome, including nonbacterial gastroenteritis, epidemic gastroenteritis, acute infectious nonbacterial gastroenteritis, and winter vomiting disease. The transmissibility of an agent by oral inoculation of human volunteers with a fecal filtrate was repeatedly demonstrated (Adler and Zickl 1969; Clarke et al. 1972; Dolin et al. 1971; Gordon et al. 1947; Jordan et al. 1953; Reimann et al. 1945). This approach established the possibility of a viral etiology, and although the natural history of this transmissible agent was comprehensively described, all attempts to isolate a bacterial pathogen or a viral agent failed.

An outbreak of epidemic gastroenteritis in a primary school in Norwalk, Ohio, USA led to confirmation of the viral etiology of winter vomiting disease (Kapikian et al. 1972). Fecal filtrates from affected children were fed to volunteers, whose stools were examined by immunoelectron microscopy. A previously undescribed virus-like particle, 27 nm in diameter, was detected and subsequently named Norwalk virus. Further studies in volunteers established Norwalk virus as the agent responsible for the original outbreak. Seroconversions or rising IgG titers, as well as virus excretion, were demonstrated in infected volunteers, and the histopathology of jejunal biopsies from those with acute disease gave new insights into the cell tropism of Norwalk virus in the small intestine (Agus et al. 1973; Schreiber et al. 1973). Further volunteer studies by American workers identified viruses morphologically similar to the Norwalk virus in two outbreaks of nonbacterial gastroenteritis. These viruses were termed Montgomery County and Hawaii, respectively, after the locations of the outbreaks. This mode of nomenclature became common (Caul 1988) and laboratories continue to name strains after the location of isolation.

Soon after the discovery of the Norwalk virus, morphologically indistinguishable viruses from clinically similar outbreaks were reported. The agents responsible for these virologically characterized outbreaks were termed Hawaii (Thornhill et al. 1977; Wyatt et al. 1974), Snow Mountain (Dolin et al. 1982; Morens et al. 1979) and Taunton (Caul et al. 1979; Pether and Caul 1983).

Volunteer studies were central to the understanding of the transmissibility, pathogenesis, and immunobiology of the Norwalk and Hawaii viruses (Parrino et al. 1977; Schreiber et al. 1973; 1974; Wyatt et al. 1974) and established a previously undescribed and poorly characterized group of related viruses as an important cause of epidemic gastroenteritis. The Norwalk-like viruses cause acute, explosive diarrhea, vomiting, or both, and are highly infective, with rapid secondary spread. Large outbreaks have been described in semiclosed communities throughout the world as a result of person-to-person spread (Caul 1988; Christensen 1989; Kaplan et al. 1982; Pether and Caul 1983). Point-source outbreaks resulting from the ingestion of sewage-contaminated water, contaminated shellfish or food (Morens et al. 1979; Murphy et al. 1982) emphasize the great public health importance of these viruses. There are major problems in controlling such outbreaks, and the economic implications, including those applicable to the food and shellfish industries, are being increasingly recognized.

The widespread application of electron microscopy (EM) to the examination of diarrheal stool samples resulted in major advances in our understanding of the etiology of nonbacterial gastroenteritis. Rotaviruses were rapidly identified as major pathogens in endemic infantile gastroenteritis, and other viruses, including 'fastidious' adenoviruses, were added to the list of enteric 'diarrhea' viruses. In addition to these distinctive viruses there were many reports of an apparently wide range of small-round viruses (SRV) approximately 30 nm in diameter. In many studies SRVs were identified by immunoelectron microscopy (IEM), which masks surface morphology, and often resulted in a confusing picture of the etiology of nonbacterial gastroenteritis. Other SRVs were identified from their classic surface structure, and detailed descriptions of the morphology of the newly described astroviruses and 'classic' caliciviruses were published (Madeley 1979).

In 1982 an 'interim classification scheme' was presented (Caul and Appleton 1982) as an to aid national surveillance within the UK and to establish which SRVs were causally related to viral gastroenteritis. The authors concluded that the causative agents of diarrheal disease were the SRVs that possessed surface morphology to which descriptive terms could be applied. These viruses included the previously described astroviruses, 'classic' caliciviruses, and a third group of viruses that shared the features of an amorphous surface structure and 'ragged'-edged virions. This third group was represented by the prototype Norwalk virus, and within the interim scheme were termed small-round structured viruses (SRSV). A prerequisite for classification under this scheme was that all viruses were examined in the absence of antibody to ensure that any surface structure would not be obscured. SRSVs emerged as the most important cause of epidemic nonbacterial gastroenteritis worldwide, with viruses of this group causing similar illnesses.

This morphological classification scheme recognized fundamental differences between astroviruses, the classic caliciviruses, and SRSVs, and was supported by epidemiological and immunological distinctions (Blacklow and Greenberg 1991; Caul 1988). The molecular characterization of these three different viruses showed that they contained positive-sense single-stranded RNA genomes. The genome structure of astroviruses, however, is very different from that of the SRSVs and 'classic' caliciviruses, and so the astroviruses have been assigned to a separate virus family and are discussed in Chapter 41, Human enteric RNA viruses: Astroviruses. SRSVs and the 'classic' caliciviruses both belong to two separate genera within the *Caliciviridae*, which from 1998 to 2002 were temporarily called Norwalk-like viruses (NLV) and Sapporo-like viruses (SLV), respectively. The ICTV has now settled on a new nomenclature for these genera, namely Noroviruses and Sapoviruses, reflecting the place of discovery of each of the prototypes. The clinical, epidemiological and pathological aspects of Noroviruses and Sapoviruses are summarized (Table 42.1).

On the basis of sequence analysis and genome organization, human enteric caliciviruses have been assigned to two separate genera within the *Caliciviridae* (Jiang et al. 1993; Lambden et al. 1993; Dingle et al. 1995). The SRSVs or Norwalk-like viruses belong to the *Norovirus* genus and the Sapporo-like or 'classic' caliciviruses are members of the *Sapovirus* genus. Two other genera are included in the family and contain viruses pathogenic for animals. The *Vesivirus* genus includes *Feline calicivirus* and *Vesicular exanthema of swine virus*. The fourth genus, *Lagovirus*, is represented by the *Rabbit hemorrhagic disease virus* (RHDV) and the closely related *European brown hare syndrome virus* (EBHSV).

NOROVIRUSES

Classification and morphology

The prototypic Norwalk virus was originally described as non-enveloped, round, 27-nm particles with a 'ragged' outer edge but lacking a definite surface structure (Kapikian et al. 1972). The low titer of virions found in stool samples, together with their small size and amorphous structure, has made them difficult to detect by direct EM. Many other Noroviruses have been described and have in common a buoyant density of 1.33–1.41 g/cm^3, an inability to propagate in vitro, and an RNA genome of positive polarity (Greenberg and Matsui 1992).

Characteristically, Noroviruses possess a single capsid protein (Greenberg et al. 1981), but lack of a cell-culture system has restricted the production of capsid antigen to recombinant heterologous expression systems. Capsid proteins expressed in insect cells using

Table 42.1 *The clinical, epidemiological and pathological aspects of Noroviruses and Sapoviruses*

Appearance	Genome structure	Clinical features	Examples
Noroviruses			

Feathery, ragged outline
No distinctive surface structure
Some preparations resemble classic calicivirus
No cell-culture system
	ssRNA, +ve polarity, polyadenylated, ca. 7.7 kb group I and 7.5 kb group II
	ORF1 nonstructural polyprotein
	ORF2 capsid
	ORF3 small basic protein
	Possible subgenomic RNA
		Winter vomiting disease
		Epidemic nausea vomiting and diarrhea
		Acquisition of antibodies is gradual, vomiters are more likely to seroconvert
		Peak illness in adults
		No immunity
		Clinical features identical for group I and group II viruses
			Group I:
			Norwalk virus:
			  (school outbreak, USA 1969)
			Southampton virus
			  (family outbreak, UK 1991)
			
			Group II:
			Hawaii virus:
			  (family outbreak, USA 1972)
			Lordsdale virus
			  (hospital outbreak, UK 1993)

Sapoviruses			

Distinctive cup-shaped surface depressions, giving classic 'Star of David' morphology
No cell-culture system
	ssRNA, +ve polarity, polyadenylated, ca. 7.3 kb
	ORF1 nonstructural polyprotein contiguous with and fused to capsid gene
	ORF2 small basic protein
	Subgenomic RNA and VPg present in animal viru
		No seasonal variance
		Predominantly pediatric illness
		Antibodies acquired at young age
		Diarrheal illness usually mild
			Group I:
			Sapporo virus:
			  outbreak in an orphanage Sapporo and Japan, 1982
			Manchester virus:
			  sporadic case of acute vomiting and diarrhea in a 6-month-old child (1993)
			
			Group II:
			Bristol virus: sporadic case 15-month -old child (1998)
			London virus:
			  8-month-old infant hospitalized for diarrhea and vomiting (1992)

baculovirus vectors spontaneously assemble to form virus-like particles and are released into the cell culture supernatant (Dingle et al. 1995; Jiang et al. 1992; Jiang et al. 1995b). These virus-like particles are larger in diameter and have the appearance of empty virions (Figure 42.1).

Cryo-electron microscopy and computer image processing techniques have determined the empty virion structure to a resolution of 2.2 nm (Rothnagel et al. 1994) (Figure 42.2). The empty capsids are composed of 90 dimers of the capsid structural protein and are 38 nm in diameter, with T = 3 icosahedral symmetry. Archlike capsomers formed from dimers of the capsid structural protein and deep depressions at the five- and three-fold axes are distinctive features. Each virus-like particle has 32 surface hollows surrounded by the protruding arches. Twelve hollows are at the icosahedral fivefold axis and have a small hump at the center. The other 20 hollows at the three-fold positions seem to be flat. This distinctive molecular architecture has also been described for a primate calicivirus (Prasad et al. 1994).

The structure of recombinant Norwalk virus capsids at near-atomic resolution has been determined by X-ray crystallography (Prasad et al. 1999, 2000). The structure of the capsid protein is organized into two domains joined by a flexible hinge (Figure 42.3). The inner shell (S) domain is composed of the N-terminal 225 residues and is involved in the formation of the icosahedral capsid shell. The shell domain also shows the classic eight-stranded β barrel structure typical of many viral capsid proteins. The protruding (P) domain forms prominent structures extending from the surface of the shell, and is formed from the C-terminal half of the protein. The P domain is further organized into two subdomains (P1 and P2), and it has been suggested that these structures may be involved in binding to cellular receptors and may also be the determinants of strain specificity (Prasad et al. 1999). Mutational analysis of the critical residues involved in VLP formation (Bertolotti-Ciarlet et al. 2002) has shown that complete removal of the P domain resulted in the formation of smooth particles with a diameter slightly less than that of the complete rNV VLPs. These studies demonstrated that the shell domain alone of the capsid protein was able to initiate spontaneous assembly into particles, but the P domain was required for particle stability.

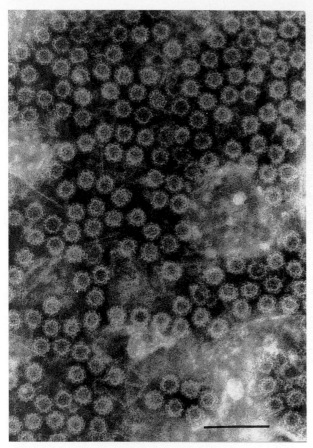

Figure 42.1 *Electron micrograph showing recombinant virus-like particles produced by expression of Southampton virus capsid protein from insect cells. Bar, 100 nm.*

Genome organization

Since the first reports of the molecular cloning of the Norwalk virus genome in 1990, rapid progress has been made in the genome analysis of Noroviruses. Virus purified from feces of volunteers infected with Norwalk virus was used to generate a library of cDNA clones representing most of the viral genome. Authentic clones were identified by hybridization to post- but not preinfection stool nucleic acid. Sequence information indicated that the Norwalk virus genome is single-stranded positive-sense RNA of about 7.5 kb and polyadenylated at the 3′ terminus (Jiang et al. 1990). In one of the viral clones a motif characteristic of viral RNA-dependent RNA polymerases was identified. Matsui and colleagues (Matsui et al. 1991) then cloned a region of the Norwalk virus genome that was immunoreactive when expressed in recombinant λ phage. Following these early studies a number of complete genome sequences of human Noroviruses (Dingle et al. 1995; Green et al. 2002; Hardy and Estes 1996; Jiang et al. 1993; Katayama et al. 2002; Lambden et al. 1993; Lambden et al. 1995; Pletneva et al. 2001; Schreier et al. 2000; Seah et al. 1999; Someya et al. 2000) have been determined, together with numerous partial sequences covering the RNA polymerase and capsid regions in the 3′ half of the genome.

Phylogenetic analyses of the RNA polymerase and capsid regions of the genome indicate that human Noroviruses are divided into two genetic groups (Ando et al. 1994; Cubitt et al. 1994; Green et al. 1994; Wang et al. 1994). The genome of group I viruses is slightly larger (7.7 kb) than the group II genome (7.5 kb), although computer analyses reveal that the reading frame usage of these two genetic groups is very similar. The genomes of both group I and group II Noroviruses (Figure 42.4) are characterized by a large 5′ open reading frame (ORF) encoding a nonstructural polyprotein of approximately 1 700 amino acids, followed by a smaller ORF encoding the capsid structural protein.

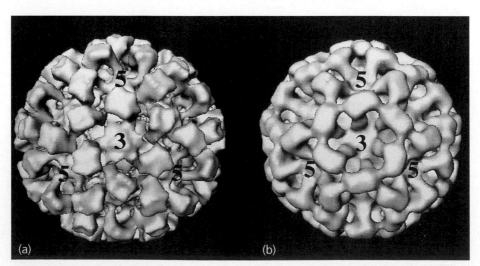

Figure 42.2 *Computer-generated images from cryo-electron microscopic preparations of **(a)** recombinant Norwalk virus capsids and **(b)** primate calicivirus. The images are viewed along the threefold axes. (Photograph courtesy of Dr B.V.V. Prasad, Baylor College of Medicine, Houston TX, USA.)*

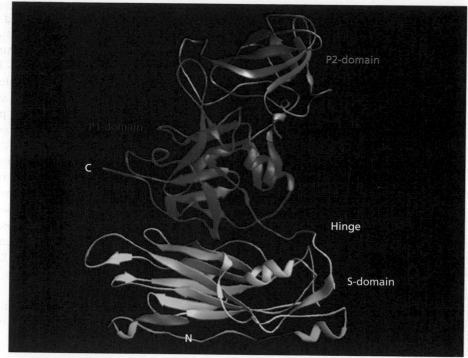

Figure 42.3 *Ribbon representation showing the structure of recombinant Norwalk virus capsid protein. The N-terminal arm, S domain, and P1/P2 subdomains are colored green, yellow, red, and blue, respectively. The N and C termini, together with the hinge region between the shell and protruding domains, are indicated. (Image courtesy of Dr B.V.V. Prasad, Baylor College of Medicine, Houston TX, USA.)*

At the 3′ end of the genome is a small ORF, predicted by computer analysis to encode a basic protein. This genome organization clearly distinguishes Noroviruses from other positive-strand RNA viruses, such as the picornaviruses.

The smaller size of the group II *Norovirus* genome is attributable to its smaller ORF1. The nucleotide (nt) sequence in the 5′ region of ORF1 shows significant diversity between the two genetic groups, although distal to this variable region both groups show the characteristic motifs of the NTPase, cysteine protease, and RNA polymerase in the same relative genomic positions. Sequence diversity at the 5′ end of the genome may reflect fundamental differences between the two groups of viruses in terms of secondary structures or regulatory signals. The first 110 nucleotides of the Norwalk virus genome have been shown to form stable complexes with several cellular proteins from HeLa and CaCo cell extracts (Gutierrez-Escolano et al. 2000). The proteins La, PCBP-2, PTB, and hnRNPL, which are required for translation in poliovirus and hepatitis C virus, may also be essential for translation of caliciviral RNA.

The capsid coding region in the *Norovirus* genome is similar to the arrangement in feline calicivirus (FCV), in which ORF2 is frame-shifted relative to ORF1 so that the N terminus of the capsid protein overlaps the C terminus of the putative RNA-dependent RNA polymerase. However, the extent of reading frame overlap

differs between the two genetic groups of Noroviruses, being 17 nt in group I and 20 nt in group II. The small 3′ ORF is also in a different reading frame from the capsid-encoding ORF2. The first residue of the initiator codon of ORF3 overlaps the last base of the terminator codon of the capsid gene. A characteristic feature of the animal caliciviruses is the production of a 3′ co-terminal polyadenylated subgenomic RNA coding for the capsid and small 3′ ORF. This subgenomic RNA is thought to provide an additional message for the production of capsid protein, and in the case of RHDV this additional RNA is packaged into mature virions (Meyers et al. 1991). It is not yet clear whether Noroviruses produce a subgenomic message, although detection of RNA of over 2 kb by Northern blot analysis of total stool RNA from a volunteer infected with Norwalk virus suggested that this virus also produces a subgenomic RNA (Jiang et al. 1993). A characteristic feature of the animal calicivirus genomic and subgenomic RNAs is that the 5′ termini are highly conserved (Lambden and Clarke 1995). The 5′ terminal sequence of ORF1 is repeated around the 5′ terminal region of ORF2, suggesting that human enteric caliciviruses, like their animal counterparts, also produce a subgenomic RNA. The 5′ genomic and subgenomic termini of both groups I and II Noroviruses begin with the sequence GU, and by analogy with the animal caliciviruses this terminal sequence is linked to the VPg

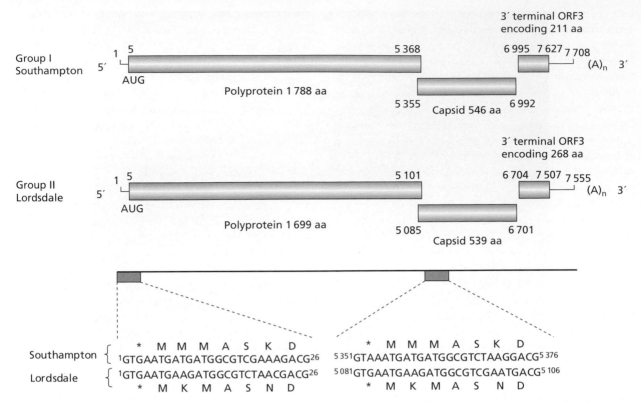

Figure 42.4 *Comparison of the genome structures of groups I and II Noroviruses. Shaded boxes represent computer-predicted open reading frames. Translation products and their sizes are indicated on the open reading frames. The conserved sequences at the 5′ genomic termini and the predicted 5′ termini of the subgenomic RNAs of groups I and II Noroviruses are aligned beneath the genome maps. Southampton virus (EMBL/GenBank Accession No. L07418); Lordsdale virus (EMBL/GenBank Accession No. X86557).*

protein. The conserved GU residues at the 5′ genomic termini appears to be a common feature of the *Caliciviridae*. The amino acid involved in the linkage between VPg and the RHDV genome has been identified as Tyr-21 (Machin et al. 2001).

Viral proteins

Highly purified Norwalk virus recovered from CsCl equilibrium density gradients contains a single protein of 59 kDa (Greenberg et al. 1981). The single capsid protein was identified by radioimmunoprecipitation of purified virions with acute and convalescent sera from infected volunteers. Similar studies with the antigenically distinct Snow Mountain agent revealed a major structural polypeptide of 62 kDa (Madore et al. 1986). In addition to the 59 kDa capsid protein of Norwalk virus, a soluble protein with a molecular weight of 30 kDa was also detected in the supernatant of fecal suspensions. It has been estimated that up to 50 percent of the excreted antigen is present as soluble protein (Jiang et al. 1992). Until recently the source of the soluble protein remained uncertain, and was suggested to be an immunogenic nonstructural protein or a cleavage product derived from the capsid protein. However, analysis of virus-like particles expressed

from insect cells infected with recombinant baculovirus demonstrated that the 30 kDa protein is a specific cleavage product of the viral capsid (Hardy et al. 1995). Recombinant Norwalk virus treated with trypsin released a 32 kDa protein, and analysis of the N-terminal sequence of this product revealed that a trypsin-specific cleavage occurred at amino acid residue 227. The 30 kDa soluble protein reacted with rabbit polyclonal antisera raised against recombinant Norwalk virus capsids, and analysis of the N-terminal sequence of the approximately 30 kDa soluble protein showed it to be identical to the 32 kDa trypsin cleavage product. In addition, it was shown that the 32 kDa proteolytic cleavage product is derived from soluble capsid protein and not intact assembled virions. These data suggest that the Norwalk virus capsid undergoes proteolytic cleavage during the course of infection. Japanese isolates antigenically related to the Hawaii virus also demonstrated immunoreactive structural proteins of 63 and 30 kDa by Western blot analysis (Hayashi et al. 1989; Oishi et al. 1992).

Several groups have described capsid gene sequences from a number of different *Norovirus* isolates that encode proteins with predicted molecular weights of approximately 60 kDa. Computer alignments of the capsid sequence data support the division of Noroviruses into two major genetic groups. The capsid proteins have approximately 68 percent amino acid sequence identity within a genetic group and 40 percent between groups. However, the *Norovirus* capsids show only limited homology with the corresponding proteins in members of the other genera. A dendrogram showing the phylogenetic relatedness of caliciviruses is shown in Figure 42.5. The prototype Norwalk virus and the antigenically distinct Southampton virus are both members of genetic group I, together with the Desert Shield virus. A UK isolate, Lordsdale virus, has been assigned to genetic group II, along with Snow Mountain agent, Hawaii virus, Toronto virus, and Mexico virus.

The first major ORF encodes a polyprotein that is presumably processed by a proteolytic cascade analogous to that of picornaviruses. Computer analysis of the ORF1 sequence data has identified conserved amino acid motifs typical of the picornaviral 2C NTPase, 3C protease, and RNA-dependent RNA polymerase. NTPase activity has been demonstrated in recombinant p41of Southampton virus expressed as an *Escherichia coli* fusion protein (Pfister and Wimmer 2001). Sequence comparisons of group I and II Noroviruses reveal, apart from the short conserved sequence motifs, extreme sequence diversity at the 5′ proximal regions of the genomes. In RHDV the genomic and subgenomic RNAs are linked at their 5′ termini to a small protein analogous to picornaviral VPg, although the caliciviral protein (approximately 15 kDa) is considerably larger than the picornaviral equivalent (22 amino acids). The presence of a VPg-like protein, encoded by ORF1 in Noroviruses, is strongly inferred by analogy with the animal caliciviruses.

Although no specific biological function has been assigned to the translation product of ORF3 it has been reported that this protein is present in mature virions (Glass et al. 2000). A role for ORF3 protein as a minor capsid protein has also been reported in vesiviruses (FCV) (Sosnovtsev and Green 2000) and lagoviruses (RHDV) (Wirblich et al. 1996). The ORF3 translation product shows considerable sequence variation both within and between genera, which is surprising if the predicted protein product has the same functional role in all caliciviruses. It has been proposed that this basic protein may play a role in RNA packaging and assembly of the mature virion.

Polyprotein processing

In common with picornaviruses, caliciviral proteins are synthesized as a large polyprotein precursor which is subsequently processed in a proteolytic cascade by the viral 3C-like protease. In vitro transcription and translation of genomic clones does not appear to generate the intact polyprotein, suggesting that proteolytic processing probably occurs cotranslationally. Using in vitro mutagenesis and expression of the active protease in *E. coli*, five cleavage sites have been identified in Southampton *Norovirus* (Figure 42.6) (Liu et al. 1996; Liu et al. 1999b). Two of the cleavages in Southampton virus are at QG dipeptides and are responsible for the release of the p48 N-terminal protein and p41 NTPase from the polyprotein. Three further cleavages at EA and EG dipeptides generate the p22 (3A), p16 (VPg), p19 (3C protease), and p57 (RNA-dependent RNA polymerase). The preference for a glutamate residue at the P1 position of the cleavage dipeptide is also evident in FCV (Sosnovtsev et al. 1998, 2002) and RHDV (Wirblich et al. 1995; Meyers et al. 2000). The amino acid at the P1′ position of the cleavage dipeptide is more variable, but there appears to be a marked preference for glycine residues. The P4 position N terminus of the scissile bond also appears to be important in efficient processing (Hardy et al. 2002).

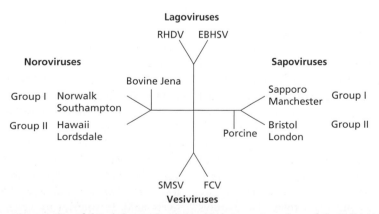

Figure 42.5 *Diagrammatic representation of the phylogenetic relationship between members of the* Caliciviridae*: adapted from (Robinson et al. 2002). Assignments are based on computer analyses of the complete amino acid sequence of the capsid proteins.* Norovirus *(Southampton, L07418; Norwalk, M87661; Lordsdale, X86557; Hawaii, U07611; Bovine, AJ011099);* Sapovirus *(Sapporo, U65427; Manchester, X86560; Bristol, AJ249939; London, U95645; Porcine, AF182760); FCV (Feline calicivirus, M86379); SMSV (San Miguel sealion virus, M87481); RHDV (Rabbit hemorrhagic disease virus, M67473); EBHSV (European brown hare syndrome virus, Z69620). The EMBL/GenBank accession numbers are shown in parentheses.*

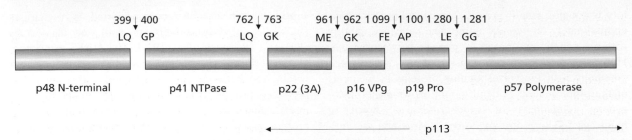

Figure 42.6 *Proteolytic cleavage map of the Southampton virus polyprotein encoded by ORF1. The shaded boxes represent the mature cleavage products of the nonstructural polyprotein. Cleavage sites are indicated between the boxes, and the amino acid coordinates at the P1/P1' cleavage dipeptide are given each side of the arrows. The calculated molecular masses and functions of the cleavage products are indicated below the boxes. The large primary cleavage product (p113) observed in in vitro translation reactions extends from amino acid 763 to the carboxy terminus of the 3D polymerase and is indicated by the arrow below the cleavage map.*

Antigenic variation

Several approaches have been used in an attempt to evaluate antigenic relationships between the Noroviruses. Using human volunteers, cross-challenge studies have demonstrated that Norwalk and Hawaii viruses are antigenically distinct (Kapikian 1994), and further volunteer studies with the Montgomery County agent identified a one-way cross-protection with Hawaii virus. There was short-term homologous immunity after challenge of humans with all three viruses (Dolin et al. 1972; Wyatt et al. 1974).

The antigenic relatedness of Norwalk, Hawaii, and Snow Mountain viruses was also studied by testing serological responses in volunteers. Using an enzyme immunoassay (EIA) variable degrees of antigenic relatedness were observed, with a two-way cross-reaction between Snow Mountain and Hawaii virus and a one-way cross-reaction between Norwalk and Snow Mountain viruses (Madore et al. 1990). These results may reflect heterologous responses and contrast with the greater specificity of IEM or solid-phase immunoelectron microscopy (SPIEM), which is based on the use of intact virions (from fecal specimens) and convalescent sera.

Four antigenic types of *Norovirus* were originally described in the UK, identified by IEM or SPIEM (Lambden et al. 1993; Lewis 1991; Lewis 1990), six in the USA (Lewis et al. 1995) and nine in Japan (Okada et al. 1990). However, all the above methods suffered from the same technical drawbacks of poorly defined and limited reagents, which meant it was not possible to compare the differently defined antigenic 'types'. Although these were useful methods in the early days of research they have largely been replaced by modern molecular methods.

A definitive approach for serotyping Noroviruses based on neutralization is not possible because there is no cell-culture system. The ability to express the capsid protein in insect cells where it assembles to form virus-like particles, first demonstrated for Norwalk virus (Jiang et al. 1992), was a significant advance that has provided a renewable source of capsid antigen for many different strains. Apart from their use in structural studies, purified VLPs have been used to raise polyclonal and monoclonal antisera for the development of new diagnostic reagents. Several antigen capture EIAs have been developed using polyclonal antisera to VLPs from different animal species. Evaluation of these assays has shown that they are highly *Norovirus* strain specific; thus EIAs for Norwalk or Mexico virus will detect only homologous antigens (Graham et al. 1994; Jiang et al. 1995a). Phylogenetic analysis of capsid sequences suggests that the clustering of strains that show high levels of sequence conservation is also reflected by immunological relationships defined by EIA. However, some caution must be exercised in interpreting the meaning of these observations, as immunological relationships defined by EIA may still mean that viruses are not serotypically related as defined by virus neutralization.

Clinical manifestations

Detailed information on the clinical, immunological, and pathological aspects of Noroviruses have been established from investigations on volunteers (Kapikian 1994), in whom infections by Norwalk virus, Hawaii agent, Montgomery County agent, and the Snow Mountain agent are clinically indistinguishable (Morens et al. 1979; Wyatt et al. 1974). Following transmission by the fecal–oral route, volunteer and epidemiological studies have established an incubation period of approximately 24 h (Kapikian 1994), with a dose-dependent range of 18–48 h (Blacklow and Herrmann 1988). Symptoms are sudden in onset and are accompanied by nausea and vomiting, which can be projectile and severe. Low-grade fever and diarrhea usually occur, the latter being relatively mild. In contrast to bacterial gastroenteritis, diarrheal stools do not contain blood, mucus, or white cells. Other symptoms include mild abdominal pain or cramps, malaise, and headaches. Vomiting may arise from a decrease in gastric motility (Meeroff et al. 1980), giving rise to a reflux action into the stomach. Respiratory involvement has not been observed, and nasopharyngeal washings from an acutely ill volunteer did not induce disease on passage to other volunteers (Dolin et al. 1972).

In general, *Norovirus* infections are self-limiting and affected patients rarely need to be hospitalized. There have, however, been occasional reports of severe dehydration that required the administration of intravenous fluids. Deaths associated with *Norovirus* infections are exceptionally rare and have not been directly attributed to this group of viruses (Kaplan et al. 1982).

Pathogenesis

Volunteer studies show that as few as 10–100 infectious particles may be needed to initiate infection. Replication is considered to occur in the mucosal epithelium of the small intestine, although direct evidence is lacking. Light microscopy of jejunal biopsies from volunteers infected with Norwalk virus showed partial flattening and broadening of the villi, with disorganization of the mucosal epithelium (Agus et al. 1973; Schreiber et al. 1973). The lamina propria was infiltrated with mononuclear cells and vacuolization of mucosal epithelium was noted. Crypt cell hyperplasia was common, and, at the ultrastructural level, mucosal epithelial cells showed dilatation of the rough and smooth endoplasmic reticulum, with an increase in multivesiculate bodies. Microvilli were significantly shortened, and amorphous electron-dense material was present in the expanded intercellular spaces. The absence of Noroviruses in damaged mucosal cells was noteworthy. The results of light and electron microscopy in volunteers infected with the Hawaii agent were similar, and, again, virus particles were not identified in biopsies (Dolin et al. 1975; Schreiber et al. 1974). In general, *Norovirus* infections seem to cause mild atrophy of the villi of the small intestine, assumed to arise from limited virus replication that damages the mucosal cells. The appearance of mucosal lesions was paralleled by a decrease in brush border enzymes, which returned to normal values during convalescence (Agus et al. 1973).

Epidemiology

Noroviruses are now established as the most important cause of epidemic nonbacterial outbreaks of gastroenteritis worldwide. National surveillance and diagnosis by EM of outbreaks of nonbacterial gastroenteritis in the UK have shown that Noroviruses are a more common cause of infective gastroenteritis than *Salmonella* or *Campylobacter* (Food Standards Agency 2000). The infectious intestinal disease study conducted in England and Wales between August 1993 and January 1996 suggested that at least 600 000 cases of gastroenteritis annually could be attributed to *Norovirus* infections (Food Standards Agency 2000). This figure is likely to be a considerable underestimate, as the relatively insensitive method of EM was chosen for *Norovirus* detection. There has also been an increasing prevalence of Noroviruses in recent years, with a strong suggestion of a winter seasonality culminating with a major epidemic in the UK in January 2002. Similarly, since October 2002 several states in the USA have reported an increase in outbreaks of *Norovirus* infection (www.cdc.gov/mmwr/PDF/wk/mm5203.pdf).

The diversity of settings associated with these economically important viruses is demonstrated by work conducted in the USA soon after the discovery of the Norwalk virus. This virus originally caused a community-wide outbreak in Norwalk, Ohio; Hawaii and Montgomery County agents were responsible for small family outbreaks (Thornhill et al. 1977), whereas the Snow Mountain agent caused an outbreak at a holiday camp in Colorado (Morens et al. 1979). The Taunton agent caused considerable disruption in a hospital in southern England (Caul et al. 1979; Pether and Caul 1983). Subsequent surveillance and investigations of outbreaks in many parts of the world identified the potential of Noroviruses for causing epidemic gastroenteritis in semiclosed or community-wide populations, for example families, healthcare institutions, holiday locations including cruise ships, educational establishments, and the catering industry. Outbreaks occur among children and adults, but rarely among neonates or very young children. Although considerable data are available on the causal role of Noroviruses in outbreaks, less is known about their role in endemic disease, perhaps because of the relative mildness of the illness. Hospitalization of individual cases is thus unusual, and opportunities to investigate sporadic cases are scarce.

Despite the lack of secondary spread by the respiratory route, it is clear that many of the explosive outbreaks described cannot be due solely to fecal–oral transmission. Noroviruses can be detected in vomitus (Greenberg et al. 1979b): the projectile vomiting associated with acute infections and the consequent formation of aerosols offers an alternative mode of spread (Caul 1994a; Chadwick and McCann 1994; Sawyer et al. 1988; Ho et al. 1989). This, in conjunction with the low infectious dose, would explain the rapid, explosive outbreaks commonly observed in semiclosed communities. The epidemiology of *Norovirus* infections should thus include not only person-to-person spread but also mechanical transmission from hand to mouth. The likelihood of spread from inhalation of aerosol by contacts in close proximity to the index case has been suggested but not proven (Caul 1994a).

In addition to these modes of transmission, Noroviruses are often associated with point-source outbreaks (Caul et al. 1993; Kapikian 1994; Okada et al. 1990). In many cases a likely vehicle of transmission has been identified, for example in the USA, contaminated water supplies – e.g. municipal water, drinking water on cruise ships, recreational swimming water (lake or pool), and commercially produced ice-cubes – have been incriminated (Blacklow and Greenberg 1991; Cukor and Blacklow 1984; Greenberg et al. 1979a). Foodborne outbreaks are well recognized, and food-specific attack rates have incriminated salads, bakery products, fresh fruit, cold foods, sandwiches, and cooked meat The source of the contamination has often been identified as a symptomatic food handler (Pether and Caul 1983; Reid et al. 1988). The secondary attack rate of point-source outbreaks is often high. In the UK, 20–25 percent of *Norovirus* outbreaks were associated with contaminated food (Caul 1994b), and 26 of 38 outbreaks in Japan were considered to be foodborne (Okada et al. 1990). The application of molecular epidemiology (RT-PCR) has increased our knowledge of such outbreaks and the role of the food handler in transmission. The secondary attack rates in outbreaks in the USA reported by the Centers for Disease Control and Prevention (CDC), Atlanta, ranged between 4 and 32 percent, but attack rates of more than 50 percent have often been reported in semiclosed communities. Outbreaks have been prolonged by the introduction of susceptible individuals into an infected environment (e.g. aboard cruise ships and in hospitals).

Contaminated shellfish are a major source of epidemic gastroenteritis (Appleton and Pereira 1977; Christopher et al. 1978; Kaplan et al. 1982; Caul 1994b; Morse et al. 1986). The most commonly reported are the bivalve molluscs (oysters, cockles, and mussels), which are filter-feeders and become infected by Noroviruses from raw sewage. Noroviruses are the major cause of viral gastroenteritis arising from eating shellfish in the UK, and both small and large outbreaks have frequently been reported around the world (Kohn et al. 1995; Le Guyader et al. 2000; Murphy et al. 1979).

Seroepidemiology

The inability to propagate Noroviruses in cell culture and the lack of a suitable animal model severely limited seroprevalence studies in the past. American workers developed a number of crude serological assays, using fecal extracts containing Norwalk virus, to assess the acquisition of Norwalk antibody in different populations (Greenberg et al. 1979a; Kapikian et al. 1978). Antibodies were acquired gradually during childhood, about 20 percent of children under 5 years old being positive. The prevalence of antibody rose rapidly to 45 percent in 18–35-year-olds, and to 55–60 percent in those aged 45–65. These findings are in accordance with the prevalence of *Norovirus* infections in older children and adults, and contrast with those of rotaviruses and *Sapovirus* in developing countries, where antibody is acquired very early in life. In Bangladesh 100 percent of children had acquired antibody by the age of 5, whereas in the former

Yugoslavia the seroprevalence rate was intermediate between that of the USA and those of less developed countries (Kapikian 1994); similar results have been reported from Taiwan and the Philippines. The prevalence of Norwalk virus antibody in blood donors in the USA, Belgium, Yugoslavia, and Switzerland ranges from 54 to 77 percent, and emphasizes the ubiquitous nature of this agent. Compelling evidence that Norwalk virus was responsible for many outbreaks throughout the world in the 1970s has been demonstrated by RIA tests (Kapikian 1994). All these studies were performed when Norwalk virus was circulating in the community.

The expression of recombinant Norwalk virus capsid protein (Jiang et al. 1992) in insect cells, and subsequently the expression of the capsid protein from a number of other Noroviruses, has allowed extensive seroepidemiological studies to be performed using defined reagents in an ELISA format. Importantly, it was shown that recombinant Norwalk virus antigen performs identically to natural Norwalk virus antigen purified from feces of infected volunteers (Green et al. 1993). Seroepidemiological studies using recombinant *Norovirus* capsid antigens have yielded generally similar results: newborn to 6-month-old children had higher serum antibody levels than children aged 6–11 months, representing the decay of maternal antibodies in the early months of life (Cubitt et al. 1998; Dimitrov et al. 1997; Gray et al. 1993; Parker et al. 1994; Pelosi et al. 1999). *Norovirus* antibody prevalence increases in the first 2 years of life, reaching 90 percent in individuals over 60 years old. The prevalence of antibodies to genogroup II Noroviruses appears to be greater, and there are some differences in the rate of antibody acquisition between studies. However, it is likely that these assays detect a range of heterologous responses to Noroviruses, rather than antibodies specific for a single virus type.

Some 20 percent of individuals appear to be resistant to *Norovirus* infections (Graham et al. 1994). Norwalk virus VLPs were used in an interesting study to investigate their binding properties to epithelial cells (Marionneau et al. 2002). This study showed that Norwalk virus VLPs attach to the surface of epithelial cells, but only for secretor phenotype individuals, who represent 80 percent of American/European populations. Inactivation of the *FUT2* gene (chromosome 19) is the predominant mutation that defines the nonsecretor phenotype. Competitive binding studies using H1 and/or H3/4 trisaccharides confirmed that Norwalk virus VLPs uses these as ligands for binding to epithelial cells of secretors, and this may in part account for the susceptibilty of the general population. A separate volunteer challenge study (Hutson et al. 2002) showed that patients with the B blood group antigen have a decreased risk of *Norovirus* infection; however, this work did not evaluate the secretor status of the individuals tested. Recently it was shown, using a human challenge model, that 29 percent of a study population was homozygous recessive for the *FUT2* gene, and that these individuals were resistant to infection following challenge. However, some individuals in the susceptible population were resistant to infection, suggesting an immune component to resistance (Lindesmith et al. 2003).

Laboratory diagnosis

VIRUS ISOLATION

There are no reports of the isolation of Noroviruses in either cell or human intestinal organ cultures. Tests with a wide range of animals have also failed to identify a suitable model (Kapikian 1994), although recently it was reported that macaques could be experimentally infected with human Noroviruses (Subekti et al. 2002). Some success has been achieved with the transmission of Norwalk virus in chimpanzees, in which serological responses and excretion of Norwalk virus antigen in stools were described (Wyatt et al. 1978). It is, however, unlikely that isolation in cell cultures will ever be used for diagnosis, as in vitro methods are too slow and labor-intensive.

ELECTRON MICROSCOPY

EM is the most commonly used laboratory diagnostic method for direct detection of Noroviruses in stools. All Noroviruses are indistinguishable on EM when examined by routine negative staining methods (1.5 percent phosphotungstic acid at pH 6.5). Virions possess an amorphous surface structure, lacking a defined symmetry, with a ragged outline (Figure 42.7a) that probably explains the wide range of particle diameters (32–38 nm) reported. It is essential that preparations of Noroviruses are examined in the absence of antibody, which can mask the surface structure and lead to incorrect identification (Caul and Appleton 1982).

Noroviruses are commonly excreted in feces as small aggregates and in very low numbers at 10^6 viruses/g of stool (relative to other enteric viral infections, e.g rotaviruses and adenoviruses). These concentrations are close to the limit of sensitivity of the EM, so careful examination of preparations is necessary. Contamination with other proteins in clinical samples often obscures Noroviruses, and can be overcome by applying SPIEM with human convalescent sera. Samples prepared in this way are superior to conventional methods of virus concentration used in EM and significantly increase the detection rate of Noroviruses. SPIEM is as sensitive as molecular methods for detecting Noroviruses (Green et al. 1995) and has the advantage of speed that is so important to the management of outbreaks. EM has the added value of being a 'catch-all' system, whereby all viruses associated with gastroenteritis can be detected. EM will probably retain an important role in the investigation of future *Norovirus* outbreaks, for which rapid diagnosis is a prerequisite.

SEROLOGICAL METHODS

The preparation of hyperimmune antisera to recombinant *Norovirus* capsid antigens has facilitated the development of an EIA for identifying naturally acquired or experimentally induced Norwalk virus antigen and antibody (Jiang et al. 1992; Treanor et al. 1993). Application of these new assays to volunteer studies has provided new insights into Norwalk virus infection (Graham et al. 1994), showing that seroconversions were highest among volunteers who experienced vomiting. The assays for Norwalk virus are highly specific, revealing more subclinical infections, longer periods of virus excretion (up to 7 days), and higher infection rates than were previously recognized (Graham et al. 1994). Subsequent to the development of the Norwalk virus EIA a range of antigen capture EIAs were developed based on polyclonal antisera from different animal species for the capture and detection of *Norovirus* antigens in human fecal specimens (Jiang et al. 1995a, b; Leite et al. 1996; Green et al. 1997; Hale et al. 1999; Vipond et al. 2000).

All these assays show a high degree of type or strain specificity, and as yet it has not been possible to develop a 'catch-all' antigen trap EIA. The EIA format for detection of Noroviruses in clinical specimens offers considerable advantages over RT-PCR. EIA is cheap, rapid, and simple, and thus easy to deploy in the routine diagnostic setting. Recently the first commercially available EIA has been brought to the diagnostic marketplace. This contains a mixture of polyclonal sera for antigen capture and monoclonal antibodies for detection, and is designed to detect a range of both genogroup I and genogroup II human Noroviruses.

RT-PCR

The characterization of the *Norovirus* genome has allowed the application of molecular techniques to the diagnosis of *Norovirus* infection. The scientific literature now abounds with RT-PCR-based studies. Most diagnostic RT-PCR approaches are based on the RNA polymerase and capsid regions of Noroviruses. Both these regions show considerable heterogeneity, allowing the division of human strains into a minimum of two genetic groups (Green et al. 1994) and many different clusters or clades. Molecular epidemiology is a powerful tool for the investigation of point-source outbreaks, particularly for examining shellfish (Atmar et al. 1993) and in monitoring the spread of Noroviruses (Green et al. 1995). These techniques are not used for routine diagnosis because of cost considerations and the need for specialized laboratory equipment (e.g. thermal cyclers), and are thus restricted to the research or reference laboratory.

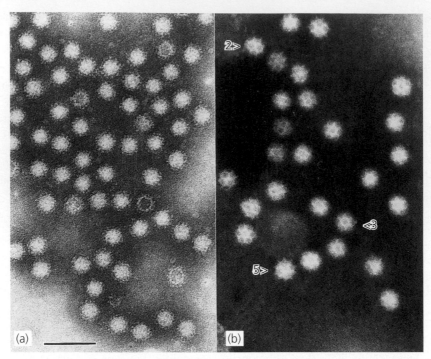

Figure 42.7 *Electron microscopic appearance of human enteric caliciviruses.* **(a)** *Noroviruses lack the distinctive surface morphology characteristic of Sapoviruses, although a ragged edge is clearly visible surrounding some of the particles.* **(b)** *The distinctive surface structures on a Sapovirus viewed along the two-, three- and fivefold (indicated) axes of symmetry. Bar, 100 nm for each panel.*

An electronic system (CaliciNet) has been developed at CDC Atlanta to fingerprint strains of Noroviruses that are associated with foodborne outbreaks (www.cdc.gov/foodsafety/fsactivities.htm).

Prevention and control

In volunteers, Noroviruses induce both short- and long-term immunity but, until the mechanisms are fully understood, it is unlikely that a vaccine can be developed (Green et al. 1995).

The high infectivity of Noroviruses and the explosive outbreaks of gastroenteritis that often occur in semi-closed communities present a major challenge to control of infection and require aggressive intervention (Caul 1994a; Chadwick and McCann 1994). Measures for interrupting the various modes of transmission (see Epidemiology) must include 'enteric' precautions, but these alone are ineffective and should be supplemented by measures to deal with patients who vomit (Chadwick et al. 2000). Symptomatic healthcare workers should be excluded from contact with patients for at least 2 days after resolution of symptoms. Effective handwashing should be routine. People caring for patients should wear disposable gloves, gowns, and masks when cleaning vomit, fecal material, or contaminated clothing. Soiled linen and clothes should be handled carefully, to minimize the generation of aerosols, and transported in plastic bags to the laundry. All potentially contaminated surfaces in toilets, bathrooms, and rooms occupied by patients should be disinfected with a chlorine-based product and cleaned with a hot detergent solution. Contact with other patients should be avoided.

Common-source outbreaks are well documented. Symptomatic food handlers have often been incriminated and must be excluded from the workplace for at least 2 days after resolution of symptoms. Decontamination of all potentially infected surfaces in the kitchens and associated rest and toilet facilities is essential (Caul et al. 1993). Suspect water supplies may require shock chlorine treatments. Shellfish are a particular problem in the transmission of Noroviruses, and the most effective preventive measure is to cultivate them in clean water, as depuration processes are not effective in eliminating Noroviruses from shellfish.

SAPOVIRUSES

Distinctive virus particles 30-40 nm in diameter and differing from both astroviruses and the Noroviruses were first recognized in fecal samples by negative staining techniques in 1976 (Madeley and Cosgrove 1976). These viruses, displaying a distinctive typical calicivirus morphology, have since been assigned to a separate genus (*Sapovirus*). Viral particles viewed along their threefold axes of symmetry possess a central stain-filled cup (calyx) surrounded by six peripheral cups, giving rise to the 'star of David' appearance. Viewed along their two-fold axes of symmetry they have four cups (Figure 42.7b). Particles viewed along their fivefold axes present as 10-pointed spheres and may not be identified so readily as the classic particles described above. Unlike astroviruses, which possess a smooth, entire edge, caliciviruses have a ragged outline which makes accurate measurement difficult, and explains the particle diameters of 31–38 nm quoted by most workers. Sapoviruses have a buoyant density of 1.37–1.38 g/cm^3 (Terashima et al. 1983). The history of these viruses has been reviewed (Chiba et al. 2000). The significance of molecular data to differentiate between classic caliciviruses and Noroviruses was first recognized in our laboratory (Lambden et al. 1994). Further extensive sequencing studies have shown that the classic caliciviruses have a different genome structure from the Noroviruses, and phylogenetic analysis clearly places them in a different genus. The prototype strain *Sapporo virus* was isolated from an orphanage in Sapporo, Japan (Chiba et al. 1979).

Detailed ultrastructural studies on caliciviruses showing the typical morphology have been performed only on animal caliciviruses (Prasad et al. 1994; Zheng et al. 2001). The three-dimensional structure of the viruses was determined by cryo-electron microscopy and computer image-processing techniques. The primate calicivirus virions are 40 nm in diameter and have a T = 3 icosahedral symmetry, with 32 surface depressions at the five- and three-fold axes of symmetry (Figure 42.2). The surface depressions are surrounded by 90 archlike capsomers, each of which is a capsid protein, in an arrangement similar to that seen in the Noroviruses.

Genome organization

Sequence analyses of isolates of Sapoviruses from the UK, USA, and Japan have been used to assign this group of viruses to a separate genus (Berke et al. 1997; Jiang et al. 1997; Lambden et al. 1994; Liu et al. 1995; Matson et al. 1995; Noel et al. 1997; Vinjé et al. 2000).

Only two complete genome sequences of human *Sapovirus* (UK/Manchester/93; UK/Bristol/98) have so far been described (Liu et al. 1995, 1997; Robinson et al. 2002), and the sequence and genome organization of these viruses support their allocation to a genus separate from the Noroviruses. The complete sequence of the Manchester isolate consists of 7 431 nt, with the first predicted in-frame AUG codon at position 13. The 3' end of the genome contains 84 untranslated nucleotides, followed by a polyadenylate tail. The genetically distinct Bristol isolate has a genome of 7 490 nt, with the predicted translation initiator codon at position 14. The 3' untranslated region of Bristol virus consists of 140 nt preceding the poly (A) tail. The small ORF overlapping the start of the capsid encoding region of the genome of Manchester virus was not present in the Bristol isolate, suggesting that this region of the genome may not encode a biologically active product. This overlapping sequence was also missing from the closely related London/92 isolate (Jiang et al. 1997). In common with all caliciviruses examined to date, Sapoviruses also possess the small 3' terminal ORF. Sequence comparisons and phylogenetic analyses suggest that the Sapoviruses form distinct genetic clusters in a manner analogous to the Noroviruses (Berke et al. 1997; Vinjé et al. 2000). A recent analysis has suggested that there may be two discrete genetic clades of human Sapoviruses, together with genetically distinct animal counterparts (Robinson et al. 2002), mirroring the situation in the *Norovirus* genus (Figure 42.5).

A fundamental difference between Noroviruses and Sapoviruses is that the region of the genome predicted to encode the structural capsid protein of Sapoviruses is in the same frame as ORF1 and contiguous with the RNA polymerase coding region, resulting in one large fused polyprotein (Figure 42.8). This genome organization is also found in the rabbit hepatotropic calicivirus, RHDV, and contrasts with those of all Noroviruses sequenced to date. The consequence of such a genome organization is that an additional proteolytic cleavage is required to release the RNA polymerase from the capsid protein.

A major feature that distinguishes the caliciviruses from the picornaviruses is the production of one or more species of subgenomic RNAs during replication. In the case of RHDV, a subgenomic RNA is also encapsidated into mature virus particles (Meyers et al. 1991; Zheng et al. 2001). The existence of a subgenomic RNA has not been established for Sapoviruses, and only indirect evidence exists for Norwalk virus. The 5' terminal sequences of the putative subgenomic RNAs share sequence homology with the 5' genomic RNA termini, although the level of sequence identity was less than the analogous conserved motifs observed both for Noroviruses and animal caliciviruses. The conservation of sequence motifs suggests an important regulatory role for these regions of the genome, perhaps serving as promoters for the synthesis of genomic and subgenomic RNAs from negative-strand intermediates.

Viral proteins

The lack of a productive cell culture system for Sapoviruses and the resistance of adults to experimental infection (Cubitt 1994) has greatly impeded analysis of the viral polypeptides. During acute infection the viruses are, however, shed in relatively high concentrations. A single fecal specimen obtained during an outbreak of acute gastroenteritis in an orphanage in Sapporo, Japan, was used for the purification of virions (Terashima et al. 1983). This study showed that classic *Sapovirus* particles contain a single polypeptide of 62 kDa that could be precipitated with convalescent (4 weeks) but not acute-phase (2 days) serum from the same patient.

The large ORF1 has a coding potential of 2 280 amino acids and includes conserved motifs typical of the 2C NTPase, 3C protease, and 3D RNA polymerase in

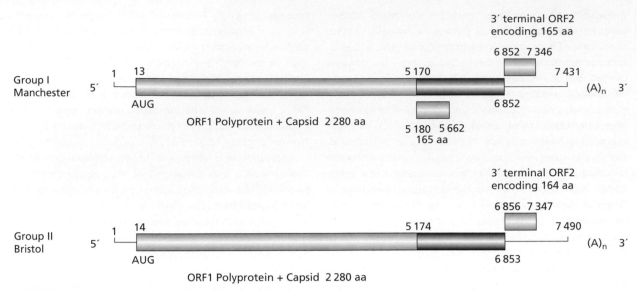

Figure 42.8 *Comparison of the genome structures of groups I and II Sapoviruses (Manchester, EMBL/GenBank Accession No. X86560; Bristol, EMBL/GenBank Accession No. AJ249939). Shaded boxes represent computer-predicted open reading frames. Translation products and their sizes are indicated on the open reading frames. The darker shaded area at the 3′ terminus of ORF1 represents the capsid coding region which is fused to the ORF1 nonstructural polyprotein. In group I Sapoviruses an additional small protein (161 aa) encoded in an alternative reading frame is predicted within the capsid coding region.*

relative genomic positions similar to those of other caliciviruses. Sequence comparisons of Sapoviruses with other caliciviruses, including the Noroviruses, show only 20–40 percent amino acid identity in the functional domains of the nonstructural polyprotein. Relatively little is known about polyprotein processing in Sapoviruses, except that in vitro protein synthesis in a coupled transcription translation reaction yields a very different cleavage pattern from the Noroviruses (Clarke and Lambden 2000). The exact cleavage dipeptide has not been experimentally determined for Sapoviruses, but it is likely that these viruses will show a similar site preference for EG residues.

Clinical manifestations

Symptomatic *Sapovirus* infection occurs most often in infants and young children, and appears indistinguishable from the milder forms of rotavirus infection (Cubitt 1987; Cubitt and McSwiggan 1981; Sakai et al. 2001; Suzuki et al. 1979). Transmission is by person-to-person spread through the fecal–oral route, and this is probably important in maintaining an endemic state in some semi-closed communities. Contaminated shellfish, cold foods, and drinking water have also been implicated as vehicles of infection (Cubitt 1988).

The incubation period is 1–3 days and symptoms persist for an average of 4 days. Diarrhea and vomiting are common, whereas fever with upper respiratory symptoms is less so. There is no evidence that Sapoviruses replicate in respiratory mucosal cells or that respiratory spread occurs. As respiratory symptoms have

been described mainly in young children, they may arise from one of the concomitant respiratory viral infections common in this age group.

Pathogenesis

In contrast to Noroviruses there have been no reports of ultrastructural studies of human *Sapovirus* infections in the gut. Analogy with all the other 'diarrhea viruses' would suggest that human Sapoviruses replicate in mucosal cells lining the villi of the small intestine. In limited adult volunteer studies the virus was administered by the nasal/oral route (Cubitt 1994). Symptoms were inapparent, or ranged from mild to moderately severe, where the latter included nausea, vomiting, diarrhea, pyrexia, and abdominal pains. These clinical features resemble those in naturally acquired infections.

Epidemiology

Most of our data on the epidemiology of Sapoviruses derives from EM observations and seroprevalence studies using purified viruses or hyperimmune sera in blocking ELISAs, although latterly some RT-PCR surveys have been conducted. When the Sapoviruses were first discovered it was not possible to assign a causal role because 20 percent of children excreting them were asymptomatic. Subsequently, an outbreak of gastroenteritis in an infant and junior school in north London was investigated and a *Sapovirus* was shown to be the causal agent (Cubitt et al. 1979) This outbreak was mistakenly described as 'winter vomiting disease,' although spread to others in the school and to home contacts was negligible, being perhaps limited by their immunity. These epidemiological and immunological features are not consistent with 'winter vomiting disease' caused by Noroviruses. Sapoviruses have since been established as enteric pathogens (Christensen 1989; Cubitt 1994). In children hospitalized with sporadic diarrhea, excretion rates of 0.9–6.6 percent have been reported (Cubitt and McSwiggan 1981; Suzuki et al. 1979). A similar excretion rate (2.9 percent) was reported in a daycare center in the USA (Matson et al. 1989). All these studies suggest that Sapoviruses are a minor cause of clinically significant disease. In contrast with infection in older children, neonatal infection is often subclinical (Matson et al. 1990). These observations are supported by data from the IID study in England and Wales which showed that Sapoviruses were found most frequently in children between the ages of 1 and 4 years, and constituted 7 percent of the viruses identified in the general practice component of this study (Food Standards Agency 2000). This is in agreement with an RT-PCR survey conducted in Japan, where 6.6 percent of patients with gastroenteritis were positive for Sapoviruses (Okada et al. 2002), and a survey of children aged 2–24 months in Finland, where 9.2 percent of stool specimens were positive (Pang et al. 2001).

Sapovirus infections are endemic in the UK, usually appearing sporadically in young children, although community and nosocomial outbreaks have also been recognized. Outbreaks have been reported in Japan (Chiba et al. 1979; Oishi et al. 1980), Australia (Grohmann et al. 1991), England (Cubitt et al. 1979, 1980; Cubitt and McSwiggan 1981; Gray et al. 1987; Humphrey et al. 1984), Canada (Spratt et al. 1978), and Scandinavia (Kjeldsberg 1977), not only among children but also among elderly patients in nursing homes, where the attack rates ranged from 50 to 70 percent. Outbreaks among adults and elderly patients are unusual and may represent infections that have arisen because of waning immunity. A distinct seasonality has not been described for *Sapovirus* infections, primarily because too few cases were reported from which to analyze seasonality.

Seroepidemiology

Progress in understanding the seroepidemiology of Sapoviruses has been dependent on using viruses from fecal specimens. Attempts at expression of the human *Sapovirus* major capsid protein in insect cells using recombinant baculoviruses have met with mixed fortunes. Whereas some laboratories have reported success in obtaining recombinant VLPs with a structure and morphology similar to those of the native virions, in most cases these VLPs are unstable. Fortunately, it has been possible to purify sufficient *Sapovirus* particles from stool samples to produce diagnostic antigen trap ELISAs. Such an ELISA was also used in a blocking assay presenting captured antigen from stool specimens to measure antibodies to Sapoviruses in 128 serum samples from an age-stratified population from the USA. This important study showed a high incidence of antibody in young children, reaching 100 percent in the 4–6-year age group (Nakata et al. 1988). Thus immunity to Sapoviruses appears to be long-lived, in sharp contrast to *Norovirus* infections, where the short-term immunity allows symptomatic reinfections (Greenberg and Matsui 1992).

In Japan, antibody to *Sapovirus* is rapidly acquired between 6 months and 2 years of age, with a prevalence of 30 percent, rising to 65 percent in 2–5-year-olds and approximately 90 percent in older children and adults (Nakata et al. 1985; Sakuma 1981). Tests on pooled γ-globulin and serum samples in all continents confirm these findings (Christensen 1989). The high seroprevalence in early childhood agrees with the reported excretion rates of Sapoviruses in young children. The paucity of reports of *Sapovirus* infection in hospitalized children with diarrhea suggests that asymptomatic – or at least clinically insignificant – disease in childhood is common.

Laboratory diagnosis

VIRUS ISOLATION

Human Sapoviruses cannot be grown in cell culture, although there is a single report of serial propagation of human *Sapovirus* in dolphin kidney and HEK cells in the presence of trypsin (Cubitt and Barrett 1984). In this work, cytoplasmic replication was demonstrated by immunofluorescence and by radiolabeling of polypeptides. This report has not been confirmed, and many other workers have failed to propagate human Sapoviruses in vitro.

ELECTRON MICROSCOPY

The unique morphology of Sapoviruses allows definitive identification by EM (Madeley 1979), and micrographs should always be checked to confirm direct observations with the EM. The characteristic morphology has been the main criterion for identifying Sapoviruses. If the morphology suggests a *Sapovirus* but is not convincing, RT-PCR analysis may confirm the diagnosis (Honma et al. 2000; Robinson et al. 2002). EM is currently the only routine method available for laboratory diagnosis, and requires skilled operators to achieve consistent results.

IMMUNOASSAYS

The need for alternative methods of identifying caliciviruses in stool samples has been generally recognized.

Nakata and co-workers (Nakata et al. 1983) found that a solid-phase RIA using a hyperimmune guinea-pig serum was more sensitive than EM. This assay was later modified to an EIA of similar sensitivity (Nakata et al. 1988). No commercially produced ELISA tests are available to the routine laboratory.

SEROLOGY

Specific IgM, seroconversions or rising titers of specific IgG have been observed following infection (Chiba et al. 1979; Cubitt et al. 1979; Cubitt et al. 1980; Cubitt et al. 1981; Nakata et al. 1985; Sakuma 1981). These techniques, although useful in epidemiological studies, are not ethically justified for diagnosing enteric 'diarrhoea virus' infections in young children because they involve taking blood samples.

PREVENTION AND CONTROL

The measures needed to prevent the spread of calicivirus infections are the same as those recommended in the previous section on Prevention and control.

ANIMAL ENTERIC CALICIVIRUSES

Following the discovery of human enteric caliciviruses similar viruses were found in cattle and swine. These viruses were either observed directly by EM or, in some cases, their presence was inferred by a positive polymerase chain reaction (PCR). With improved detection technology it is likely that other mammalian enteric caliciviruses are yet to be discovered, and although there is no evidence for cross-species infection, an animal reservoir for human infection remains a possibility.

Noroviruses

Early studies revealed the presence of viruses resembling Noroviruses in fecal specimens from cattle (Almeida et al. 1978; Granzow and Schirrmeier 1985; Günther et al. 1984; Woode and Bridger 1978). The first bovine Noroviruses were described in England and, following the tradition established for the human Noroviruses, are called Newbury agents 1 and 2 after the geographical location where they were discovered (Woode and Bridger 1978). The Newbury agent 1 (NA1), like the human Noroviruses, has a single major capsid protein (Dastjerdi et al. 2000). Following the discovery of the Newbury agents similar viruses were also found by two independent groups in the former East Germany (Granzow and Schirrmeier 1985; Günther et al. 1984). Since these early studies the application of RT-PCR to fecal specimens from farm animals has revealed the presence of *Norovirus*-like sequences in both swine (Sugieda and Nakajima 2002; Sugieda et al. 1998) and cattle (van der Poel et al. 2000).

The complete genome sequence of a bovine virus (Jena virus (JV)) has been determined (Liu et al. 1999a) and shows that the JV genome organization is very similar to that of the human Noroviruses. Sequence analysis of the capsid region of Newbury agent 2 (NA2) has confirmed the relationship of the bovine Noroviruses to the human Noroviruses, and phylogenetic analysis suggests that the bovine Noroviruses belong to a distinct genetic group (Belliot et al. 2001). Bovine Noroviruses do not grow in cell culture; however, calves have been used in an experimental setting to study infection. Newborn calves and calves up to 60 days of age are susceptible to infection with bovine Noroviruses (Bridger 1990). Virus replication occurs in the enterocytes of the small intestine, showing a similar tissue and cell tropism to that observed for human Noroviruses (Hall et al. 1984).

EM studies from the 1980s suggested that bovine Noroviruses are 'commonly found in the British calf population' (Bridger et al. 1984). Recently the capsid protein of JV has been expressed in insect cells using a recombinant baculovirus vector. The protein assembled to form VLPs, and this allowed the development of a diagnostic ELISA and an ELISA to study the seroprevalence of JV. The antigen capture ELISA was used to survey fecal specimens collected from calves in dairy herds in Germany, and showed that 8.9 percent of the samples were positive for JV infection. Seroepidemiological data from the same study indicated that 99.1 percent of cattle have antibodies to JV. The very high seroprevalence for JV suggests that bovine *Norovirus* infections are endemic, and the high antibody levels in older cattle suggests that they are constantly re-exposed to infection. These observations, coupled to the findings of RT-PCR surveillance in other countries which has identified *Norovirus* sequences in bovine and swine, confirms the widespread nature of *Norovirus* infections, and it would seem likely that Noroviruses remain to be found infecting other mammalian species. It has been suggested that animal Noroviruses could be a source of infection for humans. Although there are no data on the susceptibility of humans to animal *Norovirus* infections (with the exception of a single report), no human Noroviruses have been shown to infect and cause disease in other mammalian species. Thus the bovine system may provide an important animal model for studying the human viruses.

A bovine calicivirus morphologically indistinguishable from the Noroviruses was recently sequenced in the USA (Smiley et al. 2002). This virus (BEC NB) was originally observed in 1980, along with a coronavirus, in a fecal specimen from a calf in Nebraska, Ohio. However, the genome organization of BEC NB resembled that of the Sapoviruses, with the ORF1 polyprotein fused to and contiguous with the capsid encoding region of the genome. In experimental infections of calves, BEC NB showed similar intestinal lesions and tropism to the bovine Noroviruses. Phylogenetic analysis suggests that BEC NB may be a representative of new genus of enteric caliciviruses.

Sapoviruses

Membership of the *Sapovirus* genus is defined on the basis of phylogeny and the organization of the viral genome. An enteric calicivirus infecting swine was first described in the USA in 1980 (Saif et al. 1980). Experimental infections with this virus (Cowden PECV) using gnotobiotic piglets established a causal role in enteric disease. Infection results in villous atrophy and profuse diarrhea. The adaptation of Cowden PECV to growth in cell culture marked an important and significant breakthrough in calicivirus research, as this is the only enteric calicivirus that can be cultured. Following serial passage through gnotobiotic piglets the virus was adapted to grow in primary porcine embryonic kidney cells (Flynn and Saif 1988), and then in a continuous pig kidney cell line (Parwani et al. 1991). The key factor in this success was the incorporation of the intestinal contents of uninfected gnotobiotic piglets into the cell culture medium. The growth-promoting factors of the intestinal contents of piglets have been investigated in depth (Chang et al. 2002). Pretreatment of cells or PECV prior to infection (30 min) with intestinal contents, followed by removal, failed to support viral growth, suggesting that cells needed constant signaling/stimulation from intestinal contents to allow viral growth. Transfection with synthetic genomes of PECV (bypassing receptor binding by the virus) only produced infectious progeny when intestinal contents were continually present. However, the addition of suramin, together with other adenylate cyclase inhibitors, restricted the growth-promoting effect of intestinal contents, suggesting that replication of PECV is dependent on a cAMP signaling pathway that is induced by intestinal contents. Interestingly, the cell culture-adapted virus did not produce clinical disease in experimentally infected piglets (Guo et al. 2001b), suggesting that the cell culture adaptation process had attenuated the virus. The complete genome sequences were determined for wildtype (wt) and cell culture-adapted strains (tc) of Cowden PECV. The genome organization of Cowden PECV conforms closely with that of human Sapoviruses (see Genome organization). PECV tc showed two silent mutations and two amino acid changes in ORF1, and five nucleotide changes in the capsid that result in four amino acid changes compared to PECV wt. It was speculated that the changes in the capsid sequence are responsible for the attenuation of the cell culture-adapted virus (Guo et al. 1999) The capsid protein of Cowden PECV has been expressed in insect cells using a recombinant baculovirus, and undergoes spontaneous assembly to form virus-like particles that are morphologically and antigenically similar to the native virus (Guo et al. 2001c).

Insect cells infected by the recombinant baculovirus were used to investigate seroresponses of experimentally infected piglets, and an antigen trap ELISA was developed using hyperimmune sera raised to the VLPs. A preliminary survey using this ELISA showed that variants of PECV were circulating in local swine herds.

It seems likely that there are as yet undiscovered Sapoviruses infecting other animal species. Confirmation that a candidate calicivirus belongs to the *Sapovirus* genus requires phylogenetic and genome organization analyses. An enteric calicivirus was described in mink, but this virus could not be grown in cell culture. RT-PCR of a fragment of the *RNA polymerase* gene showed that the mink virus was closely related to PECV (Guo et al. 2001a). However, the mink from the farm where the virus was discovered had been fed raw offal from pigs, casting doubt on the precise origin of the virus.

REFERENCES

Adler, J.L. and Zickl, R. 1969. Winter vomiting disease. *J Infect Dis*, **119**, 668–73.

Agus, S.G., Dolin, R., et al. 1973. Acute infectious nonbacterial gastroenteritis: intestinal histopathology. Histologic and enzymatic alterations during illness produced by the Norwalk agent in man. *Ann Intern Med*, **79**, 18–25.

Almeida, J.D., Craig, C.R. and Hall, T.E. 1978. Multiple viruses present in the faeces of a scouring calf. *Vet Rec*, **102**, 170–1.

Ando, T., Mulders, M.N., et al. 1994. Comparison of the polymerase region of small round structured virus strains previously classified in three antigenic types by solid-phase immune electron microscopy. *Arch Virol*, **135**, 217–26.

Appleton, H. and Pereira, M.S. 1977. A possible virus ætiology in outbreaks of food-poisoning from cockles. *Lancet*, **i**, 780–1.

Atmar, R.L., Metcalf, T.G., et al. 1993. Detection of enteric viruses in oysters by using the polymerase chain-reaction. *Appl Env Microbiol*, **59**, 631–5.

Belliot, G.M., Frankhauser, R.L., et al. 2001. Characterization of 'Norwalk-like viruses' and astroviruses by liquid hybridization assay. *J Virol Meth*, **91**, 119–30.

Berke, T., Golding, B., et al. 1997. Phylogenetic analysis of the caliciviruses. *J Med Virol*, **52**, 419–24.

Bertolotti-Ciarlet, A., White, L.J., et al. 2002. Structural assembly of Norwalk virus-like particles. *J Virol*, **76**, 4044–55.

Blacklow, N.R. and Greenberg, H.B. 1991. Medical progress: viral gastroenteritis. *N Engl J Med*, **325**, 252–64.

Blacklow, N.R., Herrmann, J.E. 1988. Norwalk virus, Proceedings of the Ninth BSG SK&F International Workshop, 65–9.

Bradley, W.H. 1943. Epidemic nausea and vomiting. *Br Med J*, **1**, 309–12.

Bridger, J.C. 1990. Small viruses associated with gastroenteritis in animals. In: Saif, L.J. and Theil, K.W. (eds), *Viral diarrheas of man and animals*. Boca Raton: CRC Press, 161–82.

Bridger, J.C., Hall, G.A., et al. 1984. Characterization of a calici-like virus (Newbury agent) found in association with astrovirus in bovine diarrhea. *Infect Immun*, **43**, 133–8.

Caul, E.O. 1988. Small round human fecal viruses. In: Pattison, J.R. (ed.), *Parvoviruses and human disease*. Boca Raton: CRC Press, 139–63.

Caul, E.O. 1994a. Small round structured viruses: airborne transmission and hospital control. *Lancet*, **343**, 1240–2.

Caul, E.O. 1994b. Viruses in food. In: Spencer, R.C., Wright, E.P., et al. (eds), *Rapid methods and automation in microbiology and immunology*. Andover: Intercept, 347–54.

Caul, E.O. and Appleton, H. 1982. The electron microscopical and physical characteristics of small round human fecal viruses: an interim scheme for classification. *J Med Virol*, **9**, 257–65.

Caul, E.O., Ashley, C.R., et al. 1979. 'Norwalk'-like particles in epidemic gastroenteritis in the UK. *Lancet*, **2**, 1292.

Caul, E.O., Sellwood, N.J., et al. 1993. Outbreaks of gastroenteritis associated with SRSVs. *PHLS Microbiol Digest*, **10**, 2–8.

Chadwick, P.R. and McCann, R. 1994. Transmission of a small round structured virus by vomiting during a hospital outbreak of gastroenteritis. *J Hosp Infect*, **26**, 251–9.

Chadwick, P.R., Beards, G., et al. 2000. Management of hospital outbreaks of gastro-enteritis due to small round structured viruses. *J Hosp Infect*, **45**, 1–10.

Chang, K.O., Kim, Y., et al. 2002. Cell-culture propagation of porcine enteric calicivirus mediated by intestinal contents is dependent on the cyclic AMP signaling pathway. *Virology*, **304**, 302–10.

Chiba, S., Sakuma, Y., et al. 1979. An outbreak of gastroenteritis associated with calicivirus in an infant home. *J Med Virol*, **4**, 249–54.

Chiba, S., Nakata, S., et al. 2000. Sapporo virus: history and recent findings. *J Infect Dis*, **181**, Suppl. 2, S303–8.

Christensen, M.L. 1989. Human viral gastroenteritis. *Clin Microbiol Rev*, **2**, 51–89.

Christopher, P.J., Grohmann, G.S., et al. 1978. Parvovirus gastroenteritis – a new entity for Australia. *Med J Aust*, **1**, 121–4.

Clarke, I.N. and Lambden, P.R. 2000. Organisation and expression of calicivirus genes. *J Infect Dis*, **181**, S309–16.

Clarke, S.K.R., Cook, G.T., et al. 1972. A virus from epidemic vomiting disease. *Br Med J*, **3**, 86–9.

Cubitt, W.D. 1987. The candidate caliciviruses. *Ciba Found Symp*, **128**, 126–43.

Cubitt, W.D. 1988. *Caliciviruses*, Proceedings of the Ninth BSG SK&F International Workshop, 82–4.

Cubitt, W.D. 1994. Caliciviruses. In: Kapikian, A.Z. (ed.), 2nd edn, *Viral infections of the gastrointestinal tract*, Vol. 10. 2nd edn. New York: Marcel Dekker, 549–68.

Cubitt, W.D. and Barrett, A.D.T. 1984. Propagation of human candidate calicivirus in cell culture. *J Gen Virol*, **65**, 1123–6.

Cubitt, W.D. and McSwiggan, D.A. 1981. Calicivirus gastroenteritis in north west London. *Lancet*, **2**, 975–7.

Cubitt, W.D., McSwiggan, D.A. and Moore, W. 1979. Winter vomiting disease caused by calicivirus. *J Clin Pathol*, **32**, 786–93.

Cubitt, W.D., McSwiggan, D.A. and Arstali, S. 1980. An outbreak of calicivirus infection in a mother and baby unit. *J Clin Pathol*, **33**, 1095–8.

Cubitt, W.D., Pead, P.J. and Saeed, A.A. 1981. A new serotype of calicivirus associated with an outbreak of gastroenteritis in a residential home for the elderly. *J Clin Pathol*, **34**, 924–6.

Cubitt, W.D., Jiang, X.J., et al. 1994. Sequence similarity of human caliciviruses and small round structured viruses. *J Med Virol*, **43**, 252–8.

Cubitt, W.D., Green, K.Y. and Payment, P. 1998. Prevalence of antibodies to the Hawaii strain of human calicivirus as measured by a recombinant protein based immunoassay. *J Med Virol*, **54**, 135–9.

Cukor, G.C. and Blacklow, N.R. 1984. Human viral gastroenteritis. *Microbiol Rev*, **48**, 157–79.

Dastjerdi, A.M., Snodgrass, D.R. and Bridger, J.C. 2000. Characterisation of the bovine enteric calici-like virus, Newbury agent 1. *FEMS Microbiol Lett*, **192**, 125–31.

Dimitrov, D.H., Dashti, S.A.H., et al. 1997. Prevalence of antibodies to human caliciviruses (HuCVs) in Kuwait established by ELISA using baculovirus-expressed capsid antigens representing two genogroups of HuCVs. *J Med Virol*, **51**, 115–18.

Dingle, K.E., Lambden, P.R., et al. 1995. Human enteric *Caliciviridae*: the complete genome sequence and expression of virus-like particles from a genetic group II small round structured virus. *J Gen Virol*, **76**, 2349–55.

Dolin, R., Blacklow, N.R., et al. 1971. Transmission of acute infectious nonbacterial gastroenteritis to volunteers by oral administration of stool filtrates. *J Infect Dis*, **123**, 307–12.

Dolin, R., Blacklow, N.R., et al. 1972. Biological properties of Norwalk agent of acute infectious nonbacterial gastroenteritis. *Proc Soc Exp Biol Med*, **140**, 578–83.

Dolin, R., Levy, A.G., et al. 1975. Viral gastroenteritis induced by the Hawaii agent: jejunal histopathology and serologic response. *Am J Med*, **59**, 761–8.

Dolin, R., Reichmann, R.C., et al. 1982. Detection by immune electron microscopy of the Snow Mountain agent of acute viral gastroenteritis. *J Infect Dis*, **146**, 184–9.

Flynn, W.T. and Saif, L.J. 1988. Serial propagation of porcine enteric calicivirus-like virus in primary porcine kidney-cell cultures. *J Clin Microbiol*, **26**, 206–12.

Food Standards Agency. 2000. A report of the study of infectious intestinal disease in England.

Glass, P.J., White, L.J., et al. 2000. Norwalk virus open reading frame 3 encodes a minor structural protein. *J Virol*, **74**, 6581–91.

Gordon, I., Ingraham, H.S. and Korns, R.F. 1947. Transmission of epidemic gastroenteritis to human volunteers by oral administration of fecal filtrates. *J Exp Med*, **86**, 409–22.

Graham, D.Y., Jiang, X., et al. 1994. Norwalk virus infection of volunteers: new insights based on improved assays. *J Infect Dis*, **170**, 34–43.

Granzow, H. and Schirrmeier, H. 1985. Identification of 32 nm viruses in faeces of diarrhoeic calves by electron microscopy. *Monats Veterinarmed*, **40**, 228–9.

Gray, J.D. 1939. Epidemic nausea and vomiting. *Br Med J*, **1**, 209–11.

Gray, J.J., Wreghitt, T.G., et al. 1987. An outbreak of gastroenteritis in a home for the elderly associated with astrovirus type-1 and human calicivirus. *J Med Virol*, **23**, 377–81.

Gray, J.J., Jiang, X., et al. 1993. Prevalence of antibodies to Norwalk virus in England: detection by enzyme-linked immunosorbent assay using baculovirus-expressed Norwalk virus capsid antigen. *J Clin Microbiol*, **31**, 1022–5.

Green, K.Y., Lew, J.F., et al. 1993. Comparison of the reactivities of baculovirus-expressed recombinant Norwalk virus capsid antigen with those of the native Norwalk virus antigen in serologic assays and some epidemiologic observations. *J Clin Microbiol*, **31**, 2185–91.

Green, K.Y., Kapikian, A.Z., et al. 1997. Expression and self-assembly of recombinant capsid protein from the antigenically distinct Hawaii human calicivirus. *J Clin Microbiol*, **35**, 1909–14.

Green, K.Y., Belliot, G., et al. 2002. A predominant role for Norwalk-like viruses as agents of epidemic gastroenteritis in Maryland nursing homes for the elderly. *J Infect Dis*, **185**, 133–46.

Green, S.M., Dingle, K.E., et al. 1994. Human enteric *Caliciviridae*: a new prevalent small round-structured virus group defined by RNA-dependent RNA polymerase and capsid diversity. *J Gen Virol*, **75**, 1883–8.

Green, S.M., Lambden, P.R., et al. 1995. Polymerase chain reaction detection of small round-structured viruses from two related hospital outbreaks of gastroenteritis using inosine-containing primers. *J Med Virol*, **45**, 197–202.

Greenberg, H.B. and Matsui, S.M. 1992. Astroviruses and caliciviruses: emerging enteric pathogens. *Infect Agent Dis*, **1**, 71–91.

Greenberg, H.B., Valdesuso, J., et al. 1979a. Role of Norwalk virus in outbreaks of nonbacterial gastroenteritis. *J Infect Dis*, **139**, 564–8.

Greenberg, H.B., Wyatt, R.G. and Kapikian, A.Z. 1979b. Norwalk virus in vomitus. *Lancet*, **1**, 55.

Greenberg, H.B., Valdesuso, J.R., et al. 1981. Proteins of Norwalk virus. *J Virol*, **37**, 994–9.

Grohmann, G.S., Glass, R.I.M., et al. 1991. Outbreak of human calicivirus gastroenteritis in a day-care center in Sydney, Australia. *J Clin Microbiol*, **29**, 544–50.

Günther, H., Otto, P. and Heilman, P. 1984. Studies into diarrhoea of young calves. Sixth communication: Detection and determination of pathogenicity of a bovine corona virus and an undefined icosahedric virus. *Arch Exp Vet Med Leipzig*, **38**, 781–92.

Guo, M., Chang, K.O., et al. 1999. Molecular characterisation of a porcine enteric calicivirus genetically related to Sapporo-like human caliciviruses. *J Virol*, **73**, 9625–31.

Guo, M., Evermann, J.F. and Saif, L.J. 2001a. Detection and molecular characterization of cultivable caliciviruses from clinically normal mink and enteric caliciviruses associated with diarrhea in mink. *Arch Virol*, **146**, 479–93.

Guo, M., Hayes, J., et al. 2001b. Comparative pathogenesis of tissue culture-adapted and wildtype Cowden porcine enteric calicivirus (PEC) in gnotobiotic pigs and induction of diarrhea by intravenous inoculation of wild-type PEC. *J Virol*, **75**, 9239–51.

Guo, M., Qian, Y. and Saif, L.J. 2001c. Expression and self-assembly in baculovirus of porcine enteric calicivirus capsids into virus-like particles and their use in an enzyme-linked immunosorbent assay for antibody detection in swine. *J Clin Microbiol*, **39**, 1487–93.

Gutierrez-Escolano, A.L., Brito, Z.U., et al. 2000. Interaction of cellular proteins with the 5′ end of Norwalk virus genomic RNA. *J Virol*, **74**, 8558–62.

Hale, A.D., Crawford, S.E., et al. 1999. Expression and self-assembly of Grimsby virus: Antigenic distinction from Norwalk and Mexico viruses. *Clin Diagn Lab Immunol*, **6**, 142–5.

Hall, G.A., Bridger, J.C., et al. 1984. Lesions of gnotobiotic calves experimentally infected with a calicivirus-like (Newbury) agent. *Vet Pathol*, **21**, 208–15.

Hardy, M.E. and Estes, M.K. 1996. Completion of the Norwalk virus genome sequence. *Virus Genes*, **12**, 287–90.

Hardy, M.E., White, L.J., et al. 1995. Specific proteolytic cleavage of recombinant Norwalk virus capsid protein. *J Virol*, **69**, 1693–8.

Hardy, M.E., Crone, T.J., et al. 2002. Substrate specificity of the Norwalk virus 3C-like proteinase. *Virus Res*, **89**, 29–39.

Hayashi, Y., Ando, T., et al. 1989. Western blot (immunoblot) assay of small, round-structured virus associated with an acute gastroenteritis outbreak in Tokyo. *J Clin Microbiol*, **27**, 1728–33.

Ho, M-S, Glass, R.I.M., et al. 1989. Viral gastroenteritis aboard a cruise ship. *Lancet*, **2**, 961–4.

Honma, S., Nakata, S., et al. 2000. Evaluation of nine sets of PCR primers in the RNA dependent RNA polymerase region for detection and differentiation of members of the family *Caliciviridae*, Norwalk virus and Sapporo virus. *Microbiol Immunol*, **44**, 411–19.

Humphrey, T.J., Cruickshank, J.G. and Cubitt, W.D. 1984. An outbreak of calicivirus associated gastroenteritis in an elderly persons home. A possible zoonosis? *J Hyg Camb*, **92**, 293–9.

Hutson, A.M., Atmar, R.L., et al. 2002. Norwalk virus infection and disease is associated with ABO histo-blood group type. *J Infect Dis*, **185**, 1335–7.

Jiang, X., Graham, D.Y., et al. 1990. Norwalk virus genome cloning and characterization. *Science*, **250**, 1580–3.

Jiang, X., Wang, M., et al. 1992. Expression, self-assembly, and antigenicity of the Norwalk virus capsid protein. *J Virol*, **66**, 6527–32.

Jiang, X., Wang, M., et al. 1993. Sequence and genomic organization of Norwalk virus. *Virology*, **195**, 51–61.

Jiang, X., Cubitt, D., et al. 1995a. Development of an ELISA to detect MX virus, a human calicivirus in the Snow Mountain agent genogroup. *J Gen Virol*, **76**, 2739–47.

Jiang, X., Matson, D.O., et al. 1995b. Expression, self-assembly, and antigenicity of a Snow Mountain agent-like calicivirus capsid protein. *J Clin Microbiol*, **33**, 1452–5.

Jiang, X., Cubitt, W.D., et al. 1997. Sapporo-like human caliciviruses are genetically and antigenically diverse. *Arch Virol*, **142**, 1813–27.

Jordan, W.S., Gordan, I. and Dorrance, W.R. 1953. A study of illness in a group of Cleveland families. VII. Transmission of acute nonbacterial gastroenteritis to volunteers: evidence for two different etiologic agents. *J Exp Med*, **98**, 461–75.

Kapikian, A.Z. 1994. Norwalk and Norwalk-like Viruses. In: Kapikian, A.Z. (ed.), *Viral infections of the gastrointestinal tract*, vol. 10, 2nd edn. New York: Marcel Dekker, 471–518.

Kapikian, A.Z., Wyatt, R.G., et al. 1972. Visualization by immune electron microscopy of a 27-nm particle associated with acute infectious nonbacterial gastroenteritis. *J Virol*, **10**, 1075–81.

Kapikian, A.Z., Greenberg, H.B., et al. 1978. Prevalence of antibody to the Norwalk agent by a newly developed immune adherence hemagglutination assay. *J Med Virol*, **2**, 281–94.

Kaplan, J.E., Gary, G.W., et al. 1982. Epidemiology of Norwalk gastroenteritis and the role of Norwalk virus in outbreaks of acute nonbacterial gastroenteritis. *Ann Intern Med*, **96**, 756–61.

Katayama, K., Shirato-Horikoshi, H., et al. 2002. Phylogenetic analysis of the complete genome of 18 Norwalk-like viruses. *Virology*, **299**, 225–39.

Kjeldsberg, E. 1977. Small spherical viruses in faeces from gastroenteritis patients. *Acta Pathol Microbiol Scand*, **85**, 351–4.

Kohn, M.A., Farley, T.A., et al. 1995. An outbreak of Norwalk virus gastroenteritis associated with eating raw oysters: implications for maintaining safe oyster beds. *J Am Med Assoc*, **273**, 466–71.

Lambden, P.R. and Clarke, I.N. 1995. Genome organization in the *Caliciviridae*. *Trends Microbiol*, **3**, 261–5.

Lambden, P.R., Caul, E.O., et al. 1993. Sequence and genome organization of a human small round-structured (Norwalk-like) virus. *Science*, **259**, 516–19.

Lambden, P.R., Caul, E.O., et al. 1994. Human enteric caliciviruses are genetically distinct from small round structured viruses. *Lancet*, **343**, 666–7.

Lambden, P.R., Liu, B.L. and Clarke, I.N. 1995. A conserved sequence motif at the 5′ terminus of the Southampton virus genome is characteristic of the *Caliciviridae*. *Virus Genes*, **10**, 149–52.

Le Guyader, F., Haugarreau, L., et al. 2000. Three-year study to assess human enteric viruses in shellfish. *Appl Env Microbiol*, **66**, 3241–8.

Leite, J.P.G., Ando, T., et al. 1996. Characterization of Toronto virus capsid protein expressed in baculovirus. *Arch Virol*, **141**, 865–75.

Lewis, D.C. 1990. Three serotypes of Norwalk-like virus demonstrated by solid-phase immune electron microscopy. *J Med Virol*, **30**, 77–81.

Lewis, D. 1991. Norwalk agent and other small-round structured viruses in the UK. *J Infect*, **23**, 220–2.

Lewis, D., Ando, T., et al. 1995. Use of solid-phase immune electron microscopy for classification of Norwalk-like viruses into six antigenic groups from 10 outbreaks of gastroenteritis in the United States. *J Clin Microbiol*, **33**, 501–4.

Lindesmith, L., Moe, C., et al. 2003. Human susceptibility and resistance to Norwalk virus infection. *Nature Med*, **9**, 548–53.

Liu, B.L., Clarke, I.N., et al. 1995. Human enteric caliciviruses have a unique genome structure and are distinct from the Norwalk-like viruses. *Arch Virol*, **140**, 1345–56.

Liu, B.L., Clarke, I.N. and Lambden, P.R. 1996. Polyprotein processing in Southampton virus: Identification of 3C-like protease cleavage sites by in vitro mutagenesis. *J Virol*, **70**, 2605–10.

Liu, B.L., Clarke, I.N., et al. 1997. The genomic 5′ terminus of Manchester calicivirus. *Virus Genes*, **15**, 25–8.

Liu, B.L., Lambden, P.R., et al. 1999a. Molecular characterization of a bovine enteric calicivirus: relationship to the Norwalk-like viruses. *J Virol*, **73**, 819–25.

Liu, B.L., Viljoen, G.J., et al. 1999b. Identification of further proteolytic cleavage sites in the Southampton calicivirus polyprotein by expression of the viral protease in *E. coli*. *J Gen Virol*, **80**, 291–6.

Machin, A., Alonso, J.M.M. and Parra, F. 2001. Identification of the amino acid residue involved in rabbit hemorrhagic disease virus VPg uridylylation. *J Biol Chem*, **276**, 27787–92.

Madeley, C.R. 1979. Comparison of the features of astroviruses and caliciviruses seen in samples of feces by electron microscopy. *J Infect Dis*, **139**, 519–23.

Madeley, C.R. and Cosgrove, B.P. 1976. Caliciviruses in man. *Lancet*, **i**, 199–200.

Madore, H.P., Treanor, J.J. and Dolin, R. 1986. Characterization of the Snow Mountain agent of viral gastroenteritis. *J Virol*, **58**, 487–92.

Madore, H.P., Treanor, J.J., et al. 1990. Antigenic relatedness among the Norwalk-like agents by serum antibody rises. *J Med Virol*, **32**, 96–101.

Marionneau, S., Ruvoen, N., et al. 2002. Norwalk virus binds to histo-blood group antigens present on gastroduodenal epithelial cells of secretor individuals. *Gastroenterology*, **122**, 1967–77.

Matson, D.O., Estes, M.K., et al. 1989. Human calicivirus-associated diarrhea in children attending day care centers. *J Infect Dis*, **159**, 71–8.

Matson, D.O., Estes, M.K., et al. 1990. Asymptomatic human calicivirus infection in a day-care center. *Pediatr Infect Dis J*, **9**, 190–6.

Matson, D.O., Zhong, W.-M., et al. 1995. Molecular characterization of a human calicivirus with sequence relationships closer to animal caliciviruses than other known human caliciviruses. *J Med Virol*, **45**, 215–22.

Matsui, S.M., Kim, J.P., et al. 1991. The isolation and characterization of a Norwalk virus-specific cDNA. *J Clin Invest*, **87**, 1456–61.

Meeroff, J.C., Schreiber, D.S., et al. 1980. Abnormal gastric motor functions in viral gastroenteritis. *Ann Intern Med*, **92**, 370–3.

Meyers, G., Wirblich, C. and Thiel, H.-J. 1991. Genomic and subgenomic RNAs of rabbit hemorrhagic disease virus are both protein-linked and packaged into particles. *Virology*, **184**, 677–86.

Meyers, G., Wirblich, C., et al. 2000. Rabbit hemorrhagic disease virus: genome organisation and polyprotein processing of a calicivirus studied after transient expression of cDNA constructs. *Virology*, **276**, 349–63.

Miller, R. and Raven, M. 1936. Epidemic nausea and vomiting. *Br Med J*, **1**, 1242–4.

Morens, D.M., Zweighaft, R.M., et al. 1979. A waterborne outbreak of gastroenteritis with secondary person-to-person spread. *Lancet*, **1**, 964–6.

Morse, D.L., Guzewich, J.J., et al. 1986. Widespread outbreaks of clam- and oyster-associated gastroenteritis: role of Norwalk virus. *N Engl J Med*, **314**, 678–81.

Murphy, A.M., Grohmann, G.S., et al. 1979. An Australia-wide outbreak of gastroenteritis from oysters caused by Norwalk virus. *Med J Aust*, **2**, 329–33.

Murphy, A.M., Grohmann, G.S., et al. 1982. Norwalk virus gastroenteritis following raw oyster consumption. *Am J Epidemiol*, **115**, 348–51.

Nakata, S., Chiba, S., et al. 1983. Microtiter solid phase radio-immunoassay for detection of human calicivirus in stools. *J Clin Microbiol*, **17**, 198–201.

Nakata, S., Chiba, S., et al. 1985. Humoral immunity in infants with gastroenteritis caused by human calicivirus. *J Infect Dis*, **152**, 274–9.

Nakata, S., Estes, M.K. and Chiba, S. 1988. Detection of human calicivirus antigen and antibody by enzyme-linked immunosorbent assays. *J Clin Microbiol*, **26**, 2001–5.

Noel, J.S., Liu, B.L., et al. 1997. Parkville virus: a novel genetic variant of human calicivirus in the Sapporo virus clade, associated with an outbreak of gastroenteritis in adults. *J Med Virol*, **52**, 173–8.

Oishi, I., Maeda, A., et al. 1980. Calicivirus detected in outbreaks of acute gastroenteritis in school children. *Biken J*, **23**, 163–8.

Oishi, I., Yamazaki, K., et al. 1992. Demonstration of low molecular weight polypeptides associated with small, round-structured viruses by Western immunoblot analysis. *Microbiol Immunol*, **36**, 1105–12.

Okada, S., Sekine, S., et al. 1990. Antigenic characterization of small, round-structured viruses by immune electron microscopy. *J Clin Microbiol*, **28**, 1244–8.

Okada, M., Shinozaki, K., et al. 2002. Molecular epidemiology and phylogenetic analysis of Sapporo-like viruses – Brief report. *Arch Virol*, **147**, 1445–51.

Pang, X.L., Zeng, S.Q., et al. 2001. Effect of rotavirus vaccine on Sapporo virus gastroenteritis in Finnish infants. *Pediatr Infect Dis J*, **20**, 295–300.

Parker, S.P., Cubitt, W.D., et al. 1994. Seroprevalence studies using a recombinant Norwalk virus protein enzyme immunoassay. *J Med Virol*, **42**, 146–50.

Parrino, T.A., Schreiber, D.S., et al. 1977. Clinical immunity in acute gastroenteritis caused by Norwalk agent. *N Engl J Med*, **297**, 86–9.

Parwani, A.V., Flynn, W.T., et al. 1991. Serial propagation of porcine enteric calicivirus in a continuous cell-line effect of medium supplementation with intestinal contents or enzymes. *Arch Virol*, **120**, 115–22.

Pelosi, E., Lambden, P.R., et al. 1999. The seroepidemiology of genogroup 1 and genogroup 2 Norwalk-like viruses in Italy. *J Med Virol*, **58**, 93–9.

Pether, J.V.S. and Caul, E.O. 1983. An outbreak of food-borne gastroenteritis in two hospitals associated with a Norwalk-like virus. *J Hyg*, **91**, 343–50.

Pfister, T. and Wimmer, E. 2001. Polypeptide p41 of a Norwalk-like virus is a nucleic acid-independent nucleoside triphosphatase. *J Virol*, **75**, 1611–19.

Pletneva, M.A., Sosnovtsev, S.V. and Green, K.Y. 2001. The genome of Hawaii virus and its relationship with other members of the *Caliciviridae*. *Virus Genes*, **23**, 5–16.

Prasad, B.V.V., Matson, D.O. and Smith, A.W. 1994. Three-dimensional structure of calicivirus. *J Mol Biol*, **240**, 256–64.

Prasad, B.V.V., Hardy, M.E., et al. 1999. X-ray crystallographic structure of the Norwalk virus capsid. *Science*, **286**, 287–90.

Prasad, B.V.V., Hardy, M.E. and Estes, M.K. 2000. Structural studies of recombinant Norwalk capsids. *J Infect Dis*, **181**, S317–21.

Reid, J.A., White, D.G., et al. 1988. Role of infected food handler in hotel outbreak of Norwalk-like viral gastroenteritis: implications for control. *Lancet*, **2**, 321–3.

Reimann, H.A., Price, A.H. and Hodges, J.H. 1945. The cause of epidemic diarrhea, nausea and vomiting (viral dysentery?). *Proc Soc Exp Biol Med*, **59**, 8–9.

Robinson, S., Clarke, I.N., et al. 2002. Epidemiology of human Sapporo-like caliciviruses in the south west of England: molecular characterisation of a genetically distinct isolate. *J Med Virol*, **67**, 282–8.

Rothnagel, R., Jiang, X., et al. 1994. Three-dimensional structure of baculovirus-expressed Norwalk virus capsids. *J Virol*, **68**, 5117–25.

Saif, L.J., Bohl, E.H., et al. 1980. Rotavirus-like, calicivirus-like, and 23p nm virus-like particles associated with diarrhea in young pigs. *J Clin Microbiol*, **23**, 105–11.

Sakai, Y., Nakata, S., et al. 2001. Clinical severity of Norwalk virus and Sapporo virus gastroenteritis in children in Hokkaido, Japan. *Pediatr Infect Dis J*, **20**, 849–53.

Sakuma, Y. 1981. Studies on infantile gastroenteritis due to calicivirus. *Sapporo Med J*, **50**, 225–37.

Sawyer, L.A., Murphy, J.J., et al. 1988. 25- to 30-nm virus particle associated with a hospital outbreak of acute gastroenteritis with evidence for airborne transmission. *Am J Epidemiol*, **127**, 1261–71.

Schreiber, D.S., Blacklow, N.R. and Trier, J.S. 1973. The mucosal lesion of the proximal small intestine in acute infectious nonbacterial gastroenteritis. *N Engl J Med*, **288**, 1318–23.

Schreiber, D.S., Blacklow, N.R. and Trier, J.S. 1974. The small intestinal lesion induced by Hawaii agent acute infectious nonbacterial gastroenteritis. *J Infect Dis*, **129**, 705–8.

Schreier, E., Doring, F. and Kunkel, U. 2000. Molecular epidemiology of outbreaks of gastroenteritis associated with small round structured viruses in Germany in 1997/98. *Arch Virol*, **145**, 443–53.

Seah, E.L., Marshall, J.A. and Wright, P.J. 1999. Open reading frame 1 of the Norwalk-like virus Camberwell: Completion of sequence and expression in mammalian cells. *J Virol*, **73**, 10531–5.

Smiley, J.R., Chang, K.O., et al. 2002. Characterization of an enteropathogenic bovine calicivirus representing a potentially new calicivirus genus. *J Virol*, **76**, 10089–98.

Someya, Y., Takeda, N. and Miyamura, T. 2000. Complete nucleotide sequence of the Chiba virus genome and functional expression of the 3C-like protease in *Escherichia coli*. *Virology*, **278**, 490–500.

Sosnovtsev, S.V. and Green, K.Y. 2000. Identification and genomic mapping of the ORF3 and VPg proteins in feline calicivirus virions. *Virology*, **277**, 193–203.

Sosnovtsev, S.V., Sosnovtseva, S.A. and Green, K.Y. 1998. Cleavage of the feline calicivirus capsid precursor is mediated by a virus-encoded proteinase. *J Virol*, **72**, 3051–9.

Sosnovtsev, S.V., Garfield, M. and Green, K.Y. 2002. Processing map and essential cleavage sites of the nonstructural polyprotein encoded by ORF1 of the feline calicivirus genome. *J Virol*, **76**, 7060–72.

Spratt, H.C., Marks, M.I., et al. 1978. Nosocomial infantile gastroenteritis associated with minirotavirus and calicivirus. *J Paediatr*, **93**, 922–6.

Subekti, D.S., Tjaniadi, P., et al. 2002. Experimental infection of *Macaca nemestrina* with a Toronto Norwalk-like virus of epidemic viral gastroenteritis. *J Med Virol*, **66**, 400–6.

Sugieda, M. and Nakajima, S. 2002. Viruses detected in the caecum contents of healthy pigs representing a new genetic cluster in genogroup II of the genus 'Norwalk-like viruses'. *Virus Res*, **87**, 165–72.

Sugieda, M., Nagaoka, H., et al. 1998. Detection of Norwalk-like virus genes in the caecum contents of pigs. *Arch Virol*, **143**, 1–7.

Suzuki, H., Konno, T., et al. 1979. The occurrence of calicivirus in infants with acute gastroenteritis. *J Med Virol*, **4**, 321–6.

Terashima, H., Chiba, S., et al. 1983. The polypeptide of a human calicivirus. *Arch Virol*, **78**, 1–7.

Thornhill, T.S., Wyatt, R.G., et al. 1977. Detection by immune electron microscopy of 26- to 27-nm viruslike particles associated with two family outbreaks of gastroenteritis. *J Infect Dis*, **135**, 20–7.

Treanor, J.J., Jiang, X., et al. 1993. Subclass-specific serum antibody responses to recombinant Norwalk virus capsid antigen (rNV) in adults infected with Norwalk, Snow Mountain, or Hawaii virus. *J Clin Mjcrobiol*, **31**, 1630–4.

van der Poel, W., Vinjé, J., et al. 2000. Norwalk-like calicivirus genes in farm animals. *Emerg Infect Dis*, **6**, 36–41.

Vinjé, J., Deijl, H., et al. 2000. Molecular detection and epidemiology of Sapporo-like viruses. *J Clin Microbiol*, **38**, 530–6.

Vipond, I.B., Pelosi, E., et al. 2000. A diagnostic EIA for detection of the prevalent SRSV strain in United Kingdom outbreaks of gastroenteritis. *J Med Virol*, **61**, 132–7.

Wang, J., Jiang, X., et al. 1994. Sequence diversity of small, round-structured viruses in the Norwalk virus group. *J Virol*, **68**, 5982–90.

Wirblich, C., Sibilia, M., et al. 1995. 3C-like protease of rabbit hemorrhagic disease virus: Identification of cleavage sites in the ORF1 polyprotein and analysis of cleavage specificity. *J Virol*, **69**, 7159–68.

Wirblich, C., Thiel, H-J and Meyers, G. 1996. Genetic map of the calicivirus rabbit hemorrhagic disease virus as deduced from in vitro translation studies. *J Virol*, **70**, 7974–83.

Woode, G.N. and Bridger, J.C. 1978. Isolation of small viruses resembling astroviruses and caliciviruses from acute enteritis of calves. *J Med Microbiol*, **11**, 441–52.

Wyatt, R.G., Dolin, R., et al. 1974. Comparison of three agents of acute infectious nonbacterial gastroenteritis by cross-challenge in volunteers. *J Infect Dis*, **129**, 709–14.

Wyatt, R.G., Greenberg, H.B., et al. 1978. Experimental infection of chimpanzees with the Norwalk agent of epidemic viral gastroenteritis. *J Med Virol*, **2**, 89–96.

Zahorsky, J. 1929. Hyperemesis hiemis or the winter vomiting disease. *Arch Pediatr*, **46**, 391–5.

Zheng, D., Xue, T., et al. 2001. Three-dimensional structure of the wild-type RHDV. *Chin Sci Bull*, **46**, 1005–9.

43

Reoviruses, orbiviruses, and coltiviruses

TERENCE S. DERMODY AND ULRICH DESSELBERGER

INTRODUCTION AND GENERAL CLASSIFICATION

The *Reoviridae* family contains ten genera:

- *Orthoreovirus*, *Rotavirus*, *Orbivirus*, all infecting animals and humans
- *Coltivirus* infecting insects, rodents, and humans
- *Aquareovirus* infecting fish and molluscs
- *Cypovirus* infecting insects
- *Fijivirus*, *Phytoreovirus*, and *Oryzavirus* infecting plants and insects (Mertens et al. 2000; Nibert and Schiff 2001).
- *Seadornavirus* infecting insects and humans (Attoui et al. 2000)

In this chapter *Orthoreovirus* is called **reovirus**, the term being an acronym derived from **r**espiratory, **e**nteric, **o**rphan viruses. Only the mammalian genera are discussed; the rotaviruses are reviewed in Chapter 44, Rotaviruses.

Members of the *Reoviridae* have the following features in common:

- They contain a genome of 10–12 segments of double-stranded RNA (dsRNA).
- They form icosahedral, nonenveloped particles of approximately 70–80 nm in diameter with a double- or triple-shelled capsid.
- They replicate in the cytoplasm of cells without complete uncoating, produce 5′ end-capped, non-polyadenylated mRNAs, and form intracytoplasmic inclusion bodies.

In comparison to many other viruses, the *Reoviridae* are relatively resistant to inactivation by heat, lipid solvents, and a wide range of pH (with the exception of the orbiviruses, which lose infectivity at low pH).

Full-length sequences of the genomes of several strains of reo-, rota-, and orbiviruses are known, and the protein-coding assignments have been established. The overall genome size in bp (genomic molecular mass in kDa) is 23 540 bp (7 770 kDa) for reoviruses (type 3 reovirus), 18 555 bp (6 120 kDa) for rotaviruses (SA 11 rotavirus), and 19 218 bp (6 340 kDa) for orbiviruses [bluetongue virus type 10 (BTV 10)] (Mertens et al. 2000). The 5′ and 3′ untranslated regions (UTR) of all reovirus RNAs are short (reovirus: 5′-UTR 13–32 nt, 3′-UTR 35–83 nt; rotavirus: 5′-UTR 9–49 nt, 3′-UTR 17–182 nt; orbivirus: 5′-UTR 11–34 nt, 3′-UTR 31–116 nt).

Reoviruses have been isolated from humans but are rarely associated with disease. They cause systemic disease in rodents (mice), and the mouse model of reovirus infection has been used extensively to study mechanisms of viral pathogenesis (Virgin et al. 1997). Rotaviruses are the major cause of infantile gastro-enteritis worldwide and the causative agent of acute diarrhea in the young of many mammalian species (e.g. calves, piglets, and lambs). Orbiviruses mainly infect animals, producing severe disease (e.g. African horse sickness, epizootic hemorrhagic disease in cattle and deer, and bluetongue disease in sheep). *Coltivirus* causes Colorado tick fever in humans. Mammalian reoviruses have a broad host range and frequently contaminate water supplies. Rotaviruses are most commonly spread by the fecal–oral route, and orbiviruses are transmitted by a variety of ticks and mosquitoes.

REOVIRUSES

Genome, gene protein assignment, and structure

Orthoreoviruses (reoviruses) are found worldwide in a wide range of vertebrates. They cause hepatic and neurological disease in mice, diarrhea in cattle and sheep, and respiratory tract infections in dogs. In birds, reovirus infections are associated with hepatitis, arthritis, and diarrhea. There are three serotypes of mammalian reovirus, each represented by a prototype strain isolated from a human host: type 1 Lang (T1L), type 2 Jones (T2J), and type 3 Dearing (T3D).

The reovirus genome consists of ten segments of dsRNA that fall into three size classes, which for strain T3D are: large (L), 3 854–3 916 bp; medium (M), 2 203–2 304 bp; and small (S) 1 189–1 416 bp (Nibert and Schiff 2001). The viral proteins are designated according to size: λ for proteins encoded by large gene segments, μ by medium segments, and σ by small segments. Each gene segment is monocistronic with the exception of the *S1* gene, which encodes the viral attachment protein, $\sigma1$, and a small nonstructural protein, $\sigma1s$. Several protein products are modified post-translationally. The genome segments, their size in bp, and the size, number of molecules, and location in the virion, post-translational modifications, and some of the recognized functions of the protein products are shown in Table 43.1.

Reovirus virions consist of two concentric protein shells, called outer capsid and core. Three different types of reovirus particles are formed during the process of viral disassembly (Figure 43.1, p. 935):

1 Virions contain the full complement of eight structural proteins. These represent the infectious form of the virus and are capable of spread from host to host.
2 Infectious subvirion particles (ISVP) lack $\sigma3$, contain particle-associated cleavage fragments of $\mu1$ called δ and ϕ, and have an extended form of $\sigma1$. ISVPs are formed in the intestinal lumen or in the endocytic pathway.
3 Cores are devoid of outer-capsid proteins. These particles are enzymatically active and catalyze synthesis of viral RNA.

There are 11 reovirus proteins, eight structural proteins ($\lambda1$, $\lambda2$, $\lambda3$, $\mu1$, $\mu2$, $\sigma1$, $\sigma2$, and $\sigma3$) and three nonstructural proteins (μNS, σNS, and $\sigma1s$). Image reconstructions of cryo-electron micrographs of reovirus particles (Metcalf et al. 1991; Dryden et al. 1993, 1998) (Figure 43.1) combined with X-ray crystallographic analysis of cores (Reinisch et al. 2000) and outer-capsid proteins (Olland et al. 2001; Chappell et al. 2002; Liemann et al. 2002) have revealed the particle structure

in great detail. The core lattice is formed by 120 copies of $\lambda1$. Channels of $\lambda1$ are found at the fivefold symmetry axes of the icosahedral core particle. The $\lambda3$ (12 copies) and $\mu2$ (20 copies) proteins are located at the internal aspect of these channels. The $\lambda3$ protein is the viral RNA-dependent RNA polymerase (RdRp) and is closely associated with the ten segments of genomic dsRNA. The crystal structure of $\lambda3$ reveals a cage-like molecule, with independent channels for template and product (Tao et al. 2002). On top of the $\lambda1$ shell are 150 copies of $\sigma2$ that act as a clamp to stabilize the $\lambda1$ lattice. The $\lambda2$ protein (60 copies) forms pentamers at the fivefold symmetry axes. 'Turrets' of $\lambda2$ reach to the outer capsid. The $\lambda2$ protein plays an important role in viral RNA synthesis by serving as the capping enzyme complex. The outer shell is formed by 600 copies of $\mu1$ and 600 copies of $\sigma3$ that interact extensively to form heterohexamers (Liemann et al. 2002). The $\mu1$ protein is myristoylated at its N terminus and is involved in viral penetration of host-cell membranes. The $\sigma3$ protein serves as a protective cap for $\mu1$ and renders the virus stable in the environment. The $\sigma1$ protein (36 copies) is the viral attachment protein and forms trimers at the icosahedral vertices. The N terminus of $\sigma1$ is embedded in the turrets of $\lambda2$.

Replication

The reovirus replication cycle is entirely cytoplasmic (Figure 43.2, p. 935). Many of the features of reovirus replication are similar, though not identical, to those of rotaviruses (for further details, see Nibert and Schiff 2001 and Chapter 44, Rotaviruses).

Reovirus infection is initiated by the binding of the $\sigma1$ protein to cell-surface receptors. The $\sigma1$ protein is a trimer consisting of an elongated fibrous domain – the tail – that inserts into the virion and a virion-distal globular domain – the head (Fraser et al. 1990). Type 3 $\sigma1$ contains two receptor-binding domains, one in the head that binds to junctional adhesion molecule 1 (JAM1) (Barton et al. 2001b) and another in the tail that binds α-linked sialic acid (Chappell et al. 2000). In T3D $\sigma1$, these domains are dissociable by treatment of $\sigma1$ with intestinal proteases, such as trypsin or chymotrypsin (Nibert et al. 1995). Type 1 $\sigma1$ binds cell-surface carbohydrate as well, but this molecule has not been identified. For sialic-acid-binding reovirus strains, the initial interaction between the viral particle and the host cell is likely mediated by sialic acid due to the high surface concentration of this carbohydrate (Barton et al. 2001a). By virtue of its rapid association rate, virus binding to sialic acid likely adheres the virion to the cell surface, thereby enabling it to diffuse laterally until it encounters JAM1. Such an adhesion-strengthening mechanism of viral attachment has been shown for several other viruses including herpesviruses and lentiviruses.

Table 43.1 *Gene protein assignments and functions of mammalian reovirus proteins (T3D)*

RNA		Proteins				
Segment	Size (bp)	Designation	Size (kDa)	Number of molecules/virion	Location	Modification	Functions
L1	3 854	λ3	142	ca. 12	Core	...	RdRp
L2	3 916	λ2	145	60	Core spike (outer capsid)	...	Guanylyltransferase; methyltransferases
L3	3 901	λ1	143	120	Core	Zn metalloprotein	Binds RNA; NTPase? RNA helicase? RNA triphosphatase?[a]
M1	2 304	μ2	83	ca. 20	Inner capsid	...	Binds RNA; NTPase?
M2	2 203	μ1	76	600	Outer capsid	N-myristoylated	Role in penetration and transcriptase activation
		μ1C	72	...	...	Cleavage product of μ1	...
M3	2 241	μNS	80	...	Nonstructural	Phosphoprotein	ssRNA-binding; core binding; role in RNA assortment or replication?
		μNSC	75	...	Nonstructural	...	Unknown
S1	1 416	σ1	49	36	Outer capsid	...	Viral attachment protein; hemagglutinin; type-specifying antigen
		σ1s	14	...	Nonstructural	...	Unknown (dispensable in cell culture)
S2	1 331	σ2	47	150	Inner capsid	...	Binds ds RNA
S3	1 198	σNS	41	...	Nonstructural	...	ssRNA-binding; role in assortment or replication?
S4	1 196	σ3	41	600	Outer capsid	Zn metalloprotein, sensitive to protease degradation	dsRNA-binding; effects on translation

Modified from Nibert and Schiff 2001.
a) Possibly encoded by the M1 gene segment μ2 protein (Tao et al. 2002).

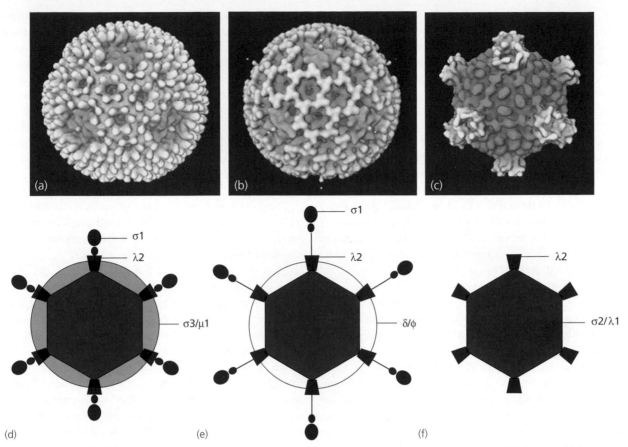

Figure 43.1 *Reovirus virions, ISVPs, and cores.* **(a–c)** *Surface-shaded views of the reovirus strain T1L* **(a)** *virion,* **(b)** *ISVP, and* **(c)** *core. The images were obtained using cryo-electron microscopy and three-dimensional image reconstruction. Each particle is viewed along a threefold axis. Figure modified from Centonze et al. 1995 with permission.* **(d–f)** *Schematic representations of reovirus* **(d)** *virion,* **(e)** *ISVP, and* **(f)** *core. Major viral structural proteins are indicated.*

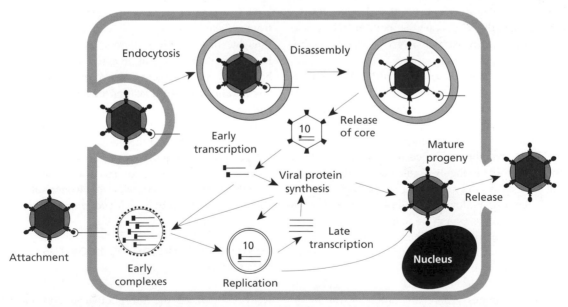

Figure 43.2 *The reovirus replication cycle. Reovirus virions attach to cellular receptors and enter cells by receptor-mediated endocytosis. Within an endocytic compartment, the viral outer capsid is removed to generate ISVPs. ISVPs penetrate membranes of endocytic vesicles and release the viral core into the cytoplasm. Transcription of the viral genome occurs within the core, and nascent mRNAs are released through turret-like openings at the viral vertices. Viral mRNAs are used as template for viral protein synthesis and replication of viral genomic dsRNA. Particles containing dsRNA segments are termed replication particles. These particles are transcriptionally active and yield additional viral mRNAs, resulting in an amplification of viral protein synthesis. Following addition of viral outer-capsid proteins to the replication particles, progeny virions are assembled and exit the cell.*

Following attachment to cell-surface receptors, reovirus enters cells by receptor-mediated endocytosis. In the endocytic compartment, virions undergo proteolysis by endocytic proteases, resulting in generation of ISVPs. The endocytic cysteine-containing proteases cathepsin B and cathepsin L convert virions to ISVPs in mouse fibroblasts (Ebert et al. 2002). ISVPs also can be formed extracellularly in the murine intestine or by treatment with intestinal proteases in vitro. During virion-to-ISVP conversion, σ3 is degraded and lost from virions, σ1 undergoes a conformational change, and μ1 is cleaved to form particle-associated fragments δ and φ (Figure 43.1). Removal of σ3 is thought to expose hydrophobic domains in μ1 that facilitate interactions of ISVPs with endosomal membranes, leading to delivery of core particles into the cytoplasm (Nibert et al. 1991; Liemann et al. 2002).

Transcription of the reovirus genome is fully conservative, i.e. both strands of the genome remain within the cores. The nature of the functional reovirus transcriptase is not fully understood. The λ1, λ2, λ3, and μ2 proteins all likely play important roles in viral RNA synthesis, with λ3 serving as the viral RdRp. Only positive-sense transcripts are produced during primary transcription, and these transcripts are capped, as the core contains virus-encoded capping enzymes. The λ2 protein has guanylyltransferase and methyltransferase activities (Luongo et al. 2000; Reinisch et al. 2000). Nascent transcripts leave the core via channels formed by pentamers of λ2 at the vertices of the fivefold symmetry axes. Transcripts are produced in a ratio according to their size; S-class RNAs are more abundant than M-class RNAs, which are in turn more abundant than L-class RNAs. Capped, full-length RNAs act as both mRNAs and templates for negative-strand RNA synthesis within progeny cores.

Replication of reovirus genomic dsRNA segments occurs within newly formed cores, although the mechanisms underlying this process are poorly understood. Plus-strand RNA is thought to be packaged during assembly of cores, where it serves as template for minus-strand synthesis. The assembly of the correct number of RNA segments into cores is highly regulated, but the process ensuring that each core receives a single copy of each RNA is unknown. Following synthesis of dsRNA, the nascent cores become transcriptionally active and enter a second round of mRNA synthesis. In contrast to the products of primary transcription, these secondary transcripts are not capped.

Both capped and uncapped RNAs serve as translational templates. There are different translation efficiencies of reovirus mRNAs, suggesting post-transcriptional control. The variability in translation is in part due to the sequence context of the initiator AUG (especially at the −3 and +4 positions) (Kozak 1981). The 3′-UTRs of some reovirus mRNAs also contain translational control sequences (Mochow-Grundy and Dermody 2001). During reovirus infection, most protein synthesis in the cell is viral in origin. Outer-capsid protein σ3 may play a central role in this process through its effects on the activity of the interferon-induced enzyme, protein kinase RNA (PKR). This effect is thought to relate to the affinity of σ3 for dsRNA and its capacity to compete with PKR for dsRNA binding (Imani and Jacobs 1988; Lloyd and Shatkin 1992; Schmechel et al. 1997). Sequestration of dsRNA by σ3 presumably attenuates PKR activation, thereby impeding the capacity of PKR to phosphorylate eIF-2a.

The morphogenesis of reovirus particles is complex. The earliest detectable newly formed particles contain single-stranded RNA (ssRNA). These particles, termed 'replicase particles,' are actively engaged in genomic dsRNA synthesis. Once dsRNA is synthesized, the replicase particles initiate secondary transcription and are termed 'transcriptase particles.' The additional uncapped transcripts lead to increased protein synthesis. Outer-capsid proteins condense onto the transcriptase particles, silencing transcription, to form mature, double-shelled reovirus virions. Viral nonstructural proteins are involved in collecting ssRNA prior to formation of replicase particles (Antczak and Joklik 1992) and may play additional roles in particle morphogenesis (Broering et al. 2000; Becker et al. 2001). A peculiar feature of reoviruses is the occurrence of oligonucleotides (di- to nonanucleotides) in viral particles. These RNA species appear to be synthesized following particle assembly and are likely to represent aborted products of transcription (5′ ends of mRNAs).

The mechanism by which progeny virions are released from infected cells has not been determined, but it is thought that reovirus egress occurs by cell lysis. However, most virus in infected cell lysates remains bound to cell fragments, which probably reflects the association of viral replication centers with cytoskeletal components. Reovirus induces apoptosis of infected cells. Thus, it is possible that virus may be released in association with membrane-bound apoptotic bodies.

Numerous attempts have been made to establish a reverse genetics system for reoviruses. Several reports describing such a system (e.g. Roner et al. 1990; Roner and Joklik 2001) await wider application.

Apoptosis induced by reovirus infection

Reovirus induces the morphological and biochemical hallmarks of apoptosis in cultured cells and in vivo. Strain-specific differences in the capacity of reovirus to induce apoptosis are determined by the σ1-encoding *S1* gene (Tyler et al. 1995). Binding of σ1 to both sialic acid (Connolly et al. 2001) and JAM1 (Barton et al. 2001b) is required to achieve maximal levels of apoptosis.

However, viral attachment is not sufficient to elicit an apoptotic response. Inhibitors of acid-dependent viral disassembly block apoptosis by reovirus (Connolly and Dermody 2002), indicating a requirement for post-attachment entry steps in apoptosis induction. Viral transcription, however, is dispensable for apoptosis by reovirus, as inhibitors of viral RNA synthesis do not diminish the capacity of reovirus to induce apoptosis (Tyler et al. 1995; Connolly and Dermody 2002). These findings suggest that apoptosis induced by reovirus is triggered by a signaling pathway initiated by early steps in the viral replication cycle.

A critical component of the signaling cascade that leads to apoptosis of reovirus-infected cells is the transcription factor NF-κB. Within hours following viral adsorption, reovirus activates NF-κB, and this activation is required to induce an apoptotic response (Connolly et al. 2000). In some cell types, reovirus infection leads to expression of death receptors DR4 and DR5 and their pro-apoptotic ligand TRAIL (Clarke et al. 2000), suggesting apoptosis is induced by an extrinsic cell-death pathway. However, mitochondrial injury during reovirus infection has been documented (Kominsky et al. 2002), providing evidence that intrinsic signals are also involved in apoptosis induced by reovirus infection.

Pathogenesis: the mouse model

The elucidation of viral genetic determinants of the pathogenesis of reovirus disease has led to the establishment of general principles of viral disease mechanisms (for reviews, see Virgin et al. 1997; Tyler 2001).

This analysis is based on two main observations:

- Different reovirus serotypes cause different disease manifestations in the CNS of newborn mice (reovirus type 1: hydrocephalus; reovirus type 3: encephalitis).
- Different reovirus serotypes have different RNA and protein migration profiles by polyacrylamide gel electrophoresis (PAGE) (Figure 43.3).

Because reovirus has a segmented genome, 'reassortant genetics' can be used to identify specific viral genes involved in various aspects of virus–host interaction. Parental virus strains that differ with respect to a given phenotype (e.g. tissue tropism) are used to generate progeny reassortant viruses containing different combinations of gene segments from each of the parents (Figure 43.4). Careful observation of mice infected with various reassortant viruses has revealed the relative contributions of individual genes or sets of genes and their products to the pathogenic process.

Viruses produce disease by interacting with the host in a discrete series of steps:

- entry into host
- primary replication
- spread through the host

- specific cell and tissue tropism
- host immune response.

Following oral inoculation, reovirus is taken up by Peyer's patches via the M cells (Wolf et al. 1981), specialized gut epithelia overlying the lymphoid tissue of the Peyer's patches. Virus then disseminates to various sites within the host including the CNS. However, not all reovirus strains are capable of growth in the intestine and systemic spread following oral inoculation. Strain T3D is neurovirulent after intracranial (Weiner et al. 1980b; Morrison et al. 1993) or intramuscular (Tyler et al. 1986) inoculation but does not infect the murine intestine after oral inoculation. By contrast, T1L produces high titers in intestinal tissue and spreads systemically (Rubin and Fields 1980; Keroack and Fields 1986; Bodkin and Fields 1989) (Table 43.2, p. 939). Using T1L × T3D reassortant viruses, it was shown that the σ1-encoding S1 gene and the λ2-encoding L2 gene are the primary determinants of strain-specific differences in reovirus growth in the intestine (Bodkin and Fields 1989).

Following oral or intramuscular inoculation, strains of both serotypes invade the CNS, yet by different routes and with distinct pathological consequences (Table 43.2). T1 reovirus spreads to the CNS hematogenously and infects ependymal cells (Weiner et al. 1980b; Tyler et al. 1986), resulting in hydrocephalus (Weiner et al. 1977). By contrast, T3 reovirus spreads to the CNS neurally and infects neurons (Weiner et al. 1980b; Tyler et al. 1986; Morrison et al. 1991), causing lethal encephalitis (Weiner et al. 1977; Tardieu et al. 1983). T1L × T3D reassortant viruses were used to show that the pathways of viral spread (Tyler et al. 1986) and tropism for neural tissues (Weiner et al. 1980b; Dichter and Weiner 1984) segregate with the σ1-encoding S1 gene (Weiner et al. 1980a; Lee et al. 1981). Thus, σ1 determines the CNS cell types that serve as targets for reovirus infection.

Reovirus pathogenesis is not restricted to the CNS. Reovirus infection causes pathology and physiological dysfunction in a wide range of organs and tissues including the hepatobiliary system, myocardium, lungs, and endocrine tissues. Reovirus hepatobiliary disease (Wilson et al. 1994) and myocarditis (Sherry et al. 1989) in mice have become particularly well-established experimental models of viral injury at these sites.

Myocarditis induced by reovirus is unusual in comparison to other viral causes of myocarditis in that the pathogenesis is not immune-mediated. Instead, reovirus cytopathicity is a direct cause of myocyte injury, which results from a complex interplay of the interferon (Sherry et al. 1998; Noah et al. 1999; Azzam-Smoak et al. 2002) and apoptotic pathways (DeBiasi et al. 2001). Efficiency of viral RNA synthesis is a key factor in determining the extent of myocardial injury (Sherry et al. 1996). Accordingly, viral gene segments encoding proteins involved in

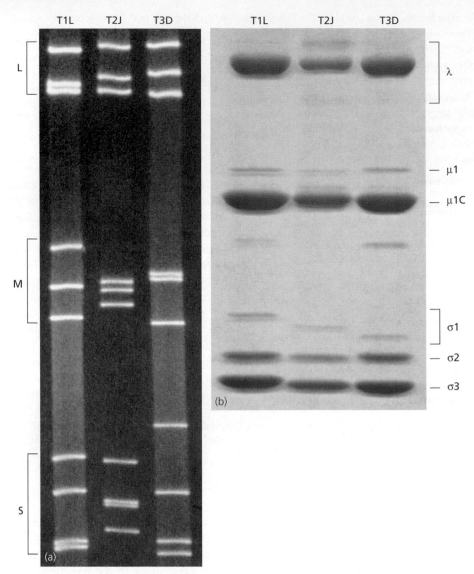

Figure 43.3 *Electrophoretic profiles of* **(a)** *genomic dsRNA and* **(b)** *structural proteins of prototype reovirus strains T1L, T2J, and T3D. Equal numbers of reovirus particles were resolved by acrylamide gel electrophoresis.* **(a)** *Viral dsRNA gene segments were visualized following staining of the gel with ethidium bromide. Gene segment size classes, large (L), medium (M), and small (S), are indicated.* **(b)** *Viral structural proteins were visualized following staining of the gel with Coomassie blue. Viral proteins are indicated. This figure was prepared with the assistance of J. Denise Wetzel, Vanderbilt University.*

viral transcription and genome replication play important roles in determining strain-specific differences in the capacity of reovirus to induce myocarditis (Sherry and Fields 1989; Sherry and Blum 1994; Sherry et al. 1998).

Illness in humans

Reoviruses are recognized and well-studied pathogens of mice and other rodents, but it has been difficult to link reovirus infections to disease in humans. Although infections of humans are common, most infections are asymptomatic. Reovirus infections are occasionally associated with enteritis, rhinitis, and CNS disease in infants and children (Tyler 2001).

Reovirus has also been linked to neonatal biliary atresia in humans (Tyler et al. 1998). While a definitive

causal relationship between reovirus infection and biliary atresia has not been established, it is quite provocative that infection of newborn mice (ND4 Swiss Webster) with a reovirus type 3 strain that utilizes sialic acid as a coreceptor was associated with viral replication in bile duct epithelium and abnormalities in hepatobiliary function very similar to those accompanying bile duct obstruction in humans, including hyperbilirubinemia, elevated levels of serum alkaline phosphatase, and steatorrhea (for details see Barton et al. 2003; for review Forrest and Dermody, 2003).

Epidemiology

By the end of childhood, most humans have antibodies against each of the three reovirus serotypes (Jackson

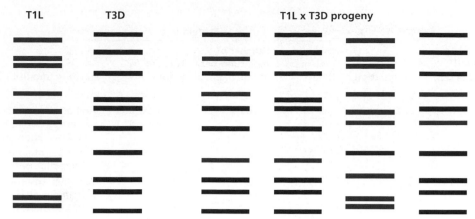

Figure 43.4 *Generation of reassortant viruses. Biological polymorphisms exhibited by different reovirus strains can be mapped to specific gene segments through the use of reassortant viruses. Reovirus strains are distinguishable by signature electrophoretic profiles of their dsRNA gene segments (i.e. electropherotypes). Co-infection of cells with different strains produces a collection of progeny reassortant viruses containing various combinations of gene segments from each parent. A phenotypic difference between two parental strains can be genetically mapped by screening the reassortant viruses in appropriate assays and correlating expression of the phenotype with a specific parental gene segment. The electropherotypes of prototype strains T1L and T3D are illustrated in this figure.*

Table 43.2 *Properties of reovirus pathogenesis attributable to σ1 protein*

Viral serotype	Functional property				
	Intestinal growth	Pathway of spread	CNS tropism	Tail receptor	Head receptor
Type 1	Yes	Hematogenous	Ependymal cells	Unknown	JAM1
Type 3	Variable[a]	Neural	Neurons	Sialic acid	JAM1

a) Some type 3 reovirus strains can infect the intestine and disseminate systemically. Others fail to infect intestinal tissue and do not spread to distant sites.

et al. 1961; Lerner et al. 1962; Leers and Rozee 1966). In a study conducted at a pediatric hospital in the USA, the incidence of anti-reovirus antibodies increased from less than 25 percent in those less than 1 year of age to greater than 70 percent in those over 3 years of age (Lerner et al. 1962). Reovirus-specific antibodies are also found in most mammals. Reovirus infections do not appear to have a seasonal distribution, although the original isolates were from patients with diarrheal illnesses occurring during the summer months. Reoviruses are commonly found in environmental water sources (Adams et al. 1982; Ridinger et al. 1982; Dahling et al. 1989), and it has been suggested that human fecal contamination is a major source of virus in water supplies (Matsuura et al. 1993).

Reovirus oncolysis

Transformed cells are substantially more permissive for reovirus infection than untransformed cells (Strong and Lee 1996). This property correlates with an activated *Ras* signaling pathway (Strong et al. 1998). Reovirus kills transformed cells in animals (Coffey et al. 1998) and is being investigated for the treatment of some forms of cancer in humans.

ORBIVIRUSES

Genome, gene protein assignment, and structure

The genome of orbiviruses consists of 10 segments of dsRNA of three size classes termed *L1–L3*, *M4–M6*, and *S7–S10*. Full-length sequences of each of the genome segments of BTV 10 have been determined (Roy 1989). Protein-coding assignments have been established for each of the BTV genes (Roy 2001). The genome segments, their size in bp, and the size, number of molecules, and location in the virion, post-translational modifications, and some of the recognized functions of the protein products are shown in Table 43.3.

With the exception of the *S10* RNA, orbivirus genes are monocistronic, encoding seven structural proteins (VP1–VP7) and four nonstructural proteins (NS1–NS3, NS3A). The 5′ and 3′ termini of the orbivirus RNA segments are conserved and have inverted complementarity (Roy 2001), theoretically allowing formation of 'panhandle' structures, a property common to other members of the *Reoviridae*.

The inner core of the virion consists of the segmented genome with which three minor proteins, VP1, VP4, and

Table **43.3** *Gene protein assignments and functions of orbivirus proteins (BTV 10)*

RNA segment		Protein				
Designation	Size (bp)	Designation	Deduced mol. mass (kDa)	Number of molecules per virion	Location in virion	Function (modification)
L1	3 954	VP1	149.6	12	Inner core	RdRp
L2	2 926	VP2	111.1	180	Outer capsid (exposed)	Viral attachment protein; hemagglutinin; type-specifying neutralization antigen
L3	2 772	VP3	103.3	120	Core (subcore layer)	Scaffold protein for VP7; interaction with genomic RNA
M4	2 011	VP4	76.4	ca. 24	Inner core	Guanylyltransferase; methyltransferases; NTPase; RNA 5'-triphosphatase; pyrophosphatase
M5	1 639	VP5	59.2	360	Outer capsid (under surface)	Glycoprotein; crossreactive antigen; not neutralization-specific; virus penetration; fusogenic; positioning of VP2?
M6	1 770	NS1	64.4	. . .	Nonstructural	Tubule formation; translocation of virus particles?
S7	1 156	VP7	38.5	780	Core surface	Group-specific antigen; core binding to insect cells
S8	1 124	NS2	41.0	. . .	Nonstructural	Phosphoprotein; binds ssRNA; morphogenesis (cytoplasmic inclusions)
S9	1 046	VP6	35.8	ca. 72	Inner core	Binds ssRNA and dsRNA; helicase; ATPase
S10	822	NS3	25.6	. . .	Nonstructural	Glycoprotein; virus release
	. . .	NS3A	24.0	. . .	Nonstructural	Function unknown

Slightly modified from Roy 2001, with permission of author and publisher.

VP6 (encoded by the *L1*, *M4*, and *S9* RNAs, respectively), are closely associated. These proteins serve as the viral RdRp, guanylyltransferase, and RNA-binding proteins, respectively. The inner core is surrounded by an inner capsid layer composed of VP3 trimers (interior of the inner capsid; encoded by the *L3* RNA), which form a scaffold for a layer of VP7 trimers (exterior of the inner capsid; encoded by the *S7* RNA). The structure containing the genome and proteins VP1, VP4, VP6, VP3, and VP7 is also referred to as the viral core. The core is surrounded by the outer capsid, which consists of VP5 (encoded by the *M5* RNA), a glycoprotein, and VP2 (encoded by the *L2* RNA). VP2 is the most variable of the BTV proteins and carries major epitopes determining serotype and neutralization specificity. VP2 is the orbivirus attachment protein and hemagglutinin (Roy 2001). Antibodies directed against VP2 protect animals from infection, but antibodies directed against VP5 do not.

There are four orbivirus nonstructural proteins:

● NS1 (encoded by the *M6* RNA)
● NS2 (encoded by the *S8* RNA)
● NS3/NS3A (encoded by the *S10* RNA, initiating from in-frame AUG codons and differing in size by 1.5 kDa).

The precise functions of the orbivirus nonstructural proteins are not fully understood (Roy 2001).

Although the three main genera of the *Reoviridae* (reo-, rota-, and orbiviruses) have unique characteristics in structure, replication, pathogenesis, and epidemiology, these viruses exhibit remarkable parallels in the functions of their structural proteins (Table 43.4). All these viruses have a virion-associated RdRp and proteins with RNA-capping activity. They also share structural proteins that act as scaffolds in several layers of the capsid and others that interact with receptors, hemagglutinate, and determine neutralization (serotype) specificity. There is increasing evidence that the nonstructural proteins have similar functions in morphogenesis, virion assembly, and release, but the parallels in the functions of these proteins are less obvious.

Replication

Orbiviruses are unusual among the *Reoviridae* in that they replicate in both mammalian and insect cells. This property reflects the capacity of these viruses to productively infect cells at very different temperatures (37°C and 22–27°C, respectively).

Table 43.4 *Functional similarities of structural proteins of reovirus, rotavirus, and* bluetongue virus[a]

Location in virion	Function	Protein designation (and coding RNA segment)					
		Reovirus		Rotavirus		Bluetongue virus	
Core (inner layer)	RdRp	λ3	(*L1*)	VP1	(1)	VP1	(*L1*)
	Guanylyltransferase, methyltransferases	λ2	(*L2*)	VP3	(3)	VP4	(*M4*)
	Scaffolding protein;	λ1/σ2	(*L3/S2*)	VP2	(2)	VP3	(*L3*)
	RNA binding	μ2	(*M1*)			VP6	(*S9*)
Inner capsid (middle layer)	Structural protein	μ1/μ1C	(*M2*)	VP6	(6)	VP7	(*S7*)
Outer capsid (outer layer)	Structural protein	σ3	(*S4*)	VP7	(7[b])	VP5	(*M5*)
	Attachment protein	σ1	(*S1*)	VP4	(4)	VP2	(*L2*)

Slightly modified from Mattion et al. 1994, with permission of authors and publisher.

a) Functional analogies of the nonstructural proteins (reovirus μNS, σNS, and σ1s; rotavirus: NS1–NS5; and bluetongue: NS1–NS3, NS3A) are difficult to define at present.

b) Depending on the strain, VP7, NSP2, and NSP3 are encoded by RNA 7, 8, or 9.

Orbiviruses attach via VP2 to sialic-acid-containing receptors on the surface of mammalian cells. It is possible that receptors in addition to sialic acid are used for viral attachment in a manner analogous to that of other members of the *Reoviridae*; however, such receptors have thus far not been identified. Core particles, which lack VP2 and VP5, adsorb well to and infect insect cells, suggesting that VP7 at the exterior of the core interacts with insect cell receptors. Virus enters mammalian cells by endocytosis, after which the outer capsid (VP2 and VP5) is removed. The resulting core particle is transcriptionally active and catalyzes synthesis of viral mRNAs. The viral RdRp has a temperature optimum in vitro of 28°C but retains activity at 37°C (Van Dijk and Huismans 1982), reflecting adaptation of viral replication to different types of host cells. VP4 mediates capping enzyme activities, resulting in the production of capped mRNAs (Martinez-Costas et al. 1998; Ramadevi et al. 1998; Ramadevi and Roy 1998). Viral proteins are synthesized from 2 to 14 hours after infection and accumulate in the cytoplasm. The viral NS1 protein forms extensive tubules throughout the cytoplasm, but their function is unknown (Eaton et al. 1990). Orbivirus release is thought to be accomplished by cell lysis.

Core-like particles (CLP) and virus-like particles (VLP) largely self-assemble when combinations of viral proteins (CLPs: VP3 and VP7; VLPs: VP2, VP3, VP5, and VP7) are overexpressed simultaneously in insect cells using baculovirus recombinants (French et al. 1990) (Figure 43.5).

Detailed morphological studies of VLPs (Hewat et al. 1994) and biochemical analyses of individual viral proteins have led to the identification of protein

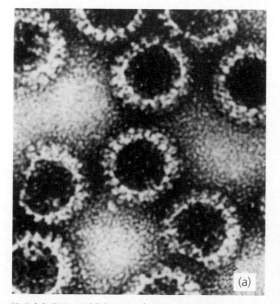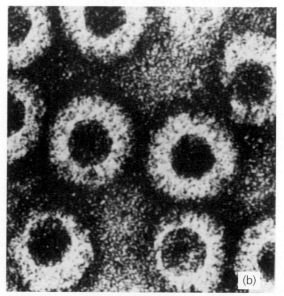

Figure 43.5 (a) *CLPs and* **(b)** *VLPs of BTV. The particles were obtained by coexpression of baculovirus recombinants in insect cells (CLPs: VP3 and VP7; VLPs: VP2, VP3, VP5, and VP7). Particles were purified and examined by cryo-electron microscopy and three-dimensional image reconstruction. (From French et al. 1990 with permission of the authors and publisher.)*

domains responsible for protein–protein and protein–RNA interactions (reviewed by Roy 2001). The structure of VP7 has been solved using X-ray crystallography, and its domain structure is known in atomic detail (Grimes et al. 1995). The structure of the BTV core also has been solved using X-ray crystallography, revealing significant insights into the nature of the enzymatic activities of the core and providing clues to mechanisms of RNA packaging (Grimes et al. 1998).

Pathogenesis

In mammals, BTV replicates mainly in the lymphoreticular system. The virus has a particular affinity for endothelial cells of capillaries, causing ischemic lesions, inflammatory changes, and edema. There is a prolonged viremia that lasts for up to 1 month, although neutralizing antibody appears 7–10 days following infection (Parsonson 1990). Different BTV serotypes are capable of gene segment reassortment in vitro and in their natural hosts (Samal et al. 1987), giving rise to considerable diversity among field isolates.

Illness

The incubation period for BTV-induced disease is 6–9 days. Illness starts with fever, followed by vomiting and hemorrhage. Bronchopneumonia occurs and can be fatal. Disease severity can vary, and many BTV infections are subclinical. Symptomatic disease is observed in 10–30 percent of infected animals, and mortality is approximately 5 percent (Parsonson 1990). Besides sheep, cattle are commonly infected, although these infections are usually asymptomatic. BTV can infect the fetus and is associated with abortions and fetal abnormalities in sheep and cattle (Parsonson 1990).

Epidemiology

BTV constitutes one of at least 14 serogroups of orbiviruses (Mertens et al. 2000) and occurs in 24 serotypes. These viruses infect sheep, cattle, goats, and wild ungulates in many countries of the tropical and subtropical zones (Parsonson 1990). Their distribution is supported by a variety of insect vectors (Culicoides midges, ticks, and mosquitoes) in which the virus replicates (Mellor 1990). Other orbivirus serogroups, such as African horse sickness virus (AHSV), occurring in horses, donkeys, and dogs, and epizootic hemorrhagic disease virus (EHDV), occurring in deer, also have diverged into serotypes. Sequence comparisons of BTV, AHSV, and EHDV indicate that there is considerable conservation of the VP3 gene product (58–79 percent). There is less conservation of the VP7 gene product (43–63 percent), the protein specifying the group antigen, and less still of the VP2 gene product (32–45 percent), which specifies viral serotype (Roy 2001).

Vaccines

Antibodies specific for BTV VP2 are neutralizing and provide effective homotypic protection (Huismans et al. 1987). Generation of CLPs and VLPs by co-expression of viral genes in insect cells infected with baculovirus recombinants (e.g. French et al. 1990) (Figure 43.5) has enabled the development of vaccine candidates (Roy et al. 1992; Roy and Sutton 1998). These particles, formulated either as mixtures derived from different serotypes or as particle chimeras, have the potential to elicit broad protective immune responses. A vaccine of inactivated particles of AHSV serotype 4 has been shown to fully protect against homologous challenge (House 1998).

COLTIVIRUSES

Coltiviruses possess a genome of 12 segments of dsRNA and are now classified as a separate genus of the *Reoviridae* (Mertens et al. 2000). Within the *Coltivirus* genus, two groups and several subgroups have been defined based on sequence comparisons of RNA segments (Attoui et al. 1998). These viruses are isolated from ticks, mosquitoes, rodents, and humans. Colorado tick fever virus (CTFV) can cause a fatal disease in humans. Different isolates of CTFV differ mostly in RNA segments 4 and 6, suggesting that protein products of these genes are located in the outer capsid and carry neutralization-specific epitopes (Bodkin and Knudson 1987).

CTFV is endemic in the Rocky Mountain region of the USA and Canada. In the insect vector, which includes ticks of many species, CTFV infects the midgut, from which it spreads to other organs including the salivary glands, allowing transmission to mammalian hosts by bite. As rodents have prolonged CTFV viremia, they may serve as a reservoir for tick infection in nature. However, a variety of other mammals (e.g. marmots, deer, elk, and sheep) can also be infected. Humans are infected by bite but are not thought to generate sufficient viremia to maintain the transmission cycle (Monath and Guirakhoo 1996).

CTFV can be isolated from the erythrocytes of humans for as long as 120 days after infection, whereas it disappears from plasma very quickly (Bowen 1988). This cell-associated viremia is likely to originate from infection of bone marrow stem cells; from these cells, virus is continuously dispersed into the periphery in maturing erythrocytes. Interestingly, the viremia persists in the presence of a strong neutralizing antibody response (Monath and Guirakhoo 1996).

After an incubation period of 4 days (range 1–19 days), humans infected with CTFV develop fever (possibly due to elevated interferon levels), leukopenia, gastrointestinal symptoms (20 percent of cases), rash (10 percent), and meningoencephalitis (3–7 percent). A severe hemorrhagic form of the disease (purpura, epistaxis, and gastrointestinal bleeding) is rarely seen. The case-fatality rate is less than 0.1 percent.

CTFV can be isolated from the blood of infected persons using continuous cell lines (e.g. Vero and BHK-21 cells), and viral antigen can be detected in erythrocytes by immunofluorescence testing (IFT). Serological diagnosis can be accomplished by IFT using infected Vero cells as antigen or by enzyme-linked immunosorbent assay (ELISA).

Treatment of Colorado tick fever is supportive. Ribavirin has been used in cases of severe hemorrhagic disease. However, controlled clinical trials to test its efficacy have not been reported.

REFERENCES

Adams, D.J., Ridinger, D.N. and Spendlove, R.S. 1982. Protamine prescription of two reovirus particle types from polluted waters. *Appl Environ Microbiol*, **44**, 589–96.

Antczak, J.B. and Joklik, W.K. 1992. Reovirus genome segment assortment into progeny genomes studied by the use of monoclonal antibodies directed against reovirus proteins. *Virology*, **187**, 760–76.

Attoui, H., Charrel, R.N., et al. 1998. Comparative sequence analysis of American, European and Asian isolates of viruses in the genus *Coltivirus*. *J Gen Virol*, **79**, 2481–9.

Attoui, H., Billoir, F., et al. 2000. Complete sequence determination and genetic analysis of Banna virus and Kadipiro virus: proposal for assignment of a new genus (Seadornavirus) within the family Reoviridae. *J Gen Virol*, **81**, 1507–15.

Azzam-Smoak, K., Noah, D.L., et al. 2002. Interferon regulatory factor-1, interferon-beta, and reovirus-induced myocarditis. *Virology*, **298**, 20–9.

Barton, E.S., Connolly, J.L., et al. 2001a. Utilization of sialic acid as a coreceptor enhances reovirus attachment by multistep adhesion strengthening. *J Biol Chem*, **276**, 2200–11.

Barton, E.S., Forrest, J.C., et al. 2001b. Junction adhesion molecule is a receptor for reovirus. *Cell*, **104**, 441–51.

Barton, E.S., Youree, B.E., et al. 2003. Utilization of sialic acid as a coreceptor is required for reovirus-induced biliary disease. *J Clin Invest*, **111**, 1823–33.

Becker, M.M., Goral, M.I., et al. 2001. Reovirus sNS protein is required for nucleation of viral assembly complexes and formation of viral inclusions. *J Virol*, **75**, 1459–75.

Bodkin, D.K. and Fields, B.N. 1989. Growth and survival of reovirus in intestinal tissue: role of the *L2* and *S1* genes. *J Virol*, **63**, 1188–93.

Bodkin, D.K. and Knudson, D.L. 1987. Genetic relatedness of Colorado tick fever virus isolates by RNA-RNA blot hybridization. *J Gen Virol*, **68**, 1199–204.

Bowen, G.S. 1988. Colorado tick fever. In: Monath, T.P. (ed.), *The arboviruses: epidemiology and ecology*. Boca Raton, FL: CRC Press, 159–76.

Broering, T.J., McCutcheon, A.M., et al. 2000. Reovirus nonstructural protein μNS binds to core particles but does not inhibit their transcription and capping activities. *J Virol*, **74**, 5516–24.

Centonze, V.E., Chen, Y., et al. 1995. Visualization of single reovirus particles by low-temperature, high-resolution scanning electron microscopy. *J Struct Biol*, **115**, 215–25.

Chappell, J.D., Duong, J.L., et al. 2000. Identification of carbohydrate-binding domains in the attachment proteins of type 1 and type 3 reoviruses. *J Virol*, **74**, 8472–9.

Chappell, J.D., Prota, A., et al. 2002. Crystal structure of reovirus attachment protein σ1 reveals evolutionary relationship to adenovirus fiber. *EMBO J*, **21**, 1–11.

Clarke, P., Meintzer, S.M., et al. 2000. Reovirus-induced apoptosis is mediated by TRAIL. *J Virol*, **74**, 8135–9.

Coffey, M.C., Strong, J.E., et al. 1998. Reovirus therapy of tumors with activated *Ras* pathway. *Science*, **282**, 1332–4.

Connolly, J.L. and Dermody, T.S. 2002. Virion disassembly is required for apoptosis induced by reovirus. *J Virol*, **76**, 1632–41.

Connolly, J.L., Rodgers, S.E., et al. 2000. Reovirus-induced apoptosis requires activation of transcription factor NF-κB. *J Virol*, **74**, 2981–9.

Connolly, J.L., Barton, E.S. and Dermody, T.S. 2001. Reovirus binding to cell surface sialic acid potentiates virus-induced apoptosis. *J Virol*, **75**, 4029–39.

Dahling, D.R., Safferman, R.S. and Wright, B.A. 1989. Isolation of enterovirus and reovirus from sewage and treated effluents in selected Puerto Rican communities. *Appl Environ Microbiol*, **55**, 503–6.

DeBiasi, R., Edelstein, C., et al. 2001. Calpain inhibition protects against virus-induced apoptotic myocardial injury. *J Virol*, **75**, 351–61.

Dichter, M.A. and Weiner, H.L. 1984. Infection of neuronal cell cultures with reovirus mimics in vitro patterns of neurotropism. *Ann Neurol*, **16**, 603–10.

Dryden, K.A., Wang, G., et al. 1993. Early steps in reovirus infection are associated with dramatic changes in supramolecular structure and protein conformation: analysis of virions and subviral particles by cryoelectron microscopy and image reconstruction. *J Cell Biol*, **122**, 1023–41.

Dryden, K.A., Farsetta, D.L., et al. 1998. Internal structures containing transcriptase-related proteins in top component particles of mammalian orthoreovirus. *Virology*, **245**, 33–46.

Eaton, B.T., Hyatt, A.D. and Brookes, S.M. 1990. The replication of bluetongue virus. *Curr Top Microbiol Immunol*, **162**, 89–118.

Ebert, D.H., Deussing, J., et al. 2002. Cathepsin L and cathepsin B mediate reovirus disassembly in murine fibroblast cells. *J Biol Chem*, **277**, 24609–17.

Forrest, J.C. and Dermody, T.S. 2003. Reovirus receptors and pathogenesis. *J Virol*, **77**, 9109–15.

Fraser, R.D.B., Furlong, D.B., et al. 1990. Molecular structure of the cell-attachment protein of reovirus: correlation of computer-processed electron micrographs with sequence-based predictions. *J Virol*, **64**, 2990–3000.

French, T.J., Marshall, J.J. and Roy, P. 1990. Assembly of double-shelled, viruslike particles of bluetongue virus by the simultaneous expression of four structural proteins. *J Virol*, **64**, 5695–700.

Grimes, J., Basak, A.K., et al. 1995. The crystal structure of bluetongue virus VP7. *Nature*, **373**, 167–70.

Grimes, J.M., Burroughs, J.N., et al. 1998. The atomic structure of the bluetongue virus core. *Nature*, **395**, 470–8.

Hewat, E.A., Booth, T.F. and Roy, P. 1994. Structure of correctly self-assembled bluetongue virus-like particles. *J Struct Biol*, **112**, 183–91.

House, J.A. 1998. Future international management of African horse sickness vaccines. *Arch Virol Suppl*, **14**, 297–304.

Huismans, H., van der Walt, N.T., et al. 1987. Isolation of a capsid protein of bluetongue virus that induces a protective immune response in sheep. *Virology*, **157**, 172–9.

Imani, F. and Jacobs, B.L. 1988. Inhibitory activity for the interferon-induced protein kinase is associated with the reovirus serotype 1 sigma 3 protein. *Proc Natl Acad Sci U S A*, **85**, 7887–91.

Jackson, G.G., Muldoon, R.L. and Cooper, R.S. 1961. Reovirus type 1 as an etiologic agent of the common cold. *J Clin Invest*, **40**, 1051.

Keroack, M. and Fields, B.N. 1986. Viral shedding and transmission between hosts determined by reovirus *L2* gene. *Science*, **232**, 1635–8.

Kominsky, D.J., Bickel, R.J. and Tyler, K.L. 2002. Reovirus-induced apoptosis requires mitochondrial release of Smac/DIABLO and involves reduction of cellular inhibitor of apoptosis protein levels. *J Virol*, **76**, 11414–24.

Kozak, M. 1981. Possible role of flanking nucleotides in recognition of the AUG initiator codon by eukaryotic ribosomes. *Nucleic Acids Res*, **9**, 5233–52.

Lee, P.W., Hayes, E.C. and Joklik, W.K. 1981. Protein σ1 is the reovirus cell attachment protein. *Virology*, **108**, 156–63.

Leers, W.D. and Rozee, K.R. 1966. A survey of reovirus antibodies in sera of urban children. *Can Med Assoc J*, **94**, 1040–2.

Lerner, A.M., Cherry, J.D., et al. 1962. Infections with reoviruses. *N Engl J Med*, **267**, 947–52.

Liemann, S., Chandran, K., et al. 2002. Structure of the reovirus membrane-penetration protein, μ1, in a complex with is protector protein, σ3. *Cell*, **108**, 283–95.

Lloyd, R.M. and Shatkin, A.J. 1992. Translational stimulation by reovirus polypeptide σ3: substitution for VA1-RNA and inhibition of phosphorylation of the α-subunit of eukaryotic initiation factor-II. *J Virol*, **66**, 6878–84.

Luongo, C.L., Reinisch, K.M., et al. 2000. Identification of the mRNA guanylyltransferase region and active site in in reovirus λ2 protein. *J Biol Chem*, **275**, 2804–10.

Martinez-Costas, J., Sutton, G., et al. 1998. Guanylyltransferase and RNA 5′-triphosphatase activities of the purified expressed VP4 protein of bluetongue virus. *J Mol Biol*, **280**, 859–66.

Matsuura, K., Ishikura, M., et al. 1993. Ecological studies on reovirus pollution of rivers in Toyama Prefecture. II. Molecular epidemiological study of reoviruses isolated from river water. *Microbiol Immunol*, **37**, 305–10.

Mattion, N.M., Cohen, J.J. and Estes, M.K. 1994. The rotavirus proteins. In: Kapikian, A.Z. (ed.), *Viral infections of the gastrointestinal tract*. New York: Marcel Dekker, 169–249.

Mellor, P.S. 1990. The replication of bluetongue virus in *Culicoides* vectors. *Curr Top Microbiol Immunol*, **162**, 143–61.

Mertens, P.P.C., Arella, M., et al. 2000. *Reoviridae*. In: Van Regenmortel, M.H.V., Fauquet, C.M., et al. (eds), *Virus taxonomy, classification and nomenclature of viruses*. San Diego, CA: Academic Press, 395–400.

Metcalf, P., Cyrklaff, M. and Adrian, M. 1991. The 3-dimensional structure of reovirus obtained by cryoelectron microscopy. *EMBO J*, **10**, 3129–36.

Mochow-Grundy, M. and Dermody, T.S. 2001. The reovirus S4 gene 3′ nontranslated region contains a translational operator sequence. *J Virol*, **75**, 6517–26.

Monath, T.P. and Guirakhoo, F. 1996. Orbiviruses and coltiviruses. In: Fields, B.N., Knipe, D.M., et al. (eds), *Fields virology*, 3rd edn. Philadelphia, PA: Lippincott-Raven, 1735–66.

Morrison, L.A., Sidman, R.L. and Fields, B.N. 1991. Direct spread of reovirus from the intestinal lumen to the central nervous system through vagal autonomic nerve fibers. *Proc Natl Acad Sci U S A*, **88**, 3852–6.

Morrison, L.A., Fields, B.N. and Dermody, T.S. 1993. Prolonged replication in the mouse central nervous system of reoviruses isolated from persistently infected cultures. *J Virol*, **67**, 3019–26.

Nibert, M.L. and Schiff, L.A. 2001. Reoviruses and their replication. In: Knipe, D.M., Howley, P.M., et al. (eds), *Fields virology*, 4th edn. Philadelphia, PA: Lippincott-Raven, 1679–728.

Nibert, M.L., Schiff, L.A. and Fields, B.N. 1991. Mammalian reoviruses contain a myristoylated structural protein. *J Virol*, **65**, 1960–7.

Nibert, M.L., Chappell, J.D. and Dermody, T.S. 1995. Infectious subvirion particles of reovirus type 3 Dearing exhibit a loss in infectivity and contain a cleaved σ1 protein. *J Virol*, **69**, 5057–67.

Noah, D.L., Blum, M.A. and Sherry, B. 1999. Interferon regulatory factor 3 is required for viral induction of beta interferon in primary cardiac myocyte cultures. *J Virol*, **73**, 10208–13.

Olland, A.M., Jané-Valbuena, J., et al. 2001. Structure of the reovirus outer capsid and dsRNA-binding protein s3 at 1.8 Å resolution. *EMBO J*, **20**, 979–89.

Parsonson, I.M. 1990. Pathology and pathogenesis of bluetongue infections. *Curr Top Microbiol Immunol*, **162**, 119–41.

Ramadevi, N. and Roy, P. 1998. Bluetongue virus core protein VP4 has nucleoside triphosphate phosphohydrolase activity. *J Gen Virol*, **79**, 2475–80.

Ramadevi, N., Burroughs, J.N., et al. 1998. Capping and methylation of mRNA by purified recombinant VP4 protein of bluetongue virus. *Proc Natl Acad Sci USA*, **95**, 13537–42.

Reinisch, K.M., Nibert, M.L. and Harrison, S.C. 2000. Structure of the reovirus core at 3.6 Å resolution. *Nature*, **404**, 960–7.

Ridinger, D.N., Spendlove, R.S., et al. 1982. Evaluation of cell lines and immunofluorescence and plaque assay procedures for quantifying reoviruses in sewage. *Appl Environ Microbiol*, **43**, 740–6.

Roner, M.R. and Joklik, W.K. 2001. Reovirus reverse genetics: Incorporation of the *CAT* gene into the reovirus genome. *Proc Natl Acad Sci U S A*, **98**, 8036–41.

Roner, M.R., Sutphin, L.A. and Joklik, W.K. 1990. Reovirus RNA is infectious. *Virology*, **179**, 845–52.

Roy, P. 1989. Bluetongue virus genetics and genome structure. *Virus Res*, **13**, 179–206.

Roy, P. 2001. Orbiviruses. In: Knipe, D.M., Howley, P., et al. (eds), *Fields virology*, 4th edn. Philadelphia, PA: Lippincott-Raven, 1835–69.

Roy, P. and Sutton, G. 1998. New generation of African horse sickness virus vaccines based on structural and molecular studies of the virus particles. *Arch Virol Suppl*, **14**, 177–202.

Roy, P., French, T. and Erasmus, B.J. 1992. Protective efficacy of virus-like particles for bluetongue disease. *Vaccine*, **10**, 28–32.

Rubin, D.H. and Fields, B.N. 1980. Molecular basis of reovirus virulence: role of the *M2* gene. *J Exp Med*, **152**, 853–68.

Samal, S.K., Livingston, C.W. Jr, et al. 1987. Analysis of mixed infection of sheep with bluetongue virus serotypes 10 and 17: evidence for genetic reassortment in the vertebrate host. *J Virol*, **61**, 1086–91.

Schmechel, S., Chute, M., et al. 1997. Preferential translation of reovirus mRNA by a sigma3-dependent mechanism. *Virology*, **232**, 62–73.

Sherry, B. and Blum, M.A. 1994. Multiple viral core proteins are determinants of reovirus-induced acute myocarditis. *J Virol*, **68**, 8461–5.

Sherry, B. and Fields, B.N. 1989. The reovirus *M1* gene, encoding a viral core protein, is associated with the myocarditic phenotype of a reovirus variant. *J Virol*, **63**, 4850–6.

Sherry, B., Schoen, F.J., et al. 1989. Derivation and characterization of an efficiently myocarditic reovirus variant. *J Virol*, **63**, 4840–9.

Sherry, B., Baty, C.J. and Blum, M.A. 1996. Reovirus-induced acute myocarditis in mice correlates with viral RNA synthesis rather than generation of infectious virus in cardiac myocytes. *J Virol*, **70**, 6709–15.

Sherry, B., Torres, J. and Blum, M.A. 1998. Reovirus induction of and sensitivity to beta interferon in cardiac myocyte cultures correlate with induction of myocarditis and are determined by viral core proteins. *J Virol*, **72**, 1314–23.

Strong, J.E. and Lee, P.W. 1996. The v-*erbB* oncogene confers enhanced cellular susceptibility to reovirus infection. *J Virol*, **70**, 612–16.

Strong, J.E., Coffey, M.C., et al. 1998. The molecular basis of viral oncolysis: usurpation of the *Ras* signaling pathway by reovirus. *EMBO J*, **17**, 3351–62.

Tao, Y., Farsetta, D.L., et al. 2002. RNA synthesis in a cage – structural studies of reovirus polymerase lambda3. *Cell*, **111**, 733–45.

Tardieu, M., Powers, M.L. and Weiner, H.L. 1983. Age-dependent susceptibility to reovirus type 3 encephalitis: role of viral and host factors. *Ann Neurol*, **13**, 602–7.

Tyler, K.L. 2001. Mammalian reoviruses. In: Knipe, D.M., Howley, P.M., et al. (eds), *Fields virology*, 4th edn. Philadelphia, PA: Lippincott-Raven, 1729–45.

Tyler, K.L., McPhee, D.A. and Fields, B.N. 1986. Distinct pathways of viral spread in the host determined by reovirus *S1* gene segment. *Science*, **233**, 770–4.

Tyler, K.L., Squier, M.K., et al. 1995. Differences in the capacity of reovirus strains to induce apoptosis are determined by the viral attachment protein s1. *J Virol*, **69**, 6972–9.

Tyler, K.L., Sokol, R.J., et al. 1998. Detection of reovirus RNA in hepatobiliary tissues from patients with extrahepatic biliary atresia and choledochal cysts. *Hepatology*, **27**, 1475–82.

Van Dijk, A.A. and Huismans, H. 1982. The effect of temperature on the in vitro transcriptase reaction of bluetongue virus, epizootic haemorrhagic disease virus and African horse sickness virus. *Onderstepoort J Vet Res*, **49**, 227–32.

Virgin, H.W., Tyler, K.L. and Dermody, T.S. 1997. Reovirus. In: Nathanson, N. (ed.), *Viral pathogenesis*. New York: Lippincott-Raven, 669–99.

Weiner, H.L., Drayna, D., et al. 1977. Molecular basis of reovirus virulence: role of the *S1* gene. *Proc Natl Acad Sci U S A*, **74**, 5744–8.

Weiner, H.L., Ault, K.A. and Fields, B.N. 1980a. Interaction of reovirus with cell surface receptors. I. Murine and human lymphocytes have a receptor for the hemagglutinin of reovirus type 3. *J Immunol*, **124**, 2143–8.

Weiner, H.L., Powers, M.L. and Fields, B.N. 1980b. Absolute linkage of virulence and central nervous system tropism of reoviruses to viral hemagglutinin. *J Infect Dis*, **141**, 609–16.

Wilson, G.A.R., Morrison, L.A. and Fields, B.N. 1994. Association of the reovirus *S1* gene with serotype 3-induced biliary atresia in mice. *J Virol*, **68**, 6458–65.

Wolf, J.L., Rubin, D.H., et al. 1981. Intestinal M cells: a pathway of entry of reovirus into the host. *Science*, **212**, 471–2.

44

Rotaviruses

ULRICH DESSELBERGER, JIM GRAY AND MARY K. ESTES

Rotaviruses were discovered in 1973 as being associated with diarrheal disease in children (Bishop et al. 1973; Flewett et al. 1973) and have since been recognized as the major cause of gastroenteritis in infants and young children and in a wide range of animal species. In humans, they cause 500 000–600 000 deaths each year (Miller and McCann 2000), and there is an urgent need for a vaccine. For reviews of other viral causes of gastroenteritis, see Blacklow and Greenberg (1991), Kapikian (1994), Hart and Cunliffe (1997), Chiba et al. (1997), Desselberger (1998a), Chadwick and Goode (2001), Cohen et al. (2002), Desselberger and Gray (2003), and Chapters 22, Adenovirus; 41, Human enteric RNA viruses: astroviruses; and 42, Human enteric RNA viruses: noroviruses and sapoviruses.

GENOME, GENE PROTEIN ASSIGNMENT, AND STRUCTURE

Rotaviruses have a genome of 11 segments of double-stranded RNA (dsRNA) which can be easily separated by polyacrylamide gel electrophoresis. The RNA segments code for six structural (VP1, VP2, VP3, VP4, VP6, VP7) and six nonstructural proteins (NSP1–NSP6) (Estes 2001). The structural proteins make up a triple-layered particle and are located in the core (inner layer; VP1–VP3), inner shell (intermediate layer; VP6) and outer shell (outer layer; VP4, VP7). The wheel-like (Latin: *rota*) appearance by electron microscopy of the triple-layered particles is diagnostic (Figure 44.1a). Figure 44.1b shows diagrammatically the gene coding assignment, the position of the structural proteins in the particles and their three-dimensional (3D) structure as obtained by image processing techniques from cryo-electron micrographs.

Further details of the 3D structure have been elucidated in a number of excellent studies by the groups of Prasad (Prasad et al. 1988, 1990, 1996; Shaw et al. 1993; Prasad and Chiu 1994; Lawton et al. 1997a, b, 1999, 2000; Prasad and Estes 1997; Crawford et al. 2001; Pesavento et al. 2001); Yeager (Yeager et al. 1990, 1994), Rey (Petitpas et al. 1998; Lepault et al. 2001; Mathieu et al. 2001) and Hewat (Thouvenin et al. 2001). According to their findings, the genome is comprised within the core shell formed by VP2. The transcription complex, consisting of VP1 and VP3, is attached at the 12 fivefold symmetry positions on the inside of the shell. The addition of VP6 (260 trimers) produces double-layered particles, and further addition of VP7 (780 molecules) and VP4 (60 dimers) leads to the formation of triple-layered particles which are the infectious virions after VP4 cleavage. The triple-layered capsid is ordered along five-, three-, and two-fold symmetry axes and is perforated by 132 aqueous channels of types I–III (located in the three symmetry positions). The type I channels play an important role in transcription (see below).

Complete gene–protein assignments have been achieved for several *Rotavirus* strains. Table 44.1, p. 948

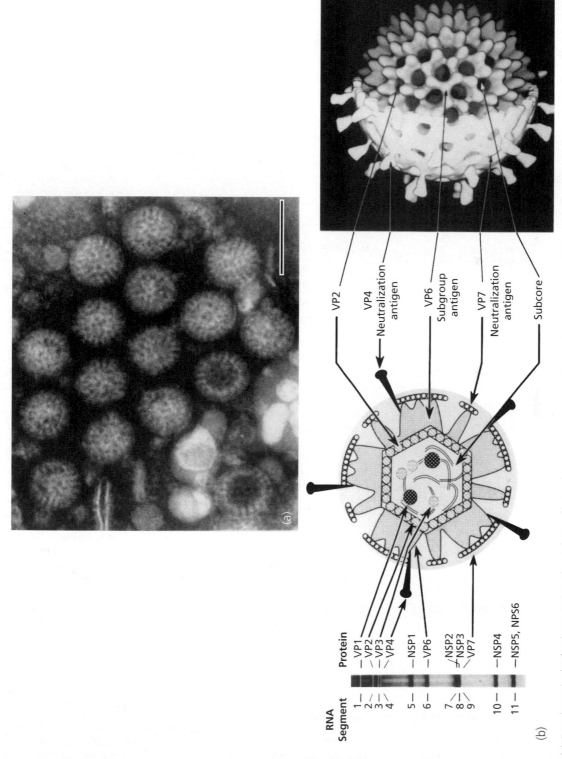

Figure 44.1 (a) Rotaviruses in the fecal suspension of an infant suffering from acute gastroenteritis. Electron micrograph, PTA stain. (Courtesy of Dr. E.A.C. Follett, Regional Virus Laboratory, Ruchill Hospital, Glasgow. Bar, 100 nm.) **(b)** RNA profile (10 percent SDS polyacrylamide gel, silver stain), protein products (gene protein assignment and particle structure (diagram and reconstruction from a cryo-electron micrograph) of rotaviruses. (From Mattion et al. 1994, with permission of the authors and publisher)

Table 44.1 *Genes, gene protein assignments, and functions of proteins of group A* Rotavirus

RNA segment No.	Size (bp)	Protein product Description	Deduced mol. mass (kDa)	Location	No. of molecules per virion	Post-translational modification	Functions
1	3 302	VP1	125.0	Inner core	12	–	RNA-dependent RNA polymerase; binds ssRNA; complex with VP3
2	2 690	VP2	94.0	Core	120	Myristylation	Binds RNA; required for replicase activity of VP1
3	2 591	VP3	88.0	Inner core	12	–	Guanylyltransferase; methyltransferase; complex with VP1
4	2 362	VP4	86.8	Outer capsid (dimer)	120	Proteolytic cleavage to VP5* and VP8*	Hemagglutinin; cell attachment; neutralization antigen (ab protective); fusogenic; protease-enhanced infectivity; virulence (mice, piglets)
5	1 611	NS53, NSP1 (VP5)	58.7	Nonstructural	NA[c]	–	Binds RNA; virulence (mice); nonessential for replication (some strains); interacts with IRF-3
6	1 356	VP6	44.8	Inner capsid (trimer)	780	Myristylation	Group- and subgroup-specific antigen; protection (intracellular neutralization)? Required for transcription
7[a]	1 059	VP9 (NSP3)	34.6	Nonstructural (dimer)	NA	–	Binds RNA (3′ end); competes with cellular PABP for interaction with eIF-4G1 (translation); inhibits host-cell translation
8[a]	1 104	NS35, NSP2 (VP8)	36.7	Nonstructural (octamer)	NA	–	Binds RNA; NTPase; helicase; involved in +strand RNA packaging; virulence (mice)
9[a]	1 062	VP7	37.4[b]	Outer capsid (trimer)	780	Cleavage of signal sequence; glycosylation	Neutralization antigen (ab protective); binds Ca^{2+}
10	751	VP12 (NSP4)	20.3	Nonstructural	NA	Glycosylation (VP10, NS28); trimming	Intracellular receptor (morphogenesis); viral enterotoxin (secreted cleavage product); protection by specific ab; virulence (mice, piglets)
11	667	VP11 (NSP5)	21.7	Nonstructural	NA	O-glycosylation, phosphorylation	Binds RNA; protein kinase; interacts with NSP2, VP2, and NSP6
		NSP6	12.0	Nonstructural	NA		Interacts with NSP5

Modified from Estes (2001).
a) This gene protein assignment is of the SA11 rotavirus strain.
b) Second in-frame initiation codon located 30 codons downstream (deduced mol. mass 33.9 kDa).
c) NA, not applicable.

lists the RNA segments and their products for the simian rotavirus SA11 strain; also noted are post-translational modifications and functions as far as known.

CLASSIFICATION INTO SUBGROUPS, SEROTYPES, AND GENOTYPES

A classification of rotaviruses has been derived from immunological characteristics of various components of the particles and from genomic composition (Estes 2001). Groups A–E can be differentiated according to lack of serological crossreactivities of the inner capsid protein VP6 with polyclonal and monoclonal antibodies. There may be two more groups, F and G (Bridger 1987). Within group A rotaviruses, subgroups (I, II, I+II, nonI, nonII) were defined according to exclusive reactivities of two VP6-specific monoclonal antibodies (Greenberg et al. 1982). Types within group A are determined by cross-neutralization studies as serotypes (Offit et al. 1986; Green and Kapikian 1992) or by sequence comparison as genotypes. (Typing of rotaviruses within other groups is rudimentary.) As the two surface proteins (VP4 and VP7) carry neutralization-specific antigens, a dual classification scheme, similar to that developed for influenza viruses, has been established, differentiating G types (for VP7 which is a **g**lycoprotein) and P types (for VP4 which is a **p**rotease-sensitive protein, being cleaved post-translationally into its subunits VP5* and VP8*). So far, 14 G types and at least 20 P types have been differentiated, indicating extensive genomic diversity within group A rotaviruses (Estes 2001). As these proteins are coded for by different RNA segments and as rotaviruses of the same group reassort readily in doubly infected cells, both in vitro (Garbarg-Chenon et al. 1984; Graham et al. 1987) and in vivo (Gombold and Ramig 1986; Ward et al. 1990), the observed diversity resulting from various combinations of VP7 and VP4 types is very large. Whilst the correlation of G serotypes and genotypes is practically complete, for many P genotypes no serotype has been established yet. Therefore P serotype and genotype are designated separately but jointly (where available), the latter in square brackets: for example, the human Wa strain is classified as G1P1A[8], the human DS-1 strain as G2P1B[4], the equine strain Eq/L338 as G13P12[18], the bovine strain Bo/993/83 as G7P[17], etc.

REPLICATION

Rotaviruses spread via the oral–fecal route and infect the small intestine after oral ingestion. Multiplication occurs in the mature epithelial cells at the tips of the villi of the small intestine. Rotaviruses grow well in secondary monkey kidney cells and in immortalized monkey kidney cell lines (MA104, BS-C1) in the presence of trypsin, and therefore their replication in vitro could be studied in detail (Estes 2001). Figure 44.2 is a diagrammatic presentation of these events. Triple-layered particles (i.e. the infectious virions) attach to the host cells via the outer-layer protein VP4 (Ludert et al. 1996). Virus entry is by receptor-mediated endocytosis or direct penetration (Cuadras et al. 1997; Gilbert et al. 1997). The cellular receptor or receptors have not been fully characterized yet, but some animal strains use sialic acid located on glycolipids (Ciarlet and Estes 1999; Ciarlet et al. 2002b). Other strains seem to recognize galactose (Jolly et al. 2001). In addition to glycolipids, several integrins have been proposed to mediate uptake, possibly in a post-attachment step, acting as co-receptors (Coulson et al. 1997; Guerrero et al. 2000; Hewish et al. 2000). The heat-shock cognate (Hsc) protein 70 may also be involved as a co-receptor (Guerrero et al. 2002). For porcine rotavirus, a ganglioside receptor has been described (Rolsma et al. 1998). Replication is exclusively in the cytoplasm. After removal of the outer capsid proteins, the viral RNA-dependent RNA polymerase (coded for by RNA 1) is activated in double-layered particles (Cohen et al. 1979), and by use of the VP1/VP2/VP3 transcription complex (Lawton et al. 2000) large numbers of positive-strand RNA molecules are transcribed and exit from the double-layered particles via their 12 aqueous channels located on the vertices of the fivefold symmetry axes. This process is ATP-dependent. Transcription is asymmetric, i.e. only positive-strand RNAs appear as transcription products. Multiple RNA molecules can be transcribed from a single actively transcribing particle. The new RNA molecules act as mRNAs, and their translation products start to accumulate in the cytoplasm. NSP3 is intimately involved in translation by binding to the 3′ end of mRNA and to the eukaryotic translation factor eIF-4G (Vende et al. 2000). Molecules of mRNA seem to be pulled through VP2 oligomers (the nascent core) by means of a complex formation with NSP2 which has NTPase activity and acts as a molecular motor (Taraporewala et al. 1999; Patton 2001; Schuck et al. 2001; Taraporewala and Patton 2001). NSP5 that interacts with VP2 and NSP2 (Berois et al. 2003) is also involved at this stage. Double-layered particles are formed, consisting of VP1, VP2, VP3, and VP6 and several of the nonstructural proteins, and containing one genome equivalent of packaged single-stranded RNA which is then replicated to form dsRNA. Double-layered particles accumulate and form pseudocrystalline aggregates termed viroplasm (= intracytoplasmic inclusion bodies). It is not clear at present how the very tight packaging control of rotaviruses (and of other *Reoviridae*) is achieved. When budding through the rough endoplasmic reticulum (RER), whereby NSP4 acts as an intracellular receptor for VP6, double-layered particles incorporate VP7 and VP4 to form the third, outer layer (a transient, RER-derived envelope is shed before complete maturation). Triple-layered infectious virions are released by cell lysis. VP4 may reach the plasma membrane through

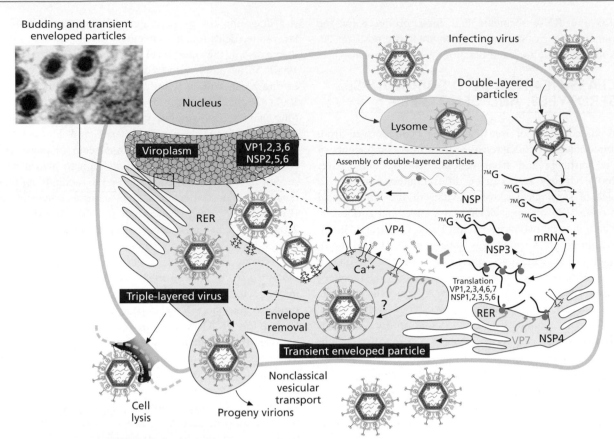

Figure 44.2 *Major features of the* Rotavirus *replication cycle. For details see text. Triple layered rotavirus particles (TLPs, i.e. infectious virions) attach to the surface of the host cell by its outer layer protein, VP4, interacting with sialic acid (in glycolipids) or other receptors on the cell surface. Virus entry is by receptor mediated endocytosis. The outer layer proteins VP4 and VP7 are removed (possibly in lysosomes). The resulting double layered particles (DLPs) are transcription active, i.e. they synthesize and extrude large numbers of mRNAs (specific for all RNA segments) that are capped but not polyadenylated. Only positive sense transcription products are made. The mRNAs are translated into proteins using the cellular machinery. This process is facilitated by the viral NSP3 interacting with the 3′ end of the mRNA and forming a complex with the eukaryotic translation factor eIF4G. Rotavirus cores are formed, consisting of VP2, VP1, and VP3, into which rotavirus mRNA molecules are incorporated. The rotavirus proteins NSP2 and NSP5 are intimately involved in this process which is ATP dependent. Within the cores the ssRNA segments are replicated to form the dsRNA genome. The early packaging process is tightly controlled. Rotavirus cores interact with VP6 to form DLPs which in turn aggregate into pseudocrystalline arrays termed 'viroplasm' (i.e. intracytoplasmic inclusion bodies). DLPs then bud through the rough endoplasmic reticulum (RER); this step is facilitated by interaction of NSP4 that has become part of the RER membranes with DLPs via VP6 (NSP4 acting as an intracellular receptor for DLPs). In the RER, DLPs acquire VP7 and VP4 to become TLPs. During this process particles are transiently enveloped; however, the envelope is shed before complete maturation (this step is a unique characteristic of rotavirus replication that is still poorly understood). TLPs are then released by the cell undergoing lysis or by a 'non-classical' vesicular transport involving interaction with lipid 'rafts' near the plasma membrane. (Redrawn from Estes 2001, with permission of the publisher)*

the microtubule network and interact with cholesterol liposphingolipid rafts, possibly promoting assembly near the plasma membrane (Nejmeddine et al. 2000; Sapin et al., 2002; not shown in Figure 44.2) (For further details of structure–function correlations and replication see Prasad and Estes 1997; Lawton et al. 2000; Estes 2001). In immunodeficient hosts and under certain experimental conditions, rotaviruses undergo genome rearrangements (for review: Desselberger 1996).

PATHOGENESIS: ANIMAL MODELS

Cell death and desquamation reduce digestion and adsorption of nutrients (primary malabsorption) and lead to villous atrophy. This is followed by a reactive crypt-cell hyperplasia accompanied by increased secretion, which is thought to contribute to the severity of diarrhea. The local pathogenesis is shown diagrammatically in Figure 44.3.

Several animal models for rotavirus infections are being explored (mice, rabbits, piglets, rats; Saif et al. 1994; Burns et al. 1995; Conner and Ramig 1996; Guérin-Danan et al. 1998; Ciarlet et al. 2002a). Of those, piglets and rats are infectable with human strains and produce diarrhea; they are therefore of particular interest. Many features of rotavirus infections, particularly pathogenicity and immune responses, have been studied in animal models to a greater extent than in man (see below).

The viral factors determining pathogenicity of rotaviruses have been investigated in several animal models

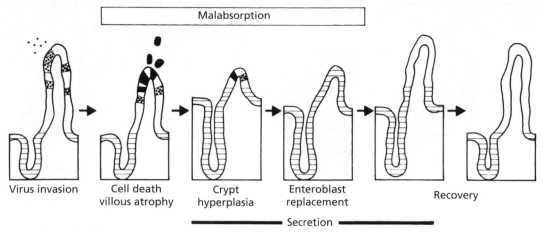

Figure 44.3 Rotavirus *pathogenesis (diagram). Development of damage to gut mucosa and ensuing diarrhea. (Redrawn from Phillips 1989, with permission of the author and publisher.)*

(piglets, mice, rabbits). The product of RNA segment 4, VP4, is likely to be a major determinant (Offit et al. 1986; Gorziglia et al. 1988; Bridger et al. 1992, 1998; Burke et al. 1994a, b), but products of other structural genes (RNA 3 coding for VP3 and RNAs 8 or 9 coding for VP7) and nonstructural genes (RNA 5, coding for NSP1, RNA 8 coding for NSP2, and RNA 10 coding for NSP4) have also been associated with pathogenicity (Table 44.2) (Broome et al. 1993; Hoshino et al. 1993, 1995; Ball et al. 1996 ; review by Burke and Desselberger 1996).

The discovery of NSP4 as an enterotoxin (Tian et al. 1994, 1995; Ball et al. 1996) has allowed the old observation that rotavirus-infected animals exhibit profuse diarrhea prior to the detection of histological lesions to be explained. NSP4 or a peptide thereof (aa 114–135) induce dose- and age-dependent diarrhea in laboratory animals (mice, rats) in the absence of histological changes (Ball et al. 1996) (Figure 44.4).

NSP4 produces an increase in intracellular Ca^{2+} concentration (Tian et al. 1994), disturbing the cellular homeostasis. Recently it was found that a peptide of NSP4, that is active as an enterotoxin is secreted from infected cells (Zhang and Zeng 2000) and is able to induce intracellular Ca^{2+} elevation and diarrhea in mice.

It is thought that the secreted protein binds to a (still hypothetical) receptor and thus affects uninfected cells (Zhang and Zeng 2000; Tafazoli et al. 2001). A model of the NSP4 action is proposed in Figure 44.5, p. 953.

Antibody to NSP4 has been shown to reduce the severity of diarrheal disease in suckling mice (Estes 2003). The effect of rotavirus infection on the enteric nervous system also may play a role in pathogenesis (Lundgren et al. 2000).

ILLNESS AND TREATMENT

After a short incubation period of 24–48 hours, the onset of illness is sudden with watery diarrhea, vomiting, and rapid dehydration. Untreated rotavirus infection is a major cause of infant death in the developing world. It should be noted, though, that the clinical symptoms of rotavirus infection may vary widely: asymptomatic infections of neonates with so-called nursery strains have been described (Hoshino et al. 1985; Gorziglia et al. 1988), but also central nervous system infections (Iturriza-Gómara et al. 2002a) and chronic infections and hepatitis in children with immunodeficiencies (Gilger et al. 1992).

Table 44.2 Rotavirus *genes implicated in pathogenicity in different hosts*

Gene segment	Gene product	Host	Reference
3	VP3	Pig	Hoshino et al. 1993, 1995
4	VP4	Mouse	Offit et al. 1986
		Human	Gorziglia et al. 1988
		Pig	Bridger et al. 1992; Burke et al. 1994a, b; Hoshino et al. 1993, 1995
5	NS53 (NSP1)	Mouse	Broome et al. 1993
7	NS35 (NSP2)	Mouse	Broome et al. 1993
7 or 8	NSP3	Mouse	Mossel and Ramig 2002, 2003
8 or 9	VP7	Pig	Hoshino et al. 1993, 1995
10	NS28 (NSP4)	Pig	Hoshino et al. 1993, 1995
		Mouse, rat	Tian et al. 1994, 1995; Ball et al. 1996; Zhang and Zeng 2000; Tafazoli et al. 2001; Yu and Langridge 2001 ; Estes 2003

Modified from Burke and Desselberger 1996.

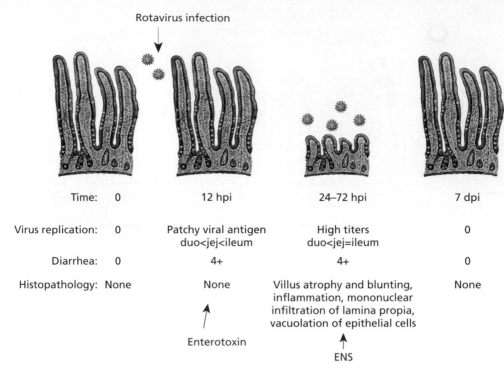

Figure 44.4 Rotavirus *pathogenesis. Correlation of virus replication, histopathology, and disease over time. Enterotoxin, NSP4; ENS, enteric nervous system. (From Estes 2001 with permission of the publisher)*

Treatment is by oral, subcutaneous, or intravenous rehydration (Bhan et al. 1994; International Study Group on Reduced-osmolarity ORS Solutions 1995; Desselberger 1999). Table 44.3 gives the WHO-approved formulae of oral rehydration solutions (ORS). There is no approved specific antiviral treatment (Desselberger 1999). Oral immunoglobulins seem to shorten the period of virus shedding and diarrhea but are not in routine therapeutic use (Guarino et al. 1994; Bass 2003).

DIAGNOSIS

The number of virus particles in the gut at the peak of the diarrhea can be as high at 10^{11}/ml of feces. Diagnosis is therefore relatively easy using electron microscopy, enzyme-linked immunosorbent assays (ELISA) or passive particle agglutination techniques.

Electron microscopy allows quick identification of the pathognomonic double- and triple-layered rotavirus particles. These particles differ morphologically from other viruses causing acute gastroenteritis: enteric adenoviruses, human caliciviruses (noro- and sapo-viruses), astroviruses, and small round viruses (SRV) (Doane 1994) (see Chapters 22, Adenovirus; 41, Human enteric RNA viruses: astroviruses; and 42, Human enteric RNA viruses: noroviruses and sapoviruses).

Serological assays to detect rotavirus antigen are used widely, mostly applying direct or indirect ELISAs. The tests can be calibrated and quantified and are easily performed. If the detecting anti-rotavirus antibody is type-specific, the test can be used for G and P typing; this, however, depends on the presence of triple-layered virus particles in the clinical specimen. Another frequently used rapid technique is a passive particle agglutination test (Ruggeri et al. 1992). Details of procedures are described by Yolken and Wilde (1994).

The viral genome can be detected easily after phenol extraction of RNA from crude or semipurified rotavirus-containing specimens and separation by polyacrylamide gel electrophoresis (PAGE) followed by silver staining (Herring et al. 1982). Nowadays, the procedure is of value mainly in outbreak investigations.

The use of rotavirus-specific oligonucleotide primers in reverse transcription-polymerase chain reactions (RT-PCR) has allowed not only sensitive detection but also subgroup determination and typing for both G and P types when the subgroup- and type-specifying sequence diversities are exploited (Gouvea et al. 1990; Gentsch et al. 1992; Iturriza-Gómara et al. 2002c, 2003b). For rotavirus typing, RT-PCR has become the method of choice (Iturriza-Gómara et al. 1999, 2000).

Human rotaviruses can be grown in vitro on monkey kidney cells in the presence of trypsin (Ward et al. 1984), but the procedure is not in routine use.

IMMUNE RESPONSE AND CORRELATES OF PROTECTION

After neonatal or primary rotavirus infection a mainly serotype-specific humoral immune response is elicited, but there is also partial protection against subsequent

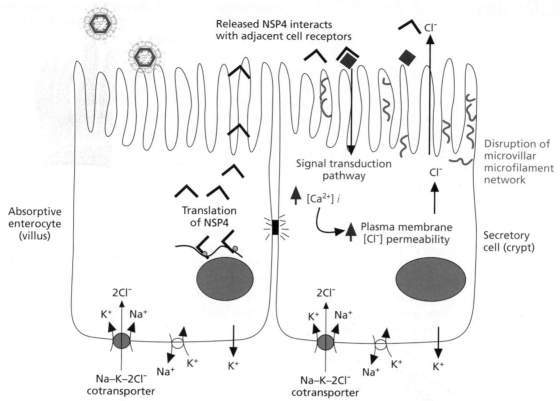

Figure 44.5 *Proposed model of NSP4 action. Rotavirus-infected enterocytes produce virus-specific proteins including NSP4. NSP4 is released from cells by lysis or secretion, and this extracellular NSP4 acts in a paracellular fashion by binding to an as yet unidentified receptor for NSP4 on adjacent cells. This triggers a rapid response involving a signal transduction pathway that mobilizes intracellular Ca^{2+} and results in increased plasma membrane Cl^- permeability. The secretory cells are likely to be crypt cells but might also be villus enterocytes. The plasma membrane permeability is age-dependent, based on studies in CFTR knock-out mice (Morris et al. 1999). Extracellular NSP4 also causes a delayed disruption of the organization of filamentous actin and transepithelial resistance (Tafazoli et al. 2001). ∧, NSP4; ◆, (putative) NSP4 receptor. (Redrawn from Estes et al. 2001)*

heterotypic infections (Bishop et al. 1983; Chiba et al. 1986; Friedman et al. 1988). The exact correlates of protection remain to be determined (Offit 1994), but the best are provided by coproantibodies of the IgA subclass (Coulson et al. 1992; Matson et al. 1993; Feng et al. 1994, 1997; Yuan et al. 1996; To et al. 1998) although not in all cases (O'Neal et al. 2000). There seems to be protection from severe disease after natural infection and vaccination (see below) even if the serotype of the

challenging virus differs from that of the first infection or vaccination (Ward et al. 1992; Offit 1994; Velazquez et al. 1996). In the mouse model, homologous protection from infection depends on the level of mucosal IgA antibodies; heterologous protection can also be achieved, but depends on dose and strain and also seems to be correlated with the ability of the heterologous strain to stimulate detectable rotavirus-specific intestinal IgA antibody (Feng et al. 1994, 1997). In mice, rotavirus VP6-specific IgA monoclonal antibodies that lack direct neutralizing activity can protect from primary infection. It has been proposed that the mechanism of protection is by intracellular viral inactivation following transcytosis of IgA (Burns et al. 1996; Herrmann et al. 1996; Feng et al. 1997; Schwartz-Cornil et al. 2002) as experimentally shown for influenza viruses (Mazanec et al. 1995), but firm data on 'intracellular neutralization' have not become available so far for rotaviruses. The extent to which heterotypic protection is efficient in humans remains unclear (Offit 1994). There are rotavirus-specific cytotoxic T-cell responses but their exact role in overcoming the infection and protecting against subsequent infections is not clear (Offit et al. 1993; Offit 1994; Franco and Greenberg 1995).

Table 44.3 *Oral rehydration solutions (ORS) for the treatment of Rotavirus-related diarrhea*

Component	Osmolarity (mmol/l)	
	WHO ORS	'ORS light'
Sodium	90	60
Potassium	20	20
Chloride	80	50
Citrate	10	10
Glucose	111	84
Total, osmolarity	**311**	**224**

Modified from Desselberger (1999).

EPIDEMIOLOGY

The epidemiology of group A rotavirus infections is complex, as at any one time and in any geographical location rotaviruses of different G types co-circulate (e.g. Noel et al. 1991; Gentsch et al. 1996; Ramachandran et al. 1998). The relative incidence of G types also changes over time in the same location. Approximately 95 percent of co-circulating strains are types G1–G4 in most places, typically G1P1A[8], G2P1B[4], G3P1A[8], and G4P1A[8], but other G types may be represented at high frequencies, particularly in tropical areas (Gentsch et al. 1996; Leite et al. 1996; Ramachandran et al. 1996; Cunliffe et al. 1999; Iturriza-Gómara et al. 2000; for review: Desselberger et al. 2001). Recently, G9 rotaviruses have been isolated as one of the predominant outbreak strains in several locations in the USA (Ramachandran et al. 1998) and in the UK (Iturriza-Gómara et al. 2002b). Group B rotaviruses have caused outbreaks of diarrhea in children and adults in China (for review see Hung 1988; Fang et al. 1989) and have been isolated from sporadic cases of gastroenteritis in Calcutta, India (Krishnan et al. 1999; Kobayashi et al. 2001). Group C rotaviruses are associated with small outbreaks in humans (Caul et al. 1990; Jiang et al. 1995).

Besides the accumulation of point mutations (genomic drift; Iturriza-Gómara et al. 2003b), gene reassortment upon dual infection with co-circulating human, or human and animal strains (genomic shift; Iturriza-Gómara et al. 2001, 2003b) is likely to play a major role in generating the increasing diversity of rotaviruses. Although reassortment of two different viruses with 11 gene segments theoretically predicts 2^{11} different progeny viruses (including the parent strains), constraints to reassortment have been identified in naturally circulating rotaviruses (Graham et al. 1987). The genes encoding the structural proteins VP6, VP7, and VP4 reassort independently, although some constraints among the genetic lineages of these proteins seem to exist (Iturriza-Gómara et al. 2001, 2003b). By contrast, the genes encoding VP4 and NSP4 are inextricably linked in progeny, possibly through their intense interaction during morphogenesis (Iturriza-Gómara et al. 2003a).

As for group A rotaviruses (Estes 2001), there is a large animal reservoir for group B rotaviruses. Whilst transmission of animal rotaviruses to man has been demonstrated, it is not clear at present to what extent animal rotaviruses can be transmitted to man (Das et al. 1993; Gentsch et al. 1996).

VACCINE DEVELOPMENT

Rotavirus infections have been recognized as a major viral infection in children worldwide (Bern and Glass 1994), and therefore development of vaccine candidates has been a major goal and has been in progress since the early 1980s. Results have been mixed for some time, owing to the enormous genomic and antigenic diversity of rotaviruses (for review see Kapikian 1994; Vesikari 1994; Desselberger 1998b). Mainly animal rotaviruses (of simian or bovine origin) have been used as live attenuated vaccines. In many cases, protection from infection and/or mild disease was only modest (40–50 percent). By contrast, 70–80 percent protection from severe disease including dehydration was recently achieved (Rennels et al. 1996; Joensuu et al. 1997; Pérez-Schael et al. 1997), particularly when applying a cocktail of viruses, for example as a tetravalent vaccine containing a rhesus monkey rotavirus (RRV) of G3 type and three monoreassortants, individually carrying the VP7 gene of human serotypes G1, G2, and G4 in the RRV genetic background. A tetravalent RRV-based reassortant vaccine (Rotashield®) received Food and Drug Administration (FDA) approval as a universal vaccine in the USA in August 1998, and recommendations for its usage have been issued (Centers for Disease Control and Prevention 1999a). More than 1.5 million doses were administered in the following 10 months. During that time cases of intussusception were observed in vaccinees, particularly within 3–7 days after the first dose with a relative risk of 27.9 (95 percent confidence interval 10.8–72.1; Murphy et al. 2001), and attributable risks of between one case of intussusception in every 4 700–9 500 children vaccinated (Murphy et al. 2001) and one case in 11 000 children vaccinated (Kramarz et al. 2001) have been calculated. These observations led the Centers for Disease Control and Prevention (CDC) and the American Academy of Pediatrics to withdraw the recommendation for use in infants (Centers for Disease Control and Prevention, 1999b, c). Recent ecological studies have failed to demonstrate an increase in the incidence of intussusception during the time of usage of the Rotashield vaccine (Chang et al. 2001; Simonsen et al. 2001), suggesting that the attributable risk may be even smaller.

However, due to the urgent need for a rotavirus vaccine, the research for its development is ongoing. There are several other live attenuated candidate vaccine strains: the bovine WC3 virus (G6P7[5]) and G1 and P1A[8] reassortants thereof (Treanor et al. 1995; Clark et al. 1996), the attenuated human strain 89-12 (G1P1A[8]: Bernstein et al. 1998, 1999), and multivalent vaccines comprising representative strains carrying G1–G4 and G9. Two live, attenuated oral rotavirus candidate vaccines, consisting of a) a pentavalent WC3-based, human reassortant vaccine (Rota-Teq™), and b) a monovalent strain 89-12-based vaccine (Rotarix™), are in advanced stages of large phase III trials (Heaton 2004, De Vos 2004), and are likely to enter the licensure process in 2005. Rotarix™ has already been approved in Mexico in early 2005.

In addition, new approaches to immunization are under investigation: applying inactivated virus or synthetic peptides (Conner et al. 1993), enhancing rotavirus immunogenicity by microencapsidation (Offit et al. 1994), using virus-like particles (VLP) obtained by co-expression of viral proteins (VP2, VP4, VP6, and VP7) from baculovirus recombinants in insect cells (Crawford et al. 1994; Conner et al. 1996; O'Neal et al. 1997; Ciarlet et al. 1998) or using DNA vaccines (Herrmann et al. 1996; Chen et al. 1997, 1998). Expression of rotavirus proteins in plants (potatoes, bananas) from vectors downstream of plant-specific promoters is also under investigation ('edible vaccines,' Arntzen 1997; Yu and Langridge 2001; Mason et al. 2002). In view of the heterotypic immune responses observed after natural infection and immunization, it must be determined which of the epidemiologically important human P and G rotaviruses are mainly required for protection (Offit 1994).

ACKNOWLEDGMENTS

The authors thank Jean Cohen for critical reading of and advice on this chapter.

REFERENCES

Arntzen, C.J. 1997. Edible vaccines. *Public Health Rep*, **112**, 190–7.

Ball, J.M., Tiang, P., et al. 1996. Age-dependent diarrhea induced by a rotaviral nonstructural glycoprotein. *Science*, **272**, 101–4.

Bass, D. 2003. Treatment of viral gastroenteritis. In Desselberger, U. and Gray, J. (eds), *Viral gastroenteritis*. Series *Perspectives in medical virology*. Amsterdam: Elsevier Science, 93–104.

Bern, C. and Glass, R.I. 1994. Impact of diarrheal diseases worldwide. In: Kapikian, A.Z. (ed.), *Viral infections of the gastrointestinal tract*, 2nd edn. New York: Marcel Dekker, 1–26.

Bernstein, D.I., Smith, V.E., et al. 1998. Safety and immunogenicity of live, attenuated human rotavirus vaccine 89-12. *Vaccine*, **16**, 381–7.

Bernstein, D.I., Sack, D.A., et al. 1999. Efficacy of live, attenuated human rotavirus vaccine 89-12 in infants: a randomized placebo-controlled trial. *Lancet*, **354**, 287–90.

Berois, M., Sapin, C., et al. 2003. Rotavirus nonstructural protein NSP5 interacts with the major core protein VP2. *J Virol*, **77**, 1757–63.

Bhan, M.K., Mahalanabis, D., et al. 1994. Clinical trials of improved oral rehydration salt formulations: a review. *Bull WHO*, **72**, 945–55.

Bishop, R.F., Davidson, G.P., et al. 1973. Virus particles in epithelial cells of duodenal mucosa from children with viral gastroenteritis. *Lancet*, **1**, 1281–3.

Bishop, R.F., Barnes, G.L., et al. 1983. Clinical immunity after neonatal rotavirus infection: a prospective longitudinal study in young children. *N Engl J Med*, **309**, 72–6.

Blacklow, N.R. and Greenberg, H.B. 1991. Viral gastroenteritis. *N Engl J Med*, **325**, 252–64.

Bridger, J.C. 1987. Novel rotaviruses in animals and man. *Ciba Found Symp*, **128**, 5–23.

Bridger, J.C., Burke, B., et al. 1992. The pathogenicity of two porcine rotaviruses differing in their in vitro growth characteristics and genes 4. *J Gen Virol*, **73**, 3011–15.

Bridger, J., Tauscher, G.I. and Desselberger, U. 1998. Viral determinant of rotavirus pathogenicity in pigs: evidence that the fourth gene of a porcine rotavirus confers diarrhea in the homologous host. *J Virol*, **72**, 6929–31.

Broome, R.L., Vo, P.T., et al. 1993. Murine rotavirus genes encoding outer capsid proteins VP4 and VP7 are not major determinants of host range restriction and virulence. *J Virol*, **67**, 2448–55.

Burke, B. and Desselberger, U. 1996. Rotavirus pathogenicity. *Virology*, **218**, 299–305.

Burke, B., Bridger, J.C. and Desselberger, U. 1994a. Temporal correlation between a single amino acid change in the VP4 of a porcine rotavirus and a marked change in pathogenicity. *Virology*, **202**, 754–9.

Burke, B., McCrae, M.A. and Desselberger, U. 1994b. Sequence analysis of two porcine rotaviruses differing in growth in vitro and in pathogenicity. Distinct VP4 sequences and conservation of *NS53*, *VP6* and *VP7* genes. *J Gen Virol*, **75**, 2205–12.

Burns, J.W., Krishnaney, A., et al. 1995. Analyses of homologous rotavirus infection in the mouse model. *Virology*, **207**, 143–53.

Burns, J.W., Siadet-Pajouh, M., et al. 1996. Protective effect of rotavirus VP6-specific IgA monoclonal antibodies that lack neutralizing activity. *Science*, **272**, 104–7.

Caul, E.O., Ashley, C.R., et al. 1990. Group C rotavirus associated with fatal enteritis in a family outbreak. *J Med Virol*, **30**, 201–5.

CDC. 1999a. Advisory Committee on Immunization Practices (ACIP). Rotavirus vaccine for the prevention of rotavirus gastroenteritis among children. *Morb Mortal Wkly Rep*, **48(RR-2)**, 1–22.

CDC. 1999b. Advisory Committee on Immunization Practices (ACIP). Intussusception among recipients of rotavirus vaccine – United States, 1998–1999. *Morb Mortal Wkly Rep*, **48**, 577–81.

CDC. 1999c. Advisory Committee on Immunization Practices (ACIP). Withdrawal of rotavirus vaccine recommendation. *Morb Mortal Wkly Rep*, **48**, 1007.

Chadwick, D. and Goode, J.A. (eds). 2001. *Gastroenteritis viruses*. Ciba Foundation Symposium 238. Chichester: John Wiley and Sons.

Chang, H.H., Smith, P.F., et al. 2001. Intussusception, rotavirus diarrhea, and rotavirus vaccine among children in New York State. *Pediatrics*, **108**, 54–60.

Chen, S.C., Fynan, E.F., et al. 1997. Protective immunity induced by rotavirus DNA vaccines. *Vaccine*, **15**, 899–902.

Chen, S.C., Jones, D.H., et al. 1998. Protective immunity induced by oral immunization with a rotavirus DNA vaccine encapsulated in microparticles. *J Virol*, **72**, 5757–61.

Chiba, S., Nakata, S., et al. 1986. Protective effect of naturally acquired homotypic and heterotypic rotavirus antibodies. *Lancet*, **2**, 417–21.

Chiba, S., Estes, M.K., et al. (eds). 1997. Viral gastroenteritis. *Arch Virol*, **142** (Suppl 12), 311 pp.

Ciarlet, M. and Estes, M.K. 1999. Human and animal rotavirus strains do not require the presence of sialic acid on the cell surface for efficient infectivity. *J Gen Virol*, **80**, 943–8.

Ciarlet, M., Crawford, S.E., et al. 1998. Subunit rotavirus vaccine administered parenterally to rabbits induces active protective immunity. *J Virol*, **72**, 9233–46.

Ciarlet, M., Conner, M.E., et al. 2002a. Group A rotavirus infection and age-dependent diarrheal disease in rats: a new animal model to study the pathophysiology of rotavirus infection. *J Virol*, **76**, 41–57.

Ciarlet, M., Ludert, J.E., et al. 2002b. Initial interaction of rotavirus strains with N-acetylneuraminic (sialic) acid residues on the cell surface correlates with VP4 genotype, not species of origin. *J Virol*, **76**, 4087–95.

Clark, H.F., Offit, P.A., et al. 1996. WC3 reassortant vaccines in children. *Arch Virol*, **12**, Suppl, 187–98.

Cohen, J., Laporte, J., et al. 1979. Activation of rotavirus RNA polymerase by calcium chelation. *Arch Virol*, **60**, 177–86.

Cohen, J., Garbarg-Chenon, A. and Pothier, C.H. (eds) 2002. *Les gastroentérites virales*. Paris: Elsevier SAS.

Conner, M.E. and Ramig, R.F. 1996. Enteric diseases. In: Nathanson, N., Ahmed, R., et al. (eds), *Viral pathogenesis*. Philadelphia, PA: Lippincott-Raven, 713–43.

Conner, M.E., Crawford, S.E., et al. 1993. Rotavirus vaccine administered parenterally induces protective immunity. *J Virol*, **67**, 6633–41.

Conner, M.E., Zarley, C.D., et al. 1996. Virus-like particles as a rotavirus subunit vaccine. *J Infect Dis*, **174**, Suppl 1, S88–92.

Coulson, B., Grimwood, K., et al. 1992. Role of coproantibody in clinical protection of children during reinfection with rotavirus. *J Clin Microbiol*, **30**, 1678–84.

Coulson, B.S., Londrigan, S.H. and Lee, D.J. 1997. Rotavirus contains integrin ligand sequences and a disintegrin-like domain implicated in virus entry into cells. *Proc Nat Acad Sci U S A*, **94**, 5389–94.

Crawford, S.E., Labbé, M., et al. 1994. Characterization of virus-like particles produced by the expression of rotavirus capsid protein in insect cells. *J Virol*, **68**, 5945–52.

Crawford, S.E., Mukherjee, S.K., et al. 2001. Trypsin cleavage stabilizes the rotavirus VP4 spike. *J Virol*, **75**, 6052–61.

Cuadras, M.A., Arias, C.F. and Lopez, S. 1997. Rotaviruses induce an early membrane permeabilization of MA104 cells and do not require a low intracellular Ca^{++} concentration to initiate their replication cycle. *J Virol*, **71**, 9065–74.

Cunliffe, N.A., Gondwe, J.S., et al. 1999. Rotavirus G and P types with acute diarrhoea in Blantyre, Malawi: predominance of novel P[6] G8 strains. *J Med Virol*, **57**, 308–12.

Das, M., Dunn, S.J., et al. 1993. Both surface proteins (VP4 and VP7) of an asymptomatic neonatal rotavirus strain (I321) have high levels of sequence identity with the homologous proteins of a serotype 10 bovine rotavirus. *Virology*, **194**, 374–9.

Desselberger, U. 1996. Genome rearrangements of rotaviruses. *Adv Virus Res*, **46**, 69–95.

Desselberger, U. 1998a. Viral gastroenteritis. *Curr Opin Infect Dis*, **11**, 565–75.

Desselberger, U. 1998b. Prospects for vaccine against rotaviruses. *Rev Med Virol*, **8**, 43–52.

Desselberger, U. 1999. Rotavirus infections: guidelines for treatment and prevention. *Drugs*, **58**, 447–52.

Desselberger, U. and Gray, J. (eds). 2003. *Viral gastroenteritis*. Series *Perspectives in medical virology*. Amsterdam: Elsevier Science.

Desselberger, U., Iturriza-Gómara, M. and Gray, J. 2001. Rotavirus epidemiology and surveillance. *Novartis Found Symp*, **238**, 125–47.

De Vos, B. 2004. Phase III evaluation of GlaxoSmithkline Biologicals' live attenuated rotavirus vaccine. In: *Program and Abstracts*, The Sixth International Rotavirus Symposium. Mexico City: p. 51.

Doane, F.W. 1994. Electron microscopy for the detection of gastroenteritis viruses. In: Kapikian, A.Z. (ed.), *Viral infections of the gastrointestinal tract*, 2nd edn. New York: Marcel Dekker, 101–30.

Estes, M.K. 2001. Rotaviruses and their replication. In: Knipe, D.M., Howley, P.M., et al. (eds), *Fields virology*, 4th edn. Philadelphia, PA: Lippincott Williams & Wilkins, 1747–85.

Estes, M.K. 2003. The rotavirus NSP4 enterotoxin: current status and challenges. In: Desselberger, U. and Gray, J. (eds), *Viral gastroenteritis*. Amsterdam: Elsevier Science, 207–24.

Estes, M.K., Kang, G., et al. 2001. Pathogenesis of rotavirus gastroenteritis. *Novartis Found Symp*, **238**, 82–96, discussion 96–100.

Fang, Z.Y., Ye, Q., et al. 1989. Investigation of an outbreak of adult diarrhoea rotavirus in China. *J Infect Dis*, **160**, 948–53.

Feng, N.G., Burns, J.W., et al. 1994. Comparison of mucosal and systemic humoral immune responses and subsequent protection in mice orally inoculated with a homologous or a heterologous rotavirus. *J Virol*, **68**, 7766–73.

Feng, N., Vo, P.T., et al. 1997. Heterotypic protection following oral immunization with live heterologous rotavirus in a mouse model. *J Infect Dis*, **175**, 330–41.

Flewett, T.H., Bryden, A.S. and Davies, H. 1973. Virus particles in gastroenteritis. *Lancet*, **2**, 1497.

Franco, M.A. and Greenberg, H.B. 1995. Role of B cells and cytotoxic T lymphocytes in clearance and immunity of rotavirus infection in mice. *J Virol*, **68**, 7800–6.

Friedman, M.G., Galil, A., et al. 1988. Two sequential outbreaks of rotavirus gastroenteritis: evidence of symptomatic and asymptomatic reinfections. *J Infect Dis*, **158**, 814–22.

Garbarg-Chenon, A., Bricout, F., et al. 1984. Study of genetic reassortment between 2 human rotaviruses. *Virology*, **139**, 358–65.

Gentsch, J.R., Glass, R.I., et al. 1992. Identification of group A rotavirus gene 4 types by polymerase chain reaction. *J Clin Microbiol*, **30**, 1365–73.

Gentsch, J.R., Woods, P.A., et al. 1996. Review of G and P typing results from a global collection of rotavirus strains: implication for vaccine developments. *J Infect Dis*, **174**, Suppl 1, S30–6.

Gilbert, J.M., Greenberg, H.B., et al. 1997. Virus-like particle induced fusion-from-without in tissue culture cells; role of outer-layer proteins VP4 and VP7. *J Virol*, **71**, 4555–63.

Gilger, M.A., Matson, D.O., et al. 1992. Extraintestinal rotavirus infections in children with immunodeficiencies. *J Pediatr*, **120**, 912–17.

Gombold, J.L. and Ramig, R.F. 1986. Analysis of reassortants of genome segments in mice mixedly infected with rotavirus SA11 and RRV. *J Virol*, **57**, 110–16.

Gorziglia, M., Green, K., et al. 1988. Sequence of the fourth gene of human rotaviruses recovered from asymptomatic or symptomatic infections. *J Virol*, **64**, 2978–84.

Gouvea, V., Glass, R.I., et al. 1990. Polymerase chain reaction amplification and typing of rotavirus nucleic acid from stool specimens. *J Clin Microbiol*, **28**, 276–82.

Graham, A., Kudesia, G., et al. 1987. Reassortment of human rotavirus possessing genome rearrangements with bovine rotavirus: evidence for host cell selection. *J Gen Virol*, **68**, 115–22.

Green, K.Y. and Kapikian, A.Z. 1992. Identification of VP7 epitopes associated with protection against human rotavirus infection or shedding in volunteers. *J Virol*, **66**, 548–53.

Greenberg, H.B., McAuliffe, V., et al. 1982. Serologic analysis of the subgroup protein of rotavirus using monoclonal antibody. *Infect Immun*, **39**, 91–9.

Guarino, A., Canani, R.B., et al. 1994. Oral immunoglobulins for treatment of acute rotaviral gastroenteritis. *Pediatrics*, **93**, 12–16.

Guérin-Danan, C., Meslin, J.C., et al. 1998. Development of a heterologous model in germfree suckling rats for studies of rotavirus diarrhea. *J Virol*, **72**, 9298–302.

Guerrero, C.A., Méndez, E., et al. 2000. Integrin $\alpha_v\beta_3$ mediates rotavirus cell entry. *Proc Natl Acad Sci USA*, **97**, 14644–9.

Guerrero, C.A., Bouyssounade, D., et al. 2002. The heat shock cognate protein 70 is involved in rotavirus cell entry. *J Virol*, **76**, 4096–102.

Hart, C.A. and Cunliffe, N.A. 1997. Viral gastroenteritis. *Curr Opin Infect Dis*, **10**, 408–13.

Heaton, P.M. 2004. Phase III evaluation of the Merck bovine rotavirus vaccine. In: *Program and Abstracts*, The Sixth International Rotavirus Symposium. Mexico City: p. 49.

Herring, A.J., Inglis, N.F., et al. 1982. Rapid diagnosis of rotavirus infection by direct detection of viral nucleic acid in silver-stained polyacrylamide gels. *J Clin Microbiol*, **16**, 473–7.

Herrmann, J.E., Chen, S.C., et al. 1996. Protection against rotavirus infection by DNA vaccination. *J Infect Dis*, **174**, Suppl 1, S93–7.

Hewish, M.J., Takada, Y. and Coulson, B.S. 2000. Integrins alpha2beta1 and alpha4beta1 can mediate SA11 rotavirus attachment and entry into cells. *J Virol*, **74**, 228–36.

Hoshino, Y., Wyatt, R.G., et al. 1985. Serotypic characterization of rotaviruses derived from asymptomatic human neonatal infections. *J Clin Microbiol*, **21**, 425–30.

Hoshino, Y., Sereno, M., et al. 1993. Genetic determinants of rotavirus virulence studied in gnotobiotic piglets. In: Ginsberg, H.S., Brown, F., et al. (eds), *Vaccines*. Cold Spring Harbor, NY: Cold Spring Harbor Laboratory Press, 277–82.

Hoshino, Y., Saif, L.J., et al. 1995. Identification of group A rotavirus genes associated with virulence of a porcine rotavirus and host range restriction of a human rotavirus in the gnotobiotic piglet model. *Virology*, **209**, 274–80.

Hung, T. 1988. Rotavirus and adult diarrhoea. *Adv Virus Res*, **35**, 193–218.

International Study Group on Reduced-osmolarity ORS Solutions, 1995. Multicentre evaluation of reduced-osmolarity oral rehydration salts solution. *Lancet*, **345**, 282-5.

Iturriza-Gómara, M., Green, J., et al. 1999. Comparison of specific and random priming in the reverse transcription polymerase chain reaction for genotyping group A rotaviruses. *J Virol Methods*, **78**, 93–103.

Iturriza-Gómara, M., Green, J., et al. 2000. Molecular epidemiology of human group A rotavirus infections in the UK between 1995 and 1998. *J Clin Microbiol*, **38**, 4394–401.

Iturriza-Gómara, M., Isherwood, B., et al. 2001. Reassortment *in vivo*: driving force for diversity of human rotavirus strains isolated in the United Kingdom between 1995 and 1999. *J Virol*, **75**, 3696–705.

Iturriza-Gómara, M., Auchterlonie, I.A., et al. 2002a. Rotavirus gastroenteritis and central nervous system (CNS) infection: characterisation of the *VP7* and *VP4* genes of rotavirus strains isolated from paired faecal and CSF samples from a child with CNS disease. *J Clin Microbiol*, **40**, 4797–9.

Iturriza-Gómara, M., Cubitt, D., et al. 2002b. Characterization of rotavirus G9 strains isolated in the UK between 1995 and 1998. *J Med Virol*, **61**, 510–17.

Iturriza-Gómara, M., Wong, C., et al. 2002c. Molecular characterisation of *VP6* genes of human rotavirus isolates: correlation of genogroups with subgroups and evidence of independent segregation. *J Virol*, **76**, 6596–601.

Iturriza-Gómara, M., Anderton, E., et al. 2003a. Evidence for genetic linkage between the gene segments encoding NSP4 and VP6 proteins in common and reassortant human rotavirus strains. *J Clin Microbiol*, **41**, 3566–73.

Iturriza-Gómara, M., Desselberger, U. and Gray, J. 2003b. Molecular epidemiology of rotaviruses: genetic mechanisms associated with diversity. In: Desselberger, U. and Gray, J. (eds), *Viral gastroenteritis*. Amsterdam: Elsevier Science, 317–44.

Jiang, B., Dennehy, P.H., et al. 1995. First detection of group C rotavirus in faecal specimens of children with diarrhea in the United States. *J Infect Dis*, **172**, 45–50.

Joensuu, J., Koskenniemi, E., et al. 1997. Randomized placebo-controlled trial of rhesus-human reassortant rotavirus vaccine for prevention of severe rotavirus gastroenteritis. *Lancet*, **351**, 1205–9.

Jolly, C.J., Beisner, B., et al. 2001. Non-lytic extraction and characterization for receptors for multiple strains of rotavirus. *Arch Virol*, **146**, 1307–23.

Kapikian, A.Z. (ed.) 1994. *Viral infections of the gastrointestinal tract*, 2nd edn. New York: Marcel Dekker.

Kobayashi, N., Naik, T.N., et al. 2001. Sequence analysis of genes encoding structural and nonstructural proteins of a human group B rotavirus detected in Calcutta, India. *J Med Virol*, **64**, 583–8.

Kramarz, P., France, E.K., et al. 2001. Population-based study of rotavirus vaccination and intussusception. *Ped Infect Dis J*, **20**, 410–16.

Krishnan, T., Sen, A., et al. 1999. Emergence of adult diarrhoea rotavirus in Calcutta, India. *Lancet*, **353**, 380–1.

Lawton, J.A., Estes, M.K. and Prasad, B.V.V. 1997a. Three-dimensional visualization of mRNA release from actively transcribing rotavirus particles. *Nat Struct Biol*, **4**, 118–21.

Lawton, J.A., Zeng, C.Q., et al. 1997b. Three-dimensional structural analysis of recombinant rotavirus-like particles with intact and amino-terminal -deleted VP2: implications for the architecture of VP2 capsid layer. *J Virol*, **71**, 7353–69.

Lawton, J.A., Estes, M.K. and Prasad, B.V. 1999. Comparative structural analysis of transcriptionally competent and incompetent rotavirus-antibody complexes. *Proc Nat Acad Sci USA*, **96**, 5428–33.

Lawton, J.A., Estes, M.K. and Prasad, B.V. 2000. Mechanism of genome transcription in segmented dsRNA viruses. *Adv Virus Res*, **55**, 185–229.

Leite, J.P.G., Alfieri, A.A., et al. 1996. Rotavirus P and G types circulating in Brazil: characterization by RT-PCR, probe hybridization and sequence analysis. *Arch Virol*, **141**, 2365–74.

Lepault, J., Petitpas, I., et al. 2001. Structural polymorphism of the major capsid protein of rotavirus. *EMBO J*, **20**, 1498–507.

Ludert, J.E., Feng, N., et al. 1996. Genetic mapping indicates that VP4 is the rotavirus cell-attachment protein *in vitro* and *in vivo*. *J Virol*, **70**, 487–93.

Lundgren, O.I., Peregrin, A.T., et al. 2000. Role of the enteric nervous system in the fluid and electrolyte secretion of rotavirus diarrhea. *Science*, **287**, 491–5.

Mason, H.S., Warzecha, H., et al. 2002. Edible plant vaccines: applications for prophylactic and therapeutic molecular medicine. *Trends Mol Med*, **8**, 324–9.

Mathieu, M., Petitpas, I., et al. 2001. Atomic structure of the major capsid protein of rotavirus: implications for the architecture of the virion. *EMBO J*, **20**, 1485–97.

Matson, D., O'Ryan, M., et al. 1993. Fecal antibody responses to symptomatic and asymptomatic rotavirus infections. *J Infect Dis*, **167**, 577–83.

Mattion, N.M., Cohen, J. and Estes, M.K. 1994. The rotavirus proteins. In: Kapikian, A.Z. (ed.), *Viral infections of the gastrointestinal tract*, 2nd edn. New York: Marcel Dekker, 169–249.

Mazanec, M.B., Coudret, C.L. and Fletcher, D.R. 1995. Intracellular neutralization of influenzavirus by immunoglobulin A anti-hemagglutinin monoclonal antibodies. *J Virol*, **69**, 1339–43.

Miller, M.A. and McCann, L. 2000. Policy analysis of the use of hepatitis B, *Haemophilus influenzae* type B-, *Streptococcus pneumoniae*-conjugate, and rotavirus vaccines in national immunisations schedules. *Health Economics*, **9**, 19–35.

Morris, A.P., Scott, J.K., et al. 1999. NSP4 elicits age-dependent diarrhea and Ca^{2+} mediated I^-influx into intestinal crypts of CF mice. *Am J Physiol*, **277**, 2 Pt 1, G431–44.

Mossel, E.C. and Ramig R.F. 2002. Rotavirus genome segment 7 (NSP3) is a determinant of extraintestinal spread in the neonatal mouse. *J Virol*, **76**, 6502–5.

Mossel, E.C. and Ramig, R.F. 2003. A lymphatic mechanism of rotavirus extraintestinal spread in the neonatal mouse. *J Virol*, **77**, 12352–6.

Murphy, T.V., Garguillo, P.M., et al. 2001. Intussusception among infants given an oral rotavirus vaccine. *N Engl J Med*, **344**, 564–72.

Nejmeddine, M., Trugnan, G., et al. 2000. Rotavirus spike protein VP4 is present at the plasma membrane and is associated with microtubules in infected cells. *J Virol*, **74**, 3313–20.

Noel, J.S., Beards, G.M. and Cubitt, W.D. 1991. An epidemiological survey of human rotavirus serotypes and electropherotypes in young children admitted to two hospitals in north east London. *J Clin Microbiol*, **29**, 2213–19.

Offit, P.A. 1994. Rotaviruses: immunological determinants of protection against infection and disease. *Adv Virus Res*, **44**, 161–202.

Offit, P.A., Blavat, G., et al. 1986. Molecular basis for rotavirus virulence: role of rotavirus gene segment 4. *J Virol*, **57**, 46–9.

Offit, P.A., Hoffenberg, E.J., et al. 1993. Rotavirus-specific humoral and cellular immune response after primary symptomatic infection. *J Infect Dis*, **167**, 1436–40.

Offit, P.A., Khouri, C.A., et al. 1994. Enhancement of rotavirus immunogenicity by microencapsidation. *Virology*, **203**, 134–43.

O'Neal, C.M., Crawford, E., et al. 1997. Rotavirus virus-like particles administered mucosally induce protective immunity. *J Virol*, **71**, 8707–17.

O'Neal, C.M., Harriman, G.R. and Conner, M.E. 2000. Protection of the villus epithelial cells of the small intestine from rotavirus infections does not require IgA. *J Virol*, **74**, 4102–9.

Patton, J.T. 2001. Rotavirus RNA replication and gene expression. *Novartis Found Symp*, **238**, 64–77.

Pérez-Schael, I., Guntiñas, M.J., et al. 1997. Efficacy of the rhesus rotavirus-based quadrivalent vaccine in infants and young children in Venezuela. *N Engl J Med*, **337**, 1181–7.

Pesavento, J.B., Lawton, J.A., et al. 2001. The reversible condensation and expansion of the rotavirus genome. *Proc Natl Acad Sci U S A*, **98**, 1381–6.

Petitpas, I., Lepault, J., et al. 1998. Crystallization and preliminary x-ray analysis of rotavirus protein VP6. *J Virol*, **72**, 7615–19.

Phillips, A.D. 1989. Mechanisms of mucosal injury: human studies. In: Farthing, M.J.G. (ed.), *Viruses and the gut*. London: Swan Press, 30–40.

Prasad, B.V.V. and Chiu, W. 1994. Structure of rotaviruses. In: Ramig, R.F. (ed.), *Rotaviruses*. Berlin: Springer-Verlag, 9–29.

Prasad, B.V.V. and Estes, M.K. 1997. Molecular basis of rotavirus replication: structure-function correlations. In: Chiu, W., Burnett, R.M. and Garcia, R.L. (eds), *Structural biology of viruses*. New York: Oxford University Press, 239–68.

Prasad, B.V.V., Wang, G.Y., et al. 1988. Three-dimensional structure of rotavirus. *J Mol Biol*, **199**, 269–75.

Prasad, B.V.V., Burns, J.W., et al. 1990. Localization of VP4 neutralization sites in rotavirus by three-dimensional cryo-electron microscopy. *Nature (Lond)*, **343**, 476–9.

Prasad, B.V.V., Rothnagel, R., et al. 1996. Visualization of ordered genomic RNA and localization of transcriptional complexes in rotavirus. *Nature*, **382**, 471–3.

Ramachandran, M., Das, B.K., et al. 1996. Unusual diversity of human G and P genotypes in India. *J Clin Microbiol*, **34**, 436–9.

Ramachandran, M., Gentsch, J., et al. 1998. Detection and characterization of novel rotavirus strains in the United States. *J Clin Microbiol*, **36**, 3223–9.

Rennels, M.B., Glass, R.I., et al. 1996. Safety and efficacy of high-dose rhesus-human reassortant rotavirus vaccines. Report of the national multicenter trial. *Pediatrics*, **97**, 7–13.

Rolsma, M.D., Kuhlenschmidt, T.B., et al. 1998. Structure and function of a ganglioside receptor for porcine rotavirus. *J Virol*, **72**, 9079–91.

Ruggeri, F.M., Marziano, M.L., et al. 1992. Laboratory diagnosis of rotavirus infection in diarrhoeal patients by immunoenzymatic and latex agglutination assays. *Microbiologica*, **15**, 249–57.

Saif, L.J., Rosen, B. and Parwani, A. 1994. Animal rotaviruses. In: Kapikian, A.Z. (ed.), *Viral infections of the gastrointestinal tract*, 2nd edn. New York: Marcel Dekker, 279–367.

Sapin, C., Colard, O., et al. 2002. Rafts promote assembly and atypical targeting of a non-enveloped virus, rotavirus, in CaCo-2 cells. *J Virol*, **76**, 4591–602.

Schuck, P., Taraporewala, Z., et al. 2001. Rotavirus nonstructural protein NSP2 self-assembles into octamers that undergo ligand-induced conformational changes. *J Biol Chem*, **276**, 9679–87.

Schwartz-Cornil, I., Bénureau, Y., et al. 2002. Heterologous protection induced by the inner capsid proteins of rotavirus requires transcytosis of mucosal immunoglobulins. *J Virol*, **76**, 8110–17.

Shaw, A.L., Rothnagel, R., et al. 1993. Three-dimensional visualization of the rotavirus hemagglutinin structure. *Cell*, **74**, 693–701.

Simonsen, L., Morens, D.M., et al. 2001. Incidence trends in infant hospitalization for intussusception: impact of the 1998–1999 rotavirus vaccination program in 10 US States. *Lancet*, **358**, 1224–9.

Tafazoli, F., Zeng, C.Q.Y., et al. 2001. The NSP4 enterotoxin of rotavirus induces paracellular leakage in polarized epithelial cells. *J Virol*, **75**, 1540–6.

Taraporewala, T.F. and Patton, J.T. 2001. Identification and characterization of the helix-destabilizing activity of rotavirus nonstructural protein NSP2. *J Virol*, **75**, 4519–27.

Taraporewala, T.F., Chen, D. and Patton, J.T. 1999. Multimers formed by the rotavirus nonstructural protein NSP2 bind to RNA and have nucleoside triphosphatase activity. *J Virol*, **73**, 9934–43.

Thouvenin, E., Schoehn, G., et al. 2001. Antibody inhibition of the transcriptase activity of the rotavirus DLP: a structural view. *J Mol Biol*, **307**, 161–72.

Tian, P., Hu, Y., et al. 1994. The nonstructural glycoprotein of rotavirus affects intracellular calcium levels. *J Virol*, **68**, 251–7.

Tian, P., Estes, M.K., et al. 1995. The rotavirus nonstructural glycoprotein NSP4 mobilizes Ca^{2+} from the endoplasmic reticulum. *J Virol*, **69**, 5763–72.

To, T.L., Ward, L.A., et al. 1998. Serum and intestinal isotype antibody responses and correlates of protective immunity to human rotavirus in a gnotobiotic pig model of disease. *J Gen Virol*, **79**, 2661–72.

Treanor, J., Clark, H.F., et al. 1995. Evaluation of the protective efficacy of a serotype 1 bovine-human rotavirus reassortant vaccine in infants. *Pediatr Infect Dis J*, **14**, 301–7.

Velazquez, F.R., Matson, D.O., et al. 1996. Rotavirus infection in infants as protection against subsequent infections. *N Engl J Med*, **335**, 1022–8.

Vende, P., Piron, M., et al. 2000. Efficient translation of rotavirus mRNA requires simultaneous interaction of NSP3 with the eukaryotic translation initiation factor eIF4G and the mRNA 3′end. *J Virol*, **74**, 7064–71.

Vesikari, T. 1994. Bovine rotavirus-based rotavirus vaccines in humans. In: Kapikian, A.Z. (ed.), *Viral infections of the gastrointestinal tract*, 2nd edn. New York: Marcel Dekker, 419–42.

Ward, R.L., Knowlton, D.R. and Pierce, M. 1984. Efficiency of human rotavirus propagation in cell culture. *J Clin Microbiol*, **19**, 748–53.

Ward, R.L., Nakagomi, O., et al. 1990. Evidence for natural reassortants of human rotaviruses belonging to different genogroups. *J Virol*, **64**, 3219–25.

Ward, R.L., Clemens, J., et al. 1992. Evidence that protection against rotavirus diarrhoea after natural infection is not dependent on serotype-specific neutralizing antibody. *J Infect Dis*, **166**, 1251–7.

Yeager, M., Dryden, K.A., et al. 1990. Three-dimensional structure of rhesus rotavirus by cryoelectron microscopy and image reconstruction. *J Cell Biol*, **110**, 2133–44.

Yeager, M., Berriman, J.A., et al. 1994. Three-dimensional structure of the rotavirus haemagglutinin VP4 by cryo-electron microscopy and difference map analysis. *EMBO J*, **13**, 1011–18.

Yolken, R.H. and Wilde, J.A. 1994. Assays for detecting human rotavirus. In: Kapikian, A.Z. (ed.), *Viral infections of the gastrointestinal tract*, 2nd edn. New York: Marcel Dekker, 251–78.

Yu, J. and Langridge, W.H. 2001. A plant-based multicomponent vaccine protects mice from enteric diseases. *Nature Biotechnol*, **19**, 548–52.

Yuan, L.Z., Ward, L.A. and Rosen, B.I. 1996. Systemic and intestinal antibody secreting cell responses and correlates of protective immunity to human rotavirus in a gnotobiotic pig model of disease. *J Virol*, **70**, 3075–83.

Zhang, M. and Zeng, C.Q.Y. 2000. A functional NSP4 enterotoxin peptide secreted from rotavirus-infected cells. *J Virol*, **74**, 11663–70.

45

Rubella

JENNIFER M. BEST, SAMANTHA COORAY, AND JANGU E. BANATVALA

HISTORICAL INTRODUCTION

Rubella was first described in the mid-eighteenth century by two German physicians, de Bergen and Orlow. At that time it was frequently known by the German name 'Röteln,' and it was due to the early interest of the German physicians and the general acceptance of a German name that the disease subsequently became known as 'German measles.' For many years, German measles was frequently confused with measles and scarlet fever, other infectious diseases presenting with rash, and at one time was considered to be a cross between them. The clinical differences between these diseases were recognized in the nineteenth century and rubella was accepted as a distinct disease by an International Congress of Medicine in London in 1881 (Smith 1881). The disease received comparatively little attention, for infection was generally mild and severe complications were rare, until the 1940s when the association between maternal infection and such congenital defects as cataract, heart disease, and hearing loss was first recognized (Gregg 1941). This report is discussed in more detail later.

Rubella virus (RUBV) was not isolated in cell culture until 1962, when Parkman and colleagues (1962) detected the presence of RUBV in primary vervet monkey kidney cell cultures by means of the interference technique and Weller and Neva (1962) reported unique cytopathic effects in primary amnion cell cultures. Tests for neutralizing and hemagglutination inhibition (HAI) antibodies were reported in 1962 (Parkman et al. 1962, 1964) and 1967 (Stewart et al. 1967) respectively.

These tests allowed seroepidemiological investigations to be conducted. The fine structure of RUBV was not determined until 1968 as it is difficult to obtain the high titers of virus required for electron microscopy (Best et al. 1967; Holmes et al. 1968). Much of the work on the molecular structure and replication of RUBV was carried out in the late 1980s and early 1990s, some time after similar work on other viruses. This was probably because RUBV is slow to grow in cell culture, high levels of virus are difficult to produce consistently and the high G+C content of the genome made sequencing difficult.

PROPERTIES OF THE VIRUS

Classification

Rubella virus, an enveloped single-stranded RNA virus, belongs to the family *Togaviridae* (Chapter 47, Togaviruses) and is probably distantly related to the alphaviruses (Frey 1994). Unlike other togaviruses, RUBV has no known invertebrate host and has been placed by itself in the genus *Rubivirus*.

Morphology and structure

The virion has a mean diameter of 58 nm with a 30 nm core (Figure 45.1) (Best et al. 1967; Holmes et al. 1968; Murphy et al. 1968). The core is surrounded by a lipoprotein envelope with surface spikes 5–8 nm in length. In thin sections of infected cells an electron-lucent zone is seen between the core and the envelope. The virion is

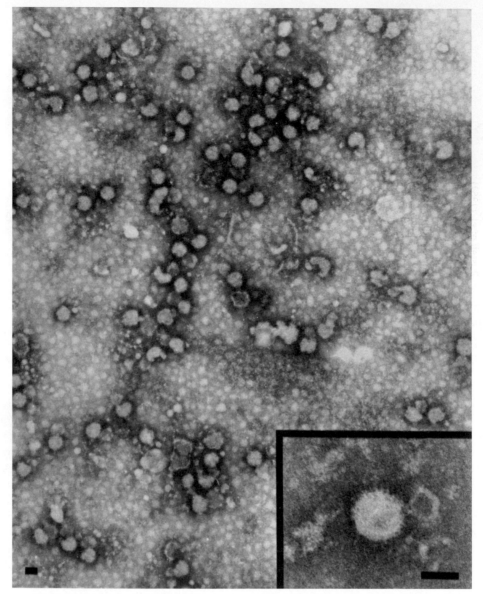

Figure 45.1 *Negatively stained preparation of rubella virus. Inset, an enlarged particle, showing spikes. Bar, 50 nm (kindly provided by Dr. I. Chrystie).*

pleomorphic, owing to the delicate nonrigid nature of the envelope. The symmetry of the nucleocapsid has been difficult to establish because of its instability, but rotational analysis of thin sections of rubella virions suggests that the core has a T = 3 icosahedral symmetry and 32 capsomers (Matsumoto and Higashi 1974).

Physical properties of RUBV are shown in Table 45.1 and were reviewed by Horzinek (1973, 1981). The stability of the virus is enhanced by the addition of proteins and MgSO$_4$ to the suspending medium. Because of the lipid content of the viral envelope, RUBV is inactivated by detergents and organic solvents. The effects of these and other chemicals have been reviewed (Parkman et al. 1964; Norrby 1969; Plotkin 1969; Horzinek 1973, 1981; Herrmann 1979).

Genome organization

The RUBV genome consists of a single strand of positive sense RNA, 9 762 nucleotides (nt) in length, which is capped at the 5′ end and polyadenylated at the 3′ end. The cap is required for efficient translation as it serves as a ribosome recognition site (Oker-Blom 1984; Frey 1994). The genome contains two nonoverlapping open reading frames (ORF) separated by a linker region of 123 nucleotides (nt) in the same translation frame. The 5′ proximal ORF extends from nt 41 to 6 388 and encodes the p200 polyprotein precursor for the nonstructural proteins (NSP) p150 and p90 (Dominguez et al. 1990; Pugachev et al. 1997a; Liang and Gillam 2000). The 3′ proximal ORF extends from nt 6 512 to 9 700, and encodes the structural proteins (SP): capsid (C), and

	Properties	Reference
Virus particle		
Diameter	40–70 nm	Reviewed by Horzinek (1973)
Buoyant density	in sucrose: 1.16–1.19 g/ml	Reviewed by Horzinek (1973)
	in CsCl$_2$: 1.20–1.23 g/ml	
Sedimentation coefficient	240S	Thomssen et al. (1968)
	342S	Russell et al. (1967)
	350 ± 50S	Bardeletti et al. (1975)
Nucleocapsid		
Diameter	30–40 nm	Reviewed by Horzinek (1973)
Symmetry	Icosahedral	Reviewed by Horzinek (1973)
Buoyant density	in CsCl$_2$: 1.4 ± 0.4 g/ml	
Sedimentation coefficient	150S	Vaheri and Hovi (1972)
Molecular weight	2 600–4 000 kDa	Kenney et al. (1969)
Nucleic acid		
Buoyant density	Single strand of RNA	Hovi and Vaheri (1970)
	1.634 g/ml	Sedwick and Sokol (1970)
Sedimentation coefficient	38–40S	
Molecular weight	3 200–3 500 kDa	
Length of surface projections	5–6 nm	Holmes et al. (1969); Smith and Hobbins (1969)
Chemical composition	RNA 2.4%	Voiland and Bardeletti (1980)
	Proteins 74.8%	
	Lipid 18.8%	
	Carbohydrate 4.0%	
Major polypeptides	Envelope	Oker-Blom et al. (1983)
	E1 58 kDa	Waxham and Wolinsky (1985)
	E2 42–47 kDa	
	C 33–35 kDa	
	Nucleocapsid	
Thermal stability		
4°C	Stable for ⩾7 days	Fabiyi et al. (1966)
37°C	Inactivated at 0.1–0.4 log$_{10}$ TCID$_{50}$/ml per h	Parkman (1965)
56°C	Inactivated at 1.5–3.5 log$_{10}$ TCID$_{50}$/0.1 ml per h	Parkman (1965)
70°C	Inactivated at 5.5 log$_{10}$ TCID$_{50}$/0.1 ml per 0.5 h	Kistler and Sapatino (1972)
−70°C	Stable	Parkman et al. (1964)
Freeze drying	Stable	Parkman et al. (1964)
pH sensitivity	Stable at pH 6.0–8.1	Schell and Wong (1966); Norrby (1969)
	Unstable at more acid and alkaline pH	
UV sensitivity	Inactivated within 40 s	Fabiyi et al. (1966)
1 350 W/cm^2	Inactivated at 7.0 log$_{10}$ TCID$_{50}$/0.1 ml per h	Kistler and Sapatino (1972)
Photosensitivity	Labile, K = 0.07/min in PBS	Booth and Stern (1972)
Sonication	Stable for ⩾9 min	Schell and Wong (1966)
Chemical sensitivity	Formaldehyde, lipid solvents, detergents e.g. SDS, Nonidet P-40, Tween 80	Parkman et al. (1964); Chantler et al. (2001)

TCID$_{50}$, 50% tissue culture infective dose.

glycoproteins E1 and E2 (Dominguez et al. 1990; Frey 1994; Yao et al. 1998). The gene order is 5'-p150–p90–C–E2–E1-3' (Forng and Frey 1995). The genomic RNA serves as the template for synthesis of a complementary negative-sense RNA strand, which in turn, is the template for synthesis of positive-sense 40S genomic and 24S subgenomic RNA, from which the SPs are translated (Figure 45.2).

The base composition of the genome is 14.9 percent A, 15.4 percent U, 30.8 percent G and 38.7 percent C, making the G+C composition 69.5 percent, the highest reported for an RNA virus. This initially made sequence determination difficult, and errors were made in the first sequences reported (Dominguez et al. 1990). Genome-length cDNA clones have been produced and used to synthesize infectious RNA transcripts (Wang et al. 1994).

Virus life cycle

ATTACHMENT AND ENTRY

RUBV can replicate in a variety of cell lines which suggests that the receptor for RUBV is a ubiquitous molecule (reviewed by Frey 1994). The receptor has not yet been identified, but as membrane lipid molecules play an essential role it may be a lipid–carbohydrate complex (Mastromarino et al. 1990). The reproductive life cycle of RUBV takes place in the cytoplasm. Like most enveloped animal viruses, RUBV probably enters cells by receptor-mediated endocytosis and uses endocytic machinery to travel within the cytoplasm (Sodeik 2000). During endocytosis, the virion is internalized in a coated vesicle, which is transported to the endosomal compartment. The low pH environment of the endosome triggers a conformational change in the envelope glycoproteins that favors the fusion of viral and endosomal membranes (Katow and Sugiura 1988; reviewed by Frey 1994). The low pH also causes the C protein to undergo a structural change which makes it more hydrophobic, and allows uncoating of nucleocapsid to occur (Mauracher et al. 1991; Lee and Bowden 2000). Both events suggest that the low pH environment mediates delivery of viral genomic RNA into the cytoplasm.

REPLICATION, TRANSCRIPTION, AND TRANSLATION

The replication cycle of RUBV in vertebrate cell cultures is slow and less efficient than that of alphaviruses. Peak virus production usually occurs at 48 h postinfection (Hemphill et al. 1988; Frey 1994). Replication of RUBV has been suggested to occur in 'replication complexes' that appear as membrane-bound cytoplasmic vacuoles, lined internally with vesicles and associated with the rough endoplasmic reticulum (RER). The vesicles within the complex appear to be the sites of viral replication, and may also protect the genomic RNA from cellular ribonucleases. The replication complexes also appear to serve as sites for nucleocapsid assembly (Lee et al. 1994; Lee and Bowden 2000). Some RUBV replication complexes are modified lysosomes, characterized by the presence of degenerating material within the vacuole. However, others may be endosomal in origin, as observed in alphavirus-infected cells (Chapter 47, Togaviruses) (Magliano et al. 1998).

Following the uncoating of capsid and release of genomic RNA into the cytoplasm, the 40S genomic RNA serves as the template for nonstructural protein (NSP) synthesis. The NSPs are translated from the 5' proximal ORF as a 2 116 amino acid polyprotein, p200 (200 kDa), which is proteolytically cleaved to produce two nonstructural proteins p150 (residues 1–1 301, 150 kDa) and p90 (residues 1 302–2 116, 90 kDa) (Marr et al. 1994; Forng and Frey 1995; Chen et al. 1996). Preceding the NSP-ORF there are three potential AUG start sites at nucleotides 3, 41, and 57. Translation of the NSP-ORF is initiated at AUG_{41}, whereas AUG_3 and AUG_{57} are in a different reading frame and terminate at nucleotides 54 and 90, respectively. Neither of these short ORFs are essential for virus replication (Pugachev et al. 1997a; Pugachev and Frey 1998a).

The cleavage of the p200 polyprotein precursor is mediated by an RUBV-encoded protease within the C-terminal region of p150, which is homologous to several other viral and cellular papain-like proteases (Gorbalenya et al. 1991; Marr et al. 1994). The catalytic dyad is formed by residues Cys-1152 and His-1273 and cleavage takes place at Gly-1301 in the sequence Gly_{1300}–Gly_{1301}–Gly_{1302} (Marr et al. 1994; Chen et al. 1996; Liang and Gillam 2000). Site-directed mutagenesis of Gly-1301 to Ala or Val, and of Gly-1300/1302 to Val abrogates cleavage and results in non-infectious virus (Chen et al. 1996; Liang and Gillam 2000).

The 40S positive-sense genomic RNA also acts as the template for the synthesis of a complementary negative-sense strand of RNA. The negative strand, which is present in double-stranded form, is in turn the template for synthesis of the positive-sense 40S genomic RNA and 24S subgenomic RNA. p200 is the principal RNA-dependent RNA polymerase (RdRp) for negative-strand RNA synthesis, and cleavage products p150/p90 are required for positive-strand (genomic and subgenomic) RNA synthesis (Liang and Gillam 2000, 2001). Thus the switch from the synthesis of negative to positive-strand RNA is regulated by NSP processing. The p150 protein has also been shown to be localized in RUBV replication complexes (Kujala et al. 1999). Negative strand RNA synthesis continues to accumulate until 10 h postinfection, and remains constant thereafter. Synthesis of positive-strand RNAs (genomic and subgenomic) begins 10 h postinfection and escalates dramatically. This replication pattern resembles that of alphaviruses where negative-strand synthesis ceases after 4–6 h and switches to positive-strand RNA synthesis (Sawicki et al. 1981; Liang and Gillam 2001).

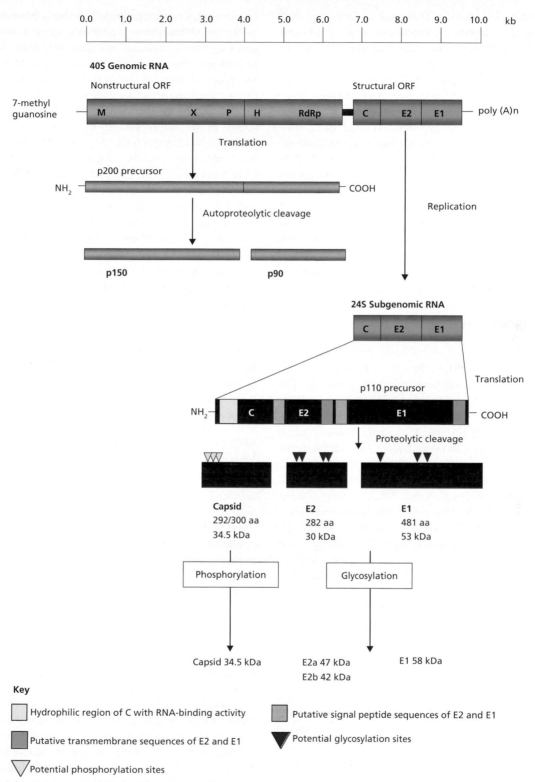

Figure 45.2 *Schematic representation of the steps involved in the replication translation, and processing of Rubella virus structural and nonstructural proteins. The RUBV genome consists of two long nonoverlapping ORFs, the 5′ ORF encodes the nonstructural proteins and the 3′ ORF encodes the structural proteins. The translation of RUBV RNA produces the p200 precursor, which is cleaved to produce the p150 and p90 nonstructural proteins. This initiates the synthesis of the full-length negative-strand RNA. The negative strand acts as a template for the synthesis of the full-length positive strand RNA for new viral progeny and the 24S subgenomic RNA. The 24S subgenomic RNA is translated into the p110 polyprotein precursor, which is proteolytically cleaved and post-translationally modified to produce the structural proteins C, E2, and E1. Within the 5′ nonstructural ORF are putative amino acid sequence motifs for methyltransferase (M), RNA-dependent RNA polymerase (RdRp), helicase (H), and papain-like cysteine protease (P) activity. The X motif indicates a region of unknown function, which has homology to alphaviruses, hepatitis E virus, and coronaviruses.*

The subgenomic RNA is translated to produce a 1 063 amino acid polyprotein precursor, p110 (110 kDa), which is proteolytically cleaved to produce the SPs C, E2, and E1 (Figure 45.2) (Kalkkinen et al. 1984; Oker-Blom 1984). The cleavage of p110 is thought to occur at signal peptide sequences that precede the amino termini of E2 and E1. The E2 and E1 signal peptides remain attached to the carboxy termini of C and E2, respectively, and direct the insertion of these proteins into the endoplasmic reticulum (ER) (Suomalainen et al. 1990; Marr et al. 1991; Baron et al. 1992). The capsid protein lacks the autoprotease activity of other alphavirus C proteins and cleavage of p110 is mediated by a host-cell signalase found within the lumen of the ER (Clarke et al. 1988; Frey and Marr 1988; Oker-Blom et al. 1990). The E2 signal peptide is required for RUBV glycoprotein-dependent localization of capsid to the juxtanuclear region and subsequent virus assembly in the golgi (Frey 1994; Qiu et al. 1994; Law et al. 2001). Retention of the E2 signal peptide on the carboxy terminus of capsid is unique to Rubella virus within the *Togaviridae* (Law et al. 2001).

Following proteolytic cleavage E1 and E2 form disulfide-linked heterodimers before they exit the ER. Heterodimerisation of E1 with E2 is required for E1 to be correctly folded and transported from the ER to the Golgi and the cell surface. Incorrectly folded proteins are retained in the ER (Frey 1994). An internal hydrophobic domain in E1 (aa 81–109) plays a major role in the formation of the E1–E2 heterodimer (Yang et al. 1998). The capsid protein forms dilsulfide linked homodimers (Waxham and Wolinsky 1983; Baron and Forsell 1991). Newly synthesized 40S genomic RNA is packaged with the RUBV capsid protein to form nucleocapsids. A 29 nt sequence (nt 347–375), within the genomic RNA has been identified as a binding domain for capsid, and a peptide region (amino acids 28–56) with specific RNA binding activity has been identified in the capsid (Liu et al. 1996; Wolinsky 1996).

DEFECTIVE INTERFERING (DI) RNAS

Serial undiluted passage of RUBV in Vero cells results in the production of DI RNAs, approximately 7 000 and 800 nt in length (Frey and Hemphill 1988). Characterization of these DI RNAs revealed that the 7 000-nt species contained a 2 500–2 700-nt deletion in the SP-ORF, and the 800 nt species was the subgenomic DI RNA synthesized from the larger species (Derdyn and Frey 1995). These are the only types of DI RNA which are continuously generated. Although DI RNAs are generated during persistent infection, their presence is not necessary to establish persistence (Frey and Hemphill 1988).

VIRUS RELEASE

Newly synthesized RUBV particles are released by budding from both the plasma membrane and internal membranes. The nucleocapsid core buds from the modified internal membranes and subsequently attains E1 and E2 glycoproteins and the host-cell lipids it requires to form the viral envelope. The mechanism by which the nucleocapsid interacts with E2–E1 heterodimers and the precise mechanism of budding is not known. However, E1 transmembrane and cytoplasmic domains have been found to be important in the late stages of virus assembly. The cytoplasmic domain of E1 may interact with the capsid protein to drive the budding process (Yao and Gillam 1999; Lee and Bowden 2000).

In vitro, virus release varies according to the type of cells infected. Vero cells release more virus into the cell culture medium than BHK-21 cells, as virus maturation only occurs at the plasma membrane and less intracellular virus is produced (Bardeletti et al. 1979). In BHK-21 virus maturation occurs both at the plasma membrane and at the Golgi and vacuoles of the cytoplasm. Wolinsky (1996) suggested that the capacity to mature within intracellular vacuoles, avoiding the host's immune system, may enable the virus to establish persistent infections in humans. Pathak et al. (1994), using immunoelectron microscopy, reported spherules (pleomorphic membrane-bound structures containing a dense thread-like structure) as well as virions budding from the surface of infected Vero cells.

EFFECT ON THE HOST CELL AND ULTRASTRUCTURAL STUDIES

RUBV infection in Vero cells does not affect total cellular RNA synthesis, and total cell protein synthesis is only modestly inhibited (Hemphill et al. 1988). However, this effect may be cell-type dependent as, in contrast, others have reported an increase in cellular metabolism (Vaheri and Cristofalo 1967; Bardeletti 1977).

In RUBV-infected cell cultures, virus-producing cells display intracellular membrane alterations and vacuolation approximately 2 days after infection. Membrane alterations included proliferation and distension, as well as the appearance of crystalline inclusions and annulate lamellae (Bardeletti et al. 1979; Pathak et al. 1994). Freeze-substitution electron microscopy of RUBV-infected cells has revealed the presence of homogeneously dense particles lacking a virus core within Golgi stacks, which coexist with mature virions, and appear to be virion precursors (Risco et al. 2003).

Large osmiophilic inclusion bodies containing myelin whorls and densely packed vesicles of varying size have been observed in the epithelial cells of human fetal nasal and tracheal organ cultures infected in vitro with RUBV (Kistler et al. 1967). The cytoplasmic ground substance as well as the extracellular space in close vicinity to the microvilli of these cells contained numerous viruslike particles with a diameter of 380–700 Å. It is possible that the inclusion bodies described by these authors correspond to the replication complexes analyzed by Lee and Bowden (2000).

RUBELLA VIRUS-INDUCED APOPTOSIS

RUBV-induced cytopathic effect has been shown to be due to caspase-dependent apoptosis in a number of susceptible cell lines (Pugachev and Frey 1998b; Megyeri et al. 1999; Hofmann et al. 1999; Duncan et al. 1999; Cooray et al. 2003; Domegan and Atkins 2002). Replicating virus is required for the induction of apoptotic cell signaling, which begins early post-infection (Megyeri et al. 1999; Cooray et al. 2003). The genetic determinants of cytopathogenicity have been mapped to the NSP-ORF (Pugachev et al. 1997b), but these have not been demonstrated to be directly involved in RUBV-induced apoptosis. Expression of the capsid protein alone was shown to induce cell death in transfected RK13 cells (Duncan et al. 2000). However, this function of the RUBV capsid is disputed by Hofmann et al. (1999), who demonstrated that expression of the entire SP-ORF reading frame did not cause apoptosis. Whether RUBV-induced apoptosis is dependent upon p53 is uncertain. Although p53 and p21 protein expression, and *p21* gene expression is detected in RUBV-infected Vero cells (Megyeri et al. 1999), p53 null neurons die in the same way as normal neurons in response to RUBV infection (Domegan and Atkins 2002). Anti-apoptotic protein Bcl-X is able to confer partial protection against RUBV infection in BHK-21 cells, but not in RK13 cells (Duncan et al. 1999).

REGULATORY ELEMENTS

The Rubella virus genome contains four regions of nucleotide sequence, which are thought to function as regulatory signals for RUBV replication, and have homology to the alphavirus genome (Dominguez et al. 1990; Frey 1994). Two of these regions are located at the 5′ and 3′ termini of the RUBV genomic RNA and are predicted to form stable stem-loop (SL) structures, and are termed the 5′ (+) SL and 3′ (+) SL, respectively. The 5′ (+) SL is located between nucleotides 15 and 65, it is preceded by a 14-nt single-stranded leader (ss-leader) sequence and consists of a terminal loop and a hinge region. A complementary equivalent of the 5′ (+) SL is present at the 3′ end of the viral minus-strand RNA (termed the 3′(−) SL), and is thought to serve as a promotor for initiation of positive-strand genomic RNA by the viral replicase (Pugachev and Frey 1998a). The 3′ (+) terminal 305 nt of the RUBV genome is predicted to form four stable SL structures. The first two SLs (SL1 and SL2) are located at the end of the the the E1 coding region, and the second two (SL3 and SL4) within the 59-nt 3′ untranslated region (UTR) that precedes the poly(A) tract. An inverted repeat sequence of 12 nt preceding the 59-nt 3′ UTR and capable of forming a SL structure, is required for initiation of negative-strand synthesis (Nakhasi et al. 1990, 1994).

Pogue et al. (1993) analyzed the transcriptional activity of the 5′ and 3′ ends of the genome by constructing chimeras of chloramphenicol acetyl transferase (CAT) RNA flanked by the 3′(+) or 5′(+) SL sequences. The translational efficiencies of the 5′(+) and 3′(+) SLs were measured by the level of CAT activity from the chimeras in transfected cells. Both 3′ and 5′(+) SLs were found to be necessary for efficient translation of CAT RNA in vitro and in vivo.

The third region of homology consists of 23 nucleotides upstream of the subgenomic (SG) RNA start site (nt −46 to −23). This site has been termed the SG promoter and synthesis of SG RNA is initiated in this region on a negative-strand copy of the genomic RNA (Frey 1994; Tzeng and Frey 2002). In contrast, the SG promoter region of alphaviruses is immediately adjacent to the RNA start site. The region necessary for synthesis of RUBV SG RNA and production of viable virus has been mapped to −28 nt upstream (5′) through to at least +6 nt downstream (3′) of the SG start site (Tzeng and Frey 2002). The predicted secondary structure around the SG promoter region consists of two stem-loop structures SLI (−20 to −47 nt) and SLII (−16 to SG start site). However only SLII lies within SG promoter region and may be necessary for promoter function (Tzeng and Frey 2002).

A fourth predicted regulatory region lies 224 nt downstream of the 5′ end and consists of a stretch of 46 nt. However, unlike alphaviruses, this region does not form a predicted double stem-loop configuration, and its functional significance is unknown.

INTERACTION OF THE RUBV GENOME WITH CELLULAR PROTEINS

Cellular host factors are often involved in RNA virus replication and translation. Cellular proteins with RNA recognition elements may contribute enzymatic, structural, and regulatory activities required for RNA synthesis. A number of cellular proteins have been identified which interact with the RUBV genome.

The SL at the 3′ (+) end of the genome is able to bind to three host-encoded cytosolic proteins (61, 63, and 68 kDa). Phosphorylation of the host proteins is necessary for this interaction (Nakhasi et al. 1990). The 61 kDa protein has been purified and identified as the simian homolog of human calreticulin (Singh et al. 1994; Nakhasi et al. 1994). Phosphorylation of calreticulin is required for RNA-binding activity and calreticulin autophosphorylates itself at Ser and Thr residues. RNA binding and autophosphorylation activities were localized to the N-terminal 180 amino acids (aa). RNA binding activity was abrogated by deletion of the first ten aa residues, whereas autophosphorylation activity was localized to aa 60–180 (Singh et al. 1994; Atreya et al. 1995). The specific binding of calreticulin to the 3′(+) is important in regulating RUBV RNA negative strand synthesis.

UV cross-linking and RNA gel shift assays were used to identify host-cell proteins which interacted with the 5′

(+) SL. Two host proteins (53 and 59 kDa) present in both RUBV infected and uninfected cells were found to interact specifically with the 5′ (+) SL. Human serum with anti-Ro/SS-A antigen specificity immunoprecipitated the 53 and 59 kDa protein-RNA complexes containing the 5′ (+) SL RNA (Pogue et al. 1993). Serum from individuals with various immune disorders, which recognized La, or Ro and La autoantigens, immunoprecipitated ribonucleoprotein complexes containing both the 3′ and 5′ (+) SL RNAs. Like Ro, the La autoantigen was found to interact specifically with the 5′ (+) SL (Pogue et al. 1996). Identification of autoantigens binding to RUBV RNA suggests they may play a role in replication and pathogenesis.

Polypeptides

The SP ORF has two closely spaced AUG initiation codons, which may both be used indiscriminantly to produce capsid protein of 292 or 300 aa in length (Clarke et al. 1988). The capsid protein is phosphorylated, nonglycosylated, and has a molecular weight of 33 kDa. The protein is highly basic due to a high proportion of proline and arginine residues, which probably contribute to dimerization and binding of the 40S genomic RNA within the viral nucleocapsid. RUBV capsid protein is phosphorylated prior to virus assembly (Garbutt et al. 1999). A number of Ser/Thr residues within the capsid are potential phosphorylation sites, but site-directed mutagenesis experiments identified Ser 46, within the RNA binding region, as the most significant (Law et al. 2003). Capsid phophorylation is not essential for virus replication, but mutation of Ser 46 to Ala impairs virus growth and cytopathic effect. Hyperphosphorylated capsid mutants bind viral RNA more efficiently than wildtype capsid, and phosphatase treatment of wildtype improved RNA binding. This suggests that the capsid undergoes a dephosphorylation step prior to interaction with genomic RNA and nucleocapsid assembly (Law et al. 2003).

Host-cell mitochondrial protein p32 has been shown to bind to the N-terminal capsid domain and may regulate nucleocapsid assembly (Garbutt et al. 1999; Mohan et al. 2002). The exact physiological function of p32 is unknown, although it was originally identified as a C1q binding protein, it is capable of binding to a wide range of cellular and viral proteins (Beatch and Hobman 2000; Mohan et al. 2002). Binding of capsid to p32 at the mitochondria and overexpression of the SPs, results in clustering of the mitochondria to the perinuclear region.

E2 is 282 aa in length, and in most RUBV strains sequenced, it contains four potential N-linked glycosylation sites (Asn-X-Ser/Thr/Cys), where X can be any residue except proline. E2 also contains O-linked carbohydrates (Lundstrom et al. 1991). More than two forms of E2 occur (42–47 kDa) which differ in their degree of glycosylation (Bowden and Westaway 1985; Waxham and Wolinsky 1985).

E1 is 481 aa in length, has a molecular weight of 58 kDa, and three potential N-linked glycosylation sites (Figure 45.2) (Kalkkinen et al. 1984; Bowden and Westaway 1985; Waxham and Wolinsky 1985). E2–E1 heterodimers are membrane-bound and exposed on the surface of the virus particle. E2 is less accessible to the action of enzymes and antibodies than E1, suggesting that E2 is buried under E1 in the E2–E1 heterodimer (Waxham and Wolinsky 1985).

The RUBV structural proteins have been expressed in *Escherichia coli* and mammalian cells using Sindbis virus and vaccinia virus vectors, and in insect cells using baculovirus-expression vectors. Recombinant proteins have been purified from all of these systems (Seppanen et al. 1991; Londesborough et al. 1992; Oker-Blom et al. 1995; Chen et al. 1995; Orellana et al. 1999; Johansson et al. 1996). E1 and E2 have been expressed in soluble form (Hobman et al. 1994c; Seto et al. 1995), and virus-like particles containing the three structural proteins have been produced in transient and stably transfected CHO and BHK-21 cells (Hobman et al. 1994a, 1994b; Qiu et al. 1994).

RUBV NSPs contain a number of motifs of functional significance (Figure 45.2). P150 contains a region of homology to alphavirus NSP3, termed the X-motif, which is located adjacent to the protease domain, between aa 834 and 940. This motif has only been found in the genomes of the alphaviruses, Rubella virus, Hepatitis E virus, and possibly coronaviruses (Dominguez et al. 1990; Gorbalenya et al. 1991; Frey 1994). The X motif is necessary for *trans* cleavage activity of the NSP protease, but the exact function is still unknown. It is speculated that the proline-rich region within the X-motif may provide a protein–protein interaction domain that enables protease to easily gain access to its *trans* substrate (Liang and Gillam 2000). A methyltransferase (MT) motif has been identified at the N-terminus of p150 (Rozanov et al. 1992). It consists of a hydrophobic segment followed by a glycine-rich loop and is believed to have a role in the capping of viral RNA (Koonin 1993).

The second NSP, p90, contains two global amino acid motifs, which are conserved among positive-sense RNA viruses: a GDD motif (aa 1 966–1 968) indicative of RdRp activity, and a GKS/T motif indicative of helicase activity (Dominguez et al. 1990; Frey 1994; Pugachev et al. 1997a). Mutation of either Asp-1967 or Asp-1968 residues to Ala within the GDD motif are lethal. Mutation of Gly-1966 to Ala blocks virus replication and impairs infectivity, demonstrating that RUBV does have RdRp catalytic activity (Wang and Gillam 2001). This supports the role of p90 in positive-strand RNA synthesis.

ANTIGENIC COMPOSITION

Antigenic properties

Only one serotype of rubella virus has been described, and the virus is serologically distinct from other toga-viruses. Early work on RUBV identified hemagglutinating (HA), complement-fixing (CF), precipitating (Le Bouvier 1969) and platelet-aggregating (PA) (Penttinen and Myllyla 1968) antigens. Kobayashi (1978) demonstrated that RUBV also has hemolytic activity.

The HA activity is associated with the surface projections on the viral envelope. It can be obtained from the supernatant fluid of infected BHK-21 cell cultures if these are maintained on serum-free medium or if nonspecific inhibitors of hemagglutination (serum lipoproteins) are first removed by kaolin treatment from the serum included in the maintenance medium (Stewart et al. 1967). Alternatively, treatment of the RUBV harvest with EDTA will separate HA from nonspecific inhibitors by removing Ca^{2+} (Furukawa et al. 1967). Rubella HA can also be prepared by alkaline extraction of infected BHK-21 or Vero cell cultures (Halonen et al. 1967). Although treatment of virus with ether destroys the HA activity, treatment with ether and Tween 80 retains this activity and increases the titer of the antigen, because of the formation of subunits. Ca^{2+} is required for the attachment of HA to erythrocytes. Optimum conditions for hemagglutination and further details of the nonspecific inhibitors of HA and methods for their removal from test sera were reviewed by Herrmann (1979).

Three CF antigens have been described: (1) a large particle antigen with a density of 1.19–1.23 g/ml in sucrose gradients and associated with the infectivity and HA activity; (2) a small particle ('soluble') antigen, which is probably a subunit of the protein coat of the virus (Schmidt and Styk 1968); and (3) a 150S particle, which appears to be associated with the ribonucleoprotein core of the virus (Vesikari 1972). High-titer preparations of RUBV can be used as CF antigens. These are usually prepared either by concentration of infected cell culture fluids or by alkaline extraction of infected cells (Herrmann 1979). BHK-21 and Vero cells are used for the production of suitable high-titer virus.

B-cell epitopes

During rubella infection, antibody responses are produced against all three structural proteins, but the E1 protein appears to be immunodominant (Table 45.2) (Cusi et al. 1989; Chaye et al. 1992a; Wolinsky et al. 1991). Studies using murine monoclonal antibodies have identified several epitopes on E1; three of these exhibit neutralizing or hemagglutinating activity, and have been mapped to residues 245–285 (Terry et al. 1988). A

further well-conserved neutralization domain has been identified within residues 211–239 (Chaye et al. 1992b; Mitchell et al. 1992b; Wolinsky et al. 1993). Human sera react with synthetic peptides comprising residues 214–285 of the E1 protein, suggesting that this region may represent a major neutralization domain. A recombinant protein containing these epitopes is recognized by most rubella antibody-positive human sera (Starkey et al. 1995). Murine and human antibody-binding domains also occur outside this region (Ilonen et al. 1992; Mitchell et al. 1993; Newcombe et al. 1994). A neutralization epitope has also been identified on the E2 glycoprotein (1–26) (Dorsett et al. 1985); other epitopes have been located between amino acids 51 and 105. At least two epitopes are present on the C protein (residues 9–29 and 64–97) (reviewed by Frey 1994). However, the epitopes that confer protection are probably conformational (Wolinsky et al. 1991) and have not yet been identified.

T-cell epitopes

Rubella virus-specific cellular immune responses have been measured in vitro by lymphoproliferation assays and lymphocyte-mediated cytotoxicity assays. All three structural proteins contain T-cell epitopes. Immunoreactive regions have been identified within capsid protein residues 9–29, 119–152, 255–280, E2 residues 54–74 and E1 residues 213–239, 273–284, 358–377, and 389–422 (Ou et al. 1993; reviewed by Chantler et al. 2001). MHC-restricted cytotoxic T-cell responses have been described (reviewed by Chantler et al. 2001). The significance of these T-cell epitopes in relation to protection is unclear.

Biological, antigenic, and nucleic acid sequence variation

Differences in the biological activity of attenuated and wild-type strains have been reported. The attenuated Cendehill strain has lower infectivity for rabbits and other laboratory animals than wild-type strains (Zygraich et al. 1971; Gill and Furesz 1973). Ohtawara and colleagues (1985) demonstrated that the growth of Japanese vaccine strains is restricted at 39°C, the body temperature of the rabbit, suggesting that the attenuated strains are temperature-sensitive mutants. Chantler and colleagues (1993) have shown that the vaccine strains RA27/3 and Cendehill differ from wild-type strains in growth characteristics, plaque morphology, and temperature sensitivity. They have suggested that the processing in the Golgi of the viral glycoproteins from the attenuated strains was slower than for wild-type strains, particularly in synovial cells (a human chondrocyte cell line and synovial membrane cells). The growth of the HPV77-DE5 vaccine strain was similar to the M33 strain

Table 45.2 *Antigenic regions of RUBV structural proteins identified as B-cell epitopes*

Structural protein	Amino acid residues	Hemagglutination activity	Neutralization activity	References
E1	157–176			Chaye et al. (1993)
	202–283	+	+	Wolinsky et al. (1991)
	208–239		+	Corboba et al. (2000)
	212–286			Starkey et al. (1995)
	213–239	+	+	Mitchell et al. (1993)
	214–233		+	Chaye et al. (1992b)
	214–240	+		Chaye et al. (1992b)
	219–233		+	Chaye et al. (1992b)
	219–239			Mitchell et al. (1993)
	221–239		+	Wolinsky et al. (1993)
	243–286		+	Starkey et al. (1995)
	245–251	+	+	Terry et al. (1988)
	250–252			Lozzi et al. (1990)
	258–277			Mitchell et al. (1993)
	260–263		+	Lozzi et al. (1990)
	260–266	+	+	Terry et al. (1988)
	274–285	+	+	Terry et al. (1988)
	374–390			Chaye et al. (1993)
E2	?		+	Green and Dorsett (1986)
	10–36			Mitchell et al. (1993)
	1–115			Wolinsky et al. (1991)
	151–170			Mitchell et al. (1993)
	244–263			Mitchell et al. (1993)
C	1–30			Ou et al. (1992)
	9–29			Wolinsky et al. (1991)
	64–97			Wolinsky et al. (1991)
	96–123			Ou et al. (1992)

from which it was derived. More recently, the slower replication of the Cendehill strain has been confirmed and both wildtype and attenuated strains have been shown to induce apoptosis (Domegan and Atkins 2002; Cooray et al. 2003).

Many studies in the late 1960s and 1970s failed to reveal any antigenic variation among RUBV strains and there was no reliable test to distinguish wild and attenuated strains. However, differences have been observed by cross-neutralization tests and neutralization kinetics (reviewed by Banatvala and Best 1990). More recent studies with monoclonal antibodies used in neutralization, HAI and enzyme immunoassay (EIA) revealed no significant differences between nine RUBV strains tested, which included the vaccine strains Cendehill, RA27/3, HPV77-DE5, and TO336 (Best et al. 1992). However, Dorsett et al. (1985) demonstrated strain-specific epitopes within the E2 glycopolypeptide when disrupted virus was used.

RUBV is genetically stable when compared to other RNA viruses. Although there is only one serotype of Rubella virus (Best et al. 1992), two genotypes have been identified (Bosma et al. 1996; Frey et al. 1998). Genotype 1 was isolated from cases in Europe, North America, and Japan between 1966 and 1996. Genotype 2 was isolated from cases in India and China in the 1990s and has more recently been detected in Italy (Zheng et al. 2003). A variable region (aa 697–800) has been identified within the gene coding for NSP1 (Hofmann et al. 2003). Nucleic acid sequencing has revealed that five characteristic nucleotide changes found within a 1 300 nucleotide sequence of the E1 coding region of the RA27/3 vaccine strain distinguishes it from other isolates of RUBV (Frey and Abernathy 1993; Frey 1994). Despite this, the deduced amino acid sequence of RUBV is remarkably stable (0.0–2.9 percent) although the amino acid sequence of E1 is more variable (Bosma et al. 1996; Frey et al. 1998; Hofmann et al. 2003).

CLINICAL AND PATHOLOGICAL ASPECTS

Introduction

In 1941, N. McAlister Gregg, an Australian ophthalmologist, published his now famous retrospective study 'Congenital cataract following german measles in the mother,' in which he showed that, if acquired in early pregnancy, rubella could cause congenital malformations

(Gregg 1941). Seventy-eight babies, all with a similar type of congenital cataract, were born in New South Wales after an extensive rubella epidemic there in 1940 and many of the mothers gave a history of rubella, usually in the first or second month of pregnancy. Congenital defects of the heart were also noted in 66 percent of cases whose cardiac condition was recorded. These findings were soon confirmed in Australia, and deafness was also noted in many congenitally infected infants. Microcephaly, dental defects, and low birth weight were also reported.

Despite confirmation of Gregg's original observation, an annotation in the *Lancet* (Editorial 1944) suggested that additional studies were required, as it could not be proved that the illness with rash experienced by these mothers was in fact rubella and that it was unlikely that such an association would have previously gone unnoticed. However, Hope-Simpson (1944) reported in the *Lancet* congenital cataract and heart defects in two babies in England after epidemic rubella. Similar defects had been noted before Gregg's original observation, but their significance had not been appreciated. Additional retrospective studies reporting congenital defects induced by rubella in early pregnancy were subsequently carried out (reviewed by Hanshaw et al. 1985).

Variable results were obtained in retrospective studies carried out before the isolation of rubella virus in 1962. When the starting point for investigations was an infant with one or more rubella-induced deformities results suggested that a very high proportion of mothers who had rubella during pregnancy were delivered of infants with congenital malformations. The outcome of pregnancies in which maternal rubella was followed by the birth of unaffected infants was not recorded. In 1940, when rubella was at its peak incidence in New South Wales, Gregg and colleagues (1945) reported that 96 percent of infants whose mothers had had rubella in early pregnancy suffered from congenital defects that were confined to cases in which maternal rubella had occurred before the 16th week of gestation.

In the period 1963–1964, within a year of the first reports of RUBV isolation and detection of rubella antibodies by neutralization tests, the USA experienced one of the most extensive outbreaks of rubella ever recorded. During this epidemic it was shown that maternal rubella could result in a generalized and persistent fetal infection and that infants excreted virus not only at birth but also for many months after this, despite developing rubella-specific antibody responses. In addition, the spectrum of anomalies was much wider than had hitherto been described. The impact of this epidemic stimulated research into the development of rubella vaccines and, following this, attenuated vaccines were licensed for use, in the USA in 1969 and in Britain in 1970. Congenitally acquired rubella, therefore, became a potentially preventable disease. National programs, which achieved high uptake rates, have recently shown a marked reduction in both postnatally and congenitally acquired rubella.

Postnatally acquired infection

CLINICAL AND VIROLOGICAL FEATURES

After an incubation period of 14–21 days, the characteristic features of rubella, rash, and lymphadenopathy may appear. In young children the onset of illness is usually abrupt. Such constitutional symptoms as fever and malaise may be present for a day or two before onset of the rash, but they usually subside rapidly after its appearance. Older children and adults may experience more pronounced constitutional symptoms 3–4 days before the rash appears, and during this prodromal phase an enanthem consisting of erythematous pinpoint lesions on the soft palate may be present. The exanthem is usually discrete, in the form of pinpoint maculopapular lesions. It appears first on the face and spreads rapidly to the rest of the body; lesions on the body may coalesce. The rash usually persists for about 3 days, occasionally longer, but may be fleeting. The mechanism by which rash is induced has not been established. Although immunopathological mechanisms may be responsible, RUBV has been isolated from skin biopsy specimens taken not only from areas with rash, but also from parts of the skin without rash and from the skin of patients with subclinical infection (Heggie 1978). Furthermore, the development of rash may be prevented by the administration of pooled human immunoglobulin, although this does not prevent viremia. Patients may complain of tender lymph nodes when or just before the rash appears. Follow-up studies of susceptible people exposed to rubella have revealed that lymphadenopathy may be present 7–10 days before the onset of rash, and sometimes for an even longer period after it has disappeared. Suboccipital, postauricular, and cervical lymph nodes are most frequently affected. Rubella is rarely associated with severe complications. Encephalitis may occur in one in 5 000–10 000 cases, but in general the prognosis is good (Krugman and Ward 1968). Very occasionally, there is clinical evidence of thrombocytopenia, which may result in purpuric rash, epistaxis, hematuria, and gastrointestinal bleeding.

The most common complication of postnatally acquired rubella is joint involvement. Although this is rare among children and adult males, it may occur in up to 60 percent of postpubertal females. Symptoms generally develop as the rash subsides and vary in severity from mild stiffness of the small joints of the hands to a frank arthritis with severe pain, joint swelling, and limitation of movement. The finger joints, wrists, knees, and ankles are most frequently affected. The duration of these symptoms is usually about 3 days, but occasionally they may persist for up to a month. Rubella-induced arthralgia is not associated with any sequelae. Arthralgia also occurs in postpubertal females after administration of rubella vaccine. The mechanism by which naturally acquired and vaccine-induced infection causes arthralgia is probably complex. Thus, joint symptoms may result from direct infection of the synovial membrane by virus, as RUBV has been isolated from the joint aspirates of vaccinees with vaccine-induced arthritis (Weibel et al. 1969). Furthermore, studies in vitro have shown that attenuated virus strains will replicate in human synovial membrane cell cultures (Grayzel and Beck 1971). However, an immune mechanism is probably also involved, because, in addition to virus, joint aspirates have been shown to contain rubella-specific IgG (Ogra and Herd 1971; Mims et al. 1985), which suggests that joint symptoms may be induced by immune complexes. It is therefore of interest that the presence of rubella antibody containing immune complexes in the serum has been associated with a high incidence of joint symptoms following rubella vaccination (Coyle et al. 1982). However, hormonal factors may also play a role, for, in addition to being common in postpubertal females, the development of joint symptoms appears to be related to the menstrual cycle. After rubella vaccination, they are most likely to occur within 7 days of the onset of the cycle (Harcourt et al. 1979).

RUBV has been suggested as a possible cause of chronic inflammatory joint disease, but studies on patients with that disease have yielded conflicting and unconfirmed results. In the 1980s it was claimed that RUBV could be detected in synovial fluid or the synovium, as well as in lymphocytes from patients with both rheumatoid arthritis and seronegative arthritis (i.e. rheumatoid factor negative), but these reports have not been confirmed. However, it is known that RUBV is able to establish persistent infection in vivo (Waxham and Wolinsky 1984), as well as in human synovial cell cultures and organ cultures (Cunningham and Fraser 1985; Miki and Chantler 1992) and that high levels of rubella antibody are found in joint fluid (Mims et al. 1985). Although there is no doubt that RUBV may be isolated from synovial fluid after naturally acquired infection or vaccination and from occasional patients with chronic inflammatory joint disease (Report 1994; Bosma et al. 1998), recent studies show that rubella vaccination is not associated with chronic inflammatory joint disease.

DIFFERENTIAL DIAGNOSIS

Rubella is often difficult to diagnose clinically because the illness may present atypically with minimal lymphadenopathy and an evanescent rash, and, conversely, typical rubelliform rashes may be induced by other viruses (Ramsay et al. 2002). Thus, such viruses as enteroviruses, human herpesviruses 6 and 7, West Nile virus and dengue virus may occasionally induce rubella-like rashes. Chikungunya virus and Ross River virus

(Chapter 47, Togaviruses) and parvovirus B 19 (Chapter 21, Parvoviruses) may induce not only a rubella-like rash, but also arthralgia. Serological studies have shown that there is poor correlation between a past history of rubella and immune status, particularly among adults (Brown et al. 1969). This is not surprising because not only may rubella present atypically, but disease without rash or subclinical infection may occur in up to 25 percent of children (Krugman and Ward 1954; Green et al. 1965).

The relation between clinical and virological features is shown in Figure 45.3. The patient is potentially infectious for a prolonged period, as pharyngeal virus excretion may occur for up to a week before onset of rash and persist thereafter for 7–10 days. Virus may also be detected in the stools and urine, but excretion occurs for a shorter time. These are not suitable specimens from which to isolate virus and do not play an important role in virus transmission. Viremia is present for about a week before the onset of rash, but as this appears rubella antibodies develop and viremia terminates.

EPIDEMIOLOGY

Rubella has a worldwide distribution. In temperate climates, before the introduction of rubella vaccination, epidemics usually occurred in spring and early summer, rubella occurring less commonly among preschool children than among schoolchildren and young adults. Women of child-bearing age were often infected as a result of exposure to their own children or at work. Seroepidemiological studies showed that the proportion of seropositive people increased progressively with age, about 50 percent of 9- to 11-year-old children being immune. Among women of child-bearing age, the proportion increased to about 80–85 percent (Dowdle et al. 1970). In industrialized parts of the world (e.g. UK, USA, Sweden, and Finland), which have achieved high uptake rates for rubella vaccine, postnatally and congenitally acquired rubella are now rare. However, in the UK, there is still a pool of rubella-susceptible males who have not been vaccinated. Many young men were infected in localized outbreaks of rubella in 1993 and 1996 (Figure 45.4), transmitting infection to some susceptible pregnant women, most of them being young primigravidae and many of whom were immigrants (Miller et al. 1997, www.hpa.org.uk/infections). Immigrants from Asia are at particular risk, as up to 23 percent may be susceptible (Tookey et al. 2002). Despite the success of the rubella vaccination program in the USA, a number of cases of congenitally acquired rubella were reported in California among immigrant women and among the Amish population in Pennsylvania in 1989/1990, this resulting from infection of unvaccinated women (Lindegren et al. 1991).

During the last few years, several studies have demonstrated that there is a considerable problem of

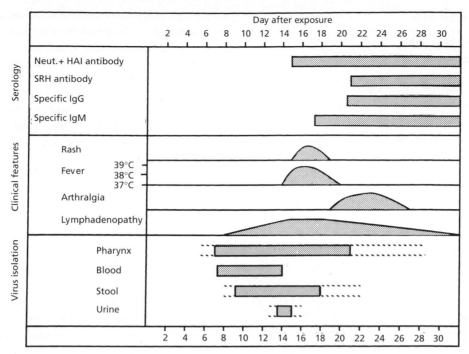

Figure 45.3 *Relationship between clinical and virological features of postnatally acquired rubella. HAI, hemagglutination inhibition; Neut., neutralizing; SRH, single radial hemolysis.*

congenital rubella in developing countries (Cutts et al. 1997; WHO 2000a, c). Such countries have an annual incidence of 0.6–4.1 cases per 1 000 live births, usually associated with rubella outbreaks. This is similar to the incidence in developed countries before the introduction of rubella vaccination. Epidemics of rubella occur every 4–7 years. The proportion of women susceptible to rubella has been shown to be 15–20 percent in many areas, although there may be considerable variation between different areas of a country, with susceptibility usually being higher in rural than in urban areas (Cutts et al. 1997). In some countries ≥25 percent are susceptible. Particularly high susceptibility rates occurred in island populations, including Jamaica and Trinidad and Tobago. An increasing number of countries are addressing this problem by including rubella vaccination in their national immunization programs (see Vaccination programs).

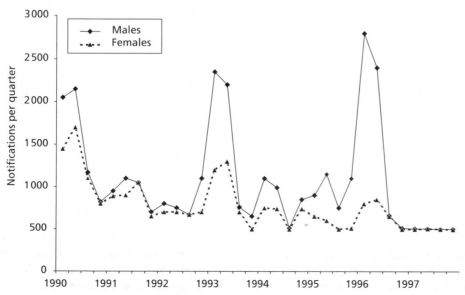

Figure 45.4 *Epidemic periodicity of rubella in males and females in England and Wales. Laboratory reports 1990 to 1997 (Miller et al. 1997).*

IMMUNE RESPONSES

Rubella-specific IgG, IgM, and IgA responses develop rapidly after the onset of rash. Rubella-specific IgG persists for life, but may decline to low levels in old age. The IgG response is predominantly IgG1. IgG3 is detected in most sera from cases of recently acquired rubella and IgG4 occasionally in sera from cases of remote rubella (Stokes et al. 1986; Thomas and Morgan-Capner 1988). Rubella-specific IgM usually appears within 4 days of onset of rash and persists for 4–12 weeks, but detection depends on the sensitivity of the technique employed. Specific IgM may sometimes persist for up to 1 year after both naturally acquired infection and rubella immunization (Pattison et al. 1975; O'Shea et al. 1985). Serum and nasopharyngeal IgA responses are detectable for at least 5 years after infection. The specific serum IgA response is exclusively IgA1. Specific IgD and IgE responses develop rapidly after onset of infection and persist for at least 6 months. The results of Mitchell and colleagues (1992a) suggest that males have a more rapid antibody response than females. Methods available for the detection and quantification of rubella antibodies are discussed under Laboratory diagnosis.

Immunoblotting for detection of polypeptide-specific antibodies is technically difficult. However, Zhang et al. (1992) demonstrated that antibodies to E1 and E2 were detected more effectively under nonreducing conditions than in the presence of 2-mercaptoethanol. The response to E1 is greater than to E2 and there is a strong response to the capsid protein (C) (Zhang et al. 1992; Nedeljkovic et al. 1999). Antibodies to E1 are essential for protection (Cusi et al. 1995). Avidity of IgG antibody to E1 matures during the 2 years after rubella infection, but IgG anti-E2 and anti-C show minimal avidity maturation (Mauracher et al. 1992).

A decrease in total leukocytes, neutrophils, and T cells, and a transient depression of lymphocyte responsiveness to mitogens and antigens such as purified protein derivative (PPD) is seen after rubella (Buimovici-Klein et al. 1976; Maller et al. 1978; Niwa and Kanoh 1979; Hyypiä et al. 1984). Cell-mediated immune responses, measured by lymphocyte proliferation assays, develop within a few days of onset of rash and persist for many years. Lymphokine secretion has also been detected (Honeyman et al. 1974; Buimovici-Klein and Cooper 1985). MHC class I-restricted CD8[+] cytotoxic T lymphocytes have been demonstrated in rubella-immune individuals (Lovett et al. 1993).

RE-INFECTION

Natural infection is followed by protection from reinfection, except in rare cases. However, evidence of reinfection may occasionally be obtained by demonstrating a significant increase in antibody concentration following natural and experimental exposure to rubella. Such reinfection is generally asymptomatic (Horstmann et al. 1970; Vesikari 1972). Reinfection in pregnancy is hazardous only if viremia occurs, and this has rarely been documented in experimental studies (O'Shea et al. 1983). Following maternal reinfection during the first 16 weeks in pregnancy, the risk of fetal infection has been estimated to be no more than 8 percent, and fetal damage is rare (Best et al. 1989; Morgan-Capner et al. 1991). Although it is possible that, in such cases, transmission of virus to the fetus may be due to a specific defect in the maternal immune response, rubella reinfection is not associated with a lack of neutralizing antibodies or persistent impairment of rubella-specific lymphoproliferative responses (O'Shea et al. 1994). Sequence changes have not been identified in the E1 ORF of isolates from cases of reinfection (Bosma et al. 1996). Further studies are required to determine whether reinfection is due to a failure to produce an immune response to the protective epitopes of the virus. Reinfection in pregnancy will be eliminated if high rates of rubella vaccination are achieved and maintained among the target groups (see Vaccination programs). Rubella reinfection has been reviewed by Best (1993) and Bullens et al. (2000).

Congenitally acquired infection

CLINICAL MANIFESTATIONS

Although the early retrospective enquiries emphasized the frequency and importance of such defects as congenital anomalies of the heart and eyes, and deafness, it was not until follow-up studies had been carried out on infants whose mothers had had rubella during the extensive 1963–1964 outbreak in the USA that it was fully appreciated that congenital rubella frequently caused widespread multisystem disease. Follow-up studies showed that congenital rubella syndrome (CRS) was not a static disease and that prolonged careful evaluation of infants at risk was necessary before some or all of the features of CRS were apparent. The broader range of anomalies described after the US 1963/1964 and subsequent outbreaks were probably not due to any change in viral virulence, but rather to more careful and prolonged observation. Careful scrutiny of the records of infants with CRS who were born before these outbreaks revealed that such anomalies as thrombocytopenic purpura and osteitis, although not reported in the literature, occurred fairly frequently.

Cooper (1975) divided clinical features associated with rubella infection into those that were transient, developmental, or permanent (Table 45.3). The pathogenesis of transient lesions is not understood, but they are usually present only during the first few weeks of life, do not recur and are not associated with the development of permanent sequelae. Intrauterine growth retardation resulting in low birth weight but at a normal gestational

Table 45.3 *Clinical features associated with congenitally acquired rubella (adapted from Cooper 1975)*

	Common	Uncommon
Transient	Low birth weight	Cloudy cornea
	Thrombocytopenic purpura	Hepatitis
	Hepatosplenomegaly	Generalized lymphadenopathy
	Bone lesions	Hemolytic anemia
	Meningoencephalitis	Pneumonitis
Developmental	Sensorineural deafness	Severe myopia
	Peripheral pulmonary stenosis	Thyroiditis
	Mental retardation	Hypothyroidism
	Central language defects	Growth hormone deficiency
	Diabetes mellitus	'Late onset disease'
Permanent	Sensorineural deafness	Severe myopia
	Peripheral pulmonary stenosis	Thyroid disorders
	Pulmonary valvular stenosis	Dermatoglyptic abnormalities
	Patent ductus arteriosus	Glaucoma
	Ventricular septal defect	Myocardial abnormalities
	Retinopathy	
	Cataract	
	Microphthalmia	
	Psychomotor retardation	
	Microcephaly	
	Cryptorchidism	
	Inguinal hernia	
	Diabetes mellitus	

age ('small for dates' babies) is among the most common of the transient features. Thus, Cooper and colleagues (1965) found that about 60 percent of infected infants fell below the tenth, and 90 percent below the 50th percentile.

A petechial or purpuric rash is also common, particularly among infants whose mothers had had maternal rubella in early pregnancy (Figure 45.5) (Cooper et al. 1965; Horstmann et al. 1965). However, low birth weight and a purpuric rash are seldom the sole manifestations of congenital rubella. These infants may have other anomalies, such as congenital heart and eye defects, although they may not always be apparent at birth. Infants with thrombocytopenic purpura generally have a platelet count ranging from 3 000 to 100 000/mm^3, this being associated with a decreased number of mega-karyocytes, but of normal morphology, in the bone marrow. In general, the platelet count rises spontaneously during the first month of life, although (rarely) some infants die from such complications as intracranial hemorrhage.

OCULAR DEFECTS

Many of the ocular defects characteristic of CRS were described by Gregg (1941), who drew particular attention to pigmented retinopathy and cataract. Pigmented retinopathy may be present in up to 50 percent of infants with CRS (Menser and Reye 1974; Vijaya-lakshmi et al. 2002) and may provide a useful aid in clinical diagnosis. The macular area of the retina is generally affected, but the lesions rarely impair vision. Cataracts may be unilateral or bilateral. Although usually present at birth, they may not be visible until several weeks later (Murphy et al. 1967). Lesions may be subtotal, consisting of a dense pearly-white central opacity (Figure 45.6) or, total with a more uniform density throughout the lens. Microphthalmus and iris hypoplasia are often associated with congenital cataract, but glaucoma is less common. However, it is important to recognize glaucoma as it can rapidly lead to blindness. Strabismus and nystagmus are also common (Vijayalakshmi et al. 2002).

Microphthalmia and glaucoma result from disturbances in organogenesis, and retinopathy and cataract result from intrauterine tissue destruction. However, delayed manifestations of congenital infection have also been recorded including lens changes, chronic uveitis, glaucoma, choroidal neovascularization, corneal hydrops, and keratoconus. Mechanisms postulated include virus persistence in the eye, resulting in RUBV-induced reduced growth rate and lifespan of cells, autoimmune phenomena or virally induced vascular damage and reactive hypervascularization (reviewed by Arnold et al. 1994).

DEAFNESS

Of the permanent defects, the most common is sensorineural deafness. This results from rubella-induced

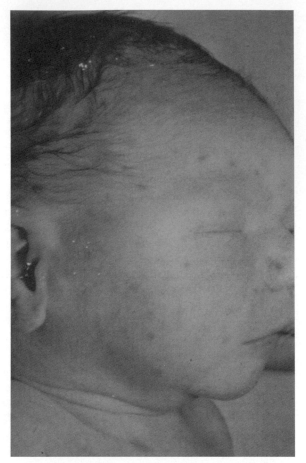

Figure 45.5 *Purpuric rash in newborn infant with congenitally acquired rubella, who was subsequently found to have congenital heart disease and cataract.*

damage to the organ of Corti. However, central auditory impairment may also occur. Hearing loss, which may be unilateral or bilateral, mild or profound, may sometimes be the only rubella-induced congenital anomaly.

Peckham (1972) followed up 218 children who were apparently normal at birth, but who had been exposed to rubella in utero. When assessed for hearing loss at the

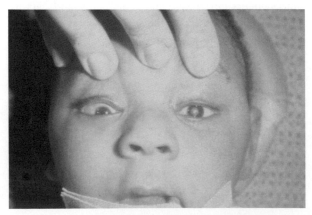

Figure 45.6 *Congenital rubella cataract in a 9-month-old infant. Cataract present in the left eye was surgically removed.*

age of 1–4 years, 50 (23 percent) were deaf. When 85 were re-examined between the ages of 6 and 8 years, further hearing defects were detected in another nine children. Of the children with hearing defects, 90 percent were seropositive. Because rubella antibodies are uncommon before the age of 4 years, it is particularly important to follow up infants with persistent rubella antibody so that hearing defects can be recognized as early as possible. Hearing defects can be detected in early infancy by testing auditory brainstem responses and otoacoustic emissions (Van Straaten et al. 1996).

HEART DISEASE

Congenital anomalies of the cardiovascular system are responsible for much of the high perinatal mortality associated with CRS. Numerous studies have shown that the most common lesions are persistence of a patent ductus arteriosus, proximal (valvular) or peripheral pulmonary artery stenosis, and a ventricular septal defect (Sperling and Verska 1966; Hastreiter et al. 1967; Cooper 1975).

Occasionally, neonatal myocarditis is found, often associated with other cardiac malformations (Korones et al. 1965). Rubella-induced damage to the intima of the arteries may result in obstructive lesions in the renal and pulmonary arteries (Rorke and Spiro 1967; Phelan and Campbell 1969).

DEFECTS IN THE CENTRAL NERVOUS SYSTEM

About 25 percent of infants who present at birth with clinical evidence of CRS have central nervous system (CNS) involvement, usually in the form of a meningo-encephalitis. Such infants are often lethargic at birth, but may become irritable and often exhibit evidence of photophobia. They have a full anterior fontanelle, pleo-cytosis, and an increased amount of protein in the cerebrospinal fluid (CSF) (Desmond et al. 1967). The outcome is variable and unpredictable. Although approximately 25 percent of infants presenting with meningoencephalitis at birth may, by the age of 18 months, be severely retarded, suffering from communication problems, ataxia, or spastic paresis, others appear to progress well neurologically despite poor development in the first 6 months of life.

Rubella panencephalitis is rare. Only about 50 cases have been reported, the majority as a consequence of congenital rubella infection, although it has also been reported following postnatally acquired disease. Most patients with CRS develop clinical signs between the ages of 8 and 20 years (reviewed by Frey 1997). RUBV has been recovered from the brain both with and without cocultivation techniques. It has also been recovered from patients' lymphocytes (Cremer et al. 1975; Wolinsky et al. 1979). Elevated levels of rubella-specific IgG and occasionally IgM may be detected in the serum.

The CSF may contain elevated concentrations of protein and immunoglobulin. Oligoclonal bands and a high CSF: serum rubella antibody ratio may be present suggesting intrathecal production of antibodies (Wolinsky et al. 1982).

Histological studies show panencephalitis with a perivascular inflammatory response, as well as a vasculitis. Rubella antigens have not been detected in brain sections by immunofluorescence. It has been postulated that post-rubella panencephalitis may be mediated by immune complexes (Waxham and Wolinsky 1984) or by virus-mediated autoreactivity to brain antigens (Martin et al. 1989).

DIABETES

Diabetes mellitus was originally believed to be a rare complication of CRS. However, follow-up studies of infants infected in utero during the Australian and US epidemics of 1940 and 1963/1964, respectively, have shown that nine of 45 (20 percent) of Australian and 30 of 242 (12.4 percent) of US children eventually developed insulin-dependent diabetes mellitus (IDDM). Up to 40 percent of CRS patients have impaired glucose tolerance (See and Tilles 1998). A long latent period is characteristic, the mean age of children developing IDDM in the US study being 9 years; all the Australian patients were in their third decade (Menser et al. 1978; Ginsberg-Fellner et al. 1985). Lymphocytic infiltration of the pancreas of an infant with CRS, but without IDDM may suggest that RUBV can initiate a train of events that subsequently results in IDDM in later life (Bunnell and Monif 1972). It seems likely that autoimmune mechanisms are involved in the pathogenesis of IDDM, because the HLA types in these patients are typical of those with autoimmune disease, there being a significant increase in prevalence of HLA-DR3, some increase in HLA-DR4 and a virtual absence of HLA-DR2. In addition, islet cell antibodies have been detected in 20 percent of these patients. These antibodies have a cytotoxic effect on cultured islet cells and predict the diabetic state. Although autoimmune responses may play an important role, the mechanism by which RUBV might trigger them remains to be established. An experimental study employing human fetal islet cells showed that RUBV induced a depression of immunoreactive secreted insulin without being cytolytic (Numazaki et al. 1990). A further study suggested that autoimmune phenomena might be involved, because immunoreactive epitopes in the RUBV capsid shared antigenicity with islet β cell protein (molecular mimicry) (Karounos et al. 1993).

BONE DEFECTS

Bone lesions may be detected by X-ray. Irregular areas of translucency are present in the metaphyseal portion of the long bones, but there is no evidence of periosteal reaction in over 20 percent of infants with congenital rubella (Cooper et al. 1965). These lesions generally resolve within 1–2 months. Cooper et al. (1965) detected these characteristic radiological changes in a fetus of 18 weeks' gestational age, suggesting that the process inducing such changes begins in early gestational life.

LATE ONSET DISEASE

Between the ages of about 3 and 12 months, some infants may present with such features as a chronic rubelliform rash, persistent diarrhea and pneumonitis. Marshall (1973) referred to this syndrome as 'late onset disease.' Although mortality is high, some infants show a dramatic response to treatment with corticosteroids. This syndrome may reflect an immunopathological phenomenon. Circulating immune complexes that appear to contain rubella antigen have been demonstrated in infants with late onset disease (Tardieu et al. 1980), and Coyle and colleagues (1982) demonstrated rubella antibody containing immune complexes in children with congenital rubella who developed new clinical problems some years after birth.

Some developmental defects may take many months or years to become apparent, but then persist permanently. Failure to recognize such defects in early infancy may not always be the result of difficulty in their detection. There is evidence which suggests that such defects as perceptive deafness, CNS anomalies and some ocular defects may actually develop or become increasingly severe some considerable time after birth. Menser and Forrest (1974) showed that it might be up to 4 years before the first rubella defects were recognized. Further defects might continue to be recognized up to the age of 8 years. The progressive nature of congenitally acquired disease is emphasized by the finding that children with previously stable congenital rubella-induced defects developed a widespread subacute progressive panencephalitis with progressive motor retardation as late as the second decade in life (Townsend et al. 1975; Weil et al. 1975).

LONG-TERM FOLLOW-UP OF CRS

As a result of the extent and severity of rubella-induced congenital malformations, children who survive will need continuous specialized management, education, and rehabilitation. However, a study carried out on 50 25-year-old patients with CRS born in Australia after the 1940/1941 epidemic showed that, although many were deaf or had eye defects, they had developed far better than had been anticipated when assessed in early childhood. Many had married and produced normal children, and all but four were employed, most patients being of average intelligence (Menser et al. 1967a). Follow-up studies so far reported on children with CRS following the 1963/1964 US rubella epidemic suggest that it may have had a more catastrophic impact on the lives of affected children than did the 1940/1941

Australian epidemic (Cooper 1975). This may be a reflection on the more modern methods of treatment available to the children born after this more recent epidemic. Many might not have survived previously.

Although congenitally acquired rubella is now rare in countries that have adopted rubella vaccination programs, a heavy burden from previous epidemics persists. A 20-year follow-up on 125 patients infected during the extensive 1963–1965 USA outbreak showed that, although many patients had multiple defects, ocular disease was the most commonly noticed disorder (78 percent) followed by sensorineural deafness (66 percent), psychomotor retardation (62 percent), and cardiac anomalies (58 percent). A 60-year follow-up of the Australian cohort has shown that the prevalence of diabetes, thyroid disorders, early menopause, and osteoporosis is higher in those with CRS than in the general population (Forrest et al. 2002).

Pathogenesis

The fetus is at risk during the period of maternal viremia, because placental infection may occur at this time. The most likely source of virus is from the maternal viremia. Virus may also be excreted via the cervix for up to 6 days after the onset of rash (Seppala and Vaheri 1974), and, because virus may exist in the genital tract for even longer, placental infection by direct contact or from ascending genital infection cannot be excluded.

After infection in early pregnancy, rubella induces a generalized and persistent virus infection in the fetus, which may result in multisystem disease. Töndury and Smith (1966) conducted histopathological studies on the products of conception from mothers clinically diagnosed as infected with rubella: anomalies were present in 68 percent of 57 fetuses when maternal rubella was contracted in the first trimester. When contracted in the first month of pregnancy, 80 percent were abnormal, sporadic foci, or cellular damage being present in the heart, inner ear, lens, skeletal muscle, and teeth. It was suggested that RUBV enters the fetus via the chorion, in which it induces necrotic changes in the epithelial cells, as well as in the endothelial lining of the blood vessels. The damaged endothelial cells are desquamated into the lumen of the vessel and then transported as virus-infected 'emboli' into the fetal circulation to settle in and infect various fetal organs. Lesions in the chorion were present as early as the tenth day after the onset of maternal rash. Fetal endothelial damage was distributed widely and probably resulted from viral replication rather than from antibody-mediated damage, because the most extensive histopathological changes were present at a gestational period before the fetal immune defense mechanism was sufficiently mature to be activated. Indeed, a characteristic feature of rubella embryopathy following maternal rubella in early gestational life is the notable absence of an inflammatory cell response (Töndury and Smith 1966).

At least three mechanisms have been suggested for inducing fetal damage: a virus-induced retardation in cell division, apoptosis (Pugachev and Frey 1998b), and tissue necrosis. Studies in vitro on embryonic cell cultures and rubella-infected fetuses suggest that RUBV may induce chromosomal damage and cause cells to divide more slowly than those that are uninfected (Plotkin et al. 1965). This may be due to a specific protein that reduces the mitotic rate of infected cells (Plotkin and Vaheri 1967). If retardation of cell division occurs during the critical phase of organogenesis, it is likely to result in congenital malformations. It has also been shown that the organs of rubella-infected infants are smaller and contain fewer cells than those of uninfected infants (Naeye and Blanc 1965). The fetal endothelial damage induced by rubella infection may cause hemorrhages in small blood vessels, leading to tissue necrosis and further damage of malformed organs over a longer period. Such organs as the liver, myocardium, and organ of Corti may be affected. Studies on the products of conception obtained from virologically confirmed cases of rubella during the first trimester have shown that the fetus is almost invariably infected, regardless of the time at which infection has occurred during this period (Rawls 1968; Thompson and Tobin 1970). It has also been suggested that RUBV may interfere with organ growth by preventing the assembly of actin and interrupt the cell cycle by binding to the tumor suppressor protein pRB (reviewed by Lee and Bowden 2000).

RUBV is isolated infrequently from neonates whose mothers developed infection after the first trimester, possibly because by then fetal immune mechanisms can effectively terminate infection. More mature fetal tissues do not have a reduced susceptibility to infection, for studies in vitro have shown that RUBV will replicate as well in organs derived from fetuses of 12–13 weeks' gestational age as in those of younger fetuses (Best et al. 1968). Nevertheless, even though severe congenital anomalies are rarely encountered following rubella after the first trimester, serological evidence of fetal infection has been shown to occur in 25–33 percent of infants whose mothers acquired maternal rubella between the 16th and 28th weeks of gestation (Cradock-Watson et al. 1980; Vejtorp and Mansa 1980).

Persistence of virus

Following intrauterine infection in early pregnancy, RUBV persists throughout gestation and can be isolated from most organs obtained at autopsy from infants who die in early infancy with severe and generalized infections. Virus may also be recovered from the nasopharyngeal secretions, urine, stools, CSF, and tears of survivors. RUBV can be isolated from nasopharyngeal secretions of most neonates with severe congenitally acquired disease, but by the age of 3 months the proportion excreting virus has declined to 50–60 percent and by 9–12 months to 10 percent (Cooper and Krugman 1967). Particularly during the first few weeks after birth, those with severe disease may excrete high concentrations of virus and readily transmit infection to rubella-susceptible contacts. RUBV may persist in infants with CRS in secluded sites for even longer. Thus, RUBV has been recovered from a cataract removed from a 3-year-old child (Menser et al. 1967b) and from the CSF of children with CNS involvement up to the age of 18 months (Desmond et al. 1967). Rubella antigen was detected in the thyroid from a 5-year-old child with Hashimoto's disease by immunofluorescence (Ziring et al. 1977), and by cocultivation techniques RUBV was recovered from the brain of a child who developed rubella panencephalitis at the age of 12 years (Cremer et al. 1975; Weil et al. 1975). Experimental studies have shown that, within the CNS, the astrocyte is the main cell type in which RUBV replicates with high concentrations of virus being expressed. Intrauterine infection involving these cells may perhaps induce focal areas of necrosis resulting in the pattern of neurological deficit observed in CRS (Chantler et al. 1995).

How RUBV persists throughout gestation and for a limited period during the first year of life has not been clearly established. Possible mechanisms include defects in cell-mediated immunity (CMI), poor interferon synthesis, and the possibility that a limited number of infected fetal cells give rise to infected clones which persist for a limited period. It has also been suggested that selective immune tolerance to the RUBV E1 protein may play a role (Mauracher et al. 1993). Studies in vitro show that RUBV replicates in T lymphocytes and macrophages and can also persist in B lymphocytes, causing inhibition of host-cell protein synthesis (Chantler and Tingle 1980; van der Logt et al. 1980). Infection of macrophages may interfere with their interactions with T cells. Postnatally acquired rubella causes a transient reduction in lymphocyte responses to phytohemagglutinin (Buimovici-Klein et al. 1976; Maller et al. 1978; Vesikari 1980), as well as a decrease in the numbers of T cells (Niwa and Kanoh 1979). CRS might be expected to cause an even greater reduction in responsiveness. Indeed, significantly diminished lymphoproliferative responses to phytohemagglutinin and rubella antigen, as well as diminished interferon synthesis, were demonstrated in 40 congenitally infected children aged 1–12 years (Buimovici-Klein et al. 1979). Impairment of CMI responses was related to the gestational age at which maternal infection occurred, and was greatest in infants whose mothers acquired rubella in the first 8 weeks of pregnancy. Hosking and colleagues (1983) suggested that children with nerve deafness due to CRS could be distinguished from those

with immunity due to postnatally acquired rubella by their failure to produce lymphoproliferative responses to rubella antigen. O'Shea and colleagues (1992) also found that 10 of 13 (80 percent) children with CRS under the age of 3 years failed to mount a lymphoproliferative response. Congenitally infected infants also have impaired natural killer cell activity (Fuccillo et al. 1974) and persistent T-cell abnormalities (Rabinowe et al. 1986). Defective CMI responses may persist into the second decade of life, well beyond the time when RUBV can be recovered from accessible sites.

Risks to the fetus

Whether maternal rubella induces fetal damage that causes intrauterine death or the birth of a malformed infant depends on the gestational age at which maternal rubella occurs, although other factors may also be involved. Maternal rubella may result in spontaneous abortion in up to 20 percent of cases (Siegel et al. 1971). This occurs most commonly when maternal infection is acquired during the first 8 weeks of pregnancy. To this must be added fetal wastage from therapeutic abortion following virologically confirmed rubella.

MATERNAL RUBELLA IN THE FIRST TRIMESTER

Many early prospective studies, the results of which are still quoted, underestimated the risks of congenital malformations, because maternal infections were included that were not rubella-induced and some rubella-infected infants were not followed up for sufficiently long. It is now known that 75–100 percent of infants born to mothers infected at this time will be congenitally infected and most of those infected will have associated defects (Enders 1982; Miller et al. 1982; Grillner et al. 1983). Many infants, although apparently normal at birth, if followed up for periods ranging from a few months to some years, may eventually be shown to have such defects as perceptive deafness or minimal CNS anomalies. Figure 45.7 relates the gestational age of maternal rubella to the clinical manifestations of congenitally acquired disease among 376 infants infected in utero during the 1964 epidemic in the USA. When maternal infection is acquired during the first 8 weeks of pregnancy – the critical phase of organogenesis – cardiac and eye defects are likely to occur. Retinopathy, hearing, and CNS defects are more evenly distributed throughout the first 16–20 weeks of gestational life.

MATERNAL RUBELLA AFTER THE FIRST TRIMESTER

RUBV is seldom isolated from infants whose mothers acquired rubella after the first trimester, although studies in vitro have shown that fetal tissues, regardless of gestational age, are susceptible to infection (Best

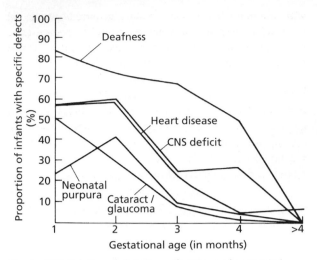

Figure 45.7 *Relation of clinical manifestations of congenital rubella to time of maternal infection, extrapolated from Cooper et al. (1969).*

et al. 1968). Indeed, serological studies confirm that a high proportion of infants are infected as a result of maternal rubella contracted after the first trimester, rubella-specific IgM being detected in 25–33 percent of infants whose mothers had rubella between the 16th and 20th weeks of pregnancy (Cradock-Watson et al. 1980). However, because organogenesis is complete by 12 weeks and in more mature fetuses immune responses may limit or terminate infection, such infants rarely have severe or multiple anomalies. Deafness and retinopathy, which per se does not affect vision, are likely to be the only anomalies commonly associated with rubella after the first trimester. When the results of four studies conducted in different countries are combined it is seen that the risk is about 17 percent when infection occurs at 13–16 weeks and about 5.9 percent after infection at 17–20 weeks (Peckham 1972; Miller et al. 1982; Grillner et al. 1983; Munro et al. 1987). Figure 45.7 shows that deafness is usually the sole clinical manifestation of fetal infection occurring between 13 and 16 weeks, and is relatively common, but that deafness or any other defects are only rarely encountered after this time.

PRECONCEPTUAL RUBELLA

Studies conducted in Germany and Britain indicate that preconceptual rubella does not result in transmission of RUBV to the fetus. Thus, Enders and colleagues (1988) found no serological or clinical evidence of intrauterine infection in 38 infants whose mothers' rashes appeared before or within 11 days after their last menstrual period (LMP). However, the fetus of a mother whose rash appeared 12 days after her LMP became infected, and all of ten mothers who developed rash 3–6 weeks after their LMP transmitted infection to their fetuses.

LABORATORY DIAGNOSIS

Rubella antibody screening

Tests for rubella antibodies are extensively used to identify susceptible women who should be offered rubella vaccination. In the UK, all antenatal patients are tested, as should women presenting to their general practitioners and 'well woman' clinics who have no history of vaccination or a previous positive antibody result (Department of Health 2003). A number of tests are available commercially. Enzyme-linked immunosorbent assay (EIA) is used widely because it is readily automated and can easily be included in automated antenatal screening. Latex agglutination (LA) has the advantage that a result is available in a few minutes. Single radial hemolysis (SRH) plates may be prepared in the laboratory with commercially available reagents. HAI is not recommended for screening since false-positive results may occur as a result of incomplete removal of β lipoprotein inhibitors of HA, and because it is more time consuming and labor intensive. These techniques have been described in detail by Best and O'Shea (1995). Vaccination should be offered to women who are seronegative or have antibody concentrations <10 IU/ml.

Rubella antibodies may be detected in oral fluid by IgG-capture radioimmunoassay (RIA) (GACRIA) (Parry et al. 1987). The use of oral fluid rather than serum has several benefits for seroepidemiological studies, especially those involving children and in developing countries, since it can be obtained by a noninvasive technique (Eckstein et al. 1996; Nokes et al. 1998).

Most rubella antibody tests use whole virus as antigen, but peptides and proteins produced by recombinant techniques have been evaluated (Mitchell et al. 1992b; Hobman et al. 1994c; Starkey et al. 1995) and some methods seem promising. One commercial test employed virus-like particles produced by expression in BHK cells (Grangeot-Keros et al. 1995).

Virus isolation and identification by RT-PCR

RUBV may be detected in clinical samples by isolation in cell culture or by reverse transcription polymerase chain reaction (RT-PCR). Preferred samples are a throat swab or oral fluid. Virus isolation techniques are rarely used for the diagnosis of postnatally acquired rubella because this may be established more reliably and rapidly by serological methods. However, virus isolation may be of value for determining the duration of excretion in congenitally infected infants, as they may transmit infection to susceptible contacts. RUBV isolates are also required to study the molecular epidemiology of the virus.

RUBV can be identified by the production of CPE in RK13, SIRC, and certain sublines of Vero cells, by interference in primary vervet monkey kidney (VMK) (Parkman et al. 1962) and other monkey kidney cultures, or by using immunofluorescence or immunoperoxidase for detection of antigen in such cells as RK13, BHK-21, and Vero. The most sensitive technique for isolation of RUBV is one or two passages in Vero cells, followed by passage in RK13 cells, in which the virus may be identified by immunofluorescence employing hyperimmune sera or monoclonal antibodies or by RT-PCR. These techniques have been described in detail by Best and O'Shea (1995). However, as virus isolation is labor intensive and a minimum of 3 weeks is required to obtain a result, this technique is available only in a few specialized laboratories.

Nested RT-PCRs for the detection of RUBV RNA employing primers from the E1 region have been described by Bosma et al. (1995b); Revello et al. (1997); Vyse and Jin (2002) and Li Jin (personal communication, 2003). Results of these assays compared well with virus isolation. RT-PCR is now used for the pre- and postnatal diagnosis of congenital rubella and is useful for detection of RUBV RNA in oral fluid when serological results are equivocal (Vyse and Jin 2002).

Laboratory diagnosis of postnatally acquired infection

A clinical diagnosis of rubella is unreliable and therefore laboratory confirmation is required, particularly for the diagnosis of rubella-like illness during pregnancy and for contacts of pregnant women. The detection of rubella-specific IgM is the method of choice. Specific IgM antibodies may be detected by indirect and M-antibody capture enzyme immunoassays. Care should be taken to ensure that the test chosen has a high degree of specificity and sensitivity (Hudson and Morgan-Capner 1996; Tipples et al. 2004). Rubella-specific IgM usually appears within 4 days of onset of rash and persists for 4–12 weeks. More than 4 weeks after onset, detection will depend on the sensitivity of the technique employed. The diagnosis should be confirmed by detecting a significant rise in antibody concentration or by testing a further serum for specific IgM. A significant rise in antibody concentration may be detected by a variety of methods, including HAI, EIA, or LA titration. Seroconversion can also be detected by SRH. Although HAI antibodies develop within a day or 2 of onset of rash, antibodies detected by EIA, LA, or SRH may be delayed until 7–8 days (Figure 45.3).

Rubella-specific IgG and IgM antibodies may be detected in oral fluid using antibody capture radioimmunoassays. Results correlate well with serum antibodies (Perry et al. 1993; Vyse et al. 1999). The optimum time for detecting specific IgM is 1–5 weeks after onset of illness. This method is particularly useful when testing children and has been used to demonstrate that many rubella-like rashes are caused by other viruses or bacteria (Ramsay et al., 1998, 2002).

RE-INFECTION

Reinfection is associated with a rise in antibody concentration, sometimes to very high levels. An IgM response may also be present, but is usually lower and more transient than that following primary infection. An accurate history of rubella contact, rubella vaccination, and previous rubella antibody screening is required in order to interpret results. It may be particularly difficult to distinguish between a primary infection and reinfection, if blood is not obtained shortly after contact or if sera taken prior to contact (e.g. for screening purposes) are not available. However, reinfection may be distinguished from primary infection by examining the antigen-binding avidity of specific IgG, because the avidity of specific IgG from cases of recent primary rubella is low compared with that from people with remote infection or reinfection (Thomas and Morgan-Capner 1991).

Testing for reinfection is not indicated in populations where most women are rubella seropositive and there is a low incidence of rubella (Morgan-Capner and Crowcroft 2002).

ASSESSMENT OF THE RISK TO WOMEN EXPOSED TO OR WHO DEVELOP RUBELLA-LIKE ILLNESS IN PREGNANCY

Precise details of the date of onset of illness, presence, and distribution of such clinical features as rash, lymphadenopathy, and arthralgia should be obtained from pregnant women who present with rubella-like clinical features. If there is a history of contact with a rubella-like illness the date, duration, and type of contact (e.g. casual or more prolonged household contact) should be obtained, in order to interpret the results of virological investigations. In addition, enquiry should be made about results of previous screening tests for rubella antibodies and history of rubella vaccination.

Patients who have been exposed to rubella should be carefully followed up serologically because retrospective studies have shown that some women who delivered infants with CRS gave no history of a rubella-like illness during pregnancy. Blood should be collected from pregnant women with rubella-like features as soon as possible after the onset of symptoms. Provided that a blood sample is obtained within the first 3–4 days, it is usually possible to detect a significant rise in antibody concentration and rubella-specific IgM in a second blood sample taken a few days later.

Although most patients develop rubella antibodies within a few days of onset of symptoms, antibody responses may very occasionally be delayed for as long as 10 days. This underlines the importance of collecting further blood samples from patients who remain seronegative. Many patients present in the postacute phase of their illness, at which time antibody concentrations are likely to have reached maximum concentrations. It must be emphasized that there is no particular concentration of antibody ascertained by any test that can be regarded as indicative of recent or current infection. Because a virological diagnosis is usually required quickly for obstetric reasons, such patients should be tested for rubella-specific IgM with minimum delay.

Women who present within the incubation period and who have antibodies may be reassured, although it is often wise to obtain a second blood sample 7–10 days later to ensure that antibody concentrations are stable. The interpretation of results may depend on the accuracy of the history given by the patient. Sometimes an earlier blood sample is available (e.g. taken at the first antenatal visit) which can be tested in parallel with a sample taken after contact. If there is no change in antibody concentration the patient can be reassured with confidence that she was already immune.

Patients presenting after an interval greater than the incubation period and who are seropositive are more difficult to assess because antibody levels may already have reached their maximum. The sera of such patients should therefore be tested for rubella-specific IgM. Detection of rubella-specific IgM in women who give no history of a rubella-like rash or contact with such a rash, should be interpreted with caution. In some patients, the specific IgM may persist for months or years after infection and vaccination (Banatvala et al. 1985; Thomas et al. 1992) and false-positive results may occur in patients with autoimmune diseases and other infections. In such cases it is necessary to use further tests, such as specific IgG avidity and western blot to determine whether recent infection has occurred (Pustowoit and Liebert 1998; Thomas et al. 1999; Best et al. 2002).

Because rubella is unlikely to be acquired as a result of casual or brief contact (e.g. while shopping or in public transport), seronegative patients who experience this type of exposure should be reassured that the risks of acquiring rubella are small. Nevertheless, it is essential to follow up such people serologically. Those exposed more closely over a longer period are at greater risk, but even they may be reassured, particularly during nonepidemic times, by being told that the clinical diagnosis of rubella is often incorrect. Anxiety may be allayed by testing the index case, in order to confirm or refute the diagnosis. Patients who have been followed up, but who remain seronegative, should be offered rubella vaccination in the immediate postpartum period.

Laboratory diagnosis of congenital rubella

POSTNATAL TESTS

The National Congenital Surveillance Programme in the UK classifies suspected cases of congenital rubella according to the criteria listed in Table 45.4. The congenital rubella syndome (CRS) case classification for the United States has been revised (Reef et al. 2000).

A diagnosis of CRS can be established by:

- Detection of rubella-specific IgM in cord serum or serum samples obtained in early infancy. An IgM antibody capture assay is generally preferred for this purpose (Chantler et al. 1982; Hudson and Morgan-Capner 1996). Specific IgM has been detected by M-antibody capture radioimmunoassay (MACRIA) in all symptomatic infants up to the age of 3 months, in 90 percent of infants aged 3–6 months, in fewer than 50 percent of infants aged 6–12 months and only occasionally in children over 1 year old (Chantler et al. 1982). However, commercially available enzyme immunoassays (indirect and M-antibody capture formats) have not been evaluated for the diagnosis of CRS and may be less sensitive. The absence of specific IgM by IgM antibody capture assays in the neonatal period virtually excludes congenital rubella.
- Detection of persistent rubella IgG antibody in serum or oral fluid at a time when maternal antibodies are no longer detectable (approximately 8 months). This may be a useful technique when patients present too late for the detection of specific IgM.
- Isolation of RUBV or detection of RUBV RNA by RT-PCR (Bosma et al. 1995b) in specimens (such as pharyngeal swabs) taken from infants during early infancy. Facilities for RUBV isolation are not widely available. RT-PCR can also be applied to lens

Table 45.4 *Congenital rubella: case classification criteria (Miller et al. 1994)*

Congenital rubella infection	No rubella defects, but congenital infection confirmed by isolation of virus, or detection of specific IgM or persistent IgG in infant
Congenital rubella syndrome	
Confirmed	Typical rubella defect(s) plus virus-specific IgM or persistent IgG in infant; or two or more rubella defects plus confirmed maternal infection in pregnancy
Compatible	Two or more rubella defects with inconclusive laboratory data, or single rubella defect plus confirmed maternal infection in pregnancy
Possible	Compatible clinical findings with inconclusive laboratory data, e.g. single defect plus probable maternal infection in pregnancy
Unclassified	Insufficient information to confirm or exclude

aspirates from cataracts in order to establish a diagnosis of CRS (Bosma et al. 1995a).

RUBV can be isolated from the stools, urine, tears, CSF, and nasopharyngeal secretions of infants with CRS. Cooper and Krugman (1967) isolated RUBV from the nasopharynx of almost all severely infected infants at birth, but by the age of 3 months the proportion declined to about 60 percent and, by 9–12 months, to approximately 10 percent. Virus excretion has not yet been tested by RT-PCR, which may detect virus excretion for longer. However, RUBV may persist at other sites for even longer (see Persistence of virus). RUBV can be isolated from most of the organs obtained at autopsy from severely infected infants who die in early infancy. Babies excreting virus may transmit infection to susceptible contacts. Therefore, until virus is no longer being excreted, women of childbearing age, some of whom may be in the early stages of pregnancy, should be dissuaded from visiting such babies until serological tests confirm that they are immune.

Rubella-specific lymphoproliferative assays (O'Shea et al. 1992) and tests for low avidity specific IgG (Thomas et al. 1993) may be of value for retrospective diagnosis of CRS in children between the ages of 1 and 3 years.

Children with CRS may lose antibodies to the E1 glycoprotein (de Mazancourt et al. 1986; Mitchell et al. 1992b; Mauracher et al. 1993; Meitsch et al. 1997) and consequently HAI antibodies may not be detected (Cooper et al. 1971; Ueda et al. 1975). Forty-one percent of 40 persons with CRS tested at 60 years of age had no rubella antibodies detectable by EIA (Forrest et al. 2002). In order to determine the immune status of such persons in later life, it may be necessary to use tests such as western blot, which detect antibodies to individual RUBV polypeptides.

PRENATAL TESTS

Prenatal diagnosis of CRS may provide a more accurate estimate of risk when the mother is reluctant to have a therapeutic abortion following rubella in the first trimester, when maternal reinfection is confirmed or suspected and when serological results are equivocal, for example when rubella-specific IgM is detected in a woman with no history of a rubella-like illness. A prenatal diagnosis may be made by testing amniotic fluid for RUBV RNA by RT-PCR, and fetal blood for RUBV RNA and rubella-specific IgM. The detection of RUBV RNA in amniotic fluid and fetal blood has sensitivities of 87.5 percent and positive predictive values of 100 percent (Enders 1998) when tested by the RT-PCR method described by Bosma et al. (1995a). Amniotic fluid can be taken after 15 weeks' gestation and ≥8 weeks after onset of maternal rubella infection. However, as false-negative results may occur, it is desirable to test further amniotic fluid, as well as fetal blood at 22–23 weeks' gestation.

As the fetus may not produce sufficient IgM before 22 weeks' gestation, fetal blood should be obtained by cordocentesis after that time. It is advisable to test fetal blood for rubella-specific IgM with more than one assay as levels may be low. Although this approach means that the patient may have to wait some time for the final test, it is possible that false-negative results may be obtained before this time (Tang et al. 2003).

Prenatal diagnosis has also been discussed by Revello et al. (1997); Enders (1998) and Katow (1998).

PREVENTION

Rubella vaccination

Rubella and congenitally acquired rubella are preventable, and the elimination of CRS in some countries with national vaccination programs results from the administration of attenuated rubella vaccines.

RUBELLA VACCINES

The first attenuated strain of rubella was developed by the National Institutes of Health in the USA. This strain was isolated from a military recruit with acute rubella and attenuated by 77 passages in VMK cell cultures. Following preliminary trials in primates in which this vaccine was shown to be protective, controlled trials were conducted among institutionalized children, the vaccine strain having been passaged a further five times in duck embryo fibroblasts. Within a short time, further vaccine strains were prepared, being attenuated in primary rabbit kidney (Cendehill) and in human diploid cell cultures (RA27/3) (Proceedings 1969). The vaccine containing the RA27/3 strain, originally isolated from the fetal kidney of a rubella-infected conceptus, is the most widely used worldwide, although a number of vaccine strains developed in Japan and China are now used in these countries (Perkins 1985). The accumulated data from trials employing rubella vaccines show that they are immunogenic, protective, and well tolerated. Vaccinees excrete virus via the nasopharynx, but infection is not transmitted to susceptible contacts. The development and properties of different rubella vaccines have been reviewed by Banatvala and Best (1989) and Best (1991). Rubella vaccine is now usually given with measles and mumps vaccines as the triple vaccine measles, mumps, and rubella (MMR) (Salisbury and Begg 1996).

VACCINATION PROGRAMS

Rubella vaccines were licensed in the USA in 1969 and in the UK in 1970. In the USA a policy of universal childhood immunization was adopted, this being aimed at interrupting transmission of virus by vaccinating preschool children, thereby reducing the risk of pregnant women being exposed to rubella. Because high uptake rates were achieved, this policy markedly reduced the incidence of postnatally acquired and CRS (Figure 45.8). However, in 1989/1990 rubella occurred among unvaccinated women in some parts of the USA, resulting in cases of CRS (Lindegren et al. 1991). Rubella vaccine is now given as the MMR vaccine at 12–15 months and 4–6 years of age. Those who miss the second dose should be offered it at 11–12 years (Centers for Disease Control and Prevention 2001a).

A selective vaccination program was initially adopted in the UK, this being directed first at prepubertal schoolgirls, women at particular risk of acquiring rubella (e.g. nurses and school teachers), and seronegative adult women identified by rubella antibody screening. Because complete vaccination of the target population was an unrealistic goal, the vaccination program was augmented in 1988 by offering rubella vaccine to preschool children of both sexes (Banatvala 1987) and rubella is now given with measles and mumps (MMR) vaccine in two doses at 12–15 months and 4–5 years of age. This resulted in a fall in the number of reported cases of rubella, congenital rubella, and of terminations of pregnancy because of rubella (Figure 45.9). Following the administration of MR vaccine to all 5- to 16-year-old school children in late 1994 to prevent a predicted measles epidemic, it was agreed to discontinue vaccination of schoolgirls, but to continue to ensure that susceptible pregnant women were vaccinated postpartum.

Although a significant proportion of young adult males remains susceptible, high rates of vaccine uptake among preschool children together with the markedly reduced susceptibility among pregnant women have resulted in CRS being rare in the UK. Thus, in contrast to 1984 in which 52 cases were reported, in 1996 only 12 cases were notified to the National Congenital Rubella Surveillance Programme. Two of the 12 mothers had acquired the infection while abroad (Tookey and Peckham 1999). Seven babies with CRS were born in the 2-year period 2000–2001. Five of the seven mothers had acquired rubella abroad (Rahi et al. 2001; P Tookey, personal communication, 2002). It will be unfortunate if CRS returns in the future, as a consequence of the fall in the uptake of MMR due to the unjustified public concern about its safety (see Vaccine reactions).

Most countries in Europe administer MMR vaccine between the first and second birthdays; and many now offer a second dose. Although uptake of rubella vaccine is poor in some countries in Europe, Sweden and Finland have eliminated rubella by use of two-dose MMR programs (Peltola et al. 1994; Böttiger and Forsgren 1997). A review published by the World Health Organization (WHO) in 1997 highlighted the problem of congenital rubella in developing countries (Cutts et al. 1997). A meeting was held in 2000 to consider methods for surveillance of rubella and congenital rubella and the use of rubella vaccines in developing countries (World Health Organization 2000a). WHO also published guidelines for the surveillance of rubella and CRS (World Health Organization 1999) and a position paper on rubella vaccines (World Health Organization 2000b). Many developing countries have introduced rubella vaccination, since it has been shown to be cost-effective (Hinman et al. 2002), and by 2002, 123 (57 percent) of all countries/territories in the world had included rubella vaccination in their national immunization programs (Figure 45.10). Forty-one of the 44 countries in the Pan American Health Organization (PAHO) had incorporated MR or MMR into their childhood immunization programmes by 2002 (World Health Organization 2003a). Although it is desirable to give rubella vaccine to children with measles (as MR or

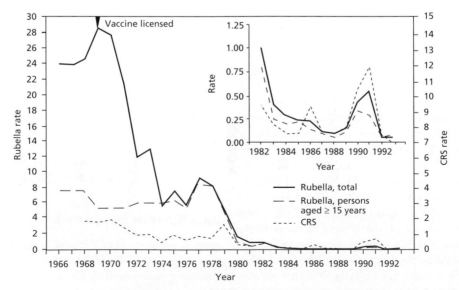

Figure 45.8 *Incidence rates of rubella and congenital rubella syndrome (CRS) in the USA, 1966–1993; cases of rubella reported to the National Notifiable Disease Surveillance System per 100 000 population; cases of CRS reported to the National CRS Registry per 100 000 live births (from Centers for Disease Control and Prevention, 1994).*

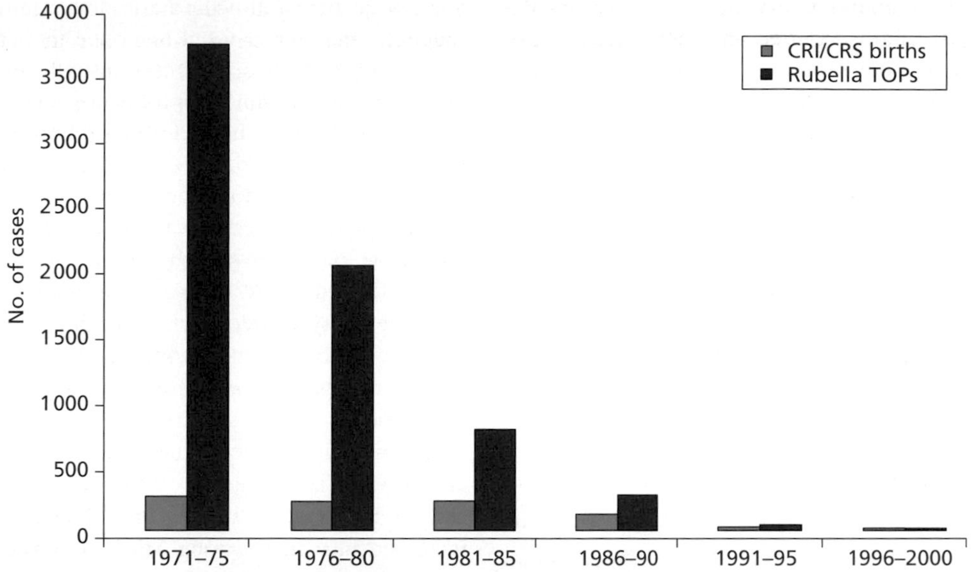

Figure 45.9 *Congenital rubella births and rubella-associated terminations of pregnancy (TOP) in England and Wales (data from National Congenital Rubella Surveillance Programme 2003, www.ich.ucl.ac.uk).*

MMR), it is also necessary to vaccinate susceptible women of child-bearing age, as childhood vaccination alone will increase the risk to susceptible adults (Robertson et al. 1997, World Health Organization 2000a, c). WHO recommend that surveillance for rubella, CRS, and rubella vaccine coverage should be monitored (World Health Organization, 1999, 2003a), since it is necessary to have a vaccine uptake of at least 80 percent among children to prevent circulation of rubella.

IMMUNE RESPONSES

About 95 percent of vaccinees develop an immune response. Serum antibodies develop between 10 and 28 days after vaccination and reach maximum levels about 6 months later. Occasionally, antibody responses may be delayed for up to 8 weeks. Failure to respond may result from concurrent infections, pre-existing low levels of antibody undetectable by less sensitive assays, or the presence of passively acquired antibody acquired maternally, via blood transfusion or administration of immunoglobulin. Failure to comply with the manufacturer's recommendations during storage or after reconstitution may result in virus inactivation and loss of potency of the vaccine.

Following vaccination, antibodies to the major structural proteins E1, E2, and C may be detected, and rubella-specific IgG, IgA and IgM responses are present. Specific IgM responses are detected in about 70 percent of vaccinees. Occasionally, rubella-specific IgM may persist at low levels for up to 4 years after vaccination (O'Shea et al. 1985). Virus-specific IgA concentrations decline more rapidly than specific IgG. There is a transient oligomeric (10S) IgA response, which is succeeded by a 7S response that may persist at low levels for 10–12 years after vaccination. The RA27/3 vaccine induces a secretory IgA response which persists for up to 5 years (O'Shea et al. 1985).

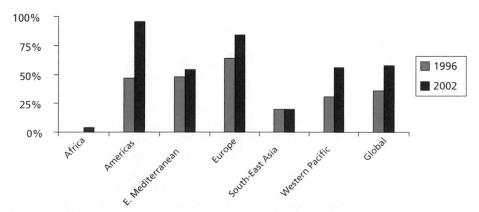

Figure 45.10 *Percentage of countries/territories, by WHO region and globally, with rubella vaccine in the national immunization system, 1996 and 2002 (Source: WHO Department of Vaccines and Biologicals, December 2002).*

Although serum antibody levels detected by HAI and SRH persist for at least 21 years in most vaccinees, in approximately 10 percent the levels decline to <15 IU/ml within 5–8 years. A small number may become completely seronegative (reviewed by Banatvala and Best 1989). However, when volunteers with low levels of antibody were challenged intranasally with high titer RA27/3 vaccine, most appeared to be protected although a transient low level of virus-specific IgM was present in four of 19 and a transient viremia was detected in one of 19 volunteers (O'Shea et al. 1983). A transient lymphoproliferative response has been detected following rubella vaccination (Buimovici-Klein and Cooper 1985).

VACCINE EFFICACY AND RE-INFECTION

The protective efficacy of rubella vaccines is about 95 percent (reviewed by Plotkin 1999). Experimental studies demonstrate that reinfection (see relevant sections on reinfection) is more likely to occur in those whose immunity is vaccine-induced than in those with naturally acquired immunity (reviewed by Best 1991). Re-infection is less likely to occur after vaccination with the RA27/3 vaccine strain, than with the Cendehill and HPV-77 vaccine strains, which is why the RA27/3 strain is now used in most rubella vaccines (see above).

Vaccination is recommended for adult women who have rubella antibodies <10 IU/ml, but some of these women will fail to mount a booster response, as seen in vaccine trials (Best 1991). Therefore, no more than two doses of vaccine are indicated for such women. However, it may be of value to test the sera from these women for rubella IgG using more than one technique (Best, 1991; Best and O'Shea 1995). Following vaccination, women may be considered immune if antibodies ≤10 IU/ml are detected by two different techniques. Survivors of CRS may fail to respond to rubella vaccine.

VIRUS EXCRETION

Rubella vaccine may be detected in nasopharyngeal secretions from most vaccinees 6–29 days after vaccination, as well as in the breast milk of lactating women vaccinated postpartum. Although lack of transmission to susceptible contacts may result from low concentrations in nasopharyngeal secretions, it is possible that attenuation may alter the biological properties of the virus, resulting in poor replication in the respiratory tract. Very occasionally, virus has been transmitted to breastfed infants, but they do not develop any clinical features of infection.

VACCINE REACTIONS

Rubella vaccine is well tolerated although lymphadenopathy, rash, and arthropathy may occur between 10 and 30 days after vaccination. In general, such reactions are less severe than following naturally acquired infection. Indeed, vaccinees may fail to notice their lymphadenopathy and, if rash occurs, it is usually macular, faint, and evanescent. Joint symptoms are related to age and gender, being rare in children of both sexes (2.5–10 percent), but occurring in up to 58 percent of post-pubertal females. Most commonly, the small joints of the hands are affected, but the knees, wrists, and ankles may also be involved. Symptoms rarely persist for longer than a week. However, a small proportion of vaccinees may develop arthritis with pain and limitation of joint movement, which may occasionally recur intermittently. Joint symptoms rarely result in absence from work.

Although it has been suggested that MMR is associated with inflammatory bowel disease and autism, several longitudinal studies have failed to confirm an increased incidence among MMR vaccinees. A number of prestigious groups and committees have examined the evidence and stated that there is no good scientific evidence to support this theory (Chief Medical Officer 2001; Institute of Medicine 2001; Miller, 2001; World Health Organization 2003b). The association is circumstantial as these diseases are first detected at about 15 months of age, the age at which MMR is given to children. However, due to the publicity generated in the media, public concern has resulted in a serious fall in the uptake of MMR in some parts of the UK, which has lead to outbreaks of measles (Jansen et al. 2003).

CONTRAINDICATIONS

As with other live vaccines, immunocompromised patients should not be vaccinated. Such people include those with malignant disease and those being treated with cytotoxic drugs, radiotherapy, or corticosteroids. Thrombocytopenic patients should not be vaccinated. HIV-positive people, with or without symptoms, are exceptions to these recommendations because they may be vaccinated with such live vaccines as MMR and polio. HIV-positive people do not react adversely to such live vaccines but, if unprotected, may experience serious complications, particularly if infected with measles.

Live vaccines may be administered concurrently, preferably at different sites (except in the case of MMR). If this is not possible, the two live vaccines should be separated by an interval of 3 weeks. A similar period should be allowed between the administration of rubella vaccine, or MMR, and BCG. If a vaccinee has a febrile illness, it is prudent to postpone rubella vaccination until the individual has recovered. The rubella vaccines may contain such antibiotics as neomycin, kanamycin, or polymyxin, and anyone with established hypersensitivity to these antibiotics should not be vaccinated. As passively acquired antibodies may interfere with vaccine-induced responses, rubella vaccination should be delayed for 3 months after blood transfusion or administration of immunoglobulin. However, the administration of anti-D immunoglobulin does not suppress vaccine-induced immune responses, although it may be prudent to confirm seroconversion 2–3 months after vaccination.

VACCINATION DURING PREGNANCY

Although wild-type strains of rubella are teratogenic, the accumulated data from studies reported in different countries, in which 661 rubella-susceptible women were vaccinated during pregnancy, have shown that this has not resulted in rubella-induced permanent fetal defects. Forty-four percent of these women were vaccinated during the high-risk period between 2 weeks before and 6 weeks after conception. Vaccine strains may, however, infect the conceptus because rubella vaccine strains have been isolated from the placenta, kidney, and bone marrow for up to 94 days after vaccination. Furthermore, rubella-specific IgM responses or antibodies persisting for up to a year have been detected in about 3 percent of infants delivered of mothers inadvertently vaccinated during early pregnancy. Among the 661 infants born to women who were inadvertently vaccinated during pregnancy, only one rubella-IgM positive infant had a heart murmur which resolved by 2 months of age (P. Tookey, personal communication 2000; reviewed by Best and Banatvala 2004).

The theoretical maximum risk of rubella vaccine-induced major malformations based on a 95 percent confidence limit of the binomial distribution has been calculated to be 1.2 percent, this being less than the 3 percent of major malformations occurring in 'normal' pregnancies (Bart et al. 1985; Enders 1985). These encouraging reports have resulted in a substantial reduction in terminations of pregnancy being carried out as a result of inadvertent vaccination in pregnancy in Britain. Nevertheless, it is still recommended that pregnant women should not be vaccinated against rubella and that pregnancy should be avoided for 1 month after vaccination (Salisbury and Begg, 1996; Centers for Disease Control and Prevention 2001b).

Passive immunization

Normal human immunoglobulin does not confer any clearcut protection (Report 1970). This preparation may reduce the incidence of clinically overt maternal infection, but subclinical infection may nevertheless occur, with a prolonged incubation period. Because inapparent infection is accompanied by viremia, fetal damage is not prevented when it is used in pregnancy. However, it is possible that the administration of normal human globulin reduces the level of fetal infection or damage, or both (Peckham 1974; Hanshaw et al. 1985).

High-titer rubella immunoglobulin has been used experimentally to determine whether infection induced by rubella vaccine can be prevented (Urquhart et al. 1978). This preparation has not been properly evaluated in the field, but may be recommended for the few susceptible pregnant women who come into contact with clinical rubella and for whom therapeutic abortion is unacceptable.

REFERENCES

Arnold, J.J., McIntosh, E.D., et al. 1994. A fifty-year follow-up of ocular defects in congenital rubella: late ocular manifestations. *Aust NZ J Ophthalmol*, **22**, 1–6.

Atreya, C.D., Singh, N.K. and Nakhasi, H.L. 1995. The rubella virus RNA binding activity of human calreticulin is localised to the N-terminal domain. *J Virol*, **69**, 3848–51.

Banatvala, J.E. 1987. Measles must go and with it rubella. *Br J Med*, **295**, 2–3.

Banatvala, J.E. and Best, J.M. 1989. Rubella vaccines. In: Zuckerman, A.J. (ed.), *Recent developments in prophylactic immunization*. Lancaster: Kluwer, 155–80.

Banatvala, J.E. and Best, J.M. 1990. Rubella. In: Collier, L.H. and Timbury, M. (eds), *Topley and Wilson's Principles of bacteriology, virology and immunity*, Vol. 4. 8th edn. London: Edward Arnold, 501–31.

Banatvala, J.E., Best, J.M., et al. 1985. Persistence of rubella antibodies following vaccination; detection of viremia following experimental challenge. *Rev Infect Dis*, **7**, Suppl. 1, S86–90.

Bardeletti, G. 1977. Respiration and ATP level in BHK2Y 135 cells during the earliest stages of rubella virus replication. *Intervirology*, **8**, 100–9.

Bardeletti, G., Kessler, N. and Aymard-Henry, M. 1975. Morphology, biochemical analysis and neuraminidase activity of rubella virus. *Arch Virol*, **49**, 175–86.

Bardeletti, G., Tektoff, J. and Gautheron, D. 1979. Rubella virus maturation and production in two host cell systems. *Intervirology*, **11**, 97–103.

Baron, M.D. and Forsell, K. 1991. Oligomerization of the structural proteins of rubella virus. *Virology*, **185**, 811–19.

Baron, M.D., Ebel, T. and Suomalainen, M. 1992. Intracellular transport of rubella virus structural proteins expressed from cloned cDNA. *J Gen Virol*, **73**, 1073–86.

Bart, S.W., Stetler, H.C., et al. 1985. Fetal risk associated with rubella vaccine: an update. *Rev Infect Dis*, **7**, Suppl. 1, S95–S102.

Beatch, M.D. and Hobman, T.C. 2000. Rubella virus capsid associates with host cell protein p32 and localizes to mitochondria. *J Virol*, **74**, 5569–76.

Best, J.M. 1991. Rubella vaccines – past, present and future. *Epidemiol Infect*, **107**, 17–30.

Best, J.M. 1993. Rubella reinfection. *Curr Med Lit: Virol*, **2**, 35–40.

Best, J.M. and Banatvala, J.E. 2004. Rubella. In: Zuckerman, A.J., Banatvala, J.E., et al. (eds), *Principles and practice of clinical virology*, 5th edn. Chichester: John Wiley.

Best, J.M. and O'Shea, S. 1995. Rubella. In: Lennette, E.H., Lennette, D.A. and Lennette, E.T. (eds), *Diagnostic procedures for viral, rickettsial and chlamydial infections*, 7th edn. Washington DC: American Public Health Association, 583–600.

Best, J.M., Banatvala, J.E., et al. 1967. The morphological characteristics of rubella virus. *Lancet*, **2**, 237–9.

Best, J.M., Banatvala, J.E. and Moore, B.M. 1968. Growth of rubella virus in human embryonic organ cultures. *J Hyg*, **66**, 407–13.

Best, J.M., Banatvala, J.E., et al. 1989. Fetal infection after maternal reinfection with rubella: criteria for defining reinfection. *Br J Med*, **299**, 773–5.

Best, J.M., Thomson, A., et al. 1992. Rubella virus strains show no major antigenic differences. *Intervirology*, **34**, 164–8.

Best, J.M., O'Shea, S., et al. 2002. Interpretation of rubella serology in pregnancy – pitfalls and problems. *Br J Med*, **325**, 147–8.

Booth, J.C. and Stern, H. 1972. Photodynamic inactivation of rubella virus. *J Med Microbiol*, **5**, 515–28.

Bosma, T.J., Corbett, K.M., et al. 1995a. Use of PCR for prenatal and postnatal diagnosis of congenital rubella. *J Clin Microbiol*, **33**, 2881–7.

Bosma, T.J., Corbett, K.M., et al. 1995b. Use of the polymerase chain reaction for the detection of rubella virus RNA in clinical samples. *J Clin Microbiol*, **33**, 1075–9.

Bosma, T.J., Best, J.M., et al. 1996. Nucleotide sequence analysis of a major antigenic domain of the E1 glycoprotein of 22 rubella virus isolates. *J Gen Virol*, **77**, 2523–30.

Bosma, T.J., Etherington, J., et al. 1998. Rubella virus and chronic joint disease: is there an association? *J Clin Microbiol*, **36**, 3524–6.

Böttiger, M. and Forsgren, M. 1997. Twenty years' experience of rubella vaccination in Sweden: 10 years of selective vaccination (of 12-year-old girls and of women postpartum) and 13 years of a general two-dose vaccination. *Vaccine*, **15**, 1538–44.

Bowden, D.S. and Westaway, E.G. 1985. Changes in glycosylation of rubella virus envelope proteins during maturation. *J Gen Virol*, **66**, 201–6.

Brown, T., Hambling, M.H. and Ansari, B.M. 1969. Rubella-neutralising and haemagglutinin-inhibiting antibodies in children of different ages. *Br J Med*, **4**, 263–5.

Buimovici-Klein, E. and Cooper, L.Z. 1985. Cell-mediated immune response in rubella infections. *Rev Infect Dis*, **7**, Suppl. 1, S123–8.

Buimovici-Klein, E., Vesikari, T., et al. 1976. Study of the lymphocyte in vitro response to rubella antigen and phytohemagglutinin by a whole blood method. *Arch Virol*, **52**, 323–31.

Buimovici-Klein, E., Lang, P.B., et al. 1979. Impaired cell mediated immune response in patients with congenital rubella: correlation with gestational age at time of infection. *Pediatrics*, **64**, 620–6.

Bullens, D., Smets, K., et al. 2000. Congenital rubella syndrome after maternal reinfection. *Clin Pediatr*, **39**, 113–16.

Bunnell, C.E. and Monif, G.R.G. 1972. Interstitial pancreatitis in the congenital rubella syndrome. *J Pediatr*, **80**, 465–6.

Centers for Disease Control and Prevention. 1994. Reported vaccine-preventable diseases – United States 1993. *MMWR*, **43**, 57–60.

Centers for Disease Control and Prevention. 2001a. Control and prevention of rubella: Evaluation and management of suspected outbreaks, rubella in pregnant women, and surveillance for congenital rubella syndrome. *MMWR*, **50** (RR-12), 1–23.

Centers for Disease Control and Prevention. 2001b. Revised ACIP recommendation for avoiding pregnancy after receiving a rubella-containing vaccine. *MMWR*, **50** (49), 1117.

Chantler, J.K. and Tingle, A.J. 1980. Replication and expression of rubella virus in human lymphocyte populations. *J Gen Virol*, **50**, 317–28.

Chantler, J.K., Smymis, L. and Tai, G. 1995. Selective infection of astrocytes in human glial cell cultures by rubella virus. *Lab Invest*, **72**, 334–40.

Chantler, J., Wolinsky, J.S. and Tingle, A. 2001. Rubella virus. In: Knipe, D.M., Howley, P.M., et al. (eds), *Fields' Virology*. Philadelphia: Lippincott, Williams & Wilkins, 963–90.

Chantler, J.K., Lund, K.D., et al. 1993. Characterisation of rubella virus strain differences associated with attenuation. *Intervirology*, **36**, 225–36.

Chantler, S., Evans, C.J., et al. 1982. A comparison of antibody capture radio- and enzyme immunoassays with immunofluorescence for detecting IgM antibody in infants with congenital rubella. *J Virol Meth*, **4**, 305–13.

Chaye, H.H., Mauracher, C.A., et al. 1992a. Cellular and humoral immune responses to rubella virus structural proteins E1, E2 and C. *J Clin Microbiol*, **30**, 2323–9.

Chaye, H., Chong, P., et al. 1992b. Localisation of the virus neutralising and hemagglutinin epitopes of E1 glycoprotein of rubella virus. *Virology*, **189**, 483–92.

Chaye, H., Ou, D., et al. 1993. Human T- and B-cell epitopes of E1 glycoprotein of rubella virus. *J Clin Immunol*, **13**, 93–100.

Chen, J.P., Miller, D., et al. 1995. Expression of the rubella virus structural proteins by an infectious Sindbis virus vector. *Arch Virol*, **140**, 2075–84.

Chen, J.P., Strauss, J.H., et al. 1996. Characterization of the rubella virus nonstructural protease domain and its cleavage site. *J Virol*, **70**, 4707–13.

Chief Medical Officer, Chief Nursing Officer, and the Chief Pharmaceutical Officer. 2001. *Current vaccine and immunisation issues*. London: Department of Health, 1–12.

Clarke, D.M., Loo, T.W., et al. 1988. Expression of rubella virus cDNA coding for the structural proteins. *Gene*, **65**, 23–30.

Cooper, L.Z. 1975. Congenital rubella in the United States. In: Krugman, S. and Gershon, A.A. (eds), *Progress in clinical and biological research*. New York: Alan R Liss, 1–22.

Cooper, L.Z. and Krugman, S. 1967. Clinical manifestations of postnatal and congenital rubella. *Arch Ophthalmol*, **77**, 434–9.

Cooper, L.Z., Green, R.H., et al. 1965. Neonatal thrombocytopenic purpura and other manifestations of rubella contracted in utero. *Am J Dis Child*, **110**, 416–27.

Cooper, L.Z., Zirling, P.R., et al. 1969. Rubella: clinical manifestations and management. *Am J Dis Child*, **118**, 18–29.

Cooper, L.Z., Forman, A.L., et al. 1971. Loss of rubella hemagglutination inhibition antibody in congenital rubella. Failure of seronegative children with congenital rubella to respond to HPV-77 rubella vaccine. *Am J Dis Child*, **122**, 397–403.

Cooray, S., Best, J.M. and Jin, L. 2003. Time-course induction of apoptosis by wild-type and attenuated strains of rubella virus. *J Gen Virol*, **84**, 1275–9.

Coyle, P.K., Wolinsky, J.S., et al. 1982. Rubella-specific immune complexes after congenital infection and vaccination. *Infect Immun*, **36**, 498–503.

Corboba, P., Grutadauria, S., et al. 2000. Neutralizing monoclonal antibody to the E1 glycoprotein epitope of rubella virus mediates virus arrest in VERO cells. *Viral Immunol*, **13**, 83–92.

Cradock-Watson, J.E., Ridehalgh, M.K.S., et al. 1980. Fetal infection resulting from maternal rubella after the first trimester of pregnancy. *J Hyg*, **85**, 381–91.

Cremer, N.E., Oshiro, L.S., et al. 1975. Isolation of rubella virus from brain in chronic progressive panencephalitis. *J Gen Virol*, **29**, 143–53.

Cunningham, A.L. and Fraser, J.R.E. 1985. Persistent rubella virus infection of human synovial cells cultured in vitro. *J Infect Dis*, **151**, 638–45.

Cusi, M.G., Metelli, R., et al. 1989. Immune responses to wild and vaccine rubella viruses after rubella vaccination. *Arch Virol*, **106**, 63–72.

Cusi, M.G., Valassina, M., et al. 1995. Evaluation of rubella virus E2 and C proteins in protection against rubella virus in a mouse model. *Virus Res*, **37**, 199–208.

Cutts, F.T., Robertson, S.E., et al. 1997. Control of rubella and congenital rubella syndrome (CRS) in developing countries. Part 1: burden of disease from CRS. *Bull World Health Organ*, **75**, 55–68.

de Mazancourt, A., Waxham, M.N., et al. 1986. Antibody responses to the rubella virus structural proteins in infants with the congenital rubella syndrome. *J Med Virol*, **19**, 111–22.

Department of Health. 2003. Screening for infectious disease in pregnancy. Standards to support the UK antenatal screening programme. London: Stationery Office. Available from www.doh.gov.uk/antenatalscreening.

Derdyn, C.A. and Frey, T.K. 1995. Characterisations of defective-interfering RNAs of rubella virus generated during serial undiluted passage. *Virology*, **206**, 216–26.

Desmond, M.M., Wilson, G.S., et al. 1967. Congenital rubella encephalitis: course and early sequelae. *J Pediatr*, **71**, 311–31.

Domegan, L.M. and Atkins, G.J. 2002. Apoptosis induction by the Therien and vaccine RA27/3 strains of rubella virus causes depletion of oligodendrocytes from rat neural cell cultures. *J Gen Virol*, **83**, 2135–43.

Dominguez, G., Wang, C.-Y. and Frey, T.K. 1990. Sequence of the genome of rubella virus. Evidence for genetic rearrangement during togavirus evolution. *Virology*, **177**, 225–38.

Dorsett, P.H., Miller, D.C., et al. 1985. Structure and function of the rubella virus proteins. *Rev Infect Dis*, **7**, Suppl 1, S150–6.

Dowdle, W.R., Ferreira, W., et al. 1970. Study on the sero-epidemiology of rubella in Caribbean and Middle and South American populations in 1968. *Bull World Health Organ*, **42**, 419–22.

Duncan, R., Muller, J., et al. 1999. Rubella virus-induced apoptosis varies among cell lines and is modulated by Bcl-XL and caspase inhibitors. *Virology*, **255**, 117–28.

Duncan, R., Esmaili, A., et al. 2000. Rubella virus capsid protein induces apoptosis in transfected RK13 cells. *Virology*, **275**, 20–9.

Eckstein, M.B., Brown, D.W.G., et al. 1996. Congenital rubella in south India: diagnosis using saliva from infants with cataract. *Br J Med*, **312**, 161.

Editorial, 1944. Rubella and congenital malformations. *Lancet*, **1**, 316.

Enders, G. 1982. Röteln-Embryopathie noch heute? *Geburtshilfe Frauenheilkd*, **42**, 403–13.

Enders, G. 1985. Rubella antibody titres in vaccinated and non-vaccinated women and results of vaccination during pregnancy. *Rev Infect Dis*, **7**, Suppl 1, S103–12.

Enders, G. 1998. Fetale Infektionen. In: Hansmann, M., Feige, A. and Saling, E. (eds), *Pränatal- und Geberutsmedizin*. Berichte vom 5 Kongress der Gesellschaft für Pränatal- und Geburtsmedizin vom 21 bis 23 Februar 1997. Meckenheim: DCM Druck Center, 76–82.

Enders, G., Nikerl-Pacher, U., et al. 1988. Outcome of confirmed periconceptional maternal rubella. *Lancet*, **1**, 1445–7.

Fabiyi, A., Sever, J.L., et al. 1966. Rubella virus: growth characteristics and stability of infectious virus and complement-fixing antigen. *Proc Soc Exp Biol Med*, **122**, 392–6.

Forng, R.Y. and Frey, T.K. 1995. Identification of the rubella virus non-structural proteins. *Virology*, **206**, 843–53.

Forrest, J.M., Turnbul, F.M., et al. 2002. Gregg's congenital rubella patients 60 years later. *Med J Aust*, **177**, 664–7.

Frey, T.K. 1994. Molecular biology of rubella virus. *Adv Virus Res*, **44**, 69–160.

Frey, T.K. 1997. Neurological aspects of rubella virus infection. *Intervirology*, **40**, 167–75.

Frey, T.K. and Abernathy, E.S. 1993. Identification of strain-specific nucleotide sequences of the RA 27/3 rubella virus chain. *J Infect Dis*, **168**, 854–64.

Frey, T.K., Abernathy, E.S., et al. 1998. Molecular analysis of rubella virus epidemiology across three continents, North America, Europe and Asia, 1961–1997. *J Infect Dis*, **178**, 642–50.

Frey, T.K. and Hemphill, M.L. 1988. Generation of defective-interfering particles by rubella virus in Vero cells. *Virology*, **164**, 22–9.

Frey, T.K. and Marr, L.D. 1988. Sequence of the region coding for virion proteins C and E2 and the carboxy terminus of the nonstructural proteins of rubella virus: comparison with alphaviruses. *Gene*, **62**, 85–99.

Fuccillo, D.A., Steele, R.W., et al. 1974. Impaired cellular immunity to rubella virus in congenital rubella. *Infect Immun*, **9**, 81–4.

Furukawa, T., Plotkin, S.A., et al. 1967. Studies on hemagglutination by rubella virus. *Proc Soc Exp Biol Med*, **126**, 745–50.

Garbutt, M., Law, L.M., et al. 1999. Role of rubella virus glycoprotein domains in assembly of virus-like particles. *J Virol*, **73**, 3524–33.

Gill, S.D. and Furesz, J. 1973. Genetic stability in humans of the rabbit immunogenic marker of Cendehill rubella vaccine virus. *Arch Gesamt Virusforsch*, **43**, 135–43.

Ginsberg-Fellner, F., Witt, M.E., et al. 1985. Diabetes mellitus and autoimmunity in patients with the congenital rubella syndrome. *Rev Infect Dis*, **7**, Suppl. 1, S170–6.

Gorbalenya, A.E., Koonin, E.V. and Lai, M.M. 1991. Putative papain-related thiol proteases of positive-strand RNA viruses. Identification of rubi- and aphthovirus proteases and delineation of a novel conserved domain associated with proteases of rubi-, alpha- and coronaviruses. *FEBS Lett*, **288**, 201–5.

Grangeot-Keros, L., Pustowoit, B. and Hobman, T. 1995. Evaluation of Cobas core rubella IgG EIA recomb, a new enzyme immunoassay based on recombinant rubella-like particles. *J Clin Microbiol*, **33**, 2392–4.

Grayzel, A.I. and Beck, C. 1971. The growth of vaccine strain of rubella virus in cultured human synovial cells. *Proc Soc Exp Biol Med*, **136**, 496–8.

Green, K.Y. and Dorsett, P.H. 1986. Rubella virus antigens: localization of epitopes involved in hemagglutination and neutralization by using monoclonal antibodies. *J Virol*, **57**, 893–8.

Green, R.H., Balsamo, M.R., et al. 1965. Studies of the natural history and prevention of rubella. *Am J Dis Child*, **110**, 348–65.

Gregg, N.Mc.A. 1941. Congenital cataract following german measles in the mother. *Trans Ophthal Soc Aust*, **3**, 35–46.

Gregg, N.Mc.A., Beavis, W.R., et al. 1945. The occurrence of congenital defects in children following maternal rubella. *Med J Aust*, **2**, 122–6.

Grillner, L., Forsgren, M., et al. 1983. Outcome of rubella during pregnancy with special reference to the 17th–24th weeks of gestation. *Scand J Infect Dis*, **15**, 321–5.

Halonen, P.E., Ryan, I.H. and Stewart, J.A. 1967. Rubella hemagglutinin prepared with alkaline extraction of virus grown in suspension culture of BHK-21 cells. *Proc Soc Exp Biol Med*, **125**, 162–7.

Hanshaw, J.B., Dudgeon, J.A. and Marshall, W.C. 1985. *Viral diseases of the fetus and newborn*, 2nd edn. Philadelphia, London, Toronto: WB Saunders.

Harcourt, G.C., Best, J.M. and Banatvala, J.E. 1979. HLA antigens and responses to rubella vaccination. *J Hyg*, **83**, 405–12.

Hastreiter, A.R., Joorabchi, B., et al. 1967. Cardiovascular lesions associated with congenital rubella. *J Pediatr*, **71**, 59–65.

Heggie, A.D. 1978. Pathogenesis of the rubella exanthem: distribution of rubella virus in the skin during rubella with and without rash. *J Infect Dis*, **137**, 74–6.

Hemphill, M.L., Forng, R.Y., et al. 1988. Time course of virus-specific macromolecular synthesis during rubella virus infection in Vero cells. *Virology*, **162**, 65–75.

Herrmann, K.L. 1979. Rubella virus. In: Lennette, E.H. and Schmidt, N.J. (eds), *Diagnostic procedures for viral, rickettsial and chlamydial infections*, 5th edn. Washington DC: American Public Health Association, 725–66.

Hinman, A.R., Irons, B., et al. 2002. Economic analyses of rubella and rubella vaccines: a global review. *Bull World Health Organ*, **80**, 264–70.

Hobman, T.C., Seto, N.O.L. and Gillam, S. 1994a. Expression of soluble forms of rubella virus glycoproteins in mammalian cells. *Virus Res*, **31**, 277–89.

Hobman, T.C., Lundstrom, M.L., et al. 1994b. Assembly of rubella virus structural proteins into virus-like particles in transfected cells. *Virology*, **202**, 574–85.

Hobman, T.C., Lündstrom, M.L., et al. 1994c. Assembly of rubella virus structural protein into virus particles in transfected cells. *Virology*, **202**, 574–85.

Hofmann, J., Pletz, M.W. and Leibert, U.G. 1999. Rubella virus-induced cytopathic effect in vitro is caused by apoptosis. *J Gen Virol*, **80**, 1657–64.

Hofmann, J., Renz, M., et al. 2003. Phylogenetic analysis of rubella virus including new genotype I isolates. *Virus Res*, **96**, 123–8.

Holmes, I.H., Wark, M.C., et al. 1968. Identification of two possible types of virus particles in rubella infected cells. *J Gen Virol*, **2**, 37–42.

Holmes, I.H., Wark, M.C. and Warburton, M.V. 1969. Is rubella an arbovirus? Ultrastructural morphology and development. *Virology*, **371**, 5–25.

Honeyman, M.C., Forrest, J.M. and Dorman, D.C. 1974. Cell-mediated immune response following natural rubella and rubella vaccination. *Clin Exp Immunol*, **17**, 665–71.

Hope-Simpson, R.E. 1944. Rubella and congenital malformations. *Lancet*, **1**, 483.

Horstmann, D.M., Banatvala, J.E., et al. 1965. Maternal rubella and the rubella syndrome in infants: epidemiologic, clinical and virologic observations. *Am J Dis Child*, **110**, 408–15.

Horstmann, D.M., Liebhaber, H., et al. 1970. Rubella: reinfections of vaccinated and naturally immune persons exposed in an epidemic. *N Engl J Med*, **283**, 771–8.

Horzinek, M.C. 1973. The structure of togaviruses. *Prog Med Virol*, **16**, 109–56.

Horzinek, M.C. 1981. *Non-arthropod-borne togaviruses*. London: Academic Press.

Hosking, C.S., Pyman, C. and Wilkins, B. 1983. The nerve deaf child – intrauterine rubella or not? *Arch Dis Child*, **58**, 327–9.

Hovi, T. and Vaheri, A. 1970. Rubella virus-specific ribonucleic acids in infected BHK21 cells. *J Gen Virol*, **6**, 77–83.

Hudson, P. and Morgan-Capner, P. 1996. Evaluation of 15 commercial enzyme immunoassays for the detection of rubella-specific IgM. *Clin Diagn Virol*, **5**, 21–6.

Hyypiä, T., Eskola, J., et al. 1984. B-cell function in vitro during rubella infection. *Infect Immun*, **43**, 589–92.

Ilonen, J., Seppanen, H., Narvanen, A., Korkolainen, M. and Salmi, A.A. 1992. Recognition of synthetic peptides with sequences of rubella virus E1 polypeptide by antibodies and T lymphocytes. *Viral Immunol*, **5**, 221–8.

Institute of Medicine. 2001. Immunization safety review: measles-mumps-rubella vaccine and autism. http://search.nap.edu/books/0309074479/html/

Jansen, V.A.A., Stollenwerk, N., et al. 2003. Measles outbreaks in a population with declining vaccine uptake. *Science*, **301**, 804.

Johansson, T., Enestam, A., et al. 1996. Synthesis of soluble rubella virus spike proteins in two lepidopteran insect cell lines: large scale production of the E1 protein. *J Biotechnol*, **50**, 171–80.

Kalkkinen, N., Oker-Blom, C. and Pettersson, R.F. 1984. Three genes code for rubella virus structural proteins E1, E2A, E2b and C. *J Gen Virol*, **65**, 1549–57.

Karounos, D.G., Wolinsky, J.S. and Thomas, J.W. 1993. Monoclonal antibody to rubella virus capsid protein recognises a beta-cell antigen. *J Immunol*, **150**, 3080–5.

Katow, S. 1998. Rubella virus genome diagnosis during pregnancy and mechanism of congenital rubella. *Intervirology*, **41**, 163–9.

Katow, S. and Sugiura, A. 1988. Low pH-induced conformational change of rubella virus envelope proteins. *J Gen Virol*, **69**, 2797–807.

Kenney, M.T., Albright, M.T., et al. 1969. Inactivation of rubella virus by gamma radiation. *J Virol*, **4**, 807–10.

Kistler, G.S. and Sapatino, V. 1972. Temperature and UV-light resistance of rubella virus infectivity. *Arch gesamt Virusforsch*, **38**, 11–16.

Kistler, G.S., Best, J.M., et al. 1967. Elektronenmikroskopische Untersuchungen an rötelninfizierten menschlichen Organkulturen. *Schweiz Med Wochenschr*, **97**, 1377–82.

Kobayashi, N. 1978. Hemolytic activity of rubella virus. *Virology*, **89**, 610–12.

Koonin, E.V. 1993. Computer-assisted identification of a putative methyltransferase domain in NS5 protein of flaviviruses and lambda 2 protein of reovirus. *J Gen Virol*, **74**, 733–40.

Korones, S.B., Ainger, L.E., et al. 1965. Congenital rubella syndrome: study of 22 infants. Myocardial damage and other new clinical aspects. *Am J Dis Child*, **110**, 434–40.

Krugman, S. and Ward, R. 1954. The rubella problem. *J Pediatr*, **44**, 489–98.

Krugman, S. and Ward, R. 1968. Rubella (german measles). In: *Infectious diseases of children*, 4th edn. St Louis, MO: CV Mosby, 279–95.

Kujala, P., Ahola, T., et al. 1999. Intracellular distribution of rubella virus nonstructural protein P150. *J Virol*, **73**, 7805–11.

Law, L.M., Duncan, R., et al. 2001. Rubella virus E2 signal peptide is required for perinuclear localization of capsid protein and virus assembly. *J Virol*, **75**, 1978–83.

Law, L.M., Everitt, J.C., et al. 2003. Phosphorylation of rubella virus capsid regulates its RNA binding activity and virus replication. *J Virol*, **77**, 1764–71.

Le Bouvier, G.L. 1969. Precipitinogens of rubella virus-infected cells. *Proc Soc Exp Biol Med*, **130**, 51–4.

Lee, J.-Y. and Bowden, D.S. 2000. Rubella virus replication and links to teratogenicity. *Clin Microbiol Rev*, **13**, 571–87.

Lee, J.Y., Marshall, J.A. and Bowden, D.S. 1994. Characterization of rubella virus replication complexes using antibodies to double-stranded RNA. *Virology*, **200**, 1, 307–12.

Liang, Y. and Gillam, S. 2000. Mutational analysis of the rubella virus nonstructural polyprotein and its cleavage products in virus replication and RNA synthesis. *J Virol*, **74**, 5133–41.

Liang, Y. and Gillam, S. 2001. Rubella virus RNA replication is cis-preferential and synthesis of negative- and positive-strand RNAs is regulated by the processing of nonstructural protein. *Virology*, **282**, 307–19.

Lindegren, M., Fehrs, L.J., et al. 1991. Update: rubella and congenital rubella syndrome, 1980–1990. *Epidemiol Rev*, **13**, 341–8.

Liu, Z., Yang, D., et al. 1996. Identification of domains in rubella virus genomic RNA and capsid protein necessary for specific interaction. *J Virol*, **70**, 2184–90.

Londesborough, P., Terry, G. and Ho-Terry, L. 1992. Reactivity of a recombinant rubella E1 antigen expressed in *E coli. Arch Virol*, **122**, 391–7.

Lovett, A.E., Chang, S.H., et al. 1993. Rubella virus-specific cytotoxic T-lymphocyte responses: identification of the capsid as a target of major histocompatiblity complex class I - restricted lysis and definition of two epitopes. *J Virol*, **67**, 5849–58.

Lozzi, L., Rustici, M., et al. 1990. Structure of rubella E1 glycoprotein epitopes established by multiple peptide synthesis. *Arch Virol*, **110**, 271–6.

Lündstrom, M.L., Mauracher, C.A. and Tingle, A.J. 1991. Characterization of carbohydrates linked to rubella virus glycoprotein E2. *J Gen Virol*, **72**, 843–50.

Magliano, D., Marshall, J.A., et al. 1998. Rubella virus replication complexes are virus-modified lysosomes. *Virology*, **240**, 57–63.

Maller, R., Fryden, A. and Soren, L. 1978. Mitogen stimulation and distribution of T- and B-lymphocytes during natural rubella infection. *Acta Pathol Microbiol Immunol Scand, Sect C, Immunol*, **86**, 93–8.

Marr, L.D., Sanchez, A., et al. 1991. Efficient in vitro translation and processing of the rubella virus structural proteins in the presence of microsomes. *Virology*, **180**, 400–5.

Marr, L.D., Wang, C.Y. and Frey, T.K. 1994. Expression of the rubella virus non-structural protein ORF and demonstration of the proteolytic processing. *Virology*, **198**, 586–92.

Marshall, W.C. 1973. *Intrauterine infections, Ciba Foundation Symposium No 10*. Amsterdam: Associated Scientific Publishers.

Martin, R., Marquardt, P., et al. 1989. Virus specific and autoreactive T cell lines isolated from cerebrospinal fluid of a patient with chronic rubella panencephalitis. *J Neuroimmunol*, **23**, 1–10.

Mastromarino, P., Cioe, L., et al. 1990. Role of membrane phospholipids and glycolipids in the Vero cell surface receptor for rubella virus. *Med Microbiol Immunol*, **179**, 105–14.

Matsumoto, A. and Higashi, M. 1974. Electron microscopic studies on the morphology and morphogenesis of togaviruses. *Annu Rep Inst Virus Res, Kyoto University*, **17**, 11–22.

Mauracher, C.A., Gillam, S., et al. 1991. pH independent solubility shift of rubella virus capsid protein. *Virology*, **181**, 773–7.

Mauracher, C.A., Mitchell, L.A. and Tingle, A.J. 1992. Differential IgG avidity to rubella virus structural proteins. *J Med Virol*, **36**, 202–8.

Mauracher, C.A., Mitchell, L.A. and Tingle, A.J. 1993. Selective tolerance to the E1 protein of rubella virus in congenital rubella syndrome. *J Immunol*, **151**, 2041–9.

Megyeri, K., Berencsi, K., et al. 1999. Involvement of a p53-dependent pathway in rubella virus-induced apoptosis. *Virology*, **259**, 74–84.

Meitsch, K., Enders, G., et al. 1997. The role of rubella-immunoblot and rubella-peptide-EIA for the diagnosis of the congenital rubella syndrome during the prenatal and newborn periods. *J Med Virol*, **51**, 280–3.

Menser, M.A. and Forrest, J.M. 1974. Rubella: high incidence of defects in children considered normal at birth. *Med J Aust*, **1**, 123–6.

Menser, M.A. and Reye, R.D.K. 1974. The pathology of congenital rubella: a review written by request. *Pathology*, **6**, 215–22.

Menser, M.A., Dods, L. and Harley, J.D. 1967a. A twenty-five year follow up of congenital rubella. *Lancet*, **2**, 1347–50.

Menser, M.A., Harley, J.D., et al. 1967b. Persistence of virus in lens for three years after prenatal rubella. *Lancet*, **2**, 387–8.

Menser, M.A., Forrest, J.M. and Bransby, R.D. 1978. Rubella infection and diabetes mellitus. *Lancet*, **1**, 57–60.

Miki, N.P.H. and Chantler, J.K. 1992. Differential ability of wild-type and vaccine strains of rubella virus to replicate and persist in human joint tissue. *Clin Exp Rheumatol*, **10**, 3–12.

Miller, E. 2001. MMR vaccine – worries are not justified. Commentary. *Arch Dis Child*, **85**, 273–4.

Miller, E., Cradock-Watson, J.E. and Pollock, T.M. 1982. Consequences of confirming maternal rubella at successive stages of pregnancy. *Lancet*, **2**, 781–4.

Miller, E., Tookey, P., et al. 1994. Rubella surveillance to June 1994: third joint report from the PHLS and the National Congenital Rubella Surveillance Programme. *Commun Dis Rep*, **199**, R146–52.

Miller, E., Waight, P., et al. 1997. The epidemiology of rubella in England and Wales before and after the 1994 measles-rubella immunization campaign: fourth joint report from the PHLS and the National Congenital Rubella Surveillance Programme. *Commun Dis Rep Rev*, **4**, R26–32.

Mims, C.A., Stokes, A. and Grahame, R. 1985. Synthesis of antibodies including antiviral antibodies in the knee joints of patients with chronic arthritis. *Ann Rheum Dis*, **44**, 734–7.

Mitchell, L.A., Zhang, T. and Tingle, A.J. 1992a. Differential antibody responses to rubella virus infection in males and females. *J Infect Dis*, **166**, 128–65.

Mitchell, L.A., Zhang, T., et al. 1992b. Characterisation of rubella virus specific antibody responses by using a new synthetic peptide based enzyme linked immunosorbent assay. *J Clin Microbiol*, **30**, 1841–7.

Mitchell, L.A., Decarie, D., et al. 1993. Identification of immunoreactive regions of rubella virus E1 and E2 envelope proteins by using synthetic peptides. *Virus Res*, **29**, 33–57.

Mohan, K.V., Ghebrehiwet, B. and Atreya, C.D. 2002. The N-terminal conserved domain of rubella virus capsid interacts with the C-terminal region of cellular p32 and overexpression of p32 enhances the viral infectivity. *Virus Res*, **85**, 151–61.

Morgan-Capner, P. and Crowcroft, N. 2002. Guidelines on the management of, and exposure to, rash illness in pregnancy (including consideration of relevant antibody screening programmes in pregnancy). *Commun Dis Public Health*, **5**, 59–71.

Morgan-Capner, P., Miller, E., et al. 1991. Outcome of pregnancy after maternal reinfection with rubella. *Commun Dis Rep*, **1**, R57–9.

Munro, N.D., Sheppard, S., et al. 1987. Temporal relations between maternal rubella and congenital defects. *Lancet*, **2**, 201–4.

Murphy, A.M., Reid, R.R., et al. 1967. Rubella cataracts. Further clinical and virologic observations. *Am J Ophthalmol*, **64**, 1109–19.

Murphy, F.A., Halonen, P.E. and Harrison, A.K. 1968. Electron microscopy of the development of rubella virus in BHK21 cells. *J Virol*, **2**, 1223–7.

Naeye, R.L. and Blanc, W. 1965. Pathogenesis of congenital rubella. *JAMA*, **194**, 1277–83.

Nakhasi, H.L., Rouault, T.A. and Haile, D.J. 1990. Specific high-affinity binding of host cell proteins to the 3′ region of rubella virus RNA. *New Biol*, **2**, 255–64.

Nakhasi, H., Singh, N.K., et al. 1994. Identification and characterisation of host factor interactions with *cis*-acting elements of rubella virus RNA. *Arch Virol*, **9**, 255–67.

Nedeljkovic, J., Jovanovic, T., et al. 1999. Immunoblot analysis of natural and vaccine-induced IgG responses to rubella virus proteins expressed in insect cells. *J Clin Virol*, **14**, 119–31.

Newcombe, J., Starkey, W., et al. 1994. Recombinant rubella E1 fusion protein for antibody screening and diagnosis. *Clin Diagn Virol*, **2**, 149–63.

Niwa, Y. and Kanoh, T. 1979. Immunological behaviour following rubella infection. *Clin Exp Immunol*, **37**, 470–6.

Nokes, D.J., Nigatu, W., et al. 1998. A comparison of oral fluid and serum for the detection of rubella-specific antibodies in a community study in Addis Ababa, Ethiopia. *Trop Med Int Health*, **3**, 258–67.

Norrby, E. 1969. Rubella virus. In: *Virology monographs*, 7th edn. Vienna, New York: Springer-Verlag, 115–74.

Numazaki, K., Goldman, H., et al. 1990. Infection by human cytomegalovirus and rubella of cultured human fetal islets of Langerhans. *In Vivo*, **4**, 49–54.

Ogra, P.L. and Herd, J.L. 1971. Arthritis associated with induced rubella infection. *J Immunol*, **107**, 810–13.

Ohtawara, M., Kobune, F., et al. 1985. Inability of Japanese rubella vaccines to induce antibody response in rabbits is due to growth restrictions at 39°C. *Arch Virol*, **83**, 217–27.

Oker-Blom, C. 1984. The gene order for rubella virus structural proteins is NH2-*C-E2-E1*-COOH. *J Virol*, **51**, 354–8.

Oker-Blom, C., Kalkkinen, N., et al. 1983. Rubella virus contains one capsid protein and three envelope glyoproteins, E1, E2a and E2b. *J Virol*, **46**, 964–73.

Oker-Blom, C., Jarvis, K.L. and Summers, M.D. 1990. Translocation and cleavage of rubella virus envelope glycoproteins: identification and role of the E2 signal sequence. *J Gen Virol*, **71**, 3047–53.

Oker-Blom, C., Blomster, M., et al. 1995. Synthesis and processing of the rubella virus p110 polyprotein in baculovirus-infected *Spodoptera frugiperda* cells. *Virus Res*, **35**, 71–9.

Orellana, A., Mottershead, D., et al. 1999. Mimicking rubella virus particles by using recombinant envelope glycoproteins and liposomes. *J Biotechnol*, **75**, 209–19.

O'Shea, S., Best, M.M. and Banatvala, J.E. 1983. Viremia, virus excretion, and antibody responses after challenge in volunteers with low levels of antibody to rubella virus. *J Infect Dis*, **148**, 639–47.

O'Shea, S., Best, J.M., et al. 1985. Development and persistence of class-specific serum and nasopharyngeal antibodies in rubella vaccinees. *J Infect Dis*, **151**, 89–98.

O'Shea, S., Best, J.M. and Banatvala, J.E. 1992. A lymphocyte transformation assay for the diagnosis of congenital rubella. *J Virol Meth*, **37**, 139–48.

O'Shea, S., Corbett, K.M., et al. 1994. Rubella reinfection; role of neutralising antibodies and cell-mediated immunity. *Clin Diagn Virol*, **2**, 349–58.

Ou, D., Chong, P., et al. 1992. Analysis of T- and B-cell epitopes of capsid protein of rubella virus by using synthetic peptides. *J Virol*, **66**, 1674–81.

Ou, D., Chong, P., et al. 1993. Mapping T-cell epitopes of rubella virus structural proteins E1, E2 and C recognised by T-cell lines and clones derived from infected and immunised populations. *J Med Virol*, **40**, 175–83.

Parkman, P.D. 1965. Biological characteristics of rubella virus. *Arch ges Virusforsch*, **16**, 401–11.

Parkman, P.D., Buescher, E.L. and Artenstein, M.S. 1962. Recovery of the rubella virus from recruits. *Proc Soc Exp Biol*, **111**, 225–30.

Parkman, P.D., Buescher, E.L., et al. 1964. Studies of rubella. 1. Properties of the virus. *J Immunol*, **93**, 595–607.

Parry, J.V., Perry, K.R. and Mortimer, P.P. 1987. Sensitive assays for viral antibodies in saliva: an alternative to tests on serum. *Lancet*, **1**, 72–5.

Pathak, S., Webb, H.E., et al. 1994. Immunoelectron microscopical study of rubella virus grown in Vero cells with special reference to membrane bound spherules. In: Jouffrey, B. and Colliex, C. (eds), *Electron microscopy 1994*. Proceedings of the 13th International Conference on Electron Microscopy, vol. 3B. Les Ulis, France: Editions de Physique, 1381–2.

Pattison, J.R., Dane, D.S. and Mace, J.E. 1975. Persistence of specific IgM after natural infection with rubella virus. *Lancet*, **1**, 185–7.

Peckham, C.S. 1972. Clinical laboratory study of children exposed in utero to maternal rubella. *Arch Dis Child*, **47**, 571–7.

Peckham, C.S. 1974. Clinical and serological assessment of children exposed in utero to confirmed maternal rubella. *Br J Med*, **2**, 259–61.

Peltola, H., Heinonen, O.P., et al. 1994. The elimination of indigenous measles, mumps, and rubella from Finland by a 12-year, two-dose vaccination program. *N Engl J Med*, **331**, 1446–7.

Penttinen, K. and Myllyla, G. 1968. Interaction in human blood platelets, viruses and antibodies. 1. Platelet aggregation test with microequipment. *Ann Med Exp Biol Fenn*, **46**, 188–92.

Perkins, F.T.C. 1985. Licensed vaccines. *Rev Infect Dis*, **7**, suppl 1, S73–8.

Perry, K.R., Brown, W.G., et al. 1993. Detection of measles, mumps and rubella antibodies in saliva using antibody capture radioimunoassay. *J Med Virol*, **40**, 235–40.

Phelan, P. and Campbell, P. 1969. Pulmonary complications of rubella embryopathy. *J Pediatr*, **75**, 202–12.

Plotkin, S.A. 1969. Rubella virus. In: Lennette, E.H. and Schmidt, N.J. (eds), *Diagnostic procedures in viral and rickettsial diseases*, 4th edn. Washington DC: American Public Health Association, 364–413.

Plotkin, S.A. 1999. Rubella vaccine. In: Plotkin, S. and Orenstein, W.A. (eds), *Vaccines*, 3rd edn. Philadelphia: WB Saunders Co, 409–39.

Plotkin, S.A. and Vaheri, A. 1967. Human fibroblasts infected with rubella virus produce a growth inhibitor. *Science*, **156**, 659–61.

Plotkin, S.A., Oski, F.A., et al. 1965. Some recently recognized manifestations of the rubella syndrome. *J Pediatr*, **67**, 182–91.

Pogue, G.P., Cao, X.-Q., et al. 1993. 5′ sequences of rubella virus RNA stimulate translation of chimeric RNAs and specifically interact with two host-encoded proteins. *J Virol*, **67**, 7106–17.

Pogue, G.P., Hoffmann, J., et al. 1996. Autoantigens interact with *cis*-acting elements of rubella virus RNA. *J Virol*, **70**, 6269–77.

Proceedings, 1969. Proceedings of the International Conference on Rubella Immunisation. *Am J Dis Child*, **118**, 2–399.

Pugachev, K.V., Abernathy, E.S. and Frey, T.K. 1997a. Genomic sequence of the RA27/3 vaccine strain of rubella virus. *Arch Virol*, **142**, 1165–80.

Pugachev, K.V., Abernathy, E.S. and Frey, T.K. 1997b. Improvement of the specific infectivity of the rubella virus (RUB) infectious clone: determinants of cytopathogenicity induced by RUB map to the nonstructural proteins. *J Virol*, **71**, 562–8.

Pugachev, K.V. and Frey, T.K. 1998a. Effects of defined mutations in the 5′ nontranslated region of rubella virus genomic RNA on virus viability and macromolecule synthesis. *J Virol*, **72**, 641–50.

Pugachev, K.V. and Frey, T.K. 1998b. Rubella virus induces apoptosis in culture cells. *Virology*, **250**, 359–70.

Pustowoit, B. and Liebert, U.G. 1998. Predictive value of serological tests in rubella virus infection during pregnancy. *Intervirology*, **41**, 170–7.

Qiu, Z., Ou, D., et al. 1994. Expression and characterisation of virus like particles containing rubella virus structural proteins. *J Virol*, **68**, 4068–91.

Rabinowe, S.L., George, K.L., et al. 1986. Congenital rubella: monoclonal antibody-defined T cell abnormalities in young adults. *Am J Med*, **81**, 779–82.

Rahi, J., Adams, G., et al. 2001. Epidemiological surveillance of rubella must continue. *Br J Med*, **323**, 112.

Ramsay, M.E., Brugha, R., et al. 1998. Salivary diagnosis of rubella: a study of notified cases in the United Kingdom, 1991–4. *Epidemiol Infect*, **120**, 315–19.

Ramsay, M., Reacher, M., et al. 2002. Causes of morbilliform rash in a highly immunised English population. *Arch Dis Child*, **87**, 202–6.

Rawls, W.E. 1968. Congenital rubella: the significance of virus persistence. *Prog Med Virol*, **10**, 238–85.

Reef, S.E., Plotkin, S., et al. 2000. Preparing for elimination of congenital rubella syndrome (CRS): Summary of a workshop on CRS elimination in the United States. *Clin Infect Dis*, **31**, 85–95.

Report of the Public Health Laboratory Working Party on Rubella. 1970. Studies on the effect of immunoglobulin on rubella in pregnancy. *Br J Med*, **2**, 497.

Report. 1994. Report of an International Meeting on rubella vaccines and vaccination, 9 August 1993, Glasgow, United Kingdom. *J Infect Dis*, **170**, 507–9.

Revello, M.G., Baldanti, F.S., et al. 1997. Prenatal diagnosis of rubella virus infection by direct detection and semiquantitation of viral RNA in clinical samples by reverse transcription-PCR. *J Clin Microbiol*, **35**, 708–13.

Risco, C., Carrascoasa, J.L. and Frey, T.K. 2003. Structural maturation of rubella virus in the Golgi complex. *Virology*, **312**, 261–9.

Robertson, S.E., Cutts, F.T., et al. 1997. Control of rubella and congenital rubella syndrome (CRS) in developing countries, part 2: vaccination against rubella. *Bull World Health Organ*, **2**, 69–80.

Rorke, L.B. and Spiro, A.J. 1967. Cerebral lesions in congenital rubella syndrome. *J Pediatr*, **70**, 243–55.

Rozanov, M.N., Koonin, E.V. and Gorbalenya, A.E. 1992. Conservation of the putative methyltransferase domain: a hallmark of the 'Sindbis-like' supergroup of positive-strand RNA viruses. *J Gen Virol*, **73**, 2129–34.

Russell, B., Selzer, G. and Goetz, H. 1967. The particle size of rubella virus. *J Gen Virol*, **1**, 305–10.

Salisbury, D.M. and Begg, N.T. (eds) 1996. *Rubella, Immunisation against infectious disease*. London: HMSO, 193–202.

Sawicki, D.L., Sawicki, S.G., et al. 1981. Specific Sindbis virus-coded function for minus-strand RNA synthesis. *J Virol*, **39**, 348–58.

Schell, K. and Wong, K.T. 1966. Stability and stage of rubella complement fixing antigen. *Nature(Lond)*, **212**, 621–2.

Schmidt, N.J. and Styk, B. 1968. Immunodiffusion reactions with rubella antigens. *J Immunol*, **101**, 210–16.

Sedwick, W.D. and Sokol, F. 1970. Nucleic acid of rubella virus and its replication in hamster kidney cells. *J Virol*, **5**, 478–87.

See, D.M. and Tilles, J.G. 1998. The pathogenesis of viral-induced diabetes. *Clin Diagn Virol*, **9**, 85–8.

Seppala, M. and Vaheri, A. 1974. Natural rubella infection of the female genital tract. *Lancet*, **1**, 46–7.

Seppanen, H., Huhtala, M., et al. 1991. Diagnostic potential of baculovirus-expressed rubella virus envelope proteins. *J Clin Microbiol*, **29**, 1877–82.

Seto, N.O., Ou, D. and Gillam, S. 1995. Expression and characterisations of secreted forms of rubella virus E2 glycoprotein in insect cells. *Virology*, **206**, 736–41.

Siegel, M., Fuerst, H.T. and Guinee, V.G. 1971. Rubella epidemicity and embryopathy. Results of a long term prospective study. *Am J Dis Child*, **121**, 469–73.

Singh, N.K., Atreya, C.D. and Nakhasi, H.L. 1994. Identification of calreticulin as a rubella virus RNA binding protein. *Proc Natl Acad Sci USA*, **91**, 12770–4.

Smith, J.L. 1881. Contributions to the study of Rötheln. *Trans Int Med Congr Phil*, **4**, 14.

Smith, K.O. and Hobbins, T.E. 1969. Physical characteristics of rubella virus. *J Immunol*, **102**, 1016–23.

Sodeik, B. 2000. Mechanisms of viral transport in the cytoplasm. *Trends Microbiol*, **8**, 465–72.

Sperling, D.R. and Verska, J.J. 1966. Rubella syndrome. *California Med*, **105**, 340–4.

Starkey, W.G., Newcombe, J., et al. 1995. Use of rubella E1 fusion proteins for the detection of rubella antibodies. *J Clin Microbiol*, **33**, 270–4.

Stewart, G.L., Parkman, P.D., et al. 1967. Rubella-virus hemagglutination-inhibition test. *N Engl J Med*, **276**, 554–7.

Stokes, A., Mims, C.A. and Grahame, R. 1986. Subclass distribution of IgG and IgA responses to rubella virus in man. *J Med Microbiol*, **21**, 283–5.

Suomalainen, M., Garoff, H., et al. 1990. The E2 signal sequence of rubella virus remains part of the capsid protein and confers membrane association in vitro. *J Virol*, **64**, 5500–9.

Tang, J.W., Aarons, E., et al. 2003. Prenatal diagnosis of congenital rubella infection in the second trimester of pregnancy. *Prenat Diagn*, **23**, 509–12.

Tardieu, M., Grospierre, B. and Durandy, A. 1980. Circulating immune complexes containing rubella antigens in late-onset rubella syndrome. *J Pediatr*, **97**, 370–3.

Terry, G.M., Ho-Terry, L.M., et al. 1988. Localisation of the rubella E1 epitopes. *Arch Virol*, **98**, 189–97.

Thomas, H.I.J., Barrett, E., et al. 1999. Simultaneous IgM reactivity by EIA against more than one virus in measles, parvovirus B19 and rubella infection. *J Clin Virol*, **14**, 107–18.

Thomas, H.I.J. and Morgan-Capner, P. 1988. Rubella-specific IgG subclass avidity: ELISA and its role in the differentiation between primary rubella and rubella re-infection. *Epidemiol Infect*, **101**, z591–8.

Thomas, H.I.J. and Morgan-Capner, P. 1991. The use of antibody avidity measurements for the diagnosis of rubella. *Rev Med Virol*, **1**, 41–50.

Thomas, H.I.J., Morgan-Capner, P., et al. 1993. Slow maturation of IgG1, avidity and persistence of specific IgM in congenital rubella: implications for diagnosis and immunopathology. *J Med Virol*, **41**, 196–200.

Thomas, H.I.J., Morgan-Capner, P., et al. 1992. Persistent rubella-specific IgM reactivity in the absence of recent primary rubella and rubella re-infection. *J Med Virol*, **36**, 188–92.

Thompson, K.M. and Tobin, J.O.'H. 1970. Isolation of rubella virus from abortion material. *Br J Med*, **2**, 264–6.

Thomssen, R., Laufs, R. and Muller, J. 1968. Physical properties and particle size of rubella virus. *Arch ges Virusforsch*, **23**, 332–45, in German.

Tipples, G.A., Hamkar, R., et al. 2004. Evaluation of rubella IgM serology assays. *J Clin Virol*, **30**, 233–8.

Töndury, G. and Smith, D.W. 1966. Fetal rubella pathology. *J Pediatr*, **68**, 867–79.

Tookey, P.A., Cortina-Borja, M. and Peckham, C.S. 2002. Rubella susceptibility among pregnant women in North London, 1996–1999. *J Public Health Med*, **24**, 211–16.

Tookey, P.A. and Peckham, C.S. 1999. Surveillance of congenital rubella in Great Britain, 1976–96. *Br J Med*, **318**, 769–70.

Townsend, J.J., Baringer, J.R., et al. 1975. Progressive rubella panencephalitis: late onset after congenital rubella. *N Engl J Med*, **292**, 990–3.

Tzeng, W.P. and Frey, T.K. 2002. Mapping the rubella virus sub-genomic promoter. *J Virol*, **76**, 3189–201.

Ueda, K., Nishida, Y., et al. 1975. Seven-year follow-up study of rubella syndrome in Ryuku with special reference to persistence of rubella hemagglutination inhibition antibodies. *Jap J Microbiol*, **19**, 181–5.

Urquhart, G.E.D., Crawford, R.J. and Wallace, J. 1978. Trial of high-titre human rubella immunoglobulin. *Br J Med*, **2**, 1331–2.

Vaheri, A. and Cristofalo, V.J. 1967. Metabolism of rubella virus BHK21 cells. *Arch ges Virusforsch*, **21**, 425–36.

Vaheri, A. and Hovi, T. 1972. Structural proteins and subunits of rubella virus. *J Virol*, **9**, 10–16.

van der Logt, J.T.M., van Loon, A.M. and van der Veen, J. 1980. Replication of rubella virus in human mono-nuclear blood cells. *Infect Immun*, **27**, 309–14.

Van Straaten, H.L., Grotte, M.E. and Oudesluys-Murphy, A.M. 1996. Evaluation of an automated auditory brainstem response infant hearing screening method in at risk neonates. *Eur J Pediatr*, **155**, 702–5.

Vejtorp, M. and Mansa, B. 1980. Rubella IgM antibodies in sera from infants born after maternal rubella, later than the 12th week of pregnancy. *Scand J Infect Dis*, **12**, 1–5.

Vesikari, T. 1972. Antibody response in rubella re-infection. *J Infect Dis*, **4**, 11–16.

Vesikari, T. 1980. Suppression of lymphocyte PHA – responsiveness after rubella vaccination with Cendehill and RA27/3 strains. *Scand J Infect Dis*, **12**, 7–11.

Vijayalakshmi, P., Kakkar, G., et al. 2002. Ocular manifestations of congenital rubella syndrome in a developing country. *Ind J Ophthalmol*, **50**, 307–11.

Voiland, A. and Bardeletti, G. 1980. Fatty acid composition of rubella virus and BHK21/13 S infected cells. *Arch Virol*, **64**, 319–28.

Vyse, A.J., Brown, D.W., et al. 1999. Detection of rubella virus-specific immunoglobulin G in saliva by an amplification-based enzyme-linked immunosorbent assay using monoclonal antibody to fluorescein isothiocyanate. *J Clin Microbiol*, **37**, 391–5.

Vyse, A.J. and Jin, L. 2002. An RT-PCR assay using oral fluid samples to detect rubella virus genome for epidemiological surveillance. *Mol Cell Probe*, **16**, 93–7.

Wang, X. and Gillam, S. 2001. Mutations in the GDD motif of rubella virus putative RNA-dependent RNA polymerase affect virus replication. *Virology*, **285**, 322–31.

Wang, C.Y., Domingeuz, G. and Frey, T.K. 1994. Construction of rubella virus genome-length cDNA clones and synthesis of infectious RNA transcripts. *J Virol*, **68**, 3550–7.

Waxham, M.N. and Wolinsky, J.S. 1983. Immunochemical identification of rubella virus haemagglutinin. *Virology*, **126**, 194–203.

Waxham, M.N. and Wolinsky, J.S. 1984. Rubella virus and its effect in the central nervous system. *Neurol Clin*, **2**, 367–85.

Waxham, M.N. and Wolinsky, J.S. 1985. A model of the structural organisation of rubella virions. *Rev Infect Dis*, **7**, Suppl. 1, S133–9.

Weibel, R.E., Stokes, J. Jr., et al. 1969. Live rubella vaccines in adults and children. HPV-77 and Merck-Benoit strains. *Am J Dis Child*, **118**, 226–9.

Weil, M.J., Itabashi, H. and Creamer, N.E. 1975. Chronic progressive panencephalitis due to rubella virus simulating subacute sclerosing panencephalitis. *N Engl J Med*, **292**, 994–8.

Weller, T.H. and Neva, F.A. 1962. Propagation in tissue culture of cytopathic agents from patients with rubella-like illness. *Proc Soc Exp Biol Med*, **111**, 215–25.

Wolinsky, J.S. 1996. Rubella. In: Fields, B.N., Knipe, D.M. and Howley, P.M. (eds), *Fields' Virology*, 3rd edn. Philadelphia, PA: Lippincott-Raven, 899–929.

Wolinsky, J.S., Dau, P.C., et al. 1979. Progressive rubella panencephalitis: immunovirological studies and results of isoprinosine therapy. *Clin Exp Immunol*, **35**, 397–404.

Wolinsky, J.S., Waxham, M.N., et al. 1982. Immunochemical features of a case of progressive rubella panencephalitis. *Clin Exp Immunol*, **48**, 359–66.

Wolinsky, J.S., McCarthy, M., et al. 1991. Monoclonal antibody defined epitope map of expressed rubella virus protein domains. *J Virol*, **65**, 3986–94.

Wolinsky, J.S., Sukholutsky, E., et al. 1993. An antibody- and synthetic peptide-defined rubella virus E1 glycoprotein neutralisation domain. *J Virol*, **67**, 961–8.

World Health Organization. 1999. Guidelines for surveillance of congenital rubella syndrome and rubella. Field test version. WHO/V&B/99.22. Geneva: WHO.

World Health Organization. 2000a. Report of a meeting on preventing congenital rubella syndrome: immunization strategies, surveillance needs. Unpublished document WHO/V&B/00; available from http://www.who.int/vaccines-documents.

World Health Organization. 2000b. Rubella vaccines. WHO position paper. *Wkly Epidemiol Rec*, **75**, 161–72.

World Health Oganization. 2000c. Preventing congenital rubella syndrome. *Wkly Epidemiol Rec*, **75**, 290-295.

World Health Organization. 2003a. Accelerated control of rubella and prevention of congenital rubella syndrome, WHO region of the Americas. *Wkly Epidemiol Rec*, **78**, 50–54.

World Health Organization. 2003b. Global Advisory Committee on Vaccine Safety, 16-17 December 2002. *Wkly Epidemiol Rec*, **78**, 17–18.

Yang, D., Hwang, D., et al. 1998. Effects of mutations in the rubella virus E1 glycoprotein on E1-E2 interaction and membrane fusion activity. *J Virol*, **72**, 8747–55.

Yao, J., Yang, D., et al. 1998. Proteolytic processing of rubella virus nonstructural proteins. *Virology*, **246**, 74–82.

Yao, J. and Gillam, S. 1999. Mutational analysis, using a full-length rubella virus cDNA clone of rubella virus E1 transmembrane and cytoplasmic domains required for virus release. *J Virol*, **73**, 4622–30.

Zhang, T., Mauracher, C.A., et al. 1992. Detection of rubella virus-specific imunoglobulins G (IgG), IgM and IgA antibodies by immunoblot assays. *J Clin Microbiol*, **30**, 824–30.

Zheng, D.-P., Zhu, H., et al. 2003. Phylogenetic analysis of rubella virus isolated during a period of epidemic transmission in Italy, 1991–1997. *J Infect Dis*, **187**, 1587–97.

Ziring, P.R., Gallo, G., et al. 1977. Chronic lymphocytic thyroiditis: identification of rubella virus antigen in the thyroid of a child with congenital rubella. *J Pediatr*, **90**, 419–20.

Zygraich, N., Peetermans, J. and Huygelen, C. 1971. In vivo properties of attenuated rubella virus 'Cendehill strain'. *Arch ges Virusforsch*, **33**, 225–33.

46

Flaviviruses

JOHN T. ROEHRIG AND DUANE J. GUBLER

PROPERTIES OF THE VIRUSES

This family of enveloped, positive-strand RNA viruses contains over 70 members, of which about 50 are arthropod-borne; many are pathogenic for humans and other vertebrates. The family name is derived from that of the type species, *Yellow fever virus* (YFV) (Latin: *flavus* = yellow).

Classification

The family *Flaviviridae* contains three genera: *Flavivirus*, *Pestivirus*, and *Hepacivirus*, and the unassigned GBV viruses (GBV-A, GBV-B, and GBV-C). All members of the *Flavivirus* genus are antigenically related. Serological crossreactions are most evident in hemagglutination-inhibition (HI) tests, and plaque reduction neutralization tests (PRNT) show the greatest specificity. Seven subgroups or complexes of flaviviruses have been defined on the basis of cross-neutralization tests (De Madrid and Porterfield 1974), and this subdivision has recently been substantially confirmed and extended in a more comprehensive study (Calisher et al. 1989). Flaviviruses can also be divided into three biological subsets based upon their mode of transmission, by mosquitoes, ticks, or by having no known arthropod vector. Table 46.1 shows the relationship between the subgroups determined by the PRNT and the mode of transmission of currently named flaviviruses.

Three pathogens of farm animals: hog cholera virus (HCV) or *Classical swine fever virus* (CSFV), bovine viral diarrhea virus (BVDV), and *Border disease virus* (BDV), constitute the *Pestivirus* genus. The mosquito cell-fusing agent is an additional member of the *Flaviviridae* but is outside the genus *Flavivirus*. Hepaciviruses as well as the unassigned GBV viruses, both agents of hepatitis, are the topic of another chapter and are not further discussed here.

Morphology and virion structure

Flaviviruses possess an isometric core, 30–35 nm in diameter, that contains a nucleocapsid or core (C) protein complexed with single-stranded positive-sense RNA. This core is surrounded by a lipid bilayer containing an envelope (E) protein and a membrane (M) protein, giving a total virion diameter of about 45 nm. The flavivirus E protein is a class II fusion protein. The M protein is first synthesized as a precursor protein, prM. The virion structure of dengue virus (DENV) virus has recently been solved using cryo-electron microscopy, and differs from the structure of recombinant subviral particles (RSP) derived from mammalian cells transfected with a plasmid containing only the genes for the prM and E proteins of tick-borne encephalitis virus (TBEV) (Ferlenghi et al. 2001; Kuhn et al. 2002). The virion envelope contains an icosahedral scaffold of 90 E protein dimers (Kuhn et al. 2002).

Pestiviruses are 40–60 nm particles that contain an electron-dense core of about 30 nm. The virion is enveloped with the E^{rns}, E1, and E2 proteins associated with envelope. Purified pestiviruses sometimes show a racquet type of morphology (Renard et al. 1985).

Genome structure and function

The genome of flaviviruses is a molecule of single-stranded, positive-sense RNA, approximately 11 kb in length containing short untranslated regions at 3′ and 5′ ends, a 5′ cap and a non-polyadenylated 3′ terminus (Figure 46.1). There is no subgenomic mRNA in flavivirus-infected cells. Complete genome sequences are known for YFV (Rice et al. 1985; Chambers et al. 1989), West Nile virus (WNV) (Castle et al. 1985; Wengler et al. 1985, 1987; Nowak et al. 1989; Lanciotti et al. 1999), all four serotypes of DENV (Hahn et al. 1988; Mackow et al. 1987; Osatomi and Sumiyoshi 1990; Fu et al. 1992), Japanese encephalitis virus (JEV) (Sumiyoshi et al. 1987), Kunjin virus (KUNV) (Coia et al. 1988), Powassan virus (POWV) (Mandl et al. 1993) and TBEV (Pletnev et al. 1990). A number of partial genome sequences, primarily of the E proteins,

Table 46.1 *Relationship between* Flavivirus *subgroup and mode of transmission*

Tick-borne viruses		No-vector viruses		Mosquito-borne viruses	
Virus	Subgroup	Virus	Subgroup	Virus	Subgroup
Karshi virus (KSIV)	1	*Carey Island virus* (CIV)	1	*Alfuy virus* (ALFV)	(3)
KFDV	1	*Phnom Penh bat virus* (PPBV)	1	*Japanese encephalitis virus* (JEV)	3
Langat virus (LGTV)	1	*Apoi virus* (APOIV)	2A	*Kedougou virus* (KEDV)	3
Louping ill virus (LIV)	1	*Bukalasa bat virus* (BBV)	2A	*Kokobera virus* (KOKV)	3(5?)
Negishi virus (NEG)V	1	*Dakar bat virus* (DBV)	2A	*Koutango virus* (KOUV)	3
Omsk hemorrhagic fever virus (OHFV)	1	*Entebbe bat virus* (ENTV)	2A	Kunjin virus (KUNV)	3
Powassan virus (POWV)	1	*Rio Bravo virus* (RBV)	2A	*Murray Valley encephalitis virus* (MVEV)	3
Royal Farm virus (RFV)	1	*Saboya virus* (SABV)	2A	*Saint Louis encephalitis virus* (SLEV)	3
Tick-borne encephalitis virus (TBEV)	1	*Cowbone Ridge virus* (CRV)	2B	Stratford virus (STRV)	3
Meaban virus (MEAV)	1A	*Jutiapa virus* (JUTV)	2B	*Usutu virus* (USUV)	3
Saumarez Reef virus (SREV)	1A	*Modoc virus* (MODV)	2B	*West Nile virus* (WNV)	3
Tyuleniy virus (TYUV)	1A	*Sal Vieja virus* (SVV)	2B	*Yaounde virus* (YAOV)	(3)[a]
Gadget's Gully virus (GGYV)	U	*San Perlita virus* (SPV)	2B	Spondweni virus (Spondweni)	4
Kadam virus (KADV)	U	*Aroa virus* (AROAV)	U	*Zika virus* (ZIKV)	4
		Batu Cave virus (BCV)	(U)[a]	*Bagaza virus* (BAGV)	5
		Cacipacore virus (CPCV)	U	*Israel turkey meningo-encephalitis virus* (ITV)	5
		Montana myotis leukoencephalitis virus (MMLV)	U	*Ntaya virus* (NTAV)	5
		Sokuluk virus (SOKV)	U	*Tembusu virus* (TMUV)	5
		Tamana bat virus (TABV)	U	*Yokose virus* (YOKV)	5
				Banzi virus (BANV)	6
				Bouboui virus (BOUV)	6
				Edge Hill virus (EHV)	6
				Potiskum virus (POTV)	(6)[a]
				Uganda S virus (UGSV)	
				Dengue virus 1 (DENV-1)	7
				Dengue virus 2 (DENV-2)	7
				Dengue virus 3 (DENV-3)	7
				Dengue virus 4 (DENV-4)	7
				Bussuquara virus (BSQV)	U
				Ilhéus virus (ILHV)	U
				Jugra virus (JUGV)	U
				Naranjal virus (NJLV)	U
				Rocio virus (ROCV)	U
				Sepik virus (SEPV)	U
				Wesselsbron virus (WESSV)	U
				Yellow fever virus (YFV)	U
Total:	14		19		36=69

Based on data from De Madrid and Porterfield 1974 and from Calisher et al. 1989.
U, unrelated to any other virus.
a) Batu Cave virus, Potiskum virus, and *Yaounde virus* were not examined in either series, but are included for completeness.

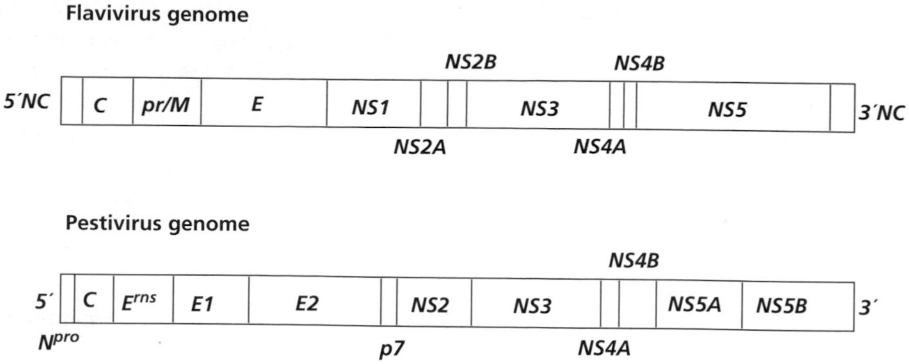

Flavivirus genome

Pestivirus genome

Figure 46.1 *Flavivirus and Pestivirus genome organization.*

are also available. A single long open reading frame (10 223 nt in the case of YFV) spans almost the entire length of the RNA. The gene order is 5′-C–prM–(M)–E–NS1–NS2A–NS2B–NS3–NS4A–NS4B–NS5-3′ (Rice et al. 1985) (Figure 46.1).

The genome of pestiviruses has been shown to be more similar to hepaciviruses than flaviviruses and is reported to be 12.5 kb in length. The 3′ end of the genomic RNA is not polyadenylated (Renard et al. 1987), and unlike flaviviruses, the pestivirus RNA lacks a 5′-cap structure (Brock et al. 1992). The pestivirus genome encodes a single open reading frame with a theoretical coding capacity of about 4 000 amino acids. Complete genome sequences have been determined for CSFV (Meyers et al. 1989; Moormann et al. 1990) and BVDV (Collett et al. 1988; Deng and Brock 1992), and BDV (Becher et al. 1994, 1998). Similar to flaviviruses, the genes encoding the structural proteins are located at the 5′ end of the genome. The gene order is 5′-Npro–C–Erns–E1–E2–p7–NS2–NS3–NS4A–NS4B–NS5A–NS5B-3′ (Collett et al. 1989).

Polypeptides: structural and nonstructural

Cell-associated flaviviruses have a C protein with a molecular mass of 12–13 kDa surrounded by a lipid bilayer containing the two membrane glycoproteins E and prM (mol. mass 50 and 22 kDa, respectively). Extracellular virions contain the shorter M protein (mol. mass 8 kDa) instead of prM. Seven nonstructural proteins have been well described (see section below on Replication). Because of the continued medical significance of the flaviviruses, the structure and function of the E protein (approximately 500 amino acids) have been intensely investigated.

Three antigenic domains (A, B, and C) have been identified on the E protein (Mandl et al. 1989; Heinz and Roehrig 1990; Roehrig et al. 1998). The A domain (amino acids 50–130 and 185–300) is a linearly discontinuous domain that is divided by the C domain (amino acids 130–185). The A-domain structure is stabilized by five disulfide

bridges and contains mostly conformationally dependent virus-neutralizing epitopes. Much of the antigenicity of the B domain (amino acids 300–400) requires a disulfide bond between Cys 11 and Cys 12. The A, B, and C domains constitute the 'head' of the E glycoprotein. A 100 amino acid stalk (approximately amino acids 400–500) that includes a 50 amino acid hydrophobic tail (amino acids 450–500) anchors the molecule in the virion envelope. Unlike other enveloped viruses, there is essentially no cytoplasmic tail on the E protein. The three-dimensional molecular structure of the amino terminal 380 amino acid tryptic fragment of the TBEV E protein homodimer has recently been solved (Rey et al. 1995). The protein folds into three distinct domains (I, II, and III), which correlate well to the previously defined domains C, A, and B. Because the locations of the E protein Cys residues are conserved among all flaviviruses, it is generally assumed that this overall structure is the same for all flaviviruses (Figure 46.2).

Three major nonstructural proteins (NS1, NS3, and NS5) can be found in flavivirus-infected cells. The NS1 protein is a membrane-bound glycoprotein whose function has not been fully determined. It is possible that this protein is involved in virion morphogenesis. The NS2A and NS3 proteins appear to function in concert as a virus-specific protease (Yusof et al. 2000; Leung et al. 2001). The NS3 protein also exhibits helicase activity (Utama et al. 2000; Matusan et al. 2001). The crystal structure of a portion of the NS3 proteins has recently been solved (Valle and Falgout 1998; Krishna Murthy et al. 1999; Murthy et al. 1999, 2000). The NS5 protein is the virus RNA-dependent RNA-polymerase.

Pestivirus proteins also appear to be synthesized as a polyprotein. Four structural proteins: C (14 kDa), and three envelope proteins – Erns (44–48 kDa), E1 (33 kDa), and E2 (55 kDa) – have been identified. The envelope glycoproteins, E1 and E2, form dimers through disulfide bridging in both infected cells and virions. The nonstructural protein Npro (23 kDa) that has autoproteolytic activity is located 5′ of the C protein. This protein has no analogue in the flaviviruses. Pestiviruses also do not

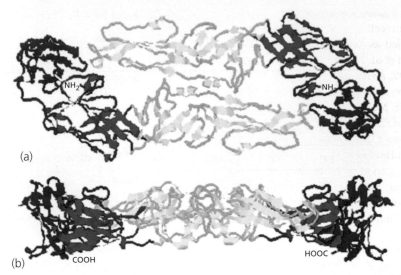

Figure 46.2 *E-glycoprotein structure. Homodimer of the TBE E protein (a.a. 1–395). Color domains: Domain I (C-domain), red; Domain II (A-domain), yellow; Domain III (B-domain), blue.* **(a)** *top view;* **(b)** *side view.*

appear to have a protein analogue of the flavivirus NS1 protein. Another nonstructural protein, NS2/NS3, is located 3′ of the envelope genes and apparently functions as a viral protease involved in polyprotein processing (Wiskerchen and Collett 1991). The NS2/NS3 protein is cleaved to NS2 and NS3 in some pestiviruses. Both the NS2/NS3 and the cleaved NS3 must have serine protease activity, even though the catalytic motif is located in the N-terminal region of NS3. At least three other nonstructural proteins have been identified: NS2, NS5A, and NS5B. The NS5B contains sequence motifs similar to flaviviral RNA polymerase.

Antigens

The E protein is the viral hemagglutinin, which also elicits neutralizing, enhancing, and protective antibodies. The C protein contributes to the group reactivity detected by the complement fixation (CF) test. The NS1 protein is responsible for inducing the soluble complement-fixing antigen detected in virus-infected cells. Monoclonal antibodies (mAb) specific for the NS1 protein can protect animals from virus challenge (Schlesinger et al. 1987; Henchal et al. 1988; Zhang et al. 1988; Falgout et al. 1990; McCown et al. 1990).

The pestivirus E^rns and E2 are primarily responsible for eliciting pestivirus neutralizing antibodies (Weiland et al. 1990, 1992). Because it is difficult to elicit virus-neutralizing antibody specific for the E1 protein, it is thought that most of this protein is buried in the virus envelope, similar to the flavivirus M protein.

Replication

Although it has not been conclusively proven, evidence is accumulating that flaviviruses infect cells by attaching to cellular receptors through the E-protein domain III (Bhardwaj et al. 2001; Crill and Roehrig 2001; Hurrelbrink and McMinn 2001). Flavivirus cellular receptor moieties have been implicated but not been identified conclusively (Chen et al. 1997; Lee and Lobigs 2000, 2002; Chu and Ng 2002; Germi et al. 2002). After endocytosis, the nucleocapsid is released into the cytoplasm by membrane fusion catalyzed by a low-pH dependent conformational change in the E protein. All flavivirus E proteins have a highly conserved sequence (amino acids 98–110) that has chemical similarities to regions shown to be responsible for cell-membrane fusion in orthomyxoviruses and paramyxoviruses.

The viral mRNA is translated as a polyprotein, which undergoes extensive co-translational and post-translational proteolytic processing and cleavage by cellular signalase(s). Cleavage generates the primary amino acid sequence of the mature structural proteins, prM and E, and the amino terminus of the following nonstructural protein, NS1. The amino-terminal portion of the polyprotein is released as a molecule, the anchored C protein, which is associated with membranes of the rough endoplasmic reticulum. The anchored C protein is converted to mature C protein by removal of the carboxyl-terminal hydrophobic segment. Cell-associated virions are constructed from the proteins C, prM, and E. The prM protein is cleaved in the Golgi vesicles, by a furin-like enzyme resulting in loss of the amino-terminal fragment of this protein and release of mature virions from infected cells. It is currently believed that the prM protein functions as an E-protein chaperone, protecting it from acid-catalyzed denaturation during virus maturation. The cleavage sites generating the nonstructural proteins NS2A, NS2B, NS4A, and NS4B have been identified.

Flavivirus infection causes virus-specific cytopathic effects in mammalian cells. Flavivirus cell killing has recently been identified as an apoptotic event (Despres et al. 1996, 1998; Liao et al. 1997, 1998; Marianneau et al. 1997, 1998a, b, c, 1999; Avirutnan et al. 1998; Couvelard et al. 1999; Kamalov et al. 1999; Balachandran et al. 2000; Jan et al. 2000; Matthews et al. 2000; Ho et al. 2001; Prikhod'ko et al. 2001, 2002; Su et al. 2001, 2002; Lin et al. 2002; Parquet et al. 2002; Sauerwald et al. 2002; Shafee and AbuBakar 2002). Cytopathic effects in flavivirus-infected arthropod cells are not as dramatic. The site of flavivirus budding is not fully defined. Nucleocapsids do not appear to accumulate at the plasma membranes, indicating that budding may be quite efficient.

The processing of the pestivirus structural proteins has been described (Rümenapf et al. 1993). The pestiviral envelope glycoproteins are produced as a precursor protein, $E^{rns}/E1/E2$, which is rapidly cleaved to $E^{rns}/E1$ and E2. The $E^{rns}/E1$ precursor is then processed to E^{rns} and E1. The E^{rns} protein has no hydrophobic anchor sequence and can be found in infected cell supernatant. This cleavage pattern is similar to that seen with the flavivirus prM/E protein.

Flavivirus vaccines

The live-attenuated YFV vaccine is historically one of the most successful virus vaccines ever developed. It has low reactogenicity and excellent immunogenicity. Recently, however, a low rate of both neurotropic and viscerotropic adverse reactions following vaccination with YFV vaccines have been documented (Vasconcelos et al. 2001; Cetron et al. 2002). These reactions have primarily been associated with vaccination of the elderly, and preliminary genomic sequence data from recovered YFV vaccine show no signs of reversion. Further study is necessary to determine the reasons behind these new observations.

Modern approaches based on recombinant DNA technology are now being applied to flavivirus vaccine development. These approaches utilize DNA copies of the viral genome or individual viral genes to prepare either attenuated chimeric flaviviruses or direct DNA vaccines. Chimeric viruses based on either the YFV or DENV genome have been prepared (Bray and Lai 1991; Guirakhoo et al. 1999, 2000, 2001, 2002; Monath et al. 1999, 2000, 2002; Butrapet et al. 2000; Huang et al. 2000; Arroyo et al. 2001). Some of these chimeric vaccines have passed preclinical testing and are being prepared for human clinical trials. DNA-based vaccines have been prepared from number of flaviviruses (Konishi et al. 1997, 2000a, b, 2001; Chang et al. 2000, 2001; Hunt et al. 2001; Konishi and Fujii 2002). Preliminary tests of a DNA vaccine for WN virus have suggested that it may be effective in horses (Davis et al. 2001).

CLINICAL AND PATHOLOGICAL ASPECTS

Diseases caused by flaviviruses: general features

The flaviviruses known to cause human disease are listed in Table 46.2, several of which may also cause disease in wild or domestic animals. For example, in South Africa, Wesselsbron virus (WESSV) causes disease in sheep, and to a lesser extent goats and cattle (Coetzer and Theodoridis 1982); Kyasanur Forest disease virus (KFDV) has killed monkeys in India (Sreenivasan et al. 1979); and YFV can kill South American monkeys in nature and Asian monkeys in the laboratory, but not African monkeys. Israel turkey meningo-encephalitis virus (ITV) has caused economic losses in turkey farms in Israel and is also present in South Africa (Barnard et al. 1980).

CLINICAL MANIFESTATIONS

Flaviviruses cause a spectrum of clinical manifestations ranging from asymptomatic infections to undifferentiated febrile illnesses, fevers with rash or arthralgia or both, to hemorrhagic fevers, hepatitis, and encephalitis, which may result in death. The same virus can cause a variety of syndromes.

ARTHROPOD VECTORS

Much is known about the epidemiology of viruses such as DENV, YFV, JEV, St. Louis encephalitis virus (SLEV), and Central European TBEV, but there are also many uncertainties about these and other flaviviruses. For example, there are substantial differences between the natural history of YFV in Africa and in the New World (Downs 1982). YFV and DENV are classic examples of mosquito-borne flaviviruses, being transmitted in urban outbreaks by *Aedes aegypti* in both Africa and the Americas (YFV) and globally in the tropics (DENV) by a variety of mosquito species in the forest cycle. DENV are the only arboviruses that have fully adapted to a human–mosquito–human cycle and no longer depend on the forest cycle for maintenance. It has also been recovered from ticks in West Africa (Germain et al. 1982), although it is not known whether these arthropods contribute to the maintenance of the virus in nature.

In general, mosquito-borne flaviviruses are more common in the tropics, whereas tickborne flaviviruses tend to be prevalent in more temperate regions. The flaviviruses without a known vector are associated with rodents and bats, and are thought to be transmitted by contact with infective secretions. Only one virus in this subset, Dakar bat virus (DBV), is known to infect humans naturally, but several other nonvector-borne flaviviruses have caused laboratory infections. Transovarial, vertical,

Table **46.2** *Flaviviruses known to cause human disease*

Virus	Geographical distribution	Other features
Mosquito-borne viruses		
Banzi virus (BANV)	S and E Africa	2 cases only
Bussuquara virus (BSQV)	Brazil, Colombia, Panama	1 case only
Dengue viruses 1–4 (DENV types 1–4)	Worldwide in the tropics	Tropics and subtropics where the virus and a *Stegomyia* vector exist
Edge Hill virus (EHV)	Australia	
Ilhéus virus (ILHV)	C and S America	
Japanese encephalitis virus (JEV)	E, SE, S Asia, W Pacific	
Kedougou virus (KEDV)	Africa	Laboratory infection
Kokobera virus (KOKV)	Australia	
Kunjin virus (KUNV)	Australia, Sarawak	
Murray Valley encephalitis virus (MVEV)	Australia, New Guinea	
Rocio virus (ROCV)	Brazil	Epidemics of encephalitis
St. Louis encephalitis virus (SLEV)	N America, Panama, Jamaica, Trinidad, Brazil, Argentina	
Sepik virus (SEPV)	New Guinea	1 case only
Spondweni virus (SPOV)	E, W & S Africa	
Usutu virus (USUV)	E, W, Central Africa, Central Europe (Austria)	Found in birds in Austria
Wesselsbron virus (WESSV)	E, W, S Africa, Thailand	
West Nile virus (WNV)	E, W, S Africa, S and SE Asia, India, Mediterranean area, N America	Large epidemic throughout USA
Yellow fever virus (YFV)	W and Central Africa, S and Central America	Periodical epidemics, e.g. Ethiopia, Nigeria
Zika virus (ZIKV)	E and W Africa, Malaysia, Philippines	1 case in Uganda
Tickborne viruses		
Absettarov virus (ABSV)	Europe	
Hanzalova virus (HANV)	Europe	
Hypr virus (HYPRV)	Europe	
Karshi virus (KSIV)	Asia	
Koutango virus (KOUV)	Africa	
Kumlinge virus (KUMV)	Europe	
Kyasanur Forest disease virus (KFDV)	Mysore, India	
Langat virus (LGTV)	Malaysia	Only experimental cases proven
Louping ill virus (LIV)	British Isles	
Negishi virus (NEGV)	Asia	
Omsk hemorrhagic fever virus (OHFV)	The former Soviet Union	
Powassan virus (POWV)	Canada and USA	
Tick-borne encephalitis		
Western equine encephalomyelitis virus (WEEV)	Europe from Scandinavia to Balkans and from Germany to the former Soviet Union	
Eastern equine encephalomyelitis virus (EEEV)	Eastern Europe and the former Soviet Union	
No known arthropod vector		
Apoi virus (APOIV)	Japan	Laboratory infection
Dakar bat virus (DBV)	W, E and Central Africa, Madagascar	2 cases only
Phnom Penh bat virus (PPBV)	Cambodia, Malaysia	
RBV	USA, Mexico	

and trans-stadial transmission have been documented with several mosquito-borne and tickborne flaviviruses (Rosen 1987).

PATHOGENESIS

Flavivirus infections in humans cause three main disease patterns – nonspecific febrile illness (pantomorphic), encephalitis (neuromorphic), and hemorrhagic fever (viseromorphic) – which generally reflect the tropisms of the viruses for different target organs (Monath 1986). Symptoms in most flavivirus infections probably result from the direct effects of virus replication in the various target organs, which include the brain, liver, skin, lymphoid tissue, and cells of the mononuclear phagocyte lineage. Most flaviviruses are pantomorphic, causing only a nonspecific febrile illness in a large proportion of infections. Some, however, have virulence and evolutionary host characteristics that make them more neuromorphic or viseromorphic, thus causing encephalitis or hemorrhagic fever, respectively.

Both viral and host factors influence the pathogenesis of flaviviral infections of humans. Many flaviviruses have been shown to vary naturally in virulence characteristics as a result of selection pressures associated with the arthropod vector and/or vertebrate host. In addition, host factors such as age, immune status, and genetic background may influence pathogenesis. A mouse model of natural resistance to flavivirus infection has been developed (Brinton et al. 1998; Sangster et al. 1998; Shellam et al. 1998; Brooks and Phillpotts 1999; Urosevic et al. 1999; Silvia et al. 2001; Mashimo et al. 2002; Perelygin et al. 2002). This resistance appears to be associated, at least in part, with the intrinsic antiviral interferon response.

IMMUNE RESPONSE

Antigenically related flaviviruses may co-exist within similar habitats. There is extensive crossreactivity between flaviviruses in serological tests, and while there is no cross-protective immunity, heterologous flavivirus antibody may modulate clinical illness. This is especially important with DENV, in that infection with a single serotype provides homotypic immunity, but may enhance infection with a heterologous DENV and increase the risk of dengue shock syndrome (DSS) or dengue hemorrhagic fever (DHF).

DIAGNOSIS

Isolation of virus provides definitive evidence of flavivirus infection. Development of rapid and sensitive assays to detect viral RNA in tissue have extended the abilities to identify virus when viral titers are too low for isolation, or specimens have not been handled properly (Briese et al. 2000; Lanciotti et al. 2000; Lanciotti and Kerst 2001; Hunt et al. 2002; Komar et al. 2002). In practice, however, infections are diagnosed most frequently on the basis of serological tests, which include the PRNT, CF, and HI, and ELISA for virus-specific IgM and IgG (Roehrig 2000). A variety of flavivirus derived murine mAbs are available for virus identification (Roehrig 2000).

CONTROL

Measures directed towards vector control provide the only practical means of limiting virus transmission for most flaviviruses. Vaccines are available for YFV, JEV, and TBEV.

IMPORTANT MOSQUITO-BORNE DISEASES

Yellow fever virus

Although yellow fever virus (YFV) is believed to have originated in Africa, the first recorded outbreak was in Mexico in 1648. This was followed during the seventeenth, eighteenth, and nineteenth centuries by numerous urban epidemics in the West Indies, Central and South America, and the eastern part of the USA as far north as New York. Epidemics in more temperate regions of the western hemisphere were the result of introductions through seaports and of transport of mosquito vectors and viruses along commercial shipping routes. The work of the US Army Commission in Cuba established that urban transmission of YFV from human to human was infected by *Ae. aegypti* mosquitoes (Reed 1902), and subsequent eradication measures against this mosquito, and immunization using a live attenuated virus vaccine (see below), effectively controlled urban YF in the Americas and West Indies, respectively. However, the disease persisted sporadically in forest areas of both Africa and South America as a consequence of sylvatic cycles involving monkeys and forest-dwelling mosquitoes, e.g. *Haemagogus* and *Sabethes* spp. in South America, *Ae. africanus* in East Africa, and a variety of *Aedes* spp. in West Africa (Strode 1951). In the past 20 years, *Ae. aegypti* has reinfested nearly all tropical American countries, putting this region at the highest risk of urban epidemics of YF in more than 50 years.

In humans, YF illness varies from an inapparent infection to a fulminating disease terminating in death; three stages (infection, remission, and intoxication) can be commonly recognized. After an incubation period of 3–10 days, there is sudden onset of fever, rigors, headache, and backache. The patient is usually intensely ill and restless with flushed face, swollen lips, bright red tongue, and congested conjunctivae; many patients suffer from nausea and vomiting. A bleeding tendency may be seen early on. This stage of active congestion is followed after 2–3 days by a brief remission and then a resumption of febrile illness. The facial edema and flushing are replaced by a dusky pallor, the gums become swollen and bleed easily, and there is a pronounced hemorrhagic tendency with black vomit, melena, and ecchymoses. The pulse rate is slow, despite the high fever, and the blood pressure falls, resulting in albuminuria, oliguria, and anuria. Death, when it occurs, is usually within 6–7 days of onset, and is rare after 10 days of illness. The jaundice, which gives the disease its name, is generally apparent only in convalescing patients. In patients with intoxication, mortality may occur in 20–50 percent. In a recent outbreak in Nigeria, mortality was over 50 percent (Nasidi et al. 1989). Most patients with severe disease will have leukopenia, thrombocytopenia, elevated liver enzymes, and coagulation defects. At autopsy the organs most affected are the liver, spleen, kidneys, and heart. Typically, midzonal necrosis is apparent in the liver, affecting cells around the periphery of the lobule and sparing areas around the central vein. Hyaline necrosis is evident and Councilman inclusion bodies are usually present.

Treatment is supportive and confined to nonspecific measures, including maintenance of fluid and electrolyte balances and replacement of any substantial amounts of blood lost through hemorrhage. Laboratory diagnosis can be made by virus isolation, serology, polymerase chain reaction (PCR), and immunohistochemistry. One dose of live-attenuated 17D vaccine provides complete protection for 10 years. A French vaccine prepared from a neurotropic strain of YFV has been widely used in Africa. It confers good protection and is cheaper than the 17D vaccine, but because it has caused adverse reactions, including a number of cases of encephalitis, its use is limited.

Dengue/dengue hemorrhagic fever (DHF)

There are four DENV serotypes: DENV-1, DENV-2, DENV-3, and DENV-4. These viruses are closely related to each other antigenically, and crossreactivity occurs in serological tests. However, there is no lasting cross-protective immunity; cross-protection between DENV serotypes lasts for only a few months. Thus, individuals can have as many as four dengue infections in their life, one with each serotype.

Major DENV epidemics have been caused by all four DENV serotypes. Generally one serotype predominates in an area until increased herd immunity decreases transmission. Then another serotype predominates. DENV changes genetically during natural transmission, and significant biological differences have been shown between strains of the same serotype (Russell and McCown 1972; Gubler and Rosen 1977; Gubler et al. 1978).

The epidemiology of the four DENV serotypes is similar (Gubler 1988, 1998). All have a worldwide distribution in the tropics and are maintained in most tropical urban centers in a mosquito–human–mosquito cycle. In many urban centers, multiple virus serotypes co-circulate (hyper-

endemicity). The principal mosquito vector is *Ae. aegypti*, an African species that was spread around the world during the seventeenth, eighteenth, and nineteenth centuries with the slave trade and shipping industry. This species became highly adapted to living in intimate association with humans and is a highly efficient epidemic vector in urban settings. Secondary vectors include other *Ae. stegomia* species such as *Ae. albopictus*, *Ae. polynesiensis*, and *Ae. scutellaris* spp. These secondary vector species can transmit outbreaks, but may be more important as maintenance vectors. DENV are also maintained in forest cycles in Asia and Africa. These are thought to be primitive cycles and involve monkeys and canopy-dwelling *Aedes* spp. mosquitoes that rarely come in contact with humans. Current evidence suggests that these forest cycles are not important in contributing to urban epidemics (Rico-Hesse 1990).

Infection with DENV causes a spectrum of clinical illness, ranging from inapparent infection to mild nonspecific viral syndrome to classical DENV fever to severe and fatal hemorrhagic disease. The clinical picture of classical DENV fever has been described in experimentally infected volunteers (Siler et al. 1926; Simmons et al. 1931). Classic DENV fever is seen in adults and older children. After an infective mosquito bite, there is an incubation period of 4–6 days (range 3–14 days), followed by the sudden onset of fever (which is often biphasic), severe headache, chills, and generalized pains in the muscles and joints. A maculopapular rash generally appears on the trunk between the third and fifth day of illness and spreads to the face and extremities. Lymphadenopathy, anorexia, constipation, and altered taste sensation are common. Occasionally, petechiae are seen on the dorsum of the feet, legs, hands, axillae, and palate late in the illness. In young children, the illness is usually mild, but may be severe. The illness generally lasts for 5–7 days, after which recovery is usually complete, although convalescence may be prolonged. There is leukopenia with a relative lymphocytosis, and thrombocytopenia may occur. Liver enzymes may be elevated and hemorrhagic manifestations may occur.

DHF is a severe form of DENV infection characterized by sudden onset of fever, usually of 2–7 days' duration, and nonspecific signs and symptoms. The critical stage of DHF occurs 24 hours before to 24 hours after the temperature falls to or below normal. During this time, hemorrhagic manifestations usually occur, and signs of circulatory failure may appear. The patient may become restless or lethargic, experience acute abdominal pain, and have cold extremities, skin congestion, and oliguria, usually on or after the third day of illness. Clinical laboratory tests at this time will show thrombocytopenia (platelet count <100 000/mm^3) and evidence of a vascular leak syndrome, which may cause hypovolemia, shock, and death. The most common hemorrhagic manifestations are skin hemorrhages, but epistaxis, bleeding gums, gastrointestinal hemorrhage, and hematuria may occur.

DHF is most commonly observed in children under the age of 15 years in Asia, but in the Pacific and Americas, DHF also occurs in adults (Gubler et al. 1978; Guzman et al. 1984a, b; Schatzmayr et al. 1986; Dietz et al. 1996). The pathogenesis of DHF is still not well understood. It is hypothesized that classical DHF with a capillary leak syndrome has a unique immunopathologic basis associated with heterologous dengue antibody-dependent enhancement of viral infection of cells of the mononuclear phagocyte lineage (Halstead 1980). Infection of these cells stimulates the release of a vasoactive mediator(s) that apparently causes increased vascular permeability; if not promptly detected and corrected, this can lead to hypovolemia, shock, and death. Although the risk of DHF is higher in children experiencing a second dengue infection, DHF also occurs in patients experiencing primary infections with DENV, suggesting that heterologous DENV antibody (previous infection) is not a necessary prerequisite for DHF. Furthermore, some strains of DENV cannot be enhanced in vitro (Rosen 1977; Gubler et al. 1978). Both field and laboratory evidence has been accumulating in recent years that supports a more prominent role of viral factors in the pathogenesis of DHF and suggesting that virus strain and serotype are also important risk factors for severe disease (Rosen 1986b, 1989; Gubler 1988, 1998; Trent et al. 1989; Rico-Hesse et al. 1997). Another complicating factor is that DEN infections with severe hemorrhage, but no evidence of a capillary leak syndrome, may have another pathogenetic mechanism (Gubler 1988). Because there is not a good animal model for DHF, a full understanding of the pathogenetic mechanism of severe dengue disease will have to await careful field studies in dengue endemic areas.

DENV infection can be diagnosed by virus isolation, serology, PCR, and immunohistochemistry. Although laboratory tests are reliable for diagnosis, they are not rapid and should not be used to make management and treatment decisions in a clinical setting. Instead clinicians should rely on clinical laboratory tests that can be used to monitor whether there is a capillary leak.

Case-fatality rates can be as high as 20–40 percent in DHF/DSS, but can be reduced with early diagnosis and proper case management using fluid replacement therapy. On average, DHF case-fatality rates are almost 5 percent. There is no vaccine for DENV/DHF, although significant progress has been made in developing both live attenuated vaccine candidates and second-generation recombinant candidate vaccines using infectious clone technology in recent years (Kinney and Huang 2001). Currently, disease prevention depends exclusively on mosquito control and avoiding mosquito bites.

Japanese encephalitis

Japanese encephalitis virus (JEV) is widespread throughout Asia, from the maritime provinces of Russia to South India and Sri Lanka (Umenai et al. 1985; Rosen 1986a). JEV is the most important cause of arboviral encephalitis globally with more than 45 000 cases reported annually. In recent years, JEV, which has been limited to Asia, has expanded its geographical distribution with outbreaks in the Pacific (Paul et al. 1993; Hanna et al. 1995). Epidemics occur in late summer in temperate regions, but the virus is enzootic and occurs throughout the year in many tropical areas of Asia. JEV is maintained in a natural enzootic cycle involving culicine mosquitoes and water birds. The virus is transmitted to man by *Culex* mosquitoes, primarily *Cx. tritaeniorhynchus*, and related species, which breed in rice fields. Pigs are the primary amplifying hosts of JEV in the peridomestic environment.

The incubation period of JE is 5–14 days. Onset of symptoms is usually sudden, with fever, headache, and vomiting. The illness resolves in 5–7 days if there is no CNS involvement. In those patients with CNS involvement, lethargy is common, faces are expressionless, and there are sensory and motor disturbances affecting speech, the eyes, and limbs. There may be confusion and delirium progressing to coma, with convulsions in children as a presenting sign. Weakness and paralysis may affect any part of the body. The lesions are generally upper motor neuron in character. Neck rigidity and a positive Kernig sign are found, and reflexes are abnormal. Initial leukocytosis is followed by leukopenia. The mortality in most outbreaks of JE is less than 10 percent, but is higher in children and has exceeded 30 percent in some outbreaks in India and in Korea (Umenai et al. 1985). Neurological sequelae in patients who recover are reported in up to 30 percent of cases.

A formalin-inactivated vaccine prepared in mice infected with the Nakayama strain of JEV is used widely in Japan, Korea, Taiwan, and Thailand; in China, an inactivated vaccine prepared in primary hamster kidney cell cultures has been given to millions of children. A live-attenuated vaccine prepared in primary hamster kidney cell culture has also given very promising results in children in China (Xin et al. 1988).

St. Louis encephalitis

St. Louis encephalitis (SLE) is one of the most important mosquito-borne encephalitides in the USA, causing periodic epidemics in the midwest and southeast. SLEV is prevalent throughout the western hemisphere from Canada to Argentina, but epidemics are unknown in South and Central America (Monath and Tsai 1987). SLEV is maintained in a culicine mosquito–bird–mosquito cycle, with periodic amplification by peridomestic birds and *Culex* mosquitoes. In Florida, the principal vector is *Cx. nigripalpus*, in the Midwest, *Cx. pipiens pipiens* and *Cx. p. quinquefasciatus* and in the western United States, *Cx. tarsalis*.

Only a small proportion of SLE infections lead to clinical illness. Onset of illness is usually insidious, with a nonspecific prodrome. The disease is generally milder in children than in adults. In those children who do have severe disease, however, there is a high rate of encephalitis. The elderly are at highest risk for severe disease and death. No vaccine is yet available, and prevention, therefore, is by mosquito-control measures.

West Nile virus

West Nile virus (WNV) is closely related to JEV, Murray Valley encephalitis virus (MVEV), and SLEV. It, like the other flaviviruses that cause encephalitis, has a natural maintenance cycle involving wild birds and mosquitoes. Historically, the geographical distribution of WNV included Africa, Central Asia, the Middle East, and Europe. In 1999, WNV was identified in the western hemisphere for the first time in New York City and has since spread throughout most of the USA, southern Canada, and the northern part of Mexico along the US boarder (Gubler et al. 2000; Marfin et al. 2001; Petersen and Roehrig 2001; Campbell et al. 2002; Petersen and Marfin 2002; Roehrig et al. 2002). Genomic sequencing studies have identified two lineages of WNV (Mathiot et al. 1990; Lanciotti et al. 1999, 2002; Scherret et al. 2001). Lineage 1 contains viruses that have caused major human outbreaks in Africa, Europe, the Middle East, and the USA. Also included as a lineage 1 WNV is the Australian flavivirus, KUNV. KUNV normally causes mostly asymptomatic infections, but occasional cases of encephalitis have been reported (Muller et al. 1986). Lineage 2 WNVs are primarily enzootic viruses that circulate in Africa and have not been associated with human epidemics. The lineage 1 North American WNV is most closely related to a genotype in Israel (Jia et al. 1999; Lanciotti et al. 1999), indicating that this was the most likely source of the North American WNV.

An interesting aspect of the North American/Israeli strain of WNV is its virulence for some of its avian reservoirs, especially members of the family *Corvidae* (e.g. crows, blue jays, etc.), humans, horses, and a number of other animal species. High virulence is not common among other strains of WNV and avian virulence in the form of dead bird surveillance has been exploited as a particularly effective method to identify WNV activity in North America (Eidson et al. 2001a, b). To date, more than 150 species of birds and 19 other mammalian species have been shown to be infected with WNV in the USA (Komar et al. 2002). Based on sero-prevalance of WNV-reactive antibodies in birds and their large populations, passerine birds appear to be major avian reservoirs for WNV in North America. Thousands of horses have been infected with WNV in the USA since 1999, with a case-fatality rate of about 25 percent. Studies suggest, however, that the horse is a dead-end host for WNV (Bunning et al. 2002). In addition, WNV morbidity and/or mortality have been documented in other mammals. A killed WNV vaccine has been developed for horses. Beginning in 2001, it has been used extensively in the USA. How, or if, this vaccination program has modified current the equine epizootic in North America is not known. A DNA vaccine also shows promise for disease prevention in horses (Davis et al. 2001).

The principal mosquito vectors belong to the genus *Culex*, including *Cx. univittatus* in Africa, *Cx. pipiens* and *Cx. modertus* in the Middle East and Europe, and the *Cx. vishnui* and *Cx. tritaeniorhynchus* complexes in Asia. While *Cx. pipiens pipiens* and *Cx. p. quinquefaciatus* appear to be primary vectors among the bird reservoirs in North America, at least 40 other species of mosquitoes have been shown to be infected with WNV, and several of them are being investigated as possible bridge vectors to humans and horses (Nasci et al. 2001; Turell et al. 2001, 2002; Dohm et al. 2002). In addition, WNV has been isolated from both soft and hard ticks, which may be involved in the maintenance cycle in some areas (Gromashevsky et al. 1973; Lvov et al. 2000).

Human infection is usually mild and generally presents as a nonspecific viral syndrome. In those cases with more severe disease, meningoencephalitis is the most common complication. In the USA, WNV encephalitis can present as a poliomyelitis-like syndrome (Glass et al. 2002; Leis et al. 2002). The incubation period can range from 2 to 15 days post-infection. A single case of hepatitis caused by WNV has been reported from Africa. The case-fatality rate in severe cases is about 10 percent, but like SLE, may be much higher in elderly people above the age of 50. The summer of 2002 in the USA saw the largest human outbreak of WNV meningo-encephalitis ever documented with more than 3 800 human cases. Results of human serosurveys in the USA suggest that 1:150 WNV infections progress to encephalitis in persons less than 65 years, but may be as high as 1:50 in older individuals (Mostashari et al. 2001).

Recent studies have also demonstrated that WNV can be transmitted through transfusion or transplantation of virus-contaminated blood or other tissues, through human breast milk, or transplacentally. While these may be infrequent events, the blood contamination may necessitate screening of blood products for the presence of WNV during intense human viral outbreaks.

There is no human vaccine for WNV. Prevention relies on mosquito control and protection from mosquito bites to reduce the risk of exposure. Definitive diagnosis can only be made using laboratory tests to isolate the virus or detect specific antibodies.

Murray Valley encephalitis

Murray Valley encephalitis (MVE) is a zoonosis that occurs only in Australia and New Guinea. The virus is closely related to JEV, WNV, SLEV, and several other flaviviruses, all of which are zoonoses and cause encephalitis in humans. MVEV, first isolated in 1951, has been and is responsible for major epidemics of encephalitis in Australia. Like other flaviviruses of this group, the virus is believed to be maintained in a natural cycle involving water birds and mosquitoes. However, this is not proven and serological evidence suggests other hosts are commonly infected. The major mosquito vector appears to be *Cx. aunutirostris*, although other species such as *Ae. normanensis* and other *Aedes* spp. may play a role, especially in the maintenance cycle. The inapparent to apparent ratio infection is about 500:1. Clinical disease is characterized by sudden onset of a nonspecific viral syndrome with fever, headache, nausea/vomiting, anorexia, and myalgias, followed by drowsiness, malaise, irritability, mental confusion, and meningismus. There is a pleocytosis and leukocytosis. In severe cases, there may be hyperactive reflexes, spastic paresis, convulsions, coma, and death. The case-fatality rate is about 20 percent; neurological sequaleae occur in a significant number of those patients that survive. All age groups are affected.

Viremia in humans has not been documented in MVEV infections, and it is likely that they are dead-end hosts. The pathological changes that occur in the central nervous system are similar to those caused by other viral zoonoses that cause encephalitis. Definitive diagnosis must rely on laboratory tests that detect specific antibody to MVEV.

There is no vaccine for MVE. Prevention relies on mosquito control and individuals taking responsibility to protect themselves against mosquito bites.

Other mosquito-borne infections

ILHÉUS VIRUS

Ilhéus virus (ILHV) is active over wide areas of Central and South America, including Trinidad, and is probably maintained in a forest cycle involving birds and mosquitoes. Most human infections are asymptomatic, but occasional cases of encephalitis are recognized.

ROCIO VIRUS

Rocio virus (ROCV) is antigenically related to SLEV and is known only from Brazil. Clinically it causes CNS disease similar to other flaviviruses that cause encephalitis. It has caused major epidemics in Brazil, principally in males 15–30 years of age (de Souza Lopes et al. 1981; Iversson 1988).

SPONDWENI VIRUS

Spondweni virus (SPOV) is present in South Africa, and has produced overt human disease in a few expatriates in West Africa (Wolfe et al. 1982).

USUTU VIRUS

The historical range of Usutu virus (USUV) is in East, West and Central Africa. Recently, however, USUV has been isolated from birds in Austria (Weissenbock et al. 2002). A single case with fever and a rash has been reported.

WESSELSBRON VIRUS

Wesselsbron virus (WESSV) has wide distribution in Africa and causes epizootics in sheep, producing abortion and death in newborn lambs and ewes, and less severe disease in goats and cattle (Coetzer and Theodoridis 1982). The virus also infects man in nature and in the laboratory (Justines and Shope 1969).

TICK-BORNE INFECTIONS

Tick-borne encephalitis

Tick-borne encephalitis (TBE) is caused by two closely related viruses that are distinct biologically. The eastern subtype causes Russian spring–summer encephalitis (RSSE) and is transmitted by *Ixodes persulcatus*. The western subtype is transmitted by *Ixodes ricinus* and causes Central European encephalitis (CEE). The latter name is somewhat misleading, since the condition occurs in foci extending from Scandinavia in the north to Yugoslavia and Greece in the south.

Of the two subtypes, RSSE is the more severe infection, having a case-fatality rate of up to 25 percent in some outbreaks, whereas mortality in CEE seldom exceeds 5 percent. Both viruses are maintained in natural cycles involving a variety of mammals and ticks; the latter serve as the main reservoir host by passing the viruses from generation to generation by transovarial and trans-stadial transmission. Human exposure occurs in the spring and summer months in temperate zones and in fall and winter in the Mediterranean, when the ticks are more active. Most human exposure is associated with work or recreational activities in enzootic areas. The incubation period is 7–14 days. Infection usually presents as a mild, influenza-type illness or as benign, aseptic meningitis, but may result in fatal meningoencephalitis. Fever is often biphasic, and there may be severe headache and neck rigidity, with transient pareses of the limbs, shoulder girdle, or, less commonly, of the respiratory musculature. A few patients are left with residual flaccid paralysis (Ackermann et al. 1986). Although the great majority of TBE infections follow exposure to ticks, infection has occurred through the ingestion of infected cows' or goats' milk.

Inactivated vaccines are available against both eastern and western subtypes of TBE. The vaccine against the western subtype is highly effective (Kunz et al. 1980). Definitive diagnosis can only be achieved by specific laboratory tests to detect antibody.

Louping ill

Louping ill (LI) is derived from an old Norse word meaning 'to leap.' Louping ill virus (LIV) is a member of the TBEV complex. It is known in the British Isles as a disease of sheep characterized by CNS manifestations, in particular, cerebellar ataxia, paralysis, and death. It has never been a serious hazard to humans: most reported cases are the result of laboratory infections. A few natural infections do occur in persons closely associated with sheep. The illness is generally biphasic with encephalitic involvement in the second stage. The vector is *I. ricinus* and the virus is maintained in rodents, deer, and ground-living birds (Reid 1988).

Powassan virus

Powassan virus (POWV) is a member of the TBEV complex. It is thought to be a rare cause of acute viral CNS disease in Canada and the USA, but is also present in the former Soviet Union, where it has been recovered from mosquitoes, ticks, and humans. It was first isolated from the brain of a 5-year-old child who died in Ontario in 1958, and has since caused a number of cases of encephalitis in Canada and the eastern USA (Artsob 1988). However, with intensified surveillance for neurological disease caused by WNV in the northeastern USA, four cases of POWV encephalitis have been documented (Centers for Disease Control and Prevention 2001). Patients who recover may have residual neurological sequelae. In addition to isolations from humans, the virus has been recovered from ticks (*I. marxi, I. cookei*, and *Dermacentor andersoni*) and from the tissues of a skunk (*Spiligale putorius*) (Johnson 1987). There is clinical and serological evidence that POWV can cause fatal encephalitis in horses, which may be confused with rabies encephalitis (Little et al. 1985).

Kyasanur Forest disease

Kyasanur Forest disease virus (KFDV) was first recognized in 1957 during a fatal epizootic affecting wild monkeys in Mysore (Karnataka) State, India. Since then, thousands of infections have occurred in forest workers with a mortality of up to 10 percent. Until recently it was found only in southwestern India. The virus has been isolated from monkeys, humans, and ticks. The principal tick vector appears to be *Haemaphysalis spinigera*; the

vertebrate reservoir host is uncertain (Banerjee 1988). Human infection with KFDV causes a spectrum of illness ranging from inapparent infection to severe hemorrhagic disease. Hemorrhagic manifestations are common and may involve the skin, gums, and gastrointestinal tract. Although CNS involvement is uncommon, there may be signs of meningeal irritation and stiff neck. An inactivated vaccine is available in Europe.

An apparent subtype of KFDV has been isolated from fatal human cases of hemorrhagic disease in Jeddah, Saudi Arabia, associated with meat handlers (Zaki 1997; Besaud 2005). The virus was subsequently isolated from other patients with illness ranging from fatal hemorrhagic disease to viral syndrome. All known human infections to date have been associated with handling meat or drinking unpasteurized camels' milk. The virus appears to be associated with sheep and camels, and to be transmitted by ticks, but no data are available on either the natural vertebrate host or the arthropod vector.

Omsk hemorrhagic fever

Omsk hemorrhagic fever virus (OHFV) is also caused by a tickborne Flavivirus. It was first isolated in association with human disease in Siberia in 1945; illness was characterized by biphasic fever with lymphadenopathy and hemorrhages from mucous membranes. OHFV is antigenically distinct from the eastern and western subtypes of TBEV. Infection may be acquired from ticks, usually *Dermacentor pictus* or *D. marginatus*, or from exposure to infected water voles or muskrats (Lvov 1988).

Other tick-borne infections

MEABAN VIRUS, SAUMAREZ REEF VIRUS, AND TYULENIY VIRUS

These viruses are associated with seabird ticks in France, Australia, and subarctic regions of the USA and the former Soviet Union (Clifford et al. 1971; Lvov et al. 1971; St George et al. 1977; Chastel et al. 1985).

NEGISHI VIRUS

Negishi virus (NEGV) has caused at least two fatal cases of encephalitis in Japan (Okuno et al. 1961). Although tick transmission has not been proven, this virus is closely related to other tick-borne flaviviruses (De Madrid and Porterfield 1974; Furuta et al. 1984; Calisher et al. 1989).

PESTIVIRUS INFECTIONS

Bovine viral diarrhea

Infection with BVDV occurs worldwide in many wild and domestic bovine species. Two clinical syndromes are recognized in cattle, namely bovine viral diarrhea and mucosal disease. The former is a mild, transient infection with high morbidity but low mortality, which is followed by immunity. Viral infection during pregnancy can result in abortion or the birth of persistently infected offspring, some of which may have teratogenic defects. Two biotypes of virus have been recognized, only one of which is cytopathic. When persistently infected, antibody negative animals carrying the noncytopathic strain virus are reinfected with a serologically related cytopathic strain, they develop mucosal disease, which carries a high mortality (Baker 1987; Brownlie et al. 1987).

Antibodies reactive with pestivirus antigens have been detected in the serum of two children with microcephaly (Potts et al. 1987). With a mAb prepared against BVDV Yolken et al. (1989) detected pestivirus antigens in the feces of infants with gastroenteritis.

Border disease

BDV of sheep, originally recognized in the Scottish border country, occurs also in New Zealand. The causative virus is closely related to that of bovine viral diarrhea (Horzinek 1981; Nettleton 1987).

Classical swine fever (hog cholera)

This important disease of pigs occurs worldwide and is associated with persistent infections, abortion, and congenital malformations (Liess 1987).

REFERENCES

Ackermann, R., Kruger, K., et al. 1986. Spread of early-summer meningo encephalitis in the Federal Republic of Germany. *Dtsch Med Wochenschr*, **111**, 927–33.

Arroyo, J., Guirakhoo, F., et al. 2001. Molecular basis for attenuation of neurovirulence of a yellow fever virus/Japanese encephalitis virus chimera vaccine (ChimeriVax-JE). *J Virol*, **75**, 934–42.

Artsob, H. 1988. Powassen encephalitis. In: Monath, T.P. (ed.), *The arboviruses: ecology and epidemiology*, vol. IV. . Boca Raton, FL: CRC Press, 29–50.

Avirutnan, P., Malasit, P., et al. 1998. Dengue virus infection of human endothelial cells leads to chemokine production, complement activation, and apoptosis. *J Immunol*, **161**, 6338–46.

Baker, J.C. 1987. Bovine viral diarrhea virus: a review. *J Am Vet Assoc*, **11**, 1449–58.

Balachandran, S., Roberts, P.C., et al. 2000. Alpha/beta interferons potentiate virus-induced apoptosis through activation of the FADD/Caspase-8 death signaling pathway. *J Virol*, **74**, 1513–23.

Banerjee, K. 1988. Kyanasur Forest disease. In: Monath, T.P. (ed.), *The arboviruses: ecology and epidemiology*. vol. III. Boca Raton, FL: CRC Press, 93–116.

Barnard, B.J.H., Buys, S.B., et al. 1980. Turkey meningo-encephalitis in South Africa. *Onderstepoort J Vet Res*, **47**, 89–94.

Becher, P., Shannon, A.D., et al. 1994. Molecular characterization of border disease virus, a pestivirus from sheep. *Virology*, **198**, 542–51.

Becher, P., Orlich, M., et al. 1998. Complete genomic sequence of border disease virus, a pestivirus from sheep. *J Virol*, **72**, 5165–73.

Bessaud, M., Grard, G. et al. 2005. Indentification and enzymatic characterization of NS2B-NS3 protease of Alkhuma virus, a class 4 flavirus. *Virus Res*, **107**, 57–62.

Bhardwaj, S., Holbrook, M., et al. 2001. Biophysical characterization and vector-specific antagonist activity of domain iii of the tick-borne flavivirus envelope protein. *J Virol*, **75**, 4002–7.

Bray, M. and Lai, C.J. 1991. Construction of intertypic chimeric dengue viruses by substitution of structural protein genes. *Proc Natl Acad Sci U S A*, **88**, 10342–6.

Briese, T., Glass, W.G., et al. 2000. Detection of West Nile virus sequences in cerebrospinal fluid. *Lancet*, **355**, 1614–15.

Brinton, M.A., Kurane, I., et al. 1998. Immune mediated and inherited defences against flaviviruses. *Clin Diagn Virol*, **10**, 129–39.

Brock, K.V., Deng, R. and Riblet, S. 1992. Nucleotide sequencing of 5′ and 3′ termini of bovine viral diarrhea virus by RNA ligation and PCR. *J Virol Methods*, **38**, 39–46.

Brooks, T.J. and Phillpotts, R.J. 1999. Interferon-alpha protects mice against lethal infection with St Louis encephalitis virus delivered by the aerosol and subcutaneous routes. *Antiviral Res*, **41**, 57–64.

Brownlie, J., Clarke, M.C., et al. 1987. Pathogenesis and epidemiology of bovine virus diarrhea infection of cattle. *Ann Rech Vét*, **18**, 157–66.

Bunning, M.L., Bowen, R.A., et al. 2002. Experimental infection of horses with West Nile virus. *Emerg Infect Dis*, **8**, 380–6.

Butrapet, S., Huang, C.Y., et al. 2000. Attenuation markers of a candidate dengue type 2 vaccine virus, strain 16681 (PDK-53), are defined by mutations in the 5′ noncoding region and nonstructural proteins 1 and 3. *J Virol*, **74**, 3011–19.

Calisher, C.H., Karabatsos, N., et al. 1989. Antigenic relationships between flaviviruses as determined by cross-neutralization tests with polyclonal antisera. *J Gen Virol*, **70**, 37–43.

Campbell, G.L., Marfin, A.A., et al. 2002. West Nile virus. *Lancet Infect Dis*, **2**, 519–29.

Castle, E., Nowak, T., et al. 1985. Sequence analysis of the viral core and the membrane associated proteins V1 and NV2 of the flavivirus West Nile virus and of the genome sequence of those proteins. *Virology*, **145**, 227.

CDC 2001. Outbreak of Powassan encephalitis – Maine and Vermont, 1999–2001. *MMWR Morbid Mortal Wkly Rep*, **50**, 761–4.

Cetron, M.S., Marfin, A.A., et al. 2002. Yellow fever vaccine. Recommendations of the advisory committee on immunization practices. *MMWR Morbid Mortal Wkly Rep Recomm Rep*, **51**, 1–11.

Chambers, T.J., McCourt, D.W. and Rice, C.M. 1989. Yellow fever virus proteins NS2A, NS2B, NS4B: identification and partial N-terminal amino acid sequence analysis. *Virology*, **169**, 100–9.

Chang, G.J., Hunt, A.R., et al. 2000. A single intramuscular injection of recombinant plasmid DNA induces protective immunity and prevents Japanese encephalitis in mice. *J Virol*, **74**, 4244–52.

Chang, G.J., Davis, B.S., et al. 2001. Flavivirus DNA vaccines: current status and potential. *Ann N Y Acad Sci*, **951**, 272–85.

Chastel, C., Main, A.J., et al. 1985. The isolation of Meaban virus, a new *Flavivirus* from the seabird tick *Ornithodoros* (*Alectorobius*) *maritimus* in France. *Arch Virol*, **83**, 129–40.

Chen, Y., Maguire, T., et al. 1997. Dengue virus infectivity depends on envelope protein binding to target cell heparan sulfate. *Nat Med*, **3**, 866–71.

Chu, J.J. and Ng, M.L. 2002. Infection of polarized epithelial cells with flavivirus West Nile: polarized entry and egress of virus occur through the apical surface. *J Gen Virol*, **83**, 2427–35.

Clifford, C.M., Yunker, C.E., et al. 1971. Isolation of a group B arbovirus from *Ixodes uriae* collected on Three Arch Rocks National Wildlife Refuge, Oregon. *Am J Trop Med Hyg*, **20**, 461–8.

Coetzer, J.A.W. and Theodoridis, A. 1982. Clinical and pathological studies in adult sheep and goats experimentally infected with Wesselsbron disease virus. *Onderstepoort J Vet Res*, **49**, 19–22.

Coia, G., Parker, M.D., et al. 1988. Nucleotide and complete amino acid sequences of Kunjin virus: definitive gene order and characteristics of the virus-specified proteins. *J Gen Virol*, **69**, 1–21.

Collett, M.S., Larson, R., et al. 1988. Proteins encoded by bovine viral diarrhea virus: the genomic organization of a pestivirus. *Virology*, **165**, 200–8.

Collett, M.S., Moennig, V. and Horzinek, M.C. 1989. Recent advances in pestivirus research. *J Gen Virol*, **70**, 253–66.

Couvelard, A., Marianneau, P., et al. 1999. Report of a fatal case of dengue infection with hepatitis: demonstration of dengue antigens in hepatocytes and liver apoptosis. *Hum Pathol*, **30**, 1106–10.

Crill, W.D. and Roehrig, J.T. 2001. Monoclonal antibodies that bind to domain III of dengue virus E glycoprotein are the most efficient blockers of virus adsorption to Vero cells. *J Virol*, **75**, 7769–73.

Davis, B.S., Chang, G.J., et al. 2001. West Nile virus recombinant DNA vaccine protects mouse and horse from virus challenge and expresses in vitro a noninfectious recombinant antigen that can be used in enzyme-linked immunosorbent assays. *J Virol*, **75**, 4040–7.

De Madrid, A.T. and Porterfield, J.S. 1974. The flaviviruses (group B arboviruses): a cross-neutralization study. *J Gen Virol*, **23**, 91–6.

Deng, R. and Brock, K.V. 1992. Molecular cloning and nucleotide sequence of a pestivirus genome, noncytopathic bovine viral diarrhea virus strain SD-1. *Virology*, **191**, 867–79.

de Souza Lopes, O., Sacchetta, L.A., et al. 1981. Emergence of a new arbovirus disease in Brazil. III. Isolation of Roccio virus from *Psorophora* Ferox (Humboldt, 1819). *Am J Epidemiol*, **113**, 122–5.

Despres, P., Flamand, M., et al. 1996. Human isolates of dengue type 1 virus induce apoptosis in mouse neuroblastoma cells. *J Virol*, **70**, 4090–6.

Despres, P., Frenkiel, M.P., et al. 1998. Apoptosis in the mouse central nervous system in response to infection with mouse-neurovirulent dengue viruses. *J Virol*, **72**, 823–9.

Dietz, V., Gubler, D.J., et al. 1996. The 1986 dengue and dengue hemorrhagic fever epidemic in Puerto Rico: epidemiologic and clinical observations. *P R Health Sci J*, **15**, 201–10.

Dohm, D.J., Sardelis, M.R., et al. 2002. Experimental vertical transmission of West Nile virus by *Culex pipiens* (Diptera: *Culicidae*). *J Med Entomol*, **39**, 640–4.

Downs, W.G. 1982. The known and the unknown in yellow fever ecology and epidemiology. *Ecol Dis*, **1**, 103–10.

Eidson, M., Komar, N., et al. 2001a. Crow deaths as a sentinel surveillance system for West Nile virus in the northeastern United States, 1999. *Emerg Infect Dis*, **7**, 615–20.

Eidson, M., Kramer, L., et al. 2001b. Dead Bird Surveillance as an early warning system for West Nile Virus. *Emerg Infect Dis*, **7**, 631–5.

Falgout, B., Bray, M., et al. 1990. Immunization of mice with recombinant vaccinia virus expressing authentic dengue virus nonstructural protein NS1 protects against lethal dengue virus encephalitis. *J Virol*, **64**, 4356–63.

Ferlenghi, I., Clarke, M., et al. 2001. Molecular organization of a recombinant subviral particle from tick-borne encephalitis virus. *Mol Cell*, **7**, 593–602.

Fu, J., Tan, B.-H., et al. 1992. Full-length cDNA sequence of dengue type virus (Singapore strain S275/90). *Virology*, 188, **1**, 953–8.

Furuta, I., Takashina, I., et al. 1984. Antigenic analysis of flaviviruses with monoclonal antibodies against Negishi virus. *Microbiol Immunol*, **28**, 1023–30.

Germain, M., Cornet, M., et al. 1982. Recent advances in research regarding sylvatic yellow fever in west and central Africa. *Bull Inst Pasteur*, **80**, 315–30.

Germi, R., Crance, J.M., et al. 2002. Heparan sulfate-mediated binding of infectious dengue virus type 2 and yellow fever virus. *Virology*, **292**, 162–8.

Glass, J.D., Samuels, O., et al. 2002. Poliomyelitis due to West Nile virus. *N Engl J Med*, **347**, 1280–1.

Gromashevsky, V.L., Lvov, D.K., et al. 1973. A complex natural focus of arboviruses on Glinyanyi Island, Baku Archipelago, Azerbaidzhan S.S.R. *Acta Virol*, **17**, 155–8.

Gubler, D.J. 1988. Dengue. In: Monath, T.P. (ed.), *Epidemiology of arthropod-borne viral disease*, vol. II. Boca Raton, FL: CRC Press, 223–60.

Gubler, D.J. 1998. Dengue and dengue hemorrhagic fever. *Clin Microbiol Rev*, **11**, 480–96.

Gubler, D.J. and Rosen, L. 1977. Quantitative aspects of replication of dengue viruses in *Aedes albopictus* (Diptera: *Culicidae*) after oral and parenteral infection. *J Med Ent*, **13**, 469–72.

Gubler, D.J., Reed, D., et al. 1978. Epidemiologic, clinical and virologic observations on dengue in the Kingdom of Tonga. *Am J Trop Med Hyg*, **27**, 581–59.

Gubler, D.J., Campbell, G.L., et al. 2000. West Nile virus in the United States: guidelines for detection, prevention and control. *Viral Immunol*, **13**, 469–75.

Guirakhoo, F., Zhang, Z.X., et al. 1999. Immunogenicity, genetic stability, and protective efficacy of a recombinant, chimeric yellow fever-Japanese encephalitis virus (ChimeriVax-JE) as a live, attenuated vaccine candidate against Japanese encephalitis. *Virology*, **257**, 363–72.

Guirakhoo, F., Weltzin, R., et al. 2000. Recombinant chimeric yellow fever-dengue type 2 virus is immunogenic and protective in nonhuman primates. *J Virol*, **74**, 5477–85.

Guirakhoo, F., Arroyo, J., et al. 2001. Construction, safety, and immunogenicity in nonhuman primates of a chimeric yellow fever-dengue virus tetravalent vaccine. *J Virol*, **75**, 7290–304.

Guirakhoo, F., Pugachev, K., et al. 2002. Viremia and immunogenicity in nonhuman primates of a tetravalent yellow fever-dengue chimeric vaccine: genetic reconstructions, dose adjustment, and antibody responses against wild-type dengue virus isolates. *Virology*, **298**, 146–59.

Guzman, M.G., Kouri, G.P., et al. 1984a. Dengue haemorrhagic fever in Cuba. I. Serological confirmation of clinical diagnosis. *Trans R Soc Trop Med Hyg*, **78**, 235–8.

Guzman, M.G., Kouri, G.P., et al. 1984b. Dengue haemorrhagic fever in Cuba. II. Clinical investigations. *Trans R Soc Trop Med Hyg*, **78**, 239–41.

Hahn, Y.S., Galler, R., et al. 1988. Nucleotide sequence of dengue 2 RNA and comparison of the encoded proteins with those of other flaviviruses. *Virology*, **162**, 167–80.

Halstead, S.B. 1980. Immunopathological parameters of togarvirus disease syndromes. In: Schleslinger, R.W. (ed.), *The Togaviruses: Biology, Structure, Replication*. New York: Academic Press, 107–74.

Hanna, J., Ritchie, S., et al. 1995. Probable Japanese encephalitis acquired in the Torres Strait. *Comm Dis Intell*, **19**, 206–8.

Heinz, F.X. and Roehrig, J.T. 1990. Flaviviruses. In: Van Regenmortel, M.H.V. and Neurath, A.R. (eds), *Immunochemistry of viruses II. The basis for serodiagnosis and vaccines*. Amsterdam: Elsevier, 289–305.

Henchal, E.A., Henchal, L.S., et al. 1988. Synergistic interactions of anti-NS1 monoclonal antibodies protect passively immunized mice from lethal challenge with dengue 2 virus. *J Gen Virol*, **69**, 2101–7.

Ho, L.J., Wang, J.J., et al. 2001. Infection of human dendritic cells by dengue virus causes cell maturation and cytokine production. *J Immunol*, **166**, 1499–506.

Horzinek, M.C. 1981. *Non-arthropod-borne togaviruses*. New York: Academic Press.

Huang, C.Y., Butrapet, S., et al. 2000. Chimeric dengue type 2 (vaccine strain PDK-53)/dengue type 1 virus as a potential candidate dengue type 1 virus vaccine. *J Virol*, **74**, 3020–8.

Hunt, A.R., Cropp, C.B., et al. 2001. A recombinant particulate antigen of Japanese encephalitis virus produced in stably-transformed cells is an effective noninfectious antigen and subunit immunogen. *J Virol Methods*, **97**, 133–49.

Hunt, A.R., Hall, R.A., et al. 2002. Detection of West Nile virus antigen in mosquitoes and avian tissues by a monoclonal antibody-based capture enzyme immunoassay. *J Clin Microbiol*, **40**, 2023–30.

Hurrelbrink, R.J. and McMinn, P.C. 2001. Attenuation of Murray Valley encephalitis virus by site-directed mutagenesis of the hinge and putative receptor-binding regions of the envelope protein. *J Virol*, **75**, 7692–702.

Iversson, L.B. 1988. In Monath, T.P. (ed.), *The arboviruses: ecology and epidemiology*, vol. IV. Boca Raton, FL: CRC Press, 77–92.

Jan, J.T., Chen, B.H., et al. 2000. Potential dengue virus-triggered apoptotic pathway in human neuroblastoma cells: arachidonic acid, superoxide anion and NF-kappaB are sequentially involved. *J Virol*, **74**, 8680–91.

Jia, X.Y., Briese, T., et al. 1999. Genetic analysis of West Nile New York 1999 encephalitis virus. *Lancet*, **354**, 1971–2.

Johnson, H.N. 1987. Isolation of Powassan virus from a spotted skunk in California. *J Wildl Dis*, **23**, 152–3.

Justines, G.A. and Shope, R.E. 1969. Wesselsbron virus infection in a laboratory worker, with virus recovery from a throat washing. *Health Lab Sci*, **6**, 46–9.

Kamalov, N.I., Novozhilova, A.P., et al. 1999. Morphological features of cell death in various types of acute tick-borne encephalitis. *Neurosci Behav Physiol*, **29**, 449–53.

Kinney, R.M. and Huang, C.Y. 2001. Development of new vaccines against dengue fever and Japanese encephalitis. *Intervirology*, **44**, 176–97.

Komar, N., Lanciotti, R., et al. 2002. Detection of West Nile virus in oral and cloacal swabs collected from bird carcasses. *Emerg Infect Dis*, **8**, 741–2.

Konishi, E. and Fujii, A. 2002. Dengue type 2 virus subviral extracellular particles produced by a stably transfected mammalian cell line and their evaluation for a subunit vaccine. *Vaccine*, **20**, 1058–67.

Konishi, E., Win, K.S., et al. 1997. Particulate vaccine candidate for Japanese encephalitis induces long-lasting virus-specific memory T lymphocytes in mice. *Vaccine*, **15**, 281–6.

Konishi, E., Yamaoka, M., et al. 2000a. Japanese encephalitis DNA vaccine candidates expressing premembrane and envelope genes induce virus-specific memory B cells and long-lasting antibodies in swine. *Virology*, **268**, 49–55.

Konishi, E., Yamaoka, M., et al. 2000b. A DNA vaccine expressing dengue type 2 virus premembrane and envelope genes induces neutralizing antibody and memory B cells in mice. *Vaccine*, **18**, 1133–9.

Konishi, E., Fujii, A., et al. 2001. Generation and characterization of a mammalian cell line continuously expressing Japanese encephalitis virus subviral particles. *J Virol*, **75**, 2204–12.

Krishna Murthy, H.M., Judge, K., et al. 1999. Crystallization, characterization and measurement of MAD data on crystals of dengue virus NS3 serine protease complexed with mung-bean Bowman-Birk inhibitor. *Acta Crystallogr D Biol Crystallogr*, **55**, 1370–2.

Kuhn, R.J., Zhang, W., et al. 2002. Structure of dengue virus: implications for flavivirus organization, maturation, and fusion. *Cell*, **108**, 717–25.

Kunz, C., Heinz, F.X. and Hoffmann, H. 1980. Immunogenicity and reactigenicity of a highly purified vaccine against tick-borne encephalitis. *J Med Virol*, **6**, 103–9.

Lanciotti, R.S. and Kerst, A.J. 2001. Nucleic acid sequence-based amplification assays for rapid detection of West Nile and St. Louis encephalitis viruses. *J Clin Microbiol*, **39**, 4506–13.

Lanciotti, R.S., Roehrig, J.T., et al. 1999. Origin of the West Nile virus responsible for an outbreak of encephalitis in the northeastern United States. *Science*, **286**, 2333–7.

Lanciotti, R.S., Kerst, A.J., et al. 2000. Rapid detection of West Nile virus from human clinical specimens, field-collected mosquitoes, and avian samples by a TaqMan reverse transcriptase-PCR assay. *J Clin Microbiol*, **38**, 4066–71.

Lanciotti, R.S., Ebel, G.D., et al. 2002. Complete genome sequences and phylogenetic analysis of West Nile virus strains isolated from the United States, Europe, and the Middle East. *Virology*, **298**, 96–105.

Lee, E. and Lobigs, M. 2000. Substitutions at the putative receptor-binding site of an encephalitic flavivirus alter virulence and host cell tropism and reveal a role for glycosaminoglycans in entry. *J Virol*, **74**, 8867–75.

Lee, E. and Lobigs, M. 2002. Mechanism of virulence attenuation of glycosaminoglycan-binding variants of Japanese encephalitis virus and Murray Valley encephalitis virus. *J Virol*, **76**, 4901–11.

Leis, A.A., Stokic, D.S., et al. 2002. A poliomyelitis-like syndrome from West Nile virus infection. *N Engl J Med*, **347**, 1279–80.

Leung, D., Schroder, K., et al. 2001. Activity of recombinant dengue 2 virus NS3 protease in the presence of a truncated NS2B co-factor, small peptide substrates and inhibitors. *J Biol Chem*, **276**, 45762–71.

Liao, C.L., Lin, Y.L., et al. 1997. Effect of enforced expression of human *bcl-2* on Japanese encephalitis virus-induced apoptosis in cultured cells. *J Virol*, **71**, 5963–71.

Liao, C.L., Lin, Y.L., et al. 1998. Antiapoptotic but not antiviral function of human *bcl-2* assists establishment of Japanese encephalitis virus persistence in cultured cells. *J Virol*, **72**, 9844–54.

Liess, B. 1987. Pathogenesis and epidemiology of hog cholera. *Ann Rech Vet*, **18**, 139–45.

Lin, C.F., Lei, H.Y., et al. 2002. Endothelial cell apoptosis induced by antibodies against dengue virus nonstructural protein 1 via production of nitric oxide. *J Immunol*, **169**, 657–64.

Little, P.B., Thorsen, J., et al. 1985. Powassan viral encephalitis: a review and experimental studies in the horse and rabbit. *Vet Pathol*, **22**, 500–7.

Lvov, D.K. 1988. Omsk hemorrhagic fever. In: Monath, T.P. (ed.), *Epidemiology of arthropod-borne viral disease*, vol. III. Boca Raton, FL: CRC Press, 205–16.

Lvov, D.K., Timopheeva, A.A., et al. 1971. Tyuleniy virus. A new group B arbovirus isolated from *Ixodes (Ceratixodes) putus* Pick.-Camb. 1878 collected on Tuleniy Island, Sea of Okhotsk. *Am J Trop Med Hyg*, **20**, 456–60.

Lvov, D.K., Butenko, A.M., et al. 2000. Isolation of two strains of West Nile virus during an outbreak in southern Russia, 1999. *Emerg Infect Dis*, **6**, 373–6.

Mackow, E., Makino, Y., et al. 1987. The nucleotide sequence of dengue 4 virus: analysis of genes coding for nonstructural proteins. *Virology*, **158**, 217–28.

Mandl, C.W., Guirakhoo, F.G., et al. 1989. Antigenic structure of the flavivirus envelope protein E at the molecular level, using tick-borne encephalitis virus as a model. *J Virol*, **63**, 564–71.

Mandl, C.W., Holzmann, H., et al. 1993. Complete genomic sequence of Powassan virus: evaluation of genetic elements in tick-borne versus mosquito-borne flaviviruses. *Virology*, **194**, 173–84.

Marfin, A.A., Petersen, L.R., et al. 2001. Widespread West Nile virus activity, eastern United States, 2000. *Emerg Infect Dis*, **7**, 730–5.

Marianneau, P., Cardona, A., et al. 1997. Dengue virus replication in human hepatoma cells activates NF-kappaB which in turn induces apoptotic cell death. *J Virol*, **71**, 3244–9.

Marianneau, P., Flamand, M., et al. 1998a. Apoptotic cell death in response to dengue virus infection: what are the consequences of viral pathogenesis? *Ann Biol Clin (Paris)*, **56**, 395–405, [in French].

Marianneau, P., Flamand, M., et al. 1998b. Induction of programmed cell death (apoptosis) by dengue virus in vitro and in vivo. *Acta Cient Venez*, **49**, 13–17.

Marianneau, P., Flamand, M., et al. 1998c. Apoptotic cell death in response to dengue virus infection: the pathogenesis of dengue haemorrhagic fever revisited. *Clin Diagn Virol*, **10**, 113–19.

Marianneau, P., Steffan, A.M., et al. 1999. Infection of primary cultures of human Kupffer cells by dengue virus: no viral progeny synthesis, but cytokine production is evident. *J Virol*, **73**, 5201–6.

Mashimo, T., Lucas, M., et al. 2002. A nonsense mutation in the gene encoding 2′–5′-oligoadenylate synthetase/L1 isoform is associated with West Nile virus susceptibility in laboratory mice. *Proc Natl Acad Sci U S A*, **99**, 11311–16.

Mathiot, C.C., Georges, A.J., et al. 1990. Comparative analysis of West Nile virus strains isolated from human and animal hosts using monoclonal antibodies and cDNA restriction digest profiles. *Res Virol*, **141**, 533–43.

Matthews, V., Robertson, T., et al. 2000. Morphological features of Murray Valley encephalitis virus infection in the central nervous system of Swiss mice. *Int J Exp Pathol*, **81**, 31–40.

Matusan, A.E., Pryor, M.J., et al. 2001. Mutagenesis of the dengue virus type 2 NS3 protein within and outside helicase motifs:

effects on enzyme activity and virus replication. *J Virol*, **75**, 9633–43.

McCown, J., Cochran, M., et al. 1990. Protection of mice against lethal Japanese encephalitis with a recombinant baculovirus vaccine. *Am J Trop Med Hyg*, **42**, 491–9.

Meyers, G., Rümenapf, T. and Theil, H.-J. 1989. Molecular cloning and nucleotide sequence of the genome of hog cholera virus. *Virology*, **171**, 555–67.

Monath, T.P. 1986. Pathobiology of the flaviviruses. In: Schlesinger, S. and Schlesinger, M.J. (eds), *The Togaviridae and Flaviviridae*. New York: Plenum, 375–440.

Monath, T.P. and Tsai, T.F. 1987. St. Louis encephalitis: lessons from the last decade. *Am J Trop Med Hyg*, **37**, 40–59S.

Monath, T.P., Soike, K., et al. 1999. Recombinant, chimaeric live, attenuated vaccine (ChimeriVax) incorporating the envelope genes of Japanese encephalitis (SA14-14-2) virus and the capsid and nonstructural genes of yellow fever (17D) virus is safe, immunogenic and protective in non-human primates. *Vaccine*, **17**, 1869–82.

Monath, T.P., Levenbook, I., et al. 2000. Chimeric yellow fever virus 17D-Japanese encephalitis virus vaccine: dose-response effectiveness and extended safety testing in rhesus monkeys. *J Virol*, **74**, 1742–51.

Monath, T.P., McCarthy, K., et al. 2002. Clinical proof of principle for ChimeriVax: recombinant live, attenuated vaccines against flavivirus infections. *Vaccine*, **20**, 1004–18.

Moormann, R.J.M., Warmerdam, P.A.M., et al. 1990. Molecular cloning and nucleotide sequence of hog cholera virus strain Brescia and mapping of the genomic region encoding envelope protein E1. *Virology*, **177**, 184–98.

Mostashari, F., Bunning, M.L., et al. 2001. Epidemic West Nile encephalitis, New York, 1999: results of a household-based seroepidemiological survey. *Lancet*, **358**, 261–4.

Muller, D., McDonald, M., et al. 1986. Kunjin virus encephalomyelitis. *Med J Aust*, **144**, 41–9.

Murthy, H.M., Clum, S., et al. 1999. Dengue virus NS3 serine protease. Crystal structure and insights into interaction of the active site with substrates by molecular modeling and structural analysis of mutational effects. *J Biol Chem*, **274**, 5573–80.

Murthy, H.M., Judge, K., et al. 2000. Crystal structure of dengue virus NS3 protease in complex with a Bowman–Birk inhibitor: implications for flaviviral polyprotein processing and drug design. *J Mol Biol*, **301**, 759–67.

Nasci, R.S., White, D.J., et al. 2001. West Nile virus isolates from mosquitoes in New York and New Jersey, 1999. *Emerg Infect Dis*, **7**, 626–30.

Nasidi, A., Monath, T.P., et al. 1989. Urban yellow fever epidemic in western Nigeria, 1987. *Trans R Soc Trop Med Hyg*, **83**, 401–6.

Nettleton, P.F. 1987. Pathogenesis and epidemiology of border disease. *Ann Rech Vét*, **18**, 147–55.

Nowak, T., Farber, P., et al. 1989. Analyses of the terminal sequences of West Nile virus structural proteins and of the in vitro translation of these proteins allow the proposal of a complete scheme of the proteolytic cleavages involved in their synthesis. *Virology*, **169**, 365–76.

Okuno, T., Oya, A. and Ho, T. 1961. The identification of Negishi virus: a presumably new member of Russian spring-summer encephalitis virus family isolated in Japan. *Jpn J Med Sci Biol*, **14**, 51–9.

Osatomi, K. and Sumiyoshi, H. 1990. Complete nucleotide sequence of dengue type 3 virus genome RNA. *Virology*, **176**, 643–7.

Parquet, M.C., Kumatori, A., et al. 2002. St. Louis encephalitis virus induced pathology in cultured cells. *Arch Virol*, **147**, 1105–19.

Paul, W.S., Moore, P.S., et al. 1993. Outbreak of Japanese encephalitis on the island of Saipan, 1990. *J Infect Dis*, **167**, 1053–8.

Perelygin, A.A., Scherbik, S.V., et al. 2002. Positional cloning of the murine flavivirus resistance gene. *Proc Natl Acad Sci U S A*, **99**, 9322–7.

Petersen, L.R. and Marfin, A.A. 2002. West Nile virus: a primer for the clinician. *Ann Intern Med*, **137**, 173–9.

Petersen, L.R. and Roehrig, J.T. 2001. West Nile virus: a reemerging global pathogen. *Emerg Infect Dis*, **7**, 611–14.

Pletnev, A.G., Yamshikov, V.F. and Blinov, V.M. 1990. Nucleotide sequence of the genome and complete amino acid sequence of the polyprotein of tick-borne encephalitis virus. *Virology*, **174**, 250–63.

Potts, B.J., Sever, J.L., et al. 1987. Possible role of pestiviruses in microcephaly. *Lancet*, **1**, 972–3.

Prikhod'ko, G.G., Prikhod'ko, E.A., et al. 2001. Infection with Langat flavivirus or expression of the envelope protein induces apoptotic cell death. *Virology*, **286**, 328–35.

Prikhod'ko, G.G., Prikhod'ko, E.A., et al. 2002. Langat flavivirus protease NS3 binds caspase-8 and induces apoptosis. *J Virol*, **76**, 5701–10.

Reed, W. 1902. Recent researches concerning etiology, propagation and prevention of yellow fever, by the United States Army Commission. *J Hyg*, **2**, 101–19.

Reid, H.W. 1988. Louping-ill. In: Monath, T.P. (ed.), *The arboviruses: ecology and epidemiology*, vol. III. Boca Raton, FL: CRC Press, 117–36.

Renard, A., Guiot, C., et al. 1985. Molecular cloning of bovine viral diarrhea viral sequences. *DNA*, **4**, 429–38.

Renard, A., Schmetz, D.A., et al. 1987. Molecular cloning of the bovine viral diarrhea virus genome RNA. *Ann Rech Vet*, **18**, 121–5.

Rey, F.A., Heinz, F.X., et al. 1995. The envelope glycoprotein from tick-borne encephalitis virus at 2 A resolution. *Nature (Lond)*, **375**, 291–8.

Rice, C.M., Lenches, E.M., et al. 1985. Nucleotide sequence of yellow fever virus: implications for flavivirus gene expression and evolution. *Science*, **229**, 726–33.

Rico-Hesse, R. 1990. Molecular evolution and distribution of dengue viruses type 1 and 2 in nature. *Virology*, **174**, 479–93.

Rico-Hesse, R., Harrison, L.M., et al. 1997. Origins of dengue type 2 viruses associated with increased pathogenicity in the Americas. *Virology*, **230**, 244–51.

Roehrig, J.T. 2000. Arboviruses. In: Specter, S., Hodinka, R. and Young, S.A. (eds), *Manual of clinical laboratory immunology*, 6th edn. Washington, DC: American Society for Microbiology, 356–73.

Roehrig, J.T., Bolin, R.A. and Kelly, R.G. 1998. Monoclonal antibody mapping of the envelope glycoprotein of the dengue 2 virus, Jamaica. *Virology*, **246**, 317–28.

Roehrig, J.T., Layton, M., et al. 2002. The emergence of West Nile virus in North America: ecology, epidemiology, and surveillance. *Curr Top Microbiol Immunol*, **267**, 223–40.

Rosen, L. 1977. The Emperor's New Clothes revisited, or reflections on the pathogenesis of dengue hemorrhagic fever. *Am J Trop Med Hyg*, **26**, 337–43.

Rosen, L. 1986a. The natural history of Japanese encephalitis. *Annu Rev Microbiol*, **40**, 395–414.

Rosen, L. 1986b. The pathogenesis of dengue hemorrhagic fever – a critical appraisal of current hypotheses. *South African Med J*, Suppl, 40–2.

Rosen, L. 1987. Overwintering mechanisms of mosquito-borne arboviruses in temperate climates. *Am J Trop Med Hyg*, **37**, 69–76S.

Rosen, L. 1989. Disease exacerbation caused by sequential dengue infections: myth or reality. *Rev Infect Dis*, **11**, Suppl 4, S840–2.

Rümenapf, T., Unger, G., et al. 1993. Processing of the envelope glycoproteins of pestivirus. *J Virol*, **67**, 3288–94.

Russell, P.K. and McCown, J. 1972. Comparison of dengue-2 and dengue-3 virus strains by neutralization tests and identification of a subtype of dengue-3. *Am J Trop Med Hyg*, **21**, 97–9.

St George, T.D., Standfast, H.A., et al. 1977. The isolation of Saumarez Reef virus, a new flavivirus, from bird ticks *Ornithodoros capensis* and *Ixodes eudyptidis* in Australia. *Aust J Exp Biol Med Sci*, **55**, 493–9.

Sangster, M.Y., Mackenzie, J.S., et al. 1998. Genetically determined resistance to flavivirus infection in wild *Mus musculus domesticus* and other taxonomic groups in the genus *Mus*. *Arch Virol*, **143**, 697–715.

Sauerwald, T.M., Betenbaugh, M.J., et al. 2002. Inhibiting apoptosis in mammalian cell culture using the caspase inhibitor XIAP and deletion mutants. *Biotechnol Bioeng*, **77**, 704–16.

Schatzmayr, H.G., Nogueira, R.M.R. and Travassos da Rosa, A.P.A. 1986. An outbreak of dengue virus at Rio de Janeiro – 1986. *Mem Inst Oswaldo Cruz*, **81**, 245–6.

Scherret, J.H., Poidinger, M., et al. 2001. The relationships between West Nile and Kunjin viruses. *Emerg Infect Dis*, **7**, 697–705.

Schlesinger, J.J., Brandriss, M.W., et al. 1987. Protection of mice against dengue 2 virus encephalitis by immunization with the dengue 2 virus non-structural glycoprotein NS1. *J Gen Virol*, **68**, 853–7.

Shafee, N. and AbuBakar, S. 2002. Zinc accelerates dengue virus type 2-induced apoptosis in Vero cells. *FEBS Lett*, **524**, 20–4.

Shellam, G.R., Sangster, M.Y., et al. 1998. Genetic control of host resistance to flavivirus infection in animals. *Rev Sci Tech*, **17**, 231–48.

Siler, J.F., Hall, M.W. and Hitchens, A.P. 1926. Dengue: its history, epidemiology, mechanisms of transmission, etiology, clinical manifestations, immunity and prevention. *Philippine J Sci*, **29**, 1–304.

Silvia, O.J., Shellam, G.R., et al. 2001. Innate resistance to flavivirus infection in mice controlled by Flv is nitric oxide-independent. *J Gen Virol*, **82**, 603–7.

Simmons, J.S., St John, J.H. and Reynolds, F.H.K. 1931. Experimental studies of dengue. *Philippine J Sci*, **44**, 1–251.

Sreenivasan, M.A., Bhat, H.R. and Rajagopalan, P.K. 1979. Studies on the transmission of Kyasanur forest disease virus by partly fed ixodid ticks. *Ind J Med Sci*, **69**, 708–13.

Strode, G.K. 1951. *Yellow fever*. New York: McGraw-Hill.

Su, H.L., Lin, Y.L., et al. 2001. The effect of human *bcl-2* and *bcl-X* genes on dengue virus-induced apoptosis in cultured cells. *Virology*, **282**, 141–53.

Su, H.L., Liao, C.L., et al. 2002. Japanese encephalitis virus infection initiates endoplasmic reticulum stress and an unfolded protein response. *J Virol*, **76**, 4162–71.

Sumiyoshi, H., Mori, C., et al. 1987. Complete nucleotide sequence of the Japanese encephalitis virus genome RNA. *Virology*, **161**, 497–510.

Trent, D.W., Grant, J.A., et al. 1989. Genetic variation and microevolution of dengue 2 virus in southeast Asia. *Virology*, **172**, 523–35.

Turell, M.J., O'Guinn, M.L., et al. 2001. Vector competence of North American mosquitoes (Diptera: *Culicidae*) for West Nile virus. *J Med Entomol*, **38**, 130–4.

Turell, M.J., Sardelis, M.R., et al. 2002. Potential vectors of West Nile virus in North America. *Curr Top Microbiol Immunol*, **267**, 241–52.

Umenai, T., Krzysko, R., et al. 1985. Japanese encephalitis: current worldwide status. *Bull WHO*, **63**, 625–31.

Urosevic, N., Silvia, O.J., et al. 1999. Development and characterization of new flavivirus-resistant mouse strains bearing Flv(r)-like and Flv(mr) alleles from wild or wild- derived mice. *J Gen Virol*, **80**, 897–906.

Utama, A., Shimizu, H., et al. 2000. Identification and characterization of the RNA helicase activity of Japanese encephalitis virus NS3 protein. *FEBS Lett*, **465**, 74–8.

Valle, R.P. and Falgout, B. 1998. Mutagenesis of the NS3 protease of dengue virus type 2. *J Virol*, **72**, 624–32.

Vasconcelos, P.F., Luna, E.J., et al. 2001. Serious adverse events associated with yellow fever 17DD vaccine in Brazil: a report of two cases. *Lancet*, **358**, 91–7.

Weiland, E., Stark, R., et al. 1990. Pestivirus glycoprotein which induces neutralizing antibodies forms part of a disulfide-linked heterodimer. *J Virol*, **64**, 3563–9.

Weiland, E., Ahl, R., et al. 1992. A second envelope glycoprotein mediates neutralization of a pestivirus. *J Virol*, **66**, 3677–82.

Weissenbock, H., Kolodziejek, J., et al. 2002. Emergence of Usutu virus, an African mosquito-borne flavivirus of the Japanese encephalitis virus group, central Europe. *Emerg Infect Dis*, **8**, 652–6.

Wengler, G., Castle, E., et al. 1985. Sequence analysis of the membrane protein V3 of the flavivirus West Nile virus and of its gene. *Virology*, **147**, 264–74.

Wengler, G., Wengler, G., et al. 1987. Analysis of the influence of proteolytic cleavage on the structural organization of the surface of the West Nile flavivirus leads to the isolation of a protease-resistant E protein oligomer from the viral surface. *Virology*, **160**, 210–19.

Wiskerchen, M. and Collett, M.S. 1991. Pestivirus gene expression: protein p80 of bovine viral diarrhea virus is a proteinase involved in polyprotein processing. *Virology*, **184**, 341–50.

Wolfe, M.S., Calisher, C.H. and McGuire, K. 1982. Spondweni virus infection in a foreign resident of Upper Volta. *Lancet*, **2**, 1306–8.

Yolken, R., Dubovi, E., et al. 1989. Infantile gastroenteritis associated with excretion of pestivirus antigens. *Lancet*, **1**, 517–20.

Yusof, R., Clum, S., et al. 2000. Purified NS2B/NS3 serine protease of dengue virus type 2 exhibits cofactor NS2B dependence for cleavage of substrates with dibasic amino acids in vitro. *J Biol Chem*, **275**, 9963–9.

Xin, Y.Y., Ming, Z.G., et al. 1988. Safety of a live-attenuated Japanese encephalitis virus vaccine (SA14-14-2) for children. *Am J Trop Med Hyg*, **39**, 214–17.

Zaki, A.M. 1997. Isolation of a flavivirus related to the tick-borne encephalitis complex from human cases in Saudi Arabia. *Trans R Soc Trop Med Hyg*, **91**, 179–81.

Zhang, Y.M., Hayes, E.P., et al. 1988. Immunization of mice with dengue structural proteins and nonstructural protein NS1 expressed by baculovirus recombinant induces resistance to dengue virus encephalitis. *J Virol*, **62**, 3027–31.

47

Togaviruses

SCOTT C. WEAVER AND ILYA V. FROLOV

CLASSIFICATION

Two decades ago the *Togaviridae* family included a wide variety of small, enveloped viruses with single-stranded RNA genomes of positive polarity of about 4×10^6 Da. These RNAs could serve directly as messenger RNA and were packaged into nucleocapsids demonstrating cubic symmetry. The family name was derived from the Latin *toga* (a Roman mantle or cloak) and refers to the lipid envelope. However, since the *Togaviridae* was first defined, its contents have changed significantly based on accumulated data about viral replication and nucleotide sequences of the genomes. Flaviviruses, pestiviruses, and arteriviruses, which were temporarily brought together with alphaviruses and rubella virus, were finally classified into different families (Weaver et al. 2000). Currently the Togaviridae is comprised of two genera, *Alphavirus* and *Rubivirus*. Twenty-eight known alphaviruses are grouped into eight complexes, the prototypes of which are *Western equine encephalitis virus* (WEEV), *Eastern equine encephalitis virus* (EEEV), *Venezuelan equine encephalitis virus* (VEEV), *Semliki Forest virus* (SFV), *Middelburg virus* (MIDV), *Ndumu virus* (NDUV), *Trocara virus* (TROCV), and *Salmon pancreas disease virus* (SPDV) (Table 47.1). Partially or completely sequenced genomes of different alphaviruses reveal at least 60 percent nucleotide sequence identity in the nonstructural and 40 percent or more identity in the structural proteins. Sequencing and phylogenetic studies have indicated that WEEV, *Highlands J virus* (HJV)

and *Fort Morgan virus* (FMV) are recombinant New World alphaviruses whose glycoproteins were derived from a Sindbis-like ancestor, the remainder of the genome being derived from an EEE-like ancestor (Figure 47.1, p. 1012). Phylogenetic studies suggest only three clearly defined virus groups: a VEE/EEE group, an SF group (including MIDV), and a Sindbis group (Powers et al. 2001).

Most alphaviruses are described as arthropod-borne, or arboviruses that are maintained in nature through biological transmission among vertebrate hosts by arthropod vectors, predominantly mosquitoes (Griffin 2001a). However, the recent finding of salmon pancreas disease and sleeping disease alphaviruses indicates that arthropod vectors may not be required for the circulation of all alphaviruses.

Alphaviruses have highly differing abilities to cause disease in humans and animals. Some of them, including VEEV, EEEV and WEEV, can cause severe epidemic encephalitis, with a high mortality rate. Infection by others usually leads to either serious, but not life-threatening, illnesses or clinically inapparent infection with mild symptoms, including headache, fever, skin rashes, and arthritis. Many alphaviruses (at least mosquito-transmitted ones) are believed to have similar lifecycles, structures of viral particles, and replication strategies (Griffin 2001a).

The genus *Rubivirus* (Chapter 45, Rubella) consists of a single known member, *Rubella virus*. Alphaviruses and rubella virus do not have significant primary sequence

Table 47.1 *List of alphaviruses*

Antigenic complex	Species (abbreviation)	Subtype	Clinical syndrome	Distribution
Barmah Forest	*Barmah Forest virus* (BFV)		Febrile illness, rash, arthritis	Australia
Eastern equine encephalitis (EEE)	EEE virus (EEEV)		Febrile illness, encephalitis (none recognized in Latin America)	North, Central, South America
Middelburg	*Middelburg virus* (MIDV)		None recognized	Africa
Ndumu	*Ndumu virus* (NDUV)		None recognized	Africa
Semliki Forest	*Semliki Forest virus* (SFV)		Febrile illness	Africa
	Chikungunya virus (CHIKV)		Febrile illness, rash, arthritis	Africa
	O'nyong-nyong virus (ONNV)		Febrile illness, rash, arthritis	Africa
	Getah virus (GETV)		None recognized	Asia
	Bebaru virus (BEBV)		None recognized	Malaysia
	Ross River virus (RRV)	Sagiyama	Febrile illness, rash, arthritis	Australia, Oceania
	Mayaro virus (MAYV)		Febrile illness, rash, arthritis	South and Central America, Trinidad
	Una virus (UNAV)		None recognized	South America
Venezuelan equine encephalitis (VEE)	VEE virus (VEEV)	IAB	Febrile illness, encephalitis	North, Central, South America
		IC	Febrile illness, encephalitis	South America
		ID	Febrile illness, encephalitis	South America, Panama
		IE	Febrile illness, encephalitis	Central America, Mexico
	Everglades virus (EVEV)		Febrile illness, encephalitis	Florida (USA)
	Mucambo virus (MUCV)		Febrile illness, myalgia	South America, Trinidad
		strain 71D1252	Unknown	Peru
	Tonate virus (TONV)		Febrile illness, encephalitis	Brazil, Colorado (USA)
	Pixuna virus (PIXV)		Febrile illness, myalgia	Brazil
	Cabassou virus (CABV)		None recognized	French Guiana
	AG80-663 virus (AGV)		Febrile illness, myalgia	Argentina
	Mosso das Pedras virus (MDPV)		None recognized	Brazil
Western equine encephalitis (WEE)	*Sindbis virus* (SINV)		Febrile illness, rash, arthritis	Africa, Europe, Asia, Australia
		Babanki	Febrile illness, rash, arthritis	Africa
		Ockelbo	Febrile illness, rash, arthritis	Europe
		Kyzylagach	None recognized	Azerbaijan, China
	Whataroa virus (WHAV)		None recognized	New Zealand
	Aura virus (AURAV)		None recognized	South America
	WEEV	Several	Febrile illness, encephalitis	Western North, South America
	Highlands J virus (HJV)			Eastern North America
	Fort Morgan virus (FMV)	Buggy Creek	None recognized	Western North America
Trocara	*Trocara virus* (TROV)		None recognized	South America
Salmon pancreas disease (SPD)	SPD virus (SPDV)		Pancreatic disease (salmon)	Atlantic Ocean and tributaries
		Sleeping disease virus	Sleeping disease (trout)	Worldwide

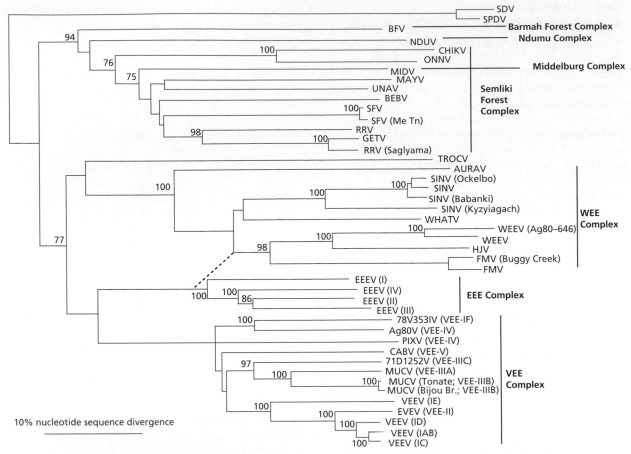

Figure 47.1 *Phylogenetic tree of all* Alphavirus *species, and selected subtypes and variants (in parentheses). Virus abbreviations are found in Table 47.1. Numbers refer to bootstrap values for clades defined by the adjacent node.*

homology in structural and nonstructural proteins. However, the coding strategies, their genomes, mechanisms of replication and structure of viral particles demonstrate a number of similarities, suggesting a common ancestry and supporting their inclusion in the same family *Togaviridae*.

VIRION STRUCTURE

Alphavirus virions are about 70 nm in diameter and are composed of an icosahedral nucleocapsid with T = 4 symmetry, surrounded by a lipid envelope containing glycoprotein spikes. The three-dimensional organization of viral particles has been determined for Ross River virus (RRV), Sindbis virus (SINV), and VEEV, which represent three different *Alphavirus* complexes. Electron cryomicroscopy and image reconstruction demonstrated that for these viruses the envelope glycoproteins are arranged on the outer surface of particles in a very similar way. The 240 heterodimers of E1 and E2 are combined into 80 trimers forming glycoprotein spikes that are distributed on the surface of viral particles in a T = 4 icosahedral lattice that mirrors the symmetry of the nucleocapsid. The regularity of spike distribution is determined by the direct interaction of glycoprotein

heterodimers with capsid protein subunits. The E1 glycoprotein, which is structurally homologous to the envelope glycoprotein of flaviviruses, appears to lie parallel to the lipid envelope (Lescar et al. 2001), whereas the E2 glycoprotein projects outward from the virion to form the spikes.

GENOME STRUCTURE AND REPLICATION

The *Alphavirus* genome is a single-stranded RNA molecule of positive polarity nearly 12 000 nucleotides in length, with a sedimentation coefficient of ca. 42–49S (Schlesinger and Schlesinger 2001; Strauss and Strauss 1994). The genomic RNA mimics the structure of cellular messenger RNA: it contains a 5′ methylguanylate cap structure and a 3′ polyadenylate sequence. The nonstructural viral proteins coded by the 5′ two-thirds of the genome are translated directly from this RNA immediately following its introduction to the cytosol. Structural proteins are coded by the subgenomic RNA that corresponds to the 3′ one-third of the genome. The subgenomic 26S RNA, transcribed from the subgenomic promoter located on the minus-strand intermediate of the viral genome, is also capped and polyadenylated. The full-length minus-strand intermediate is synthesized on the template of viral genomic RNA and serves as a template for both subgenomic and genomic RNAs. The general scheme of *Alphavirus* replication is demonstrated in Figure 47.2. Synthesis of all three RNAs is asymmetric and highly regulated. Minus-strand synthesis is detectable only within the first 4 h post infection, whereas later only plus-strand RNAs (genome and subgenome) are being synthesized. This regulation is achieved via the sequential processing of the nonstructural proteins. Initially they are synthesized for different alphaviruses as two polypeptides, P123 and P1234, or just single P1234. This difference in synthesis of nonstructural proteins depends on the presence of the opal codon at the end of nsP3. Some alphaviruses contain this terminating codon, and P1234 can be synthesized only upon readthrough of the UGA that occurs with 5–20 percent efficiency. Other alphaviruses contain arginine or cysteine codons in place of UGA, and only P1234 is translated. This polyprotein comprises sequences of all four nonstructural proteins, nsP1, nsP2, nsP3, and nsP4, and its processing is mediated by the protease domain of nsP2. First autoproteolytic cleavage

is performed in *cis* and results in the release of P123 and nsP4. These two proteins form the viral component of the replicative complex, and this replicative complex is active for minus-strand synthesis but is inefficient in generating the plus-strand genome and subgenomic RNAs. Further cleavage of nsP1/nsP2 and nsP2/nsP3 junctions is also performed by nsP2 protease, this time in *trans*, which changes the template specificity of replicative complex by making it incapable of minus-strand RNA synthesis and significantly increasing its activity in plus-strand RNAs production. The time of genomic and subgenomic RNA synthesis concurs with the most efficient release of viral particles, which requires high-level production of viral genomes and structural proteins for packaging. In spite of a great deal of progress in understanding *Alphavirus* genome replication, the detailed mechanism of viral nonstructural protein functioning is not completely understood. nsP1 possesses both guanine-7-methyltransferase and guanyltransferase activities required for capping of both genomic and subgenomic RNA. This protein also appears to be involved in binding of the replicative complexes to the membranes. nsP2 has a number of activities. Its amino terminal domain is considered to have helicase function,

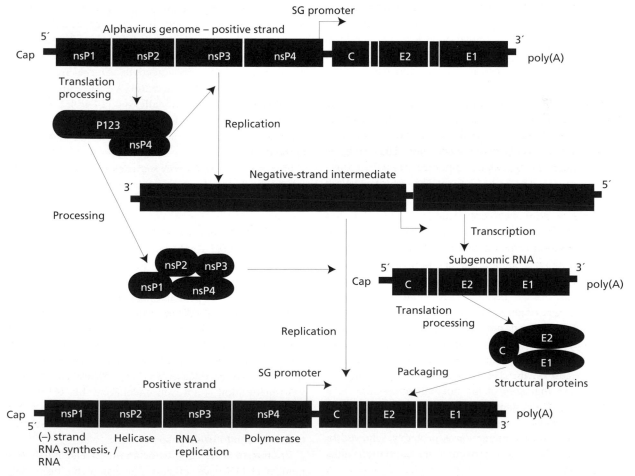

Figure 47.2 *Organization of the* Alphavirus *genome and schematic presentation of* Alphavirus *replication*

and the carboxy terminal part of the protein is a protease that orchestrates the processing of nonstructural proteins. Point mutations in this protein or in the nsP2/nsP3 cleavage site change the ratio of genome/subgenome RNA synthesis, suggesting that this protein is involved in the functioning of the subgenomic promoter. This protein accumulates in infected cells in a ten-fold excess to nsP4, and a significant fraction is transported to the nucleus. A number of mutations in this protein convert cytopathic alphaviruses, SINV and SFV into noncytopathic variants, which can persist in some cell lines of vertebrate origin (Frolova et al. 2002). These facts suggest that, in addition to its role in RNA replication, nsP2 may have additional functions in virus–host cell interactions. nsP3 is the least-studied protein, with unidentified functions. It can tolerate extensive deletions in C-terminal sequence that have very low sequence identity among alphaviruses, but mutations in the other fragments can make virus replication temperature sensitive. nsP4 is the RNA polymerase and contains the characteristic GDD motif found in all RNA-dependent polymerases. Mutations in this protein can make replicative complexes incapable of both minus- and plus-strand RNAs synthesis.

Alphavirus genomes contain a number of conserved sequences, so-called *cis*-acting elements that are required for replication. These short sequences include a 19-nt conserved sequence element (CSE), which immediately precedes the 3′ terminal poly(A) tract. The location of the 19-nt CSE suggests that it is an important element of the promoter for minus-strand RNA synthesis. Mutations in this sequence are either lethal or significantly alter virus replication. Another conserved sequence, 24-nt CSE, was identified as a promoter for transcription of the subgenomic RNA that functions on the minus-strand replicative intermediate. The 5′ termini of viral genomes appear to contain at least two functional elements. The 51-nt CSE (nt 155–205 of SINV) is located inside the nsP1-coding sequence and is predicted to form two short stem-loop structures. This CSE was shown to function as a replicational enhancer that operates in a host-dependent manner. Point mutations in this element alter virus replication in more mosquito cells than in cells of mammalian origin. The 5′UTR of alphaviruses was always believed to contain a promoter element that is required for initiation of the plus-strand RNA synthesis, and mutations in the 5′UTR significantly downregulate virus replication. The 5′ *cis*-acting elements not only determine plus-strand RNA synthesis when present on the 3′ end of minus-strand replicative intermediate, but control the minus-strand synthesis as well. The compelling evidence suggests that the 5′ and 3′ ends of *Alphavirus* genome RNAs interact to initiate replication, and this interaction is probably achieved by bringing them into close proximity via translation initiation factors.

STRUCTURAL PROTEINS

Alphavirus structural proteins are translated from the subgenomic RNA. Like the nonstructural proteins, they are synthesized as a single polypeptide that is cleaved both co- and post-translationally. Structural proteins are coded in the order capsid (C), E3, E2, 6K, and E1. The capsid is 260–270 amino acids in length (30–34 kDa), and the crystal structure has been solved for Sindbis virus. The capsid protein is synthesized first, possesses a serine protease activity, but in contrast to the nonstructural protease, the nsP2, it acts only in *cis* and cleaves itself from the polypeptide chain that is still being translated. This cleavage releases the signal peptide from the E3 (10 kDa) protein, leading to translocation of both E3 and E2 (PE2, sometimes called P62) into the endoplasmic reticulum (ER). PE2 remains attached to membranes via hydrophobic amino acids in the carboxy terminal part that function as a membrane anchor. The very end of the PE2 contains a signal sequence for translocation into the ER of the amino terminal part of the next short protein, 6K, whose role in virus particle formation is not well understood. In turn, the C-terminal part of 6K serves as the signal peptide required for transport of the last protein, E1, into ER. The latter protein also possesses a hydrophobic anchor on the C terminus. Proteolytic cleavages between PE2 and 6K, as well as between 6K and E1, are performed by cell signalases. The last, very critical, cleavage in the E3/E2 cleavage site is accomplished by a furin-type protease and is required for viral infectivity. During transport to the plasma membrane in secretory vesicles, the envelope proteins are postranslationally modified: E2 (420–424 amino acids) and E1 (438–442 amino acids) acquire oligosaccharides, become palmitoylated, and form heterodimers.

Formation of *Alphavirus* particles is based on specific RNA–protein and protein–protein interactions. The nucleocapsid protein is capable of selectively packaging viral genomes. It recognizes the encapsidation signal(s) located in the sequence of the nonstructural proteins in the viral genomic RNA and, after further oligomerization, 240 molecules of the capsid protein form an icosahedral nucleocapsid. During the final steps of viral replication, the capsid protein molecules in completely or partially assembled nucleocapsids interact with the cytoplasmic domain of E2 in E1–E2 heterodimers on the cell membrane. This leads to envelopment of the nucleocapsid by the plasma membrane containing glycoprotein spikes, and to the release of virus particles. This stage of virus maturation is not well understood, but it has been demonstrated that nucleocapsids undergo conformational changes and heterodimers of glycoproteins appear to assemble into trimeric spikes.

Because of their close association, E1 and E2 share a number of biological functions and antigenic properties.

The glycoprotein spike functions both in attachment to cellular receptors and in fusion with cellular membranes. The E2 glycoprotein elicits high-titer virus-specific neutralizing antibody. Two domains capable of eliciting neutralizing antibody have been identified in the E2 glycoprotein: amino acids 114–120, 180–220 (or 230–250 for RRV) using monoclonal antibody neutralization escape variants and rapid penetration variants. Antibodies to the carboxyl-proximal domain neutralize virus infectivity by blocking virion attachment to susceptible cells. Antibodies to the E2 glycoprotein can also block virus hemagglutination, presumably because of its close association with E1. The amino terminal 25 amino acids of the VEEV E2 glycoprotein protect mice from virus challenge. Mutations in the E2 glycoprotein have been associated with differences in virulence and the ability to infect and replicate in mosquitoes.

The E1 glycoprotein contains a highly conserved amino acid sequence (amino acids 80–96), which has sequence and chemical similarities to regions responsible for cell membrane fusion in orthomyxoviruses and paramyxoviruses. Mutation of this region alters the fusion characteristics of the virus. Because cell-membrane fusion seems, therefore, to be mediated by the E1 glycoprotein, it is not surprising that this glycoprotein elicits potent hemagglutination-inhibiting antibody. Virus-neutralizing anti-E1 antibodies have also been identified. Binding of these antibodies has been associated with E1 amino acid 132 using monoclonal antibody neutralization escape variants. Anti-E1 antibodies are usually not serotype specific and fix complement well.

Many of the biologically important epitopes on both the E1 and the E2 glycoproteins are conformational. This result makes mimicking these antigens in subunit or peptide vaccines difficult. The C protein elicits broadly cross-reactive antibody and is also a major complement-fixing antigen.

VIRUS–HOST CELL INTERACTIONS

Most data on *Alphavirus* replication in vitro were derived from experiments on relatively nonpathogenic members of the genus, SINV and SFV, but are probably applicable to most members of the genus. In general, alphaviruses can infect a wide variety of hosts and cell lines of vertebrate and invertebrate origin. Infection is initiated by virion attachment to cellular receptors. Their broad host range strongly indicates that alphaviruses can either attach to multiple receptors on the cell surface or use a very conserved protein as a receptor. Both of these assumptions appear to be correct. Several receptors have been identified for SINV in different cells (reviewed by Strauss and Strauss 1994). At the same time, it was unambiguously demonstrated that after adaptation of SINV or VEEV to BHK-21 cells that are traditionally used for their propagation, both viruses

accumulate point mutations in structural glycoprotein E2, causing them to bind efficiently to heparan sulfate-like molecules (Griffin 2001a). The E2 is a protein that interacts directly with cell receptors. It is generally believed that amino acids 180–220 are directly involved in this interaction, because a considerable fraction of antibodies with neutralizing activity are specific to this peptide. Alphaviruses enter the cells via the endocytic pathway. Next, internalized virus-containing vesicles transform into endosomes, and an acidic pH leads to conformational changes in the glycoprotein spikes, trimerization of the E1 subunits, and fusion of viral and endosomal membranes. The E1 glycoprotein contains a very conserved peptide (amino acids 80–96) that was suggested to have fusogenic activity. It was recently demonstrated that the three-dimensional structure of E protein of tick-borne encephalitis virus (*Flavivirus* genus) and E1 of SFV have a number of similarities, particularly in the position of their fusogenic domains (Lescar et al. 2001). Fusion of the membranes leads to the release of nucleocapsids into the cytoplasm, and the next steps of virus disassembly are performed by ribosomes. *Alphavirus* capsid proteins have a very high affinity to ribosomes, and translocation of capsids to ribosomes results in uncoating of viral genomes and initiation of replication.

Replication of alphaviruses profoundly affects the metabolism of vertebrate cells with the inhibition of protein, RNA, and DNA synthesis playing the central role. Replication appears to activate two competing processes. First, viruses change the cellular environment to meet the needs of their propagation. At the same time, cells respond to virus replication by downregulating virus growth and activating signaling pathways, followed by secretion of cytokines that prevent dissemination of the infection. The balance between these two mechanisms appears to determine the outcome of infection on the cellular level. In spite of very extensive investigation, it is still undetermined as to what mechanism or combination of different mechanisms defines the five- to ten-fold inhibition of translation that takes place 4–8 h post-infection. However, the translational shutoff is specific to cellular mRNAs. Alphavirus subgenomic RNA is translated very efficiently in this significantly changed intracellular environment owing to the unique structural element, a translational enhancer, located downstream from the initiating AUG. This enhancer and high concentration of the subgenomic RNA make this template the only RNA translated in the cells during the late stage of the infection.

Downregulation of transcription is the second major event in alphavirus-infected cells (Frolova et al. 2002). Both messenger and ribosomal RNAs are synthesized less efficiently, if at all, in permissive cell lines. Transcriptional shutoff may play an important role in the inhibition of interferon (IFN) production by infected cells and a more efficient dissemination of the infection. Owing to dramatic changes in the intracellular environment, cells die within 24–48 h of infection, and their death is usually accompanied by apoptotic changes (Griffin 2001a).

TRANSMISSION CYCLES AND DISTRIBUTION

Most alphaviruses are **ar**thropod-**bo**rne, or **arbo**viruses, and are maintained in nature through biological transmission between susceptible vertebrate hosts by hematophagous arthropods. Arboviruses multiply and produce viremia in the vertebrate, replicate in the tissues of arthropods – obligately in the midgut and salivary glands – and are transmitted to new vertebrates when the arthropod takes a subsequent blood meal after a period of extrinsic incubation. The term arbovirus has no taxonomic significance and encompasses a heterogeneous group of viruses in seven taxonomic families, including the *Togaviridae* (alphaviruses only).

All alphaviruses are zoonotic and have at least two hosts, one a vertebrate and the other a hematophagous arthropod. The majority of alphaviruses are maintained in complex lifecycles involving one or more nonhuman vertebrate reservoir hosts and one or more arthropod vectors; an example is EEEV (Figure 47.3). These cycles remain undetected until humans or domesticated animals encroach on an enzootic focus, or the virus escapes the primary cycle via a secondary vector or vertebrate host as the result of some ecological or genetic change. Humans and domestic animals generally become involved only after the virus is brought into the peridomestic environment by a bridge vector, or after they enter an enzootic transmission focus. Humans and domestic animals, which frequently develop clinical illness, are usually considered 'dead-end' hosts because they do not produce viremia sufficient to infect vector arthropods and contribute to the transmission cycle, or because they are not bitten by a sufficient number of vectors when viremic. Many alphaviruses have several different vertebrate hosts and some are capable of

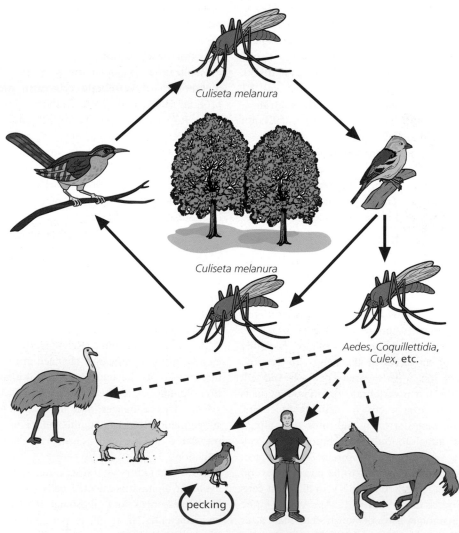

Figure 47.3 *Transmission cycle of Eastern equine encephalitis virus. Dashed arrows indicate dead-end transmission to hosts that generally do not infect additional vectors or vertebrates.*

transmission by more than one vector. A few alphaviruses, such as Chikungunya virus (CHIKV) and potentially VEEV, cause sufficient viremia in humans to be transmitted in a human–arthropod–human cycle. Transovarial transmission in nature has been demonstrated for SINV and RRV, and may facilitate maintenance of these alphaviruses in nature.

Every *Alphavirus* has its own distinct ecology. For some, such as SINV, EEEV (Figure 47.3) and WEEV (Figure 47.4), birds are the principal reservoir host, and others such as VEEV rely principally on rodents. The reservoir hosts of many alphaviruses are not known with certainty. Several, including CHIKV, EEEV, WEEV, VEEV, and SINV, have been isolated from bats, and these hosts deserve further study. All alphaviruses infecting humans are mosquito-borne. Several alphaviruses, including MIDV, CHIKV, and SINV, have also been isolated from ticks, but the significance of these findings is unknown. FMV and Bijou Bridge (a variant of

Tonate virus in the VEE complex) are believed to use as their vectors cimicid bugs that occupy bird nests.

Alphaviruses have a nearly worldwide geographical distribution. Previously only the Antarctic area was believed to be *Alphavirus*-free, but a recent discovery of southern elephant seal *Alphavirus* (La Linn et al. 2001) indicates that our knowledge of their distribution is probably far from complete. The majority of alphaviruses are found in tropical developing countries. The greatest number have been described from Africa and South America, where the flora and fauna are diverse and extensive ecological and epidemiological studies have been conducted. The smaller number of viruses described from Asia, which has ecological diversity comparable to that of Africa and tropical America, may simply reflect the lack of surveillance in that region. The geographical distribution of each *Alphavirus* is limited by the ecological parameters governing its transmission cycle, including temperature, rainfall patterns,

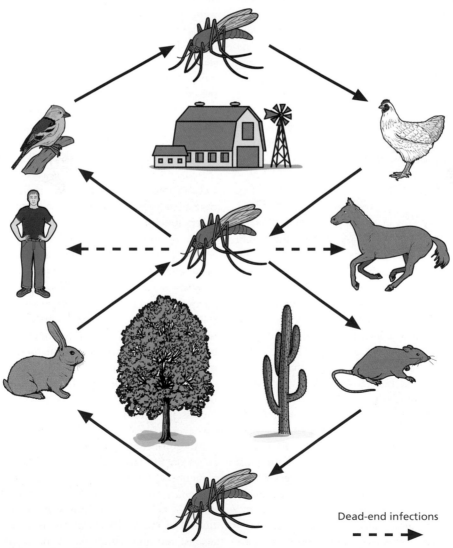

Dead-end infections

Figure 47.4 *Transmission cycles of Western equine encephalitis virus*

distribution of the arthropod vector(s), and vertebrate reservoir host(s).

Mosquitoes are by far the most important *Alphavirus* vectors, and bugs (*Cimicidae*) are also involved in the transmission of some alphaviruses. In addition to arthropod transmission, several alphaviruses, such as VEEV, are highly infectious by aerosol and numerous laboratory infections have occurred. Because of their aerosol infectivity, stability, and high degree of virulence, VEEV, EEEV, and WEEV are considered potential agents of biological warfare and terrorism.

DISEASES CAUSED BY ALPHAVIRUSES

Of the 28 currently described alphavirus species, at least 13 are known to cause disease in humans (Table 47.1). The majority of *Alphavirus* infections in humans cause a nonspecific febrile illness that is easily mistaken for infection by a respiratory virus such as influenza, or for dengue in the tropics. Onset is usually sudden, with fever, headache, myalgias, malaise, and occasionally prostration. The same virus can cause a variety of clinical syndromes. Infection with some alphaviruses, such as VEEV, EEEV, and WEEV, may lead to more severe disease, such as encephalitis, often with a fatal outcome or permanent neurological sequelae. These and some other alphaviruses are also responsible for disease in animals, notably *Equidae*. Often only a small proportion of people infected with these potentially encephalitic arboviruses progress to overt encephalitis; most develop only the prodromal, nonspecific stage of the infection, which may even be asymptomatic.

PATHOGENESIS

In vertebrates, initial sites of replication include skeletal muscle (EEEV, WEEV, SFV, RRV, SINV, and Getah virus (GETV)), and Langerhans' cells in the skin, leading to infection of the draining lymph node (VEEV, and probably others) (Griffin, 2001a; 2001b; Tsai et al. 2002). Plasma viremia is probably the main form of dissemination to other tissues and organs. Viruses such as RRV that cause a rash replicate in the skin, and RRV and CHIKV are also believed to replicate in striated muscle. Experimental studies have shown that invasion of the central nervous system (CNS), when this occurs, generally follows initial virus replication in various peripheral sites and a period of viremia exceeding a threshold for CNS entry. Entry to the CNS through the olfactory tract has been demonstrated for VEEV in a mouse model, but has not been investigated for most alphaviruses, and pathogenesis in humans is very poorly understood. CNS invasion may also occur through endothelial cells.

Alphaviruses can also cause pathology in their mosquito vectors, though vector pathogenesis has only been investigated thoroughly in a few cases. WEEV and EEEV kill midgut epithelial cells, their initial sites of replication, and this pathology may hasten dissemination of virus from the midgut to the salivary glands by facilitating passage through the basal lamina. Although mosquito pathology reduces the survival of mosquitoes infected with EEEV, the late timing of mortality may result in little effect on virus transmission.

IMMUNE RESPONSE AND DIAGNOSIS

Alphaviruses are highly immunogenic, and both cellular and humoral immune mechanisms contribute to recovery following natural or experimental infection. Humoral immunity is believed to be more important for protection (Tsai et al. 2002).

Alphavirus infections are diagnosed on the basis of either immunoglobulin M (IgM) and immunoglobulin G (IgG) serological responses, or by isolation of virus from acute-phase serum. Serological tests commonly employed include IgM or IgG ELISA, plaque reduction neutralization, hemagglutination inhibition, or complement fixation. Virus isolation is readily accomplished using a variety of vertebrate cells, such as Vero or baby hamster kidney (BHK), or using mosquito cells such as C6/36. Intracranial inoculation of newborn mice is more sensitive than cell culture for some alphaviruses. Alphaviruses are seldom recovered from the CNS, including the cerebrospinal fluid (CSF), except from fatal cases. A large array of antialphavirus murine monoclonal antibodies is available for virus identification.

CONTROL OF ALPHAVIRAL DISEASE

Because most alphaviruses are maintained in zoonotic transmission cycles, little can be done in an ecologically acceptable manner to control levels of virus circulation. The interruption of transmission to humans by mosquito control provides the only effective approach to control most alphaviral diseases. Control of some alphaviral diseases such as EEE relies on early detection of enzootic amplification in reservoir hosts (e.g. birds), followed by mosquito control to reduce vector populations in inhabited regions. Sentinel animals can also be used to detect virus circulation, or testing of potential mosquito vector pools for virus infection. For equine encephalitides such as EEE and VEE, equine cases usually precede human infection by a few weeks, and are useful indicators of the need for vector control (Weaver 2001a, b).

Mosquito control to reduce vector populations usually relies on the large-scale application of adulticides – or sometimes larvicides – in regions of enzootic or epidemic transmission. The inaccessibility of many enzootic habitats necessitates aerial insecticide applications. For many alphaviral diseases, personal protection against mosquito bites is the most effective means of human disease prevention. This is especially important for individuals who reside, work, or recreate near habitats known or suspected of harboring enzootic transmission. Diethylmethylbenzamide (DEET) (35 percent formulations recommended; 10 percent for children) is the most effective mosquito repellent generally approved for use on the skin, and permethrin can be applied to clothing and camping gear to enhance protection. Education of persons likely to contact enzootic habitats is also important for preventing human infection.

There are no licensed human alphavirus vaccines. Equine vaccines are available for EEEV, WEEV, VEEV, and GETV. For some alphaviruses, such as VEEV, that require equines for efficient amplification to infect large numbers of people, equine vaccination can be effective in limiting human disease.

ENCEPHALITIS AND OTHER IMPORTANT ALPHAVIRUS DISEASES

Eastern equine encephalitis

HISTORY AND DISTRIBUTION

EEEV was first isolated in 1933 from the brain of an infected horse, and in Argentina in 1930 (identified retrospectively). EEEV occurs in hardwood swamp habitats near the eastern seaboard, the Gulf coast, and at some inland midwestern locations of the USA, and in Canada, some Caribbean Islands, Mexico, and Central and South America (Scott and Weaver 1989; Weaver 2001a). Small outbreaks of human disease have occurred in the USA, the Dominican Republic, Cuba, and Jamaica. More extensive equine epizootics are common during the summer in temperate areas of the USA and Argentina, and as far north as Québec, Ontario, and Alberta in Canada. Four distinct antigenic variants representing distinct genetic lineages of EEEV have been delineated; three occur in Latin America and do not appear to cause human disease. The fourth is represented by all strains from North America and the Caribbean, and is highly virulent for people.

TRANSMISSION CYCLES

EEEV circulates nearly continuously in tropical and subtropical locations, and appears to overwinter in temperate areas of the USA by an unknown mechanism (Weaver 2001a). In North America, enzootic circulation involves passerine bird reservoir hosts and *Culiseta melanura*, an ornithophilic mosquito that is found in hardwood swamp habitats (Figure 47.3). The distribution of EEEV closely approximates that of *Cs. melanura*, suggesting that it is the principal enzootic vector. Larvae of *Cs. melanura* develop at the base of trees or under roots in swampy, peat soils. Because humans, equines,

and most other animals apart from passerine birds are believed to be dead-end hosts, and *Cs. melanura* is probably by far the most efficient vector, human and equine cases are generally found in close proximity to swamp habitats; epizootic transmission probably involves bridge vectors such as *Coquillettidia perturbans*, *Ochlerotatus canadensis*, and *Oc. sollicitans*, which feed on both birds and mammals and can transmit to humans, horses, and other hosts. Other species, such as *Aedes vexans* in temperate regions and *Oc. taeniorhynchus*, *Culex taeniopus*, and *Cx. nigripalpus* in the tropics, may be involved in transmission to humans and equines. The EEEV transmission cycle in Latin America is poorly characterized, but probably involves enzootic vectors in the subgenus *Culex (Melanoconion)*, and possibly birds and rodents as reservoir hosts.

DISEASE AND VIRAL GENETICS

Although not well documented, rates of inapparent (encephalitis) infection suggest that most human EEEV infections result in a nonspecific prodromal illness characterized by fever, headache, myalgias, photophobia, and dysesthesias (Tsai et al. 2002). The incubation period is 4–10 days, and the prodromal phase evolves over several days to longer than a week before the onset of encephalitis in some patients, especially young children and the elderly. The development of encephalitis is typically accompanied by severe frontal headache, dizziness, vomiting, lethargy, and later, neck stiffness, confusion, delirium, and drowsiness, sometimes leading to coma. Patients may have other neurological disorders, such as abnormal reflexes, spasticity, paralysis, and cranial nerve palsies, and infants may have convulsions and bulging fontanelles. The CSF is under pressure, has elevated protein, and pleocytosis is common. EEEV infection is also accompanied by visceral and pulmonary congestion. In the brain, loss of neurons, perivascular cuffing, microglial proliferation, and focal inflammatory infiltration are the most typical findings of human encephalitis. Vascular lesions are also common, with thrombi and extravasation of red cells, and necrosis and demyelinization also occur. Apoptosis occurs in glial and inflammatory cells, but is less commonly associated with neuronal cell death. Overall mortality rates during more recent outbreaks have averaged about 33 percent.

An EEEV vaccine is not available for general human use, although formalin-inactivated vaccines are effective in horses if administered frequently.

Genetically and antigenically, EEEV is highly conserved in North America, where a single, highly conserved lineage has evolved since 1933 (Weaver 2001a). The North American strains have also caused outbreaks as far south as Mexico and the Caribbean. EEEV strains isolated in Latin America are more genetically and antigenically diverse. There is no evidence that Central/South American strains of EEEV cause human encephalitis, or even a febrile illness. Detection of human antibodies in South America suggests that the explanation for the lack of human encephalitis cases there is related to a difference in human virulence between the North and South/Central American virus lineages.

Western equine encephalitis

HISTORY AND DISTRIBUTION

WEEV was first isolated in California in 1930 from the brain of a horse, and remains an important cause of encephalitis in *Equidae* and in humans in North America, mainly in western parts of the USA and Canada (Reisen 2001; Reisen and Monath 1988). Sporadic cases also occur in Central and South America.

TRANSMISSION CYCLES

In the western USA the enzootic cycle of WEEV occurs mainly during the summer and involves passerine birds, in which the infection is inapparent. *Cx. tarsalis*, a mosquito associated with agriculture and irrigation systems, is the principal vector (Figure 47.4). A summer cycle involving jackrabbits and *Ae. melanimon* or *Oc. dorsalis* mosquitoes has also been documented in desert environments. The mechanism of WEEV overwintering in temperate climates is unknown, but chronic infection of birds has been observed after experimental infection. WEEV has also been isolated from snakes and from a variety of mammal species. In Argentina, *Oc. albifasciatus* is a probable mosquito vector.

DISEASE AND VIRAL GENETICS

Human WEE cases are usually first seen in June or July in the northern hemisphere. Most WEEV infections are asymptomatic or present as mild, nonspecific illness with fever, headache, and fatigue. Patients with clinically apparent illness usually have a sudden onset, with fever, headache, chills, nausea, myalgia, vomiting, anorexia, and malaise, followed by altered mental status, weakness, dizziness, vomiting, and signs of meningeal irritation (Tsai et al. 2002). Some patients progress to neck stiffness, weakness, and generalized tremulousness, and occasionally stupor or coma. Children, especially those under 1 year old, are affected more severely than adults and may be left with permanent sequelae, which are seen in 5–10 percent of patients. Overall mortality in apparent cases is 4 percent and is highest among the elderly.

Several genetic lineages and antigenic subtypes of WEEV have been delineated. Interestingly, unlike EEEV, some lineages of WEEV range in distribution from North to South America, and others appear to be limited to the tropics or subtropics. Virulence differ-

ences have been detected in mice, but it is unknown whether there are differences in virulence for humans.

Venezuelan equine encephalitis

HISTORY AND DISTRIBUTION

VEEV was first isolated in Venezuela in 1938 from the brain of a horse; like EEEV and WEEV, it causes encephalitis in Equidae and humans. VEE is an important veterinary and public health problem in Central and South America because equines remain important for agriculture and transportation in many regions (Walton and Grayson 1988; Weaver 2001b). Focal outbreaks occur periodically, with some spreading over large areas and causing up to hundreds-of-thousands of equine and human cases. A large epizootic that began in Guatemala and El Salvador in 1969 reached Texas in 1971; it was estimated that over 200 000 horses died in that outbreak, which was controlled by a massive equine vaccination programme using the live-attenuated TC-83 vaccine. Several thousand human infections were documented. A more recent VEE epidemic occurred in the fall of 1995 in Venezuela and Colombia, with an estimated 100 000 human infections.

TRANSMISSION CYCLES

Epizootic transmission involves horses, mules, and donkeys as amplification hosts, and a variety of mosquitoes in the genera *Ochlerotatus*, *Psorophora*, and others as vectors. Although infected people become viremic and capable of amplification by infection of mosquito vectors, epidemiological evidence (lack of any major epidemics in the absence of equine amplification) indicates that they are not as efficient as equines; this is probably due to the fewer mosquitoes sustained by viremic persons than by equines. Although most human VEE cases occur during equine epizootics, endemic transmission also occurs in communities in close proximity to sylvatic enzootic cycles in the absence of any equine disease.

DISEASE AND VIRAL GENETICS

VEEV is one of several alphaviruses in the VEE antigenic complex (Table 47.1; Figure 47.1). Only VEEV and Everglades virus (genetically a variant of VEEV in subtype ID) are associated with encephalitis in humans, but other VEE complex viruses, such as Mucambo, can cause febrile illness. All major human and equine VEE outbreaks have involved subtype IAB and IC strains of VEEV, which are capable of efficient equine amplification via the production of high-titered viremia (Figure 47.5). These equine-virulent strains apparently evolve periodically from equine-avirulent enzootic strains in subtype ID. Some outbreaks from the 1940s to

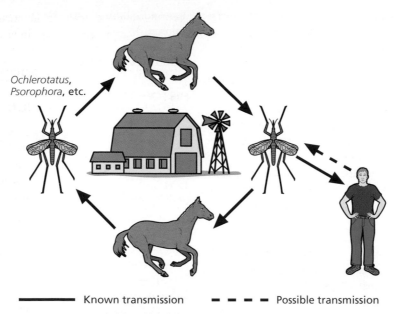

Ochlerotatus, Psorophora, etc.

———— Known transmission   – – – – Possible transmission

Figure 47.5 *Epizootic transmission cycle of Venezuelan equine encephalitis virus*

1973 may have been caused by the use of incompletely inactivated vaccines made from equine-virulent subtype IAB strains.

Enzootic strains (subtypes ID, and IE) of VEEV and all other members of the VEE complex occur in swamp or sylvatic habitats, ranging from southern Mexico to Argentina. These viruses are generally maintained in cycles involving forest-dwelling rodents and *Culex (Melanoconion)* spp. mosquito vectors. Occasional human cases or small outbreaks of human febrile illness occur when people come into contact with these enzootic cycles. The enzootic strains can also occasionally cause human encephalitis, and there may be no difference in human virulence between the epizootic (serotypes IAB and IC) and enzootic (serotypes ID and IE) VEEV strains.

In adults, VEEV infection typically leads to a nonspecific febrile illness accompanied by severe headache, fever, chills, myalgia, prostration, vomiting, diarrhea, and lymphopenia. Some patients, especially children, progress to neurological disease characterized by convulsions, disorientation, drowsiness, mental depression, seizures, and behavioral changes; permanent sequelae are common. Teratogenic effects and fetal death occur following infection in pregnant women. Infection is accompanied by diffuse congestion and edema, with hemorrhage in the brain, gastrointestinal tract, and lungs. Severe necrosis and vasculitis occur in lymph nodes, spleen, and the gastrointestinal tract, along with hepatocellular degeneration and interstitial pneumonia. During epidemics, overall mortality rates average about 0.5 percent. Although humans shed virus in the throat and are potentially infectious, epidemiological studies have failed to yield evidence of direct human–human transmission in households or healthcare settings.

Chikungunya

HISTORY AND DISTRIBUTION

Chikungunya virus (CHIKV) was first isolated from human patients and mosquitoes during an epidemic in the Newala district of Tanzania in 1952/53. The native name, which means 'that which bends up,' is derived from the main symptom of excruciating joint pains (Woodall 2001a; Jupp and McIntosh 1988). Chikungunya virus has frequently been isolated from humans and mosquitoes during epidemics in India, southeast Asia, southeast Africa and sub-Saharan Africa. The largest epidemics in recent years have been in India and Indonesia.

TRANSMISSION CYCLES

CHIKV is transmitted in Africa primarily by sylvatic *Aedes* spp., whereas *Ae. aegypti* transmits the virus in urban centres of India and southeast Asia. No vertebrate host other than humans has been discovered, although monkeys are probable reservoir hosts in Africa.

DISEASE AND VIRAL GENETICS

After an incubation period of 2–4 days there is a sudden onset of fever and crippling joint pains, which may incapacitate the patient, accompanied by chills, flushed face, headache, myalgias, backache, photophobia, and rash in ca. 80 percent of patients (Tsai et al. 2002). There may be conjunctival injection, and patients often have anorexia and constipation. The acute phase of illness lasts for 2–4 days, with recovery in 5–7 days; the fever may be biphasic. Arthralgia is the most striking sign or symptom, occurring in about 70 percent of cases. The areas affected include the metacarpophalangeal joints, wrists, elbows, shoulders, knees, ankles, and metatarsal joints. Arthralgia may affect one or several joints. Reddening and swelling may occur, and arthralgias may persist for months in a small proportion of cases. The clinical picture resembles that of dengue fever, with which it is often confused. Differential diagnosis should include dengue, SINV, and West Nile virus.

In India and southeast Asia, Chikungunya virus has been implicated in outbreaks of hemorrhagic fever, often in association with dengue viruses. A careful review of the clinical presentation of CHIKV infection in Asia, however, suggests that, although mild hemorrhagic manifestations may occur in a small proportion of cases, Chikungunya is not a cause of severe hemorrhagic disease. Hemorrhagic complications have not been reported in association with Chikungunya infections in Africa. Phylogenetic studies and historical observations have suggested that CHIKV originated in Africa and spread to Asia from eastern Africa. Two distinct CHIKV lineages have been delineated: one contains all isolates from western Africa, and the second comprises all southern and East African strains, as well as isolates from Asia.

O'nyong-nyong

HISTORY AND DISTRIBUTION

This virus caused a major epidemic that began in Uganda in 1959 and quickly spread to Kenya, Sudan, Congo, Tanzania, Mozambique, and Malawi, affecting an estimated 2 million people and 90 percent of the population in affected areas (Woodall 2001b). A 1996 epidemic in Uganda affected more than 1 million people. The name O'nyong-nyong was given by the Acholi people and means 'joint breaker.' Igbo-ora virus, isolated in Nigeria, the Central African Republic, and the Ivory Coast during the 1960s, where it caused small outbreaks, is considered a genetic variant of O'nyong-nyong virus (ONNV). ONNV is closely related to CHIKV, and the diseases produced by the two agents are very similar. However, ONNV has a geographically limited distribution in Africa.

TRANSMISSION CYCLES

O'nyong-nyong virus is transmitted by *Anopheles gambiae* and *An. funestus* mosquitoes during outbreaks (it is the only anopheline-borne alphavirus), both of which also transmit malaria. The interepidemic maintenance cycle and reservoir hosts of ONNV have not been described, but the virus has been isolated from sentinel mice in Senegal in the absence of human disease (although human serosurveys indicated a prevalence of 55 percent there).

DISEASE AND VIRAL GENETICS

Infection with ONNV is clinically indistinguishable from that with CHIKV, and is accompanied by fever, chills, severe headache, myalgia, arthralgia, and the formation of a morbilliform rash. No human mortality has been reported.

Ross River fever

HISTORY AND DISTRIBUTION

Ross River virus (RRV) is the most common human arboviral pathogen in Australia, and over 38 000 human cases were reported between 1991 and 1998. Epidemics of benign polyarthritis have been recognized there since 1928, but the causative agent, RRV, was not isolated until 1959 from *Oc. vigilax* mosquitoes collected along the Ross River (Mackenzie 2001b; Kay and Aaskov 1988). Epidemics of polyarthritis involving several thousand cases have occurred regularly in Australia, and the virus is endemic in most coastal regions of the country, as well as inland, especially along waterways and rivers. Since the early 1980s RRV has possibly expanded its geographic distribution into the Pacific, with outbreaks in New Guinea, Fiji, American Samoa, Raratonga, Tonga, and New Caledonia.

TRANSMISSION CYCLES

The natural transmission cycle of RRV is not well understood. Serological surveys suggest that a diverse group of wild and domestic animals may be involved as reservoir hosts. Humans have significant viremia, and the virus in some epidemics has been maintained in a human–mosquito transmission cycle. In coastal regions, *Oc. vigilax* in the north and *Oc. camptorhynchus* in the south and west are important mosquito vectors. *Cx. annulirostris* is also considered an important vector in Australia. In the Pacific islands, *Ae. polynesiensis*, *Oc. vigilax* and *Ae. aegypti* are important vectors. Macropods (kangaroos) are believed to be the principal reservoir hosts in Australia, but other mammals, including flying foxes and rabbits, may also be involved.

DISEASE AND VIRAL GENETICS

Disease occurs most commonly in persons 20–50 years of age and is rare in children; women are affected more often than men. The incubation period is 5–21 (typically 7–9) days; patients with polyarthritis present with fever, arthralgia of the small joints of the hands and feet, myalgia, maculopapular or vesicular rash, paresthesiae of the palms and the soles, lethargy, and headache. Photophobia, anorexia, and lymphadenopathy may also occur. The painful arthritis frequently persists for several weeks, occasionally relapsing a year or more later, but recovery is complete and no fatalities have been reported. Subclinical infections also appear to be common. The persistence of IgM antibodies for several months after infection, and the detection of viral RNA in the synovial lining fluid by RT-PCR, suggest that replication may persist in joints, possibly associated with macrophages.

No vaccine is available. Prevention and control measures are directed at the mosquito population, and at health education on how to protect against mosquito bites. Two major RRV lineages have been identified phylogenetically, in eastern and western Australia, respectively; the eastern lineage caused the Pacific outbreaks in 1979–1980.

Other alphavirus infections

BARMAH FOREST VIRUS

First isolated in Australia from *Cx. annulirostris* mosquitoes, this virus accounts for about 10 percent of epidemic polyarthritis cases there and is second only to RRV as a human arboviral pathogen. The virus appears to be restricted to Australia, where it causes a disease characterized by fever, fatigue, arthritis, arthralgia, and rash that is clinically similar to that caused by RRV. Human infection with Barmah Forest virus (BFV) was first reported in 1986, and the first epidemic of human disease occurred in 1992 in the Northern Territory (Mackenzie 2001a). BFV cross-reacts with other alphaviruses, including RRV, by hemaglutination inhibition tests, but is distinct by complement fixation and neutralization tests.

Mammals, including marsupials, are believed to be the reservoir hosts and the virus has been isolated from a wide range of mosquito species: *Cx. annulirostris* appears to be the most widespread vector. In coastal regions, *Oc. vigilax* and *Oc. camptorynchus* are believed to be major vectors. Human infection occurs sporadically, with the majority of cases being reported from Queensland.

GETAH VIRUS

This virus was originally isolated in Malaysia from *Cx. gelidus* mosquitoes and *Cx. tritaeniorhynchus*. It is closely related to Sagiyama, Bebaru, and RR viruses, which are considered to be subtypes of Getah (Kumanomido 2001; Powers et al. 2001). Getah virus (GETV) is found throughout southeast Asia, including Japan, the Philippines, and Australia, but serological cross-reaction with RRV makes interpretation of serosurvey data difficult. GETV has not been associated with human disease, but causes severe encephalitis in horses in Japan. Antibodies have also been detected in humans, horses, and pigs, but the virus is not known to cause disease in the former two hosts. Pigs may serve as amplifying hosts during equine epizootics. GETV has been isolated from a wide variety of mosquito species, especially *Culex* spp. in Asia and Australia, and from *Aedes* spp. in Siberia.

MAYARO VIRUS

Mayaro virus (MAYV) is closely related to Chikungunya and O'nyong-nyong viruses and causes a similar illness characterized by fever, chills, headache, myalgia, and arthralgia, followed by a maculopapular rash. Arthralgia may persist for weeks or even months (Powers et al. 2001; Tesh et al. 1999). Isolated first in Trinidad from human serum in 1954, it was subsequently isolated from humans in Brazil, Colombia, French Guiana, Venezuela, Bolivia, Surinam, and Peru. Serological surveys also suggest that it occurs in Guyana, Panama, and Costa Rica. Little is known about the natural history of MAYV, but it has been isolated numerous times from *Haemagogus* spp. mosquitoes, suggesting a monkey–*Haemagogus* mosquito sylvatic transmission cycle. Evolutionary studies indicate that an ancestor of Una virus and MAYV, sister species, was introduced from the Old World, where all other members of the Semliki Forest antigenic complex occur (Powers et al. 2001).

SINDBIS VIRUS

Sindbis virus (SINV) has been designated as the prototype *Alphavirus*. It was first isolated in Egypt in 1953 but has a wide distribution in Africa, India, tropical Asia, Australia, and Europe (Griffin 2001b). Three major virus lineages have been identified by phylogenetic studies: a Paleoarctic/Ethiopian lineage, an Oriental/Australian lineage, and a distinct lineage from southwestern Australia. It rarely causes overt disease, but has been associated with febrile illnesses in Africa and India. SINV has a number of variants that have caused outbreaks of human illness in Sweden (Ockelbo disease), Finland (Pogosta disease), Russia (Karelian fever), and West and Central Africa (Babanki). Ockelbo, a SINV variant, causes fever characterized by rash. The disease is described under the names of Ockelbo disease in Scandinavia, Pogosta disease in Finland, and Karelian fever in the USSR. A single case with hemorrhagic manifestations and joint pains has been reported from Australia. SINV is maintained in enzootic cycles involving a variety of birds and mosquitoes of the genera *Culex*, *Aedes*, and *Culiseta*.

SEMLIKI FOREST VIRUS

Semliki forest virus (SFV) was isolated from *Aedes* mosquitoes collected in the course of yellow fever field studies in Uganda. Zingilamo (isolated from birds in the Central African Republic) and Me Tri (isolated from humans in Vietnam) viruses are considered strains of SFV. The virus has been used widely in laboratory studies and was regarded as nonpathogenic until it caused a single, fatal infection in a laboratory worker. Antibodies to SFV are commonly found in human serum collected from both East and West Africa, but no overt disease was recognized until 1987, when it caused a large outbreak of mild febrile illness in Bangui, Central African Republic. SFV may be maintained in a monkey–*Aedes* mosquito cycle, and ticks may also be involved (Pfeffer 2001).

REFERENCES

Frolova, E.I., Fayzulin, R.Z., et al. 2002. Roles of nonstructural protein nsP2 and alpha/beta interferons in determining the outcome of Sindbis virus infection. *J Virol*, **76**, 22, 11254–64.

Griffin, D.E. 2001a. Alphaviruses. In: Knipe, D.M. and Howley, P.M. (eds), *Fields' virology*, 4th edn. New York: Lippincott, Williams & Wilkins, 917–62.

Griffin, D.E. 2001b. Sindbis virus. In: Service, M.W. (ed.), *The encyclopedia of arthropod-transmitted infections*. Wallingford, UK: CAB International, 469–73.

Jupp, P.G. and McIntosh, B.M. 1988. Chikungunya virus disease. In: Monath, T.P. (ed.), *The arbovirus: epidemiology and ecology*, Vol. II. Boca Raton, Florida: CRC Press, 137–57.

Kay, B.H. and Aaskov, J.G. 1988. Ross River virus (epidemic polyarthritis). In: Monath, T.P. (ed.), *The arboviruses: epidemiology and ecology*, Vol. IV. Boca Raton, Florida: CRC Press, 93–112.

Kumanomido, T. 2001. Getah virus. In: Service, M.W. (ed.), *The encyclopedia of arthropod-transmitted infections*. Wallingford, UK: CAB International, 194–5.

La Linn, M., Gardner, J., et al. 2001. Arbovirus of marine mammals: a new alphavirus isolated from the elephant seal louse, *Lepidophthirus macrorhini*. *J Virol*, **75**, 9, 4103–9.

Lescar, J., Roussel, A., et al. 2001. The fusion glycoprotein shell of Semliki Forest virus: an icosahedral assembly primed for fusogenic activation at endosomal pH. *Cell*, **105**, 1, 137–48.

Mackenzie, J.S. 2001a. Barmah Forest virus disease. In: Service, M.W. (ed.), *The encyclopedia of arthropod-transmitted infections*. Wallingford, UK: CAB International, 67–9.

Mackenzie, J.S. 2001b. Ross River virus and Ross River virus disease. In: Service, M.W. (ed.), *The encyclopedia of arthropod-transmitted infections*. Wallingford, UK: CAB International, 443–7.

Pfeffer, M. 2001. Semliki Forest virus. In: Service, M.W. (ed.), *The encyclopedia of arthropod-transmitted infections*. Wallingford, UK: CAB International, 462–4.

Powers, A.M., Brault, A.C., et al. 2001. Evolutionary relationships and systematics of the alphaviruses. *J Virol*, **75**, 21, 10118–31.

Reisen, W.K. 2001. Western equine encephalitis. In: Service, M.W. (ed.), *The encyclopedia of arthropod-transmitted infections*. Wallingford, UK: CAB International, 558–63.

Reisen, W.K. and Monath, T.P. 1988. Western equine encephalomyelitis. In: Monath, T.P. (ed.), *The arboviruses: epidemiology and ecology*, Vol. V. Boca Raton, Florida: CRC Press, 89–137.

Schlesinger, S. and Schlesinger, M.J. 2001. *Togaviridae:* The viruses and their replication. In: Knipe, D.M. and Howley, P.M. (eds), *Fields' virology*, 4th edn. New York: Lippincott, Williams & Wilkins, 895–916.

Scott, T.W. and Weaver, S.C. 1989. Eastern equine encephalomyelitis virus: epidemiology and evolution of mosquito transmission. *Adv Virus Res*, **37**, 277–328.

Strauss, J.H. and Strauss, E.G. 1994. The alphaviruses: gene expression, replication, and evolution. *Microbiol Rev*, **58**, 3, 491–562.

Tesh, R.B., Watts, D.M., et al. 1999. Mayaro virus disease: an emerging mosquito-borne zoonosis in tropical South America. *Clin Infect Dis*, **28**, 1, 67–73.

Tsai, T.F., Weaver, S.C. and Monath, T.P. 2002. Alphaviruses. In: Richman, D.D., Whitley, R.J. and Hayden, F.G. (eds), *Clinical virology*. Washington, DC: ASM Press, 1177–210.

Walton, T.E. and Grayson, M.A. 1988. Venezuelan equine encephalomyelitis. In: Monath, P. (ed.), *The arboviruses: epidemiology and ecology*, Vol. IV. Boca Raton, Florida: CRC Press, 203–31.

Weaver, S.C. 2001a. Eastern equine encephalitis. In: Service, M.W. (ed.), *The encyclopedia of arthropod-transmitted infections*. Wallingford, UK: CAB International, 151–9.

Weaver, S.C. 2001b. Venezuelan equine encephalitis. In: Service, M.W. (ed.), *The encyclopedia of arthropod-transmitted infections*. Wallingford, UK: CAB International, 539–48.

Weaver, S.C., Dalgarno, L., et al. 2000. Family *Togaviridae*. In: van Regenmortel, M.H.V. and Fauquet, C.M. (eds), *Virus taxonomy: classification and nomenclature of viruses. Seventh Report of the International Committee on Taxonomy of Viruses*. San Diego: Academic Press, 879–89.

Woodall, J. 2001a. Chikungunya virus. In: Service, M.W. (ed.), *The encyclopedia of arthropod-transmitted infections*. Wallingford, UK: CAB International, 115–19.

Woodall, J. 2001b. O'nyong-nyong virus. In: Service, M.W. (ed.), *The encyclopedia of arthropod-transmitted infections*. Wallingford, UK: CAB International, 388–90.

48

Bunyaviridae

ALAN D.T. BARRETT AND ROBERT E. SHOPE

PROPERTIES OF THE VIRUSES

Introduction

Viruses of the family *Bunyaviridae* are enveloped, single-stranded RNA viruses with a tripartite genome. Approximately 300 distinct viruses are included in five genera of the family: *Orthobunyavirus*, *Hantavirus*, *Nairovirus*, *Phlebovirus*, and *Tospovirus*. Viruses of the same genus share structural, genetic, and antigenic characteristics, and often similar epidemiology. Many are arboviruses (arthropod-borne viruses), transmitted between vertebrate hosts (or plants in the case of tospoviruses) by blood-feeding mosquitoes, ticks, gnats, or thrips. A significant exception is the genus *Hantavirus*, whose known members are maintained in nature by chronically infected rodents, especially of the family *Muridae*, and are thought to be transmitted most commonly among rodents by bite and aerosol, and to humans by aerosol. Among the noteworthy hantaviruses are *Hantaan virus* and *Sin Nombre virus*, which were the first viruses known to cause hemorrhagic fever with renal syndrome and hantavirus pulmonary syndrome, respectively. Other human diseases caused by viruses within the family include California encephalitis and La Crosse encephalitis (*Orthobunyavirus*), sandfly fever and Rift Valley fever (*Phlebovirus*), Crimean–Congo hemorrhagic fever (*Nairovirus*), Oropouche fever (*Orthobunyavirus*), and others. Viruses of the genus *Tospovirus* are presently known only as plant pathogens. More than 360 plant species belonging to 50 families are known to be susceptible to infection with tospoviruses.

The history of viruses of the family *Bunyaviridae* parallels that of arbovirology. Before 1950, many viruses were investigated because of their ability to cause human disease. Thus, during the Second World War, much was discovered about sandfly fever viruses, because these viruses were responsible for significant morbidity among Allied troops stationed in the Middle East (Hertig and Sabin 1964). Sandfly (or phlebotomus) fever virus later became the prototype member of the genus *Phlebovirus*. A second complex of viruses destined to become a genus within the family also has links to military medicine. Viruses now known to be members of the genus *Hantavirus* played major roles in military campaigns in Asia, Yugoslavia, and Scandinavia during the Second World War, and again during the Korean conflict. Indeed, today these viruses continue to infect soldiers in the Balkans and elsewhere. Likewise, university researchers in California isolated the prototype strain of California encephalitis in the mid-1940s, setting the stage for the discovery of many other closely related viruses, including significant human pathogens like La Crosse virus. Investigations of the California antigenic group of bunyaviruses led to the discovery of many of the fundamental characteristics of the family: the pathogenic potential of some viruses, transovarial transmission as a method of epidemiological maintenance, and the molecular basis for our current understanding of the group (LeDuc 1987).

The type species of the family, *Bunyamwera virus*, was first isolated in Uganda from a pool of *Aedes* mosquitoes collected during studies of yellow fever (Smithburn et al. 1946). *Bunyamwera virus* was clearly unrelated either to *Yellow fever virus* or to any other arbovirus then known, but subsequent studies showed that it shares structural and biochemical properties with many other viruses that now make up the family (Smithburn et al. 1946; Murphy et al. 1973; Bishop et al. 1980; Elliott 1990). In the 1950s, the Rockefeller Foundation founded a series of international research stations dedicated to the study of viral diseases of humans, and during this time many of the viruses now recognized as members of the family were first discovered. For example, the laboratory in Belem, Brazil, was the source of many viruses then grouped antigenically as the 'group C' arboviruses through the classic work of Clarke and Casals (group A viruses evolved to the genus *Alphavirus*, in the family *Togaviridae*, while the group B viruses have become the genus *Flavivirus* in the family *Flaviviridae*). The Bunyamwera, group C, *Guama*, *Simbu*, and other arboviruses were known for a time as the 'Bunyamwera supergroup,' then finally linked structurally and biochemically to form the genus *Bunyavirus*, family *Bunyaviridae*. Recently, the Bunyaviridae subcommittee of the International Committee of the Taxonomy of Viruses (ICTV) has proposed that the genus *Bunyavirus* be renamed *Orthobunyavirus* and this will be included in the Eighth Report of the ICTV due to be published in 2004. The Rockefeller Foundation-sponsored laboratories in Africa and India further contributed to the growing number of then known 'bunyaviruses'. Even today, newly recognized viruses isolated from arthropods or vertebrates are often found to be members of the family.

Classification

Viruses of the family *Bunyaviridae* are classified according to structural similarities, antigenic characteristics, common biochemical properties and, more recently, genetic homology. Five genera are now recognized, the largest being the genus *Orthobunyavirus*, with approximately 170 different viruses assigned to 18 groups (Table 48.1). The genus *Hantavirus* takes its name from *Hantaan virus*, the cause of hemorrhagic fever with renal syndrome. The hantaviruses are rapidly expanding in number, many 'new' viruses being identified by polymerase chain reaction (PCR) amplification of viral RNA obtained from field samples, but in several cases the actual viruses have yet to be isolated in a tractable form. At present, at least 26 serologically and/or genetically unique hantaviruses have been described, with many others almost certainly awaiting discovery (Table 48.2, p. 1029). The genus *Nairovirus* is named after the virus of Nairobi sheep disease (Montgomery 1917), and contains more than 30 viruses in seven groups. The genus *Phlebovirus* has recently been expanded to include an earlier distinct genus, *Uukuvirus*, now merged with the phleboviruses on the basis of a common replication strategy and genetic similarities (Elliott et al. 1992). The most recent addition to the family is the genus *Tospovirus*, which takes its name from tomato spotted wilt virus. At present, this genus is limited to plant viruses and is transmitted by thrips (Thysanoptera). The *Tospovirus* genus encompasses at least 13 viruses, 11 of which are divided into two serogroups and two others that are serologically unrelated (Table 48.3, p. 1030).

Within each genus, viruses were historically divided on serological characteristics into group, complex, virus, and subtype. 'Subtype' refers to viruses that can be serologically distinguished only with difficulty; named viruses can be easily distinguished; 'complex' refers to assemblies of viruses that are significantly cross-reactive; and 'group' or 'serogroup' encompasses complexes that are distantly related by serological activity (Peters and LeDuc 1991). More recent classification schemes have included the concept of a virus species, defined as a polythetic class of viruses. The interpretation of what constitutes a virus species is not consistent for each genus of the family, or among virus families in general.

Morphology and structure

Virions generally seem, by electron microscopy (EM), to be 80–120 nm spherical particles. Although pleomorphic particles are commonly observed by EM, such irregularity may be the result of desiccation, which occurs during specimen preparation, rather than inherent properties of viruses in the family (Hewlett and Chiu 1991). External features of the virions include a distinct bilaminar membrane, approximately 5 nm thick, and a fringe of surface projections approximately 5–10 nm long, comprised of the viral envelope glycoproteins, G1 and G2 (von Bonsdorff and Pettersson 1975; Hewlett and Chiu 1991) (Figure 48.1, p. 1030). Recently, the *Bunyaviridae* subcommittee of the ICTV has proposed that G1 and G2 be renamed Gn and Gc due to difficulties in a common nomeclature across the different genera in the *Bunyaviridae*. As this nonemcalture has not been adopted yet, the glycoproteins will be termed G1 and G2 in this chapter. Because of differences in the G1 and G2 proteins of viruses in each genus, the characteristic appearance of virions varies. The surface area of the bunyavirus, La Crosse virus, was calculated to be able to accommodate from 4 700 to 12 000 tightly packed G1 and G2 proteins; however, estimates from EM studies suggest that only 270–1 400 proteins are present on a virion (Hewlett and Chiu 1991). The arrangement of the proteins, therefore, must include wide spacing between each heterodimer of G1 and G2. The most comprehensive study of surface structure and chemical composition for a virus in the family was performed with the phlebovirus Uukuniemi virus. The virion surface units of Uukuniemi virus appeared as penton–hexon clusters with a $T = 12$, $P = 3$ icosahedral surface lattice and with hexon–hexon distances of approximately 12.5–16 nm for stained viral particles and 17 nm for freeze-etched samples

Table 48.1 *Viruses of the* Bunyaviridae *known to cause disease in humans or domestic animals and their geographic distribution and principal vectors*

	Geographic distribution	Associated illness	Principal vector
Genus *Bunyavirus*			
Anopheles A group (12)			
Tacaiuma	S America	Human	Mosquitoes
Bunyamwera group (32)			
Bunyamwera	Africa	Human	Mosquitoes
Cache valley	N America	Human, sheep, cattle	Mosquitoes
Fort Sherman	C America	Human	Mosquitoes
Garissa	Africa	Human	Not known
Germiston	Africa	Human	Mosquitoes
Ilesha	Africa	Human	Mosquitoes
Kairi	S America	Equine	Mosquitoes
Main Drain	N America	Equine	Mosquitoes, culicoid flies
Shokwe	Africa	Human	Mosquitoes
Wyeomyia	S America	Human	Mosquitoes
Xingu	S America	Human	Mosquitoes
Bwamba group (2)			
Bwamba	Africa	Human	Mosquitoes
Pongola	Africa	Human	Mosquitoes
Group C (14)			
Apeu	S America	Human	Mosquitoes
Caraparu	S and N America	Human	Mosquitoes
Itaqui	S America	Human	Mosquitoes
Madrid	N America	Human	Mosquitoes
Marituba	S America	Human	Mosquitoes
Murutucu	S America	Human	Mosquitoes
Nepuyo	S and N America	Human	Mosquitoes
Oriboca	S America	Human	Mosquitoes
Ossa	N America	Human	Mosquitoes
Restan	S America	Human	Mosquitoes
California group (14)			
California encephalitis	N America	Human	Mosquitoes
Guaroa	S and N America	Human	Mosquitoes
Inkoo (Jamestown Canyon)	Europe, N America	Human	Mosquitoes
La Crosse	N America	Human	Mosquitoes
Snowshoe hare	N America	Human	Mosquitoes
Tahyna	Europe	Human	Mosquitoes
Guama group (12)			
Catu	S America	Human	Mosquitoes
Guama	S and N America	Human	Mosquitoes
Nyando group (2)			
Nyando	Africa	Human	Mosquitoes
Simbu group (24)			
Akabane	Africa, Asia, Australia	Cattle	Mosquitoes, culicoid flies
Ingwavuma	Africa, Asia	Pigs	Mosquitoes
Oropouche	S America	Human	Culicoid flies, mosquitoes
Genus *Hantavirus* (26)			
Andes	S America	Human	Rodent
Bayou	N America	Human	Rodent
Black Creek Canal	N America	Human	Rodent
Dobrava-Belgrade	Europe	Human	Rodent
Hantaan	Asia, Europe	Human	Rodent
Laguna negra	S America	Human	Rodent
New York	N America	Human	Rodent

(Continued over)

Table 48.1 *Viruses of the* Bunyaviridae *known to cause disease in humans or domestic animals and their geographic distribution and principal vectors (Continued)*

	Geographic distribution	Associated illness	Principal vector
Puumala	Europe, Asia	Human	Rodent
Seoul	Worldwide	Human	Rodent
Sin Nombre	N America	Human	Rodent
Genus *Nairovirus* (34)			
Crimean–Congo haemorrhagic fever (CCHF) group (3)			
CCHF	Africa, Asia, Europe	Human	Ticks
Hughes group (10)			
Hughes	N and S America	Sea birds	Ticks
Nairobi sheep disease group (2)			
Dugbe	Africa	Human, cattle	Ticks, culicoid flies, mosquitoes
Nairobi sheep disease	Africa, Asia	Human, cattle	Ticks, mosquitoes
Genus *Phlebovirus* (51)			
Sandfly fever group (23)			
Candiru complex			
Alenquer	S America	Human	?
Candiru	S America	Human	?
Punta Toro complex			
Punta Toro	N, S, and C America	Human	Phlebotomine flies
Rift Valley fever complex			
Rift Valley fever	Africa	Human, cattle	Mosquitoes
Sandfly fever Naples complex			
Sandfly fever Naples	Europe, Africa, Asia	Human	Phlebotomine flies
Toscana	Europe	Human	Phlebotomine flies
No complex assigned in sandfly fever group (16)			
Chagres	C America	Human	Phlebotomine flies
Sandfly fever Sicilian	Europe, Africa, Asia	Human	Phlebotomine flies
Uukuniemi group (12)			
St. Abbs head	Europe	Sea birds	Ticks
Grouped but unassigned viruses of *Bunyaviridae* (19)			
Bhanja group (3)			
Bhanja	Africa, Asia, Europe	Human	Ticks
Kasokero	Africa	Human	?
Yogue	Africa	Human	?
Ungrouped and unassigned viruses of *Bunyaviridae* (23)			
Bangui	Africa	Human	Mosquitoes
Issyk–Kul (Keterah)	Asia	Human	Mosquitoes, ticks
Tamdy	Asia	Human	Ticks
Tataguine	Africa	Human	Mosquitoes
Wanowrie	Africa, Asia	Human	Mosquitoes, ticks

Numbers in parenthesis indicate the total viruses within that taxon.

(von Bonsdorff and Pettersson 1975). The biochemical composition of Uukuniemi virus was estimated to be 2 percent RNA, 58 percent protein, 33 percent lipid, and 7 percent carbohydrate (Obijeski and Murphy 1977).

All viruses in the family have tripartite, single-stranded RNA genomes, with segments designated large (L), medium (M), and small (S). Each RNA is complexed with many copies of the viral nucleocapsid protein (N) to form three distinct ribonucleocapsids, which seem to be helical (von Bonsdorff et al. 1970; von Bonsdorff and Pettersson 1975). Terminal, complementary, nucleotide sequences are conserved on the L, M, and S segments for viruses within a particular genus and differ from those of viruses in other genera (Patterson et al. 1983; Collett et al. 1985; Schmaljohn et al. 1986a; Rönnholm and Pettersson 1987; Schmaljohn et al. 1987;

Table 48.2 *Serologically or genetically distinct viruses in the genus* Hantavirus

Virus	Abbreviation	Original source	Geographic distribution	Location of rodent host[a]	Human disease
***Murinae* subfamily-associated viruses**					
Hantaan	HTN	*Apodemus agrarius*	Korea	Asia, Europe	HFRS[b]
Seoul	SEO	*Rattus norvegicus, R. rattus*	Korea	Asia, Europe, the Americas	HFRS
Dobrava-Belgrade	DOB	*Apodemus flavicollis*	Slovenia	Europe, Middle East	HFRS
Thai-749	THAI	*Bandicota indica*	Thailand	Asia	unknown
***Arvicolinae* subfamily-assocated viruses**					
Puumala	PUU	*Clethrionomys glareolus*	Finland	Europe, Asia	HFRS
Prospect Hill	PH	*Microtus pennsylvanicus*	Maryland	N America	Unknown
Tula	TUL	*Microtus arvalis*	Russia	Europe	Unknown
Khabarovsk	KHA	*Microtus fortis*	Russia	Asia	Unknown
Topografov	TOP	*Lemmus sibiricus*	Siberia	Russia, Asia, N America	Unknown
Isla Vista	ISLA	*Microtus californicus*	California	N America	Unknown
***Sigmodontinae* subfamily-associated viruses**					
Sin Nombre	SN	*Peromyscus maniculatus*	New Mexico	N America	HPS[c]
New York	NY	*Peromyscus leucopus*	New York	N America	HPS
Black Creek Canal	BCC	*Sigmodon hispidus*	Florida	The Americas	HPS
Bayou	BAY	*Oryzomys palustris*	Louisiana	Southeastern	HPS
Andes	AND	*Oligoryzomys longicaudatus*	Argentina	S America	HPS
Caño Delgadito	CANO	*Sigmodon alstoni*	Venezuela	S America	Unknown
Rio Mamore	RIOM	*Olygoryzomys microtis*	Bolivia, Peru	S America	Unknown
Laguna negra	LAN	*Calomys laucha*	Paraguay	S America	HPS
Muleshoe[d]	MULE	*Sigmodon hispidus*	Texas	N America	Unknown
El Moro Canyon[d]	ELMC	*Reithrodontomys megalotis*	California	N America	Unknown
Rio Segundo[d]	RIOS	*Reithrodontomys mexicanus*	Costa Rica	Mexico, Central America	Unknown
Limestone Canyon	LSC	*Peromyscus boylii*	Arizona	N America	Unknown
Calabazo[d]		*Zygodontomys brevicauda*	Panama	S America	Unknown
Choclo[d]		*Oligoryzomys fulvesens*	Panama	S America	HPS
Araraquara[d]	ARA	*Bolomys lasiurus*	Brazil	S America	HPS
Juquitiba[d]		*Unknown*	Brazil		HPS
Castelo dos Sonhos	CAS	*Unknown*	Brazil		HPS
Maporal	MAP	*Oecomys bicolor*	Venezuela	S America	Unknown
Insectivore-associated virus					
Thottapalayam	TPM	*Suncus murinus*	India	Asia	Unknown
Other possible species and hosts (limited sequence; no other information available)					
Monongahela	MON	*Peromyscus maniculatus*	W Virginia	N America	HPS
Blue River	BR	*Peromyscus leucopus*	Oklahoma	N America	Unknown
Oran	ORN	*Oligoryzomys longicaudatus*	Argentina	S America	Unknown
Lechiguanas	LEC	*Oligoryzomys flavescens*	Argentina	S America	HPS
Bermejo	BER	*Oligoryzomys chacoensis*	Argentina	S America	Unknown
Maciel	MAC	*Bolomys obscurus*	Argentina	S America	Unknown
Pergamino	PER	*Akadon azarae*	Argentina	S America	Unknown

Data from Carey et al. (1971); Lee et al. (1978, 1982); Elwell et al. (1985); Schmaljohn et al. (1985, 1995); Avsic-Zupanc et al. (1992a, b); Elliot et al. (1994); Plyusnin et al. (1994, 1996); Song et al. (1994, 1995a, b); Rollin et al. (1995); Torrez-Martinez and Hjelle (1995); Torrez-Martinez et al. (1995); Lopez et al. (1996); Rawlings et al. (1996); Bharadwaj et al. (1997); Fulhorst et al. (1997); Johnson et al. (1997); Milazzo and Eyzaguirre (2002); Sanchez et al. (2001); Johnson and DeSouza (1999); Powers et al. (1999); Vincent et al. (2000).
a) Given as approximate distribution; many rodent species occur focally, many others have widespread distributions.
b) HFRS, haemorrhagic fever with renal syndrome.
c) HPS, hantavirus pulmonary syndrome.
d) Cell culture isolate has not been reported.

Table 48.3 *Serologically distinct viruses in the genus* Tospovirus

Genus *Tospovirus*	Abbreviation	Vector	Reference
Tomato spotted wilt group			
Tomato spotted wilt	TSWV	*F. occidentalis, F. schultzei, F. intonsa, F. fusca, F. bispinosa, T. tabaci, T. setosus, T. palmi*	de Haan et al. (1992a)
Groundnut ringspot	GRSV	*F. occidentalis, F. schultzei, F. intonsa*	de Ávila et al. (1993)
Tomato chlorotic spot	TCSV	*F. accidentalis F. schultzei, F. intonsa*	de Ávila et al. (1993)
Chrysanthemum stem necrosis	CSNV	*F. schultzei, F. occidentalis*	de Ávila et al. (1993)
Zucchini lethal chlorosis	ZLCV	*F. zucchini*	de Ávila et al. (1993)
Impatiens necrotic spot	INSV	*F. accidentalis, F. schultzei, F. intonsa*	Law et al. (1991)
Watermelon silver mottle group			
Watermelon silver mottle	WSMV	*T. palmi*	Yeh and Chang (1995)
Watermelon bud necrosis	WBNV	*T. palmi*	Jain et al. (1998)
Peanut bud necrosis	PBNV	*T. palmi*	Satyanarayana et al. (1996)
Melon yellow spot[a]	MYSV	*T. palmi*	Kato et al. (2000)
Iris yellow spot	IYSV	*T. tabaci*	Cortes et al. (1998)
Ungrouped			
Peanut yellow spot	PYSV	*S. dorsalis*	Satyanarayana et al. (1998)
Peanut chlorotic fan-spot	PCFV	*S. dorsalis*	Yeh et al. (1998)

a) Previously referred to as physalis severe mottle virus (Cortes et al. 1998, 2001).

de Haan et al. 1990, 1991; Elliott et al. 1991; Kormelink et al. 1992a) (Table 48.4). Base pairing of these RNAs to form panhandle structures (Figure 48.2, p. 1032) can result in noncovalently closed circular RNAs and nucleocapsids (Pettersson and Bonsdorf 1975; Obijeski et al. 1976; Hewlett et al. 1977; Raju and Kolakofsky 1989) (see Figure 48.1).

At least one each of the L, M, and S ribonucleocapsids are required for viral infectivity. However, equal numbers of nucleocapsids may not always be packaged

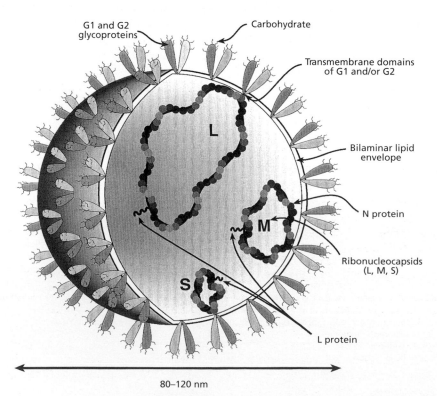

80–120 nm

Figure 48.1 *Structure of a typical virus particle in the family* Bunyaviridae. *Individual components of the virus are described in the text.*

Table **48.4** *Consensus 3′ terminal nucleotide sequences of the L, M and S genome segments of representative members of the* Bunyaviridae

Genus	Virus	Genome segment	Gene size (nucleotides)	Nucleotide sequence[a]	GenBank No.
Orthobunyavirus	Bunyamwera	S	961	3′-UCAUCACAUGAGGUG	D00353
		M	4458	3′-UCAUCACAUGAUGGC	M11852
		L	6875	3′-UCAUCACAUGAGGAU	X14383
Hantavirus	Hantaan	S	1696	3′-AUCAUCAUCUGAGGG	M14626
		M	3616	3′-AUCAUCAUCUGAGGC	M14627
		L	6533	3′-AUCAUCAUCUGAGGG	X55901
Nairovirus	Dugbe	S	1712	3′-AGAGUUUCUGUUUGC	M25150
		M	4888	3′-AGAGUUUCUGUAUGG	M94133
		L	12255	3′-AGAGUUUCUGUAGUU	U15018
Phlebovirus	Rift Valley fever	S	1690	3′-UGUGUUUCGAGGGAUC	X53771
		M	3884	3′-UGUGUUUCUGCCACGU	M11157
		L	6404	3′-UGUGUUUCUGGCGGGU	X56464
Tospovirus	Tomato spotted wilt	S	2916	3′-UCUCGUUAGCACAGUU	D00645
		M	4821	3′-UCUCGUUAGUCACGUU	S48091
		L	8897	3′-UCUCGUUAGUCCAUUU	D10066

a) Sequences identical on all three genome segments are underlined.

in mature virions (Bishop and Shope 1979). Differing complements of ribonucleocapsids were suggested to be related to virion size differences noted by EM (Talmon et al. 1987). Varying amounts of virus complementary-sense RNAs (cRNAs) were also identified in virions, but the significance, if any, of this finding is not known (Raju and Kolakofsky 1989; Simons et al. 1990; Kormelink et al. 1992a).

In addition to N, G1, and G2, virions also contain a polymerase protein (L) that is needed to copy the negative-sense viral genome into messenger-sense RNA(s) (Ranki and Pettersson 1975; Bouloy and Hannoun 1976; Schmaljohn and Dalrymple 1983; Patterson and Kolakofsky 1984; Gerbaud et al. 1987a; Adkins et al. 1995) (see Figure 48.1). The exact placement of the L protein within virions is not known, but it is believed to be associated with each of the ribonucleocapsids.

Genome structure and function

The expression strategies of the L, M, and S segments of viruses in the five genera of the family *Bunyaviridae* include both similarities and marked differences (Figure 48.3, p. 1033). All viruses encode their structural proteins (N, G1/G2, and L) in the S, M, and L cRNA, respectively. Viruses in each genus, except for those in the genus *Hantavirus*, also encode nonstructural proteins in their M and/or S segment vRNA or cRNA. The G1 and G2 proteins of all viruses are believed to be encoded as a polyprotein precursor that is cleaved cotranslationally, although direct evidence for this has been obtained only for phleboviruses (Ulmanen et al. 1981; Rönnholm and Pettersson 1987; Suzich and Collett 1988; Andersson et al. 1997a). The L segments of all

viruses described to date encode only the L protein and have <200 nucleotides of noncoding information (Elliott 1989; Schmaljohn 1990; de Haan et al. 1991; Muller et al. 1991). There is no evidence for additional coding regions in either the L segment cRNA or the vRNA but see Nairoviruses below.

ORTHOBUNYAVIRUSES

Orthobunyaviruses produce both N and a nonstructural protein, NS_S, from overlapping reading frames found in the S segment cRNA (Gentsch and Bishop 1978; Cash et al. 1979; Bishop et al. 1982; Fuller and Bishop 1982; Akashi and Bishop 1983; Cabradilla et al. 1983; Fuller et al. 1983; Akashi et al. 1984; Bouloy et al. 1984; Elliott 1985; Gerbaud et al. 1987b). Only one S segment mRNA species was detected for the orthobunyaviruses; thus, a single mRNA must be used for translation of both N and NS_S (Bouloy et al. 1984; Patterson and Kolakofsky 1984; Eshita et al. 1985; Saeed et al. 2000). The orthobunyavirus M segment encodes an NS_M protein between coding information for G2 and G1 (Eshita and Bishop 1984; Lees et al. 1986; Grady et al. 1987; Fazakerly et al. 1988; Nakitare and Elliott 1993).

HANTAVIRUSES

Hantaviruses seem to have the simplest genome expression strategy of viruses in the family bunyaviridae, in that there is no clear evidence that nonstructural proteins are generated. The S segments of certain hantaviruses have an overlapping reading frame within N, which could encode a protein similar in size to that of the bunyavirus NS_S protein. However, such a protein has not yet been found (Parrington and Kang 1990;

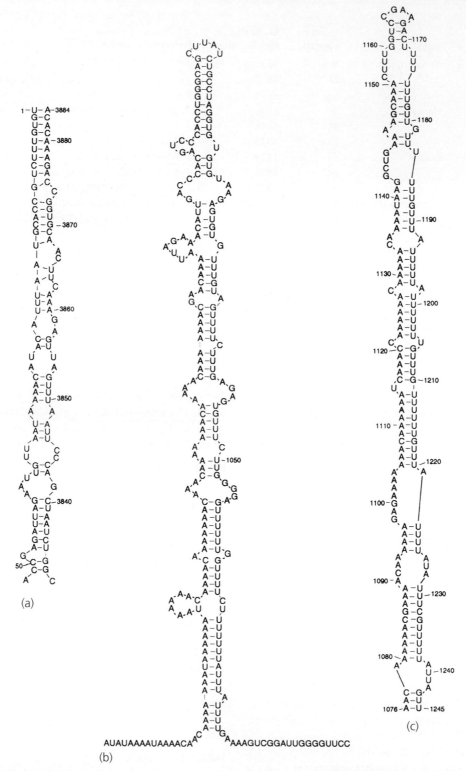

Figure 48.2 *Predicted panhandle structures formed by base-pairing of complementary sequences.* **(a)** *Terminal sequences of the M genome segment of the* Phlebovirus *Rift Valley fever virus (data from Collett et al. 1985).* **(b)** *Intergenic region of the ambisense S genome segment of the* Phlebovirus *Punta Toro virus (data from Emery 1987).* **(c)** *Intergenic region of the M genome segment of the* Tospovirus *Tomato spotted wilt virus (data from Kormelink et al. 1992b).*

Settergren et al. 1990; Stohwasser et al. 1990; Spiropoulou et al. 1994; Li et al. 1995). Certain of the New World hantaviruses have very large S segment 3′ noncoding regions; i.e. >700 bases for Sin Nombre virus as compared to <400 bases for prototype hantaan virus. Numerous repeated nucleotide sequences found in the

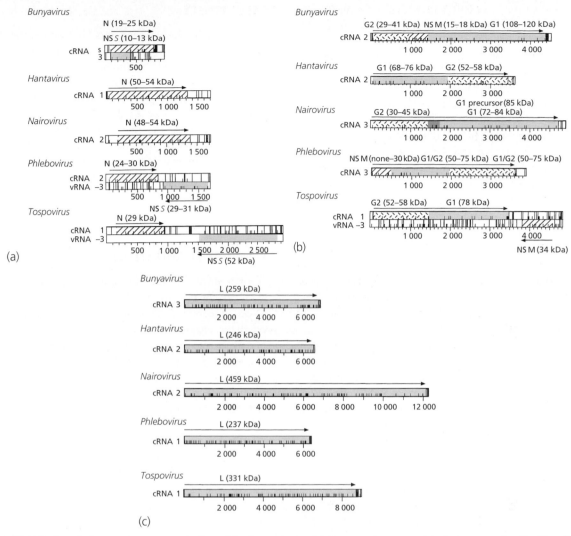

Figure 48.3 *Coding strategy and gene organization of the bunyaviruses. (a) S segment open reading frames encoding the N and NS$_S$ proteins are indicated by striped and stippled boxes, respectively. (b) M segment open reading frames encoding G1, G2, and NS$_M$ are indicated by stippled, cross-hatched and striped boxes, respectively. (c) L segment open reading frames encoding the L protein are indicated by stippled boxes. Translation initiation codons are represented by short hatch marks and stop codons are indicated by long hatch marks. The reading frame used, with respect to complementary sense RNA (cRNA, frames 1, 2, 3) or virus sense RNA (vRNA, frames −1, −2, −3) are listed to the left of the boxes. Nucleotide sequence numbers, with respect to the 5′ terminus of cRNA are shown below the boxes. Arrows indicate the direction of translation, 5′ to 3′, and predicted molecular weights of the gene products are shown above or below the arrows.*

Sin Nombre virus noncoding region are suggested to result from polymerase slippage, but a functional importance for their presence has not been discovered (Spiropoulou et al. 1994; Li et al. 1995; Morzunov et al. 1995; Ravkov et al. 1995). The M segments of hantaviruses have only a short potential intergenic region (e.g. ⩽34 amino acids for Hantaan virus) between the sequences encoding G1 and G2, as well as little additional 5′ or 3′ noncoding information (Schmaljohn et al. 1987).

PHLEBOVIRUSES

Phleboviruses use an ambisense coding strategy to produce an NS$_S$ polypeptide. That is, NS$_S$ is encoded in vRNA in a reading frame that does not overlap the cRNA sequences encoding N (Ihara et al. 1984; Overton

et al. 1987; Marriott et al. 1989; Simons et al. 1990; Giorgi et al. 1991). The existence of NS$_S$ was verified in cells infected with numerous phleboviruses, including Uukuniemi virus, Rift Valley fever virus, Punta Toro virus, and Karimabad virus (Parker and Hewlett 1981; Ulmanen et al. 1981; Smith and Pifat 1982; Struthers and Swanepoel 1982; Overton et al. 1987). In vitro translation studies and northern blot analyses with viral RNAs demonstrated that N and NS$_S$ are generated from separate, subgenomic messages (Ulmanen et al. 1981; Parker et al. 1984; Ihara et al. 1985b; Marriott et al. 1989; Simons et al. 1990). The M segment of some, but not all, phleboviruses encodes an NS$_M$ in cRNA in the same reading frame but preceding the coding information for G1 and G2 (Collett et al. 1985). For example, the cRNA open reading frame of Rift Valley fever virus has five in-frame translation initiation codons. Use of the first ATG resulted in production of uncleaved NS$_M$ G2 as well as G1, whereas use of the second ATG resulted in distinct NS$_M$ of approximately 14 kDa, G2 and G1 proteins (Collett et al. 1985; Suzich and Collett 1988; Kakach et al. 1989; Schmaljohn et al. 1989; Suzich et al. 1990). Both the NS$_M$ G2 fusion protein and the NS$_M$ protein are readily observed in cell cultures infected with Rift Valley fever virus. An even larger potential NS$_M$ protein (approximately 30 kDa) with 13 inframe initiation codons is predicted from the M segment nucleotide sequence of Punta Toro virus. However, no polypeptide of this has been identified in cells infected with Punta Toro virus (Ihara et al. 1985a). There is no apparent homology between the Rift Valley fever virus and Punta Toro virus NS$_M$ proteins, and both Rift Valley fever virus and Punta Toro virus G1 and G2 proteins can be efficiently produced in vitro in the absence of the NS$_M$ coding information (Matsuoka et al. 1988; Suzich and Collett 1988; Suzich et al. 1990).

In contrast to those of Punta Toro virus and Rift Valley fever virus, the M segment of the phlebovirus, Uukuniemi virus, has no preglycoprotein coding region, and the amino terminus of G1 is located 17 amino acids downstream of the first (and only) initiation codon (Rönnholm and Pettersson 1987). Thus, Uukuniemi virus G1 seems to be similar to the Rift Valley fever virus NS$_M$ G2 fusion protein. Cleavage of the G1/G2 precursor of Uukuniemi virus takes place cotranslationally in the endoplasmic reticulum, shortly after synthesis of G2 begins, and the G2 signal sequence remains attached to the carboxy terminus of G1 (Andersson et al. 1997a).

NAIROVIRUSES

The S segment of nairoviruses, like that of hantaviruses, encodes only a large N protein and has no known nonstructural protein coding information (Cash 1985; Ward et al. 1990; Marriott and Nuttall 1992). The M segment of the nairovirus, Dugbe virus, seems to encode only G2 and G1, although G1 was suggested to arise from post-translational cleavage of a slightly larger precursor (Marriott et al. 1992). The L segment of *Dugbe virus* is the largest gene of any member of the family bunyaviridae. Until recently it was not known why nairoviruses might need a polymerase protein almost twice the size of some of the other viruses in the family. Nucleotide sequencing of the L RNA of Crimean-Congo hemorrhagic fever virus revealed the segment is 12 164 nucleotides in length and encodes 3 944 amino acids. The amino terminus of the L protein encodes an ovarian tumorlike cysteine protease motif suggesting that the L polyprotein is autoproteolytically cleaved or involved in deubiquitination (Honig et al. 2004; Kinsella et al. 2004).

TOSPOVIRUSES

Both the S and the M segments of tospoviruses have ambisense coding strategies and separate subgenomic messages to generate structural and nonstructural proteins (de Haan et al. 1990; Kormelink et al. 1992a; Law et al. 1992). Unlike the NS$_S$ of phleboviruses, which is about the same size as N, that of tospoviruses is approximately twice the size of N (Figure 48.3). Thus, the L segment of tospoviruses is the only one of the three gene segments that uses a strictly negative-sense coding strategy (de Haan et al. 1991).

Replication

ATTACHMENT AND ENTRY

One or both of the integral viral envelope proteins, G1 and G2, are believed to mediate attachment of virions to host-cell receptors. This was first demonstrated by proteolytic enzyme treatment of purified La Crosse virus, which resulted in 'spikeless' virus particles and a concomitant 5 log$_{10}$ reduction in infectivity (Obijeski et al. 1976). For most viruses in the family, it is not known which of the envelope glycoproteins mediates attachment. To attempt to answer that question for bunyaviruses, La Crosse virus was treated with bromelain or Pronase, which degraded portions of G1, but left G2 uncleaved. Such treatment resulted in its complete loss of infectivity (Kingsford and Hill 1981). La Crosse virus G1 was also implicated as the attachment protein for mammalian cells because affinity-purified G1 protein could competitively inhibit attachment of radiolabeled G1 to Vero cells (Ludwig et al. 1991). In contrast, G2 did not bind to Vero cells, but did bind to cultured mosquito cells and midguts. To competitively inhibit binding of G2, both G1 and G2 were required, which led to the speculation that the G1 protein might be the viral attachment protein for vertebrates, whereas G2 is used for arthropod infection (Ludwig et al. 1991). Confirmation of this as a general feature of the bunyaviruses is needed. Although no similar information exists for viruses in other genera, there is evidence that neutralizing and hemagglutination-inhibiting (HI) sites are present on both the G1 and G2 proteins of phleboviruses (Keegan and Collett 1986; Pifat et al. 1988) and hantaviruses (Dantas et al. 1986; Arikawa et al. 1989), so it is possible that either or both of these proteins may be involved in attachment. Although cellular receptors have not been clearly identified for most viruses in the family, for two hantaviruses which cause hantavirus pulmonary syndrome, Sin Nombre virus and New York virus, integrins expressed on endothelial cells were implicated as specific receptors (Gavrilovskaya et al. 1998).

Fusion of infected cells at acidic pH has been reported for viruses in the *Bunyaviridae* (Gonzalez-Scarano et al. 1984; Arikawa et al. 1985; Gonzalez-Scarano 1985;

Gonzalez-Scarano et al. 1985). Such pH-dependent fusion is generally believed to relate to early events in internalization of viral particles. Electron microscopy of the infection process of Rift Valley fever virus revealed that virions seem to enter cells in phagocytic vacuoles (Ellis et al. 1988). This observation is consistent with a mode of entry similar to that first described for alphaviruses in which the virus is endocytosed in coated vesicles which subsequently become acidified (Marsh and Helenius 1980; Tycko and Maxfield 1982). The acidification triggers a fusion of viral membranes and endosomal membranes, and results in the release of the viral nucleocapsid into the cell cytoplasm. Whether one or both of the envelope proteins are necessary for fusion has not been determined for most members of the family. For the orthobunyavirus La Crosse virus, there is ample information to indicate that the G1 protein is involved in fusion. For example, it is known that monoclonal antibodies to G1 inhibit fusion, that G1 undergoes a conformational change at the pH of fusion and that a virus mutant with a defective G1 does not cause fusion (Gonzalez-Scarano 1985; Gonzalez-Scarano et al. 1985, 1987). Consistent with this, expression of G1 in the absence of G2 with recombinant vaccinia viruses resulted in cell fusion in vitro (Jacoby et al. 1993). These functions defined for the G1 and G2 proteins of bunyaviruses do not imply like functions for viruses in other genera.

TRANSCRIPTION

After uncoating of viral genomes, primary transcription of negative-sense vRNA to complementary mRNA occurs through interaction of the virion-associated polymerase (L protein) and the three viral RNA templates (Ranki and Pettersson 1975; Bouloy and Hannoun 1976). Transcription occurs entirely in the cytoplasm and there is no requirement for ongoing cellular transcription, as indicated by the resistance of viruses in the family to actinomycin D, an inhibitor of DNA-dependent RNA polymerases, such as host-cell DNA-dependent RNA polymerase II (Obijeski and Murphy 1977). Only the L and N proteins of Bunyamwera virus (Dunn et al. 1995) and Rift Valley fever virus (Lopez et al. 1995; Prehaud et al. 1997) were found to be necessary to reconstitute transcription in vitro. The L protein is believed to function first as an endonuclease to cleave capped oligonucleotides from host mRNAs to serve as transcription primers (Figure 48.4). This priming results in the presence of 5′ terminal extensions of approximately 10–18 heterogeneous nucleotides on the termini of viral mRNAs (Bishop et al. 1983; Bishop et al. 1984; Patterson and Kolakofsky 1984; Eshita et al. 1985; Ihara et al. 1985b; Collett 1986; Bouloy et al. 1990; Simons and Pettersson 1991; Kormelink et al. 1992c; Dobbs and Kang 1993; Jin and Elliott 1993a, b). For phleboviruses and tospoviruses, which have ambisense coding strategies, both the N and the NS_S subgenomic mRNA have heterogeneous, nonviral, 5′ terminal extensions (Ihara et al. 1985b; Simons and Pettersson 1991; Kormelink et al. 1992b).

Direct evidence for the presence of capped structures on the termini of the extensions was obtained by using anticap antibodies to immunoselect mRNAs (Hacker 1990; Vialat and Bouloy 1992). That the cleavage of capped oligonucleotides may not be an entirely random process is indicated by a preference for specific mono-, di- or trinucleotides at the −1 to −3 positions with respect to the 5′ terminus of mRNAs of particular viruses. For example, almost all cDNA clones of the S mRNA of the orthobunyavirus Germiston virus displayed U or G at the −1 position (Bouloy et al. 1990). Similarly, Bunyamwera virus preferred UG, but snowshoe hare virus was found to have A most commonly as the 3′ terminal nucleotide of the S mRNA extensions (Bishop et al. 1983; Eshita et al. 1985; Jin and Elliott 1993a). For phleboviruses, C was found most often at the −1 position of the M mRNA of Rift Valley fever virus and also at the −1 position of the N and NS_S mRNAs of Uukuniemi virus (Collett 1986; Simons and Pettersson 1991). For Hantaan virus, the preferred −1 nucleotide was G (Dobbs and Kang 1993; Garcin et al. 1995) and for the nairovirus Dugbe virus, C (Jin and Elliott 1993b). The reason for such preferences could imply that a restricted or specific subset of host mRNAs is used for primers, perhaps because of a need for limited base pairing with the viral genome.

Studies on the orthobunyaviruses Germiston virus and Bunyamwera virus revealed the insertion of U or GU between the primer and the 5′ terminal viral sequence. It was also noted that the 3′ most terminal nucleotides of the stolen host sequences were often similar to the 5′ terminal viral sequences, leading to the hypothesis that the insertions might arise from partial reiteration of the 5′ terminal sequences owing to a backward slippage of the viral polymerase after the first two or three nucleotides are transcribed (Vialat and Bouloy 1992; Jin and Elliott 1993a). In addition to such insertions, for orthobunyavirus and phlebovirus mRNAs, but not for the nairovirus mRNAs studied, the +1 nucleotide in the mRNA transcript is sometimes missing (Bishop et al. 1983; Bouloy et al. 1990; Simons and Pettersson 1991; Jin and Elliott 1993a, b), and for hantavirus RNAs the first three nucleotides are often absent (Dobbs and Kang 1993).These findings suggest that transcription initiation at nucleotides other than the terminal one may occur. For hantaviruses, a prime-and-realign-model for transcription was proposed which explains many of the experimental observations (Garcin et al. 1995). According to the model, priming by host oligonucleotides, with a terminal G residue would initiate transcription by aligning at the third nucleotide of the viral RNA template (C residue). After synthesis of a few oligonucleotides, the nascent RNA could realign by slipping backwards two nucleo-

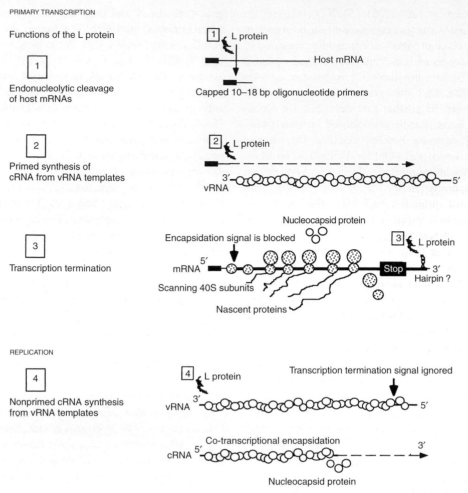

Figure 48.4 *Transcription and replication of the bunyaviruses. (1) The L protein cleaves capped oligonucleotides from host cell mRNAs. (2) The capped oligonucleotides are used to prime transcription of cRNA from vRNA templates. (3) Transcription is terminated at signals that may involve secondary structure or primary sequence of the vRNA template. mRNAs are not encapsidated, perhaps owing to the presence of scanning 40S ribosomes or the caps. (4) For replication to proceed, the L protein must use nonprimed synthesis and must ignore transcription termination signals to produce complete cRNA templates for further vRNA synthesis. The mechanism(s) of the switch from transcription to replication are not well defined.*

tides on the repeated terminal sequences (AUCAU-CAUC), such that the G becomes the first nucleotide of the nontemplated, 5′ extensions. The frequent deletion of one or two of the triplet repeats in hantaviral mRNA supports this sort of slippage mechanism and suggests that sometimes the initial priming might start at the C residue of the third triplet in the conserved sequence rather than at the C of the second triplet. A prime-and-realign model was also suggested for transcription of hantaviral vRNA and cRNA, except that transcription is postulated to initiate with pppG alignment at the third nucleotide (C residue) of the template RNA. After synthesis of several nucleotides, the polymerase slips, allowing the nascent RNA to realign such that the initial priming G residue is overhanging. The L protein was suggested to act as an endonuclease to remove the G, leaving a monophosphorylated U residue at the nascent 5′ end. The presence of the monophosphorylated U on hantaan virus RNA was experimentally demonstrated (Garcin et al. 1995).

For the phlebovirus Rift Valley fever virus, a reconstituted transcription system was used to experimentally demonstrate that the minimal signal for transcription is the 13 3′-terminal nucleotides of the S segment vRNA or cRNA (Prehaud et al. 1997). One of the two repeated dinucleotides at the temini (UGUG) could be removed without deleterious effect on transcription, thus providing indirect support for the prime-and-realign model for phleboviruses, as well as hantaviruses. Whether this model holds for all viruses in the family remains to be determined.

At present, it is not clear what host functions are important for primary transcription of viruses in the family *Bunyaviridae*. Conflicting data concerning the need for ongoing host protein synthesis for primary transcription (as defined by the inability to achieve full length transcripts in the presence of drugs, such as cycloheximide and puromycin) were reported for viruses in the genus *Orthobunyavirus* (Abraham and Pattnaik 1983; Patterson and Kolakofsky 1984; Eshita et al. 1985;

Raju and Kolakofsky 1986, 1987a, 1989; Bellocq et al. 1987). If there is a need for ongoing protein synthesis, it may be at the level of ribosome scanning, rather than translation. This speculation was based on the finding that transcription was not inhibited by edeine, a drug that prevents 40S and 60S ribosomal subunits from complexing (Vialat and Bouloy 1992). These data are consistent with an earlier hypothesis that scanning ribosomes prevent premature termination by preventing base-pairing between the template RNA and the transcript, which would cause the polymerase to halt and terminate prematurely (Bellocq et al. 1987).

Termination of primary transcripts (i.e. mRNAs) occurs approximately 100 nucleotides from the $5'$ terminus of the vRNA template, resulting in mRNAs that are truncated at their $3'$ termini, as compared to cRNA (Figure 48.4) (Cash et al. 1979; Pattnaik and Abraham 1983; Bouloy et al. 1984; Patterson and Kolakofsky 1984; Eshita et al. 1985; Pettersson et al. 1985; Collett 1986; Raju and Kolakofsky 1987b; Bouloy et al. 1990). Potential transcription termination sites have been proposed for the S segments of La Crosse virus (Patterson and Kolakofsky 1984) and snowshoe hare virus (Eshita and Bishop 1984; Eshita et al. 1985) at or near the genomic sequence $3'$-G/CUUUUU. Proposed U-rich transcription termination sites also are found on the M and S segments of Germiston virus ($3'$-AUGUUUUGUU and $3'$-GGGGUUUGUU, respectively) (Bouloy et al. 1990). Although such transcription termination sites are similar to those resulting in polyadenylation of mRNAs of other viruses, mRNAs of viruses in the family Bunyaviridae are not known to be polyadenylated (Ulmanen et al. 1981; Pattnaik and Abraham 1983; Pettersson et al. 1985). Moreover, transcription termination sites without the homopolymeric U_5 or U_6 tract have been proposed for the S and M segment mRNAs of another orthobunyavirus, snowshoe hare virus ($5'$-GGUGGGGGGUGGGG and $5'$-GGUGGGGGGUGGGG, respectively) (Eshita and Bishop 1984) and the M segments of the phleboviruses Rift Valley fever virus and Punta Toro virus ($5'$-UGGG-GUGGUGGGGU and $5'$-GGUGAGAGUGUA-GAAAG, respectively) (Collett 1986). Comparing the S segment sequences of a number of phleboviruses revealed that G-rich sequences and similar sequence motifs were found in the intergenic regions of some, but not all, phleboviruses (Giorgi et al. 1991).

Transcription termination of ambisense genes to yield structural and nonstructural protein mRNAs may occur through recognition of RNA secondary structure rather than a specific gene sequence. For example, the transcription termination sites for both the N and the NS_S mRNAs of Punta Toro virus were mapped to within 40 nucleotides of one another, and predicted hairpin structures were found in this intergenic region, as well as in the intergenic regions of the S segments of certain other phleboviruses and in both the S and the M segments of

tospoviruses (de Haan et al. 1990; Kormelink et al. 1992b; Law et al. 1992) (see Figure 48.3). For the S segment of the phlebovirus Uukuniemi virus, although there is a noncoding region of 70 nucleotides between the N and the NS_S genes, hybridization studies demonstrated that the $3'$ ends of the subgenomic messages overlap one another by about 100 nucleotides. Thus the $3'$ end of the NS_S mRNA extends into the coding region of N and the $3'$ end of the N mRNA terminates just before the coding sequences for N. A short palindromic sequence in the intergenic region (including the $3'$ ends of each mRNA) is predicted to allow formation of an A/U-rich hairpin structure (Simons and Pettersson 1991). Such structures could affect transcription termination only if they can form while the genome is complexed with N. To date there is no direct evidence that this occurs.

Although the mechanism of transcription termination is not known, studies performed with the L protein of Bunyamwera virus expressed by vaccinia virus recombinants resulted infrequently in correct transcription termination, suggesting that an additional factor (or factors), of viral or cellular origin, may be required for consistent transcription termination (Jin and Elliott 1993a). One such factor might include interaction between the transcriptase and a newly synthesized viral protein, such as NS_S (Vialat and Bouloy 1992; Jin and Elliott 1993a). This could not be a familial characteristic, however, because hantaviruses and nairoviruses are not known to encode NS_S proteins. Also, for viruses using ambisense coding to produce NS_S, the kinetics of synthesis of N and NS_S, as well as the finding that only N mRNA can be detected in the presence of cycloheximide, suggest that replication of full-length, encapsidated cRNA must occur before synthesis of the NS_S mRNA. Thus, because NS_S appears relatively late in infection, it is unlikely to have a role in primary transcription, unless it can be generated in small amounts directly by translation of the vRNA (Simons et al. 1992).

GENOME REPLICATION

The switch from primary transcription to genome replication requires the L protein to switch from primed synthesis, by using capped host-cell oligonucleotides, to a process of independently initiating transcription at the precise $3'$ end of the template and producing an encapsidated, full-length transcript. The factors dictating that vRNA and cRNA should complex with N to form nucleocapsid structures, while mRNAs should not, are not known, but it has been suggested that the added capped host cell sequences on the $5'$ ends of viral messages may somehow prevent encapsidation (Raju and Kolakofsky 1989).

Unlike primary transcription, secondary transcription is clearly sensitive to inhibitors of protein synthesis, such as cycloheximide. The need for ongoing protein synthesis for replication to proceed is likely to be due to the need for continued viral protein synthesis rather than host cell protein synthesis. Although the factors that dictate that the L protein should begin genome replication are not known for viruses in the family *Bunyaviridae*, a mechanism similar to that proposed for rhabdoviruses and paramyxoviruses seems plausible: accumulating a sufficient quantity of N seems to trigger encapsidation and to serve as an antitermination signal, thus allowing full-length genome synthesis (Blumberg et al. 1983; Wertz 1983; Patton et al. 1984a, 1984b; Arnheiter et al. 1985; Banerjee 1987; Vidal and Kolakofsky 1989). Nonstructural proteins were suggested to control the availability of the N protein of rhabdoviruses, and where available, they could possibly do the same for the *Bunyaviridae*. A model for transcription and replication based on information detailed above is presented in Figure 48.4.

SYNTHESIS AND PROCESSING OF VIRAL PROTEINS

S segment gene products

As described above (Orthobunyaviruses, Phleboviruses, Tospoviruses), the N and NS_S proteins encoded by the vRNA and cRNA of the S segments of bunyaviruses, phleboviruses, and tospoviruses do not originate from precursor polypeptides, and therefore processing of proteins is not required. Hantaviruses and nairoviruses encode only one product in their S segments. Post-translational modifications (e.g. phosphorylation or amidation) have not generally been defined for S segment products except for the NS_S of Rift Valley fever virus. For Rift Valley fever virus, the NS_S protein was reported to be phosphorylated (Parker et al. 1984) and to accumulate in the nuclei of infected cells where they seemed to aggregate as filamentous structures (Struthers and Swanepoel 1982). Although this is not known to be a general finding for phleboviruses, very few of them have been examined with immune sera specific for the NS_S protein. The NS_S of the tospovirus tomato spotted wilt virus was seen in association with fibrous structures in the cytoplasm of infected plants. However, it was not clear if the proteins actually formed the filaments or were just associated with them (Kormelink et al. 1991).

The NS_S protein has been found to function as an interferon antagonist and also inhibit host-cell protein synthesis (Bouloy et al. 2001; Bridgen et al. 2001). A detailed description of its function can be found in the Antigens, immune responses, and virulence section below.

M segment gene products

Historically, the designation of glycoproteins G1 and G2 comes from their relative migrations when analyzed by sodium dodecyl sulfate polyacrylamide gel electrophoresis (SDS-PAGE). G1 is the more slowly migrating polypeptide. These designations, based on apparent polypeptide size, do not always correlate with the gene order, structure or function of G1 and G2. For example, for the two phleboviruses Rift Valley fever virus and Punta Toro virus, it is known that G1 of Rift Valley fever virus is related to G2 of Punta Toro virus and vice versa (see Figure 48.3). Thus, the terms Gn and Gc have been proposed by the *Bunyaviridae* subcommittee of the ICTV to overcome problems with nomenclature, but have yet to be universally adopted.

Cotranslational cleavage of G1 and G2 (and in the *Bunyavirus* and *Phlebovirus* genera, NS_M) is believed to be mediated by a cellular signalase-like enzyme. Except for the *Nairovirus* Dugbe virus, which may encode G1 as a precursor, all predicted polyprotein precursors have hydrophobic regions preceding both G1 and G2 that are consistent with signal sequences that allow transport of the nascent proteins through membranes. The precursors also have variable numbers of potential transmembrane regions, and a hydrophobic sequence at the carboxy terminus, indicative of a membrane anchor region (Eshita and Bishop 1984; Collett et al. 1985; Schmaljohn et al. 1987; Fazakerley and Ross 1989; Law et al. 1992; Marriott et al. 1992). Thus, these proteins are assumed to be typical class 1 membrane proteins, i.e. with the amino terminus exposed on the surface of the virion and the C terminus anchored in the membrane.

A common property of all M segment gene products predicted from cDNA sequences studied so far is their high cysteine content (4–7 percent) and, in related viruses, the conservation of the position of the cysteine residues (Ihara et al. 1985a; Lees et al. 1986; Grady et al. 1987; Rönnholm and Pettersson 1987; Antic et al. 1992b; Kormelink et al. 1992b; Law et al. 1992; Marriott et al. 1992). These findings suggest that extensive disulfide bridge formation may occur and that the positions may be crucial for determining correct polypeptide folding. The secondary structure of the proteins can also play a role in immunogenicity, in that neutralizing or protective epitopes are often conformational and nonlinear (Battles and Dalrymple 1988; Wang et al. 1993).

All of the envelope proteins examined to date possess *N*-linked oligosaccharides. The gene sequences that define a potential *N*-linked glycosylation site are those that encode Asn–X–Ser/Thr, where X is not Pro (Hubbard and Ivatt 1981). The number of potential glycosylation sites found in the predicted M segment gene product range from four sites for certain hantaviruses to nine sites for some tospoviruses (Antic et al. 1992b; Law et al. 1992). The number of sites actually used in mature virion proteins has not been defined for most viruses. However, G2 of the phlebovirus Rift Valley fever virus was demonstrated to be glycosylated at its single available site and at least three of four possible G1 sites (Kakach et al. 1989). Analysis of the predicted amino acid sequences of the envelope proteins of the bunyavirus snowshoe hare virus (Eshita and Bishop 1984; Fazakerly et al. 1988) and examination of glycosylated tryptic oligopeptides (Vorndam and Trent 1979) suggest that all three potential glycosylation sites on G2 are used and at least one of two sites on G1. The single glycosylation site available in the G2 protein of hantaan virus is used, and this site is conserved among numerous other hantaviruses (Schmaljohn et al. 1986b; Antic et al. 1992a). Where studied, the oligosaccharides attached to the G1 and G2 proteins were mostly high-mannose glycans, although complex and novel intermediate-type oligosaccharides were also identified on the G1 protein of Uukuniemi virus (Madoff and Lenard 1982; Pesonen et al. 1982; Schmaljohn et al. 1986b; Antic et al. 1992a; Ruusala et al. 1992).

Although not studied extensively, the NS$_M$ proteins of the bunyavirus Bunyamwera virus and the phlebovirus Rift Valley fever virus were found not to be glycosylated (Lees et al. 1986; Collett et al. 1989; Kakach et al. 1989). For Rift Valley fever virus, however, another M segment gene product consisting of an uncleaved form of the NS$_M$ protein and G2 is also routinely generated, and the NS$_M$ portion of that fusion protein is glycosylated (Kakach et al. 1989). The NS$_M$ protein of tospoviruses is not a membrane protein. It is encoded in the ambisense and is translated from a subgenomic message. Because this protein has no counterpart in any of the other genera of the family, it was suggested to be a genetic adaption of these viruses for survival in plant hosts (Kormelink et al. 1994; Storms et al. 1995).

L segment gene products

No post-translational modifications of L proteins for viruses in the *Bunyaviridae* have been described. The L protein is a multifunctional enzyme. For Bunyamwera virus and Rift Valley fever virus, the L and N proteins are essential and sufficient for transcriptase activity (Dunn et al. 1995; Lopez et al. 1995). The Bunyamwera virus L protein transcribes a synthetic template in concert with the N proteins of closely related bunyaviruses, but only inefficiently with more dissimilar orthobunyavirus N proteins (Dunn et al. 1995). The complementary terminal nucleotide sequences of viruses in the family *Bunyaviridae* that are predicted to form panhandle structures have been suggested as possible polymerase recognition structures. Although only limited information exists, in one study a point mutation resulting in disruption of the base-paired structure was found to drastically reduce Bunyamwera virus L transcriptase activity in vitro (Dunn et al. 1995).

Comparison of L protein sequences of viruses in the family *Bunyaviridae* with other RNA polymerases revealed the presence of four conserved 'polymerase motifs' (Poch et al. 1989; Jin and Elliott 1992). Mutational analysis of cDNA representing Bunyamwera virus

L within these conserved regions was used to demonstrate that amino acid residues that are highly conserved among viruses in the family could not be changed, but that changes in nonconserved amino acids did not generally reduce the ability of the expressed L protein to transcribe authentic viral nucleocapsid templates in an in vitro assay (Jin and Elliott 1992; Dunn et al. 1995).

TRANSPORT

One of the earliest notable features found to distinguish bunyaviruses from all other negative-strand RNA viruses was that the viral particles are formed intracellularly by a budding process at smooth surface vesicles in the Golgi area (von Bonsdorff et al. 1970; Lyons and Heyduk 1973; Murphy et al. 1973; Bishop and Shope 1979). Recent studies with Uukuniemi virus indicated that viruses mature not only in the Golgi stacks, but also in the pre-Golgi intermediate compartment (Jäntti and Hilden 1997). Because the virus particles are too large to be transported in the 60-nm vesicles postulated to function in the intra-Golgi transport network, it was suggested that the Golgi cisternae themselves may be involved in virion transport (Jäntti and Hilden 1997). The site of virus maturation, be it either the intermediate compartment or the Golgi stacks, is at least partly dictated by the accumulation and retention of a sufficient concentration of the viral envelope proteins. The factors involved in Golgi transport and retention have been studied for viruses in the genera *Phlebovirus*, *Hantavirus*, and *Orthobunyavirus*. For most of these viruses, it appears that dimerization of the two envelope proteins in the endoplasmic reticulum must occur before they are transported to the Golgi. For Punta Toro virus, kinetic studies indicated that heterodimerization occurs between newly synthesized G1 and G2 within 3 min after protein synthesis and that the dimers are linked by disulfide bonds (Chen and Compans 1991).

For phleboviruses, orthobunyaviruses, and some hantaviruses, if dimerization does not occur, then only one protein can move to the Golgi (Matsuoka et al. 1988, 1991; Chen and Compans 1991; Rönnholm 1992; Ruusala et al. 1992). For example, in the absence of G1, G2 of Punta Toro virus was transported out of the ER and expressed on the cell surface. Removal of the carboxy-terminal anchor sequence of G1 resulted in secretion of this protein. When both proteins were expressed, however, both G1 and G2 were found in the Golgi. These studies suggest that the Golgi transport and retention signal is located on the G1 protein of Punta Toro virus (Chen et al. 1991). Similar results were obtained with the phlebovirus Uukuniemi virus, in that expression of G1 and G2 independently in COS cells resulted in translocation of only G1 to the Golgi, while G2 remained in the ER, suggesting that the signal for transport resides on G1 and that G2 is transported only by association with G1 (Rönnholm 1992).

Conclusive evidence that the region of the cytoplasmic tail adjacent to the transmembrane domain is the Golgi retention signal for phleboviruses was obtained by expression of truncated and chimeric G1 proteins of Punta Toro (Matsuoka et al. 1994, 1996) and Uukuniemi viruses (Andersson et al. 1997b). In these studies, deleting or replacing the cytoplasmic tail of G1 resulted in cell surface expression, rather than Golgi retention. Also, addition of the cytoplasmic domain to proteins normally expressed at the plasma membrane effected Golgi retention. For Punta Toro virus, the retention signal was found to be located within the first ten amino acids of the cytoplasmic domain (Matsuoka et al. 1996). Similar studies have yet to be reported for viruses in other genera of the *Bunyaviridae*.

Although Golgi retention is the norm for G1 and G2 proteins of viruses in the family, some viruses mature at cell surface membranes. For two New World hantaviruses, Sin Nombre virus and Black Creek Canal virus, envelope glycoproteins were detected on the cell surface, and virus budding from the plasma membrane was observed by electron microscopy (Goldsmith et al. 1995; Ravkov et al. 1997). Likewise, even though the phlebovirus Rift Valley fever virus matures in the Golgi in continuous cell lines, in primary rat hepatocytes budding was observed at the plasma membrane in addition to Golgi membranes (Anderson and Smith 1987). The molecular basis for these observations has not yet been determined.

For bunyaviruses and phleboviruses, which express an NS_M protein in addition to G1 and G2, all three proteins localize in the Golgi. However, NS_M is not needed for transport, as indicated by targeting of G1 and G2 to the Golgi even when they were expressed from an M segment from which the NS_M coding region had been deleted (Matsuoka et al. 1988; Wasmoen et al. 1988; Lappin et al. 1994).

The transport of tospovirus proteins within plant cells and insect cells has not been studied extensively. These viruses replicate in insects (Ullman et al. 1993; Wijkamp et al. 1993), as well as plants. Therefore, in addition to possessing the transport mechanisms described for other arthropod-borne viruses in this family, tospoviruses must also be able to traverse the plant cell wall. For tomato spotted wilt virus, the NS_M protein was found to be associated with nucleocapsid aggregates and was postulated to be involved in cell-to-cell movement of nonenveloped ribonucleocapsids (Kormelink et al. 1994). The NS_M protein was further shown to assemble into tubulelike structures that were postulated to penetrate the plasmodesmata, allowing transport of the free, nonenveloped ribonucleocapsids from cell to cell (Storms et al. 1995). The association of NS_M only with nucleocapsids, but never with mature enveloped particles (Kormelink et al. 1994) supports this hypothesis. Thus it is likely that the G1 and G2 proteins (and envelope) of tospoviruses are required for replication in their insect vectors, but not in plants (Verkleij and Peters 1983; de Resende et al. 1991).

PROTEIN INTERACTIONS IN VIRUS ASSEMBLY AND RELEASE

Unlike viruses in families such as the *Rhabdoviridae*, *Orthomyxoviridae*, and *Paramyxoviridae*, which utilize their matrix (M) protein to act as a nucleating step for assembly and to bridge the gap between the integral viral envelope proteins and their nucleocapsids, bunyaviruses that do not have an M protein must rely on direct interaction of the envelope proteins and ribonucleocapsids to trigger assembly (Smith and Pifat 1982). Because viral ribonucleocapsids and spike structures have been observed only on portions of Golgi vesicle membranes directly involved in the budding process and not on adjacent areas of the same membranes, it is likely that some sort of transmembranal recognition between the viral glycoproteins and the N protein is required for budding. Direct evidence for transmembrane regions of G1 and G2 was obtained by enzymatic digestion of exposed proteins of the phlebovirus Karimabad. In this study, it was determined that approximately 12 percent of G1 or G2, or both, was exposed on the cytoplasmic face of membranes in infected cells and was accessible to digestion. A large protease-resistant fragment was identified, which was presumably sequestered in the membrane in a manner that rendered it safe from enzymatic digestion (Smith and Pifat 1982). Candidate transmembrane regions have been predicted from hydropathic characteristics of derived amino acid sequences representing the envelope proteins of all members of the *Bunyaviridae* examined to date. For Uukuniemi virus, it has been suggested that the cytoplasmic tail of G1 (which is at least 70 residues long) is a logical candidate for interaction with the nucleocapsids (Rönnholm and Pettersson 1987; Pettersson 1991).

This cytoplasmic tail was found to be palmitylated. Although removal of palmitylation sites (cysteine residues) had no effect on the transport of G1 to the Golgi, it is conceivable that such fatty acid acylation of the cytoplasmic domain could play a role in virus assembly, perhaps by facilitating interaction with N, but this remains to be experimentally determined (Andersson et al. 1997b).

It is believed that, after the particles bud into the Golgi cisternae, they are released in individual small vesicles in a manner analogous to secretory granules of other cell types (Broadwell and Oliver 1981; Rothman 1981; Smith and Pifat 1982). The release of virus from infected cells presumably occurs when the cytoplasmic, virus-containing vesicles fuse with the cellular plasma membrane, i.e. by normal exocytosis.

Host factors involved in transport of viral proteins have not been clearly defined. However, for Black Creek Canal virus, an interaction of nucleocapsid protein with cellular actin filaments was identified and was suggested to play a role in virus assembly or release (Ravkov et al. 1998). Because this virus is atypical of most other viruses in the family (i.e. it buds at the plasma membrane instead of in the Golgi), it is not known if this finding will prove relevant to other members of the *Bunyaviridae*.

The morphogenesis of tospoviruses in their insect vector, thrips, seems to be similar to that observed with other viruses in the family (Wijkamp et al. 1993). Differences, however, are seen in plants and plant cells. As indicated above, it is likely that the tospovirus envelope is needed only for replication in insects, and not in plants. Nonenveloped tospovirus particles are commonly seen in infected plants (Kitajima et al. 1992); defective tomato spotted wilt virus isolates, which are defective in glycoprotein synthesis and lack the lipid envelope, were found to retain the ability to spread through plant tissues at the same rate as nondefective viruses (Verkleij and Peters 1983; de Resende et al. 1991). These findings, as well as the small pore size (approximately 3 nm) of plants' plasmodesmata, suggest that infectious ribonucleocapsids, rather than complete tospovirus virions, are transported through the plant plasmodesmata (Kormelink et al. 1994).

Antigens, immune responses, and virulence

The major viral antigens are the structural proteins, N, G1, and G2. Generally, the N protein is highly antigenic, and is usually the prominent antigen detected in serological assays such as complement fixation and ELISA of infected cell-culture lysates. The G1 and G2 proteins are the basis for serological assays such as hemagglutination inhibition and plaque-reduction neutralization.

For all animal-infecting bunyaviruses, the envelope glycoproteins, G1 and G2, are presumed to be the major antigens involved in induction of immunity. Three lines of evidence support this assumption: (1) monoclonal antibodies to G1 or G2 or both, but not to N, can neutralize viral infectivity in vitro; (2) passive transfer of neutralizing, but not nonneutralizing, monoclonal antibodies or monospecific polyclonal sera to G1 or G2 or both, protects animals from challenge with homologous viruses; and (3) immunization of animals with recombinant viruses expressing G1 or G2 (or both) results in protective immunity (Dantas et al. 1986; Collett et al. 1987; Pifat et al. 1988; Arikawa et al. 1989, 1992; Dalrymple et al. 1989; Schmaljohn et al. 1990; Pekosz et al. 1995). For some viruses, such as the phlebovirus Rift Valley fever virus, although monoclonal antibodies to both G1 and G2 will neutralize virus in cell culture, only those specific for G2 were able to passively protect animals. Passively transferred polyclonal, monospecific sera to G2 were also found to be protective, but sera to G1 were not (Dalrymple et al. 1981, 1989; Keegan and

Collett 1986; Smith et al. 1987). This finding was substantiated in mice immunized with recombinant vaccinia or baculoviruses expressing either G1 or G2, in that only the G2 recombinants induced a protective immune response in the animals (Dalrymple et al. 1989; Schmaljohn et al. 1989). These findings suggest that a humoral response alone to one or both of the envelope glycoproteins may be sufficient for protection from infection with viruses in the family.

Little information is available concerning the importance of cell-mediated immune responses to members of the *Bunyaviridae*. For the hantavirus, Hantaan virus-specific cytotoxic T lymphocytes (CTL) were demonstrated after restimulation of immune mouse lymphocytes with Haantan virus antigen in vitro. The CTL response was also suggested to be involved in cross-reactive protection among hantaviruses. Evidence for this was obtained by restimulating, with Hantaan virus, spleen cells from mice immunized with heterologous hantaviruses. In one instance of cross-protection (i.e. immunization with Puumala virus and protection against Hantaan virus), evidence suggested that T cells may be particularly relevant (Asada et al. 1987, 1988, 1989). A non-neutralizing, presumably cell-mediated, protective immune response was also demonstrated in hamsters immunized with baculovirus-expressed Hantaan virus and challenged with virulent Hantaan virus (Schmaljohn et al. 1990).

Recent studies have investigated the early immune response to bunyavirus infection. The type I interferon system, that includes protein kinase R (PKR), $2'-5'$ oligoadenylate synthetase/RNase L and Mx proteins, has been shown to be important for antiviral activity by blocking transcription, translation, and replication of viral RNA, including sequestion of the N protein by the Mx protein (Frese et al. 1996; Kanerva et al. 1996; Jin et al. 2001; Kochs et al. 2002; Bridgen et al. 2004) and interferon knockout mice are susceptible to La Crosse virus infection, whereas wild-type mice are not (Hefti et al. 1999). Investigation of the function of the NSs protein of phleboviruses and orthobunyaviruses has shown that this viral protein is an interferon antagonist and has a critical function of suppressing the production of interferon in virus-infected cells. Initial studies with Rift Valley fever virus showed that a strain containing a deletion in the NSs gene was attenuated and a good interferon inducer, while wild-type virus was virulent and a poor interferon inducer (Vialat et al. 2000; Bouloy et al. 2001). Thus, NSs is an important virulence factor for members of the *Bunyaviridae*. Subsequent studies using reverse genetics of Bunyamwera virus showed that mutation of NSs resulted in a virus that induced high levels of interferon, whereas wild-type virus did not (Bridgen et al. 2001; Weber et al. 2002). These studies also suggested a role for NSs in the shutoff of host-cell protein synthesis that has been substantiated by Colon-Ramos et al. (2003) who have shown the orthobunyavirus NSs has sequence and functional activities similar to Reaper, a proapoptotic protein from *Drosophila*, including inhibition of host-cell protein synthesis. Investigation of the mechanism of action of NSs shows that NSs blocks an early step in interferon induction, namely activation of interferon transcription factors NF-κB and interferon regulatory factor 3 (IRF-3) by double-stranded RNA (dsRNA) (Weber et al. 2000; Weber et al. 2002). Kohl et al. (2003) showed that virus lacking a functional NSs induces apoptotic cell death more rapidly than wild-type virus. Although both wild-type and NSs mutant viruses activated proapoptotic transcription factor IRF-3, only wild-type virus suppressed signaling downstream of IRF-3, thus delaying cell death via IFR-3-mediated apoptosis. However, although Bunyamwera virus NSs blocks induction of interferon by dsRNA, unlike other interferon antognists, it does not appear to involve the dsRNA-activated PKR and RNase L systems (Streitenfeld et al. 2003).

In recent years animal models have been developed for hantavirus pulmonary syndrome (Hooper et al. 2001b; Milazzo and Eyzaguirre 2002) and phlebovirus hemorrhagic fever (Fisher and Tesh 2003) that will be important in elucidating the pathogenesis of bunyavirus diseases.

For tospoviruses, resistance to infection was achieved by transforming plants with viral nucleoprotein (*N*) gene sequences (de Haan et al. 1992b; Vaira et al. 1995). This protection was demonstrated to be RNA-mediated, i.e. gene silencing owing to the presence of *N* gene sequences rather than to the presence of N protein (de Haan et al. 1992b; Pang et al. 1997). In addition to immunogenicity, the viral envelope glycoproteins are also most frequently associated with virulence, although this asssociation is not absolute. By using reassortant viruses, it was demonstrated that both mouse virulence and mosquito infectivity correlated with the M segment gene products of the bunyavirus, La Crosse virus (Gonzalez-Scarano et al. 1988). However, a study of reassortants of the phlebovirus Rift Valley fever virus revealed that attenuating mutations (for mice) were present in a vaccine strain virus on all three of the genome segments (Saluzzo and Smith 1990).

CLINICAL AND PATHOLOGICAL ASPECTS

Clinical manifestations

Over 60 viruses of the family *Bunyaviridae* are known to cause disease in humans or animals. Most human infections are silent, and are detectable only by the appearance of specific antibodies. When clinical disease occurs, manifestation of infection ranges from self-limited febrile disease to potentially fatal fulminant hemorrhagic fever or encephalitis. Acute undifferentiated illness is often characterized by an abrupt onset of fever, usually accompanied by chills. Myalgia, arthralgia, headache with or without photophobia, malaise, anorexia, and nausea are common; occasionally vomiting also occurs. Gastrointestinal symptoms rarely dominate the clinical picture, however, nor are respiratory symptoms often seen, although some patients may have sore throat, cough, or even pulmonary infiltrates. A notable exception is hantavirus pulmonary syndrome. Physical examination may reveal conjunctival injection, mild adenopathy, and some abdominal tenderness. Clinical laboratory findings usually indicate a normal, decreased, or moderately elevated white blood count. The typical duration of uncomplicated illness is 2–4 days, perhaps extending to a week. A second wave of fever may occur ('saddle-back fever'), but there is no residual illness seen, although convalescence may require several days.

More severe infections may include a maculopapular rash on the trunk appearing after the onset of illness and lasting a few days (Bwamba, Oropouche, and others), bleeding (most severe in Crimean–Congo hemorrhagic fever, Garissa fever, and Rift Valley fever), encephalitis (Bhanja, California group and Rift Valley fever), hepatitis (hantaviruses and Rift Valley fever), acute kidney failure (hantaviruses), aseptic meningitis (Bwamba, Oropouche, and others), respiratory distress due to acute pulmonary edema (New World hantaviruses) and retinal vasculitis (unique to Rift Valley fever). Fatal infections have often been associated with California group viruses, especially La Crosse virus in children, Crimean–Congo hemorrhagic fever, hantaviral infections, especially hantavirus pulmonary syndrome in which case fatality rates approach 50 percent, and Rift Valley fever virus.

The most important veterinary pathogens are akabane virus, the cause of congenital malformations and abortions in cattle, sheep, and goats in Japan, Australia, South Africa, and Israel (Parsonson and McPhee 1985), Aino, Cache Valley, and Nairobi sheep disease viruses, the cause of malformations and abortions in sheep and/or cattle. Rift Valley fever virus, in addition to human infections, also causes abortion and death in domestic animals. Rift Valley fever virus is commonly found throughout subSaharan Africa, with periodic epizootic/epidemic transmission in Egypt (Meegan 1979), Yemen, and Saudi Arabia (Shoemaker et al. 2002).

IMPORTANT INFECTIONS

California encephalitis and related viruses

California encephalitis was until 2000, the most important arboviral disease seen in the USA, the vast majority of cases being detected among children infected with La Crosse virus. For example, in 1996–1997, of the 286 confirmed or probable arboviral infections, 252 (88 percent) were caused by California group viruses. In those years, the greatest number of cases occurred in

West Virginia (139 cases) with 11 other states having at least one case (Report 1998). Other pathogenic California group viruses include prototype California encephalitis virus, Guaroa, Inkoo (Jamestown Canyon), snowshoe hare virus and Tahyna virus. With the exception of Inkoo and Tahyna viruses, California group viruses are found predominantly in North America where they are transmitted by mosquitoes. Inkoo and Tahyna viruses are found in Europe, and there is serological evidence to suggest that viruses similar or identical to snowshoe hare virus are present in Asia. Tahyna-related viruses have been found in Africa. California group viruses are widely distributed, being found from the tropical zones to above the Arctic Circle (reviewed in LeDuc 1979).

The incubation period for California encephalitis patients is about 3–7 days after an infectious mosquito bite. Onset is abrupt with fever, headache, and lethargy; nausea and vomiting are common. Rash, diarrhea and arthralgia are uncommon. In milder cases, recovery occurs within a week, the only indication of neurological involvement being meningeal signs and perhaps disorientation. More severe cases develop seizures, convulsions, and loss of consciousness, with coma in some instances. Mild neurological signs, which may still be present at discharge, manifest as irritability and other conditions, but usually resolve over the course of several weeks, with little in the way of permanent illness being reported. Of 166 cases reported, two died and two had lasting hemiparesis. Patients with seizures during acute disease are at greater risk for subsequent convulsions, usually seen within a year after recovery. Intellectual and social functions do not seem to be disturbed among recovered children (Matthews et al. 1968; Sabatino and Cramblett 1968; Grabow et al. 1969; Rie et al. 1973). La Crosse encephalitis is usually a disease of children, whereas Jamestown Canyon encephalitis is found in adults.

Tahyna virus is found primarily in Europe, with a related or identical virus being found in Africa (Lumbovirus). Antibodies in humans have been found in Sri Lanka, China, and Russia. Human infection ranges from a mild febrile disease to aseptic meningitis. Pharyngitis, pulmonary involvement, or gastrointestinal disturbances, such as nausea and vomiting may be common. Although CNS involvement has been documented, serious illness or death has not been associated with Tahyna virus infections (Peters and LeDuc 1991).

Akabane virus

Akabane virus is an important veterinary pathogen causing congenital malformations, arthrogryposis, hydranencephaly, and other deformities, as well as abortions in cattle, sheep, and goats in Japan, Australia, South Africa, and Israel (Parsonson and McPhee 1985). Antibodies to akabane virus have been found in sera collected from 25 of 41 wildlife species in 11 subSaharan African countries (Al Busaidy et al. 1987). Both *Culex* mosquitoes and *Culicoides* are implicated in transmission.

Oropouche fever virus

Oropouche virus was first isolated in Trinidad from the blood of a forest worker with a mild febrile illness. Although never common in Trinidad, the virus has become a major cause of rural and urban epidemics in the Amazon region of South America, a large percentage of the resident population being infected during outbreaks. More than 500 000 cases have been recorded, primarily from the Brazilian states of Para, Amazonas, Maranhao, and Goias and more recently from Peru, Panama, Bolivia, and Costa Rica (Vasconcelos et al. 1989, 1994; Watts et al. 1997; Saeed et al. 2000). The disease is characterized by headache, fever, myalgia, arthralgia, photophobia, retrobulbar pain, nausea, and dizziness. Rash occurs in less than 10 percent of the confirmed cases. Symptoms may recur in more than half those clinically ill, usually within 1–2 weeks of the initial onset. No deaths have been reported for Oropouche fever, but meningitis or meningismus has been reported. Patients are often debilitated and prostration is common (reviewed in LeDuc and Pinheiro 1988).

Hantavirus infections

Hemorrhagic fever with renal syndrome (HFRS) has long been recognized clinically in Asia, Russia, and Scandinavia, but the etiology of the syndrome has been known only since the late 1970s. Over 200 synonyms have been used to describe HFRS, including Korean hemorrhagic fever, epidemic hemorrhagic fever, nephropathia epidemica, epidemic nephrosonephritis, and many others, often referring to geographic locations. It was not until 1978, however, that the causative agent, hantaan virus, was isolated from the lungs of the striped fieldmouse, *Apodemus agrarius* (Lee et al. 1978). Unlike other members of the family *Bunyaviridae*, the hantaviruses that infect humans are maintained in nature by chronically infected rodents. No arthropod vector is involved in their transmission cycle. Hantaan virus was named after the Hantaan River, near the demilitarized zone dividing the Korean peninsula, where the infected field mice were first captured.

Subsequent studies have demonstrated that hantaan virus represents an antigenically and genetically novel virus among the *Bunyaviridae* and was thus the prototype member for a new genus within the family (Schmaljohn and Dalrymple 1983; Schmaljohn et al. 1985). Subsequently, additional serologically related viruses have been isolated, many of which are known to cause human disease. Previously, human disease was thought to be limited to febrile illness followed by varying degrees of kidney failure. Recently, however, a new clinical presentation has been documented: hantavirus pulmonary syndrome (Duchin et al. 1994). This syndrome is characterized by acute onset of febrile disease, followed by an often fatal respiratory distress syndrome. Recent studies have shown this new disease to be caused also by hantaviral infections, but with a unique group of antigenically and genetically related viruses found only in the Americas. Thus, it appears that two basic lineages of hantaviruses have evolved, one occurring predominantly in the Old World, specifically evolving with rodent species found there, and leading to hemorrhagic fever with renal syndrome presentations, and one in the New World causing hantavirus pulmonary syndrome, maintained in nature by New World rodent species (Figure 48.5; and see Table 48.2). Phylogenetic studies suggest that the hantaviruses can be divided into three main groups: the Hantaan-like viruses that are carried by Murinae rodents (Old World mice and rats), Puumala-like viruses that are carried by Arvicolinae rodents (lemmings and voles), and Sin Nombre-like viruses that are carried by Sigmodontinae rodents (New World mice and rats) (Plyusnin 2002). However, a number of these 'viruses' are classified solely on genetic data for a portion of the genome in the absence of virus isolation and few serologic studies (see Table 48.2). No

doubt more detailed studies on these viruses will become available in the future.

The most severe form of HFRS occurs in Asia and is caused by prototype hantaan virus. It is associated with a case-fatality rate of approximately 5 percent, although this may be much higher in certain rural areas. This disease is characterized by an abrupt onset of fever, chills, malaise, myalgia, headache, dizziness, and anorexia after a variable incubation period of 2–42 days, but most often of 2–4 weeks. During this initial febrile phase, severe abdominal and back pain appear, accompanied by increasing nausea and vomiting, tenderness over the lower back, flushing of the face, neck and chest, and injection of the conjunctivae, palate, and pharynx. Petechiae may appear on the axillae, face, neck, chest, and soft palate, and hemorrhages into the conjunctivae may occur. Clinical laboratory studies reveal normal or slightly elevated white blood cell counts, decreased platelets and rising hematocrit (packed cell volume) values. Proteinuria may appear towards the end of this phase of the disease (McKee et al. 1985).

Defervescence occurs after 3–7 days and marks the start of the hypotensive phase, which may last from several hours to a few days. This phase is characterized by tachycardia, falling arterial pressure, and narrowing pulse pressure, mental changes and, in severe cases, classic shock. Bleeding tendencies continue with capillary hemorrhage and rising hematocrit values. Leukocytosis with a left shift, thrombocytopenia, and prolonged bleeding times are seen; there are high levels of proteinuria and oliguria begins. About one-third of the fatalities occur during this phase. The oliguric phase follows and lasts for 3–7 days, during which blood pressure returns to normal or is slightly elevated due to relative hypervolemia. The fall in urinary output is accompanied by elevated serum creatinine and blood urea nitrogen and other evidence of renal failure. Pulmonary edema may occur and care must be taken in fluid management. Rash and facial flushing disappear during this phase, although nausea and vomiting may continue. Severe hemorrhagic manifestations may occur, gastrointestinal or CNS bleeding being especially serious. Almost half the deaths occur during this phase, often due to pulmonary edema or infection, electrolyte imbalance, late shock, or hemorrhage into the brain. Clinical recovery begins during the diuretic phase, with the normalization of clotting and return of renal function. For the next few hours or days there is diuresis, with outputs of 3–6 liters daily. Strength and appetite improve, but fluid management must be maintained to prevent negative fluid balances which may lead to shock. The convalescent phase may require several months, and hyposthenuria may persist for months to years (McKee et al. 1985). Although complete recovery has been assumed, recent studies with Seoul virus have called this assumption into question (Glass et al. 1993). Specific therapy is not available, and careful supportive care is

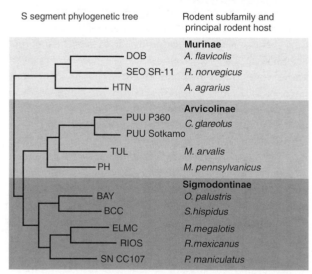

S segment phylogenetic tree / Rodent subfamily and principal rodent host

Murinae
DOB — *A. flavicolis*
SEO SR-11 — *R. norvegicus*
HTN — *A. agrarius*

Arvicolinae
PUU P360 — *C. glareolus*
PUU Sotkamo
TUL — *M. arvalis*
PH — *M. pennsylvanicus*

Sigmodontinae
BAY — *O. palustris*
BCC — *S. hispidus*
ELMC — *R. megalotis*
RIOS — *R. mexicanus*
SN CC107 — *P. maniculatus*

Figure 48.5 *Relationships of hantaviruses and their rodent hosts. Phylogenetic relationship of the complete S segments of hantaviruses is represented in a single most parsimonious tree derived by using PAUP 3.1.1 software. Horizontal lengths of branches are proportional to nucleotide sequence differences. Abbreviations for viruses and accession numbers for the S segment viral sequences are: Dobrava virus, DOB, L41916; Seoul virus, SEO, M34881; Hantaan virus, HTN, M14626; Puumala virus, PUU virus (strain P360), L11347; PUU (strain Sotkamo), X61035; Tula virus, TUL, Z30941; Prospect Hill virus, PH, X55128; Bayou virus, BAY, L36929; Black Creek Canal virus, BCC, L39949; El Moro Canyon virus, ELMC, U11427; Rio Segundo virus, RIOS, U18100; Sin Nombre virus (strain CC107) SN, L33683.*

essential to improving survival. Care must be consistent with the phase of the disease, careful attention being paid to fluid management. Recent studies have demonstrated that ribavirin is efficacious in treating HFRS if administered early in the course of illness (Huggins et al. 1991). Treated patients had significantly fewer deaths than those untreated, and they spent less time in each phase of the disease and were more likely to skip entire phases altogether.

Other Old World hantaviruses cause diseases similar to, though generally less severe than, classic hantaan virus infections. These include Puumala virus, the cause of nephropathia epidemica of western Europe, Scandinavia, and the western portions of Russia. Nephropathia epidemica may follow the same phases as classic HFRS, but is fatal in less than 1 percent of cases.

The severity of the clinical course of HFRS caused by Puumala virus was found to correlate statistically with specific HLA haplotypes, indicating that host, as well as virus, factors can dictate the outcome of hantaviral infection (Mustonen et al. 1996, 1998). In the Balkan region of Europe, Puumala virus overlaps in many areas with both classic hantaan virus and local strains that are capable of causing very severe disease with mortality rates at least as high as those seen in Asia. The severe HFRS of the Balkans has been associated with Dobrava virus, also reported as Belgrade virus (now known to be the same viruses) and is indistinguishable clinically from HFRS of Asia (Gligic et al. 1992; Avsic-Zupanc et al. 1992a, 1992b, 1995; Taller et al. 1993). Seoul virus, associated with *Rattus norvegicus* (brown rat), probably originated in Asia, but is now found throughout the world wherever large populations of rats exist (LeDuc et al. 1986). It causes a less severe form of HFRS that is characterized by greater liver involvement than classic Hantaan infections, and in general a lower case-fatality rate, although deaths have been recorded. Seoul virus infections are especially common in China, but have been documented in many parts of the world, including Europe and the Americas. In the USA, careful studies have associated past Seoul virus infection with an increased risk of hypertensive renal disease (Glass et al. 1993), an observation that could have significant economic implications for many developed countries (LeDuc et al. 1992).

Hantavirus pulmonary syndrome was first recognized in 1993, when an outbreak of an apparently new and highly fatal form of severe respiratory illness occurred in southwestern USA. As a result of subsequent field and laboratory investigations, the epidemiology and clinical characteristics of this new disease were described, and the name hantavirus pulmonary syndrome was proposed. It was caused by a previously unknown hantavirus, later named Sin Nombre virus (also reported as Four Corners or Muerto Canyon virus). The overall case-fatality rate was 52 percent and examination of the first 100 cases found they were distributed between 21 states. Further-

more the disease had been recognized since at least 1959 (Khan et al. 1996).

Hantavirus pulmonary syndrome has a prodrome of fever and myalgia (all of 17 patients originally described), with cough or dyspnea (76 percent), gastrointestinal symptoms (76 percent) and headache (71 percent) (Duchin et al. 1994). Physical characteristics seen among these original 17 cases include tachypnea (100 percent), tachycardia (94 percent), and hypotension (50 percent). Laboratory findings reflect leukocytosis, increased hematocrit, thrombocytopenia, prolonged prothrombin, and partial thromboplastin times, elevated serum lactate dehydrogenase, decreased serum protein concentrations, and proteinuria. Fifteen (88 percent) cases rapidly progressed to acute pulmonary edema, and 13 (76 percent) died. Predictors of death included increases in hematocrit and partial thromboplastin time, and all deaths occurred with profound hypotension (Duchin et al. 1994). Despite laboratory evidence strongly suggestive of disseminated intravascular coagulopathy, clinical signs of hemorrhage have rarely been reported (Zaki et al. 1995). Radiographic examination reveals bilateral pulmonary infiltrates in virtually all hospitalized patients, and pleural effusions in many. At postmortem examination, copious pleural effusions are often found (Zaki et al. 1995). Multiorgan involvement was found in all of 44 fatal cases examined, with generalized vascular congestion. The primary histopathological features were seen in the lung where microscopic examination revealed mild to moderate interstitial pneumonitis with variable degrees of congestion, edema, and mononuclear cell infiltrates (Zaki et al. 1995). Immunohistochemical examination of postmortem tissue from 44 fatal cases revealed viral antigen-positive cells widely distributed in various tissues, but seen predominantly within endothelial cells of capillaries and small vessels. The most intensive and extensive endothelial staining was in tissues of the lungs, where viral antigen was abundant and uniformly distributed. It involved most of the pulmonary microvasculature, although high densities of viral antigens were also observed in lymphoid follicles of the spleen and, to a lesser extent, in lymph node follicles (Zaki et al. 1995). The magnitude and extent, however, of pulmonary endothelial involvement reflect the difficulty experienced by clinicians in attempting to manage the often terminal shock syndrome.

Treatment has been prompt hospitalization, aggressive clinical management, and early pulmonary support. Ribavirin, which can be efficacious in the treatment of HFRS patients, has been administered to hantavirus pulmonary syndrome patients, but at present there are insufficient data to indicate efficacy clearly.

Crimean–Congo hemorrhagic fever virus

Crimean–Congo hemorrhagic fever (CCHF) is a severe, tickborne, acute hemorrhagic fever found throughout much of Africa, extending northward to Albania, the former Yugoslavia, Crimea, and elsewhere in the former Soviet Union, Iraq, and much of the Middle East, and eastward into Pakistan and western China. Clinical disease has been well described from cases seen in the former Soviet Union, and nosocomial outbreaks have been common among hospitalized patients, especially those undergoing surgery. The case–fatality rate originally described for cases occurring in Crimea was 15–30 percent (Chumakov 1946); other outbreaks have had case–fatality rates as high as 40 percent (Hoogstraal 1979). Cases usually occur singly among shepherds or others with rural exposure who have been fed on by ticks, or as small clusters among individuals involved in the slaughter of an infected animal (Swanepoel et al. 1985). Nosocomial outbreaks have occurred in the former Soviet Union, the former Yugoslavia, South Africa, and the Middle East (Burney et al. 1976). They typically involve a severely ill patient with hemorrhage and a suspected acute abdomen, perforated ulcer or other diagnosis leading to surgical intervention. Inevitably the patient dies, and often the medical team, family members, or both, are infected, often with a fatal outcome.

The clinical picture of CCHF is an initial influenza-like illness followed by severe headache, joint and back pains, fever, nausea, vomiting, and photophobia. The incubation period is typically 3–6 days in nosocomial infections, and 3–12 days following tick exposure. Initial symptoms may be followed by circulatory collapse, shock, and a variety of hemorrhagic manifestations, such as epistaxis, hemoptysis, hematemesis, melena, and skin hemorrhage. Bleeding into the intestinal tract may cause the patient to present with acute abdominal pain, leading to surgical intervention and increased risk of nosocomial spread. Involvement of the central nervous system indicates a poor prognosis. Clinical laboratory data include leukopenia from the onset of illness, neutropenia, thrombocytopenia, and falling hemoglobin and erythrocyte counts in severely ill patients. The clinically apparent attack rate was estimated to be five infections per case of hemorrhagic fever in the former Soviet Union (Goldfarb et al. 1980).

Nairobi sheep disease virus

This acute, hemorrhagic gastroenteritis affecting sheep and goats in East Africa was described by Montgomery (1917), who correctly attributed transmission to the tick, *Rhipicephalus appendiculatus*. The case–fatality rate may be 70–90 percent in sheep, but goats are less seriously affected. Herdsmen tending infected animals may develop a mild, febrile illness, and laboratory infections with this virus have occurred (Swanepoel 1995). In India, Ganjam virus was isolated from ticks collected from sheep and goats in Orissa state (Karabatsos 1985). Ganjam virus is now considered to be synonymous with

Nairobi sheep disease virus (Davies et al. 1978). Dugbe virus, another virus of the genus *Nairovirus*, has been isolated many times from cattle ticks in Nigeria (Kemp et al. 1971), and there have been a few Dugbe virus isolations from febrile humans.

Rift Valley fever virus

Epizootics of Rift Valley fever virus were first reported at the beginning of the twentieth century, but the virus was first isolated in the 1930s in the Rift Valley of Kenya, where sheep suffered fatal hepatic necrosis and abortion. Since then, there have been many epizootics throughout subSaharan Africa, and associated human disease has been described. In 1977, Rift Valley fever was first documented outside subSaharan Africa, when an outbreak occurred in Egypt (Hoogstraal 1979; Laughlin et al. 1979; Meegan 1979). Extensive human and animal disease occurred in Egypt, including the Nile delta region, between 1977 and 1979, but adjacent countries were spared. Transmission appears to have ceased in 1979. In 1993, however, Rift Valley fever once again appeared in Egypt, initially in Upper Egypt near Aswan, and subsequently in the Nile delta (WHO 1994). This presumed importation has likewise not spread beyond Egypt's borders, and may have been contained or eliminated by an aggressive vaccination campaign.

The disease appeared in Mauritania and Senegal in 1987 when an estimated 224 patients died in Mauritania, and many abortions occurred in sheep and goats. This epidemic was associated with flooding at the Diama Dam near the mouth of the Senegal River (Digoutte and Peters 1989). In 2000, the virus was detected in Yemen and Saudi Arabia where nearly 2 000 cases were reported with an estimated 245 deaths. Genetic studies of the virus were consistent with the theory that infection was introduced from East Africa (Shoemaker et al. 2002).

Sheep, cattle, and goats suffer 10–30 percent mortality from Rift Valley fever virus, and a large percentage of infected pregnant animals abort. Disease and death are most frequent in young animals. Native ungulates seem to be more resistant to lethal infection. Disease in humans is characterized by acute onset of fever, headache and myalgia with incapacitating prostration. The incubation period is typically 2–6 days; in most patients the illness resolves after 2–3 days' rest, although symptoms may persist for a week. A small proportion, perhaps 1 percent, of cases develop hemorrhagic fever, encephalitis, or retinal vasculitis. Hemorrhagic disease begins as typical Rift Valley fever, but patients develop gastrointestinal bleeding, become jaundiced, and may die in shock. Disseminated vascular damage and hepatic failure may contribute to the cause of death. Fatal encephalitis may also follow Rift Valley fever, which typically develops a few days to 1–2 weeks after initial recovery from classic disease. Patients develop headache, confusion, return of fever, and various neurological signs that may lead to residual illness or death. Similarly, ocular complications appear up to 3 weeks after acute disease, presenting with rapid onset of decreased visual acuity due to retinal hemorrhage, exudates, and macular edema. Vision returns as the edema and exudates resolve, but about half the patients suffer some degree of permanent visual loss.

Sandfly fever and related viruses

Sandfly fever, also known as pappataci fever or phlebotomus fever, has been recognized as a militarily important disease since the Napoleonic Wars (Hertig and Sabin 1964). During both World Wars, foreign troops suffered significant incidence rates of sandfly fever in the Mediterranean theaters. These viruses are transmitted by the bite of infectious sandflies (genus *Phlebotomus*, thus 'phlebotomus fever'), and take their names from the sites of their original isolation. Sabin was the first to demonstrate that these two distinct viruses could cause virtually identical diseases in humans (Sabin 1951). The clinical syndrome after infections with either Naples virus or Sicilian virus is characterized by abrupt onset of fever lasting 2–4 days, headache, eye pain, photophobia, pain in the back and joints, anorexia, and malaise. Nausea and vomiting, other abdominal symptoms, sore throat, drowsiness, dizziness, and saddleback fever may also be seen, but rash or meningeal signs are uncommon (Sabin 1951; Hertig and Sabin 1964; Bartelloni and Tesh 1976). No deaths have been documented among several hundred cases studied, and no sequelae are recognized. Life-long homologous protection probably follows infection, but there is no crossprotection between Naples and Sicilian viruses.

Toscana virus was isolated in 1971 from sandflies (*Phlebotomus pernicious*) captured in the Tuscany region of central Italy (Verani et al. 1980). Subsequent investigations there have shown it to be the causative agent in many cases of summertime aseptic meningitis (Verani and Nicoletti 1995). Serological surveys have found antibodies to Toscana virus in other southern European countries as well, although its health impact in these areas is less well characterized (Balducci et al. 1985).

New World sandfly fever viruses

Alenquer, Candiru, Chagres, and Punta Toro are all New World sandfly fever viruses originally isolated from febrile patients. The clinical disease following infection with any of these viruses is virtually indistinguishable from that seen in Naples or Sicilian infections. Human cases are not common owing to the secretive nature of their New World sandfly vectors (genus *Lutzomyia*), which inhabit tropical forests and are unlikely to come into contact with large numbers of humans. Even so,

antibody prevalence rates ranging from 2 to 34 percent for Punta Toro virus were detected in serological surveys of residents of rural Panama, and about half those rates for Chagres virus (LeDuc et al. 1980).

Other infections

Bangui virus causes a febrile illness with rash in the Central African Republic. It has also been recovered from a bird in the same country (Digoutte et al. 1980).

Bhanja virus was first isolated in India from *Haemaphysalis intermedia* ticks collected from goats in Ganjam district, Orissa (Shah and Work 1969). Other isolations have been made from cattle and goat ticks in West Africa, and from blood samples collected there from cattle, sheep, ground squirrels, and hedgehogs. Bhanja infection of goats is widespread in the former Czechoslovakia, Italy, and the former Yugoslavia; and many animal sera collected in Sri Lanka have antibodies against this virus. Infection of humans caused severe neurological disease and death in at least two cases in the former Yugoslavia, and laboratory infections have occurred (Vesenjak-Hirjan et al. 1980).

Bwamba virus was first isolated from acutely ill febrile patients in Bwamba County, Uganda (Smithburn et al. 1941). Later serological studies have found high prevalence rates of antibodies to this and closely related viruses throughout East, Central, West, and South Africa. Bwamba virus seems to be a common cause of febrile illness in humans in Africa, causing a self-limiting disease accompanied by rash and prostration, often with meningeal signs (Georges et al. 1980). Bwamba and a closely related virus, Pongola, have been isolated from various mosquito species, but little is known about their natural history. Kasokero virus has been isolated from bats in Uganda, where it may cause fever in humans (Kaluda et al. 1986). Laboratory infections have occurred.

Cache Valley virus has been associated with congenital malformations in sheep and cattle, and serological surveys have frequently found antibodies in domestic animals and humans throughout the Americas. Human disease is uncommon. However, a recent report of severe encephalitis and multiorgan failure attests to its ability to cause life-threatening illness (Edwards et al. 1989; Sexton et al. 1997).

Garissa virus is a reassortant bunyavirus. It was isolated from acute hemorrhagic fever cases during an epidemic of Rift Valley fever in Kenya and southern Somalia in 1997 and early 1998. Initial studies indicated that the sequences of the L and S RNA segments were nearly identical to those of Bunyamwera virus, whereas the sequence of the M segment was very different (33 percent nucleotide and 28 percent amino acid differences from Bunyamwera virus). Acute sera of 14 hemorrhagic fever cases yielded either virus isolation or PCR evidence of infection (Bowen et al. 2001). Very recent studies have shown that Garissa and Ngari virus M segments are nearly identical in sequence while the L and S segments of Bunyamwera virus are very similar to Ngari virus. These data indicate that Garissa virus is not a reassortant but is an isolate of Ngari virus, which is a reassortant of Bunyamwera virus (Gerrard et al. 2004). Previously, Ngari virus has not been considered a cause of hemorrhagic fever and further studies are required to investigate the pathogenesis and epidemiology of Ngari virus.

Keterah virus, isolated in Malaysia from Argas ticks and from bats, is indistinguishable from Issyk–kul virus, which has been isolated from *Aedes caspius* mosquitoes and from bats (*Nyctalus noctula*, *Myotis blythii* and *Vespertilio serotinus*) and ticks (*Argasvespertilionsis*) in Kirghiz SSR, the former USSR. It has since been associated with epidemics of febrile disease in humans in that region (Lvov et al. 1984).

Nyando virus was isolated from mosquitoes in Kenya, and from humans in the Central African Republic, where it caused fever, myalgia, and vomiting (Digoutte et al. 1980).

Tamdy virus is a tick-borne virus causing a febrile illness in humans in the Asiatic regions of the former USSR (Lvov et al. 1976).

Tataguine virus is a mosquito-borne virus that causes fever, joint pains, and rash in humans in Africa (Digoutte et al. 1980).

Wanowrie virus was isolated from *Hyalomma marginatum isaaci* ticks collected from sheep in India, and from the brain of a 17-year-old girl who died in Sri Lanka after a 2-day fever with abdominal pain and vomiting (Pavri et al. 1976). The virus is also present in Egypt and Iran (Sureau and Klein 1980).

Epidemiology

GENERAL CONSIDERATIONS

Viruses of the family *Bunyaviridae* are maintained in nature in a complex life cycle, usually involving an arthropod vector and a vertebrate host. The exceptions are viruses of the genus *Hantavirus*, which are maintained by chronic infection of rodents and other small mammals. In general, each virus is specifically associated with a particular arthropod species that serves to transmit the virus, and one or more species of vertebrate hosts that serve to amplify the virus following infection through a transient viremia. Arthropod vectors, especially mosquitoes, are often seasonally abundant, which results in seasonal transmission of the viruses they transmit. During periods of adverse weather conditions, virus survival is often maintained by vertical or transovarial transmission whereby an infected female passes the viral infection on to the next generation of vectors. The virus survives in association with the dormant egg and, with hatching and subsequent development, virus

transmission to vertebrate hosts takes place during blood feeding. Viruses may also be transmitted venereally from infected males to uninfected female vectors during mating. Vertebrate hosts serve to amplify the amount of virus in circulation by means of a viremia of varying intensity and duration. Uninfected vector species become infected when ingesting a viremic bloodmeal. Following an extrinsic incubation period of a few days' duration, during which the virus replicates and is disseminated throughout the vector, the newly infected vectors are then able to transmit the virus at subsequent blood feeding. Mosquitoes are the most important group of arthropod vectors, but ticks, sandflies, and biting midges (*Culicoides* spp.) are also important vectors for certain viruses.

Most of the bunyaviruses are zoonotic in nature, and humans are usually only accidental hosts that generally do not facilitate amplification of the virus in nature. Exceptions are Oropouche virus and perhaps sandfly fever viruses, in which humans seem to be important sources of virus for uninfected vectors. Selected examples of the transmission cycles of representative viruses are presented below to demonstrate their complexity.

IMPORTANT INFECTIONS

California encephalitis due to La Crosse virus

Most viruses of the genus *Bunyavirus* are transmitted by mosquitoes, and California encephalitis due to La Crosse virus may serve as an example of one of the better understood transmission cycles (see Calisher and Thompson 1983, for overview). The mosquito *Aedes triseriatus* is the principal vector of La Crosse virus. This species is common in the hardwood forests of the upper midwestern United States, where it breeds primarily in tree holes. It survives the harsh winters in the egg stage. In late spring or early summer the first adults emerge, mate, and begin to seek a blood meal. La Crosse virus is transmitted transovarially from infected adult female *Ae. triseriatus* to the next generation of eggs, so a proportion of those newly emerging adults are already infected with the virus (Watts et al. 1973, 1974). These infected females transmit the virus to susceptible vertebrate hosts at blood feeding, beginning the amplification cycle each year, whereas infected males may pass the virus to uninfected females during mating. (Male mosquitoes do not feed on blood, and thus cannot transmit the virus directly to an amplifying vertebrate host.) *Ae. triseriatus* females typically feed during the day, most frequently on squirrels, chipmunks, foxes, and rabbits, and on humans if present. Susceptible squirrels and chipmunks circulate the virus in high enough titer to infect other *Ae. triseriatus*, thus serving to amplify the prevalence of virus in the vector population. Foxes, with their larger range, may both amplify the virus among local vector populations and also disseminate it to more distant vector populations (Yuill 1983). Humans are infected when they enter the woods for recreation or work, most clinical cases being seen among children less than 15 years old. As *Ae. triseriatus* breeds equally well in discarded tyres or other items that retain water, infected mosquito populations may flourish in close proximity to dwellings, increasing the risk of infection to residents. Prevention of California encephalitis due to La Crosse virus can be facilitated by clean-up campaigns to reduce the availability of mosquito breeding sites, but elimination of all breeding is probably impossible owing to the abundance of natural breeding sites (Francy 1983).

Oropouche virus

Although most viruses of the genus *Orthobunyavirus* are transmitted by mosquitoes, some, such as Oropouche and other members of the *Simbu* serogroup, are transmitted by biting midges (family *Ceratopogonidae*, genus *Culicoides*). Oropouche virus was first described from Trinidad, but in the past two decades has become a major public health problem in northern Brazil and adjacent Amazon Basin nations (for an overview, see LeDuc and Pinheiro 1988). This increase is almost certainly a result of the changing ecology of the Amazon Basin, deforestation leading to human settlements and large plantations of banana and cacao, with the organic waste from these and other crops serving as ideal breeding sites for the vector *Culicoides*. This has led to tremendous population densities of *C. paraensis* in many parts of the Amazon Basin. Oropouche virus is thought to be maintained in two distinct transmission cycles: silent sylvatic transmission involving nonhuman primates, sloths, and perhaps other vertebrate hosts, and an urban cycle in which humans are the primary amplifying and disseminating host and *C. paraensis* serving as the primary vector (Pinheiro et al. 1981). This species lives in close association with humans and readily feeds during daylight hours. Epidemics occur when midge populations are large, the majority of the human population is susceptible and Oropouche virus is introduced from the silent sylvatic cycle into the urban setting. Although only a small percentage of the midges are able to transmit the virus, it seems that the populations are often so abundant that transmission is sustained until the majority of those humans susceptible have been infected. Humans circulate virus in sufficiently high titers to infect feeding *C. paraensis*, and consequently may serve to introduce the virus to new areas through their travel. With the increasing deforestation of the Amazon Basin, epidemics of Oropouche and other previously uncommon viruses found there are likely to increase.

Hantaan and related hantaviruses

Unlike other viruses of the family *Bunyaviridae*, arthropod vectors do not seem to play a significant role in the transmission of the hantaviruses. It seems that the hantaviruses, perhaps like other members of the family, represent an excellent example of co-evolution of the virus with a specific vertebrate host. As information about each of the genetically unique hantaviruses accumulates, it is increasingly apparent that each virus is specifically linked to a particular species of rodent host. These associations are shown in Table 48.2. The virus lineages closely follow the origin of the rodent hosts. Within the rodent family *Muridae*, three subfamilies exist: *Murinae*, *Arvicolinae*, and *Sigmodontinae*; the hantaviruses maintained by rodent species of each of these subfamilies are genetically most closely related to each other, and less so to those of viruses associated with rodents of the other subfamilies (see Figure 48.5) (for an overview, see LeDuc 1995). Transmission of hantaviruses between rodent hosts is thought to occur by aerosol from infectious excreta, and perhaps by saliva (Glass et al. 1988; Nuzum et al. 1988). Biting may play an important role in transmission of hantaviruses among rodents as territories are set and mating occurs (Glass et al. 1988). Studies have failed to demonstrate direct transmission from infected parent rodents to their offspring. Humans are infected when they come into contact with infected rodent hosts. There is thus a strong occupational association with the risk of hantaviral infection, farmers, woodcutters, soldiers, and others with significant rural exposure being most often infected. Hantaviral infections are seasonal. They occur frequently in warmer months when recreational activities and outdoor work bring people into close contact with infected rodents. Infections caused by hantaan and Puumala virus peak in prevalence also in late fall and early winter in Asia and Europe, respectively. In cold seasons, the rodents seek shelter in homes and sheds, infecting not only male workers, but also children and women.

Crimean–Congo hemorrhagic fever virus

Crimean–Congo hemorrhagic fever (CCHF) virus serves as an excellent example of two aspects of the epidemiology of viruses in the family *Bunyaviridae*: the threat of nosocomial or other direct transmission from infected blood to susceptible humans, and transmission by ticks (for overviews, see Hoogstraal 1979; Watts et al. 1989; Swanepoel 1995). CCHF virus is widely distributed from eastern Europe to Asia and Africa. In general, its distribution follows closely that of the primary tick vectors of the genus *Hyalomma*. Immature ticks acquire infection during feeding on viremic hosts, often small mammals, or by vertical transmission from infected females to the progeny. As ticks develop, the virus may be transmitted transstadially to subsequent developmental stages, and infected ticks may pass the virus to uninfected females during mating. Adult females, including those infected venereally, may then pass the virus to subsequent generations transovarially (Gonzalez et al. 1992). Viremia occurs after infection of small mammals as well as of domestic ruminants, which may serve to infect uninfected tick vectors. The proportion of uninfected ticks that becomes infected when feeding on a viremic host generally increases with the intensity of viremia. In addition, nonviremic transmission, as described for Dugbe virus, is also thought to occur with CCHF (Jones et al. 1987; Jones et al. 1989).

Humans become infected either through the bite of an infected tick or through direct contact with infectious blood from an infected animal. The original outbreak of CCHF, described from the Crimean peninsula in 1944–1946, involved large numbers of people exposed to ticks during post-war conditions, clearing agricultural lands that had been fallow. Today, however, most cases are seen among individuals in Bulgaria, Albania, and adjacent parts of the former Yugoslavia, sporadically in the Middle East, and as isolated cases in Africa, especially in South Africa where the virus is well known and studied. Clusters of cases occur in hospitals, especially in remote or ill-equipped clinics and surgeries, where the disease may not be recognized initially, and staff are infected by direct contact with infectious bodily fluids. Transmission of CCHF virus to workers in the laboratory setting has also occurred, leading to severe disease and fatalities.

Pathogenesis, pathology, and immune response

Human infection with a bunyavirus generally follows the bite of an infectious vector or, less frequently, inhalation of infectious virus. After an incubation period, a brief viremia often occurs, which corresponds to the period of acute illness. Signs and symptoms probably result from direct effects of virus on target organs, such as the liver or brain. Immunohistochemical analysis has found widespread hantaviral antigens in endothelial cells of the microvasculature of hantavirus pulmonary syndrome patients, which may reflect similar targets of infection with other hantaviruses (Zaki et al. 1995). Disseminated intravascular coagulopathy may occur in severe disease with hemorrhagic manifestations such as HFRS, CCHF or Rift Valley fever. A typical humoral immune response leads to cessation of viremia and clinical recovery in most cases, with immunoglobulin M (IgM) predominating initially, followed by immunoglobulin G (IgG). The cellular immune response to bunyavirus infections is not well defined, nor is the role of cytokines. A brief discussion of the pathogenesis, pathology, and immune response of selected diseases is presented in Clinical manifestations.

Diagnosis

Diagnosis is based on demonstration of the specific virus causing infection, by isolation, by detection of viral antigen or nucleic acids, or by acquisition of antibody specific for the infecting virus. Classic virus isolation techniques such as inoculation of suckling mice or cell cultures of mammalian or insect origin have been often used with considerable success. Likewise, routine serological techniques such as hemagglutination inhibition, complement fixation, immunofluorescent antibody assays, neutralization tests in mice or cell culture have been used to demonstrate rising or falling titers of antibody in paired sera from patients. These techniques are generally time consuming and expensive, and do not offer a definitive diagnosis soon enough to influence clinical management. Recently, more rapid diagnostic procedures have been developed that can offer a presumptive diagnosis within a few hours of receipt of a single acute serum sample. With enzyme immunoassays, viral antigen may be detected directly, or virus-specific IgM antibody demonstrated, generally in time to influence clinical management. For example, patients with HFRS due to hantaan virus are often positive for IgM antibodies at the time of hospital admission (LeDuc et al. 1990). Confirmation of the specific etiology helps in forecasting the course of the illness and initiating antiviral therapy such as ribavirin, which is efficacious in the treatment of HFRS (Huggins et al. 1991). Direct detection of viral nucleic acid, most often through reverse transcriptase-polymerase chain reaction amplification, and subsequent sequencing or endonuclease digestion of amplified products, has recently been applied for diagnosis, especially of hantavirus infections (Nichol et al. 1993). Acute specimens and autopsy tissues have both been used successfully to establish the diagnosis. However, the value of the technique is limited by the need for specially designed primers and very careful laboratory techniques to minimize the risk of contamination (Grankvist et al. 1992; Feldmann et al. 1993; Nichol et al. 1993). At present, these techniques are limited to research or reference laboratories and not widely available.

Prevention and control

Diseases caused by bunyaviruses have, with few exceptions, a low incidence of human infection and thus do not justify development of vaccines. An exception is HFRS, especially that due to hantaan virus in Asia, where several candidate vaccines are in development, under field trials or, in at least one case, commercially available (Lee et al. 1990; Schmaljohn et al. 1994). Most current candidates are inactivated whole virus vaccines that require multiple inoculations and boosters to ensure protection. However, recombinant candidates are also under development. In particular, DNA vaccines appear to have significant promise for Hantaan and related viruses (Hooper et al. 2001a; Custer et al. 2003). Development of live-attenuated vaccines for hantavirus infections has been hampered by the absence of a suitable animal model that would faithfully mimic human disease (WHO 1995), although recent studies suggest some animal models may have utility (Hooper et al. 2001b; Milazzo and Eyzaguirre 2002; Fisher and Tesch 2003). Vaccines for Rift Valley fever virus have also been developed, with both inactivated and live attenuated products available for veterinary use, and an inactivated vaccine available on a limited basis for humans (Smithburn 1949; Eddy et al. 1981; Kark et al. 1982; Morrill et al. 1987, 1991). A live-attenuated candidate vaccine for humans is now in early clinical trails. Observational studies indicate that ribavirin has a beneficial effect in CCHF infections. Thus it may be that oral prophylactic treatment of exposed persons is warranted (Mardani et al. 2003).

Most often, however, prevention and control of bunyaviruses are based on avoidance of human contact with infected arthropod or small mammal vectors. Infection usually occurs when people enter into the ecological setting where viruses are being transmitted silently among infected vectors and wild vertebrate hosts. In these situations, personal protective measures, such as the liberal use of insect repellants and wearing appropriate clothing, may reduce the risk of infection. Likewise, care should be taken to ensure that houses, vacation cabins, or campsites do not attract or support breeding potential vectors. Thus, using screens on windows and doors and removing potential mosquito breeding sites, such as used tyres or other water-holding containers, will help prevent infections. In the case of rodentborne hantaviruses, special precautions are needed to rodent-proof homes and to maintain clean campsites.

ACKNOWLEDGMENTS

This chapter was written shortly before the death of Bob Shope. Bob's friendship and knowledge is greatly missed by all of us who work on arboviruses.

REFERENCES

Abraham, G. and Pattnaik, A. 1983. Early RNA synthesis in Bunyamwera virus-infected cells. *J Gen Virol*, **64**, 1277–90.

Adkins, S., Quadt, R., et al. 1995. An RNA-dependent RNA polymerase activity associated with virions of tomato spotted wilt virus, a plant- and insect-infecting bunyavirus. *Virology*, **207**, 308–11.

Akashi, H. and Bishop, D. 1983. Comparison of the sequences and coding of La Crosse and snowshoe hare bunyavirus S RNA species. *J Virol*, **45**, 1155–8.

Akashi, H., Gay, M., et al. 1984. Localized conserved regions of the S RNA gene products of bunyaviruses are revealed by sequence analysis of the Simbu serogroup Aino viruses. *Virus Res*, **1**, 51–63.

Al Busaidy, S., Hamblin, C. and Taylor, W. 1987. Neutralising antibodies to Akabane virus in free-living wild animals in Africa. *Trop Anim Health Prod*, **19**, 197–202.

Anderson, G.W. Jr. and Smith, J.F. 1987. Immunoelectron microscopy of Rift Valley fever morphogenesis in primary rat hepatocytes. *Virology*, **161**, 91–100.

Andersson, A.M., Melin, L., et al. 1997a. Processing and membrane toplogy of the spike proteins G1 and G2 of Uukuniemi virus. *J Virol*, **71**, 218–25.

Andersson, A.M., Melin, L., et al. 1997b. A retention signal necessary and sufficient for Golgi localization maps to the cytoplasmic tail of a *Bunyaviridae* (Uukuniemi virus) membrane glycoprotein. *J Virol*, **71**, 4717–27.

Antic, D., Wright, K. and Kang, C. 1992a. Maturation of Hantaan virus glycoproteins G1 and G2. *Virology*, **189**, 324–8.

Antic, D., Kang, C., et al. 1992b. Comparison of the deduced gene products of the L, M and S genome segments of hantaviruses. *Virus Res*, **24**, 35–46.

Arikawa, J., Takashima, I. and Hashimoto, N. 1985. Cell fusion by haemorrhagic fever with renal syndrome (HFRS) viruses and its application for titration of virus infectivity and neutralizing antibody. *Arch Virol*, **86**, 303–13.

Arikawa, J., Schmaljohn, A., et al. 1989. Characterization of Hantaan virus envelope glycoprotein antigenic determinants by monoclonal antibodies. *J Gen Virol*, **70**, 615–24.

Arikawa, J., Yao, J., et al. 1992. Protective role of antigenic sites on the envelope protein of Hantaan virus defined by monoclonal antibodies. *Arch Virol*, **126**, 271–81.

Arnheiter, H., Davis, N., et al. 1985. Role of the nucleocapsid proteins in regulating vesicular stomatitis virus RNA synthesis. *Cell*, **41**, 259–67.

Asada, H., Tamura, M., et al. 1987. Role of T lymphocyte subsets in protection and recovery from Hantaan virus infection in mice. *J Gen Virol*, **68**, 1961–9.

Asada, H., Tamura, M., et al. 1988. Cell-mediated immunity to virus causing haemorrhagic fever with renal syndrome: generation of cytotoxic T lymphocytes. *J Gen Virol*, **69**, 2179–88.

Asada, H., Balachandra, K., et al. 1989. Cross-reactive immunity among different serotypes of virus causing haemorrhagic fever with renal syndrome. *J Gen Virol*, **70**, 819–25.

Avsic-Zupanc, T., Poljak, M. et al. 1992a. Antigenic variation of hantavirus isolates from Slovenia. 2nd International Conference on Haemorrhagic Fever with Renal Syndrome, Beijing, China, October 26–28 (Abstract).

Avsic-Zupanc, T., Xiao, S., et al. 1992b. Characterization of Dobrava virus: a hantavirus from Slovenia, Yugoslavia. *J Med Virol*, **38**, 132–7.

Avsic-Zupanc, T., Toney, A.R., et al. 1995. Genetic and antigenic properties of Dobrava virus: a unique member of the *Hantavirus* genus, family *Bunyaviridae*. *J Gen Virol*, **76**, 2801–8.

Balducci, M., Fausto, A., Verani, P. 1985. Phlebotomus-transmitted viruses in Europe. In Pozzi, E.L. (ed.), Proceedings of the International Congress for Infectious Diseases, Rome.

Banerjee, A. 1987. Transcription and replication of rhabdoviruses. *Microbiol Rev*, **51**, 66–87.

Bartelloni, P. and Tesh, R. 1976. Clinical and serologic responses of volunteers infected with phlebotomus fever virus (Sicilian type). *Am J Trop Med Hyg*, **25**, 456–62.

Battles, J. and Dalrymple, J. 1988. Genetic variation among geographic isolates of Rift Valley fever virus. *Am J Trop Med Hyg*, **39**, 617–31.

Bellocq, C., Raju, R., et al. 1987. Translational requirement of La Crosse virus S-mRNA synthesis: in vitro studies. *J Virol*, **61**, 87–95.

Bharadwaj, M., Botten, J., et al. 1997. Rio Mamore virus: genetic characterization of a newly recognized hantavirus of the pygmy rice rat, *Oligoryzomys microtis*, from Bolivia. *Am J Trop Med Hyg*, **57**, 368–74.

Bishop, D. and Shope, R. 1979. *Bunyaviridae*. In: Fraenkel-Conrat, H. and Wagner, R.R. (eds), *Comprehensive virology*, Vol. 14. New York: Plenum Press, 1–156.

Bishop, D., Calisher, C., et al. 1980. Bunyaviridae. *Intervirology*, **14**, 125–43.

Bishop, D., Gould, K., et al. 1982. The complete sequence and coding content of snowshoe hare bunyavirus small (S) viral RNA species. *Nucleic Acids Res*, **10**, 3703–13.

Bishop, D., Gay, M. and Matsuoko, Y. 1983. Nonviral heterogeneous sequences are present at the 5′ ends of one species of snowshoe hare bunyavirus S complementary RNA. *Nucleic Acids Res*, **11**, 6409–19.

Bishop, D., Rud, E., et al. 1984. Genome structure, transcription, and genetics. In: Compans, R.D. and Bishop, D. (eds), *Segmented negative strand viruses, Arenavirus, Bunyaviruses and Orthomyxoviruses*. Orlando, FL: Academic Press, 3–11.

Blumberg, B., Giorgi, C. and Kolakofsky, D. 1983. N protein of vesicular stomatitis virus selectively encapsidates leader RNA in vitro. *Cell*, **32**, 559–67.

Bouloy, M. and Hannoun, C. 1976. Studies on Lumbo virus replication. I. RNA-dependent RNA polymerase associated with virions. *Virology*, **69**, 258–64.

Bouloy, M., Vialat, M., et al. 1984. A transcript from the S segment of the Germiston bunyavirus is uncapped and codes for the nucleoprotein and a nonstructural protein. *J Virol*, **49**, 717–23.

Bouloy, M., Pardigon, N., et al. 1990. Characterization of the 5′ and 3′ ends of viral messenger RNAs isolated from BHK21 cells infected with Germiston virus (Bunyavirus). *Virology*, **175**, 50–8.

Bouloy, M., Janzen, C., et al. 2001. Genetic evidence that for an interferon-antagonistic function of Rift Valley fever virus nonstructural protein NSs. *J Virol*, **75**, 1371–7.

Bowen, M.D., Trappier, S.G., et al. 2001. A reassortant bunyavirus isolated from acute hemorrhagic fever cases in Kenya and Somalia. *Virology*, **291**, 185–90.

Bridgen, A., Weber, F., et al. 2001. Bunyamwera bunyavirus nonstructural protein NSs is a nonessential gene product that contributes to viral pathogenesis. *Proc Natl Acad Sci USA*, **98**, 664–9.

Bridgen, A., Dalrymple, A., et al. 2004. Inhibition of Dugbe nairovirus replication by human MxA protein. *Virus Res*, **99**, 47–50.

Broadwell, R. and Oliver, C. 1981. Golgi apparatus, GERL, and secretory granule formation within neurons of the hypothalamo-neurohypophysial system of control and hyperosmotically stressed mice. *J Cell Biol*, **90**, 474–84.

Burney, M., Ghafoor, A., et al. 1976. Nosocomial outbreak of viral hemorrhagic fever caused by Crimean hemorrhagic fever-Congo virus in Pakistan. *Am J Trop Med Hyg*, **29**, 941–7.

Cabradilla, C., Holloway, B. and Obijeski, J. 1983. Molecular cloning and sequencing of the La Crosse virus S RNA. *Virology*, **128**, 463–8.

Calisher, C. and Thompson, W. 1983. *California serogroup viruses*. New York: Alan R Liss.

Carey, D., Reuben, R., et al. 1971. Thottapalayam virus: a presumptive arbovirus isolated from a shrew in India. *Indian J Med Res*, **59**, 1758–60.

Cash, P. 1985. Polypeptide synthesis of Dugbe virus, a member of the *Nairovirus* genus of the *Bunyaviridae*. *J Gen Virol*, **66**, 141–8.

Cash, P., Vezza, A., et al. 1979. Genome complexities of the three mRNA species of snowshoe hare bunyavirus and in vitro translation of S mRNA to viral N polypeptide. *J Virol*, **31**, 685–94.

Chen, S. and Compans, R. 1991. Oligomerization, transport and Golgi retention of Punta Toro virus glycoproteins. *J Virol*, **65**, 5902–9.

Chen, S., Matsuoka, Y. and Compans, R. 1991. Golgi complex localization of the Punta Toro virus G2 protein requires its association with the G1 protein. *Virology*, **183**, 351–65.

Chumakov, M. 1946. *Vestnik Akademii Nauk SSSR*, **2**, 19.

Collett, M.S. 1986. Messenger RNA of the M segment RNA of Rift Valley fever virus. *Virology*, **151**, 151–6.

Collett, M.S., Purchio, A.F., et al. 1985. Complete nucleotide sequence of the M RNA segment of Rift Valley fever virus. *Virology*, **144**, 228–45.

Collett, M., Keegan, K., et al. 1987. Protective subunit immunogens to Rift Valley fever virus from bacteria and recombinant vaccinia virus. In: Mahy, B.W.J. and Kolakofsky, D. (eds), *The biology of negative strand viruses*. Amsterdam: Elsevier, 321–9.

Collett, M.S., Kakach, L., et al. 1989. Protein structure and function. In: Mahy, B.W.J. and Kolakofsky, D. (eds), *Genetics and pathogenicity of negative strand viruses*. Amsterdam: Elsevier, 49–57.

Colon-Ramos, D.A., Irusta, P., et al. 2003. Inhibition of translation and induction of apoptosis by bunyaviral nonstructural proteins bearing sequence similarity to Reaper. *Mol Biol Cell*, **14**, 4162–72.

Cortes, I., Pereira, A., et al. 1998. An RT-PCR procedure to amplify S RNA sequences of distinct tospoviruses. In: Peters, D. and Goldbach, R. (eds), *Recent progress in tospovirus and thrips research*. The Netherlands: Waginengen.

Cortez, I., Saaijer, J., et al. 2001. Identification and characterization of a novel tospovirus species using a new RT-PCR approach. *Arch Virol*, **146**, 265–78.

Custer, D.M., Thompson, E., et al. 2003. Active and passive vaccination against hantavirus pulmonary syndrome with Andes virus M genome segment-based DNA vaccine. *J Virol*, **77**, 9894–905.

Dalrymple, J., Peters, C., et al. 1981. Bunyaviruses. In: Bishop, D.H.L. and Compans, R.W. (eds), *The replication of negative strand viruses*. New York: Elsevier, 167–72.

Dalrymple, J., Hasty, S., et al. 1989. Mapping protective determinants of Rift Valley fever virus using recombinant vaccinia virus. In: Brown, F., Chanock, R.M., et al. (eds), *Vaccines 89*. Cold Spring Harbor, NY: Cold Spring Harbor Laboratory, 371–5.

Dantas, J.R., Okuno, Y., et al. 1986. Characterization of glycoproteins of virus causing hemorrhagic fever with renal syndrome (HFRS) using monoclonal antibodies. *Virology*, **151**, 379–84.

Davies, F., Casals, J., et al. 1978. The serological relationships of Nairobi sheep disease virus. *J Comp Pathol*, **88**, 519–23.

de Ávila, A., de Haan, P., et al. 1993. Classification of tospoviruses based on phylogeny of nucleoprotein gene sequences. *J Gen Virol*, **74**, 153–9.

de Haan, P., Wagemakers, L., et al. 1990. The S RNA segment of tomato spotted wilt virus has an ambisense character. *J Gen Virol*, **71**, 1001–7.

de Haan, P., Kormelink, R., et al. 1991. Tomato spotted wilt virus L RNA encodes a putative RNA polymerase. *J Gen Virol*, **72**, 2207–16.

de Haan, P., de Ávila, A.C., et al. 1992a. The nucleotide sequence of the S RNA of Impatiens necrotic spot virus, a novel tospovirus. *FEBS Lett*, **306**, 27–32.

de Haan, P., Gielen, J., et al. 1992b. Characterization of RNA-mediated resistance to tomato spotted wilt virus in transgenic tobacco plants. *BioTechnology*, **10**, 1133–7.

de Resende, R.O., de Haan, P., et al. 1991. Generation of envelope and defective interfering RNA mutants of tomato spotted wilt virus by mechanical passage. *J Gen Virol*, **72**, 2375–83.

Digoutte, J.-P. and Peters, C.J. 1989. General aspects of the 1987 Rift Valley fever epidemic in Mauritania. *Res Virol*, **140**, 27–30.

Digoutte, J.-P., Salaum, J.-J., et al. 1980. Les arboviroses mineures en Afrique Centrale et Occidentale. *Med Trop*, **40**, 523–33.

Dobbs, M., Kang, C.Y. 1993. Hantaan virus mRNAs contain non-viral 5′ end sequences and lack poly(A) at the 3′ end. IXth International Congress of Virology, Abstract P44-16: 280.

Duchin, J.S., Koster, F.T., et al. 1994. Hantavirus pulmonary syndrome: a clinical description of 17 patients with a newly recognized disease. *N Engl J Med*, **330**, 949–55.

Dunn, E.F., Pritlove, D.C., et al. 1995. Transcription of a recombinant bunyavirus RNA template by transiently expressed bunyavirus proteins. *Virology*, **211**, 133–43.

Eddy, G., Peters, C., et al. 1981. Rift Valley fever vaccine for humans. *Contrib Epidemiol Biostat*, **3**, 124–41.

Edwards, J.F., Livingston, C.W., et al. 1989. Ovine arthrogryposis and central nervous system malformations associated with in utero Cache Valley infection: spontaneous disease. *Vet Pathol*, **26**, 33–9.

Elliot, L.H., Ksiazek, T.G., et al. 1994. Isolation of the causative agent of hantavirus pulmonary syndrome. *Am J Trop Med Hyg*, **51**, 102–8.

Elliott, R.M. 1985. Identification of nonstructural proteins encoded by viruses of the bunyamwera serogroup (family *Bunyaviridae*). *Virology*, **143**, 119–26.

Elliott, R.M. 1989. Nucleotide sequence analysis of the large (L) genomic RNA segment of bunyamwera virus, the prototype of the family *Bunyaviridae*. *Virology*, **173**, 426–36.

Elliott, R.M. 1990. Molecular biology of the *Bunyaviridae*. *J Gen Virol*, **71**, 501–22.

Elliott, R.M., Schmaljohn, C.S. and Collett, M.S. 1991. *Bunyaviridae* genome structure and gene expression. *Curr Top Microbiol Immunol*, **169**, 91–141.

Elliott, R.M., Dunn, E., et al. 1992. Nucleotide sequence and coding strategy of the Uukuniemi virus L RNA segment. *J Gen Virol*, **73**, 1745–52.

Ellis, D.S., Shirodaria, P.V., et al. 1988. Morphology and development of Rift Valley fever virus in Vero cell cultures. *J Med Virol*, **24**, 161–74.

Elwell, M.R., Ward, G.S., et al. 1985. Serologic evidence of Hantaan-like virus in rodents and man in Thailand. *Southeast Asian J Trop Med Public Health*, **16**, 349–54.

Emery, V.C. 1987. Characterization of Punta Toro S mRNA species and identification of an inverted complementary sequence in the intergenic region of Punta Toro phlebovirus ambisense S RNA that is involved in mRNA transcription termination. *Virology*, **156**, 1–11.

Eshita, Y. and Bishop, D.H.L. 1984. The complete sequence of the M RNA of snowshoe hare bunyavirus reveals the presence of internal hydrophobic domains in the viral glycoprotein. *Virology*, **137**, 227–40.

Eshita, Y., Ericson, B., et al. 1985. Analyses of the mRNA transcription processes of snowshoe hare bunyavirus S and M RNA species. *J Virol*, **55**, 681–9.

Fazakerley, J.K. and Ross, A.M. 1989. Computer analysis suggests a role for signal sequences in processing polyproteins of enveloped RNA viruses and as a mechanism of viral fusion. *Virus Genes*, **2**, 223–39.

Fazakerly, J.K., Gonzalez-Scarano, F., et al. 1988. Organization of the middle RNA segment of snowshoe hare bunyavirus. *Virology*, **167**, 422–32.

Feldmann, H., Sanchez, A., et al. 1993. Utilization of autopsy RNA for the synthesis of the nucleocapsid antigen of a newly recognized virus associated with hantavirus pulmonary syndrome. *Virus Res*, **30**, 351–67.

Fisher, A. and Tesh, R.B. 2003. Induction of severe disease in hamsters by two sandfly fever group viruses, Punta toro and Gabek Forest (Phlebovirus, *Bunyaviridae*), similar to that caused by Rift Valley fever virus. *Am J Trop Med Hyg*, **69**, 269–76.

Francy, D. 1983. Mosquito control for prevention of California (La Crosse) encephalitis. In: Calisher, C. and Thompson, W. (eds), *California serogroup viruses*. New York: Alan R Liss, 365–75.

Frese, M., Kochs, G., et al. 1996. Inhibition of bunyaviruses, phleboviruses, and hantaviruses by human MxA protein. *J Virol*, **70**, 915–23.

Fulhorst, C.F., Monroe, M.C., et al. 1997. Isolation, characterization and geographic distribution of Caño Delgadito virus, a newly discovered South American hantavirus (family *Bunyaviridae*). *Virus Res*, **521**, 159–71.

Fuller, F., Bhown, A.S. and Bishop, D.H.L. 1983. Bunyavirus nucleoprotein, N, and a non-structural protein, NS$_S$, are coded by overlapping reading frames in the S RNA. *J Gen Virol*, **64**, 1705–14.

Fuller, F. and Bishop, D.H.L. 1982. Identification of virus-coded nonstructural polypeptides in bunyavirus-infected cells. *J Virol*, **41**, 643–8.

Garcin, D., Lezzi, M., et al. 1995. The 5′ ends of Hantaan virus (*Bunyaviridae*) RNAs suggest a prime-and-realign mechanism for the initiation of RNA synthesis. *J Virol*, **69**, 5754–62.

Gavrilovskaya, I.N., Shepley, M., et al. 1998. B$_3$ integrins mediate the cellular entry of hantaviruses that cause respiratory failure. *Proc Natl Acad Sci USA*, **95**, 7074–9.

Gentsch, J.R. and Bishop, D.H.L. 1978. Small viral RNA segment of bunyaviruses codes for viral nucleocapsid protein. *J Virol*, **28**, 417–19.

Georges, A., Saluzzo, J., et al. 1980. Arboviruses from Central African Republic: incidence, diagnosis in human pathology. *Med Trop*, **40**, 561–8.

Gerbaud, S., Pardigon, N., et al. 1987a. Gene expression, transcription and genome replication. In: Kolakofsky, D. and Mahy, B.W.J. (eds), *The biology of negative strand viruses*. Amsterdam: Elsevier, 191–8.

Gerbaud, S., Vialat, P., et al. 1987b. The S segment of the Germiston virus RNA genome can code for three proteins. *Virus Res*, **8**, 1–13.

Gerrard, S.R., Li, L., et al. 2004. Ngari virus is a Bunyamwera virus reassortant that can be associated with large outbreaks of hemorrhagic fever in Africa. *J Virol*, **78**, 8922–6.

Giorgi, C., Accardi, L., et al. 1991. Sequences and coding strategies of the S RNAs of Toscana and Rift Valley fever viruses compared to those of Punta Toro, Sicilian sandfly fever and Uukuniemi viruses. *Virology*, **180**, 738–53.

Glass, G., Childs, J., et al. 1988. Association of intraspecific wounding with hantaviral infection in wild rats (*Rattus norvegicus*). *Epidemiol Infect*, **101**, 459–72.

Glass, G.E., Watson, A.J., et al. 1993. Infection with a rat-borne hantavirus in United States residents is consistently associated with hypertensive renal disease. *J Infect Dis*, **167**, 614–20.

Gligic, A., Dimkovic, N., et al. 1992. Belgrade virus: a new hantavirus causing severe hemorrhagic fever with renal syndrome in Yugoslavia. *J Infect Dis*, **166**, 113–20.

Goldfarb, L., Chumakov, M., et al. 1980. An epidemiological model of Crimean hemorrhagic fever. *Am J Trop Med Hyg*, **29**, 260–4.

Goldsmith, C.S., Elliott, L.H., et al. 1995. Ultrastructural characteristics of Sin Nombre virus, causative agent of hantavirus pulmonary syndrome. *Arch Virol*, **140**, 2107–22.

Gonzalez, J., Le-Guenno, B., et al. 1992. Serological evidence in sheep suggesting phlebovirus circulation in a Rift Valley fever enzootic area in Burkina Faso. *Trans R Soc Trop Med Hyg*, **86**, 680–2.

Gonzalez-Scarano, F. 1985. La Crosse virus G1 glycoprotein undergoes a conformational change at the pH of fusion. *Virology*, **140**, 209–16.

Gonzalez-Scarano, F., Pobjecky, N. and Nathanson, N. 1984. La Crosse bunyavirus can mediate pH-dependent fusion from without. *Virology*, **132**, 222–5.

Gonzalez-Scarano, F., Janssen, R.S., et al. 1985. An avirulent G1 glycoprotein variant of La Crosse bunyavirus with defective fusion function. *J Virol*, **54**, 757–63.

Gonzalez-Scarano, F., Pobjecky, N. and Nathanson, N. 1987. Virus–membrane interactions. In: Kolakofsky, D. and Mahy, B.W.J. (eds), *The biology of negative strand viruses*. New York: Elsevier, 33–9.

Gonzalez-Scarano, F., Beaty, B., et al. 1988. Genetic determinants of the virulence and infectivity of La Crosse virus. *Microb Pathog*, **4**, 1–7.

Grabow, J., Matthews, C., et al. 1969. The electroencephalogram and clinical sequelae of California arbovirus encephalitis. *Neurology*, **19**, 394–404.

Grady, L.J., Sanders, M.L. and Campbell, W.P. 1987. The sequence of the M RNA of an isolate of La Crosse virus. *J Gen Virol*, **68**, 3057–71.

Grankvist, O., Juto, P., et al. 1992. Detection of nephropathia epidemica virus RNA in patient samples using a nested primer-based polymerase chain reaction. *J Infect Dis*, **165**, 934–7.

Hacker, D. 1990. Anti-mRNAS in La Crosse bunyavirus-infected cells. *J Virol*, **64**, 5051–7.

Hefti, H.P., Frese, M., et al. 1999. Human MxA protein protects mice lacking a functional alpha/beta interferon system against La Crosse virus and other lethal viral infections. *J Virol*, **73**, 6984–91.

Hertig, M. and Sabin, A. 1964. Sandfly fever (Papatasi, Phlebotomus, three-day fever). In: Coates, J., Hoff, E. and Hoff, P. (eds), *Preventive medicine in World War II*. Washington DC: Office of the Surgeon General, 109–74.

Hewlett, M.J. and Chiu, W. 1991. Virion structure. *Curr Top Microbiol Immunol*, **169**, 79–90.

Hewlett, M.J., Petterson, R.F. and Baltimore, D. 1977. Circular forms of Uukuniemi virion RNA: an electron microscopic study. *J Virol*, **21**, 1085–93.

Honig, J.E., Osborne, J.C. and Nichol, S.T. 2004. Crimean-Congo hemorrhagic fever virus L RNA segment and encoded protein. *Virology*, **321**, 29–35.

Hoogstraal, H. 1979. The epidemiology of tick-borne Crimean-Congo haemorrhagic fever in Asia, Europe and Africa. *J Med Entomol*, **15**, 307–417.

Hooper, J.W., Custer, D.M., et al. 2001a. DNA vaccination with the Hantaan virus M gene protects hamsters against three of four HFRS hantaviruses and elicits a high-titer neutralizing antibody response in rhesus monkeys. *J Virol*, **75**, 8469–77.

Hooper, J.W., Larsen, T., et al. 2001b. A lethal disease model for hantavirus pulmonary syndrome. *Virology*, **289**, 6–14.

Hubbard, S. and Ivatt, R. 1981. Synthesis and processing of asparagine-linked oligosaccharides. *Annu Rev Biochem*, **50**, 55–83.

Huggins, J.W., Hsiang, C.M., et al. 1991. Prospective, double-blind, concurrent, placebo-controlled clinical trial of intravenous ribavirin therapy of hemorrhagic fever with renal syndrome. *J Infect Dis*, **164**, 1119–27.

Ihara, T., Akashi, H. and Bishop, D. 1984. Novel coding strategy (ambisense genomic RNA) revealed by sequence analysis of Punta Toro phlebovirus S RNA. *Virology*, **136**, 293–306.

Ihara, T., Dalrymple, J.M. and Bishop, D.H.L. 1985a. Complete sequences of the glycoprotein and M RNA of Punta Toro phlebovirus compared to those of Rift Valley fever virus. *Virology*, **144**, 246–59.

Ihara, T., Matsuura, Y. and Bishop, D.H.L. 1985b. Analysis of the mRNA transcription processes of Punta Toro phlebovirus (*Bunyaviridae*). *Virology*, **147**, 317–25.

Jacoby, D., Cooke, C., et al. 1993. Expression of the La Crosse M segment proteins in a recombinant vaccinia expression system mediates pH-dependent cellular fusion. *Virology*, **193**, 993–6.

Jain, R.K., Pappu, H.R., et al. 1998. Watermelon bud necrosis tospovirus in a distinct virus species. *Arch Virol*, **143**, 1637–44.

Jäntti, J. and Hilden, P. 1997. Immunocytochemical analysis of Uukuniemi virus budding compartments. *J Virol*, **71**, 1162–72.

Jin, H. and Elliott, R. 1992. Mutagenesis of the L protein encoded by bunyamwera virus and production of monospecific antibodies. *J Gen Virol*, **73**, 2235–44.

Jin, H. and Elliott, R.M. 1993a. Characterization of bunyamwera virus S RNA that is transcribed and replicated by the L protein expressed from recombinant vaccinia virus. *J Virol*, **67**, 1396–404.

Jin, H. and Elliott, R.M. 1993b. Non-viral sequences at the 5′ ends of Dugbe nairovirus S mRNAs. *J Gen Virol*, **74**, 2293–7.

Jin, H.K., Yoshimatsu, K., et al. 2001. Mouse Mx2 protein inhibits hantavirus but not influenza virus replication. *Arch Virol*, **146**, 41–9.

Johnson, A.M. and de Souza, L.T. 1999. Genetic investigation of novel hantaviruses causing fatal HPS in Brazil. *J Med Virol*, **59**, 527–35.

Johnson, A.M., Bowen, M.D., et al. 1997. Laguna Negra virus associated with HPS in western Paraguay and Bolivia. *Virology*, **238**, 115–27.

Jones, L., Davies, C., et al. 1987. A novel mode of arbovirus transmission involving a nonviremic host. *Science*, **237**, 775–7.

Jones, L., Hodgson, E. and Nuttall, P. 1989. Enhancement of virus transmission by tick salivary glands. *J Gen Virol*, **70**, 1895–8.

Kakach, L.T., Suzich, J.A. and Collett, M.S. 1989. Rift Valley fever virus M segment: phlebovirus expression strategy and protein glycosylation. *Virology*, **170**, 505–10.

Kaluda, M., Mukwaya, L., et al. 1986. Kasokero virus: a new human pathogen from bats (*Rousettus aegyptiacus*) in Uganda. *Am J Trop Med Hyg*, **35**, 387–92.

Kanerva, M., Melen, K., et al. 1996. Inhibition of puumala and tula hantaviruses in Vero cells by MxA protein. *Virology*, **224**, 55–62.

Karabatsos, N. 1985. *International catalog of arboviruses including certain other viruses of vertebrates*. San Antonio: American Society of Tropical Medicine and Hygiene.

Kark, J.D., Aynor, Y., et al. 1982. A serological survey of Rift Valley fever antibodies in the northern Sinai. *Trans R Soc Trop Med Hyg*, **76**, 427–30.

Kato, K., Hanada, K. and Kameya-Iwaki, M. 2000. Melon yellow spot virus: a distinct species of the genus *Tospovirus* isolated from melon. *Phytopathology*, **90**, 422–6.

Keegan, K. and Collett, M.S. 1986. Use of bacterial expression cloning to define the amino acid sequences of antigenic determinants on the G2 glycoprotein of Rift Valley fever virus. *J Virol*, **58**, 263–70.

Kemp, G., Causey, O. and Causey, C. 1971. Virus isolations from trade cattle, sheep, goats and swine at Ibadan, Nigeria, 1964–68. *Bull Epizootic Dis Afr*, **19**, 131–5.

Khan, A.S., Khabbaz, R.F., et al. 1996. Hanta virus pulmonary syndrome: the first 100 US cases. *J Inf Dis*, **173**, 1297–303.

Kingsford, L. and Hill, D.W. 1981. The effects of proteolytic enzymes on structure and function of La Crosse G1 and G2 glycoproteins. In: Bishop, D. and Compans, R. (eds), *The replication of negative strand viruses*. New York: Elsevier, 111–16.

Kinsella, E., Martin, S.G., et al. 2004. Sequence determination of the Crimean-Congo hemorrhagic fever virus L segment. *Virology*, **321**, 23–8.

Kitajima, E.W., de Avila, A.C., et al. 1992. Comparative cytological and immunogold labelling studies on different isolates of tomato spotted wilt virus. *J Submicrosc Cytol Pathol*, **24**, 1–4.

Kochs, G., Janzen, C., et al. 2002. Antivirally active MxA protein sequesters La Crosse virus nucleocapsid protein into perinclear complexes. *Proc Natl Acad Sci USA*, **99**, 3153–8.

Kohl, A., Clayton, R., et al. 2003. Bunyamwera virus nonstructural protein NSs counteracts interferon regulatory factor 3-mediated induction of early cell death. *J Virol*, **77**, 7999–8008.

Kormelink, R., Kitajima, E.W., et al. 1991. The nonstructural protein (NS$_S$) encoded by the ambisense S RNA segment of tomato spotted wilt virus is associated with fibrous structures in infected plant cells. *Virology*, **181**, 459–68.

Kormelink, R., de Haan, P., et al. 1992a. The nucleotide sequence of the M RNA segment of tomato spotted wilt virus, a bunyavirus with two ambisense RNA segments. *J Gen Virol*, **73**, 2795–804.

Kormelink, R., de Haan, P., et al. 1992b. Viral RNA synthesis in tomato spotted wilt virus-infected *Nicotiana rustica* plants. *J Gen Virol*, **73**, 687–93.

Kormelink, R., Van Poelwijk, F., et al. 1992c. Non-viral heterogeneous sequences at the 5′ ends of tomato spotted wilt virus mRNAs. *J Gen Virol*, **73**, 2125–8.

Kormelink, R., Storms, M., et al. 1994. Expression and subcellular location of the NS$_M$ protein of tomato spotted wilt virus (TSWV), a putative viral movement protein. *Virology*, **200**, 56–65.

Lappin, D.F., Nakitare, G.W., et al. 1994. Localization of Bunyamwera bunyavirus G1 glycoprotein to the Golgi requires association with G2 but not with NS$_M$. *J Gen Virol*, **75**, 3441–51.

Laughlin, L.W., Meegan, J.M., et al. 1979. Epidemic Rift Valley fever in Egypt: observations of the spectrum of human illness. *Trans R Soc Trop Med Hyg*, **73**, 630–3.

Law, M.D., Speck, J. and Moyer, J.W. 1991. Nucleotide sequence of the 3′ non-coding region and N gene of the S RNA of a serologically distinct tospovirus. *J Gen Virol*, **72**, 2597–601.

Law, M.D., Speck, J. and Moyer, J.W. 1992. The M RNA of impatiens necrotic spot tospovirus (*Bunyaviridae*) has an ambisense genomic organization. *Virology*, **188**, 732–41.

LeDuc, J. 1979. The ecology of California group viruses. *J Med Entomol*, **16**, 1–17.

LeDuc, J.W. 1987. Epidemiology and ecology of the California serogroup viruses. *Am J Trop Med Hyg*, **37**, 60S–8S.

LeDuc, J. 1995. Hanta virus infections. In: Porterfield, J. (ed.), *Kass handbook of infectious diseases, exotic viral infections*. Oxford: Chapman & Hall Medical, 261–84.

LeDuc, J. and Pinheiro, F. 1988. *The arboviruses: epidemiology and ecology*. Boca Raton, FL: CRC Press.

LeDuc, J.W., Cuevas, M. and Garcia, M. 1980. The incidence and prevalence of Phlebotomus fever group virus in Panama. In: Pinheiro, F.P. (ed.) Proceedings of International Symposium on Tropical Arboviruses and Hemorrhagic Fevers. Rio de Janeiro: Academia Brasileira de Ciencias, 385–90.

LeDuc, J.W., Smith, G.A., et al. 1986. Global survey of antibody to Hantaan-related viruses among peridomestic rodents. *Bull WHO*, **64**, 139–44.

LeDuc, J.W., Ksiazek, T.G., et al. 1990. A retrospective analysis of sera collected by the Hemorrhagic Fever Commission during the Korean Conflict. *J Infect Dis*, **162**, 1182–4.

LeDuc, J.W., Childs, J.E. and Glass, G.E. 1992. The hantaviruses, etiologic agents of hemorrhagic fever with renal syndrome: a possible cause of hypertension and chronic renal disease in the United States. *Annu Rev Public Health*, **13**, 79–98.

Lee, H.W., Lee, P.W. and Johnson, K.M. 1978. Isolation of the etiologic agent of Korean hemorrhagic fever. *J Infect Dis*, **137**, 298–308.

Lee, H., Baek, L. and Johnson, K. 1982. Isolation of Hantaan virus, the etiologic agent of Korean hemorrhagic fever, from wild urban rats. *J Infect Dis*, **146**, 638–44.

Lee, H., Ahn, C., et al. 1990. Field trial of an inactivated vaccine against hemorrhagic fever with renal syndrome in humans. *Arch Virol Suppl*, **1**, 35–47.

Lees, J.F., Pringle, C.R. and Elliott, R.M. 1986. Nucleotide sequence of the bunyamwera virus M RNA segment: conservation of structural features in the bunyavirus glycoprotein gene product. *Virology*, **148**, 1–14.

Li, D., Schmaljohn, A.L., et al. 1995. Complete nucleotide sequences of the M and S segments of two hantavirus isolates from California: evidence for reassortment in nature among viruses related to hantavirus pulmonary syndrome. *Virology*, **206**, 973–83.

Lopez, N., Muller, R., et al. 1995. The L protein of Rift Valley fever virus can rescue viral ribonucleoproteins and transcribe synthetic genome-like RNA molecules. *J Virol*, **69**, 3972–9.

Lopez, N., Padula, P., et al. 1996. Genetic identification of a new hantavirus causing severe pulmonary syndrome in Argentina. *Virology*, **220**, 223–6.

Ludwig, G.V., Israel, B.A., et al. 1991. Role of La Crosse virus glycoproteins in attachment of virus to host cells. *Virology*, **181**, 564–71.

Lvov, D., Sidorova, G., et al. 1976. Virus 'Tandy' – a new arbovirus, isolated in the Uzbec SSR and Turkmen SSR from ticks *Hyalamma asiaticum asiaticum* Schulce et Schlottke, 1929 and *Hyalomma plumbeum plumbeum* Panzer, 1796. *Arch Virol*, **51**, 15–21.

Lvov, D., Kostyukov, M., et al. 1984. An outbreak of arbovirus infection in the Tajik SSR caused by Issyk-kyl virus (Issyk-kul fever). *Vopr Virusol*, **29**, 89–92.

Lyons, M.J. and Heyduk, J. 1973. Aspects of the developmental morphology of California encephalitis virus in cultured vertebrate and arthropod cells and in mouse brain. *Virology*, **54**, 37–52.

Madoff, D.H. and Lenard, J. 1982. A membrane glycoprotein that accumulates intracellularly: cellular processing of the large glycoprotein of La Crosse virus. *Cell*, **28**, 821–9.

Mardani, M., Keshtkar Jahrome, M., et al. 2003. The efficacy of oral ribavirin in the treatment of Crimean-Congo hemorrhagic fever in Iran. *Clin Infec Dis*, **36**, 1613–18.

Marriott, A.C. and Nuttall, P.A. 1992. Comparison of the S RNA segments and nucleoprotein sequences of Crimean-Congo hemorrhagic fever, Hazara and Dugbe viruses. *Virology*, **189**, 795–9.

Marriott, A., Ward, V. and Nuttall, P. 1989. The S RNA segment of sandfly fever Sicilian virus: evidence for an ambisense genome. *Virology*, **169**, 341–5.

Marriott, A., El-Ghorr, A. and Nuttall, P. 1992. Dugbe nairovirus M RNA: nucleotide sequence and coding strategy. *Virology*, **190**, 606–15.

Marsh, M. and Helenius, A. 1980. Adsorptive endocytosis of Semliki Forest virus. *J Mol Biol*, **142**, 439–54.

Matsuoka, Y., Ihara, T., et al. 1988. Intracellular accumulation of Punta Toro virus glycoproteins expressed from cloned cDNA. *Virology*, **167**, 251–60.

Matsuoka, Y., Chen, S.Y. and Compans, R.W. 1991. Bunyavirus protein transport and assembly. *Curr Top Microbiol Immunol*, **169**, 161–79.

Matsuoka, Y., Chen, S.Y. and Compans, R.W. 1994. A signal for Golgi retention in the bunyavirus G1 glycoprotein. *J Biol Chem*, **269**, 22565–73.

Matsuoka, Y., Chen, S.Y., et al. 1996. Molecular determinants of Golgi retention in the Punta Toro virus G1. *Arch Biochem Biophys*, **336**, 184–9.

Matthews, C., Chun, R. and Grabow, J. 1968. Psychological sequelae in children following California arbovirus encephalitis. *Neurology*, **18**, 1023–30.

McKee, K. Jr., MacDonald, C., et al. 1985. Hemorrhagic fever with renal syndrome, a clinical perspective. *Milit Med*, **150**, 640–7.

Meegan, J. 1979. The Rift Valley fever epizootic in Egypt 1977–78. I. Description of the epizootic and virological studies. *Trans R Soc Trop Med Hyg*, **73**, 618–23.

Milazzo, M.L. and Eyzaguirre, E.J. 2002. Maporal viral infection in the Syrian golden hamster: a model of hantavirus pulmonary syndrome. *J Inf Dis*, **186**, 1390–5.

Montgomery, R. 1917. On a tick-borne gastro-enteritis of sheep and goats occurring in British East Africa. *J Comp Pathol*, **30**, 28–57.

Morrill, J.C., Jennings, G.B., et al. 1987. Pathogenicity and immunogenicity of a mutagen-attenuated Rift Valley fever virus immunogen in pregnant ewes. *Am J Vet Res*, **48**, 1042–7.

Morrill, J.C., Carpenter, L., et al. 1991. Further evaluation of a mutagen-attenuated Rift Valley fever vaccine in sheep. *Vaccine*, **9**, 35–41.

Morzunov, S.P., Feldmann, H., et al. 1995. A newly recognized virus associated with a fatal case of hantavirus pulmonary syndrome in Louisiana. *J Virol*, **69**, 1980–3.

Muller, R., Argentini, C., et al. 1991. Completion of the genome sequence of Rift Valley fever phlebovirus indicates that the L RNA is negative sense or ambisense and codes for a putative transcriptase-replicase. *Nucleic Acids Res*, **19**, 5433.

Murphy, F.A., Harrison, A.K. and Whitfield, S.G. 1973. Morphologic and morphogenetic similarities of bunyamwera serological supergroup viruses and several other arthropod-borne viruses. *Intervirology*, **1**, 297–316.

Mustonen, J., Partanen, J., et al. 1996. Genetic susceptibility to severe course of nephropathia epidemica caused by Puumala hantavirus. *Kidney Int*, **49**, 217–21.

Mustonen, J., Partanen, J., et al. 1998. Association of HLA B27 with benign clinical course of nephropathia. *Scan J Immunol*, **47**, 277–9.

Nakitare, G.W. and Elliott, R.M. 1993. Expression of the bunyamwera virus M genome segment and intracellular localization of NS_M. *Virology*, **195**, 511–20.

Nichol, S.T., Spiropoulou, C.F., et al. 1993. Genetic identification of a novel hantavirus associated with an outbreak of acute respiratory illness in the southwestern United States. *Science*, **262**, 914–17.

Nuzum, E.O., Rossi, C.A., et al. 1988. Aerosol transmission of Hantaan and related viruses to laboratory rats. *Am J Trop Med Hyg*, **38**, 636–40.

Obijeski, J.F. and Murphy, F.A. 1977. *Bunyaviridae*: recent biochemical developments. *J Gen Virol*, **37**, 1–14.

Obijeski, J.F., Bishop, D.H.L., et al. 1976. Segmented genome and nucleocapsid of LaCrosse virus. *J Virol*, **20**, 664–75.

Overton, H.A., Ihara, T. and Bishop, D.H. 1987. Identification of the N and NS_S proteins coded by the ambisense S RNA of Punta Toro phlebovirus using monospecific antisera raised to baculovirus expressed N and NS_S proteins. *Virology*, **157**, 338–50.

Pang, S.Z., Jan, F.J. and Gonsalves, D. 1997. Nontarget DNA sequences reduce the transgene length necessary for RNA-mediated tospovirus resistance in transgenic plants. *Proc Natl Acad Sci USA*, **94**, 8261–6.

Parker, M.D. and Hewlett, M.J. 1981. Bunyaviruses. In: Bishop, D. and Compans, R. (eds), *Replication of negative strand viruses*. New York: Elsevier, 125–45.

Parker, M.D., Smith, J.F. and Dalrymple, J.M. 1984. Genome structure, transcription and genetics. In: Compans, R. and Bishop, D. (eds), *Segmented negative strand viruses*. Orlando, FL: Academic Press, 21–8.

Parrington, M.A. and Kang, C.Y. 1990. Nucleotide sequence analysis of the S genomic segment of Prospect Hill virus: comparison with the prototype hantavirus. *Virology*, **175**, 167–75.

Parsonson, I. and McPhee, D.A. 1985. Bunyavirus pathogenesis. *Adv Virus Res*, **30**, 279–316.

Patterson, J.L. and Kolakofsky, D. 1984. Characterization of La Crosse virus small-genome segment transcripts. *J Virol*, **49**, 680–5.

Patterson, J.L., Kolakofsky, D., et al. 1983. Isolation of the ends of La Crosse virus small RNA as a double-stranded structure. *J Virol*, **45**, 882–4.

Pattnaik, A.K. and Abraham, G. 1983. Identification of four complementary RNA species in Akabane virus-infected cells. *J Virol*, **47**, 452–62.

Patton, J.T., Davis, N.L. and Wertz, G.W. 1984a. N protein alone satisfies the requirement for protein synthesis during RNA replication of vesicular stomatitis virus. *J Virol*, **49**, 303–9.

Patton, J.T., Davis, N.L. and Wertz, G.W. 1984b. Transcription and replication. In: Bishop, D. and Compans, R. (eds), *Nonsegmented negative strand viruses. Paramyxoviruses and rhabdoviruses*. Orlando FL: Academic Press, 147–52.

Pavri, R., Anandarajah, M., et al. 1976. Isolation of Wanowrie virus from brain of a fatal human case from Sri Lanka. *Indian J Med Res*, **64**, 557–61.

Pekosz, A., Griot, C., et al. 1995. Protection from La Crosse virus encephalitis with recombinant glycoproteins: role of neutralizing anti-G1 antibodies. *J Virol*, **69**, 3475–81.

Pesonen, M., Kuismanen, E. and Pettersson, R.F. 1982. Monosaccharide sequence of protein-bound glycans of Uukuniemi virus. *J Virol*, **41**, 390–400.

Peters, C. and LeDuc, J. 1991. Bunyaviruses, phleboviruses and related viruses. In: Belshe, R. (ed.), *Textbook of human virology*. St Louis, MO: Mosby Year Book, 571–614.

Pettersson, R.F. 1991. Protein localization and virus assembly at intracellular membranes. *Curr Top Microbiol Immunol*, **170**, 67–106.

Pettersson, R.F. and Bonsdorf, C.H. 1975. Ribonucleoproteins of Uukuniemi virus are circular. *J Virol*, **15**, 386–92.

Pettersson, R.F., Kuismanen, E., et al. 1985. mRNAs of Uukuniemi virus, a bunyavirus. In: Becker, Y. (ed.), *Viral messenger RNA transcription, processing, splicing, and molecular structure. Developments in molecular virology*, Vol. 7. Boston, MA: Martinus Nijhoff, 283–300.

Pifat, D.Y., Osterling, M.C. and Smith, J.F. 1988. Antigenic analysis of Punta Toro virus and identification of protective determinants with monoclonal antibodies. *Virology*, **167**, 442–50.

Pinheiro, F.P., Travassos da Rosa, A.P.A. and Travassos da Rosa, J.F.S. 1981. Oropouche virus. I. A review of clinical, epidemiological and ecological findings. *Am J Trop Med Hyg*, **30**, 149–60.

Plyusnin, A. 2002. Genetics of hantaviruses: implications to taxonomy. *Arch Virol*, **147**, 665–82.

Plyusnin, A., Vapalahti, O., et al. 1994. Tula virus: a newly detected hantavirus carried by European common voles. *J Virol*, **68**, 7833–9.

Plyusnin, A., Vapalahti, O., et al. 1996. Newly recognised hantavirus in Siberian lemmings. *Lancet*, **347**, 1835, letter.

Poch, O., Sauvaget, I., et al. 1989. Identification of four conserved motifs among the RNA-dependent polymerase encoding elements. *EMBO J*, **8**, 3867–75.

Powers, A.M., Mercer, D.J., et al. 1999. Isolation and genetic characterization of a hantavirus (*Bunyaviridae*: Hantavirus) from a rodent, *Oligoryzomys microtis* (*Muridae*), collected in northeastern Peru. *Am J Trop Med Hyg*, **61**, 92–8.

Prehaud, C., Lopez, N., et al. 1997. Analysis of the 3′ terminal sequence recognized by the Rift Valley fever virus transcription complex in its ambisense S segment. *Virology*, **227**, 189–97.

Raju, R. and Kolakofsky, D. 1986. Inhibitors of protein synthesis inhibit both La Crosse virus S-mRNA and S genome syntheses in vivo. *Virus Res*, **5**, 1–9.

Raju, R. and Kolakofsky, D. 1987a. Translational requirement of La Crosse virus S-mRNA synthesis. *J Virol*, **63**, 122–8.

Raju, R. and Kolakofsky, D. 1987b. Unusual transcripts in La Crosse virus-infected cells and the site for nucleocapsid assembly. *J Virol*, **61**, 667–72.

Raju, R. and Kolakofsky, D. 1989. The ends of La Crosse virus genome and antigenome RNAs within nucleocapsids are base paired. *J Virol*, **63**, 122–8.

Ranki, M. and Pettersson, R.F. 1975. Uukuniemi virus contains an RNA polymerase. *J Virol*, **16**, 1420–5.

Ravkov, E.V., Rollin, P.E., et al. 1995. Genetic and serologic analysis of Black Creek Canal virus and its association with human disease and *Sigmodon hispidus* infection. *Virology*, **210**, 482–9.

Ravkov, E.V., Nichol, S.T. and Compans, R.W. 1997. Polarized entry and release in epithelial cells of Black Creek Canal virus, a New World hantavirus. *J Virol*, **71**, 1147–54.

Ravkov, E.V., Nichol, S.T., et al. 1998. Role of action microfilaments in Black Creek Canal virus morphogenesis. *J Virol*, **72**, 2865–70.

Rawlings, J.A., Torrez-Martinez, N., et al. 1996. Cocirculation of multiple hantaviruses in Texas, with characterization of the small (S) genome of a previously undescribed virus of cotton rats (*Sigmodon hispidus*). *Am J Trop Med Hyg*, **55**, 672–9.

Report. 1998. Arboviral infections of the central nervous system – United States, 1996–1997. *Morb Mortal Wkly Rep*, **47**, 517–22.

Rie, H., Hilty, M. and Cramblet, H. 1973. Intelligence and coordination following California encephalitis. *Am J Dis Child*, **125**, 824–7.

Rollin, P.E., Ksiazek, T.G., et al. 1995. Isolation of Black Creek Canal virus, a new hantavirus from *Sigmodon hispidus* in Florida. *J Med Virol*, **46**, 35–9.

Rönnholm, R. 1992. Localization to the Golgi complex of Uukuniemi virus glycoproteins G1 and G2 expressed from cloned cDNAs. *J Virol*, **66**, 4525–31.

Rönnholm, R. and Pettersson, R.F. 1987. Complete nucleotide sequence of the M RNA segment of Uukuniemi virus encoding the membrane glycoproteins G1 and G2. *Virology*, **160**, 191–202.

Rothman, J.E. 1981. The Golgi apparatus: two organelles in tandem. *Science*, **213**, 1212–18.

Ruusala, A., Persson, R., et al. 1992. Coexpression of the membrane glycoproteins G1 and G2 of Hantaan virus is required for targeting to the Golgi complex. *Virology*, **186**, 53–64.

Sabatino, D. and Cramblett, H. 1968. Behavioral sequelae of California encephalitis virus infection in children. *Dev Med Child Neurol*, **10**, 331–7.

Sabin, A. 1951. Experimental studies on phlebotomus (pappataci, sandfly) fever during World War II. *Arch Virusforsch*, 367–410.

Saeed, M.F., Wang, H., et al. 2000. Nucleotide sequence determination and phylogeny of the nucleocapsid gene of Oropouche virus. *J Gen Virol*, **81**, 743–8.

Saluzzo, J.F. and Smith, J.F. 1990. Use of reassortant viruses to map attenuating and temperature -sensitive mutations of the Rift Valley fever virus MP-12 vaccine. *Vaccine*, **8**, 369–75.

Sanchez, A.J., Abbott, K.D. and Nichol, S.T. 2001. Genetic identification and characterization of limestone canyon virus, a unique *Peromyscus*-borne hantavirus. *Virology*, **286**, 345–53.

Satyanarayan, T., Mitchell, S.E., et al. 1996. The complete nucleotide sequence and genome organization of the M RNA segment of peanut bud necrosis tospovirus and comparison with other tospoviruses. *J Gen Virol*, **77**, 2347–52.

Satyanarayan, T., Gowda, S., et al. 1998. Peanut yellow spot virus is a member of a new serogroup of Tospovirus genus based on small (S) RNA sequence and organization. *Arch Virol*, **143**, 353–64.

Schmaljohn, C. 1990. Nucleotide sequence of the L genome segment of hantaan virus. *Nucleic Acids Res*, **18**, 6728.

Schmaljohn, C.S. and Dalrymple, J.M. 1983. Analysis of Hantaan virus RNA: evidence for a new genus of *Bunyaviridae*. *Virology*, **131**, 482–91.

Schmaljohn, C.S., Hasty, S.E., et al. 1985. Antigenic and genetic properties of viruses linked to hemorrhagic fever with renal syndrome. *Science*, **227**, 1041–4.

Schmaljohn, C.S., Schmaljohn, A.L. and Dalrymple, J.M. 1987. Hantaan virus M RNA: coding strategy, nucleotide sequence, and gene order. *Virology*, **157**, 31–9.

Schmaljohn, C.S., Hasty, S.E., et al. 1986a. Hantaan virus replication: effects of monensin, tunicamycin and endoglycosidases on the structural glycoproteins. *J Gen Virol*, **67**, 707–17.

Schmaljohn, C.S., Jennings, G.B., et al. 1986b. Coding strategy of the S genome of Hantaan virus. *Virology*, **155**, 633–43.

Schmaljohn, C.S., Parker, M.D., et al. 1989. Baculovirus expression of the M genome segment of Rift Valley fever virus and examination of antigenic and immunogenic properties of the expressed proteins. *Virology*, **170**, 184–92.

Schmaljohn, C.S., Chu, Y.K., et al. 1990. Antigenic subunits of Hantaan virus expressed by baculovirus and vaccinia virus recombinants. *J Virol*, **64**, 3162–70.

Schmaljohn, C., Dalrymple, J., et al. 1994. Preclinical trials of recombinant vaccinia for HTN virus, cause of hemorrhagic fever with renal syndrome. In: Talwar, G., Rao, K. and Chauha, V. (eds), *Recombinant and synthetic vaccines*. New Delhi: Narosa Publishing, 332–9.

Schmaljohn, A.L., Li, D., et al. 1995. Isolation and initial characterization of a new found hantavirus from California. *Virology*, **206**, 963–72.

Settergren, B., Juto, P., et al. 1990. Molecular characterization of the RNA S segment of nephropathia epidemica virus strain Hallnas B1. *Virology*, **174**, 79–86.

Sexton, D.J., Rollin, P.E., et al. 1997. Life-threatening Cache Valley virus infection. *New Engl J Med*, **336**, 547–9.

Shah, K. and Work, T. 1969. Bhanja virus: a new arbovirus from ticks *Haemaphysalis intermedia* Warburton and Nuttall, 1909, in Orissa, India. *Indian J Med Res*, **57**, 793–8.

Shoemaker, T., Boulianne, C., et al. 2002. Genetic analysis of viruses associated with emergence of Rift Valley fever in Saudi Arabia and Yemen, 2000–01. *Emerg Infec Dis*, **8**, 1415–20.

Simons, J.F. and Pettersson, R.F. 1991. Host-derived 5′ ends and overlapping complementary 3′ ends of the two mRNAs transcribed from the ambisense S segment of Uukuniemi virus. *J Virol*, **65**, 4741–8.

Simons, J.F., Hellman, U. and Pettersson, R.F. 1990. Uukuniemi virus S RNA segment: ambisense coding strategy, packaging of complementary strands into virions, and homology to members of the genus *Phlebovirus*. *J Virol*, **64**, 247–55.

Simons, J.F., Persson, R. and Pettersson, R.F. 1992. Association of the nonstructural protein NS$_S$ of Uukuniemi virus with the 40S ribosomal subunit. *J Virol*, **66**, 4233–41.

Smith, J.F. and Pifat, D.Y. 1982. Morphogenesis of sandfly viruses (*Bunyaviridae* family). *Virology*, **121**, 61–81.

Smith, J.F., Hodson, L. et al. 1987. Induction of neutralizing antibodies to Rift Valley fever virus with synthetic peptides. VIIth International Congress of Virology, Edmonton, Alberta, Canada, 65 (abstract).

Smithburn, K. 1949. Rift Valley fever: the neurotropic adaptation of the virus and the experimental use of this modified virus as a vaccine. *Br J Exp Pathol*, **30**, 1–16.

Smithburn, K., Mahaffy, A. and Paul, J. 1941. Bwamba fever and its causative virus. *Am J Trop Med Hyg*, **21**, 75–90.

Smithburn, K., Haddow, A. and Mahaffy, A. 1946. A neurotropic virus isolated from *Aedes* mosquitoes caught in the Semliki Forest. *Am J Trop Med Hyg*, **21**, 189–208.

Song, J.W., Baek, L.J., et al. 1994. Isolation of pathogenic hantavirus from white-footed mouse (*Peromyscus leucopus*). *Lancet*, **344**, 1637, Letter.

Song, W., Quintana, M. et al. 1995a. High genetic complexity of hantavirus radiation of New World microtine voles (*Rodentia microtus*). 3rd International Conference on HFRS and Hantaviruses, Helsinki, Finland (Abstract).

Song, W., Torrez-Martinez, N., et al. 1995b. Isla Vista virus: a genetically novel hantavirus of the California vole *Microtus californicus*. *J Gen Virol*, **76**, 3195–9.

Spiropoulou, C.F., Morzunov, S., et al. 1994. Genome structure and variability of a virus causing hantavirus pulmonary syndrome. *Virology*, **200**, 715–23.

Stohwasser, R., Giebel, L.B., et al. 1990. Molecular characterization of the RNA S segment of nephropathia epidemica virus strain Hallnas B1. *Virology*, **174**, 79–86.

Storms, M.M., Kormelink, R., et al. 1995. The nonstructural NSm protein of tomato spotted wilt virus induces tubular structures in plant and insect cells. *Virology*, **214**, 485–93.

Streitenfeld, H., Boyd, A., et al. 2003. Activation of PKR by Bunyamwera virus is independent of the viral interferon antagonist NSs. *J Virol*, **77**, 5507–11.

Struthers, J.K. and Swanepoel, R. 1982. Identification of a major non-structural protein in the nuclei of Rift Valley fever virus-infected cells. *J Gen Virol*, **60**, 381–4.

Sureau, P. and Klein, J.-M. 1980. Arbovirus en Iran. *Med Trop*, **40**, 549–54.

Suzich, J.A. and Collett, M.S. 1988. Rift Valley fever virus M segment: cell-free transcription and translation of virus-complementary RNA. *Virology*, **164**, 478–86.

Suzich, J.A., Kakach, L.T. and Collett, M.S. 1990. Expression strategy of a phlebovirus: biogenesis of proteins from the Rift Valley fever virus M segment. *J Virol*, **64**, 1549–55.

Swanepoel, R. 1995. Nairovirus infections. In: Porterfield, J. (ed.), *Kass handbook of infectious diseases, exotic viral infections*. Oxford: Chapman & Hall Medical, 285–93.

Swanepoel, R., Shepherd, A., et al. 1985. A common-source outbreak of Crimean-Congo haemorrhagic fever on a dairy farm. *S Afr Med J*, **68**, 635–7.

Taller, A.M., Xiao, S.Y., et al. 1993. Belgrade virus, a cause of hemorrhagic fever with renal syndrome in the Balkans, is closely related to Dobrava virus of field mice. *J Infect Dis*, **168**, 750–3.

Talmon, Y., Prasad, B.V., et al. 1987. Electron microscopy of vitrified-hydrated La Crosse virus. *J Virol*, **61**, 2319–21.

Torrez-Martinez, N. and Hjelle, B. 1995. Enzootic of Bayou hantavirus in rice rats (*Oryzomys palustris*) in 1983. *Lancet*, **346**, 780–1, Letter.

Torrez-Martinez, N., Song, W. and Hjelle, B. 1995. Nucleotide sequence analysis of the M genomic segment of El Moro Canyon hantavirus: antigenic distinction from Four Corners hantavirus. *Virology*, **211**, 336–8.

Tycko, B. and Maxfield, F.R. 1982. Rapid acidification of endocytic vesicles containing alpha-2-macroglobulin. *Cell*, **28**, 643–51.

Ullman, D.E., German, T.L., et al. 1993. Tospovirus replication in insect vector cells: immunocytochemical evidence that the nonstructural protein encoded by the S RNA of tomato spotted wilt tospovirus is present in thrips vector cells. *Phytopathology*, **83**, 456–63.

Ulmanen, I., Seppala, P. and Pettersson, R.F. 1981. In vitro translation of Uukuniemi virus-specific RNAs: identification of a nonstructural protein and a precursor to the membrane glycoproteins. *J Virol*, **37**, 72–9.

Vaira, A.M., Semeria, L., et al. 1995. Resistance to tospoviruses in *Nicotiana benthamiana* transformed with the N gene of tomato spotted wilt virus: correlation between transgene expression and protection in primary transformants. *Mol Plant Microbe Interact*, **8**, 66–73.

Vasconcelos, P.F., Travassos da Rosa, J.F., et al. 1989. 1st register of an epidemic caused by Oropouche virus in the states of Maranhao and Goias. *Rev Inst Med Trop Sao Paulo*, **31**, 271–8.

Vasconcelos, P., Travassos da Rosa, J. and Travassos da Rosa, A. In: Travassos da Rosa, A. and Ishak, R. (eds) Virologica 91: II Simposio Internacional Soubre Arbovirus dos Tropicos e Febres Hemorragicas. Brazil: Instituto Evandro Chagas/Universidade Federal do Para/ Sociedade Brasileira de Virologia, 347–60.

Verani, P. and Nicoletti, L. 1995. In: Porterfield, J. (ed.), *Kass handbook of infectious diseases, exotic viral infections*. Oxford: Chapman & Hall Medical, 295–317.

Verani, P., Lopes, M. et al. 1980. Arboviruses in the Mediterranean countries. *Zentralbl Bakteriol Mikrobiol Hyg*, 195–201.

Verkleij, F.N. and Peters, D. 1983. Characterization of a defective form of tomato spotted wilt virus. *J Gen Virol*, **64**, 677–86.

Vesenjak-Hirjan, J., Calisher, C., et al. 1980. Arboviruses in the Mediterranean countries. *Zentralblatt Bakteriol Parasit Infect Hyg*, **1 Abt**, 297–301.

Vialat, P. and Bouloy, M. 1992. Germiston virus transcriptase requires active 40S ribosomal subunits and utilizes capped cellular RNAs. *J Virol*, **66**, 685–93.

Vialat, P., Billecoq, A., et al. 2000. The S segment of Rift Valley fever Phlebovirus (*Bunyaviridae*) carries determinants for attenuation and virulence in mice. *J Virol*, **74**, 1538–43.

Vidal, S. and Kolakofsky, D. 1989. Modified model for the switch from Sendai virus transcription to replication. *J Virol*, **63**, 1951–8.

Vincent, M.J., Quirez, E., et al. 2000. Hantavirus pulmonary syndrome in Panama: identification of novel hantaviruses and their likely reservoirs. *Virology*, **277**, 14–19.

von Bonsdorff, C.-H. and Pettersson, R. 1975. Surface structure of Uukuniemi virus. *J Virol*, **95**, 1–7.

von Bonsdorff, C.-H., Saikku, P. and Oker-Blom, N. 1970. Electron microscopy study on development of Uukuniemi virus. *Acta Virol*, **14**, 109–14.

Vorndam, A.V. and Trent, D.W. 1979. Oligosaccharides of the California encephalitis viruses. *Virology*, **95**, 1–7.

Wang, M.W., Pennock, D.G., et al. 1993. Epitope mapping studies with neutralizing and non-neutralizing monoclonal antibodies to the G1 and G2 envelope glycoproteins of Hantaan virus. *Virology*, **197**, 757–66.

Ward, V.K., Marriott, A.C., et al. 1990. Coding strategy of the S RNA segment of Dugbe virus (*Nairovirus*; *Bunyaviridae*). *Virology*, **175**, 518–24.

Wasmoen, T.L., Kakach, L.T. and Collett, M.S. 1988. Rift Valley fever virus M segment: cellular localization of M segment-encoded proteins. *Virology*, **166**, 275–80.

Watts, D., Pantuwatana, S., et al. 1973. Transovarial transmission of La Crosse virus (California encephalitis group) in the mosquito, *Aedes triseriatus*. *Science*, **182**, 123–30.

Watts, D., Thompson, W., et al. 1974. Overwintering of La Crosse virus in *Aedes triseriatus*. *Am J Trop Med Hyg*, **23**, 694–700.

Watts, D., Ksiazek, T., et al. 1989. Crimean–Congo hemorrhagic fever. In: Monath, T. (ed.), *The arboviruses: epidemiology and ecology*. Vol. 2. Boca Raton, FL: CRC Press, 177–222.

Watts, D.M., Philips, I., et al. 1997. Oropouche virus transmission in the Amazon River basin of Peru. *Am J Trop Med Hyg*, **56**, 148–52.

Weber, F., Bridgen, A., Elliott, R.M. 2000. The Bunyamwera virus nonstructural protein NSs is a repressor of the viral polymerase and confers interferon-antagonistic function. Eleventh International Conference on Negative Strand Viruses. Quebec, Canada.

Weber, F., Bridgen, A., et al. 2002. Bunyamwera nonstructural protein NSs counteracts the induction of alpha/beta interferon. *J Virol*, **76**, 7949–55.

Wertz, G.W. 1983. Replication of vesicular stomatitis virus defective interfering particle RNA in vitro: transition from synthesis of defective interfering leader RNA to synthesis of full-length defective interfering RNA. *J Virol*, **46**, 513–22.

WHO. 1994. Weekly epidemiological record. *Wkly Epidemiol Rec*, 197–204.

WHO. 1995. *Report of a meeting on hantavirus vaccine development*. Geneva: World Health Organization.

Wijkamp, I., van Lent, J., et al. 1993. Multiplication of tomato spotted wilt virus in its insect vector, *Frankliniella occidentalis*. *J Gen Virol*, **74**, 341–9.

Yeh, S.D. and Chang, T.F. 1995. Nucleotide sequence of the N gene of watermelon silvermottle virus, a proposed new member of the genus *Tospovirus*. *Phytopathology*, **85**, 58–64.

Yeh, S.D., Peng, Y.C., et al. 1998. Peanut chlorotic fan-spot virus is serologically and phylogenetically distinct from other tospoviruses. In: Peters, D. and Goldbach, R. (eds), *Recent progress in tospovirus and thrips research*. The Netherlands: Waginengen.

Yuill, T. 1983. The role of mammals in the maintenance and dissemination of La Crosse virus. In: Calisher, C. and Thompson, C. (eds), *California serogroup viruses*. New York: Alan R Liss, 77–88.

Zaki, S.R., Greer, P.W., et al. 1995. Hantavirus pulmonary syndrome. Pathogenesis of an emerging infectious disease. *Am J Pathol*, **146**, 552–79.

49

Arenaviruses

MARIA S. SALVATO AND JUAN D. RODAS

PROPERTIES OF THE ARENAVIRUSES

INTRODUCTION

The arenaviruses are enveloped, single-stranded RNA viruses that are primarily carried by rodents and occasionally transmitted to humans. Old World and New World arenaviruses have been isolated on the African and American continents respectively (see Table 49.1). The arenaviruses are important clinically as human pathogens and experimentally as models for persistent infection and cellular immune responses. The prototype virus, lymphocytic choriomeningitis virus (LCMV), was first isolated from a human diagnosed with St. Louis encephalitis; tissue homogenates passaged through monkeys and mice caused fever and aseptic meningitis (Armstrong and Lillie 1934). A year later, a filterable agent was isolated from the cerebrospinal fluids of two patients; this agent elicited similar symptoms in mice (Rivers and Scott 1935). At the same time, Traub (1935) discovered a contaminant virus in the mouse colony of the Rockefeller Laboratories. Viruses were exchanged between the three laboratories and their identity was confirmed by neutralization in vitro and cross-protection in vivo (Rivers and Scott 1936). LCMV has frequently been found as a contaminant of laboratory mice, rats, and hamsters in North America and Europe, and may

have entered North America via mice from Europe. Studies of murine LCMV infection have contributed to a wealth of information on the mechanisms of viral persistence and the interactions of viruses with host immune systems (see section entitled Immune response).

In 1956, the nonpathogenic Tacaribe virus was isolated from Caribbean fruit bats (Downs et al. 1963). With the agricultural expansion in South America, two pathogenic arenaviruses emerged: Junin, isolated from humans with Argentine hemorrhagic fever (Parodi et al. 1958); and Machupo, isolated from humans with Bolivian hemorrhagic fever (Johnson et al. 1965). Collaboration between field workers, the Yale Arbovirus Laboratories and the Rockefeller Laboratories documented the morphology and antigenicity of the 'Tacaribe group' of viruses. A nonpathogenic member of this group, Pichinde virus, was isolated during a trapping programme in Colombia, and has since served in many biochemical studies (Trapido and Sanmartin 1971; Cosgriff et al. 1987; Liu et al. 1986; Qian et al. 1991). More recently, other arenaviruses have been discovered in Argentina (Oliveros virus, Bowen et al. 1996), Brazil (Cupixi, Charrel et al. 2002), Venezuela (Pirital virus, Charrel et al. 2001a), Peru (Allpahuayo virus, Moncayo et al. 2001) and the US (Whitewater Arroyo virus, Charrel et al. 2001b; Bear Canyon virus, Fulhorst et al. 2002).

Table 49.1 Arenaviridae: *carriers and geographical distribution (modified from Clegg 2002)*

Virus	Virus carrier	Geographical distribution	Potential for human disease
New World			
Allpahuayo	*Oecomys* spp.	Peru	None reported
Amapari	*Oryzomys goeldii*	Brazil	None reported
	Neacomys guinae	Brazil	
Bear Canyon	*Peromyscus californicus*	California, USA	None confirmed
Cupixi	*Oryzomys* spp.	Brazil	None reported
Flexal	*Neacomys* spp.	Brazil	None reported
Guanarito	*Oryzomys* spp.	Venezuela	Severe
Junin	*Calomys laucha*	Argentina	Severe
	Calomys musculinus	Argentina	
	Akodon azarae	Argentina	
Latino	*Calomys callosus*	Bolivia	None reported
Machupo	*Calomys callosus*	Bolivia	Severe
Oliveros	*Bolomys obscures*	Argentina	None reported
Parana	*Oryzomys buccinatus*	Paraguay	None reported
Pichinde	*Oryzomys albigularis*	Colombia	None
	Thomasomys fuscatus	Colombia	
Pirital	*Sigmodon alstoni*	Venezuela	None reported
Sabía	Not known	Brazil	Severe
Tacaribe	*Artibeus literatus*	Trinidad	None reported
	Artibeus jamaicensis	Trinidad	
Tamiami	*Sigmodon hispidus*	Florida, USA	None reported
Whitewater Arroyo	*Neotoma* spp.: *albigula, cinerea, mexicana, micropus*	New Mexico, USA	Three fatalities had a virus, 87 percent identical to WWA
Old World			
LCM	*Mus musculus*	Worldwide	Mild to severe
Lassa	*Mastomys natalensis*	West Africa	Severe, often fatal
Mopeia	*Mastomys natalensis*	Mozambique Zimbabwe	None reported
Mobala	*Praomys jacksoni*	Central African Republic	None reported
Ippy	*Mastomys natalensis*	Central African Republic	None reported

It was not until the late 1960s that the morphological similarities between LCMV and the Tacaribe group of viruses were noted: both were enveloped viruses with a granular or sandy appearance. Serological tests later confirmed the relationship and they were named arenaviruses after the Latin *arena* for 'sandy' (Johnson et al. 1965; Dalton et al. 1968; Rowe et al. 1970). When Lassa fever virus emerged in Africa, it was quickly identified as an arenavirus on morphological and serological criteria (Murphy 1975). Arenaviruses are considered 'emerging pathogens' because new isolates are coming to our attention with great frequency (Coimbra and Nassar 1994). The following publications contain more details about the arenaviruses: Oldstone (2002); Bishop (1990); McCormick (1990); Salvato (1993a); Southern (1996); Buchmeier et al. (2001), and Peters (1997).

CLASSIFICATION

The *Arenaviridae* are one of seven families of negative-strand RNA viruses, the others being *Filoviridae*, *Rhabdoviridae*, *Paramyxoviridae*, *Orthomyxoviridae*, *Bunya-*viridae, and *Bornaviridae*. These viruses are characterized by single-stranded, non-infectious genomic RNA that requires a virus-encoded RNA transcriptase to initiate replication. Arenaviruses have been classified by a combination of morphological characteristics, biochemical analyses, and immunological tests (Pfau 1974) and are the only family of negative-strand RNA viruses with a bisegmented genome (Pedersen 1979). Under the Old World and New World groupings are at least 22 species of arenaviruses (Table 49.1) with the probable addition of further viruses as surveillance continues. Genetic relationships among the arenaviruses can be depicted by a phylogenetic tree based on the sequence differences between viral nucleocapsid proteins (Figure 49.1). A recent comparison (Bowen et al. 2000) found the broadest range of sequences within the *Lassa* species, i.e. up to 24.1 percent nucleotide divergence and up to 12 percent amino acid divergence. However, two distinct species of New World arenaviruses, *Junin virus* and *Machupo virus*, were relatively similar to each other with 23.3 percent nucleotide divergence and 13.7 percent amino acid divergence.

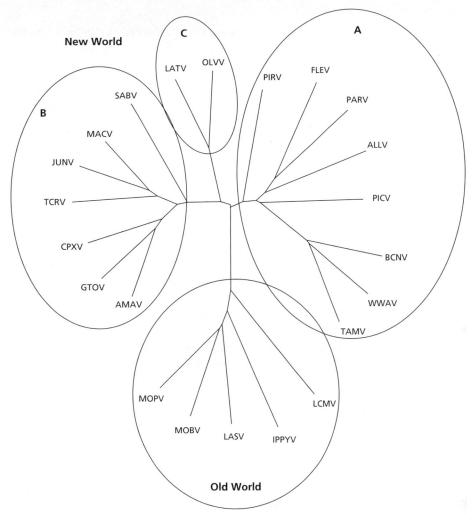

Figure 49.1 *Phylogenetic relationships among the* Arenaviridae. *Partial N gene nucleotide sequences corresponding to nt 1770–2418 of* Tacaribe virus *S RNA sequence (GenBank accession no. M20304) were aligned (Clustal X 1.81) and analyzed by Jukes–Cantor algorithm and neighbor-joining method using the MEGA v2.1 software program (modified from Bowen et al. 2000).*

Considering that picornaviruses have as much as 30 percent amino acid divergence within species (Dahourou et al. 2002), the arenaviruses are considerably subdivided. In addition to sequence criteria, classification of arenaviruses is influenced by the ability of viruses to reassort with one another, i.e. intraspecies reassortment should be possible and interspecies reassortment, as between *Lassa virus* and *Mopeia virus* (Lukashevich 1992), is rare.

DISTRIBUTION

The worldwide distribution of arenaviruses follows the distribution of their natural reservoir hosts, primarily rodents (Figure 49.2). Occasionally, infected humans have traveled extensively, resulting in movement of the viruses (Holmes et al. 1990).

Although there are over 30 families of rodents, the arenaviruses are associated with only two major families: the *Muridae* (e.g. house mice and rats) and the *Cricetidae* (e.g. voles, deer mice, and gerbils). The *Muridae*

inhabit human dwellings and food stores, in contrast to the *Cricetidae* that live in the open grasslands. Muridae include *Mastomys*, that carries the Lassa-like viruses; *Praomys*, that carries Mobala; and *Mus*, that spread from the Old World to the rest of the globe, simultaneously dispersing LCMV. The cottonrat, *Sigmodon hispidus*, from which Tamiami virus was isolated in the USA, is related to the *Cricetidae*: *Calomys, Akadon, Oryzomys*, and *Neocomys* of South America and *Peromyscus* of North America. Tacaribe virus is an exception in that it was isolated from the fruit bat, *Artibeus*. It is notable that infections follow seasonal associations between humans and carriers; for example, the harvest season in Argentina, April to June, is also the peak time for the occurrence of Argentine hemorrhagic fever.

MORPHOLOGY AND STRUCTURE

The envelope composition of an arenavirus derives from host-cell membranes during maturation from the cell

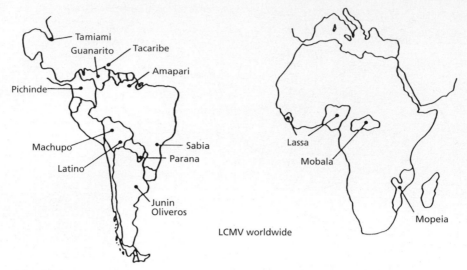

Figure 49.2 *Map of the distribution of Old World and New World arenaviruses. The Old World viruses originated on the European and African continents and the New World viruses originated in the Americas.*

surface (Figure 49.3a). The envelope is sensitive to organic solvents and detergents; treatment with these reagents can be used to separate viral cores from their envelopes. Virions are also sensitive to UV and gamma-irradiation, to heating at 56°C, and to pH outside the range of 5.5–8.5. Acid or high salt treatment of LCMV causes one of the envelope glycoprotein chains, GP-1, to dissociate from the virion surface, whereas the other chain, GP-2, remains anchored in the envelope (Di Simone et al. 1994). Acid treatment of LCMV decreases its Vero cell infectivity, which is due to virus aggregation or the loss of GP-1. Virions are generally purified from the media surrounding infected cells by a combination of precipitation with 7 percent polyethylene glycol and centrifugation: buoyant densities are 1.9–1.2 g/cm^3 in cesium chloride, 1.17–1.18 g/cm^3 in sucrose and 1.14 g/cm^3 in amidotrizoate (Buchmeier et al. 1978).

Originally, electron micrographs showed arenaviruses as highly pleiomorphic, probably because of their instability during fixation procedures. More recently, cryo-electron micrographs have revealed spherical particles with an average diameter of 90–110 nm (Burns and Buchmeier 1993) (Figure 49.3c, d). Glycoproteins on the surface of the virion form T-shaped spikes extending 7–10 nm from the envelope. Electron-dense granules within arenaviruses, from which the name 'arena' derives, are ribonucleoprotein particles. These include ribosomal RNA, and perhaps whole ribosomes, and more of such particles are present in late viral harvests than in early harvests (Farber and Rawls 1975; Pedersen 1979; Dutko and Oldstone 1983; Southern et al. 1987). With Pichinde virus, virion-associated ribosomes are not essential for the infectious process; viruses produced in cells containing *ts* ribosomes are infectious even at the nonpermissive temperature (Leung and Rawls 1977). Electron microscopy of disrupted virions reveals circu-

larized strings of ribonucleoproteins (Palmer et al. 1977) that may have resulted from the self-annealing of the RNA termini that encode approximately 20 bases of complementary nucleotides.

Arenaviruses produce defective interfering (DI) particles (reviewed by Buchmeier et al. 1980a). DI particles are generated rapidly during infection of tissue cultures with LCMV, and render the cells resistant to super-infection with LCMV, less resistant to Pichinde and entirely susceptible to heterologous viruses (Lehmann-Grube et al. 1969; Welsh and Buchmeier 1979). DI particles sediment to a lower density than infectious virus and have a smaller target size for UV inactivation, and their concentration can be measured by cytopathogeni-city-reduction assays. DI particles of Pichinde lack conventional S RNA (Dutko et al. 1976).

GENOME STRUCTURE AND FUNCTION

The arenaviruses contain single-stranded RNA that consists of 2 RNA segments, L ca. 7000 bases and S ca. 3400 bases. Complete sequences are now available for LCMV, Lassa, Tacaribe, and Pichinde, and partial sequences for Junin, Mopeia, and other arenaviruses (Romanowski et al. 1985; Auperin et al. 1986; Auperin and McCormick 1989; Iapalucci et al. 1989; Salvato and Shimomaye 1989; Salvato et al. 1989; Ghiringhelli et al. 1991; Harnish et al. unpublished; reviewed in Clegg 1993). Four open reading frames have been identified: a gene for the envelope glycoprotein is encoded at the 5′ end of the S RNA segment, and, in the negative sense, a gene for the nucleocapsid protein is encoded at the 3′ end of the S RNA. A gene for a small zinc-binding protein is encoded at the 5′ end of the L RNA, and, in the negative sense, a gene for the viral RNA polymerase is encoded at the 3′ end of the L RNA (Figure 49.4).

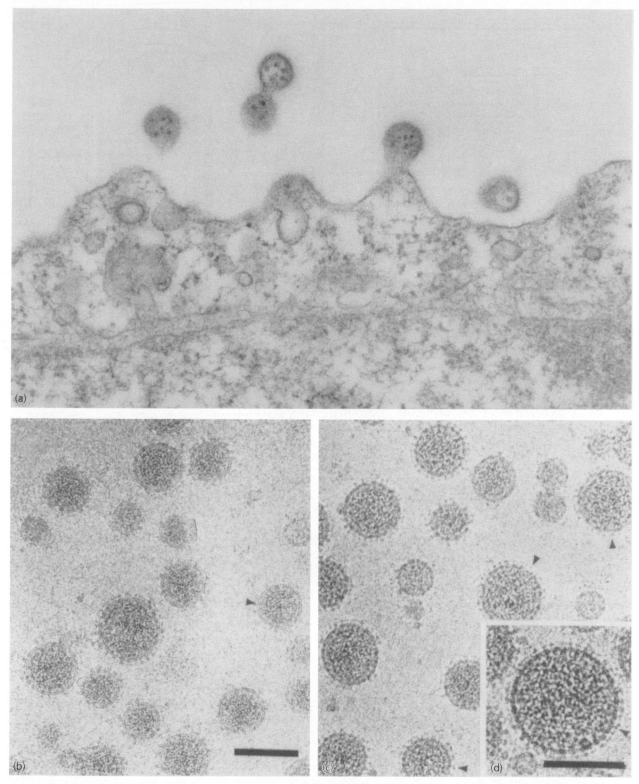

Figure 49.3 *Electron micrographs of LCM virions.* **(a)** *Thin section showing virions budding from infected BHK-21 cells. Typical 110 nm virions containing 20 nm electron-dense particles are evident.* **(b)** *Cryo-electron micrograph of unstained LCM virions at the 1.5 μm defocus level to emphasize lipid bilayer (see arrow) and in* **(c)** *cryo-electron micrograph of LCM at the 3 μm defocus level to emphasize surface topography. Bars = 100 nm. (Microscopy by R Milligan, Scripps Clinic and Research Foundation, San Diego. Reproduced from Burns and Buchmeier 1993.)*

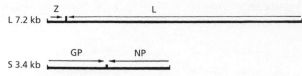

Figure 49.4 *The two arenavirus RNA segments, L and S, are depicted with the four encoded genes: Z (zinc-binding protein), L (polymerase), GP (envelope glycoprotein) and NP (nucleocapsid protein). (Reproduced from Salvato 1993b)*

A hallmark of the arenaviruses is their 'ambisense' coding strategy (Auperin et al. 1984). Each RNA segment encodes a gene in the positive (mRNA) sense and an additional nonoverlapping gene in the negative sense, i.e. the latter gene must first be transcribed to obtain the mRNA sense. The viruses are classified as negative strand, because the mRNA sense genes cannot function in translation directly from the genomic RNA; subgenomic mRNA copies of these genes must first be produced by transcription (Figure 49.5).

Strong secondary structures can be predicted for arenavirus genomic RNAs: stem–loops in the intergenic regions and base-paired 'panhandles' at the termini of the RNA segments. The terminal 20 bases of the arenavirus genomic RNA are conserved between genera and are almost identical within one arenavirus strain. It is possible to form intra- and extramolecular complexes, i.e. the 3′ and 5′ termini of the S RNA can anneal with each other or the 3′ of the S RNA can anneal with the 5′ of the L RNA, and so on. It has been suggested that this conserved terminal structure may represent a binding site for the viral RNA polymerase (Salvato 1993b) (Figure 49.6).

Reassortment of the two genomic RNA segments has been used to map functions to one segment or the other. Production of reassortant viruses involves infection of cultured cells with two virus isolates at once and screening for progeny virus by nucleic acid hybridization, reverse transcriptase polymerase chain reaction (RT-PCR), or by limited sequence analysis. Reassortant

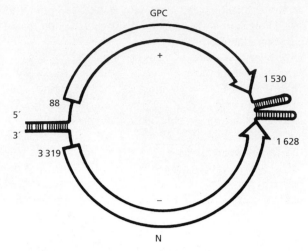

Figure 49.6 *The S RNA segment of Junin virus can be predicted to form strong secondary structures at the RNA terminus (a panhandle of the 3′ and 5′ ends) and at the intergenic region (a double stem–loop structure). The glycoprotein (GP-C) and the nucleocapsid protein (N) open reading frames are in opposite coding sense on either side of the intergenic stem–loops. (Reproduced from Romanowski 1993)*

viruses that contain the S RNA of one parental virus and the L RNA of the other can usually be isolated. This approach was used to show that the virulence of LCMV WE for guinea-pigs mapped to the L RNA (Riviere 1986), that the S RNA of LCMV Armstrong is associated both with diminished growth in C3H mice (Oldstone et al. 1985) and with the emergence of insulin-dependent diabetes in nonobese diabetic mice (Oldstone et al. 1990), and that the persistence of an LCMV Armstrong isolate depends on the L RNA (Matloubian et al. 1993). The latter case illustrates one shortcoming of this approach in that the persistent phenotype is likely to be pleiotropic, with essential genetic components on both RNAs (Salvato et al. 1991). Likewise, reassortant viruses between the Old World arenaviruses Mopeia and Lassa allowed mapping of the ability of Lassa S segment to protect against a lethal intracerebral inoculation of Lassa virus in the murine model (Lukashevich 1992).

A reverse genetics system developed by the de la Torre laboratory indicates a transcription inhibitory function for Z protein (Lee and de la Torre 2002)

REPLICATION

Tropism and virus entry

Arenaviruses replicate in a broad range of mammalian hosts and in almost every tissue of the host, reaching high titers in brain, kidney, liver, and secondary lymphoid organs (see Figure 49.9). Virus replication is restricted in lymphocytes, macrophages, and terminally differentiated neurons, probably because of the absence

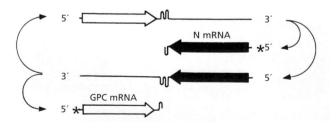

Figure 49.5 *The ambisense coding strategy of the arenaviruses is illustrated for the S RNA segment of Junin virus. First, the subgenomic nucleocapsid mRNA (N mRNA) is made and then the full-length antigenomic RNA is made (this is a 'replication intermediate'); finally, the subgenomic glycoprotein mRNA (GP-C mRNA) is made. For the L RNA a similar sequence occurs with the L and Z subgenomic mRNAs. (Reproduced from Romanowski 1993)*

of host cell factors (Borrow et al. 1991; de la Torre et al. 1993; Polyak et al. 1995a). Arenaviruses are often propagated in adherent cell lines such as BHK-21 cells, mouse L cells or Vero cells. The broad range of mammalian cells that can be infected suggests that the receptor for virus entry is fairly well conserved. In attempts to find the receptor for LCMV, Borrow and Oldstone (1992) used a virus overlay blot assay to identify a 160 kDa glycoprotein from rodent fibroblasts. Further studies of this protein made it clear that several arenaviruses bind to a 120–140 kDa cellular glycoprotein identified as α-dystroglycan (Cao et al. 1998). However, variations in binding affinity to α-dystroglycan were observed among the LCMV strains, with LCMV Cl –13 and WE strains being typical of high affinity binders while Arm binds at low affinity. Other arenaviruses (i.e. Lassa, Mobala, Oliveros) also bind to this glycoprotein, but Guanarito virus does not, suggesting that more than one cellular protein may serve as a receptor for arenaviruses (Buchmeier 2002).

Arenavirus entry into cultured cells is sensitive to lysosomotropic agents (Pichinde: Mifune et al. 1971; Lassa and Mopeia: Glushakova and Lukashevich 1989, Glushakova et al. 1992; LCMV: Borrow and Oldstone 1994; Di Simone et al. 1994). In the case of LCMV, this uptake was not affected by cytochalasins, so does not require clathrin-coated pits and takes place in smooth-walled vesicles by 'viropexis.' Once the virus is in the cell, the life cycle of uncoating, mRNA transcription, translation, and genome replication takes place in the cytoplasm,

with some contribution from host-cell components for transcription and translation (Figure 49.7).

Arenavirus gene expression

The ambisense coding arrangement of the arenavirus genome provides a mechanism for temporal regulation of gene expression: NP and L mRNAs can be transcribed from the incoming genomic RNA, whereas GP and Z mRNAs are transcribed only from RNA antigenomic templates that also function as replication intermediates. Kinetic analysis of LCMV replication shows simultaneous accumulation of NP and GP mRNA (Fuller-Pace and Southern 1988), but in Tacaribe virus, newly synthesized NP mRNA accumulates before the onset of RNA replication. Furthermore, inhibition of protein synthesis during early infection prevents RNA replication but allows the continued synthesis of NP mRNA (Lopez and Franze-Fernandez 1985; Franze-Fernandez et al. 1987). For LCMV, it has been shown that the Z mRNA is included in the virion, unlike mRNAs for the other viral genes, and may be essential at an early stage of the viral life cycle (Salvato and Shimomaye 1989). Further work with inhibitors of transcription and translation will be necessary to characterize the sequence of events in arenavirus replication.

Arenavirus mRNA transcription begins with 3–7 nontemplated nucleotides: this has been demonstrated for the 5′ terminus of the NP mRNA in Tacaribe virus (Raju et al. 1990), the NP and GP mRNAs in LCMV

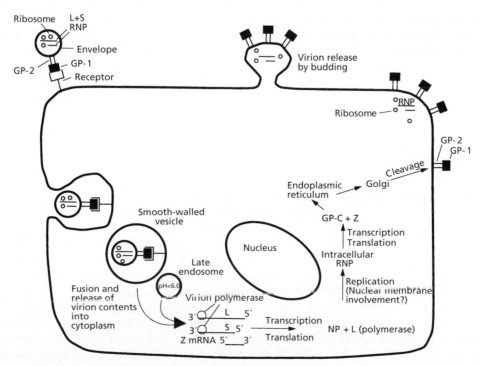

Figure 49.7 *Arenavirus life cycle. L, large RNA segment; S, small RNA segment; RNP, ribonucleoprotein. RNP complexes in the virion contain viral genomic RNA, Z mRNA, viral proteins, and host components such as ribosomal proteins.*

(Meyer and Southern 1993) and the NP and GP mRNAs in Pichinde virus (Polyak et al. 1995b). Genome and antigenomes generally have one nontemplated base. These may arise either by de novo synthesis or by a cap stealing mechanism as has been described for the *Orthomyxoviridae* and the *Bunyaviridae* (Garcin and Kolakofsky 1990).

The noncoding regions of arenavirus genomic RNA have the potential to form several stem–loop structures that are well placed to regulate transcription and translation. LCMV, Lassa, and Pichinde viruses each have single intergenic stem–loops on the S RNA, whereas Mopeia, Tacaribe, and Junin viruses each predict double stem–looped structures (reviewed by Clegg 1993). Translation termination codons have been described on the proximal side of the intergenic stem–loops on the S RNA and L RNA. Transcription terminations for Tacaribe virus NP, GP, Z, and L mRNAs have been described at the distal portion of each stem–loop, indicating that the secondary structure is not acting to stop transcription. Furthermore, since transcription termination has been described at multiple positions on the stem, it is likely that the polymerase is displaced from the RNA by an extragenomic factor rather than by a feature of the genome structure (Franze-Fernandez et al. 1993; Meyer and Southern 1993). Thus, since it appears that the intergenic stem–loops may help stop translation, in conjunction with the encoded stop codons, they are unlikely to serve as terminators or attenuators of transcription, and they may serve as recognition or nucleation points for virus assembly and encapsidation.

Recent studies using a LCMV RNA analogue, showed clearly that L and NP are the minimal viral factors required for efficient RNA synthesis mediated by the LCMV polymerase (Lee et al. 2000). In addition, this system allowed tests for the *cis*-elements required for transcription and replication of LCMV genome in vitro (Lee et al. 2002).

Virus–host interactions during arenavirus replication

LCMV infections in carrier mice (covered more extensively in the section entitled Clinical and pathological aspects) can persist in a broad range of tissues, without detectable cellular damage or inflammation (see Figure 49.9). However, some terminally differentiated cell functions or 'luxury functions' can be abolished by the presence of replicating virus. For example, a reduction of macrophage lymphokines, growth hormone, thyroid hormones, and acetylcholinesterase have been observed in persistently infected murine systems (Jacobs and Cole 1976; Oldstone et al. 1977, 1982, 1985; Rodriguez et al. 1983; Klavinskis and Oldstone 1987). The ability of LCMV to affect differentiated functions of the immune, neural, and endocrine systems depends on the genetic background of the host.

In tissue culture at low multiplicity of infection (i.e. moi <0.1) arenavirus replication is not detected for 6 h, after which cell-associated virus increases exponentially. The titer of extracellular virus reaches a maximum 36–48 h after infection. Infected cells undergo only limited cytopathic change during virus production with little or no change in the level of host protein synthesis. Long-term virus cultures are readily established.

Although arenavirus replication takes place in the host-cell cytoplasm, enucleated cells fail to support virus production. Specifically, the host-cell nucleus is required during the first 10 h of Pichinde virus infection of BHK-21 cells (Banerjee et al. 1976). Either enucleation removes a site of virus replication near the nuclear membrane or host nuclear products are required for viral replication. The latter is supported by the finding that α-amanitin, an inhibitor of host RNA polymerase II that is responsible for mRNA and hnRNA synthesis, prevents arenavirus replication. In contrast, actinomycin D, which primarily inhibits rRNA synthesis, has a lesser effect on Pichinde replication.

Host-cell ribosomes that become incorporated into nascent virions retain their capacity to catalyse protein synthesis, but are not necessary for virus replication (Leung and Rawls 1977). In Pichinde virus, hybrid molecules between viral RNA and host-cell ribosomal RNA have been observed (Shivraprakesh et al. 1988) but their functional significance is unclear. Host-cell ribosomal proteins and translation factors are definitely incorporated within virus but may simply be remnants of assembly complexes rather than the package of complete ribosome (Borden et al. 1998b).

Host-cell enzymes are essential for the maturation of arenavirus envelope glycoproteins. These are translated as a long precursor (GP-C) that undergoes glycosylation, transport, and proteolysis involving host-cell enzymes (Buchmeier and Oldstone 1979; reviewed in Burns and Buchmeier 1993). Initially, for LCMV, a 58-residue signal peptide is cleaved from the N terminus of GP-C. Further cleavage depends on glycosylation of the precursor in the Golgi or post-Golgi compartments with 5–6 N-linked glycosylations for the N-terminal portion of GP-C (to become GP-1) and 2 N-linked glycosylations for the C-terminal portion of GP-C (to become GP-2) (Wright et al. 1989). Cleavage by a furinlike protease occurs at Arg_{262}–Arg_{263}. This cleavage is followed by trimming of the N-terminal portion of GP-2 (Burns and Buchmeier 1993). A protein kinase activity capable of phosphorylating the nucleocapsid protein has been identified in preparations of LCMV (Howard and Buchmeier 1983), but it is not known whether this is a cellular or viral enzyme or if it has any essential function. Recently, it has also been shown that Lassa Gp precursor is cleaved in endoplasmic reticulum by the cellular subtilase SKI-1/S1P, an enzyme that has been observed to be involved in cholesterol metabolism (Lenz et al. 2001). Moreover, since apparently only the cleaved glycoprotein is incorporated into virions, this cellular enzyme is necessary for the formation of infectious virus. Lassa GP-C is the first viral glycoprotein known to be processed by SKI-1/S1P and its tissue expression pattern in rats revealed highest levels of activity in liver, spleen, and adrenal glands and low levels in brain (Seidah et al. 1999). Accordingly, in human Lassa fever cases, higher viral titers are recovered from liver, spleen, lungs, kidneys, and adrenal but not from brain (Walker et al. 1982a). This finding suggests that specific inhibitors for SKI-1/S1P mediated cleavage of Lassa virus GP-C might lead to new therapeutical approaches for Lassa fever (Lenz et al. 2001).

POLYPEPTIDES: STRUCTURE AND FUNCTION

Arenavirus proteins include the 250-kDa RNA polymerase (L), the 11–14-kDa zinc-binding protein (Z) encoded on the L RNA, the 63-kDa nucleocapsid protein (N or NP) and the 75-kDa glycoprotein precursor (GP-C) encoded on the S RNA (see Figure 49.4). These four proteins account for the coding capacity of the virus without overlap (Salvato and Shimomaye 1989). The stoichiometry of proteins in the LCM virion has been determined by metabolic labeling (Salvato et al. 1992). Per virion, there are about 30 copies of L protein, 1500 copies of NP, 650 copies of GP-1, 650 copies of GP-2 and 450 copies of Z protein (Figure 49.8). According to cross-linking studies, NP and Z are associated (Salvato et al. 1992) and NP and GP-2 are associated (Burns and Buchmeier 1991). Recent immunoprecipitation and genetic studies reveal Z:L binding that explains the ability of Z to inhibit transcription (Jacamo et al. 2003).

NP is the most abundant virion protein as well as the most stable and abundant viral protein in infected cells. There are ca. 1500–2000 copies of NP per virion, or one copy per 10–20 bases of viral genomic RNA (Bishop 1990). Among the negative-strand viruses, the nucleocapsid proteins usually function as the primary structural protein of viral cores and in mediating the interaction of the RNA polymerase with the viral RNA. A phosphorylated form of NP has been detected late in acute infection and in greater abundance in persistently infected cells (Bruns et al. 1986), leading to the suggestion that phosphorylation of NP is associated with attenuation of virus production and persistence. Breakdown products of NP have also been detected both in infected cells and in virions. It is conceivable, but not yet demonstrated, that fragments of NP serve as minor structural proteins (Coto et al. 1993). A 28 kDa degradation product of NP has been identified within the nuclei of Pichinde virus-infected cells, but no significance can yet be assigned to this (Howard 1993).

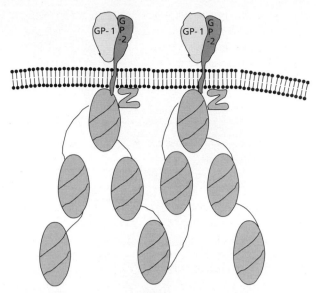

Figure 49.8 *Hypothetical scheme for the association of structural proteins in the LCM virion. The viral RNA is represented as a string winding around the beads that are the nucleocapsid protein molecules. The Z protein is depicted as a Z associated with the nucleocapsid proteins. GP-2 is anchored in the viral envelope and associated with NP. GP-1 is loosely associated with the surface of the virion. In each virion the proportions of Z, GP-1, and GP-2 in the virion are roughly equivalent, whereas NP is 3- to 5-fold more abundant. The polymerase or L protein accounts for only 30 molecules per virion. (Reproduced from Salvato 1993b)*

For LCMV, the envelope glycoprotein (GP) is synthesized as a 73-kDa precursor and cleaved into 43-kDa (GP-1) and 35-kDa (GP-2) polypeptides (Buchmeier and Oldstone 1979). Cleavage and maturation of the arenavirus glycoproteins, using host enzymes, has been described in the previous section. All arenaviruses that have been examined so far have potential cleavage sites in the glycoprotein precursor and two cleavage products that can be identified in protein gels. Tamiami and Tacaribe viruses are an exception in which only one cleavage product is observed in gels; however, the situation was clarified for Tacaribe virus when it was shown that the two cleavage products comigrate on gels but can be detected by analysis of the peptide termini (Burns and Buchmeier 1993).

The spikes of the virion are composed of GP-1 and GP-2: GP-2 is anchored in the membrane and associated with the nucleocapsid core through its C terminus and GP-1 is loosely attached to the virion surface through ionic interactions. Cross-linking studies indicate that GP-1 and GP-2 are present as homotetramers (Burns and Buchmeier 1991). Sequence analysis and antigenic cross-reactivity indicate that GP-2 contains a highly conserved sequence, whereas GP-1 contains the most variable sequence among the *Arenaviridae* (Weber and Buchmeier 1988; Clegg 1993). With Junin virus, rabbits and guinea-pigs inoculated with GP-2 produce neutralizing antibodies against the infectious virus (reviewed in

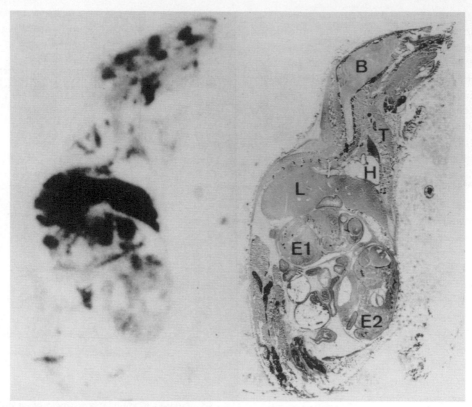

Figure 49.9 *Sagittal section of a pregnant mouse infected with LCMV. On the left is an autoradiograph of radioactive probes hybridizing to viral RNA within the section. On the right is the stained section: B, brain; E1, one embryo; E2, another embryo; H, heart; L, liver; T, thymus. (Reproduced from Southern et al. 1984)*

Martinez Peralta et al. 1993). In contrast, for LCMV, neutralizing antibodies predominately recognize conformational epitopes within GP-1 (Parekh and Buchmeier 1986) and this recognition depends on glycosylation and retention of disulphide bonds (Wright et al. 1989). It is likely that conformational changes of GP-1 expose domains on the spike glycoprotein that mediate virus entry into host cells (Di Simone et al. 1994).

The arenavirus L protein is the viral RNA-dependent RNA polymerase, is encoded in the 3′ ORF of the L RNA segment and has a molecular mass of 180–250 kDa. The L protein is a component of nucleocapsids since polymerase activity has been associated with these structures. The LAS L protein contains six motifs of conserved amino acids that have been found among arenavirus L proteins and core RNA-dependent RNA polymerase (RdRp) of other segmented negative-stranded (SNS) viruses (*Arena-*, *Bunya-*, and *Orthomyxoviridae*). (Lukashevich et al. 1997). Two regions found in the polymerases of arenaviruses and bunyaviruses are conserved in arenaviruses L proteins.

The zinc-binding protein of 11–14 kDa has a strongly conserved 'ring finger' motif in LCMV, Tacaribe, and Pichinde (Iapalucci et al. 1989; Salvato and Shimomaye 1989; Harnish et al. unpublished). This motif is characterized by the classic zinc-binding residues described in TFIIIA, and additional cysteine and histidine residues that help the molecule form a ring, i.e. C–X2–C–X(9–27)–

C–X(1–3)–H–Y2–C–X2–C–X(4–48)–C–X2–C (Freemont 1993). Ring finger proteins generally have *trans*-regulatory functions and have been involved in protein–protein, protein–membrane and protein–nucleic acid interactions. The LCMV Z protein is a significant structural component of the virion and is able to bind isotopic zinc (Salvato and Shimomaye 1989; Salvato et al. 1992). Z protein has been detected in cytoplasm and nucleus of LCMV-infected cells and recent studies revealed that interacts with a nuclear oncoprotein, promyelocyte leukemia protein (PML), modulating the interferon response as well as ribosomal proteins (P0, P1, and P2) and transcription factors (eIF4E) performing regulatory functions in infected cells (Borden et al. 1997, 1998a, b; Campbell Dwyer et al. 2000; Djavani et al. 2001b). Garcin et al. (1993) showed that immunoprecipitation of Tacaribe Z protein blocked transcription whereas de la Torre's minigenome transcription system was inhibited by addition of excess of Z (Cornu and de la Torre, 2001, 2002). Also, the protein Z had a positive role on virus assembly using the same system (Lee and de la Torre 2002) Thus, the Z protein of the arenaviruses is most likely to be a matrix protein.

ANTIGENS

Highly accurate nucleic acid technologies (i.e. sequencing and RT-PCR) have recently superseded the use of viral antigens in identification and classification of arenaviruses. Nevertheless, complement fixation (CF), immunodiffusion (ID), immunofluorescence (IF), enzyme-linked immunosorbent assay (ELISA), and neutralization/plaque-reduction assays have all been instrumental in the detection, diagnosis, characterization, and classification of arenaviruses (Bro-Jorgensen 1971; Brown and Kirk 1969; Chastel 1970; Geshwender et al. 1976; Simon 1970).

CF shows a strong relationship between Tacaribe, Junin, and Machupo viruses, and distant cross-reactivities between Pichinde and Tamiami viruses (Casals 1975; Casals et al. 1975; Rawls and Buchmeier 1975). By the CF test, LCMV and Lassa viruses are related to each other, but very distantly related to the New World arenaviruses. The complement-fixing antigen is probably a portion of the nucleocapsid protein (Howard 1993; Rawls and Leung 1979).

IF with antisera raised against heterologous viral antigens afforded the first evidence that Tacaribe and LCMV are related. Serological cross-reactivities between the 'type-specific' envelope proteins have been determined by IF assays in which unfixed cells, displaying viral envelope antigens, are suspended with antisera. Cross-reactivities between 'group-specific' nucleocapsid proteins are determined from acetone-fixed cells, because the primary antigen within infected cells is NP. Serological cross-reactions in patients with Bolivian and Argentine hemorrhagic fevers are detected by IF tests with fixed cultures. Acute phase and early convalescent sera have been particularly valuable. A great deal of cross-reactivity can be seen between Machupo and Junin viruses, closely followed by Tacaribe virus (Buchmeier et al. 1977).

IF has played an important role in arenavirus diagnosis. In the case of Lassa fever virus, infected cells have been fixed to glass slides that are stable for months and can be used for field work in Africa (McCormick 1987). Infected cells on slides can be treated with UV and γ-irradiation and with acetone to ensure that they are not infectious. ELISA has also been useful for diagnosis in the field, but requires more viral antigen than the fixed-cell slides.

Cross-neutralization is the most specific test of antigen relatedness between arenaviruses. Neutralizing antibodies to Lassa appear late in convalescent sera, but are usually too specific or too weak to be detected in cross-neutralization (Peters 1984). High titer animal sera can effect cross-neutralization between Junin, Tacaribe, and Machupo viruses, but cross-neutralization has not been observed between Junin and Machupo viruses with human convalescent sera, even though these are positive in CF assays. The sensitivity of the neutralization test can be increased for LCMV by adding complement or anti-γ-globulin to the test system. The incorporation of antibodies into the overlay for a plaque assay can also be used to detect neutralizing antibodies; for example, plaque size reduction was described for Pichinde virus (Chanas et al. 1980).

With the advent of monoclonal antibodies, many useful and specific reagents against arenavirus antigens became available. Initially they were used to demonstrate the relatedness or conservation of arenavirus antigens. Panels of monoclonal antibodies against LCMV and Pichinde virus showed distinct cross-reactivities with Lassa and Mopeia viruses (Buchmeier et al. 1981). Antibodies against GP-2 and NP are more broadly cross-reactive than antibodies against GP-1, which react only against a subset of the strains. For example, one LCMV GP-2 monoclonal cross-reacted with both Old World (LCMV, Lassa, Mopeia, and Mobala) and New World (Pichinde, Junin, Tacaribe, Amapari, Parana, and Machupo) viruses (Weber and Buchmeier 1988). In a similar comparison, monoclonals raised to Lassa virus were tested against Mopeia and Mobala viruses, and GP-2 cross-reactivity once again was notable (Gonzalez et al. 1984). Cross-reactivity of NP epitopes between Lassa and Mopeia has been confirmed, along with lesser reactivity to the envelope glycoprotein (Clegg and Lloyd 1984). Broad cross-reactivities observed between epitopes on Pichinde and Old World arenaviruses demonstrate that several surface antigens are conserved between the Old World and New World arenaviruses (Buchmeier et al. 1980b).

In recent studies, monoclonal and monospecific antibodies have been invaluable in determining the molecular structure and function of arenaviruses. For example, nucleic acid sequences have been confirmed to encode proteins by the use of peptide-specific antisera (Southern et al. 1987; Salvato et al. 1989), neutralizing antisera have been used to identify the viral structural proteins involved in neutralization (Burns and Buchmeier 1993, Martinez Peralta et al. 1993).

CLINICAL AND PATHOLOGICAL ASPECTS

CLINICAL MANIFESTATIONS

In animals

All arenaviruses establish persistent infection in the natural rodent host after virus infection in utero or within a few days of birth. Adult mice inoculated intracerebrally with LCMV develop tremor with characteristic extensor spasm of the legs and they finally go into convulsions and die (Oldstone 1987b). When adult mice are inoculated peripherally, the outcome is variable with a marked loss of body weight. Lassa virus causes a silent persistent infection in its natural reservoir *Mastomys natalensis,* in the same way that LCMV infects mice. In hamsters, LCMV causes symptoms similar to those in mice. Guinea-pigs infected with Junin virus develop hemorrhagic disease with extensive necrosis of lymphatic tissue and a late development of neurological disease (Weissenbacher et al. 1975; Molinas et al. 1978). Guanarito virus causes mortality in suckling mice and adult guinea-pigs, but not in adult mice (Tesh et al. 1994). In rhesus and cynomolgus monkeys, LCMV and Lassa virus cause fever, anorexia, severe petechial rash on the face, progressive wasting and death within about 2 weeks, with a course similar to Lassa fever in humans (Jahrling et al. 1980; Peters et al. 1987). Similar manifestations have recently been described after the intravenous inoculation of rhesus macaques with a low dose (1 000 plaque forming units) of the LCMV WE strain (Lukashevich et al. 2002). Junin and Machupo virus infections of nonhuman primates simulate the disease in humans, with fever, anorexia, weight loss, and gastrointestinal symptoms. The animals die with cachexia and severe dehydration (Eddy et al. 1975; Kastello et al. 1976; Weissenbacher et al. 1979; Avila et al. 1987).

In humans

Arenavirus infections in humans range from a febrile disease with aseptic meningitis with LCMV (Armstrong and Sweet 1939) and Tacaribe (anecdotal laboratory-acquired infection in 1976; see Martinez Paralta et al. 1993) to total collapse and death with circulatory and respiratory failure with the hemorrhagic fever viruses: Lassa fever virus (Rose 1956; Buckley et al. 1970; Frame et al. 1970), Junin virus, Argentine hemorrhagic fever (Maiztegui 1975) and Machupo virus Bolivian hemorrhagic fever (Mackenzie et al. 1964; Johnson et al. 1965), Guanarito virus Venezuelan hemorrhagic fever (Peters et al. 1974) and Sabía virus infection (Coimbra and Nassar 1994). The arenavirus hemorrhagic fevers are often severe, generalized febrile diseases with multi-organ involvement and fatality rates of about 16–30 percent in untreated hospitalized patients, characterized by tissue and pulmonary edema with prominent hypovolemic shock and acute respiratory distress syndrome (Fisher-Hoch 1993). Several of the South American arenaviruses have been found by screening rodent populations but are not associated with human disease; for example, Oliveros virus is carried by 20–30 percent of *Bolomys obscuras* in the Argentine hemorrhagic fever areas (Mills et al. 1996).

LCMV infection may be asymptomatic, mild or moderately severe with central nervous system (CNS) manifestation. Lymphocytic choriomeningitis begins with fever, malaise, weakness, myalgia, and headache associated with photophobia. Anorexia, nausea, and dizziness are common (Farmer and Janeway 1942). It has also been reported that LCMV has teratogenic capacity (Baldridge et al. 1993; Barton et al. 1995)

The onset of Lassa fever is characterized by generalized symptoms, including high fever, joint pain, back pain, and severe headache, leading on to dry cough and exudative pharyngitis. In severe cases, patients have raised hematocrit (packed cell volume), vomiting and diarrhea (Fisher-Hoch et al. 1985; Johnson et al. 1987; McCormick et al. 1987a; Walker et al. 1982a). Edema and bleeding may occur together or independently. Acute neurological manifestations ranging from unilateral or bilateral deafness to moderate or severe diffuse encephalopathy with or without seizures are common in Lassa fever. A febrile, systemic illness typically progresses in 4 days to subacute or chronic neuropsychiatric syndromes, including generalized seizures, dystonia, and memory difficulties or seizures, agitation with personality and cognitive changes (McCormick et al. 1987a; Solbrig 1993). In pregnant women, Lassa fever is severe, especially during the third trimester, and fetal/neonatal loss is 87 percent (Price et al. 1988). In children, Lassa virus infection has been associated with a 'swollen baby syndrome' consisting of widespread edema, abdominal distension, and bleeding (Monson et al. 1987).

Argentine hemorrhagic fever, Bolivian hemorrhagic fever, Venezuelan hemorrhagic fever, and the newly isolated Sabía virus infection are clinically very similar (Mackenzie et al. 1964; Johnson et al. 1965; Peters et al. 1974; Maiztegui 1975; Weissenbacher et al. 1987; Coimbra and Nassar 1994). Symptoms include malaise, high fever, severe myalgia, arthralgia, anorexia, relative bradycardia, lumbar pain, epigastric pain, abdominal tenderness, conjunctivitis and retro-orbital pain, with photophobia. In severe cases there is nausea, vomiting, diarrhea, tremor, and convulsions (Vainrub and Salas 1994). Proteinuria, microscopic hematuria with subsequent oliguria, and uremia are common. Fatal cases show hemorrhagic disorders due to vascular collapse with hypotensive shock, hypothermia, and pulmonary edema. In contrast to Lassa fever, bleeding with severe thrombocytopenia is more common in Argentine and Bolivian hemorrhagic fevers (Fisher-Hoch 1993).

EPIDEMIOLOGY

Arenaviruses are zoonotic agents maintained within rodent hosts in a chronic carrier state. The majority of the rodents associated with arenaviruses are commensals or semi-commensals, living within human dwellings or in cultivated fields. The habitat preferences of each species dictate the epidemiological patterns of the diseases they cause in humans with regard to occupational, sexual, or seasonal bias (reviewed by Childs and Peters 1993).

In the case of LCMV, vertical transmission in utero is the major mechanism of viral maintenance in *Mus musculus* at the population level. Transmission through the gastrointestinal tract is the other possibility (Montali et al. 1993; Rai et al. 1996). Rodent-to-human infections probably occur through aerosols or contact with rodent blood, droplets, and fomites. Nosocomial spread of LCMV has not been reported. A longitudinal study in the USA from 1941 to 1958 implicated LCMV infections in about 8 percent of the patients diagnosed with suspected viral meningitis, and serological studies have suggested an incidence of LCMV infection in the general population of up to 10–15 percent (Childs and Peters 1993). Most of these infections are probably mild or subclinical. Laboratory infections with LCMV are relatively common.

Human-to-human spread has been reported for Lassa fever in the community and in hospital settings (McCormick et al. 1987b), whereas only a few cases of nosocomial transmission have been reported for Bolivian hemorrhagic fever (Peters et al. 1974) and none for Argentine hemorrhagic fever virus. There have been reports suggestive of sexual transmission of Lassa and Machupo viruses from convalescing patients (Douglas et al. 1965). Aerosol spread and direct contact are the most likely routes of infection between humans. Neonates are at risk of infection through their mother's milk.

The aerosol stability of arenaviruses seems to be high. Studies with Lassa virus indicate a biological half-life of 55 min at 25°C and 30 percent relative humidity or 18 min at 25°C and 80 percent relative humidity (Stephenson et al. 1984). Arenaviruses are susceptible to heat and desiccation.

In natural primary hosts, arenaviruses can establish at least two types of chronic infections. LCMV, Junin, Machupo, and Lassa viruses can establish persistent infections resulting in long-term viremia with few signs of disease in carriers. Other arenaviruses such as Latino virus and Tamiami virus cause chronic infections without persistent viremia (Jennings et al. 1970; Webb et al. 1973). Strain and passage history of arenaviruses inoculated into experimental animals have a marked effect on lethality, tissue tropism, and development of persistent infection (Traub 1938; Dutko and Oldstone 1983). The dose of arenavirus in conjunction with the route of exposure and age of the host can have a critical effect on the type of infection that results (Webb et al. 1975).

PATHOGENESIS

In animals

Adult mice infected intracerebrally with LCMV develop an acute inflammatory leptomeningitis, and choroiditis leading to death within 6–10 days (Oldstone 1987a). When adult mice are inoculated peripherally, viremia peaks about 4–5 days after inoculation, usually causing widespread immune-mediated damage to the meninges, choroid plexus, and ependyma (Cole and Johnson 1975). LCMV is known to infect and replicate in virtually every organ examined, particularly in the spleen, liver, kidney, brain, lung, uterus, thymus, and lymph nodes (Figure 49.9). Immunopathology char-

acteristic of acute murine infection with LCMV is described in the section entitled Immune response. In newborn mice, LCMV inoculation by any route leads to persistent infection. After replication in the brain, virus enters the circulation to reach tissues, serum, and urine. The pathogenesis of Lassa virus in mice is minimal and similar to infection by LCMV, whereas Junin and Machupo viruses may cause either illness and death or may induce persistence in newborn mice (Webb et al. 1975; Sabattini et al. 1977). Junin and Machupo viruses in their natural rodent hosts, Calomys spp., cause up to 50 percent fatality of infected suckling animals. Machupo virus renders the animals sterile, causes fetal mortality, and also induces hemolytic anemia with significant splenomegaly.

Histological studies of LCMV infection in hamsters and guinea-pigs show that the virus is pantropic, with high titers of virus and little evidence of histological damage. In guinea-pigs, Lassa virus causes myocarditis, pulmonary edema, and hepatocellular damage (Walker et al. 1975; Jahrling et al. 1982). Junin virus is mainly viscerotropic in guinea-pigs without evidence of an immunopathological mechanism. The animals develop hemorrhagic disease with extensive necrosis of lymphatic tissue (Weissenbacher et al. 1975; Molinas et al. 1978). Monkeys infected with Lassa virus have mild hepatic focal necrosis, pulmonary interstitial pneumonitis with interstitial edema, and focal adrenal cortical necrosis (Walker et al. 1982a). In rhesus and cynomolgus monkeys the infection causes death in 10–15 days due to vascular collapse and shock, with mild hemorrhage into mucosal surfaces (Fisher-Hoch et al. 1987). A primate model showing similar hemorrhagic fever was developed for the hepatotropic LCMV strain WE (Lukashevich et al., 2002, 2003).

In humans

The arenavirus hemorrhagic fevers in humans are often severe, generalized febrile diseases with multi-organ involvement. The hemostatic defect in these infections is characterized by platelet dysfunction and loss of integrity of the capillary bed. This presumably causes the leakage of fluids and macromolecules into the extravascular spaces and subsequent hemoconcentration, hypoalbuminemia, and hypovolemic shock. There is no evidence for major hepatorenal failure or organ destruction by direct viral replication. Renal damage in Argentine and Bolivian hemorrhagic fevers is characterized by structural damage in the distal tubular cells and collecting ducts (Cossio et al. 1975). Lungs show large areas of intra-alveolar or bronchial hemorrhage. Microscopic examinations reveal a general alteration in endothelial cells and mild edema of the vascular walls, with capillary swelling and perivascular hemorrhage (reviewed by Fisher-Hoch 1993). Necropsy findings from a single case of Sabía virus infection show diffuse pulmonary edema and congestion with intraparenchymal hemorrhages, hepatic congestion with focal hemorrhage and necrosis, renal edema and acute tubular necrosis, splenic enlargement and congestion, and massive gastrointestinal hemorrhage (Coimbra and Nassar 1994).

The pathogenesis of CNS disease in arenavirus infections is poorly understood. Seizures, delirium, memory difficulties, and abnormal movements are the final common pathways of many metabolic changes. Failure of postmortem examinations to detect specific pathological changes in the brain of Lassa virus-infected individuals along with lower viral titers than other organs suggests that some of the neurological manifestations of these infections may not result from a direct viral effect but are due to some indirect cause (reviewed by Solbrig 1993). In 1998, Lukashevich et al. showed that Lassa virus could suppress inflammatory response in primates and in human cell cultures (Lukashevich et al. 1999). This is in contrast to guinea-pig studies (Maiztegui 1975) and in support of human studies showing that fatal infection tended to have less TNF, IP-10, and IL-8 (Mahanty et al. 2001)

IMMUNE RESPONSE

The LCMV murine model has proved to be invaluable for the study of acute and persistent infections in a natural host and has also brought to light several principles of viral immunobiology and viral immunopathology. As many of the studies on arenavirus immunology have been done in the LCMV murine model, the virus-specific immune responses in the LCMV context are summarized here.

Adult immunocompetent mice inoculated with LCMV either succumb to the disease or survive with permanent immunity. Neonatally infected mice or immunosuppressed mice inoculated with LCMV develop a life-long persistent infection. Anti-LCMV antibodies are detectable by day 4 and LCMV-specific cytotoxic T lymphocytes (CTL) peak around 7–9 days after infection (Hotchin 1971; Lehmann-Grube 1971; Bro-Jorgensen and Volkert 1974).

Protection against an acute LCMV infection is mediated almost exclusively by CD8[+] CTLs (Zinkernagel and Doherty 1979; Buchmeier et al. 1980a; Lehmann-Grube et al. 1988). The same CTLs may also cause immunopathology (Hotchin 1962; Cole et al. 1972; Doherty and Zinkernagel 1974; Zinkernagel and Doherty 1979; Leist et al. 1988). The kinetics of viral spread and the T-cell response are important factors that affect the outcome of the disease (Hotchin 1962; Buchmeier et al. 1980a). After intracerebral infection, the T-cell immune response is protective only when a large number of T cells are recruited early, while relatively few choriomeningeal cells are infected. When virus spreads rapidly

and too many choriomeningeal cells are infected, immune T cells cause extensive lysis and therefore lethal immunopathological disease (Oehen et al. 1991; Battegay et al. 1992).

During the acute LCMV infection, the H-2-restricted, LCMV-specific CD8[+] CTL response peaks at 7–9 days after infection (Marker and Volkert 1973; Zinkernagel and Doherty 1974). These responses are accompanied by and depend on high levels of *IL-2* gene transcription, IL-2 production and expression of the high affinity form of the IL-2 receptor (Kasaian and Biron 1990). A secondary stimulation of LCMV-immune mice with homologous virus results in a memory CTL response peaking earlier than in primary infections (Lehmann-Grube and Lohler 1981). The magnitude of secondary CTL response is often less than the acute response, probably because the virus is cleared so rapidly. CD8[+] cells have a functional autonomy during the immune response to LCMV infection and do not depend on the presence of the majority of CD4[+] cells to sustain either activation or proliferation in vivo (Kasaian et al. 1991).

In contrast to the fatal meningitis mediated by CD8[+] T cells, CD4[+] T cells mediate a less severe form of choriomeningitis in response to intracerebral LCMV infection. Evaluation of the immune response against LCMV in CD8-defective mice reveals a CD4[+] T cell-dependent immunopathology after intracerebral infection with LCMV and the clearance of LCMV by mechanisms independent of CD8[+] T cells (Fung-Leung et al. 1991).

Mice persistently infected with LCMV by congenital infection or neonatal inoculation do not develop a detectable CTL response and can be regarded as 'tolerant' at the level of CTLs. The characteristically subclinical persistent infections of these animals have given rise to the notion that persistence requires B-cell tolerance (Hotchin 1971). However, these mice are not completely tolerant to LCMV, because they make antibodies to all the LCMV structural proteins (Oldstone and Dixon 1967; Buchmeier et al. 1978).

LCMV infection in the mouse has been important for the study of CD8[+] T cells because it induces a large T-cell response that can be identified using ex vivo cytolytic assays and, more recently, Elispot and Tetramer assays, to confirm the size and specificity of the early expansion of T-cell populations. Tetrameric peptide–MHC-class-I complexes (tetramers) allow antigen-specific T cells to be tracked in time and space, as well as a detailed analysis of their surface phenotype (Altman et al. 1996).

Of all the potential peptides, one dominant epitope elicits a response up to 30 percent of the CD8[+] T cells in the spleen with little evidence of bystander activation (Klenerman et al. 2002). In several strains different epitopes have been identified with similarly dominant T-cell responses (Murali-Krishna et al. 1998; Gallimore et al. 1998).

The response of T cells to antigen during LCMV infection in the mouse seems to follow a bell-shaped curve with increasing antigen leading to increased T-cell activation. In conditions of extreme or prolonged antigenic stimulation, tetramer-positive T cells lose their function and then decline in number. This situation is reversible and cells recover if antigen load decreases. Lack of help, lack of costimulation and other factors might contribute to T-cell deletion as well (Ou et al. 2001).

In Lassa fever there is a substantial macrophage response, with little if any lymphocytic infiltrate. The antibodies directed against the glycoprotein and nucleocapsid protein appear early in the illness in Lassa fever, with a classic primary IgG and IgM response. The antibodies are present simultaneously with viremia in humans and primates (Fisher-Hoch et al. 1987; Johnson et al. 1987). Thus, though the antibodies are markers of acute illness, they are not involved in recovery. Neutralizing antibodies are found in only a minority of patients several months after the clearance of virus (Jahrling et al. 1980; Jahrling and Peters 1984). Thus, clearance of virus presumably depends on cell-mediated immunity. In contrast, IgG antibodies to Junin and Machupo viruses appear 12–30 days after onset and are usually associated with clinical improvement and virus clearance, and the therapeutic efficacy of immune plasma in patients with Junin infection is directly associated with the titer of neutralizing antibodies in the donor plasma (Peters et al. 1973; Enria et al. 1984). The role of cell-mediated immunity in viral clearance and subsequent protection from Junin and Machupo virus infections is not known.

IMMUNOPATHOLOGY

Efficient cell-mediated immunity is crucial for the recovery of a host from acute LCMV infection (Zinkernagel and Doherty 1979; Buchmeier et al. 1980a). In infections with a noncytopathic virus such as LCMV, the balance between the virus spread and the T-cell immune response determines whether either virus elimination (protection) or cell and tissue damage (immunopathology) predominates or whether a virus carrier state (no virus elimination, no cell and tissue damage) results. Acute LCM disease, chronic LCM-wasting disease and LCM carrier status in mice (Hotchin 1962; Zinkernagel and Doherty 1979; Buchmeier et al. 1980a) are examples of these varying equilibrium conditions between virus and immune response.

Effectors of immunopathology

Intraperitoneal or intravenous infection of adult mice with LCMV usually results in a virus-specific CTL response that clears the virus with long-lasting immunity, whereas intracerebral inoculation results in a lethal leptomeningitis associated with virus replication in the brain and an intense mononuclear cell infiltrate. Death and the associated meningitis are blocked if the mice are treated with thymectomy, immunosuppressive irradiation or immunosuppressive drugs such as cyclophosphamide; this led to the suggestion that the disease is mediated by the immune response (Haas and Stewart 1956; Rowe et al. 1963; Gilden et al. 1972). Subsequent investigations have supported the hypothesis that the pathology in acute LCMV disease is mediated by cellular immunity (Volkert and Lundstedt 1968; Cole et al. 1972; Gilden et al. 1972).

Interferon (IFN) increases the susceptibility of LCMV-infected fibroblasts to lysis by H-2-restricted CTLs (Bukowski and Welsh 1985). This enhanced lysis correlates with increased cell surface expression of MHC antigens but not of LCMV antigen. IFN-γ is an especially potent inducer of MHC expression in most cell types (Wong et al. 1984). This indicates that the limiting component in the lytic interaction is the histocompatibility antigen and that physiological influences on the expression of antigen may affect the progress of host-mediated disease. Treatment of adult mice infected intracerebrally with LCMV with antibody to IFN prevents their death, whereas untreated control mice succumb to the same dose of lethal LCMV, thus showing the role of IFN in the pathogenesis of cell damage in murine LCM (Pfau et al. 1983). The promyelocytic leukemia protein (PML) is a mediator of arenavirus sensitivity to IFN (Djavani et al. 2001a; Bonilla et al. 2002).

Murine LCMV infection is also considered the classic example of virus-induced immune complex disease. Persistent LCMV infection with circulating non-neutralizing antibodies in ratios and quantities that favor binding of complement and deposition in tissues results in immunopathology. This state is affected by host and viral genetic factors (Oldstone et al. 1983). Large quantities of deposited immune complexes along with IFN-γ seem to cause development of glomerulonephritis (Walker and Murphy 1987). Strains of mice characterized as intermediate IFN responders, such as outbred Swiss mice, have higher levels of circulating immune complexes and develop much more severe immune complex-associated glomerulonephritis than strains of low IFN responder mice, such as BALB/c mice, after LCMV infection (Woodrow et al. 1982). Antibodies to IFN diminish glomerular damage without affecting levels of circulating immune complexes (Pfau et al. 1983).

Progress of central nervous system pathology

CD8[+] T cells along with macrophages are thought to be the main cells that contribute to meningeal inflammation after LCMV infection (Allan et al. 1987). In addition, natural killer (NK) cells, CD4$^+$ T cells, neutrophils, and B cells are also present at the site of inflammation (Johnson et al. 1978). Large numbers of white blood cells, including CTLs, NK cells, and macrophages, are found in the cerebrospinal fluid (CSF), brain tissue, and meningeal exudate. Although the integrity of the blood–brain barrier is destroyed, the relatively non-lytic LCMV itself is unlikely to disrupt the barrier (Doherty 1973; Doherty and Zinkernagel 1974). It is more likely that the virus-induced IFN-γ initiates the infiltration of inflammatory cells across the blood–brain barrier.

The presence of CTLs in CSF has been shown by functional studies and by immunocytochemistry (Zinkernagel and Doherty 1973). CTL activity is also present in the CSF 3 days after immune-cell transfer to LCMV-infected, immunosuppressed animals. After CNS infection with LCMV, high levels of NK-cell activity are detected in CSF and cervical lymph nodes. However, meningitis presumably does not occur before development of T cell response, as NK cells probably do not play an essential role in LCMV-induced immunopathology (Allan and Doherty 1986). NK cells do not influence LCMV synthesis in vivo, but do decrease the level of Pichinde virus (Welsh 1987; Brutkiewicz and Welsh 1995).

The CTLs present in cyclophosphamide-suppressed LCMV-infected mice after passive transfer of immune cells are of donor and not of recipient origin. So CD8$^+$ T cells also seem to be essential for triggering infiltration into the CNS. Presumably, for a maximal inflammatory process to occur, MHC class I-restricted CD8$^+$ T cells proliferate first in the peripheral lymphoid tissue and then enter the brain after recognition of MHC class I-compatible infected cells at the blood–CSF barrier (reviewed by Allan et al. 1987).

Immunosuppressed mice that survive an ordinarily lethal dose of LCMV develop acute LCM disease and die when reconstituted with syngeneic LCMV-specific immune T cells (Gilden et al. 1972). Thus, it is possible to imitate the immunopathology observed in acute LCMV infection by inoculating LCMV-specific H-2-restricted CTLs into carrier mice, which in turn cause either viral clearance and recovery or CTL-mediated immunopathology and death (Allan and Doherty 1985). CD8$^+$ T cells act directly rather than by the recruitment of circulating monocytes. Lethal LCM can be prevented in the uninfected mouse by intracerebral inoculation of cloned CD8$^+$ T cells together with the virus (Baenziger et al. 1986). The co-injected CD8$^+$ T cells gradually eliminate virus-infected cells without causing the massive inflammation associated with acute LCM disease. Severe meningitis ensues in adoptive transfer of LCMV-specific CTLs only when there is matching of MHC class I antigens between donor and recipient mice. In comparison, compatibility of MHC class II antigens is less important (Doherty et al. 1976; Allan and Doherty 1985).

Immunosuppression

MECHANISM OF IMMUNOSUPPRESSION

Acute infection of adult mice with LCMV leads to a general suppression of the immunological and mitogenic responses in vivo and in vitro, which persists for 2–3 months after infection (Mims and Wainwright 1968; Bro-Jorgensen and Volkert 1972; Jacobs and Cole 1976; Brenan and Zinkernagel 1983). Although different mechanisms have been postulated to explain this phenomenon, it is still poorly defined. LCMV infects different types of lymphocytes (Gartner et al. 1986; Rosenthal et al. 1986; Ahmed et al. 1987b) and macrophages (Mims and Subrahmanyan 1966; Zinkernagel and Doherty 1979). The ability of LCMV to induce a virus carrier state conatally or neonatally and in adult mice may be due to these particular tropisms of LCMV (Ahmed et al. 1987b). Depending on the virus isolate, the virus dose, the time after infection, and the mouse strain infected, LCMV can cause a severe immune deficiency, rendering the mice more susceptible to secondary infections.

Mice persistently infected with LCMV are deficient in generating LCMV-specific CTLs and delayed type hypersensitivity responses and also make low levels of antibodies against LCMV (Buchmeier et al. 1980a). LCMV-specific immune responses are inhibited by a lack of appropriate T-helper cells, because although deletion of CD4$^+$ T cells in a transgenic mouse model does not impair the primary CD8$^+$ LCMV-specific CTL response (Rahemtulla et al. 1991) it does impair T-cell memory (Matloubian et al. 1994). The different levels of cytokines in the brain and sera of acutely and persistently infected mice indicate that the two types of infections probably activate different types of cells.

A mechanism for generalized immunosuppression has been elucidated in the case of a particular LCMV isolate. For this isolate, LCMV Armstrong clone 13 (Ahmed et al. 1984), virus replicates to high titer in the spleen, causing immune-mediated destruction of dendritic cells; hence loss of the cells needed for immune responses to other pathogens (Tishon et al. 1993; Borrow et al. 1995). Clonal deletion of LCMV-specific CTLs may occur subsequently (Moskophidis et al. 1993). The long-term effect of clone 13 infection is that reduced immune response capacity allows the virus to persist, in contrast to infection with other isolates of this strain that are cleared within weeks by a vigorous cellular immune response (Salvato et al. 1991). The persistent and rapidly cleared isolates of LCMV Armstrong are analogous to the Docile (viscerotropic) and Aggressive (neurotropic) isolates of LCMV UBC in which docility is associated with the tendency for high titer replication in the viscera that leads to suppression of the CTL response and persistent infection (Thomsen and Pfau 1993). It is important to note that viral tropism is crucial to the pathogenesis in these cases. The different tropisms of LCMV Armstrong and its variant isolate, clone 13, are shown in Figure 49.10.

Suppression of cell-mediated immunity

LCMV infection causes suppression of responses to T-dependent antigens in vivo (Mims and Wainwright 1968) and to allografts (Lehmann-Grube et al. 1972; Guttler et al. 1975). This may be due to a decreased number of mature T lymphocytes in lymphoid organs as a result of an alteration of T-progenitor cells in the bone marrow (Bro-Jorgensen and Volkert 1972; Thomsen et al. 1982). Alternatively, it is suggested that the immunosuppression may be related to the lysis of infected T lymphocytes and macrophages by virus-specific CTLs (Silberman et al. 1978). In addition to unresponsiveness to antigens, the proliferative response to T- and B-cell mitogens is also depressed and a virus-induced macrophage defect is probably responsible for the abortive collaboration with T lymphocytes (Jacobs and Cole 1976).

Suppression of humoral immunity

The suppression of T-independent IgM and a strictly T help-dependent IgG immune response against a second infectious agent is observed in immunocompetent adult mice infected with LCMV but not in tolerant LCMV carrier mice or LCMV-infected mice that have been depleted of CD8[+] T cells with monoclonal antibodies. Thus, the immune suppression is due not to LCMV itself nor to IFN induced by it but rather to the CD8[+] T cell-dependent immune response against LCMV (Leist et al. 1988).

Studies of the kinetics of T cell-mediated immunosuppressive effects of LCMV infection on primary and secondary antibody responses (to Vesicular stomatitis virus (VSV)) show that LCMV-WE induced immunosuppression is absolute for primary IgG responses induced during a limited time between days 2 and 11 after LCMV infection. The kinetics of induction of the T cell-independent IgM responses closely follow that of a normal CTL response to LCMV-WE (Roost et al. 1988). LCMV infection on the same day or before (but not after) VSV infection leads to suppression of IgG responses to VSV. However, primed IgG responses are not suppressed by a subsequent LCMV-WE infection and immunosuppression is not antigen specific but general (Ruedi et al. 1990). LCMV-induced suppression is absolute to the extent that priming does not occur, since subsequent challenge with the identical VSV serotype triggers a strictly primary response.

The severity and duration of immunosuppressiveness depend on the virus dose, the virus isolate, and the mouse strain used. LCMV-WE and LCMV Docile are the most and LCMV Armstrong the least immunosuppressive. Mouse strains differ considerably with respect to extent of suppression, depending on both the MHC and non-MHC genes. H-2q and H-2k mice seem to be more susceptible to immune suppression than H-2b or H-2d mice (Roost et al. 1988).

DIAGNOSIS

Diagnosis of arenavirus infection relies mainly on isolation and subsequent identification of the virus. Serological tests can also be used to detect specific antibodies or antigens.

Virus can be isolated mainly from the blood or serum. In addition, throat swabs, CSF, urine, breast milk, or other tissues taken by biopsy or at necropsy can also be used (Monath et al. 1974; Walker et al. 1982b; Johnson et al. 1987). The most successful system for isolating arenaviruses has proved to be cell culture. In addition to cell culture, laboratory animals such as suckling mice, guinea-pigs, and hamsters can also be used, although they are more expensive and increased safety precautions are necessary. The probability and timing of virus isolation vary with each arenavirus (Table 49.2).

Differential diagnosis for arenavirus infections, especially for Lassa fever, includes bacterial septicemia, typhoid, paratyphoid, typhus, trypanosomiasis,

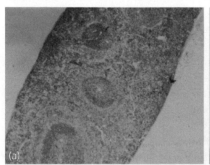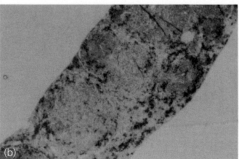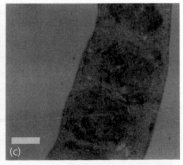

Figure 49.10 *Localization of LCMV nucleic acids in murine spleen by in situ hybridization with* [35]*S riboprobe specific for NP mRNA.* **(a)** *Spleen section from an uninfected control mouse (BALB/c ByJ).* **(b)** *Spleen section from a mouse infected IV with LCMV Armstrong for 3 days.* **(c)** *Spleen section from a mouse infected IV with the clone 13 variant of LCMV Armstrong for 3 days. (Reproduced from Borrow et al. 1995.)*

Table 49.2 *Arenavirus isolation from tissue specimens at different stages of illness*

Virus	Tissue specimen	Stage of illness
LCMV	Blood	Initial febrile stage
	CSF	During acute illness
Junin	Blood	Up to 8 days in milder cases, up to 2 weeks in severely ill patients
	Throat swab	During acute illness
	Breast milk	During acute illness
Machupo	Blood	Up to 2 weeks (intermittent viremia)
	Throat swabs	Sporadic detection
Lassa	Blood	3–5 days in milder cases, up to 4 weeks in severely ill patients
	Throat swabs	Days 5–12 of illness
	Breast milk	During acute illness
	CSF	During acute illness
	Pleural transudate	During acute illness
	Pericardial transudate	During acute illness
	Urine	Up to 1– 2 months

Data adapted from McCormick (1990).

streptococcal pharyngitis, leptospirosis, malignant malaria, and other viral hemorrhagic fevers (Howard and Simpson 1990). Nucleic acid amplification by RT-PCR along with Southern blot hybridization with virus-specific DNA probe can be used as an early, rapid, and sensitive method for detecting arenavirus nucleic acid in peripheral blood mononuclear cells (PBMC) as well as from other tissues. Studies with Junin virus-infected PBMCs and tissues have shown that this assay allows detection of Junin virus RNA in RNA extracted from 100 μl of whole blood by guanidinium thiocyanate disruption and acid phenol extraction. As little as 0.01 pfu of Junin virus can be detected in a blood sample by this assay (Bockstahler et al. 1992; Lozano et al. 1993). In situ hybridization by viral sequence-specific radioactive probes can be done directly on biopsy or autopsy specimens to detect viral RNA and has proved to be highly sensitive in experimental LCMV infections of mice (see Figure 49.9).

Antibodies to arenaviruses can be detected in serum by a variety of serological methods, including IF assay, ELISA, immunoperoxidase labeling, radioimmunoassay, reverse phase hemagglutination assay, and hemagglutination inhibition tests. The complement fixation test is now rarely used because it is less sensitive than other methods (serological tests and antibody levels in arenavirus infections have been reviewed by McCormick 1990). IF is often used in serological diagnoses to detect arenavirus antigens in cell monolayers that have been exposed to suspect sera. At present, ELISA is increasingly used for the diagnosis of arenavirus infections. Alternatively, known antiserum or monoclonal antibodies can be used to detect viral antigens in biopsy or necropsy materials by immunohistochemical techniques.

PROPHYLAXIS

The development of a safe and effective vaccine for arenavirus infections of humans has proved difficult.

Several killed and live-attenuated vaccines have been tested for Lassa, Junin, and Machupo viruses, none of which has proved suitable for widespread human use. Many of these vaccines are still in the stage of animal trials. A new live-attenuated Junin virus vaccine, Candid:1, has been developed which has been shown to be safe and immunogenic in nonhuman primates (Barrera Oro and McKee 1991; Contigiani et al. 1991; McKee et al. 1993). Laboratory animals infected with various avirulent viruses serologically related to Lassa virus, including LCMV, Mopeia, and Mobala viruses, survived a subsequent challenge with virulent Lassa virus (Walker et al. 1982a; Jahrling and Peters 1986). Similar strategies for protection against Junin virus with heterologous live vaccines have repeatedly demonstrated protection against Junin virus in guinea-pigs and hamsters (reviewed by Barrera Oro and McKee 1991). Other vaccine trials with inactivated Lassa and Machupo viruses have given mixed results, although they are immunogenic. Immunization with inactivated Lassa virus protects *Papio hamadryas* monkeys from a subsequent challenge with Lassa virus (Krasnianski et al. 1993), but fails to protect rhesus monkeys even though there is a secondary, high titer antibody response to the major structural proteins of Lassa virus in these vaccinated monkeys (McCormick et al. 1992).

For Lassa virus, a killed antigen vaccine has proved ineffective and an attenuated virus vaccine is not available, so a live recombinant virus vaccine provides a very attractive alternative. Recombinant vaccinia virus vaccines, which express either the Lassa virus nucleoprotein or the glycoprotein gene, successfully protect guinea pigs from a lethal Lassa virus infection, but offer incomplete protection in primates (Auperin et al. 1988; Morrison et al. 1989; Auperin 1993). Fisher-Hoch et al. (2000) have tested a variety of Lassa vaccines delivered to nonhuman primates via the NYBH vaccinia vector. In this study, the authors described the outcome after the vaccination of 44 monkeys with Mopeia or with vaccinia expressing Lassa S segment genes (*G1*, *G2*, *N*, *G1+G2* or combinations of them). A third of the monkeys were Cynomolgus macaques and the remainder were rhesus and all of them were challenged with a lethal dose (10^5 pfu) of Lassa (Josiah strain). The data indicate that vaccines delivering all genes of the Lassa S RNA (both *N* and *G*) are more protective than vaccines with only the glycoprotein genes and, later, these are more protective than vaccines with only the *N* gene. From these experiments it is apparently clear that animals with high titers of neutralizing antibodies are not protected whereas others that survived did not show high levels of neutralizing antibodies, this finding supports the need for cellular immune response to protect against the Lassa challenge (Fisher-Hoch et al. 2000). A weak but measurable cross-protection against LCMV intracranial challenge can be mediated by Lassa-specific CD4$^+$ T cells (La Posta et al. 1993; Djavani et al. 2000, 2001b). Vaccine trials so far have suggested that cell-mediated immune response must be activated to protect against challenge with arenaviruses.

Immunization with recombinant vaccinia virus that expresses the LCMV glycoprotein (VV GP) or nucleoprotein (VV NP) protects mice from LCM disease by induction of a protective CTL response in an H-2 haplotype-dependent manner (Hany and Oehen 1989; Klavinskis et al. 1990; Oehen et al. 1991). Mice can be specifically protected by subcutaneous inoculation of recombinant LCMV proteins (GP or NP) or just the T-cell epitope of the LCMV nucleoprotein as an unmodified free synthetic peptide in incomplete Freund's adjuvant (Schulz et al. 1991; Bachmann et al. 1994). Vaccination with DNA encoding the LCMV nucleoprotein or the glycoprotein also confers protection against lethal LCMV challenge and against persistent LCMV infection in an MHC-dependent manner by priming CD8$^+$ cytotoxic lymphocytes (Martins et al. 1995; Yokoyama et al. 1995).

In certain circumstances however, immunization with VV GP or VV NP aggravates disease. For example, BALB/C mice infected with a high dose of the LCMV Docile isolate usually survive, unless they are pre-injected with VV NP or VV GP (Oehen et al. 1991). This suggests that low level immunization may accelerate development of disease. Vaccination may shift the balance from low (i.e. late) to high (i.e. early) responder status and may therefore prevent immunopathologically mediated disease, or it may shift the balance only slightly from a nonresponsive asymptomatic carrier to a low or intermediate responder status to cause immunopathology. Thus, as well as illustrating the potential value of CTL vaccines, these vaccine studies also highlight the limitations of subunit vaccines. To protect an outbred population in an MHC-restricted fashion, it will be necessary to make a vaccine that consists of a cocktail of relevant peptides and to ensure that none of its components aggravates the disease in a subsequent virus challenge.

TREATMENT

Immunotherapy

LCMV-induced persistent infection in mice is a classic example of viral persistence and serves as a model to study basic principles of immune clearance in persistent and disseminated infections in general. This model system makes it possible to test the potential of specific immune therapy to clear virus from a chronically infected host and to study the effector mechanisms responsible for clearing such infections.

Volkert (1963) was the first to show that the adoptive transfer of spleen cells from LCMV-challenged immune adult mice results in reduction of infectious virus in carrier mice. This has been confirmed by a number of workers (Gilden et al. 1972; Allan and Doherty 1985; Baenziger et al. 1986). Distinct patterns of viral clearance and histopathology are observed in different organs after adaptive immunotherapy of persistently infected (carrier) mice. The clearance of viral materials from the CNS is distinct in pattern and timing with clearance from other organs. Clearance from the liver, lung, spleen, lymph nodes, pancreas etc. occurs within 30 days, whereas in the brain, infectious virus is eliminated but viral antigen persists up to 90 days after immunotherapy (Ahmed et al. 1987a). The urinary system is the most resistant to immunotherapy, and the viral antigen is localized within the renal tubules in the form of antigen–antibody complexes (Oldstone and Dixon 1967).

Clearance of viral materials (infectious virus, viral nucleic acid and proteins) from several organs of persistently infected mice probably occurs by reconstitution of LCMV-specific CTLs that have malfunctioned or have been deleted during viral infection. By using mice that are recombinant in the H-2 region and by selective depletion of lymphocyte subpopulations, it has been shown that viral clearance is mediated by cooperation between virus-specific CD8$^+$ T cells and nonspecific bone marrow-derived mononuclear cells from the carrier host (Ahmed et al. 1987b). The effector mechanisms responsible for eliminating the persistent and disseminated LCMV infection of mice are dependent on the lytic ability of CTLs, because perforin-negative transgenic mice are unable to clear infection (Kagi et al. 1994).

Early success of Lassa virus immune plasma in the treatment of Lassa fever (Leifer et al. 1970) and immunotherapy of Machupo virus infections in primates (Eddy et al. 1975) showed promise for the treatment of arenavirus infections in humans. Convalescent phase plasma from Junin virus patients reduced mortality from 16 to 1 percent in those who were treated in the first 8 days of illness (Maiztegui et al. 1979), and the efficacy of the plasma seemed to be directly related to the concentration of neutralizing antibodies of the plasma. However, a better understanding of the limitations of this approach and reduced success in subsequent cases have restricted its use. A late neurological syndrome developed 4–6 weeks after the onset of acute illness in about 10 percent of the cases treated with Junin virus immune plasma. Passive antibody therapy depends on collection of plasma from people known to have had the disease, testing the plasma or screening the donor for antibodies to bloodborne agents such as hepatitis, and proper storage of plasma until it is used. In addition, the existence of HIV and other retroviral diseases transmissible by blood products has made the further screening of plasma mandatory before use. A study of combined antibody and ribavirin therapy has been performed in the mouse model (Seiler et al. 2000).

Antiviral agents

The antiviral drug ribavirin has proved effective in the treatment of Lassa fever in laboratory animals (Jahrling et al. 1980; Jahrling et al. 1984) and in humans (McCormick et al. 1986), especially when administered during the first 6 days after the onset of illness. Later, the pathogenesis of the infection is less reversible. Patients presenting late in disease require more effective clinical management of physiological dysfunction and need other drugs which may be used to stabilize the state of shock sufficiently long to facilitate recovery and survival. Ribavirin is perhaps more effective if given intravenously than orally (McCormick et al. 1986; McCormick 1990). It is the drug of choice for treatment and for prophylaxis in cases of possible exposure to Lassa virus, in laboratory or hospitals. Studies with Junin virus infections indicate that ribavirin may also have beneficial effect in Argentine hemorrhagic fever (Enria and Maiztegui 1994). A single case of laboratory-acquired Sabía virus infection was successfully treated with intravenous ribavirin (Barry et al. 1995) at a dosage recommended by the Centers for Disease Control and Prevention (CDC) for other arenavirus infections (a loading dose of 30 mg/kg body weight, followed by a dose of 15 mg/kg every 6 h for 4 days, and then by a dose of 7.5 mg/kg 3 times daily for 6 days).

In addition, fluid, electrolyte, and osmotic imbalances must be corrected in anticipation of the development of clinical shock and broad spectrum antibiotics administered to prevent secondary bacterial infections. However, even vigorous support of this kind may be insufficient to prevent fatal progression of disease.

REFERENCES

Ahmed, R., Jamieson, B.D. and Porter, D.D. 1987a. Immune therapy of a persistent and disseminated viral infection. *J Virol*, **61**, 3920–9.

Ahmed, R., King, C.-C. and Oldstone, M.B.A. 1987b. Virus-lymphocyte interaction: T cells of the helper subset are infected with lymphocytic choriomeningitis virus during persistent infection *in vivo. J Virol*, **61**, 1571–6.

Ahmed, R.A., Salmi, A., et al. 1984. Selection of genetic variants of lymphocytic choriomeningitis virus in spleens of persistently infected mice: role in suppression of cytotoxic T lymphocyte response and viral persistence. *J Exp Med*, **160**, 521–40.

Allan, J.E. and Doherty, P.C. 1985. Consequences of cyclophosphamide treatment in murine lymphocytic choriomeningitis: evidence for cytotoxic T cell replication in vivo. *Scand J Immunol*, **22**, 367–74.

Allan, J.E. and Doherty, P.C. 1986. Natural killer cells contribute to inflammation but do not appear to be essential for the induction of clinical lymphocytic choriomeningitis. *Scand J Immunol*, **24**, 153–62.

Allan, J.E., Dixon, J.E. and Doherty, P.C. 1987. Nature of the inflammatory process in the central nervous system of mice infected with LCMV. *Curr Top Microbiol Immunol*, **134**, 131–43.

Altman, J., Moss, P.A., et al. 1996. Direct visualization and phenotypic analysis of virus-specific T lymphocytes in HIV-infected individuals. *Science*, **274**, 94–6.

Armstrong, C. and Lillie, R.D. 1934. Experimental lymphocytic choriomeningitis of monkeys and mice produced by a virus encountered in studies of the 1993 St Louis encephalitis epidemic. *Pub Health Rep (Washington)*, **49**, 1019–27.

Armstrong, C. and Sweet, L.K. 1939. Lymphocytic choriomeningitis. *Pub Health Rep (Washington)*, **54**, 673–84.

Auperin, D.D. 1993. Construction and evaluation of recombinant virus vaccines for Lassa fever. In: Salvato, M.S. (ed.), *The Arenaviridae*. New York: Plenum Press, 259–80.

Auperin, D.D., Romanowski, V., et al. 1984. Sequence studies of Pichinde arenavirus S RNA indicate a novel coding strategy, ambisense viral S RNA. *J Virol*, **52**, 897–904.

Auperin, D.D., Sasso, D.R. and McCormick, J.B. 1986. Nucleotide sequence of the glycoprotein gene and intergenic region of the Lassa virus S genome RNA. *Virology*, **154**, 155–67.

Auperin, D.D., Esposito, J.J. and Lange, J.V. 1988. Construction of a recombinant vaccinia virus expressing the Lassa virus glycoprotein gene and protection of guinea pigs from a lethal Lassa virus infection. *Virus Res*, **9**, 233–43.

Auperin, D.D. and McCormick, J.B. 1989. Nucleotide sequence of the Lassa virus (Josiah strain) S genome RNA and amino acid sequence comparison of the N and GPC proteins to other arenaviruses. *Virology*, **156**, 421–5.

Avila, M.M., Samailovich, S.R., et al. 1987. Protection of Junin virus infected marmosets by passive administration of immune serum: association with late neurologic signs. *J Med Virol*, **21**, 67–74.

Bachmann, M.F., Kundig, T.M., et al. 1994. Induction of protective cytotoxic T cells with viral proteins. *Eur J Immunol*, **24**, 2228–36.

Baenziger, J., Hengartner, H., et al. 1986. Induction or prevention of immunopathological disease by cloned cytotoxic T cell lines specific for LCMV. *Eur J Immunol*, **16**, 387–93.

Banerjee, S.N., Buchmeier, M. and Rawls, W.E. 1976. Requirement of a cell nucleus for the replication of an arenavirus. *Intervirology*, **6**, 190–6.

Baldridge, J.R., Pearce, B.D., et al. 1993. Teratogenic effects of neonatal arenavirus infection on the developing rat cerebellum are abrogated by passive immunotherapy. *Virology*, **197**, 669–77.

Barton, L.L., Peters, C.J. and Ksiazek, T.G. 1995. Lymphocytic choriomeningitis virus: an unrecognized teratogenic pathogen. *Emerg Infect Dis*, **1**, 152–3.

Barrera Oro, J.G. and McKee, K.T. Jr 1991. Toward a vaccine against Argentine hemorrhagic fever. *Bull Pan Am Hlth Org*, **25**, 118–26.

Barry, M., Russi, M., et al. 1995. Brief report: treatment of a laboratory-acquired Sabía virus infection. *N Engl J Med*, **333**, 294–6.

Battegay, M., Oehen, S., et al. 1992. Vaccination with a synthetic peptide modulates LCMV-mediated immunopathology. *J Virol*, **66**, 1199–201.

Bishop, D.H.L. 1990. *Arenaviridae* and their replication. In: Fields, B.N. and Knipe, D.M. (eds), *Fields' virology*. New York: Raven Press, 1231–43.

Bockstahler, L.E., Carney, P.G., et al. 1992. Detection of Junin virus by the polymerase chain reaction. *J Virol Methods*, **39**, 231–5.

Bonilla, W.V., Pinschewer, D.D., et al. 2002. Effects of promyelocytic leukemia protein on virus-host balance. *J Virol*, **76**, 3810–18.

Borden, K.L., Campbell Dwyer, E.J. and Salvato, M.S. 1998a. An arenavirus RING (zinc-binding) protein binds the oncoprotein promyelocyte leukemia protein (PML) and relocates PML nuclear bodies to the cytoplasm. *J Virol*, **72**, 758–66.

Borden, K.L., Campbell Dwyer, E.J., et al. 1998b. Two RING finger proteins, the oncoprotein PML and the arenavirus Z protein, colocalize with the nuclear fraction of the ribosomal P proteins. *J Virol*, **72**, 3819–26.

Borden, K.L., Campbell Dwyer, E.J. and Salvato, M.S. 1997. The promyelocytic leukemia protein PML has a pro-apoptotic activity mediated through its RING domain. *FEBS Lett*, **418**, 30–4.

Borrow, P. and Oldstone, M.B.A. 1992. Characterization of lymphocytic choriomeningitis virus-binding receptor protein(s): a candidate cellular receptor of the virus. *J Virol*, **66**, 7270–81.

Borrow, P. and Oldstone, M.B.A. 1994. Mechanism of lymphocytic choriomeningitis virus entry into cells. *Virology*, **198**, 1–9.

Borrow, P., Tishon, A. and Oldstone, M.B.A. 1991. Infection of lymphocytes by a virus that aborts cytotoxic T lymphocyte activity and establishes persistent infection. *J Exp Med*, **174**, 203–12.

Borrow, P., Evans, C.F. and Oldstone, M.B.A. 1995. Virus-induced immunosuppression: immune system-mediated destruction of virus-infected dendritic cells results in generalized immunosuppression. *J Virol*, **69**, 1059–70.

Bowen, M.D., Peters, C.J., et al. 1996. Oliveros virus: a novel arenavirus from Argentina. *Virology*, **217**, 362–6.

Bowen, M.D., Rollin, P.E., et al. 2000. Genetic diversity among Lassa virus strains. *J Virol*, **74**, 6992–7004.

Brenan, M. and Zinkernagel, R.M. 1983. Influence of one virus infection on a second concurrent primary in vivo antiviral cytotoxic T cell response. *Infect Immun*, **41**, 470–5.

Bro-Jorgensen, K. 1971. Characterization of virus specific antigen in cell culture infected with lymphocytic choriomeningitis virus. *Acta Pathol Microbiol Scand (B) Microbiol Immunol*, **79**, 466–74.

Bro-Jorgensen, K. and Volkert, M. 1972. Haemopoietic defects in mice infected with lymphocytic choriomeningitis virus. *Acta Pathol Microbiol Scand*, **80**, 853–62.

Bro-Jorgensen, K. and Volkert, M. 1974. Defects in the immune system of mice infected with LCMV. *Infect Immun*, **9**, 605–14.

Brown, W.J. and Kirk, B.I. 1969. Complement fixing antigen from BHK-21 cell cultures infected with lymphocytic choriomeningitis virus. *Appl Microbiol*, **18**, 496–9.

Bruns, M., Zeller, W., et al. 1986. Lymphocytic choriomeningitis virus. 9. Properties of the nucleocapsid. *Virology*, **151**, 77–85.

Brutkiewicz, R.R. and Welsh, R.M. 1995. Major histocompatibility complex class I antigens and the control of viral infections by natural killer cells. *J Virol*, **69**, 3967–71.

Buchmeier, M.J. 2002. Arenaviruses: protein structure and function. *CTMI*, **262**, 159–74.

Buchmeier, M.J. and Oldstone, M.B.A. 1979. Protein structure of lymphocytic choriomeningitis virus: evidence for a cell-associated precursor of the virion glycopeptides. *Virology*, **99**, 111–20.

Buchmeier, M.J., Gee, S.R., et al. 1977. Antigens of Pichinde virus I. Relationship of soluble antigens derived from infected BHK-21 cells to the structural components of the virion. *J Virol*, **22**, 175–86.

Buchmeier, M.J., Elder, J.H. and Oldstone, M.B.A. 1978. Protein structure of lymphocytic choriomeningitis virus: identification of the virus structural and cell-associated polypeptides. *Virology*, **89**, 133–45.

Buchmeier, M.J., Welsh, R.M., et al. 1980a. The virology and immunobiology of lymphocytic choriomeningitis virus infection. *Adv Immunol*, **30**, 275–331.

Buchmeier, M.J., Lewicki, H.A., et al. 1980b. Monoclonal antibodies to lymphocytic choriomeningitis virus react with pathogenic arenaviruses. *Nature (London)*, **288**, 486–7.

Buchmeier, M.J., Lewicki, H.A., et al. 1981. Monoclonal antibodies to lymphocytic choriomeningitis and Pichinde virus: generation, characterization, and cross-reactivity with other arenaviruses. *Virology*, **113**, 73–85.

Buchmeier, M.J., Bowen, M.D. and Peters, C.J. 2001. Arenaviridae: the viruses and their replication. In: Knipe, D.M. and Howley, P.M. (eds), *Fields' virology*, 4th edn. Philadelphia: Lippincott Williams and Wilkins, 1635–68.

Buckley, S.M., Casals, J. and Downs, W.G. 1970. Isolation and antigenic characterization of Lassa virus. *Nature (London)*, **227**, 174–6.

Bukowski, J.F. and Welsh, R.M. 1985. Inability of interferon to protect virus-infected cells against lysis by natural killer (NK) cells correlates with NK cell-mediated antiviral effects in vivo. *J Immunol*, **135**, 3537–41.

Burns, J.W. and Buchmeier, M.J. 1991. Protein–protein interactions in lymphocytic choriomeningitis virus. *Virology*, **183**, 620–9.

Burns, J.W. and Buchmeier, M.J. 1993. Glycoproteins of the arenaviruses. In: Salvato, M.S. (ed.), *The Arenaviridae*. New York: Plenum Press, 17–35.

Campbell Dwyer, E.J., Lai, H., et al. 2000. The lymphocytic choriomeningitis virus RING protein Z associates with eukaryotic initiation factor 4E and selectively represses translation in a RING-dependent manner. *J Virol*, **74**, 3293–300.

Cao, W., Henry, M.D., et al. 1998. Identification of alpha-dystroglycan as a receptor for lymphocytic choriomeningitis virus and Lassa fever virus. *Science*, **282**, 1999–2000.

Casals, J. 1975. Arenaviruses. *Yale J Biol Med*, **48**, 115–40.

Casals, J., Buckley, S.M. and Cedeno, R. 1975. Antigenic properties of the arenaviruses. *Bull WHO*, **52**, 421–5.

Chanas, A.C., Young, P.R., et al. 1980. Evaluation of plaque size reduction as a method for the detection of Pichinde virus antibody. *Arch Virol*, **65**, 157–67.

Charrel, R.N., de Lamballerie, X., et al. 2001a. Nucleotide sequence of the pirital virus (family *Arenaviridae*) small genomic segment. *Biochem Biophys Res Commun*, **280**, 1402–7.

Charrel, R.N., de Lamballerie, X. and Fulhorst, C.F. 2001b. The Whitewater Arroyo virus: natural evidence for genetic recombination among Tacaribe serocomplex viruses (family *Arenaviridae*). *Virology*, **283**, 161–6.

Charrel, R.N., Feldmann, H., et al. 2002. Phylogeny of New World arenaviruses based on the complete coding sequences of the small genomic segment identified an evolutionary lineage produced by intra-segmental recombination. *Biochem Biophys Res Commun*, **296**, 1118–24.

Chastel, C. 1970. Immunodiffusion studies on a fluorocarbon-extracted antigen of lymphocytic choriomeningitis virus. *Acta Virol (Praha)*, **14**, 507–9.

Childs, J.E. and Peters, C.J. 1993. Ecology and epidemiology of arenaviruses and their hosts. In: Salvato, M.S. (ed.), *The arenaviridae*. New York: Plenum Press, 331–84.

Clegg, J.C.S. 1993. Molecular phylogeny of the arenaviruses and guide to published sequence data. In: Salvato, M.S. (ed.), *The Arenaviridae*. New York: Plenum Press, 175–87.

Clegg, J.C.S. 2002. Molecular phylogeny of the Arenavirus. In Oldstone, M.B.A. (ed.), *Arenavirus I, The epidemiology, molecular and cell biology of the arenaviruses, CTMI*, **262**, 1–24.

Clegg, J.C.S. and Lloyd, G. 1984. The African arenaviruses Lassa and Mopeia: biological and immunochemical comparisons. In: Compans, R.W. and Bishop, D.H.L. (eds), *Segmented negative strand RNA viruses*. Orlando FL: Academic Press, 341–7.

Coimbra, T.L.M. and Nassar, E.S. 1994, New arenavirus isolated in Brazil. *Lancet*, **343**, 391–2.

Cole, G.A. and Johnson, E.D. 1975. Immune responses to LCM virus infection *in vivo* and *in vitro*. *Bull WHO*, **52**, 465–70.

Cole, G.A., Nathanson, N. and Pendergast, R.A. 1972. Requirements for theta-bearing cells: lymphocytic choriomeningitis virus induced central nervous system disease. *Nature (London)*, **238**, 335–7.

Cornu, T.I. and de la Torre, J.C. 2001. RING finger Z protein of lymphocytic choriomeningitis virus (LCMV) inhibits transcription and RNA replication of an LCMV S-segment minigenome. *J Virol*, **75**, 9415–26.

Cornu, T.I. and de la Torre, J.C. 2002. Characterization of the arenavirus RING finger Z protein regions required for Z-mediated inhibition of viral RNA synthesis. *J Virol*, **76**, 6678–88.

Cosgriff, T., Jarling, P.B., et al. 1987. Studies of the coagulation system in arenaviral hemorrhagic fever: experimental infection of strain 13 guinea pigs with Pichinde virus. *Am J Trop Med Hyg*, **36**, 416–23.

Contigiani, M.S., Medeot, S.I., et al. 1991. Rapid vascular clearance of two strains of Junin virus in *Calomys musculinus*: selective macrophage clearance. *Acta Virol*, **35**, 144–51.

Cossio, P.M., Laguens, R.P., et al. 1975. Ultrastructural and immunohistochemical study of the human kidney in Argentine hemorrhagic fever. *Virchows Arch*, **368**, 1–9.

Coto, C.E., Damonte, E.B., et al. 1993. Genetic variation in Junin virus. In: Salvato, M.S. (ed.), *The Arenaviridae*. New York: Plenum Press, 85–101.

Dahourou, G., Guillot, S., et al. 2002. Genetic recombination in wild-type poliovirus. *J Gen Virol*, **83**, 3103–10.

Dalton, A.J., Rowe, W.P., et al. 1968. Morphological and cytochemical studies on lymphocytic choriomeningitis virus. *J Virol*, **2**, 1465–78.

de la Torre, J.C., Rall, G., et al. 1993. Replication of LCMV is restricted in terminally differentiated neurons. *J Virol*, **67**, 7350–9.

Di Simone, C., Zandonatti, M.A. and Buchmeier, M.J. 1994. Acidic pH triggers LCMV membrane fusion activity and conformational change in the glycoprotein spike. *Virology*, **198**, 455–65.

Djavani, M., Yin, C., et al. 2000. Murine immune responses to mucosally delivered Salmonella expressing Lassa fever virus nucleoprotein. *Vaccine*, **18**, 1543–54.

Djavani, M., Yin, C., et al. 2001a. Mucosal immunization with Salmonella typhimurium expressing Lassa virus nucleocapsid protein cross-protects mice from lethal challenge with lymphocytic choriomeningitis virus. *J Hum Virol*, **4**, 103–8.

Djavani, M., Rodas, J.D., et al. 2001b. Role of the promyelocytic leukemia protein PML in the interferon sensitivity of lymphocytic choriomeningitis virus. *J Virol*, **75**, 6204–8.

Doherty, P.C. 1973. Quantitative studies of the inflammatory process in fatal viral meningoencephalitis. *Am J Pathol*, **73**, 607–22.

Doherty, P.C. and Zinkernagel, R.M. 1974. T-cell mediated immunopathology in viral infections. *Transplant Rev*, **19**, 89–120.

Doherty, P.C., Dunlop, M.B.C., et al. 1976. Inflammatory process in murine lymphocytic choriomeningitis is maximal in H-2K or H-2D compatible interactions. *J Immunol*, **117**, 187–90.

Douglas, G.R., Wiebenga, N.H. and Couch, R.B. 1965. Bolivian hemorrhagic fever probably transmitted by personal contact. *Am J Epidemiol*, **82**, 85–91.

Downs, W.G., Anderson, C.R., et al. 1963. Tacaribe virus: a new agent isolated from Artibeus bats and mosquitoes in Trinidad, West Indies. *Am J Trop Med Hyg*, **12**, 640–6.

Dutko, F. and Oldstone, M.B.A. 1983. Genomic and biological variation among commonly used lymphocytic choriomeningitis virus strains. *J Gen Virol*, **64**, 1689–98.

Dutko, F.J., Wright, E.A. and Pfau, C.J. 1976. The RNAs of the defective interfering Pichinde virus. *J Gen Virol*, **31**, 417–27.

Eddy, G.A., Scott, S.K., et al. 1975. Pathogenesis of Machupo virus infection in primates. *Bull WHO*, **52**, 517–21.

Enria, D.A. and Maiztegui, J.I. 1994. Antiviral treatment of Argentine hemorrhagic fever. *Antiviral Res*, **23**, 23–31.

Enria, D., Brigiler, A.M., et al. 1984. Importance of dose of neutralizing antibodies in treatment of Argentine hemorrhagic fever with immune plasma. *Lancet*, **2**, 255–6.

Farber, R.E. and Rawls, W.E. 1975. Isolation of ribosome-like structures from Pichinde virus. *J Gen Virol*, **26**, 21–31.

Farmer, T.W. and Janeway, C.A. 1942. Infections with the virus of lymphocytic choriomeningitis. *Medicine*, **21**, 1–64.

Fisher-Hoch, S.P. 1993. Arenavirus pathophysiology. In: Salvato, M.S. (ed.), *The Arenaviridae*. New York: Plenum Press, 299–323.

Fisher-Hoch, S.P., Price, M.J., et al. 1985. Safe intensive care management of a severe case of Lassa fever using simple barrier nursing techniques. *Lancet*, **2**, 1227–9.

Fisher-Hoch, S.P., Mitchell, S.W., et al. 1987. Physiologic and immunologic disturbances associated with shock in Lassa fever in a primate model. *J Infect Dis*, **155**, 465–74.

Fisher-Hoch, S.P., Hutwagner, L., et al. 2000. Effective vaccine for Lassa Fever. *J Virol*, **74**, 6777–83.

Frame, J.D., Baldwin, M.N., et al. 1970. Lassa fever: a new virus disease of man from West Africa. 1. Clinical description and pathological findings. *Am J Trop Med Hyg*, **73**, 219–24.

Franze-Fernandez, M.T., Zetina, C., et al. 1987. Molecular structure and early events in the replication of Tacaribe arenavirus S RNA. *Virus Res*, **7**, 309–24.

Franze-Fernandez, M.-T., Iapalucci, S., et al. 1993. Subgenomic RNAs of Tacaribe virus. In: Salvato, M.S. (ed.), *The Arenaviridae*. New York: Plenum Press, .

Freemont, P.S. 1993. The ring finger: a novel protein sequence motif related to the zinc finger. *Ann NY Acad Sci*, **47**, 174–84.

Fulhorst, C.F., Bennett, S.G., et al. 2002. Bear Canyon virus: an arenavirus naturally associated with the California mouse (*Peromyscus californicus*). *Emerg Infect Dis*, **8**, 717–21.

Fuller-Pace, F.V. and Southern, P.J. 1988. Temporal analysis of transcription and replication during acute infection with lymphocytic choriomeningitis virus. *Virology*, **162**, 260–3.

Fung-Leung, W.P., Kundig, T.M., et al. 1991. Immune response against LCMV infection in mice without CD8 expression. *J Exp Med*, **174**, 1425–9.

Gallimore, A., Glitherto, A., et al. 1998. Induction and exhaustion of lymphocytic-choriomeningitis – virus-specific cytotoxic T lymphocytes visualized using soluble tetrameric major histocompatibility complex class-I-peptide complexes. *J Exp Med*, **187**, 1383–93.

Garcin, D. and Kolakofsky, D. 1990. A novel mechanism for the initiation of Tacaribe arenavirus genome replication. *J Virol*, **64**, 6196–203.

Garcin, D., Rochat, S. and Kolakofsky, D. 1993. The Tacaribe Arenavirus small zinc finger protein is required for both mRNA synthesis and genome replication. *J Virol*, **67**, 807–12.

Gartner, S., Markovits, P., et al. 1986. The role of mononuclear phagocytes in HTLV-III/LAV infection. *Science*, **233**, 215–19.

Geshwender, H.H., Rutter, G., et al. 1976. Lymphocytic choriomeningitis virus. II. Characterization of extractable complement-fixing activity. *Med Microbiol Immunol (Berl)*, **162**, 119–31.

Ghiringhelli, P.E., Rivera-Pomar, R.V., et al. 1991. Molecular organization of Junin virus S RNA: complete nucleotide sequence, relationship with other members of the Arenaviridae and unusual secondary structures. *J Gen Virol*, **72**, 2129–41.

Gilden, D.H., Cole, G.A., et al. 1972. Immunopathogenesis of acute central nervous system disease produced by lymphocytic choriomeningitis virus. 1. Cyclophosphamide-mediated induction of virus-carrier state in adult mice. *J Exp Med*, **135**, 860–73.

Glushakova, S.E. and Lukashevich, I.S. 1989. Early events in arenavirus replication are sensitive to lysosomotropic compounds. *Arch Virol*, **104**, 157–61.

Glushakova, S., Omelyanenko, V., et al. 1992. The fusion of artificial lipid membranes induced by the synthetic arenavirus 'fusion peptide'. *Biochim Biophys Acta*, **1110**, 202–8.

Gonzalez, J.P., Buchmeier, M.J., et al. 1984. Comparative analysis of Lassa and Lassa-like arenavirus isolates from Africa. In: Compans, R.W. and Bishop, D.H.L. (eds), *Segmented negative strand RNA viruses*. Orlando FL: Academic Press, 210–18.

Guttler, F., Bro-Jorgensen, K. and Jorgensen, P.N. 1975. Transient impaired cell-mediated tumor immunity after acute infection with lymphocytic choriomeningitis virus. *Scand J Immunol*, **4**, 327–36.

Haas, V.H. and Stewart, S.E. 1956. Sparing effect of amethopterin and guanazolo in mice with the virus of lymphocytic choriomeningitis. *Virology*, **2**, 511–16.

Hany, M. and Oehen, S. 1989. Anti-viral protection and prevention of lymphocytic choriomeningitis or of the local footpad swelling reaction in mice by immunization with vaccinia-recombinant virus expressing LCMV-WE nucleoprotein or glycoprotein. *Eur J Immunol*, **19**, 417–24.

Holmes, G.P., McCormick, J.B., et al. 1990. Lassa fever in the United States. *N Engl J Med*, **323**, 1120–3.

Hotchin, J. 1962. The foot pad reaction of mice to lymphocytic choriomeningitis virus. *Virology*, **17**, 214–16.

Hotchin, J. 1971. Tolerance to lymphocytic choriomeningitis virus. 3. Persistent tolerant infection of LCM and other oncogenic viruses. *Ann NY Acad Sci*, **181**, 159–82.

Howard, C.R. 1993. Antigenic diversity among the arenaviruses. In: Salvato, M.S. (ed.), *The Arenaviridae*. New York: Plenum Press, 37–41.

Howard, C. and Buchmeier, M.J. 1983. A protein kinase activity in lymphocytic choriomeningitis virus and identification of the phosphorylated product using monoclonal antibody. *Virology*, **126**, 538–47.

Howard, C.R. and Simpson, D.I.H. 1990. Arenaviruses. In: Collier, L.H. and Timbury, M.C. (eds), *Topley and Wilson's principles of bacteriology, virology and immunity*, Vol. 4. 8th edn. London: Edward Arnold, 593–607.

Iapalucci, S., Lopez, N., et al. 1989. The 5′ region of Tacaribe virus L RNA encodes a protein with a potential metal binding domain. *Virology*, **173**, 357–61.

Jacamo, R., Lopez, N., Wilda, M., and Franze-Fernandez, M.T. 2003. Tacaribe virus Z protein interacts with the L polymerase protein to inhibit viral RNA synthesis. *J Virol*, **77**, 10383–93.

Jacobs, R.P. and Cole, G.A. 1976. Lymphocytic choriomeningitis virus-induced immunosuppression: a virus-induced macrophage defect. *J Immunol*, **117**, 1004–9.

Jahrling, P.B. and Peters, C.J. 1984. Passive antibody therapy of Lassa fever in cynomolgus monkeys: importance of neutralizing antibody and Lassa virus strain. *Infect Immun*, **44**, 528–33.

Jahrling, P.B. and Peters, C.J. 1986. Serology and virulence diversity among Old World arenaviruses, and the relevance to vaccine development. *Med Microbiol Immunol*, **175**, 165–7.

Jahrling, P.B., Hesse, R.A., et al. 1980. Lassa virus infection of rhesus monkeys: pathogenesis and treatment with ribavirin. *J Infect Dis*, **141**, 580–9.

Jahrling, P.B., Smith, S., et al. 1982. Pathogenesis of Lassa virus infection in guinea pigs. *Infect Immun*, **37**, 771–8.

Jahrling, P.B., Peters, C.J. and Stephens, E.L. 1984. Enhanced treatment of Lassa fever by immune plasma combined with ribavirin in cynomolgus monkeys. *J Infect Dis*, **149**, 420–7.

Jennings, W.L., Lewis, A.L., et al. 1970. Tamiami virus in the Tampa Bay area. *Am J Trop Med Hyg*, **19**, 527–36.

Johnson, E.D., Monjan, A.A. and Morse, H.C. 1978. Lack of B cell participation in acute LCM disease of CNS. *Cell Immunol*, **36**, 143–50.

Johnson, K.M., Wiebenga, N.H., et al. 1965. Virus isolation from human cases of hemorrhagic fever in Bolivia. *Proc Soc Exp Biol Med*, **118**, 113–18.

Johnson, K.M., McCormick, J.B., et al. 1987. Lassa fever in Sierra Leone: clinical virology in hospitalized patients. *J Infect Dis*, **155**, 456–64.

Kagi, D., Ledermann, B., et al. 1994. Cytotoxicity mediated by T cells and natural killer cells is greatly impaired in perforin-deficient mice. *Nature (London)*, **369**, 31–7.

Kasaian, M.T. and Biron, C.A. 1990. Cyclosporin A inhibition of IL-2 gene expression, but not NK cell proliferation, after interferon induction in vivo. *J Exp Med*, **171**, 745–62.

Kasaian, M.T., Leite-Morris, K.A. and Biron, C.A. 1991. The role of CD4+ cells in sustaining lymphocyte proliferation during LCMV infection. *J Immunol*, **146**, 1955–63.

Kastello, M.D., Eddy, G.A. and Kuehne, R.W. 1976. A rhesus monkey model for the study of Bolivian hemorrhagic fever. *J Infect Dis*, **133**, 57–62.

Klavinskis, L.S. and Oldstone, M.B.A. 1987. Lymphocytic choriomeningitis virus can persistently infect thyroid epithelial cells and perturb thyroid hormone production. *J Gen Virol*, **68**, 1867–73.

Klavinskis, L.S., Whitton, J.L., et al. 1990. Vaccination and protection from a lethal viral infection: identification, incorporation, and use of a cytotoxic T lymphocyte glycoprotein epitope. *Virology*, **178**, 393–8.

Klenerman, P., Cerundolo, V. and Dunbar, R. 2002. Tracking T cells with tetramers: new tales from new tools. *Nature Rev Immunol*, **2**, 263–72.

Krasnianski, V.P., Potryvaeva, N.V., et al. 1993. A trial to produce an inactivated Lassa fever vaccine. *Vopr Virusol*, **38**, 276–9.

La Posta, V., Auperin, D.D., et al. 1993. Cross-protection against lymphocytic choriomeningitis virus mediated by a CD4+ T-cell clone specific for an envelope glycoprotein epitope of Lassa virus. *J Virol*, **67**, 3497–506.

Lee, K.G., de la Torre, J.C. 2002. Reverse genetics of arenaviruses. In *Arenavirus I, the epidemiology, molecular and cell biology of arenaviruses, CTMI*, **262**, 175–93.

Lee, K.J., Novella, I.S., et al. 2000. NP and L proteins of lymphocytic choriomeningitis virus (LCMV) are sufficient for efficient transcription and replication of LCMV genomic RNA analogs. *J Virol*, **74**, 3470–7.

Lee, K.J., Perez, M., et al. 2002. Identification of the Lymphocytic Choriomeningitis Virus (LCMV) proteins required to rescue LCMV RNA analogs into LCMV-like particles. *J Virol*, **76**, 6393–7.

Lehmann-Grube, F. 1971. Lymphocytic choriomeningitis virus. *Virol Monogr*, **10**, 1–173.

Lehmann-Grube, F. and Lohler, J. 1981. Immunopathologic alterations of lymphatic tissues of mice infected with lymphocytic choriomeningitis virus. 2. Pathogenetic mechanism. *Lab Invest*, **44**, 205–13.

Lehmann-Grube, F., Slenczka, W. and Tees, R. 1969. A persistent and inapparent infection of L cells with the virus of lymphocytic choriomeningitis. *J Gen Virol*, **5**, 63–81.

Lehmann-Grube, F., Niemeyer, I.P. and Lohler, J. 1972. Lymphocytic choriomeningitis of the mouse. 4. Depression of the allograft reaction. *Med Microbiol Immunol*, **158**, 16–25.

Lehmann-Grube, F., Moskophidis, D. and Lohler, J. 1988. Recovery from acute virus infection: role of cytotoxic T lymphocytes in the elimination of lymphocytic choriomeningitis virus from spleens of mice. *Ann NY Acad Sci*, **532**, 238–56.

Leifer, E., Goecke, D.J. and Bourne, H. 1970. Lassa fever: a new virus disease of man from West Africa. 2. Report of a laboratory acquired infection treated with plasma from a person recently recovered from the disease. *Am J Trop Med Hyg*, **19**, 677–9.

Leist, T.P., Ruedi, E. and Zinkernagel, R.M. 1988. Virus-triggered immune suppression in mice caused by virus-specific cytotoxic T cells. *J Exp Med*, **167**, 1749–54.

Lenz, O., Ter Meulen, J., et al. 2001. The Lassa virus glycoprotein precursor GP-C is proteolytically processed by subtilase SKI-1/S1P. *Proc Natl Acad Sci USA*, **98**, 12701–5.

Leung, W.C. and Rawls, W.E. 1977. Virion associated ribosomes are not required for the replication of Pichinde virus. *Virology*, **81**, 174–6.

Liu, C.T., Jarling, P.B. and Peters, C.J. 1986. Evidence for the involvement of sulfidopeptide leukotrienes in the pathogenesis of pichinde virus infection in strain 13 guinea pigs. *Prostaglandins Leukotrienes Med*, **24**, 129–38.

Lopez, R. and Franze-Fernandez, M.-T. 1985. Effect of Tacaribe virus infection on host cell protein and nucleic acid synthesis. *J Gen Virol*, **66**, 1753–61.

Lozano, M.E., Ghiringhelli, P.D., et al. 1993. A simple nucleic acid amplification assay for the rapid detection of Junin virus in whole blood samples. *Virus Res*, **27**, 37–53.

Lukashevich, I.S. 1992. Generation of reassortants between African arenaviruses. *Virology*, **188**, 600–5.

Lukashevich, I.S., Djavani, M., et al. 1997. The Lassa fever virus L gene: nucleotide sequence, comparison, and precipitation of a predicted 250 kDa protein with monospecific antiserum. *J Gen Virol*, **78**, 547–51.

Lukashevich, I.S., Maryankova, R., et al. 1999. Lassa and Mopeia virus replication in human monocytes/macrophages and in endothelial cells: different effects on IL-8 and TNF-alpha gene expression. *J Med Virol*, **59**, 552–60.

Lukashevich, I.S., Djavani, M., et al. 2002. Hemorrhagic fever occurs after intravenous, but not after intragastric, inoculation of rhesus macaques with lymphocytic choriomeningitis virus. *J Med Virol*, **67**, 171–86.

Lukashevich, I.S., Tikkonov, I., et al. 2003. Arenaviruses mediated pathology: acute LCMV infection of Rhesus macaques is characterized by high IL-6 expression and hepatocyte proliferation. *J Virol*, **77**, 1727–37.

Mackenzie, R.B., Beye, H.K., et al. 1964. Epidemic hemorrhagic fever in Bolivia. 1. A preliminary report of the epidemiologic and clinical findings in a new epidemic area South America. *Am J Trop Med Hyg*, **13**, 620–5.

Mahanty, S., Bausch, D.G., et al. 2001. Low levels of interleukin-8 and interferon-inducible protein-10 in serum are associated with fatal infections in acute Lassa fever. *J Infect Dis*, **183**, 1713–21.

Maiztegui, J.I. 1975. Clinical and epidemiological patterns of Argentine hemorrhagic fever. *Bull WHO*, **52**, 567–75.

Maiztegui, J.I., Fernandez, N.J. and de Damilano, A.J. 1979. Efficacy of immune plasma in treatment of Argentine hemorrhagic fever and association between treatment and a late neurological syndrome. *Lancet*, **2**, 1216–17.

Marker, O. and Volkert, M. 1973. Studies on cell mediated immunity to lymphocytic choriomeningitis virus in mice. *J Exp Med*, **137**, 1511–25.

Martinez Peralta, L.A., Coto, C.E. and Weissenbacher, M.C. 1993. The Tacaribe complex: the close relationship between a pathogenic (Junin) and nonpathogenic (Tacaribe) arenavirus. In: Salvato, M.S. (ed.), *The Arenaviridae*. New York: Plenum Press, 281–98.

Martins, L.P., Lau, L.L., et al. 1995. DNA vaccination against persistent viral infection. *J Virol*, **69**, 2574–82.

Matloubian, M., Kohlhekar, S.R., et al. 1993. Molecular determinants of macrophage tropism and virus persistence: importance of single amino acid changes in the polymerase and glycoprotein of lymphocytic choriomeningitis virus. *J Virol*, **67**, 7340–9.

Matloubian, M., Concepcion, R.J. and Ahmed, R. 1994. CD4[+] T cells are required to sustain CD8[+] cytotoxic T-cell responses during chronic viral infection. *J Virol*, **68**, 8056–63.

McCormick, J.B. 1987. Epidemiology and control of Lassa fever. *Curr Top Microbiol Immunol*, **134**, 69–78.

McCormick, J.B. 1990. Arenaviruses. In: Fields, B.N. and Knipe, D.M. (eds), *Fields' virology*. New York: Raven Press, 1245–67.

McCormick, J.B., King, I.J. and Webb, P.A. 1986. Lassa fever: effective therapy with ribavirin. *N Engl J Med*, **314**, 202–26.

McCormick, J.B., King, I.J., et al. 1987a. Lassa fever: a case control study of the clinical diagnosis and course. *J Infect Dis*, **155**, 445–55.

McCormick, J.B., Webb, P.A., et al. 1987b. A prospective study of the epidemiology and ecology of Lassa fever. *J Infect Dis*, **155**, 437–44.

McCormick, J.B., Mitchell, S.W., et al. 1992. Inactivated Lassa virus elicits a non protective immune response in rhesus monkeys. *J Med Virol*, **37**, 1–7.

McKee, K.T.J., Oro, J.G., et al. 1993. Safety and immunogenicity of a live attenuated Junin (Argentine hemorrhagic fever) vaccine in rhesus macaques. *Am J Trop Med Hyg*, **48**, 403–11.

Meyer, B.J. and Southern, P.J. 1993. Concurrent sequence analysis of 5′ and 3′ RNA termini by intramolecular circularization reveals 5′ nontemplated bases and 3′ terminal heterogeneity for lymphocytic choriomeningitis mRNAs. *J Virol*, **67**, 2621–7.

Mifune, K., Carter, M. and Rawls, W. 1971. Characterization of the Pichinde virus – a member of the arenavirus group. *Proc Soc Exp Biol Med*, **136**, 637–44.

Mills, J.N., Barrera Oro, J.G., et al. 1996. Characterization of Oliveros virus, a new member of the Tacaribe complex (*Arenaviridae*: arenavirus). *Am J Trop Med Hyg*, **54**, 399–404.

Mims, C.A. and Subrahmanyan, T.P. 1966. Immunofluorescence study of the mechanism of resistance to superinfection in mice carrying the LCMV. *J Pathol Bacteriol*, **91**, 403–15.

Mims, C.A. and Wainwright, S. 1968. The immunodepressive action of lymphocytic choriomeningitis virus in mice. *J Immunol*, **101**, 717–24.

Molinas, F.C., Paz, R.A., et al. 1978. Studies of blood coagulation and pathology in experimental infection of guinea pigs with Junin virus. *J Infect Dis*, **137**, 740–6.

Monath, T.P., Maher, M., et al. 1974. Lassa fever in the eastern province of Sierra Leone, 1970–1972. 2. Clinical observations and virological studies on selected hospital cases. *Am J Trop Med Hyg*, **23**, 1140–9.

Moncayo, A.C., Hice, C.L., et al. 2001. Allpahuayo virus: a newly recognized arenavirus (*Arenaviridae*) from arboreal rice rats (*Oecomys bicolor* and *Oecomys paricola*) in northeastern Peru. *Virology*, **284**, 277–86.

Monson, M.H., Cole, A.D., et al. 1987. Pediatric Lassa fever: a review of 33 Liberian cases. *Am J Trop Med Hyg*, **36**, 408–15.

Montali, R.J., Scanga, C.A., et al. 1993. A common source outbreak of callitrichid hepatitis in captive tamarins and marmosets. *J Infect Dis*, **167**, 946–50.

Morrison, H.G., Bauer, S.P., et al. 1989. Protection of guinea pigs from Lassa fever by vaccinia virus recombinants expressing the nucleoprotein or the envelope glycoproteins of Lassa virus. *Virology*, **171**, 179–88.

Moskophidis, D., Lechner, F., et al. 1993. Virus persistence in acutely infected immunocompetent mice by exhaustion of antiviral cytotoxic effector T cells. *Nature (London)*, **362**, 758–61.

Murali-Krishna, K., Altman, J.D., et al. 1998. Counting antigen-specific CD8 T cells: a reevaluation of bystander activation during viral infection. *Immunity*, **8**, 177–87.

Murphy, F.A. 1975. Arenavirus taxonomy: a review. *Bull WHO*, **52**, 389–91.

Oehen, S., Hengartner, H. and Zinkernagel, R.M. 1991. Vaccination for disease. *Science*, **251**, 195–8.

Oldstone, M.B.A. 1987a. Arenaviruses – an introduction. *Curr Top Microbiol Immunol*, **134**, 1–4.

Oldstone, M.B.A. 1987b. Immunotherapy for virus infection. *Curr Top Microbiol Immunol*, **134**, 212–29.

Oldstone, M.B.A. 2002. Biology and pathogenesis of lymphocytic chroriomeningitis virus infection. *Curr Top Microbiol Immunol*, **262**, 83–118.

Oldstone, M.B.A. and Dixon, F.J. 1967. Lymphocytic choriomeningitis: production of antibody by 'tolerant' infected mice. *Science*, **158**, 1193–5.

Oldstone, M.B.A., Holmstoen, J. and Welsh, R.M. 1977. Alterations of acetylcholine enzymes in neuroblastoma cells persistently infected with lymphocytic choriomeningitis virus. *J Cell Physiol*, **91**, 459–72.

Oldstone, M.B.A., Sinha, Y.N., et al. 1982. Virus induced alterations in homeostasis: alterations in differentiated functions of infected cells in vivo. *Science*, **218**, 1125–7.

Oldstone, M.B.A., Tishon, A. and Buchmeier, M.J. 1983. Virus induced immune complex disease: genetic control of C1q binding complexes in the circulations of mice persistently infected with LCMV. *J Immunol*, **130**, 912–18.

Oldstone, M.B.A., Ahmed, R., et al. 1985. Perturbation of differentiated functions during viral infection in vivo. 1. Relationship of lymphocytic choriomeningitis virus and host strains to growth hormone deficiency. *Virology*, **142**, 158–74.

Oldstone, M.B.A., Ahmed, R. and Salvato, M. 1990. Viruses as therapeutic agents. 2. Viral reassortants map prevention of insulin-dependent diabetes mellitus to the small RNA of lymphocytic choriomeningitis virus. *J Exp Med*, **171**, 2091–100.

Ou, R., Zhou, S., et al. 2001. Critical role for α/β and γ interferons in persistence of LCMV by clonal exhaustion of CTL. *J Virol*, **75**, 8407–23.

Palmer, E.L., Obijeski, J.F., et al. 1977. The circular segmented nucleocapsid of an arenavirus, Tacaribe virus. *J Gen Virol*, **36**, 541–5.

Parekh, B.S. and Buchmeier, M.J. 1986. Proteins of lymphocytic choriomeningitis virus: antigenic topography of the viral glycoproteins. *Virology*, **153**, 168–78.

Parodi, A.S., Greenway, D.J., et al. 1958. Sobre la etiologia del bute epidemico de Junin. *Diagn Med*, **30**, 2300–2.

Pedersen, I.R. 1979. Structural components and replication of arenaviruses. *Adv Virus Res*, **24**, 277–330.

Peters, C.J. 1984. Arenaviruses. In: Belshe, R.B. (ed.), *Textbook of human virology*. Littleton MA: PSG, 513–45.

Peters, C.J. 1997. Viral hemorrhagic fevers. In: Nathanson, N. (ed.), *Viral pathogenesis*. NY: Lippincott-Raven, 779–99.

Peters, C.J., Webb, P.A. and Johnson, K.M. 1973. Measurement of antibodies to Machupo virus by the indirect fluorescent technique. *Proc Soc Exp Biol Med*, **142**, 526–31.

Peters, C.J., Kuehne, R.W., et al. 1974. Hemorrhagic fever in Cochabamba, Bolivia, 1971. *Am J Epidemiol*, **99**, 425–32.

Peters, C.J., Jahrling, P.B., et al. 1987. Experimental studies of arenaviral hemorrhagic fevers. *Curr Top Microbiol Immunol*, **134**, 5–68.

Pfau, C.J. 1974. Biochemical and biophysical properties of the arenaviruses. *Progr Med Virol*, **18**, 64–80.

Pfau, C.J., Gresser, I. and Hunt, K.D. 1983. Lethal role of interferon in lymphocytic choriomeningitis virus induced encephalitis. *J Gen Virol*, **64**, 1827–32.

Polyak, S.J., Zheng, S. and Harnish, D.G. 1995a. Analysis of Pichinde arenavirus transcription and replication in human THP-1 monocytic cells. *Virus Res*, **36**, 37–48.

Polyak, S.J., Zheng, S. and Harnish, D.G. 1995b. 5′ termini of Pichinde arenavirus S RNAs and mRNAs contain nontemplated nucleotides. *J Virol*, **69**, 3211–15.

Price, M.E., Fisher-Hoch, S.P., et al. 1988. Lassa fever in pregnancy. *Br Med J*, **297**, 584–8.

Qian, C., Liu, C.T. and Peters, C.J. 1991. Metabolism of platelet-activating factor in neutrophils isolated from Pichinde virus-infected guinea pigs. *J Leuko Biol*, **51**, 210–13.

Rahemtulla, A., Fung-Leung, W.P., et al. 1991. Normal development and function of CD8+ cells but markedly decreased helper cell activity in mice lacking CD4+. *Nature (London)*, **353**, 180–4.

Rai, S.K., Cheung, D.S., et al. 1996. Murine infection with LCMV following gastric inoculation. *J Virol*, **70**, 7213–18.

Raju, R., Raju, L., et al. 1990. Nontemplated bases at the 5′ ends of Tacaribe virus mRNAs. *Virology*, **174**, 53–9.

Rawls, W.E. and Buchmeier, M. 1975. Arenaviruses: purification and physicochemical nature. *Bull WHO*, **52**, 393–401.

Rawls, W.E. and Leung, W.C. 1979. Arenaviruses. *Compr Virol*, **14**, 157–92.

Rivers, T.M. and Scott, T.F.M. 1935. Meningitis in man caused by a filterable virus. *Science*, **81**, 439–40.

Rivers, T.M. and Scott, T.F.M. 1936. Meningitis in man caused by a filterable virus. 2. Identification of the etiological agent. *J Exp Med*, **63**, 415–32.

Riviere, Y. 1986. Mapping arenavirus genes causing virulence. *Curr Top Microbiol Immunol*, **133**, 59–66.

Rodriguez, M., von Wedel, R.J., et al. 1983. Pituitary dwarfism in mice persistently infected with lymphocytic choriomeningitis virus. *Lab Invest*, **49**, 48–53.

Romanowski, V. 1993. Genetic organization of Junin virus, the etiological agent of Argentine hemorrhagic fever. In: Salvato, M.S. (ed.), *The Arenaviridae*. New York: Plenum Press, 51–83.

Romanowski, V., Matsuura, Y. and Bishop, D.H.L. 1985. Complete sequence of the S RNA of lymphocytic choriomeningitis virus (WE strain) compared to that of Pichinde arenavirus. *Virus Res*, **3**, 101–14.

Roost, H., Charan, S., et al. 1988. An acquired immune suppression in mice caused by infection with lymphocytic choriomeningitis virus. *Eur J Immunol*, **18**, 511–18.

Rose, J.R. 1956. A new clinical entity? *Lancet*, **2**, 197–9.

Rosenthal, K.L., Zinkernagel, R.M., et al. 1986. Persistence of vesicular stomatitis virus in cloned interleukin-2 dependent NK cell lines. *J Virol*, **60**, 539–47.

Rowe, W.P., Black, P.H. and Lercy, R.H. 1963. Protective effect of neonatal thymectomy on mouse LCM infection. *Proc Soc Exp Biol Med*, **114**, 248–51.

Rowe, W.P., Murphy, F.A., et al. 1970. Arenaviruses: proposed name for a newly defined virus group. *J Virol*, **5**, 651–2.

Ruedi, E., Hengartner, H. and Zinkernagel, R.M. 1990. Immunosuppression in mice by lymphocytic choriomeningitis virus infection: time dependence during primary and absence of effects on secondary antibody responses. *Cell Immunol*, **130**, 501–12.

Sabattini, M.S., de Rios, L.E.G., et al. 1977. Natural and experimental infection of rodents with Junin virus. *Medicina (Buenos Aires)*, **37**, 149–61.

Salvato, M.S. 1993a. *The Arenaviridae*. New York: Plenum Press.

Salvato, M.S. 1993b. Molecular biology of the prototype arenavirus, lymphocytic choriomeningitis virus. In: Salvato, M.S. (ed.), *The Arenaviridae*. New York: Plenum Press, 133–56.

Salvato, M.S. and Shimomaye, E.M. 1989. The completed sequence of lymphocytic choriomeningitis virus reveals a unique RNA structure and a gene for a zinc finger protein. *Virology*, **173**, 1–10.

Salvato, M.S., Shimomaye, E.M. and Oldstone, M.B.A. 1989. The primary structure of the lymphocytic choriomeningitis virus L gene encodes a putative RNA polymerase. *Virology*, **169**, 377–84.

Salvato, M., Borrow, P., et al. 1991. Molecular basis of viral persistence: a single amino acid change in the glycoprotein of lymphocytic choriomeningitis virus is associated with suppression of the antiviral cytotoxic T lymphocyte response and establishment of persistence. *J Virol*, **65**, 1863–9.

Salvato, M.S., Schweighofer, K.J., et al. 1992. Biochemical and immunological evidence that the 11 kDa zinc-binding protein of lymphocytic choriomeningitis virus is a structural component of the virus. *Virus Res*, **22**, 185–98.

Schulz, M., Aichele, P., et al. 1991. Major histocompatibility complex binding and T cell recognition of a viral nonapeptide containing a minimal tetrapeptide. *Eur J Immunol*, **21**, 1181–6.

Seidah, N.G., Mowla, S.J., et al. 1999. Mammalian subtilisin/kexin isozyme SKI-1: A widely expressed proprotein convertase with a unique cleavage specificity and cellular localization. *Proc Natl Acad Sci USA*, **96**, 1321–6.

Seiler, P., Senn, B.M., et al. 2000. Additive effect of neutralizing antibody and antiviral drug treatment in preventing virus escape and persistence. *J Virol*, **74**, 5896–90.

Shivraprakesh, M., Harnish, D. and Rawls, W.E. 1988. Characterization of temperature-sensitive mutants of Pichinde virus. *J Virol*, **62**, 4037–43.

Silberman, S.L., Jacobs, R.P. and Cole, G.A. 1978. Mechanisms of hemopoietic and immunological dysfunction induced by lymphocytic choriomeningitis virus. *Infect Immun*, **19**, 533–9.

Simon, M. 1970. Multiplication of lymphocytic choriomeningitis virus in various systems. *Acta Virol*, **14**, 369–76.

Solbrig, M.V. 1993. Lassa virus and central nervous system diseases. In: Salvato, M.S. (ed.), *The Arenaviridae*. New York: Plenum Press, 325–30.

Southern, P.J. 1996. *Arenaviridae*: the viruses and their replication. In: Fields, B.N., Knipe, D.M., et al. (eds), *Fields' virology*, 3rd edn. New York: Raven Press, 1505–19.

Southern, P.J., Blount, P. and Oldstone, M.B.A. 1984. Analysis of persistent virus infections by in situ hybridization to whole-mouse sections. *Nature (London)*, **312**, 555–8.

Southern, P.J., Singh, M.K., et al. 1987. Molecular characterization of the genomic S RNA segment from lymphocytic choriomeningitis virus. *Virology*, **157**, 145–50.

Stephenson, E.H., Larson, E.W. and Dominik, J.W. 1984. Effect of environmental factors on aerosol-induced Lassa virus infection. *J Med Virol*, **14**, 295–303.

Tesh, R.B., Jahrling, P.B., et al. 1994. Description of Guanarito virus (*Arenaviridae*: Arenavirus), the etiologic agent of Venezuelan hemorrhagic fever. *Am J Trop Med Hyg*, **50**, 452–9.

Thomsen, A.R. and Pfau, C.J. 1993. Influence of host genes on the outcome of murine lymphocytic choriomeningitis infection: a model for studying genetic control of virus-specific immune responses. In: Salvato, M.S. (ed.), *The Arenaviridae*. New York: Plenum Press, 199–224.

Thomsen, A.R., Bro-Jorgensen, K. and Jensen, B.L. 1982. Lymphocytic choriomeningitis induced immunosuppression: evidence for viral interference with T cell maturation. *Infect Immun*, **37**, 981–6.

Tishon, A., Borrow, P., et al. 1993. Virus induced immunosuppression. 1. Age at infection relates to a selective or generalized defect. *Virology*, **195**, 397–405.

Trapido, H. and Sanmartin, C. 1971. Pichinde virus, A new virus of the Tacaribe group from Colombia. *Am J Trop Med Hyg*, **20**, 631–41.

Traub, E. 1935. A filterable virus recovered from white mice. *Science*, **81**, 298–9.

Traub, E. 1938. Factors influencing the persistence of choriomeningitis virus in the blood of mice after clinical recovery. *J Exp Med*, **68**, 229–50.

Vainrub, B. and Salas, R. 1994. Latin American hemorrhagic fever. *Infect Dis Clin North Am*, **8**, 47–59.

Volkert, M. 1963. Studies on immunological tolerance to LCMV. 2. Treatment of virus carrier mice by adoptive immunization. *Acta Pathol Microbiol Scand*, **57**, 465–87.

Volkert, M. and Lundstedt, C. 1968. The provocation of latent LCMV infections in mice by treatment with anti-lymphocytic serum. *J Exp Med*, **127**, 327–39.

Walker, D.H. and Murphy, F.A. 1987. Pathology and pathogenesis of arenavirus infections. *Curr Top Microbiol Immunol*, **133**, 89–113.

Walker, D.H., Wolff, H., et al. 1975. Comparative pathology of Lassa virus infection in monkeys, guinea pigs and *Mastomys natalensis*. *Bull WHO*, **52**, 523–34.

Walker, D.H., Johnson, K.M., et al. 1982a. Experimental infection of rhesus monkeys with Lassa virus and a closely related arenavirus, Mozambique virus. *J Infect Dis*, **146**, 360–80.

Walker, D.H., McCormick, J.B. and Johnson, K.M. 1982b. Pathologic and virologic study of fatal Lassa fever in man. *Am J Pathol*, **107**, 349–56.

Webb, P.A., Johnson, K.M., et al. 1973. Behavior of Machupo and Latino viruses in *Calomys callosus* from two geographic areas of Bolivia. In: Lehmann-Grube, F. (ed.), *Lymphocytic choriomeningitis virus and other arenaviruses*. New York: Springer Verlag, 314–22.

Webb, P.A., Justines, G. and Johnson, K.M. 1975. Infection of wild and laboratory animals with Machupo and Latino viruses. *Bull WHO*, **52**, 493–9.

Weber, E.B. and Buchmeier, M.J. 1988. Fine mapping of a peptide sequence containing an antigenic site conserved among arenaviruses. *Virology*, **164**, 30–8.

Weissenbacher, M.C., de Guerrero, L.B. and Boxaca, M.C. 1975. Experimental biology and pathogenesis of Junin virus infection in animals and in man. *Bull WHO*, **52**, 507–15.

Weissenbacher, M.C., Calello, M.A., et al. 1979. Argentine hemorrhagic fever: a primate model. *Intervirology*, **11**, 363–7.

Weissenbacher, M.C., Laguens, R.P. and Coto, C.E. 1987. Argentine hemorrhagic fever. *Curr Top Microbiol Immunol*, **133**, 79–116.

Welsh, R.M. 1987. Regulation and role of large granular lymphocytes in arenavirus infections. *Curr Top Microb Immunol*, **134**, 185–209.

Welsh, R.M. and Buchmeier, M.J. 1979. Protein analysis of defective interfering lymphocytic choriomeningitis virus and persistently infected cells. *Virology*, **96**, 503–15.

Wong, G.H.W., Bartlett, P.F., et al. 1984. Inducible expression of H-2 and Ia antigens in brain cells. *Nature (London)*, **310**, 688–91.

Woodrow, D., Ronco, P., et al. 1982. Severity of glomerulonephritis induced in different strains of suckling mice by infection with LCMV: correlation with amounts of endogenous interferon and circulating immune complexes. *J Pathol*, **138**, 325–36.

Wright, K.E., Salvato, M.S. and Buchmeier, M.J. 1989. Neutralizing epitopes of lymphocytic choriomeningitis virus are conformational and require both glycosylation and disulfide bonds for expression. *Virology*, **171**, 417–26.

Yokoyama, M., Zhang, J. and Whitton, J.L. 1995. DNA immunization confers protection against lethal lymphocytic choriomeningitis virus infection. *J Virol*, **69**, 2684–8.

Zinkernagel, R.M. and Doherty, P.C. 1973. Cytotoxic thymus derived lymphocytes in cerebrospinal fluid of mice with lymphocytic choriomeningitis. *J Exp Med*, **138**, 1266–9.

Zinkernagel, R.M. and Doherty, P.C. 1974. Restriction of *in vitro* T cell-mediated cytotoxicity in LCMV with a syngeneic or semiallogeneic system. *Nature (London)*, **248**, 701–2.

Zinkernagel, R.M. and Doherty, P.C. 1979. MHC-restricted cytotoxic T cells: studies on the biological role of polymorphic major transplantation antigens determining T-cell restriction-specificity, function and responsiveness. *Adv Immunol*, **27**, 51–177.

50

Filoviruses

HEINZ FELDMANN AND HANS-DIETER KLENK

PROPERTIES OF FILOVIRUSES

Introduction

In 1967, an outbreak of viral hemorrhagic fever occurred among laboratory workers in Europe exposed to tissues and blood from African green monkeys (*Cercopithecus aethiops*) imported from Uganda (Siegert et al. 1967; Martini and Siegert 1971). The virus, which had been isolated from a number of patients, has been called Marburg virus (MARV), after the city with the first reported cases. This episode marked the first identified outbreak of disease caused by a member of a group of viruses that have been classified in the family *Filoviridae*.

It was nearly a decade later, in 1976, when two other major filovirus outbreaks occurred in southern Sudan and northern Zaire (now Democratic Republic of the Congo). These outbreaks occurred simultaneously, but involved two biologically distinct species, Sudan ebolavirus (SEBOV) and Zaire ebolavirus (ZEBOV), of a new filovirus, Ebola virus (EBOV) (World Health Organization 1978a, 1978b; McCormick et al. 1983). In 1989, a third species of Reston ebolavirus (REBOV) emerged as the causative agent of an epizootic among a group of cynomolgus monkeys (*Macaca fascicularis*) imported from the Philippines into the United States (Jahrling et al. 1990). A similar epizootic occurred in 1992 when cynomolgus monkeys were imported into Italy from the same supplier who shipped the 1989 monkeys to the USA (World Health Organization 1992). In contrast to other human filoviruses, REBOV seemed to be less pathogenic, and no disease occurred in four humans who were infected with this species of EBOV (Peters et al.

1993). This is also reflected in a lower pathogenicity for nonhuman primates (Fisher-Hoch and Brammer 1992). EBOV was also detected in western Africa (Ivory Coast) in 1994, when a single human case was identified and a novel species Côte d'Ivoire ebolavirus (CIEBOV) was isolated (LeGuenno et al. 1995). This person was presumed to have been infected with EBOV while she was performing a necropsy on a wild chimpanzee, whose troop had undergone increased mortality, presumably due to EBOV disease.

In the past years EBOV and MARV have caused several major outbreaks of hemorrhagic fever in Central Africa. In 1995 EBOV re-emerged in the Democratic Republic of the Congo, causing a severe outbreak of hemorrhagic fever in the city of Kikwit and surrounding villages in Bandundu Province. A total of 315 cases of EBOV hemorrhagic fever were reported, of whom 244 died (77 percent) (World Health Organization 1995a). Molecular analyses identified the causative agent as ZEBOV, the glycoprotein gene differing by only 1.6 percent from the virus that caused the 1976 outbreak in northern Zaire (Democratic Republic of the Congo) (Sanchez et al. 1996). From 1994 to 1997 Gabon has suffered from three EBOV epidemics that occurred in the northeastern part of the country (Makokou). Virus isolation and sequence analysis demonstrated that all epidemics were caused by ZEBOV (Georges et al. 1999). In 1998, MARV emerged in the northern part of the Democratic Republic of the Congo near the border to Uganda and Sudan. More than 100 cases were reported with a mortality of about 70 percent (Muyembe-Tamfum 2000; Nichol 2000; Bausch et al. 2003). In October 2000, EBOV emerged in northeastern Uganda. The virus has been identified as species

SEBOV. Four hundred and twenty-five cases were confirmed with 224 deaths (World Health Organization 2001). There is currently (spring 2003) an EBOV outbreak ongoing in Congo-Brezaville that has so far claimed more than 100 human lives and has killed large parts of the local gorilla and chimpanzee population.

In addition to the major outbreaks described above, sporadic cases of filovirus hemorrhagic fever in humans have occurred in various parts of Africa. Incidences of filovirus disease in humans that have been confirmed by virus isolation are summarized in Table 50.1.

Classification

Filoviruses are classified in the order *Mononegavirales*, a large group of viruses that have nonsegmented negative-strand (NNS) RNA as their genomes. The family *Filoviridae* was created on the basis of unique morphologic, morphogenetic, physicochemical, and biological features of its members (Kiley et al. 1982). The family harbors two genera, *Marburgvirus* and *Ebolavirus*. The genus *Marburgvirus* is more homogeneous and consists of only a single species, but at least two different genetic lineages co-exist (Kiley et al. 1988; van Regenmortel et al. 2000; Sanchez et al. 1998a). The genus *Ebolavirus*, however, can be subdivided into four species: *Côte d'Ivoire*, *Reston*, *Sudan*, and *Zaire* (CIEBOV, REBOV, SEBOV, ZEBOV) (Feldmann et al. 1997; Sanchez et al. 1996; Feldmann et al. 2004). Nucleotide sequence comparison between MARV and EBOV shows only scattered similarities, which is in contrast to strong similarities seen between amino acid sequences of the structural proteins. Despite this amino acid similarity, there is no indication that there is any significant serological (antigenic) cross-reactivity between EBOV and MARV, but the species of EBOV share common epitopes (Richman et al. 1983; Feldmann et al. 1994). It may be that the nucleotide sequences of these agents diverged at some point in the distant past but the structural proteins have maintained similar structures and functions. Significant differences within the genus *Ebolavirus* were first noted from peptide and oligonucleotide mapping (Buchmeier et al. 1983; Cox et al. 1983), and have been confirmed by sequence analysis of the glycoprotein genes (Sanchez et al. 1996). The study by Sanchez et al. showed that all four species differ from each other to a comparable extent (37–41 percent nucleotide differences). This suggests that filoviruses have evolved into specific niches and may reflect a similar divergence in the natural hosts, assuming they have co-evolved.

Molecular analyses of the genomes of filoviruses have clearly demonstrated a close genetic relationship to the other families of the order, especially the *Rhabdoviridae* and *Paramyxoviridae*. All NNS RNA viruses share a similar genome organization: the more conserved genes that encode core and L proteins are located at the 3′ and 5′ ends, respectively, of the genomic RNA. In between these conserved areas is a more variable region that generally contains genes encoding envelope and certain membrane-associated proteins. The only exception occurs in the genomes of filoviruses, which contain a minor nucleocapsid-associated protein (VP30) in this region (Figure 50.1). Filovirus genomes are more complex than those of rhabdoviruses, and their organization is more like those of members of the genera *Respovirus* and *Morbillivirus* of *Paramyxoviridae*. This relationship was confirmed by comparisons of the deduced amino acid sequences of the nucleoprotein and L protein (Feldmann et al. 1993; Sanchez et al. 1993).

In terms of biohazard classification, filoviruses are classified as 'Biosafety Level 4' agents on the basis of their high mortality rate, person-to-person transmission, potential aerosol infectivity and absence of vaccines or chemotherapeutic agents. Maximum containment is required for all laboratory work with infectious material (Centers for Disease Control and Prevention 1993).

Morphology and structure

Filovirus virions are bacilliform in shape, but particles can also appear as branched, circular, U or 6-shaped and long filamentous forms. This morphology is unusual for viruses and has been important in the classification and nomenclature (Latin *filum*: thread) (Figure 50.1a,b). Virions vary greatly in length but show a uniform diameter of approximately 80 nm. Family members differ in length of virion particles but seem to be very similar in morphology. Peak infectivity has been associated with particles of 665 nm for MARV and 805 nm for EBOV. Virions are composed of a central core formed by a nucleocapsid or ribonucleoprotein (RNP) complex, which is surrounded by a lipid envelope derived from the host cell plasma membrane. Electron micrographs reveal an axial channel (10–15 nm in diameter) that is surrounded by a central dark layer (20 nm in diameter) and an outer helical layer (50 nm in diameter) with cross-striations of 5 nm intervals. Spikes, approximately 7 nm in diameter and spaced at intervals of approximately 10 nm are seen as globular structures on the surface of virions (Siegert et al. 1967; Peters et al. 1971; Murphy et al. 1978; Kiley et al. 1982).

The RNP complex is composed of a genomic RNA molecule and four of the seven virion structural proteins: the nucleoprotein (NP), virion structural protein (VP) 30, VP35, and the large (L) protein (Becker et al. 1998) (see Figure 50.1b). The genomic RNA has a molecular weight of 4 200 kDa and constitutes 1.1 percent of the virion mass (Regnery et al. 1980). The three remaining structural proteins are membrane-associated; the glycoprotein (GP) shows a type I transmembrane protein profile (Will et al. 1993; Sanchez et al. 1998b), while the VP24 and VP40 are probably located at the inner side of the

Table 50.1 *Outbreaks of filoviral hemorrhagic fever*

Location	Year	Virus/species	Cases (mortality)	Reference	Epidemiology
Germany/Yugoslavia	1967	MARV	32 (23%)[a]	Martini and Siegert (1971)	Imported monkeys from Uganda source of most human infections
Zimbabwe	1975	MARV	3 (33%)	Gear et al. (1975)	Unknown origin; index case infected in Zimbabwe; secondary cases were infected in South Africa
Southern Sudan	1976	SEBOV	284 (53%)	World Health Organization (1978a)	Unknown origin; spread mainly by close contact; nosocomial transmission and infection of medical staff
Northern Democratic Republic of the Congo	1976	ZEBOV	318 (88%)	World Health Organization (1978b)	Unknown origin; spread by close contact and by use of contaminated needles and syringes in hospitals
Tandala, Democratic Republic of the Congo	1977	ZEBOV	1 (100%)	Heymann et al. (1980)	Unknown origin; single case in missionary hospital; other cases may have occurred nearby
Southern Sudan	1979	SEBOV	34 (65%)	Baron et al. (1983)	Unknown origin; recurrent outbreak at the same site as the 1976 outbreak
Kenya	1980	MARV	2 (50%)	Smith et al. (1982)	Unknown origin; index case infected in western Kenya died, but physician secondarily infected survived
Kenya	1987	MARV	1 (100%)	Johnson et al. (1996)	Unknown origin; expatriate traveling in western Kenya
USA	1989/90	REBOV	4 (0%)	Jahrling et al. (1990)	Introduction of virus with imported monkeys from the Philippines; four humans asymptomatically infected
Italy	1992	REBOV	0 (0%)	World Health Organization (1992)	Introduction of virus with imported monkeys from the Philippines; no human infections associated
Ivory Coast	1994	CIEBOV	1 (0%)	LeGuenno et al. (1995)	Contact with chimpanzees; single case
Gabon	1994	ZEBOV	Unknown	Georges et al. (1999)	Several laboratory confirmed cases; outbreak associated with the death of nonhuman primates
Kikwit, Democratic Republic of the Congo	1995	ZEBOV	315 (77%)	World Health Organization (1995a)	Unknown origin; course of outbreak as in 1976
Gabon	1996	ZEBOV	50 (50%)	Georges et al. (1999)	Outbreak was linked to the butchering, transport and preparation for consumption of a dead chimpanzee
USA	1996	REBOV	0 (0%)	Rollin et al. (1999)	Introduction of virus with imported monkeys from the Philippines; no human infections associated
Gabon	1996/97	ZEBOV	60 (75%)	Georges et al. (1999)	Outbreak associated with the death of nonhuman primates
South Africa	1996	ZEBOV	2 (50%)	Richards et al. (2000)	Disease was introduced from Gabon
Northern Democratic Republic of the Congo	1998–2000	MARV	>100 (70%)	Bausch et al. (2003)	Outbreak with several introductions; cases are associated with illegal gold mining
Uganda	2000/01	SEBOV	425 (53%)	World Health Organization (2001)	Unknown origin; ongoing outbreak around Gulu close to the border to the Democratic Republic of the Congo
Congo-Brazzaville	2002	Ebola	>100 (90%)		Originating from large outbreak among gorillas and chimpanzees

a) Numbers include a primary case that has been diagnosed some years after the epidemic (Slenczka et al. unpublished data).

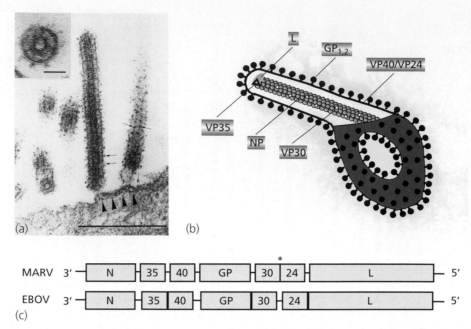

Figure 50.1 *Structure of filovirus particles.* **(a)** *Ultrathin sections obtained from primary cultures of human endothelial cells 3 days after infection with MARV analyzed by transmission electron microscopy. Particles consist of a nucleocapsid surrounded by a membrane in which spikes are inserted (arrows). The nucleocapsid contains a central channel (inset). The plasma membrane of infected cells is often thickened at locations where budding occurs (arrowheads) (bar, 0.5 μm; bar inset, 50 nm).* **(b)** *Schematic illustration of a filoviral particle. Four proteins are involved in nucleocapsid formation: polymerase or large (L) protein, nucleoprotein (NP), virion structural protein (VP) 30 and VP35. The glycoprotein (GP$_{1,2}$) is a type 1 transmembrane protein and anchored with the carboxy-terminal part in the virion membrane. Homotrimers of GP form the spikes on the virion surface (arrows in panel a). VP40 and VP24 are membrane-associated.* **(c)** *Schematic illustration of the filoviral genome. The genome consists of a single, negative-stranded, linear RNA molecule. G, glycoprotein gene; L, polymerase (L) gene; N, nucleoprotein gene; 24/30/35/40, virion structural protein (VP) genes; asterisk, gene overlap (altered from Feldmann and Kiley, 1999).*

membrane. Virus particles have a molecular weight of 3–6×10^8 and a density in potassium tartrate of 1.14 g/cm^3 (Kiley et al. 1988).

Genome structure and function

Genomes of filoviruses consist of a single negative-stranded linear RNA molecule (Kiley et al. 1982; Regnery et al. 1980). The RNA is non-infectious, does not contain a poly(A) tail, and upon entry into the cytoplasm of host cells is transcribed to generate poly-adenylated subgenomic mRNA species (Kiley et al. 1982; Feldmann et al. 1992; Sanchez et al. 1993). The complete nucleic acid sequences of two different isolates of MARV (Feldmann et al. 1992; Bukreyev et al. 1995), the Mayinga isolate of ZEBOV and two isolates of REBOV (Sanchez et al. 1993; Volchkov et al. 1999, 2000a) have been elucidated. Filovirus genomes are approximately 19 kb long (MARV, 19.1 kb; EBOV, 18.9 kb) and are significantly larger than those of other *Mononegavirales*. Genes have been delineated by transcriptional signals at their 3′ and 5′ ends that have been identified by their conservation and by analysis of mRNA sequences. The following order is characteristic for filoviruses: 3′-(leader)-N-VP35–VP40–GP–VP30-VP24-L-(trailer)-5′ (Figure 50.1c).

Genes of filoviruses are usually separated from one another by intergenic regions that vary in length and nucleotide composition. However, some genes overlap, especially those of EBOV, and the positions and numbers of overlaps vary among filoviruses. ZEBOV possesses three overlaps, between the VP35 and VP40, GP and VP30, and VP24 and L genes, whereas MARV isolates have only one overlap, involving the VP30 and VP24 genes (Figure 50.1c). The length of the overlaps is centered on five highly conserved nucleotides within the transcriptional signals (3′-UAAUU-5′) that are found at the internal ends of the conserved sequences. Transcriptional start signals are conserved among filoviruses, and the sequence 3′-CUNCNUNUAAUU-5′ represents the consensus motif. Transcriptional stop signals are identical for all genes (3′-UAAUUCUUUUU-5′) except the *VP40* gene of MARV (Feldmann et al. 1992) and the *L* gene of ZEBOV (Volchkov et al. 1999) (see Figure 50.3). Most genes tend to possess long noncoding sequences at their 3′ and/or 5′ ends which contribute to the increased length of the genome. Extragenic sequences are found at the 3′ (leader) and 5′ (trailer) ends of the genome. Those leader and trailer sequences are complementary to one another at the extreme ends (Kiley et al. 1986; Feldmann et al. 1992; Feldman and Kiley 1999; Volchkov et al. 1999), a feature that is shared by all NNS RNA viruses.

Polypeptides

NUCLEOPROTEIN

The nucleoprotein (NP) is encoded by the 3'-most end of the linear RNA genome. The NP from various filoviruses differ slightly in their electrophoretic mobility patterns, ranging from 95 kDa (MARV) to 105 kDa (ZEBOV). The molecular weight calculated from the deduced amino acid sequences of the corresponding genes of MARV (695 amino acids) and EBOV (739 amino acids) are 78 kDa and 83 kDa, respectively, and the differences in their lengths is related to the variable C termini of the protein (Sanchez and Kiley 1989; Sanchez et al. 1992). The NP proteins possess an unusually high molecular weight compared to other NNS virus nucleocapsid proteins which range from 42 to 62 kDa. The NP protein is the major structural phosphoprotein, and only the phosphorylated form of the protein is incorporated into virions. This implies that phosphorylation is needed to form stable virion RNP complexes (Elliott et al. 1985; Elliott et al. 1993b; Becker et al. 1994). NP is the major component of the RNP complex and is tightly bound to it (see Figure 50.1b).

VP35: POLYMERASE COFACTOR (PHOSPHOPROTEIN EQUIVALENT)

The *VP35* gene encodes a protein that ranges from 329 amino acids for MARV to 340 for ZEBOV (Feldmann et al. 1992; Bukreyev et al. 1993; Sanchez et al. 1993). The association of this protein in the RNP complex is much weaker than that of the NP and VP30 (Elliott et al. 1985; Kiley et al. 1988). Within the complex VP35 interacts with NP and L (see Figure 50.1b) and the three proteins seem to be the key component of the transcription and replication machinery (Becker et al. 1998). Hydropathy plots of MARV and EBOV VP35 showed similar profiles and a prominent common hydrophilic domain in close proximity to the N-termini. This region may be involved in template binding. Data obtained with an artificial replication system revealed that VP35 is functionally equivalent to a phosphoprotein of *Mononegavirales* (Mühlberger et al. 1998, 1999). In contrast to other phosphoproteins of paramyxoviruses and rhabdoviruses, however, this protein is only weakly phophorylated (Becker and Mühlberger 1999). Finally, VP35 has been shown to function as a type I interferon antagonist (Basler et al. 2000) by interfering with IRF3 phosphorylation (Basler et al. 2003).

VP40: MATRIX PROTEIN

The VP40 of filoviruses is 303 and 326 amino acids long for MARV and ZEBOV, respectively (Feldmann et al. 1992; Sanchez et al. 1993; Bukreyev et al. 1993). This protein, which is abundant in virion particles, is not associated with the RNP complex and behaves like a membrane-associated protein when analyzed after nonionic detergent treatment of virion particles (Elliott et al. 1985; Kiley et al. 1988). VP40 is nonglycosylated, shows a predominantly hydrophobic profile, and functions as the matrix protein (see Figure 50.1b). VP40 is essential for assembly, and its crystal structure shows that it is composed of two structurally similar β-sandwich domains (Dessen et al. 2000; Ruigrok et al. 2000). The monomeric form of VP40 can be induced to change its conformation into oligomeric ring-like structures, which may play an important role in virus assembly and budding (Scianimanico et al. 2000). VP40 octamers have specific RNA-binding properties suggesting that this protein has additional functions in the life cycle besides promoting virion formation (Gomis Rüth et al. 2003).

GLYCOPROTEIN

The glycoprotein (GP) is encoded in the fourth gene, and is the only glycosylated structural protein of virions (Figure 50.1b). GP of MARV and ZEBOV are 681 and 676 amino acids in length, respectively (Will et al. 1993; Sanchez et al. 1993; Volchkov et al. 1995). They are type I transmembrane proteins and can be subdivided into a large ectodomain, a lipid membrane spanning domain of approximately 30 amino acids, and a short cytoplasmic tail of four (EBOV) and eight amino acids (MARV). GP undergoes a complex sequence of processing events in the endoplasmic reticulum (ER). This includes the removal of the signal peptide (Will et al. 1993; Sanchez et al. 1998b), N-glycosylation (Feldmann et al. 1991, 1994; Becker et al. 1996; Sanchez et al. 1998b), and oligomerization (Feldmann et al. 1991; Sanchez et al. 1998b). ER processing is followed by acylation in a pre-Golgi compartment (Funke et al. 1995; Ito et al. 2001), and by O-glycosylation and maturation of N-glycans in the Golgi apparatus (Feldmann et al. 1991, 1994; Geyer et al. 1992; Will et al. 1993; Becker et al. 1996). Depending on the host cell, there are wide variations in the amount of neuraminic acid present on MARV GP (Feldmann et al. 1994). Finally, GP is proteolytically cleaved into a larger amino (GP_1) and smaller carboxy-terminal (GP_2) subunit in the trans-Golgi network by a subtilisin-like proprotein convertase, most likely furin (Volchkov et al. 1998a, 2000b) (see Figure 50.2).

The mature envelope glycoprotein ($GP_{1,2}$) is able to form spikes on membrane surfaces without the need of other viral proteins in this maturation process (Volchkov et al. 1998b). It is anchored in the membrane via a carboxy-terminal hydrophobic domain of GP_2. The middle region of $GP_{1,2}$ is variable, extremely hydrophilic, and carries the bulk of N- and O-glycans that account for more than one third of the molecular weight of the mature protein (Geyer et al. 1992; Will et al. 1993; Feldmann et al. 1991; Becker et al. 1996). Oligosaccharide side chains differ in their terminal sialylation patterns, which seem to be isolate-, as well as cell line-dependent (Feldmann et al. 1994). Detailed structural analyses of carbohydrates are available for MARV only

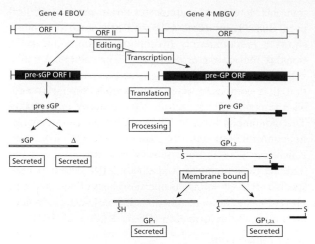

Figure 50.2 *Transcription and expression strategies of the glycoprotein genes of filoviruses. In contrast to MARV, the EBOV surface glycoprotein GP is encoded in two overlapping reading frames (ORF I and II), and expression of GP occurs through transcriptional editing. ORF I encodes for the precursor of the secreted small glycoprotein (pre-sGP) that is expressed from unedited transcripts and post-translationally cleaved into the soluble products sGP and Δ-peptide. Mature GP (GP$_{1,2}$) consists of the disulfide-linked (S–S) subunits GP$_1$ and GP$_2$. Significant amounts of GP$_1$, sGP, Δ-peptide, and GP$_{1,2Δ}$ are released from cells, in soluble form (altered from Klenk et al. 1998).*

(Geyer et al. 1992). Comparison of amino acid sequences shows conservation at the amino- and carboxy-terminal ends in which the two hydrophobic

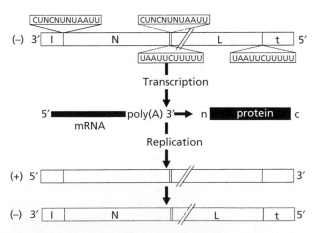

Figure 50.3 *The mode of transcription and replication of filoviruses, based on the data available to date. Each gene on the linear arranged nonsegmented (−)-sense genome is flanked by conserved transcriptional start (3'-CUNCNUNUAAUU-5'; indicated above) and termination signals (3'-UAAUUCUUUUU-5'; indicated underneath). Transcription starts at the 3' end of the (−)-sense genome and leads to polyadenylated mRNA species. For replication a full-length (+)-sense antigenome is synthesized which serves as the template for the synthesis of progeny (−)-sense RNA. c, carboxy-terminal end of proteins; l, 3' untranslated region (leader); L, viral RNA-dependent RNA polymerase; n, amino-terminal end of proteins; N, nucleoprotein; poly(A), polyadenylation of mRNA species; t, 5' untranslated region (trailer).*

domains (signal peptide, membrane anchor) and most of the highly conserved cysteine residues are located. The two most carboxy-terminal cysteine residues seem to be acylated (Funke et al. 1995; Ito et al. 2001). GP$_2$ contains a sequence of several uncharged and hydrophobic amino acids at a distance of 22 (EBOV) or 91 (MARV) amino acids from the cleavage site which bears some structural similarity to the fusion peptides of retroviruses (Gallaher 1996; Volchkov et al. 2000b). The special arrangement of the cysteine residues in the molecule allows an intramolecular disulfide bridge formation between the two cleavage products which results in a stem region consisting of GP$_1$ and GP$_2$ and a crownlike domain on the top formed by GP$_1$ carrying the mass of the carbohydrate side chains (Jeffers et al. 2002). Mature GP$_{1,2}$ is a trimer consisting of disulfide-bonded GP$_{1,2}$ molecules (Feldmann et al. 1991; Sanchez et al. 1998b). X-ray crystallography demonstrated that the central structural feature of the GP$_2$ ectodomain is a long triple-stranded coiled coil followed by a disulfide-bonded loop which reverses the chain direction and connects to an α helix packed antiparallel to the core helices (Weissenhorn et al. 1998a, 1998b; Malashkevich et al. 1999). During maturation GP$_1$ is partly shed in monomeric form after release of its disulfide linkage to the transmembrane subunit GP$_2$ (Volchkov et al. 1998b). Cleavage by the metalloprotease TACE results in shedding of the entire ectodomain (GP$_{1,2Δ}$) (Dolnik et al. 2004).

In general, filovirus GPs lack significant homologies with envelope proteins of other viruses. However, a region of 26 amino acids (and less conserved surrounding sequences) in the external domain in close proximity to the transmembrane region shows significant homology to an immunosuppressive domain in envelope proteins of several retroviruses (Volchkov et al. 1992; Will et al. 1993; Bukreyev et al. 1995). This region is also the most conserved sequence in the GPs of MARV and EBOV. It is not known whether this sequence in filovirus GPs has immunosuppressive properties. As the only surface protein of virions GP functions in receptor binding and fusion (see Virus entry). Furthermore, GP is discussed (see Immune responses) as an important target for the host immune response.

VP30: MINOR NUCLEOPROTEIN

The fifth gene encodes VP30, a protein intimately associated with the RNP complex (Elliott et al. 1985; Kiley et al. 1988) (Figure 50.1b). The protein has a length of 260 and 281 amino acids with ZEBOV and MARV, respectively (Feldmann et al. 1992; Sanchez et al. 1993). VP30 is the second strongest phosphorylated protein of virions (Elliott et al. 1985, 1993b; Becker and Mühlberger 1999). Using an artificial reverse genetic system (Mühlberger et al. 1999), it was shown that VP30 is essential for EBOV-specific transcription, but not replication. VP30 seems to be involved in transcription initiation, most likely by inhibiting pausing of the transcription complex at the RNA structure of the first transcription start site. For transcription of the following genes VP30 seems to be nonessential (Weik et al. 2002).

VP24: MEMBRANE-ASSOCIATED PROTEIN OF UNKNOWN FUNCTION

VP24 is expressed from the sixth gene, and is 253 and 251 amino acids long in MARV and ZEBOV, respectively (Feldmann et al. 1992; Sanchez et al. 1993). Unlike VP40, VP24 is not completely removed from the RNP complex under isotonic conditions (Elliott et al. 1985; Kiley et al. 1988). VP24 presumably serves as a second matrix protein (see Figure 50.1b).

LARGE PROTEIN (RNA-DEPENDENT RNA POLYMERASE)

The large (L) protein is encoded at the 5′ end of the linear genome and has a predicted molecular weight of 267 kDa (2 331 amino acids) for MARV (Mühlberger et al. 1992) and 253 kDa (2 212) for ZEBOV (Volchkov et al. 1999). Computer-assisted comparison revealed significant homologies to L proteins of other NNS RNA viruses. Homologies are mainly located in the amino-terminal half of the protein and concentrated within three common motifs, named boxes A, B, and C. Other common features are a high content of leucine and isoleucine residues, a large positive net charge, clusters of basic amino acids interspersed with nonbasic ones, putative ATP-binding sites, two neighboring cysteine residues located in the C-terminal half of the protein, and the genome localization of the encoding gene. A highly conserved peptide motif, -GDNQ-, is located at the carboxy-terminal end of domain B and is flanked by hydrophobic amino acid residues. Similar motifs with alterations in the first amino acid have been described and discussed as catalytic sites for some RNA-dependent RNA polymerases of plant, animal, and bacterial viruses. Studies using an artificial reverse genetic system (Mühlberger et al. 1998, 1999) identified the L protein as the viral RNA-dependent RNA polymerase (see Figure 50.1b).

NONSTRUCTURAL GLYCOPROTEINS

The secreted glycoprotein precursor (pre-sGP) is the primary expression product of gene 4 of EBOV (Volchkov et al. 1995; Sanchez et al. 1996). For ZEBOV it has a length of 364 amino acids and shares the amino-terminal 294 amino acids with the transmembrane GP. The different carboxy terminus (69 amino acids) contains many charged residues, as well as conserved cysteine residues. sGP undergoes several co- and posttranslational processing events, such as signal peptide cleavage, glycosylation, oligomerization, and proteolytic cleavage. The limiting step during maturation and transport seems to be oligomerization in the ER (Volchkova et al. 1998, 1999). After oligomerization sGP is transported into the Golgi compartments where glycosy-

lation is completed and posttranslational cleavage by furin into the mature form sGP and a small peptide, called Δ-peptide, occurs (Volchkova et al. 1999). Due to the lack of a transmembrane anchor mature sGP is efficiently secreted from infected cells, a process which is independent of proteolytic cleavage. sGP appears as a disulfide-linked homodimer which shows an antiparallel orientation (Sanchez et al. 1998b; Volchkova et al. 1998). Dimerization is due to an intermolecular disulfide linkage between the amino and carboxy-terminal cysteine residues at positions 53 and 306, respectively. The remaining four highly conserved cysteine residues at the amino-terminus seem to be involved in the intramolecular folding of monomers (Volchkova et al. 1998).

Δ-peptide, the small cleavage product of pre-sGP, varies in length between 40 and 48 amino acids for the different EBOV. Its molecular mass of approximately 10 to 14 kDa is significantly larger than the one predicted from the amino acid sequence (approximately 4.7 kDa). The difference is due to the attachment of several O-glycans that carry terminal sialic acids. In this respect it differs from sGP which seems to mainly carry N-linked carbohydrates. As with mature sGP the peptide is secreted from infected cells (Volchkova et al. 1999).

The small secreted glycoprotein (ssGP) of EBOV resembles a natural carboxy-terminal truncated variant of sGP and is generated from gene 4 by transcriptional editing. Due to the lack of a transmembrane anchor and carboxy-terminal cysteine residues ssGP is secreted in monomeric form (Volchkov et al. 1995; Volchkova et al. 1998).

FILOVIRUS REPLICATION

Virus growth in cell cultures

The Vero cell line, especially the E6 clone, is most widely used for virus isolation and propagation. Primary virus isolation has also been successful in MA-104 and SW13 cells (McCormick et al. 1983; Jahrling et al. 1990). A variety of other cells have been tested as substrates for filovirus replication (van der Groen et al. 1978; McCormick et al. 1983; Peters et al. 1992). These include human microvascular endothelial cells (HMEC-1), primary cultures of human umbilical cord vein endothelial cells (HUVEC), and human peripheral blood monocytes/macrophages (Schnittler et al. 1993; Feldmann et al. 1996a).

MARV and ZEBOV cause lytic infections in cell culture. SEBOV and REBOV replicate more slowly upon primary isolation, and the cytopathic effect (CPE) is not as prominent as with ZEBOV. The course of infection in tissue culture can be monitored by an indirect immunofluorescence assay (IFA) or by plaque assay. In cases of little or no CPE, reverse transcriptase-polymerase chain reaction (RT-PCR) on viral RNA isolated from infected cells and tissue culture supernatants can be helpful for quantification (Schnittler et al. 1993; Sanchez and Feldmann 1996).

Viral subgenomic RNA synthesis in tissue culture is detectable as early as 3 h after infection, reaches a maximum by 18 h, and declines thereafter. CPE is not seen before 48 h after infection. The first subgenomic RNA to be detected is NP-specific which reaches levels sufficient to produce protein by 7 h after infection. All proteins are detectable by in vitro translation of poly-adenylated RNA isolated 18 h after infection, thereafter the yield of translation products decreases. Polymerase chain reaction (PCR) assays of genomic RNA of MARV particles in supernatants of infected cells indicated that the replication cycle is approximately 12 h (Sanchez and Kiley 1987; Schnittler et al. 1993; Mühlberger et al. 1996).

Virus entry

The filovirus GP mediates receptor binding and subsequent fusion with susceptible cells (Takada et al. 1997; Wool-Levis and Bates 1998; Yang et al. 1998; Chan et al. 2000b). There is evidence that MARV uses the asialo glycoprotein receptor to infect hepatocytes (Becker et al. 1995). For EBOV, it was suggested that integrins, especially the beta 1 group, might interact with the glycoprotein and perhaps be involved in virus entry (Takada et al. 2000). Other studies indicate that the folate receptor alpha serves as cofactor for entry of EBOV and MARV (Chan et al. 2001). A similar role has been postulated for C-type lectins (Alvarez et al. 2002). Fusion activity has never been experimentally demonstrated using standard methodology. Early post-infection filovirus particles are associated with coated pits along the plasma membrane indicating endocytosis as a possible mechanism for entry (Geisbert and Jahrling 1995). This is supported by studies which employed lysosomotropic agents (Mariyankova et al. 1993; Chan et al. 2000b). A fusion peptide was postulated for ZEBOV in a distance of 22 amino acids from the cleavage site (amino acids 524–539) (Gallaher 1996). Recently it was demonstrated that the same peptide induces fusion with liposomes (Ruiz-Argüello et al. 1998). This together with mutational analysis of the putative fusion domain (Ito et al. 1999) offers compelling support for a fusion peptide role for this conserved hydrophobic region in the EBOV GP. For MARV a similar putative fusion domain can be found at a distance of 91 amino acids from the cleavage site (Volchkov et al. 2000b). Receptor binding and fusion are followed by uncoating, a mechanism which is unknown.

Transcription, translation, and genome replication

Filovirus transcription and replication take place in the cytoplasm of infected cells, and the mechanisms resemble those of other NNS RNA viruses. As with other members of the order *Mononegavirales*, transcription is believed to start at the extreme 3′ end, leading to the synthesis of a short (+)-leader sequence that is terminated when the first transcription start site is encountered (Figure 50.3). The seven structural genes are subsequently transcribed to produce seven mono-cistronic polyadenylated subgenomic RNA species. There is no evidence for larger amounts of bi- or multi-cistronic subgenomic RNA species (Sanchez and Kiley 1987; Feldmann et al. 1992; Sanchez et al. 1993). Analyses of MARV mRNA species have shown that the 5′ ends of the transcripts are two bases shorter than previously published (Mühlberger et al. 1996). All start signals of filovirus genes contain the consensus sequence 3′-CUNCNUNUAAUU-5′. The 3′ ends of the transcripts carry a poly(A) tail generated by a stuttering mechanism of the viral polymerase at a run of five to six uridine residues located at the 5′ end of all transcription stop signals. Therefore, the sequence 3′-UAAUU-CUUUUU(U)-5′ serves as a transcription stop and poly-adenylation signal. Both signals carry the pentamer 3′-UAAUU-5′, a unique feature among NNS RNA viruses. The function of the pentamer is unknown, but it could serve as the recognition site for positioning the polymerase complex. The surrounding semiconserved sequences may then mediate the exact initiation of transcription and termination/polyadenylation events.

Filovirus transcripts start precisely at the first nucleotide of the highly conserved transcriptional start signal. They contain unusually long untranslated regions especially at the 3′ ends. The 5′ end untranslated regions can build a stable secondary structure with the conserved nucleotides located in the stem region of a hairpin. Nucleotide substitutions in the conserved 5′ regions are accompanied by compensatory mutations of the complementary nucleotide thus leading to conservation of the secondary structure. Hairpin formation might play a role in transcript stability and ribosome binding (Sanchez et al. 1993; Mühlberger et al. 1996). The role of gene overlaps in regulation of transcription is unknown. Sanchez et al. (1993) proposed that, following mRNA synthesis, transcription is reinitiated by reposition of the polymerase at the downstream start site. This 'back up' mechanism is supported by the finding that attenuation of filovirus genes with start sites in overlaps does not occur to any higher degree, as has been noted for a much larger overlap found in the respiratory syncytial virus genome. Alternatively, the polymerase may occasionally terminate transcription without polyadenylation at the overlap and initiate transcription of the downstream gene, but there is no evidence for detectable levels of transcripts lacking poly(A) tails (see Figure 50.3).

The switch mechanism between transcription and replication is unknown, but as with other NNS viruses, synthesis of the NP protein could be a key factor.

Encapsidation and polymerase complex entry sites are probably located on the leader sequence, and the fact that the ends of the genome are complementary suggests a single identical encapsidation site on genome and antigenome. This would function for both transcription as well as replication (Feldmann et al. 1992). Replication involves a full-length (+)-strand antigenome which serves as the template for synthesis of (−)-strand genome molecules. Encapsidated genomic RNA forms nucleocapsids that go into the formation of new infectious virions at the cell surface (Figure 50.3).

In the past years artificial replication systems have been developed for MARV and EBOV which allowed more detailed study of the requirements for transcription and replication (Mühlberger et al. 1998, 1999). It could be demonstrated that NP, VP35, and L are essential and sufficient for transcription, as well as replication and encapsidation of MARV monocistronic monigenomes, whereas EBOV-specific transcription was also dependent on the presence of VP30 systems (see Polypeptides). Recently, the successful generation of infectious clones for ZEBOV was reported which will finally allow the determination of the critical steps in virus replication (Volchkov et al. 2001; Neumann et al. 2002).

The organization and transcription of the GP genes of EBOV is unusual, and involves transcriptional editing. EBOV GP genes possess two overlapping reading frames (Figure 50.2). Full-length GP is expressed by the addition of a single nontemplated adenosine residue at a run of seven uridine residues on the vRNA template (Volchkov et al. 1995; Sanchez et al. 1996). The primary gene product is a small nonstructural glycoprotein (sGP) that is secreted from infected cells (see Nonstructural glycoproteins). In addition, virus variants have been found after passaging in tissue culture and animals that express full-length GP from a single open reading frame. Those variants acquired a mutation that added a single uridine nucleotide at the editing site connecting the GP open reading frame (Sanchez et al. 1993; Volchkov et al. 1995). The MARV GP is expressed in a single frame and the gene does not contain sequences favoring mechanisms such as editing or frameshifting (Will et al. 1993; Bukreyev et al. 1995).

Virus assembly and exit

Virions usually bud at the plasma membrane, and the budding process is probably mediated at membrane locations where GP is incorporated. The cytoplasmic tail of GP is thought to interact with VP40 or VP24, or both. VP40 or VP24 may mediate the linkage between the RNP complexes and the transmembrane protein GP (see also Polypeptides). Particles mature preferentially in a vertical mode, but budding via the longitudinal axis has also been observed. In macrophages, budding has also been observed at intracytoplasmic

membranes surrounding vacuoles which form during infection (Feldmann et al. 1996a). VP40 appears to be targeted by 'late domains' to multivesicular bodies that may play an important role in virus assembly (Kolesnikova et al. 2002; Jasenosky and Kawaoka 2004).

CLINICAL AND PATHOLOGICAL ASPECTS

Epidemiology

It is generally accepted that human filovirus outbreaks are of a zoonotic nature. Guinea pigs, primates, bats, and hard ticks have been suspected to be natural hosts, but the search for filoviruses in these and many other wild species was unsuccessful. Studies on experimentally infected wild animals have shown that fruit and insectivorous bats support replication and circulation of high titers of EBOV without necessarily becoming ill, indicating that bats could serve as the reservoir host (Swanepoel et al. 1996).

MARV and the SEBOV and ZEBOV appear to be indigenous to the African continent, and both EBOV species have been isolated from human patients only in Africa. MARV has been isolated from human patients in Africa and Europe, though the European cases were caused by a virus originating from Africa (Martini and Siegert 1971). The REBOV outbreak provided the first evidence for the presence of a filovirus outside Africa (Hayes et al. 1992). Serological studies (IFA) among captive macaques in the Philippines indicated that the source of REBOV might be wild nonhuman primates. However, IFA-detected antibodies seem to be spurious, and latent infections in nonhuman primates have never been observed (Fisher-Hoch et al. 1992).

Serological studies suggest that filoviruses are endemic in many central African regions (summarized in Feldmann et al. 1996b, 2003). Serosurveys in other countries, such as Germany, the United States, and the Philippines, have identified antibodies to filoviruses in humans as well. Serological data based on IFA are of only limited reliability, as nonspecific reactivity has been observed when filovirus antigens are used. Nevertheless, it is possible that subclinical infections caused by known or unknown filoviruses or a closely related virus (paramyxovirus?) may be responsible for a certain amount of the seropositivity detected in human populations.

Clinical manifestation

MODE OF TRANSMISSION

Person-to-person transmission by intimate contact is the main route of infection in human outbreaks. The EBOV outbreaks in 1976 and 1995 and the MARV outbreak in 1967 all involved nosocomial transmission via contaminated syringes and needles. Therefore, extreme care should be taken with blood, secretions, and excretions from infected patients. On the basis of experiences from these episodes, isolation of patients, use of strict barrier nursing procedures (e.g. protective clothing, respirator), and measures to handle and disinfect contaminated material promptly are sufficient to prevent transmission to healthcare workers. Transmission by droplets and small-particle aerosols have been observed in outbreaks among experimentally infected and quarantined imported monkeys. This is confirmed by identification of filovirus particles in alveoli of naturally and experimentally infected monkeys and humans (Peters et al. 1991; Pokhodyaeu et al. 1991; Geisbert et al. 1992; Zaki and Peters 1997; Zaki and Goldsmith 1999). Epidemiological studies of human outbreaks, however, indicate that aerosols and droplets do not seem to be an important route of transmission.

CLINICAL SYNDROME

The onset of the disease is sudden with fever, chills, headache, myalgia, and anorexia. This may be followed by symptoms such as abdominal pain, sore throat, nausea, vomiting, cough, arthralgia, diarrhea, and pharyngeal and conjunctival injection (Figure 50.4). Patients are dehydrated, apathetic, disoriented, and may develop a characteristic, nonpuritic, maculopapular centripetal rash associated with varying degrees of erythema and desquamate by day 5–7 of the illness. Hemorrhagic

manifestations develop during the peak of the illness; they are of prognostic value for the disease. Bleeding into the gastrointestinal tract is most prominent beside petechia and hemorrhages from puncture wounds and mucous membranes. Laboratory parameters are less characteristic, but the following findings are associated with the disease: leukopenia (as low as 1 000/μl), left shift with atypical lymphocytes, thrombocytopenia (50 000–100 000/μl), markedly elevated serum transaminase levels (AST typically exceeding ALT), hyperproteinemia, and proteinuria. Prothrombin and partial thromboplastin times are prolonged and fibrin split products are detectable. In a later stage, secondary bacterial infection may lead to elevated white blood counts.

Nonfatal cases have fever for about 5–9 days; fatal cases develop clinical signs early during infection and death commonly occurs between day 6 and 16, due to hemorrhage and hypovolemic shock. Mortality is high and varies between 22 and 88 percent depending on the virus. The highest rate has been reported for ZEBOV; REBOV seems to possess a very low pathogenicity for humans or may even be apathogenic.

Convalescence is prolonged and sometimes associated with myelitis, recurrent hepatitis, psychosis, or uveitis. There is an increased risk of abortion for pregnant women, and clinical observations indicate a high death rate for children of infected mothers (Martini and Siegert 1971; Pattyn 1978; Baron et al. 1983; Peters et al. 1996; Peters and LeDuc 1999; Sanchez et al. 2001).

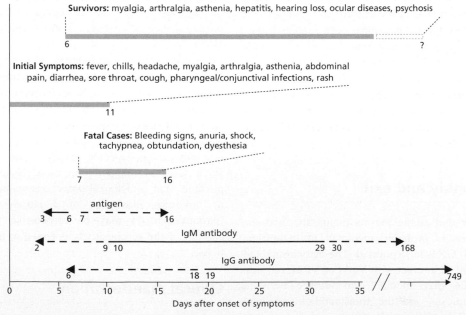

Figure 50.4 *Clinical course of filoviral hemorrhagic fever. The scheme presents an average clinical course of Ebola hemorrhagic fever. Key: gray bars, time interval of symptoms; black lines, period in which clinical samples are most likely be tested positive (antigen, IgM, or IgG antibodies); dashed lines, period in which a mix of positive and negative results can be obtained (antigen, IgM or IgG antibodies); numbers, days post onset of symptoms (adapted from Bwaka et al. (1999) and Rowe et al. (1999)).*

Pathology

PATHOLOGY IN EXPERIMENTAL ANIMALS

Monkeys, guinea pigs, suckling mice, and hamsters have been experimentally infected with filoviruses. MARV and ZEBOV are highly virulent for most of these species. SEBOV and REBOV are less virulent, often causing a self-limited infection in guinea pigs and monkeys.

The incubation period for rhesus and African green monkeys inoculated with MARV and ZEBOV is 4–16 days. High titers of virus can be detected in liver, spleen, lymph nodes, and lungs by onset of clinical symptoms. All these organs, especially liver, show severe necrosis due to virus replication in parenchymal cells. Little inflammatory response at those sites is typical. Interstitial hemorrhage occurs and is most prominent in the gastrointestinal tract. In infected nonhuman primates, thrombocytopenia has been found accompanied by aggregation disorders of the remaining platelets in response to agonists such as ADP and collagen (Murphy et al. 1971; Fisher-Hoch et al. 1985). Histopathological damage of the target organs is at odds with serum transferase levels showing increases in AST and ALT (AST:ALT = 7:1). This argues against hepatocellular dysfunction and raises the question for extrahepatic targets (Peters et al. 1996). Morphologic studies on REBOV-infected monkeys revealed extensive virus replication in tissue macrophages, interstitial fibroblasts of many organs, circulating monocytes/macrophages and less frequently in endothelial cells, hepatocytes, adrenal corticoid cells, and renal tubular epithelium (Geisbert et al. 1992). Similar results have been reported from monkeys experimentally infected with MARV and ZEBOV (Ryabchikova et al. 1999).

PATHOLOGY IN HUMANS

In fatal cases, generalized hemorrhage is found macroscopically in most organ systems. Microscopic changes include focal necrosis in liver, lymphatic organs, kidneys, testes, and ovaries. The liver, although always involved with large eosinophilic intracytoplasmic inclusion bodies in hepatocytes and Councilman-like bodies within necrotic foci, is not the site of massive, potentially fatal necrosis. Generalized lymphoid necrosis is characteristic for the disease, and renal tubular necrosis is commonly found in agonal stages. A diffuse encephalitis, as described for many viral infections, has been observed. In addition, focal hemorrhages have been observed. The clotting system is activated and intravascular fibrin thrombi have been observed. Viral antigen can be detected in many organs, predominantly in liver, kidneys, spleen, and adrenal glands. Viral persistence has been demonstrated for filoviruses by antigen/RNA detection or isolation from liver biopsy material, anterior chamber of the eye (4–5 weeks), and semen (12 weeks), despite an apparently normal immune response (e.g. Martini and Siegert 1971; Pattyn 1978; Peters et al. 1996; Rowe et al. 1999; Sanchez et al. 2001).

Pathophysiology

Pathophysiological changes that make filovirus infections so devastating are only partially understood. Clinical and biochemical findings support the anatomical observations of extensive liver involvement, renal damage, changes in vascular permeability, and activation of the clotting cascade. The visceral organ necrosis is a consequence of virus replication in parenchymal cells. However, no organ, not even the liver, shows sufficient damage to account for death. The role of disseminated intravascular coagulation (DIC) in pathogenesis is still controversial, because laboratory confirmation of DIC in human infections has never been demonstrated. In nonhuman primates the intrinsic clotting pathway is most affected, whereas the extrinsic pathway is spared.

Laboratory parameters in the crucial early stage of filovirus hemorrhagic fever, such as high AST/ALT ratio, normal bilirubin levels, and marked lymphopenia followed by a dramatic neutrophilia with left shift, suggest extrahepatic targets in the infection (Peters et al. 1996). As with some hemorrhagic fever with renal syndrome, dengue hemorrhagic fever, and Lassa fever, fluid distribution problems and platelet abnormalities are dominant clinical manifestations indicating dysfunction or damage of endothelial cells and platelets. Post mortem, there is little monocyte/macrophage infiltration in sites of parenchymal necrosis suggesting that also a dysfunction of white blood cells, such as macrophages, occurs. Morphological studies on REBOV-infected monkeys from the 1989 epizootic (Geisbert et al. 1992) and monkeys experimentally infected with ZEBOV (Ryabchikova et al. 1999) showed that monocytes/macrophages and fibroblasts are the preferred sites of virus replication in early stages, whereas other cell types may become involved as the disease progresses. Human macrophages in culture are also sensitive to infection resulting in massive production of infectious virus and cell lysis (Feldmann et al. 1996a). Although the studies on infected nonhuman primates did not identify endothelial cells as sites of massive virus replication, in vitro studies and investigations on human cases with EBOV hemorrhagic fever clearly demonstrated that endothelial cells are suitable targets for virus replication (Schnittler et al. 1993). Here, infection leads to complete cell lysis indicating that damage of endothelial cells may occur during infection. Recently cell destruction upon expression of EBOV glycoprotein was reported (Chan et al. 2000a; Yang et al. 2000).

Supernatants of MARV-infected monocyte/macrophage cultures can increase paraendothelial permeability in an in vitro model (Feldmann et al. 1996a). Examination for mediators in those supernatants revealed increased levels of secreted cytokines and chemokines, especially TNF-α. These data support a mechanism of a mediator-induced vascular instability that leads to increased permeability and a shock syndrome that is seen in severe cases. Hemorrhagic manifestations, however, are also likely to be caused in part by the damage inflicted upon the reticuloendothelial system as a direct result of massive virus replication. Hemorrhages occur later in infection and could be due to an extended damage which cannot be repaired by wound-healing mechanisms. The bleeding tendency is reinforced by a decrease in blood pressure as a common consequence of shock. The combination of viral replication in endothelial cells and virus-induced cytokine release from macrophages may also promote a distinct proinflammatory endothelial phenotype that then triggers the coagulation cascade (Schnittler and Feldmann 1999).

Immune responses

The mechanisms of recovery from filovirus infections in humans and wild as well as laboratory animals are not well understood. In contrast to survivors and asymptomatic cases that show IgM and IgG antibody responses to filovirus antigens, fatal filovirus infections usually end with high viremia and little evidence of a humoral immune response (Baize et al. 1999; Ksiazek et al. 1999; Leroy et al. 2000). Neutralizing anti-GP antibodies were shown to have protective and therapeutic properties in animal models (Maruyama et al. 1999; Wilson et al. 2000). Protection by convalescence sera has been reported anecdotally, but has not been evaluated in controlled clinical trials to date (Mupapa et al. 1999).

Immunosuppression, in general, seems to be an important factor in the pathogenesis of filoviral hemorrhagic fever. The mechanisms, however, leading to the immunosuppressed status of the hosts are unknown and currently being investigated. In humans and monkeys, there is extensive disruption of the parafollicular regions in the spleen and lymph nodes, and proliferation of filoviruses in macrophages (cytolytic in vitro) has been demonstrated (Murphy et al. 1971; Baskerville et al. 1985; Geisbert et al. 1992; Feldmann et al. 1996a; Ryabchikova et al. 1999). For EBOV, it has been reported that sGP interacts with the host immune response by binding to neutrophils through CD16b, the neutrophil-specific form of the Fcγ receptor III. Subsequently, sGP binding appears to inhibit early activation of these cells (Yang et al. 1998; Kindzelskii et al. 2000). This concept, however, has been challenged by a report from Maruyama and colleagues (1998). Relatively high amounts of GP_1 are released into the medium of filovirus-infected cells, and it has been discussed that this soluble glycoprotein as well as sGP may effectively bind antibodies that might otherwise be protective (Sanchez et al. 1996; Volchkov et al. 1998b; Ito et al. 2001). In addition, filovirus transmembrane glycoprotein molecules possess a sequence close to the carboxy terminus resembling a presumptive immunosuppressive domain found in retrovirus glycoproteins (Volchkov et al. 1992; Will et al. 1993; Bukreyev et al. 1995). Peptides synthesized according to this 26 amino acid long region inhibited the blastogenesis of lymphocytes in response to mitogens, inhibited production of cytokines, and decreased proliferation of mononuclear cells in vitro (Ignatyev 1999). It is not yet known, however, if the immunosuppressive domain on the GP is functional on mature molecules.

There is also evidence that filoviruses interfere with innate immunity which is generally believed to play an important role in viral replication and which, therefore, allows the cellular and the humoral arm of the immune system to clear the virus in later stages of the infection. Recent studies with EBOV have shown that VP35 blocks dsRNA- and virus-mediated induction of an IFN-responsive promoter and the IFN-β promoter. VP35 is therefore likely to function as an inhibitor of the type I IFN response in EBOV-infected cells and may be an important determinant in EBOV pathogenicity (Basler et al. 2000).

Diagnosis

In tropical settings identification of a filovirus hemorrhagic fever may be difficult, because the most common causes of severe, acute, febrile disease are malaria and typhoid fever. A wide range of infectious disease must be considered next, such as shigellosis, meningococcal septicemia, plague, leptospirosis, anthrax, relapsing fever, typhus, murine typhus, yellow fever, Chikungunya fever, Rift Valley fever, hemorrhagic fever with renal syndrome, Crimean–Congo hemorrhagic fever, Lassa fever, and fulminant viral hepatitis. Travel, treatment in local hospitals, contact with sick persons or wild and domestic monkeys are useful historical features in returning travelers, especially from Africa. Diagnosis of single cases is extremely difficult, but the occurrence of clusters of cases with prodromal fever followed by cases of hemorrhagic diatheses and person-to-person transmission are suggestive of viral hemorrhagic fever, and containment procedures have to be initiated. In filoviral hemorrhagic fever prostration, lethargy, wasting, and diarrhea seem to be more severe than observed in patients with other viral hemorrhagic fevers. The rash is characteristic and useful in differential diagnosis.

Laboratory diagnosis can be achieved in two ways: measurement of the host-specific immune response to the infection; and detection of viral antigen and genomic RNA in the infected host (Table 50.2, Figure 50.4). Antigen detection ELISA (Ksiazek et al. 1992, 1999) and reverse transcriptase-polymerase chain reaction (Sanchez and Feldmann 1996; Sanchez et al. 1999) are the primary tests to diagnose an acute infection. For antibody detection the most commonly used assays are

Table 50.2 *Laboratory diagnosis*

Test	Target	Source	Remarks
Indirect immunofluorescence assay (IFA)	Virus-specific antibodies	Serum	Simple to perform, but prone to false positives and subjective interpretation
Enzyme-linked immunosorbent assay (ELISA)	Virus-specific antibodies	Serum	Specific and sensitive, but initial response slower than IFA
Immunoblot	Virus-specific antibodies	Serum	Protein-specific, but interpretation sometimes difficult
Antigen ELISA	Viral antigen	Blood, serum, tissues	Rapid and sensitive, but requires special equipment
Immunohistochemistry	Viral antigen	Tissues (e.g. skin, liver)	Inactivated material, but requires time
Fluorescence assay (FA)	Viral antigen	Tissues (e.g. liver)	Rapid and easy, but interpretation is subjective
Polymerase chain reaction (PCR)	Viral nucleic acid	Blood, serum, tissues	Rapid and sensitive, but requires special equipment
Electron microscopy	Viral particle	Blood, tissues	Unique morphology (immunostaining possible), but insensitive and requires expensive equipment
Virus isolation	Viral particle	Blood, tissues	Virus available for studies, but requires time

A surveillance assay based on formalin-fixed skin specimens has been established for the field (Lloyd et al. 1999).

direct IgG and IgM enzyme-linked immunosorbent assays (ELISA) (Ksiazek 1991; Becker et al. 1992), and IgM capture assay (Ksiazek et al. 1999). Confirmatory tests include Western blot (Becker et al. 1992; Elliott et al. 1993a) and the indirect immunofluorescence assay on acetone-fixed infected cells inactivated by γ-radiation. Electron microscopy has been particulary useful in diagnosis of filovirus infections (Siegert et al. 1967; Murphy et al. 1978; Jahrling et al. 1990). Viral structures can be visualized in culture fluid from initial passage cell cultures by negative staining, and in thin sections of any infected material. Immunohistochemistry on formalin-fixed material and paraffin-embedded tissues can be used for detection of filoviruses (Jahrling et al. 1990), as well as immunofluorescence on impression smears of tissues (Rollin et al. 1990).

Viral antigen can be detected in blood from day 3 up to 7–16 days after the onset of symptoms. With the development of more sensitive tests, such as the direct IgG and and the IgM capture ELISA (Ksiazek et al. 1999) antibody detection became more valuble in early diagnosis. Based on data from Kikwit, IgM antibodies appear between 2 and 9 days after the onset of symptoms and disappear between 30 and 168 days after onset. IgG-specific antibodies develop between day 6 and 18 after onset and persist (Rowe et al. 1999) (Figure 50.4).

Attempts to isolate virus from serum or other clinical material should be performed using Vero or MA-104 cells (monkey kidney cells). However, most filoviruses do not cause extensive cytopathic effect on primary isolation. Guinea pigs can be used for primary isolation of those filoviruses that initially do not grow well in tissue culture. Several passages are usually required to produce a uniformly fatal disease.

Patient management and control

Vaccination and chemotherapy for human application do not exist yet. Supportive therapy should be directed towards maintenance of effective blood volume and electrolyte balance. Shock, cerebral edema, renal failure, coagulation disorders, and secondary bacterial infection have to be managed and may be life-saving. Heparin treatment should only be considered in cases with clear evidence for DIC. Human convalescence plasma has been used to successfully treat patients (Mupapa et al. 1999). However, its general usefulness remains unconfirmed. Recently neutralizing anti-GP antibodies could be generated from different species, including human, which were immunized or infected with EBOV. The neutralizing antibodies showed protective and therapeutic properties in animal models (Maruyama et al. 1999; Wilson et al. 2000). Filoviruses are resistant to the antiviral effects of interferon, and interferon administration to monkeys has failed to increase survival rate or achieve a reduction in virus titer. Ribavirin has no effect on filoviruses in vitro and is probably of no therapeutic value.

Isolation of patients is recommended, and protection of medical and nursing staff is required. This can be achieved by strict barrier nursing techniques and the use of high-efficiency particulate air (HEPA) filter respirators for protection against aerosols when feasible. Detailed information has been published regarding management of patients with suspected filoviral hemorrhagic fever and ways to minimize spread of virus in outbreaks, especially in Africa (Centers for Disease Control and Prevention 1988; World Health Organization 1995b).

A protective vaccine would be extremely valuable for at-risk medical personnel in Africa and researchers working with infectious filoviruses. Crossprotection among different EBOV subtypes in experimental animal systems has been reported, suggesting a general value of vaccines (Bowen et al. 1980; Fisher-Hoch and Brammer 1992). Inactivated vaccines have been developed with formalin or heat treatment of cell culture-propagated MARV and EBOV (species Sudan and Zaire) (Lupton et al. 1980; Agafonov et al. 1992). Because of the biohazard of filoviruses and the general lack of knowledge as to the pathogenic processes involved in filovirus diseases, it would be difficult to insure the safety of attenuated strains of MARV or EBOV. The transmembrane glycoprotein GP is assumed to be the major antigenic molecule of virion particles. The successful use of this protein in different immunization approaches has clearly demonstrated its immunogenic and protective properties in small animal models and nonhuman primates (Hevey et al. 1998; Vanderzanden et al. 1998; Xu et al. 1998; Pushko et al. 2000; Sullivan et al. 2000; Sullivan et al. 2003; Garbutt et al. 2004).

The importation of wild-caught monkeys is an important factor in the introduction of filoviruses into foreign human populations (Martini and Siegert 1971; Jahrling et al. 1990; World Health Organization 1992). Quarantine of imported nonhuman primates and professional handling and testing of these animals will help to minimize the risk of filovirus outbreaks in humans. Guidelines have been published for quarantine and proper handling of monkeys in medical research (Centers for Disease Control and Prevention 1990).

Filovirus infectivity is quite stable at room temperature (20°C), but is destroyed in 30 min at 60°C. Infectivity is also destroyed by ultraviolet and γ-irradiation, formalin (1 percent), lipid solvents (deoxycholate, ether), β-propiolactone, and hypochloric and phenolic disinfectants (Elliott et al. 1982; Centers for Disease Control and Prevention 1988, 1993).

REFERENCES

Agafonov, A.P., Ignatyev, G.M., et al. 1992. The immunogenic properties of Marburg virus proteins. *Voprosy Virusol*, **37**, 58–61.

Alvarez, C.P., Losala, F., et al. 2002. C-type lectins DC-SIGN and L-SIGN mediate cellular entry by Ebola virus in cis and in trans. *J Virol*, **76**, 6841–4.

Baize, S., Leroy, E.M., et al. 1999. Defective humoral response and extensive intravascular apoptosis are associated with fatal outcome of Ebola virus-infected patients. *Nat Med*, **5**, 373–4.

Baron, R.C., McCormick, J.B. and Zubeir, O.A. 1983. Ebola haemorrhagic fever in southern Sudan: hospital dissemination and intrafamilial spread. *Bull WHO*, **61**, 997–1003.

Barrientos, L.G., Martin, A.M., et al. 2004. Disulfide bond assignment of the Ebola secreted glycoprotein sGP. *Biochem Biophys Res Comm*, **323**, 696–702.

Baskerville, A., Fisher-Hoch, S.P., et al. 1985. Ultrastructural pathology of experimental Ebola haemorrhagic fever virus infection. *J Pathol*, **147**, 199–209.

Basler, C., Wang, X., et al. 2000. The Ebola virus VP35 protein functions as a type I IFN antagonist. *Proc Natl Acad Sci USA*, **97**, 12289–94.

Basler, C.F., Mikulasova, A., et al. 2003. The Ebola virus VP35 protein inhibits activation of interferon regulatory factor 3. *J Virol*, **77**, 7945–56.

Bausch, D.G., Borchert, M., et al. 2003. Risk factors for Marburg hemorrhagic fever, Democratic Republic of the Congo. *Emerg Infect Dis*, **9**, 1531–7.

Becker, S. and Mühlberger, E. 1999. Co- and posttranslational modifications and functions of Marburg virus proteins. *Curr Top Microbiol Immunol*, **235**, 23–34.

Becker, S., Feldmann, H., et al. 1992. Evidence for occurrence of filovirus antibodies in humans and imported monkeys: do subclinical filovirus infections occur worldwide? *Med Microbiol Immunol*, **181**, 43–55.

Becker, S., Huppertz, S., et al. 1994. The nucleoprotein of Marburg virus is phosphorylated. *J Gen Virol*, **75**, 809–18.

Becker, S., Spiess, M. and Klenk, H.D. 1995. The asialoglycoprotein receptor is a potential liver-specific receptor for Marburg virus. *J Gen Virol*, **76**, 393–9.

Becker, S., Klenk, H.D. and Mühlberger, E. 1996. Intracellular transport and processing of the Marburg virus surface protein in vertebrate and insect cells. *Virology*, **225**, 145–55.

Becker, S., Rinne, C., et al. 1998. Interactions of Marburg virus nucleocapsid proteins. *Virology*, **249**, 406–17.

Bowen, E.T.W., Platt, G.S., et al. 1980. A comparative study of strains of Ebola virus isolated from southern Sudan and northern Zaire in 1976. *J Med Virol*, **6**, 129–38.

Buchmeier, M.J., DeFries, R., et al. 1983. Comparative analysis of the structural polypeptides of Ebola virus from Sudan and Zaire. *J Infect Dis*, **147**, 276–81.

Bukreyev, A.A., Volchkov, V.E., et al. 1993. The VP35 and VP40 proteins of filoviruses: homology between Marburg and Ebola viruses. *FEBS Lett*, **322**, 41–6.

Bukreyev, A.A., Volchkov, V.E., et al. 1995. The nucleotide sequence of the Popp (1967) strain of Marburg virus: a comparison with the Musoke (1980) strain. *Arch Virol*, **140**, 1589–600.

Bwaka, M.A., Bonnet, M.J., et al. 1999. Ebola hemorrhagic fever in Kikwit, Democratic Republic of the Congo: clinical observations in 103 patients. *J Infect Dis*, **179**, Suppl. 1, S1–7.

Centers for Disease Control and Prevention. 1988. Management of patients with suspected viral haemorrhagic fever. *Morb Mortal Wkly Rep*, 37 (Suppl. 3), 1–16.

Centers for Disease Control and Prevention. 1990. Update: Ebola-related filovirus infection in nonhuman primates and interim guidelines for handling nonhuman primates during transit and quarantine. *Morb Mortal Wkly Rep*, 39, 22–24, 29–30.

Centers for Disease Control and Prevention. 1993. Biosafety in microbiology and biomedical laboratories. US Department of Health and Human Services (HHS), publication No. (CDC) 93-8395. Washington DC: US Government Printing Office.

Chan, S.Y., Ma, M.C. and Goldsmith, M.A. 2000a. Differential induction of cellular detachment by envelope glycoproteins of Marburg and Ebola (Zaire) viruses. *J Gen Virol*, **81**, 2155–9.

Chan, S.Y., Speck, R.F., et al. 2000b. Distinct mechanisms of entry by envelope glycoproteins of Marburg and Ebola (Zaire) viruses. *J Virol*, **74**, 4933–7.

Chan, S.Y., Empig, C.J., et al. 2001. Folate receptor-α is a cofactor for cellular entry by Marburg and Ebola viruses. *Cell*, **106**, 117–26.

Cox, N.J., McCormick, J.B., et al. 1983. Evidence for two subtypes of Ebola virus based on oligonucleotide mapping of RNA. *J Infect Dis*, **147**, 272–5.

Dessen, A., Volchkov, V., et al. 2000. Crystal structure of the matrix protein of Ebola virus. *EMBO J*, **19**, 4228–36.

Dolnik, O., Volchkova, V., et al. 2004. Ectodomain shedding of the glycoprotein GP of Ebola virus. *EMBO J*, **23**, 2175–84.

Elliott, L.H., McCormick, J.B. and Johnson, K.M. 1982. Inactivation of Lassa, Marburg and Ebola viruses by gamma irradiation. *J Clin Microbiol*, **16**, 704–8.

Elliott, L.H., Kiley, M.P. and McCormick, J.B. 1985. Descriptive analysis of Ebola virus proteins. *Virology*, **147**, 169–76.

Elliott, L.H., Bauer, S.P., et al. 1993a. Improved specificity of testing methods for filovirus antibodies. *J Virol Meth*, **43**, 85–100.

Elliott, L.H., Sanchez, A., et al. 1993b. Ebola protein analysis for the determination of genetic organization. *Arch Virol*, **133**, 423–36.

Feldmann, H. and Kiley, M.P. 1999. Classification, structure, and replication of filoviruses. *Curr Top Microbiol Immunol*, **235**, 1–21.

Feldmann, H., Will, C., et al. 1991. Glycosylation and oligomerization of the spike protein of Marburg virus. *Virology*, **182**, 353–6.

Feldmann, H., Mühlberger, E., et al. 1992. Marburg virus, a filovirus: messenger RNAs, gene order, and regulatory elements of the replication cycle. *Virus Res*, **24**, 1–19.

Feldmann, H., Klenk, H.D. and Sanchez, A. 1993. Molecular biology and evolution of filoviruses. *Arch Virol*, **7**, Suppl., 81–100.

Feldmann, H., Nichol, S.T., et al. 1994. Characterization of filoviruses based on differences in structure and antigenicity of the virion glycoprotein. *Virology*, **199**, 469–73.

Feldmann, H., Bugany, H., et al. 1996a. Filovirus-induced endothelial leakage triggered by infected monocytes/macrophages. *J Virol*, **70**, 2208–14.

Feldmann, H., Slenczka, W. and Klenk, H.D. 1996b. Emerging and reemerging of filoviruses. *Arch Virol*, **11**, Suppl., 77–100.

Feldmann, H., Volchkov, V.E. and Klenk, H.D. 1997. Filovirus Ebola et Marburg. *Ann Pasteur*, **8**, 2, 285–96.

Feldmann, H., Jones, S., et al. 2003. Ebola virus: from discovery to vaccine. *Nat Rev Immunol*, **3**, 677–85.

Feldmann, H., Geisbert, T.W., et al. 2004. *Filoviridae*. In: Fauquet, C.M., Mayo, M.A., et al. (eds), *Virus taxonomy*, VIIIth Report of the ICTV. London: Elsevier/Academic Press, 645–53.

Fisher-Hoch, S.P. and Brammer, L. 1992. Pathogenic potential of filoviruses: role of geographic origin of primate host and virus strain. *J Infect Dis*, **166**, 753–63.

Fisher-Hoch, S.P., Platt, G.S., et al. 1985. Pathophysiology of shock and hemorrhage in a fulminating viral infection (Ebola). *J Infect Dis*, **152**, 887–94.

Fisher-Hoch, S.P., Perez-Oronoz, G.I., et al. 1992. Filovirus clearance in non-human primates. *Lancet*, **340**, 451–3.

Funke, C., Becker, S., et al. 1995. Acylation of the Marburg virus glycoprotein. *Virology*, **208**, 289–97.

Gallaher, W.R. 1996. Similar structural models of the transmembrane proteins of Ebola and avian sarcoma viruses. *Cell*, **85**, 477–8, letter.

Garbutt, M., Liebscher, R., et al. 2004. Properties of replication-competent vesicular stomatitis virus vectors expressing glycoproteins of filoviruses and arenaviruses. *J Virol*, **78**, 5458–65.

Gear, J.S.S., Cassel, G.A., et al. 1975. Outbreak of Marburg virus disease in Johannesburg. *Br Med J*, **4**, 489–93.

Geisbert, T.W. and Jahrling, P.B. 1995. Differentiation of filoviruses by electron microscopy. *Virus Res*, **39**, 129–50.

Geisbert, T.W., Jahrling, P.B., et al. 1992. Association of Ebola-related Reston virus particles and antigen with tissue lesions of monkeys imported to the United States. *J Comp Path*, **106**, 137–52.

Georges, A.J., Leroy, E.M., et al. 1999. Ebola hemorrhagic fever outbreaks in Gabon, 1994–1997: epidemiology and health control issues. *J Infect Dis*, **179**, Suppl. 1, S65–75.

Geyer, H., Will, C., et al. 1992. Carbohydrate structure of Marburg virus glycoprotein. *Glycobiology*, **2**, 299–312.

Gomis-Rüth, F.X., Dessen, A., et al. 2003. The matrix protein VP40 from Ebola virus octamerizes into pore-like structures with specific RNA-binding proteins. *Structure*, **11**, 423–33.

Hayes, C.G., Burans, J.P., et al. 1992. Outbreak of fatal illness among captive macques in the Philippines caused by an Ebola-related filovirus. *Am J Trop Med Hyg*, **46**, 664–71.

Hevey, M., Negley, D., et al. 1998. Marburg virus vaccines based upon alphavirus replicons protect guinea pigs and nonhuman primates. *Virology*, **251**, 28–37.

Heymann, D.L., Weisfeld, J.S., et al. 1980. Ebola haemorrhagic fever: Tandala Zaire, 1977–78. *J Infect Dis*, **142**, 372–6.

Ignatyev, G.M. 1999. Immune response to filovirus infections. *Curr Top Med Microbiol Immunol*, **235**, 205–17.

Ito, H., Watanabe, S., et al. 1999. Mutational analysis of the putative fusion domain of Ebola virus glycoprotein. *J Virol*, **73**, 8907–12.

Ito, H., Watanabe, S., et al. 2001. Ebola virus glycoprotein: proteolytic processing, acylation, cell tropism, and detection of neutralizing antibodies. *J Virol*, **75**, 1576–80.

Jahrling, P.B., Geisbert, T.W., et al. 1990. Preliminary report: isolation of Ebola virus from monkeys imported to USA. *Lancet*, **335**, 502–5.

Jasenosky, L.D. and Kawaoka, Y. 2004. Filovirus budding. *Virus Res*, **106**, 181–8.

Jeffers, S.A., Sanders, D.A. and Sanchez, A. 2002. Covalent modifications of the Ebola virus glycoprotein. *J Virol*, **76**, 12463–72.

Johnson, E.D., Johnson, B.K., et al. 1996. Characterization of a new Marburg virus isolated from a 1987 fatal case in Kenya. *Arch Virol*, **11**, Suppl., 101–14.

Kiley, M.P., Bowen, E.T.W., et al. 1982. Filoviridae: a taxonomic home for Marburg and Ebola viruses? *Intervirology*, **18**, 24–32.

Kiley, M.P., Wilusz, J., et al. 1986. Conservation of the 3' terminal nucleotide sequence of Ebola and Marburg viruses. *Virology*, **149**, 251–4.

Kiley, M.P., Cox, N.J., et al. 1988. Physicochemical properties of Marburg virus: evidence for three distinct virus strains and their relationship to Ebola virus. *J Gen Virol*, **69**, 1957–67.

Kindzelskii, A.L., Yang, Z., et al. 2000. Ebola virus secretory glycoprotein (sGP) diminishes Fc(RIIIB-to-CR3 proximity on neutrophils. *J Immunol*, **164**, 953–8.

Kolesnikova, L., Bugany, H., et al. 2002. VP40, the matrix protein of Marburg virus, is associated with membranes of the late endosomal compartment. *J Virol*, **76**, 1825–38.

Klenk, H.D., Volchkov, V.E. and Feldmann, H. 1998. Two strings to the bow of Ebola virus. *Nature Med*, **4**, 388–9.

Ksiazek, T.G. 1991. Laboratory diagnosis of filovirus infections in non-human primates. *Lab Animal*, **20**, 34–46.

Ksiazek, T.G., Rollin, P.E., et al. 1992. Enzyme immunosorbent assay for Ebola virus antigens in tissues of infected primates. *J Clin Micro*, **30**, 947–50.

Ksiazek, T.G., Rollin, P.E., et al. 1999. Clinical virology of Ebola hemorrhagic fever (EHF): virus, virus antigen, and IgG and IgM antibody findings among EHF patients in Kikwit, Democratic Republic of the Congo, 1995. *J Infect Dis*, **179**, Suppl. 1, S177–87.

LeGuenno, B., Formentry, P., et al. 1995. Isolation and partial characterization of a new strain of Ebola virus. *Lancet*, **345**, 1271–4.

Leroy, E.M., Baize, S., et al. 2000. Human asymptomatic Ebola infection and strong inflammatory response. *Lancet*, **355**, 2210–15.

Lloyd, E.S., Zaki, S.R., et al. 1999. Long-term disease surveillance in Bandundu region, Democratic republic of the Congo: a model for early detection and prevention of Ebola hemorrhagic fever. *J Infect Dis*, **179**, Suppl. 1, S274–80.

Lupton, H.W., Lambert, R.D., et al. 1980. Inactivated vaccine for Ebola virus efficacious in guinea pig model. *Lancet*, **2**, 1294–5.

Malashkevich, V.N., Schneider, B.J., et al. 1999. Core structure of the envelope glycoprotein GP2 from Ebola virus at 1.9-Å resolution. *Proc Natl Acad Sci USA*, **96**, 2662–7.

Mariyankova, R.F., Giushakowa, S.E., et al. 1993. Marburg virus penetration into eukaryotic cells. *Vopr Virusol*, **2**, 74–6.

Martini, G.A. and Siegert, R. 1971. *Marburg virus disease*, 1st edn. New York: Springer, 1–230.

Maruyama, T., Buchmeier, M.J., et al. 1998. Ebola virus, neutrophils and antibody specificity. *Science*, **282**, 845a.

Maruyama, T., Rodriguez, L.L., et al. 1999. Ebola virus can be effectively neutralized by antibody produced in natural human infection. *J Virol*, **73**, 6024–30.

McCormick, J.B., Bauer, S.P., et al. 1983. Biological differences between strains of Ebola virus from Zaire and Sudan. *J Infect Dis*, **147**, 264–7.

Mühlberger, E., Sanchez, A., et al. 1992. The nucleotide sequence of the L gene of Marburg virus, a filovirus: homologies with paramyxoviruses and rhabdoviruses. *Virology*, **187**, 534–47.

Mühlberger, E., Trommer, S., et al. 1996. Termini of all mRNAs species of Marburg virus: sequence and secondary structure. *Virology*, **223**, 376–80.

Mühlberger, E., Lotfering, B., et al. 1998. Three of the four nucleocapsid proteins of Marburg virus, NP, VP35 and L, are sufficient to mediate replication and transcription of Marburg virus-specific monocistronic minigenomes. *J Virol*, **72**, 8756–64.

Mühlberger, E., Weik, M., et al. 1999. Comparison of the transcription and replication strategies of Marburg virus and Ebola virus by using artificial replication systems. *J Virol*, **73**, 2333–42.

Mupapa, K.D., Massamba, M., International Scientific and Technical Committee, et al. 1999. Treatment of Ebola hemorrhagic fever with blood transfusions from convalescent patients. *J Infect Dis*, **179**, Suppl. 1, S18–23.

Murphy, F.A., Simpson, D.I.H., et al. 1971. Marburg virus infection in monkeys. *Lab Invest*, **24**, 279–91.

Murphy, F.A., van der Groen, G., et al. 1978. Ebola and Marburg virus morphology and taxonomy. In: Pattyn, S.R. (ed.), *Ebola virus haemorrhagic fever*, 1st edn. Amsterdam: Elsevier/North-Holland, 61–84.

Muyembe-Tamfum, J.J. 2000. *Marburg hemorrhagic fever Watsa/Burba, DRC: an endemo-epidemic phenomenon*. Symposium on Marburg and Ebola Viruses, Marburg, Germany.

Neumann, G., Feldmann, H., et al. 2002. Reverse genetics demonstrates that proteolytic processing of the Ebola virus glycoprotein is not essential for replication in cell culture. *J Virol*, **76**, 406–10.

Nichol, S.T. 2000. *Multiple introduction of genetically diverse Marburg viruses into the human population during the hemorrhagic fever outbreak in Durba, Democratic Republic of the Congo, 1998–2000*. Symposium on Marburg and Ebola Viruses, Marburg, Germany.

Pattyn, S.R. 1978. *Ebola virus haemorrhagic fever*, 1st edn. Amsterdam: Elsevier/North-Holland, 1–436.

Peters, C.J. and LeDuc, J.W. 1999. Ebola: the virus and the disease. *J Infect Dis*, **179**, Suppl. 1, S1–S288.

Peters, C.J., Johnson, E.D. and McKee, K.T. 1991. Filoviruses and management and viral haemorrhagic fevers. In: Belshe, R.B. (ed.), *Textbook of human virology*. St Louis: Mosby Year Book, 699–712.

Peters, C.J., Jahrling, P.B., et al. 1992. Filovirus contamination of cell cultures. *Dev Biol Stand*, **76**, 267–74.

Peters, C.J., Johnson, E.D., et al. 1993. Filoviruses. In: Morse, S.S. (ed.), *Emerging viruses*. Oxford: Oxford University Press, 159–75.

Peters, C.J., Sanchez, A., et al. 1996. Filoviridae: Marburg and Ebola viruses. In: Fields, B.N. and Knipe, D.M. (eds), *Virology*, 3rd edn. Philadelphia: Raven Press, 1161–76.

Peters, D., Müller, G. and Slenczka, W. 1971. Morphology, development, and classification of Marburg virus. In: Martini, G.A. and Siegert, R. (eds), *Marburg virus disease*, 1st edn. New York: Springer, 68–83.

Pokhodyaeu, V.A., Gonchar, N.I. and Pshenichnov, V.A. 1991. Experimental study of Marburg virus contact transmission. *Vopr Virusol*, **36**, 506–8.

Pushko, P., Bray, M., et al. 2000. Recombinant RNA replicons derived from attenuated Venezuelan equine encephalitis virus protect guinea pigs and mice from Ebola hemorrhagic fever virus. *Vaccine*, **19**, 142–53.

Regnery, R.L., Johnson, K.M. and Kiley, M.P. 1980. Virion nucleic acid of Ebola virus. *J Virol*, **36**, 465–9.

Richards, G.A., Murphy, S., et al. 2000. Unexpected Ebola virus in a tertiary setting: clinical and epidemiological aspects. *Crit Care Med*, **28**, 284–5.

Richman, D.D., Cleveland, P.H., et al. 1983. Antigenic analysis of strains of Ebola viruses: identification of two Ebola virus subtypes. *J Infect Dis*, **147**, 268–71.

Rollin, P.E., Ksiazek, T.G., et al. 1990. Detection of Ebola-like viruses by immunofluorescence. *Lancet*, **336**, 8730, 1591.

Rollin, P.E., Williams, R.J., et al. 1999. Ebola (subtype Reston) virus among quarantine nonhuman primates recently imported from the Philippines to the United Staes. *J Infect Dis*, **179**, Suppl. 1, S108–14.

Rowe, A.K., Bertolli, J., et al. 1999. Clinical, virologic, and immunologic follow-up of convalescent Ebola hemorrhagic fever patients and their household contacts, Kikwit, Democratic Republic of the Congo. Commission de Lutte contre les Epidemies a Kikwit. *J Infect Dis*, **179**, Suppl. 1, S28–35.

Ruigrok, R.W.H., Schoehn, G., et al. 2000. Structural characterization and membrane binding properties of the matrix protein VP40 of Ebola virus. *J Mol Biol*, **300**, 103–12.

Ruiz-Agüello, M.B., Goni, F.M., et al. 1998. Phosphatidylinositol-dependent membrane fusion induced by a putative fusogenic sequence of Ebola virus. *J Virol*, **72**, 1775–81.

Ryabchikova, E., Kolesnikova, L.V. and Luchko, S.V. 1999. An analysis of features of pathogenesis in two animal models of Ebola virus infection. *J Infect Dis*, **179**, Suppl. 1, S199–202.

Sanchez, A. and Feldmann, H. 1996. Detection of Marburg and Ebola virus infections by polymerase chain reaction assays. In: Becker, Y. and Darai, G. (eds), *Frontiers in virology – diagnosis of human viruses by polymerase chain reaction technology*. Berlin, Heidelberg, New York: Springer, 411–18.

Sanchez, A. and Kiley, M.P. 1987. Identification and analysis of Ebola virus messenger RNAs. *Virology*, **157**, 414–20.

Sanchez, A. and Kiley, M.P. 1989. The nucleoprotein gene of Ebola virus: cloning, sequencing, and in vitro expression. *Virology*, **170**, 81–91.

Sanchez, A., Kiley, M.P., et al. 1992. Sequence analysis of the Marburg virus nucleoprotein gene: comparison to Ebola virus and other non-segmented negative-strand RNA viruses. *J Gen Virol*, **73**, 347–57.

Sanchez, A., Kiley, M.P., et al. 1993. Sequence analysis of the Ebola virus genome: organization, genetic elements, and comparison with the genome of Marburg virus. *Virus Res*, **29**, 215–40.

Sanchez, A., Trappier, S.G., et al. 1996. The virion glycoprotein of Ebola viruses are encoded in two reading frames and are expressed through transcriptional editing. *Proc Natl Acad Sci USA*, **93**, 3602–7.

Sanchez, A., Trappier, S.G., et al. 1998a. Variation in the glycoprotein and VP35 genes of Marburg virus strains. *Virology*, **240**, 138–46.

Sanchez, A., Yang, Z.Y., et al. 1998b. Biochemical analysis of the secreted and virion glycoproteins of Ebola virus. *J Virol*, **72**, 6442–7.

Sanchez, A., Ksiazek, T.G., et al. 1999. Detection and molecular chracterization of Ebola viruses causing disease in human and non-human primates. *J Infect Dis*, **179**, Suppl. 1, S164–9.

Sanchez, A., Khan, A.S., et al. 2001. Filoviridae: Marburg and Ebola viruses. In: Knipe, D.M., Howley, P.M., et al. (eds), *Field's virology*. Vol. 1. Philadelphia: Lippincott Williams & Wilkins, 1279–304.

Schnittler, H.J. and Feldmann, H. 1999. Molecular pathogenesis of filovirus infections: role of macrophages and endothelial cells. *Curr Top Microbiol Immunol*, **235**, 175–204.

Schnittler, H.J., Mahner, F., et al. 1993. Replication of Marburg virus in human endothelial cells. A possible mechanism for the development of viral haemorrhagic disease. *J Clin Invest*, **91**, 1301–9.

Scianimanico, S., Schoehn, G., et al. 2000. Membrane association induces a conformational change in the Ebola virus matrix protein. *EMBO J*, **19**, 6732–41.

Siegert, R., Shu, H.-L., et al. 1967. Zur Ätiologie einer unbekannten von Affen ausgegangenen Infektionskrankheit. *Dtsch Med Wochenschr*, **92**, 2341–3.

Smith, D.H., Johnson, B.K., et al. 1982. Marburg-virus disease in Kenya. *Lancet*, **1**, 816–20.

Sullivan, N.J., Sanchez, A., et al. 2000. Development of a preventive vaccine for Ebola virus infection in primates. *Nature*, **408**, 605–9.

Sullivan, N.J., Geisbert, T.W., et al. 2003. Accelerated vaccination for Ebola virus haemorrhagic fever in non-human primates. *Nature*, **424**, 681–4.

Swanepoel, R., Leman, P.A., et al. 1996. Experimental inoculation of plants and animals with Ebola virus. *Emerg Infect Dis*, **2**, 321–5.

Takada, A., Robison, C., et al. 1997. A system for functional analysis of Ebola virus glycoprotein. *Proc Natl Acad Sci USA*, **94**, 14764–9.

Takada, A., Watanabe, S., et al. 2000. Downregulation of beta 1 integrins by Ebolavirus glycoprotein: implications for virus entry. *Virology*, **278**, 20–6.

van der Groen, G., Johnson, K.M., et al. 1978. Results of Ebola antibody survey in various population groups. In: Pattyn, S.R. (ed.), *Ebola virus haemorrhagic fever*, 1st edn. Amsterdam: Elsevier/North-Holland, 203–8.

Vanderzanden, L., Bray, M., et al. 1998. DNA vaccines expressing either the GP or NP genes of Ebola virus protect mice from lethal challenge. *Virology*, **246**, 134–44.

Volchkov, V.E., Blinov, V.M. and Netesov, S.V. 1992. The envelope glycoprotein of Ebola virus contains an immunosuppressive-like domain similar to oncogenic retroviruses. *FEBS Lett*, **305**, 181–4.

Volchkov, V.E., Becker, S., et al. 1995. GP mRNA of Ebola virus is edited by the Ebola virus polymerase and by T7 and vaccinia virus polymerases. *Virology*, **214**, 421–30.

Volchkov, V.E., Feldmann, H., et al. 1998a. Processing of the Ebola virus glycoprotein by the proprotein convertase furin. *Proc Natl Acad Sci USA*, **95**, 5762–7.

Volchkov, V.E., Volchkova, V.A., et al. 1998b. Release of viral glycoproteins during Ebola virus infection. *Virology*, **245**, 110–19.

Volchkov, V.E., Volchkova, V.A., et al. 1999. Characterization of the L gene and 5′trailer region of Ebola virus. *J Gen Virol*, **80**, 355–62.

Volchkov, V.E., Chepurnov, A.A., et al. 2000a. Molecular characterization of guinea-pig-adapted variants of Ebola virus. *Virology*, **277**, 147–55.

Volchkov, V.E., Volchkova, V.A., et al. 2000b. Proteolytic processing of Marburg virus glycoprotein. *Virology*, **268**, 1–6.

Volchkov, V.E., Volchkova, V.A., et al. 2001. Recovery of infectious Ebola virus from cDNA: transcriptional RNA editing of the GP gene controls viral cytotoxicity. *Science*, **291**, 1965–9.

Volchkova, V., Klenk, H.D. and Volchkov, V.E. 1999. Delta-peptide is the carboxy-terminal cleavage fragment of the nonstructural small glycoprotein sGP of Ebola virus. *Virology*, **265**, 164–71.

Volchkova, V.A., Feldmann, H., et al. 1998. The nonstructural small glycoprotein of Ebola virus is secreted as an antiparallel-orientated homodimer. *Virology*, **250**, 408–14.

Weik, M., Modrof, J., et al. 2002. Ebola virus VP30-mediated transcription is regulated by RNA secondary structure formation. *J Virol*, **76**, 8532–9.

Weissenhorn, W., Calder, L.J., et al. 1998a. The central structural feature of the membrane fusion protein subunit from the Ebola virus glycoprotein is a long triple-stranded coiled coil. *Proc Natl Acad Sci USA*, **95**, 6032–6.

Weissenhorn, W., Carfi, A., et al. 1998b. Crystal structure of the Ebola virus membrane fusion subunit, GP2, from the envelope glycoprotein ectodomain. *Mol Cell*, **2**, 605–16.

Will, C., Mühlberger, E., et al. 1993. Marburg virus gene 4 encodes the virion membrane protein, a type I transmembrane glycoprotein. *J Virol*, **67**, 1203–10.

Wilson, J.A., Hevey, M., et al. 2000. Epitopes involved in antibody-mediated protection from Ebola virus. *Science*, **287**, 1664–6.

Wool-Levis, R.J. and Bates, P. 1998. Characterization of Ebola virus entry by using pseudotyped viruses: identification of receptor-deficient cell lines. *J Virol*, **72**, 3155–60.

World Health Organization. 1978a. Ebola haemorrhagic fever in Sudan, 1976. *Bull WHO*, **56**, 247–70.

World Health Organization. 1978b. Ebola haemorrhagic fever in Zaire, 1976. *Bull WHO*, **56**, 271–93.

World Health Organization. 1992. Viral haemorrhagic fever in imported monkeys. *Wkly Epidemiol Rep*, **67**, 142-43.

World Health Organization. 1995a. Ebola haemorrhagic fever. *Wkly Epidemiol Rec*, **70**, 241–42

World Health Organization. 1995b. Viral haemorrhagic fever – management of suspected cases. *Wkly Epidemiol Rec*, **70**, 249–56.

World Health Organization. 2001. Outbreak of Ebola hemorrhagic fever, Uganda, August 2000–January 2001. *Wkly Epidemiol Rec*, **76**, 41–46.

Xu, L., Sanchez, A., et al. 1998. Immunization for Ebola virus infection. *Nature Med*, **4**, 37–42.

Yang, Z., Delgado, R., et al. 1998. Distinct cellular interactions of secreted and transmembrane Ebola virus glycoproteins. *Science*, **279**, 1034–6.

Yang, Z., Duckers, H.J., et al. 2000. Identification of the Ebola virus glycoprotein as the main viral determinant of vascular cell cytotoxicity and injury. *Nature Med*, **6**, 886–9.

Zaki, S.R. and Goldsmith, C.S. 1999. Pathologic features of filovirus infections in humans. *Curr Top Microbiol Immunol*, **235**, 97–116.

Zaki, S.R. and Peters, C.J. 1997. Viral hemorrhagic fevers. In: Connor, D.H., Schwartz, D.A., et al. (eds), *Diagnostic pathology of infectious diseases*. Stamford, CT: Appleton and Lange, 347–64.

51

Rhabdoviruses: rabies

NOËL TORDO, PIERRE-EMMANUEL CECCALDI, YVES GAUDIN, AND
ALEX I. WANDELER

INTRODUCTION

The family *Rhabdoviridae* (from Greek *rhabdos*: rod) contains hundreds of viruses whose hosts vary widely among vertebrates, invertebrates, and plants (Murphy et al. 1995; Tordo et al. 2004) in which they give rise to various diseases (Figure 51.1). This variability contrasts strongly with their striking similarity in morphology, structure, and mechanisms of replication. Another common feature is that all members present a danger to humans, not only from direct disease but also from livestock and crop losses.

Arthropods are their most frequent vectors and probable original reservoirs, from which they adapted to plants and vertebrates. Traces of this evolution still exist: the sigma virus exclusively infects the fruit fly *Drosophila*; the plant rhabdoviruses have mixed arthropod–plant cycles; vesiculoviruses, ephemeroviruses, and possibly lyssaviruses undergo mixed insect–mammal cycles; and some evidence even suggests that an aquatic arthropod could be involved in the transmission of fish rhabdovirus. Several insect species replicate both vertebrate and plant rhabdoviruses, but a triple insect–plant–vertebrate cycle has not so far been observed. Finally, rabies and rabies-related viruses became more narrowly adapted and now infect only mammals. The vast majority of rhabdoviruses are transmitted mechanically: in plants by injury or through arthropod or worm vectors and in vertebrates by aerosols, contact, bite, or sexual transmission. A few viruses (e.g. the sigma virus of *Drosophila*) are vertically transmitted.

For historical reasons, studies on rabies virus contributed greatly to the development of vaccines, pathology, and analysis of the immune response. Studies on vesicular stomatitis virus, which is comparatively safe to handle and replicates readily in most cell types, have provided much useful biochemical, biophysical, and molecular data. The fish, plant, and cattle rhabdoviruses, long neglected, have recently attracted increased attention because of their economic importance.

PROPERTIES OF THE VIRUSES

The *Rhabdoviridae*

The family *Rhabdoviridae* belongs to the order *Mononegavirales*, which also embraces the families *Paramyxoviridae*, *Filoviridae* and *Bornaviridae*. These viruses share a linear nonsegmented RNA genome of negative polarity embedded within a helical ribonucleoprotein complex (RNP). The criteria for *Rhabdovirus* classification have been progressively sharpened, taking into account physical, chemical, and structural properties, antigenicity and, finally, genetics. The viruses were first grouped into genera or other groups by serological cross-reactions between internal antigens and their antibodies. Subdivision into serotypes was performed by cross-reaction between envelope antigens (Schneider et al. 1973). The use of monoclonal antibodies (mAbs) further refined the classification (Rupprecht et al. 1991). Molecular biology techniques permitted phylogenetic

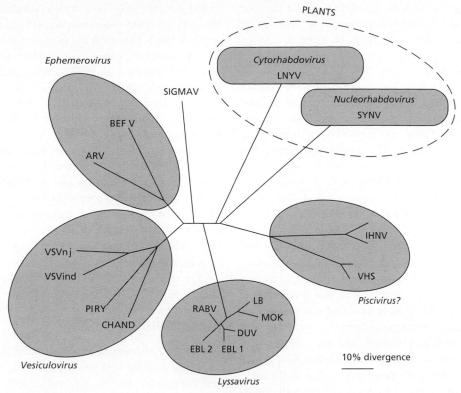

Figure 51.1 *Radial phylogenetic tree of the* Rhabdoviridae *family established from N protein sequence alignment using the ClustalW program (neighbor joining method). Gray circles outline the genera. ARV, Adelaide River virus; BEFV, bovine ephemeral fever virus; CHPV, Chandipura virus; DUVV, Duvenhage virus; EBLV-1 and EBLV-2, European bat Lyssavirus, types 1 and 2; IHNV, infectious hematopoietic necrosis virus; LBV, Lagos bat virus; LNYV, lettuce necrotic yellow virus; MOKV, Mokola virus; PIRYV, piry virus; RABV, rabies virus; SIGMAV, sigma virus; SYNV, sonchus yellow net virus; VHSV, viral hemorrhagic septicemia; VSIV, vesicular stomatitis virus, Indiana; VSNJ, vesicular stomatitis virus, New Jersey.*

studies and the definition of genotypes (Badrane et al. 2001; Bourhy et al. 1993a; Morzunov et al. 1995; Tordo et al. 1995; Wang et al. 1995; Tordo et al. 2004 and references herein). However, a considerable number of rhabdoviruses remain, classified only roughly on the basis of morphology, host or geographical distribution, or pathological features. Further analysis is needed to justify their inclusion in existing groups or the creation of new ones.

GENUS *VESICULOVIRUS*

The main member of the genus *Vesiculovirus* (Latin *vesicula*: blister) is vesicular stomatitis virus (VSV), which is frequently designated as the prototype of the entire family *Rhabdoviridae*. Eight species have been characterized, of which Indiana and New Jersey are the most recent (Murphy et al. 1995; Tordo et al. 2004). VSV causes a febrile illness in cattle, horses, and pigs, characterized by the appearance of blisters in the mouth, which rapidly ulcerate (see Clinical and pathological aspects: vesiculovirus infection). Other 'vesicular viruses,' which include members of other families, cause similar lesions: for example, *Picornaviridae* (foot-and-mouth disease and swine vesicular disease) and *Caliciviridae* (vesicular exanthema virus). These viruses, of

great economic importance for farming, are readily distinguished by morphological or serological criteria.

GENUS *LYSSAVIRUS*

Until 1956 and the first isolations of rabies-related viruses in Africa (King et al. 1994) and Europe (Schneider and Cox 1994), rabies virus (RABV) was believed to be antigenically unique. This warranted the creation of the genus *Lyssavirus* (Greek *lyssa*: rabies) for viruses responsible for rabies-like encephalitis. The genus was at first divided into four serotypes by antigenic crossreactivity with sera and mAbs, but European bat lyssavirus (EBLV) isolates remained unclassified (Dietzschold et al. 1988; Rupprecht et al. 1991; WHO 1992). Phylogenetic analysis of the nucleoprotein and glycoprotein genes further delineated six genotypes, the first four of which matched the serotypes (1) rabies, (2) Lagos bat, (3) Mokola, and (4) Duvenhage. The other two genotypes are EBL types 1 (5) and 2 (6) (Bourhy et al. 1993a).

Genotype 1 corresponds to classic RABV. It encompasses laboratory strains used for vaccine seed or control (challenge virus standard (CVS)) and many viruses isolated from various rabid domestic or wild animals worldwide. Members of genotypes 2–6 are rabies-related viruses, which so far have been isolated only in the Old World. They have a narrower geographical distribution than rabies and, although they occasionally infect humans and domestic animals, they seem to infect preferentially certain specific host species. Lagos bat virus, Molokai virus, and Duvenhage virus were isolated in sub-Saharan Africa, principally from frugivorous bats, small mammals (shrews and rodents), and insectivorous bats, respectively (King et al. 1994). EBLV-1 and EBLV-2 are spreading widely in Europe, from the former USSR to Spain, and mainly infect insectivorous bats of the *Eptesicus* and *Myotis* species, respectively (Bourhy et al. 1992, 1993a; Schneider and Cox 1994; Amengual et al. 1997; Serra-Cobo et al. 2002).

In May 1996, a new lyssavirus was isolated from fruit-eating bats (flying foxes, *Pteropus alecto*) on the eastern coast of Australia, a country considered to be rabies-free since 1867. The same virus was also isolated from two other species of *Pteropus*, and from an insectivorous bat. Within the two following years, two fatal cases of human encephalitis caused by this new Australian bat lyssavirus (ABLV) were confirmed. Genetic and antigenic analysis of the virus, as well as cross-seroneutralization suggested that ABLV is closer to genotype 1, but sufficiently distinct to justify a new genotype (7) (Guyatt et al. 2003). The current seven genotypes are distributed in two phylogroups with distinct pathological and immunological properties: phylogroup I includes genotypes 1 and 4 to 7; phylogroup II comprises genotypes 2 and 3 (Badrane et al. 2001; Nadin-Davis et al. 2002). This classification is however bound to evolve, particularly as surveillance for bat lyssaviruses is re-enforced (Arguin et al. 2002; Reynes et al. 2004). Already, four additional divergent lyssaviruses have been isolated in bats of Central Asia, East Siberia, and the Black Sea region and are proposed as new genotypes: Aravan virus (ARAV), Khujand virus (KHUV), Irkut virus (IRKV), and West-Caucasian bat virus (WCBV) (Botvinkin et al. 2003; Kuzmin et al. 2003).

From the epizootiological point of view, rabies is maintained and transmitted by mammalian species serving as reservoirs and vectors (Baer 1991) (see section on Epizootiology and epidemiology below). They are distinguished from other mammals, which, although susceptible to infection, constitute epidemiological cul-de-sacs. Rabies exists in two major epidemiological forms: (1) canine rabies, of which stray dogs are the vectors, is responsible for >95 percent of the human cases in developing countries (Plotkin 1993; Meslin et al. 1994); and (2) sylvatic rabies, which involves wildlife worldwide. The wild vectors vary geographically and include terrestrial mammals, mainly carnivores, and bats. The last are vectors for six out of seven *Lyssavirus* genotypes characterized so far, and the exclusive vector in five of them. Phylogenetic analysis supports the evolution of lyssaviruses in bat vectors with occasional but regular spill over and host switching to carnivore vectors

to extend the virus host range (Badrane and Tordo 2001). Polymerase chain reaction (PCR) technology has revolutionized the analysis of lyssavirus field isolates (Benmansour et al. 1992; Sacramento et al. 1992; Smith et al. 1992; Tordo et al. 1992a, 1993a, 1995; Bourhy et al. 1993a, b; Nadin-Davis et al. 1993, 1994; Kissi et al. 1995; Nel et al. 1993; Smith et al. 1993 and many others). In particular, phylogenetic analysis revealed that each genotype comprises variants with distinct genetic patterns typical of the geographical area and/or the species of isolation. In addition, in genotype 1 (classical rabies), a cosmopolitan lineage illustrates human influence in the worldwide spread of variant, probably transmitted by dogs present in Europe in earlier centuries (Kissi et al. 1995; Smith et al. 1992; Badrane and Tordo 2001). This variant has undergone successful adaptation to other wildlife species. Most of the current rabies vaccine strains derive from a wild strain of genotype 1 isolated by Pasteur (Tordo 1996).

GENUS *EPHEMEROVIRUS*

The genus *Ephemerovirus* was created to accommodate viruses in tropical and subtropical areas transmitted by hematophagous insects to cattle and water buffalo (Walker et al. 1992, 1994; Fu et al. 1994a). The name came from the prototype bovine ephemeral fever virus (BEFV), which was initially reported to cause a brief, transient fever. However, ephemeroviruses have also been isolated from healthy insects and cattle, as well as from cattle with acute febrile illnesses of major economic importance. BEFV has been found in Australia, Japan, China, the Middle East, and South Africa. Adelaide river virus (ARV), Kimberley virus, and *Berrimah virus* have been isolated in Australia, *Makalal virus* in Kenya, and *Puchong virus* in Malaysia (Calisher et al. 1989; Tordo et al. 2004).

Ephemeroviruses are genetically closer to vesiculoviruses (Wang et al. 1995) but are antigenically related to: (1) the unclassified rhabdoviruses Obodhiang virus, Kotonkan virus, and Kolongo virus that were isolated from, respectively, mosquitoes in the Sudan, midges in Nigeria, and birds in the Central African Republic; and (2) the rabies-related Lagos bat virus (Calisher et al. 1989). Obodhiang virus and Kotonkan virus are in turn serologically linked to the rabies-related Molokai virus (Calisher et al. 1989), which is the only lyssavirus replicating in *Aedes albopictus* cell cultures (Buckley 1975). Taken together, these data suggest that Obodhiang virus and Kotonkan virus may occupy an intermediate position between the genus *Lyssavirus*, adapted to mammals, and the genus *Ephemerovirus*, which has maintained a mixed arthropod–mammal cycle.

PLANT RHABDOVIRUSES

Although more than 100 plant viruses are listed as possible rhabdoviruses, their poor immunogenicity has hampered serological grouping and classification was established at the genetic level (Jackson et al. 1999; Tordo et al. 2004). They are named according to the lesions they cause (e.g. necrosis, yellowing, and mosaic). Most are still classified according to the type of arthropod vector (aphid, leafhopper, etc.) (Jackson et al. 1987). Their transmission is mechanical, via arthropod or worm vectors, and most of those examined replicate efficiently in these vectors (Jackson et al. 1987). Two genera have so far been distinguished on replicative criteria. Members of the genus *Cytorhabdovirus* (prototype: lettuce necrotic yellows virus (LNYV)) replicate in the cytoplasm in association with viroplasms, and their morphogenesis takes place in vesicles of the endoplasmic reticulum. Members of the genus *Nucleorhabdovirus* (prototype: potato yellow dwarf virus (PYDV)) replicate in the nucleus, morphogenesis takes place at the inner nuclear envelope and virions accumulate in the perinuclear spaces (Murphy et al. 1995; Jackson et al. 1999).

FISH RHABDOVIRUSES

The rhabdoviruses of fish cause hematopoietic necrosis, hemorrhagic septicemia, dropsy, swim bladder inflammation and hydrocephalus, diseases of major economic importance to the fish farming industry. Several are similar to vesiculoviruses based on structural similarities in protein composition and size. Phylogenetic analyses suggest placing these viruses in a separate genus, *Novirhabdovirus* (Benmansour et al. 1994; Morzunov et al. 1995; Schütze et al. 1995; Tordo et al. 2004). Fish rhabdoviruses grow in cell cultures at the ambient temperature of fish. They may be transmitted by an aquatic arthropod.

SIGMA VIRUS

Sigma virus is unique among the rhabdoviruses. It is a hereditary factor endemic in 20 percent of natural populations of the fruit fly *Drosophila*, in which it is propagated via the gametes. Sigma virus is not cytopathic and only slightly pathogenic in the infected flies, except that it confers sensitivity to CO_2. Replication is partly under the control of an antiviral host gene, *ref(2)P*, which is also required for male fertility (Dezélée et al. 1989). It has been suggested that sigma was a rhabdovirus trapped by a nonbiting fly and behaved as a hereditary factor to ensure its own survival (Brun 1984).

BIRD RHABDOVIRUSES

There have been rare isolations of rhabdoviruses from birds in America, Central Africa, and India. Very little is known from them, except that they replicate quite efficiently in insect cells (Zeller and Mitchell 1989; Travassos da Rosa et al. 2002).

Morphology and chemical composition

MORPHOLOGY

Under the electron microscope (Figure 51.2), animal rhabdoviruses are usually bullet-shaped with one round end and the other flat; plant rhabdoviruses are more frequently bacilliform (Figures 51.2 and 51.3); a few examples of conical forms have been observed in Obhodiang virus, Kotonkan virus, and bovine ephemeral fever virus and sometimes in RABV. The virion diameter is almost constant (50–100 nm), but lengths vary (100–430 nm), depending on the species or on the presence of defective interfering (DI) particles, which appear when the multiplicity of infection is high. The DI particles possess a truncated genome, are therefore defective in various viral functions, and must depend on infectious virions to complement their deficiency (Lazzarini et al. 1981). Their smaller genomes compete efficiently with normal genomes for replication and packaging into virions. Although their role during natural infection remains unclear, these subgenomic deletion mutants have been mimicked extensively to generate non-infectious recombinant viruses for reverse genetic studies (reviewed by Conzelmann 1996).

The virion is composed of two structural units (Figure 51.4). One is a central cylinder 50 nm in diameter with characteristic cross-striations composed of a tightly coiled RNP with helical symmetry. This is contained within the second unit, a lipoprotein membrane that is provided by the cell membrane during budding, and through which protrudes an array of knobbed glycoprotein spikes of about 10 nm in length.

CHEMICAL COMPOSITION

The chemical composition is approximately 74 percent proteins, 20 percent lipids (composition dependent on the host cell), 3 percent carbohydrates, and 3 percent RNA. The RNA is a single molecule of negative polarity (i.e. non-infectious). There are five major viral proteins with post-translational modifications that have been assigned either to the envelope or to the RNP structures by biochemical dissection of the virion with proteases and detergents (Delagneau et al. 1981; Tordo and Poch 1988b). From outside to inside:

- The membrane-anchored glycoprotein forms a trimer (Doms et al. 1987; Gaudin et al. 1992) that is glycosylated, and acylated with palmitic acid (Schmidt and Schlesinger 1979; Gaudin et al. 1991b). It constitutes the protruding spikes that are detected at the virion surface in electron microscopy (Delagneau et al. 1981; Gaudin et al. 1992).
- The central RNP is formed by an intimate association between the nucleoprotein (phosphorylated in RABV) and the RNA genome, which is thereby rendered insensitive to nucleases. The heavily phosphorylated

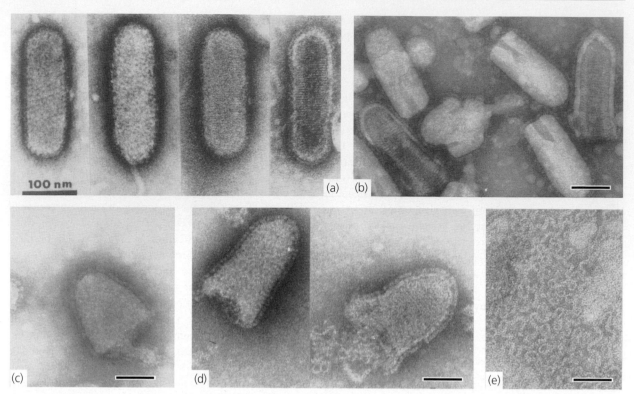

Figure 51.2 *Electron micrographs of rhabdoviruses.* **(a)** *Plant rhabdoviruses (courtesy of A.O. Jackson).* **(b)** *Vesiculovirus.* **(c)** *Lyssavirus (rabies virus, PV strain).* **(d)** *Lyssavirus (Mokola); one damaged virion with ribonucleocapsid protruding from the base).* **(e)** *Ribonucleocapsid RNP. All scale bars, 100 nm.*

phosphoprotein and the large protein (polymerase) are also bound to the RNP, although less intimately.

- The exact position of the matrix protein remains controversial. It is unclear if it is embedded in the inner layer of the membrane, in the central axial channel of the RNP, or both (Barge et al. 1993; Gaudin et al. 1995a). RABV matrix protein is palmitoylated (Gaudin et al. 1991a), whereas VSV matrix protein is phosphorylated (Kaptur et al. 1995). A subpopulation of M protein is ubiquitinylated in order to recruit the cellular machinery necessary for budding (Harty et al. 2001).

For historical reasons, the nomenclature of the five basic proteins differs between viruses; reports of their relative number per virion also vary owing to the different assay techniques used (reviewed by Coll 1995). Despite these discrepancies, the proteins have similar functions and similar molecular weights. We shall use the conventional abbreviations N for nucleoprotein (50–55 kDa), P for phosphoprotein (35–40 kDa), M for matrix protein (25 kDa), G for glycoprotein (60–70 kDa), and L for the large polymerase (approximately 200 kDa).

Besides these main viral proteins, several rhabdoviruses have developed additional polypeptides for specific functions (see section on Implications for the structure of the genome below, and Figure 51.7). These additional proteins are rarely found in the viral particle, suggesting their involvement in replicative functions or interaction with the host cell. Conversely, several cellular proteins are reported as being packaged in the RABV and VSV virions, for example cellular kinases playing a major role in activation of the phosphoprotein for replicative functions (Gao and Lenard 1995b; Gupta et al. 1995) and heat shock proteins (Sagara and Kawai 1992). Cytoskeleton-associated proteins such as actin-binding proteins (from the ezrin–radizin–moesin family) are closely associated with the membrane glycoprotein and thereby promote incorporation of actin into the virion (Sagara et al. 1995). Their involvement in virion formation during the budding process is likely but the exact role of the cytoskeleton in the replication/assembly process remains unclear.

Infection cycle in the cell

Except for the sigma virus of *Drosophila*, which is passed vertically, the vast majority of rhabdoviruses are transmitted mechanically by injury, contacts, bite, or aerosols. Tissue tropisms and pathogenicity vary with individual viruses. The main steps of cell infection, shared by all the rhabdoviruses, will now be described (Figure 51.5). It should be noted that the data come mainly from studies on VSV and to some extent on RABV; current researches on other rhabdoviruses may reveal variations.

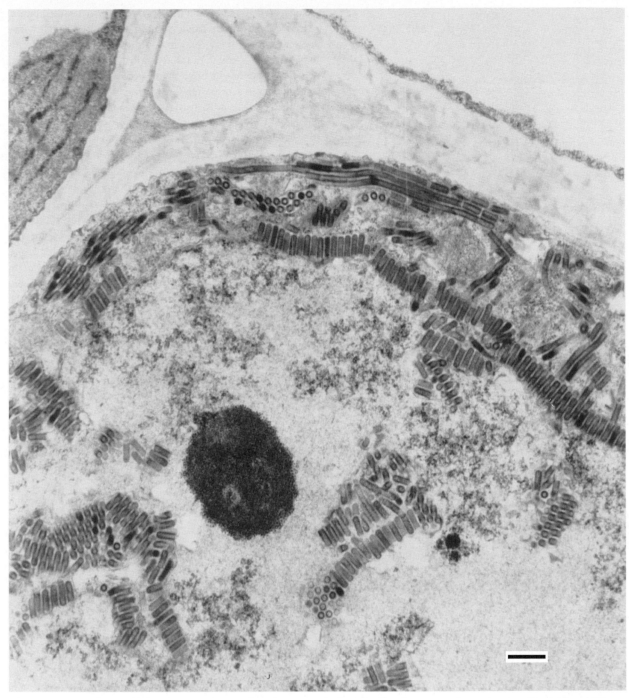

Figure 51.3 *Eggplant mottle dwarf virus within a cell nucleus. Note the long bacillary forms near the nuclear membrane. Bar, 4.5 μm (courtesy of R. Hull).*

PENETRATION INTO THE CELL

The attachment of the virus to the susceptible cell membrane is mediated by the glycoprotein, which recognizes specific receptors (Coll 1995). The nature of these receptors remains a matter of debate and the accumulated data reveal the complexity of the problem. In addition, most of the studies have been performed on strains that have been adapted for multiplication in established cell lines. For example, RABV isolates multiply and propagate exclusively inside neurons. Although adaptation does not abolish neurotropism, it renders the virus able to grow in nonneuronal cells. This adaptation may be due to the capability of fixed RABV strains to use ubiquitous receptors present on every cell type investigated to date. Ubiquitous receptors could be molecules such as phospholipids (Superti et al. 1984), gangliosides (Conti et al. 1988; Superti et al. 1986) or proteins (Wunner et al. 1984; Broughan and Wunner 1995; Gastka et al. 1996).

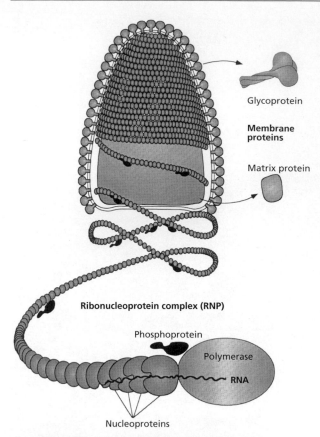

Glycoprotein

Membrane proteins

Matrix protein

Ribonucleoprotein complex (RNP)

Phosphoprotein

Polymerase

RNA

Nucleoproteins

Figure 51.4 *Structure of the virion.*

Several studies indicated that the nicotinic acetylcholine receptor (nAChR) is a receptor for RABV (for a review, see Baer and Lentz 1991). Nevertheless, as the nAChR is located mainly on muscle cells and as RABV infects neurons that do not express nAChR (McGehee and Lorca 1995), it has been proposed that, in animals, this receptor enbles street RABV to multiply locally in myotubes only at the site of inoculation (Burrage et al. 1985). This would facilitate subsequent penetration into neurons. More recently, the neuronal cell adhesion molecule (NCAM) has been shown to facilitate viral entry in established laboratory cell lines (Thoulouze et al. 1998) and, thus, has been proposed to be another receptor for RABV. Finally, an expression cloning approach using soluble RABV glycoprotein led to the identification of the murine p75 neurotropin receptor as another putative RABV receptor (Tuffereau et al. 1998). Subsequent examination of other lyssaviruses' genotypes revealed that the glycoprotein from European bat lyssavirus 2 (but not that of the other genotypes) could also bind p75 (Tuffereau et al. 2001).

Phosphatidylserine has been proposed to be a receptor for VSV (Schlegel et al. 1983). Nevertheless, the absence of this lipid in the outer leaflet of cells (except when they are apoptotic) suggests that this putative receptor has to be considered with caution.

Very few things are known concerning the receptor of other members of the family. Recently, it has been suggested that fibronectin is a receptor for viral hemorrhagic septicemia virus (VHSV), a salmonid rhabdovirus (Bearzotti et al. 1999). This putative receptor was identified using mAbs generated against rainbow trout gonad cells. These mAbs have been selected for their ability to protect cells from VHSV infection. The blocking activity of these mAbs was also effective against other nonantigenically related fish rhabdoviruses. Interestingly, Broughan and Wunner (1995) had also suggested an involvement of fibronectin for RABV entry in BHK21 cells. Thus, fibronectin might play a general role in rhabdovirus entry.

Once bound, the virus is internalized into a cellular endosome. Then, as the pH decreases within the endosome, the viral membrane fuses with the vesicle one and the RNP is freed into the cytoplasm. Fusion of rabies virus with liposomes has been studied in detail (Perrin et al. 1982; Gaudin et al. 1991b, 1993). Fusion is only triggered at low pH and does not require any specific composition of the target membrane. It is optimal around pH 6, and is not detected above pH 6.4. These pH values are very similar to those determined for VSV (White et al. 1981; Carneiro et al. 2003) and for a fish rhabdovirus (Gaudin et al. 1999). Preincubation of rhabdoviruses at low pH in the absence of a target membrane leads to inhibition of viral fusion properties. However, loss of fusion properties can be reversed by readjusting the pH to above 7. This is the main difference between rhabdoviruses and other viruses fusing at low pH for which low pH-induced fusion inactivation is irreversible (reviewed in Gaudin 2000a).

Low pH-induced conformational changes of RABV glycoprotein and their relationships with fusion activity have been studied. At the virion surface, G can assume at least three different states that have been characterized by electron microscopy, sensitivity to proteases, and monoclonal antibody assays (Gaudin et al. 1991b, 1993, 1995b; Roche and Gaudin 2002). The native (N) state is detected at the viral surface at pH above 7. The activated (A) hydrophobic state is detected immediately after acidification. It interacts with the target membrane as a first step of the fusion process (Durrer et al. 1995). After prolonged incubation at low pH, G is in a fusion inactive conformation (I) that is antigenically distinct from the N state. There is a pH-dependent equilibrium between these states which is shifted toward the I state at low pH (Roche and Gaudin 2002). Similar results have been obtained for VSV G (Clague et al. 1990; Doms et al. 1987; Pak et al. 1997; Carneiro et al. 2003). Finally, the results obtained so far suggest that, for rhabdoviruses, the sequence of events leading to membrane fusion are very similar to that of other enveloped viruses (Gaudin 2000b) and that the fusion complex is made of several trimers (Roche and Gaudin 2002).

Once delivered into the cytoplasm the RNP is ready to serve as a template for gene expression. In the

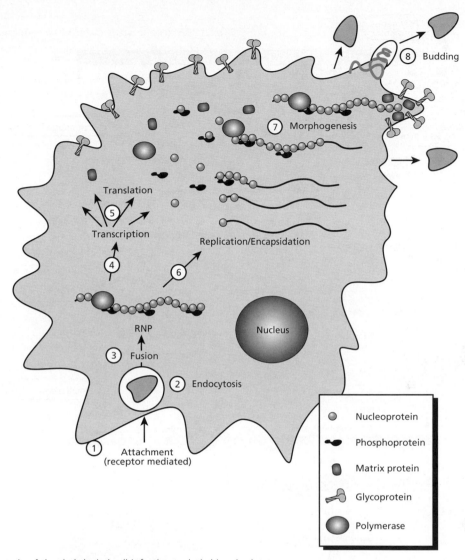

Figure 51.5 *Example of the rhabdoviral cell infection cycle (rabies virus).*

particular case of neuron infection by RABV, the RNP is first transported by retrograde axonal flow and replicates only in the perikaryon. Recently, it has been demonstrated that the phosphoprotein of lyssaviruses binds the LC8 light chain of the dynein motor suggesting that dynein might play a role in the transport of the RNP (Raux et al. 2000; Jacob et al. 2000). Nevertheless, as an RABV mutant, having a mutated phosphoprotein unable to bind LC8, behaves as wild-type virus even in animals, the exact role of this interaction is not clear (Mebatsion 2001).

Gene expression takes place exclusively in the cytoplasm and only a limited number of viral transcripts or proteins reach the nucleus where their exact role is not clear. In the case of vesiculoviruses, M protein, by interacting with nuclear pores, enhances the availability of the cellular translation machinery by inhibiting the export of cellular mRNAs from the nucleus (Her et al. 1997; Petersen et al. 2000; von Kobbe et al. 2000). In the

case of RABV, the *P* gene products are able to interact with the nuclear PML bodies. As these nuclear structures are involved in the resistance of many cells to viral infection, this interaction is supposed to modulate the cellular innate immune response (Blondel et al. 2002).

Mechanism of genome expression

Mechanisms of rhabdovirus genome expression have been more extensively explored on the VSV model (reviews: Banerjee 1987; Tordo and Poch 1988b; Vidal and Kolakofsky 1989; Banerjee and Barik 1992; Tordo and Kouznetzoff 1993; Barr et al. 2002; Kolakofsky et al. 2004; Whelan et al. 2004). Because the rhabdovirus genome has negative polarity, it must be transcribed to produce the complementary positive-strand mRNAs. The RNP serves as template for two successive RNA synthetic functions (Figure 51.6): transcription then

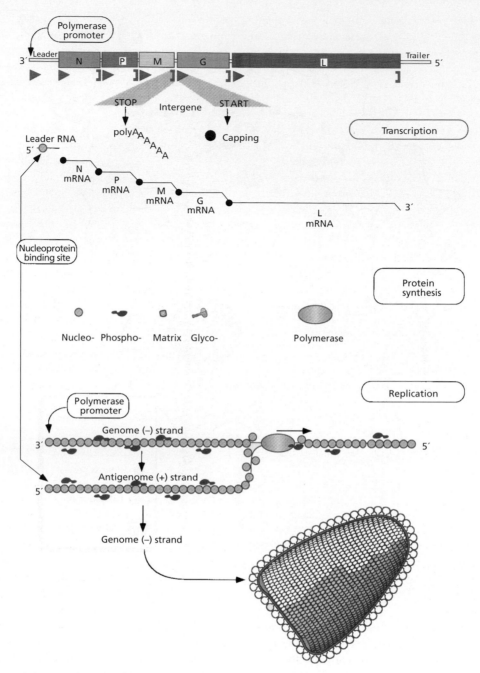

Figure 51.6 *Transcription, translation, and replication mechanisms of rhabdoviruses.*

replication. For both, the viral polymerase recognizes a promoter at the 3′ end of the encapsidated genome, and proceeds towards the 5′ end. There is still a debate whether there is a single 3′or two different promoters for transcription and replication. The difference between transcription and replication is determined by the processivity of the polymerase, that influences the way it progresses either sequentially or continuously. Transcription gives rise to mostly monocistronic transcripts: first a short noncapped, nonpolyadenylated leader RNA, then five (or more) mRNAs coding for the viral proteins (Figure 51.6). This sequential progression depends on the recognition of short conserved *cis*-acting signals,

bordering the cistrons, which initiate start (and capping) and stop (and polyadenylation) of the mRNAs. When the transcriptase stops transcribing at one polyadenylation signal, it scans in both directions for the nearby (re)start mRNA signal. This strategy results in sequential transcription from the 3′ to the 5′ cistrons, associated with a progressive attenuation due to the cumulative probability of the polymerase to fall off the template during scanning. Thus, the length of the scanned intergenic region influences the efficiency of re-initiation. Bidirectional scanning permits overlapping cistrons when the polymerase backtracks and restarts within the cistron upstream.

In contrast, the replicase acts continuously and generates a full-length positive-strand antigenome that is in turn replicated into negative-strand genomes for the progeny virions. To become functional templates, the genomes and antigenomes must be encapsidated into RNP, which protects them from the action of nuclease. This is why viral protein synthesis is a prerequisite for replication. There is an entry site for the nucleoprotein at its 5′ end to promote the concomitant encapsidation of the growing RNA. During the transcription step, leader RNA carrying this entry site is released. During replication, the 5′ end remains linked to the growing RNA genome, which is progressively encapsidated.

The main event influencing continuous synthesis by the polymerase and its switch from transcription to replication mode is the concomitant (anti)genome encapsidation. Here, the amount of nucleoprotein available is decisive (Vidal and Kolakofsky 1989; Horikami et al. 1992). At low levels, the polymerase stops at the end of the leader RNA and immediately re-initiates at the start signal of the first mRNA. This initiation prevents encapsidation of the mRNAs and causes a shift to the sequential transcription mode, in which elongation is independent of encapsidation. This results in an increase in viral protein. At high levels of nucleoprotein, the concomitant encapsidation prevents the polymerase stopping at the end of the leader RNA, causing a switch into the processive mode and the replicase becomes unable to recognize the following start and stop signals.

The translation step separating transcription from replication is ensured by cellular mechanisms. The classic scanning model (Kozak 1989), predicting that ribosomes bind to the capped 5′ end of the mRNA and scan downstream, is generally accepted. Thus, most of the viral proteins start at the first AUG codon along the mRNA. Exceptions to this rule have, however, been noted during translation of the P mRNA. In addition to the normal P protein, VSV encodes two other polypeptides starting at distal AUGs, one in the same open reading frame (ORF) (Herman 1986) and one in another ORF (Spiropoulou and Nichol 1993). By contrast, RABV uses at least four AUGs in the same ORF. Translation of these proteins is initiated by a leaky scanning mechanism (Chenik et al. 1995). The resulting polypeptides are either cytoplasmic or nuclear, depending on the accessibility of corresponding export and import signals, and thereby interact with various cellular partners (Blondel et al. 2002). All the viral proteins are expressed in the cytosol by free polyribosomes, except the glycoprotein which is synthesized as a transmembrane protein by polyribosomes associated with membranes of the rough endoplasmic reticulum (RER). It is then transported to the cytoplasmic membrane via the Golgi apparatus. Because of the acidity of the RER and Golgi compartments, the glycoprotein is synthesized in a conformation inactive for fusion, thus impairing its interaction with viral cellular

membranes during transport. Once at the cell surface, the pH increases and the conformation reverts to the native type (Gaudin et al. 1995b, c).

Several viruses have developed variations on this general model of expression. The ephemeroviruses use a polycistronic strategy to express both structural and regulatory genes (Wang and Walker 1993; Wang et al. 1994). In the case of vaccine strains of RABV (PV, ERA, SAD), there are alternative terminations for the matrix and glycoprotein cistrons (Tordo and Poch 1988a, Morimoto et al. 1989; Sacramento et al. 1992, Tordo et al. 1992b; Tordo and Kouznetzoff 1993). Two consecutive stop (polyadenylation) signals are alternatively recognized by the transcriptase to produce either a small or a large mRNA. It has been proposed that alternative termination, by modifying the length of the scanned intergenic region, could influence the transcription level of the distal cistron, resulting in a regulation tool for genome expression (Tordo and Poch 1988a; Tordo et al. 1992b; Tordo and Kouznetzoff 1993). This regulation could be partly under the control of specific cellular factors, reinforcing the importance of the intracellular environment for cell susceptibility noted above, and suggesting that it might be worthwhile to study rabies neurotropism at the transcriptional level.

Implications for the structure of the genome

The genome of rhabdoviruses varies in length between 11 kb (*Vesiculovirus*) and 15 kb (*Ephemerovirus*) (see Figure 51.7). Its structure subserves a typical expression mechanism. For both the minus-strand genome and the plus-strand antigenome the promoter for the polymerase is located at the 3′ end (Smallwood and Moyer 1993); the entry site of the nucleoprotein for encapsidation is at the 5′ end (Moyer et al. 1991) (Figure 51.6). As the minus-strand genome is template for either transcription or replication, while the plus-strand antigenome is only template for replication, the promoter for replication of the plus-strand antigenome is logically much stronger than that of the minus-strand genome (Barr et al. 2002; Le Mercier et al. 2003; Whelan et al. 2004). The consequence of the preservation of these important signals is that the extremities of both positive and negative strands are complementary, although a hairpin structure was never evidenced in vivo. Indeed, a minigenome consisting of only 50 residues from each end is sufficient to ensure transcription, replication, encapsidation, and envelopment (Pattnaik et al. 1995). In addition, when the complementarity between extremities is increased by mutagenesis, replication rather than transcription is favored (Wertz et al. 1994; Whelan et al. 2004). It is interesting that most of the DI particles effectively mimic such minigenomes; those with extensive complementary ends are the most efficient for interference.

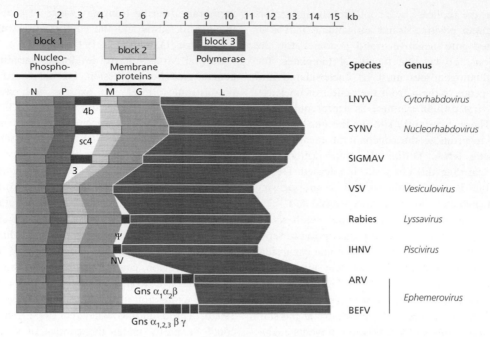

Figure 51.7 *Structural comparison of the rhabdovirus genomes. ARV, Adelaide River virus; BEFV, bovine ephemeral fever virus; IHNV, infectious hematopoietic necrosis virus; LNYV, lettuce necrotic yellows virus; SYNV, sonchus yellow net virus; VSV, vesicular stomatitis virus.*

Besides the conserved extremities, the genome possesses a modular structure with the juxtaposition of cistrons independently controlled by signal sequences. Indeed, the progressive decrease in the rate of transcription from the 3′ to the 5′ end implies that the position of a cistron directly influences its rate of expression. This explains why rhabdoviruses have conserved very similar genome organizations into three blocks (Figure 51.7) (Tordo et al. 1992a). Block 1 at the 3′ end encodes proteins required in large quantities (N, P), particularly the nucleoprotein that balances the switch between transcription and replication. Block 2 encodes the membrane proteins (M, G). Block 3 at the 5′ end encodes the viral polymerase (L), required in limited amounts. This modular structure accepts some flexibility, and in several viruses typical genes are inserted that are adapted to their particular biology. Between blocks 1 and 2, the plant rhabdoviruses encode a protease-like protein (sc4, 4b) that corresponds to the movement protein needed for passage of the virus through plasmodesmata, thus allowing cell-to-cell transmission despite the presence of the cell wall (Scholthof et al. 1994). At the same position the sigma virus encodes a protein related to the reverse transcriptase of retro-elements (ORF 3) (Landès-Devauchelle et al. 1995). Between blocks 2 and 3, the ephemeroviruses encode a second heavily glycosylated glycoprotein (Gns) which probably arose from a sequence duplication of the *G* gene (Wang and Walker 1993). Gns is nonstructural and of unknown function, as are the additional small proteins (α, β, γ) encoded consecutively (Wang et al. 1994) and the NV protein of the fish rhabdovirus IHNV (Morzunov et al. 1995; Kurath et al.

1997). It is interesting that, at the same position between blocks 2 and 3, lyssaviruses conserve a large noncoding area initially termed 'pseudogene' ψ because it could represent a vestige of the multiple changes occurring in this region during rhabdovirus evolution (Tordo et al. 1986, 1992b; Ravkov et al. 1995).

Exit from the cell

Before viral budding, transcription and replication are inhibited and, simultaneously, the RNP becomes intensively condensed and coiled. A considerable body of evidence suggests that this morphological role during virion assembly is played by the matrix protein (see Morphology and chemical composition above). In parallel, glycoproteins are concentrated in particular regions of the plasma membrane (Brown and Lyles 2003). After the cytoplasmic maturation step, the virion leaves the cell by budding, the lipid envelope being provided by the host cell membrane. Most rhabdoviruses bud from the plasma membrane and some from internal cell membranes. The plant rhabdoviruses bud either from the endoplasmic reticulum (cytorhabdoviruses) or from the inner nuclear envelope (nucleorhabdoviruses) and accumulate in perinuclear spaces (Jackson et al. 1987).

Functional role of the viral polypeptides

The advances in genetic manipulation of negative-strand RNA viruses have greatly facilitated the functional dissection of viral genes and proteins by reverse genetics (see Conzelmann 1996 for a review, and also Lawson et al. 1995; Whelan et al. 1995; Kretzschmar et al. 1996; Schnell et al. 1996; Le Mercier et al. 2002). The use of these viruses has greatly improved the understanding of viral pathogenesis and has provided stable vectors to express foreign genes and develop new vaccines (Schnell et al. 1996; Dietzschold et al. 2003; McKenna et al. 2003; Faber et al. 2004). In addition, studies of the interactions between the proteins and the backbone RNA genome are being pursued by various physical (electron microscopy and crystallography), biochemical, and immunological methods.

THE RIBONUCLEOCAPSID COMPLEX (RNP)

The RNP is the minimum structure needed to mediate RNA synthesis. The N protein RNA is the template whereas the polymerase function is catalyzed by the L and P proteins (Conzelmann and Schnell 1994). Minus-strand as well as plus-strand genomic templates are so tightly complexed with the N protein that they are resistant to both RNases and post-translational gene silencing by short interfering RNA (Bitko and Barik 2001). The RNP complex possesses a typical helical form (Schoehn et al. 2001). Chemical probing experiments on VSV RNP showed that the N protein binds to the sugar–phosphate backbone, exposes the Watson–Crick positions of the bases to the solvent and modifies their reactivity (Iseni et al. 2000). Indeed, the nucleoprotein melts secondary RNA structure (helical activity) and favors transcription/replication without the need for dissociation. L is the RNA-dependent RNA polymerase that possesses most of the required enzymatic activities: RNA synthesis (De and Banerjee 1984); mRNA capping and methylation (Horikami and Moyer 1982); mRNA polyadenylation (Hunt et al. 1984; Hunt and Hutchinson 1993); and possibly kinase activity on the P protein (Barik and Banerjee 1992). P is a regulatory cofactor for which various functions have been proposed: mediating interaction between L and the N-RNA template (Isaac and Keene 1982; De and Banerjee 1984); transiently displacing the N protein to gain access to the RNA (Hudson et al. 1986); complexing the soluble N to maintain it in a replication-competent form for encapsidation (Masters and Banerjee 1988; Howard and Wertz 1989; La Ferla and Peluso 1989; Mavrakis et al. 2003).

The nucleoprotein N appears as a two-modular protein, with a large, compact (resistant to proteases) and well-conserved NH_2-terminal core binding the RNA, and a smaller, flexible and variable COOH tail which is exposed and ensures contact with the P protein (Banerjee et al. 1989; Iseni et al., 1998; Schoehn et al. 2001). RNA-binding sites with noncanonical motifs have been tentatively identified for RABV and viral hemorrhagic septicemia virus (Kouznetzoff et al. 1998; Said et al. 1998). Site-directed and deletion mutagenesis and

two-hybrid method suggested domains important for N–N and N–P interactions (Chenik et al. 1994; Jacob et al. 2001; Schoehn et al. 2001). The rabies virus N protein N is phosphorylated (unlike VSV). The role for this phosphorylation due to a cellular kinase is unclear; phosphate hydrolysis could produce free energy for transcription and replication (Wu et al. 2002, 2003).

The interaction network of the P protein within the RNP has been extensively studied, (Chenik et al. 1994, 1998; Fu et al. 1994b; Gao and Lenard 1995a; Jacob et al. 2001; Takacs and Banerjee 1995). The rabies virus P protein seems to be composed of two independent domains that nicely outline its intermediate position between the L and N–RNA template. The NH_2 half encompasses the L binding site close to the N terminus (amino acids (aa) 1–52 particularly 1–19) as well as a weak N-binding site (aa 1–185 particularly 69–138) which probably interacts and maintains the soluble N in an encapsidation-competent form (Mavrakis et al, 2003). The COOH half comprises a strong N-binding site (aa 176–297), which likely binds the N–RNA template. The atomic structure of the COOH half (186–297) has been determined and the residues important for N–RNA binding mapped (Mavrakis et al. 2004). The COOH half is a monomer and the oligomerization of P rather involves the NH_2 half (particularly aa 52–189). The phosphorylation of P is essential for regulating its activity in transcription (Barik and Banerjee 1992; Beckes and Perrault 1992; Gao and Lenard 1995a) and replication (Chang et al. 1994). P subspecies varying in degree of phosphorylation and in physical state (soluble, multimeric, or complexed with N or L) have different activities in relation to both functions (Tuffereau et al. 1985; Gao and Lenard 1995a; Richardson and Peluso 1996). The P phosphorylation step is ensured at precise sites by different cellular kinases packaged in the virion: the casein kinase-II and an L-associated kinase (LAK) for VSV (Barik and Banerjee 1992; Beckes and Perrault 1992; Chen et al. 1997; Gao and Lenard 1995a, 1995b; Gupta et al. 1995); the protein kinase C (isomers α, β, and γ and another cellular rabies specific phosphokinase (RVPK) for rabies virus. It is interesting that protein kinase Cγ is mostly found in nerve tissue, and could provide another tissue-specific element in the regulation of rabies transcription. Phosphorylation is thought to promote conformational changes. Phosphorylation is required for oligomerization of the VSV but not of the rabies P protein (Gao and Lenard 1995b, Gigant et al. 2000). The small C and C' basic proteins encoded in a second ORF on the P gene (Spiropoulou and Nichol 1993; Kretzschmar et al. 1996) are unnecessary for VSV growth in tissue culture (Kretzschmar et al. 1996). It has been suggested that they play a role in viral pathogenesis or transmission by insect vectors (Kretzschmar et al. 1996).

Due to very limited amounts in the virion as well as in infected cell, less is known on the structure–function of the L polymerase. The region binding the P protein is located at the COOH side: in aa 1638–1873 for VSV (Canter and Perrault 1996); in the C-terminal 566 aa for rabies virus (Chenik et al. 1998). The sequence alignment of L proteins from *Mononegavirales* has provided a structure that is consistent with its multifunctional nature: six conserved domains (probably carrying the catalytic activities) are concatenated by variable hinge regions (Poch et al. 1990). The domains seem to be autonomous as suggested by complementation between L mutants (Flamand 1980). Putative functions have been tentatively assigned to several domains (Poch et al. 1990). In particular, domain III possesses four or five hyperconserved motifs similar in structure and position to those found in all RNA-dependent polymerases (Poch et al. 1989; Müller et al. 1994) and also in DNA-dependent polymerases, although more distantly (Delarue et al. 1990). Distant from this 'polymerase module,' domain VI (500 aa toward the COOH side) is typical from 2′-*O*-ribose-methyltransferases (Bujnicki and Rychlewski 2002; Ferron et al. 2002) and could be involved in the methylation during mRNA capping (Abraham et al. 1975; Gupta et al. 2002). This predictive analysis has guided the first trials of site-directed mutagenesis, which basically confirmed the functional importance of the predicted motifs (Sleat and Banerjee 1993; Schnell and Conzelmann 1995). A more systematic analysis by extensive sequence comparison between wildtype and mutant strains of VSV suggests that residues in the interdomain V–VI are essential for polyadenylation and thermosensitivity (Hunt and Hutchinson 1993). In addition, it was suggested that host factor(s) might be required for the activity of the L protein (Mathur et al. 1996).

MEMBRANE PROTEINS

M is a small protein (slightly more than 200 amino acid residues) comprising a positively charged amino terminal part (Poch et al. 1988). For VSV, this amino terminal part can be removed by proteolysis (Ogden et al. 1986). Cleavage of VSV M by thermolysin provided a resistant core (Mth) composed of two noncovalently associated fragments (residues 48–121 and 122–(or 123 or 124 depending on the thermolysin cleavage site) 229) (Gaudier et al. 2001) that could be crystallized allowing the determination of its structure (Gaudier et al. 2002).

The M protein is involved in the late steps of the infectious cycle. It condenses the RNP into a tightly coiled helical structure (Newcomb et al. 1982). This tightly coiled structure seems to be formed near cellular membranes where M is bound (Odenwald et al. 1986; Flood and Lyles 1999). Strong evidence that M plays a major role in VSV budding comes from studies of VSV temperature-sensitive mutants affected in budding that were shown to be mutated in the *M* gene and were complemented by wild-type plasmid-derived M

(Flamand 1970; Lyles et al. 1996). More recently, an M-deficient RABV mutant has been obtained using reverse genetic (Mebatsion et al. 1999). In the absence of M, infectious particles were mainly cell associated and the yield of cellfree infectious virus was largely reduced demonstrating the role of RABV M in virus budding. Supernatants from cells infected with the M-deficient RABV did not contain the typical bullet-shaped rhabdovirus particles, but instead contained long, rod-shaped virions, showing severe impairment of the virus formation.

Two biochemical properties of VSV M have been studied, auto-association and membrane-binding VSV. M self-associates into large multimers at physiological NaCl concentration (McCreedy et al. 1990), a process initiated by trypsin-sensitive nucleation sites that is reversed by increasing the salt concentration (Gaudin et al. 1995a). M self-association could be important for nucleocapsid compaction and may constitute a driving force for budding. VSV M cell membrane association is also necessary for budding. This interaction was proved to be extremely stable in vivo as it is not destabilized by harsh treatments such as 2M KCl or pH 11 (Bergmann and Fusco 1988; Chong and Rose 1993, 1994). The regions of the protein involved in membrane association are not completely defined: hydrophobic photolabeling has identified the amino-terminal region of the protein (Lenard and Vanderoef 1990), but M mutants deleted from the amino-terminal domain still interact with cellular membranes, suggesting that another domain of the protein is involved (Chong and Rose 1994; Ye et al. 1994). Indeed, the structure of Mth revealed a hydrophobic patch at the surface of the protein. This patch is located close to a hydrophobic loop containing the cleavage site of thermolysin and surrounded by basic residues (two arginines and three lysines). The combined presence of hydrophobic and basic residues suggests that it is a likely candidate for being a region interacting with membranes (Gaudier et al. 2002).

The amino-terminal part of the matrix protein contains two short motifs (PPxY and PSAP) that are supposed to recruit the cellular partners involved in the ultimate step of the budding process (i.e. the fission step). The PPxY motif has been shown to be recognized by an E3 ubiquitin ligase (Harty et al. 2001) and to influence budding efficiency (Jayakar et al. 2000). The exact role of the PSAP motif remains to be determined.

The functions of M are not limited to viral assembly and budding. Both VSV and RABV M inhibits the transcription of the viral genome (Clinton et al. 1978; De et al. 1982; Finke et al. 2003). RABV M acts also as a replication stimulatory factor (Finke et al. 2003). For RABV M, a mutation has been identified that affect the function of M only in regulation of RNA synthesis, but not in assembly and budding, providing evidence that these functions are genetically separable (Finke and Conzelmann 2003).

Finally, VSV M expression causes the rounding of cells, a phenotype characteristic of VSV infection (Blondel et al. 1990; Melki et al. 1994) that is probably a consequence of M-induced apoptosis (Kopecky et al. 2001; Kopecky and Lyles 2003). As mentioned above, it also inhibits the export of RNAs from the nucleus (Her et al. 1997; Petersen et al. 2000; von Kobbe et al. 2000). This export inhibition may be the cause of M-induced inhibition of host-cell transcription (Black et al. 1993; Black and Lyles 1992). It has also been proposed that host transcription shut-off is induced by an effect of M on the transcription factor TFIID, which was found to be ineffective in the cells where M is expressed (Yuan et al. 1998). All these cytopathic effects of M protein explain why VSV is deleterious to all types of cell.

The glycoprotein (reviewed by Coll 1995) has the typical structure of group I transmembrane proteins. An NH_2 terminal signal peptide of about 20 amino acids (aa) in length serves the translocation of nascent protein through the RER membrane and is cleaved in the mature protein. A hydrophobic transmembrane segment (approximately 20 aa) remains embedded in the viral envelope. It separates the 'cytoplasmic' COOH domain (about 50 aa), interacting with internal viral proteins, from the glycosylated NH_2 ectodomain (approximately 450 aa). The glycosylation and palmitoylation sites have been mapped (Rose et al. 1984; Gaudin et al. 1991a; Shakin-Eshleman et al. 1992). The role of glycosylation in correct folding of G ectodomain has been studied in detail (Machamer and Rose 1988; Hammond and Helenius 1994; Mathieu et al. 1996; Gaudin 1997). A map of the disulfide bridges of the ectodomain of VHSV G has also been established (Einer-Jensen et al. 1998) that has allowed a general model for the rhabdoviral G (Walker and Kongsuwan 1999). It has to be noted that VSV G and some of its thermosensitive mutants have been used as model glycoproteins to elucidate how membrane proteins are transported all along the secretory pathway. Particularly, VSV G has been used to study the quality control mechanisms that operate in the endoplasmic reticulum (ER) and the downstream compartments to ensure that only proteins that are correctly folded are transported (e.g. Hammond and Helenius 1994; Cannon et al. 1996).

The important functions of the ectodomain have also been mapped. Based on sequence similarity with snake venom curare-mimetic neurotoxins (Lentz et al. 1984; Rustici et al. 1993; Tordo et al. 1993b) and further studies using anti-idiotypic antibodies (Hanham et al. 1993), the 190–203 aa sequence of rabies glycoprotein ectodomain has been implicated in the recognition of the nicotinic AChR. By selection of RABV mutants that were not neutralized by a soluble form of p75, the domain of interaction with this receptor has been shown to implicate aa 318 and 352 (Langevin and Tuffereau 2002). The region involved in fusion has also been searched by insertion and directed mutagenesis. Different sites modified the ectodomain structure in such a way that fusion activity was blocked or modified (Li et al. 1993; Zhang and Ghosh 1994; Fredericksen and Whitt 1995, 1996). However, the exact locations of the fusion peptide were mapped by photolabeling to the following sequences: aa 102–179 for RABV, 58–221 for VSV (Durrer et al. 1995). Taken together, these data suggest that a sequence corresponding to aa 118-136 of VSV enriched in prolines and aromatic residues might constitute G fusion peptide. However, the data obtained during these studies have also indicated that a second region of the protein, located in the carboxy-terminal part of the ectodomain (around aa 400), controls the low pH-induced conformational changes of G (Gaudin et al. 1996; Shokralla et al. 1998). Finally, several residues of the ectodomain seem to play a crucial role in pathogenicity and virulence (Tordo et al. 1993b). For RABV, neurovirulence is directly linked to the maintenance of a basic residue in position 333 (Tuffereau et al. 1989) that may be involved in p75 recognition (Tuffereau et al. 1998). Mutation at this residue reduced the categories of neurons sensitive to infection (Coulon et al. 1994).

Antigens

In the case of RABV, several hundred mAbs have been used to characterize the antigenic structure of G making this protein one of the best known viral antigens (Raux et al. 1995; Benmansour et al. 1991; Préhaud et al. 1988; Seif et al. 1985; Lafon et al. 1983; Wiktor and Koprowski 1980). RABV G has two major antigenic sites that are antigenic sites II and III. Antigenic site II is located between positions 34 and 42 and positions 198 and 200 (Préhaud et al. 1988). These peptides are joined by a disulfide bridge and maintained together in the tertiary structure of G (Dietzschold et al. 1982). Antigenic site III extends from amino acids 330 to 338 (Seif et al. 1985). Beside these major antigenic sites, one minor antigenic site and a few isolated epitopes have been described (Lafay et al. 1996; Raux et al. 1995; Benmansour et al. 1991; Dietzschold et al. 1990).

The immune response against lyssaviruses is complex; the response to RABV has been extensively studied. Although all the viral proteins are antigenic, their roles in protection vary (Lafon 1994; Xiang et al. 1995; Drings et al. 1999). Their respective importance has been defined by recombinant DNA techniques (Tordo 1991; Perrin et al. 2001). Two of them, G and N, are of primary importance, the phosphoprotein P being of less significance. Purified G protein protects against intracerebral challenge with RABV, and is the only antigen that consistently induces virus-neutralizing antibody (Wiktor et al. 1973). This property mainly depends on the preservation of its three-dimensional structure, although a linear neutralizing epitope has been identified (Bunschoten et al. 1989; Benmansour et al. 1991; Ni et al. 1995). On the other hand, the glycoprotein shares with the N and P proteins of RNP the capacity to induce a cellular immune response, involving, respectively, T helper cells (Th) and cytotoxic T cells (Tc) (Lafon 1994; Xiang et al. 1995). Purified RNP protects against challenge by peripheral routes, probably through a cross-help mechanism between N-specific Th lymphocytes and G-specific B lymphocytes producing neutralizing antibodies (Dietzschold et al. 1987; Lodmell et al. 1991; Lodmell et al. 1993). An effective role of the Tc response in protection remains to be clearly demonstrated (Xiang et al. 1995). It is interesting that the G and N antigens conserve their immunogenic properties when administered orally (Hooper et al. 1994). This property is used extensively in large vaccination campaigns with vaccinia or adenoviruses expressing recombinant G protein (see Control).

Most of the current rabies vaccine strains derive from a wild strain isolated by Pasteur (Tordo 1991). This was initially passaged intracerebrally in rabbits until the incubation period shortened and became 'fixed' at 5–8 days. From this, multiple passages in animal brain and cell culture were performed. Vaccine strains belong to genotype 1 (causing classic rabies) and protect against homologous isolates (Lodmell et al. 1995), but do not protect efficiently against rabies-related viruses in genotypes 2–6 that also pose possible threats to humans (Bahloul et al. 1998; Badrane et al. 2001). Work is in progress to improve the protection offered by the vaccine by increasing the number of genotypes against which it is effective. The conserved N protein, a strong inducer of Th cells, may be important in this respect. It behaves as a superantigen in humans and BALB/c mice, activating Vβ8 and Vβ6 T cells, respectively (Lafon et al. 1992; Lafon 1994). The antigenic sites for B and T cell responses have been extensively mapped along the G, N, and P viral antigens by sequencing mutants resistant to neutralizing antibodies or by measuring the reactivity of chemically cleaved or synthetic peptides (Bunschoten et al. 1989; Benmansour et al. 1991; Ertl et al. 1991; Minamoto et al. 1994; Goto et al. 1995). The vast majority of the G protein antigenic sites seem to be conformational, sometimes involving regions that are distant from each other in the primary structure, but which are brought in proximity by protein folding and disulfide bridges. Taking into account the recent modifications in rabies epidemiology and especially the growing importance of bats in human transmission, an important effort has been done to enlarge the protection spectrum of vaccines, from anti-rabies to anti-lyssavirus status. Novel strategies have been elaborated using the versatility permitted by DNA-based immunization (Bahloul et al. 1998; Jallet et al. 1999). Plasmids expressing chimeric G proteins were constructed by fusing the COOH half of one genotype with the NH_2 half of another genotype. Upon intra-muscular injection in mice, protection was obtained against the two parental genotypes but also against other genotypes, demonstrating the possibility of increasing the spectrum from antirabies to anti-lyssavirus vaccines. Protection was also obtained by intramuscular vaccination of dogs (Perrin et al. 2000). Finally, the capability of the lyssavirus G protein to carry foreign epitopes/antigens was also demonstrated in the perspective of a future DNA multivalent vaccine against various zoonoses for carnivores (Desmezières et al. 1999).

CLINICAL AND PATHOLOGICAL ASPECTS: VESICULOVIRUS INFECTION

Vesicular stomatitis

The interest in vesicular stomatitis viruses as models for basic studies in virology and molecular biology has tended to overshadow their natural history and their role as agents of disease. The disease was first reported in livestock in the USA in 1821 (Hanson 1981). It is largely confined to the western hemisphere and reports of its occurrence elsewhere are considered to be either of importations from the West or of doubtful authenticity (Brown and Crick 1979). The virus was first isolated by Cotton (1927) and its morphology established by Chow and co-workers (Chow et al. 1954).

Disease in animals

The clinical manifestations in horses and cattle are fever, development of vesicles on the tongue, gums, and lips, and excessive salivation. Teats of milking cows may be infected and, less commonly, lesions may be seen on the feet. Animals have difficulty in eating and walking, and lose weight; milking cows stop lactating. The disease is rarely lethal except in pigs. Epizootics of vesicular stomatitis are sudden in onset (within approximately 2 weeks) and quickly involve many animals in a herd but often do not spread to adjacent farms. In the USA it occurs in the summer months in approximately 10-year cycles. In Central America, outbreaks are more frequent and possibly associated with the change from wet to dry seasons.

Disease in humans

The virus can also infect humans, usually causing a mild influenzalike illness, although more severe forms are reported. The incubation period is 1–9 days after exposure and symptoms may last 3–4 days; occasionally there may be a relapse (Sellers 1984). Infections of humans have mostly been reported in laboratory workers after aerosol inhalation or accidental contamination of eyes or abrasions. However, in some areas of North and Central

America 25–90 percent of farmers have antibody to VSV (Hanson 1981).

Transmission

The virus is found in vesicle fluid and epithelium and does not persist after recovery. It is not excreted in urine, feces, or milk. Spread by direct contact with vesicle fluid is possible, and transfer from teat lesions by milkers and milking equipment is occasionally reported. However, experimental studies have failed to demonstrate direct animal-to-animal transmission, and Sellers (1984) noted many outbreaks in which the disease did not spread to neighboring animals on the same farm. The bites of infected blood-sucking arthropods seem to be the most likely mode of transmission, demonstrated experimentally with several strains of the virus. In addition, many vesiculoviruses have been isolated in nature from mosquitoes, sandflies, midges, mites, and ticks. There are no overt pathological signs in arthropods, and how they become infected is obscure. The disease in animals being brief, with minimal and transient viremia, they are unlikely natural reservoirs of the virus. It has been suggested that some strains may be plant viruses and that animals are infected either directly, by eating infected plants, or by the bites of insects that have fed on such plants.

Vaccines

Vaccines ranging from live unmodified virus to vaccinia recombinants specific for the G protein have been used with poor success. Their development has not been pursued vigorously, both because of the self-limiting nature of the disease and because the durability of the immune response is uncertain. However, the potential of reverse genetic methods could give new perspectives in this domain (Barr et al. 2002).

CLINICAL AND PATHOLOGICAL ASPECTS: RABIES INFECTION

Although the clinical signs of rabies have been recognized for many centuries, it is mainly since the late nineteenth century that significant progress has been made in laboratory diagnosis, human postexposure treatment, control of animal rabies, and studies of the epidemiology, pathogenesis, and immune response. Currently, in most of the industrialized world, diagnostic systems are well organized, rapid, and efficient; human postexposure treatment is very effective; host species are principally wildlife; and technologically, there are excellent prospects for control or eradication of the disease in large geographical areas. In spite of these remarkable advances, rabies is still a serious problem with significant economic losses and human deaths in large parts of Africa, Asia, and South America.

Clinical aspects

FACTORS DETERMINING CLINICAL MANIFESTATIONS

The fact that not every rabid animal bite could result in clinical rabies and death has pointed out the existence of factors that could determine the clinical manifestations and lethal outcome of the disease (Hemachudha 1989). First, different species have different levels of susceptibility, latency, and infectivity (Hemachudha and Mitrabhakdi 2000). Thus, it has been possible to place species into different groups of low (e.g. opossums), moderate (e.g. nonhuman primates), high (e.g. cattle), and extremely high susceptibilities (e.g. fox) (WHO 1973). Other determinant factors are the severity of the wounds, the site of exposure, and the virus content of the saliva. For example, the incubation period is generally shorter following bite wounds to the head region than after those at the extremities, with grossly an inverse correlation between the length of the incubation period and the dose of virus. It is thought that a specific pattern of clinical manifestations could not be associated with a particular rabies virus variant, as reported by Hemachudha et al. (2003). Taken together, a combination of these factors results in the fact that the incubation period in animals may vary widely, with an usual range from 2 to 12 weeks with periods much longer than 3 months (Charlton et al. 1987), and also in the fact that in human rabies mortality after rabid animal bites varies from 35 to 57 percent (Hemachudha and Phuapradit 1997), with a few recorded cases of incubation periods of several years (Fishbein 1991; Smith et al. 1991).

CLINICAL MANIFESTATIONS IN HUMANS

Rabies is mainly transmitted through bite exposure; however, contamination can occur through aerosol, as reported in caves inhabited by rabid bats or in laboratory accidents with infected aerosolized rabid tissues. Rarely, transmission of rabies may also be associated with handling of infected carcasses, or exposure of the mucous membranes and skin abrasion to virus-laden saliva, and corneal transplantation. The transplacental route has been rarely reported in humans (Hemachudha and Mithrabhakdi 2000).

The incubation period in humans may vary from 20 to 90 days (Jackson 2003), with incubation periods as long as years that had been reported (Smith et al. 1991). The early symptoms are frequently nonspecific and may include general malaise, fever, chills, nausea, vomiting, diarrhea, headache, anxiety, apprehension, and irritability, often accompanied with itching and pruritus at the site of animal bite. After a period ranging from 2 to 10 days, neurological signs appear and the disease may then develop according to either a furious ('encephalitic') or paralytic ('dumb') form, which may not be distinguished from magnetic resonance imaging (Laothamatas et al. 2003). Fever and proximal weakness with loss of deep tendon reflexes and urinary incontinence are universal findings. Sensory function remains intact in all modalities (Hemachudha and Phuapradit 1997).

The general features accompanying the disease are fluctuating body temperature, probably due to the effect of rabies virus infection on the hypothalamic center, myocarditis, and cerebral hypoxia due to respiratory compromise that can cause intracranial pressure, seizures, and coma (Hemachudha 1994; Warell 1976). In the furious form, signs of irritation of the central nervous system predominate, with hyperactivity (hallucinations, agitation), which can be aggravated by internal or external stimuli such as noise or light. Hydrophobia may occur in up to 50 percent of the patients (Mrak and Young 1994). Periods of hyperactivity may be interspersed with periods of calm and lucidity. Unless the patient dies early, the 'encephalitic symptoms' progress to paralysis and coma. If the disease presents as dumb (paralytic) rabies, the prodrome may be similar but the main feature is paralysis. Unless intensive care is given, patients with encephalitic rabies usually die within 7 days; those with paralytic rabies may survive as long as 2–3 weeks. A very few cases of recovery have been reported in the literature: only four patients with rabies have been reported to survive; none of them had cardinal features of rabies and were regarded as atypical rabies cases (Hemachudha and Mitrabhakdi 2000).

CLINICAL MANIFESTATIONS IN ANIMALS

It is noteworthy that most of the clinical signs of rabies are expressions of neurological dysfunctions rather than neural cell lysis (Charlton 1994). Although the clinical signs in animals are variable and may be nonspecific in the early stages of the disease, the prodromal period is generally accompanied in animals by behavioral changes. For example, during the initial prodromic phase, the dog appears as anxious and nervous (Chomel 1999) and the cat shows gait abnormality and a strange look in the eyes (Fogelman et al. 1993). Most animals become disorientated and wander aimlessly without regard for the social organization of the species.

Although there is variability in many clinical signs, the range in length of illness in most species is 1–10 days. Paralysis is fairly consistent, and is seen in nearly all cases unless death occurs early. In the dog, a furious form can be observed for 1–7 days, characterized by irritability, aggression, hypersensitivity, disorientation, and seizures (Barnes et al. 2003). In the paralytic or dumb form, which lasts 1–10 days, paralysis will affect one or more limbs, and then progresses to affect the

entire nervous system, especially the cranial nerves and larynx (Chomel 1999). In horses, a predominant feature is weakness or paralysis of the hindquarters, which may be accompanied by lameness and colic (Green et al. 1992). In cattle, foamy hypersalivation and loss of appetite, voice modification, paralysis, and paresis occurred 2 days after initial signs; presence of the three major symptoms: hypersalivation, loss of appetite, and frequent mooing, should always suggest rabies infection (Chomel 1999). In wildlife, aggressive behavior is observed in up to 50 percent of the rabid raccoons, and the clinical signs are quite similar to those observed in infected skunks. In these latter, it has been shown that experimentally infected animals, after restlessness in the early stages, develop paralysis in a few days and die usually within a week (Charlton 1988, 1994; Charlton et al. 1991). Aggressive behavior has also been well documented in foxes and mongooses, which are often seen attacking domestic animals (Everard and Everard 1992). In bats, rabid animals are generally found lying on the ground, unable to fly; an experimental model of rabies virus infection has allowed to demonstrate that stable variants of the fixed rabies virus strain CVS-24 induced clinical signs such as paresis, ataxia, and inability to fly for one, whereas the second did not induce neurological signs (Reid and Jackson 2001).

Epizootiology and epidemiology

FACTORS AFFECTING THE EPIZOOTIOLOGY OF RABIES

Different species of the orders Carnivora and Chiroptera (bats) support independent epizootic cycles of different *Lyssavirus* variants. A particular species may serve as a principal host only in a limited part of its geographical distribution. The disease is transmitted regularly to a number of other mammalian species in addition to the species recognized as the principal host. The occurrence of rabies in these other species may have little or no influence on the course of an epizootic; however, their role is often not readily defined. Each principal host species has its specific pattern population biology and specific modes of social interaction. These host qualities determine which virus variants are capable of survival in this species. It is essential that an infected animal transmit the virus during a period of virus excretion to an adequate number of other susceptible individuals. For this to occur, *Lyssavirus* strains must be adapted to the physiological traits and population biology of their hosts (Bacon 1985; Wandeler 1991a; Wandeler et al. 1994). They must have a host-specific pathogenicity and pathogenesis (length of incubation period, duration and magnitude of virus excretion, duration and extent of clinical illness). We assume that each principal host has its own virus variants adapted for persistence in its populations. Thus, within the area of a principal host, there is little virus variation among the isolates, even if they are performed in a species that is the principal host in another area. With the development of molecular and monoclonal antibody technologies it became possible to demonstrate that indeed antigenically distinct variants exhibiting phylogenetic relationships, circulate in different host populations (Rupprecht et al. 1991; Benmansour et al. 1992; Sacramento et al. 1992; Smith et al. 1992; Bourhy et al. 1993a, b; King et al. 1994; Kissi et al. 1995; Nadin-Davis et al. 1993, 1994; Nel et al. 1993; Smith et al. 1993; Tordo et al. 1993a).

TRANSMISSION OF INFECTION

Transmission of the disease usually requires bite-inflicted deposition of virus-laden saliva into tissues of the recipient animal. Virus may be excreted several days before the onset of clinical signs. The maximum recorded times are: fox, 5 days; skunk, 6 days; dog, 7 days with a Mexican isolate and 13 days with an Ethiopian isolate; cat, 3 days; bat (*Tadarida brasiliensis mexicana*), 12 days (for a review, see Charlton 1988). Excretion of virus before signs of illness is the justification for quarantine (usually 10–14 days) of clinically normal dogs and cats that have bitten humans. Occasionally, excretion of virus may be intermittent. Virus may not be isolated from glands of animals that had previously shed virus in saliva. Because of these features and the patchy nature of antigen-containing cells in salivary glands, examinations of saliva or salivary glands at the time of death may not be reliable indicators of virus transmitted in an earlier exposure to a rabid animal. There are very few data on the dose of virus received in natural infections. The carrier is defined as a clinically normal animal that secretes virus in saliva (not the immediately prodromal excretion of virus just described). There is no convincing evidence of the carrier state in field cases in North America. Most of the reports of rabies transmission by apparently healthy animals (usually dogs) and prolonged secretion in saliva are from Africa and Asia (for a review, see Fedaku 1991).

RABIES IN DOGS

One can readily distinguish between areas of the world in which dogs are the predominant hosts and those where rabies is maintained in wild animals and in which only 0.1–5.0 percent of the rabies cases reported annually are in dogs. In large parts of Asia, Africa, and Latin America, rabies in dogs is much more common, making up 95 percent or more of all diagnosed cases. Even though dog rabies is often termed 'urban rabies,' it is clearly a rural problem in many developing countries (Fedaku 1991; Bingham et al. 1999a; Wandeler and Bingham 2000). Dogs are kept and tolerated at very high numbers in most human societies, sometimes reaching densities of several thousand/km^2; this is considerably more than any wild carnivore population

ever achieves (for a review, see Wandeler et al. 1993). Such high densities could facilitate enzootic canine rabies, although it is sometimes suspected that rabies in dogs is linked with wildlife rabies. There is no doubt that rabid dogs are the major source of human infection (Beran 1991). In industrialized countries of North America and Europe, where the epizootic is maintained and spread by wild carnivores, three factors may account for the low incidence of rabies in dogs: most dogs are restricted in their movements; they are kept indoors or in enclosures and leashed when outside; dog vaccination is strongly recommended or even compulsory.

RABIES IN WILD CARNIVORA

The principal rabies hosts of the order Carnivora are small- to medium-size (0.4–20 kg) omnivores, scavenging and foraging on small vertebrates, invertebrates, fruit, and refuse produced by humans. They reach high population densities (often several individuals/km^2) in and near human settlements. High intrinsic population growth rates allow rapid recovery of populations reduced by persecution or disease. They are all able to support initial epidemics of high case density and thereafter an oscillating prevalence over many years (Wandeler 1991a).

Areas for which associations of RABV variants with populations of wild Carnivora are well documented are limited to North America, Europe, parts of southern Africa, and some Caribbean islands. The red fox (*Vulpes vulpes*) is the principal rabies host in subarctic and northeastern North America, in all of central and eastern Europe, and in subarctic and temperate zones of Asia (Blancou et al. 1991). In arctic regions of North America and Asia, the arctic fox (*Alopex lagopus*) is the predominant rabies host (Crandall 1991). The viruses isolated from red and arctic foxes from fox rabies areas of North America are all closely related, but distinct from European fox isolates. Jackals (*Canis* spp.) are the principal hosts in southern Africa (Foggin 1985; Bingham et al. 1999b) and are probably involved in much larger areas in Africa and Asia. Other wildlife species that maintain independent cycles of distinct RABV variants in southern Africa are various viverrids, especially the yellow mongoose (*Cynictis penicillata*), and possibly the bat-eared fox (*Otocyon megalotis*) (King et al. 1994). The striped skunk (*Mephitis mephitis*) is the species most often diagnosed rabid in large areas of Canada and the USA (Charlton et al. 1991). Raccoon (*Procyon lotor*) rabies is at present confined to the USA, but is spreading in the southeastern and in mid-Atlantic states (Winkler and Jenkins 1991). Mongooses (*Herpestes auropunctatus*) introduced to some Caribbean islands are now the principal reservoir there (Everard and Everard 1985). Gray foxes (*Urocyon cinereoargenteus*) in some North American areas (Carey et al.

1978) and raccoon dogs (*Nyctereutes procyonides*) introduced to eastern and subarctic Europe (Cherkasskiy 1988) are sometimes suspected of supporting independent epizootics.

RABIES IN BATS

The African bat *Lyssavirus* isolates are of genotypes (serotypes) 2 and 4, while those from bats in Europe were identified as genotypes 5 and 6. Isolates from Australian Megachiroptera and from insectivorous bats are called Australian bat lyssaviruses. They form a distinct clade (genotype 7) in phylogenetic analysis (for a review, see McColl et al. 2000). American bat rabies viruses have been categorized as genotype 1, but a more detailed analysis of the large diversity of distinct isolates offers some surprises. Chiroptera have life history traits that are quite different from those of carnivorous rabies hosts: they are small, long-lived, have low intrinsic population growth rates, and are ecological specialists. The properties of lyssaviruses adapted to bats must therefore be different from those of Carnivora rabies. This statement remains a hypothesis because the population biology and epidemiology of bat rabies is insufficiently explored. A notable exception is rabies in vampire bats as described by Lord et al. (1975). An interesting feature of bat rabies is the vast antigenic diversity of isolates. In Canada alone, 12 distinct variants are recognized with mAbs. Several variants occur in a single species, and the geographical distribution of variants is overlapping (Nadin-Davis et al. 2001). This is in sharp contrast to the pattern of rabies in Carnivora, where very little epitope variation is recognized over very large areas (Nadin-Davis et al. 1999).

INCIDENCE OF RABIES IN HUMANS

In industrialized countries, rabies in humans is rare owing to low rates of exposure, high standards of health education and relatively easy access to postexposure treatment with potent vaccines. However, an estimated 35 000–60 000 people die from rabies every year worldwide. The number of people receiving postexposure treatment – mostly after dog bites – is about 3.5 million per year (Bögel and Motschwiller 1986; Bögel and Meslin 1990). Almost all deaths of humans from rabies and the vast majority of treated bite exposures occur in developing countries (Acha and Arambulo 1985). This may in part be due to a high rate of exposure to biting rabid dogs, but even if this assumption is correct, it does not fully explain the high number of rabies casualties. In view of the efficacy of modern postexposure treatment, nearly all cases of rabies in humans must be considered as failures of the medical system. For various reasons, including lack of availability or ignorance, the correct treatment was not applied or not applied in time (Wandeler et al. 1993).

PATHOGENESIS AND PATHOLOGY

Rabies virus spread

INOCULATION SITE

After contamination, it has been shown that rabies virus might infect the cells located within the site of inoculation, generally the myocytes (Figure 51.8) (Murphy et al. 1973; Charlton and Casey 1979). The data are confirmed by in vitro models of infection of cultured myotubes, where infection and replication of street rabies virus can be demonstrated (Tsiang et al. 1986). These data can provide an explanation for the long incubation that can be observed during natural rabies virus infection (Charlton et al. 1997). However, classical experiments have shown that in some cases rabies virus was able to leave the site within a few hours following inoculation, in agreement with a mouse model of infection where direct infection of the nerve endings without prior replication in the muscle has been demonstrated (Shankar et al. 1991).

VIRUS SPREAD TO THE CENTRAL NERVOUS SYSTEM

Whichever are the first host cells to be infected, rabies virus enters both sensory and motor fibers (Coulon et al. 1989; Lafay et al. 1991) probably through a receptor-mediated endocytosis (for the putative receptors see section on Epizootiology and epidemiology above). Studies in cultured neuronal cells indicate that after entry in axon terminals (or somatodendritic domain), rabies virus can be detected in endosomes shortly after uptake (Lewis and Lentz 1998; Lewis et al. 1998).

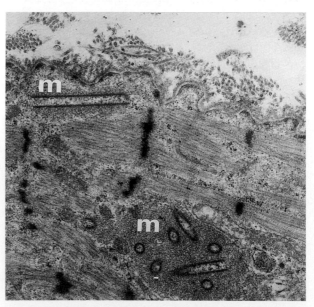

Figure 51.8 *Electron micrograph of two bodies of matrix (m) and anomalous tubular structures in a muscle cell of a skunk at the site of inoculation of street RABV (×2 000).*

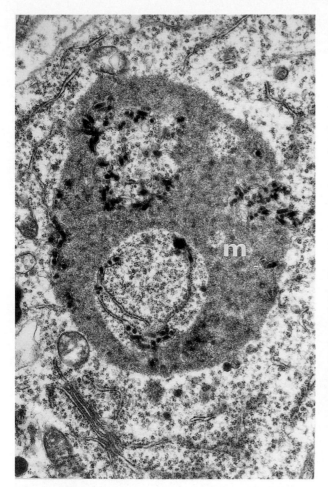

Figure 51.9 *Electron microscopic structure of Negri body in a neuron in skunk brain. Note the body of matrix (m) with entrapped rough endoplasmic reticulum, free ribosomes and virions (×15 000).*

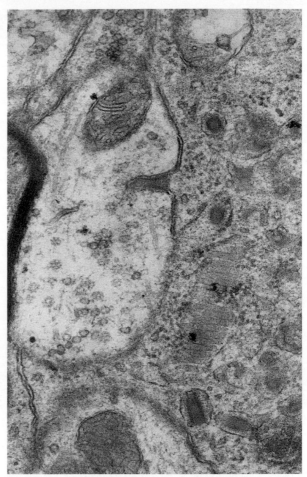

Figure 51.10 *Electron micrograph of skunk brain. Virion budding on neuronal plasma membrane and simultaneous endocytosis by an adjacent axon terminal (×25 000).*

Rabies virus is then transported through axonal transport in the peripheral nervous system toward the central nervous system. This transport is dependent on the microtubule network, as shown by inhibition produced by microtubule-disrupting colchicine and vinblastine (Bijlenga and Heany, 1978; Tsiang 1979). By using cultured sensory neurons in two-compartments devices, it has been demonstrated that rabies virus used the retrograde axonal transport to disseminate within the neuron, at a rate of 25–50 mm/day at least, which is compatible with a fast microtubule-based retrograde transport (Lycke and Tsiang 1987; Tsiang et al. 1991). These properties of rabies virus have been used for retrograde transneuronal tracing studies within the peripheral nervous system (Tang et al. 1999) (Figures 51.9 and 51.10).

SPREAD WITHIN THE CENTRAL NERVOUS SYSTEM

Once rabies virus has reached the spinal cord or brainstem neurons, it disseminates rapidly throughout the central nervous system. Analysis of postmortem brains of naturally infected humans indicate that almost all the brain areas may be infected: thalamus, spinal cord, pons, medulla oblongata, cerebellum, hippocampus, and striatum (Bingham and van der Merwe 2002; Vural et al. 2001). Rabies virus replication occurs primarily in the neurons (Tsiang et al. 1983; Gillet et al. 1986; Kelly and Strick 2000), although some rabies virus strains in some species have been reported to be able to infect significantly other neural cells, such as Bergmann glia (Jackson et al. 2000). The spread of rabies within the central nervous system occurs from neuron to neuron by combination of axonal transport and transsynaptic passage.

The transsynaptic passage has been studied by stereotactic inoculation experiments in the rat (Gillet et al. 1986; Ceccaldi et al. 1989), which have shown that rabies virus uptake occurs mainly at the axon terminal, following the neuroanatomical connections. This is compatible with electron microscopy studies in the skunk, showing viral budding at the postsynaptic membrane (Charlton and Casey 1979). The viral glycoprotein G is required for this transsynaptic transfer (Etessami et al. 2000) and is responsible for the diverse distribution patterns of the different rabies virus strain in the brain (Yan et al. 2002).

The retrograde axonal transport of rabies virus in the brain has also been demonstrated by stereotactic inoculation experiments (Gillet et al. 1986; Ceccaldi et al. 1989; Etessami et al. 2000) and by neuroanatomical studies (Kucera et al. 1985). More recently, the retrograde axonal transport, transsynaptic transfer and its low cytopathic effect of rabies virus has been used for neuroanatomical tracing studies within the monkey brain (Kelly and Strick 2000). Rabies virus transport within the central nervous system is dependent on the integrity of the microtubule network (Ceccaldi et al. 1989; Ceccaldi et al. 1990). In the past few years, the molecular basis for axonal transport of rabies virus has been extensively studied since two independent groups demonstrated a strong interaction between the rabies virus phosphoprotein P and the light chain (so-called LC8 of the cytoplasmic dynein) (Jacob et al. 2000; Raux et al. 2000). These results are confirmed by reverse genetic studies showing that abolishing the P–LC8 interaction by deletion of the conserved LC8-interacting motif (K/RXTQT) in the rabies virus phosphoprotein P is able to reduce the efficiency of peripheral spread of an attenuated rabies virus strain SAD D-19 (with replacement at the Arg at position 333) (Mebatsion 2001). However, this deletion has no effect in intracranial inoculation, suggesting that other mechanisms could act together with P–LC8 interaction for rabies virus spread, although recombinant *P*-gene-deficient rabies viruses are apathogenic in adult and suckling mice, even when inoculated intracranially (Shoji et al. 2004).

Events within the central nervous system

HISTOPATHOLOGY

Relatively mild neuropathological changes are generally observed in the central nervous system of infected hosts (Iwasaki and Tobita 2002), and neuronal cell death does not seem to be prominent during the course of rabies (Ceccaldi 1999; Jackson 2003; Kelly and Strick 2000). However, according to the viral strains that are concerned, mild to severe histopathological can be observed, although they are not constant. They can vary from moderate perivascular cuffing with mononuclear cells (Foley and Zachary 1995), focal and regional gliosis, slight neuronophagia, and presence of inflammatory cells in the meninges (Charlton 1988; Perl and Good 1991) to extensive neuronal degeneration and neuronophagia, associated with widespread inflammation (Fekadu et al. 1982).

Spongiform lesions in rabies were first described by Charlton (1984) in experimentally infected skunks and red foxes, and were further found in natural infections and in other species (Foley and Zachary 1995). The

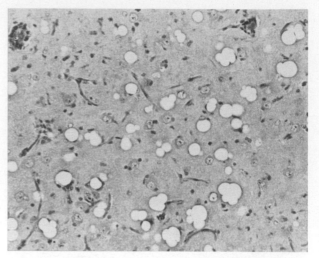

Figure 51.11 *Spongiform lesions in neurophil of thalamus of a skunk experimentally infected with street RABV (H & E, ×160) (reproduced, with permission of the publisher, from Charlton 1984).*

thalamus (all nuclei) and cerebral cortex are the most frequently and severely affected regions (Figure 51.11). Vacuolation seems to develop rapidly, probably in <2–3 days, occurs after infection by several street virus variants, and is independent of the immune response, route of inoculation, or viral preparation (Charlton et al. 1987) (Figure 51.12). In affected regions of the brain, the degree of vacuolation was not correlated with the amount of antigen accumulation, suggesting that spongiform change in rabies is probably an indirect effect, such as neurotransmitter imbalance.

NEURAL DYSFUNCTIONS

The fact that brain damage may be relatively limited and that neuronal death is not pronounced during rabies

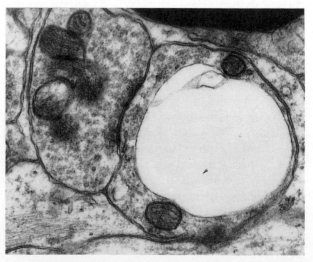

Figure 51.12 *Electron micrograph of a membrane-bound vacuole in the dendrite of a neuron in skunk brain (×30 000) (reproduced, with permission of the publisher, from Charlton 1984).*

has rapidly led to the hypothesis that rabies disease would be mostly due to neural dysfunction rather than neuronal cell lysis (Tsiang et al. 1983; Jackson 2002). Clinically, some data have been provided recently by magnetic resonance imaging of the brain where some patients show multifocal lesions in the brainstem and hypothalamus, with high signals on T2-weighted images in the medulla, pontine tegmentum, and hypothalamus (Pleasure and Fischbein 2000). Experimentally, it has been shown that rabies virus was able to alter the neuronal physiology at different levels, in cultured neural cells as well as in murine models. These alterations concern the release and uptake of neurotransmitters, as shown for GABA whose uptake is reduced (45 percent) in rabies virus-infected cells (Ladogana et al. 1994), or serotonin release (Bouzamondo et al. 1993). Changes in the number of receptors to neurotransmitters have also been described (Ceccaldi et al. 1993). Abnormalities are also detected in the modulation of neural receptors, such as α2-adrenoreceptors whose modulation is prevented by rabies virus, but not muscarinic receptors, of Ca^{2+} channels in neuroblastoma cells (Iwata et al. 2000). Nitric oxide neurotoxicity has been hypothesized to mediate neuronal dysfunction in rabies, since induction of inducible nitric oxide synthase mRNA and increased quantities of nitric oxide in brains of experimentally infected rodents have been reported (Koprowski et al. 1993; Hooper et al. 1995). Interestingly, inducible nitric oxide synthase inhibition is able to delay death of rabies virus-infected mice (Ubol et al. 2001).

More recently, regulation of neuronal gene expression has been described in experimentally infected murine models of rabies virus. These works report activation of immediate–early genes mRNA expression (correlated with an increase in rabies RNA (Fu et al. 1993), upregulation of nine genes during rabies virus infection (Egr1, STAT1) (Saha and Rangarajan 2003) and dysregulation of expression of 39 genes during infection; these included genes involved in regulation of cell metabolism, protein synthesis, synaptic activity, and cell growth and differentiation (Prosniak et al. 2001).

APOPTOSIS

Apoptosis can be observed during rabies infection both in vivo in mice (Thoulouze et al. 1997), and in virus-infected mouse neuroblastoma cells which undergo chromatin condensation and DNA fragmentation within 48 h postinfection (Ubol et al. 1998). Interestingly, a bat strain and a primary canine rabies virus isolate were both able to induce apoptosis in infected mice and reactivate a developmentally down-regulated gene, *Nedd-2*, which may be required for apoptotic elimination of cells damaged by infection (Ubol and Kasisith 2000). Apoptosis could play a role during nonfatal rabies infection, where the levels of viral replication and primary degeneration of infected neurons by apoptosis could be responsible for the infiltration of T lymphocytes capable of inducing secondary degeneration of neural cells (Galelli et al. 2000). The pro-apoptotic properties of the different virus strains being dependent on the viral glycoprotein G (Préhaud et al. 2003) as well as matrix protein M (Kassis et al. 2004).

However, the fact that a silver-haired bat rabies virus variant does not induce apoptosis in the brain of experimentally infected mice suggests that apoptosis would not be an essential pathogenic mechanism for the outcome of a rabies virus infection. Furthermore other pathological processes may contribute to the profound neuronal dysfunction characteristic of street rabies (Yan et al. 2001), although numerous apoptotic neurons could be identified in the brain stem and hippocampus of the brain of a rabies- (and HIV-)infected patient (Adle-Biassette et al. 1996).

PERIPHERAL SPREAD OF VIRUS AND INFECTION OF NONNERVOUS TISSUE

While rabies virus disseminates and replicates within the central nervous system, a subsequent viral transport to peripheral tissues occurs. This transport allows infection of nonnervous tissues such as muscle, myocardium, kidney, lung, pancreas, and lacrymal glands. In a study performed in 11 human rabies confirmed cases, it has been shown that rabies virus antigens could always be found in the adrenal glands, heart, pancreas, and gastrointestinal tract (Jogai et al. 2002). In a murine experimental model of infection, Tsiang demonstrated that the mechanism for such a centrifugal spread was microtubule dependent and involved the axonal transport (Tsiang 1979). The infection of salivary glands is of particular relevance to further transmit the disease for many species (Figures 51.13 and 51.14).

IMMUNE RESPONSES

An important concern is the extent to which the expressions of the naturally occurring disease are the result of the immune response. Although conclusive evidence from natural infections is rather sparse, several reports of experimental studies suggest that the immune response can influence the susceptibility, incubation, and morbidity periods, the type of clinical signs, excretion of virus, and recovery from infection (before or, rarely, after clinical signs). In addition, these effects frequently depend on interactions of the immune response with other factors, such as animal species and age, viral strain, route of inoculation, and dose of virus.

NEUTRALIZING ANTIBODIES

Virus-neutralizing antibodies (VNA) are a critical component of immune resistance. They are produced in response to RABV glycoprotein; production is T-cell dependent, requiring $CD4^+$ T cells, as well as B cells. They are considered to be most effective in the early

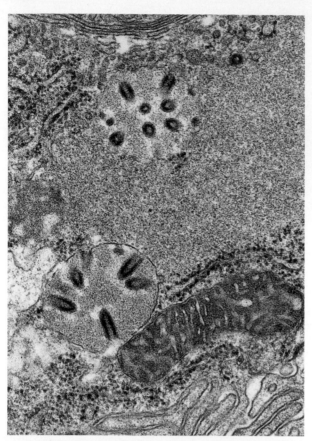

Figure 51.13 *Electron micrograph of rabies virions in acinar lumen of submandibular salivary gland (skunk) (×30 000).*

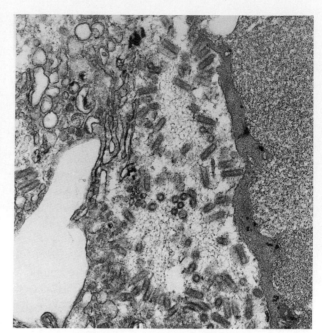

Figure 51.14 *Electron micrograph of mucous cell of submandibular salivary gland of skunk infected with street RABV. Viral budding on the inner surface of secretory granules (×37 500).*

stages of infection, i.e. before viral entrance into peripheral nerves. However, some weakly pathogenic strains can be cleared from the central nervous system (CNS) by VNA. Apparently, protection resides primarily with IgG rather than IgM (for reviews, see Turner 1990; Lafon 1994). Measurement of serum VNA has been and continues to be the predominant method for estimating immune resistance to rabies infection in humans, and in conjunction with challenge is frequently used in efficacy tests of vaccines in other animals.

Generally, VNA is not detected in infected humans until after the onset of clinical signs (for reviews, see Fishbein 1991; Hemachudha 1994). In animal experiments, the relation of neutralizing antibody to outcome of infection is variable. There are several reports of VNA in a small proportion of apparently healthy foxes, skunks, and raccoons in rabies enzootic areas, presumably because of previous exposure to the virus (for reviews, see McLean 1975; Winkler 1975; Blancou et al. 1991; Winkler and Jenkins 1991; Wandeler et al. 1994). The prevalence of VNA in mongooses in enzootic areas in Grenada may be high (up to 40 percent), and fluctuates with changes in the incidence of rabies. High titers of VNA may be indicative either of advanced CNS infection or of recovery. Evidence that the VNA response can influence susceptibility to rabies comes mainly from work with inbred strains of mice inoculated intraperitoneally with street RABV (for review, see Lodmell 1988): resistant and susceptible strains were, respectively, good or poor responders in terms of VNA production.

N PROTEIN

Recent advances include the demonstration, originally by Dietzschold and co-workers (1987), that N protein can induce an immune response sufficient to protect animals against challenge in the absence of detectable VNA. Priming with N protein can augment the production of VNA on subsequent inoculation of live vaccines (for review, see Fu et al. 1994). A recent study indicates that the nucleoprotein of RABV is a superantigen (Lafon et al. 1992). The significance of this in immune resistance has not yet been determined (Lafon 1994).

IMMUNOSUPPRESSION AND CELL-MEDIATED IMMUNITY

Various features of rabies have been studied by immunosuppression or other manipulations of immune mechanisms in experimental animals. The findings include an increase or a decrease in the incubation period due to immunosuppression (Tignor et al. 1974; Smith et al. 1982; Charlton et al. 1984); early death in mice due to antibody and not to immune T cells (Prabhakar and Nathanson 1981); optimum clearance of RABV from the nervous system requires both B and T lymphocytes (Kaplan et al. 1975; Miller et al. 1978; Prabhakar et al. 1981; Smith 1981); immunosuppression-facilitated centrifugal neural migration of virus (Smith et al. 1982); and dissemination to the salivary glands (Charlton et al. 1987).

Cytotoxic T cells can be induced by rabies glycoprotein, nucleocapsid, N protein, and NS protein (for review, see Lafon 1994). The precise role of cytotoxic T cells in immunoprotection has not been resolved. Under certain circumstances, they may be critical for host defense (Nathanson and Gonzalez-Scarano 1991). Lafon (1994) has indicated that, in the absence of neutralizing antibodies, cytotoxic T cells are not sufficient to protect the host; however, their participation in combination with other immune effector mechanisms cannot be excluded. Alternatively, they may contribute to immune injury in rabies.

INFLUENCE OF IMMUNE RESPONSE ON TYPE OF RABIES

The role of the immune response in the type of clinical signs, especially encephalitic versus paralytic rabies, is now being studied. As described above, in skunks inoculated with street virus, early spread in the CNS included ventral motor neurons in the lumbar cord, the motor cortex, and other brain nuclei relevant to motor control of skeletal muscle. Assuming its deleterious effect on infected neurons, an early immune response might be more likely to induce paralytic rather than encephalitic signs. In fact, several studies do support a role for the immune response in paralytic rabies (Tignor et al. 1974; Iwasaki et al. 1977; Smith et al. 1982; Sugamata et al. 1992; Weiland et al. 1992; Lafon et al. 1994). However, Hemachudha et al. (1988) suggested that in humans, lymphocyte proliferative responses are associated with encephalitic rabies, and that paralysis in mice infected with the CVS strain of RABV did not depend on the T-cell system (Hovanessian et al. 1988). Still other studies suggest that the immune response has little effect on the type of clinical signs (Gourmelon et al. 1991; Charlton 1994).

Diagnosis

Rabies diagnosis serves epidemiological surveillance, the monitoring of disease control efforts, and to educate postexposure prophylaxis (PEP) in exposed people. Because almost all human infections result from bites by rabid animals, the decision to initiate or continue PEP often depends on the results of laboratory diagnostic tests on the animal of concern. Diagnostic programs require efficient and well-organized field inspection, specimen collection, and submission systems, adequately equipped laboratories and well-trained laboratory personnel, and effective reporting systems. Details of the laboratory procedures are contained in several excellent reviews (Webster and Casey 1988; Sureau et al. 1991; Trimarchi and Debbie 1991; Bourhy et al. 1992; Meslin et al. 1995).

NEGRI BODIES

The inclusion bodies discovered by Negri (1903) in the cytoplasm of rabies-infected neurons served as exclusive pathognomonic lesions for half a century until immunofluorescence methods were introduced in the late 1950s and early 1960s (Goldwasser and Kissling 1958). The Negri body methods are rapid, but there is a fairly high rate of false negatives (10–20 percent) when compared to antigen detection by immunofluorescence or virus isolation.

IMMUNOFLUORESCENCE

During the 1960s, the fluorescent antibody test (FAT) rapidly became the method of choice. The method can be performed on smears of brain tissue, produces results in a few hours, and, most importantly, is highly specific. With improvements in conjugates and microscopes, the rate of false-negatives has gradually decreased to about 0.1 percent. Most laboratories use immunofluorescence as a primary test. It is recommended that negative FAT results on brains from animals with a history of human exposure be subjected to a confirmatory test, such as a cell culture or mouse inoculation test.

MOLECULAR BIOLOGICAL TECHNIQUES

The 1992 WHO Expert Committee on Rabies did not recommend PCR for routine rabies diagnosis because of the obvious difficulties in preventing cross-contaminations in diagnostic laboratory settings. However, molecular techniques are becoming rapidly more accessible and sophisticated and have potential for diagnostic applications (Sacramento et al. 1991; Tordo et al. 1992b, 1995; Kamolvarin et al. 1993), particularly for antemortem confirmation of suspect human cases (Tordo et al. 1995) and for material that is not suitable for FAT.

OTHER METHODS

The rapid rabies enzyme immunodiagnosis (RREID) test has a high degree of accuracy, and has been advocated for laboratories (e.g. in developing countries) having difficulties in using the FA test, and for screening large numbers of specimens in epidemiological studies. It can be performed on heat-inactivated specimens but not on formalin-fixed specimens. Immunohistochemical (immunoperoxidase) methods and in situ hybridization (Nadin-Davis et al. 2003) are suitable when only formalin-fixed specimens are available.

Antemortem diagnosis is occasionally requested for humans with suspected rabies. Corneal impressions and skin biopsies (back of the neck above the hairline) are recommended for immunofluorescence and oral fluids for virus isolation and PCR detection of viral RNA.

IDENTIFICATION OF VIRUS VARIANTS

Molecular analysis has largely replaced serological methods for the classification of viruses. The characterization of selected parts of viral genomes permits reconstructing evolutionary relationships. These can be displayed as phylogenetic trees. Likelihood values can be calculated for different conceivable branching topologies. Molecular epidemiology is the reconstruction of the history of an epidemic using these powerful tools (Nadin-Davis et al. 1999). Monoclonal antibodies recognize phenotypic aspects of viral proteins and can therefore not provide phylogenetic information with the same accuracy. However, they bind to molecular surface structures recognized by a host's immune system, structures that are likely to have functional properties on which natural selection may act. While molecular studies remain fairly laborious and costly processes, the antigenic characterization with mAbs is an inexpensive 'workhorse' approach to identify large numbers of virus isolates in a diagnostic laboratory setting. Though the binding of a larger number of mAbs can be studied on infected cell cultures, it is important that the tests can be conducted on the original brains in order to remain low in cost and efforts. A panel of mAbs must discriminate between the different species and variants occurring in an area. Variants should be defined as members of a clade (branch) in a phylogenetic tree.

Control

The ultimate purpose of rabies control is the protection of humans from both infection and economic loss. In humans, rabies can be controlled by prophylactic vaccination and postexposure treatment, by reducing the risk of human exposure, or, conclusively, by eradication.

CONTROL OF RABIES IN DOMESTIC ANIMALS

Control measures may include immunization, movement restrictions, reproduction control, habitat control, and removal of stray dogs (Wandeler and Bingham 2000; Meslin et al. 2000).

Immunization

An effective way of reducing the incidence of human infection is by prophylactic immunization of those domestic animals that are the most common sources of human exposure. Rabies has a high incidence in dogs in enzootic areas where dog populations reach high densities. Well-planned and -executed vaccination campaigns drastically reduce rabies incidence in dogs and may even eliminate the disease in areas where it is not maintained by wildlife. Elimination of the disease should be the goal rather than a temporary reduction in incidence. The most economical way to achieve it is by mass vaccination performed in accordance with a comprehensive national plan. Vaccinations should be done by parenteral inoculation of a product approved by the national authorities, usually an inactivated vaccine conferring 2 years of immunity after one injection. When the appropriate technology and resources are available, the immunization of individual domestic animals should be verifiable by certification, preferably in the form of an implanted microchip.

Whenever possible, modern inactivated cell culture vaccines should be used for the immunization of dogs and other domestic animals. They combine safety with high immunogenicity. Cell lines and primary cell cultures are used as substrates for a number of different virus strains. Several manufacturers include a variety of different antigens (distemper, adenovirus, leptospirosis, parainfluenza, parvovirus) in combined vaccines. The use of live-attenuated vaccines is no longer recommended for dog immunization, except for special situations (e.g. national campaigns under economic constraints). Live recombinant vaccines and other products of genetic engineering are now becoming available.

Quarantine

Many countries have legislation for destroying or quarantining for several weeks domestic animals after possible contact with a suspect animal. A ten-day quarantine is recommended for dogs and cats that have bitten a person. The quarantined animal is killed and submitted for laboratory diagnosis if it develops suspicious symptoms during this observation period.

A number of countries that are free from rabies in wild carnivores and dogs have prevented the importation of terrestrial mammal rabies by rigorous enforcement of quarantine measures; for example, a 6-month quarantine period for imported cats and dogs in the UK. This approach is now considered unnecessary, given the availability of effective vaccines for pet animal immunization and tests for verifying an adequate antibody response.

IMMUNIZATION OF WILD ANIMALS

Control of wildlife rabies by reducing population densities of host species has been attempted repeatedly. However, the resilience of these opportunistic Carnivora to persecution, their reproductive potential, and high carrying capacities of both rural and urban habitats often nullify such efforts. A more promising approach is mass vaccination of the main hosts. Immunization of free-living wild animals is not an easy task. The wild mammal has to be lured into vaccinating itself. The methods have to be simple and efficient, so that it becomes technically and economically possible to establish the herd immunity required to eliminate rabies. Oral rabies immunization became attainable in the early 1970s when it was found that ingested attenuated rabies vaccine, ERA, immunized foxes (Black and Lawson 1970; Baer et al. 1971). This discovery suggested the possibility of administering an oral rabies vaccine to wild carnivores by bait.

Wandeler (1991b) detailed the requirements for vaccines to be used for oral immunization of free-living wild animals. Currently only live-attenuated or live recombinant vaccines are available for oral immunization. They have to infect host cells for eliciting a protective immune response. A high residual pathogenicity is a severe weakness of the initially applied ERA/SAD vaccines. The most important qualities of baits for proper vaccine delivery are that they should, as far as possible, be attractive for the target species and not for others. The delivery system must ensure mass immunization of the target species. Technical resources, administrative structures and labor needs, as well as constraints imposed by safety requirements, terrain, climate, etc., have to be taken into account.

The development of oral immunization of wildlife as an instrument for rabies control has been described by Winkler (1992). Aubert et al. (1994) have reported the extent of wildlife rabies vaccination in Europe, and Campbell (1994) has given an account of the North American situation. The first field trial with foxes was carried out in Switzerland in 1978 (Steck et al. 1982). Most areas in Switzerland and later, large areas of other European countries and Canada became free from rabies after oral immunization campaigns with ERA/SAD vaccines. Newer genetically engineered recombinant vaccines have great potential for wildlife rabies control (Blancou et al. 1986; Rupprecht et al. 1986; Yarosh et al. 1996). A vaccinia–rabies glycoprotein recombinant (V–RG) has been used successfully in Belgium (Brochier et al. 1991), Luxembourg, and in parts of France (Aubert et al. 1994). V–RG is applied in North America in attempts to control rabies in raccoons (Robbins et al. 1998), coyotes, and gray foxes.

The most important conclusion from the field applications of oral vaccination is that it appears to be possible to immunize sufficient host individuals to stop the spread of the disease into rabiesfree areas and to eliminate it from enzootic areas in terrestrial mammals. In Europe, rabies did not reappear spontaneously from an undetected reservoir after fox vaccination campaigns were discontinued, but was occasionally able to reinvade a fox population from infected contiguous areas. However, caution has to be applied when interpreting prevalence data from field studies that have no adequate controls and that cannot be repeated (Wandeler 2000).

RABIES PROPHYLAXIS IN HUMANS

The history of rabies vaccines and of postexposure treatment in humans from the time of Louis Pasteur to the modern era has been well described (Vodopija and Clark 1991; Thraenhart et al. 1994). Highly efficacious vaccines that usually provoke only minimal or no side effects are now available and can be used for pre- and postexposure immunization. All of them contain RABV antigens in a concentrated and partially purified form. Preparations widely used are the human diploid cell strain (HADES) or the Vero cell strain, which are inactivated with β-propiolactone. Unfortunately, because of economic considerations, the cheaper brain tissue-derived vaccines are still predominant in large parts of the world. These vaccines are of inferior potency and may induce severe allergic reactions that can occasionally be difficult to distinguish from clinical rabies (Hemachudha 1989).

Pre-exposure prophylaxis

Pre-exposure immunization is generally encouraged only for people at potentially high risk of exposure; for example, laboratory personnel working with rabies, veterinarians, and animal control and wildlife officers. Pre-exposure immunization consists of a series of inoculations (usually three) within 21–180 days with an approved and potent inactivated vaccine. Serum antibody titers should be monitored. For people at continuing high risk of exposure, it is recommended that booster injections are given when the serum antibody titer falls below 0.5 IU/ml (WHO 1992).

Postexposure prophylaxis

People bitten or licked by a mammal acting abnormally in a geographic area where rabies might occur must be considered as exposed and postexposure treatment should begin as soon as possible. Properly administered, it is highly effective. It consists of passive immunization with rabies immunoglobulin, and vaccination (WHO 1992). Instant thorough washing of bite and scratch wounds with water and soap or detergent is most important; the use of disinfectants is also recommended. Purified rabies immunoglobulin, of equine or, preferably, human origin (HRIG), and the first dose of a potent vaccine must be administered with as little delay as possible. Additional doses of vaccine at the officially specified intervals are necessary. Tetanus prophylaxis should also be given to people without definite evidence of recent immunization. Recommendations on what has to be considered an exposure, what vaccines to use, routes of vaccine administration, treatment schedules, and the application of immunoglobulins vary from country to country; the guidelines of the national health authority must be consulted.

REFERENCES

Abraham, G., Rhodes, D.P. and Banerjee, A.K. 1975. The 5′ terminal structure of the methylated mRNA synthesized *in vitro* by vesicular stomatitis virus. *Cell*, **5**, 51–8.

Acha, P.N. and Arambulo, P.V. 1985. Rabies in the tropics: history and current status. In: Kuwert, E., Mérieux, C., et al. (eds), *Rabies in the tropics*. Berlin: Springer-Verlag, 343–59.

Adle-Biassette, H., Bourhy, H., et al. 1996. Rabies encephalitis in a patient with AIDS: a clinicopathological study. *Acta Neuropathol*, **92**, 415–20.

Amengual, B., Whitby, J.E., et al. 1997. Evolution of European bat lyssaviruses. *J Gen Virol*, **78**, 2319–28.

Arguin, P.M., Murray-Lillibridge, K., et al. 2002. Serologic evidence of Lyssavirus infections among bats, the Philippines. *Emerg Infect Dis*, **8**, 258–62.

Aubert, M.F.A., Masson, E., et al. 1994. Oral wildlife rabies vaccination field trials in Europe, with recent emphasis on France. In: Rupprecht, C.E., Dietzschold, B. and Koprowski, H. (eds), *Lyssaviruses*. Berlin: Springer-Verlag, 219–43.

Bacon, P.J. 1985. A systems analysis of wildlife rabies epizootics. In: Bacon, P.J. (ed.), *Population dynamics of rabies in wildlife*. London: Academic Press, 109–30.

Badrane, H. and Tordo, N. 2001. Host-switching in lyssavirus history from chiroptera to carnivora orders. *J Virol*, **75**, 8096–104.

Badrane, H., Bahloul, C., et al. 2001. Evidence of two lyssavirus phylogroups with distinct pathogenicity and immunogenicity. *J Virol*, **75**, 3268–76.

Baer, G.M. 1991. *The natural history of rabies*. Boca Raton, FL: CRC Press.

Baer, G.M. and Lentz, T.L. 1991. Rabies pathogenesis to the central nervous system. In: Baer, G.M. (ed.), *The natural history of rabies*, 2nd edn. Boca Raton, FL: CRC Press, 105–20.

Baer, G.M., Abelseth, M.K. and Debbie, J.G. 1971. Oral vaccination of foxes against rabies. *Am J Epidemiol*, **93**, 487–90.

Bahloul, C., Jacob, Y., et al. 1998. DNA-based immunisation for exploring the enlargement of immunological cross-reactivity against the lyssaviruses. *Vaccine*, **16**, 417–25.

Banerjee, A.K. 1987. Transcription and replication of rhabdoviruses. *Microbiol Rev*, **51**, 66–87.

Banerjee, A.K. and Barik, S. 1992. Gene expression of vesicular stomatitis virus genome RNA. *Virology*, **188**, 417–28.

Banerjee, A.K., Masters, P.S., et al. 1989. Specific interaction of vesicular stomatitis capsid protein (N) with the phosphoprotein (NS) prevents its binding with non-specific RNA. In: Kolakofsky, D. and Mahy, B.W.J. (eds), *Genetics and pathogenicity of negative strand viruses*. New York: Elsevier, 121–8.

Barge, A., Gaudin, Y., et al. 1993. Vesicular stomatitis virus M protein may be inside the ribonucleocapsid coil. *Virology*, **67**, 7246–53.

Barik, S. and Banerjee, A.K. 1992. Sequential phosphorylation of the phosphoprotein of vesicular stomatitis virus by cellular and viral protein kinases is essential for transcription activation. *J Virol*, **66**, 1109–18.

Barnes, H.L., Chrisman, C.L., et al. 2003. Clinical evaluation of rabies virus meningoencephalomyelitis in a dog. *J Am Anim Hosp Assoc*, **39**, 547–50.

Barr, J.N., Whelan, S.P. and Wertz, G.W. 2002. Transcriptional control of the RNA-dependent RNA polymerase of vesicular stomatitis virus. *Biochim Biophys Acta*, **1577**, 337–53.

Bearzotti, M., Delmas, B., et al. 1999. Fish rhabdovirus cell entry is mediated by fibronectin. *J Virol*, **73**, 7703–9.

Beckes, J.D. and Perrault, J. 1992. Stepwise phosphorylation of vesicular stomatitis virus P protein by virion-associated protein kinases and uncoupling of second step from in vitro transcription. *Virology*, **188**, 606–17.

Benmansour, A., Leblois, H., et al. 1991. Antigenicity of rabies virus glycoprotein. *J Virol*, **65**, 4198–203.

Benmansour, A., Brahimi, M., et al. 1992. Rapid sequence evolution of street rabies glycoprotein is related to the heterogeneous nature of the viral population. *Virology*, **187**, 33–45.

Benmansour, A., Paubert, G., et al. 1994. The polymerase-associated protein (M1) and the matrix protein (M2) from a virulent and avirulent strain of viral hemorrhagic septicemia virus (VHSV), a fish rhabdovirus. *Virology*, **198**, 602–12.

Beran, G.W. 1991. Urban rabies. In: Baer, G.M. (ed.), *The natural history of rabies*, 2nd edn. Boca Raton, FL: CRC Press, 427–43.

Bergmann, J.E. and Fusco, P.J. 1988. The M protein of vesicular stomatitis virus associates specifically with the basolateral membranes of polarized epithelial cells independently of the G protein. *J Cell Biol*, **107**, 1707–15.

Bijlenga, G. and Heany, T. 1978. Post-exposure local treatment of mice infected with rabies with two axonal flow inhibitors, colchicine and vinblastine. *J Gen Virol*, **39**, 381–5.

Bingham, J. and van der Merwe, M. 2002. Distribution of rabies antigen in infected brain material: determining the reliability of different regions of the brain for the rabies fluorescent antibody test. *J Virol Meth*, **101**, 85–94.

Bingham, J., Foggin, C.M., et al. 1999a. The epidemiology of rabies in Zimbabwe. 1. Rabies in dogs (*Canis familiaris*). *Onderstepoort J Vet Res*, **66**, 1–10.

Bingham, J., Foggin, C.M., et al. 1999b. The epidemiology of rabies in Zimbabwe. 2. Rabies in jackals (*Canis adustus* and *Canis mesomelas*). *Onderstepoort J Vet Res*, **66**, 11–23.

Bitko, V. and Barik, S. 2001. Phenotypic silencing of cytoplasmic genes using sequence-specific double-stranded short interfering RNA and its application in the reverse genetics of wild type negative-strand RNA viruses. *BMC Microbiol*, **1**, 34.

Black, J.G. and Lawson, K.F. 1970. Sylvatic rabies studies in the silver fox (*Vulpes vulpes*): susceptibility and immune responses. *Can J Comp Med*, **34**, 309–11.

Black, B.L. and Lyles, D.S. 1992. Vesicular stomatitis virus matrix protein inhibits host cell-directed transcription of target genes in vivo. *J Virol*, **66**, 4058–64.

Black, B.L., Rhodes, R.B., et al. 1993. The role of vesicular stomatitis virus matrix protein in inhibition of host-directed gene expression is genetically separable from its function in virus assembly. *J Virol*, **67**, 4814–21.

Blancou, J., Kieny, M.P., et al. 1986. Oral vaccination of the fox against rabies using a live recombinant vaccinia virus. *Nature (London)*, **322**, 373–5.

Blancou, J., Aubert, M.F.A. and Artois, M. 1991. Fox rabies. In: Baer, G.M. (ed.), *The natural history of rabies*, 2nd edn. Boca Raton, FL: CRC Press, 257–90.

Blondel, D., Harmison, G.G. and Schubert, M. 1990. Role of matrix protein in cytopathogenesis of vesicular stomatitis virus. *J Virol*, **64**, 1716–25.

Blondel, D., Regad, T., et al. 2002. Rabies virus P and small P products interact directly with PML and reorganize PML nuclear bodies. *Oncogene*, **21**, 7957–70.

Bögel, K. and Meslin, F. 1990. Economics of human and canine rabies elimination: guidelines for programme orientation. *Bull WHO*, **68**, 281–91.

Bögel, K. and Motschwiller, E. 1986. Incidence of rabies and post-exposure treatment in developing countries. *Bull WHO*, **64**, 883–7.

Botvinkin, A.D., Poleschuk, E.M., et al. 2003. Novel lyssaviruses isolated from bats in Russia. *Emerg Infect Dis*, **9**, 1623–5.

Bourhy, H., Kissi, B., et al. 1992. Antigenic and molecular characterization of bat rabies virus in Europe. *J Clin Microbiol*, **30**, 2419–26.

Bourhy, H., Kissi, B. and Tordo, N. 1993a. Molecular diversity of the *Lyssavirus* genus. *Virology*, **194**, 70–81.

Bourhy, H., Kissi, B. and Tordo, N. 1993b. Taxonomy and evolutionary studies on lyssaviruses with special reference to Africa. *Onderstepoort J Vet Res*, **60**, 277–82.

Bouzamondo, E., Ladogana, A. and Tsiang, H. 1993. Alteration of of potassium evoked 5-HT release from virus-infected rat cortical synaptosomes. *Neuroreport*, **4**, 555–8.

Brochier, B., Kieny, M.P., et al. 1991. Large scale eradication of rabies using recombinant vaccinia-rabies vaccine. *Nature (London)*, **354**, 520–2.

Broughan, J.H. and Wunner, W.H. 1995. Characterization of protein involvement in rabies virus binding to BHK-21 cells. *Arch Virol*, **140**, 75–93.

Brown, F. and Crick, J. 1979. Natural history of rhabdoviruses of vertebrates and invertebrates. In: Bishop, D.H.L. (ed.), *The rhabdoviruses*, Vol. 1. Boca Raton, FL: CRC Press, 1–22.

Brown, E.L. and Lyles, D.S. 2003. Organization of the vesicular stomatitis virus glycoprotein into membrane microdomains occurs independently of intracellular viral components. *J Virol*, **77**, 3985–92.

Brun, G. 1984. Host-range mutants of Pincy virus, a new type of mutant in drosophila. In: Bishop, D.H.L. and Compans, R.W. (eds), *Non-segmented negative strand viruses*. Orlando, FL: Academic Press, 921–6.

Buckley, S.M. 1975. Arbovirus infection of vertebrate and insect cell cultures, with special emphasis on Mokola, Obodhiang and Kotonkan viruses of the rabies serogroup. *Ann NY Acad Sci*, **266**, 241–50.

Bujnicki, J.M. and Rychlewski, L. 2002. In silico identification, structure prediction and phylogenetic analysis of the 2′-O-ribose (cap 1) methyltransferase domain in the large structural protein of ssRNA negative-strand viruses. *Protein Eng*, **15**, 101–8.

Bunschoten, H., Gore, M., et al. 1989. Characterization of a new virus-neutralization epitope that denotes a sequential determinant on rabies virus glycoprotein. *J Gen Virol*, **70**, 291–8.

Burrage, T.G., Tignor, G.H. and Smith, A.L. 1985. Rabies virus binding at neuromuscular junctions. *Virus Res*, **2**, 273–89.

Calisher, C.H., Karabatsos, N., et al. 1989. Antigenic relationships among rhabdoviruses from vertebrates and hematophagous arthropods. *Intervirology*, **49**, 241–57.

Campbell, J.B. 1994. Oral rabies immunization of wildlife and dogs: challenges to the Americas. In: Rupprecht, C.E., Dietzschold, B. and Koprowski, H. (eds), *Lyssaviruses*. Berlin: Springer-Verlag, 245–66.

Cannon, K.S., Hebert, D.N. and Helenius, A. 1996. Glycan-dependent and -independent association of vesicular stomatitis virus G protein with calnexin. *J Biol Chem*, **271**, 14280–4.

Canter, D.M. and Perrault, J. 1996. Stabilization of vesicular stomatitis virus L polymerase protein by P protein binding: a small deletion in the C-terminal domain of L abrogates binding. *Virology*, **219**, 376–86.

Carey, A.B., Giles, R.H. and McLean, R.G. 1978. The landscape epidemiology of rabies in Virginia. *Am J Trop Med Hyg*, **27**, 573–80.

Carneiro, F.A., Stauffer, F., et al. 2003. Membrane fusion induced by vesicular stomatitis virus depends on histidine protonation. *J Biol Chem*, **278**, 13789–94.

Ceccaldi, P.E. 1999. The pathogenesis of rabies. In *Rabies guidelines for medical professionals*. Trenton: Veterinary Learning Systems, 12–19.

Ceccaldi, P.E., Gillet, J.P. and Tsiang, H. 1989. Inhibition of the transport of rabies virus in the central nervous system. *J Neuropathol Exp Neurol*, **48**, 620–30.

Ceccaldi, P.E., Ermine, A. and Tsiang, H. 1990. Continuous delivery of colchicine in the rat brain with osmotic pumps for inhibition of rabies virus transport. *J Virol Meth*, **28**, 79–84.

Ceccaldi, P.E., Fillion, M.P., et al. 1993. Rabies virus selectively alters 5-HT receptors subtypes in rat brain. *Eur J Pharmacol*, **245**, 129–38.

Chang, T.L., Reiss, C.S. and Huang, A.S. 1994. Inhibition of vesicular stomatitis virus RNA synthesis by protein hyperphosphorylation. *J Virol*, **68**, 4980–7.

Charlton, K.M. 1984. Rabies: spongiform lesions in the brain. *Acta Neuropathol (Berl)*, **63**, 198–202.

Charlton, K.M. 1988. The pathogenesis of rabies. In: Campbell, J.B. and Charlton, K.M. (eds), *Rabies*. Boston, MA: Kluwer Academic, 101–50.

Charlton, K.M. 1994. The pathogenesis of rabies and other lyssaviral infections. In: Rupprecht, C.E., Dietzschold, B. and Koprowski, H. (eds), *Lyssaviruses*. Berlin: Springer-Verlag, 95–119.

Charlton, K.M. and Casey, G.A. 1979. Experimental rabies in skunks: immunofluorescent, light and electron microscopic studies. *Lab Invest*, **41**, 36–44.

Charlton, K.M., Casey, G.A. and Campbell, J.B. 1984. Experimental rabies in skunks: effects of immunosuppression induced by cyclophosphamide. *Can J Comp Med*, **48**, 72–7.

Charlton, K.M., Casey, G.A. and Campbell, J.B. 1987. Experimental rabies in skunks: immune response and salivary gland infection. *Comp Immunol Microbiol Infect Dis*, **10**, 227–35.

Charlton, K.M., Webster, W.A. and Casey, G.A. 1991. Skunk rabies. In: Baer, G.M. (ed.), *The natural history of rabies*, 2nd edn. Boca Raton, FL: CRC Press, 307–24.

Charlton, K.M., Nadin-Davis, S., et al. 1997. The long incubation period in rabies. Delayed progression of infection in muscle at the inoculation site. *Acta Neuropathol*, **94**, 73–7.

Chen, J.L., Das, T. and Banerjee, A.K. 1997. Phosphorylated states of vesicular stomatitis virus P protein in vitro and in vivo. *Virology*, **228**, 200–12.

Chenik, M., Chebli, K., et al. 1994. In vivo interaction of rabies virus phosphoprotein (P) and nucleoprotein (N): existence of two N-binding sites on P protein. *J Gen Virol*, **75**, 2889–96.

Chenik, M., Chebli, K. and Blondel, D. 1995. Translation initiation at alternate in-frame AUG codons in the rabies virus phosphoprotein mRNA is mediated by a ribosomal leaky scanning mechanism. *J Virol*, **69**, 707–12.

Chenik, M., Schnell, M., et al. 1998. Mapping the interacting domains between the rabies virus polymerase and phosphoprotein. *J Virol*, **72**, 1925–30.

Cherkasskiy, B.L. 1988. Roles of the wolf and the raccoon dog in the ecology and epidemiology of rabies in the USSR. *Rev Infect Dis*, **10**, S634–6.

Chomel, B.B. 1999. Rabies exposure and clinical disease in animals. In *Rabies guidelines for medical professionals*. Trenton: Veterinary Learning Systems, 20–6.

Chong, L.D. and Rose, J.K. 1993. Membrane association of functional vesicular stomatitis virus matrix protein in vivo. *J Virol*, **67**, 407–14.

Chong, L.D. and Rose, J.K. 1994. Interactions of normal and mutant vesicular stomatitis matrix proteins with the plasma membrane and nucleocapsids. *J Virol*, **68**, 441–7.

Chow, T.L., Chow, F.H. and Hanson, R.P. 1954. Morphology of vesicular stomatitis virus. *J Bacteriol*, **68**, 724–6.

Clague, M.J., Schoch, C., et al. 1990. Gating kinetics of pH-activated membrane fusion of vesicular stomatitis virus with cells: stopped-flow measurements by dequenching of octadecylrhodamine fluorescence. *Biochemistry*, **29**, 1303–8.

Clinton, G.M., Little, S.P., et al. 1978. The matrix (M) protein of vesicular stomatitis virus regulates transcription. *Cell*, **15**, 1455–62.

Coll, J.M. 1995. The glycoprotein G of rhabdoviruses. *Arch Virol*, **140**, 827–51.

Conti, C., Hauttecoeur, B., et al. 1988. Inhibition of rabies virus infection by a soluble membrane fraction from the rat central nervous system. *Arch Virol*, **98**, 73–86.

Conzelmann, K.K. 1996. Genetic manipulation of non-segmented negative-strand RNA viruses. *J Gen Virol*, **77**, 381–9.

Conzelmann, K. and Schnell, M. 1994. Rescue of synthetic genomic RNA analogs of rabies virus by plasmid-encoded proteins. *J Virol*, **68**, 713–19.

Coulon, P., Derbin, C., et al. 1989. Invasion of the peripheral nervous systems of adult mice by the CVS strain of rabies virus and its avirulent derivative Av01. *J Virol*, **63**, 3550–4.

Coulon, P., Lafay, F., et al. 1994. The molecular basis for altered pathogenicity of lyssavirus variants. In: Rupprecht, C.E., Dietzschold, B. and Koprowski, H. (eds), *Lyssaviruses*. Berlin: Springer-Verlag, 69–84.

Crandall, R.A. 1991. Arctic fox rabies. In: Baer, G.M. (ed.), *The natural history of rabies*. Boca Raton, FL: CRC Press, 291–306.

De, B.P. and Banerjee, A.K. 1984. Specific interactions of vesicular stomatitis virus L and NS proteins with heterologous genome ribonucleoprotein template lead to mRNA synthesis in vitro. *J Virol*, **51**, 628–34.

De, B.P., Thornton, G.B., et al. 1982. Purified matrix protein of vesicular stomatitis virus blocks viral transcription in vitro. *Proc Natl Acad Sci USA*, **79**, 7137–41.

Delagneau, J.F., Perrin, A. and Atanasin, P. 1981. Structure of the rabies virus: spatial relationships of the proteins 6, M_1, M_2 and N. *Ann Virol (Inst Pasteur)*, **132E**, 473–93.

Delarue, M., Poch, O., et al. 1990. An attempt to unify the structure of polymerases. *Protein Eng*, **3**, 461–7.

Desmezières, E., Jacob, Y., et al. 1999. Lyssavirus glycoproteins expressing immunologically potent B cell and cytotoxic T lymphocyte epitopes as prototypes for multivalent vaccines. *J Gen Virol*, **80**, 2343–51.

Dezélée, S., Bras, F., et al. 1989. Molecular analysis of *ref(2)p*, a *Drosophila* gene implicated in sigma rhabdovirus multiplication and necessary for male fertility. *EMBO J*, **8**, 3437–46.

Dietzschold, B., Wiktor, T.J., et al. 1982. Antigenic structure of rabies virus glycoprotein: ordering and immunological characterization of the large CNBr cleavage fragments. *J Virol*, **44**, 595–602.

Dietzschold, B., Wang, H., et al. 1987. Induction of protective immunity against rabies by immunization with rabies virus ribonucleoprotein. *Proc Natl Acad Sci USA*, **84**, 9165–9.

Dietzschold, B., Rupprecht, C.E., et al. 1988. Antigenic diversity of the glycoprotein and nucleocapsid proteins of rabies and rabies-related viruses: implications for epidemiology and control of rabies. *Rev Infect Dis*, **10**, S785–98.

Dietzschold, B., Gore, M., et al. 1990. Structure and immunological characterization of a linear virus-neutralizing epitope of the rabies virus glycoprotein and its possible use in a synthetic vaccine. *J Virol*, **64**, 3804–9.

Dietzschold, B., Faber, M. and Schnell, M.J. 2003. New approaches to the prevention and eradication of rabies. *Expert Rev Vaccines*, **2**, 399–406.

Doms, R.W., Keller, D.S., et al. 1987. Role for adenosine triphosphate in regulating the assembly and transport of vesicular stomatitis virus G protein trimers. *J Cell Biol*, **105**, 1957–69.

Drings, A., Jallet, C., et al. 1999. Is there an advantage to including the nucleoprotein in a rabies glycoprotein subunit vaccine. *Vaccine*, **17**, 1549–57.

Durrer, P., Gaudin, Y., et al. 1995. Photolabeling identifies a putative fusion domain in the envelope glycoprotein of rabies and vesicular stomatitis virus. *J Biol Chem*, **270**, 17575–81.

Einer-Jensen, K., Krogh, T.N., et al. 1998. Characterization of intramolecular disulfide bonds and secondary modifications of the glycoprotein from viral hemorrhagic septicemia virus, a fish rhabdovirus. *J Virol*, **72**, 10189–96.

Ertl, H.C.J., Dietzschold, B. and Otvos, J. 1991. T-helper cell epitopes of rabies virus nucleoprotein defined by tri- and tetrapeptides. *Eur J Immunol*, **21**, 1–10.

Etessami, R., Conzelmann, K.K., et al. 2000. Spread and pathogenic characteristics of a G-deficient rabies virus recombinant: an in vitro and in vivo study. *J Gen Virol*, **81**, 2147–53.

Everard, C.O.R. and Everard, J.D. 1985. Mongoose rabies in Grenada. In: Bacon, P.J. (ed.), *Population dynamics of rabies in wildlife*. London: Academic Press, 43–69.

Everard, C.O. and Everard, J.D. 1992. Mongoose rabies in the Caribbean. *Ann NY Acad Sci*, **653**, 356–66.

Faber, M., Pulmanausahakul, R., et al. 2004. Identification of viral genomic elements responsible for rabies virus neuroinvasiveness. *Proc Natl Acad Sci USA*, **101**, 16328–32.

Fedaku, M. 1991. Canine rabies. In: Baer, G.M. (ed.), *The natural history of rabies*, 2nd edn. Boca Raton, FL: CRC Press, 367–87.

Fekadu, M., Chandler, F.W. and Harrison, A.K. 1982. Pathogenesis of rabies in dogs inoculated with an Ethiopian rabies virus strain. Immunofluorescence, histologic and ultrastructural studies of the central nervous system. *Arch Virol*, **71**, 109–26.

Ferron, F., Longhi, S., et al. 2002. Viral RNA-polymerases: a predicted 2′-O-ribose methyltransferase domain shared by all Mononegavirales. *Trends Biochem Sci*, **27**, 222–4.

Finke, S. and Conzelmann, K.K. 2003. Dissociation of rabies virus matrix protein functions in regulation of viral RNA synthesis and virus assembly. *J Virol*, **77**, 12074–82.

Finke, S., Mueller-Waldeck, R. and Conzelmann, K.K. 2003. Rabies virus matrix protein regulates the balance of virus transcription and replication. *J Gen Virol*, **84**, 1613–21.

Fishbein, D.B. 1991. Rabies in humans. In: Baer, G.M. (ed.), *The natural history of rabies*, 2nd edn. Boca Raton, FL: CRC Press, 519–49.

Flamand, A. 1970. Genetic study of vesicular stomatitis virus: classification of spontaneous thermosensitive mutants into complementation groups. *J Gen Virol*, **8**, 187–95.

Flamand, A. 1980. Rhabdovirus genetics. In: Bishop, D.H.L. (ed.), *Rhabdoviruses*. Boca Raton, FL: CRC Press, 115–39.

Flood, E.A. and Lyles, D.S. 1999. Assembly of nucleocapsids with cytosolic and membrane-derived matrix proteins of vesicular stomatitis virus. *Virology*, **261**, 295–308.

Fogelman, V., Fischman, H.R., et al. 1993. Epidemiologic and clinical characteristics of rabies in cats. *J Am Vet Med Assoc*, **202**, 1829–33.

Foggin, C.M. 1985. The epidemiological significance of jackal rabies in Zimbabwe. In: Kuwert, E. and Mérieux, C. (eds), *Rabies in the tropics*. Berlin: Springer-Verlag, 399–405.

Foley, G.L. and Zachary, J.F. 1995. Rabies-induced spongiform change and encephalitis in a heifer. *Vet Pathol*, **32**, 309–11.

Fredericksen, B.L. and Whitt, M.A. 1995. Vesicular stomatitis virus glycoprotein mutations that affect membrane fusion activity and abolish virus infectivity. *J Virol*, **69**, 1435–43.

Fredericksen, B.L. and Whitt, M.A. 1996. Mutations at two conserved acidic amino acids in the glycoprotein of vesicular stomatitis virus affect pH-dependent conformational changes and reduce the pH threshold for membrane fusion. *Virology*, **217**, 49–57.

Fu, Z.F., Weihe, E., et al. 1993. Differential effects of rabies and Borna disease viruses on immediate–early response and late-response gene expression in brain tissues. *J Virol*, **67**, 6674–81.

Fu, Z.F., Wunner, W.H. and Dietzschold, B. 1994a. Immunoprotection by rabies virus nucleoprotein. In: Rupprecht, C.E., Dietzschold, B. and Koprowski, H. (eds), *Lyssaviruses*. Berlin: Springer-Verlag, 161–72.

Fu, Z.F., Zengh, Y., et al. 1994b. Both the N- and the C-terminal domains of the nominal phosphoprotein of rabies virus are involved in the binding to the N protein. *Virology*, **200**, 590–7.

Galelli, A., Baloul, L. and Lafon, M. 2000. Abortive rabies virus central nervous infection is controlled by T lymphocyte local recruitment and induction of apoptosis. *J Neurovirol*, **6**, 359–72.

Gao, Y. and Lenard, J. 1995a. Cooperative binding of multimeric phosphoprotein (P) of vesicular stomatitis virus to polymerase (L) and template: pathway and assembly. *J Virol*, **69**, 7718–23.

Gao, Y. and Lenard, J. 1995b. Multimerization and transcriptional activation of the phosphoprotein (P) of vesicular stomatitis virus by casein kinase-II. *EMBO J*, **14**, 1240–7.

Gastka, M., Horvath, J., et al. 1996. Rabies virus binding to the nicotinic acetylcholine receptor alpha subunit demonstrated by virus overlay protein binding assay. *J Gen Virol*, **77**, 2437–40.

Gaudier, M., Gaudin, Y. and Knossow, M. 2001. Cleavage of vesicular stomatitis virus matrix protein prevents self-association and leads to crystallization. *Virology*, **288**, 308–14.

Gaudier, M., Gaudin, Y. and Knossow, M. 2002. Crystal structure of vesicular stomatitis virus matrix protein. *EMBO J*, **21**, 2886–92.

Gaudin, Y. 1997. Folding of rabies virus glycoprotein: epitope acquisition and interaction with endoplasmic reticulum chaperones. *J Virol*, **71**, 3742–50.

Gaudin, Y. 2000a. Reversibility in fusion protein conformational changes. The intriguing case of rhabdovirus-induced membrane fusion. *Subcell Biochem*, **34**, 379–408.

Gaudin, Y. 2000b. Rabies virus-induced membrane fusion pathway. *J Cell Biol*, **150**, 601–12.

Gaudin, Y., Tuffereau, C., et al. 1991a. Fatty acylation of rabies virus proteins. *Virology*, **184**, 441–4.

Gaudin, Y., Tuffereau, C., et al. 1991b. Reversible changes and fusion activity of the rabies virus glycoprotein. *J Virol*, **65**, 4853–9.

Gaudin, Y., Ruigrok, R.W.H., et al. 1992. Rabies virus glycoprotein is a trimer. *Virology*, **187**, 627–32.

Gaudin, Y., Ruigrok, R.W.H., et al. 1993. Low-pH conformational changes of rabies virus glycoprotein and their role in membrane fusion. *J Virol*, **67**, 1365–72.

Gaudin, Y., Barge, A., et al. 1995a. Aggregation of VSV M protein is reversible and mediated by nucleation sites: implications for viral assembly. *Virology*, **206**, 28–37.

Gaudin, Y., Tuffereau, C., et al. 1995b. Biological function of the low-pH, fusion-inactive conformation of rabies virus glycoprotein (G): G is transported in a fusion-inactive state-like conformation. *J Virol*, **69**, 5528–34.

Gaudin, Y., Ruigrok, R.W.H. and Brunner, J. 1995c. Low-pH induced conformational changes in viral fusion proteins: implications for the fusion mechanism. *J Gen Virol*, **76**, 1541–56.

Gaudin, Y., Raux, H., et al. 1996. Identification of amino acids controlling the low-pH-induced conformational change of rabies virus glycoprotein. *J Virol*, **70**, 7371–8.

Gaudin, Y., de Kinkelin, P. and Benmansour, A. 1999. Mutations in the glycoprotein of viral haemorrhagic septicaemia virus that affect virulence for fish and the pH threshold for membrane fusion. *J Gen Virol*, **80**, 1221–9.

Gigant, B., Iseni, F., et al. 2000. Neither phosphorylation nor the amino-terminal part of rabies virus phosphoprotein is required for its oligomerization. *J Gen Virol*, **81**, 1757–61.

Gillet, J.P., Derer, P. and Tsiang, H. 1986. Axonal transport of rabies virus in the central nervous system of the rat. *J Neuropathol Exp Neurol*, **45**, 619–34.

Goldwasser, R.A. and Kissling, R.E. 1958. Fluorescent antibody staining of street and fixed rabies virus antigen. *Proc Soc Exp Biol Med*, **98**, 219–23.

Goto, H., Nimamoto, N., et al. 1995. Expression of the nucleoprotein of rabies virus in *Escherichia coli* and mapping of antigenic sites. *Arch Virol*, **140**, 1061–74.

Gourmelon, P., Briet, D., et al. 1991. Sleep alterations in experimental street rabies virus infection occur in the absence of major EEG abnormalities. *Brain Res*, **554**, 159–65.

Green, S.L., Smith, L.L., et al. 1992. Rabies in horses: 21 cases (1970–1990). *J Am Vet Med Assoc*, **200**, 1133–7.

Gupta, A.K., Das, T. and Banerjee, A.K. 1995. Casein kinase II is the protein phosphorylating cellular kinase associated with the ribonucleoprotein complex of purified vesicular stomatitis virus. *J Gen Virol*, **76**, 365–72.

Gupta, A.K., Mathur, M. and Banerjee, A.K. 2002. Unique capping activity of the recombinant RNA polymerase (L) of vesicular stomatitis virus: association of cellular capping enzyme with the L protein. *Biochem Biophys Res Commun*, **293**, 264–8.

Guyatt, K.J., Twin, J., et al. 2003. A molecular epidemiological study of Australian bat lyssavirus. *J Gen Virol*, **84**, 485–96.

Hammond, C. and Helenius, A. 1994. Folding of VSV G protein: sequential interaction with BiP and calnexin. *Science*, **266**, 456–8.

Hanham, C.A., Zhao, F. and Tignor, G.H. 1993. Evidence from the anti-idiotypic network that the acetylcholine receptor is a rabies virus receptor. *J Virol*, **67**, 530–42.

Hanson, R.P. 1981. *Virus diseases of food animals*, Vol. 2, Gibbs E.P.J. (ed.), London: Academic Press.

Harty, R.N., Brown, M.E., et al. 2001. Rhabdoviruses and the cellular ubiquitin-proteasome system: a budding interaction. *J Virol*, **75**, 10623–9.

Hemachudha, T. 1989. Rabies. In: Vinken, P.J., Bruyn, G.W. and Klawans, H.L. (eds), *Handbook of clinical neurology*. Amsterdam: Elsevier Science, 383–404.

Hemachudha, T. 1994. Human rabies: clinical aspects, pathogenesis and potential therapy. In: Rupprecht, C.E., Dietzschold, B. and Koprowski, H. (eds), *Lyssaviruses*. Berlin: Springer-Verlag, 121–43.

Hemachudha, T. and Mitrabhakdi, E. 2000. Rabies. In: Davis, L.E. and Kennedy, P.G.E. (eds), *Infectious diseases of the nervous system*. Oxford: Elsevier, 401–44.

Hemachudha, T. and Phuapradit, P. 1997. Rabies. *Curr Opin Neurol*, **10**, 260–7.

Hemachudha, T., Phanuphak, P., et al. 1988. Immunologic study of human encephalitic and paralytic rabies. *Am J Med*, **84**, 673–7.

Hemachudha, T., Wacharapluesadee, S., et al. 2003. Sequence analysis of rabies virus in humans exhibiting encephalitic or paralytic rabies. *J Infect Dis*, **188**, 960–6.

Her, L.S., Lund, E. and Dahlberg, J.E. 1997. Inhibition of Ran guanosine triphosphatase-dependent nuclear transport by the matrix protein of vesicular stomatitis virus. *Science*, **276**, 1845–8.

Herman, R.C. 1986. Internal initiation of translation on the vesicular stomatitis virus phosphoprotein mRNA yields a second protein. *J Virol*, **58**, 797–804.

Hooper, D.C., Pierard, I., et al. 1994. Rabies ribonucleocapsid as an oral immunogen and immunological enhancer. *Proc Natl Acad Sci USA*, **91**, 10908–12.

Hooper, D.C., Ohnishi, S.T., et al. 1995. Local nitric oxide production in viral and autoimmune diseases of the central nervous system. *Proc Natl Acad Sci USA*, **92**, 5213–316.

Horikami, S.M. and Moyer, S.A. 1982. Host range mutants of vesicular stomatitis virus defective in in vitro RNA methylation. *Proc Natl Acad Sci USA*, **79**, 7694–8.

Horikami, S.M., Curran, J., et al. 1992. Complexes of Sendai virus NP-P and P-L proteins are required for defective interfering particle genome replication in vitro. *J Virol*, **66**, 4901–8.

Hovanessian, A.R., Marcovistz, R., et al. 1988. Production and action of interferon in rabies virus infection. In: Smith, R.A. (ed.), *Interferon treatment of neurologic disorders*. New York: Marcel Dekker, 157–86.

Howard, M. and Wertz, G. 1989. Vesicular stomatitis virus RNA replication: a role for the NS protein. *J Gen Virol*, **70**, 2683–94.

Hudson, L.D., Condra, C. and Lazzarini, R.A. 1986. Cloning and expression of viral phosphoprotein: structure suggests vesicular stomatitis virus NS may function by mimicking an RNA template. *J Virol*, **67**, 1571–9.

Hunt, D.M. and Hutchinson, K. 1993. Amino acid changes in the L polymerase protein of vesicular stomatitis virus which confer aberrant polyadenylation and temperature-sensitive phenotypes. *Virology*, **193**, 786–93.

Hunt, D.M., Smith, E.F. and Buckley, D.W. 1984. Aberrant polyadenylation by a vesicular stomatitis virus mutant is due to an altered L protein. *J Virol*, **52**, 515–21.

Isaac, C.L. and Keene, J.D. 1982. RNA polymerase-associated interactions near template promoter sequences of defective interfering particles of vesicular stomatitis virus. *J Virol*, **43**, 241–9.

Iseni, F., Barge, A., et al. 1998. Characterization of rabies virus nucleocapsids and recombinant nucleocapsid-like structures. *J Gen Virol*, **79**, 2909–19.

Iseni, F., Baudin, F., et al. 2000. Structure of the RNA inside the vesicular stomatitis virus nucleocapsid. *RNA*, **6**, 270–81.

Iwasaki, Y. and Tobita, M. 2002. Pathology. In: Jackson, A.C. and Wunner, W.H. (eds), *Rabies*. San Diego: Academic Press, 283–306.

Iwasaki, Y., Gerhard, W. and Clark, H.F. 1977. Role of the host immune response in the development of either encephalitic or paralytic disease after experimental rabies infection in mice. *Infect Immun*, **18**, 220–5.

Iwata, M., Unno, T., et al. 2000. Rabies virus infection prevents the modulation by α_2-adrenoceptors, but not muscarinic receptors, of Ca^{2+} channels in NG108-15 cells. *Eur J Pharmacol*, **404**, 79–88.

Jackson, A.C. 2002. Update on rabies. *Curr Opin Neurol*, **15**, 327–31.

Jackson, A.C. 2003. Rabies virus infection: An update. *J Neurovirol*, **9**, 253–8.

Jackson, A.O., Francki, R.I.B. and Zuidema, D. 1987. Biology, structure, and replication of plant rhabdoviruses. In: Wagner, R.R. (ed.), *The rhabdoviruses*. New York: Plenum Press, 427–508.

Jackson, A.C., Phelan, C.C. and Rossiter, J.P. 2000. Infection of Bergmann glia in the cerebellum of a skunk experimentally infected with street rabies virus. *Can J Vet Res*, **64**, 226–8.

Jackson, A.O., Goodin, M., et al. 1999. Plant rhabdoviruses. In: Granoff, A. and Webster, R.G. (eds), *Encyclopedia of virology*. New York: Academic Press, 1531–41.

Jacob, Y., Badrane, H., et al. 2000. Cytoplasmic dynein LC8 interacts with lyssavirus phosphoprotein. *J Virol*, **74**, 10217–22.

Jacob, Y., Real, E. and Tordo, N. 2001. Functional interaction map of lyssavirus phosphoprotein: identification of the minimal transcription domains. *J Virol*, **75**, 9613–22.

Jallet, C., Jacob, Y., et al. 1999. Chimeric lyssavirus glycoproteins with increased immunological potential. *J Virol*, **73**, 225–33.

Jayakar, H.R., Murti, K.G. and Whitt, M.A. 2000. Mutations in the PPPY motif of vesicular stomatitis virus matrix protein reduce virus budding by inhibiting a late step in virion release. *J Virol*, **74**, 9818–27.

Jogai, S., Radotra, B.D. and Banerjee, A.K. 2002. Rabies viral antigen in extracranial organs: a post-mortem study. *Neuropathol Appl Neurobiol*, **28**, 334–8.

Kamolvarin, N., Tirawatnpong, T., et al. 1993. Diagnosis of rabies by polymerase chain reaction with nested primers. *J Infect Dis*, **167**, 207–10.

Kaplan, M.M., Wiktor, T.J. and Koprowski, H. 1975. Pathogenesis of rabies in immunodeficient mice. *J Immunol*, **114**, 1761–5.

Kaptur, P.E., McKenzie, M.O., et al. 1995. Assembly functions of vesicular stomatits virus matrix protein are not disrupted by mutations at major sites of phosphorylation. *Virology*, **206**, 894–903.

Kassis, R., Larrous, F., et al. 2004. Lyssavirus matrix protein induces apoptosis by a TRAIL-dependent mechanism involving caspase-8 activation. *J Virol*, **78**, 6543–55.

Kelly, R.M. and Strick, P.L. 2000. Rabies as a transneuronal tracer of circuits in the central nervous system. *J Neurosci Meth*, **103**, 63–71.

King, A.A., Meredith, C.D. and Thomson, G.R. 1994. The biology of southern African Lyssavirus variants. In: Rupprecht, C.E., Dietzschold, B. and Koprowski, H. (eds), *Lyssaviruses*. Berlin: Springer-Verlag, 267–95.

Kissi, B., Tordo, N. and Bourhy, H. 1995. Genetic polymorphism in the rabies virus nucleoprotein gene. *Virology*, **209**, 526–37.

Kolakofsky, D., Le Mercier, P., et al. 2004. Viral DNA polymerase scanning and the gymnastics of Sendai virus RNA synthesis. *Virology*, **318**, 463–73.

Kopecky, S.A. and Lyles, D.S. 2003. The cell-rounding activity of the vesicular stomatitis virus matrix protein is due to the induction of cell death. *J Virol*, **77**, 5524–8.

Kopecky, S.A., Willingham, M.C. and Lyles, D.S. 2001. Matrix protein and another viral component contribute to induction of apoptosis in cells infected with vesicular stomatitis virus. *J Virol*, **75**, 12169–81.

Koprowski, H., Zheng, Y.M., et al. 1993. In vivo expression of inducible nitric oxide synthase in experimentally induced neurologic diseases. *Proc Natl Acad Sci USA*, **90**, 3024–7.

Kozak, M. 1989. The scanning model of translation: an update. *J Cell Biol*, **108**, 229–41.

Kouznetzoff, A., Buckle, M. and Tordo, N. 1998. Identification of a region of the rabies virus N protein involved in direct binding to the viral RNA. *J Gen Virol*, **79**, 1005–13.

Kretzschmar, E., Peluso, R., et al. 1996. Normal replication of vesicular stomatitis virus without C proteins. *Virology*, **216**, 309–16.

Kucera, P., Dolivo, M., et al. 1985. Pathways of the early propagation of virulent and avirulent rabies strains from the eye to the brain. *J Virol*, **55**, 158–62.

Kurath, G., Higman, K.H. and Bjorklund, H.V. 1997. Distribution and variation of NV genes in fish rhabdoviruses. *J Gen Virol*, **78**, 113–17.

Kuzmin, I.V., Orciari, L.A., et al. 2003. Bat lyssaviruses (Aravan and Khujand) from Central Asia: phylogenetic relationships according to N, P and G gene sequences. *Virus Res*, **97**, 65–79.

Ladogana, A., Bouzamondo, E., et al. 1994. Modification of tritiated g-amino-n-butyric acid transport in rabies virus-infected primary cortical cultures. *J Gen Virol*, **75**, 623–7.

Lafay, F., Coulon, P., et al. 1991. Spread of CVS strain of rabies virus and of the avirulent mutant AV01 along the olfactory pathways of the mouse after intranasal inoculation. *Virology*, **183**, 320–30.

Lafay, F., Benmansour, A., et al. 1996. Immunodominant epitopes defined by a yeast-expressed library of random fragments of the rabies virus glycoprotein map outside major antigenic sites. *J Gen Virol*, **77**, 339–46.

La Ferla, F. and Peluso, R. 1989. The 1:1 N-NS protein complex of vesicular stomatitis virus is essential for efficent genome replication. *J Virol*, **63**, 3852–7.

Lafon, M., Wiktor, T.J. and Macfarlan, R.I. 1983. Antigenic sites on the CVS rabies virus glycoprotein: analysis with monoclonal antibodies. *J Gen Virol*, **64**, 843–51.

Lafon, M. 1994. Immunobiology of lyssaviruses: the basis for immunoprotection. In: Rupprecht, C.E., Dietzschold, B. and Koprowski, H. (eds), *Lyssaviruses*. Berlin: Springer-Verlag, 145–60.

Lafon, M., Lafage, M., et al. 1992. Evidence in humans of a viral superantigen. *Nature (London)*, **358**, 507–9.

Lafon, M., Scott-Algara, D., et al. 1994. Neonatal deletion and selective expansion of mouse T-cells by exposure to rabies virus nucleocapsid superantigen. *J Exp Med*, **180**, 1207–15.

Landès-Devauchelle, C., Bras, F., et al. 1995. Gene 2 of the sigma rhabdovirus genome encodes the PO protein, and gene 3 encodes a protein related to the reverse transcriptase of retroelements. *Virology*, **213**, 300–12.

Langevin, C. and Tuffereau, C. 2002. Mutations conferring resistance to neutralization by a soluble form of the neurotrophin receptor (p75NTR) map outside of the known antigenic sites of the rabies virus glycoprotein. *J Virol*, **76**, 10756–65.

Laothamatas, J., Hemachudha, T., et al. 2003. MR imaging in human rabies. *Am J Neuroradiol*, **24**, 1102–9.

Lawson, D.L., Stillman, E.A., et al. 1995. Recombinant vesicular stomatitis viruses from DNA. *Proc Natl Acad Sci USA*, **92**, 4477–81.

Lazzarini, R.A., Keene, J.D. and Schubert, M. 1981. The origins of defective interfering particles of the negative strand RNA viruses. *Cell*, **26**, 145–54.

Le Mercier, P., Jacob, Y., et al. 2002. A novel expression cassette of lyssavirus shows that the distantly related Mokola virus can rescue a defective rabies virus genome. *J Virol*, **76**, 2024–7.

Le Mercier, P., Garcin, D., et al. 2003. Competition between the Sendai virus N mRNA start site and the genome 3'-end promoter for viral RNA polymerase. *J Virol*, **77**, 9147–55.

Lenard, J. and Vanderoef, R. 1990. Localization of the membrane-associated region of vesicular stomatitis virus M protein at the N terminus, using the hydrophobic, photoreactive probe 125I-TID. *J Virol*, **64**, 3486–91.

Lentz, T.L., Wilson, P.T., et al. 1984. Amino acid sequence similarity between rabies virus glycoprotein and snake venom curaremimetic neurotoxins. *Science*, **226**, 847–8.

Lewis, P. and Lentz, T.L. 1998. Rabies virus entry into cultured rat hippocampal neurons. *J Neurocytol*, **27**, 559–73.

Lewis, P., Fu, Y. and Lentz, T.L. 1998. Rabies virus entry into endosomes in IMR-32 human neuroblastoma cells. *Exp Neurol*, **153**, 65–73.

Li, Y., Drone, C., et al. 1993. Mutational analysis of the vesicular stomatitis virus glycoprotein G for membrane fusion domains. *J Virol*, **67**, 4070–7.

Lodmell, D.L. 1988. Genetic control of resistance to rabies. In: Campbell, J.B. and Charlton, K.M. (eds), *Rabies*. Boston, MA: Kluwer Academic, 151–61.

Lodmell, D.L., Sumner, J.W., et al. 1991. Raccoon poxvirus recombinants expressing the rabies virus nucleoprotein protect mice against lethal rabies virus infection. *J Virol*, **65**, 3400–5.

Lodmell, D.L., Esposito, J.J. and Ewalt, L.C. 1993. Rabies virus antinucleoprotein antibody protects against rabies challenge in vivo and inhibits rabies virus replication in vitro. *J Virol*, **67**, 6080–6.

Lodmell, D.L., Smith, J.S., et al. 1995. Cross-protection of mice against a global spectrum of rabies virus variants. *J Virol*, **69**, 4957–62.

Lord, R.D., Fuenzalida, E., et al. 1975. Observations on the epizootiology of vampire bat rabies. *Bull Pan Am Health Org*, **9**, 189–95.

Lycke, E. and Tsiang, H. 1987. Rabies virus infection of cultured rat sensory neurons. *J Virol*, **61**, 2733–41.

Lyles, D.S., McKenzie, M.O., et al. 1996. Complementation of M gene mutants of vesicular stomatitis virus by plasmid-derived M proteins converts spherical extracellular particles into native bullet shapes. *Virology*, **217**, 76–87.

Machamer, C.E. and Rose, J.K. 1988. Vesicular stomatitis virus G proteins with altered glycosylation sites display temperature-sensitive intracellular transport and are subject to aberrant intermolecular disulfide bonding. *J Biol Chem*, **263**, 5955–60.

Masters, P.S. and Banerjee, A.K. 1988. Complex formation with vesicular stomatitis virus phosphoprotein NS prevents binding of nucleocapsid protein N to nonspecific RNA. *J Virol*, **62**, 2658–64.

Mathieu, M.E., Grigera, P.R., et al. 1996. Folding, unfolding, and refolding of the vesicular stomatitis virus glycoprotein. *Biochemistry*, **35**, 4084–93.

Mathur, M., Das, T. and Banerjee, A.K. 1996. Expression of the L protein of vesicular stomatitis virus Indiana serotype from recombinant baculovirus in insect cells: requirement of host factor(s) for its biological activity in vitro. *J Virol*, **70**, 2252–9.

Mavrakis, M., Iseni, F., et al. 2003. Isolation and characterisation of the rabies virus N°–P complex produced in insect cells. *Virology*, **305**, 406–14.

Mavrakis, M., McCarthy, A.A., et al. 2004. Structure and function of the C-terminal domain of the polymerase cofactor of rabies virus. *J Mol Biol*, **343**, 819–31.

McColl, K.A., Tordo, N. and Aguilar Setién, A. 2000. Bat lyssavirus infections. *Rev Sci Tech Off Int Epiz*, **19**, 177–96.

McCreedy, B.J. Jr., McKinnon, K.P. and Lyle, D.S. 1990. Solubility of vesicular stomatitis virus M protein in the cytosol of infected cells or isolated from virions. *J Virol*, **64**, 902–6.

McGehee, D.S. and Lorca, L.W. 1995. Physiological diversity of nicotinic acetylcholine receptors expressed by vertebrate cells. *Annu Rev Physiol*, **57**, 521–46.

McKenna, P.M., McGettigan, J.P., et al. 2003. Recombinant rhabdoviruses as potential vaccines for HIV-1 and other diseases. *Curr HIV Res*, **1**, 229–37.

McLean, R.G. 1975. Racoon rabies. In: Baer, G.M. (ed.), *The natural history of rabies*, Vol. 2. . New York: Academic Press, 53–77.

Mebatsion, T. 2001. Extensive attenuation of rabies virus by simultaneously modifying the dynein light chain binding site in the P protein and replacing Arg333 in the G protein. *J Virol*, **75**, 11496–502.

Mebatsion, T., Weiland, F. and Conzelmann, K.K. 1999. Matrix protein of rabies virus is responsible for the assembly and budding of bullet-shaped particles and interacts with the transmembrane spike glycoprotein G. *J Virol*, **73**, 242–50.

Melki, R., Gaudin, Y. and Blondel, D. 1994. Interaction between tubulin and the matrix protein of vesicular stomatitis virus: possible implications in the viral cytopathic effect. *Virology*, **202**, 339–47.

Meslin, F.-X., Fishbein, D.B. and Matter, H.C. 1994. Rationale and prospects for rabies elimination in developing countries. In: Rupprecht, C.E., Dietzschold, B. and Koprowski, H. (eds), *Lyssaviruses*. Berlin: Springer-Verlag, 1–26.

Meslin, F.X., Kaplan, M.M. and Koprowski, H. 1995. *Laboratory techniques in rabies*, 4th edn. Geneva: WHO.

Meslin, F.X., Miles, M.A., et al. 2000. Zoonoses control in dogs. In: Macpherson, C.N.L., Meslin, F.X. and Wandeler, A.I. (eds), *Dogs, zoonoses and public health*. Wallingford: CABI Publishing, 333–72.

Miller, A., Morse, H.C., et al. 1978. The role of antibody in recovery from experimental rabies. I. Effect of depletion of B and T cells. *J Immunol*, **121**, 321–6.

Minamoto, N., Tanaka, H., et al. 1994. Linear and conformational-dependent antigenic sites on the nucleoprotein of rabies virus. *Microbiol Immunol*, **38**, 449–55.

Morimoto, K., Ohkubo, A. and Kawai, A. 1989. Structure and transcription of the glycoprotein gene of attenuated HEP-Flury strain of rabies virus. *Virology*, **173**, 465–77.

Morzunov, S.P., Winton, J.R. and Nichol, S.T. 1995. The complete genome structure and phylogenetic relationships of infectious hematopoietic necrosis virus. *Virus Res*, **38**, 175–92.

Moyer, S.A., Smallwood-Kentro, S., et al. 1991. Assembly and transcription of synthetic vesicular stomatitis virus nucleocapsids. *J Virol*, **65**, 2170–8.

Mrak, R.E. and Young, L. 1994. Rabies encephalitis in humans: pathology, pathogenesis, and pathophysiology. *J Neuropathol Exp Neurol*, **53**, 1–10.

Müller, R., Poch, O., et al. 1994. Rift valley fever virus L segment: correction of the sequence and possible functional role of newly identified regions conserved in RNA-dependent polymerases. *J Gen Virol*, **75**, 1345–52.

Murphy, F.A., Bauer, S.P., et al. 1973. Comparative pathogenesis of rabies and rabies-like virus. Viral infection and transit from inoculation site to the central nervous system. *Lab Invest*, **28**, 361–76.

Murphy, F.A., Fauquet, C.M., et al. 1995. *Virus taxonomy*. Vienna: Springer-Verlag.

Nadin-Davis, S.A., Casey, G.A. and Wandeler, A. 1993. Identification of regional variants of the rabies virus within the Canadian province of Ontario. *J Gen Virol*, **74**, 829–37.

Nadin-Davis, S.A., Casey, G.A. and Wandeler, A.I. 1994. A molecular epidemiological study of rabies virus in central Ontario and western Quebec. *J Gen Virol*, **75**, 2575–83.

Nadin-Davis, S.A., Sampath, M.I., et al. 1999. Phylogeographic patterns exhibited by Ontario rabies virus variants. *Epidemiol Infect*, **123**, 325–36.

Nadin-Davis, S.A., Huang, W., et al. 2001. Antigenic and genetic divergence of rabies viruses from bat species indigenous to Canada. *Virus Res*, **74**, 139–56.

Nadin-Davis, S.A., Abdel-Malik, M., et al. 2002. Lyssavirus P gene characterisation provides insights into the phylogeny of the genus and identifies structural similarities and diversity within the encoded phosphoprotein. *Virology*, **298**, 286–305.

Nadin-Davis, S.A., Sheen, M. and Wandeler, A.I. 2003. Use of discriminatory probes for strain typing of formalin-fixed, rabies virus-infected tissues by in situ hybridization. *J Clin Microbiol*, **41**, 4343–52.

Nathanson, N. and Gonzalez-Scarano, F. 1991. Immune response to rabies virus. In: Baer, G.M. (ed.), *The natural history of rabies*. Boca Raton, FL: CRC Press, 145–61.

Negri, A. 1903. Beitrag zum Studium der Aetiologie der Tollwuth. *Z Hyg Infectionskr*, **43**, 507–27.

Nel, L.H., Thomson, G.R. and Von Teicham, B.F. 1993. Molecular epidemiology of rabies virus in South Africa. *Onderstepoort J Vet Res*, **60**, 301–6.

Newcomb, W.W., Tobin, T.J., et al. 1982. In vitro reassembly of vesicular stomatitis virus skeletons. *J Virol*, **41**, 1055–62.

Ni, Y., Tominaga, Y., et al. 1995. Mapping and characterization of a sequential epitope on the rabies virus glycoprotein which is recognized by a neutralizing monoclonal antibody RG719. *Microbiol Immunol*, **39**, 693–702.

Odenwald, W.F., Arnheiter, H., et al. 1986. Stereo images of vesicular stomatitis virus assembly. *J Virol*, **57**, 922–32.

Ogden, J.R., Pal, R. and Wagner, R.R. 1986. Mapping regions of the matrix protein of vesicular stomatitis virus which bind to the ribonucleocapsids, liposomes, and monoclonal antibodies. *J Virol*, **58**, 860–8.

Pak, C.C., Puri, A. and Blumenthal, R. 1997. Conformational changes and fusion activity of vesicular stomatitis virus glycoprotein: [125I]iodonaphthyl azide photolabeling studies in biological membranes. *Biochemistry*, **36**, 8890–6.

Pattnaik, A.K., Ball, A.L., et al. 1995. The termini of VSV DI particle RNAs are sufficient to signal encapsidation, replication, and budding to generate infectious particles. *Virology*, **206**, 760–4.

Perl, D.P. and Good, P.F. 1991. The pathology of rabies in the CNS. In: Baer, G.M. (ed.), *The natural history of rabies*. Boca Raton, FL: CRC Press, 163–90.

Perrin, P., Portmoi, D. and Sureau, P. 1982. Étude de l'adsorption et de la pénétration du virus rabique: interactions avec les cellules BHK21 et des membranes artificielles. *Ann Virol (Inst Pasteur)*, **133E**, 403–22.

Perrin, P., Jacob, Y., et al. 2000. Immunization of dogs with a DNA vaccine induces protection against rabies virus. *Vaccine*, **18**, 479–86.

Perrin, P., Jacob, Y., et al. 2001. New recombinant vaccines against lyssaviruses. In: Dodet, D. (ed.), *Reflexions bioéthiques: rabies control in Asia*. Paris: John Libbey Eurotext, 156–70.

Petersen, J.M., Her, L.S. and Dahlberg, J.E. 2000. Multiple vesiculoviral matrix proteins inhibit both nuclear export and import. *Proc Natl Acad Sci USA*, **98**, 8590–5.

Pleasure, S.J. and Fischbein, N.J. 2000. Correlation of clinical and neuroimaging findings in a case of rabies encephalitis. *Arch Neurol*, **57**, 1765–9.

Plotkin, S.A. 1993. Vaccination in the 21st century. *J Infect Dis*, **168**, 29–57.

Poch, O., Tordo, N. and Keith, G. 1988. Sequence of the 3386 3′ nucleotides of the genome of the Av01 strain rabies virus: structural similarities of the protein regions involved in transcription. *Biochimie*, **70**, 1019–29.

Poch, O., Sauvaget, I., et al. 1989. Identification of four conserved motifs among the RNA-dependent polymerase encoding elements. *EMBO J*, **8**, 3867–74.

Poch, O., Blumberg, B.M., et al. 1990. Sequence comparison of five polymerases (L proteins) of unsegmented negative-strand RNA viruses: theoretical assignments of functional domains. *J Gen Virol*, **71**, 1153–62.

Prabhakar, B.S. and Nathanson, N. 1981. Acute rabies death mediated by antibody. *Nature (London)*, **290**, 590–1.

Prabhakar, B.S., Fischman, H.R. and Nathanson, N. 1981. Recovery from experimental rabies by adoptive transfer of immune cells. *J Gen Virol*, **56**, 25–31.

Préhaud, C., Coulon, P., et al. 1988. Antigenic site II of the rabies virus glycoprotein: structure and role in viral virulence. *J Virol*, **62**, 1–7.

Préhaud, C., Lay, S., et al. 2003. Glycoprotein of nonpathogenic rabies viruses is a key determinant of human cell apoptosis. *J Virol*, **77**, 10537–47.

Prosniak, M., Hooper, D.C., et al. 2001. Effect of rabies virus infection on gene expression in mouse brain. *Proc Natl Acad Sci USA*, **98**, 2758–63.

Raux, H., Coulon, P., et al. 1995. Monoclonal antibodies which recognize the acidic configuration of the rabies glycoprotein at the surface of the virion can be neutralizing. *Virology*, **210**, 400–8.

Raux, H., Flamand, A. and Blondel, D. 2000. Interaction of the rabies virus P protein with the LC8 dynein light chain. *J Virol*, **74**, 10212–16.

Ravkov, E.V., Smith, J.S. and Nichol, S.T. 1995. Rabies virus glycoprotein gene contains a long 3′ noncoding region which lacks pseudogene properties. *Virology*, **206**, 718–23.

Reid, J.E. and Jackson, A.C. 2001. Experimental rabies virus infection in *Artibeus jamaicensis* bats with CVS-24 variants. *J Neurovirol*, **7**, 511–17.

Reynes, J.M., Molia, S., et al. 2004. Serologic evidence of lyssavirus infection in bats, Cambodia. *Emerg Infect Dis*, **10**, 2231–4.

Richardson, J.C. and Peluso, R.W. 1996. Inhibition of VSV genome RNA replication but not transcription by monoclonal antibodies specific for the viral P protein. *Virology*, **216**, 26–34.

Robbins, A.H., Borden, M.D., et al. 1998. Prevention of the spread of rabies to wildlife by oral vaccination of raccoons in Massachusetts. *JAMA*, **213**, 1407–17.

Roche, S. and Gaudin, Y. 2002. Characterization of the equilibrium between the native and fusion-inactive conformation of rabies virus glycoprotein indicates that the fusion complex is made of several trimers. *Virology*, **297**, 128–35.

Rose, J.K., Adams, G.A. and Gallione, C.J. 1984. The presence of cysteine in the cytoplasmic domain of the vesicular stomatitis virus glycoprotein is required for palmitate addition. *Proc Natl Acad Sci USA*, **81**, 2050–4.

Rupprecht, C.E., Wiktor, T.J., et al. 1986. Oral immunization and protection of raccoons (*Procyon lotor*) with a vaccinia-rabies glycoprotein recombinant virus vaccine. *Proc Natl Acad Sci USA*, **83**, 7947–50.

Rupprecht, C.E., Dietzschold, B., et al. 1991. Antigenic relationships of lyssaviruses. In: Baer, G.M. (ed.), *The natural history of rabies*, 2nd edn. Boca Raton, FL: CRC Press, 69–100.

Rustici, M., Bracci, L., et al. 1993. A model of the rabies glycoprotein active site. *Biopolymers*, **3**, 961–9.

Sacramento, D., Bourhy, H. and Tordo, N. 1991. PCR technique as an alternative method for diagnosis and molecular epidemiology of rabies virus. *Mol Cell Probes*, **6**, 229–40.

Sacramento, D., Badrane, H., et al. 1992. Molecular epidemiology of rabies in France: comparison with vaccinal strains. *J Gen Virol*, **73**, 1149–58.

Sagara, J. and Kawai, A. 1992. Identification of heat shock protein 70 in the rabies virion. *Virology*, **190**, 845–8.

Sagara, J., Tsukita, S., et al. 1995. Cellular actin-binding ezrin-radixin-moesin (ERM) family proteins are incorporated into the rabies virion and closely associated with viral envelope proteins in the cell. *Virology*, **206**, 485–94.

Saha, S. and Rangarajan, P.N. 2003. Common host genes are activated in mouse brain by Japanese encephalitis and rabies viruses. *J Gen Virol*, **84**, 1729–35.

Said, T., Bruley, H., et al. 1998. An RNA-binding domain in the viral haemorrhagic septicaemia virus nucleoprotein. *J Gen Virol*, **79**, 47–50.

Schlegel, R., Tralka, M., et al. 1983. Inhibition of VSV binding and infectivity by phosphatidylserine: is phosphatidylserine a VSV-binding site? *Cell*, **32**, 639–46.

Schmidt, M.F. and Schlesinger, M.J. 1979. Fatty acid binding to vesicular stomatitis virus glycoprotein: a new type of post-translational modification of the viral glycoprotein. *Cell*, **17**, 813–19.

Schneider, L.G. and Cox, J.H. 1994. Bat lyssaviruses in Europe. In: Rupprecht, C.E., Dietzschold, B. and Koprowski, H. (eds), *Lyssaviruses*. Berlin: Springer-Verlag, 207–18.

Schneider, L.G., Dietzschold, B., et al. 1973. Rabies group-specific ribonucleoprotein antigen and a test system for grouping and typing of rhabdoviruses. *J Virol*, **11**, 748–55.

Schnell, M. and Conzelmann, K.K. 1995. Polymerase activity of in vitro mutated rabies virus L protein. *Virology*, **214**, 522–30.

Schnell, M.J., Buonocore, L., et al. 1996. The minimal conserved transcription stop-start signal promotes stable expression of a foreign gene in vesicular stomatitis virus. *J Virol*, **70**, 2318–23.

Schoehn, G., Iseni, F., et al. 2001. Structure of recombinant rabies virus N-RNA and identification of the phosphoprotein binding site. *J Virol*, **75**, 490–8.

Scholthof, K.B.G., Hillman, B., et al. 1994. Characterization and detection of sc4: a sixth gene encoded by sonchus yellow net virus. *Virology*, **204**, 279–88.

Schütze, H., Enzmann, P.-J., et al. 1995. Complete genomic sequence of the fish rhabdovirus infectious haematopoietic necrosis virus. *J Gen Virol*, **76**, 2519–27.

Seif, I., Coulon, P., et al. 1985. Rabies virulence: effect on pathogenicity and sequence characterization of rabies virus mutations affecting antigenic site III of the glycoprotein. *J Virol*, **53**, 926–34.

Sellers, R.F. 1984. Vesicular viruses. In: Brown, F. and Wilson, G.S. (eds), *Topley and Wilson's principles of bacteriology, virology and immunity*, Vol. 4. 7th edn. London: Edward Arnold, 213–32.

Serra-Cobo, J., Amengual, B., et al. 2002. European bat lyssavirus infection in Spanish bat populations. *Emerg Infect Dis*, **8**, 413–20.

Shakin-Eshleman, S.H., Remaley, A.T., et al. 1992. N-linked glycosylation of rabies virus glycoprotein. Individual sequons differ in their glycosylation efficiencies and influence on cell surface expression. *J Biol Chem*, **267**, 10690–8.

Shankar, V., Dietzschold, B. and Koprowski, H. 1991. Direct entry of rabies virus into the central nervous system without prior local replication. *J Virol*, **65**, 2736–8.

Shokralla, S., He, Y., et al. 1998. Mutations in a carboxy-terminal region of vesicular stomatitis virus glycoprotein G that affect membrane fusion activity. *Virology*, **242**, 39–50.

Shoji, Y., Inoue, S., et al. 2004. Generation and charcterization of P-gene deficient rabies virus. *Virology*, **318**, 295–305.

Sleat, D.E. and Banerjee, A.K. 1993. Transcriptional activity and mutational analysis of recombinant vesicular stomatitis virus RNA polymerase. *J Virol*, **67**, 1334–9.

Smallwood, S. and Moyer, S.A. 1993. Promoter analysis of vesicular stomatitis virus RNA polymerase. *Virology*, **192**, 254–63.

Smith, J.S. 1981. Mouse model for abortive rabies infection of the central nervous system. *Infect Immun*, **31**, 297–308.

Smith, J.S., Fishbein, D.B., et al. 1991. Unexplained rabies in three immigrants in the United States. *New Engl J Med*, **324**, 205–11.

Smith, J.S., McClelland, C.L., et al. 1982. Dual role of the immune response in street rabies virus infection of mice. *Infect Immun*, **35**, 213–21.

Smith, J.S., Orciari, L.A., et al. 1992. Epidemiologic and historical relationships among 97 rabies virus isolates as determined by limited sequence analysis. *J Infect Dis*, **166**, 296–307.

Smith, J.S., Yager, P.A. and Orciari, L.A. 1993. Rabies in wild and domestic carnivores of Africa: epidemiological and historical associations determined by limited sequence analysis. *Onderstepoort J Vet Res*, **60**, 307–14.

Spiropoulou, C.F. and Nichol, S.T. 1993. A small highly basic protein is encoded in overlapping frame within the P gene of vesicular stomatitis virus. *J Virol*, **67**, 3103–10.

Steck, F., Wandeler, A., et al. 1982. Oral immunization of foxes against rabies: a field study. *Zentralbl Veterinär-Med B*, **29**, 372–96.

Sugamata, M., Miyazawa, M., et al. 1992. Paralysis of street rabies virus-infected mice is dependent on T lymphocytes. *J Virol*, **66**, 1252–60.

Superti, F., Seganti, L., et al. 1984. Role of phospholipids in rhabdovirus attachment to CER cells. Brief report. *Arch Virol*, **81**, 321–8.

Superti, F., Hauttecoeur, B., et al. 1986. Involvement of gangliosides in rabies virus infection. *J Gen Virol*, **67**, 47–56.

Sureau, P., Ravisse, P. and Rollin, P.E. 1991. Rabies diagnosis by animal inoculation, identification of Negri bodies, or ELISA. In: Baer, G.M. (ed.), *The natural history of rabies*. Boca Raton, FL: CRC Press, 203–17.

Takacs, A.M. and Banerjee, A.K. 1995. Efficient interaction of the vesicular stomatitis virus P protein or the N protein in cell expressing the recombinant proteins. *Virology*, **208**, 821–6.

Tang, Y., Rampin, O., et al. 1999. Spinal and brain circuits to motoneurons of the bulbospongiosus muscle: retrograde transneuronal tracing with rabies virus. *J Comp Neurol*, **414**, 167–92.

Thoulouze, M.I., Lafage, M., et al. 1997. Rabies virus infects mouse and human lymphocytes and induces apoptosis. *J Virol*, **71**, 7372–80.

Thoulouze, M.I., Lafage, M., et al. 1998. The neural cell adhesion molecule is a receptor for rabies virus. *J Virol*, **72**, 7181–90.

Thraenhart, O., Marcus, I. and Kreuzfelder, E. 1994. Current and future immunoprophylaxis against rabies: reduction of treatment failure and errors. In: Rupprecht, C.E., Dietzschold, B. and Koprowski, H. (eds), *Lyssaviruses*. Berlin: Springer-Verlag, 173–94.

Tignor, G.H., Shope, R.E., et al. 1974. Immunopathologic aspects of infection with Lagos bat virus of the rabies serogroup. *J Immunol*, **112**, 260–5.

Tordo, N. 1991. Contribution of molecular biology to vaccine development and molecular epidemiology of rabies disease. *Mem Inst Butantan*, **53**, 31–51.

Tordo, N. 1996. Characteristic and molecular biology of the rabies virus. In: Meslin, F.X. and Bögel, K. (eds), *Laboratory techniques in rabies*. Geneva: World Health Organization, 28–51.

Tordo, N. and Kouznetzoff, A. 1993. The rabies virus genome: an overview. *Onderstepoort J Vet Res*, **60**, 263–9.

Tordo, N. and Poch, O. 1988a. Strong and weak transcription signals within the rabies genome. *Virus Res Suppl*, **2**, 30.

Tordo, N. and Poch, O. 1988b. The structure of rabies virus. In: Campbell, J.B. and Charlton, K.M. (eds), *Rabies*. Boston, MA: Kluwer Academic, 25–45.

Tordo, N., Poch, O., et al. 1986. Walking along the rabies genome: is the large G-L intergenic region a remnant gene? *Proc Natl Acad Sci USA*, **83**, 3914–18.

Tordo, N., Bourhy, H. and Sacramento, D. 1992a. Polymerase chain reaction technology for rabies virus. In: Becker, Y. and Darai, G. (eds), *Frontiers in virology*. Berlin: Springer-Verlag, 389–405.

Tordo, N., De Haan, P., et al. 1992b. Evolution of negative-stranded RNA genomes. *Semin Virol*, **3**, 311–417.

Tordo, N., Badrane, H., et al. 1993a. Molecular epidemiology of lyssaviruses: focus on the glycoprotein and pseudogenes. *Onderstepoort J Vet Res*, **60**, 315–23.

Tordo, N., Bourhy, H., et al. 1993b. Structure and expression in the baculovirus of the Mokola virus glycoprotein: an efficient recombinant vaccine. *Virology*, **194**, 59–69.

Tordo, N., Bourhy, H. and Sacramento, D. 1995. PCR technology for lyssavirus diagnosis. In: Clewley, J.P. (ed.), *The polymerase chain reaction for human diagnosis*. Boca Raton, FL: CRC Press, 125–45.

Tordo, N., Benmansour, A., et al. 2004. Rhabdoviridae. In: Fauquet, M., Mayo, M.A., et al. (eds), *Virus taxonomy, VIIIth Report of the ICTV*. London: Elsevier/Academic Press, 623–44.

Travassos da Rosa, J.F.S., Mather, T.N., et al. 2002. Two new rhabdoviruses (Rhabdoviridae) isolated from birds during surveillance for arboviral encephalitis, Northeastern United States. *Emerg Inf Dis*, **8**, 614–18.

Trimarchi, C.V. and Debbie, J.G. 1991. The fluorescent antibody in rabies. In: Baer, G.M. (ed.), *The natural history of rabies*, 2nd edn. Boca Raton, FL: CRC Press, 219–33.

Tsiang, H. 1979. Evidence for an intraaxonal transport of fixed and street rabies virus. *J Neuropathol Exp Neurol*, **38**, 286–96.

Tsiang, H., de la Porte, S., et al. 1986. Infection of rat myotubes and neurons from the spinal cord by rabies virus. *J Neuropathol Exp Neurol*, **45**, 28–42.

Tsiang, H., Koulakoff, A., et al. 1983. Neurotropism of rabies virus, an in vitro study. *J Neuropathol Exp Neurol*, **42**, 439–52.

Tsiang, H., Ceccaldi, P.E. and Lycke, E. 1991. Rabies virus infection and transport in human sensory dorsal root ganglia neurons. *J Gen Virol*, **72**, 1191–4.

Tuffereau, C., Fischer, S. and Flamand, A. 1985. Phosphorylation of the N and M1 proteins of rabies virus. *J Gen Virol*, **66**, 2285.

Tuffereau, C., Leblois, H., et al. 1989. Arginine or lysine in position 333 of ERA and CVS glycoprotein is necessary for rabies virulence in adult mice. *Virology*, **172**, 206–12.

Tuffereau, C., Benejean, J., et al. 1998. Low-affinity nerve-growth factor receptor (P75NTR) can serve as a receptor for rabies virus. *EMBO J*, **17**, 7250–9.

Tuffereau, C., Desmezieres, E., et al. 2001. Interaction of lyssaviruses with the low-affinity nerve-growth factor receptor p75NTR. *J Gen Virol*, **82**, 2861–7.

Turner, G.S. 1990. Rhabdoviridae and rabies. In: Collier, L.H. and Timbury, M.C. (eds), *Topley & Wilson's principles of bacteriology, virology and immunity*, Vol. 4. 8th edn. London: Edward Arnold, 479–98.

Ubol, S. and Kasisith, J. 2000. Reactivation of Nedd-2, a developmentally down-regulated apoptotic gene, in apoptosis induced by a street strain of rabies virus. *J Med Microbiol*, **49**, 1043–6.

Ubol, S., Sukwattanapan, C. and Utaisincharoen, P. 1998. Rabies virus replication induces Bax-related, caspase dependent apoptosis in mouse neuroblastoma cells. *Virus Res*, **56**, 207–15.

Ubol, S., Sukwattanapan, C. and Maneerat, Y. 2001. Inducible nitric oxide synthase inhibition delays death of rabies virus-infected mice. *J Med Microbiol*, **50**, 238–42.

Vidal, S. and Kolakofsky, D. 1989. Modified model for the switch from Sendai virus transcription to replication. *J Virol*, **63**, 1951–8.

Vodopija, I. and Clark, H.F. 1991. Human vaccination against rabies. In: Baer, G.M. (ed.), *The natural history of rabies*, 2nd edn. Boca Raton FL: CRC Press, 571–95.

von Kobbe, C., van Deursen, J.M., et al. 2000. Vesicular stomatitis virus matrix protein inhibits host cell gene expression by targeting the nucleoporin Nup98. *Mol Cell*, **6**, 1243–52.

Vural, S.A., Alcigir, G. and Berkin, S. 2001. Immunohistochemical and histopathological studies of fixed rabies virus in goats. *Onderst J Vet Res*, **68**, 83–9.

Walker, P.J. and Kongsuwan, K. 1999. Deduced structural model for animal rhabdovirus glycoproteins. *J Gen Virol*, **80**, 1211–20.

Walker, P.J., Byrne, K.E., et al. 1992. The genome of bovine ephemeral fever rhabdovirus contains two related glycoproteins. *Virology*, **191**, 49–61.

Walker, P.J., Wang, Y., et al. 1994. Structural and antigenic analysis of the nucleoprotein of bovine ephemeral fever rhabdovirus. *J Gen Virol*, **75**, 1889–99.

Wandeler, A.I. 1991a. Carnivore rabies: ecological and evolutionary aspects. *Hystrix*, **3**, 121–35.

Wandeler, A.I. 1991b. Oral immunization of wildlife. In: Baer, G.M. (ed.), *The natural history or rabies*, 2nd edn. Boca Raton, FL: CRC Press, 485–503.

Wandeler, A.I. 2000. Oral immunization against rabies: afterthoughts and foresight. *Schweiz Arch Tierheilk*, **142**, 455–62.

Wandeler, A.I. and Bingham, J. 2000. Dogs and rabies. In: Macpherson, C.N.L., Meslin, F.X. and Wandeler, A.I. (eds), *Dogs, zoonoses and public health*. Wallingford: CABI Publishing, 63–90.

Wandeler, A.I., Matter, H.C., et al. 1993. The ecology of dogs and canine rabies: a selective review. *Rev Sci Tech*, **12**, 51–71.

Wandeler, A.I., Nadin-Davis, S.A., et al. 1994. Rabies epidemiology: some ecological and evolutionary perspectives. In: Rupprecht, C.E., Dietzschold, B. and Koprowski, H. (eds), *Lyssaviruses*. Berlin: Springer-Verlag, 297–324.

Wang, Y. and Walker, P.J. 1993. Adelaide river rhabdovirus expresses consecutive glycoprotein genes as polycistronic mRNAs: new evidence of gene duplication as an evolutionary process. *Virology*, **195**, 719–31.

Wang, Y., Cowley, J.A. and Walker, P.J. 1995. Adelaide river virus nucleoprotein gene: analysis of phylogenetic relationships of ephemeroviruses and other rhabdoviruses. *J Gen Virol*, **76**, 995–9.

Wang, Y., McWilliam, S.M., et al. 1994. Complex genome organization in the Gns-L intergenic region of Adelaide river rhabdovirus. *Virology*, **203**, 63–72.

Warell, D.A. 1976. The clinical picture of rabies in man. *Trans R Soc Trop Med Hyg*, **70**, 188–95.

Webster, W.A. and Casey, G.A. 1988. Diagnosis of rabies infection. In: Campbell, J.B. and Charlton, K.M. (eds), *Rabies*. Boston, MA: Kluwer Academic, 201–22.

Weiland, F., Cox, J.H., et al. 1992. Rabies virus neuritic paralysis: immunopathogenesis of non fatal paralytic rabies. *J Virol*, **66**, 5096–9.

Wertz, G.W., Whelan, S., et al. 1994. Extent of terminal complementarity modulates the balance between transcription and replication of vesicular stomatitis virus RNA. *Proc Natl Acad Sci USA*, **91**, 8587–91.

Whelan, S.P.J., Ball, L.A., et al. 1995. Efficient recovery of infectious vesicular stomatitis virus entirely from cDNA clones. *Proc Natl Acad Sci USA*, **92**, 8388–92.

Whelan, S.P., Barr, J.N. and Wertz, G.W. 2004. Transcription and replication of nonsegmented negative-strand RNA viruses. *Curr Top Microbiol Immunol*, **283**, 61–119.

White, J., Matlin, K. and Helenius, A. 1981. Cell fusion by Semliki Forest, influenza, and vesicular stomatitis viruses. *J Cell Biol*, **89**, 674–9.

WHO. 1973. *WHO Expert Committee on Rabies – sixth report*. Geneva: WHO.

WHO. 1992. *WHO Expert Committee on Rabies – eighth report*. Geneva: WHO.

Wiktor, T.J. and Koprowski, H. 1980. Antigenic variants of rabies virus. *J Exp Med*, **152**, 99–112.

Wiktor, T.J., Gyorgy, E., et al. 1973. Antigenic properties of rabies virus components. *J Immunol*, **110**, 269–76.

Winkler, W.G. 1975. Fox rabies. In: Baer, G.M. (ed.), *The natural history of rabies*, Vol. 2. New York: Academic Press, 3–22.

Winkler, W.G. 1992. A review of the development of the oral vaccination technique for immunizing wildlife against rabies. In: Bögel, K., Meslin, F.-X. and Kaplan, M. (eds), *Wildlife rabies control*. Chapel Place: Wells Medical, 82–96.

Winkler, W.G. and Jenkins, S.R. 1991. Racoon rabies. In: Baer, G.M. (ed.), *The natural history of rabies*, 2nd edn. Boca Raton, FL: CRC Press, 325–40.

Wu, X., Gong, X., et al. 2002. Both viral transcription and replication are reduced when the rabies virus nucleoprotein is not phosphorylated. *J Virol*, **76**, 4153–61.

Wu, X., Lei, X. and Fu, Z.F. 2003. Rabies virus nucleoprotein is phosphorylated by cellular casein kinase II. *Biochem Biophys Res Commun.*, **304**, 333–8.

Wunner, W.H., Reagan, K.J. and Koprowski, H. 1984. Characterization of saturable binding sites for rabies virus. *J Virol*, **50**, 691–7.

Xiang, Z.Q., Spitalnik, S.L., et al. 1995. Immune responses to nucleic acids vaccines to rabies virus. *Virology*, **209**, 569–79.

Yan, X., Prosniak, M., et al. 2001. Silver-haired bat rabies virus variant does not induce apoptosis in the brain of experimentally infected mice. *J Neurovirol*, **7**, 518–27.

Yan, X., Mohankumar, P.S., et al. 2002. The rabies virus glycoprotein determines the distribution of different rabies virus strains in the brain. *J Neurovirol*, **8**, 345–52.

Yarosh, O.K., Wandeler, A.I., et al. 1996. Human adenovirus type 5 vectors expressing rabies glycoprotein. *Vaccine*, **14**, 4321257–64.

Ye, Z., Sun, W., et al. 1994. Membrane-binding domains and cytopathogenesis of the matrix protein of vesicular stomatitis virus. *J Virol*, **68**, 7386–96.

Yuan, H., Yoza, B.K. and Lyles, D.S. 1998. Inhibition of host RNA polymerase II-dependent transcription by vesicular stomatitis virus results from inactivation of TFIID. *Virology*, **251**, 383–92.

Zeller, H.G. and Mitchell, C.J. 1989. Replication of certain recently classified viruses in toxorhynchites amboinensis mosquitoes and in mosquito and mammalian cell lines, with implications for their arthropod-borne status. *Res Virol*, **140**, 563–70.

Zhang, L. and Ghosh, H.P. 1994. Characterization of the putative fusogenic domain in vesicular stomatitis virus glycoprotein G. *J Virol*, **68**, 2186–93.

52

Borna disease virus

THOMAS BRIESE, MADY HORNIG, AND W. IAN LIPKIN

GENERAL FEATURES

Borna disease virus (BDV) is the prototype of the family *Bornaviridae*, genus *Bornavirus*, within the nonsegmented, negative-strand (NNS) RNA viruses (order *Mononegavirales*). The name Borna refers to the city of Borna, Germany, which was the site of an equine epidemic in 1895–1896 that crippled the Saxon cavalry. This neurotropic virus appears to be distributed worldwide and has the potential to infect most, if not all, warmblooded hosts. At the time of writing it is the only known example of the family *Bornaviridae*. BDV is similar in genomic organization to other NNS RNA viruses; however, its genome (about 8.9 kb) is substantially smaller than those of *Rhabdoviridae* (about 11–15 kb), *Paramyxoviridae* (about 15–16 kb) or *Filoviridae* (about 19 kb), and BDV is distinctive in its nuclear localization of replication and transcription. Although this feature is shared with the plant nucleorhabdoviruses (Martins et al. 1998), it is unique among NNS RNA animal viruses. Genome organization and gene expression of BDV are remarkable for the overlap of open reading frames (ORF), transcription units, and transcription signals; readthrough of transcription termination signals; and differential use of translation initiation codons. There is precedent for the use of each of these strategies by the *Mononegavirales*. The concurrent use by BDV of such a diversity of strategies for the regulation of its gene expression is unprecedented in NNS RNA viruses. Furthermore, BDV uses the cellular splicing machinery to generate some of its mRNAs. Although splicing is found in *Orthomyxoviridae* (segmented, negative-strand RNA viruses), it is novel in an NNS RNA virus.

Virion molecular weight and the $S_{20,\omega}$ are not known. Partially purified BDV infectious particles have a buoyant density in CsCl of 1.16–1.22 g/cm^3, in sucrose of 1.22 g/cm^3, and in renografin of 1.13 g/cm^3. Virions are stable at 37°C and lose only minimal infectivity after 24 h of incubation in the presence of serum. Virus infectivity is rapidly lost by heat treatment at 56°C, exposure to pH 5.0, organic solvents, detergents, chlorine, formaldehyde, or UV radiation (Ludwig et al. 1988). Several complete genomic BDV sequences are now reported, including strain V (Briese et al. 1994), He/80 (Cubitt et al. 1994a), CRNP5 (a rat-passaged strain with altered pathogenicity) (Nishino et al. 2002), and No/98 (Nowotny et al. 2000; Pleschka et al. 2001). No/98, an Austrian isolate, is unusual in that it differs from other isolates by more than 15 percent at the nucleotide level; other known BDV isolates, including those where only partial sequence data are available, differ generally by less than 6 percent.

MOLECULAR BIOLOGY OF BDV

BDV genome organization

Independent cloning experiments in two laboratories, using either ribonucleoprotein (RNP) preparations or viral particles obtained from infected cultured cells with high salt release techniques, revealed a negative-polarity single-stranded RNA genome comprising approximately 8.9 kb (Briese et al. 1994; Cubitt et al. 1994a). The BDV genome is remarkably compact, encoding six major ORFs in three transcription units framed by complementary termini similar to those of other NNS RNA viruses (Figure 52.1) (Briese et al. 1994; Wehner et al. 1997). The first transcription unit reveals a simple pattern with only one coded protein (nucleoprotein, N, p38/40). The second transcription unit encodes proteins X (p10) and P (phosphoprotein, p23) in overlapping ORFs. The third unit contains coding sequence for the matrix protein (M, p16), type I membrane glycoprotein (G, p57, gp94), and polymerase (L, p190). Elaboration of these proteins is dependent upon a variety of mechanisms for transcriptional, posttranscriptional, and translational control of expression, including alternative transcriptional initiation, readthrough of termination signals, splicing, and leaky ribosomal scanning (reviewed in Schneemann et al. 1995).

Replication and transcription

Replication and transcription of the BDV genome occur in the cell nucleus. Although nuclear replication and transcription are found in segmented negative-strand RNA viruses and nucleorhabdoviruses (NNS RNA viruses of plants), BDV is the only NNS RNA virus of animals with this property (Briese et al. 1992).

The 5′ and 3′ terminal nontranscribed sequences of NNS RNA viruses typically encode promoters that serve for both replication and transcription of the genome. BDV contains a 42 nucleotide untranslated region (UTR) at the 3′ end of the genome, which presumably functions as a promoter for expression of the viral (+) sense antigenome and viral transcripts, and a 54 nucleotide UTR at the 5′ end, presumably initiating

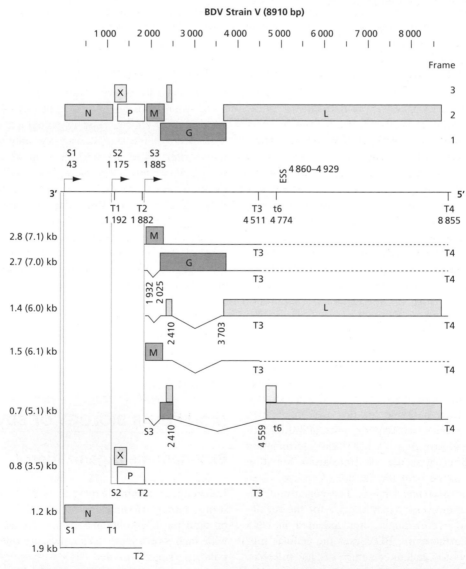

Figure 52.1 *BDV genomic map and transcripts. Abbreviations: S1 through S3, initiation sites of transcription; T1 through T4, and t6, termination sites of transcription. Readthrough at termination signals T2 and T3 is indicated by dashed lines; ESS, exon splicing suppressor.*

transcription of the (–) sense genome during replication (Schneemann et al. 1994). In other NNS RNA viruses the ratio or abundance of viral proteins during the replication cycle in the cell regulates the switch from transcription to production of full-length viral antigenome and genome from the same promoter sequences, rather than from different promoters. However, in vitro replication/transcription and reverse genetic systems are not yet established for BDV; thus, there are no direct data concerning how BDV regulates transcription and replication.

Transcription of the BDV genome results in the synthesis of at least six primary, polyadenylated, subgenomic RNAs with chain lengths of 0.8, 1.2, 1.9, 2.8, 3.5, and 7.1 kb (Briese et al. 1994; Cubitt et al. 1994a). The 7.1 kb RNA and 2.8 kb RNA are modified by splicing of two introns of approximately 0.1 and 1.3 kb to yield RNAs of 7.0/6.1/6.0 and 2.7/1.5/1.4 kb, respectively (Figure 52.1) (Cubitt et al. 1994b; Schneider et al. 1994b). The 7.1 or 7.0 kb RNAs can be further modified by alternative choice of the splice acceptor site of intron 2, generating a third intron of approximately 2.1 kb and yielding RNAs of 6.5 or 0.7 kb (or 6.6/0.8 kb if intron 1 is not spliced) (Tomonaga et al. 2000; Cubitt et al. 2001). The 1.9 kb RNA is fundamentally different from the other transcripts. It starts at the 3′ terminus of the genome rather than at the first transcription initiation signal, is not capped, and is only partly polyadenylated (Schneemann et al. 1994). Whether it represents an analog of leader-containing subgenomic RNAs found in other NNS RNA viruses or an abortive replication intermediate with a stop at the second termination signal is unknown.

The molar abundance of the individual BDV mRNAs in infected cultured cells and tissues resembles that of rhabdoviruses and paramyxoviruses, where transcription by the endogenous nucleocapsid-associated viral RNA polymerase complex occurs sequentially from the 3′ end of the genome following the order of the genes (Briese et al. 1994; Cubitt et al. 1994a). NNS RNA viruses typically contain signal sequences in the noncoding intergenic regions of the genome that specify transcriptional termination/polyadenylation and initiation by the viral polymerase complexes (Banerjee 1987). RNA circularization, followed by RT-PCR over the ligated ends and sequencing, revealed that BDV contains three semiconserved, U-rich initiation motifs that are unique to BDV, and four stop signals that, similar to other NNS RNA viruses, contain an A followed by six or seven U residues (Schneemann et al. 1994). However, the gene junctions are atypical for NNS RNA viruses as they cannot be clearly divided into discrete regions corresponding to a termination signal for one transcription unit, an intergenic region, and an initiation signal for the next transcription unit. The first and the second transcription units overlap, such that the second initiation signal, S2, lies upstream of the first termination signal,

T1 (Figure 52.1). A similar organization is postulated to serve as an attenuation signal for control of polymerase expression in respiratory syncytial virus (Collins et al. 1987); however, in BDV, attenuation appears not to take place, as the two transcription units are expressed at similar levels (Briese et al. 1994). The second and third transcription units are separated by only two nucleotides, with the second termination signal, T2, fully contained within the third initiation signal, S3. The initiation signal S3 gives rise to two different primary transcripts: the first terminates at the third termination signal T3, whereas the second is expressed by readthrough of T3 and termination at T4 (Figure 52.1). Indeed, readthrough of T3 in BDV is essential for the expression of p190, the polymerase protein. Transcriptional readthrough may provide a means for regulating the expression of the BDV polymerase, a protein only needed in catalytic amounts. Consistent with this notion is the observation that levels of the 7.1 kb transcript are lower than those of the 2.8 kb transcript (Briese et al. 1994).

Splicing of BDV mRNAs

Splicing is an intriguing feature of BDV that allows for efficient use of its genome, controls the expression of three ORFs comprising the third transcription unit, and may have implications for neurotropism and pathogenesis. Introns are located at nucleotides (nt) 1932–2025 (intron 1) and 2410–3703 (intron 2) (Cubitt et al. 1994b; Schneider et al. 1994b) (Figure 52.1). Differential splicing and the potential for either termination or readthrough at the termination signal T3 allows for the expression of six additional RNAs (Schneider et al. 1994b). Differential splicing of the two introns regulates expression of the M, G, and L proteins. Splicing of intron 1 places the 13th amino acid (aa) residue of the M ORF in frame with a stop codon. Whereas this abrogates M expression, the resulting 13 aa minicistron facilitates G expression by ribosomal reinitiation (Schneider et al. 1997b). Preliminary data suggest that the 13 aa minicistron which facilitates G expression by ribosomal reinitiation also facilitates L expression. Splicing of intron 2 fuses 17 nt of an upstream, AUG-containing sequence with a continuous ORF comprising the remainder of the L coding sequence (nt 3703–8819) (Briese et al. 1994; Schneider et al. 1994b; Walker et al. 2000). Recently, an alternative splice acceptor site has been identified at nt 4559 (Figure 52.1) that is controlled by an exon splicing repressor downstream (Tomonaga et al. 2000). Splicing of intron 3 (nt 2410–4559) and transcriptional readthrough to t6 (Briese et al. 1994) may result in the expression of two additional BDV specified proteins (Tomonaga et al. 2000; Cubitt et al. 2001). In one potential product, the upstream L exon would be fused to a short ORF terminating at t6 to yield an 8.4 kDa polypeptide. In the other, the N-terminal portion of G would be fused to the truncated L ORF to yield a 165 kDa polypeptide. Splice junctions associated with the three introns are homologous to mammalian splice junction consensus sequences and can be processed by the host-cell splicing machinery. However, the splice acceptor side at nt 4559 is not strictly conserved throughout sequenced BDV isolates; the lack of conservation in No/98 (Pleschka et al. 2001) indicates that potential protein products are not likely to be essential to the basic lifecycle of the virus.

Viral proteins

NUCLEOPROTEIN

The first ORF of the BDV antigenome codes for a protein of 40 kDa. Although participation in RNP complex formation and binding to RNA has yet to be demonstrated, its position in the viral genome, its size, and its relative abundance in infected cells suggests that it corresponds to the BDV nucleoprotein (N).

This protein, together with BDV P, comprises the soluble antigen (s antigen), a complex found in the noninfectious supernatant obtained after high-speed centrifugation of sonicated, infected brain, or cultured cells. The s antigen was a cornerstone for diagnosis of infection prior to the advent of molecular probes and recombinant proteins, and provided the first evidence for interaction of BDV proteins (von Sprockhoff 1956; Wagner et al. 1968; Ludwig et al. 1973; Haas et al. 1986; Bause-Niedrig et al. 1992).

The nucleoprotein exists as either a 40 kDa or a 38 kDa isoform. Whereas p40 uses the entire ORF, p38 initiates at the second in-frame AUG and lacks 13 aa at the amino terminus (Figure 52.2). It is unknown whether p38 and p40 are translated from a single transcript, although an RNA has been found that initiates downstream of S1 and encodes p38 (Pyper and Gartner 1997). Immunohistochemical and cell fractionation experiments with cells transfected for expression of p40 or p38 revealed that, whereas p40 is primarily nuclear, p38 is primarily cytoplasmic. This difference in the subcellular distribution of p40 and p38 reflects the presence in p40 of an amino terminal nuclear localization signal (NLS) ($_3$PKRRLVDDA$_{11}$) (Kobayashi et al. 1998; Pyper and Gartner 1997). The in vivo significance of the two isoforms of N is unknown. Both p38 and p40 bind the BDV phosphoprotein (P). P contains a potent NLS; thus, it is conceivable that the 38 kDa isoform may enter the nucleus through interaction with P. Interaction with P is facilitated by two motifs located in the N-terminal half of N (K_{51}–Y_{100}, and L_{131}–I_{158}; Figure 52.2) (Berg et al. 1998; Kobayashi et al. 2001). p38 and p40 also contain an internal leucine-rich nuclear export signal (NES) (L_{128}TELEISSIFSHCC$_{141}$) (Kobayashi et al.

2001) that overlaps with the P binding motif. It is hypothesized that the NLS-lacking p38 isoform of N, possibly in complex with mature RNPs, may redistribute to the cytosol after dissociation of bound P (Kobayashi et al. 2001).

X-PROTEIN

Unlike the first transcription unit, which is monocistronic and encodes only two isoforms of N, the second transcription unit is bicistronic and encodes two polypeptides expressed from different ORFs, X and P. X is expressed from an ORF that initiates upstream of P and overlaps with the P ORF in a +1 frame shift (Wehner et al. 1997). X and P interact in mammalian two-hybrid and coimmunoprecipitation experiments (Schwemmle et al. 1998). The site of binding on X has been localized to the N-terminal motif S_3DLRLTLLELVRRL$_{16}$ (Malik et al. 2000; Wolff et al. 2000). X is both nuclear and cytoplasmic. It has been suggested that nuclear localization of X is a result of its binding to P. Similarity of the leucine-rich N-terminal motif to NESs of several cellular and viral export proteins, such as HIV-1 Rev or PKI (see Figure 52.2, leucines underlined), led to speculation that X may mediate nucleocytoplasmic shuttling through its interaction with the viral RNP via P. However, recent data suggest that this motif functions as an NLS rather than an NES (Figure 52.2, R_6LTLLELVRRNGN$_{19}$ (Wolff et al. 2002)). X transport through the nuclear pore complex is mediated by direct binding to importin α. The role of X in the BDV lifecycle is unknown.

PHOSPHOPROTEIN

The phosphoprotein is expressed from the second ORF of the second transcription unit of the BDV genome. There is no evidence of splicing to eliminate the first AUG initiating translation of X (Briese et al. 1994; Cubitt et al. 1994a); thus, it is likely that P is expressed through a leaky scanning mechanism. The phosphoproteins of NNS RNA viruses are essential cofactors for virus transcription and replication. Their phosphorylation by cellular kinases influences the ability of phosphoproteins to form homomultimers, bind other viral proteins, and serve as transcriptional activators. Although there are no direct data concerning the function of P, it is postulated by analogy to be similar to other viral phosphoproteins. P contains two strong NLSs at its N and C termini (Figure 52.2) (Shoya et al. 1998; Schwemmle et al. 1999b). Mammalian two-hybrid and coimmunoprecipitation experiments indicate that P interacts with itself, X, and N. Analysis of P truncation mutants led to the identification of three nonoverlapping regions important for homo-oligomerization (aa 135–172), binding to X (aa 33–115), and to N (aa 197–201) (Figure 52.2) (Schwemmle et al. 1998).

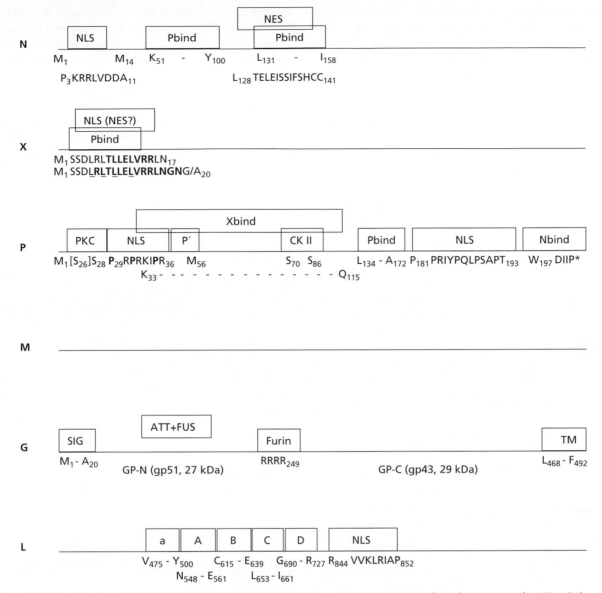

Figure 52.2 *Functional motifs identified in BDV proteins. Abbreviations: a, A, B, C, D, conserved L-polymerase motifs; ATT + FUS, attachment and fusion domain; CK II, casein kinase II phosphorylation; Furin, Furin cleavage site; M1 and M14 in N, and M1 and M56 in P indicate start sites of p40 and p38, or P and P', respectively; Nbind, site of interaction with N; NES, nuclear export signal; NLS, nuclear localization signal; Pbind, site of interaction with P; PKCϵ, protein kinase Cϵ phosphorylation; SIG, signal peptide; TM, transmembrane domain; Xbind, site of interaction with X.*

Investigation of the phosphorylation sites of P revealed a complex phosphorylation pattern that is unusual for NNS RNA viruses. P is phosphorylated predominantly by protein kinase Cϵ (PKCϵ) and, to a lesser extent, by casein kinase II (CK II). Peptide mapping studies identified Ser28 (and Ser26, which is not present in all strains) as site(s) for PKCϵ, and Ser70 and Ser86 as sites for CK II phosphorylation (Schwemmle et al. 1997). In other viral systems, sequential phosphorylation by different kinases may be associated with conformational changes that influence protein–protein interactions (Barik and Banerjee 1992). Whereas the PKCϵ phosphorylation site(s) of P overlap with the NLS, the CK II phosphorylation sites overlap with the region of interaction with X (Figure 52.2). Thus, it is conceivable that the status of P phosphorylation may influence nuclear trafficking of P (and possibly X through its interaction with P). PKCϵ is highly concentrated in limbic circuitry (Saito et al. 1993). This observation is intriguing, given the limbic distribution of BDV, and suggests that phosphorylation events may be important in BDV neurotropism.

MATRIX PROTEIN

The first ORF of the third transcription unit predicts a protein with a molecular weight of 16 kDa (p16, M). This protein was characterized as a viral product prior to the advent of genetic analysis of BDV when a 14.5 kDa protein was isolated from the brains of neonatally infected rats (Schädler et al. 1985). Later, protein microsequencing identified this protein as the product of the 16 kDa ORF (Kliche et al. 1994). Early studies indicated oligosaccharide modification of extracted protein, and a neutralizing activity of p16-specific antibodies led to the speculation that p16 might be an unusual, glycosylated matrix protein (Kliche et al. 1994; Hatalski et al. 1995; Stoyloff et al. 1997). However, more recent work indicates that p16 is a nonglycosylated matrix protein (Kraus et al. 2001). In light of these data, the neutralizing activity of p16-specific antibodies may represent reactivity with RNPs, which are thought to be involved in the spread of BDV during infection (Cubitt and de la Torre 1994; Gosztonyi et al. 1993).

GLYCOPROTEIN

The second ORF of the third transcription unit predicts a protein with a molecular weight of 57 kDa. Post-translational modification by N-glycosylation with high-mannose oligosaccharides yields a full-length type 1 membrane protein of 94 kDa (G, gp94) (Schneider et al. 1997a; Richt et al. 1998; Kiermayer et al. 2002) that is proteolytically processed by the cellular protease furin (Richt et al. 1998). Carboxyterminal cleavage of arginine$_{249}$ yields two fragments, GP-N (27 kDa nonglycosylated) and GP-C (29 kDa nonglycosylated) (Kiermayer et al. 2002; Richt et al. 1998) (Figure 52.2). Whereas precursor gp94 accumulates in the endoplasmic reticulum, the GP-C product is transferred to the cellular membrane, anchored by its C-terminal transmembrane domain. Both gp94 and glycosylated GP-C (43 kDa, gp43) are incorporated into infectious particles (Gonzalez-Dunia et al. 1997). The extensively glycosylated GP-N product (51 kDa, gp51) was recently demonstrated in infected cells and infectious particles (Kiermayer et al. 2002). Analysis of the N-glycans in gp43 and gp51 revealed maturation of the oligosaccharide chains. Whereas precursor gp94 carries only high-mannose glycans, gp43 and gp51 both contain a mixture of high-mannose and complex type glycans (Kiermayer et al. 2002).

In other viral systems glycoproteins typically mediate attachment and entry, and it has been suggested that BDV enters the cell through endocytosis followed by membrane fusion in the acidic environment of the endosome (Gonzalez-Dunia et al. 1998). Several lines of evidence indicate a role for G in BDV attachment and entry. Neutralization activity of sera from infected animals is reduced following immunoadsorption with gp94 protein; preincubation of susceptible cells with G protein interferes with infectivity (Schneider et al. 1997a); and sera raised against a bacterially expressed, truncated protein (starting at M$_{150}$) neutralizes BDV (Gonzalez-Dunia et al. 1997). Protease inhibitor studies

indicate that cleavage of the precursor gp94 is essential for infectivity (Richt et al. 1998). Pseudotyping experiments implicate the N-terminal portion of the BDV G protein in attachment and entry (Perez et al. 2001). In view of recent data indicating the presence of GP-N in virions (Kiermayer et al. 2002), it seems likely that critical residues are positioned C-terminal of M$_{150}$.

Although G may be expressed from unspliced transcripts by leaky ribosomal scanning, intron 1 spliced transcripts are more likely to serve as messages for G in vivo (Schneider et al. 1997b).

POLYMERASE

The most 5′ gene of BDV occupies more than half of the BDV genome and is thought to represent the viral RNA-dependent RNA polymerase, analogous to other NNS RNA virus L polymerases. A continuous ORF with a coding capacity of 190 kDa is formed by RNA splicing of intron 2, which fuses a small upstream ORF to the large downstream ORF (Briese et al. 1994; Schneider et al. 1994b). The product of this splicing event is considered to represent the active BDV polymerase, though no functional data are currently available (Walker et al. 2000). The protein contains the known conserved L-polymerase motifs (Briese et al. 1994; Cubitt et al. 1994a) (Figure 52.2) and, similar to other L polymerases, it interacts with P and is phosphorylated by cellular kinases (Walker et al. 2000). The protein localizes to the nuclear compartment of infected cells (Walker et al. 2000), mediated by a strong NLS mapped to a R$_{844}$VVKLRIAP$_{852}$ motif in the middle of the ORF shortly after the conserved L polymerase motif D (Walker and Lipkin 2002).

PATHOGENESIS AND EPIDEMIOLOGY OF BDV

Hosts and epidemiology

A syndrome of progressive meningoencephalitis of horses and sheep consistent with BDV infection (von Sind 1767) was recognized 100 years before the disease received its name from an equine outbreak near the town Borna in Germany. Although this clinical pattern is still considered to represent classic Borna disease (BD), infection may also result in asymptomatic carrier status, subtle disturbances in learning and memory, profound disorders of behavior and movement (Narayan et al. 1983a; Carbone et al. 1989, 1991a; Rott and Becht 1995), or death. Emerging epidemiologic data, including reports of asymptomatic, naturally infected animals (Matthias 1954; Ihlenburg and Brehmer 1964; Lange et al. 1987; Kao et al. 1993; Nakamura et al. 1995, 1996; Bahmani et al. 1996; Hagiwara et al. 1997a, 2001; Reeves et al. 1998; Berg et al. 1999, 2001; Nishino et al.

1999; Yamaguchi et al. 1999; Dauphin et al. 2001; Helps et al. 2001; Horii et al. 2001; Vahlenkamp et al. 2002; Inoue et al. 2002; Yilmaz et al. 2002), suggest that the host range and geographic distribution of BDV are larger than previously appreciated (Table 52.1). Natural infection has been reported in a wide variety of hosts, including horses, donkeys, sheep, cattle, dogs, cats, rabbits, lynxes, foxes, and birds. Experimental infection has been achieved in many of these species, and also in rodents and primates. Whether BDV naturally infects humans remains controversial; however, there is consensus that all warmblooded animals are likely to be susceptible to infection. Although Central Europe has the highest reported prevalence of Borna disease, natural infection has been described throughout Europe, in Asia, and in North America. It is unclear whether the apparent increase in host and geographic range of BDV is due to spread of the virus, or enhanced awareness of the agent and improved diagnostic reagents.

Neither the reservoir nor the mode of transmission of natural infection is known. Natural infection of horses and sheep is typically sporadic and peaks in the spring months; epidemics of disease are infrequent (reviewed in Dürrwald and Ludwig 1997). An olfactory route of transmission has been proposed because intranasal infection is efficient and the olfactory bulbs of naturally infected horses show inflammation and edema early in the course of disease (Joest and Degen 1911; Ludwig et al. 1988). One outbreak in a zoo has been attributed to inadvertent inoculation of BDV during vaccine administration (H. Müller, personal communication). Experimental infection of neonatal rats results in virus persistence and is associated with the presence of viral gene products in saliva, urine, and feces (Sierra-Honigmann et al. 1993). Such secreta/excreta are known to be important in the transmission of other pathogenic viruses (for example, lymphocytic choriomeningitis virus, hantaviruses). Normal adult rats housed in cages separate from but adjacent to those of neonatally infected rats can become infected, suggesting the possibility of aerosol transmission (M. Hornig, M. V. Solbrig, and T. Briese, personal communication). Reports of BDV nucleic acid and proteins in peripheral blood mononuclear cells (PBMC) also indicate a potential for hematogenous transmission (Sierra-Honigmann et al. 1993; Rubin et al. 1995). The observations that rodents can be persistently infected with BDV and excrete virus suggest that they have the potential to serve as both natural reservoirs and vectors for virus dissemination. However, naturally infected rodents have not been found (Tsujimura et al. 1999; Hagiwara et al. 2001); thus, the significance of rodents for the transmission of BDV to other domesticated animals and humans remains speculative. An alternative avian reservoir is suggested by studies indicating the presence of BDV nucleic acids in the feces of wild mallards and jackdaws (Berg et al. 2001).

Natural infections

Although infection may be asymptomatic, symptomatic disease typically follows a predictable course. Clinical signs at the onset of disease in horses and sheep are nonspecific: excited or depressed behavior, hyperthermia, anorexia, jaundice, constipation, and colic (Rott and Becht 1995). Classic disease becomes apparent within 1–2 weeks. Animals maintain an upright, wide-based stance, with the head extended. Repetitive behaviors are common and may include vacuous chewing, circular ambulation, and running into obstacles. In the terminal phases of disease, horses become paretic. A distinctive decubitus posture associated with paddling movements of the legs has been described. Frequently, in late disease, the virus migrates centrifugally along the optic nerve to cause retinopathy and visual impairment. Acute mortality may be as high as 80–100 percent in horses and 50 percent in sheep (Rott and Becht 1995). Sheep that survive may have permanent neurologic deficits. Recurrence of acute disease has been described in sheep (Heinig 1969). Natural symptomatic infection with a fatal outcome has also been reported in cattle (Bode et al. 1994; Caplazi et al. 1994), cats (Lundgren and Ludwig 1993; Lundgren et al. 1995a, b; Nakamura et al. 1999b), rabbits (Metzler et al. 1978), and dogs (Weissenbock et al. 1998; Okamoto et al. 2002). Epidemics of paresis in ostriches were attributed to BDV infection; however, these data have not been confirmed (Malkinson et al. 1995).

Viral persistence without apparent disease has been described in naturally infected horses (Ihlenburg and Brehmer 1964; Lange et al. 1987; Nakamura et al. 1995; Berg et al. 1999; Hagiwara et al. 2002), sheep (Matthias 1954; Hagiwara et al. 1997a; Vahlenkamp et al. 2002), and cats (Nakamura et al. 1996; Reeves et al. 1998; Nishino et al. 1999; Helps et al. 2001; Horii et al. 2001) in Europe and Asia. There is one report indicating subclinical infection of horses in North America (Kao et al. 1993). Vertical transmission of BDV has been described in horses (Hagiwara et al. 2000).

Experimental models of bornavirus infection

A wide range of animal species has been experimentally infected with BDV. Rats (Nitzschke 1963; Hirano et al. 1983; Narayan et al. 1983a), mice (Kao et al. 1984; Rubin et al. 1993; Hallensleben et al. 1998), rabbits (Zwick and Seifried 1925; Krey et al. 1979a, b), guinea pigs (Zwick and Seifried 1925), gerbils (Nakamura et al. 1999a; Watanabe et al. 2001), tree shrews (Sprankel et al. 1978), rhesus monkeys (Zwick et al. 1927; Pette and Környey 1935; Cervos-Navarro et al. 1981; Stitz et al. 1981; Krey et al. 1982), and chickens (Zwick et al. 1926; Ludwig et al. 1988) are all susceptible to classic disease; however, the

Table 52.1 *Animal species reported to be infected with BDV*

Host and sample type	Country	Seropositive	Viral protein/RNA	Seropositive and viral protein/RNA	References
Horse					
Normal	USA	3–6% (8–18/295)			Kao et al. 1993
CNS disease (B)	Germany	38% (3/8)	RNA 100% (8/8)	38% (3/8)	Zimmermann et al. 1994
CNS disease (B)	Germany	100% (4/4)	RNA 100% (4/4)	100% (4/4)	Binz et al. 1994
Normal (PBMC)	Japan	26% (15/57)	RNA 30% (17/57)	18% (10/57)	Nakamura et al. 1995
Normal (PBMC)	Iran	16.7% (12/72)	23.6% (17/72)	12.5% (9/72)	Bahmani et al. 1996
CNS disease (B)	Japan	66.7% (4/6)	66.7% (4/6)	66.7% (4/6)	Hagiwara et al. 1997b
Normal	Japan	17.8% (16/90)			Yamaguchi et al. 1999
Normal (PBMC)	Sweden	24.5% (13/53)	RNA 1.9% (1/53)	0% (0/53)	Berg et al. 1999
CNS disease (PBMC)	Sweden	57.7% (15/26)	RNA 26.9% (7/26)	19.2% (5/26)	Berg et al. 1999
Various (B)	France		RNA 4% (3/75)		Dauphin et al. 2001
Various (PBMC)	France		RNA 63.6% (14/22)		Dauphin et al. 2001
Normal	China	75% (15/20)			Hagiwara et al. 2001
Various	Japan	32% (8/25)			Yamaguchi et al. 2001
Normal	Turkey	25% (82/323)			Yilmaz et al. 2002
Various	Japan	46.4% (58/125)			Hagiwara et al. 2002
Normal	Japan	26.9% (35/130)			Inoue et al. 2002
Donkey					
CNS disease (B)	Germany	50% (1/2)	RNA 50% (1/2)	50% (1/2)	Zimmermann et al. 1994
CNS disease (B)	Germany	100% (1/1)	RNA 100% (1/1)	100% (1/1)	Binz et al. 1994
Cattle					
Normal (PBMC)	Japan	20% (15/74)	RNA 11% (8/74)		Hagiwara et al. 1996
Various (B)	France		RNA 9.7% (3/31)		Dauphin et al. 2001
Normal	China	0% (0/20)			Hagiwara et al. 2001
Sheep					
CNS disease (B)	Germany	50% (1/2)	RNA 100% (2/2)	50% (1/2)	Zimmermann et al. 1994
CNS disease (B)	Germany	100% (1/1)	RNA 100% (1/1)	100% (1/1)	Binz et al. 1994
Normal (PBMC)	Japan	36.7% (11/30)			Hagiwara et al. 1996
Normal	China	50% (10/20)			Hagiwara et al. 2001
Normal (PBMC)	Germany	11.5–19.4% (3/26–13/67)	RNA 0–14.9% (0/26–10/67)		Vahlenkamp et al. 2002

(Continued over)

Table 52.1 *Animal species reported to be infected with BDV (Continued)*

Host and sample type	Country	Seropositive	Viral protein/ RNA	Seropositive and viral protein/RNA	References
Cat					
CNS disease	Germany	7% (12/173)			Lundgren et al. 1993
CNS disease	Sweden	46% (11/24)			Lundgren et al. 1993
Various (PBMC)	Japan	8% (7/83)	RNA 13% (11/83)	0% (0/83)	Nakamura et al. 1996
CNS disease	Japan	66.7% (10/15)	RNA 53.3% (8/15)		Nakamura et al. 1999b
Normal (PBMC)	Japan	18.75% (6/32)	RNA 6.25% (2/32)	3.1% (1/32)	Nishino et al. 1999
CNS disease (PBMC)	UK		RNA 80% (4/5)		Reeves et al. 1998
Various (B)	UK		RNA 33% (6/18)		Reeves et al. 1998
FIV+	Germany	33.8% (22/68)			Huebner et al. 2001
Normal, FIV−	Germany	17.2% (32/186)			Huebner et al. 2001
CNS disease	Japan	46.2% (24/52)			Ouchi et al. 2001
Normal	Japan	23.7% (36/152)			Ouchi et al. 2001
Various	Turkey	42.5% (34/80)			Helps et al. 2001
Various	Japan	3.1% (12/383)			Horii et al. 2001
Various	Philippines	3.8% (2/53)			Horii et al. 2001
Various	Indonesia	2.0% (1/51)			Horii et al. 2001
CNS disease (B)	Sweden	40% (4/10)	RNA 100% (10/10)	40% (4/10)	Johansson et al. 2002
Lynx					
CNS disease (B)	Sweden		Protein/RNA 100% (1/1)		Degiorgis et al. 2000
Fox					
Unknown (B)	France		RNA 6.8% (4/59)		Dauphin et al. 2001
Dog					
CNS disease (B)	Austria		Protein/RNA 100% (1/1)		Weissenböck et al. 1998
CNS disease (B)	Japan	100% (1/1)	100% (1/1)	100% (1/1)	Okamoto et al. 2002
Ostrich					
CNS disease (B)	Israel		Protein 53.8% (7/13)		Malkinson et al. 1993
Birds					
Normal (F)	Sweden		RNA 33% (2/6)		Berg et al. 2001
Rodents					
Normal	China	0% (0/165)			Hagiwara et al. 2001
Normal	Japan	0% (0/106)			Tsujimura et al. 1999

Tissue examined for protein/RNA: (PBMC) peripheral blood mononuclear cells; (B) brain tissue; (F) fecal matter.

incubation period, mortality, and severity of disease vary considerably between species, between strains within a species, and depend on the immune status of the host. Whereas, in immunocompetent adult hosts, infection results in dramatic immune-mediated meningoencephalitis consistent with the classic syndrome observed in naturally infected horses and sheep, animals tolerant of infection owing to immature or compromised immune systems have a more subtle course.

ADULT RAT MODEL

Susceptibility to disease varies with the host rat strain. Wistar rats and black-hooded (BH) rats can be produc-

tively infected but have less severe disease than Lewis rats, a strain with a lesion in the hypothalamopituitary–adrenal axis associated with enhanced susceptibility to immune-mediated disorders, such as experimental allergic encephalomyelitis and adjuvant-induced arthritis (Cizza and Sternberg 1994; Sternberg et al. 1990). One report found that resistance to BD was inherited as a dominant trait in Lewis and BH hybrids that was independent of major histocompatibility complex (MHC) genes (Herzog et al. 1991). The virulence of viral strains for rats may be enhanced by serial passage of the virus in rat brain (Nitzschke 1963).

Infection is most rapidly achieved with intracranial and intranasal inoculations. Nonetheless, any route of inoculation that allows virus access to nerve terminals (for example, intramuscular, intraperitoneal, or footpad injection) ultimately results in central nervous system (CNS) infection and classic disease. Viremia is unlikely to play a significant role in BDV dissemination and pathogenesis. Although viral gene products have been found in PBMCs of infected animals (Steinbach 1994), intravascular inoculation only infrequently results in productive infection. Several observations indicate that BDV disseminates primarily via neural networks: (1) viral proteins and nucleic acids can be traced centripetally and transsynaptically after olfactory, ophthalmic, or intraperitoneal inoculation (Carbone et al. 1987; Morales et al. 1988); (2) the onset of disease is delayed with distance of the inoculation site to the CNS (Carbone et al. 1987); and (3) migration of virus to the CNS after footpad infection can be prevented by sciatic nerve transection (Carbone et al. 1987). Irrespective of the route of inoculation, clinical disease begins coincidentally with the appearance of viral proteins in hippocampal neurons and the onset of meningitis (Carbone et al. 1987; Richt et al. 1989). It has been proposed that BDV, like rabies virus, is likely to spread as an RNP complex within neural networks (Gosztonyi et al. 1993). Although structures consistent with RNPs have been described in neurons of experimentally infected animals (Cervos-Navarro et al. 1981; Sasaki and Ludwig 1993), the form of disseminating virus is unknown.

Infection of adult Lewis rats produces a prominent neurobehavioral disorder and is characterized by pronounced immunopathology. In the acute phase (4–8 weeks post infection), cellular infiltrates (CD4$^+$ and CD8$^+$ T cells, natural killer (NK) cells, and macrophages) and Th1-type cytokines are prominent in perivascular and parenchymal regions of CNS; in the chronic phase (15 weeks post-infection and beyond), a decline in infiltrates is accompanied by an increase in Th2-type cytokines and a shift to a humoral immune response (Hatalski et al. 1998a). Although antibodies to N and P generated during the acute phase of disease are nonneutralizing (Furrer et al. 2001), antibodies with neutralizing capacity increase dramatically after the acute phase (Hatalski et al. 1995) and probably participate in restriction of the virus to neural tissues (Stitz et al. 1998a). Mechanisms contributing to viral persistence are as yet uncertain. Altered viral gene expression is an unlikely explanation as there is little substantive change in CNS over the course of disease in viral titers (Narayan et al. 1983b; Carbone et al. 1987), transcripts coding for BDV proteins, or levels of BDV N and P proteins (Hatalski 1996). Modulation of immune responses as BD progresses to the chronic phase may exert some influence on BDV persistence.

The distinct clinical and behavioral features of the immune-mediated adult rat model closely parallel the CNS pathology of the acute and chronic phases. In the acute phase, coinciding with monocyte infiltration in CNS regions of early viral burden, such as the hippocampus, amygdala, and other limbic structures (Carbone et al. 1987), animals demonstrate exaggerated startle responses and hyperactivity. As animals enter the chronic phase of infection, high-grade stereotyped motor behaviors (continuous repetition of behavioral elements, including sniffing, chewing, scratching, grooming, and self-biting), dyskinesias, dystonias, and flexed seated postures appear (Solbrig et al. 1994), in parallel with the spread of virus throughout limbic and prefrontal circuits. Up to 10 percent of animals become obese, achieving body weights up to 300 percent of normal (Ludwig et al. 1988).

Disorders of movement and behavior in adult-infected rats are associated with dysfunction in dopamine (DA) circuits (Solbrig et al. 1994, 1995, 1996a, b, 1998), as seen in many neuropsychiatric disorders (Cooper et al. 1991; Kane and Marder 1993; Anderson 1994; Hamner and Diamond 1996; Kelsoe et al. 1996; Partonen 1996; Ernst et al. 1997), and may be further linked to serotonin (5HT) abnormalities (Solbrig et al. 1995). Enhanced sensitivity of central DA systems of adult-infected BD animals to DA agonists, antagonists, and DA reuptake inhibitors is observed. Administration of the mixed-acting DA agonist dextroamphetamine (Solbrig et al. 1994), or of cocaine, a DA reuptake inhibitor, to adult-infected rats elicits increased locomotor and stereotypic behavior, indicating dose-dependent potentiation of DA neurotransmission (Solbrig et al. 1998). Low presynaptic autoreceptor doses of the direct DA agonist apomorphine reduce hyperactivity, whereas higher doses increase locomotion. Both pre- and postsynaptic sites of the DA transmitter system appear to be damaged in striatum: DA reuptake sites, as measured by mazindol binding, are reduced in caudate-putamen (Solbrig et al. 1998) and nucleus accumbens (Solbrig et al. 1996b); and postsynaptic D2, but not D1, receptor binding is markedly reduced in caudate-putamen, whereas D2 and D3 receptor binding is reduced in nucleus accumbens (Solbrig et al. 1994, 1996a, b). In contrast, postsynaptic DA receptors (D1, D2, D3) remain intact in prefrontal cortex (Solbrig et al. 1996a). Further support for D2-selective losses and resultant D1 hypersensitivity as mediators of neurobehavioral disturbances in adult BD is found in the ability to reverse locomotor hyperactivity through the administration of D1 receptor blocking agents, such as the D1 antagonist SCH23390, or clozapine, an atypical antipsychotic with mixed D1, D2, D3, and D4 antagonist activity, but not through the administration of D2-selective antagonists (e.g. raclopride) (Solbrig et al. 1994).

Neurochemical studies further support a lesion in DA transmission consistent with partial DA deafferentation and compensatory metabolic hyperactivity in nigrostriatal and mesolimbic DA systems. Decreases in DA levels exceed those in dihydroxyphenylacetic acid (DOPAC, the major metabolite of DA) levels in high performance liquid chromatography (HPLC) analysis of tissues from striatum, nucleus accumbens, and olfactory tubercle (Solbrig et al. 1994), whereas in prefrontal cortex marked increases are noted in DOPAC (Solbrig et al. 1996a). Depletion of tyrosine hydroxylase (TH)-immunoreactive cells in substantia nigra, ventral tegmental area (Solbrig et al. 1994), and striatum (Solbrig et al. 2000), and a decrease TH protein content in striatum but not in substantia nigra pars compacta, are nonetheless accompanied by an increase in TH functional activity (Solbrig et al. 2000). Increased gene expression of neurotrophic factors that support the growth of DA-producing cells in vitro, including BDNF, NT-3, NT-4, and CNTF, may also contribute to the sensitivity to DA agonist action in adult BD (Solbrig et al. 2000).

Additional neuromodulator abnormalities are also noted in the adult model. The expression of genes for neuromodulatory substances and their associated synthesizing enzymes, including somatostatin, cholecystokinin, and glutamic acid decarboxylase, is greatly reduced during the acute phase and recovers toward normal in the chronic phase of adult BD (Lipkin et al. 1988). The cholinergic system, a major participant in sensorimotor processing, learning, and memory, is similarly affected, with a decrease in choline acetyltransferase-positive fibers as early as day 6 post-infection, progressing to nearly complete loss of these fibers in hippocampus and neocortex by day 15 (Gies et al. 1998). Preliminary work on the dysregulation of 5HT and norepinephrine (NE) systems suggests metabolic hyperactivity of 5HT, with a modest increase in the metabolite 5-hydroxyindoleacetic acid in striatum, and of NE, as evidenced by a small increase in the NE metabolite, 3-methoxy-4-hydroxyphenethyleneglycol, in prefrontal and anterior cingulate cortex regions (Solbrig et al. 1995). These changes may reflect compensatory upregulation or heterotypic sprouting following partial loss of DA afferents to these brain regions. Selective effects of BDV on 5HT and NE pre- or post-synaptic receptors have not yet been investigated. Pharmacologic and neurotransmitter-specific molecular probes have also been used to characterize endogenous opioid systems in the adult rat model. Infected animals respond abnormally to the opiate antagonist naloxone, with hyperkinesis and seizures, and also demonstrate increases in striatal preproenkephalin mRNA at 14 and 21 days (Fu et al. 1993b), and 6 weeks after BDV infection (Solbrig et al. 2002a). BDV and met-enkephalin immunoreactivity also coincide in a high percentage of cells (Solbrig et al. 2002a). Induction of the enkephalin system in adult BD may relate to increased levels of phosphorylated cyclic AMP response element binding (phosphoCREB) protein through activation by BDV of the mitogen-activated protein (MAP) kinase pathway, thus stimulating transcription factors that regulate enkephalin expression in striatum (Konradi et al. 1993). However, the mechanisms by which these changes in endogenous opioid systems occur are unclear. The marked CNS inflammation in adult-infected rats confounds the role of direct effects of the virus, virus effects on resident cells of the CNS, and cellular immune responses to viral gene products in the production of monoamine, cholinergic, and opiatergic dysfunction in BD.

NEONATAL RAT MODEL

The neonatal rat model does not show overt immunopathology; instead, despite a high virus load in the brain and lifelong persistence, animals infected within the first 12 h of life develop a milder behavioral syndrome and restricted neuropathology that may provide a more intriguing model for neuropsychiatric disorders. The cerebellar and hippocampal dysgenesis observed in neonatally infected animals is consistent with the more subtle neurodevelopmental abnormalities reported by some investigators in autism (Kemper and Bauman 1993), schizophrenia (Altshuler et al. 1987; Fish et al. 1992), and affective disorders (Soares and Mann 1997). Neonatally infected animals display a wide range of physiologic and neurobehavioral disturbances. They are smaller than uninfected littermates (Carbone et al. 1991b; Bautista et al. 1994), with no demonstrable alteration of glucose, growth hormone, or insulin-like growth factor-1 (Bautista et al. 1994) or amount of food ingested (Bautista et al. 1995); display an enhanced preference for salt solutions; and exhibit altered circadian rhythms (Bautista et al. 1994). Behavioral and cognitive changes in rats infected in the neonatal period include abnormal early locomotor development (Hornig et al. 1999), spatial and aversive learning deficits (Dittrich et al. 1989; Rubin et al. 1999), increased motor activity (Bautista et al. 1994; Hornig et al. 1999), abnormal anxiety responses (Dittrich et al. 1989; Hornig et al. 1999; Pletnikov et al. 1999a), stereotypic behaviors (Hornig et al. 1999), and reduced initiation of, and response to, nondominance-related play interactions (Pletnikov et al. 1999b). Thus, the neuropathologic, physiologic, and neurobehavioral features of BDV infection of neonates indicate that it not only provides a useful model for exploring the mechanisms by which viral and immune factors may damage developing neurocircuitry, but also has significant links to the range of biologic, neurostructural, locomotor, cognitive, and social deficits observed in a wide range of human neuropsychiatric illnesses.

CNS dysfunction in neonatally infected animals has been proposed to be linked to direct viral effects on morphogenesis of the hippocampus and cerebellum, two structures that in rodents continue to mature postnatally. Although overall architecture is maintained, granule cells of the dentate gyrus (Hornig et al. 1999; Rubin et al. 1999) and Purkinje cells of the cerebellum are lost (Eisenman et al. 1999; Hornig et al. 1999) through apoptosis (Hornig et al. 1999). The extent of neuronal loss in the dentate gyrus is correlated with the severity of spatial learning and memory deficiencies in neonatally infected Lewis rats (Rubin et al. 1999). Testing of cerebellar function demonstrates deficits in motor coordination and postural stability (Hornig et al. 1999; Pletnikov et al. 2001), consistent with Purkinje cell losses. Further studies are needed to evaluate the mechanisms by which early postnatal exposure to BDV induces apoptotic losses and functional damage in cerebellar and limbic circuitry.

Although the cellular inflammatory response to BDV following neonatal infection is restricted, a phenomenon ascribed to the immaturity of rat postnatal immune function, a brief surge in mononuclear cell infiltrates occurs (Hornig et al. 1999), along with elevations in the expression of proinflammatory cytokine (Hornig et al. 1999; Sauder and de la Torre 1999), chemokine (Sauder et al. 2000), and chemokine receptor (Rauer et al. 2002) transcripts. However, this transient immune response does not colocalize with sites of neuropathologic damage (Weissenböck et al. 2000). Neuropathology instead parallels regions and the time course of microglial proliferation and expression of MHC class I and class II, ICAM, CD4, and CD8 molecules (Weissenböck et al. 2000). Humoral immune response to BDV in neonatally infected animals is also curtailed, with anti-BDV antibody titers remaining below 1:10 through 133 days post infection (Carbone et al. 1991b).

Reduced levels of neurotrophic factor mRNAs occur in the neonatal model (Hornig et al. 1999; Zocher et al. 2000). However, these changes are restricted to the hippocampus; thus, a different mechanism must be invoked to account for losses of Purkinje cells in cerebellum. It is conceivable that abnormal regulation of apoptosis – either failure of normal apoptotic sequences to be curtailed with age, or excess activation of apoptotic cell programs – may contribute to abnormal CNS architecture in neonatal infections with BDV or other neurotropic viruses. Excitotoxic stimulation, including activation of glutamatergic circuitry, is one factor that might trigger neuronal apoptosis. Complex alterations in mRNAs for apoptosis mediators, including increased levels of mRNAs for FAS and ICE (caspase-1), two promotors of apoptosis, and decreased mRNA for bcl-x, a factor that inhibits apoptosis, have been identified in hippocampus, amygdala, prefrontal cortex, nucleus accumbens, and cerebellum, and are consistent with the promotion of apoptosis throughout the brains of rats neonatally infected with BDV (Hornig et al. 1999).

Recent studies in tissue culture systems are providing insights into mechanisms for viral damage that may illuminate pathogenesis in neonatal infection. Inhibition of cell-to-cell spread of BDV by a MAPK/ERK kinase (MEK) inhibitor in cell culture (Planz et al. 2001b) and analyses of neuronal differentiation of PC12 cells (Hans et al. 2001) indicate an interaction of BDV with cellular MAP kinase signaling pathways. Infected PC12 cells demonstrate constitutive phosphorylation of MEK,

ERK, and the transcriptional activator Elk-1; however, nuclear translocation of ERK is impaired, and cells fail to differentiate with NGF treatment (Hans et al. 2001). Inhibition of neurite outgrowth is also reported in other infected cell lines, and has been ascribed to interference by BDV P with the normal interaction between the neurite outgrowth factor, amphoterin, and its receptor, RAGE (*R*eceptor for *A*dvanced *G*lycation *End*-products). Complex formation between amphoterin and P leads to altered intracellular distribution of amphoterin in infected cells, with reduced levels of amphoterin and of RAGE activation at growth cones of extending cells (Kamitani et al. 2001).

MOUSE MODEL

Mice are readily infected and have high titers of virus in the brain (Kao et al. 1984). Until recently mice were considered to be relatively resistant to disease; however, two reports indicate that disease can be induced by adaptation of virus through multiple passages in mice (Rubin et al. 1993) or infection of specific host strains during the neonatal period (Hallensleben et al. 1998). As in rats, severe clinical disease is mediated by MHC class I-restricted cytotoxic T cells (Hallensleben et al. 1998; Hausmann et al. 1999). The immunopathological process mediated by CD8[+] T cells in a CD4[+] T cell-dependent fashion is most obvious in mouse strains carrying the H-2^k allele of the MHC. In H-2^k mice the BDV N peptide T$_{129}$ELEISSI$_{136}$ has been identified as the dominant cytotoxic T-cell epitope that sensitizes cells for lysis (Schamel et al. 2001).

TREE SHREWS

Little is known about BDV pathogenesis in phylogenetically higher species such as nonhuman primates and the prosimian tree shrew (*Tupaia glis*). Intracerebral inoculation of tree shrews leads to persistent infection and a disorder characterized primarily by hyperactivity and alterations in sociosexual behavior, rather than motor dysfunction (Sprankel et al. 1978). Disturbances in breeding and social behavior were most profound in animals caged in mating pairs. Females, rather than males, initiated mating, and infected animals failed to reproduce despite increased sexual activity. Although detailed neuroanatomic studies were not performed, the syndrome was interpreted to be due to neuropathological changes in the limbic system.

NONHUMAN PRIMATES

The only reported studies of experimentally infected primates employed adult Rhesus macaques (*Macaca mulatta*). These animals were initially hyperactive and subsequently became apathetic and hypokinetic. Pathology was remarkable for meningoencephalitis and retinopathy (Stitz et al. 1981).

Immune response and BDV persistence in the CNS

Neurotropism affords BDV an opportunity to persist in an environment characterized by a restricted immune response. However, this does not reflect a failure to induce an immune response. Indeed, humoral immunity appears to play a role of confinement of infection to the CNS (Stitz et al. 1998a), and cellular immunity is essential to the expression of classic disease. Early studies of BD reported a correlation between the severity of meningoencephalitis and the clinical manifestations of disease (Zwick 1939). The first direct evidence for the role of the immune response in the pathogenesis of BD emerged from studies in which splenectomized Rhesus monkeys became persistently infected but had prolonged incubation periods and less severe disease than immune competent animals (Cervos-Navarro et al. 1981; Stitz et al. 1981). Experiments with infected athymic rats or adult rats immunosuppressed by treatment with cyclophosphamide and cyclosporin A (Stitz 1991; Narayan et al. 1983a; Herzog et al. 1985; Stitz et al. 1989) provided further evidence that BD is immune mediated.

In acute BD, CNS infiltrates are comprised of macrophages, CD4$^+$ T lymphocytes, CD8$^+$ T lymphocytes, NK cells and, to a lesser extent, plasma cells (Deschl et al. 1990; Bilzer et al. 1995). Antibodies to CD4 and CD8 markers were initially used to deplete these cells and investigate their individual contributions to immunopathogenesis. Although depletion of either CD4$^+$ or CD8$^+$ T lymphocytes resulted in amelioration of the inflammatory response in brain and the severity of acute clinical disease (Stitz et al. 1992; Planz et al. 1995), only depletion of CD8$^+$ cells was found to reduce brain atrophy (Bilzer and Stitz 1994). Although these data may suggest that CD4$^+$ T lymphocytes are not important in BD pathogenesis, others demonstrated that the recruitment of CD8$^+$ cells is dependent on CD4$^+$ T lymphocytes (Nöske et al. 1998). It has been argued that neuronal cells express little or no MHC class I surface markers and should not be susceptible to CD8$^+$ CTL lysis (Joly et al. 1991); however, both neurons and astrocytes in BDV-infected rats have been shown to express MHC class I protein (Bilzer and Stitz 1994; Planz et al. 1993). Furthermore, lymphocytes isolated from BD rat brain were found to lyse infected target cells in an MHC class I-restricted manner (Planz et al. 1993). Adoptive transfer experiments have been pursued with N protein-specific CD4$^+$ T lymphocytes. Immunosuppressed, persistently infected rats so treated had a neurological disease that was similar but not identical to BD (Richt et al. 1989). The cellular immune response to BDV in the rat seems to be restricted to N, and the N peptide A$_{230}$SYAQMTTY$_{238}$ has been identified as the relevant T-cell epitope naturally recognized in the context of MHC class I in Lewis rats (Planz et al. 2001a; Planz and Stitz 1999).

In animals that progress to chronic BD there is a pronounced decrease in CNS infiltration. The numbers of macrophages, CD4$^+$ T lymphocytes, and CD8$^+$ T lymphocytes in brain are markedly reduced; however, numbers of plasma cells are increased. In contrast to the immunopathogenesis of acute BD, which has been extensively studied by several investigators, little is known about the basis for the decline in CNS infiltration in chronic infection. Potential mechanisms include altered viral gene expression or modulation of the immune response. The first possibility is unlikely because viral titers do not change substantially over the course of disease (Narayan et al. 1983a). In addition, brain levels of N and P, the only BDV proteins that can be readily quantified, and of RNAs coding for M, G, and L (Hatalski 1996), are similar in early and late disease. There is, however, evidence for modulation of the immune response over the course of BD, manifest as induction of BDV-specific type 1 T lymphocyte (Th1) tolerance. Whereas lymphocytes isolated from the brains of acutely infected rats have potent cytolytic activity, lymphocytes from brains of chronically infected rats do not lyse BDV-infected target cells (Sobbe et al. 1997). Induction of BDV-specific tolerance in chronic infection may reflect the time course for presentation of viral antigens in the thymus (Rubin et al. 1995). Alternatively, Th1 cells may become anergic or undergo apoptosis owing to the presentation of BDV antigens in brain without essential co-stimulatory signals (Schwartz 1992; Karpus et al. 1994; Khoury et al. 1995). Support for this hypothesis is found in the observation that apoptosis of perivascular inflammatory cells is most apparent at 5–6 weeks post infection, coincident with the onset of decline in encephalitis (Hatalski et al. 1998a).

Variability in cytokine expression in brain over the course of BD may also be important for modulation of the immune response. Cytokine mRNA levels have been measured in rat brain at different times post infection by RT-PCR (Shankar et al. 1992), RNase protection assay, or Northern hybridization (Hatalski et al. 1998a). Interferon-γ (IFN-γ), tumor necrosis factor-α (TNF-α), interleukin (IL)-1α, and IL-6 mRNAs are transiently expressed in the acute phase of disease (Shankar et al. 1992; Hatalski et al. 1998a). Message for another proinflammatory cytokine, IL-2, was detected by RT-PCR experiments throughout infection (Shankar et al. 1992); however, RNase protection assays revealed that IL-2 mRNA peaks in the acute phase of infection and declines thereafter (Hatalski et al. 1998a). IL-2 and IFN-γ are produced by Th1 cells for the recruitment and activation of CTL and the stimulation of antigen-presenting cells (Mosmann and Coffman 1989). The peak in CNS levels of these proinflammatory cytokine mRNAs in acute BD is temporally correlated with the peak of immune cell infiltration. Cytokines produced by type 2 T lymphocytes (Th2), such as IL-4, have the potential to down-regulate the cellular immune response. IL-4 mRNA levels are elevated throughout the course of BD, but increased in the chronic phase of infection (Hatalski et al. 1998a). IL-10 mRNA peaks in the acute phase of BD and declines thereafter (Hatalski 1996). As in experimental allergic encephalomyelitis (Kennedy et al. 1992), the peak in IL-10 mRNA expression is correlated with a shift away from CNS recruitment of immune cells. The high levels of IL-4, IL-6, and IL-10 mRNAs observed in acute BD are likely to contribute to B-cell activation. Indeed, in rats, progression toward the chronic phase of disease is accompanied by an increase in brain levels of BDV-specific antibodies (Hatalski et al. 1998b).

The cytokine profile in chronic BD is consistent with modulation of the CNS immune response to reduce Th1 T-cell activation and increase the Th2 humoral response. TGF-β mRNA expression is elevated in BD rat brain from the onset of acute disease forward (Hatalski et al. 1998a), and its presence in chronic BD is compatible with a Th2 response. TGF-β has the potential to mediate inhibition of the proinflammatory effects of TNF-α, suppression of T- and B-cell growth, reduction of free radical formation, and inhibition of antibody production and CTL activity (Barnard et al. 1990; Fontana et al. 1992). Experimental administration of TGF-β to BD rats reduced the severity of encephalitis but did not prevent the onset of acute disease; thus, the role of TGF-β in BD pathogenesis remains unclear (Stitz et al. 1991).

The basis for the Th1 to Th2 switch in BD is a matter only for speculation. There are no data to indicate whether presentation of antigen on MHC class I is insufficient or activation of the Th1 cells is inefficient owing to inadequate costimulation. However, the result of this switch is consistent with the induction of Th1 down-regulation, an event that would allow survival of the host and foster viral persistence.

BDV and human disease

Recognition of BDV's broad experimental host range and the observation that disturbances in behavior in experimentally infected animals are reminiscent of some aspects of human neuropsychiatric diseases, including major depressive disorder, bipolar disorder, schizophrenia, and autism, led to the proposal that BDV might be implicated in their pathogenesis. Although there is consensus that humans are likely to be susceptible to BDV infection, the epidemiology and clinical consequences of human infection remain controversial. There have been no large controlled prevalence studies. Furthermore, methods for the diagnosis of human infection are not standardized; thus, it is difficult to pursue

meta-analysis. Most reports suggesting an association between BDV and human disease have focused on neuropsychiatric disorders, including unipolar depression, bipolar disorder, or schizophrenia; however, BDV has also been linked to chronic fatigue syndrome, AIDS encephalopathy, multiple sclerosis, motor neuron disease, and brain tumors (glioblastoma multiforme) (Tables 52.2 and 52.3). The improbably broad spectrum of candidate disorders has led some investigators to propose that infection is ubiquitous, and that in some disorders elevation of serum antibody titers or the presence of viral transcripts in peripheral blood mononuclear cells or neural tissues reflects generalized (AIDS) or localized (glioblastoma multiforme) immunosuppression.

There are only infrequent reports where infectious virus has been isolated from humans (Bode et al. 1996; Nakamura 1998; Planz et al. 1999; Nakamura et al. 2000), and only two reports in which BDV gene products were found in human brain by in situ hybridization and immunohistochemistry (de la Torre et al. 1996; Nakamura et al. 2000). Methods most commonly used for serologic diagnosis of infection include indirect immunofluorescence with infected cells and Western immunoblot or enzyme-linked immunosorbent assays (ELISA) with extracts of infected cells or recombinant proteins. One study found that the majority of human serum antibodies binding BDV proteins in these assays did so with low avidity; the authors suggested, therefore, that cross-reactivity accounts for much of the seroprevalence data in BDV epidemiology (Allmang et al. 2001). However, more detailed analyses of the same sera using peptide arrays representing BDV N and P sequence, indicated that some low-avidity sera also contain low levels of high-avidity antibodies (Billich et al. 2002). Another explanation for the erratic performance of serologic assays in the Borna system may be that antibodies are bound in circulating immune complexes (CIC). In the one study based on the use of this serologic method, CICs were detected in more than 90 percent of subjects with major depressive disorder or bipolar disorder, versus 30 percent of healthy controls (Bode et al. 2001).

Infection has also been diagnosed through the demonstration of BDV transcripts and proteins in tissues or peripheral blood mononuclear cells (reviewed in Hatalski et al. 1997). Most frequently, detection of viral RNA has been achieved through nested reverse transcription-polymerase chain reaction (nRT-PCR). Although sensitive, this method is prone to artifacts because of the inadvertent introduction of template from laboratory isolates or cross-contamination of samples (Schwemmle et al. 1999a). Amplification products representing bona fide isolates are difficult to distinguish from artifacts by sequence analysis. As noted earlier, BDV is characterized by extraordinary sequence conservation. Studies of N and P sequence from widely

Table 52.2 *Serum immunoreactivity to BDV in subjects with various diseases.*

Disease	Prevalence		Assay	References
	Disease	Control		
Psychiatric (various)	0.6% (4/694)	0% (0/200)	IFA	Rott et al. 1985
	2% (13/642)	2% (11/540)	IFA	Bode et al. 1988
	4–7% (200–350/5000)	1% (10/1000)	WB/IFA	Rott et al. 1991
	12% (6/49)		IFA	Bode et al. 1993
	30% (18/60)		WB	Kishi et al. 1995b
	14% (18/132)	1.5% (3/203)	WB	Sauder et al. 1996
	24% (13/55)	11% (4/36)	IFA	Igata-Yi et al. 1996
	0% (0/44)	0% (0/70)	IFA/WB	Kubo et al. 1997
	2.8% (35/1260)	1.1% (10/917)	ECLIA	Yamaguchi et al. 1999
	9.8% (4/41)		IFA	Bachmann et al. 1999
	14.8% (4/27)	0% (0/13)	IFA	Vahlenkamp et al. 2000
	0% (0/89)	0% (0/210)	IFA/WB	Tsuji et al. 2000
	1.1–5.5% (1 or 5/90)	0% (0/45)	WB (N or P)	Fukuda et al. 2001
	2.1% (17/816)		ELCIA	Rybakowski et al. 2001a
	2.4% (23/946)	1.0% (4/412)	ECLIA	Rybakowski et al. 2001b, 2002
	12.6% (11/87)	15.5% (45/290)	IFA	Lebain et al. 2002
Affective disorders	4.5% (12/265)	0% (0/105)	IFA	Amsterdam et al. 1985
	4% (12/285)	0% (0/200)	IFA	Rott et al. 1985
	38 or 12% (53 or 17/138)	16 or 4% (19 or 5/117)	WB (N or P)	Fu et al. 1993a
	37% (10/27)		IFA	Bode et al. 1993
	12% (6/52)	1.5% (3/203)	WB	Sauder et al. 1996
	0–0.8% (0–1/122)	0% (0/70)	IFA/WB	Kubo et al. 1997
	2% (1/45)	0% (0/45)	WB	Fukuda et al. 2001
	92.6% (26/28)	32.3% (21/65)	CIC	Bode et al. 2001
Schizophrenia	25% (1/4)		IFA	Bode et al. 1993
	9–28% (8 or 25/90)	0–20% (0 or 4/20)	WB (N or P)	Waltrip et al. 1995
	17% (15/90)	15% (3/20)	IFA	Waltrip et al. 1995
	14% (16/114)	1.5% (3/203)	WB	Sauder et al. 1996
	20% (2/10)		WB	Richt et al. 1997
	0–1% (0-2/167)	0% (0/70)	IFA/WB	Kubo et al. 1997
	14% (9/64)	0% (0/20)	WB	Waltrip et al. 1997
	17.9 or 35.8% (12 or 24/67)	0% (0/26)	WB (N or P)	Iwahashi et al. 1997
	12.1% (38/276)		WB	Chen et al. 1999b
	10.3% (3/29)	23.1% (6/26)	IFA	Selten et al. 2000
	9% (4/45)	0% (0/45)	WB	Fukuda et al. 2001
	12.6% (11/87)	15.5% (45/290)	IFA	Lebain et al. 2002
CFS	24% (6/25)		WB	Nakaya et al. 1996
	34% (30/89)		WB	Kitani et al. 1996, Nakaya et al. 1997
	0% (0/69)	0% (0/62)	WB	Evengard et al. 1999
	100% (7/7)	33% (1/3)	WB	Nakaya et al. 1999
MS	13% (15/114)	2.3% (11/483)	IP/IFA	Bode et al. 1992
	0% (0/50)		IFA	Kitze et al. 1996
Mental health care workers	9.8% (8/82)	2.9% (8/277)	WB	Chen et al. 1999b
Family of schizophrenic patients	12.1% (16/132)	2.9% (8/277)	WB	Chen et al. 1999b
Live near horse farms	2.6–14.8% (2/78–16/108)	1% (1/100)	ELISA	Takahashi et al. 1997
Ostrich exposure	46% (19/41)	10% (4/41)	ELISA	Weisman et al. 1994

Abbreviations: CFS, chronic fatigue syndrome; CIC, circulating immune complexes; ELCIA, electrochemiluminescence immunoassay; ELISA, enzyme-linked immunosorbent assay; IFA, immunofluorescence assay; IP, immunoprecipitation; MS, multiple sclerosis; N, nucleoprotein; P, phosphoprotein; WB, western immunoblot.

Table 52.3 *BDV RNA, virus or protein in subjects with various diseases*

Disease	Tissue	Prevalence Disease	Prevalence Controls	Divergence[a]	References
Psychiatric (various)	PBMC	67% (4/6)	0% (0/10)	0–3.6%	Bode et al. 1995
	PBMC	37% (22/60)			Kishi et al. 1995b
	PBMC	42% (5/12)	0% (0/23)	0–4.0%	Sauder et al. 1996
	PBMC-coculture	9% (3/33)	0% (0/5)	0.07–0.83%	Bode et al. 1996
	PBMC	2% (2/106)	0% (0/12)		Kubo et al. 1997
	PBMC	0% (0/24)	0% (0/4)		Richt et al. 1997
	PB	0% (0/159)			Lieb et al. 1997a
	Blood	(1/1)			Planz et al. 1998
	PBMC	4% (5/126)	2.4% (2/84)		Iwata et al. 1998
	PBMC	20% (3/15)	0% (0/3)		Planz et al. 1999
	PBMC	0% (0/81)			Kim et al. 1999
	PBMC	0% (0/27)			Bachmann et al. 1999
	CSF	0% (0/27)			Bachmann et al. 1999
	PBMC	1.8% (1/56)	0.6% (1/173)		Tsuji et al. 2000
	PBMC	37% (10/27)	15.4% (2/13)		Vahlenkamp et al. 2000
	PBMC	1.1% (1/90)	0% (0/45)		Fukuda et al. 2001
Affective disorders	PBMC	33% (1/3)	0% (0/23)		Sauder et al. 1996
	PBMC	17% (1/6)	0% (0/36)		Igata-Yi et al. 1996
	Brain	40% (2/5)	0% (0/10)		Salvatore et al. 1997
	PBMC	4% (2/49)	2% (2/84)	0–5.1%	Iwata et al. 1998
	CSF	5% (3/65)	0% (0/69)	[Protein][a]	Deschle et al. 1998
	PBMC	2% (1/45)	0% (0/45)		Fukuda et al. 2001
Schizophrenia	Brain	0% (0/3)	0% (0/3)		Sierra-Honigmann et al. 1995
	CSF	0% (0/8)	0% (0/8)		Sierra-Honigmann et al. 1995
	PBMC	0% (0/7)	0% (0/7)		Sierra-Honigmann et al. 1995
	PBMC	64% (7/11)	0% (0/23)		Sauder et al. 1996
	PBMC	10% (5/49)	0% (0/36)		Igata-Yi et al. 1996
	PBMC	100% (3/3)		4.2–9.3%	Kishi et al. 1996
	PBMC	0% (0/10)	0% (0/10)		Richt et al. 1997
	Brain	53% (9/17)	0% (0/10)		Salvatore et al. 1997
	PBMC	9.8% (6/61)	0% (0/26)		Iwahashi et al. 1997
	PBMC	4% (3/77)	2% (2/84)	0–5.1%	Iwata et al. 1998
	PBMC	14% (10/74)	1.4% (1/69)		Chen et al. 1999a
	Brain	25% (1/4)		[RNA, virus, protein][a]	Nakamura et al. 2000
	PBMC	13.8% (4/29)	34.6% (9/26)		Selten et al. 2000
	PBMC	0% (0/45)	0% (0/45)		Fukuda et al. 2001
CFS	PBMC	12% (3/25)		6.0–14%	Nakaya et al. 1996
	PBMC	12% (7/57)	4.9% (8/172)		Kitani et al. 1996, Nakaya et al. 1997
	PBMC	0% (0/18)			Evengard et al. 1999
FMS	CSF	0% (0/18)	0% (0/6)		Wittrup et al. 2000
Hippocampal sclerosis	Brain	80% (4/5)			de la Torre et al. 1996
	Brain	15% (3/20)	0% (0/85)		Czygan et al. 1999
MS	CSF	11% (2/19)	0% (0/69)	[Protein][a]	Deuschle et al. 1998
	PBMC	0% (0/34)	0% (0/40)		Haase et al. 2001
Mental health care workers	PBMC	15% (7/45)	1.4% (1/69)		Chen et al. 1999a
Normal controls	PBMC		5% (8/172)		Kishi et al. 1995a
	Brain		6.7% (2/30)		Haga et al. 1997

Abbreviations: CFS, chronic fatigue syndrome; CSF, cerebrospinal fluid; FMS, fibromyalgia syndrome; MS, multiple sclerosis; PB, peripheral blood; PBMC, peripheral blood mononuclear cells.

a) Divergence of P-gene nucleotide sequence from common BDV isolates (strain V and He/80); [Protein], [virus, protein] indicates antigen analysis, or virus and antigen analysis.

disparate BDV isolates revealed variability of up to 4.1 percent at the nucleotide level and 1.5–3 percent at the predicted amino acid level (Schneider et al. 1994a); only a single sequence has been identified that shows greater divergence (Nowotny et al. 2000). Thus, similarities in sequence between putative new isolates and confirmed isolates cannot be used to exclude the former as artifacts.

VACCINES AND ANTIVIRALS

Lapinized BDV 'Dessau' was used as a vaccine for horses in regions of endemic infection in Germany for decades. Concerns about the efficacy and safety of this vaccine led to its abandonment in the western states of Germany in 1980, and in the eastern states of Germany in 1992 (Dürrwald and Liebermann 1991; Richt and Rott 2001). There are two published reports of efforts to develop vaccines in rodent models using strain He/80. In one study rats were inoculated with either high or low doses of virus attenuated by multiple passages in MDCK cells. Low-dose recipients had classic T-cell-mediated disease and succumbed to encephalitis (although with a longer course); high-dose recipients had high antibody titers to BDV and only mild disease (Oldach et al. 1995). In another study, rats were infected with a recombinant vaccinia virus expressing BDV nucleoprotein and subsequently challenged with BDV. Although vaccination resulted in enhanced viral clearance, disease was aggravated (Lewis et al. 1999). No studies are described for vaccines based on BDV G; however, results of passive immunotherapy experiments wherein a monoclonal antibody directed against G was protective suggest that this approach might be effective (Furrer et al. 2001).

Three compounds are described as having antiviral efficacy against BDV: amantadine, ribavirin, and 1-β-D-arabinofuranosylcytosine (ARA-C). Findings with amantadine are controversial. The drug was found to inhibit replication of some human BDV isolates in cell culture and improve the clinical course in some subjects with affective disorders (Bode et al. 1997; Dietrich et al. 2000). The antidepressant response to amantadine has been variously attributed to drug effects on viral replication (Bode et al. 1997; Bode and Ludwig 2001) or on brain levels of neurotransmitters implicated in depression (Lieb et al. 1997b). Interestingly, tests of animal isolates indicated no antiviral effect in vitro or in vivo (Cubitt and de la Torre 1997; Hallensleben et al. 1997; Stitz et al. 1998b). The sensitivities of the other human isolates, RW98 (Planz et al. 1999) and HuP2br (Nakamura et al. 2000), are unknown. Ribavirin inhibits transcription and replication of both He/80 and strain V BDV in a variety of cell lines (Mizutani et al. 1998; Jordan et al. 1999). In addition to its antiviral effects through the depletion of cellular GTP pools, interference with mRNA capping, and direct interaction with

viral polymerases, ribavirin can promote a Th1-type immune response (Hultgren et al. 1998; Tam et al. 1999). This led to concerns that enhancement of cellular immunity might aggravate the immunopathology of BD (Sobbe et al. 1997; Hatalski et al. 1998a; Lewis et al. 1999). The efficacy of ribavirin was assessed in the rat model, wherein the drug was administered directly to the brain by intraventricular injection. Although ribavirin had no effect on viral load, treated animals had less inflammation and milder disease, presumably owing to antimitotic effects on microglia (Solbrig et al. 2002b). Ara-C, a nucleoside analog that inhibits DNA polymerase enzymes, also inhibits BDV replication. The mechanism of action remains unclear, but is postulated to be direct inhibition of the viral polymerase rather than an indirect effect mediated by host cell factors (Bajramovic et al. 2002).

The establishment of two functional BDV minireplicon assays (Perez et al. 2003; Schneider et al. 2003) was recently reported. The importance of N:P protein stoichiometry was demonstrated in both.

REFERENCES

Allmang, U., Hofer, M., et al. 2001. Low avidity of human serum antibodies for Borna disease virus antigens questions their diagnostic value. *Mol Psychiatry*, **6**, 329–33.

Altshuler, L.L., Conrad, A., et al. 1987. Hippocampal pyramidal cell orientation in schizophrenia: a controlled neurohistologic study of the Yakovlev Collection. *Arch Gen Psychiatry*, **44**, 1094–8.

Amsterdam, J.D., Winokur, A., et al. 1985. Borna disease virus. A possible etiologic factor in human affective disorders? *Arch Gen Psychiatry*, **42**, 1093–6.

Anderson, G.M. 1994. Studies on the neurochemistry of autism. In: Kemper, T.L. (ed.), *The neurobiology of autism*. Baltimore: Johns Hopkins University Press, 227–42.

Bachmann, S., Caplazi, P., et al. 1999. Lack of association between Borna disease virus infection and neurological disorders among HIV-infected individuals. *J Neurovirol*, **5**, 190–5.

Bahmani, M.K., Nowrouzian, I., et al. 1996. Varied prevalence of Borna disease virus infection in Arabic, thoroughbred and their cross-bred horses in Iran. *Virus Res*, **45**, 1–13.

Bajramovic, J.J., Syan, S., et al. 2002. 1-β-D-arabinofuranosylcytosine inhibits Borna disease virus replication and spread. *J Virol*, **76**, 6268–76.

Banerjee, A.K. 1987. Transcription and replication of rhabdoviruses. *Microbiol Rev*, **51**, 66–87.

Barik, S. and Banerjee, A.K. 1992. Sequential phosphorylation of the phosphoprotein of vesicular stomatitis virus by cellular and viral protein kinases is essential for transcription activation. *J Virol*, **66**, 1109–18.

Barnard, J.A., Lyons, R.M. and Moses, H.L. 1990. The cell biology of transforming growth factor beta. *Biochim Biophys Acta*, **1032**, 79–87.

Bause-Niedrig, I., Jackson, M., et al. 1992. Borna disease virus-specific antigens. II. The soluble antigen is a protein complex. *Vet Immunol Immunopathol*, **31**, 361–9.

Bautista, J.R., Schwartz, G.J., et al. 1994. Early and persistent abnormalities in rats with neonatally acquired Borna disease virus infection. *Brain Res Bull*, **34**, 31–40.

Bautista, J.R., Rubin, S.A., et al. 1995. Developmental injury to the cerebellum following perinatal Borna disease virus infection. *Brain Res Dev Brain Res*, **90**, 45–53.

Berg, M., Ehrenborg, C., et al. 1998. Two domains of the Borna disease virus p40 protein are required for interaction with the p23 protein. *J Gen Virol*, **79**, 2957–63.

Berg, A.L., Dorries, R. and Berg, M. 1999. Borna disease virus infection in racing horses with behavioral and movement disorders. *Arch Virol*, **144**, 547–59.

Berg, M., Johansson, M., et al. 2001. Wild birds as a possible natural reservoir of Borna disease virus. *Epidemiol Infect*, **127**, 173–8.

Billich, C., Sauder, C., et al. 2002. High-avidity human serum antibodies recognizing linear epitopes of Borna disease virus proteins. *Biol Psychiatry*, **51**, 979–87.

Bilzer, T. and Stitz, L. 1994. Immune-mediated brain atrophy. CD8+ T cells contribute to tissue destruction during borna disease. *J Immunol*, **153**, 818–23.

Bilzer, T., Planz, O., et al. 1995. Presence of CD4+ and CD8+ T cells and expression of MHC class I and MHC class II antigen in horses with Borna disease virus-induced encephalitis. *Brain Pathol*, **5**, 223–30.

Binz, T., Lebelt, J., et al. 1994. Sequence analyses of the p24 gene of Borna disease virus in naturally infected horse, donkey and sheep. *Virus Res*, **34**, 281–9.

Bode, L. and Ludwig, H. 2001. Borna disease virus – a threat for human mental health? In: Rowlands, D.J. (ed.), *New challenges to health: the threat of virus infection. Society for General Microbiology, Symposium 60*. Cambridge: Cambridge University Press, 269–310.

Bode, L., Riegel, S., et al. 1988. Borna disease virus-specific antibodies in patients with HIV infection and with mental disorders. *Lancet*, **2**, 689.

Bode, L., Riegel, S., et al. 1992. Human infections with Borna disease virus: seroprevalence in patients with chronic diseases and healthy individuals. *J Med Virol*, **36**, 309–15.

Bode, L., Ferszt, R. and Czech, G. 1993. Borna disease virus infection and affective disorders in man. *Arch Virol*, **7**, 159–67.

Bode, L., Durrwald, R. and Ludwig, H. 1994. Borna virus infections in cattle associated with fatal neurological disease. *Vet Rec*, **135**, 283–4.

Bode, L., Zimmermann, W., et al. 1995. Borna disease virus genome transcribed and expressed in psychiatric patients. *Nature Med*, **1**, 232–6.

Bode, L., Dürrwald, R., et al. 1996. First isolates of infectious human Borna disease virus from patients with mood disorders. *Mol Psychiatry*, **1**, 200–12.

Bode, L., Dietrich, D.E., et al. 1997. Amantadine and human Borna disease virus in vitro and in vivo in an infected patient with bipolar depression. *Lancet*, **349**, 178–9.

Bode, L., Reckwald, P., et al. 2001. Borna disease virus-specific circulating immune complexes, antigenemia, and free antibodies – the key marker triplet determining infection and prevailing in severe mood disorders. *Mol Psychiatry*, **6**, 481–91.

Briese, T. and de la Torre, J.C. 1992. Borna disease virus, a negative-strand RNA virus, transcribes in the nucleus of infected cells. *Proc Natl Acad Sci USA*, **89**, 11486–9.

Briese, T., Schneemann, A., et al. 1994. Genomic organization of Borna disease virus. *Proc Natl Acad Sci USA*, **91**, 4362–6.

Caplazi, P., Waldvogel, A., et al. 1994. Borna disease in naturally infected cattle. *J Comp Pathol*, **111**, 65–72.

Carbone, K.M., Duchala, C.S., et al. 1987. Pathogenesis of Borna disease in rats: evidence that intra-axonal spread is the major route for virus dissemination and the determinant for disease incubation. *J Virol*, **61**, 3431–40.

Carbone, K.M., Trapp, B.D., et al. 1989. Astrocytes and Schwann cells are virus-host cells in the nervous system of rats with Borna disease. *J Neuropathol Exp Neurol*, **48**, 631–44.

Carbone, K.M., Moench, T.R. and Lipkin, W.I. 1991a. Borna disease virus replicates in astrocytes, Schwann cells and ependymal cells in persistently infected rats: location of viral genomic and messenger RNAs by in situ hybridization. *J Neuropathol Exp Neurol*, **50**, 205–14.

Carbone, K.M., Park, S.W., et al. 1991b. Borna disease: association with a maturation defect in the cellular immune response. *J Virol*, **65**, 6154–64.

Cervos-Navarro, J., Roggendorf, W., et al. 1981. Die BORNA-Krankheit beim Affen unter besonderer Berücksichtigung der encephalitischen Reaktion. *Verh Dtsch Ges Path*, **65**, 208–12.

Chen, C.H., Chiu, Y.L., et al. 1999a. Detection of Borna disease virus RNA from peripheral blood cells in schizophrenic patients and mental health workers. *Mol Psychiatry*, **4**, 566–71.

Chen, C.H., Chiu, Y.L., et al. 1999b. High seroprevalence of Borna virus infection in schizophrenic patients, family members and mental health workers in Taiwan. *Mol Psychiatry*, **4**, 33–8.

Cizza, G. and Sternberg, E.M. 1994. The role of the hypothalamic-pituitary-adrenal axis in susceptibility to autoimmune/inflammatory disease. *Immunomethods*, **5**, 73–8.

Collins, P.L., Olmsted, R.A., et al. 1987. Gene overlap and site-specific attenuation of transcription of the viral polymerase L gene of human respiratory syncytial virus. *Proc Natl Acad Sci USA*, **84**, 5134–8.

Cooper, J.R., Bloom, F.E. and Roth, R.H. 1991. *The biochemical basis of neuropharmacology*. New York: Oxford University Press.

Cubitt, B. and de la Torre, J.C. 1994. Borna disease virus (BDV), a nonsegmented RNA virus, replicates in the nuclei of infected cells where infectious BDV ribonucleoproteins are present. *J Virol*, **68**, 1371–81.

Cubitt, B. and de la Torre, J.C. 1997. Amantadine does not have antiviral activity against Borna disease virus. *Arch Virol*, **142**, 2035–42.

Cubitt, B., Oldstone, C. and de la Torre, J.C. 1994a. Sequence and genome organization of Borna disease virus. *J Virol*, **68**, 1382–96.

Cubitt, B., Oldstone, C., et al. 1994b. RNA splicing contributes to the generation of mature mRNAs of Borna disease virus, a nonsegmented negative strand RNA virus. *Virus Res*, **34**, 69–79.

Cubitt, B., Ly, C. and de la Torre, J.C. 2001. Identification and characterization of a new intron in Borna disease virus. *J Gen Virol*, **82**, 641–6.

Czygan, M., Hallensleben, W., et al. 1999. Borna disease virus in human brains with a rare form of hippocampal degeneration but not in brains of patients with common neuropsychiatric disorders. *J Infect Dis*, **180**, 1695–9.

Dauphin, G., Legay, V., et al. 2001. Evidence of Borna disease virus genome detection in French domestic animals and in foxes (*Vulpes vulpes*). *J Gen Virol*, **82**, 2199–204.

de la Torre, J.C. and Bode, L. 1996. Sequence characterization of human Borna disease virus. *Virus Res*, **44**, 33–44.

de la Torre, J.C., Gonzalez-Dunia, D., et al. 1996. Detection of Borna disease virus antigen and RNA in human autopsy brain samples from neuropsychiatric patients. *Virology*, **223**, 272–82.

Degiorgis, M.P., Berg, A.L., et al. 2000. Borna disease in a free-ranging lynx (*Lynx lynx*). *J Clin Microbiol*, **38**, 3087–91.

Deschl, U., Stitz, L., et al. 1990. Determination of immune cells and expression of major histocompatibility complex class II antigen in encephalitic lesions of experimental Borna disease. *Acta Neuropathol (Berlin)*, **81**, 41–50.

Dietrich, D.E., Kleinschmidt, A., et al. 2000. Word recognition memory before and after successful treatment of depression. *Pharmacopsychiatry*, **33**, 221–8.

Dittrich, W., Bode, L., et al. 1989. Learning deficiencies in Borna disease virus-infected but clinically healthy rats. *Biol Psychiatry*, **26**, 818–28.

Dürrwald, R. and Liebermann, H. 1991. Die Bornasche Krankheit-Überblick über neuere Erkenntnisse (Übersichtsreferat). *Monatsh Vet-Med*, **46**, 608–13.

Dürrwald, R. and Ludwig, H. 1997. Borna disease virus (BDV), a (zoonotic?) worldwide pathogen. A review of the history of the disease and the virus infection with comprehensive bibliography. *Zentralbl Veterinarmed [B]*, **44**, 147–84.

Eisenman, L.M., Brothers, R., et al. 1999. Neonatal Borna disease virus infection in the rat causes a loss of Purkinje cells in the cerebellum. *J Neurovirol*, **5**, 181–9.

Ernst, M., Zametkin, A.J., et al. 1997. Low medial prefrontal dopaminergic activity in autistic children. *Lancet*, **350**, 638.

Evengard, B., Briese, T., et al. 1999. Absence of evidence of Borna disease virus infection in Swedish patients with chronic fatigue syndrome. *J Neurovirol*, **5**, 495–9.

Fish, B., Marcus, J., et al. 1992. Infants at risk for schizophrenia: sequelae of a genetic neurointegrative defect: a review and replication analysis of pandysmaturation in the Jerusalem Infant Development Study. *Arch Gen Psychiatry*, **49**, 221–35.

Fontana, A., Constam, D.B., et al. 1992. Modulation of the immune response by transforming growth factor beta. *Int Arch Allergy Immunol*, **99**, 1–7.

Fu, Z.F., Amsterdam, J.D., et al. 1993a. Detection of Borna disease virus-reactive antibodies from patients with affective disorders by western immunoblot technique. *J Affect Disord*, **27**, 61–8.

Fu, Z.F., Weihe, E., et al. 1993b. Differential effects of rabies and borna disease viruses on immediate-early- and late-response gene expression in brain tissues. *J Virol*, **67**, 6674–81.

Fukuda, K., Takahashi, K., et al. 2001. Immunological and PCR analyses for Borna disease virus in psychiatric patients and blood donors in Japan. *J Clin Microbiol*, **39**, 419–29.

Furrer, E., Bilzer, T., et al. 2001. Neutralizing antibodies in persistent borna disease virus infection: prophylactic effect of gp94-specific monoclonal antibodies in preventing encephalitis. *J Virol*, **75**, 943–51.

Gies, U., Bilzer, T., et al. 1998. Disturbance of the cortical cholinergic innervation in Borna disease prior to encephalitis. *Brain Pathol*, **8**, 39–48.

Gonzalez-Dunia, D., Cubitt, B., et al. 1997. Characterization of Borna disease virus p56 protein, a surface glycoprotein involved in virus entry. *J Virol*, **71**, 3208–18.

Gonzalez-Dunia, D., Cubitt, B. and de la Torre , J.C. 1998. Mechanism of Borna disease virus entry into cells. *J Virol*, **72**, 783–8.

Gosztonyi, G., Dietzschold, B., et al. 1993. Rabies and borna disease. A comparative pathogenetic study of two neurovirulent agents. *Lab Invest*, **68**, 285–95.

Haas, B., Becht, H. and Rott, R. 1986. Purification and properties of an intranuclear virus-specific antigen from tissue infected with Borna disease virus. *J Gen Virol*, **67**, 235–41.

Haase, C.G., Viazov, S., et al. 2001. Borna disease virus RNA is absent in chronic multiple sclerosis. *Ann Neurol*, **50**, 423–4.

Haga, S., Yoshimura, M., et al. 1997. Detection of Borna disease virus genome in normal human brain tissue. *Brain Res*, **770**, 307–9.

Hagiwara, K., Nakaya, T., et al. 1996. Borna disease virus RNA in peripheral blood mononuclear cells obtained from healthy dairy cattle. *Med Microbiol Immunol (Berlin)*, **185**, 145–51.

Hagiwara, K., Kawamoto, S., et al. 1997a. High prevalence of Borna disease virus infection in healthy sheep in Japan. *Clin Diagn Lab Immunol*, **4**, 339–44.

Hagiwara, K., Momiyama, N., et al. 1997b. Demonstration of Borna disease virus (BDV) in specific regions of the brain from horses positive for serum antibodies to BDV but negative for BDV RNA in the blood and internal organs. *Med Microbiol Immunol (Berlin)*, **186**, 19–24.

Hagiwara, K., Kamitani, W., et al. 2000. Detection of Borna disease virus in a pregnant mare and her fetus. *Vet Microbiol*, **72**, 207–16.

Hagiwara, K., Asakawa, M., et al. 2001. Seroprevalence of Borna disease virus in domestic animals in Xinjiang, China. *Vet Microbiol*, **80**, 383–9.

Hagiwara, K., Okamoto, M., et al. 2002. Nosological study of Borna disease virus infection in race horses. *Vet Microbiol*, **84**, 367–74.

Hallensleben, W., Zocher, M. and Staeheli, P. 1997. Borna disease virus is not sensitive to amantadine. *Arch Virol*, **142**, 2043–8.

Hallensleben, W., Schwemmle, M., et al. 1998. Borna disease virus-induced neurological disorder in mice: infection of neonates results in immunopathology. *J Virol*, **72**, 4379–86.

Hamner, M.B. and Diamond, B.I. 1996. Plasma dopamine and norepinephrine correlations with psychomotor retardation, anxiety, and depression in nonpsychotic depressed patients: a pilot study. *Psychiatry Res*, **64**, 209–11.

Hans, A., Syan, S., et al. 2001. Borna disease virus persistent infection activates mitogen-activated protein kinase and blocks neuronal differentiation of PC12 cells. *J Biol Chem*, **276**, 7258–65.

Hatalski, C.G. 1996. Alterations in the immune response within the central nervous system of rats infected with Borna disease virus: potential mechanisms for viral persistence. *PhD Thesis, University of California Irvine*. University of California Irvine: Irvine, CA.

Hatalski, C.G., Kliche, S., et al. 1995. Neutralizing antibodies in Borna disease virus-infected rats. *J Virol*, **69**, 741–7.

Hatalski, C.G., Lewis, A.J. and Lipkin, W.I. 1997. Borna disease. *Emerg Infect Dis*, **3**, 129–35.

Hatalski, C.G., Hickey, W.F. and Lipkin, W.I. 1998a. Evolution of the immune response in the central nervous system following infection with Borna disease virus. *J Neuroimmunol*, **90**, 137–42.

Hatalski, C.G., Hickey, W.F. and Lipkin, W.I. 1998b. Humoral immunity in the central nervous system of Lewis rats infected with Borna disease virus. *J Neuroimmunol*, **90**, 128–36.

Hausmann, J., Hallensleben, W., et al. 1999. T cell ignorance in mice to Borna disease virus can be overcome by peripheral expression of the viral nucleoprotein. *Proc Natl Acad Sci USA*, **96**, 9769–74.

Heinig, A. 1969. Die Bornasche Krankheit der Pferde und Schafe. In: Röhrer, H. (ed.), *Handbuch der Virusinfektionen bei Tieren*. Jena: VEB G. Fischer, 83–148.

Helps, C.R., Turan, N., et al. 2001. Detection of antibodies to Borna disease virus in Turkish cats by using recombinant p40. *Vet Rec*, **149**, 647–50.

Herzog, S., Wonigeit, K., et al. 1985. Effect of Borna disease virus infection on athymic rats. *J Gen Virol*, **66**, 503–8.

Herzog, S., Frese, K. and Rott, R. 1991. Studies on the genetic control of resistance of black hooded rats to Borna disease. *J Gen Virol*, **72**, 535–40.

Hirano, N., Kao, M. and Ludwig, H. 1983. Persistent, tolerant or subacute infection in Borna disease virus-infected rats. *J Gen Virol*, **64**, 1521–30.

Horii, Y., Garcia, N.P., et al. 2001. Detection of anti-Borna disease virus antibodies from cats in Asian countries, Japan, Philippines and Indonesia using electrochemiluminescence immunoassay. *J Vet Med Sci*, **63**, 921–3.

Hornig, M., Weissenbock, H., et al. 1999. An infection-based model of neurodevelopmental damage. *Proc Natl Acad Sci USA*, **96**, 12102–7.

Huebner, J., Bode, L. and Ludwig, H. 2001. Borna disease virus infection in FIV-positive cats in Germany. *Vet Rec*, **149**, 152.

Hultgren, C., Milich, D.R., et al. 1998. The antiviral compound ribavirin modulates the T helper (Th) 1/Th2 subset balance in hepatitis B and C virus-specific immune responses. *J Gen Virol*, **79**, 2381–91.

Igata-Yi, R., Yamaguchi, K., et al. 1996. Borna disease virus and the consumption of raw horse meat. *Nature Med*, **2**, 948–9.

Ihlenburg, H. and Brehmer, H. 1964. Beitrag zur latenten Borna-Erkrankung des Pferdes. *Monatsh Vet Med*, **19**, 463–5.

Inoue, Y., Yamaguchi, K., et al. 2002. Demonstration of continuously seropositive population against Borna disease virus in Misaki feral horses, a Japanese strain: a four-year follow-up study from 1998 to 2001. *J Vet Med Sci*, **64**, 445–8.

Iwahashi, K., Watanabe, M., et al. 1997. Clinical investigation of the relationship between Borna disease virus (BDV) infection and schizophrenia in 67 patients in Japan. *Acta Psychiatr Scand*, **96**, 412–15.

Iwata, Y., Takahashi, K., et al. 1998. Detection and sequence analysis of Borna disease virus p24 RNA from peripheral blood mononuclear cells of patients with mood disorders or schizophrenia and of blood donors. *J Virol*, **72**, 10044–9.

Joest, E. and Degen, K. 1911. Untersuchungen über die pathologische Histologie, Pathogenese und postmortale Diagnose der seuchenhaften Gehirn-Rückenmarksentzündung (Bornasche Krankheit) des Pferdes. *Zeitschr Infkrankh Haustiere*, **9**, 1–98.

Johansson, M., Berg, M. and Berg, A.L. 2002. Humoral immune response against Borna disease virus (BDV) in experimentally and naturally infected cats. *Vet Immunol Immunopathol*, **90**, 23–33.

Joly, E., Mucke, L. and Oldstone, M.B. 1991. Viral persistence in neurons explained by lack of major histocompatibility class I expression. *Science*, **253**, 1283–5.

Jordan, I., Briese, T., et al. 1999. Inhibition of Borna disease virus replication by ribavirin. *J Virol*, **73**, 7903–6.

Kamitani, W., Shoya, Y., et al. 2001. Borna disease virus phosphoprotein binds a neurite outgrowth factor, amphoterin/HMG-1. *J Virol*, **75**, 8742–51.

Kane, J. and Marder, J. 1993. Psychopharmacologic treatments of schizophrenia. *Schizophrenia Bull*, **19**, 287–302.

Kao, M., Ludwig, H. and Gosztonyi, G. 1984. Adaptation of Borna disease virus to the mouse. *J Gen Virol*, **65**, 1845–9.

Kao, M., Hamir, A.N., et al. 1993. Detection of antibodies against Borna disease virus in sera and cerebrospinal fluid of horses in the USA. *Vet Rec*, **132**, 241–4.

Karpus, W.J., Peterson, J.D. and Miller, S.D. 1994. Anergy in vivo: down regulation of antigen-specific CD4+ Th1 but not Th2 cytokine responses. *Int Immunol*, **6**, 721–30.

Kelsoe, J.R., Savodnick, A.D., et al. 1996. Possible locus for bipolar disorder near the dopamine transporter on chromosome 5. *Am J Med Genet*, **67**, 533–40.

Kemper, T.L. and Bauman, M.L. 1993. The contribution of neuropathologic studies to the understanding of autism. *Neurol Clin North Am*, **11**, 175–87.

Kennedy, M.K., Torrance, D.S., et al. 1992. Analysis of cytokine mRNA expression in the central nervous system of mice with experimental autoimmune encephalomyelitis reveals that IL-10 mRNA expression correlates with recovery. *J Immunol*, **149**, 2496–505.

Khoury, S.J., Akalin, E., et al. 1995. CD28-B7 costimulatory blockade by CTLA4Ig prevents actively induced experimental autoimmune encephalomyelitis and inhibits Th1 but spares Th2 cytokines in the central nervous system. *J Immunol*, **155**, 4521–4.

Kiermayer, S., Kraus, I., et al. 2002. Identification of the amino terminal subunit of the glycoprotein of Borna disease virus. *FEBS Lett*, **531**, 255–8.

Kim, Y.K., Kim, S.H., et al. 1999. Failure to demonstrate Borna disease virus genome in peripheral blood mononuclear cells from psychiatric patients in Korea. *J Neurovirol*, **5**, 196–9.

Kishi, M., Nakaya, T., et al. 1995a. Prevalence of Borna disease virus RNA in peripheral blood mononuclear cells from blood donors. *Med Microbiol Immunol (Berlin)*, **184**, 135–8.

Kishi, M., Nakaya, T., et al. 1995b. Demonstration of human Borna disease virus RNA in human peripheral blood mononuclear cells. *FEBS Lett*, **364**, 293–7.

Kishi, M., Arimura, Y., et al. 1996. Sequence variability of Borna disease virus open reading frame II found in human peripheral blood mononuclear cells. *J Virol*, **70**, 635–40.

Kitani, T., Kuratsune, H., et al. 1996. Possible correlation between Borna disease virus infection and Japanese patients with chronic fatigue syndrome. *Microbiol Immunol*, **40**, 459–62.

Kitze, B., Herzog, S., et al. 1996. No evidence of Borna disease virus-specific antibodies in multiple sclerosis patients in Germany. *J Neurol*, **243**, 660–2.

Kliche, S., Briese, T., et al. 1994. Characterization of a Borna disease virus glycoprotein, gp18. *J Virol*, **68**, 6918–23.

Kobayashi, T., Shoya, Y., et al. 1998. Nuclear targeting activity associated with the amino terminal region of the Borna disease virus nucleoprotein. *Virology*, **243**, 188–97.

Kobayashi, T., Kamitani, W., et al. 2001. Borna disease virus nucleoprotein requires both nuclear localization and export activities for viral nucleocytoplasmic shuttling. *J Virol*, **75**, 3404–12.

Konradi, C., Kobierski, L.A., et al. 1993. The cAMP-response-element-binding protein interacts, but Fos protein does not interact, with the proenkephalin enhancer in rat striatum. *Proc Natl Acad Sci USA*, **90**, 7005–9.

Kraus, I., Eickmann, M., et al. 2001. Open reading frame III of Borna disease virus encodes a nonglycosylated matrix protein. *J Virol*, **75**, 12098–104.

Krey, H., Ludwig, H. and Rott, R. 1979a. Spread of infectious virus along the optic nerve into the retina in Borna disease virus-infected rabbits. *Arch Virol*, **61**, 283–8.

Krey, H.F., Ludwig, H. and Boschek, C.B. 1979b. Multifocal retinopathy in Borna disease virus infected rabbits. *Am J Ophthalmol*, **87**, 157–64.

Krey, H.F., Stitz, L. and Ludwig, H. 1982. Virus-induced pigment epithelitis in rhesus monkeys. Clinical and histological finds. *Ophthalmologica*, **185**, 205–13.

Kubo, K., Fujiyoshi, T., et al. 1997. Lack of association of Borna disease virus and human T-cell leukemia virus type 1 infections with psychiatric disorders among Japanese patients. *Clin Diagn Lab Immunol*, **4**, 189–94.

Lange, H., Herzog, S., et al. 1987. Seroepidemiologische Untersuchungen zur Bornaschen Krankheit (ansteckende Gehirn-Rückenmarkentzündung) der Pferde. *Tierärztl Umsch*, **42**, 938–46.

Lebain, P., Vabret, A., et al. 2002. Borna disease virus and psychiatric disorders. *Schizophrenia Res*, **57**, 303–5.

Lewis, A.J., Whitton, J.L., et al. 1999. Effect of immune priming on Borna disease. *J Virol*, **73**, 2541–6.

Lieb, K., Hallensleben, W., et al. 1997a. No Borna disease virus-specific RNA detected in blood from psychiatric patients in different regions of Germany. The Bornavirus Study Group. *Lancet*, **350**, 1002.

Lieb, K., Hufert, F.T., et al. 1997b. Depression, Borna disease, and amantadine. *Lancet*, **349**, 958.

Lipkin, W., Carbone, K., et al. 1988. Neurotransmitter abnormalities in Borna disease. *Brain Res*, **475**, 366–70.

Ludwig, H., Bode, L. and Gosztonyi, G. 1988. Borna disease: a persistent virus infection of the central nervous system. *Prog Med Virol*, **35**, 107–51.

Ludwig, T.H., Becht, H. and Groh, L. 1973. Borna disease (BD), a slow virus infection. Biological properties of the virus. *Med Microbiol Immunol (Berlin)*, **158**, 275–89.

Lundgren, A.L. and Ludwig, H. 1993. Clinically diseased cats with nonsuppurative meningoencephalomyelitis have Borna disease virus-specific antibodies. *Acta Vet Scand*, **34**, 101–3.

Lundgren, A.L., Czech, G., et al. 1993. Natural Borna disease in domestic animals other than horses and sheep. *Zentralbl Veterinarmed [B]*, **40**, 298–303.

Lundgren, A.L., Lindberg, R., et al. 1995a. Immunoreactivity of the central nervous system in cats with a Borna disease-like meningoencephalomyelitis (staggering disease). *Acta Neuropathol (Berlin)*, **90**, 184–93.

Lundgren, A.L., Zimmermann, W., et al. 1995b. Staggering disease in cats: isolation and characterization of the feline Borna disease virus. *J Gen Virol*, **76**, 2215–22.

Malik, T.H., Kishi, M. and Lai, P.K. 2000. Characterization of the P protein-binding domain on the 10-kilodalton protein of Borna disease virus. *J Virol*, **74**, 3413–17.

Malkinson, M., Weisman, Y., et al. 1993. Borna disease in ostriches. *Vet Rec*, **133**, 304.

Malkinson, M., Weisman, Y., et al. 1995. A Borna-like disease of ostriches in Israel. *Curr Topics Microbiol Immunol*, **190**, 31–8.

Martins, C.R., Johnson, J.A., et al. 1998. Sonchus yellow net rhabdovirus nuclear viroplasms contain polymerase-associated proteins. *J Virol*, **72**, 5669–79.

Matthias, D. 1954. Der Nachweis von latent infizierten Pferden, Schafen und Rindern und deren Bedeutung als Virusreservoir bei der Bornaschen Krankheit. *Arch Exp Vet-Med*, **8**, 506–11.

Metzler, A., Ehrensperger, F. and Wyler, R. 1978. [Natural borna virus infection in rabbits]. *Zentralbl Veterinarmed [B]*, **25**, 161–4.

Mizutani, T., Inagaki, H., et al. 1998. Inhibition of Borna disease virus replication by ribavirin in persistently infected cells. *Arch Virol*, **143**, 2039–44.

Morales, J.A., Herzog, S., et al. 1988. Axonal transport of Borna disease virus along olfactory pathways in spontaneously and experimentally infected rats. *Med Microbiol Immunol (Berlin)*, **177**, 51–68.

Mosmann, T.R. and Coffman, R.L. 1989. TH1 and TH2 cells: different patterns of lymphokine secretion lead to different functional properties. *Annu Rev Immunol*, **7**, 145–73.

Nakamura, Y. 1998. [Isolation of Borna disease virus from the autopsy brain of a schizophrenia patient]. *Hokkaido Igaku Zasshi*, **73**, 287–97.

Nakamura, Y., Kishi, M., et al. 1995. Demonstration of Borna disease virus RNA in peripheral blood mononuclear cells from healthy horses in Japan. *Vaccine*, **13**, 1076–9.

Nakamura, Y., Asahi, S., et al. 1996. Demonstration of borna disease virus RNA in peripheral blood mononuclear cells derived from domestic cats in Japan. *J Clin Microbiol*, **34**, 188–91.

Nakamura, Y., Nakaya, T., et al. 1999a. High susceptibility of Mongolian gerbil (*Meriones unguiculatus*) to Borna disease virus. *Vaccine*, **17**, 480–9.

Nakamura, Y., Watanabe, M., et al. 1999b. High prevalence of Borna disease virus in domestic cats with neurological disorders in Japan. *Vet Microbiol*, **70**, 153–69.

Nakamura, Y., Takahashi, H., et al. 2000. Isolation of Borna disease virus from human brain tissue. *J Virol*, **74**, 4601–11.

Nakaya, T., Takahashi, H., et al. 1996. Demonstration of Borna disease virus RNA in peripheral blood mononuclear cells derived from Japanese patients with chronic fatigue syndrome. *FEBS Lett*, **378**, 145–9.

Nakaya, T., Kuratsune, H., et al. 1997. [Demonstration on Borna disease virus in patients with chronic fatigue syndrome]. *Nippon Rinsho*, **55**, 3064–71.

Nakaya, T., Takahashi, H., et al. 1999. Borna disease virus infection in two family clusters of patients with chronic fatigue syndrome. *Microbiol Immunol*, **43**, 679–89.

Narayan, O., Herzog, S., et al. 1983a. Behavioral disease in rats caused by immunopathological responses to persistent borna virus in the brain. *Science*, **220**, 1401–3.

Narayan, O., Herzog, S., et al. 1983b. Pathogenesis of Borna disease in rats: immune-mediated viral ophthalmoencephalopathy causing blindness and behavioral abnormalities. *J Infect Dis*, **148**, 305–15.

Nishino, Y., Funaba, M., et al. 1999. Borna disease virus infection in domestic cats: evaluation by RNA and antibody detection. *J Vet Med Sci*, **61**, 1167–70.

Nishino, Y., Kobasa, D., et al. 2002. Enhanced neurovirulence of Borna disease virus variants associated with nucleotide changes in the glycoprotein and L polymerase genes. *J Virol*, **76**, 8650–8.

Nitzschke, E. 1963. Untersuchungen über die experimentelle Bornavirus-Infektion bei der Ratte. *Zentrabl Vet-Med [B]*, **10**, 470–527.

Nöske, K., Bilzer, T., et al. 1998. Virus-specific CD4+ T cells eliminate Borna disease virus from the brain via induction of cytotoxic CD8+ T cells. *J Virol*, **72**, 4387–95.

Nowotny, N., Kolodziejek, J., et al. 2000. Isolation and characterization of a new subtype of Borna disease virus. *J Virol*, **74**, 5655–8.

Okamoto, M., Kagawa, Y., et al. 2002. Borna disease in a dog in Japan. *J Comp Pathol*, **126**, 312–17.

Oldach, D., Zink, M.C., et al. 1995. Induction of protection against Borna disease by inoculation with high-dose-attenuated Borna disease virus. *Virology*, **206**, 426–34.

Ouchi, A., Kishi, M., et al. 2001. Prevalence of circulating antibodies to p10, a nonstructural protein of the Borna disease virus in cats with ataxia. *J Vet Med Sci*, **63**, 1279–85.

Partonen, T. 1996. Dopamine and circadian rhythms in seasonal affective disorder. *Med Hyp*, **47**, 191–2.

Perez, M., Sanchez, A., et al. 2003. A reverse genetics system for Borna disease virus. *J Gen Virol*, **84**, 3099–104.

Perez, M., Watanabe, M., et al. 2001. N-terminal domain of Borna disease virus G (p56) protein is sufficient for virus receptor recognition and cell entry. *J Virol*, **75**, 7078–85.

Pette, H. and Környey, S. 1935. Über die Pathogenese und die Histologie der Bornaschen Krankheit im Tierexperiment. *Dtsch Zeitschr Nervenheilkd*, **136**, 20–63.

Planz, O. and Stitz, L. 1999. Borna disease virus nucleoprotein (p40) is a major target for CD8[+]-T-cell-mediated immune response. *J Virol*, **73**, 1715–18.

Planz, O., Bilzer, T., et al. 1993. Lysis of major histocompatibility complex class I-bearing cells in Borna disease virus-induced degenerative encephalopathy. *J Exp Med*, **178**, 163–74.

Planz, O., Bilzer, T. and Stitz, L. 1995. Immunopathogenic role of T-cell subsets in Borna disease virus-induced progressive encephalitis. *J Virol*, **69**, 896–903.

Planz, O., Rentzsch, C., et al. 1998. Persistence of Borna disease virus-specific nucleic acid in blood of psychiatric patient. *Lancet*, **352**, 623.

Planz, O., Rentzsch, C., et al. 1999. Pathogenesis of Borna disease virus: granulocyte fractions of psychiatric patients harbor infectious virus in the absence of antiviral antibodies. *J Virol*, **73**, 6251–6.

Planz, O., Dumrese, T., et al. 2001a. A naturally processed rat major histocompatibility complex class I-associated viral peptide as target structure of Borna disease virus-specific CD8+ T cells. *J Biol Chem*, **276**, 13689–94.

Planz, O., Pleschka, S. and Ludwig, S. 2001b. MEK-specific inhibitor U0126 blocks spread of Borna disease virus in cultured cells. *J Virol*, **75**, 4871–7.

Pleschka, S., Staeheli, P., et al. 2001. Conservation of coding potential and terminal sequences in four different isolates of Borna disease virus. *J Gen Virol*, **82**, 2681–90.

Pletnikov, M.V., Rubin, S.A., et al. 1999a. Persistent neonatal Borna disease virus (BDV) infection of the brain causes chronic emotional abnormalities in adult rats. *Physiol Behav*, **66**, 823–31.

Pletnikov, M.V., Rubin, S.A., et al. 1999b. Developmental brain injury associated with abnormal play behavior in neonatally Borna disease virus-infected Lewis rats: a model of autism. *Behav Brain Res*, **100**, 43–50.

Pletnikov, M.V., Rubin, S.A., et al. 2001. Neonatal Borna disease virus infection (BDV)-induced damage to the cerebellum is associated with sensorimotor deficits in developing Lewis rats. *Brain Res Dev Brain Res*, **126**, 1–12.

Pyper, J.M. and Gartner, A.E. 1997. Molecular basis for the differential subcellular localization of the 38- and 39-kilodalton structural proteins of Borna disease virus. *J Virol*, **71**, 5133–9.

Rauer, M., Pagenstecher, A., et al. 2002. Upregulation of chemokine receptor gene expression in brains of Borna disease virus (BDV)-infected rats in the absence and presence of inflammation. *J Neurovirol*, **8**, 168–79.

Reeves, N.A., Helps, C.R., et al. 1998. Natural Borna disease virus infection in cats in the United Kingdom. *Vet Rec*, **143**, 523–6.

Richt, J.A. and Rott, R. 2001. Borna disease virus: a mystery as an emerging zoonotic pathogen. *Vet J*, **161**, 24–40.

Richt, J.A., Stitz, L., et al. 1989. Borna disease, a progressive meningoencephalomyelitis as a model for CD4+ T cell-mediated immunopathology in the brain. *J Exp Med*, **170**, 1045–50.

Richt, J.A., Alexander, R.C., et al. 1997. Failure to detect Borna disease virus infection in peripheral blood leukocytes from humans with psychiatric disorders. *J Neurovirol*, **3**, 174–8.

Richt, J.A., Furbringer, T., et al. 1998. Processing of the Borna disease virus glycoprotein gp94 by the subtilisin-like endoprotease furin. *J Virol*, **72**, 4528–33.

Rott, R. and Becht, H. 1995. Natural and experimental Borna disease in animals. *Curr Topics Microbiol Immunol*, **190**, 17–30.

Rott, R., Herzog, S., et al. 1985. Detection of serum antibodies to Borna disease virus in patients with psychiatric disorders. *Science*, **228**, 755–6.

Rott, R., Herzog, S., et al. 1991. Borna disease, a possible hazard for man? *Arch Virol*, **118**, 143–9.

Rubin, S.A., Waltrip, R.W., et al. 1993. Borna disease virus in mice: host-specific differences in disease expression. *J Virol*, **67**, 548–52.

Rubin, S.A., Sierra-Honigmann, A.M., et al. 1995. Hematologic consequences of Borna disease virus infection of rat bone marrow and thymus stromal cells. *Blood*, **85**, 2762–9.

Rubin, S.A., Sylves, P., et al. 1999. Borna disease virus-induced hippocampal dentate gyrus damage is associated with spatial learning and memory deficits. *Brain Res Bull*, **48**, 23–30.

Rybakowski, F., Sawada, T. and Yamaguchi, K. 2001a. Borna disease virus-reactive antibodies and recent-onset psychiatric disorders. *Eur Psychiatr*, **16**, 191–2.

Rybakowski, F., Yamaguchi, K., et al. 2001b. [Detection of anti-Borna disease virus antibodies in patients hospitalized in psychiatric hospitals located in the mid-Western region of Poland]. *Psychiatr Pol*, **35**, 819–29.

Rybakowski, F., Sawada, T., et al. 2002. Borna disease virus-reactive antibodies in Polish psychiatric patients. *Med Sci Monit*, **8**, CR642–646.

Saito, N., Itouji, A., et al. 1993. Cellular and intracellular localization of ε-subspecies of protein kinase C in the rat brain; presynaptic localization of the εsubspecies. *Brain Res*, **607**, 241–8.

Salvatore, M., Morzunov, S., et al. 1997. Borna disease virus in brains of North American and European people with schizophrenia and bipolar disorder. Bornavirus Study Group. *Lancet*, **349**, 1813–14.

Sasaki, S. and Ludwig, H. 1993. In borna disease virus infected rabbit neurons 100 nm particle structures accumulate at areas of Joest-Degen inclusion bodies. *Zentralbl Veterinarmed [B]*, **40**, 291–7.

Sauder, C. and de la Torre , J.C. 1999. Cytokine expression in the rat central nervous system following perinatal Borna disease virus infection. *J Neuroimmunol*, **96**, 29–45.

Sauder, C., Muller, A., et al. 1996. Detection of Borna disease virus (BDV) antibodies and BDV RNA in psychiatric patients: evidence for high sequence conservation of human blood-derived BDV RNA. *J Virol*, **70**, 7713–24.

Sauder, C., Hallensleben, W., et al. 2000. Chemokine gene expression in astrocytes of Borna disease virus-infected rats and mice in the absence of inflammation. *J Virol*, **74**, 9267–80.

Schädler, R., Diringer, H. and Ludwig, H. 1985. Isolation and characterization of a 14500 molecular weight protein from brains and tissue cultures persistently infected with borna disease virus. *J Gen Virol*, **66**, 2479–84.

Schamel, K., Staeheli, P. and Hausmann, J. 2001. Identification of the immunodominant H-2K^k-restricted cytotoxic T-cell epitope in the Borna disease virus nucleoprotein. *J Virol*, **75**, 8579–88.

Schneemann, A., Schneider, P.A., et al. 1994. Identification of signal sequences that control transcription of Borna disease virus, a nonsegmented, negative-strand RNA virus. *J Virol*, **68**, 6514–22.

Schneemann, A., Schneider, P.A., et al. 1995. The remarkable coding strategy of borna disease virus: a new member of the nonsegmented negative strand RNA viruses. *Virology*, **210**, 1–8.

Schneider, P.A., Briese, T., et al. 1994a. Sequence conservation in field and experimental isolates of Borna disease virus. *J Virol*, **68**, 63–8.

Schneider, P.A., Schneemann, A. and Lipkin, W.I. 1994b. RNA splicing in Borna disease virus, a nonsegmented, negative-strand RNA virus. *J Virol*, **68**, 5007–12.

Schneider, P.A., Hatalski, C.G., et al. 1997a. Biochemical and functional analysis of the Borna disease virus G protein. *J Virol*, **71**, 331–6.

Schneider, P.A., Kim, R. and Lipkin, W.I. 1997b. Evidence for translation of the Borna disease virus G protein by leaky ribosomal scanning and ribosomal reinitiation. *J Virol*, **71**, 5614–19.

Schneider, U., Naegele, M., et al. 2003. Active Borna disease virus polymerase complex requires a distinct nucleoprotein-to-phosphoprotein ratio but no viral X protein. *J Virol*, **77**, 11781–9.

Schwartz, R.H. 1992. Costimulation of T lymphocytes: the role of CD28, CTLA-4 and B4/BB1 in interleukin-2 production and immunotherapy. *Cell*, **71**, 1065–8.

Schwemmle, M., De, B., et al. 1997. Borna disease virus P-protein is phosphorylated by protein kinase Cε and casein kinase II. *J Biol Chem*, **272**, 21818–23.

Schwemmle, M., Salvatore, M., et al. 1998. Interactions of the Borna disease virus P, N and X proteins and their functional implications. *J Biol Chem*, **273**, 9007–12.

Schwemmle, M., Jehle, C., et al. 1999a. Sequence similarities between human bornavirus isolates and laboratory strains question human origin. *Lancet*, **354**, 1973–4.

Schwemmle, M., Jehle, C., et al. 1999b. Characterization of the major nuclear localization signal of the Borna disease virus phosphoprotein. *J Gen Virol*, **80**, 97–100.

Selten, J.P. and van Vliet, K. 2000. Borna disease virus and schizophrenia in Surinamese immigrants to the Netherlands. *Med Microbiol Immunol (Berlin)*, **189**, 55–7.

Shankar, V., Kao, M., et al. 1992. Kinetics of virus spread and changes in levels of several cytokine mRNAs in the brain after intranasal infection of rats with Borna disease virus. *J Virol*, **66**, 992–8.

Shoya, Y., Kobayashi, T., et al. 1998. Two proline-rich nuclear localization signals in the amino- and carboxyl-terminal regions of the Borna disease virus phosphoprotein. *J Virol*, **72**, 9755–62.

Sierra-Honigmann, A.M., Rubin, S.A., et al. 1993. Borna disease virus in peripheral blood mononuclear and bone marrow cells of neonatally and chronically infected rats. *J Neuroimmunol*, **45**, 31–6.

Sierra-Honigmann, A.M., Carbone, K.M. and Yolken, R.H. 1995. Polymerase chain reaction (PCR) search for viral nucleic acid sequences in schizophrenia. *Br J Psychiatry*, **166**, 55–60.

Soares, J.C. and Mann, J.J. 1997. The anatomy of mood disorders – review of structural neuroimaging studies. *Biol Psychiatry*, **41**, 86–106.

Sobbe, M., Bilzer, T., et al. 1997. Induction of degenerative brain lesions after adoptive transfer of brain lymphocytes from Borna disease virus-infected rats: presence of CD8+ T cells and perforin mRNA. *J Virol*, **71**, 2400–7.

Solbrig, M.V., Koob, G.F., et al. 1994. Tardive dyskinetic syndrome in rats infected with Borna disease virus. *Neurobiol Dis*, **1**, 111–19.

Solbrig, M.V., Fallon, J.H. and Lipkin, W.I. 1995. Behavioral disturbances and pharmacology of Borna disease. *Curr Topics Microbiol Immunol*, **190**, 93–101.

Solbrig, M.V., Koob, G.F., et al. 1996a. Prefrontal cortex dysfunction in Borna disease virus (BDV)-infected rats. *Biol Psychiatry*, **40**, 629–36.

Solbrig, M.V., Koob, G.F., et al. 1996b. A neural substrate of hyperactivity in Borna disease: changes in brain dopamine receptors. *Virology*, **222**, 332–8.

Solbrig, M.V., Koob, G.F. and Lipkin, W.I. 1998. Cocaine sensitivity in Borna disease virus-infected rats. *Pharmacol Biochem Behav*, **59**, 1047–52.

Solbrig, M.V., Koob, G.F., et al. 2000. Neurotrophic factor expression after CNS viral injury produces enhanced sensitivity to psychostimulants: potential mechanism for addiction vulnerability. *J Neurosci*, **20**, RC104.

Solbrig, M.V., Koob, G.F. and Lipkin, W.I. 2002a. Key role for enkephalinergic tone in cortico-striatal–thalamic function. *Eur J Neurosci*, **16**, 1819–22.

Solbrig, M.V., Schlaberg, R., et al. 2002b. Neuroprotection and reduced proliferation of microglia in ribavirin-treated Bornavirus-infected rats. *Antimicrob Agents Chemother*, **46**, 2287–91.

Sprankel, H., Richarz, K., et al. 1978. Behavior alterations in tree shrews (*Tupaia glis*, Diard 1820) induced by Borna disease virus. *Med Microbiol Immunol (Berlin)*, **165**, 1–18.

Steinbach F (1994) Isolierung und Charakterisierung equiner peripherer Blutmonozyten und ihre Bedeutung für Herpes-(EHV-1-) und Borna-(BDV-) Virusinfektionen. Inaugural Dissertation (Dr med vet) Freie Universität Berlin, Germany

Sternberg, E.M., Wilder, R.L., et al. 1990. A defect in the central component of the immune system – hypothalamic-pituitary-adrenal axis feedback loop is associated with susceptibility to experimental arthritis and other inflammatory diseases. *Ann NY Acad Sci*, **594**, 289–92.

Stitz, L. 1991. [Immune intervention in Borna disease]. *Tierarztl Prax*, **19**, 509–14.

Stitz, L., Krey, H. and Ludwig, H. 1981. Borna disease in rhesus monkeys as a model for uveo-cerebral symptoms. *J Med Virol*, **6**, 333–40.

Stitz, L., Soeder, D., et al. 1989. Inhibition of immune-mediated meningoencephalitis in persistently Borna disease virus-infected rats by cyclosporine A. *J Immunol*, **143**, 4250–6.

Stitz, L., Planz, O., et al. 1991. Transforming growth factor-β modulates T cell-mediated encephalitis caused by Borna disease virus. Pathogenic importance of CD8+ cells and suppression of antibody formation. *J Immunol*, **147**, 3581–6.

Stitz, L., Sobbe, M. and Bilzer, T. 1992. Preventive effects of early anti-CD4 or anti-CD8 treatment on Borna disease in rats. *J Virol*, **66**, 3316–23.

Stitz, L., Nöske, K., et al. 1998a. A functional role for neutralizing antibodies in Borna disease: influence on virus tropism outside the central nervous system. *J Virol*, **72**, 8884–92.

Stitz, L., Planz, O. and Bilzer, T. 1998b. Lack of antiviral effect of amantadine in Borna disease virus infection. *Med Microbiol Immunol (Berlin)*, **186**, 195–200.

Stoyloff, R., Strecker, A., et al. 1997. The glycosylated matrix protein of Borna disease virus is a tetrameric membrane-bound viral component essential for infection. *Eur J Biochem*, **246**, 252–7.

Takahashi, H., Nakaya, T., et al. 1997. Higher prevalence of Borna disease virus infection in blood donors living near thoroughbred horse farms. *J Med Virol*, **52**, 330–5.

Tam, R.C., Pai, B., et al. 1999. Ribavirin polarizes human T cell responses towards a type 1 cytokine profile. *J Hepatol*, **30**, 376–82.

Tomonaga, K., Kobayashi, T., et al. 2000. Identification of alternative splicing and negative splicing activity of a nonsegmented negative-strand RNA virus, Borna disease virus. *Proc Natl Acad Sci USA*, **97**, 12788–93.

Tsuji, K., Toyomasu, K., et al. 2000. No association of borna disease virus with psychiatric disorders among patients in northern Kyushu, Japan. *J Med Virol*, **61**, 336–40.

Tsujimura, K., Mizutani, T., et al. 1999. A serosurvey of Borna disease virus infection in wild rats by a capture ELISA. *J Vet Med Sci*, **61**, 113–17.

Vahlenkamp, T.W., Enbergs, H.K. and Muller, H. 2000. Experimental and natural borna disease virus infections: presence of viral RNA in cells of the peripheral blood. *Vet Microbiol*, **76**, 229–44.

Vahlenkamp, T.W., Konrath, A., et al. 2002. Persistence of Borna disease virus in naturally infected sheep. *J Virol*, **76**, 9735–43.

von Sind, J.B. 1767. *Der im Feld und auf der Reise geschwind heilende Pferdearzt, welcher einen gründlichen Unterricht von den gewöhnlichsten Krankheiten der Pferde im Feld und auf der Reise wie auch einen auserlesenen Vorrath der nützlichsten und durch Erfahrung bewährtesten Heilungsmitteln eröffnet., 2. Auflage edn.* Frankfurt und Leipzig, Germany: Heinrich Ludwig Bönner.

Von Sprockhoff, H. 1956. Zur biologischen Charakterisierung des Borna-s-Antigens. *Scand J Immunol*, **4**, 203–8.

Wagner, K., Ludwig, H. and Paulsen, J. 1968. Fluoreszenzserologischer Nachweis von Borna-virus Antigen. *Berl Munch Tierarztl Wschr*, **81**, 395–6.

Walker, M.P. and Lipkin, W.I. 2002. Characterization of the nuclear localization signal of the Borna disease virus polymerase. *J Virol*, **76**, 8460–7.

Walker, M.P., Jordan, I., et al. 2000. Expression and characterization of the Borna disease virus polymerase. *J Virol*, **74**, 4425–8.

Waltrip, R.W., Buchanan, R.W., et al. 1995. Borna disease virus and schizophrenia. *Psychiatry Res*, **56**, 33–44.

Waltrip, R.W., Buchanan, R.W., et al. 1997. Borna disease virus antibodies and the deficit syndrome of schizophrenia. *Schizophrenia Res*, **23**, 253–7.

Watanabe, M., Lee, B.J., et al. 2001. Neurological diseases and viral dynamics in the brains of neonatally Borna disease virus-infected gerbils. *Virology*, **282**, 65–76.

Wehner, T., Ruppert, A., et al. 1997. Detection of a novel Borna disease virus-encoded 10 kDa protein in infected cells and tissues. *J Gen Virol*, **78**, 2459–66.

Weisman, Y., Huminer, D., et al. 1994. Borna disease virus antibodies among workers exposed to infected ostriches. *Lancet*, **344**, 1232–3.

Weissenböck, H., Nowotny, N., et al. 1998. Borna disease in a dog with lethal meningoencephalitis. *J Clin Microbiol*, **36**, 2127–30.

Weissenböck, H., Hornig, M., et al. 2000. Microglial activation and neuronal apoptosis in Bornavirus infected neonatal Lewis rats. *Brain Pathol*, **10**, 260–72.

Wittrup, I.H., Christensen, L.S., et al. 2000. Search for Borna disease virus in Danish fibromyalgia patients. *Scand J Rheumatol*, **29**, 387–90.

Wolff, T., Pfleger, R., et al. 2000. A short leucine-rich sequence in the Borna disease virus p10 protein mediates association with the viral phospho- and nucleoproteins. *J Gen Virol*, **81**, 939–47.

Wolff, T., Unterstab, G., et al. 2002. Characterization of an unusual importin alpha binding motif in the Borna disease virus p10 protein that directs nuclear import. *J Biol Chem*, **277**, 12151–7.

Yamaguchi, K., Sawada, T., et al. 1999. Detection of Borna disease virus-reactive antibodies from patients with psychiatric disorders and from horses by electrochemiluminescence immunoassay. *Clin Diagn Lab Immunol*, **6**, 696–700.

Yamaguchi, K., Sawada, T., et al. 2001. Synthetic peptide-based electrochemiluminescence immunoassay for anti-Borna disease virus p40 and p24 antibodies in rat and horse serum. *Ann Clin Biochem*, **38**, 348–55.

Yilmaz, H., Helps, C.R., et al. 2002. Detection of antibodies to Borna disease virus (BDV) in Turkish horse sera using recombinant p40. Brief report. *Arch Virol*, **147**, 429–35.

Zimmermann, W., Durrwald, R. and Ludwig, H. 1994. Detection of Borna disease virus RNA in naturally infected animals by a nested polymerase chain reaction. *J Virol Meth*, **46**, 133–43.

Zocher, M., Czub, S., et al. 2000. Alterations in neurotrophin and neurotrophin receptor gene expression patterns in the rat central nervous system following perinatal Borna disease virus infection. *J Neurovirol*, **6**, 462–77.

Zwick, W. 1939. Bornasche Krankheit und Enzephalomyelitis der Tiere. In: Waldmann, O. (ed.), *Handbuch der Viruskrankheiten, 2 Band.* Jena: G. Fischer, 254–354.

Zwick, W. and Seifried, O. 1925. Uebertragbarkeit der seuchenhaften Gehirn- und Rückenmarksentzündung des Pferdes (Borna'chen Krankheit) auf kleine Versuchstiere (Kanninchen). *Berl Tierärztl Wschr*, **41**, 129–32.

Zwick, W., Seifried, O. and Witte, J. 1926. Experimentelle Untersuchungen über die seuchenhafte Gehirn- und Rückenmarksentzündung der Pferde (Bornasche Krankheit). *Z Infkrankh Haustiere*, **30**, 42–136.

Zwick, W., Seifried, O. and Witte, J. 1927. Weitere Untersuchungen über die Gehirn-Rückenmarksentzündung der Pferde (Bornasche Krankheit). *Zeitschr Inf Krkh Haustiere*, **32**, 150–79.

53

Hepatitis A and E

BETTY ROBERTSON

INTRODUCTION

Enterically transmitted viral hepatitis

Although descriptions of epidemic jaundice go back to earliest recorded human history, the infectious nature of hepatitis was not widely appreciated until this century. Investigations during the Second World War led to the first clear recognition that there were distinct forms of transmissible hepatitis: one that was acquired through ingestion of contaminated food or water ('infectious jaundice') and another that was associated with the administration of blood or blood products ('homologous serum jaundice') (Havens 1944; Barker et al. 1945). MacCallum and Bradley (1944) classified these as type A and type B hepatitis, setting in place a classification scheme that still exists. The distinguishing epidemiological features of these infectious diseases and the lack of cross-protection engendered by their respective agents were confirmed by Krugman and his associates in a classic series of studies carried out among institutionalized children (Krugman and Ward 1958; Ward et al. 1958; Krugman et al. 1960). However, the modern era of hepatitis A virology began with the identification of virus particles in human fecal samples (Feinstone et al. 1973).

The subsequent development of an immune electron microscopy assay for virus-aggregating antibodies resulted in a variety of increasingly sophisticated diagnostic tests for hepatitis A virus (HAV) infection. Widespread application of these new serologies, coupled with recently developed assays for hepatitis B virus (HBV) and its related antibody responses, led to the recognition that there were at least two additional human viruses

responsible for reported cases of non-A, non-B (NANB) hepatitis. One type of NANB hepatitis, now recognized to be due to infection with Hepatitis C virus (HCV), resembled hepatitis B in that it was frequently associated with chronic liver disease and often transmitted by transfusion or other parenteral blood exposures (Choo et al. 1989). However, a distinctive agent responsible for waterborne or enterically transmitted NANB hepatitis was recognized to be the cause of large outbreaks of acute hepatitis in the Indian subcontinent and subsequently elsewhere (Khuroo 1980). These outbreaks included an epidemic in Delhi in 1955 that involved over 30 000 people and was associated with a breach in the city's sanitary water supply system. Although for many years this epidemic was considered to be due to type A 'infectious' hepatitis, serological tests carried out in the late 1970s indicated otherwise (Wong et al. 1980). The responsible agent, Hepatitis E virus (HEV), was identified by Balayan et al. (1983) in human fecal samples.

Similar and contrasting properties of HAV and HEV

HAV and HEV share a number of physical and biological characteristics (Table 53.1). Both are non-enveloped, RNA viruses with single-stranded genomes of positive polarity. Both display strong tropism for the liver (hepatocytes) and typically cause self-limited infections associated with acute hepatic inflammation. Above all, however, it is the fecal–oral transmission of HAV and HEV that distinguishes these viruses from other human hepatitis viruses, including HBV, hepatitis delta virus (HDV) and HCV. Both HAV and HEV are shed

Table 53.1 *Similar and contrasting properties of HAV and HEV*

Common properties		
Particle shape	Icosahedral	
Particle size	27–32 nm	
Chloroform sensitivity	Resistant	
Genome	ss (+)[a] 7.5 kb RNA	
Predominant transmission	Fecal–oral	
Liver disease	Acute, self-limited	
Unique properties	**HAV**	**HEV**
$S_{20,w}$	157S	183S
Bouyant density (g/cc^3)	1.33	1.29
Polypeptides	3–4 structural, 7 nonstructural	1–2 structural, 4–5 nonstructural
Stability	60°C, 1 h	Unknown
ORF	Single ORF	3 overlapping ORFs
5′ End structure	VPg	5′ Methylated cap

a) ss (+), single-stranded, positive-sense.

at high titers in the feces of infected individuals. In each case, the virus present in feces is replicated primarily in the liver and reaches the intestinal tract following secretion from the hepatocytes into biliary canaliculi and passage through the bile ducts. The absence of a lipid envelope is an important factor in this process, as it renders both HAV and HEV stable when suspended in bile. In contrast, the other human hepatitis viruses possess an outer lipid envelope and are likely to be rapidly inactivated in bile. Therefore, newly replicated HAV and HEV particles have a direct route to the outside environment that is denied the other hepatitis viruses. This allows HAV and HEV to cause explosive outbreaks of disease that are not seen with other types of hepatitis. However, neither HAV nor HEV causes persistent infections in humans and thus, unlike HBV and HCV, they have no association with chronic viral hepatitis or hepatocellular carcinoma.

Despite these similarities, HAV and HEV are very different viruses with a number of distinguishing features that result in their classification within different virus families (Table 53.1). These differences include fundamental aspects of virion structure and genome organization, as well as molecular mechanisms of translation and RNA replication.

HEPATITIS A VIRUS

Classification

On the basis of several features that distinguish HAV from other picornaviruses (Table 53.2), it is classified as the only member of the *Hepatovirus* genus of the *Picornaviridae* family (Minor 1991). Unique attributes of HAV include its tropism for the liver, its unusually slow and usually noncytolytic replication cycle, and its lack of close genetic relatedness to any other picornavirus.

Morphology of the HAV particle

The HAV virion appears as a relatively smooth, 27–30 nm rounded particle when viewed by electron microscopy in negatively stained preparations (Figure 53.1). Icosahedral symmetry is evident in many particles, but information concerning finer aspects of the capsid structure is limited. Infectious virions have a sedimentation constant of ca. 157S and band in CsCl at ca. 1.325 g/cm^3 (Lemon et al. 1985). Most virus preparations contain a large proportion of empty 70S capsids that are antigenically identical to virions.

Genome organization

The genomic RNA is single-stranded, ca. 7.5 kb in length and of positive polarity. The extreme 5′ end of the virion RNA is covalently coupled to a small viral protein, 3B (VPg), which is presumed to be removed from the RNA after its release from the capsid. The organization of the genome is similar to that of all picornaviruses (Figure 53.2, p. 1163) (Najarian et al. 1985; Cohen et al. 1987c), but there are several unique features. There are at least three functionally separate domains: the 5′ and 3′ nontranslated RNA (NTR) and a single, intervening, long open reading frame (ORF) which encodes the viral polyprotein.

5′ NONTRANSLATED RNA

The 5′ NTR is approximately 735 nt long and contains an extensive secondary and tertiary RNA structure (Figure 53.3, p. 1163). The segment from nucleotides 1–94 contains a 5′ terminal hairpin followed by 2 RNA pseudoknots (Brown et al. 1991; Shaffer et al. 1994) that, on the basis of studies of the corresponding cloverleaf-like RNA structure in poliovirus, probably play a controlling role in the initiation of positive-strand RNA

Table 53.2 *Properties of hepatoviruses and other picornaviral genera*

	Hepatoviruses	Aphthoviruses	Cardioviruses	Enteroviruses	Rhinoviruses
Primary host	Humans and higher primates	Cloven-hoofed mammals	Mammals	Higher primates	Mammals
Host-species restriction	Strict	Relatively strict	Relatively broad	Strict	Strict
Primary target organ	Liver (gut)	Systemic	CNS, liver	CNS, muscle (gut)	Respiratory mucosa
Dominant mode of transmission	Fecal–oral	Respiratory	??	Fecal–oral and respiratory	Respiratory
Serotypes	1	7	2	>70	>100
Particle size	27–30 nm	23–25 nm	24–30 nm	22–28 nm	24–30 nm
Buoyant density	1.33 g/cm^3	1.44 g/cm^3	1.34 g/cm^3	1.34 g/cm^3	1.41 g/cm^3
Stability <pH 7.0	pH 1.0	Nil	pH 3.0	pH 3.0	Nil
Stability >60°C	+	−	−	−	−
Genome RNA	7.5 kb	8.4 kb	7.8 kb	7.4 kb	7.2 kb
Sequence relatedness[a]	None	Cardioviruses	Aphthoviruses	Rhinoviruses	Enteroviruses
% G+C content	38	43	50	47	40
5′ poly(Y) tract	Poly(UUCC)	Poly(C)	Poly(C)	No	No
IRES structure	Type II	Type II	Type II	Type I	Type I
Leader (L) protein	Probably not	Yes	Yes	No	No
2A protease	No	Yes	Yes	Yes	Yes
Replication cycle	Very slow	Very fast	Very fast	Fast	Fast

a) to other *Picornaviridae*; Palmenberg (1989).

synthesis (Andino et al. 1993). At nucleotides 95–154 there is a unique pyrimidine-rich tract (pY1) that contains a series of repetitive (U)UUCC(C) sequence motifs assuming a poorly defined higher ordered structure, followed by a short, single-stranded domain (Shaffer et al. 1994). Both in location and in base composition, the pY1 domain resembles the much longer, nearly pure poly(C) tracts of the cardioviruses and aphthoviruses, other genera within the *Picornaviridae*. It seems that the pY1 tract is dispensable for viral

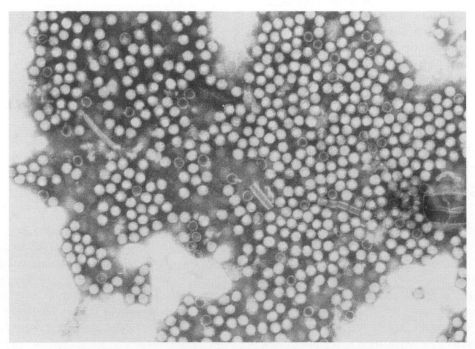

Figure 53.1 *Hepatitis A particle morphology demonstrated by electron microscopy. Negative-stained preparation.*

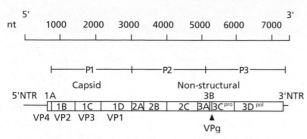

Figure 53.2 *Organization of the single-stranded positive-sense RNA genome of HAV.*

replication, both in primates in vivo and in cultured cells (Shaffer et al. 1994, 1995). The single-stranded domain located at nucleotides 135–155 seems to play a functional role in viral RNA replication, as deletion mutations in this region confer a temperature-sensitive viral replication phenotype due to a defect in RNA synthesis (Shaffer and Lemon 1995). Further downstream, the segment of 155–735 nt contains several complex stem–loops that comprise an internal ribosomal entry site (IRES) and direct the cap-independent translation of the long ORF (pp 696 and 699) (Brown et al. 1991, 1994; Glass and Summers 1992).

LONG ORF

The long ORF encodes a large polyprotein of c. 2200 amino acid residues that is proteolytically cleaved cotranslationally and post-translationally to generate mature viral proteins. As illustrated in Figure 53.2, the polyprotein can be functionally divided into three segments, P1, P2, and P3, as defined for other picornaviruses (Rueckert and Wimmer 1984). The P1 segment contains the structural proteins that form the viral capsid: 1A (also known as VP4), which is very small and not yet demonstrated to be a component of the HAV virion; 1B (VP2); 1B (VP3); and 1D (VP1). The P2 segment contains three nonstructural polypeptides, 2A, 2B, and 2C. The 2A protein appears to play a role in viral assembly and is present in immature virions as uncleaved VP1/2A (Borovec and Anderson 1993), while 2B and 2C have functions related to RNA replication (see section on Replication of HAV). The P3 segment contains four additional nonstructural proteins, including 3A (which probably helps anchor replication complexes to cellular membranes), 3B (VPg, the genome-linked protein), 3C^{pro} (a cysteine protease), and 3D^{pol} (an RNA-dependent RNA polymerase). As in poliovirus infections, some intermediate precursor proteins (e.g. 3AB, 3ABC, or 3CD) appear to have functions distinct from their processed end products (see section on Replication of HAV).

3′ NONTRANSLATED RNA

The 3′ NTR is ca. 60 nt in length and is polyadenylated at its 3′ terminus. Little is known about the functions of

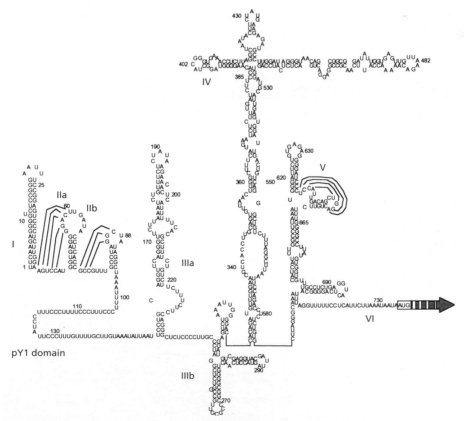

Figure 53.3 *Secondary and tertiary structure within the 5′ nontranslated RNA of HAV (Brown et al. 1991).*

the 3′ NTR sequence in virus replication. As with the 5′ NTR, the 3′ NTR is suspected to have substantial secondary structure and to interact with specific viral or host-cell proteins (Nuesch et al. 1993).

GENETIC VARIATION AMONG HAV STRAINS

Although the nucleotide sequences of different HAV strains have a relatively high degree of conservation, there is sufficient sequence heterogeneity to distinguish distinct phylogenetic lineages (Jansen et al. 1990; Robertson et al. 1991, 1992). A comparison of the sequences of a 168-nt segment near the VP1/2A junction of 152 different strains of HAV revealed seven distinct 'genotypes' that differed from each other at >15 percent of base positions (Figure 53.4) (Robertson et al. 1992). Representatives of three of these genotypes (I, II, VII) have been recovered only from human sources, whereas another genotype (III) contains viruses isolated both from humans and from captive Panamanian owl monkeys. The remaining three genotypes (IV, V, VI) are represented by single strains of simian HAV recovered from nonhuman primates (African green and cynomologus monkeys). Genotypes I and III include the vast majority of identified human strains and each contains two subgroups that differ at >7.5 percent of base positions. These have been designated subgenotypes IA and IB, IIIA and IIIB. Recently, the full genome sequences for representatives of human genotypes II (CF53/Berne, Lu et al. 2004), and VII (SLF88, Ching et al. 2002) have been determined, and the data indicate these two strains

represent two subtypes of the same genotype and have been proposed to be subgenotypes IIA and IIB within genotype II (BH Robertson, unpublished observations). Similar conclusions were derived by Costa-Mattioli and coworkers (2002) based upon their evaluation of the complete VP1 region of 81 strains from France, Kosovo, Chile, Argentina, and Uruguay.

The molecular epidemiology of HAV using sequence comparison has characterized patterns of virus spread within different regions of the world and transmission patterns in outbreaks (Jansen et al. 1990; Robertson et al. 1991, 1992, 2000; Hutin et al. 1999; Diaz et al. 2001; Bruisten et al. 2001; Taylor 1997; de Paula et al. 2002; Costa-Mattioli et al. 2001a, b; Arauz-Ruiz et al. 2001; Mbayed et al. 2002). For example, multiple genotype IA virus strains recovered in China, North and Central America, and Cuba comprise separate, phylogenetically and geographically-related clusters within genotype IA while in South America no consistent pattern of virus derivation is apparent. In contrast, most HAV strains recovered in Europe show extensive genetic divergence, suggesting the absence of a dominant circulating virus and consistent with a large proportion of European cases being caused by virus strains imported from other regions (Jansen et al. 1990; Robertson et al. 1992; Costa-Mattioli et al. 2001b; Bruisten et al. 2001). Sequence analysis has identified identical sequences within common source and community wide outbreaks (Niu et al. 1992; Hutin et al. 1999; Robertson et al. 2000) and provided the ability to

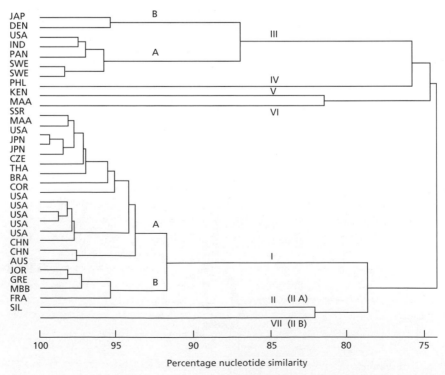

Figure 53.4 *Phylogenetic analysis of RNA sequences near the VP1/2A junctions of hepatovirus strains recovered from human sources in different geographic regions (genotypes I, II, III, and VII) or simian sources (genotypes IV, V, and VI) (Robertson et al. 1992).*

discriminate between outbreaks in the same city with different sources of transmission (Dentinger et al. 2001).

Structure of HAV

STRUCTURAL POLYPEPTIDES

The structural (capsid) proteins of HAV are encoded by the most 5′ (P1) region of the long ORF. The primary proteolytic cleavage of the nascent viral polyprotein seems to occur between the 2A and 2B polypeptides (Almela et al. 1991; Cho and Ehrenfeld 1991; Winokur et al. 1991; Borovec and Anderson 1993). The site of this cleavage, which is mediated by the viral protease 3C^{pro}, was recently shown to occur at residue 867 of the polyprotein, making 2B considerably larger than in other picornaviruses (Martin et al. 1995). Subsequent cleavage of the P1-2A precursor at the VP2/VP3 and VP3/VP1 junctions by 3C^{pro} results in 1A1B (also known as VP0), VP3 and VP1-2A (otherwise known as PX). VP1-2A seems to be an intermediate in virus assembly, as it can be detected within infected cells in pentameric subunits and possibly in some early virions (Borovec and Anderson 1993).

The VP4 sequence, located at the extreme amino terminus of the polyprotein, includes two potential methionine initiation codons (codons 1 and 3) which precede a consensus myristylation signal (GxxxT/S) (Chow et al. 1987). This has led to speculation that 'VP4' might be cleaved during replication to place the myristylation signal at the N terminus of the polyprotein, as such a signal is present at the amino terminus of the VP4 proteins of enteroviruses and rhinoviruses. Moreover, in the genera *Aphthovirus* and *Cardiovirus* of the *Picornaviridae*, a 'leader' (L) protein, located at the amino terminus of the polyprotein, is proteolytically removed to yield the free amino end of VP4, which is then myristylated (Chow et al. 1987). Thus, the VP4 proteins of all other picornaviruses are N terminally myristylated. However, despite numerous attempts, no one has yet been able to demonstrate the presence of VP4 within the HAV particle, or to determine by labeling experiments whether any of the viral capsid proteins are myristylated. In addition, site-directed mutagenesis of the two potential initiator methionines resulted in a change in the size of VP0, proving that there is no early cleavage within the sequence of VP4 and strongly suggesting that HAV VP4 is not myristylated (Tesar et al. 1992, 1993). Thus, although myristylation of VP4 seems to be important for the assembly of other picornaviruses, it does not seem to be necessary for HAV morphogenesis.

As in other picornaviruses, cleavage of VP0 to VP4 and VP2 occurs after the encapsidation of viral RNA (Bishop and Anderson 1993), resulting in a difference in the protein profile of empty capsids and complete virions. However, this cleavage occurs slowly with HAV, a feature that might be important to pathogenesis as it may prevent the infection of intestinal epithelial cells by virus secreted in the bile into the upper intestinal tract. The precise arrangement of the polypeptides within the assembled capsid is not known, as the hepatoviruses represent the only genus of the *Picornaviridae* for which the capsid structure has not been solved by X-ray crystallography. A hypothetical structure has been proposed, modeled after the structures of mengo virus and rhinovirus (Luo et al. 1988). However, this model does not correlate particularly well with experimental data obtained from biochemical and enzymatic studies, or with analysis of neutralization-resistant escape mutants (see below). Extended incubation of virus (up to 24 h) in the presence of large amounts of protease (1–10 mg/ml) results in the cleavage of VP2 by chymotrypsin and of VP1 and VP2 by trypsin. However, protease digestion has no effect on infectivity or antigenicity of the virus (Lemon et al. 1991a). Chemical iodination of exposed tyrosine residues occurs at two surface sites, one involving VP1 and the other, VP2. The VP1 residue is located between amino acids 233 and 273, whereas the VP2 site was at Tyr^{100} (Robertson et al. 1989).

ANTIGENIC STRUCTURE

Available evidence indicates that HAV strains comprise a single serotype, and that infection or immunization with any one strain confers protection against all others (LeDuc et al. 1983; Lemon and Binn 1983a; Lemon et al. 1992a). Although antigenic differences between human and simian viruses can be detected with a selected monoclonal antibody (mAb) (Nainan et al. 1991; Tsarev et al. 1991), the simian viruses react with other mAbs as well as polyclonal antibodies raised to human strains. The dominant antigenic determinants of HAV are highly conformational, as mAbs to the virus fail to recognize any capsid polypeptide in immunoblot assays. In addition, the antigenicity of the virus is curiously monotonic. Many mAbs are able to inhibit competitively by >50 percent the binding of polyclonal antibodies to the virus, and mAbs can be classified into several different groups on the basis of their ability to block the binding of two reference monoclonals (Stapleton and Lemon 1987; Ping and Lemon 1992; Schofield et al. 2002). Some mAbs recognize antigenic determinants common to 70S empty particles and 14S pentamer subunits (which are formed by five copies of the VP2–VP3–VP1 protomer subunit), whereas others recognize an antigenic determinant that is present only on 70S particles and is thus likely to span pentamer–pentamer interfaces (Stapleton et al. 1993). With few exceptions, mAbs to the virus are able to neutralize infectivity (Ping and Lemon 1992). No monoclonal antibodies have been identified that are directed toward the binding site for the putative HAV receptor, HAVcr-1 (see section on Replication of HAV).

Neutralization-resistant HAV mutants have been produced by successive rounds of neutralization and passage of virus in the presence of mAb (Stapleton and Lemon 1987). These mutants have only a limited number of amino substitutions, all in VP3 or VP1 (Ping et al. 1988; Ping and Lemon 1992; Nainan et al. 1992). Most, if not all, of these amino acid substitutions are likely to be at residues that interact directly with the complementarity-determining regions of the cognate mAb. They thus serve to map the neutralizing epitopes of the virus. The most frequently identified mutations are at Asp^{70} of VP3, but escape mutations have also been found at Pro^{65}, Ser^{71}, and Glu^{74} of this protein. Mutation at Asp^{70} profoundly alters the antigenicity of the virus, significantly reducing the reactivity of the virus with most polyclonal antibodies (Lemon et al. 1991b; Ping and Lemon 1992). Several different amino acid substitutions have been identified at this residue. Other neutralization escape mutants have substitutions within the VP1 sequence, at Ser^{102}, Asp^{104}, Lys^{105}, Val^{171}, Ala^{176}, or Lys^{221}. Except for several mutants with different amino acid substitutions at Lys^{221} of VP1 (all of which determine resistance to a single mAb), most escape mutants demonstrate extensive cross-resistance to multiple mAbs (Ping and Lemon 1992). The simian strains of HAV all contain an Asp^{70} mutation that results in lack of recognition of these viruses by monoclonal antibodies against human HAV (Nainan et al. 1992). These data suggest that residues 65–74 of VP3 (centering on Asp^{70}) and 102–105 and 171–176 of VP1 contribute to a single immunodominant antigenic site that contains a limited number of closely related and overlapping epitopes. This interpretation is consistent with the monotonicity of the polyclonal antibody response to the virus noted above.

There is also limited evidence for a neutralization epitope located near the amino terminus of VP1. Antibodies raised against a synthetic peptide representing residues 13–24 of VP1 generated neutralizing antibodies (Emini et al. 1985), and low levels of neutralizing antibodies were found in some animals immunized with a chimeric poliovirus containing this segment of the HAV VP1 molecule placed within an antigenic surface loop of poliovirus VP1 (Lemon et al. 1992b). Because the amino terminal domain of VP1 is located internally within the crystallographically determined structures of other picornaviruses, it is likely that this epitope becomes exposed only after interaction of the virus with its putative cellular receptor.

Consistent with the conformational nature of HAV epitopes, individual recombinant HAV capsid proteins generally fail to elicit antibody responses that are reactive with the viral capsid. However, such proteins may prime for B cell responses in small animals (Johnston et al. 1988). Epitope(s) responsible for such priming reside within the carboxy terminal 156 residues of VP1 (Harmon et al. 1993). Also consistent with the confor-

mational nature of HAV epitopes, a large number of synthetic peptides representing different segments of the HAV capsid proteins have been shown not to express any relevant HAV antigenic activity (Lemon et al. 1991c). There is data suggesting that a synthetic peptide 'mimotope' selected using a combinatorial approach may be able to stimulate production of antibodies that are reactive with the virus capsid (Mattioli et al. 1995).

Five antigenic domains over the entire HAV polyprotein using 237 overlapping 20mer peptides were identified using convalescent antisera (Khudyakov et al. 1999). These domains, probably composed of linear epitopes, include amino acids 57–90 (within VP2); amino acids 767–842 at the VP1–2A junction; amino acids 1403–1456 encompassing the P2C–P3A junction; amino acids 1500–1519 comprising the entire P3B protein; and amino acids 1719–1764 which encodes the P3C–P3D junction. In general, the nonstructural proteins have not proved to be adequate targets for antibody detection. Studies using expressed 3C protease for antibody detection demonstrated the presence of these antibodies after the acute phase of the illness, but they declined more rapidly than antibodies directed toward the capsid (Robertson et al. 1993; Stewart et al. 1997).

Replication of HAV

PROPAGATION OF VIRUS IN CULTURED CELLS

Replication of wild-type HAV is very slow and inefficient in cell culture, typically taking days to weeks to reach maximum virus yields (Provost and Hilleman 1979; Daemer et al. 1981; Binn et al. 1984). However, with patience and continued passage, virus yields are increased and the otherwise lengthy replication period is shortened. HAV variants that have been adapted to cell culture will replicate in many primate cell lines, but certain cell lines derived from African green monkey (BS-C-1 or CV-1) or fetal rhesus monkey kidney (FRhK-4) seem to be most permissive for virus growth (Provost and Hilleman 1979; Daemer et al. 1981; Binn et al. 1984). Other mammalian cell types are also permissive for limited replication of the virus (Dotzauer et al. 1994). Thus there does not seem to be a strict host species requirement in cell culture. Viruses that are well adapted to growth in monkey kidney cell cultures are often highly attenuated when inoculated into susceptible primates or humans (Provost et al. 1982; Karron et al. 1986) (see below).

The specific cell culture infectivity (cell culture infectious units per genome copy) of one virus variant (HM175/P16) that had been adapted to growth in cultured cells during 16 sequential passages in African green monkey kidney cells was >3 000 times that of the related wild-type virus (Jansen et al. 1988). However, even virus isolates that are well adapted to growth in cultured cells replicate much more slowly than picorna-viruses such as encephalomyocarditis virus (EMCV) or poliovirus (Lemon et al. 1991b). Most HAV strains fail to induce a cytopathic effect in cultured cells, although cytopathic variants have been selected from strains that are highly adapted to growth in cultured cells (Anderson 1987; Cromeans et al. 1987; Robertson et al. 1988; Lemon et al. 1991b). Such cytopathic variants may reach maximum yields in <24 h under one-step growth conditions (Lemon et al. 1991b). However, even these strains of HAV do not induce a specific shutdown in host cell macromolecular synthesis. To a considerable extent, the poor growth of HAV in cultured cells has limited investigations of the replication cycle.

In most cases, the replication of HAV in cell cultures can be detected only by immunological techniques or demonstration of the viral RNA by nucleic acid hybridization. The quantal, radioimmunofocus assay allows accurate titration of viral infectivity by immunostaining of viral replication foci developing beneath an agarose overlay over a period of 6–14 days (Lemon et al. 1983).

HAV CELL RECEPTOR

Recently, a putative receptor for HAV has been identified as a mucinlike class I integral membrane glycoprotein. This molecule (HAVcr-1) was identified by two independent groups using AGMK cells (Kaplan et al. 1996) and a marmoset–Vero cell hybrid (Ashida and Hamada 1997). It consists of an N-terminal Cys-rich region with homology to the immunoglobulin superfamily followed by a threonine, serine, proline-rich region which is similar to mucinlike proteins. The human homologue (huHAVcr-1) was cloned from human kidney and liver cDNA and determined to be 79 percent identical to the AGMK derived receptor, excluding three insertions/deletions within the mucinlike domain (Feigelstock et al. 1998). The huHAVcr-1 molecule does not appear to be liver specific, as it has been identified in all organs evaluated, with highest levels within kidney and testis. Evaluation of deletion mutants of the HAVcr-1 revealed that the Cys-rich region and the N-terminal N-glycosylation site is required for binding of HAV (Thompson et al. 1998); evaluation using immunoadhesins also revealed that it neutralizes bound HAV (Silberstein et al. 2001). Interestingly, a related protein from mice (Tim-1) and rats (Kim-1), expressed on T cells, is associated with airway hyperreactivity within inbred mice (McIntire et al. 2001).

In contrast to these findings, Dotzauer et al. (2000), have presented evidence that an alternative mechanism can be used by the virus to target it to liver cells. They propose that in addition to other host-derived materials found associated with HAV virions, IgA molecules bound to virus can serve to target virions to the liver using the asialoglycoprotein receptor. Initial infection

would be from ingested IgA–virus complexes or the result of local IgA stimulated within the small intestine.

CAP-INDEPENDENT TRANSLATION OF THE VIRAL POLYPROTEIN

The first step in replication following the uncoating of the viral RNA is the cap-independent translation of the viral polyprotein. The initiation of translation is carried out under direction of the IRES located between nucleotides 155 and 735 of the 5' NTR (Brown et al. 1991, 1994). Although the IRES shares several structural features with that of EMCV, it is ca. 50–100-fold less active in directing translation than the EMCV IRES, even in HAV permissive cells (Brown et al. 1994; Whetter et al. 1994; Schultz et al. 1996b). It is likely that weak IRES activity contributes to the slow and noncytopathic growth of HAV, because studies indicate that translation is rate limiting in infection of cultured African green monkey kidney cells with wild-type virus (Schultz et al. 1996b).

The IRES of HAV binds specifically to several cellular proteins, including polypyrimidine tract-binding protein (PTB) and glyceraldehyde-3-phosphate dehydrogenase (GAPDH) (p39) (Chang et al. 1993; Schultz et al. 1996a). Experimental data indicate that the binding of GAPDH destabilizes RNA secondary structure and is thus likely to be detrimental to IRES-directed translation (Schultz et al. 1996a). PTB and GAPDH compete with each other for binding to certain stem–loop structures within the 5' NTR, and the relative levels of these cellular proteins may be important in determining the translational activity of the HAV IRES (Yi et al. 2000). Specific hepatocyte factors may enhance translation directed by the HAV IRES (Glass and Summers 1993).

REPLICATION FUNCTIONS ASSOCIATED WITH NONSTRUCTURAL PROTEINS

The nonstructural proteins of HAV are responsible for proteolytic processing of the polyprotein and replication of the viral RNA. There are at least seven distinct nonstructural proteins: 2A, 2B, 2C, 3A, 3B (the genome-linked protein, VPg, which is covalently attached to the 5' end of virion RNA), 3C^{pro} (the viral protease) and 3D^{pol} (the RNA-dependent RNA polymerase). Many of the specific functions of these proteins are not well understood.

Although the 2A proteins of other picornaviruses have protease activities and are responsible for the primary cis-active cleavage of the polyprotein (at either VP1/2A or 2A/2B), this is not the case for HAV. The HAV 2A protein shares no sequence identity with these other picornaviral 2A proteins and does not have proteolytic activity. Unlike other picornaviruses, primary cleavage of the HAV polyprotein precursor occurs between 2A and 2B, resulting in a P1–2A intermediate. While the 2A/2B cleavage site has been identified as

Gln^{836}/Ala^{837} and is mediated by $3C^{pro}$ (Martin et al. 1995), the cleavage of VP1–2A has been more difficult to determine. Early data suggested that this junction was cleaved by the $3C^{pro}$ (Schultheiss et al. 1994; Schultheiss et al. 1995); Probst et al. (1997) also concluded that $3C^{pro}$ is responsible for the maturation cleavage of VP1/2A between amino acids Val^{272}-Glu^{273} and Ser^{274}. In contrast, two studies provide evidence that $3C^{pro}$ is not involved in this cleavage – mutation of the only sites possible for $3C^{pro}$ cleavage did not abolish infectivity or virus maturation (Martin et al. 1999). This conclusion was supported by identification of the C-terminal amino acids of VP1 (Graff et al. 1999); the C terminus was found to be heterogeneous and composed of Leu^{270}-Pro^{271}-Thr^{272}/Glu^{273}/Ser^{274}. The predominant terminal amino acid was Ser^{274}, but with detectable amounts of Glu^{273} and Thr^{272}. This process had been proposed to be mediated by an unknown cellular protease. Cohen et al. (2002) created deletion mutants within the 2A region, and found that deletion of the amino terminal 40 percent abolished infectivity, while deletions in the carboxy terminal 60 percent resulted in small plaque phenotype. However, earlier studies of large (15 amino acid) deletions within 2A were found not to impair virus growth in cultured cells (Harmon et al. 1995). The N-terminal deletions would alter the VP1–2A cleavage that occurs after pentamer assembly, thereby affecting virus maturation. These studies have lead to the conclusion that there are two domains within 2A; an amino terminal molecular chaperon-like domain that directs the folding of the capsid precursor for proper 3C processing, while the C terminal domain is needed for non-$3C^{pro}$-mediated processing of the VP1–2A precursor to generate mature VP1.

The 2B and 2C proteins of HAV have functions related to replication of the viral RNA and, on the basis of studies with poliovirus, presumably play essential roles in directing the assembly of a membrane-based replicase complex (Bienz et al. 1992; Cho et al. 1994). Since mutations in 2B and 2C are important for adaptation of wild-type HAV to replication in cultured cells (Emerson et al. 1992a; Emerson et al. 1993), it is very likely that these proteins interact in an as yet undefined but highly specific fashion with cellular proteins or other components of the intracellular membrane. 2C contains a 'DEAD' motif, suggesting that it may have RNA helicase activity, and has been shown to be an NTPase. The HAV 2B and 2C proteins most probably function as a complex, as mutations in these proteins which play an important role in defining the replication properties of rapidly replicating, cytopathic viruses act in a highly cooperative fashion (Zhang et al. 1995). The 2C proteins of HAV and poliovirus are clearly related phylogenetically, and mutations that confer resistance of poliovirus to guanidine (an inhibitor of poliovirus RNA replication) map to the 2C protein. HAV replication has been suggested to be sensitive to guanidine (Cho and Ehrenfeld 1991), but this has not been found to be the case by other investigators (Siegl and Eggers 1982).

The function of the 3A protein in viral replication is also poorly defined, but it is likely to serve as an anchor for 3AB or 3ABCD within the membranous replication complexes. Mutations in 3A may play a role in determining the cytopathic phenotype, as multiple cytopathic strains that have been sequenced in this region contain deletions of one or more amino acids near the amino terminus of 3A (Lemon et al. 1991b; Beneduce et al. 1995). However, any role that mutations in 3A may play in determining this phenotype is of secondary importance to the role played by mutations in 2BC (Zhang et al. 1995). The 3B (VPg) protein is covalently attached to the 5′ nucleotide of the virion RNA (Weitz et al. 1986). Studies with other picornaviruses suggest that it is removed shortly after uncoating of the viral RNA, and that it is also likely to be present at the 5′ end of newly synthesized minus-strand RNAs. Its precise functions may include a role in priming for RNA synthesis, or possibly in cleavage of the RNA if negative-strand synthesis originates from a snap-back, self-priming mechanism.

$3C^{pro}$ is clearly the best studied of the nonstructural proteins of HAV because its three-dimensional structure has been determined by X-ray crystallography (Allaire et al. 1994). It is a cysteine protease with both structural and functional relatedness to chymotrypsin and the serine proteases. $3C^{pro}$ seems to be responsible for each of the proteolytic cleavages of the viral polyprotein (Harmon et al. 1992; Kusov et al. 1992; Schultheiss et al. 1994; Tesar et al. 1994), with the exception of the VP4/VP2 cleavage (Bishop and Anderson 1993) and the VP1/2A as indicated above. The substrate specificity of the $3C^{pro}$ enzyme has been studied extensively using synthetic peptide substrates (Jewell et al. 1992; Malcolm et al. 1992). The dipeptide sequences present at the various HAV cleavage sites are considerably more variable than in other picornaviruses. Studies with poliovirus suggest that $3C^{pro}$ has specific RNA-binding activity and interacts with the 5′ NTR during initiation of plus-strand RNA synthesis; structural studies indicate that the RNA-binding site is located on the opposite side of the molecule from the protease active site. Poliovirus $3C^{pro}$ has also been considered to contribute to host cell shutdown at the transcriptional level by directing cleavage of the human TATA-binding protein (Clark et al. 1993; Das and Dasgupta 1993). However, either the HAV $3C^{pro}$ protein lacks this activity or it is expressed at much lower levels during viral replication, because HAV infection has never been shown specifically to impair host cell metabolic processes. The putative RNA-dependent RNA polymerase activity of $3D^{pol}$ is suggested by the presence of a conserved 'GDD' amino acid motif. Thus far, however, attempts to express an active polymerase have resulted in an insoluble product with no detectable activity.

GENETIC CHANGES ASSOCIATED WITH ADAPTATION TO GROWTH IN CULTURED CELLS

The genetic changes associated with adaptation of the HM175 and GBM strains of HAV to growth in cell culture have been identified by comparisons of the nucleotide sequences of wild-type and cell culture-adapted variants (Cohen et al. 1987a; Jansen et al. 1988; Ross et al. 1989; Graff et al. 1994). These studies are important because cell culture-adapted viruses are often highly attenuated and have been used as candidate vaccines in humans. The HM175 strain has been studied intensively, with complete genomic sequences determined for three independently isolated, cell culture-adapted viruses (Cohen et al. 1987a; Jansen et al. 1988; Ross et al. 1989). The mutations associated with cell culture adaptation are scattered throughout the genome, but tend to concentrate in the 5′ NTR and P2 domains.

Several individual mutations are present in multiple, independent cell culture-adapted isolates, signifying their importance to efficient replication in cell culture. The construction of an infectious cDNA clone of the HM175 virus (Cohen et al. 1987b) has allowed a detailed molecular genetics analysis of mutations that are associated with the adaptation of HAV to growth in cultured cells. Emerson and colleagues (1991, 1992a, b) found that mutations within the P2 region (2B and 2C proteins) are necessary for efficient growth in cultured cells. A relatively conservative Val^{216} to Ala^{216} substitution in 2B (nucleotide 3889) seems to be the most important single mutation with respect to growth in cultured cells. These P2 mutations probably facilitate interactions between these viral proteins and a host cell-specific factor(s) required for replication, but further details are lacking.

Mutations within the 5′ NTR, strongly associated with host-cell restricted growth, have been demonstrated in virus grown in CV-1, BS-C-1, MRC-5, HEK, and HFS cells lines. Analogous host restricted mutations are not necessary for growth in FRhK4 cells (Emerson et al. 1991, 1992a; Funkhouser et al. 1994; Graff et al. 1994; Graff et al. 1997). The mutations responsible for this effect (Day et al. 1992) are located in or near the viral IRES, and enhance cap-independent translation (Schultz et al. 1996b). These results indicate that there are cell type-specific factors that influence the efficiency of translation directed by the HAV IRES in certain cell lines. Differing cytoplasmic levels of GAPDH and PTB may play an important role in determining the activity of these 5′ NTR mutations, as these two cellular proteins compete for binding to the 5′ NTR with opposing effects on viral translation (Chang et al. 1993; Schultz et al. 1996a).

In contrast, BS-C-1-adapted HAV was grown in guinea-pig embryo cells for five passages, and selected regions (5′ NTR, 2ABC3AB, and the 3′ NTR) were amplified and sequenced. Only two nucleotides within these regions were changed; 2B nucleotide 3679, and 2C nucleotide 4419 (Frings and Dotzauer 2001). Under these circumstances, host-cell growth restriction is not regulated by interaction of cellular factors with 5′ NTR sequences. Likewise, replication of a subgenomic replicon containing luciferase in the place of the capsid proteins within Huh-7 cells was enhanced by mutations within the P2 and P3 regions, especially mutations at 2B nucleotide 3889, while the 5′ NTR region had no effect within this system (Yi and Lemon 2002).

The nearly complete nucleotide sequences have been determined for three rapidly replicating, cytopathic variants (*rr/cpe*+) recovered from cells that were persistently infected with the HM175 virus (Lemon et al. 1991b). These clonally isolated variants contained identical mutations within the 5′ and 3′ NTRs as well as within the RNA encoding the P2 and P3 proteins (2B, 2C, 3A, and 3D), while the intervening genomic sequences contained unique silent and nonsilent mutations. This suggested that the mutations that were common to the three cytopathic variants were likely to be responsible for the *rr/cpe*+ phenotype. To determine which mutations are responsible for the *rr/cpe*+ phenotype, infectious cDNA chimeras were constructed that contained various segments of one of these cytopathic variants (HM175/18f) in the genetic background of a noncytopathic virus (Zhang et al. 1995). Analysis of the chimeric viruses demonstrated that complete expression of the *rr/cpe*+ phenotype required the cooperative effects of multiple mutations in 2B, 2C, the 5′ NTR and the P3 regions of the genome. Thus, the *rr/cpe*+ phenotype represents a super-adaptation of HAV to growth in cell culture, and reflects changes in multiple virus functions.

Clinical and pathological aspects of HAV infection

PATHOGENESIS OF HEPATITIS A

To a considerable extent, present understanding of the pathogenesis of hepatitis a derives from studies of HAV infections in several species of susceptible nonhuman primates: chimpanzees, certain species of tamarins, and New World owl monkeys (Dienstag et al. 1975; Dienstag et al. 1976; Bradley et al. 1977; Cohen et al. 1989). Although these primate species can be infected either by oral or by intravenous challenge with virus, HAV infection typically follows oral exposure to the virus in humans, due either to close personal contact with an infected individual or to the ingestion of fecally contaminated water or food. Viral replication occurs primarily within hepatocytes, and the secretion of virus into bile results in large quantities of virus being shed in the feces. The titer of virus excreted in stools may be at least as high as 10^8 particles or 10^6 infectious virions/g (Purcell et al. 1984; Lemon et al. 1990). A sustained viremia throughout the incubation period and the early stages of acute liver disease parallels the fecal shedding of virus, but at titers that are 100–1000-fold lower (Cohen et al. 1989; Lemon et al. 1990) (Figure 53.5). Early studies demonstrated viral antigen within the liver, in hepatocytes and Kupffer cells, as well as in splenic macrophages and along the glomerular basement membrane in the kidney (Dienstag et al. 1976; Mathiesen et al. 1978a, 1980; Shimizu et al. 1982). However, it is not clear whether the presence of viral antigen in phagocytic cells reflects nonspecific trapping of viral antigen or replication of virus.

The genetic basis of pathogenesis has been evaluated by Emerson and coworkers (2002) by generating 14 chimeric viruses from clonal wild-type and attenuated sequences of HM-175 which contained 19 individual nucleotide changes over the whole genome. The resulting chimeras were evaluated in tamarins for their ability to cause disease. Nucleotides 3025 and 3196 within the VP1–2A junction and nucleotides 4043, 4087, 4222, and 4563 within the 2C genome region were necessary for expression of virulence within tamarins and were associated with severity of acute hepatitis. The mutations within the 2C protein, combined with a mutation at nucleotide 3889 within 2B controlled efficient replication in cultured cells.

The relationship between pathogenesis and the infected host species was approached by inoculating simian HAV (AGM27 from African green monkeys) into five different primate species (Emerson et al. 1996). The results revealed that different clinical patterns are seen depending upon the host. The most severe disease pattern was seen in African green monkeys and marmosets while infection of rhesus monkeys and cynomologus monkeys resulted in less severe symptoms; infection of chimpanzees did not result in detectable biochemical changes or histopathology, and seroconversion was delayed until 5–6 weeks after inoculation. Cross-challenge with a standard challenge dose of wild-type human HAV HM-175 in animals who had been exposed to AGM-27 revealed that all the animals were protected from acute infection, consistent with protection due to

the presence of antibodies generated by the AGM-27 infection.

Although most if not all of the virus found in feces and blood is likely to be replicated within hepatocytes, there are limited data that indicate that HAV also infects intestinal epithelial cells in vivo. The early events in hepatitis A infection and the mechanism by which the virus reaches the liver remained poorly defined. HAV antigen has been identified within intestinal epithelial cells of experimentally infected tamarins (Karayiannis et al. 1986) as well as orally inoculated owl monkeys (Asher et al. 1995). In owl monkeys, viral antigen was observed in epithelial cells lining crypts in the small intestine within 3 days of inoculation. These findings in vivo are supported by studies demonstrating the growth of cell culture-adapted HAV in polarized cultures of colonic carcinoma cells (CaCo-2) grown on semi-permeable membranes (Blank et al. 2000). Such cells could be infected only from their apical surface, and released progeny virus in a vectorial fashion only from the apical surface. Infectious virus has also been detected at low levels within pharyngeal secretions, but later in infection when viremia was also present (Cohen et al. 1989; Asher et al. 1995). It is difficult to be certain whether this reflects virus produced locally or simply secretion of virus into saliva from the blood.

The light microscopic findings in acute hepatitis A include features common to all forms of acute viral hepatitis, including inflammatory cell infiltration, hepatocellular necrosis, and liver cell regeneration. Studies in chimpanzees demonstrated that the early histological lesions of hepatitis A infection involve periportal liver cell necrosis with relative sparing of the perivenular area of the lobule (Dienstag et al. 1976). These histological observations have been confirmed in humans undergoing biopsies at different stages of the acute disease. Portal infiltration by lymphocytes, plasma cells and periodic acid–Schiff (PAS)-positive macrophages are prominent features in early biopsies. These features are more pronounced in later biopsies (Abe et al. 1982; Teixera et al. 1982). Some biopsies taken during acute hepatitis A infection demonstrate extension of the inflammatory infiltrate from the periportal region into the hepatic parenchyma, with significant erosion of the limiting plate. Although this histological picture is more suggestive of chronic hepatitis, the histopathological features of hepatitis A are reversible and generally resolve completely given sufficient time.

CELLULAR IMMUNE RESPONSE TO HAV INFECTION

Because infection of cultured cells with wildtype HAV does not result in the cytopathic effects observed with many other well characterized picornaviruses, it is generally assumed that HAV infection is also noncytopathic in vivo and that hepatitis A is an immunopathologically mediated disease. This is probably correct, as virus repli-

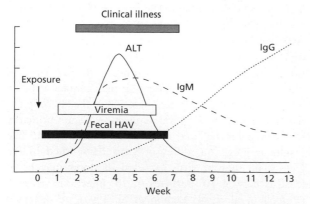

Figure 53.5 *Virological and pathological events during a typical infection with HAV.*

cation and fecal virus shedding are maximal in the late incubation period, before the onset of symptoms or biochemical evidence of liver injury. Thus, liver injury and viral clearance are closely related. CD8⁺, MHC class I-dependent, cytotoxic T cells that are capable of lysing autologous HAV infected cells, but not of controlling uninfected cells, are present both in the circulation and in the liver at the site of disease (Vallbracht et al. 1986; Vallbracht et al. 1989; Fleischer et al. 1990). These virus-specific T cells also produce interferon-γ (Maier et al. 1988). It is likely that interferon-γ and other cytokines secreted by virus-specific CD8⁺ cells serve to recruit additional, less specific, inflammatory cells to the site of the infection that may be responsible for much of the liver injury. The exact mechanism by which the infection is cleared is inadequately defined, but this process probably involves a combination of antibody-mediated neutralization of infection, interferon-mediated inhibition of viral replication, and cytotoxic T cell-induction of cellular apoptosis. A prominent feature of this response may be the upregulation of the normally low levels of MHC class I markers displayed by hepatocytes in response to interferon-γ and other cytokines. Specific T-cell epitopes of HAV have not been identified.

HUMORAL IMMUNE RESPONSE TO HAV

In addition to the cellular immune responses described above, there is a vigorous antibody response to the virus during the later stages of infection. These antibodies are directed against conformational epitopes that are displayed by intact virions as well as empty viral capsids. Serum-neutralizing antibodies provide protection against reinfection with HAV, whereas cell-mediated immunity seems to be involved in viral clearance once infection has been established. Serum antibody responses are first noted at the onset of symptoms and include virus-specific IgM as well as IgG and IgA. IgM anti-HAV is detected concurrently with the onset of clinical symptoms, but IgG is also present during the acute symptomatic phase of the infection (Locarnini et al. 1979; Lemon et al. 1980). Both IgM and IgG antibodies have virus-neutralizing activities (Lemon and Binn 1983b; Lemon 1985b). The IgG response is durable and provides longstanding protection against reinfection. However, there are suggestions that it may decline to low and potentially nondetectable levels after many decades, particularly in people infected early in life. Upon re-exposure, such individuals may experience asymptomatic reinfections associated with anamnestic IgG antibody responses in the absence of detectable IgM (Villarejos et al. 1982). Although coproantibodies have been detected by immunoassay, saliva and stool do not contain virus-specific neutralizing antibodies (Locarnini et al. 1980; Stapleton et al. 1991). These data suggest that secretory antibody plays little if any role in protection against hepatitis A.

Sensitive and specific immunoassays are widely available for the detection of total and IgM-specific antibodies to HAV. However, measurements of virus-neutralizing antibody are tedious and labor intensive. The radioimmunofocus reduction assay (Lemon and Binn 1983b) or HAV antigen reduction assay (Krah et al. 1991) are the most accurate methods available for determination of virus-neutralizing antibody. In addition to antibodies directed against the virus capsid, antibodies reactive with nonstructural proteins (especially 3C^{pro}) have also been detected. The presence of such antibodies may differentiate immunity due to natural infection from that gained by immunization with inactivated HAV vaccine (Robertson et al. 1993; Stewart et al. 1997).

CLINICAL MANIFESTATIONS

HAV causes an acute, self-limiting infection that does not progress to a chronic phase. Manifestations of the disease are generally restricted to the liver. However, although extrahepatic manifestations suggesting involvement of the central nervous system or kidneys are rare, their occurrence is well documented (Bromberg et al. 1982; Hammond et al. 1982; Malbrain et al. 1994; Ogawa et al. 1994; Zikos et al. 1995). The typical clinical course of type A hepatitis is shown in Figure 53.5. Following exposure, an incubation period of 15–45 days precedes the development of clinical symptoms. However, virus is present in the blood and shed in the stools within a few days of exposure (Asher et al. 1995; Ward et al. 1958; Krugman et al. 1962; Bower et al. 2000). The magnitude of the viremia and the amount of virus shed in the feces continues to increase until just before the onset of symptoms. Symptoms typically occur abruptly, with liver injury heralded by fever, myalgia, malaise, nausea, anorexia, and vomiting, accompanied occasionally by abdominal pain in the right upper quadrant. More distinctive signs of hepatitis and the disruption of normal hepatobiliary metabolism appear rapidly thereafter, including the passage of dark, 'Coca-Cola'-like urine, light, clay-colored stools, and frank icterus. These clinical findings coincide with the appearance of characteristic biochemical abnormalities, including abnormal elevations of serum levels of the liver-derived enzymes alanine aminotransferase (ALT), alkaline phosphatase (AST), and γ-glutamyl transpeptidase (GGTP), as well as increased levels of serum bilirubin. All these events signal the host immune response to the infection, including the appearance of virus-specific neutralizing antibodies (Lemon and Binn 1983b). Resolution is marked by slow recovery and often a prolonged period of convalescence. Nevertheless, serum enzyme levels are almost always normal by 6–12 months after onset of the disease, often much sooner. Rarely, however, HAV infection may trigger the onset of a chronic, autoimmune hepatitis (Vento et al. 1991).

The severity of symptoms associated with HAV infection is closely correlated with age. Acute, symptomatic, icteric infections seem to be the rule in older adolescents and adults (Lednar et al. 1985). On the other hand, infection in children under 2 years of age is almost never recognized clinically as hepatitis (Hadler et al. 1980). Most people with antibodies to HAV have no history of acute hepatitis, probably reflecting infection at an early age many years previously. Individuals over 50 years of age at the time of infection are at substantially increased risk of developing fulminant hepatitis, and clinical evidence of hepatic failure such as ascites, bleeding diathesis or hepatic coma (Forbes and Williams 1990; Hadler 1991; Lemon and Shapiro 1994). A systematic study has not been done, but patients with pre-existing chronic liver disease due to any cause may be at increased risk of fulminant disease when infected with HAV. Fortunately, fulminant hepatitis A is relatively rare, and accounts for fewer than 100 deaths annually in the USA (Lemon and Shapiro 1994).

Cholestatic hepatitis A and relapsing hepatitis A represent two less severe complications of type A hepatitis. Cholestatic hepatitis is characterized by persistent jaundice associated with pruritus, anorexia, and weight loss. Patients eventually recover after several weeks to months, but may recover more rapidly following a brief course of corticosteroids (Gordon et al. 1984). Such therapy should be attempted with caution, and only when there is no doubt about the diagnosis. There are many reports of clinical relapses 1–3 months after apparent recovery from acute hepatitis A. Relapsing hepatitis A is characterized by secondary rises in levels of serum enzyme, persistence of IgM anti-HAV, and possibly recurrent viremia and fecal virus shedding (Sjogren et al. 1987; Glikson et al. 1992). The pathogenesis of relapsing hepatitis A is unknown, but may involve viral escape from immune surveillance.

DIAGNOSIS

The diagnosis of acute viral hepatitis is usually suggested by the presence of the typical constellation of signs and symptoms associated with elevation of serum ALT activities. However, in the absence of a specific epidemiological setting suggestive of hepatitis A, the clinical manifestations of HAV infection are not sufficiently different from those of other types of acute viral hepatitis to allow a virus-specific diagnosis to be made without serological testing. Generally, the diagnosis is confirmed by the demonstration of IgM antibodies to the virus, which are almost always present at the onset of symptoms and which persist for up to 6 months following infection. These antibodies are usually measured by solid phase, IgM-capture immunoassays (Lemon et al. 1980; Decker et al. 1981). Competitive-inhibition immunoassays allow non-isotype-specific detection of viral antibodies (Mathiesen et al. 1978b; Decker et al. 1979). When such tests are positive in the absence of IgM antibodies, they are considered indicative of the presence of IgG anti-

bodies to the virus. This result is consistent with immunity due to prior infection or immunization against HAV.

Epidemiology of hepatitis A

TRANSMISSION OF HEPATITIS A

Almost all transmission occurs by the fecal–oral route. Within the USA, the most common risk factor for infection is close contact with a person with hepatitis A (Centers for Disease Control 1994). Person-to-person transmission accounts for most infections among household contacts as well as institutionalized individuals and children and staff in preschool daycare centers (Hadler et al. 1980). Handlers of nonhuman primates may be at risk for similar reasons. Not surprisingly, sexual behavior can influence the spread of infection, particularly among male homosexuals (Corey and Holmes 1980). Food- and waterborne transmission of HAV is also common, facilitated by the stability of the HAV virion and its relative resistance to drying (Siegl et al. 1984). Foodborne transmission of HAV may follow contamination of uncooked foods by infected food handlers, and is not infrequently implicated in common source outbreaks of disease. However, fresh produce may also be contaminated at its source, before distribution (Rosenblum et al. 1990). Finally, infection may occur following ingestion of raw or partially cooked filter-feeding shellfish collected from polluted waters, as these organisms have the ability to concentrate the virus. All these modes of transmission pose risks for travelers to HAV-endemic regions.

Although uncommon, parenteral transmission of the virus is also possible. Injecting drug users have represented a substantial proportion of cases of hepatitis A in some studies, and there is little doubt that they are at increased risk of HAV infection (Widell et al. 1983; Centers for Disease Control 1988). These infections are probably related to sharing of contaminated needles and thus to parenteral transmission of the virus, given that a relatively high level viremia is present for several weeks throughout the asymptomatic incubation period of the hepatitis A (Lemon et al. 1990). This conclusion is strongly supported by remarkable concurrent declines in the incidence of drug use-associated cases of hepatitis A, hepatitis B, and hepatitis C in the USA since 1988. This would be unexpected if cases of hepatitis A among drug users related primarily to poor sanitation. Transmission of virus by blood and blood products is also well documented, although it is much less common than with other hepatitis agents. Many such infections have been recognized in neonates who may receive split units of blood (Rosenblum et al. 1991), but transfusion-related infections have also been observed rarely in adults (Hollinger et al. 1983; Sherertz et al. 1984). Parenterally transmitted infections have been described in hemophiliacs receiving high-purity, solvent-detergent inactivated factor VIII (Mannucci et al. 1994; Robertson et al. 1994b), and cancer patients who received IL-2 produced in LAK cells maintained in 'normal human serum' (Weisfuse et al. 1990). With the possible exception of infections among drug users, however, parenteral transmission of HAV does not contribute significantly to the overall spread of the infection.

PREVALENCE OF HEPATITIS A

The prevalence of HAV infection varies widely by geographical region and depends on factors such as population density and the quality of public health sanitation and sewage disposal (Lemon and Shapiro 1994). It may be greatly increased during periods of social upheaval and war. The poorest of developing countries are characterized by the type I seroprevalence curve shown in Figure 53.6. In these countries, including many in Africa, Asia, and Central America, infections occur predominantly in very young children and are thus generally clinically inapparent. As a result, most children have antibodies against HAV by the age of 5–10 years, and disease is very infrequent in older people. With improved sanitary conditions, as found in the emerging economies of eastern Europe, the republics of the former Soviet Union and China, HAV infections tend to occur at a somewhat older age, resulting in the type II seroprevalence curve in Figure 53.6. In these regions, the probability of exposure and infection remains relatively high, but an increase in the mean age at infection results in a greater disease burden as adolescents and young adults are more likely to experience clinical symptoms when infected (Szmuness et al. 1977; Frosner et al. 1979; Lemon 1985a). In recent decades, improving economic conditions have resulted in changing epidemiological patterns in many developing nations (Innis

et al. 1991), with the result that epidemics of hepatitis A among older children, adolescents, and young adults, previously unheard of, are now becoming apparent. Older adults and the elderly are protected from infection by virtue of the antibody they carry from infections acquired in earlier, more endemic periods.

This trend continues in relatively well developed countries such as the USA and much of western Europe, where young children are no longer commonly infected (except in the setting of daycare centers), and the burden of disease is found among adolescents and young adults (Szmuness et al. 1977; Frosner et al. 1979; Lemon and Shapiro 1994). In these countries, symptomatic HAV infections in older individuals result in substantial absence from work and associated medical expenses. The major sources of infection in these populations are community-wide outbreaks, daycare centers, and common source outbreaks. Relatively high seroprevalence in the older age groups (Figure 53.6) signifies not continued risk of infection over time, but rather a cohort effect from infection in previous decades when HAV infections were more prevalent (Frosner et al. 1978). Finally, in highly developed regions such as the Scandinavian countries, seroprevalence tends to follow the type IV curve shown in Figure 53.6. There is little endemic transmission of the virus, and disease occurs primarily in travelers to other regions and in certain high risk groups such as intravenous drug users (Frosner et al. 1979; Siebke et al. 1982; Widell et al. 1983). Despite this convenient classification, it is important to note that prevalence patterns do not follow political as much as socioeconomic borders. For example, within the USA there are communities that would fit each of the type II, III, and IV patterns.

Prevention of hepatitis A

To a considerable extent, hepatitis A can be prevented by good personal hygiene, adequate disposal and treatment of human waste, and provision of safe drinking water. As indicated above, HAV is rarely transmitted endemically in countries where these standards are met. However, specific measures are also available for the prevention of hepatitis A. These include passive immunoprophylaxis with pooled human immunoglobulin (IG) and active immunization with hepatitis A vaccines.

POOLED HUMAN IMMUNOGLOBULIN

Postexposure prophylaxis is generally accomplished with human IG (0.2 ml/kg), which should be given to people who are household members or sexual contacts of an infected individual (Gellis et al. 1945; Winokur and Stapleton 1992 Immunization Practices Advisory Committee 1990). Postexposure prophylaxis with IG may not prevent infection but it is remarkably effective in reducing or eliminating symptoms. It probably exerts

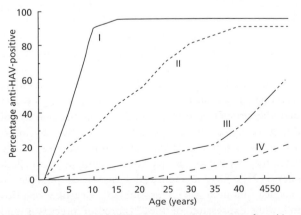

Figure 53.6 *Typical age-related seroprevalence curves found in populations residing in regions with high (I), intermediate (II) or low (III) endemicity for HAV infections, and in regions such as Scandinavia where endogenous transmission of HAV is now very uncommon (IV).*

this effect by reducing the level of viremia, thereby reducing spread of virus within the liver (Lemon 1985a). To be optimally effective, it must be given within 2 weeks of exposure to the virus. IG is also useful for pre-exposure prophylaxis (0.2–0.5 ml/kg) and has been administered routinely to individuals traveling to HAV-endemic regions. If given before exposure, IG prevents disease for up to 4–6 months (Conrad and Lemon 1987). In this setting it is more likely to prevent infection as well as symptoms of hepatitis A, but this depends on the dose administered, the time elapsed between administration of IG and exposure to the virus, as well as the magnitude of the viral inoculum. Except for very limited travel, the use of inactivated hepatitis A vaccine is preferable and is largely replacing pre-exposure prophylaxis with IG.

HEPATITIS A VACCINES

Inactivated whole virus vaccines contain purified HAV particles (both complete virions and empty capsids) produced in cell culture and inactivated with formalin (Binn et al. 1986; Andre et al., 1990; Lewis et al. 1991). Several inactivated vaccines are licensed in their countries of origin and elsewhere, making inactivated HAV vaccine available worldwide. Most of these vaccines are adsorbed with alum (aluminium hydroxide) and all seem to be very immunogenic when administered by intramuscular injection. They are generally safe, and two have been shown in well designed clinical trials to provide a high level of protection against symptomatic hepatitis A in children (Werzberger et al. 1992; Innis et al. 1994; Lemon 1994). Antibody levels exceeding that produced by a single injection of IG are often present within 2–4 weeks of the first vaccine dose. Booster doses, given as early as one month following primary immunization, enhance the titer of neutralizing antibody and thus are likely to extend the duration of protection. Although the minimal protective level of antibody is not well defined, it is very low (<45 mIU/ml) (Stapleton et al. 1985; Werzberger et al. 1992). Although inactivated vaccines do not produce detectable secretory antibody, the prevention of intrahepatic virus replication is likely to prevent or substantially reduce the fecal shedding of virus. Thus, in contrast to inactivated poliovirus vaccines, immunization with inactivated hepatitis A vaccines should render an individual unable to transmit the infection if exposed to the virus.

The major shortcoming of inactivated HAV vaccines is that they are quite expensive and thus not available for the control of hepatitis A on a population-wide basis in countries where immunization is most needed. Although inactivated vaccines are likely to be more effective than IG in controlling community-wide outbreaks of disease (Werzberger et al. 1992; Lemon and Shapiro 1994; Prikazsky et al. 1994), the use of the vaccine in this setting is also likely to be limited by cost.

Although data are limited, immunization may provide some level of protection against hepatitis A if it is administered immediately after exposure to the virus (Werzberger et al. 1992; Robertson et al. 1994a).

Several candidate attenuated HAV vaccines have been evaluated in clinical trials (Provost et al. 1986; Midthun et al. 1991; Sjogren et al. 1992). The virus strains included in these vaccines have been attenuated by passage in cell culture and require parenteral injection to initiate infection uniformly in human recipients. In general, the immune response to these candidate vaccines has been disappointing with slow, low magnitude antibody responses. This probably reflects the fact that these virus strains are highly restricted in their ability to replicate in human hosts. Although they seem quite safe in clinical trials involving limited numbers of people and are likely to be effective clinically, these candidate attenuated vaccines have generally been abandoned by commercial manufacturers in favor of the development of more profitable inactivated vaccines. However, one such vaccine has been used extensively in China (Mao et al. 1989, 1991).

A fresh approach to the selection of candidate attenuated HAV vaccine strains is likely to be required for the development of highly immunogenic attenuated vaccines. One such approach has been the creation of large deletion mutations within the 5′ NTR of a virulent, but minimally cell culture-adapted, variant of HAV (Shaffer et al. 1994). Some of these mutants have a strongly temperature-sensitive replication phenotype. However, there is no evidence thus far that these large 5′ NTR deletions result in significant attenuation of the virus in primates (Shaffer et al. 1995). A more promising alternative approach is to consider the use of simian strains of HAV, which seem to be naturally restricted in their ability to cause disease in chimpanzees (Purcell 1991), or virus chimeras containing selected sequences of human and simian HAVs. Recent data using chimeras derived from cell-adapted HM-175 (HAV/7) and the simian AGM-27 strain suggest that chimeras containing the HAV/7 background and the C terminus of the AGM-27 2C are attenuated for chimpanzees and may provide an alternative for development of an attenuated vaccine (Raychaudhuri et al. 1998).

Similarly, there has been little success in developing recombinant hepatitis A vaccines. This reflects the fact that the protective epitopes present on the surface of this picornavirus are conformationally defined by interactions between the individual capsid proteins in the assembled virus particle. However, Winokur and colleagues (1991) have demonstrated that it is possible to produce immunogenic, assembled viruslike capsids following expression of the P1 protein precursor and 3C^{pro} by recombinant vaccinia virus. Moreover, preliminary studies with synthetic peptide mimotopes (Mattioli et al. 1995) indicate that certain peptide motifs may successfully mimic the conformational, immunodominant antigenic site of HAV, suggesting the ultimate feasibility of a synthetic peptide-based vaccine.

HEPATITIS E VIRUS

Classification

On the basis of the morphology of the hepatitis E virus (HEV) particle, the absence of a lipid envelope, the type and length of its nucleic acid and the general organization of its genome, HEV was originally classified within the *Caliciviridae* (Cubitt et al. 1995) (Table 53.3). However, a phylogenetic analysis of the nucleotide sequence of HEV shows that it is related more closely to the alphavirus superfamily of positive-strand RNA viruses, in particular the rubiviruses (Koonin et al. 1992) and it has subsequently been removed from the *Caliciviridae* and reassigned to an unclassified genus termed 'hepatitis E-like virus' (Berke and Matson 2000). Hepatitis E-like viruses have been identified in humans, swine, and chickens and all have similar genetic arrangements. The swine derived virus does not appear to cause any overt clinical symptoms in the pigs; in contrast, the avian HEV-like virus is associated with a hepatitis-splenomegaly syndrome in chickens within the United States. (Haqshenas et al. 2001)

Morphology and structure

As with many other features of HEV, the exact structure of the virion remains elusive owing to the absence of a reliable cell culture system that is permissive for its replication and to difficulties in obtaining large quantities of stable particles from human and nonhuman primate samples. The HEV particle is chloroform-resistant and has a morphology resembling that of human caliciviruses and Norwalk virus (Figure 53.7; and see Table 53.1). Although early reports suggested the diameter of HEV particles to be ca. 27 nm (Balayan et al. 1983), subsequent studies have shown the average diameter to be closer to 32 nm (Bradley et al. 1988). Smaller particles may result from proteolytic degradation as the virus passes through the intestine, as both particle sizes have been observed in single stool suspensions (Bradley et al. 1987). HEV-specific antibodies recognize both forms. The characteristic cup-like surface of caliciviruses is less prominent in HEV, but Markham rotational enhancement clearly indicates surface projections and valleys (Ticehurst 1991). Cryoelectron microscopy of a recombinant baculovirus expressed ORF2 product (amino acids 112–660) revealed spherical structures approximately 27 nm in diameter. These structures contained 60 copies of the recombinant ORF2, with a T = 1 lattice of icosahedral symmetry (Xing et al. 1999). However, X-ray diffraction data on the surface structure of the virus itself which is predicted to have a T = 3 lattice composed of 180 molecules is not available since sufficient amounts cannot be obtained from cell culture growth.

GENOME ORGANIZATION

The genome of HEV is a single-stranded, 7.5-kb, positive-sense RNA that is polyadenylated at its 3′ terminus (Reyes et al. 1990; Tam et al. 1991). It contains three separate ORFs flanked by short 5′ and 3′ NTRs of 27 and 68 nt, respectively (Figure 53.8). The presence of a methyltransferase motif within the nonstructural proteins encoded by the most 5′ ORF (ORF1) closest to the 5′ terminus is consistent with the presence of a methylated cap structure (Koonin et al. 1992) on the 5′ end of the RNA. Experimental studies have confirmed the presence of such a structure (Zhang et al. 2001b;

Table 53.3 *Properties of Hepatitis E virus, Calicivirus, and Rubivirus*

	Calicivirus	Hepatitis E virus	Rubivirus
Morphology	Icosahedral	Icosahedral	Spherical
Envelope	No	No	Yes
Size	35–39 nm	27–32 nm	60 nm
Bouyant density	1.33–1.39 g/cm^3	1.29 g/cm^3	1.2 g/cm^3 (?)
S$_{20,w}$	170–183S	183S	280S (?)
RNA genome:	ss (+) RNA	ss (+) RNA	ss (+) RNA
5′ structure	VPg	5′ methylated cap (?)	5′ methylated cap
3′ structure	Poly(A)	Poly(A)	Poly(A)
Length	8.2 kb	7.5 kb	9.8 kb
Subgenomic RNAs	2	2	1
Structural proteins	1 capsid protein	2 (?) (1 glycosylated)	1 capsid protein 2 glycoproteins
Nonstructural proteins	Picorna-like protease RDRP	Papain-like protease RDRP Methyltransferase	Papain-like protease RDRP Methyltransferase

RDRP, RNA-dependent RNA polymerase; ss (+), single-stranded, positive-sense.

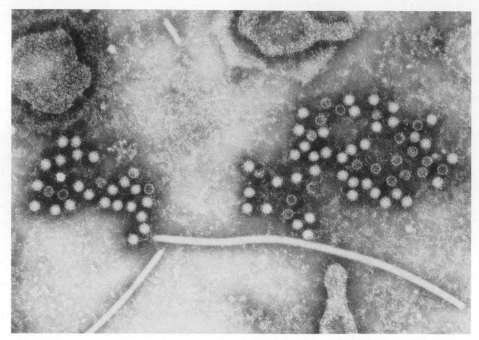

Figure 53.7 *Morphology of HEV particles demonstrated by electron microscopy.*

Kabrane-Lazizi et al. 1999a), identified the viral encoded capping enzyme (Magden et al. 2001) and verified that the capped structure is necessary for infectivity (Emerson et al. 2001). The ORF closest to the 3′ terminus (ORF2) is thought to encode the major structural protein. There is an additional short ORF (ORF3), which overlaps ORF1 by a single nucleotide and ORF2 by most of its length. ORF3 encodes a small protein that appears to be phosphorylated and is associated with the cytoskeleton (Zafrullah et al. 1997). The 5′ end of HEV RNA may contain a secondary structure analogous to that predicted to be present in alphaviruses. In addition, the sequence between 150 and 208 nt of HEV resembles

a conserved 51 nt alphavirus sequence, whilst homology at 3602–3632 nt of HEV and junction sequences of alphaviruses suggests that this region may contain a promoter for transcription of a subgenomic RNA.

HEV PROTEINS

Most information about the proteins of HEV has been obtained from analysis of the nucleotide sequence of the virus. ORF1 encodes a relatively large polyprotein that contains consensus motifs for a methyltransferase, a papain-like cysteine protease, a helicase (NTP-binding site), and an RNA-dependent RNA polymerase similar to those found in the alphaviruses (Koonin et al. 1992).

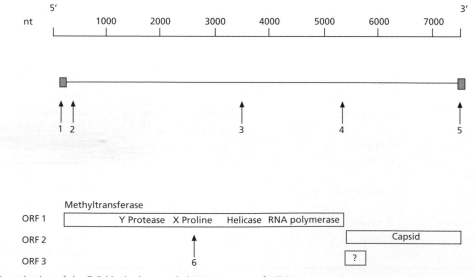

Figure 53.8 *Organization of the 7.5-kb single-stranded RNA genome of HEV.*

Also present in the ORF1 polyprotein is a polyproline 'hinge,' which is also found in rubiviruses, and a conserved 'X' domain, which is of unknown function but is found flanking the papain-like protease domain in other positive-strand RNA viruses. Although this polyprotein is almost certainly proteolytically cleaved into 4–5 individual polypeptides with distinct functions in replication, the details of this process are not understood and a preliminary study was unable to detect self-cleavage products using two different expression systems (Ropp et al. 2000). Several unusual features of this polyprotein distinguish HEV from members of the *Alphavirus* genus (Koonin et al. 1992). For example, a peculiar domain ('Y' domain) located downstream of the methyltransferase motif has no equivalent in the alphaviruses, although a similar domain is found in the plant virus, beet necrotic yellow vein virus. The function of this domain is unknown. Near the 'proline hinge' region, a 'hypervariable' region has also been noted whose function is not known (Fry et al. 1992, C.-C. Huang et al. 1992; Tsarev et al. 1992; Yin et al. 1993).

ORF2 encodes a 72 kDa capsid polypeptide and contains a signal peptide sequence and three potential glycosylation sites (Tam et al. 1991; Yarbough et al. 1991). The amino half of the ORF2 protein is rich in arginine residues, suggesting that it may associate with viral RNA. Cloning and expression of this product indicate that it is translocated in the endoplasmic reticulum, cleaved by signal peptidase and glycosylated (Jameel et al. 1996; Zafrullah et al. 1999). Subsequent studies have determined that ORF2 is present in both glycosylated and nonglycosylated forms but only the nonglycosylated form is stable in mammalian cells (Torresi et al. 1999). A portion of this molecule lacking the first 100 amino acids self assembles into viruslike particles (Li et al. 1997; Xing et al. 1999), and generates antibodies that are protective (Tsarev et al. 1994a; Zhang et al. 2001a). From an immunologic perspective, the ORF2 amino acids 452–617 are responsible for generating neutralizing antibodies that react with all four genotypes (Meng et al. 2001). An additional immunoreactive site is located at the amino terminus, but this site is not accessible using intact virions (Schofield et al. 2003). Although the ORF2 protein is found on the cell surface (Zafrullah et al. 1999), it is important to note that any surface lipid components of the virus would be unstable and almost certainly removed during passage of the virus through the bile.

Overlapping ORF1 and ORF2 is a small open reading frame (ORF3) that encodes a 13 kDa, cysteine-rich polypeptide that is immunoreactive with many patient sera. The genotype I ORF3 product has been shown to be a cytoskeleton-associated phosphoprotein (Zafrullah et al. 1997), with Ser[80] serving as the phosphorylation site. Subsequent studies using a yeast two hybrid system suggests that the phosphorylated form of this protein associates with the nonglycosylated form of the ORF2 product and therefore may be involved in capsid assembly (Tyagi et al. 2002). However, the analogous product for genotype III does not contain a Ser[80], and large deletions have been described within this ORF in viruses recovered from two separate epidemics in India (Ray et al. 1992).

REPLICATION OF HEV

Although there are reports of HEV replication in conventional cell cultures (Huang et al. 1992; Kazachkov et al. 1992), they have not been confirmed. However, replication has been documented recently in primary cultures of hepatocytes taken from cynomolgus monkeys infected in vivo (Tam et al. 1996). The absence of a well characterized and readily available permissive cell culture system has severely limited studies of the molecular mechanisms of replication. The nonstructural proteins are presumably translated from newly uncoated RNA by a 5′ cap-dependent mechanism, providing the enzymes required for subsequent synthesis of both negative- and positive-strand RNAs. The 3′ end of the viral genome binds the viral RNA dependent RNA polymerase thereby providing a mechanism for viral RNA replication (Agrawal et al. 2001) while the ORF2 protein binds to the first 76 nt of the 5′ region of the viral RNA (Surjit et al. 2004). Two 3′ co-terminal, subgenomic messenger RNAs of 3.7 and 2.0 kb seem to be transcribed from the full-length negative-strand RNA, with the 2.0-kb message present in greater abundance than the 3.7-kb product (Tam et al. 1991). However, the role of these subgenomic RNAs in directing translation of the ORF2 and ORF3 proteins remains unclear. There is no understanding of how these processes are regulated.

GENETIC AND ANTIGENIC VARIANTS OF HEV

HEV strains seem to comprise a single serotype of antigenically related viruses, as all well-characterized strains share cross-reacting epitopes. Several studies have examined the reactivity of acute or convalescent sera with synthetic peptides or recombinant proteins expressed from ORF2 and ORF3 of different HEV strains (Yarbough et al. 1991; Kaur et al. 1992; Khudyakov et al. 1993; Li et al. 1994). Antigenic epitopes have been identified at the carboxy termini of both ORF2 and ORF3 protein products. The ORF3 epitope seems to differ between eastern and western hemisphere strains (Yarbough et al. 1991), however, the biological relevance of this finding is unclear. Multiple studies have identified that the carboxy terminal portion of ORF2 (approximately amino acids 270–660) is responsible for generating neutralizing antibodies, and that recombinant constructs containing these amino acids self assemble into viruslike particles (Li et al. 1997; Xing et al. 1999). Riddell et al. (2000), were the first to identify amino acids 394–457 as part of the immunodominant capsid epitope using mouse monoclonal antibodies. Subsequently, Meng et al. (2001) used a PCR-based in vitro neutralization assay to evaluate the ability of synthetic peptides to inhibit binding of virus to PLC/PRF/5 cells and identified amino acids 452–617 as part of the neutralization epitope. A subsequent study characterized monoclonal antibodies derived from a chimpanzee experimentally infected with a construct including amino acids 112–607 (Schofield et al. 2003). Two antigenic reactive sites were identified in this study. One site, associated with neutralization, was localized to amino acids 452–617, while the second site was located between amino acids 112 and 150.

Despite the homogeneous antigenic reactivity, this group of viruses has a wide range of genetic diversity. Four distinct genotypes can be defined based upon complete genome sequences. Up to nine genotypes have been proposed based upon limited sequencing of 287 nucleotides within the OFR1 region (Schlauder and Mushahwar 2001) although this region has not been demonstrated to be representative of the complete genome. Genotype I contains human HEV strains recovered from endemic regions in the Far East and Central Asia – India, Myanmar, Nepal, Pakistan, China, Uzbekistan (Arankalle et al. 1999; Tam et al. 1991; Nakai et al. 2001; Gouvea et al. 1997; Shrestha et al. 2003; van Cuyck-Gandre et al. 2000; Li et al. 2002; Chatterjee et al. 1997) and African nations – Namibia, Algeria, Morocco, Chad, Egypt, and Tunisia (He et al. 2000; van Cuyck-Gandre et al. 1997; Meng et al. 1999; Tsarev et al. 1999; Chatterjee et al. 1997). These strains form a monophyletic cluster with individual branches being much more closely related genetically to each other (about 90 percent identity) than to strains representing viruses from other parts of the world. Genotype II is represented by a single sequence from Mexico (C.-C. Huang et al. 1992), although limited sequence of strains from Nigeria also appear to belong to genotype II (Buisson et al. 2000). Genotype III has been identified from human and swine sources in the United States, Japan, and the The Netherlands (Schlauder et al. 1998; Meng et al. 1997; Takahashi et al. 2001, 2003a, b; Okamoto et al. 2001; van der Poel et al. 2001; Widdowson et al. 2003); sporadic human cases in Greece, Spain, Italy, and the United Kingdom (Schlauder et al. 1999; Pina et al. 2000; Wang et al. 2001) and in swine populations in India and New Zealand (Arankalle et al. 2002, 2003; Garkavenko et al. 2001). Genotype IV strains have been characterized from human and swine sources in Taiwan, Japan, and China (Hsieh et al., 1998, 1999; Nishizawa et al. 2003; Takahashi et al. 2001, 2003a, b; Li et al. 2002; Wang et al. 2002), while human cases with this genotype have been identified in Vietnam (Hijikata et al. 2002). The tight genetic clustering observed within genotype I is not seen in the available sequences from these other strains.

Many of these sequences are derived from swine sources, and it has become obvious that there is a wide array of swine HEV sequences all over the world. However, the direct relationship between swine HEV and human disease is not obvious. Individuals with occupational exposures to swine do have a higher seroprevalence of antibodies against HEV, but this does not reflect disease (Drobeniuc et al. 2001; Meng et al. 2002). Other animal reservoirs including rats, mice, cows, sheep, goats, dogs, cats, wild boar, and deer have also been proposed based upon seroprevalence studies or virological studies (Balayan et al. 1990; Favorov et al. 1996, 2000; Kabrane-Lazizi et al., 1999b; Wang et al. 2002; Matsuda et al. 2003; Tei et al. 2003). In addition, avian HEV strains genetically related to swine and human HEV, have been characterized from chickens with hepatitis – splenomegaly syndrome in the United States (Haqshenas et al. 2001) and Australian big liver and spleen disease virus (Payne et al. 1999; Haqshenas et al. 2001).

Clinical and pathological aspects of HEV infection

PATHOGENESIS OF HEPATITIS E

Chimpanzees and several species of monkeys are susceptible to HEV infection and have served as experimental models of hepatitis E in humans (Bradley et al. 1987; Ticehurst et al. 1992; Tsarev et al. 1993a). In addition, swine, rats, and possibly other mammalian species may support replication of the virus as discussed above. The most reliable experimental animal models have been the rhesus and cynomolgus macaques, and much of our understanding of the pathogenesis of this disease is derived from experimental infections of these animals. Following intravenous inoculation of cynomolgus macaques, there is an incubation period of 2–6 weeks, which precedes the development of raised liver enzymes (Figure 53.9). During this period there are viremia and fecal excretion of virus, reflecting replication of virus within hepatocytes. Antibodies to HEV develop just before elevations of liver enzymes, coincident with resolution of the viremia and fecal virus shedding and reductions in the quantity of viral antigen present in the liver. A biphasic pattern of liver disease has been observed in some animals, the initial period of enzyme elevation occurring within the first 2 weeks after inoculation. Pathological changes in the liver are consistent with acute viral hepatitis (Longer et al. 1993), but not specific for any etiological agent, and include hepatocyte necrosis and inflammatory cell infiltration. In general, the overall pattern and severity of disease do not seem to be as dramatic as in humans. Although limited evidence supports the theory of replication of the virus within the gastrointestinal tract of swine, an inoculum containing $10^{6.8}$ infectious units by intravenous inocula-

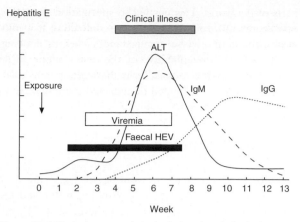

Figure 53.9 *Typical course of virological and pathological events during infection with HEV.*

tion failed to initiate infection when administered orally to macaques (Tsarev et al. 1994b).

There are few data about virological events in infected humans. In one of two reported human volunteer infections, raised liver enzymes and jaundice persisted for 3 months (Chauhan et al. 1993). Viremia was first detected at day 22, and terminated at day 46 when liver enzymes reached their peak value. Antibodies against HEV were first detected at day 41; their appearance was followed by declining levels of liver enzyme. Excretion of virus in stool samples was detected by RT-PCR between 30 and 50 days after ingestion. Disease was limited to a 1 month period in the other reported experimental human infection (Balayan et al. 1983). Examination of liver specimens from patients involved in outbreaks of disease attributed to HEV in Delhi, the Kashmir and (putatively) Ghana have revealed two general types of histopathological change (Gupta and Smetana 1955; Morrow et al. 1968; Khuroo 1980). A cholestatic pattern is characterized by prominent bile stasis within canaliculi and a unique glandlike transformation of parenchymal cells. There is portal and, to a lesser extent, parenchymal infiltration of lymphocytes and polymorphonuclear leucocytes. A second histopathological pattern is similar to that found in other types of acute hepatitis, and includes ballooning degeneration of hepatocytes and formation of acidophilic bodies.

IMMUNE RESPONSE TO HEV INFECTION

Antibodies to HEV develop during convalescence from the disease and are reactive with both linear and conformational epitopes of the virus. A wide variety of assays has been developed for detection of these antibodies, including various ELISAs using recombinant proteins (Goldsmith et al. 1992; He et al. 1993; Tsarev et al. 1993b) or combinations of peptides and recombinant antigens (Sallie et al. 1992; Paul et al. 1994) as antigen synthetic peptides (Coursaget et al. 1994; Favorov et al. 1994). In addition, immunoblot assays have been devel-

oped using recombinant antigens (Favorov et al. 1992; Li et al. 1994). These assays seem to vary considerably in their sensitivity and specificity, with relatively low overall concordance between results in a recent collaborative study. Synthetic peptides representing linear epitopes within the protein products of all three ORFs seem to react with serum from infected individuals (Kaur et al. 1992; Favorov et al. 1994), but peptide-based assays performed poorly over all against a reference panel of anti-HEV serum. A baculovirus-expressed, nearly complete ORF2 product forms viruslike particles and is a superior antigen because it displays conformation-dependent epitopes (Tsarev et al. 1993b). The early antibody response to this antigen includes both IgM and IgG antibodies to the virus (Tsarev et al. 1993b, 1994a), although the IgM response is variable. Antibody to the ORF2 protein was detectable in immunoblots for more than 12 months after infection, whereas antibody to ORF3 disappeared following resolution of the disease (Li et al. 1994). Nothing is known of the cellular immune responses, and there is controversy regarding the longevity of natural immunity after infection with HEV (Bryan et al. 1994; Arankalle et al. 1995). A number of early studies (Paul et al. 1994; Dawson et al. 1992; Mast et al. 1997) suggested that a measurable proportion of the population within nonendemic regions had evidence of antibodies to HEV (1.2–13 percent). Subsequent seroprevalence studies have revealed that individuals who are exposed to pigs in an occupational setting (farm workers, veterinarians) are more likely to be anti-HEV positive than a control population unexposed to pigs (Drobeniuc et al. 2001; Meng et al. 2002); likewise individuals who have increased exposure to rats have increased seropositivity against HEV (Smith et al. 2002).

CLINICAL MANIFESTATIONS OF HEPATITIS E

HEV, like HAV, causes an acute, self-limited disease that does not progress to a chronic phase. As shown in Figure 53.9, the incubation period is somewhat longer than that for HAV, averaging ca. 40 days. The prodromal symptoms of infection are similar to hepatitis A, including malaise, anorexia, and abdominal discomfort. A 15–20 percent case-fatality rate has been observed among women who become infected during the third trimester of pregnancy (Khuroo et al. 1981), although the clinical features of fatal disease are not well described. Fulminant disease also occurs in other settings. About 60 percent of sporadic cases of fulminant hepatitis in India are due to HEV infection (Nanda et al. 1994). The much less frequent involvement of HEV in fulminant hepatitis in developed countries (Liang et al. 1993; Sallie et al. 1994) reflects the rarity of the infection in these regions.

DIAGNOSIS

Serological diagnosis of acute infection is relatively straightforward with the assays currently available.

Detection of IgG anti-HEV in the absence of markers of other types of acute viral hepatitis is generally indicative of HEV infection. Tests for IgM antibodies have marginal sensitivity and are therefore of limited usefulness. In the past, lack of standardization and poor concordance between peptide based and recombinant ORF2 based assays for IgG anti-HEV severely limited their usefulness in population-based studies and epidemiological investigations. However, it is currently accepted that assays using the recombinant ORF2 antigen most clearly indicate evidence of infection in humans and other species.

Epidemiology of HEV

The earliest documented outbreak of hepatitis E occurred in Delhi, India, in 1955, after heavy flooding of the Yamuna River (Viswanathan 1957). Subsequent outbreaks of disease and sporadic cases of hepatitis E have been confirmed in a wide variety of tropical and developing regions, including India, China, Nepal, Pakistan, Myanmar, Indonesia, the Central Asian region of the former Soviet Union, Egypt, Ethiopia, Jordan, Algeria, the Ivory Coast, Chad, Sudan, Somalia, Ethiopia, and Mexico. In most outbreaks, contaminated drinking water has been incriminated as the source of infection. However, sporadic cases of hepatitis E also occur in these regions (Hyams et al. 1992a, b; Bile et al. 1994), suggesting that the virus is endemic. Clinically apparent hepatitis E generally occurs in individuals 25–40 years of age (Bradley 1992; Jameel et al. 1992), and the mean age at infection with HEV seems to differ markedly from the mean age of infection with HAV in regions that are endemic for both viruses. Surveys of sera collected over an interval of 10 years from an HEV-endemic region of India demonstrated that most HAV infections occurred before the age of 5 years, whereas HEV infections generally occurred after the age of 16 years (Arankalle et al. 1995). The reason for this difference is not known; serologically determined rates of infection are similar in children and adults during disease outbreaks, although adults are more likely to develop clinical evidence of hepatitis (Mast et al. 1993). Hepatitis E is an extraordinarily rare disease in the USA and Europe, although seroprevalence studies with currently available assays indicate that limited exposure to HEV or a closely related virus may indeed occur. In these regions of the world, almost all reported cases have been in travelers who have recently returned from endemic regions.

The apparent low level, endemic circulation of the virus in some regions contrasts with the fact that person-to-person transmission of HEV is unusual during epidemics (Mast et al. 1993; Aggarwal and Naik 1994). The recent data indicating markers of HEV infection in multiple animal species (pigs, deer, boar, rats, macaques) suggests that this family of viruses is ubiquitous in many parts of the world. This has led to speculation that HEV may represent a zoonotic pathogen, confined to its ecological niche until adverse circumstances, such as flooding, result in fecal contamination of the water supply (Bile et al. 1994). Another possibility is that certain individuals may shed virus for extended periods and thereby serve as reservoirs of infection (Nanda et al. 1995).

Control of hepatitis E

As with HAV, primary prevention of HEV infection rests with the provision of safe drinking water and the sanitary disposal of human waste (Bile et al. 1994), but most cases of hepatitis E occur in regions of the world where these conditions are difficult to achieve. Data concerning the protective efficacy of IG are limited and difficult to interpret (Joshi et al. 1985; Khuroo and Dar 1992). However, it is likely that anti-HEV is not present in significant titers in IG prepared from plasma collected in well developed, industrialized countries. Passive immunoprophylaxis of nonhuman primates with hyperimmune globulin has prevented biochemical and histological evidence of hepatitis although it did not prevent infection (Tsarev et al. 1994a). Both viremia and fecal virus excretion were documented in animals receiving hyperimmune globulin.

Because HEV cannot be propagated efficiently in cell culture, vaccine development has focused on recombinant immunogens. Preliminary studies suggested that immunization of cynomolgus monkeys with a recombinant, partial ORF2 protein product may have provided protection against disease, but not virus replication following challenge with a heterologous inoculum (Purdy et al. 1993). Subsequent studies have revealed that the partial recombinant ORF2 product with a molecular weight of 53 kd provides protection against disease (Tsarev et al. 1994a; Zhang et al. 2001a, 2002; Purcell et al. 2003), but not necessarily infection (depending upon the titer of the challenge inoculum) (Tsarev et al. 1997). These data are encouraging for the development of a vaccine.

REFERENCES

Abe, H., Beninger, P.R., et al. 1982. Light microscopic findings of liver biopsy specimens from patients with hepatitis type A and comparison with type B. *Gastroenterology*, **82**, 938–47.

Aggarwal, R. and Naik, S.R. 1994. Hepatitis E: intrafamilial transmission versus waterborne spread. *J Hepatol*, **21**, 718–23.

Agrawal, S., Gupta, D. and Panda, S.K. 2001. The 3′ end of hepatitis E virus (HEV) genome binds specifically to the viral RNA-dependent RNA polymerase (RdRp). *Virology*, **282**, 87–101.

Allaire, M., Chernala, M.M., et al. 1994. Picornaviral 3C cysteine proteinases have a fold similar to chymotrypsin-like serine proteinases. *Nature (London)*, **369**, 72–6.

Almela, M.J., González, M.E. and Carrasco, L. 1991. Inhibitors of poliovirus uncoating efficiently block the early membrane permeabilization induced by virus particles. *J Virol*, **65**, 2572–7.

Anderson, D.A. 1987. Cytopathology, plaque assay, and heat inactivation of hepatitis A virus strain HM175. *J Med Virol*, **22**, 35–44.

Andino, R., Rieckhof, G.E., et al. 1993. Poliovirus RNA synthesis utilizes an RNP complex formed around the 5′ end of viral RNA. *EMBO J*, **12**, 3587–98.

Andre, F.E., Hepburn, A. and D'Hondt, E. 1990. Inactivated candidate vaccines for hepatitis A. *Prog Med Virol*, **37**, 72–95.

Arankalle, V.A., Tsarev, S.A., et al. 1995. Age-specific prevalence of antibodies to hepatitis A and E viruses in Pune, India, 1982 and 1992. *J Infect Dis*, **171**, 447–50.

Arankalle, V.A., Paranjape, S., et al. 1999. Phylogenetic analysis of hepatitis E virus isolates from India (1976–1993). *J Gen Virol*, **80**, 1691–700.

Arankalle, V.A., Chobe, L.P., et al. 2002. Human and swine hepatitis E viruses from Western India belong to different genotypes. *J Hepatol*, **36**, 417–25.

Arankalle, V.A., Chobe, L.P., et al. 2003. Swine HEV infection in south India and phylogenetic analysis (1985–1999). *J Med Virol*, **69**, 391–6.

Arauz-Ruiz, P., Sundqvist, L., et al. 2001. Presumed common source outbreaks of hepatitis A in an endemic area confirmed by limited sequencing within the VP1 region. *J Med Virol*, **65**, 449–56.

Asher, L.V.S., Binn, L.N., et al. 1995. Pathogenesis of hepatitis A in orally inoculated owl monkeys (*Aotus trivergatus*). *J Med Virol*, **47**, 260–8.

Ashida, M. and Hamada, C. 1997. Molecular cloning of the hepatitis A virus receptor from a simian cell line. *J Gen Virol*, **78**, 1565–9.

Balayan, M.S., Andzhaparidze, A.G., et al. 1983. Evidence for a virus in non-A, non-B hepatitis transmitted via the fecal-oral route. *Intervirology*, **20**, 23–31.

Balayan, M.S., Usmanov, R.K., et al. 1990. Brief report: experimental hepatitis E infection in domestic pigs. *J Med Virol*, **32**, 58–9.

Barker, M.H., Capps, R.B. and Allen, F. 1945. Acute infectious hepatitis in the Mediterranean theater: including acute hepatitis without jaundice. *JAMA*, **128**, 997–1003.

Beneduce, F., Pisani, G., et al. 1995. Complete nucleotide sequence of a cytopathic hepatitis A virus strain isolated in Italy. *Virus Res*, **36**, 299–309.

Berke, T. and Matson, D.O. 2000. Reclassification of the *Caliciviridae* into distinct genera and exclusion of hepatitis E virus from the family on the basis of comparative phylogenetic analysis. *Arch Virol*, **145**, 1421–36.

Bienz, K., Egger, D., et al. 1992. Structural and functional characterization of the poliovirus replication complex. *J Virol*, **66**, 2740–7.

Bile, K., Isse, A., et al. 1994. Contrasting roles of rivers and wells as sources of drinking water on attack and fatality rates in a hepatitis E epidemic in Somalia. *Am J Trop Med Hyg*, **51**, 466–74.

Binn, L.N., Lemon, S.M., et al. 1984. Primary isolation and serial passage of hepatitis A virus strains in primate cell cultures. *J Clin Microbiol*, **20**, 28–33.

Binn, L.N., Bancroft, W.H., et al. 1986. Preparation of a prototype inactivated hepatitis A virus vaccine from infected cell cultures. *J Infect Dis*, **153**, 749–56.

Bishop, N.E. and Anderson, D.A. 1993. RNA-dependent cleavage of VP0 capsid protein in provirions of hepatitis A virus. *Virology*, **197**, 616–23.

Blank, C.D., Anderson, D.A., et al. 2000. Infection of polarized cultures of human intestinal epithelial cells with hepatitis A virus: vectorial release of progeny virions through apical cellular membranes. *J Virol*, **74**, 6476–84.

Borovec, S.V. and Anderson, D.A. 1993. Synthesis and assembly of hepatitis A virus-specific proteins in BS-C-1 cells. *J Virol*, **67**, 3095–102.

Bower, W.A., Nainan, O.V., et al. 2000. Duration of viremia in hepatitis A virus infection. *J Infect Dis*, **182**, 12–17.

Bradley, D.W. 1992. Hepatitis E: epidemiology, aetiology and molecular biology. *Rev Med Virol*, **2**, 19–28.

Bradley, D.W., Gravelle, C.R., et al. 1977. Cyclic excretion of hepatitis A virus in experimentally infected chimpanzees: biophysical characterization of the associated HAV particles. *J Med Virol*, **1**, 133–8.

Bradley, D.W., Krawczynski, K., et al. 1987. Enterically transmitted non-A, non-B hepatitis: serial passage of disease in cynomolgus macaques and tamarins and recovery of disease-associated 27- to 34-nm viruslike particles. *Proc Natl Acad Sci USA*, **84**, 6277–81.

Bradley, D., Andjaparidze, A., et al. 1988. Aetiological agent of enterically transmitted non-A, non-B hepatitis. *J Gen Virol*, **69**, 731–8.

Bromberg, K., Newhall, D.N. and Peter, G. 1982. Hepatitis A and meningoencephalitis. *JAMA*, **247**, 815.

Brown, E.A., Day, S.P., et al. 1991. The 5′ nontranslated region of hepatitis A virus: secondary structure and elements required for translation in vitro. *J Virol*, **65**, 5828–38.

Brown, E.A., Zajac, A.J. and Lemon, S.M. 1994. In vitro characterization of an internal ribosomal entry site (IRES) present within the 5′ nontranslated region of hepatitis A virus RNA: comparison with the IRES of encephalomyocarditis virus. *J Virol*, **68**, 1066–74.

Bruisten, S.M., van Steenbergen, J.E., et al. 2001. Molecular epidemiology of hepatitis A virus in Amsterdam, the Netherlands. *J Med Virol*, **63**, 88–95.

Bryan, J.P., Tsarev, S.A., et al. 1994. Epidemic hepatitis E in Pakistan: patterns of serologic response and evidence that antibody to hepatitis E virus protects against disease. *J Infect Dis*, **170**, 517–21.

Buisson, Y., Grandadam, M., et al. 2000. Identification of a novel hepatitis E virus in Nigeria. *J Gen Virol*, **81**, 903–9.

Centers for Disease Control, 1988. Hepatitis A among drug abusers. *MMWR*, **37**, 297–305.

Centers for Disease Control, 1994. *Hepatitis Surveillance Report No 55*. Atlanta GA: Centers for Disease Control and Prevention.

Chang, K.H., Brown, E.A. and Lemon, S.M. 1993. Cell type-specific proteins which interact with the 5′ nontranslated region of hepatitis A virus RNA. *J Virol*, **67**, 6716–25.

Chatterjee, R., Tsarev, S., et al. 1997. African strains of hepatitis E virus that are distinct from Asian strains. *J Med Virol*, **53**, 139–44.

Chauhan, A., Jameel, S., et al. 1993. Hepatitis E virus transmission to a volunteer. *Lancet*, **341**, 149–50.

Ching, K.Z., Nakano, T., et al. 2002. Genetic characterization of wild-type genotype VII hepatitis A virus. *J Gen Virol*, **83**, 53–60.

Cho, M.W. and Ehrenfeld, E. 1991. Rapid completion of the replication cycle of hepatitis A virus subsequent to reversal of guanidine inhibition. *Virology*, **180**, 770–80.

Cho, M.W., Teterina, N., et al. 1994. Membrane rearrangement and vesicle induction by recombinant poliovirus 2C and 2BC in human cells. *Virology*, **202**, 129–45.

Choo, Q.-L., Kuo, G., et al. 1989. Isolation of a cDNA clone derived from a blood-borne non-A, non-B viral hepatitis genome. *Science*, **244**, 359–62.

Chow, M., Newman, J.F.E., et al. 1987. Myristylation of picornavirus capsid protein VP4 and its structural significance. *Nature (London)*, **327**, 482–6.

Clark, M.E., Lieberman, P.M., et al. 1993. Direct cleavage of human TATA-binding protein by poliovirus protease 3C in vivo and in vitro. *Mol Cell Biol*, **13**, 1232–7.

Cohen, J.I., Rosenblum, B., et al. 1987a. Complete nucleotide sequence of an attenuated hepatitis A virus: comparison with wild-type virus. *Proc Natl Acad Sci USA*, **84**, 2497–501.

Cohen, J.I., Ticehurst, J.R., et al. 1987b. Hepatitis A virus cDNA and its RNA transcripts are infectious in cell culture. *J Virol*, **61**, 3035–9.

Cohen, J.I., Ticehurst, J.R., et al. 1987c. Complete nucleotide sequence of wild-type hepatitis A virus: comparison with different strains of hepatitis A virus and other picornaviruses. *J Virol*, **61**, 50–9.

Cohen, J.I., Feinstone, S. and Purcell, R.H. 1989. Hepatitis A virus infection in a chimpanzee: duration of viremia and detection of virus in saliva and throat swabs. *J Infect Dis*, **160**, 887–90.

Cohen, L., Benichou, D. and Martin, A. 2002. Analysis of deletion mutants indicates that the 2A polypeptide of hepatitis A virus participates in virion morphogenesis. *J Virol*, **76**, 7495–505.

Conrad, M.E. and Lemon, S.M. 1987. Prevention of endemic icteric viral hepatitis by administration of immune serum globulin. *J Infect Dis*, **156**, 56–63.

Corey, L. and Holmes, K.K. 1980. Sexual transmission of hepatitis A in homosexual men: incidence and mechanism. *N Engl J Med*, **302**, 435–8.

Costa-Mattioli, M., Ferre, V., et al. 2001a. Genetic variability of hepatitis A virus in South America reveals heterogeneity and co-circulation during epidemic outbreaks. *J Gen Virol*, **82**, 2647–52.

Costa-Mattioli, M., Monpoeho, S., et al. 2001b. Genetic analysis of hepatitis A virus outbreak in France confirms the co-circulation of subgenotypes IA, IB and reveals a new genetic lineage. *J Med Virol*, **65**, 233–40.

Costa-Mattioli, M., Cristina, J., et al. 2002. Molecular evolution of hepatitis A virus: a new classification based on the complete VP1 protein. *J Virol*, **76**, 9516–25.

Coursaget, P., Depril, N., et al. 1994. Hepatitis type E in a French population: detection of anti-HEV by a synthetic peptide-based enzyme-linked immunosorbent assay. *Res Virol*, **145**, 51–7.

Cromeans, T., Sobsey, M.D. and Fields, H.A. 1987. Development of a plaque assay for a cytopathic, rapidly replicating isolate of hepatitis A virus. *J Med Virol*, **22**, 45–56.

Cubitt, D., Bradley, D.W. et al. 1995. *Caliciviridae*. Virus Taxonomy: Classification and Nomenclature of Viruses, Murphy, F.A., Fauquet, C.M. et al. (eds). *Arch Virol Suppl*, **10**, 359–63.

Daemer, R.J., Feinstone, S.M., et al. 1981. Propagation of human hepatitis A virus in African green monkey kidney cell culture: primary isolation and serial passage. *Infect Immun*, **32**, 388–93.

Das, S. and Dasgupta, A. 1993. Identification of the cleavage site and determinants required for poliovirus 3C^Pro-catalyzed cleavage of human TATA-binding transcription factor TBP. *J Virol*, **67**, 3326–31.

Dawson, G.J., Chau, K.H., et al. 1992. Solid-phase enzyme-linked immunosorbent assay for hepatitis E virus IgG and IgM antibodies utilizing recombinant antigens and synthetic peptides. *J Virol Methods*, **38**, 1006–11.

Day, S.P., Murphy, P., et al. 1992. Mutations within the 5' nontranslated region of hepatitis A virus RNA which enhance replication in BS-C-1 cells. *J Virol*, **66**, 6533–40.

Decker, R.H., Overby, L.R., et al. 1979. Serologic studies of transmission of hepatitis A in humans. *J Infect Dis*, **139**, 74–82.

Decker, R.H., Kosakowski, S.M., et al. 1981. Diagnosis of acute hepatitis A by HAVAB^(R)-M, a direct radioimmunoassay for IgM anti-HAV. *Am J Clin Path*, **76**, 140–7.

Dentinger, C.M., Bower, W.A., et al. 2001. An outbreak of hepatitis A associated with green onions. *J Infect Dis*, **183**, 1273–6.

de Paula, V.S., Baptista, M.L., et al. 2002. Characterization of hepatitis A virus isolates from subgenotypes IA and IB in Rio de Janeiro, Brazil. *J Med Virol*, **66**, 22–7.

Diaz, B.I., Sariol, C.A., et al. 2001. Genetic relatedness of Cuban HAV wild-type isolates. *J Med Virol*, **64**, 96–103.

Dienstag, J.L., Feinstone, S.M., et al. 1975. Experimental infection of chimpanzees with hepatitis A virus. *J Infect Dis*, **132**, 532–45.

Dienstag, J.L., Popper, H. and Purcell, R.H. 1976. The pathology of viral hepatitis types A and B in chimpanzees. *Am J Pathol*, **85**, 131–44.

Dotzauer, A., Feinstone, S.M. and Kaplan, G. 1994. Susceptibility of nonprimate cell lines to hepatitis A virus infection. *J Virol*, **68**, 6064–8.

Dotzauer, A., Gebhardt, U., et al. 2000. Hepatitis A virus-specific immunoglobulin A mediates infection of hepatocytes with hepatitis A virus via the asialoglycoprotein receptor. *J Virol*, **74**, 10950–7.

Drobeniuc, J., Favorov, M.O., et al. 2001. Hepatitis E virus antibody prevalence among persons who work with swine. *J Infect Dis*, **184**, 1594–7.

Emerson, S.U., McRill, C., et al. 1991. Mutations responsible for adaptation of hepatitis A virus to efficient growth in cell culture. *J Virol*, **65**, 4882–6.

Emerson, S.U., Huang, Y.K., et al. 1992a. Mutations in both the 2B and 2C genes of hepatitis A virus are involved in adaptation to growth in cell culture. *J Virol*, **66**, 650–4.

Emerson, S.U., Huang, Y.K., et al. 1992b. Molecular basis of virulence and growth of hepatitis A virus in cell culture. *Vaccine*, **10**, suppl 1, S36–9.

Emerson, S.U., Huang, Y.K. and Purcell, R.H. 1993. 2B and 2C mutations are essential but mutations throughout the genome of HAV contribute to adaptation to cell culture. *Virology*, **194**, 475–80.

Emerson, S.U., Tsarev, S.A., et al. 1996. A simian strain of hepatitis A virus , AGM-27, functions as an attenuated vaccine for chimpanzees. *J Infect Dis*, **173**, 592–7.

Emerson, S.U., Zhang, M., et al. 2001. Recombinant hepatitis E virus genomes infectious for primates: importance of capping and discovery of a cis-reactive element. *Proc Natl Acad Sci USA*, **98**, 15270–5.

Emerson, S.U., Huang, Y.K., et al. 2002. Identification of VP1/2A and 2C as virulence genes of hepatitis A virus and demonstration of genetic instability of 2C. *J Virol*, **76**, 8551–9.

Emini, E.A., Hughes, J.V., et al. 1985. Induction of hepatitis A virus-neutralizing antibody by a virus-specific synthetic peptide. *J Virol*, **55**, 836–9.

Favorov, M.O., Fields, H.A., et al. 1992. Serologic identification of hepatitis E virus infections in epidemic and endemic settings. *J Med Virol*, **36**, 246–50.

Favorov, M.O., Khudyakov, Y.E., et al. 1994. Enzyme immunoassay for the detection of antibody to hepatitis E virus based on synthetic peptides. *J Virol Methods*, **46**, 237–50.

Favorov, M.O., Nazarova, O.K. et al. 1996. Cattle as a possible reservoir of hepatitis E virus infection [Abstract A140] Ninth Triennial International Symposium on Viral Hepatitis and Liver Disease (Rome) 21–25 April.

Favorov, M.O., Kosoy, M.Y., et al. 2000. Prevalence of antibody to hepatitis E virus among rodents in the United States. *J Infect Dis*, **181**, 34–40.

Feigelstock, D., Thompson, P., et al. 1998. The human homolog of HAV cr-1 codes for a hepatitis A virus cellular receptor. *J Virol*, **72**, 6621–8.

Feinstone, S.M., Kapikian, A.Z. and Purcell, R.H. 1973. Hepatitis A: detection by immune electron microscopy of a viruslike antigen associated with acute illness. *Science*, **182**, 1026–8.

Fleischer, B., Fleischer, S., et al. 1990. Clonal analysis of infiltrating T lymphocytes in liver tissue in viral hepatitis A. *Immunology*, **69**, 14–19.

Forbes, A. and Williams, R. 1990. Changing epidemiology and clinical aspects of hepatitis A. *Br Med Bull*, **46**, 303–18.

Frings, W. and Dotzauer, A. 2001. Adaptation of primate cell-adapted hepatitis A virus strain HM174 to growth in guinea pig cells is independent of mutations in the 5' nontranslated region. *J Gen Virol*, **82**, 597–602.

Frosner, G.G., Willers, H., et al. 1978. Decrease in incidence of hepatitis A infections in Germany. *Infection*, **6**, 259–60.

Frosner, G.G., Papaevangelou, G., et al. 1979. Antibody against hepatitis A in seven European countries. I. Comparison of prevalence data in different age groups. *Am J Epidemiol*, **110**, 63–9.

Fry, K.E., Tam, A.W., et al. 1992. Hepatitis E virus (HEV): strain variation in the nonstructural gene region encoding a consensus RNA-dependent RNA polymerase and a helicase domain. *Virus Genes*, **6**, 173–85.

Funkhouser, A.W., Purcell, R.H., et al. 1994. Attenuated hepatitis A virus: genetic determinants of adaptation to growth in MRC-5 cells. *J Virol*, **68**, 148–57.

Garkavenko, O., Obriadina, A., et al. 2001. Detection and characterization of swine hepatitis E virus in New Zealand. *J Med Virol*, **65**, 525–9.

Gellis, S.S., Stokes, J. Jr, et al. 1945. The use of human immune serum globulin (gamma globulin) in infectious (epidemic) hepatitis in the Mediterranean theater of operations. I. Studies on prophylaxis in two epidemics of infectious hepatitis. *JAMA*, **128**, 1062–3.

Glass, M.J. and Summers, D.F. 1992. A cis-acting element within the hepatitis A virus 5′-non-coding region required for in vitro translation. *Virus Res*, **26**, 15–31.

Glass, M.J. and Summers, D.F. 1993. Identification of a trans-acting activity from liver that stimulates hepatitis A virus translation in vitro. *Virology*, **193**, 1047–50.

Glikson, M., Galun, E., et al. 1992. Relapsing hepatitis A. Review of 14 cases and literature survey. *Medicine (Baltimore)*, **71**, 14–23.

Goldsmith, R., Yarbough, P.O., et al. 1992. Enzyme-linked immunosorbent assay for diagnosis of acute sporadic hepatitis E in Egyptian children. *Lancet*, **339**, 328–31.

Gordon, S.C., Reddy, K.R., et al. 1984. Prolonged intrahepatic cholestasis secondary to acute hepatitis A. *Ann Intern Med*, **101**, 635–7.

Gouvea, V., Snellings, N., et al. 1997. Hepatitis E virus in Nepal: similarities with the Burmese and Indian variants. *Virus Res*, **52**, 87–96.

Graff, J., Normann, A., et al. 1994. Nucleotide sequence of wild-type hepatitis A virus GBM in comparison with two cell culture-adapted variants. *J Virol*, **68**, 548–54.

Graff, J., Normann, A. and Flehmig, B. 1997. Influence of the 5′noncoding region of hepatitis A virus strain GBM on its growth in different cell lines. *J Gen Virol*, **78**, 1841–9.

Graff, J., Richards, O.C., et al. 1999. Hepatitis A virus capsid protein VP1 has a heterogeneous C terminus. *J Virol*, **73**, 6015–23.

Gupta, D.N. and Smetana, H.F. 1955. The histopathology of viral hepatitis as seen in Delhi epidemic. *Indian J Med Res*, **45**, suppl:, 101–13.

Hadler, S.C. 1991. Global impact of hepatitis A virus infection: changing patterns. In: Hollinger, F.B., Lemon, S.M. and Margolis, H.S. (eds), *Viral hepatitis and liver disease*. Baltimore MD: Williams & Wilkins, 14–20.

Hadler, S.C., Webster, H.M., et al. 1980. Hepatitis A in day-care centers: a community-wide assessment. *N Engl J Med*, **302**, 1222–7.

Hammond, G.W., MacDougall, B.K., et al. 1982. Encephalitis during the prodromal stage of acute hepatitis A. *Can Med Assoc J*, **126**, 269–70.

Haqshenas, G., Shivaprasad, H.L., et al. 2001. Genetic identification and characterization of a novel virus related to human hepatitis E virus from chickens with hepatitis-splenomegaly syndrome in the United States. *J Gen Virol*, **82**, 2449–62.

Harmon, S.A., Updike, W., et al. 1992. Polyprotein processing in cis and in trans by hepatitis A virus 3C protease cloned and expressed in Escherichia coli. *J Virol*, **66**, 5242–7.

Harmon, S.A., Broman, B., et al. 1993. Localization of priming epitope to the C-terminal portion of hepatitis A virus VP1. *J Infect Dis*, **167**, 990–2.

Harmon, S.A., Emerson, S.U., et al. 1995. Hepatitis A viruses with deletions in the 2A gene are infectious in cultured cells and marmosets. *J Virol*, **69**, 5576–81.

Havens, W.P. Jr 1944. Infectious hepatitis in the Middle East: a clinical review of 200 cases seen in a military hospital. *JAMA*, **126**, 17–23.

He, J., Tam, A.W., et al. 1993. Expression and diagnostic utility of hepatitis E virus putative structural proteins expressed in insect cells. *J Clin Microbiol*, **31**, 2167–73.

He, J., Binn, L.N., et al. 2000. Molecular characterization of a hepatitis E virus isolate from Namibia. *J Biomed Sci*, **7**, 334–8.

Hijikata, M., Hayashi, S., et al. 2002. Genotyping of hepatitis E virus from Vietnam. *Intervirology*, **45**, 101–4.

Hollinger, F.B., Khan, N.C., et al. 1983. Posttransfusion hepatitis type A. *JAMA*, **250**, 2313–17.

Hsieh, S.Y., Yang, P.Y., et al. 1998. Identification of a novel strain of hepatitis E virus responsible for sporadic acute hepatitis in Taiwan. *J Med Virol*, **55**, 300–4.

Hsieh, S.Y., Meng, X.Y., et al. 1999. Identify of a novel swine hepatitis E virus in Taiwan forming a monophyletic group with Taiwan isolates of human hepatitis E virus. *J Clin Microbiol*, **37**, 3828–34.

Huang, C.-C., Nguyen, D., et al. 1992. Molecular cloning and sequencing of the Mexico isolate of hepatitis E virus (HEV). *Virology*, **191**, 550–8.

Huang, R.T., Li, D.R., et al. 1992. Isolation and identification of hepatitis E virus in Xinjiang, China. *J Gen Virol*, **73**, 1143–8.

Hutin, Y.J., Pool, V., et al. 1999. A multistate, foodborne outbreak of hepatitis A. National Hepatitis A Investigation Team. *N Engl J Med*, **340**, 595–602.

Hyams, K.C., McCarthy, M.C., et al. 1992a. Acute sporadic hepatitis E in children living in Cairo, Egypt. *J Med Virol*, **37**, 274–7.

Hyams, K.C., Purdy, M.A., et al. 1992b. Acute sporadic hepatitis E in Sudanese children: analysis based on a new Western blot assay. *J Infect Dis*, **165**, 1001–5.

Immunization Practices Advisory Committee, 1990. Protection against viral hepatitis. *MMWR*, **39**, 1–26.

Innis, B.L., Snitbhan, R., et al. 1991. The declining transmission of hepatitis A in Thailand. *J Infect Dis*, **163**, 989–95.

Innis, B.L., Snitbhan, R., et al. 1994. Protection against hepatitis A by an inactivated vaccine. *JAMA*, **271**, 1328–34.

Jameel, S., Durgapal, H., et al. 1992. Enteric non-A, non-B hepatitis: epidemics, animal transmission, and hepatitis E virus detection by the polymerase chain reaction. *J Med Virol*, **37**, 263–70.

S., Zafrullah, M., et al. 1996. Expression in animal cells and characterization of the hepatitis E virus structural proteins. *J Virol*, **70**, 207–16.

Jansen, R.W., Newbold, J.E. and Lemon, S.M. 1988. Complete nucleotide sequence of a cell culture-adapted variant of hepatitis A virus: comparison with wild-type virus with restricted capacity for in vitro replication. *Virology*, **163**, 299–307.

Jansen, R.W., Siegl, G. and Lemon, S.M. 1990. Molecular epidemiology of human hepatitis A virus defined by an antigen-capture polymerase chain reaction method. *Proc Natl Acad Sci USA*, **87**, 2867–71.

Jewell, D.A., Swietnicki, W., et al. 1992. Hepatitis A virus 3C proteinase substrate specificity. *Biochemistry*, **31**, 7862–9.

Johnston, J.M., Harmon, S.A., et al. 1988. Antigenic and immunogenic properties of a hepatitis A virus capsid protein expressed in *Escherichia coli. J Infect Dis*, **157**, 1203–11.

Joshi, Y.K., Babu, S., et al. 1985. Immunoprophylaxis of epidemic non-A non-B hepatitis. *Indian J Med Res*, **81**, 18–19.

Kabrane-Lazizi, Y., Fine, B.J., et al. 1999a. Evidence for widespread infection of wild rats with hepatitis E virus in the United States. *Am J Trop Med Hyg*, **61**, 331–5.

Kabrane-Lazizi, Y., Meng, X.J., et al. 1999b. Evidence that the genomic RNA of hepatitis E virus is capped. *J Virol*, **73**, 8848–50.

Kaplan, G., Totsuka, A., et al. 1996. Identification of a surface glycoprotein on African green monkey kidney cells as a receptor for hepatitis A virus. *EMBO J*, **15**, 4282–96.

Karayiannis, P., Jowett, T., et al. 1986. Hepatitis A virus replication in tamarins and host immune response in relation to pathogenesis of liver cell damage. *J Med Virol*, **18**, 261–76.

Karron, R.A., Ticehurst, J.R. et al. 1986. Evaluation of attenuation of hepatitis A virus in primates, *Abstracts of the 1986 Interscience Conference on Antimicrobial Agents and Chemotherapy*, American Society for Microbiology, Washington, 278.

Kaur, M., Hyams, K.C., et al. 1992. Human linear B-cell epitopes encoded by the hepatitis E virus include determinants in the RNA-dependent RNA polymerase. *Proc Natl Acad Sci USA*, **89**, 3855–8.

Kazachkov, Y., Balayan, M.S., et al. 1992. Hepatitis E virus in cultivated cells. *Arch Virol*, **127**, 399–402.

Khudyakov, Y.E., Khudyakova, N.S., et al. 1993. Epitope mapping in proteins of hepatitis E virus. *Virology*, **194**, 89–96.

Khudyakov, Y.E., Lopareva, E.N., et al. 1999. Antigenic epitopes of the hepatitis A virus polyprotein. *Virology*, **260**, 260–72.

Khuroo, M.S. 1980. Study of an epidemic of non-A, non-B hepatitis: possibility of another human hepatitis virus distinct from post-transfusion non-A, non-B type. *Am J Med*, **68**, 818–24.

Khuroo, M.S., Teli, M.R., et al. 1981. Incidence and severity of viral hepatitis in pregnancy. *Am J Med*, **70**, 252–5.

Khuroo, M.S. and Dar, M.V. 1992. Hepatitis E: evidence for person-to-person transmission and inability of low dose immune serum globulin from an Indian source to prevent it. *Indian J Gastroenterol*, **11**, 109–12.

Koonin, E.V., Gorbalenya, A.E., et al. 1992. Computer-assisted assignment of functional domains in the nonstructural polyprotein of hepatitis E virus: delineation of an additional group of positive-strand RNA plant and animal viruses. *Proc Natl Acad Sci USA*, **89**, 8259–63.

Krah, D.L., Amin, R.D., et al. 1991. A simple antigen-reduction assay for the measurement of neutralizing antibodies to hepatitis A virus. *J Infect Dis*, **163**, 634–7.

Krugman, S. and Ward, R. 1958. Clinical and experimental studies of infectious hepatitis. *Pediatrics*, **22**, 1016–22.

Krugman, S., Ward, R., et al. 1960. Infectious hepatitis: studies on the effect of gammaglobulin and on the incidence of inapparent infection. *JAMA*, **174**, 323–30.

Krugman, S., Ward, R. and Giles, J.P. 1962. The natural history of infectious hepatitis. *Am J Med*, **32**, 717–28.

Kusov, Y.Y., Sommergruber, W., et al. 1992. Intermolecular cleavage of hepatitis A virus (HAV) precursor protein P1-P2 by recombinant HAV proteinase 3C. *J Virol*, **66**, 6794–6.

Lednar, W.M., Lemon, S.M., et al. 1985. Frequency of illness associated with epidemic hepatitis A virus infections in adults. *Am J Epidemiol*, **122**, 226–33.

LeDuc, J.W., Lemon, S.M., et al. 1983. Experimental infection of the New World owl monkey (*Aotus trivirgatus*) with hepatitis A virus. *Infect Immun*, **40**, 766–72.

Lemon, S.M. 1985a. IgM neutralizing antibody to hepatitis A virus. *J Infect Dis*, **152**, 1353–4.

Lemon, S.M. 1985b. Type A viral hepatitis: new developments in an old disease. *N Engl J Med*, **313**, 1059–67.

Lemon, S.M. 1994. Inactivated hepatitis A vaccines. *JAMA*, **271**, 1363–4.

Lemon, S.M. and Binn, L.N. 1983a. Antigenic relatedness of two strains of hepatitis A virus determined by cross-neutralization. *Infect Immun*, **42**, 418–20.

Lemon, S.M. and Binn, L.N. 1983b. Serum neutralizing antibody response to hepatitis A virus. *J Infect Dis*, **148**, 1033–9.

Lemon, S.M. and Shapiro, C.N. 1994. The value of immunization against hepatitis A. *Infect Agents Dis*, **3**, 38–49.

Lemon, S.M., Brown, C.D., et al. 1980. Specific immunoglobulin M response to hepatitis A virus determined by solid-phase radioimmunoassay. *Infect Immun*, **28**, 927–36.

Lemon, S.M., Binn, L.N. and Marchwicki, R.H. 1983. Radioimmunofocus assay for quantitation of hepatitis A virus in cell cultures. *J Clin Microbiol*, **17**, 834–9.

Lemon, S.M., Jansen, R.W. and Newbold, J.E. 1985. Infectious hepatitis A virus particles produced in cell culture consist of three distinct types with different buoyant densities in CsCl. *J Virol*, **54**, 78–85.

Lemon, S.M., Binn, L.N., et al. 1990. In vivo replication and reversion to wild-type of a neutralization-resistant variant of hepatitis A virus. *J Infect Dis*, **161**, 7–13.

Lemon, S.M., Amphlett, E. and Sangar, D. 1991a. Protease digestion of hepatitis A virus: disparate effects on capsid proteins, antigenicity, and infectivity. *J Virol*, **65**, 5636–40.

Lemon, S.M., Murphy, P.C., et al. 1991b. Antigenic and genetic variation in cytopathic hepatitis A virus variants arising during persistent infection: evidence for genetic recombination. *J Virol*, **65**, 2056–65.

Lemon, S.M., Ping, L.-H., et al. 1991c. Immunobiology of hepatitis A virus. In: Hollinger, F.B., Lemon, S.M. and Margolis, H.S. (eds), *Viral hepatitis and liver disease*. Baltimore MD: Williams & Wilkins, 20–4.

Lemon, S.M., Jansen, R.W. and Brown, E.A. 1992a. Genetic, antigenic, and biologic differences between strains of hepatitis A virus. *Vaccine*, **10**, S40–4.

Lemon, S.M., Barclay, W., et al. 1992b. Immunogenicity and antigenicity of chimeric picornaviruses which express hepatitis A virus (HAV) peptide sequences: evidence for a neutralization domain near the amino terminus of VP1 of HAV. *Virology*, **188**, 285–95.

Lewis, J.A., Armstrong, M.E., et al. 1991. Use of a live attenuated hepatitis A vaccine to prepare a highly purified, formalin-inactivated hepatitis A vaccine. In: Hollinger, F.B., Lemon, S.M. and Margolis, H.S. (eds), *Viral hepatitis and liver disease*. Baltimore MD: Williams & Wilkins, 94–7.

Li, F., Zhuang, H., et al. 1994. Persistent and transient antibody responses to hepatitis E virus detected by Western immunoblot using open reading frame 2 and 3 and glutathione *S*-transferase fusion proteins. *J Clin Microbiol*, **32**, 2060–6.

Li, K., Zhuang, H. and Zhu, W. 2002. Partial nucleotide sequencing of hepatitis E viruses detected in sera of patients wit hepatitis E from 14 cities in China. *Chin Med J*, **115**, 1058–63.

Li, T.C., Yamakawa, Y., et al. 1997. Expression and self-assemble of empty virus-like particles of hepatitis E virus. *J Virol*, **71**, 7207–13.

Liang, T.J., Jeffers, L., et al. 1993. Fulminant or subfulminant non-A, non-B viral hepatitis: the role of hepatitis C and E viruses. *Gastroenterology*, **104**, 556–62.

Locarnini, S.A., Coulepis, A.G., et al. 1979. Solid-phase enzyme-linked immunosorbent assay for detection of hepatitis A-specific immunoglobulin M. *J Clin Microbiol*, **9**, 459–65.

Locarnini, S.A., Coulepis, A.G., et al. 1980. Coproantibodies in hepatitis A: detection of enzyme-linked immunosorbent assay and immune electron microscopy. *J Clin Microbiol*, **11**, 710–16.

Longer, C.F., Denny, S.L., et al. 1993. Experimental hepatitis E: pathogenesis in cynomolgus macaques (*Macaca fascicularis*). *J Infect Dis*, **168**, 602–9.

Lu, L., Ching, K.Z., et al. 2004. Characterization of the complete genomic sequence of genotype II hepatitis A virus (CF53/Berne isolate). *J Gen Virol*, **85**, 2943–52.

Luo, M., Rossmann, M.G. and Palmenberg, A.C. 1988. Prediction of three-dimensional models for foot-and-mouth disease virus and hepatitis A virus. *Virology*, **166**, 503–14.

MacCallum, F.O. and Bradley, W.H. 1944. Transmission of infective hepatitis to human volunteers. *Lancet*, **2**, 228.

Magden, J., Takeda, N., et al. 2001. Virus specific mRNA capping enzyme encoded by hepatitis E virus. *J Virol*, **75**, 6249–55.

Maier, K., Gabriel, P., et al. 1988. Human gamma interferon production by cytotoxic T lymphocytes sensitized during hepatitis A virus infection. *J Virol*, **62**, 3756–63.

Malbrain, M.L.N.G., Lambrecht, G.L.Y., et al. 1994. Acute renal failure in non-fulminant hepatitis A. *Clin Nephrol*, **41**, 180–1.

Malcolm, B.A., Chin, S.M., et al. 1992. Expression and characterization of recombinant hepatitis A virus 3C proteinase. *Biochemistry*, **31**, 3358–63.

Mannucci, P.M., Gdovin, S., et al. 1994. Transmission of hepatitis A to patients with hemophilia by factor VIII concentrates treated with organic solvent and detergent to inactivate viruses. *Ann Intern Med*, **120**, 1–7.

Mao, J.S., Dong, D.X., et al. 1989. Primary study of attenuated live hepatitis A vaccine (H2 strain) in humans. *J Infect Dis*, **159**, 621–4.

Mao, J.S., Dong, D.X., et al. 1991. Further studies of attenuated live hepatitis A vaccine (H2 strain) in humans. In: Hollinger, F.B., Lemon, S.M. and Margolis, H.S. (eds), *Viral hepatitis and liver disease*. Baltimore MD: Williams & Wilkins, 110–11.

Martin, A., Escriou, N., et al. 1995. Identification and site-direct mutagenesis of the primary (2A/2B) cleavage site of the hepatitis A virus polyprotein: functional impact on the infectivity of HAV transcripts. *Virology*, **213**, 213–22.

Martin, A., Benichou, D., et al. 1999. Maturation of the hepatitis A virus capsid protein VP1 is not dependent on processing by the 3Cpro proteinase. *J Virol*, **73**, 6220–7.

Mast, E.E., Polish, L.B., et al. 1993. Hepatitis E among refugees in Kenya: minimal apparent person-to-person transmission, evidence for age-dependent disease expression and new serologic assays. In: Nishioka, K., Suzuki, H., et al. (eds), *Viral hepatitis and liver disease*. Tokyo: Springer-Verlag, 375–8.

Mast, E.E., Kuramoto, I.K., et al. 1997. Prevalence of and risk factors for antibody to hepatitis E virus seroreactivity among blood donors in Northern California. *J Infect Dis*, **176**, 34–40.

Mathiesen, L.R., Drucker, J., et al. 1978a. Localization of hepatitis A antigen in marmoset organs during acute infection with hepatitis A virus. *J Infect Dis*, **138**, 369–77.

Mathiesen, L.R., Feinstone, S.M., et al. 1978b. Enzyme-linked immunosorbent assay for detection of hepatitis A antigen in stool and antibody to hepatitis A antigen in sera: comparison with solid-phase radioimmunoassay, immune electron microscopy, and immune adherence hemagglutination assay. *J Clin Microbiol*, **7**, 184–93.

Mathiesen, L.R., Moller, A.M., et al. 1980. Hepatitis A virus in the liver and intestine of marmosets after oral inoculation. *Infect Immun*, **28**, 45–8.

Matsuda, H., Okada, K., et al. 2003. Severe hepatitis E virus infection after ingestion of uncooked liver from a wild boar. *J Infect Dis*, **188**, 944.

Mattioli, S., Imberti, L., et al. 1995. Mimicry of the immunodominant conformation-dependent antigenic site of hepatitis A virus by motifs selected from synthetic peptide libraries. *J Virol*, **69**, 5294–9.

Mbayed, V.A., Sookoian, S., et al. 2002. Genetic characterization of hepatitis A virus isolates from Buenos Aires, Argentina. *J Med Virol*, **68**, 168–74.

McIntire, J.J., Umetsu, S.E., et al. 2001. Identification of Tapr (an airway hyperreactivity regulatory locus) and the linked Tim gene family. *Nat Immunol*, **2**, 1109–16.

Meng, X.J., Purcell, R.H., et al. 1997. A novel virus in swine is closely related to the human hepatitis E virus. *Proc Natl Acad Sci USA*, **94**, 9860–5.

Meng, J., Cong, M., et al. 1999. Primary structure of open reading frame 2 and 3 of the hepatitis E virus isolated from Morocco. *J Med Virol*, **57**, 126–33.

Meng, J., Dai, X., et al. 2001. Identification and characterization of the neutralization epitope(s) of the hepatitis E virus. *Virology*, **288**, 203–11.

Meng, X.J., Wiseman, B., et al. 2002. Prevalence of antibodies to hepatitis E virus in veterinarians working with swine and in normal blood donors in the United States and other countries. *J Clin Microbiol*, **40**, 117–20.

Midthun, K., Ellerbeck, E., et al. 1991. Safety and immunogenicity of a live attenuated hepatitis A virus vaccine in seronegative volunteers. *J Infect Dis*, **163**, 735–9.

Minor, P.D. 1991. *Picornaviridae*. Classification and Nomenclature of Viruses: the Fifth Report of the International Committee on Taxonomy of Viruses, Francki, R.I.B., Fauquet, C.M. et al. (eds). *Arch Virol Suppl*, **2**, 320–6.

Morrow, R.H., Smetana, H.F., et al. 1968. Unusual features of viral hepatitis in Accra, Ghana. *Ann Intern Med*, **68**, 1250–64.

Nainan, O.V., Margolis, H.S., et al. 1991. Sequence analysis of a new hepatitis A virus naturally infecting cynomolgus macaques (*Macaca fascicularis*). *J Gen Virol*, **72**, 1685–9.

Nainan, O.V., Brinton, M.A. and Margolis, H.S. 1992. Identification of amino acids located in the antibody binding sites of human hepatitis A virus. *Virology*, **191**, 984–7.

Najarian, R., Caput, D., et al. 1985. Primary structure and gene organization of human hepatitis A virus. *Proc Natl Acad Sci USA*, **82**, 2627–31.

Nakai, K., Winn, K.M., et al. 2001. Molecular characteristic-based epidemiology of hepatitis B, C and E viruses and GB virus C/hepatitis G virus in Myanmar. *J Clin Microbiol*, **39**, 1536–9.

Nanda, S.K., Yalcinkaya, K., et al. 1994. Etiological role of hepatitis E virus in sporadic fulminant hepatitis. *J Med Virol*, **42**, 133–7.

Nanda, S.K., Ansari, I.H., et al. 1995. Protracted viremia during acute sporadic hepatitis E virus infection. *Gastroenterology*, **108**, 225–30.

Nishizawa, T., Takahashi, M., et al. 2003. Characterization of Japanese swine and human hepatitis E virus isolates of genotype IV with 99 percent identity over the entire genome. *J Gen Virol*, **85**, 1245–51.

Niu, M.T., Polish, L.B., et al. 1992. Multistate outbreak of hepatitis A associated with frozen strawberries. *J Infect Dis*, **166**, 518–24.

Nuesch, J.P., Weitz, M. and Siegl, G. 1993. Proteins specifically binding to the 3′ untranslated region of hepatitis A virus RNA in persistently infected cells. *Arch Virol*, **128**, 65–79.

Ogawa, M., Hori, J., et al. 1994. A fatal case of acute renal failure associated with non-fulminant hepatitis A. *Clin Nephrol*, **42**, 205–6.

Okamoto, H., Takahashi, M., et al. 2001. Analysis of the complete genome of indigenous swine hepatitis E virus isolated in Japan. *Biochem Biophys Res Commun*, **289**, 929–36.

Palmenberg, A.C. 1989. Sequence alignments of picornavirus capsid proteins. In: Semler, B.L. and Ehrenfeld, E. (eds), *Molecular aspects of picornavirus infections and detections*. Washington: American Society for Microbiology, 211–41.

Paul, D.A., Knigge, M.F., et al. 1994. Determination of hepatitis E virus seroprevalence by using recombinant fusion proteins and synthetic peptides. *J Infect Dis*, **169**, 801–6.

Payne, C.J., Ellis, T.M., et al. 1999. Sequence data suggests big liver and spleen disease virus (BLSV) is genetically related to hepatitis E virus. *Vet Microbiol*, **68**, 119–25.

Pina, S., Buti, M., et al. 2000. HEV identified in serum from humans with acute hepatitis and in sewage of animal origin in Spain. *J Hepatol*, **33**, 826–33.

Ping, L.-H. and Lemon, S.M. 1992. Antigenic structure of human hepatitis A virus defined by analysis of escape mutants selected against murine monoclonal antibodies. *J Virol*, **66**, 2208–16.

Ping, L.-H., Jansen, R.W., et al. 1988. Identification of an immunodominant antigenic site involving the capsid protein VP3 of hepatitis A virus. *Proc Natl Acad Sci USA*, **85**, 8281–5.

Prikazsky, V., Olear, V., et al. 1994. Interruption of an outbreak of hepatitis A in two villages by vaccination. *J Med Virol*, **44**, 457–9.

Probst, C., Jecht, M. and Gauss-Muller, V. 1997. Proteinase 3C-mediated processing of VP1-2A of two hepatitis A virus strains: in vivo evidence for cleavage at amino acid position 273/274 of VP1. *J Virol*, **71**, 3288–92.

Provost, P.J. and Hilleman, M.R. 1979. Propagation of human hepatitis A virus in cell culture in vitro. *Proc Soc Exp Biol Med*, **160**, 213–21.

Provost, P.J., Banker, F.S., et al. 1982. Progress toward a live, attenuated human hepatitis A vaccine. *Proc Soc Exp Biol Med*, **170**, 8–14.

Provost, P.J., Bishop, R.P., et al. 1986. New findings in live, attenuated hepatitis A vaccine development. *J Med Virol*, **20**, 165–75.

Purcell, R.H. 1991. Approaches to immunization against hepatitis A virus. In: Hollinger, F.B., Lemon, S.M. and Margolis, H.S. (eds), *Viral hepatitis and liver disease*. Baltimore MD: Williams & Wilkins, 41–6.

Purcell, R.H., Feinstone, S.M., et al. 1984. Hepatitis A virus. In: Vyas, G.N., Dienstag, J.L. and Hoofnagle, J.H. (eds), *Viral hepatitis and liver disease*. Orlando FL: Grune & Stratton, 9–22.

Purcell, R.H., Nguyen, H., et al. 2003. Preclinical immunogenicity and efficacy trial of a recombinant hepatitis E vaccine. *Vaccine*, **21**, 2607–15.

Purdy, M.A., McCaustland, K.A., et al. 1993. Preliminary evidence that a *trpE*-HEV fusion protein protects cynomolgus macaques against challenge with wild-type hepatitis E virus (HEV). *J Med Virol*, **41**, 90–4.

Ray, R., Jameel, S. and Manivel, V. 1992. Indian hepatitis E virus shows a major deletion in the small open reading frame. *Virology*, **189**, 359–62.

Raychaudhuri, G., Govindarajan, S., et al. 1998. Utilization of chimeras between human (HM-175) and simian (AGM-27) strains of hepatitis A virus to study the molecular basis of virulence. *J Virol*, **72**, 7467–75.

Reyes, G.R., Purdy, M.A., et al. 1990. Isolation of a cDNA from the virus responsible for enterically transmitted non-A, non-B hepatitis. *Science*, **247**, 1335–9.

Riddell, M.A., Li, F. and Anderson, D.A. 2000. Identification of immunodominanat and conformational epitopes in the capsid protein of hepatitis E virus by using monoclonal antibodies. *J Virol*, **74**, 8011–17.

Robertson, B.H., Khanna, B., et al. 1988. Large scale production of hepatitis A virus in cell culture: effect of type of infection on virus yield and cell integrity. *J Gen Virol*, **69**, 29–34.

Robertson, B.H., Brown, V.K., et al. 1989. Structure of the hepatitis A virion: identification of potential surface-exposed regions. *Arch Virol*, **104**, 117–28.

Robertson, B.H., Khanna, B., et al. 1991. Epidemiologic patterns of wild-type hepatitis A virus determined by genetic variation. *J Infect Dis*, **163**, 286–92.

Robertson, B.H., Jansen, R.W., et al. 1992. Genetic relatedness of hepatitis A virus strains recovered from different geographic regions. *J Gen Virol*, **73**, 1365–77.

Robertson, B.H., Jia, X.-Y., et al. 1993. Antibody response to nonstructural proteins of hepatitis A virus following infection. *J Med Virol*, **40**, 76–82.

Robertson, B.H., D'Hondt, E.H., et al. 1994a. Effect of postexposure vaccination in a chimpanzee model of hepatitis A virus infection. *J Med Virol*, **43**, 249–51.

Robertson, B.H., Friedberg, D., et al. 1994b. Sequence variability of hepatitis A virus and factor VIII associated hepatitis A infections in hemophilia patients in Europe. An update. *Vox Sang*, **67**, suppl 1, 39–46.

Robertson, B.H., Averhoff, F., et al. 2000. Genetic relatedness of hepatitis A virus isolates during a community-wide outbreak. *J Med Virol*, **62**, 144–50.

Ropp, S.L., Tam, A.W., et al. 2000. Expression of the hepatitis E virus ORF1. *Arch Virol*, **145**, 1321–37.

Rosenblum, L.S., Mirkin, I.R., et al. 1990. A multifocal outbreak of hepatitis A traced to commercially distributed lettuce. *Am J Public Health*, **80**, 1075–9.

Rosenblum, L.S., Villarino, M.E., et al. 1991. Hepatitis A outbreak in a neonatal intensive care unit: risk factors for transmission and evidence of prolonged viral excretion among preterm infants. *J Infect Dis*, **164**, 476–82.

Ross, B.C., Anderson, R.N., et al. 1989. Nucleotide sequence of high-passage hepatitis A virus strain HM175: comparison with wild-type and cell culture-adapted strains. *J Gen Virol*, **70**, 2805–10.

Rueckert, R.R. and Wimmer, E. 1984. Systematic nomenclature of picornavirus proteins. *J Virol*, **50**, 957–9.

Sallie, R., Rayner, A., et al. 1992. Detection of hepatitis 'C' virus in formalin-fixed liver tissue by nested polymerase chain reaction. *J Med Virol*, **37**, 310–14.

Sallie, R., Silva, A.E., et al. 1994. Hepatitis C and E in non-A non-B fulminant hepatic failure: a polymerase chain reaction and serological study. *J Hepatol*, **20**, 580–8.

Schlauder, G.G. and Mushahwar, I.K. 2001. Genetic heterogeneity of hepatitis E virus. *J Med Virol*, **65**, 282–92.

Schlauder, G.G., Dawson, G.J., et al. 1998. The sequence and phylogenetic analysis of a novel hepatitis E virus isolated from a patient with acute hepatitis reported in the United States. *J Gen Virol*, **79**, 447–56.

Schlauder, G.G., Desai, S.M., et al. 1999. Novel hepatitis E virus (HEV) isolates from Europe: evidene for additional genotypes of HEV. *J Med Virol*, **57**, 243–51.

Schofield, D.J., Satterfield, W., et al. 2002. Four chimpanzee monoclonal antibodies isolated by phage display neutralize hepatitis A virus. *Virology*, **292**, 127–36.

Schofield, D.J., Purcell, R.H., et al. 2003. Monoclonal antibodies that neutralize HEV recognize an antigenic site at the carboxyterminus of an ORF2 protein vaccine. *Vaccine*, **22**, 257–67.

Schultheiss, T., Kusov, Y.Y. and Gauss-Müller, V. 1994. Proteinase 3C of hepatitis A virus (HAV) cleaves the HAV polyprotein P2-P3 at all sites including VP1/2A and 2A/2B. *Virology*, **198**, 275–81.

Schultheiss, T., Sommergruber, W., et al. 1995. Cleavage specificity of purified recombinant hepatitis A virus 3C proteinase on natural substrates. *J Virol*, **9**, 1727–33.

Schultz, D.E., Hardin, C.C. and Lemon, S.M. 1996a. Specific interaction of glyceraldehyde 3-phosphate dehydrogenase with the 5′ nontranslated RNA of hepatitis A virus. *J Biol Chem*, **271**, 14134–42.

Schultz, D.E., Honda, M., et al. 1996b. Mutations within the 5′ nontranslated RNA of cell culture-adapted hepatitis A virus which enhance cap-independent translation in cultured African green monkey kidney cells. *J Virol*, **70**, 1041–9.

Shaffer, D.R. and Lemon, S.M. 1995. Temperature-sensitive hepatitis A virus mutants with deletions downstream of the first pyrimidine-rich tract of the 5′ nontranslated RNA are impaired in RNA synthesis. *J Virol*, **69**, 6498–506.

Shaffer, D.R., Brown, E.A. and Lemon, S.M. 1994. Large deletion mutations involving the first pyrimidine-rich tract of the 5′ nontranslated RNA of hepatitis A virus define two adjacent domains associated with distinct replication phenotypes. *J Virol*, **68**, 5568–78.

Shaffer, D.R., Emerson, S.U., et al. 1995. A hepatitis A virus deletion mutant which lacks the first pyrimidine-rich tract of the 5′ nontranslated RNA remains virulent in primates following direct intrahepatic nucleic acid transfection. *J Virol*, **69**, 6600–4.

Sherertz, R.J., Russell, B.A. and Reuman, P.D. 1984. Transmission of hepatitis A by tranfusion of blood products. *Arch Intern Med*, **144**, 1579–80.

Shimizu, Y.K., Shikata, T., et al. 1982. Detection of hepatitis A antigen in human liver. *Infect Immun*, **36**, 320–4.

Shrestha, S.M., Shrestha, S., et al. 2003. Molecular investigation of hepatitis E virus infection in patients with acute hepatitis in Kathmandu, Nepal. *J Med Virol*, **69**, 207–14.

Siebke, J.C., Degre, M., et al. 1982. Prevalence of hepatitis A antibodies in a normal population and some selected groups of patients in Norway. *Am J Epidemiol*, **115**, 185–91.

Siegl, G. and Eggers, H.J. 1982. Failure of guanidine and 2-(α-hydroxybenzyl)benzimidazole to inhibit replication of hepatitis A virus in vitro. *J Gen Virol*, **61**, 111–14.

Siegl, G., Weitz, M. and Kronauer, G. 1984. Stability of hepatitis A virus. *Intervirology*, **22**, 218–26.

Silberstein, E., Dveksler, G. and Kaplan, G.G. 2001. Neutralization of hepatitis A virus (HAV) by an immunoadhesin containing the cysteine-rich region of HAV cellular receptor-1. *J Virol*, **75**, 717–25.

Sjogren, M.H., Tanno, H., et al. 1987. Hepatitis A virus in stool during clinical relapse. *Ann Intern Med*, **106**, 221–6.

Sjogren, M.H., Purcell, R.H., et al. 1992. Clinical and laboratory observations following oral or intramuscular administration of a live, attenuated hepatitis A vaccine candidate. *Vaccine*, **10**, suppl 1, S135–7.

Smith, H.M., Reporter, R., et al. 2002. Prevalence study of antibody to ratborne pathogens and other agents among patients using a free clinic in downtown Los Angeles. *J Infect Dis*, **186**, 1637–76.

Stapleton, J.T. and Lemon, S.M. 1987. Neutralization escape mutants define a dominant immunogenic neutralization site on hepatitis A virus. *J Virol*, **61**, 491–8.

Stapleton, J.T., Jansen, R.W. and Lemon, S.M. 1985. Neutralizing antibody to hepatitis A virus in immune serum globulin and in the sera of human recipients of immune serum globulin. *Gastroenterology*, **89**, 637–42.

Stapleton, J.T., Lange, D.K., et al. 1991. The role of secretory immunity in hepatitis A virus infection. *J Infect Dis*, **163**, 7–11.

Stapleton, J.T., Raina, V., et al. 1993. Antigenic and immunogenic properties of recombinant hepatitis A virus 14S and 70S subviral particles. *J Virol*, **67**, 1080–5.

Stewart, D.R., Morris, T.S., et al. 1997. Detection of antibodies to the nonstructural 3C proteinase of hepatitis A virus. *J Infect Dis*, **176**, 593–601.

Surjit, M., Jameel, S. and Lal, S.K. 2004. The ORF2 protein of hepatitis E binds the 5′ region of viral RNA. *J Virol*, **78**, 320–8.

Szmuness, W., Dienstag, J.L., et al. 1977. The prevalence of antibody to hepatitis A antigen in various parts of the world: a pilot study. *Am J Epidemiol*, **106**, 392–8.

Takahashi, K., Iwata, K., et al. 2001. Full genome nucleotide sequence of a hepatitis E virus strain that may be indigenous to Japan. *Virology*, **287**, 9–12.

Takahashi, K., Kang, J.H., et al. 2003a. Full-length sequences of six hepatitis E virus isolates of genotypes III and IV from patients with sporadic acute or fulminant hepatitis in Japan. *Intervirology*, **46**, 308–18.

Takahashi, K., Nishizawa, T. and Okamoto, H. 2003b. Identification of a genotype III swine hepatitis E virus that was isolated from a Japanese pig born in 1990 and that is most closely related to Japanese isolates of human hepatitis E virus. *J Clin Microbiol*, **41**, 1342–3.

Tam, A.W., Smith, M.M., et al. 1991. Hepatitis E virus (HEV): molecular cloning and sequencing of the full-length viral genome. *Virology*, **185**, 120–31.

Tam, A.W., White, R., et al. 1996. In vitro propagation and production of hepatitis E virus from in vivo infected primary macaque hepatocytes. *Virology*, **215**, 1–9.

Taylor, M.B. 1997. Molecular epidemiology of South African strains of hepatitis A virus: 1982–1996. *J Med Virol*, **51**, 273–9.

Tei, S., Kitajima, N., et al. 2003. Zoonotic transmission of hepatitis E virus from deer to human beings. *Lancet*, **362**, 371–3.

Teixera, M.R. Jr, Weller, I.V.D., et al. 1982. The pathology of hepatitis A in man. *Liver*, **2**, 53–60.

Tesar, M., Harmon, S.A., et al. 1992. Hepatitis A virus polyprotein synthesis initiates from two alternative AUG codons. *Virology*, **186**, 609–18.

Tesar, M., Jia, X.-Y., et al. 1993. Analysis of a potential myristoylation site in hepatitis A virus capsid protein VP4. *Virology*, **194**, 616–26.

Tesar, M., Pak, I., et al. 1994. Expression of hepatitis A virus precursor protein P3 in vivo and in vitro: polyprotein processing of the 3CD cleavage site. *Virology*, **198**, 524–33.

Thompson, P., Lu, J. and Kaplan, G.G. 1998. The Cys-rich region of hepatitis A virus cellular receptor is required for binding of hepatitis A virus and protective monoclonal antibody 190/4. *J Virol*, **72**, 3751–61.

Ticehurst, J. 1991. Identification and characterization of hepatitis E virus. In: Hollinger, F.B., Lemon, S.M. and Margolis, H.S. (eds), *Viral hepatitis and liver disease*. Baltimore MD: Williams & Wilkins, 501–13.

Ticehurst, J., Rhodes, L.L., et al. 1992. Infection of owl monkeys (*Aotus trivirgatus*) and cynomolgus monkeys (*Macaca fascicularis*) with hepatitis E virus from Mexico. *J Infect Dis*, **165**, 835–45.

Torresi, J., Li, F., et al. 1999. Only the non-glycosylated fraction of hepatitis E virus capsid (open reading frame 2) protein is stable in mammalian cells. *J Gen Virol*, **80**, 1185–8.

Tsarev, S.A., Emerson, S.U., et al. 1991. Simian hepatitis A virus (HAV) strain AGM-27: comparison of genome structure and growth in cell culture with other HAV strains. *J Gen Virol*, **72**, 1677–83.

Tsarev, S.A., Emerson, S.U., et al. 1992. Characterization of a prototype strain of hepatitis E virus. *Proc Natl Acad Sci USA*, **89**, 559–63.

Tsarev, S.A., Emerson, S.U., et al. 1993a. Variation in course of hepatitis E in experimentally infected cynomolgus monkeys. *J Infect Dis*, **167**, 1302–6.

Tsarev, S.A., Tsareva, T.S., et al. 1993b. ELISA for antibody to hepatitis E virus (HEV) based on complete open-reading frame-2 protein expressed in insect cells: identification of HEV infection in primates. *J Infect Dis*, **168**, 369–78.

Tsarev, S.A., Tsareva, T.S., et al. 1994a. Successful passive and active immunization of cynomolgus monkeys against hepatitis E. *Proc Natl Acad Sci USA*, **91**, 10198–202.

Tsarev, S.A., Tsareva, T.S., et al. 1994b. Infectivity titration of a prototype strain of hepatitis E virus in cynomolgus monkeys. *J Med Virol*, **43**, 135–42.

Tsarev, S.A., Tsareva, T.S., et al. 1997. Recombinant vaccine against hepatitis E: dose response and protection against heterologous challenge. *Vaccine*, **15**, 1834–8.

Tsarev, S.A., Binn, L.N., et al. 1999. Phylogenetic analysis of hepatitis E virus isolates from Egypt. *J Med Virol*, **57**, 68–74.

Tyagi, S., Korkaya, H., et al. 2002. The phosphorylated form of the ORF3 protein of hepatitis E virus interacts with its non-glycosylated form of the major capsid protine, ORF2. *J Biol Chem*, **277**, 22759–67.

Vallbracht, A., Gabriel, P., et al. 1986. Cell-mediated cytotoxicity in hepatitis A virus infection. *Hepatology*, **6**, 1308–14.

Vallbracht, A., Maier, K., et al. 1989. Liver-derived cytotoxic T cells in hepatitis A virus infection. *J Infect Dis*, **160**, 209–17.

van Cuyck-Gandre, H., Zhang, H.Y., et al. 1997. Characterization of hepatitis E virus (HEV) from Algeria and Chad by partial genome sequence. *J Med Virol*, **53**, 340–7.

van Cuyck-Gandre, H., Zhang, H.Y., et al. 2000. Short report: phylogenetically distinct hepatitis E viruses in Pakistan. *Am J Trop Med Hyg*, **62**, 187–9.

van der Poel, W.H., Verschoor, F., et al. 2001. Hepatitis E virus sequences in swine related to sequences in humans, The Netherlands. *Emerg Infect Dis*, **7**, 970–6.

Vento, S., Garofano, T., et al. 1991. Identification of hepatitis A virus as a trigger for autoimmune chronic hepatitis type 1 in susceptible individuals. *Lancet*, **337**, 1183–7.

Villarejos, V.M., Serra, J., et al. 1982. Hepatitis A virus infection in households. *Am J Epidemiol*, **115**, 577–86.

Viswanathan, R. 1957. Epidemiology [of an 'explosive' epidemic of infectious hepatitis in Delhi during Dec–Jan, 1955–56]. *Indian J Med Res*, **45**, suppl, 1–29.

Wang, Y., Levine, D.F., et al. 2001. Partial sequence analysis of indigenous hepatitis E virus isolated in the United Kingdom. *J Med Virol*, **65**, 706–9.

Wang, Y.C., Zhang, H.Y., et al. 2002. Prevalence, isolation, and partial sequence analysis of hepatitis E virus from domestic animals in China. *J Med Virol*, **67**, 516–21.

Ward, R., Krugman, S., et al. 1958. Infectious hepatitis: studies of its natural history and prevention. *N Engl J Med*, **258**, 407–16.

Weisfuse, I.B., Graham, D.J., et al. 1990. An outbreak of hepatitis A among cancer patients treated with interleukin-2 and lymphokine activated killer cells. *J Infect Dis*, **161**, 647–52.

Weitz, M., Baroudy, B.M., et al. 1986. Detection of a genome-linked protein (VPg) of hepatitis A virus and its comparison with other picornaviral VPgs. *J Virol*, **60**, 124–30.

Werzberger, A., Mensch, B., et al. 1992. A controlled trial of a formalin-inactivated hepatitis A vaccine in healthy children. *N Engl J Med*, **327**, 453–7.

Whetter, L.E., Day, S.P., et al. 1994. Low efficiency of the 5′ nontranslated region of hepatitis A virus RNA in directing cap-independent translation in permissive monkey kidney cells. *J Virol*, **68**, 5253–63.

Widdowson, M.A., Jaspers, W.J., et al. 2003. Cluster of cases of acute hepatitis associated with hepatitis E virus infection acquired in the Netherlands. *Clin Infect Dis*, **36**, 29–33.

Widell, A., Hansson, B.G., et al. 1983. Increased occurrence of hepatitis A with cyclic outbreaks among drug addicts in a Swedish community. *Infection*, **11**, 198–200.

Winokur, P.L. and Stapleton, J.T. 1992. Immunoglobulin prophylaxis for hepatitis A. *Clin Infect Dis*, **14**, 580–6.

Winokur, P.L., McLinden, J.H. and Stapleton, J.T. 1991. The hepatitis A virus polyprotein expressed by a recombinant vaccinia virus undergoes proteolytic processing and assembly into viruslike particles. *J Virol*, **65**, 5029–36.

Wong, D.C., Purcell, R.H., et al. 1980. Epidemic and endemic hepatitis A in India: evidence for a non-A, non-B hepatitis virus etiology. *Lancet*, **2**, 876–9.

Xing, L., Kato, K., et al. 1999. Recombinant hepatitis E capsid protein self-assembles into a dual-domain T=1 particle presenting native virus epitopes. *Virology*, **265**, 35–45.

Yarbough, P.O., Tam, A.W., et al. 1991. Hepatitis E virus: identification of type-common epitopes. *J Virol*, **65**, 5790–7.

Yi, M. and Lemon, S.M. 2002. Replication of subgenomic hepatitis A virus RNAs expressing firefly luciferase is enhanced by mutations associated with adaptation of virus to growth in cultured cells. *J Virol*, **76**, 1171–80.

Yi, M., Schultz, D.E. and Lemon, S.M. 2000. Functional significance of the interaction of hepatitis A virus RNA with glyceraldehyde 3-phosphate dehydrogenase (GAPDH): Opposing effects of GAPDH and polypyrimidine tract binding protein on internal ribosome entry site function. *J Virol*, **74**, 6459–68.

Yin, S., Tsarev, S.A., et al. 1993. Partial sequence comparison of eight new Chinese strains of hepatitis E virus suggests the genome sequence is relatively stable. *J Med Virol*, **41**, 230–41.

Zafrullah, M., Ozdener, M.H., et al. 1997. The ORF3 protein of hepatitis E virus is a phosphoprotein that associates with the cytoskeleton. *J Virol*, **71**, 9045–53.

Zafrullah, M., Ozdener, M.H., et al. 1999. Mutational analysis of glycosylation, membrane translocation, and cell surface expression of the hepatitis E virus ORF2 protein. *J Virol*, **73**, 4074–82.

Zhang, H., Chao, S.-F., et al. 1995. An infectious cDNA clone f a cytopathic hepatitis A virus: genomic regions associated with rapid replication and cytopathic effect. *Virology*, **212**, 686–97.

Zhang, M., Emerson, S.U., et al. 2001a. Immunogenicity and protective efficacy of a vaccine prepared from 53Kda truncated hepatitis E virus capsid protein expressing in insect cells. *Vaccine*, **20**, 853–7.

Zhang, M., Purcell, R.H. and Emerson, S.U. 2001b. Identification of the 5′ terminal sequence of the SAR-55 and MEX-14 strains of hepatitis E virus and confirmation that the genome is capped. *J Med Virol*, **65**, 293–5.

Zhang, M., Emerson, S.U., et al. 2002. Recombinant vaccine against hepatitis E: duration of protective immunity in rhesus macaques. *Vaccine*, **20**, 3285–91.

Zikos, D., Grewal, K.S., et al. 1995. Nephrotic syndrome and acute renal failure associated with hepatitis A virus infection. *Am J Gastroenterol*, **90**, 295–8.

54

Hepatitis C virus

PETER SIMMONDS AND DAVID MUTIMER

INTRODUCTION

Since its discovery 15 years ago (Choo et al. 1989; Kuo et al. 1989), hepatitis C virus (HCV) has been the subject of intense research and clinical investigations as its major role in human disease emerged. Globally, HCV is estimated to infect 170 million people, 3 percent of the world's population, and creates a huge disease burden from chronic progressive liver disease. HCV has become a major cause of liver cancer and one of the most common indication for liver transplantation (reviewed in Pawlotsky (2003b), Hoofnagle (2002), and Seeff (2002)). HCV infection can be treated, but currently requires long-term medical support and follow up; current therapies are impractical for the majority of HCV carriers worldwide. The development of a protective vaccine remains a distant prospect.

Discovery of HCV

The discovery of HCV in 1989 was the dramatic end to a major research endeavor to find the causes of post-transfusion hepatitis. In the 1970s, several groups produced evidence for an infectious agent, distinct from the hepatitis A virus (HAV) and hepatitis B virus (HBV), that caused chronic hepatitis and was frequently transmitted by blood and blood products (Prince et al. 1974; Feinstone et al. 1975; Alter et al. 1975). Typically, non-A, non-B hepatitis (NANBH) was a mild disease that caused jaundice in fewer than half of cases, and was frequently asymptomatic. In its clinical features, it differed in several respects from acute HAV and HBV infection with a longer incubation period from exposure to liver function abnormalities, around 8 weeks, than is usually observed for HAV (4 weeks), but shorter than that for HBV (12 weeks). There was a high rate of chronicity following acute infection (at least 50 percent of cases, compared with around 5 percent for adult HBV infection). While chronic infection was almost invariably asymptomatic at first, a large proportion of cases eventually progressed to cirrhosis.

Progress towards identifying the cause of NANBH was hampered by the difficulty in culturing the agent in cell or organ culture, and the eventual characterization of the infectious agent of NANBH was made possible after the successful transmission of the agent into chimpanzees. Experimental data were then obtained that the agent passed through a 80-nm filter and was inactivated by lipid solvents such as chloroform; together these data suggested a small enveloped virus. Examination of liver biopsies from patients with NANBH and of experimentally infected chimpanzees helped to define the histologic features of acute and chronic disease and to differentiate it from other causes of hepatitis. Passaging and titration of the NANBH agent in chimpanzees eventually provided high titer stocks of virus that were necessary for the eventual cloning and sequence analysis of the infectious agent (Bradley et al. 1979; Bradley and Maynard 1986).

Nucleic acid (both DNA and RNA) was extracted following ultracentrifugation from a large volume of a plasma sample with a high infectivity titer in chimpanzees (approximately 10^6 infectious units/ml). The nucleic acid was reverse-transcribed and the resulting DNA fragments cloned into the λ-gt11 bacteriophage. The DNA sequences in the resulting library were expressed as fusion proteins during replication of the bacteriophage in *Escherichia coli*. Immunoscreening of large numbers of bacteriophage plaques with antisera from patients with NANBH led to the eventual identification of an immunoreactive clone (designated 5-1-1) that appeared to be specific for the NANBH agent (Choo et al. 1989). This clone showed no similarity with any human or *E. coli* genomic sequences and produced a protein that was consistently recognized by sera from patients with NANBH, but not by sera from control individuals, or those with hepatitis of other etiologies (Kuo et al. 1989).

The 5-1-1 clone was then used as a probe to identify overlapping sequences in the λgt-11 library and this led to the assembly of a nearly complete nucleotide sequence of the NANBH agent (Choo et al. 1991). Knowledge of the length, nucleic acid composition, and genome organization of HCV has led to its classification in the *Flaviviridae* family (see Relationship of HCV to other flaviviruses) and its method of replication (see Replication of the HCV genome). From the sequence of HCV it was possible to design hybridization probes and primers for amplification of the HCV genome by polymerase chain reaction (PCR) that can be used to detect HCV RNA in sera and liver biopsies from hepatitis patients (see Diagnostic tests for HCV infection). The original 5-1-1 clone, together with an overlapping clone, c100-3, and more recently with clones from other parts of the genome, has been used to manufacture recombinant proteins for assays for antibody to HCV. This has enabled effective screening of blood donors for HCV infection to be adopted worldwide.

RELATIONSHIP OF HCV TO OTHER VIRUSES

Relationship to positive-strand RNA viruses

The sequence of the HCV genome shares several features with other positive-strand RNA viruses. Most striking is the existence of a single continuous open reading frame that occupies almost the entire genome. After translation, this is cleaved into individual proteins that are enzymes necessary for virus replication or are structural components of the virion (Figure 54.1). In overall genome organization and likely method of replication, HCV is most similar to members of the *Flaviviridae*, and indeed the roles of the different proteins encoded by HCV have been inferred by comparison with homologues in other flaviviruses. Although there is

still no suitable method developed for the in vitro culture of HCV, expression of cloned HCV sequences in prokaryotic and eukaryotic systems, and the recently developed replicon has also allowed the replication functions of several nonstructural proteins of HCV to be identified (Figure 54.1) (described in detail below in the section Nonstructural proteins).

Other members of the *Flaviviridae* have many features in common with HCV. They have a similar genome size to HCV (YFV: 10 862 bases (Rice et al. 1985), compared with 9 379 of HCV (Choo et al. 1991)), and the virus envelope contains a viral encoded glycoprotein (E1). However, the homologue of HCV E2 in flaviviruses (also a membrane-bound glycoprotein: NS1) is not incorporated into the virion, being expressed only on the infected cell surface. Like HCV, the polyprotein of flaviviruses is cleaved by a combination of viral and host-cell proteases. Although there is no close sequence similarity between HCV and other flaviviruses, there are at least two regions with conserved amino acid residues that demonstrate enzymatic functions. The NS5B protein of HCV contains the GDD (glycine–aspartate–aspartate) motif that forms part of the active site in virus RNA-dependent RNA polymerases (RdRp) of positive-strand RNA viruses (Miller and Purcell 1990; Koonin 1991). Similarly, the NS3 protein contains domains associated with helicase and serine protease activity (Miller and Purcell 1990) (see Nonstructural proteins).

Shared features of HCV with pestiviruses

An important difference between members of the *Flaviviridae* is the structure of the 5′ and 3′ untranslated regions (UTR). These parts of the genome are involved in replication (see below), and in the initiation of translation of the virus genome by cellular ribosomes. Both pestiviruses and HCV have highly structured 5′ UTRs, in which internal base-pairing produces a complex set of stem–loop structures that interact with various host-cell and virus proteins during replication and translation (Smith et al. 1995; Tsukiyama Kohara et al. 1992; Wang et al. 1994; Poole et al. 1995). In both viruses, there is evidence for internal initiation of translation, in which binding to the host-cell ribosome directs translation to an internal methionine (AUG) codon (see HCV translation). This contrasts strongly with translation of flavivirus genomes which act much like cellular mRNAs, in which ribosomal binding occurs at the capped 5′ end of the RNA, followed by scanning of the sequence in the 5′ to 3′ direction with translation commencing at the first AUG codon.

Structurally, HCV is also more similar to the pestiviruses than flaviviruses, with a low buoyant density in sucrose (see Physicochemical properties), similar to that reported for pestiviruses and attributable in both cases

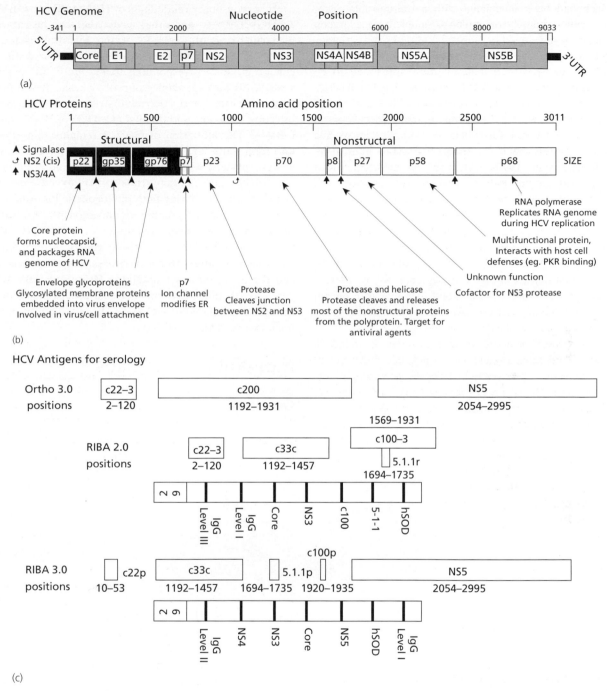

Figure 54.1 *Organization of HCV genome.* **(a)** *The coding sequences from structural and nonstructural proteins, and the 5' and 3' untranslated regions.* **(b)** *The sizes and summaries of functional properties of the mature proteins cleaved from the translated polyprotein, with the positions and enzymes responsible for the cleavage reaction indicated.* **(c)** *Regions of the genome expressed as recombinant antigens for serological assays. Nucleotide and amino acid positions numbered as in Choo et al. (1991).*

to extensively glycosylated proteins in the virus envelope. By contrast, flavivirus envelope glycoproteins contain few sites for *N*-linked glycosylation, and the virion itself is relatively dense (1.2 g/cm³). Finally, the arrangement and number of cleavage sites of the HCV polyprotein is more similar to pestiviruses, particularly in the cleavage of NS5 into two subunits, with NS5B corresponding to the RNA polymerase.

Relationship of HCV to other flaviviruses

Shortly after the discovery of HCV, a number of new flaviviruses was found to infect humans, old and new world primate species. The most closely related virus to HCV was GB virus B (GBV-B), found to cause acute, resolving infections in captive tamarins (*Sanguinis* spp.), which had been inoculated with a transmissible agent originally passaged from a plasma sample from a surgeon who had developed a hepatitis of unknown etiology (Simons et al. 1995). Remarkably, tamarins exposed to this in vitro passaged material were also found to be infected with a second, largely unrelated flavivirus, described as GB virus A (GBV-A). While a range of wild caught South American primate species show frequent evidence for infection with species-specific variants of GBV-A (Leary et al. 1997; Erker et al. 1998; Bukh and Apgar 1997), current surveys had not provided clear evidence for either active or past infection with GBV-B in New World primates, and its origin in the passaged material is therefore currently unclear. What has become apparent is that neither virus infected the human whose plasma originated the passaged material (both GBV-A and GBV-B were probably picked up at some point during passage through a number of different New World primate species), and they therefore do not represent human viruses. However, with knowledge of the sequences of GBV-A, it has proved possible to detect viruses distantly related to GBV-A found in humans and chimpanzees; two groups independently but simultaneously discovered in 1995 the human homolog, described as hepatitis G virus (HGV) or GB virus-C (Leary et al. 1996; Linnen et al. 1996). Shortly afterwards, a virus related to HGV/GBV-C was found to be widely distributed in chimpanzees (Adams et al. 1998; Birkenmeyer et al. 1998).

The evolutionary relatedness of HCV, GBV-B, GBV-A, HGV/GBV-C, and other flaviviruses can be shown by comparison of a region of the highly conserved RdRp (Figure 54.2). Flaviviruses fall into four distinct genetic groups, corresponding to (1) HCV; (2) pestiviruses; (3) an expanded group of tick and mosquito-borne viruses and nonvector-transmitted viruses infecting rodents; and finally (4) HGV/GBV-C and GBV-A. The affiliation of GBV-B remains somewhat uncertain, although most methods of phylogenetic analysis place it within the HCV group, and it resembles HCV more closely than other flaviviruses in genome structure. Using both phylogenetic information and comparisons of genome organization, the International Committee on the Taxonomy of Viruses (ICTV) has now formally classified these genetic groups into three named genera, the flaviviruses, the pestiviruses, and the hepaciviruses (containing HCV and GBV-B), and a fourth, currently unnamed and provisional genus that contains HGV/GBV-C, GBV-A, and other primate homologues (Thiel et al. 2000).

PROPERTIES OF THE VIRUS

Genome

The genome of HCV is single-stranded RNA of positive (protein coding) polarity. As with other positive-strand

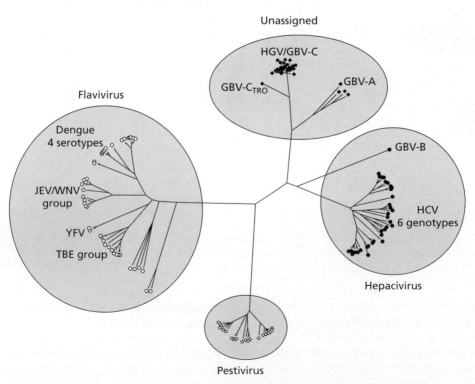

Figure 54.2 *Genera within the family* Flaviviridae. *Phylogenetic analysis of a conserved region of the RNA polymerase gene of flaviviruses reveals four well-defined genetic groups. These correspond to three of the current classified genera of flaviviruses, while the fourth group contains the currently unassigned HGV/GBV-C viruses and homologues in New World primates.*

RNA viruses, genomic RNA of HCV is infectious on experimental inoculation into chimpanzees (Yanagi et al. 1997). More than 98 percent of the HCV genome codes for virus proteins (9 033 of 9 397 bases of the HCV-PT genome (Choo et al. 1991)), with noncoding regions at both 5' and 3' ends. The 5' UTR is 341–344 bases long, with no evidence for chemical modification of the ends, such as capping with a methyl[7]guanosine residue as found in members of the genus *Flavivirus* and in eukaryotic mRNAs.

The 3' untranslated region contains three domains, 25–30 poorly conserved nucleotides. a homopolymeric region comprising mainly uridine/cytosine residues, and finally, a highly conserved 'X-region' that forms a stable RNA structure comprising three juxtaposed stem–loops. There is no evidence for any covalent modifications to the genomic RNA of HCV.

Morphology

HCV remains difficult to visualize by electron microscopy. Without an efficient in vitro culture system for HCV, most attempts at visualization have used negative-staining of HCV of high titer plasma (Figure 54.3). In the example shown (Kaito et al. 1994), HCV forms viruslike particles of diameter 55–65 nm (Figure 54.3) with 6-nm spikelike projections that may correspond to the envelope glycoproteins

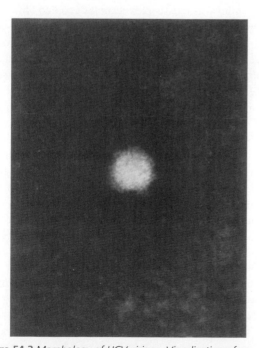

Figure 54.3 *Morphology of HCV virions. Visualization of an isolated virus particle of HCV by surface staining using 2 percent phosphotungstic acid, pH 6.5 (Kaito et al. 1994). Fine spikelike projections can be seen around the edge of the virus particle of approximate measured diameter of 60 nm. This figure was kindly provided by the authors.*

on the virion surface. The envelope glycoproteins of HCV show several potential sites for *N*-linked glycosylation (four sites in E1, 11 sites in E2) and it is likely that the addition of relatively large carbohydrate groups contribute structurally to the outer surface of the virion, and influences the ability of antibody to neutralize infectivity.

Physicochemical properties

The density of HCV is difficult to measure accurately because of its binding to various factors in plasma (the only available source of virion particles to study). For example, it associates to a variable extent with β-lipoprotein that reduces its density (Bradley et al. 1991; Thomssen et al. 1992). In samples from seropositive individuals, it may also be immune complexed with antibody creating a second density band of up to 1.20–1.25 g/cm^3 (Bradley et al. 1991; Miyamoto et al. 1992; Hijikata et al. 1993b; Carrick et al. 1992).

HCV is inactivated by exposure to chloroform, ether, and other organic solvents and by detergents. It is inactivated by dry heat treatment at 80°C or wet-heat treatment at 60°C, organic solvents (n-heptane) and detergents used in the manufacture of plasma-derived blood products (Mannucci 1993).

REPLICATION OF HCV

Culture of HCV in vitro

Despite considerable efforts, little progress has yet been made towards the development of a system for the culture of HCV in vitro. HCV does not produce obvious cytopathology, and the amounts of HCV released from cells infected in vitro are often low (Shimizu et al. 1992, 1993; Carloni et al. 1993; Shimizu and Yoshikura 1994; Kato et al. 1995). This may be because the cells used for culture are not representative of those infected in vivo, or because productive infection requires a combination of cytokines and growth factors found in the liver that is not reproduced in cell culture.

Transfection of full length DNA sequences of the HCV genome might be expected to initiate the full replicative cycle of HCV, as it does when similar experiments are carried out with picornavirus sequences. However, while HCV proteins are translated and can be processed into structural and nonstructural proteins, there is no evidence for replication of genomic RNA, nor the assembly of virion particles. Despite considerable efforts, the reason for this block is still not understood, and has led to alternative strategies to study the HCV replication cycle. Of these, the most successful has been the development of subgenomic or full-length genomic replicons of HCV (Lohmann et al. 1999; Ikeda et al. 2002; Blight et al. 2003; Pietschmann et al. 2002). The original clone was constructed as a dicistronic vector containing the nonstructural genes (NS3–NS5B) and the 3′ UTR from a genotype 1b clone whose expression was driven by a powerful IRES from encephalomyocarditis virus (EMCV). Upstream was a selectable marker (*neo*) and a 5′ terminus comprising the HCV 5′ UTR (Lohmann et al. 1999). Under neomycin selection, this replicon replicates at selfsustaining levels, although this is limited to specific cell lines such as certain clones of the Huh-7 hepatoma cell line. Replication is enhanced by the appearance of a number of 'adaptive' amino acid changes in the NS3 and NS5B regions (Bartenschlager et al. 2003), even though these play no role in natural infections and actually attenuate replication in experimentally infected chimpanzees (Bukh et al. 2002).

Since this pioneering work was carried out, several groups have developed replicons based on other genotype 1b isolates (Ikeda et al. 2002) and other genotypes (e.g. 1a, 2a; (Blight et al. 2003; Kato et al. 2003)). It is also possible to create viable replicons containing the structural proteins (Pietschmann et al. 2002; Blight et al. 2003), even though these still require selection and do not generate infectious viral particles. Clearly much remains to be discovered about the cell line restrictions, the requirement for 'adaptive,' nonphysiological sequence changes, and the underlying reasons why infectious virus does not appear to be produced in any of the available systems. Nevertheless replicons are useful in studying many aspects of the replication of HCV genomic RNA; they are also increasingly used to discover more about the mode of action of interferons used for human therapy (see Antiviral treatment), and the action and development of resistance to other antiviral agents, such as protease and RNA polymerase inhibitors (Blight et al. 2000; Frese et al. 2001; Lanford et al. 2003; Wang et al. 2003; Lu et al. 2004).

Animal models

The chimpanzee is the only animal model for HCV with demonstrated susceptibility to HCV infection, and which show a course of infection resembling that in humans. In particular, exposed chimpanzees may become persistently infected, with incubation periods, seroconversion profiles, and elevation of liver enzymes (such as alanine aminotransferase) broadly similar to that of human infections. Unfortunately, the later events in HCV infection in humans, such as the development of cirrhosis and hepatocellular carcinoma typically occurring over periods of 20–30 years, make it difficult to conduct natural history studies of the main disease outcomes of HCV infection in chimpanzees (Walker 1997).

One frequently observed difference between humans and chimpanzees lies in the immune response to infection. Inoculated chimpanzees generally show a delayed, weaker, and less broadly reactive antibody response to infection (Choo et al. 1994), while the appearance of strong T-cell responses is associated with clearance of infection (Cooper et al. 1999). These differences complicate the use of the chimpanzee as a model for vaccine development (see Immunization).

With the possible exception of the gorilla (for which there are few or no data available), HCV does not infect other primates in the wild (Makuwa et al. 2003), nor can they be infected experimentally (Bukh et al. 2001; Abe et al. 1993). There is, however, one report of the unexpected ability of HCV to replicate in the tupaia (Xie et al. 1998). It is not known whether the apparent species-specificity of HCV for human and higher apes is determined at the level of entry, by intracellular blocks in the replication cycle of HCV in cells of other species, or by missing cellular factors for virus assembly and release. The current problems associated with establishing HCV in a cell culture system make this issue experimentally difficult to resolve at present.

Replication of the HCV genome

In common with other positive-strand RNA viruses, HCV replicates its RNA genome through the production of a minus-strand replication intermediate, that is an RNA copy of the complete genome that is synthesized by the activity of a virus encoded RdRp (NS5B) (Figure 54.1). The minus-strand copy becomes the template for the generation of positive-strand copies. Because template can be transcribed several times, many minus-strand copies can be copied from the infecting positive strand, and each of these transcripts used several times to produce positive-strand progeny sequences. In this way, a single input sequence could be amplified several thousand-fold during the course of replication within a cell.

Using a highly strand-specific PCR method, antisense HCV RNA sequences have been detected in the liver of HCV-infected individuals, directly demonstrating replication of HCV via its replication intermediate (Lanford et al. 1994). Transcription initiation is dependent on possession of intact termini to the 5′ and 3′ UTRs. It has also been recently shown that replication in the replicon system requires RNA structures in the NS5B coding region (You et al. 2004; Lee et al. 2004). While the details of its role and of adjacent RNA structures in NS5B remain to be established, it is clear from other virus systems that transcription initiation and its regulation with translation are likely to be complex, and to involve multiple long-range interactions within HCV genomic RNA and with a range of cellular proteins and RNA sequences.

HCV translation

The 5′ UTR is an essential component in the initiation and regulation of translation of the large open reading frame (ORF) of HCV. The region is between 341 and 344 bases in length, and a combination of computer analysis, nuclease mapping experiments, and studies of covariance has allowed the RNA secondary structure to be accurately predicted (Tsukiyama Kohara et al. 1992; Wang et al. 1995; Smith et al. 1995). Similar structures have been predicted for pestiviruses (Smith et al. 1995; Wang et al. 1995) and GBV-B (Grace et al. 1999) despite their frequent lack of nucleotide sequence similarities with HCV.

Evidence that the 5′ UTR can direct the internal initiation of translation was originally obtained by in vitro translation of reporter genes downstream from the 5′ UTR sequence placed in mono- or dicistronic vectors (Wang et al. 1993, 1994; Fukushi et al. 1994). The IRES activity of the 5′ UTR directs translation from the AUG methionine codon at position 341, through binding to the 40S ribosomal subunit (Pestova et al. 1998). There is no evidence for translation from any of the variable number of AUG triplets upstream from this site. As the structure of the IRES extends into the coding region, its activity is influenced by these downstream sequences. For example, the efficiency of IRES-mediated translation is inversely related to the stability of a short stem loop (designated stem–loop IV; nucleotides −12 to +12 with respect to the initiation codon) (Honda et al. 1996). It has also been demonstrated that the first 28–42 nucleotides of the core sequence must lack RNA secondary structure to allow positioning of the ribosome at the start of the coding sequence (Rijnbrand et al. 2001).

The synthesis of HCV proteins occurs through translation and cotranslational or subsequent proteolytic cleavage of the large potential polyprotein encoded by the open reading frame (Figure 54.1), and is intimately connected to the formation of a replication complex of HCV that remains closely associated with the endoplasmic reticulum (ER). Initial translation of the core gene leads to a protein on the cytoplasmic side of the ER with an amino terminus embedded in the ER membrane. This hydrophobic tail is subsequently cleaved to release the core protein, and directs synthesis of the E1 glycoprotein to the luminal side of the ER. A second hydrophobic region sequence embeds E1 to the ER membrane by forming a trans-membrane anchor. A second, host-cell signal peptidase (signalase)-mediated cleavage reaction separates it from E2. Signalase subsequently mediates cleavage of E2 from p7 and p7 from NS2. The remainder of the HCV proteins are produced on the cytoplasmic side of the ER. Cleavage of NS2 from NS3 is carried out autoproteolytically by a cis-acting zinc-dependent protease formed by the uncleaved NS2/NS3 precursor protein (Figure 54.1). Subsequent translation leads to the synthesis of NS3/NS4A serine protease that mediates cleavage between NS3 and NS4A in cis, and trans-cleavage of sites between NS4A and NS4Bb, between NS4B and NS5A, and between NS5A and NS5B (Figure 54.1).

Virus entry, uncoating, assembly, and release

Currently there is uncertainty about the nature of the cellular receptor for HCV and the mechanism by which it enters the cell. It has been found that CD81, a tetra-spanin molecule that plays a role in the conformational ordering of signaling complexes, bound to the E2 protein of HCV, and that this interaction was blocked by neutralizing antibodies to HCV (Pileri et al. 1998). More recently, using a pseudotype system in which HCV envelope proteins were co-expressed with enveloped–deleted proviral clones of human immunodeficiency virus type 1 (HIV-1) to generate infectious particles, it was shown that expression of CD81 was absolutely required for infection of hepatocytes by HCV (Zhang et al. 2004). However, CD81 is widely distributed on a variety of human cell types, and does not therefore account for apparent highly specific cellular tropism of HCV for primary hepatocytes of the HCV/HIV-1 pseudotype. It is therefore likely that CD81 represents a coreceptor for HCV and that other cell surface molecules, perhaps with a liver-specific pattern of expression, are required for essential steps in HCV-binding or -fusion reactions. Of several candidate molecules, most attention has been paid to the low density lipoprotein (LDL) receptor, as its expression is restricted to the liver, and HCV purified from plasma of HCV-infected individuals is known to associate with LDL (Agnello et al. 1999; Wunschmann et al. 2000).

Replication of HCV within the cell occurs in the cytoplasm, in membrane-bound replication complexes, containing most of the nonstructural proteins of HCV and viral RNA (Lin et al. 1997; Ishido et al. 1998; Egger et al. 2002; El Hage and Luo 2003). At present, there is little information on the process of HCV virion assembly, maturation, and release from the cell, because virus particle formation is not achievable with currently used replicons of HCV, even those that express the full complement of structural proteins. However, core, E1, and E2 proteins expressed from transfected expression vectors have been shown to localize to the endoplasmic reticulum, intermediate compartment, and the cis-Golgi, likely representing steps in their maturation (such as glycosylation), and ultimately, particle assembly (Martire et al. 2001; Blanchard et al. 2002). There is currently no evidence for expression of HCV proteins on the surface of infected cells.

PROTEINS OF HCV

The genome of HCV is thought to encode at least ten proteins, of which three are structural (core, E1, and E2) and six nonstructural (NS2, NS3, NS4A, NS4B, NS5A, and NS5B) (Figure 54.1). HCV also expresses p7, a membrane-associated ion channel that may function during virus assembly or infection. Most information about the function and enzymatic activities of the nonstructural proteins has been obtained by expression of DNA sequences corresponding to the different proteins, and by direct observations of the cellular distributions and properties of HCV proteins detected in liver or plasma in vivo.

Structural proteins

The structural proteins of HCV are encoded by sequences at the 5′ end of the genome and so are translated first (Figure 54.1). Expression of this part of the genome in cells (Selby et al. 1993; Ralston et al. 1993; Grakoui et al. 1993c), or in reticulocyte lysate containing microsomal membranes (Hijikata et al. 1991b; Santolini et al. 1994) leads to the synthesis of a polyprotein followed by proteolytic cleavage into the core, E1, and E2 proteins. Cleavage between the capsid protein and E1, E1 and E2, and E2 and NS2 are dependent upon the addition of microsomal membranes, implying the role of the host-cell signalase in these processing steps.

CORE

The core or capsid protein has a size of 21–22 kDa, smaller than predicted from its coding sequence of 191 amino acids, the result of cleavage of the final 17–18 amino acids post-translationally to produce the mature protein. The N terminus contains several positively charged amino acid residues, that bind to viral RNA and which are presumably involved in the virus packaging reaction. It is not known how core proteins bind together to form the HCV nucleocapsid, although nucleocapsid formation is thought to drive the budding process in the ER that leads to the formation of fully-assembled virions. It has been proposed that the core protein of HCV can be functionally divided into three domains (Hope and McLauchlan 2000): domain 1 (amino acids 1–117) forms the nucleocapsid of the virus, while domain 3 represents the final 10–12 amino acid hydrophobic leader sequence that is cleaved after translation. Domain 2 has been shown to be the region of core responsible for its targeting to lipid droplets, a process which potentially interferes with lipid metabolism within the infected hepatocyte, and which may play a role in the development of steatosis as a complication of HCV infection (Perlemuter et al. 2002). Interestingly, domain 2 is highly conserved between HCV and GBV-B, while only the capsid region (domain 1) is obviously homologous with the capsid regions of pesti- and flaviviruses (Hope et al. 2002).

ENVELOPE (E1, E2)

The envelope proteins of HCV (E1, E2) are synthesized in mammalian cells as proteins with sizes ranging from 31–35 kDa and 68–72 kDa, respectively (Hijikata et al. 1991b; Selby et al. 1993; Grakoui et al. 1993c; Ralston et al. 1993; Santolini et al. 1994). E1 and E2 are extensively glycosylated after translation at a large number of N-linked glycosylation sites in the extracellular domains of the proteins. Interactions between E1 and E2 have been demonstrated by immunoprecipitation experiments, in which antibody to E1 or E2 could precipitate both proteins under nondenaturing conditions (Ralston et al. 1993; Grakoui et al. 1993c; Dubuisson et al. 1994). E1 and E2 are thought to form heterodimeric structures in the virus envelope through a noncovalent interaction (Dubuisson et al. 1994; Matsuura et al. 1994; Selby et al. 1994).

The envelope proteins are likely to form the principal target of antibody-mediated neutralization of virus infectivity, although investigation of this phenomenon has been hampered by the lack of an in vitro infectivity assay, and of a suitable animal model. Recently, however, it has been possible to demonstrate neutralizing antibody responses directed at the E1 and E2 glycoproteins through the use of pseudotyped virus, comprising the envelope glycoproteins from HCV and a capsid from either HIV or a murine retrovirus (Bartosch et al. 2003; Logvinoff et al. 2004). The E2 protein contains hypervariable regions (HVR) in the N-terminal region, which evolve much more rapidly during the course of persistent infection than other regions of the genome. This variability may arise through selection of amino acid changes that allow immune escape from neutralizing antibody; persistence may therefore be accompanied by continuous virus sequence change to keep ahead of developing B-cell responses (Kumar et al. 1993; Taniguchi et al. 1993; Weiner et al. 1992; Farci et al. 2000; Kantzanou et al. 2003) (see Immune escape).

P7

The small p7 protein lies between E2 and NS2 proteins of the virus polyprotein and is thus at the junction of the structural and nonstructural gene regions (Lin et al. 1994; Mizushima et al. 1994), although it is not known whether p7 is a virion component. The 63 amino acid protein is highly hydrophobic and remains embedded in the ER membrane on translation through a transmembrane anchor of two predicted alpha helices (Carrere-Kremer et al. 2002). Recently it has been shown that p7 oligomerizes to create ion channels within membranes (Griffin et al. 2003). These pores allow transport of cations across membranes, comparable to the activity of viral viroporins, such as M2 in influenza virus. Similarly, to M2, the activity of p7 is inhibited by amantadine (Carrere-Kremer et al. 2002), an observation that suggests a new strategy to treat HCV infection. It is currently unknown at what stage in the replication cycle p7 is active or required, nor whether it is an integral component in the envelope of the mature virus particle.

Nonstructural proteins

In vitro translation of the rest of the genome leads to the production of proteins of sizes 23, 70–72, 4, 27, 56–58, and 66 kDa, corresponding to NS2, NS3, NS4A, NS4B, NS5A, and NS5B, respectively (Figure 54.1).

NS2

The NS2 protein is cleaved from p7 at its N terminus by ER-associated signalase. NS2 remain membrane bound, with its C terminus located through the ER membrane, and the N terminus in the cytoplasm (Santolini et al. 1995). The only function assigned to NS2 is to form one domain of a protease in combination with the first 180 amino acid residues at the N terminus of NS3 (Hijikata et al. 1993a; Grakoui et al. 1993a). This protease activity autocatalytically excises the NS2 protein from NS3 in a *cis*-cleavage reaction through a currently unclear mechanism. The dependence of the NS2/NS3 protease on Zn^{++} and its inhibition by ethylenediaminetetraacetic acid (EDTA) (that chelates divalent cations) suggests that it might be a zinc protease. However, mutation of what would be functionally cysteine and histidine amino acids in the catalytic dyad of a cysteine protease also abolished protease activity of NS2/NS3 (Hijikata et al. 1993a). The NS2 protein is widely conserved across the flavivirus family; it is possible that it plays other roles in virus replication or assembly beyond that of a self-excising protein that detaches itself from the rest of the replication complex.

NS3

The NS3 protein has a variety of enzyme activities that participate in both RNA replication and in processing of the viral polyprotein. The mature form of NS3 migrates as a protein of 67 kDa, and is generated through NS2/NS3-mediated cleavage from NS2, and NS3/NS4B-mediated cleavage from NS4A. Although not cleaved internally when expressed in mammalian cells or during virus replication, the NS3 protein can be conceptualized as comprising two independent domains with different enzymatic activities.

The first 181 amino acid residues at the N terminus of NS3 show two different protease activities. As described in the previous section, it forms part of the NS2/NS3 protease, and forms a separate, functionally distinct serine protease after cleavage (Tanji et al. 1994). The serine protease shows *cis*-acting activity in cleavage of the NS3/NS4A junction, and *trans*-activity in the cleavage of NS4A from 4B, 4B from 5A, and 5B from 5A (Eckart et al. 1993; Hijikata et al. 1993a; Grakoui et al. 1993b; Bartenschlager et al. 1993; Tomei et al. 1993). The *trans*-activity of NS3 requires NS4A as a cofactor; recent crystallographic studies have shown that NS3 and NS4A form a tightly bound protease complex (Kim et al. 1996), with extensive interactions between residues 21 and 32 of NS4A with the β-sheet of the NS3 protease core. This interaction with NS4A may chaperone or stabilize the folding of NS3 into an active conformation. The hydrophobic, predicted membrane spanning N terminus of NS4A may, in turn, anchor the protease complex to membranes and thus link it to other components of the viral replication complex. NS3 contains a structural zinc-binding site through binding with a histidine and three cysteine residues, and which supplies electrons to the catalytic site in the enzyme complex.

The substrate specificity and mechanism of action of the NS3/NS4A protease has been extensively investigated because of the possibility of developing inhibitors that could be used to treat HCV infection (see Antiviral treatment). Each of the cleavage sites in different variants of HCV conform closely to the consensus sequence D/E – X–X–X–X–C/T // S/A (where // represents the cleavage site) (Komoda et al. 1994; Kolykhalov et al. 1994; Bartenschlager et al. 1995; Leinbach et al. 1994). There is some evidence for a less stringent requirement for specific amino acids around the *cis* cleavage site (NS3/NS4A) than those cleaved in *trans* (Bartenschlager et al. 1995). Inhibitors of NS3/NS4A have now been developed that mimic the recognition sequence, and competitively inhibit the processing of the HCV polyprotein (De Francesco et al. 2003); BILN 2061 is currently in clinical trials (Lamarre et al. 2003). While the primary function of the protease domain of NS3 is processing of the HCV polyprotein, it has recently been shown that the NS3/4A protease blocks the phosphorylation and signaling function of the antiviral interferon regulatory factor 3 (Foy et al. 2003). Blocking of this cell defense pathway may contribute to the ability of HCV to persist in vivo, and to resist exogenous interferon therapy.

The much longer second enzymatic domain of NS3 shows helicase and NTPase activities. Helicases displace base-paired RNA or DNA sequences from a template strand usually in a 3′ to 5′ direction. This process requires the presence of Mg^{++} ions and energy provided by hydrolysis of ATP by a NTPase activity of the enzyme and these are combined in an energy-dependent unwinding process of template and copied RNA sequences during virus genome replication (Gwack et al. 1997; Tai et al. 1996). Several sequence motifs in NS3 (such as the DEXH box) are shared with corresponding proteins in other positive-strand RNA viruses, suggesting a degree of functional equivalence on which the HCV helicase might be modeled (Suzich et al. 1993).

NS4A

As described above, NS4A functions as part of the NS3/NS4A protease complex, with an additional role in localizing the complex to membranes. No other function of NS4A has been determined to date.

NS4B

The function of NS4B is not fully understood. After cleavage, NS4B is membrane-associated in the ER

(Hugle et al. 2001) with at least two predicted membrane-spanning domains (Hugle et al. 2001; Lundin et al. 2003), and participates in the formation of a membranous web that may act as a structural platform for HCV replication complex (Egger et al. 2002). Recently, NS4B has been shown to possess a GTPase activity that is required for replication of the HCV replicon; this finding suggests an additional enzymatic role for NS4B in the replication complex (Einav et al. 2004; Piccininni et al. 2002).

NS5A

The NS5A protein is a 56–58-kDa nonstructural protein. Although for many years after the discovery of HCV the function of NS5A was unknown, more recent research has revealed a key role for NS5A in a variety of interactions with host-cell defense mechanisms that may be associated with the ability of the virus to persist in vivo and to resist interferon therapy. On cleavage from NS4B and NS5B, NS5A is bound to the ER by the N-terminal amphipathic helix (Figure 54.4) and becomes associated with the viral replicase complex on the cytoplasmic side of the ER; binding to NS5B may be required for the RNA polymerase activity of the replication complex (Shimakami et al. 2004). NS5A becomes phosphorylated after translation, at one or more of several targeted serine or threonine residues at the center and C terminus of the protein. The number and position of NS5A phosphorylation sites varies between genotypes (Hirota et al. 1999; Reed et al. 1997). NS5A may additionally become hyperphosphorylated within a serine-rich region at the center of the protein (Figure 54.4), although this form of NS5A is not present in the replication complex, and mutations that prevent phosphorylation at positions 2 197 and 2 204 actually enhance the replication ability of the HCV replicon (see Replication of the HCV genome).

While NS5A is a necessary part of the viral replication complex, it shows a number of additional activities that are broadly aimed at combating the innate cell defenses, thus potentially contributing to the persistence of HCV and its resistance to interferon. These include the binding to and inactivation of PKR (Gale et al. 1997), blocking apoptotic pathways through sequestering p53, modulation of intracellular calcium levels, and binding to growth factor receptor-bound protein 2 (Grb-2) (Majumder et al. 2001; Gong et al. 2001; Tan et al. 1999), and induction of anti-inflammatory interleukin-8 (IL-8) secretion (Polyak et al. 2001) (recently reviewed in Macdonald and Harris 2004). Many of these interactions block the apoptotic cellular response to persistent HCV infection, while the induction of IL-8 may potentiate viral replication and inhibit intracellular IFN-responsive antiviral pathways. These different functions have been mapped to a number of different domains in the NS5A protein (Figure 54.4).

Interferon therapy has been shown to lead to the appearance of a number of amino acid changes in the region of NS5A that interacts with PKR (Figure 54.4). An association was also found between treatment response and possession of the so-called 'prototype' NS5A sequence in the region where mutations occurred (Enomoto et al. 1995). These original findings have since been confirmed in recent meta-analyses of all the available data which demonstrated a clear correlation between possession of the prototype interferon-sensitivity determining region (ISDR) sequence and treatment resistance, and a large number of diverse amino acid changes in nonresponders (Witherell and Beineke 2001; Pascu et al. 2004). It has also been shown that the same differential response exists in genotype 2a and 2b infections (Murakami et al. 1999). Prototype ISDR sequences have also been shown to be associated with higher circulating virus loads in untreated patients (Watanabe et al. 2003). It is therefore possible that PKR evasion is a key determinant in the persistence of HCV and potentially other aspects of the virus/host interaction.

NS5B

NS5B is an RNA-dependent RNA polymerase, and is responsible for the copying of the HCV genome during replication. NS5B is cleaved at its N terminus from the rest of the HCV polyprotein by the NS3/NS4A protease. NS5B remains membrane bound through a hydrophobic,

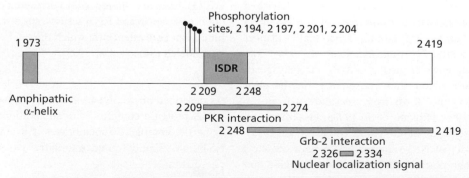

Figure 54.4 *Diagram of the NS5A gene. This shows the positions of the ER-binding amphipathic helix, the interferon-sensitivity determining region (ISDR), and regions of the protein known to interact with PKR and other cellular pathways associated with innate cell defenses against viruses. Identified sites of hyperphosphorylation found in the 58-kDa form of the protein localize to the ISDR.*

membrane-inserted anchor sequence at the carboxyl terminus of the protein. The mature form of NS5B is 68 kDa in size, is phosphorylated, and forms part of the replication complex along with other nonstructural proteins that participate in genome replication. The recently determined crystal structure (Lesburg et al. 1999) has shown NS5B to have a typical thumb/palm/finger arrangement of domains that encircle the RNA template strand, and that contains catalytic residues, such as the GDD motif characteristic of RNA polymerase of other positive-strand RNA viruses. Determining the structure of NS5B has been important for the design and optimization of activity of new classes of antiviral agents that inhibit RNA polymerase function (see Antiviral treatment). In vitro, NS5B requires a nucleic acid primer to initiate polymerization (Oh et al. 1999). The mechanism of strand initiation during genome copying is unknown, although it has recently been demonstrated that replication required one or more RNA stem–loops in the terminal NS5B region (You et al. 2004), to which NS5B directly binds (Lee et al. 2004; Cheng et al. 1999). Whether strand initiation of the opposite strand occurs through a similar mechanism, and whether there is post-transcriptional editing or modification of the newly synthesized genomic and antigenomic strands is unknown.

HCV GENETIC VARIABILITY

Nucleotide sequence variation

The first indication of the genetic heterogeneity of HCV came from comparisons of nucleotide sequences of HCV variants from Japan with that of the prototype HCV variant obtained from the USA, HCV-PT (Choo et al. 1991). For example, the complete genome sequences of HCV-J (Kato et al. 1990) and -BK (Takamizawa et al. 1991) from Japan showed 92 percent similarity to each other, but only 79 percent with HCV-PT. At that time, the former were referred to as the 'Japanese' type (or type II), while those from the USA (HCV-PT and -H) were classified as type I. However, far more divergent variants of HCV have since been found in Japan (Okamoto et al. 1992b, 1991) and elsewhere (Mori et al. 1992; Chan et al. 1992), leading to the adoption of an extended classification of HCV into types and subtypes.

Comparison of nucleotide sequences of variants recovered from infected individuals in different risk groups for infection and from different geographical regions has revealed the existence of six major genetic groups. Over the complete genome, these differ in 30–35 percent of nucleotide sites, with more variability concentrated in regions such as the E1 and E2 glycoproteins, while sequences of the core gene and some of the nonstructural protein genes, such as NS3, are more conserved. Least sequence variability between genotypes is found in the 5′ untranslated region, the 5′ end of the core gene and the 99 base pair X-tail in the 3′ UTR, where specific sequences and RNA secondary structures are required for replication and translation functions. Despite the sequence diversity of HCV, all genotypes share an identical complement of colinear genes of similar or identical size.

Each of the six major genetic groups of HCV contain a series of more closely related subtypes, typically different from each other by 20 percent in nucleotide sequences compared with the >30 percent between genotypes (Figure 54.5) (Simmonds et al. 1993a). Some, such as genotypes 1a, 1b, and 3a have become very widely distributed as a result of transmission through blood transfusion and needle sharing between infecting drug users (IDU) over the past 30–70 years, and now represent the vast majority of infections in western countries (Figure 54.5a) (see Geographical distribution of HCV genotypes). These are the genotypes most commonly encountered clinically, and for which most information has been collected on response to interferon and other antiviral treatments (see Biological differences between HCV genotypes).

A different pattern of sequence diversity is observed in parts of Africa and South East Asia. Here, there are close associations between genotypes and specific geographical regions (Figure 54.5b). For example, infections in western Africa are predominantly by genotype 2 (Jeannel et al. 1998; Mellor et al. 1995; Wansbrough Jones et al. 1998; Ruggieri et al. 1996; Candotti et al. 2003), while those in central Africa, such as the Democratic Republic of Congo (DRC) and Gabon are by genotype 1 and 4 (Bukh et al. 1993a; Fretz et al. 1995; Stuyver et al. 1993b; Menendez et al. 1999; Xu et al. 1994; Ndjomou et al. 2003; Mellor et al. 1995). In both regions, there is a remarkable diversity of subtypes; for example, 20 of 23 HCV-seropositive blood donors in Ghana (west Africa) were infected by genotype 2, but each corresponded to different and previously undescribed subtypes (Candotti et al. 2003). Similar diversity was found in Guinea, Benin, and Burkina Faso (west central Africa), where 18 different subtypes of genotypes 1 and 2 infected 41 HCV-infected individuals (Jeannel et al. 1998). These field observations reflect both the huge genetic diversity of genotypes 1, 2, and 4, and also its likely long-term presence in human populations in these parts of Africa. Taking this geographical mapping further, genotypes 3 and 6 show similar genetic diversity in south and eastern Asia (Tokita et al. 1994a, b, 1995; Mellor et al. 1995).

The model suggested by these genotype distributions is that HCV has been endemic in sub-Saharan Africa and South East Asia for a considerable time, and the occurrence of infection in western and other nontropical countries represents a relatively recent emergence of infection in new risk groups for infection (Simmonds

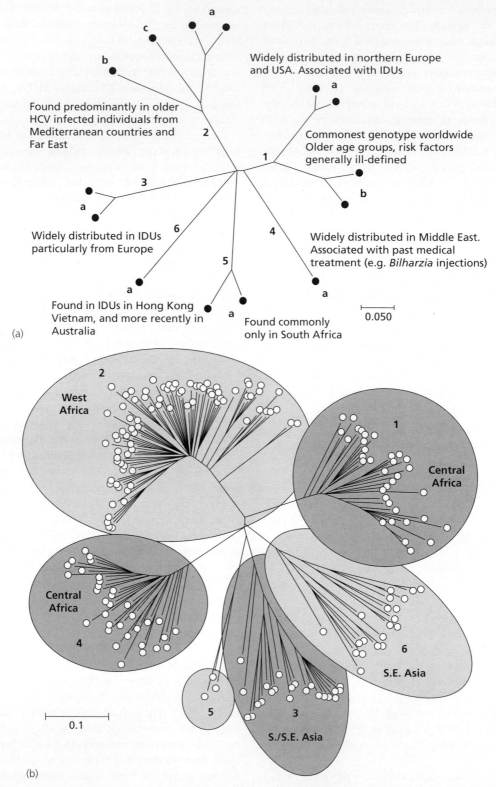

Figure 54.5 (a) *Evolutionary tree of the principal genotypes of HCV found in industrialized countries. Phylogenetic analysis was carried out on complete genome sequences of genotypes of HCV found in the main identified risk groups for HCV infection (IDUs, recipients of unscreened blood or blood products, other parenteral exposures). These represent the main variants believed to have become prevalent over the course of the twentieth century.* **(b)** *Evolutionary tree of all available NS5B sequences for different subtypes and genotypes HCV. This phylogenetic analysis demonstrates that HCV variants still fall into six distinct genotypes, but each contains numerous novel variants discovered in high diversity areas in sub-Saharan Africa and South East Asia. (The trees were constructed using the phylogeny program neighbor-joining implemented in the MEGA package, using Jukes-Cantor corrected distances.)*

2001; Ndjomou et al. 2003). In the twentieth century, parenteral exposure to bloodborne viruses became frequent through the widespread adoption of blood transfusion since the 1940s, the medical use of often unsterilized needles for injections and vaccinations (a practice that continues in many developing countries) and most specifically to industrialized countries, injecting drug use, and the sharing of injection equipment. These new routes for transmission plausibly account for the epidemiological and genetic evidence for recent epidemic spread of HCV over the past 50 years in Europe, Egypt, and elsewhere (Cochrane et al. 2002; Pybus et al. 2001, 2003; Ndjomou et al. 2003). However, the original routes of HCV transmission in endemic, high diversity areas are not understood, as transmission by either sexual contact or from mother to child is inefficient (Wasley and Alter 2000; Pradat and Trepo 2000; Thomas 2000), and there is little evidence historically for the widespread parenteral exposure that fueled the recent epidemic in western countries.

Nomenclature of HCV genotypes

The six main genetic groups or 'clades' of HCV have been designated as genotypes (Figure 54.5). Following previous proposals (Mellor et al. 1995; Mizokami et al. 1996; de Lamballerie et al., 1997), 'new' genotypes (such as 7a, 8a, 9a, and 11a) have been assigned as members of genotype 6, and genotype 10a into genotype 3. An advisory group is currently cataloging a full listing of recognized genotypes and subtypes, and resolving any inconsistencies (such as the labeling of two HCV variants with the same subtype name) for publication in 2005. The new standardized nomenclature will be adopted by public access databases that allow access to fully annotated sequences deposited on GenBank, EMBL, or DDBJ. It has also been decided not to pursue the designation of all variants within genotypes as individual subtypes. In high diversity areas such as central Africa, there may an indefinite number of 'subtypes' that would be of little value to catalog. Future assignment of subtype names will only be carried out for those where a new variant is found in three or more epidemiologically unlinked infections, thus restricting formal classification to those that are more widely distributed, and which may show specific geographical, risk group, or other epidemiological associations.

Recombination

Recombination occurs in many families of RNA viruses, its occurrence requiring both epidemiological opportunity and biological compatibility. Recombination occurs within cells infected with two or more genetically distinct variants of HCV, and thus requires both coinfection of the same individual with more than one such variant, and substantial overlaps in their geographical distributions of different genotypes to enable recombinant forms to be detected. The wide range of genotypes circulating in the main risk groups for HCV in western countries, such as 1a and 3a in IDUs, provides opportunities for recombination, as does the nature of HCV risk behavior, frequently involving multiple exposures around the time of primary infection (e.g. repeated needle-sharing with several infected individuals). Recombination may also be facilitated by the absence of protective immunity from reinfection in chronic HCV infection (Farci et al. 1992; Kao et al. 1993; Jarvis et al. 1994; Lai et al. 1994).

A convincing example of a viable, and rapidly spreading recombinant form of HCV contains structural genes from genotype 2k, a recombination point in NS2 and nonstructural genes from genotype 1b, and has been recovered from several IDUs in St Petersburg (Kalinina et al. 2002, 2004). The existence of widespread recombination would place a considerable limitation on the use of genotyping assays for HCV, as the genotype identified in the region used in the assay, such as the 5' UTR or core gene may not correspond to the genotype of other parts of the genome which may be more relevant for determining treatment response (see Biological differences between HCV genotypes).

Biological differences between HCV genotypes

The major features of HCV structure, replication, transmission, and ability to establish persistent infection are shared between all known variants. Infection with each genotype has become widespread in human populations, and indicates that they are equally capable of maintaining infections in human populations. Despite this obvious evidence for phenotypic similarity, there is growing evidence for genotype-specific differences in persistence and interactions with innate cell defenses and the immune system that have important repercussions for current and likely future therapy.

The extensive amino acid sequence variability found in both structural and nonstructural proteins would be expected to modify profoundly immunological recognition by both antibody and T-cell receptors. For example, the envelope proteins of different genotypes differ in amino acid sequence from each other by between 34–40 and 26–29 percent for E1 and E2. By analogy, this degree of sequence variability would be sufficient to prevent neutralization of one subtype by antibody elicited by a heterologous serotype, a prediction that has been borne out in recent studies using HCV chimeras (see Replication of the HCV genome). There is also clear evidence for antigenic differences between recombinant proteins or peptides from different genotypes in enzyme-linked immunosorbent assays (McOmish et al.

1993; Simmonds et al. 1993c; Tsukiyama Kohara et al. 1993; Mondelli et al. 1994). Antigenic differences between genotypes have implications for the development of vaccines for HCV and for the optimal design of serological screening and confirmatory assays for HCV (see Diagnostic tests for HCV infection).

The most clinically apparent difference between genotypes is in their susceptibility to treatment with interferon (IFN) monotherapy or IFN/ribavirin (RBV) combination therapy. Typically, only 10–20 and 40–50 percent individuals with chronic infection with genotype 1 on monotherapy and combination therapy, respectively, exhibit complete and permanent clearance of virus infection. This long-term response rate is much lower than the 50 and 70–80 percent observed on treatment of genotype 2 or 3 infections (comprehensively reviewed in Zeuzem (2004) and Pawlotsky (2003a)). This difference has proved to be highly significant in patient management, and has led to the use of higher doses and longer durations of treatment for type 1 (and type 4) infections to achieve acceptable efficacy. In numerous multivariate analyses, genotype-specific differences in treatment response have been shown to be independent of host variables, such as stage of disease progression, age, duration of infection, sex, and HIV and other virus coinfections. It is similarly independent of virus-specific factors, such as pretreatment viral load, although this also independently correlates (inversely) with response. The underlying mechanism of these differences in response is currently unknown.

Enzymatic studies and preliminary data from clinical trials provide consistent evidence for frequent genotype-specific differences in susceptibility to recently developed protease and RNA polymerase inhibitors for HCV therapy (De Francesco et al. 2003). Antiviral agents whose modeling, screening, and optimization was based on enzymatic studies of genotype 1 protease or RNA polymerase have since been found to be poorly inhibitory against other genotypes (Holland-Staley et al. 2002). For example, the protease inhibitor, BILN 2061, showed nearly 2 logs weaker binding affinity to genotype 2 and 3 proteases than to genotype 1 (Thibeault et al. 2004). These enzymatic differences may be clinically significant; in a recent efficacy trial, nongenotype 1-infected individuals were nonresponsive or only weakly responsive to short-term treatment with the BILN 2061 protease inhibitor (Reiser 2004), in contrast to its efficacy in genotype 1 (Lamarre et al. 2003).

In contrast to the clear-cut differences between genotypes in their response to antiviral therapy, it has proven much more difficult to obtain reliable data on the differences in the natural history and pathogenicity between HCV genotypes. This is because it is difficult to obtain prospective and/or case–controlled data on the outcomes of HCV infection over the exceptionally long time over which complications of HCV infection present clinically. Biased recruitment of study cohorts towards the minority with clinically apparent disease lack the community denominator and information on durations of infection with which to estimate the time course of disease development. Longitudinal studies have shown that genotype 1 invariably appeared more likely to establish persistence, and in carriers, to be associated with more severe liver disease compared with genotypes 2 and 3 (Mazzeo et al. 2003; Yee et al. 2000; Resti et al. 2003; Franchini et al. 2001). The underlying mechanism for the greater persistence of genotype 1 infections may be related to the greater treatment resistance of this genotype (see above). Most evidence supports the hypothesis that genotype 1 is more likely to cause hepatocellular carcinoma (Di Bisceglie 1997). However, infections with genotype 3 are associated with a higher incidence of steatosis (Adinolfi et al. 2001; Rubbia-Brandt et al. 2000), thought to result from direct cytopathic damage to hepatocytes from a block in lipoprotein secretion (Serfaty et al. 2001).

CLINICAL AND PATHOLOGICAL ASPECTS

Clinical and pathological features of HCV infection

Hepatitis C infection causes an indolent and slowly progressive liver disease that is asymptomatic until the development of decompensated liver disease and, often, liver cancer. The following sections review the clinical and pathological features associated with acute and chronic hepatitis, the replication of HCV in liver and possibly at extrahepatic sites, and describes proposed mechanisms of liver damage and of persistence.

Acute hepatitis

Percutaneous exposure to HCV usually results in an asymptomatic infection (not associated with jaundice), and most people become chronic carriers of the virus (Figure 54.6). This contrasts strongly with the observation that few adults infected with HBV become chronically infected. The period from exposure to the development of hepatitis has been measured in a number of investigations of post-transfusional hepatitis. Most studies have reported an interval of about 8 weeks to the development of abnormal liver function tests (such as alanine aminotransferase (ALT) levels), although viremia can be detected earlier (Figure 54.6). Only 5 percent of individuals with acute HCV infection have symptomatic disease, although in some cases it may be severe. HCV is very rarely associated with acute fulminant hepatic failure (Wright et al. 1991; Mutimer et al. 1995a). HCV may be more likely to cause acute liver failure in the patient who is a carrier of hepatitis B and in those who acquire hepatitis B and HCV

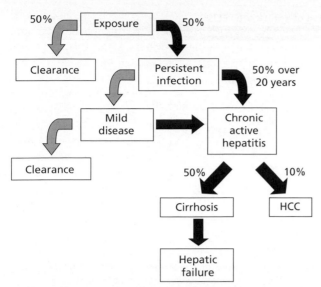

Figure 54.6 *Outcome of infection with HCV. Hepatitis can be detected by blood tests approximately 2 months after exposure to HCV. Most infections are asymptomatic, and a minority of patients develop jaundice. Approximately 50 percent of infected patients have persistent infection, i.e. they become HCV carriers. Of these, a proportion will progress to chronic active hepatitis, and may eventually progress to cirrhosis or hepatocellular carcinoma. The frequencies of the various outcomes are provided only as a very approximate guide, and are greatly influenced by host (particularly patient age) and viral factors (such as infecting genotype).*

simultaneously. Clinically, hepatitis caused by HCV is indistinguishable from that caused by other hepatitis viruses; jaundice may develop, but more usually symptoms are nonspecific such as fatigue, anorexia, and nausea. Most HCV-infected individuals cannot recall a history of jaundice, and HCV accounts for a small proportion of clinically apparent hepatitis cases in the community.

Viremia can be detected by PCR in the early stages of acute hepatitis, appearing at the same time or slightly earlier than abnormal levels of ALT (Figure 54.7). In contrast, seroconversion for antibody may be delayed for several weeks or months after the onset of hepatitis (Lelie et al. 1992), although second- and third-generation assays have closed this 'window' period to some extent. Nevertheless, reliable identification of HCV as a cause of acute hepatitis depends on the use of PCR, in contrast to acute HAV infection where IgM is generally detectable at the onset of clinical hepatitis. Histological features of acute HCV are similar to those associated with acute HAV and HBV infection; liver biopsy is rarely indicated to make a diagnosis of acute HCV infection.

Chronic hepatitis

The frequency of chronic infection following exposure to HCV is high, although there are difficulties in estimating a precise figure. For example, HCV may be identified

more frequently in those with symptomatic primary infection or those with post-transfusion hepatitis (Kiyosawa et al. 1990; Gilletterver et al. 1995), both of which may be associated with an increased likelihood of chronic infection (Gordon et al. 1993; Mutimer et al. 1995b).

Individuals infected through blood transfusion and hemophiliacs, many of whom have been repeatedly exposed to HCV through the use of nonvirally inactivated clotting factor concentrates, have a high rate of persistent infection associated with active liver disease (60–80 percent). In contrast, lower rates of chronic infection and more slowly progressive disease are observed in individuals with lesser exposure to HCV. For example, only 50 percent of women exposed to a particular batch of anti-D immunoglobulin had persistent infection (Meisel et al. 1995), whereas in a similar outbreak in Ireland, also associated with the use of anti-D (Power et al. 1994), viremia was detected by PCR in only 50 percent of people remaining seropositive 17 years after exposure. Given the tendency for antibody to become undetectable following clearance of viremia, the true frequency of persistent infection in these two cohorts may be even lower.

Persistent infection with HCV is generally associated with persistent and progressive hepatitis. Chronically infected individuals generally have fluctuating or continuously abnormal levels of ALT and are viremic. However, it has been difficult to establish a correlation between the level of viremia and the severity of liver disease. For example, HCV RNA levels in asymptomatic blood donors are similar to those found in patients treated for liver disease (Smith et al. 1996; Lau et al. 1995a). Moreover, several studies have failed to document any association between the degree of viremia and level of ALT or other biochemical abnormalities associated with hepatitis.

Histological features

HCV infection causes a range of characteristic histological changes in the liver, although none allows a specific diagnosis of HCV infection to be made. The most striking feature of HCV infection of the liver is the presence of lymphoid follicles within the portal tracts (Figure 54.8); these are less often observed in hepatitis from other viral causes. Biopsies also typically reveal a dense periportal inflammatory process, associated with the infiltration of lymphocytes and plasma cells. Bile duct damage is often found in association with the infiltration, with vacuolization and ballooning of epithelial cells lining small bile ducts. Another common observation is the appearance of lobular hepatitis, with lymphocyte infiltration within sinusoids surrounding the hepatocytes. Steatosis is a frequent histological feature of HCV infection. It may be more commonly observed in those patients with HCV genotype 3 infection and

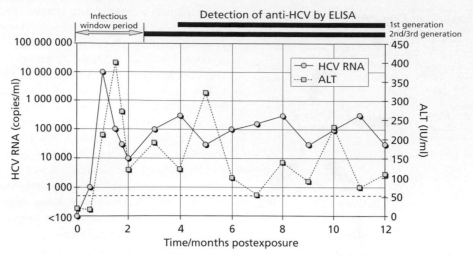

Figure 54.7 *Virological and biochemical markers of acute HCV infection. HCV RNA (solid line) and abnormal ALT levels (dotted line) appear approximately 50 days after exposure to HCV in a typical individual. The subsequent development of chronic hepatitis is indicated by persistent viremia and by fluctuating abnormal ALT levels. Antibody to HCV first appears after the onset of acute hepatitis, in this example leading to 'infectious window periods' of up to 60–80 days in currently used serological assays. The antibody profile elicited by infection is highly variable between individuals, although antibody to c33c is normally the first to appear.*

may resolve (along with other features of chronic hepatitis) in response to successful antiviral therapy.

The extent of histological abnormalities within biopsies can be summarized by descriptions such as lobular, chronic persistent hepatitis (CPH), and chronic active hepatitis (CAH), with or without cirrhosis, although more informative scoring systems such as the Knodell and Ishak scores have also been devised (Knodell et al. 1981; Ishak 1994). A spectrum of milder disease is generally observed in studies of asymptomatic individuals, such as those identified by blood donor screening, possibly reflecting a shorter duration of infection.

Despite sporadic publication of in situ histological demonstrations of HCV RNA and/or encoded proteins, most histopathologists struggle to demonstrate HCV in tissue sections and convincing reproducible studies using commercially available reagents are lacking.

Progression of disease

The percentage of chronically infected individuals who progress to cirrhosis and liver failure is not known. Progression to clinically significant liver damage is almost invariably very slow, although it may be faster in the context of immunosuppression. Particularly aggressive liver disease associated with HCV has been observed in immunosuppressed recipients of organ transplants and in patients with inherited immunodeficiency states (Healey et al. 1994). Studies of post-transfusion HCV highlight the following important clinical features. Many transfusion recipients are elderly (often suffering significant nonhepatic diseases) and die within two decades of infection, but not as a consequence of HCV infection. HCV-related mortality is rare within 20 years of infection; in one study, no excess mortality

of HCV-infected individuals was observed over a period of 17 years (Figure 54.9) (Seeff et al. 1992). Cirrhosis is rarely observed within 10 years of infection, and as few as 20 percent of infected patients have cirrhosis after 20 years' follow-up. Risk factors for progression of chronic hepatitis to cirrhosis include age at time of infection (more rapid progression observed when infection occurs at older age), male gender, and concurrent alcohol consumption (Poynard et al. 1997). Recent analyses have highlighted the potential adverse impact of hepatic steatosis (and patient body mass index (BMI)) on fibrosis progression and on response to antiviral therapy. Cirrhosis may be complicated by hepatocellular carcinoma, but this rarely develops within 15 years of HCV infection (see Hepatocellular carcinoma). Some patients have asymptomatic infection, with normal liver function tests and mild hepatitis, despite 30 years of infection.

HCV may be associated with more aggressive liver disease in older than in younger people. Prognosis may also depend on viral genotype, although this is interrelated with other factors such as age at acquisition. For example, most transfusion recipients are elderly, and HCV genotype 1b is most commonly isolated from the serum of patients with transfusion-associated infection (Mahaney et al. 1994). Although it is not possible to estimate long-term prognosis at the time of infection, it is more feasible for patients with a known long duration of infection. For instance, when a 30-year-old patient has cirrhosis within 10 years of infection, there is a high likelihood that liver failure will eventually develop. However, for a 70-year-old patient with mild hepatitis despite 30 years' duration of infection, HCV is unlikely to cause death. Assessment of prognosis is an important aspect of selecting patients for treatment.

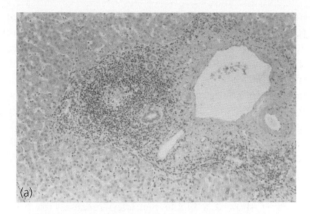

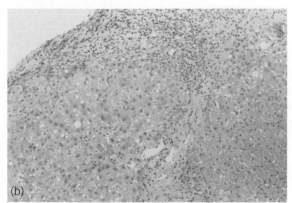

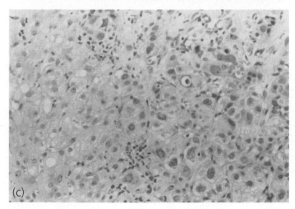

Figure 54.8 *Typical histopathological feature of HCV infection of the liver. (a) Typical HCV hepatitis with a large lymphoid aggregate within a portal tract showing reactive germinal center formation. Although the aggregate is close to a bile duct and adjacent to the limiting plate of the tract, there is little evidence of bile duct damage and none of interface hepatitis (piecemeal necrosis). Plasma cells and macrophages are also commonly present. (b) Cirrhosis. This is characterized by coarse fibrous septa separating nodules of regenerating hepatocytes. (c) Hepatocellular carcinoma. Tumor cells (right) are pleomorphic and hyperchromatic adjacent to regenerating hepatocytes in a cirrhotic nodule. There is a patchy chronic inflammatory infiltrate at the interface between them (sections kindly provided by Professor D.J. Harrison, Department of Pathology, University of Edinburgh).*

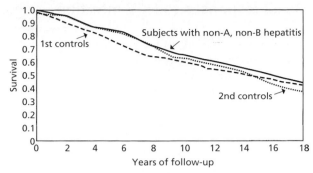

Figure 54.9 *Mortality associated with chronic post-transfusion hepatitis. The authors studied patients with transfusion-related non-A, non-B hepatitis (principally hepatitis C) who had been identified in five major prospective studies conducted in the USA between 1967 and 1980. Each index case was matched with two groups of noninfected transfusion recipients (first and second), and mortality rates from all causes were determined during an average follow up of 18 years. Mortality from all causes was high (about 50 percent in all groups), and the survival curves for the three groups were the same (reproduced from Seeff et al. (1992). Death from liver disease was low in all three groups, but was significantly higher in those originally given a diagnosis of non-A, non-B hepatitis (data not shown).*

be manifest as hepatic encephalopathy, variceal hemorrhage, or ascites. Clinical manifestations of liver failure are not specific for HCV-induced liver disease, but are common to all forms of cirrhosis. Hepatocellular carcinoma may develop in an HCV-infected liver, but is very rarely observed in the absence of cirrhosis (see below).

In summary, most HCV infection is asymptomatic; when symptoms do develop, they are the nonspecific symptoms of liver failure.

Hepatocellular carcinoma

Hepatocellular carcinoma (HCC) is a frequent complication of long-standing HCV infection. In many western countries such as Spain and Italy, as well as in Japan, HCV infection is found in 60–90 percent of cases of HCC. HCC develops slowly, typically appearing 30 years after infection, and being rare within 15 years (Kiyosawa et al. 1990). In most studies, HCC usually, although not invariably (Demitri et al. 1995), occurs in patients with pre-existing cirrhosis.

For these reasons, the mechanism by which HCV causes HCC is generally considered to be indirect, arising as a consequence of chronic damage and inflammation of liver cells. Unlike HBV, replication of HCV does not produce DNA sequences that could be integrated into the host genome, nor is there any evidence for transforming activity of any of the HCV gene products. Treatment of hepatitis C patients with interferon-α has been reported to greatly reduce the subsequent risk of developing HCC, even in those conventionally regarded as 'non-responders,' in whom long-term normalization of ALT was not achieved (Nishiguchi et al. 1995).

After many years, liver failure may develop in patients with cirrhosis (also known as decompensated cirrhosis) (Fattovich et al. 1997). Decompensation may

B-cell responses to HCV infection

Infection with HCV elicits humoral and T-cell-mediated immune responses. Antibody reactivity to several HCV proteins can be detected in most infected individuals, although the response is highly variable and generally weak compared with antibody responses to other viruses. There seems to be no specific pattern of antibody response that is predictive of the long-term outcome of infection.

HCV antibody has been found to rapidly decline in titer after clearance of viremia in those who spontaneously resolve infection and in those who respond to HCV therapy. For example, ten women with documented exposure to HCV infection through treatment with contaminated anti-D immunoglobulin in East Germany were found to be seropositive 10 years after exposure, but five became completely seronegative in the following 10 years, while antibody titers in the remainder fell to close to the cut-off the HCV serological assay (Takaki et al. 2000).

Until recently it has been difficult to assess the protective effect of the serological response to HCV infection. It is now possible to investigate neutralization of HCV in vitro through the production of virus pseudotypes, in which a different virus from HCV is packaged inside an HCV envelope, and whose infectivity can be more readily quantified than HCV (Flint et al. 2004; Bartosch et al. 2003; Hsu et al. 2003) (see Structural proteins). Neutralizing antibody responses can be detected in HCV-infected individuals; titers are initially low and highly strain-specific, but increase and broaden in reactivity on development of chronic infection (Logvinoff et al. 2004). Neutralizing antibody was found targeted to epitopes in the hypervariable region of the E2 envelope protein and elsewhere in the viral envelope (Bartosch et al. 2003). Neutralizing antibodies elicited by infection with genotype 1a was able to cross-neutralize pseudotypes generated from other strains of genotype 1a, as well as of genotype 1b. Despite these new observations, it remains unclear whether B-cell responses are important in controlling HCV replication in vivo, and contribute to virus clearance on initial infection or subsequently.

T-cell responses to HCV infection

A vigorous cellular immune response to HCV can be detected in infected individuals. T-helper cells obtained from peripheral blood of most HCV-infected people proliferate when exposed to recombinant HCV proteins, such as core, E1, E2, NS3, NS4, and NS5 (Botarelli et al. 1993; Ferrari et al. 1994; Schupper et al. 1993). Indeed, unlike B-cell responses, recovery from infection is associated with stronger and more sustained cytotoxic T lymphocyte (CTL) responses around the time of primary infection than in those who become persistently infected (Cooper et al. 1999; Thimme et al. 2001; Lechner et al. 2000). Proliferative responses were detected more frequently in individuals who had cleared infection, suggesting that the cellular immune response is important in the control of virus replication in vivo. In the East German women who lost HCV antibody reactivity on resolution of active infection (see previous section), all retained HCV-specific helper and cytotoxic T-cell responses more than 10 years after clearance of viremia (Takaki et al. 2000).

Proliferative responses of T-helper cells obtained from the liver showed a highly restricted reactivity to NS4, compared with the responses found in mononuclear cells of peripheral blood (Minutello et al. 1993). CTLs from the liver and peripheral blood of HCV-infected individuals react with a wide range of epitopes from both structural and nonstructural proteins (Koziel et al. 1992, 1993; Cerny et al. 1995b; Battegay et al. 1995). CTLs are likely to be important in both the control of, and recovery from, HCV infection and in the pathogenesis of liver disease.

Mechanism of persistence

Although humoral and cellular immune responses to HCV occur upon infection, these seem to be unable to clear the infection (see Chronic hepatitis) or to protect an individual from reinfection. For example, it is possible to reinfect chimpanzees repeatedly with the same strain of HCV (Prince et al. 1992; Farci et al. 1992), producing hepatitis de novo similar to that observed on primary infection. However, chimpanzees who have cleared previous infection are partly or completely resistant to reinfection with the homologous or heterologous genotypes of HCV (Lanford et al. 2004), possibly the result of strong T-cell memory responses characteristic of resolved infections. Repeated exposure of humans to HCV may also produce recurrent episodes of infection, observed for example in thalassemic patients transfused with HCV-contaminated blood (Lai et al. 1994). Infection with more than one HCV genotype is frequently observed in other multiply exposed individuals, such as hemophiliacs (Jarvis et al. 1994). Persistence of HCV and the observed susceptibility of individuals to reinfection occur despite the existence of neutralizing antibody responses to HCV, that which often shows cross-reactivity to other HCV genotypes.

Immune escape

Several observations suggest that many of the amino acid changes that occur during HCV infection are driven sequentially by selection pressures that prevent peptide binding to MHC class I or II alleles, or prevent neutralization by antibody responses to the virus. The envelope proteins are the principal targets of humoral immune responses, and it has been hypothesized that changes in E1 and E2 alter the antigenic properties of the proteins, thereby allowing the virus to 'escape' from neutralizing antibodies (Weiner et al. 1992). In this model, persistent virus replication is achieved by continuous diversification of HCV in regions particularly sensitive to neutralizing antibody; this hypothesis is supported by the observation that much of the variability in the *E2* gene is concentrated in discrete 'hypervariable' regions (Weiner et al. 1992; Hijikata et al. 1991a; Kato et al. 1992), that may be in close proximity to parts of the protein involved in virus/cellular receptor interactions, as in influenza A virus. Supporting this hypothesis is the observation that sequence change was slower in individuals with defects in B-cell immunity (Booth et al. 1998), where there would be reduced immune selection on B-cell epitopes. Similarly, the strong and sustained CTL responses in primary HCV infection may drive sequence change in those who became chronic carriers (Chang et al. 1997; Cantaloube et al. 2003; Sheridan et al. 2004). Immune selection may also underlie the high degree of sequence variability between and within genotypes in the envelope and other regions of the genome such as NS5A.

Mechanism of liver damage

It is likely that direct cytopathic infection of cells in the liver, as well as damage secondary to the inflammatory process contributes to HCV-associated liver disease. Evidence that HCV replication itself is directly cytopathic includes the clinical observation of more severe and rapidly progressive liver disease in individuals who are immunosuppressed and who have high levels of viremia. Secondly, there is generally a direct correlation between clearance of viremia and normalization of ALT levels in people who respond to interferon treatment (see Progression of disease), implying that it is virus replication itself that is responsible for the hepatitis. These observations contrast with HBV, in which successful treatment with interferon is thought to result from augmenting CTL activity in the liver and is associated with elevated ALT levels and a transient exacerbation of hepatitis.

Immunopathology may result from cytotoxic T cell reactivity against HCV-infected cells, or the process of HCV infection might trigger an autoimmune disease in which uninfected cells become the targets. The development of an immune response to the cellular protein, GOR, in association with HCV infection could be an example of this process (Mishiro et al. 1991). Understanding the mechanism of liver disease would assist the rational development of HCV treatment (see Antiviral treatment). Standard antiviral treatment schedules including interferon-α have been shown to clear hepatitis in some individuals (Davis et al. 1989; Di Bisceglie et al. 1989), although it is not known whether it acts as a virucidal agent or if its action depends on its immunomodulatory properties such as the upregulating expression of MHC class I on hepatocytes.

Extrahepatic manifestations

In a few infected patients, HCV may be responsible for extrahepatic clinical manifestations and disease (Martin 1993). The underlying pathogenic mechanisms for these extrahepatic manifestations are varied and often poorly understood. There are at least three mechanisms by which HCV could cause such disease. First, it is possible that HCV is capable of cytopathic replication in cell types outside the liver. Secondly, HCV may trigger an autoimmune process that is directed against antigens expressed on nonhepatic cells. Thirdly, persistent HCV infection could lead to immune-complex formation with antibodies followed by deposition in small vessels.

Methods to detect extrahepatic replication of HCV include the detection of HCV protein expression by immunocytochemistry and the detection of replication intermediates by strand-specific PCR. Simple detection of HCV RNA sequences is generally insufficient evidence, as HCV may nonspecifically associate or bind to cells such as macrophages or B lymphocytes in the peripheral circulation. The detection of HCV in tissues may reflect a process of immune-complex deposition rather than replication.

Many published studies reporting the detection of replication intermediates (complementary RNA sequences) in a range of cell types used methods that were insufficiently specific. However, using a PCR-based method for detection of sequences from the core region, Lerat and co-workers (1996) reported that replication may occur in certain lymphoid cells. In contrast, no evidence for extrahepatic replication was observed in chimpanzees, using a similar assay (Lanford et al. 1995). In other studies, HCV was detected in lymphocytes infiltrating the liver by immunocytochemical and hybridization methods (Blight et al. 1994).

HCV infection is clearly associated with certain types of vasculitis and glomerulonephritis, which are caused by immune complex deposition. In southern Europe, HCV infection seems to be associated with porphyria cutanea tarda, a potentially disfiguring skin condition associated with an acquired deficiency of the liver enzyme uroporphyrinogen decarboxylase (Herrero et al. 1993). There is a putative association of HCV with other nonhepatic conditions, including Sjögren's syndrome, rheumatoid arthritis, pulmonary fibrosis, corneal ulceration, aplastic anemia, and non-Hodgkin's lymphoma. Vasculitis and glomerulonephritis are more frequent in patients with established cirrhosis.

HCV is classically associated with the small vessel vasculitis known as 'essential mixed cryoglobulinemia' (Agnello et al. 1992) (also observed in patients with chronic HBV infection). Laboratory features include the presence of rheumatoid factor activity in serum, the presence of a cryoprecipitate, complement activation, and proteinuria/hematuria. The most important clinical manifestation is purpura, which is nearly always present, and 25–50 percent of patients have renal disease. Most patients have constitutional symptoms, especially weakness and arthralgia; Raynaud's phenomenon, Sjögren's syndrome, and neuritis may also be present. Purpura may resolve with interferon-α therapy (Misiani et al. 1994).

HCV infection is also associated with membranoproliferative glomerulonephritis (MPGN) type 1 (Johnson et al. 1993), which is a consequence of immune complex deposition in the glomerular capillaries. It is associated with serum rheumatoid factor positivity, with complement activation, and with cryoglobulinemia. MPGN is classically associated with heavy proteinuria, often in the nephrotic range (more than 3.5 g per 24 h), whilst creatinine clearance is modestly impaired. Treatment with interferon-α reduces urinary protein loss, but the impact of treatment on renal outcome is uncertain (Johnson et al. 1993). It should be emphasized that HCV infection is a relatively common cause of mixed essential cryoglobulinemia and MPGN, but that HCV infection is rarely complicated by these conditions.

EPIDEMIOLOGY

Parenteral routes of transmission

In western Europe, Australia, and North America, most HCV-infected patients have a history of percutaneous exposure to the virus, and most are (or have been) injecting drug users. The seroconversion rate of IDUs has been estimated at 20 percent per year, so long-term drug users are almost invariably HCV-infected. Drug use was uncommon before the 1960s, so drug users tend to be younger than patients infected through transfusion and are also more likely to be infected with genotypes other than type 1b. Most drug users have asymptomatic infection with no history of jaundice, but have chronic hepatitis whereas some have developed cirrhosis and a few have progressed to liver failure. Since drug use is usually associated with HCV acquisition at a fairly young age (in comparison with transfusion-acquired infection) and thus with a slower rate of progression to cirrhosis, few IDUs would progress to liver failure within two (or even three) decades of infection. However, because of the lower average age of IDUs, their life expectancy from the time of infection is five or six decades; despite less aggressive infection, many will survive long enough to develop significant liver disease.

In the 1960s, clotting factor concentrates became more widely used and most patients with coagulation disorders became infected with HCV. Thousands of donors contribute to each factor concentrate, so contamination with HCV and HIV was very likely. Many recipients were young, and most developed liver disease. Some have progressed to liver failure, and died or undergone liver transplantation (Telfer et al. 1994), although for many the prognosis may have been affected by HIV coinfection. Since the introduction of effective virus inactivation for blood products in the 1980s, factor concentrates have not transmitted HCV infection.

Repeated exposure to blood and blood products (in the absence of serological screening and/or heat treatment) is clearly associated with a high risk of HCV exposure and infection. The risk associated with exposure to a single donor product (e.g. one unit of blood) was already diminishing before the availability of specific serological tests for HCV, but varied significantly from country to country. Mercenary donors are more likely to be HCV-infected, and the prevalence of donor seropositivity was significantly reduced when 'self-exclusion' policies were introduced to combat the risk of HIV transmission. For example, by the mid-1980s fewer than 1 percent of UK donors were HCV-positive (Contreras et al. 1991).

Screening of blood donors for antibodies to HCV was introduced by most blood transfusion services in 1990 and 1991. Blood donors are clearly not representative of the entire population, but scrutiny of HCV-positive donors provides some insights into the epidemiology of this infection (Alter 1995; Mansell and Locarnini 1995). The lowest seroprevalence is observed in Scandinavia and in the UK with slightly higher prevalence in North America, western Europe, and Australia. Prevalence is intermediate in eastern and southern European countries, even higher in Japan, and most prevalent in Middle Eastern (especially Egyptian) blood donors. When donor seroprevalence is low, the seropositive donor is more likely to have an identifiable risk factor for parenteral exposure (Mutimer et al. 1995b), but as donor seroprevalence increases, prior parenteral exposure becomes more difficult to identify (Esteban et al. 1991).

In countries of low and intermediate seroprevalence, seropositive donors frequently admit to prior intravenous drug use; sometimes a single exposure, 20–30 years previously. Investigation of seropositive donors confirms that the majority are viremic, and that many have chronic hepatitis and cirrhosis (Esteban et al. 1991; Irving et al. 1994; Mutimer et al. 1995b). As seropositive donors are excluded from the blood donor panels, the frequency of seropositivity falls; in the UK, for instance, true seropositivity fell from an initial rate of 0.60 to 0.15 percent. To further reduce the already small risk for transfusion-associated infection, some blood transfusion organizations have introduced nucleic acid testing of donated products for HCV RNA (see Blood donor screening by PCR and related methods).

Transplanted organs may also transmit HCV infection, and studies in the USA and UK suggest that organ donors have a higher seropositivity rate than blood donors (Pereira et al. 1992; Wreghitt et al. 1994). The majority of high-risk blood donors are subject to self-exclusion, an option that is not available to the brain-dead organ donor. In one study, six of 554 (1.08 percent) British organ donors were HCV-seropositive in the screening assay, and four of these six infected an organ recipient.

Other routes of transmission

Most studies (and this discussion) have focused on groups at risk for HCV infection as a result of percutaneous exposure. These groups include IDUs, transfusion recipients (especially recipients of pooled plasma products such as factor VIII, anti-D) (Power et al. 1995), immunoglobulin (Healey et al. 1994), transplant recipients, hemodialysis patients, and healthcare workers (Zuckerman et al. 1994; Klein et al. 1991). Tattooing and acupuncture may also be responsible for some percutaneous exposure, and in countries of high prevalence the use of unsterilized needles for cultural rituals, medical treatment, or vaccination programs may result in HCV infection. For example, bilharzia treatment using reusable and unsterile needles in the past has frequently been suggested as a cause for the very high population prevalence of HCV infection in Egypt.

However, for many people, overt percutaneous exposure cannot be identified. For example, detailed questioning failed to identify such a cause of infection in approximately one-third of HCV-infected Scottish blood donors (Crawford et al. 1994), and this has prompted the search for other routes of transmission. There seems to be a low risk of infection associated with sexual contact with an HCV carrier. Evidence suggesting that sexual transmission may occur includes the observation that HCV seems to be more common in people who have multiple sexual partners, such as prostitutes and male homosexuals (Tedder et al. 1991; Buchbinder et al. 1994). Large-scale studies of sexual partners of HCV-positive people generally show a slightly increased likelihood of HCV infection compared with the background population (Daikos et al. 1994; Soto et al. 1994; Cerny et al. 1995a; Utsumi et al. 1995), although in two studies (both of wives of hemophiliacs) no transmissions were documented (Bresters et al. 1993a; Hallam et al. 1993). Other sexually transmitted diseases may facilitate sexual transmission of HCV, as is the case for HIV.

Barrier methods of contraception/protection are likely to prevent transmission of HCV. For casual sexual contact, such precautions are mandatory (for mutual protection from all sexually transmitted infection).

When one member of a long-term sexual partnership is identified as a carrier of HCV, both members should be counseled appropriately. The other partner might request serological testing. It seems likely that most couples will not elect to change their sexual practices. HIV/HCV coinfection may increase the risk for sexual transmission of HCV, and this may be a function of the higher HCV titer which is measured in the blood of HIV coinfected patients. In this setting, barrier methods of protection are clearly appropriate.

Early studies documented a low but detectable rate (5–15 percent) of mother-to-child transmission of HCV (Novati et al. 1992; Lam et al. 1993; Wejstal et al. 1992). However, it remains unclear whether this is true vertical transmission (in utero or during birth) or if it occurs through close contact (and possibly unapparent parenteral exposure) during the postnatal period. The risk of infant infection seems to be increased when the mother is HIV/HCV coinfected, and again this may be secondary to higher virus loads associated with immunosuppression (Ohto et al. 1994). HCV transmission may also occur as a result of 'household' contact. In this setting, it is almost impossible to distinguish vertical and sexual transmission from other 'household' contact. The parents of an index case are most likely to be infected. Relative risk is lower for spouses and siblings, and lowest for children of the index case.

In western Europe, most patients with liver failure will be referred for liver transplantation. Examination of the liver transplant experience during the 1980s and 1990s suggests that HCV has been an uncommon cause of liver failure in the UK. This observation suggests the relatively recent introduction of this virus into the western European population. It is evident that HCV infection was rare in western Europe and in North America before the emergence of intravenous drug use in the 1960s. However, it is calculated that the USA experienced an annual incidence of 15 cases per 100 000 population during the 1980s (Alter 1995), predicting a national reservoir of HCV carriers of as many as 3.5 million people. That HCV currently poses less of a clinical problem in the USA and northern Europe than in southern Europe, Japan, and the Middle East is probably due to its later introduction in these populations. In the future, all countries can expect higher rates of significant liver disease from HCV, including liver cancer.

Geographical distribution of HCV genotypes

Some genotypes of HCV (types 1a, 2a, 2b) show a broad worldwide distribution, while others such as type 5a and 6a are only found in specific geographical regions. HCV infected blood donors and patients with chronic hepatitis from countries in western Europe and the USA is frequent with genotypes 1a, 1b, 2a, 2b, and 3a, although the relative frequencies of each may vary, such as the trend for more frequent infection with type 1b in southern and eastern Europe. In many European countries, genotype distributions vary with age of patients, reflecting rapid changes in genotype distribution with time within a single geographic area.

A striking geographical change in genotype distribution is apparent between south east Europe and Turkey (both mainly type 1b) and several countries in the Middle East and parts of north and central Africa where type 4 predominates. For example, a high frequency of HCV infection is found in Egypt (20–30 percent (Saeed et al. 1991; Darwish et al. 1993; Kamel et al. 1992)), of which almost all correspond to type 4a (Simmonds et al. 1993b; McOmish et al. 1994). HCV genotype 5a is frequently found amongst NANBH patients and blood donors in South Africa, but is found only rarely in other parts of Africa or elsewhere.

In Japan and Taiwan and probably parts of China, genotypes 1b, 2a, and 2b are the most frequently found. Infection with type 1a in Japan appears to be confined to hemophiliacs who have received commercial blood products, such as factor VIII and IX clotting concentrates, provided in the USA. A genotype with a highly restricted geographical range is type 6a which was originally found in Hong Kong, where approximately one-third of anti-HCV-positive blood donors are infected with this genotype, as are an equivalent proportion in neighboring Macau and Vietnam.

Molecular epidemiology of HCV infection

Persistent infection with HCV entails continuous replication of HCV over years or decades and the large number of replication cycles, combined with the relatively error-prone RNA-dependent RNA polymerase leads to measurable sequence drift of HCV over time. For example, over an 8-year interval of persistent infection in a chimpanzee, the rate of sequence change for the genome as a whole was 0.144 percent per site per year (Okamoto et al. 1992a), similar to the rate observed in the 5′ half of the genome over 3 years in a human carrier (0.192 percent (Ogata et al. 1991)). Using this molecular clock, it is in principle possible to calculate times of divergence between HCV variants, and therefore establish their degree of epidemiological relatedness. Similarly, phylogenetic analysis of sequences from individuals exposed to HCV can be used as evidence for a common source of infection. Sequence comparisons in variable regions of the HCV genome, such as E2 and NS-5, have been used to document transmission between individuals, and to explore the possibility of nonparenteral routes of transmission such as mother to child (Weiner et al. 1993), within families (Honda et al. 1993), and by sexual contact (Rice et al.

1993; Setoguchi et al. 1994; Healey et al. 1995). For example, clustering of HCV sequences into a single phylogenetic group amongst recipients of an HCV-contaminated blood product (anti-D immunoglobulin) was still apparent 17 years after exposure (Power et al. 1995).

DIAGNOSTIC TESTS FOR HCV INFECTION

Antigens

Antibody reactivity can be detected to several linear and conformational epitopes present on both structural and nonstructural proteins of HCV. Recombinant proteins or peptides containing these antigenic regions are used for serological tests for antibody to HCV (see Figure 54.1), and much of our current knowledge of antibody responses to HCV has arisen from research aimed at improving antibody tests to enable effective screening of blood donors and diagnosis in patients. Cytotoxic T-cell and proliferative responses have also been detected to several peptides or recombinant proteins.

NS4

The original HCV-specific clone isolated from chimpanzee plasma was expressed in *E. coli*, the derived protein of 42 amino acids (1 694–1 735) being encoded by the NS4 region of the genome (see Figure 54.1). A larger clone (c100-3) assembled from several overlapping clones was expressed in yeast and formed the basis of the first commercial tests for HCV antibody. The antigen was derived from amino acids 1 569–1 931, thus spanning a small section of the NS3 region, as well as almost all of 4a and 4b. Despite its being a somewhat unnatural hybrid, use of the antigen in screening assays provided the first evidence of the importance and widespread occurrence of HCV infection. Antigen from NS4 is present in all current screening enzyme-linked immunosorbent assays (ELISA), whether singly, in combination with NS3 or in synthetic peptide form. Likewise, all commercial supplementary immunoblot assays contain NS4 components either as recombinant antigens (Chiron RIBA-2, Murex western blot, Abbott Matrix) or as synthetic peptides (Chiron RIBA-3, Organon Liatek III), which show improved specificity.

Many of the antigenic determinants in the NS4 region show considerable amino acid sequence variability between genotypes of HCV; serological reactivity to the 5-1-1 protein is absent or weak in samples from individuals infected with types 2 or 3 (Chan et al. 1991; McOmish et al. 1993). Indeed, type-specific reactivity to NS4 forms the basis for serological typing assays that can differentiate between the antibody responses elicited by different genotypes (Simmonds et al. 1993c; Tanaka et al. 1994; Bhattacherjee et al. 1995).

CORE

Infection with HCV elicits a strong humoral antibody response to the core protein, predominantly to a series of linear epitopes at the N terminus of the protein (Nasoff et al. 1991; Sallberg et al. 1992). The incorporation of either recombinant proteins or synthetic peptides from the core region led to a great improvement in the sensitivity of HCV screening assays for HCV antibody (Chiba et al. 1991; Hosein et al. 1991; Ishida et al. 1993). Commercial screening assays have mainly used recombinant antigen (c22) comprising a major portion of the core region (Ortho 3.0, amino acids 2–120; Abbott 3.0 amino acids 1–150, Murex VK47/48), but the Sanofi Pasteur New Antigen ELISA instead uses two synthetic peptides. Similarly the most recent version of the Chiron RIBA supplementary test, RIBA-3, replaces the recombinant antigen of RIBA-2 with one synthetic peptide utilizing amino acids 10–53 resulting in much improved specificity. Liatek III incorporates two peptides from the core region, while the Murex and Matrix blots retain recombinant antigen. The amino acid sequence of the core region is highly conserved between different genotypes of HCV and consequently, most epitopes are cross-reactive, with similar reactivity observed for individuals infected with different genotypes. Those differences that do exist have been exploited in a typing assay to distinguish antibody to type 1 and type 2 (Tsukiyama Kohara et al. 1993), although the core proteins of types 1, 3, 4, 5, and 6 are probably too similar to allow this assay to be extended further.

NS3

Antibody to epitopes in the NS3 region of HCV is produced early in infection and is the first detectable in many seroconversions while in established infections, it is as common as core antibody and more frequently seen than antibody to c100 or NS5. Several manufacturers were slow to realize the benefits of incorporating antigen from this region in their screening tests and some early tests had either none or too little to be effective, thus missing viremic samples (Dow et al. 1993; Courouce et al. 1995). All current screening assays contain recombinant antigen either singly or in combination with NS4 sequences (Ortho 3.0) or c22 sequences (Abbott 3.0). In Ortho 3.0, the NS3 antigen has been modified biochemically to give increased sensitivity for NS3 antibody enabling earlier detection of seroconversions (Courouce et al. 1994) and the detection of chronically infected patients with low levels of NS3 antibody (Dow et al. 1996). All supplementary immunoblots utilize recombinant antigen from the NS3 region. Changes in the concentration of the coating antigen, c33c, in RIBA-3

have made this test particularly sensitive to NS3 antibody (Courouce et al. 1994).

NS5

Recombinant antigen from the NS5 region was incorporated in the first Wellcozyme/Murex ELISA, but appeared in the Abbott and Ortho tests only with the third generation. Both Abbott and Ortho tests use recombinant antigen from almost the whole NS5 region (amino acids 2 054–2 995), whereas in the Murex assay the size of the recombinant protein has been reduced with each succeeding test and the present Murex test contains protein from only a small segment of the NS5a region. Of the current supplementary tests, RIBA-3 and Murex blot incorporate recombinant antigen, whilst in Liatek III it is a peptide. The contribution of NS5 antigens to improved specificity and sensitivity in screening tests has been difficult to quantify. Seroconversions in which antibody to NS5 occurs first are rare, and no chronically infected patient has been found with NS5 antibody as the only marker. Specificity is not enhanced, as these tests produce significant numbers of a new population of RIBA-3, NS5 indeterminates, that are all PCR-negative; it is generally agreed that improvements in sensitivity with third generation ELISAs are associated with improved NS3 antibody detection. Inclusion in supplementary tests may have value in providing extra evidence of positivity, but the poorer specificity of NS5 antigens in these tests may compromise interpretation.

The battery of antigens used in current screening and supplementary tests will detect the vast majority of chronic, established infections. Where improvement is required is in earlier detection of seroconversion. In addition, manufacturers will need to address the problems associated with antigenic variation between different genotypes. All current screening tests are based on genotype 1 antigens, and while this genotype is widely distributed throughout the world, it is not the only, nor predominant, genotype in many countries. Diminished sensitivity to genotype 3 is seen in RIBA-2 (Damen et al. 1995) and to a lesser extent RIBA-3 (Dow et al. 1996), and this may also be reflected in the sensitivity of screening ELISAs (Neville et al. 1997). Future tests will need to incorporate antigens from various genotypes to ensure an optimal sensitivity for all (response to all).

First generation tests

The first test to specifically detect antibody to HCV was based on the c100-3 antigen (Kuo et al. 1989). Use of this simple, single antigen test in ELISA format confirmed that HCV was the major cause of post-transfusion non-A, non-B hepatitis in the USA and elsewhere (Alter et al. 1989; Esteban et al. 1990; Hopf et al. 1990; van der Poel et al. 1990), and that prevalence of antibody to the c100-3 antigen was high in hemophiliacs (Brettler et al. 1990), drug abusers (Esteban et al. 1990), and in patients with hepatocellular carcinoma (Colombo et al. 1989; Bruix et al. 1989; Nishioka et al. 1991). The simple first generation tests for anti-HCV were valuable in establishing the importance of HCV infection worldwide, its identity with non-A, non-B hepatitis and its wider spread in the community usually via drug abuse.

Second generation tests

Once the HCV genome had been fully sequenced and the structural and nonstructural regions identified (Choo et al. 1991), several manufacturers developed second generation tests which included antigen to the core region (c22c) and one or more further nonstructural regions NS3 (c33), NS4 (c100-3), or NS5. The most widely used tests, those manufactured by Ortho Diagnostics and Abbott Laboratories, contained four antigens (5-1-1, c100-3, c22, and c33c). These tests were significantly more sensitive and specific than their first generation equivalents and their use for screening blood donations virtually eliminated post-transfusion HCV infection as a complication of transfusion (Aach et al. 1991). The improved sensitivity allowed earlier detection of seroconverting patients by some weeks (van der Poel et al. 1992) (Figure 54.7), and the detection of HCV antibody positivity in donors and patients previously screened as negative in the first generation assays (Yuki et al. 1992; Aoki et al. 1994).

The same series of antigens present in the second generation Ortho and Abbott tests were incorporated in an improved RIBA test by Chiron, RIBA-2 – often referred to as 4-RIBA in early reports. In this test, two bands were required for positivity, one band was termed an indeterminate result. This test was very effective in identifying ELISA false positives in first generation tests where it represented a truer confirmatory test in that it incorporated new antigens (c33c and c22) not present in the ELISA screening test (van der Poel et al. 1991; Courouce et al. 1991). There was a strong correlation between RIBA-2 positivity and viremia as detected by PCR tests (Garson et al. 1992; Larsen et al. 1992; Bresters et al. 1993b; Yun et al. 1993). The interpretation of the RIBA-2 indeterminate result, of which there were significant numbers in low risk populations such as blood donors, and the advice to give the patient/donor has proved controversial. Only PCR testing could clearly define the association with HCV infection, but few PCR-positive indeterminate individuals were found in low risk groups (Follett et al. 1991), and these were almost always associated with the c22 or c33 band (Bresters et al. 1993b). Most of the indeterminate reactivity to c22 could be shown to be due to nonspecific cross-reactivity to restricted N-terminal regions of the core antigen

(Tobler et al. 1994). RIBA-2 is less likely to 'confirm' samples from individuals infected with type 1 genotypes (Damen et al. 1995; Dow et al. 1996) due to the predominantly type-specific reactivity to the NS3 and particularly NS4 proteins.

Third generation tests

Current tests for HCV antibody omit the original 5-1-1 antigen and include the NS5 antigen, although the value of this addition is questionable. Third generation ELISAs are more sensitive and detect seroconversions significantly earlier (Courouce et al. 1994; Uyttendaele et al. 1994; Vrielink et al. 1995b), but this improvement is associated with an improved reactivity of the c33 antigen component, and not with the presence of the NS5 antigen (Barrera et al. 1995; Lee et al. 1995; Courouce et al. 1995). Counterbalancing this improvement in sensitivity is some loss in specificity related to a new population of indeterminate samples associated with the NS5 antigen; NS5 indeterminate samples are invariably PCR-negative.

Significant changes were made in the updated RIBA test, RIBA-3 introduced in Europe in 1994. As well as incorporating NS5 recombinant antigen, RIBA-3 incorporates synthetic peptides for c22 and c100 replacing the recombinant antigens of RIBA-2. Improved sensitivity is again apparent and associated with the NS3 component (Courouce et al. 1994; Zaaijer et al. 1994). Specificity is greatly enhanced and use of RIBA-3 resolves many of the nonspecific problems associated with RIBA-2 (Dow et al. 1993; Zaaijer et al. 1994). Viremia and RIBA-3 positivity are strongly associated when three and four bands are present but much less so for two-band positives (Dow et al. 1996). Care is required with all PCR-negative, two-band positives, and further ELISA and supplementary tests are necessary before equating such reactivity with HCV infection, as false positives are known (Damen et al. 1995; Dow et al. 1996). Although RIBA-3 has improved sensitivity for genotypes 2 and 3 compared to RIBA-2, some lack of sensitivity to type 3 is still apparent (Dow et al. 1996).

Alternative antigen tests

Manufacturers of HCV serological assays use recombinant proteins and peptides from type 1a, although some in the USA and Europe have cloned HCV independently and produced commercial products based upon differently sourced HCV antigens. These produce tests which show different nonspecific reactivity on screening from that produced by the Chiron-based tests. Consequently, using one such test to screen ELISA reactives from an alternatively sourced antigen test could help to resolve many of the specificity problems associated with HCV ELISAs (Craske et al. 1993). However, patent regulations have forced the removal of these tests from the marketplace and only two commercially available ELISAs with independently sourced antigen are widely available (Murex, Sanofi-Pasteur).

Alternative supplementary tests to the Chiron RIBA products are produced by several manufacturers based either on the Chiron isolate (Abbott Matrix) or independently sourced antigen (Murex Western Blot, Organon Liatek line immunoassay, Diagnostic Biotechnology blot assay). The Liatek assay most closely approaches RIBA-3 for sensitivity and specificity (Zaaijer et al. 1994). A new antigen from the E2/NS1 region of the genome incorporated into this test did not contribute to earlier detection of HCV antibody in seroconversion. Whether use of recombinant envelope antigens is helpful must await further studies. All these supplementary tests can be valuable when investigating a doubtful ELISA or RIBA result.

Genome detection

Detection of the HCV genome is indispensable for the accurate diagnosis and the complete characterization of HCV infection in a patient. Our knowledge of HCV infection has benefited immensely from use of the PCR for HCV RNA. A PCR test or equivalent is the only method of confirming HCV infection in equivocal ELISA reactives such as RIBA indeterminates, and is the only method for distinguishing between chronic and resolved infections. Retrospective studies on recipients of blood donations known to be RIBA positive or indeterminate indicate that transmission is only associated with PCR positivity (Vrielink et al. 1995a).

Detection of the virus genome is the only reliable method of following the effect of treatment with antiviral drugs on patients with chronic infection since normalization of biochemical liver function tests is not always associated with virus clearance. Similarly, chronic HCV infection with associated disease is known in patients with normal liver functions tests (Nalpas et al. 1995). Patients in early seroconversion and patients with an impaired immune response can appear falsely negative in current HCV ELISA tests and PCR is necessary for complete diagnosis in such cases (Bukh et al. 1993b). In chimpanzees, viremia can be detected by PCR within the first week after infection (Beach et al. 1992; Shimizu et al. 1990) providing a long window period when the blood is infectious but no antibody can be detected.

Blood donor screening by PCR and related methods

One of the most used applications for HCV PCR and related nucleic acid amplification tests (NAT), such as transcript-mediated amplification (TMA), has been its adoption for routine testing of blood donors in addition

to serological tests. The introduction of NAT allows acutely infected donors to be detected before their seroconversion for antibody to HCV (Figure 54.7), and thus further reducing or eliminating the potential for transfusion-transmitted HCV infections. The introduction of NAT screening was prompted by estimates that between one in 100 000–200 000 donations would be intercepted by NAT in this 'window' period, thus preventing large numbers of transfusion-transmitted infections (Courouce and Pillonel 1996; Schreiber et al. 1996). The introduction of very large-scale NAT screening in the USA, other western countries, and Japan has led to impressive progress in establishing the infrastructure and laboratory facilities for testing, as well as driving the evolution of pooled testing in which donations are combined into small pools before testing, and positives resolved by the creation of cross-pools. In practice, donor yield has proved divergent from original estimates, with incidences of less than one per million HCV NAT-positive, seronegative donations being found in most countries. Despite the scope for HCV NAT to be combined with NAT-detection methods for other viruses currently screened for in blood donors by serology methods, the cost-effectiveness of this further testing is highly questionable (Roth and Seifried 2001; Marshall et al. 2004; Jackson et al. 2003; Simmonds et al. 2002).

HCV viral load measurement

A large number of methods have been developed in-house and commercially for the measurement of HCV viral loads in plasma, and potentially in other samples such as liver biopsy. The PCR can be made semi-quantitative by 'limiting dilution' of the test sample, in which titration of nucleic acid yields an endpoint that reflects the original concentration of HCV sequence in the original sample. These techniques require calibration against agreed HCV RNA standards (Saldanha et al. 1999), and can be time-consuming and impractical for large numbers of samples. Improvement in accuracy and practicality has been achieved through the development of competitive PCR, where the test sample is co-amplified with known amounts of a separate target sequence; the ratio of amplified HCV sequences to those of the competitive target can provide an accurate quantitation of HCV (Ravaggi et al. 1995). Because of the limited quantitative range of most tube-based quantitation methods, and the rapid plateauing of product quantity when amplification proceeds beyond the exponential phase, HCV quantitation may be more effectively carried out by real-time PCR methods (such as the LightCycler from Roche, and the TaqMan method from Perkin Elmer). These assays quantify target sequences through monitoring of product accumulation at each cycle of the amplification reaction. Product detection methods generally involve the specific detection of amplified target sequences through hybridization to fluorimetric probes. For example, in the Lightcycler assay, two hybridization probes bind to adjacent sequences within the amplicon leaving one base in between, thus allowing fluorescence resonance energy transfer (FRET) between the donor fluor on the 3′ end of one probe and the acceptor fluor on the 5′ end of the other one. The TaqMan assay uses a single hybridization probe labeled with a reporter dye and an adjacent 'quencher' molecule that absorbs fluorescence. On binding to amplified sequences during PCR, the probe becomes degraded by exonuclease activity of *Taq* polymerase during copying, and releases the quencher and the reporter dyes into solution. Increases in the amount of amplified target therefore destroy quenching of the reporter dye, and lead to increases in fluorescent emission intensity.

For HCV, a non-amplification based method is widely used that uses highly sensitive branched DNA (bDNA) synthetic oligonucleotide probes which binds to viral RNA in the test sample that has been immobilized on a solid phase. The bDNA probes enable multiple copies of the alkaline phosphatase-labeled probe hybridize to each amplifier probe on the immobilized complex, which is detected by addition of a chemiluminescent substrate. Viral loads in the range from 1 000–10 million RNA copies/ml can be detected by this method.

The measurement of HCV viral load in plasma has a number of clinical applications and commercially available assays are widely used for prediction of treatment response, in combination with genotype determination (see Antiviral treatment). However, HCV viral loads do not predict the current severity of liver disease in infected individuals, or their likelihood of progression to clinically significant liver disease (Poynard et al. 1997). Viral load is, however, predictive of transmission risk in certain settings; for example, mother-to-infant transmission is strongly associated with higher viral loads. In the original study (Ohto et al. 1994), women who transmitted infection showed a significantly higher viral load ($10^{6.4\pm0.5}$ RNA copies/ml) than nontransmitters ($10^{4.4\pm1.5}$ RNA copies/ml).

HCV genotyping assays

Genotyping of HCV has become important in the treatment of infection (see Antiviral treatment), and for epidemiology tracing in studies of virus transmission. Genotyping assays are usually based upon the analysis of an amplified segment of the genome (such as the 5′ UTR, commonly used for virus detection and viral load monitoring; see Genome detection and HCV viral load measurement). The sequence of the 5′ UTR is highly conserved between genotypes, but genotype-specific differences comprising one or more substitutions can detected by probe hybridization (Stuyver et al. 1993a;

Maertens and Stuyver 1998), by changes in restriction endonuclease sites (McOmish et al. 1993; Davidson and Simmonds 1998), or by direct sequencing of the 5′ UTR (Ross et al. 2000). As described above (see Recombination), few recombinant forms have been described to date, and for practical purposes it can be assumed that the 5′ UTR sequence predicts the genotype of the whole virus. Should more circulating recombinant forms be detected, then this assumption may have to be re-examined.

In general, the 5′ UTR is highly predictive of the genotype of the rest of the virus, reflected by the high concordance between the results of genotyping assays that use the 5′ UTR and the genotype identified by nucleotide sequencing in NS5B or other coding regions of the genome (Simmonds et al. 1993c; Tanaka et al. 1994; Lau et al. 1995a; Bhattacherjee et al. 1995; Zheng et al. 2003; Gault et al. 2003; Dansako et al. 2003). However, 5′ UTR-based assays have some limitations. For example, some genotype 6 variants found in South East Asia have 5′ UTR sequences identical to those of genotype 1a or 1b (Tokita et al. 1994a, 1995; Mellor et al. 1996), although their geographical restriction is therefore not a major problem for assays carried out for clinical purposes in the USA, other western countries, and Japan. More problematic is the inability of 5′ UTR-based assays to reliably differentiate different subtypes, such as 1a from 1b, and 2a from 2c. While such information may be relevant for epidemiological purposes, the major clinical use of genotyping assays is, however, for pretreatment prediction of response and dose scheduling of interferon therapy (see Antiviral treatment). For this application, differentiation of genotype 1 from 2 or 3 is generally all that is required, and existing assays are acceptably accurate. Serological typing methods are based upon the detection of type-specific antibody to epitopes of HCV that differ between genotypes (Bhattacherjee et al. 1995; Simmonds et al. 1993c). Such assays may show high sensitivity and reproducibility, although antigenic similarity currently precludes the separate identification of subtypes, such as 1a and 1b or 2a and 2b using the NS4 peptides alone. Serological typing assays provide the only method to determine the originally infecting genotype of individuals who have cleared viremia.

Commonly used commercially available assays for HCV genotype include the VERSANT HCV genotype assay, the TRUGENE HCV 5′ NC genotyping kit (both from Bayer) and the Murex HC03 serotyping assay. The VERSANT assay is a hybridization assay using line probes immobilized on to nitrocellulose strips that capture labeled target sequences in a number of simultaneous highly sequence-specific hybridization reactions (InnoLipa II) (Stuyver et al. 1993a; Maertens and Stuyver 1998). The TRUGENE assay automates the direct sequencing of amplicons from the 5′ UTR, although this approach can in principle be extended to other regions of the genome that may be more informative if reliable identification of different subtypes is required. The HC03 serotyping assay identifies type-specific antibody to genotypes 1–6 by ELISA using peptide from regions in the NS4A and 4B regions.

CONTROL OF HCV INFECTION

Antiviral treatment

Since the introduction of serological screening of blood products, acute HCV infection is seldom encountered in clinical practice. Small studies show that treatment with interferon (interferon-α and -β have been used) during the acute phase may be beneficial, and substantially reduces the risk of chronic infection (Omata et al. 1991; Lampertico et al. 1994; Jaeckel et al. 2001).

Combination antiviral therapy with interferon-α and ribavirin can cure a substantial proportion of patients with chronic HCV infection (Figure 54.10). Most clinicians now use a pegylated form of interferon-α. 'Pegylation' involves the covalent attachment of a molecule of polyethylene glycol to an interferon-alpha molecule. This alters the pharmacological properties of the interferon-alpha to prolong the plasma half-life. As a consequence, pegylated interferons are administered only once weekly. In comparison to the combination of nonpegylated inter-

feron and ribavirin, the use of pegylated interferon and ribavirin is associated with significantly enhanced cure rates (Manns et al. 2001; Fried et al. 2002). Favorable predictors of response to antiviral treatment include HCV genotype (good response for types 2 and 3, inferior for type 1), low pretreatment viral titer, no or minimal liver fibrosis, female gender, and low BMI. In clinical trials, cure rates of approximately 50 percent have been achieved for genotype 1 patients and 80 percent for genotypes 2 and 3. Response to treatment can be monitored by quantitative HCV serum measurements.

Interferon-α and ribavirin may also be indicated for the treatment of extrahepatic manifestations of HCV infection, such as essential cryoglobulinemia and glomerulonephritis.

The mechanism by which different genotypes might differ in responsiveness to treatment remains obscure, particularly as it is still unclear whether interferon acts as an antiviral or as an immunomodulatory agent. Infection with genotypes 1, 2, and 3 all cause progressive liver disease with no evidence that type 1 is significantly more pathogenic than other variants. Similarly, studies of both blood donors and patients have indicated that virus loads are similar among individuals infected with different genotypes (Lau et al. 1995b). It is therefore unlikely that the greater response rates achieved with types 2 and 3 are simply secondary to differences in disease severity. Sequence comparisons demonstrated a

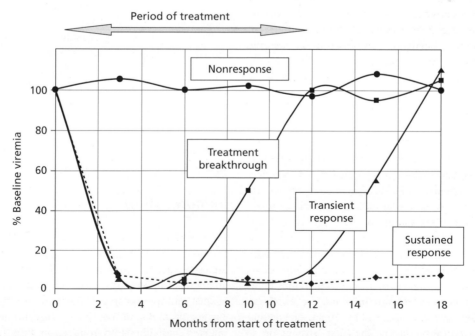

Figure 54.10 *Pattern of virological responses to interferon-α/ribavirin therapy. The response to HCV therapy is highly variable between individuals. A proportion of individuals, particularly those with genotype 1 infection will show no clearance of viremia after institution of therapy. Of those that clear viremia, three outcomes are commonly observed. Some individuals will relapse during treatment (treatment breakthrough), or after the end of the treatment schedule (transient response). Individuals who clear viremia and remain nonviremic in plasma over 6 months follow up (sustained response, dotted line) have cleared infection permanently. Clearance of viremia is almost invariably associated with normalization of biochemical markers of liver disease, such as ALT.*

cluster of amino acids in the NS5A region that consistently differed between responders and nonresponders to interferon treatment (Enomoto et al. 1995) (see Nonstructural proteins, NS5A).

The prospects for effective treatment of HCV is further enhanced by current progress in the development of several series of new antiviral agents that target the viral protease and RNA polymerase (De Francesco et al. 2003; Carroll et al. 2003; Sarisky 2004). The development of these small molecule inhibitors of HCV replication has been possible following the development of the HCV replicon culturing system, which allows large-scale screening of potential antiviral agents, and structure optimization by chemical modifications. Currently, the protease inhibitor, BILN2061 (Lamarre et al. 2003), and RNA polymerase inhibitors, NM283 and JT003 are in phase II clinical trial, while several more are in phase I or laboratory development. There are many parallels between the development strategy of HCV antivirals with those used for HIV-1 therapy. For example, some inhibitors of HCV RNA polymerase, such as 2-C-methyladenosine (Olsen et al. 2004), may act as chain terminating nucleoside analogue inhibitors, while nonnucleoside inhibitors, such as benzothiadiazines and benzimadoles bind noncatalytic sites in NS5B, and inhibit enzymatic activity though alterations in protein configuration (Sarisky 2004). Unfortunately, parallels with HIV therapy extend to the finding of large numbers of resistance mutations to all of the protease and RNA polymerase inhibitors developed to date (Nguyen et al. 2003; Lu et al. 2004); these spontaneously emerge after relatively short passaging of the replicon in the presence of antivirals in vitro. In the future, therapy with 2 or 3 antivirals targeting different enzymes may be effectively combined to reduce the frequency of treatment resistance.

Liver transplantation

Liver transplantation is indicated for patients with decompensated HCV cirrhosis and for some patients with hepatocellular carcinoma complicating HCV infection. In many countries, HCV-associated liver disease has become the most common indication for liver transplantation. Liver transplantation does not cure HCV infection, and reinfection of the graft is probably inevitable (Wright et al. 1992). Recurrence may be associated with hepatitis of the graft, which typically occurs within 6 months of transplantation. Short- and intermediate-term outcomes of graft infection are excellent, and reinfection has no discernible effect on patient morbidity or mortality during the first 3 years or so after transplantation. Liver disease is more aggressive in the setting of immunosuppression. There is a need to develop strategies for the treatment of HCV reinfection of the transplanted liver, which might also be applied to the treatment of other immunosuppressed patients (e.g.

renal transplant patients) with hepatitis due to HCV infection.

It is clear that pegylated interferon and the combination of interferon and ribavirin can cure a proportion of patients with recurrent HCV after liver transplantation (Bizollon et al. 1997). As observed for the nontransplant patient, viral genotype appears to be the most important determinant of response to treatment. Unfortunately, antiviral treatment is poorly tolerated by post-transplant patients who are more likely to experience the adverse hematological side-effects of both interferon and ribavirin. Thus, compliance with therapy may be poor in this setting, and results (on an intention-to-treat analysis) are disappointing.

Prevention

Screening of blood donors has proved to be effective in preventing transmission of HCV infection through blood transfusion. For example, the incidence of post-transfusion hepatitis fell from 10.7 to 1.9 percent in Spain (Gonzalez et al. 1995) and from 7.7 to 2.1 percent in Japan (Japanese Red Cross Non-A, Non-B Hepatitis Research Group 1991) following the introduction of first-generation screening assays. Most of the donations that were missed using this initial test would have been identified as positive by second- or third-generation assays (Aach et al. 1991; Gonzalez et al. 1995; Yuki et al. 1992; Aoki et al. 1994). A combination of blood donor screening and virus inactivation has virtually eliminated HCV transmission by blood products, such as clotting factor concentrates and immunoglobulins.

The main continuing risks for HCV transmission are intravenous drug abuse and the use of unsterile needles for medical and dental procedures, tattooing, and other percutaneous exposures. Much of this could be prevented by education, greater availability of disposable needles and, for drug abusers, needle exchange programs. Many of the public health measures adopted to prevent transmission of HIV by parenteral routes will assist efforts at controling HCV.

Immunization

The development of a vaccine for HCV faces a series of formidable obstacles. HCV is highly heterogeneous, and effective vaccines may need to be multivalent in a way analogous to poliovirus vaccine in order to be protective against multiple serotypes. Furthermore, the high rate of chronicity and the continued susceptibility of HCV-infected individuals to reinfection (see Chronic hepatitis) had suggested that a protective immune response may be difficult to achieve by immunization. However, the protection from rechallenge observed in chimpanzees with resolved genotype 1 infections may be more analogous to the immune status of a vaccine, and provides some optimism that antigens that provoke T-cell responses of similar intensity to natural infection may be protective, not only from homologous challenge, but also from infections with other genotypes.

Vaccine development has been relatively slow, partly because chimpanzees are the only in vivo model to investigate the efficacy of different putative HCV vaccines, making experiments and trials extremely expensive, and placing severe limitations on the number of immunization and challenge experiments that can be carried out. Despite these difficulties, encouraging results have been obtained using recombinant envelope proteins (E1 and E2) expressed in mammalian cells as immunogens. These induce a short-lived specific anti-E1 and E2 response in immunized chimpanzees, and a partially protective effect from challenge with low titers of the homologous virus (Choo et al. 1994; Houghton et al. 1998). Chimpanzees that became infected showed reduced levels of viremia on seroconversion, and greater likelihood of spontaneously clearing infection. In recognition of the likelihood that effective vaccines may have to contain immunogens that stimulate T-cell responses rather than just neutralizing antibody, many of the more recently developed candidate vaccines have used antigenic components from the core gene in the form of immune-stimulating complexes, virosomes, or liposomes (Polakos et al. 2001; Hunziker et al. 2002). Rather than immunize with viral proteins, T-cell responses may be more effectively induced with live vectors, such as rabies virus (Siler et al. 2002) or the alphavirus, Semliki Forest virus (Brinster et al. 2002). DNA-based vectors have also been used, designed to express HCV core or envelope coding sequences in situ after immunization (Brinster and Inchauspe 2001; Major et al. 1995; Forns et al. 2000; Geissler et al. 1998). These potently induce both T-cell responses and antibody reactivity to the immunizing proteins, and where tested, induce partial protection in experimentally challenged chimpanzees, with comparable modification to the course of infection noted for the original E1/E2 vaccines. While the lack of sterilizing immunity in chimpanzees induced by vaccination is somewhat less than originally hoped for, HCV vaccines do have potential prophylactic value in preventing a significant proportion of exposed individuals from developing chronic infection. If the vaccines can be manufactured on a large scale and at low economic cost, there is clearly future scope for large-scale prevention of HCV-induced liver disease on a worldwide scale.

ACKNOWLEDGMENTS

This chapter is updated and expanded from Simmonds, P., Mutimer, M. and Follett, E.A.C. 1998. Hepatitis C. In Mahy, B.W.J and Collier, L. (eds), *Topley & Wilson's microbiology and microbial infections*. Vol. 1. Virology, 9th edn. London: Edward Arnold, 717–44.

REFERENCES

Aach, R.D., Stevens, C.E., et al. 1991. Hepatitis C virus infection in post-transfusion hepatitis. An analysis with first- and second-generation assays. *N Engl J Med*, **325**, 1325–9.

Abe, K., Kurata, T., et al. 1993. Lack of susceptibility of various primates and woodchucks to hepatitis C virus. *J Med Primatol*, **22**, 433–4.

Adams, N.J., Prescott, L.E., et al. 1998. Detection of a novel flavivirus related to hepatitis G virus/GB virus C in chimpanzees. *J Gen Virol*, **79**, 1871–7.

Adinolfi, L.E., Gambardella, M., et al. 2001. Steatosis accelerates the progression of liver damage of chronic hepatitis C patients and correlates with specific HCV genotype and visceral obesity. *Hepatology*, **33**, 1358–64.

Agnello, V., Chung, R.T. and Kaplan, L.M. 1992. A role for hepatitis C virus infection in type-II cryoglobulinemia. *N Engl J Med*, **327**, 1490–5.

Agnello, V., Abel, G., et al. 1999. Hepatitis C virus and other flaviviridae viruses enter cells via low density lipoprotein receptor. *Proc Natl Acad Sci USA*, **96**, 12766–71.

Alter, H.J., Holland, P.V., et al. 1975. Clinical and serological analysis of transfusion-associated hepatitis. *Lancet*, **ii**, 838–41.

Alter, H.J., Purcell, R.H., et al. 1989. Detection of antibody to hepatitis C virus in prospectively followed transfusion recipients with acute and chronic non-A, non-B hepatitis. *N Engl J Med*, **321**, 1494–500.

Alter, M.J. 1995. Epidemiology of hepatitis C in the west. *Semin Liver Dis*, **15**, 5–14.

Aoki, S.K., Kuramoto, I.K., et al. 1994. Evidence that use of a second-generation hepatitis C antibody assay prevents additional cases of transfusion-transmitted hepatitis. *J Viral Hepat*, **1**, 73–7.

Barrera, J.M., Francis, B., et al. 1995. Improved detection of anti-HCV in post-transfusion hepatitis by a third-generation ELISA. *Vox Sang*, **68**, 15–18.

Bartenschlager, R., Ahlbornlaake, L., et al. 1993. Nonstructural protein-3 of the hepatitis C virus encodes a serine-type proteinase required for cleavage at the NS3/4 and NS4/5 junctions. *J Virol*, **67**, 3835–44.

Bartenschlager, R., Ahlbornlaake, L., et al. 1995. Substrate determinants for cleavage in cis and in trans by the hepatitis C virus NS3 proteinase. *J Virol*, **69**, 198–205.

Bartenschlager, R., Kaul, A. and Sparacio, S. 2003. Replication of the hepatitis C virus in cell culture. *Antiviral Res*, **60**, 91–102.

Bartosch, B., Bukh, J., et al. 2003. In vitro assay for neutralizing antibody to hepatitis C virus: evidence for broadly conserved neutralization epitopes. *Proc Natl Acad Sci USA*, **100**, 14199–204.

Battegay, M., Fikes, J., et al. 1995. Patients with chronic hepatitis C have circulating cytotoxic t cells which recognize hepatitis C virus-encoded peptides binding to HLA-a2.1 molecules. *J Virol*, **69**, 2462–70.

Beach, M.J., Meeks, E.L., et al. 1992. Temporal relationships of hepatitis C virus RNA and antibody responses following experimental infection of chimpanzees. *J Med Virol*, **36**, 226–37.

Bhattacherjee, V., Prescott, L.E., et al. 1995. Use of NS-4 peptides to identify type-specific antibody to hepatitis C virus genotypes 1, 2, 3, 4, 5 and 6. *J Gen Virol*, **76**, 1737–48.

Birkenmeyer, L.G., Desai, S.M., et al. 1998. Isolation of a GB virus-related genome from a chimpanzee. *J Med Virol*, **56**, 44–51.

Bizollon, T., Palazzo, U., et al. 1997. Pilot study of the combination of interferon alfa and ribavirin as therapy of recurrent hepatitis C after liver transplantation. *Hepatology*, **26**, 500–4.

Blanchard, E., Brand, D., et al. 2002. Hepatitis C virus-like particle morphogenesis. *J Virol*, **76**, 4073–9.

Blight, K., Lesniewski, R.R., et al. 1994. Detection and distribution of hepatitis C-specific antigens in naturally infected liver. *Hepatology*, **20**, 553–7.

Blight, K.J., Kolykhalov, A.A. and Rice, C.M. 2000. Efficient initiation of HCV RNA replication in cell culture. *Science*, **290**, 1972–4.

Blight, K.J., McKeating, J.A., et al. 2003. Efficient replication of hepatitis C virus genotype 1a RNAs in cell culture. *J Virol*, **77**, 3181–90.

Booth, J.C., Kumar, U., et al. 1998. Comparison of the rate of sequence variation in the hypervariable region of E2/NS1 region of hepatitis C virus in normal and hypogammaglobulinemic patients. *Hepatology*, **27**, 223–7.

Botarelli, P., Brunetto, M.R., et al. 1993. Lymphocyte-T response to hepatitis C virus in different clinical courses of infection. *Gastroenterology*, **104**, 580–7.

Bradley, D.W. and Maynard, J.E. 1986. Etiology and natural history of post-transfusion and enterically transmitted non-A, non-B hepatitis. *Semin Liver Dis*, **6**, 56–66.

Bradley, D.W., Cook, E.H., et al. 1979. Experimental infection of Chimpanzees with antihemophilic (factor VIII) materials: recovery of virus-like particles associated with non-A, non-B hepatitis. *J Med Virol*, **3**, 253–69.

Bradley, D., McCaustland, K., et al. 1991. Hepatitis C virus: buoyant density of the factor VIII-derived isolate in sucrose. *J Med Virol*, **34**, 206–8.

Bresters, D., Mauserbunschoten, E.P., et al. 1993a. Sexual transmission of hepatitis C virus. *Lancet*, **342**, 210–11.

Bresters, D., Zaaijer, H.L., et al. 1993b. Recombinant immunoblot assay reaction patterns and hepatitis C virus RNA in blood donors and non-A, non-B hepatitis patients hepatitis patients. *Transfusion*, **99**, 1054–60.

Brettler, D.B., Alter, H.J., et al. 1990. Prevalence of hepatitis C virus antibody in a cohort of hemophilia patients. *Blood*, **76**, 254–6.

Brinster, C. and Inchauspe, G. 2001. DNA vaccines for hepatitis C virus. *Intervirology*, **44**, 143–53.

Brinster, C., Chen, M., et al. 2002. Hepatitis C virus non-structural protein 3-specific cellular immune responses following single or combined immunization with DNA or recombinant Semliki Forest virus particles. *J Gen Virol*, **83**, 369–81.

Bruix, J., Barrera, J.M., et al. 1989. Prevalence of antibodies to hepatitis C virus in Spanish patients with hepatocellular carcinoma and hepatic cirrhosis. *Lancet*, **2**, 1004–6.

Buchbinder, S.P., Katz, M.H., et al. 1994. Hepatitis C virus infection in sexually active homosexual men. *J Infect*, **29**, 263–9.

Bukh, J. and Apgar, C.L. 1997. Five new or recently discovered (GBV-A) virus species are indigenous to new world monkeys and may constitute a separate genus of the *Flaviviridae*. *Virology*, **229**, 429–36.

Bukh, J., Purcell, R.H. and Miller, R.H. 1993a. At least 12 genotypes of hepatitis C virus predicted by sequence analysis of the putative E1 gene of isolates collected worldwide. *Proc Natl Acad Sci USA*, **90**, 8234–8.

Bukh, J., Wantzin, P., et al. 1993b. High prevalence of hepatitis C virus (HCV) RNA in dialysis patients – failure of commercially available antibody tests to identify a significant number of patients with HCV infection. *J Infect Dis*, **168**, 1343–8.

Bukh, J., Apgar, C.L., et al. 2001. Failure to infect rhesus monkeys with hepatitis C virus strains of genotypes 1a, 2a or 3a. *J Viral Hepatol*, **8**, 228–31.

Bukh, J., Pietschmann, T., et al. 2002. Mutations that permit efficient replication of hepatitis C virus RNA in Huh-7 cells prevent productive replication in chimpanzees. *Proc Natl Acad Sci USA*, **99**, 14416–21.

Candotti, D., Temple, J., et al. 2003. Frequent recovery and broad genotype 2 diversity characterize hepatitis C virus infection in Ghana, West Africa. *J Virol*, **77**, 7914–23.

Cantaloube, J.F., Biagini, P., et al. 2003. Evolution of hepatitis C virus in blood donors and their respective recipients. *J Gen Virol*, **84**, 441–6.

Carloni, G., Iacovacci, S., et al. 1993. Susceptibility of human liver cell cultures to hepatitis C virus infection. *Arch Virol*, **130**, 31–9.

Carrere-Kremer, S., Montpellier-Pala, C., et al. 2002. Subcellular localization and topology of the p7 polypeptide of hepatitis C virus. *J Virol*, **76**, 3720–30.

Carrick, R.J., Schlauder, G.G., et al. 1992. Examination of the buoyant density of hepatitis-C virus by the polymerase chain reaction. *J Virol Meth*, **39**, 279–90.

Carroll, S.S., Tomassini, J.E., et al. 2003. Inhibition of hepatitis C virus RNA replication by 2'-modified nucleoside analogs. *J Biol Chem*, **278**, 11979–84.

Cerny, A., Fowler, P., et al. 1995a. Induction in vitro of a primary human antiviral cytotoxic T cell response. *Eur J Immunol*, **25**, 627–30.

Cerny, A., McHutchison, J.G., et al. 1995b. Cytotoxic T lymphocyte response to hepatitis C virus-derived peptides containing the HLA a2.1 binding motif. *J Clin Invest*, **95**, 521–30.

Chan, S.-W., Simmonds, P., et al. 1991. Serological reactivity of blood donors infected with three different types of hepatitis C virus. *Lancet*, **338**, 1391.

Chan, S.W., McOmish, F., et al. 1992. Analysis of a new hepatitis C virus type and its phylogenetic relationship to existing variants. *J Gen Virol*, **73**, 1131–41.

Chang, K.M., Rehermann, B., et al. 1997. Immunological significance of cytotoxic T lymphocyte epitope variants in patients chronically infected by the hepatitis C virus. *J Clin Invest*, **100**, 2376–85.

Cheng, J.C., Chang, M.F. and Chang, S.C. 1999. Specific interaction between the hepatitis C virus NS5B RNA polymerase and the 3' end of the viral RNA. *J Virol*, **73**, 7044–9.

Chiba, J., Ohba, H., et al. 1991. Serodiagnosis of hepatitis C virus (HCV) infection with an HCV core protein molecularly expressed by a recombinant baculovirus. *Proc Natl Acad Sci USA*, **88**, 4641–5.

Choo, Q.L., Kuo, G., et al. 1989. Isolation of a cDNA derived from a blood-borne non-A, non-B hepatitis genome. *Science*, **244**, 359–62.

Choo, Q.L., Richman, K.H., et al. 1991. Genetic organization and diversity of the hepatitis C virus. *Proc Natl Acad Sci USA*, **88**, 2451–5.

Choo, Q.L., Kuo, G., et al. 1994. Vaccination of chimpanzees against infection by the hepatitis C virus. *Proc Natl Acad Sci USA*, **91**, 1294–8.

Cochrane, A., Searle, B., et al. 2002. A genetic analysis of hepatitis C virus transmission between injection drug users. *J Infect Dis*, **186**, 1212–21.

Colombo, M., Kuo, G., et al. 1989. Prevalence of antibodies to hepatitis C virus in Italian patients with hepatocellular carcinoma. *Lancet*, **2**, 1006–8.

Contreras, M., Barbara, J.A., et al. 1991. Low incidence of non-A, non-B post-transfusion hepatitis in London confirmed by hepatitis C virus serology. *Lancet*, **337**, 753–7.

Cooper, S., Erickson, A.L., et al. 1999. Analysis of a successful immune response against hepatitis C virus. *Immunity*, **10**, 439–49.

Courouce, A.M. and Pillonel, J. 1996. Transfusion-transmitted viral infections. *N Engl J Med*, **335**, 1609–10.

Courouce, A. and Janot, C. Hepatitis Study Group, F.S.B.T, 1991. Recombinant immunoblot assay first and second generations on 732 blood donors reactive for antibodies to hepatitis C virus by ELISA. *Vox Sang*, **61**, 177–80.

Courouce, A.M., Lemarrec, N., et al. 1994. Anti-hepatitis C virus (anti-HCV) seroconversion in patients undergoing hemodialysis: comparison of second- and third-generation anti-HCV assays. *Transfusion*, **34**, 790–5.

Courouce, A.M., Barin, F., et al. 1995. A comparitive evaluation of the sensitivity of seven anti-hepatitis C virus screening tests. *Vox Sang*, **69**, 213–16.

Craske, J., Paver, W.K. and Farmer, D. 1993. An algorithm for confirming screen reactivity in blood donors in enzyme immunoassays for antibodies to hepatitis C virus. *J Immunol Meth*, **160**, 227–35.

Crawford, R.J., Gillon, J., et al. 1994. Prevalence and epidemiological characteristics of hepatitis C in Scottish blood donors. *Transfus Med*, **4**, 121–4.

Daikos, G.L., Lai, S. and Fischl, M.A. 1994. Hepatitis C virus infection in a sexually active inner city population – the potential for heterosexual transmission. *Infection*, **22**, 72–6.

Damen, M., Zaaijer, H.L., et al. 1995. Reliability of the third-generation recombinant immunoblot assay for hepatitis C virus. *Transfusion*, **35**, 745–9.

Dansako, H., Naganuma, A., et al. 2003. Differential activation of interferon-inducible genes by hepatitis C virus core protein mediated by the interferon stimulated response element. *Virus Res*, **97**, 17–30.

Darwish, M.A., Raouf, T.A., et al. 1993. Risk factors associated with a high seroprevalence of hepatitis C virus infection in Egyptian blood donors. *Am J Trop Med Hyg*, **49**, 440–7.

Davidson, F. and Simmonds, P. 1998. Determination of HCV genotypes by RFLP. In: Lau, J.Y.N. (ed.), *Hepatitis C protocols*. Totowa: Humana Press Inc, 175–81.

Davis, G.L., Balart, L.A., Hepatitis Interventional Therapy Group, et al. 1989. Treatment of chronic hepatitis C with recombinant interferon alfa. A multicenter randomized, controlled trial. *N Engl J Med*, **321**, 1501–6.

De Francesco, R., Tomei, L., et al. 2003. Approaching a new era for hepatitis C virus therapy: inhibitors of the NS3-4A serine protease and the NS5B RNA-dependent RNA polymerase. *Antiviral Res*, **58**, 1–16.

de Lamballerie, X., Charrel, R.N., et al. 1997. Classification of hepatitis C virus variants in six major types based on analysis of the envelope 1 and nonstructural 5B genome regions and complete polyprotein sequences. *J Gen Virol*, **78**, 45–51.

Demitri, M.S., Poussin, K., et al. 1995. HCV-associated liver cancer without cirrhosis. *Lancet*, **345**, 413–15.

Di Bisceglie, A.M. 1997. Hepatitis C and hepatocellular carcinoma. *Hepatology*, **26**, 34S–8S.

Di Bisceglie, A.M., Martin, P., et al. 1989. Recombinant interferon alfa therapy for chronic hepatitis C. A randomized, double-blind, placebo-controlled trial. *N Engl J Med*, **321**, 1506–10.

Dow, B.C., Coote, I., et al. 1993. Confirmation of hepatitis C virus antibody in blood donors. *J Med Virol*, **41**, 215–20.

Dow, B.C., Munro, H., et al. 1996. Third-generation recombinant immunoblot assay: comparison of reactivities according to hepatitis C virus genotype. *Transfusion*, **36**, 547–51.

Dubuisson, J., Hsu, H.H., et al. 1994. Formation and intracellular localization of hepatitis C virus envelope glycoprotein complexes expressed by recombinant vaccinia and sindbis viruses. *J Virol*, **68**, 6147–60.

Eckart, M.R., Selby, M., et al. 1993. The hepatitis C virus encodes a serine protease involved in processing of the putative nonstructural proteins from the viral polyprotein precursor. *Biochem Biophys Res Commun*, **192**, 399–406.

Egger, D., Wolk, B., et al. 2002. Expression of hepatitis C virus proteins induces distinct membrane alterations including a candidate viral replication complex. *J Virol*, **76**, 5974–84.

Einav, S., Elazar, M., et al. 2004. A nucleotide binding motif in hepatitis C virus (HCV) NS4B mediates HCV RNA replication. *J Virol*, **78**, 11288–95.

El Hage, N. and Luo, G. 2003. Replication of hepatitis C virus RNA occurs in a membrane-bound replication complex containing nonstructural viral proteins and RNA. *J Gen Virol*, **84**, 2761–9.

Enomoto, N., Sakuma, I., et al. 1995. Comparison of full-length sequences of interferon-sensitive and resistant hepatitis C virus 1b-sensitivity to interferon is conferred by amino acid substitutions in the NS5a region. *J Clin Invest*, **96**, 224–30.

Erker, J.C., Desai, S.M., et al. 1998. Genomic analysis of two GB virus A variants isolated from captive monkeys. *J Gen Virol*, **79**, 41–5.

Esteban, J.I., Gonzalez, A., et al. 1990. Evaluation of antibodies to hepatitis C virus in a study of transfusion-associated hepatitis. *N Engl J Med*, **323**, 1107–12.

Esteban, J.I., Lopez Talavera, J.C., et al. 1991. High rate of infectivity and liver disease in blood donors with antibodies to hepatitis C virus. *Ann Intern Med*, **115**, 443–9.

Farci, P., Alter, H.J., et al. 1992. Lack of protective immunity against reinfection with hepatitis C virus. *Science*, **258**, 135–40.

Farci, P., Shimoda, A., et al. 2000. The outcome of acute hepatitis C predicted by the evolution of the viral quasispecies. *Science*, **288**, 339–44.

Fattovich, G., Giustina, G., et al. 1997. Morbidity and mortality in compensated cirrhosis type C: a retrospective follow-up study of 384 patients. *Gastroenterology*, **112**, 463–72.

Feinstone, S.M., Kapikian, A.Z. and Purcell, R.H. 1975. Transfusion-associated hepatitis not due to viral hepatitis A or B. *N Engl J Med*, **292**, 767–70.

Ferrari, C., Valli, A., et al. 1994. T-cell response to structural and nonstructural hepatitis C virus antigens in persistent and self-limited hepatitis C virus infections. *Hepatology*, **19**, 286–95.

Flint, M., Logvinoff, C., et al. 2004. Characterization of infectious retroviral pseudotype particles bearing hepatitis C virus glycoproteins. *J Virol*, **78**, 6875–82.

Follett, E.A.C., Dow, B.C., et al. 1991. HCV confimatory testing of blood donors. *Lancet*, **338**, 1024.

Forns, X., Payette, P.J., et al. 2000. Vaccination of chimpanzees with plasmid DNA encoding the hepatitis C virus (HCV) envelope E2 protein modified the infection after challenge with homologous monoclonal HCV. *Hepatology*, **32**, 618–25.

Foy, E., Li, K., et al. 2003. Regulation of interferon regulatory factor-3 by the hepatitis C virus serine protease. *Science*, **300**, 1145–8.

Franchini, M., Rossetti, G., et al. 2001. The natural history of chronic hepatitis C in a cohort of HIV-negative Italian patients with hereditary bleeding disorders. *Blood*, **98**, 1836–41.

Frese, M., Pietschmann, T., et al. 2001. Interferon-alpha inhibits hepatitis C virus subgenomic RNA replication by an MxA-independent pathway. *J Gen Virol*, **82**, 723–33.

Fretz, C., Jeannel, D., et al. 1995. HCV infection in a rural population of the Central African Republic (CAR): evidence for three additional subtypes of genotype 4. *J Med Virol*, **47**, 435–7.

Fried, M.W., Shiffman, M.L., et al. 2002. Peginterferon alfa-2a plus ribavirin for chronic hepatitis C virus infection. *N Engl J Med*, **347**, 975–82.

Fukushi, S., Katayama, K., et al. 1994. Complete 5′ noncoding region is necessary for the efficient internal initiation of hepatitis C virus RNA. *Biochem Biophys Res Commun*, **199**, 425–32.

Gale, M.J., Korth, M.J., et al. 1997. Evidence that hepatitis C virus resistance to interferon is mediated through repression of the PKR protein kinase by the nonstructural 5A protein. *Virology*, **230**, 217–27.

Garson, J.A., Clewley, J.P., et al. 1992. Hepatitis C viraemia in United Kingdom blood donors – a multicentre study. *Vox Sang*, **62**, 218–23.

Gault, E., Soussan, P., et al. 2003. Evaluation of a new serotyping assay for detection of anti-hepatitis C virus type-specific antibodies in serum samples. *J Clin Microbiol*, **41**, 2084–7.

Geissler, M., Tokushige, K., et al. 1998. Differential cellular and humoral immune responses to HCV core and HBV envelope proteins after genetic immunizations using chimeric constructs. *Vaccine*, **16**, 857–67.

Gilletterver, M.N., Modiano, P., et al. 1995. Periarthrite nodosa revealing chronic active hepatitis. *Presse Med*, **24**, 1221.

Gong, G., Waris, G., et al. 2001. Human hepatitis C virus NS5A protein alters intracellular calcium levels, induces oxidative stress, and activates STAT-3 and NF-kappa B. *Proc Natl Acad Sci USA*, **98**, 9599–604.

Gonzalez, A., Esteban, J.I., et al. 1995. Efficacy of screening donors for antibodies to the hepatitis C virus to prevent transfusion-associated hepatitis: final report of a prospective trial. *Hepatology*, **22**, 439–45.

Gordon, S.C., Elloway, R.S., et al. 1993. The pathology of hepatitis C as a function of mode of transmission – blood transfusion vs intravenous drug use. *Hepatology*, **18**, 1338–43.

Grace, K., Gartland, M., et al. 1999. The 5′ untranslated region of GB virus B shows functional similarity to the internal ribosome entry site of hepatitis C virus. *J Gen Virol*, **80**, 2337–41.

Grakoui, A., McCourt, D.W., et al. 1993a. A second hepatitis C virus-encoded proteinase. *Proc Natl Acad Sci USA*, **90**, 10583–7.

Grakoui, A., McCourt, D.W., et al. 1993b. Characterization of the hepatitis C virus-encoded serine proteinase – determination of proteinase-dependent polyprotein cleavage sites. *J Virol*, **67**, 2832–43.

Grakoui, A., Wychowski, C., et al. 1993c. Expression and identification of hepatitis C virus polyprotein cleavage products. *J Virol*, **67**, 1385–95.

Griffin, S.D., Beales, L.P., et al. 2003. The p7 protein of hepatitis C virus forms an ion channel that is blocked by the antiviral drug, Amantadine. *FEBS Lett*, **535**, 34–8.

Gwack, Y., Kim, D.W., et al. 1997. DNA helicase activity of the hepatitis C virus nonstructural protein 3. *Eur J Biochem*, **250**, 47–54.

Hallam, N.F., Fletcher, M.L., et al. 1993. Low risk of sexual transmission of hepatitis C virus. *J Med Virol*, **40**, 251–3.

Healey, C.J., Sabharwal, N.K., et al. 1994. Outbreak of acute hepatitis C following intravenous immunoglobulin therapy. *Hepatology*, **20**, 249A.

Healey, C.J., Smith, D.B., et al. 1995. Acute hepatitis C infection after sexual exposure. *Gut*, **36**, 148–50.

Herrero, C., Vicente, A., et al. 1993. Is hepatitis C virus infection a trigger of porphyria cutanea tarda. *Lancet*, **341**, 788–9.

Hijikata, M., Kato, N., et al. 1991a. Hypervariable regions in the putative glycoprotein of hepatitis C virus. *Biochem Biophys Res Commun*, **175**, 220–8.

Hijikata, M., Kato, N., et al. 1991b. Gene mapping of the putative structural region of the hepatitis C virus genome by in vitro processing analysis. *Proc Natl Acad Sci USA*, **88**, 5547–51.

Hijikata, M., Mizushima, H., et al. 1993a. Two distinct proteinase activities required for the processing of a putative nonstructural precursor protein of hepatitis C virus. *J Virol*, **67**, 4665–75.

Hijikata, M., Shimizu, Y.K., et al. 1993b. Equilibrium centrifugation studies of hepatitis C virus – evidence for circulating immune complexes. *J Virol*, **67**, 1953–8.

Hirota, M., Satoh, S., et al. 1999. Phosphorylation of nonstructural 5A protein of hepatitis C virus: HCV group-specific hyperphosphorylation. *Virology*, **257**, 130–7.

Holland-Staley, C.A., Kovari, L.C., et al. 2002. Genetic diversity and response to IFN of the NS3 protease gene from clinical strains of the hepatitis C virus. *Arch Virol*, **147**, 1385–406.

Honda, M., Kaneko, S., et al. 1993. Risk of hepatitis C virus infections through household contact with chronic carriers – analysis of nucleotide sequences. *Hepatology*, **17**, 971–6.

Honda, M., Brown, E.A. and Lemon, S.M. 1996. Stability of a stem-loop involving the initiator AUG controls the efficiency of internal initiation of translation on hepatitis C virus RNA. *RNA*, **2**, 955–68.

Hoofnagle, J.H. 2002. Course and outcome of hepatitis C. *Hepatology*, **36**, S21–9.

Hope, R.G. and McLauchlan, J. 2000. Sequence motifs required for lipid droplet association and protein stability are unique to the hepatitis C virus core protein. *J Gen Virol*, **81**, 1913–25.

Hope, R.G., Murphy, D.J. and McLauchlan, J. 2002. The domains required to direct core proteins of hepatitis C virus and GB virus-B to lipid droplets share common features with plant oleosin proteins. *J Biol Chem*, **277**, 4261–70.

Hopf, U., Moller, B., et al. 1990. Long-term follow-up of posttransfusion and sporadic chronic hepatitis non-A, non-B and frequency of circulating antibodies to hepatitis C virus (HCV). *J Hepatol*, **10**, 69–76.

Hosein, B., Fang, C.T., et al. 1991. Improved serodiagnosis of hepatitis C virus infection with synthetic peptide antigen from capsid protein. *Proc Natl Acad Sci USA*, **88**, 3647–51.

Houghton, M., Choo, Q.-L., et al. 1998. Development of a recombinant HCV subunit vaccine. *5th International Meeting on HCV and Related Viruses*. Abstract.

Hsu, M., Zhang, J., et al. 2003. Hepatitis C virus glycoproteins mediate pH-dependent cell entry of pseudotyped retroviral particles. *Proc Natl Acad Sci USA*, **100**, 7271–6.

Hugle, T., Fehrmann, F., et al. 2001. The hepatitis C virus nonstructural protein 4B is an integral endoplasmic reticulum membrane protein. *Virology*, **284**, 70–81.

Hunziker, I.P., Grabscheid, B., et al. 2002. In vitro studies of core peptide-bearing immunopotentiating reconstituted influenza virosomes as a non-live prototype vaccine against hepatitis C virus. *Int Immunol*, **14**, 615–26.

Ikeda, M., Yi, M., et al. 2002. Selectable subgenomic and genome-length dicistronic RNAs derived from an infectious molecular clone of the HCV-N strain of hepatitis C virus replicate efficiently in cultured Huh7 cells. *J Virol*, **76**, 2997–3006.

Irving, W.L., Neal, K.R., et al. 1994. Chronic hepatitis in United Kingdom blood donors infected with hepatitis C virus. *Br Med J*, **308**, 695–6.

Ishak, K.G. 1994. Chronic hepatitis: morphology and nomenclature. *Mod Pathol*, **7**, 690–713.

Ishida, C., Matsumoto, K., et al. 1993. Detection of antibodies to hepatitis C virus (HCV) structural proteins in anti-HCV-positive sera by an enzyme-linked immunosorbent assay using synthetic peptides as antigens. *J Clin Microbiol*, **31**, 936–40.

Ishido, S., Fujita, T. and Hotta, H. 1998. Complex formation of NS5B with NS3 and NS4A proteins of hepatitis C virus. *Biochem Biophys Res Commun*, **244**, 35–40.

Jackson, B.R., Busch, M.P., et al. 2003. The cost-effectiveness of NAT for HIV, HCV and HBV in whole-blood donations. *Transfusion*, **43**, 721–9.

Jaeckel, E., Cornberg, M., et al. 2001. Treatment of acute hepatitis C with interferon alfa-2b. *N Engl J Med*, **345**, 1452–7.

Japanese Red Cross Non-A, Non-B Hepatitis Research Group. 1991. Effect of screening for hepatitis C virus antibody and hepatitis B virus core antibody on the incidence of post-transfusion hepatitis. *Lancet*, **338**, 1040–1.

Jarvis, L.M., Watson, H.G., et al. 1994. Frequent reinfection and reactivation of hepatitis C virus genotypes in multitransfused hemophiliacs. *J Infect Dis*, **170**, 1018–22.

Jeannel, D., Fretz, C., et al. 1998. Evidence for high genetic diversity and long-term endemicity of hepatitis C virus genotypes 1 and 2 in West Africa. *J Med Virol*, **55**, 92–7.

Johnson, R.J., Gretch, D.R., et al. 1993. Membranoproliferative glomerulonephritis associated with hepatitis C virus infection. *N Engl J Med*, **328**, 465–70.

Kaito, M., Watanabe, S., et al. 1994. Hepatitis C virus particle detected by immunoelectron microscopic study. *J Gen Virol*, **75**, 1755–60.

Kalinina, O., Norder, H., et al. 2002. A natural intergenotypic recombinant of hepatitis C virus identified in St Petersburg. *J Virol*, **76**, 4034–43.

Kalinina, O., Norder, H. and Magnius, L.O. 2004. Full-length open reading frame of a recombinant hepatitis C virus strain from St Petersburg: proposed mechanism for its formation. *J Gen Virol*, **85**, 1853–7.

Kamel, M.A., Ghaffar, Y.A., et al. 1992. High HCV prevalence in Egyptian blood donors. *Lancet*, **340**, 427.

Kantzanou, M., Lucas, M., et al. 2003. Viral escape and T cell exhaustion in hepatitis C virus infection analysed using class I peptide tetramers. *Immunol Lett*, **85**, 165–71.

Kao, J.H., Chen, P.J., et al. 1993. Superinfection of heterologous hepatitis C virus in a patient with chronic type C hepatitis. *Gastroenterology*, **105**, 583–7.

Kato, N., Hijikata, M., et al. 1990. Molecular cloning of the human hepatitis C virus genome from Japanese patients with non-A, non-B hepatitis. *Proc Natl Acad Sci USA*, **87**, 9524–8.

Kato, N., Ootsuyama, Y., et al. 1992. Marked sequence diversity in the putative envelope proteins of hepatitis C viruses. *Virus Res*, **22**, 107–23.

Kato, N., Nakazawa, T., et al. 1995. Susceptibility of human T-lymphotropic virus type 1 infected cell line MT-2 to hepatitis C virus infection. *Biochem Biophys Res Commun*, **206**, 863–9.

Kato, T., Date, T., et al. 2003. Efficient replication of the genotype 2a hepatitis C virus subgenomic replicon. *Gastroenterology*, **125**, 1808–17.

Kim, J.L., Morgenstern, K.A., et al. 1996. Crystal structure of the hepatitis C virus NS3 protease domain complexed with a synthetic NS4A cofactor peptide. *Cell*, **87**, 343–55.

Kiyosawa, K., Sodeyama, T., et al. 1990. Interrelationship of blood transfusion, non-A, non-B hepatitis and hepatocellular carcinoma: analysis by detection of antibody to hepatitis C virus. *Hepatology*, **12**, 671–5.

Klein, R.S., Freeman, K., et al. 1991. Occupational risk for hepatitis C virus infection among New York City dentists. *Lancet*, **338**, 1539–42, see comments.

Knodell, R.G., Ishak, K.G., et al. 1981. Formulation and application of a numerical scoring system for assessing histological activity in asymptomatic chronic active hepatitis. *Hepatology*, **1**, 431–5.

Kolykhalov, A.A., Agapov, E.V. and Rice, C.M. 1994. Specificity of the hepatitis C virus NS3 serine protease: effects of substitutions at the 3/4a, 4a/4b, 4b/5a, and 5a/5b cleavage sites on polyprotein processing. *J Virol*, **68**, 7525–33.

Komoda, Y., Hijikata, M., et al. 1994. Substrate requirements of hepatitis C virus serine proteinase for intermolecular polypeptide cleavage in *Escherichia coli. J Virol*, **68**, 7351–7.

Koonin, E.V. 1991. The phylogeny of RNA-dependent RNA polymerases of positive-strand RNA viruses. *J Gen Virol*, **72**, 2197–206.

Koziel, M.J., Dudley, D., et al. 1992. Intrahepatic cytotoxic T lymphocytes specific for hepatitis-C virus in persons with chronic hepatitis. *J Immunol*, **149**, 3339–44.

Koziel, M.J., Dudley, D., et al. 1993. Hepatitis C virus (HCV)-specific cytotoxic T lymphocytes recognize epitopes in the core and envelope proteins of HCV. *J Virol*, **67**, 7522–32.

Kumar, U., Brown, J., et al. 1993. Sequence variation in the large envelope glycoprotein (E2/NS1) of hepatitis C virus during chronic infection. *J Infect Dis*, **167**, 726–30.

Kuo, G., Choo, Q.L., et al. 1989. An assay for circulating antibodies to a major etiologic virus of human non-A, non-B hepatitis. *Science*, **244**, 362–4.

Lai, M.E., Mazzoleni, A.P., et al. 1994. Hepatitis C virus in multiple episodes of acute hepatitis in polytransfused thalassaemic children. *Lancet*, **343**, 388–90.

Lam, J.P.H., McOmish, F., et al. 1993. Infrequent vertical transmission of hepatitis C virus. *J Infect Dis*, **167**, 572–6.

Lamarre, D., Anderson, P.C., et al. 2003. An NS3 protease inhibitor with antiviral effects in humans infected with hepatitis C virus. *Nature*, **426**, 186–9.

Lampertico, P., Rumi, M., et al. 1994. A multicenter randomized controlled trial of recombinant interferon-alpha 2b in patients with acute transfusion-associated hepatitis C. *Hepatology*, **19**, 19–22.

Lanford, R.E., Sureau, C., et al. 1994. Demonstration of in vitro infection of chimpanzee hepatocytes with hepatitis C virus using strand-specific RT/PCR. *Virology*, **202**, 606–14.

Lanford, R.E., Chavez, D., et al. 1995. Lack of detection of negative-strand hepatitis C virus RNA in peripheral blood mononuclear cells and other extrahepatic tissues by the highly strand-specific rTth reverse transcriptase PCR. *J Virol*, **69**, 8079–83.

Lanford, R.E., Guerra, B., et al. 2003. Antiviral effect and virus-host interactions in response to alpha interferon, gamma interferon, poly(I)-poly(C), tumor necrosis factor alpha, and ribavirin in hepatitis C virus subgenomic replicons. *J Virol*, **77**, 1092–104.

Lanford, R.E., Guerra, B., et al. 2004. Cross-genotype immunity to hepatitis C virus. *J Virol*, **78**, 1575–81.

Larsen, J., Skaug, K. and Maeland, A. 1992. Second generation and anti-HCV tests predict infectivity. *Vox Sang*, **63**, 39–42.

Lau, J.Y.N., Mizokami, M., et al. 1995a. Application of six hepatitis C virus genotyping systems to sera from chronic hepatitis C patients in the United States. *J Infect Dis*, **171**, 281–9.

Lau, J.Y.N., Simmonds, P. and Urdea, M.S. 1995b. Implications of variations of 'conserved' regions of hepatitis C virus genome. *Lancet*, **346**, 425–6.

Leary, T.P., Muerhoff, A.S., et al. 1996. Sequence and genomic organization of GBV-C: A novel member of the flaviviridae associated with human non-A-E hepatitis. *J Med Virol*, **48**, 60–7.

Leary, T.P., Desai, S.M., et al. 1997. The sequence and genomic organization of a GB virus A variant isolated from captive tamarins. *J Gen Virol*, **78**, 2307–13.

Lechner, F., Wong, D.K., et al. 2000. Analysis of successful immune responses in persons infected with hepatitis C virus. *J Exp Med*, **191**, 1499–512.

Lee, H., Shin, H., et al. 2004. *Cis*-acting RNA signals in the NS5B C-terminal coding sequence of the hepatitis C virus genome. *J Virol*, **78**, 10865–77.

Lee, S.R., Wood, C.L., et al. 1995. Increased detection of hepatitis C virus infection in commercial plasma donors by a third-generation screening assay. *Transfusion*, **35**, 845–9.

Leinbach, S.S., Bhat, R.A., et al. 1994. Substrate specificity of the NS3 serine proteinase of hepatitis C virus as determined by mutagenesis at the NS3/NS4a junction. *Virology*, **204**, 163–9.

Lelie, P.N., Cuypers, H.T.M., et al. 1992. Patterns of serological markers in transfusion-transmitted hepatitis-C virus infection using 2nd-generation HCV assays. *J Med Virol*, **37**, 203–9.

Lerat, H., Berby, F., et al. 1996. Specific detection of hepatitis C virus minus strand RNA in hematopoietic cells. *J Clin Invest*, **97**, 845–51.

Lesburg, C.A., Cable, M.B., et al. 1999. Crystal structure of the RNA-dependent RNA polymerase from hepatitis C virus reveals a fully encircled active site. *Nat Struct Biol*, **6**, 937–43.

Lin, C., Lindenbach, B.D., et al. 1994. Processing in the hepatitis C virus e2-NS2 region: identification of p7 and two distinct e2-specific products with different C termini. *J Virol*, **68**, 5063–73.

Lin, C., Wu, J.W., et al. 1997. The hepatitis C virus NS4A protein: interactions with the NS4B and NS5A proteins. *J Virol*, **71**, 6465–71.

Linnen, J., Wages, J., et al. 1996. Molecular cloning and disease association of hepatitis G virus: a transfusion-transmissible agent. *Science*, **271**, 505–8.

Logvinoff, C., Major, M.E., et al. 2004. Neutralizing antibody response during acute and chronic hepatitis C virus infection. *Proc Natl Acad Sci USA*, **101**, 10149–54.

Lohmann, V., Korner, F., et al. 1999. Replication of subgenomic hepatitis C virus RNAs in a hepatoma cell line. *Science*, **285**, 110–13.

Lu, L., Pilot-Matias, T.J., et al. 2004. Mutations conferring resistance to a potent hepatitis C virus serine protease inhibitor in vitro. *Antimicrob Agents Chemother*, **48**, 2260–6.

Lundin, M., Monne, M., et al. 2003. Topology of the membrane-associated hepatitis C virus protein NS4B. *J Virol*, **77**, 5428–38.

Macdonald, A. and Harris, M. 2004. Hepatitis C Virus NS5A: tales of a promiscuous protein. *J Gen Virol*, **85**, 2485–502.

Maertens, G. and Stuyver, L. 1998. HCV genotyping by the line probe assay INNO-LiPA HCV II. In: Lau, J.Y.N. (ed.), *Hepatitis C protocols*. Totowa: Humana Press Inc, 183–98.

Mahaney, K., Tedeschi, V., et al. 1994. Genotypic analysis of hepatitis C virus in American patients. *Hepatology*, **20**, 1405–11.

Major, M.E., Vitvitski, L., et al. 1995. DNA-based immunization with chimeric vectors for the induction of immune responses against the hepatitis C virus nucleocapsid. *J Virol*, **69**, 5798–805.

Majumder, M., Ghosh, A.K., et al. 2001. Hepatitis C virus NS5A physically associates with p53 and regulates p21/waf1 gene expression in a p53-dependent manner. *J Virol*, **75**, 1401–7.

Makuwa, M., Souquiere, S., et al. 2003. Occurrence of hepatitis viruses in wild-born non-human primates: a 3 year (1998–2001) epidemiological survey in Gabon. *J Med Primatol*, **32**, 307–14.

Manns, M.P., McHutchison, J.G., et al. 2001. Peginterferon alfa-2b plus ribavirin compared with interferon alfa-2b plus ribavirin for initial treatment of chronic hepatitis C: a randomised trial. *Lancet*, **358**, 958–65.

Mannucci, P.M. 1993. Clinical evaluation of viral safety of coagulation factor VIII and IX concentrates. *Transfusion*, **64**, 197–203.

Mansell, C.J. and Locarnini, S.A. 1995. Epidemiology of hepatitis C in the east. *Semin Liver Dis*, **15**, 15–32.

Marshall, D.A., Kleinman, S.H., et al. 2004. Cost-effectiveness of nucleic acid test screening of volunteer blood donations for hepatitis B, hepatitis C and human immunodeficiency virus in the United States. *Vox Sang*, **86**, 28–40.

Martin, P. 1993. Hepatitis C – more than just a liver disease. *Gastroenterology*, **104**, 320–3.

Martire, G., Viola, A., et al. 2001. Hepatitis C virus structural proteins reside in the endoplasmic reticulum as well as in the intermediate compartment/cis-Golgi complex region of stably transfected cells. *Virology*, **280**, 176–82.

Matsuura, Y., Suzuki, T., et al. 1994. Processing of E1 and E2 glycoproteins of hepatitis C virus expressed in mammalian and insect cells. *Virology*, **205**, 141–50.

Mazzeo, C., Azzaroli, F., et al. 2003. Ten year incidence of HCV infection in northern Italy and frequency of spontaneous viral clearance. *Gut*, **52**, 1030–4.

McOmish, F., Chan, S.W., et al. 1993. Detection of three types of hepatitis C virus in blood donors: investigation of type-specific differences in serological reactivity and rate of alanine aminotransferase abnormalities. *Transfusion*, **33**, 7–13.

McOmish, F., Yap, P.L., et al. 1994. Geographical distribution of hepatitis C virus genotypes in blood donors – an international collaborative survey. *J Clin Microbiol*, **32**, 884–92.

Meisel, H., Reip, A., et al. 1995. Transmission of hepatitis C virus to children and husbands by women infected with contaminated anti-D immunoglobulin. *Lancet*, **345**, 1209–11.

Mellor, J., Holmes, E.C., International Collaborators, et al. 1995. Investigation of the pattern of hepatitis C virus sequence diversity in different geographical regions: implications for virus classification. *J Gen Virol*, **76**, 2493–507.

Mellor, J., Walsh, E.A., et al. 1996. Survey of type 6 group variants of hepatitis C virus in southeast Asia by using a core-based genotyping assay. *J Clin Microbiol*, **34**, 417–23.

Menendez, C., Sancheztapias, J.M., et al. 1999. Molecular evidence of mother-to-infant transmission of hepatitis G virus among women without known risk factors for parenteral infections. *J Clin Microbiol*, **37**, 2333–6.

Miller, R.H. and Purcell, R.H. 1990. Hepatitis C virus shares amino acid sequence similarity with pestiviruses and flaviviruses as well as members of two plant virus supergroups. *Proc Natl Acad Sci USA*, **87**, 2057–61.

Minutello, M.A., Pileri, P., et al. 1993. Compartmentalization of T lymphocytes to the site of disease – intrahepatic CD4+ T-cells specific for the protein NS4 of hepatitis C virus in patients with chronic hepatitis C. *J Exp Med*, **178**, 17–25.

Mishiro, S., Takeda, K., et al. 1991. An autoantibody cross-reactive to hepatitis C virus core and a host nuclear antigen. *Autoimmunity*, **10**, 269–73.

Misiani, R., Bellavita, P., et al. 1994. Interferon alfa-2a therapy in cryoglobulinemia associated with hepatitis C virus. *N Engl J Med*, **330**, 751–6.

Miyamoto, H., Okamoto, H., et al. 1992. Extraordinarily low density of hepatitis C virus estimated by sucrose density gradient centrifugation and the polymerase chain reaction. *J Gen Virol*, **73**, 715–18.

Mizokami, M., Gojobori, T., et al. 1996. Hepatitis C virus types 7, 8 and 9 should be classified as type 6 subtypes. *J Hepatol*, **24**, 622–4.

Mizushima, H., Hijikata, M., et al. 1994. Two hepatitis C virus glycoprotein e2 products with different C termini. *J Virol*, **68**, 6215–22.

Mondelli, M.U., Cerino, A., et al. 1994. Hepatitis C virus (HCV) core serotypes in chronic HCV infection. *J Clin Microbiol*, **32**, 2523–7.

Mori, S., Kato, N., et al. 1992. A new type of hepatitis C virus in patients in Thailand. *Biochem Biophys Res Commun*, **183**, 334–42.

Murakami, T., Enomoto, N., et al. 1999. Mutations in nonstructural protein 5A gene and response to interferon in hepatitis C virus genotype 2 infection. *Hepatology*, **30**, 1045–53.

Mutimer, D., Shaw, J., et al. 1995a. Failure to incriminate hepatitis B, hepatitis C, and hepatitis E viruses in the aetiology of fulminant non-A non-B hepatitis. *Gut*, **36**, 433–6.

Mutimer, D.J., Harrison, R.F., et al. 1995b. Hepatitis C virus infection in the asymptomatic british blood donor. *J Viral Hepatit*, **2**, 47–53.

Nalpas, B., Romeo, R., et al. 1995. Serum hepatitis C virus (HCV) RNA: a reliable tool for evaluating HCV-related liver disease in anti-HCV positive blood donors with persistently normal alanine aminotransferase values. *Transfusion*, **35**, 750–3.

Nasoff, M.S., Zebedee, S.L., et al. 1991. Identification of an immunodominant epitope within the capsid protein of hepatitis C virus. *Proc Natl Acad Sci USA*, **88**, 5462–6.

Ndjomou, J., Pybus, O.G. and Matz, B. 2003. Phylogenetic analysis of hepatitis C virus isolates indicates a unique pattern of endemic infection in Cameroon. *J Gen Virol*, **84**, 2333–41.

Neville, J.A., Prescott, L.E., et al. 1997. Antigenic variation of core, NS3 and NS5 proteins among genotypes of hepatitis C virus. *J Clin Microbiol*, **35**, 3062–70.

Nguyen, T.T., Gates, A.T., et al. 2003. Resistance profile of a hepatitis C virus RNA-dependent RNA polymerase benzothiadiazine inhibitor. *Antimicrob Agents Chemother*, **47**, 3525–30.

Nishiguchi, S., Kuroki, T., et al. 1995. Randomised trial of effects of interferon-alpha on incidence of hepatocellular carcinoma in chronic active hepatitis C with cirrhosis. *Lancet*, **346**, 1051–5.

Nishioka, K., Watanabe, J., et al. 1991. A high prevalence of antibody to the hepatitis C virus in patients with hepatocellular carcinoma in Japan. *Cancer*, **67**, 429–33.

Novati, R., Thiers, V., et al. 1992. Mother-to-child transmission of hepatitis C virus detected by nested polymerase chain reaction. *J Infect Dis*, **165**, 720–3.

Ogata, N., Alter, H.J., et al. 1991. Nucleotide sequence and mutation rate of the H strain of hepatitis C virus. *Proc Natl Acad Sci USA*, **88**, 3392–6.

Oh, J.W., Ito, T. and Lai, M.M.C. 1999. A recombinant hepatitis C virus RNA-dependent RNA polymerase capable of copying the full-length viral RNA. *J Virol*, **73**, 7694–702.

Ohto, H., Terazawa, S., et al. 1994. Transmission of hepatitis C virus from mothers to infants. *N Engl J Med*, **330**, 744–50.

Okamoto, H., Okada, S., et al. 1991. Nucleotide sequence of the genomic RNA of hepatitis C virus isolated from a human carrier: comparison with reported isolates for conserved and divergent regions. *J Gen Virol*, **72**, 2697–704.

Okamoto, H., Kojima, M., et al. 1992a. Genetic drift of hepatitis C virus during an 8.2 year infection in a chimpanzee: variability and stability. *Virology*, **190**, 894–9.

Okamoto, H., Kurai, K., et al. 1992b. Full-length sequence of a hepatitis C virus genome having poor homology to reported isolates: comparative study of four distinct genotypes. *Virology*, **188**, 331–41.

Olsen, D.B., Eldrup, A.B., et al. 2004. A 7-deaza-adenosine analog is a potent and selective inhibitor of hepatitis C virus replication with excellent pharmacokinetic properties. *Antimicrob Agents Chemother*, **48**, 3944–53.

Omata, M., Yokosuka, O., et al. 1991. Resolution of acute hepatitis C after therapy with natural beta interferon. *Lancet*, **338**, 914–15.

Pascu, M., Martus, P., et al. 2004. Sustained virological response in hepatitis C virus type 1b infected patients is predicted by the number of mutations within the NS5A-ISDR: a meta-analysis focused on geographical differences. *Gut*, **53**, 1345–51.

Pawlotsky, J.M. 2003a. Mechanisms of antiviral treatment efficacy and failure in chronic hepatitis C. *Antiviral Res*, **59**, 1–11.

Pawlotsky, J.M. 2003b. The nature of interferon-alpha resistance in hepatitis C virus infection. *Curr Opin Infect Dis*, **16**, 587–92.

Pereira, B.J.G., Milford, E.L., et al. 1992. Prevalence of hepatitis-C virus RNA in organ donors positive for hepatitis-C antibody and in the recipients of their organs. *N Engl J Med*, **327**, 910–15.

Perlemuter, G., Sabile, A., et al. 2002. Hepatitis C virus core protein inhibits microsomal triglyceride transfer protein activity and very low density lipoprotein secretion: a model of viral-related steatosis. *FASEB J*, **16**, 185–94.

Pestova, T.V., Shatsky, I.N., et al. 1998. A prokaryotic-like mode of cytoplasmic eukaryotic ribosome binding to the initiation codon during internal translation initiation of hepatitis C and classical swine fever virus RNAs. *Gene Dev*, **12**, 67–83.

Piccininni, S., Varaklioti, A., et al. 2002. Modulation of the hepatitis C virus RNA-dependent RNA polymerase activity by the non-structural (NS) 3 helicase and the NS4B membrane protein. *J Biol Chem*, **277**, 45670–9.

Pietschmann, T., Lohmann, V., et al. 2002. Persistent and transient replication of full-length hepatitis C virus genomes in cell culture. *J Virol*, **76**, 4008–21.

Pileri, P., Uematsu, Y., et al. 1998. Binding of hepatitis C virus to CD81. *Science*, **282**, 938–41.

Polakos, N.K., Drane, D., et al. 2001. Characterization of hepatitis C virus core-specific immune responses primed in rhesus macaques by a nonclassical ISCOM vaccine. *J Immunol*, **166**, 3589–98.

Polyak, S.J., Khabar, K.S., et al. 2001. Hepatitis C virus nonstructural 5A protein induces interleukin-8, leading to partial inhibition of the interferon-induced antiviral response. *J Virol*, **75**, 6095–106.

Poole, T.L., Wang, C.Y., et al. 1995. Pestivirus translation initiation occurs by internal ribosome entry. *Virology*, **206**, 750–4.

Power, J.P., Lawlor, E., et al. 1994. Hepatitis C viraemia in recipients of Irish intravenous anti-D immunoglobulin. *Lancet*, **344**, 1166–7.

Power, J.P., Lawlor, E., et al. 1995. Molecular epidemiology of an outbreak of infection with hepatitis C virus in recipients of anti-D immunoglobulin. *Lancet*, **345**, 1211–13.

Poynard, T., Bedossa, P. and Opolon, P. 1997. Natural history of liver fibrosis progression in patients with chronic hepatitis C. *Lancet*, **349**, 825–32.

Pradat, P. and Trepo, C. 2000. HCV: epidemiology, modes of transmission and prevention of spread. *Baill Best Pract Res Clin Gastroenterol*, **14**, 201–10.

Prince, A.M., Brotman, B., et al. 1974. Long incubation post-transfusion hepatitis with evidence of exposure to hepatitis B virus. *Lancet*, **ii**, 241–6.

Prince, A.M., Brotman, B., et al. 1992. Immunity in hepatitis C infection. *J Infect Dis*, **165**, 438–43.

Pybus, O.G., Charleston, M.A., et al. 2001. The epidemic behaviour of hepatitis C virus. *Science*, **22**, 2323–5.

Pybus, O.G., Drummond, A.J., et al. 2003. The epidemiology and iatrogenic transmission of hepatitis C virus in Egypt: a Bayesian coalescent approach. *Mol Biol Evol*, **20**, 381–7.

Ralston, R., Thudium, K., et al. 1993. Characterization of hepatitis C virus envelope glycoprotein complexes expressed by recombinant vaccinia viruses. *J Virol*, **67**, 6753–61.

Ravaggi, A., Zonaro, A., et al. 1995. Quantification of hepatitis C virus RNA by competitive amplification of RNA from denatured serum and hybridization on microtiter plates. *J Clin Microbiol*, **33**, 265–9.

Reed, K.E., Xu, J. and Rice, C.M. 1997. Phosphorylation of the hepatitis C virus NS5A protein in vitro and in vivo: properties of the NS5A-associated kinase. *J Virol*, **71**, 7187–97.

Reiser, M. 2004. Antiviral effect of BILN-2061, a novel HCV serine protease inhibitor, after oral treatment over 2 days in patients with chronic hepatitis C, non-genotype 1. *54th Annual Meeting of the American Association for the Study of Liver Diseases, 24–28 October 2003, Boston, MA.* Abstract.

Resti, M., Jara, P., et al. 2003. Clinical features and progression of perinatally acquired hepatitis C virus infection. *J Med Virol*, **70**, 373–7.

Rice, C.M., Lenches, E.M., et al. 1985. Nucleotide sequence of yellow fever virus: implications for flavivirus gene expression and evolution. *Science*, **229**, 726–33.

Rice, P.S., Smith, D.B., et al. 1993. Heterosexual transmission of hepatitis C virus. *Lancet*, **342**, 1052–3.

Rijnbrand, R., Bredenbeek, P.J., et al. 2001. The influence of downstream protein-coding sequence on internal ribosome entry on hepatitis C virus and other flavivirus RNAs. *RNA*, **7**, 585–97.

Ross, R.S., Viazov, S.O., et al. 2000. Genotyping of hepatitis C virus isolates using CLIP sequencing. *J Clin Microbiol*, **38**, 3581–4.

Roth, W.K. and Seifried, E. 2001. Yield and future issues of nucleic acid testing. *Transfus Clin Biol*, **8**, 282–4.

Rubbia-Brandt, L., Quadri, R., et al. 2000. Hepatocyte steatosis is a cytopathic effect of hepatitis C virus genotype 3. *J Hepatol*, **33**, 106–15.

Ruggieri, A., Argentini, C., et al. 1996. Heterogeneity of hepatitis C virus genotype 2 variants in west Central Africa (Guinea Conakry). *J Gen Virol*, **77**, 2073–6.

Saeed, A.A., al Admawi, A.M., et al. 1991. Hepatitis C virus infection in Egyptian volunteer blood donors in Riyadh. *Lancet*, **338**, 459–60.

Saldanha, J., Lelie, N. and Heath, A. WHO Collaborative Study Group, 1999. Establishment of the first international standard for nucleic acid amplification technology (NAT) assays for HCV RNA. *Vox Sang*, **76**, 149–58.

Sallberg, M., Ruden, U., et al. 1992. Immunodominant regions within the hepatitis C virus core and putative matrix proteins. *J Clin Microbiol*, **30**, 1989–94.

Santolini, E., Migliaccio, G. and Lamonica, N. 1994. Biosynthesis and biochemical properties of the hepatitis C virus core protein. *J Virol*, **68**, 3631–41.

Santolini, E., Pacini, L., et al. 1995. The NS2 protein of hepatitis C virus is a transmembrane polypeptide. *J Virol*, **69**, 7461–71.

Sarisky, R.T. 2004. Non-nucleoside inhibitors of the HCV polymerase. *J Antimicrob Chemother*, **54**, 14–16.

Schreiber, G.B., Busch, M.P., et al. 1996. The risk of transfusion-transmitted viral infections. *N Engl J Med*, **334**, 1685–90.

Schupper, H., Hayashi, P., et al. 1993. Peripheral-blood mononuclear cell responses to recombinant hepatitis C virus antigens in patients with chronic hepatitis C. *Hepatology*, **18**, 1055–60.

Seeff, L.B. 2002. Natural history of chronic hepatitis C. *Hepatology*, **36**, S35–46.

Seeff, L.B., Buskell-Bales, Z. and Wright, E.C. 1992. Long term mortality after transfusion-associated non-A, non-B hepatitis. *N Engl J Med*, **327**, 1906–11.

Selby, M.J., Choo, Q.L., et al. 1993. Expression, identification and subcellular localization of the proteins encoded by the hepatitis C viral genome. *J Gen Virol*, **74**, 1103–13.

Selby, M.J., Glazer, E., et al. 1994. Complex processing and protein:protein interactions in the E2: NS2 region of HCV. *Virology*, **204**, 114–22.

Serfaty, L., Andreani, T., et al. 2001. Hepatitis C virus induced hypobetalipoproteinemia: a possible mechanism for steatosis in chronic hepatitis C. *J Hepatol*, **34**, 428–34.

Setoguchi, Y., Kajihara, S., et al. 1994. Analysis of nucleotide sequences of hepatitis C virus isolates from husband-wife pairs. *J Gastroenterol Hepatol*, **9**, 468–71.

Sheridan, I., Pybus, O.G., et al. 2004. High-resolution phylogenetic analysis of hepatitis C virus adaptation and its relationship to disease progression. *J Virol*, **78**, 3447–54.

Shimakami, T., Hijikata, M., et al. 2004. Effect of interaction between hepatitis C virus NS5A and NS5B on hepatitis C virus RNA replication with the hepatitis C virus replicon. *J Virol*, **78**, 2738–48.

Shimizu, Y.K. and Yoshikura, H. 1994. Multicycle infection of hepatitis C virus in cell culture and inhibition by alpha and beta interferons. *J Virol*, **68**, 8406–8.

Shimizu, Y.K., Weiner, A.J., et al. 1990. Early events in hepatitis C virus infection of chimpanzees. *Proc Natl Acad Sci USA*, **87**, 6441–4.

Shimizu, Y.K., Iwamoto, A., et al. 1992. Evidence for in vitro replication of hepatitis C virus genome in a human T-cell line. *Proc Natl Acad Sci USA*, **89**, 5477–81.

Shimizu, Y.K., Purcell, R.H. and Yoshikura, H. 1993. Correlation between the infectivity of hepatitis C virus in vivo and its infectivity in vitro. *Proc Natl Acad Sci USA*, **90**, 6037–41.

Siler, C.A., McGettigan, J.P., et al. 2002. Live and killed rhabdovirus-based vectors as potential hepatitis C vaccines. *Virology*, **292**, 24–34.

Simmonds, P. 2001. 2000 Fleming lecture. The origin and evolution of hepatitis viruses in humans. *J Gen Virol*, **82**, 693–712.

Simmonds, P., Holmes, E.C., et al. 1993a. Classification of hepatitis C virus into six major genotypes and a series of subtypes by phylogenetic analysis of the NS-5 region. *J Gen Virol*, **74**, 2391–9.

Simmonds, P., McOmish, F., et al. 1993b. Sequence variability in the 5′ non coding region of hepatitis C virus: identification of a new virus type and restrictions on sequence diversity. *J Gen Virol*, **74**, 661–8.

Simmonds, P., Rose, K.A., et al. 1993c. Mapping of serotype-specific, immunodominant epitopes in the NS-4 region of hepatitis C virus (HCV) – use of type-specific peptides to serologically differentiate infections with HCV type 1, type 2, and type 3. *J Clin Microbiol*, **31**, 1493–503.

Simmonds, P., Kurtz, J. and Tedder, R.S. 2002. The UK blood transfusion service: over a (patent) barrel. *Lancet*, **359**, 1713–14.

Simons, J.N., Pilot-Matias, T.J., et al. 1995. Identification of two flavivirus-like genomes in the GB hepatitis agent. *Proc Natl Acad Sci USA*, **92**, 3401–5.

Smith, D.B., Mellor, J., et al. 1995. Variation of the hepatitis C virus 5′ non-coding region: implications for secondary structure, virus detection and typing. *J Gen Virol*, **76**, 1749–61.

Smith, D.B., Davidson, F., et al. 1996. Levels of hepatitis C virus in blood donors infected with different viral genotypes. *J Infect Dis*, **173**, 727–30.

Soto, B., Rodrigo, L., et al. 1994. Heterosexual transmission of hepatitis C virus and the possible role of coexistent human immunodeficiency virus infection in the index case – a multicentre study of 423 pairings. *J Intern Med*, **236**, 515–19.

Stuyver, L., Rossau, R., et al. 1993a. Typing of hepatitis C virus isolates and characterisation of new subtypes using a line probe assay. *J Gen Virol*, **74**, 1093–102.

Stuyver, L., Rossau, R., et al. 1993b. Typing of hepatitis C virus isolates and characterization of new subtypes using a line probe assay. *J Gen Virol*, **74**, 1093–102.

Suzich, J.A., Tamura, J.K., et al. 1993. Hepatitis C virus NS3 protein polynucleotide-stimulated nucleoside triphosphatase and comparison with the related pestivirus and flavivirus enzymes. *J Virol*, **67**, 6152–8.

Tai, C.L., Chi, W.K., et al. 1996. The helicase activity associated with hepatitis C virus nonstructural protein 3 (NS3). *J Virol*, **70**, 8477–84.

Takaki, A., Wiese, M., et al. 2000. Cellular immune responses persist and humoral responses decrease two decades after recovery from a single-source outbreak of hepatitis C. *Nature Med*, **6**, 578–82.

Takamizawa, A., Mori, C., et al. 1991. Structure and organization of the hepatitis C virus genome isolated from human carriers. *J Virol*, **65**, 1105–13.

Tan, S.L., Nakao, H., et al. 1999. NS5A, a nonstructural protein of hepatitis C virus, binds growth factor receptor-bound protein 2 adaptor protein in a Src homology 3 domain/ligand-dependent manner and perturbs mitogenic signaling. *Proc Natl Acad Sci USA*, **96**, 5533–8.

Tanaka, T., Tsukiyamakohara, K., et al. 1994. Significance of specific antibody assay for genotyping of hepatitis C virus. *Hepatology*, **19**, 1347–53.

Taniguchi, S., Okamoto, H., et al. 1993. A structurally flexible and antigenically variable N-terminal domain of the hepatitis C virus e2/NS1 protein – implication for an escape from antibody. *Virology*, **195**, 297–301.

Tanji, Y., Hijikata, M., et al. 1994. Identification of the domain required for trans-cleavage activity of hepatitis C viral serine proteinase. *Gene*, **145**, 215–19.

Tedder, R.S., Gilson, R.J.C., et al. 1991. Hepatitis C virus: evidence for sexual transmission. *Br Med J*, **302**, 1299–302.

Telfer, P., Sabin, C., et al. 1994. The progression of HCV-associated liver disease in a cohort of haemophilic patients. *Br J Haematol*, **87**, 555–61.

Thibeault, D., Bousquet, C., et al. 2004. Sensitivity of NS3 serine proteases from hepatitis C virus genotypes 2 and 3 to the inhibitor BILN 2061. *J Virol*, **78**, 7352–9.

Thiel, H.J., Collett, M.S., et al. 2000. Flaviviridae. In van Regenmortel, M.H.V., Fauquet, C.M. (eds), *Virus taxonomy, VIIth report of the ICTV*. San Diego: Academic Press.

Thimme, R., Oldach, D., et al. 2001. Determinants of viral clearance and persistence during acute hepatitis C virus infection. *J Exp Med*, **194**, 1395–406.

Thomas, D.L. 2000. Hepatitis C epidemiology. *Curr Topic Microbiol Immunol*, **242**, 25–41.

Thomssen, R., Bonk, S., et al. 1992. Association of hepatitis c virus in human sera with beta-lipoprotein. *Med Microbiol Immunol (Berl)*, **181**, 293–300.

Tobler, L.H., Busch, M.P., et al. 1994. Evaluation of indeterminate c22-3 reactivity in volunteer blood groups. *Transfusion*, **34**, 130–4.

Tokita, H., Okamoto, H., et al. 1994a. Hepatitis C virus variants from Vietnam are classifiable into the seventh, eighth, and ninth major genetic groups. *Proc Natl Acad Sci USA*, **91**, 11022–6.

Tokita, H., Shrestha, S.M., et al. 1994b. Hepatitis C virus variants from Nepal with novel genotypes and their classification into the third major group. *J Gen Virol*, **75**, 931–6.

Tokita, H., Okamoto, H., et al. 1995. Hepatitis C virus variants from Thailand classifiable into five novel genotypes in the sixth (6b), seventh (7c, 7d) and ninth (9b, 9c) major genetic groups. *J Gen Virol*, **76**, 2329–35.

Tomei, L., Failla, C., et al. 1993. NS3 is a serine protease required for processing of hepatitis C virus polyprotein. *J Virol*, **67**, 4017–26.

Tsukiyama Kohara, K., Iizuka, N., et al. 1992. Internal ribosome entry site within hepatitis C virus RNA. *J Virol*, **66**, 1476–83.

Tsukiyama Kohara, K., Yamaguchi, K., et al. 1993. Antigenicities of group I and group II hepatitis C virus polypeptides – molecular basis of diagnosis. *Virology*, **192**, 430–7.

Utsumi, T., Hashimoto, E., et al. 1995. Heterosexual activity as a risk factor for the transmission of hepatitis C virus. *J Med Virol*, **46**, 122–5.

Uyttendaele, S., Claeys, H., et al. 1994. Evaluation of third-generation screening and confirmatory assays for HCV antibodies. *Vox Sang*, **66**, 122–9.

van der Poel, C.L., Reesink, H.W., et al. 1990. Infectivity of blood seropositive for hepatitis C virus antibodies. *Lancet*, **335**, 558–60.

van der Poel, C.L., Cuypers, H.T., et al. 1991. Confirmation of hepatitis C virus infection by new four-antigen recombinant immunoblot assay. *Lancet*, **337**, 317–19.

van der Poel, C.L., Bresters, D., et al. 1992. Early anti-hepatitis C virus response with 2nd generation C200/C22 ELISA. *Vox Sang*, **62**, 208–12.

Vrielink, H., Vanderpoel, C.L., et al. 1995a. Look-back study of infectivity of anti-HCV ELISA-positive blood components. *Lancet*, **345**, 95–6.

Vrielink, H., Zaaijer, H.L., et al. 1995b. Comparison of two anti-hepatitis C virus enzyme-linked immunosorbent assays. *Transfusion*, **35**, 601–4.

Walker, C.M. 1997. Comparative features of hepatitis C virus infection in humans and chimpanzees. *Springer Semin Immunopathol*, **19**, 85–98.

Wang, C., Pflugheber, J., et al. 2003. Alpha interferon induces distinct translational control programs to suppress hepatitis C virus RNA replication. *J Virol*, **77**, 3898–912.

Wang, C.Y., Sarnow, P. and Siddiqui, A. 1993. Translation of human hepatitis C virus RNA in cultured cells is mediated by an internal ribosome-binding mechanism. *J Virol*, **67**, 3338–44.

Wang, C.Y., Sarnow, P. and Siddiqui, A. 1994. A conserved helical element is essential for internal initiation of translation of hepatitis C virus RNA. *J Virol*, **68**, 7301–7.

Wang, C.Y., Le, S.Y., et al. 1995. An RNA pseudoknot is an essential structural element of the internal ribosome entry site located within the hepatitis C virus 5′ noncoding region. *RNA*, **1**, 526–37.

Wansbrough Jones, M.H., Frimpong, E., et al. 1998. Prevalence and genotype of hepatitis C virus infection in pregnant women and blood donors in Ghana. *Trans R Soc Trop Med Hyg*, **92**, 496–9.

Wasley, A. and Alter, M.J. 2000. Epidemiology of hepatitis C: geographic differences and temporal trends. *Semin Liver Dis*, **20**, 1–16.

Watanabe, H., Nagayama, K., et al. 2003. Sequence elements correlating with circulating viral load in genotype 1b hepatitis C virus infection. *Virology*, **311**, 376–83.

Weiner, A.J., Geysen, H.M., et al. 1992. Evidence for immune selection of hepatitis C virus (HCV) putative envelope glycoprotein variants: potential role in chronic HCV infections. *Proc Natl Acad Sci USA*, **89**, 3468–72.

Weiner, A.J., Thaler, M.M., et al. 1993. A unique, predominant hepatitis C virus variant found in an infant born to a mother with multiple variants. *J Virol*, **67**, 4365–8.

Wejstal, R., Widell, A., et al. 1992. Mother-to-infant transmission of hepatitis-C virus. *Ann Intern Med*, **117**, 887–90.

Witherell, G.W. and Beineke, P. 2001. Statistical analysis of combined substitutions in nonstructural 5A region of hepatitis C virus and interferon response. *J Med Virol*, **63**, 8–16.

Wreghitt, T.G., Gray, J.J., et al. 1994. Transmission of hepatitis C virus by organ transplantation in the United Kingdom. *J Hepatol*, **20**, 768–72.

Wright, T.L., Hsu, H., et al. 1991. Hepatitis C virus not found in fulminant non-A, non-B hepatitis. *Ann Intern Med*, **115**, 111–12.

Wright, T.L., Donegan, E., et al. 1992. Recurrent and acquired hepatitis C viral infection in liver transplant recipients. *Gastroenterology*, **103**, 317–22.

Wunschmann, S., Medh, J.D., et al. 2000. Characterization of hepatitis C virus (HCV) and HCV E2 interactions with CD81 and the low-density lipoprotein receptor. *J Virol*, **74**, 10055–62.

Xie, Z.C., Riezuboj, J.I., et al. 1998. Transmission of hepatitis C virus infection to tree shrews. *Virology*, **244**, 513–20.

Xu, L.Z., Larzul, D., et al. 1994. Hepatitis c virus genotype 4 is highly prevalent in Central Africa (Gabon). *J Gen Virol*, **75**, 2393–8.

Yanagi, M., Purcell, R.H., et al. 1997. Transcripts from a single full-length cDNA clone of hepatitis C virus are infectious when directly transfected into the liver of a chimpanzee. *Proc Natl Acad Sci USA*, **94**, 8738–43.

Yee, T.T., Griffioen, A., et al. 2000. The natural history of HCV in a cohort of haemophilic patients infected between 1961 and 1985. *Gut*, **47**, 845–51.

You, S., Stump, D.D., et al. 2004. A *cis*-acting replication element in the sequence encoding the NS5B RNA-dependent RNA polymerase is required for hepatitis C virus RNA replication. *J Virol*, **78**, 1352–66.

Yuki, N., Hayashi, N., et al. 1992. Improved serodiagnosis of chronic hepatitis C in Japan by a 2nd-generation enzyme-linked immunosorbent assay. *J Med Virol*, **37**, 237–40.

Yun, Z.B., Lindh, G., et al. 1993. Detection of hepatitis C virus (HCV) RNA by PCR related to HCV antibodies in serum and liver histology in Swedish blood donors. *J Med Virol*, **39**, 57–61.

Zaaijer, H.L., Vrielink, H., et al. 1994. Confirmation of hepatitis C infection: a comparison of five immunoblot assays. *Transfusion*, **34**, 603–7.

Zeuzem, S. 2004. Heterogeneous virologic response rates to interferon-based therapy in patients with chronic hepatitis C: who responds less well? *Ann Intern Med*, **140**, 370–81.

Zhang, J., Randall, G., et al. 2004. CD81 is required for hepatitis C virus glycoprotein-mediated viral infection. *J Virol*, **78**, 1448–55.

Zheng, X., Pang, M., et al. 2003. Direct comparison of hepatitis C virus genotypes tested by INNO-LiPA HCV II and TRUGENE HCV genotyping methods. *J Clin Virol*, **28**, 214–16.

Zuckerman, J., Clewley, G., et al. 1994. Prevalence of hepatitis C antibodies in clinical health-care workers. *Lancet*, **343**, 1618–20.

55

Hepatitis B

WOLFRAM H. GERLICH AND MICHAEL KANN

INTRODUCTION

Epidemic jaundice was described by the Babylonians, but the infectious nature of the disease and the involvement of the liver were not recognized until the late nineteenth century. In general it was believed that bad living conditions, particularly during wars, generated the catarrhal jaundice. In 1885, Lürmann observed an outbreak of jaundice 2–8 months after people had been given smallpox vaccine. This outbreak was probably caused by hepatitis B virus, since the vaccine had been prepared from human lymph. A larger outbreak of hepatitis caused by vaccination occurred in 1937 when soldiers developed severe jaundice after receiving a yellow fever vaccine containing human serum (Findlay and MacCallum 1937). On the basis of epidemiological studies, two types of agents were suggested: type A, causing large outbreaks via the fecal–oral route, and type B, transmitted mainly by human serum. Hepatitis B was therefore also called homologous serum hepatitis. During the 1970s it became apparent that more than one virus species may transmit hepatitis predominantly by the parenteral route (hepatitis C virus and hepatitis delta virus), but the first identified virus of parenterally transmissible hepatitis was called hepatitis B virus (HBV).

Early efforts to identify HBV failed because it did not grow in tissue cultures or the usual experimental animals. Only humans and higher primates (hominoidae), for example, chimpanzees, are reliably susceptible to HBV. Eventually, the surface protein of HBV was accidentally discovered in 1965 during the search by the anthropologist B.S. Blumberg for polymorphic serum proteins as genetic markers in the blood of an Australian aborigine (Blumberg et al. 1965), and was called Australia antigen. Two years later, the association between the occurrence of the Australia antigen and serum hepatitis infection was recognized (Blumberg et al. 1967). Australia antigen was exposed at the surface of pleomorphic, spherical or filamentous particles of 17–25 nm diameters, which did not contain nucleic acid and were therefore most likely not infectious agents. Among these more numerous particles, Dane and colleagues (1970) detected some larger double-shelled viruslike particles 42 nm in diameter (Figure 55.1). The surface of these so-called Dane particles cross-reacted with antibodies against Australia antigen. Their significance as the potential viral agent of hepatitis B was confirmed by the detection of antibodies against the inner shell, termed core or nucleocapsid, of the Dane particle in patients with acute hepatitis B. The core antigen was called HBcAg; the Australia antigen was called hepatitis B surface antigen (HBsAg). These antigens induce the corresponding antibodies anti-HBc and anti-HBs. Anti-HBc is a serological marker for previous and current HBV infections, whereas HBsAg is a marker for a current HBV infection. Using these epidemiological markers, it became apparent that HBV is a common human pathogen that causes acute and chronic liver disease throughout the world, particularly in Southeast Asia and sub-Saharan Africa. Chronic illness develops in 5–10 percent of infected adolescents or adults, but in up to 90 percent of infected neonates. Chronic HBV infection is a major cause of liver cirrhosis and primary liver cell carcinoma (Beasley et al. 1981). About half of the world's population has had contact with HBV.

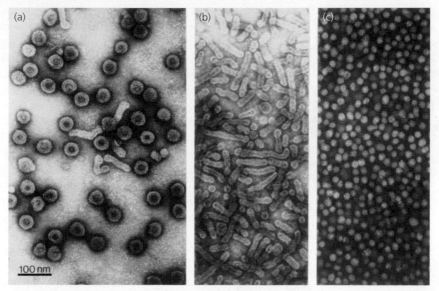

Figure 55.1 *Electron microscopy of* **(a)** *hepatitis B virus (Dane particles),* **(b)** *HBs filaments and* **(c)** *20-nm particles purified from HBV carrier plasma. Note the double-shelled structure of the HBV particles.*

PROPERTIES OF THE VIRUS

Classification

In 1973, an endogenous DNA polymerase activity (i.e. an enzyme that incorporates nucleotides into DNA without addition of an exogenous template) was discovered within Dane particles (Kaplan et al. 1973). The endogenous template was a circular partially double-stranded DNA of ca. 3 200 nucleotides (nt) (Landers et al. 1977). It was found that the DNA strand of negative polarity was transcribed inside the core particle from an encapsidated RNA template, suggesting a replication strategy similar to retroviruses (Summers and Mason 1982).

The observation that liver carcinoma occurred in the Eastern woodchuck (a marmot of the North American east coast) led to the discovery of the HBV-like *Woodchuck hepatitis B virus* (WHV), the closely related *Ground squirrel hepatitis virus* (GSHV), and recently in a variety of primates including chimpanzees, orangutans, gorillas, gibbons, and woolly monkeys. HBV-like virus species were also found in Peking ducks (*Duck hepatitis B virus* (DHBV)), gray herons *Heron hepatitis B virus* (HHBV), and other waterfowl. All these viruses are highly species specific; for example, the heron HBV does not infect ducks, and the woodchuck virus does not infect ground squirrels. Some of these animal models are very useful for elucidating the replication and pathogenesis of HBV. The great molecular and biological similarity of these viruses led to the definition of a common virus family, *Hepadnaviridae* (from *hepar*, liver, and DNA, for the type of the genome) (Mason et al. 2005). The mammalian viruses form the genus *Orthohepadnavirus* (HBV, WHV, GSHV). Because of significant

structural differences the avian viruses form a separate genus, *Avihepadnavirus* (for example, DHBV, HHBV).

Although the genome organization, biology, and replication of hepadnaviruses are quite different from those of the *Retroviridae*, the common strategy of reverse transcription places them and the *Caulimoviridae* of plants (Toh et al. 1983) into one class of viruses. *Hepadnaviridae* and *Caulimoviridae*, with their DNA genomes, have also been called pararetroviruses, in contrast to the orthoretroviruses with an RNA genome.

Morphology and structure

All well-characterized hepadnavirus species appear after negative staining in the electron microscope as double-shelled particles of ca. 42 nm diameter (Figure 55.1). In mammalian hepadnaviruses the surface of the virions consists of several hundred (possibly 240) subunits comprising three different membrane-spanning polypeptides, termed L(arge), M(iddle), and S(mall) surface (HBs) proteins (Figure 55.2; and see Figure 55.6, below). These proteins are carboxy-terminally co-terminal and differ in additional amino-terminal domains. Thus, LHBs consists of an S domain and a preS domain (i.e. preS1 plus preS2 domain) (Heermann et al. 1984). The preS domain of LHBs can be localized externally or internally (Bruss et al. 1994; Lambert and Prange 2003). MHBs contains only the preS2 and the S domain whereas SHBs consists only of the S domain (Figure 55.2 and Figure 55.6). Because all HBs proteins can be glycosylated at one or two positions, six different proteins, GP42, P39, GP36, GP33, GP27, and P24, can be distinguished whereby G indicates glycosylation and the number the molecular weight (kDa). Compared with the amount of core particles, these HBs proteins are

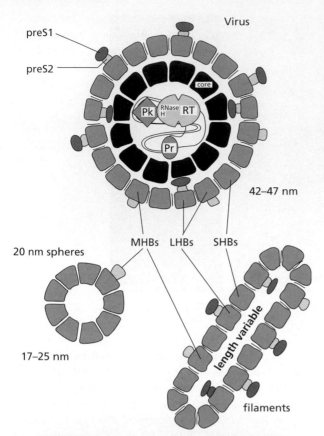

Figure 55.2 *Schematic presentation of hepatitis B virus and subviral HBsAg particles. DNA is drawn as a single or double line. Structural proteins: the viral polymerase is depicted in gray with a priming domain (Pr), the catalytic domain (RT), and RNase H. The nucleocapsid (core or HBc) is shown in black. Each block represents a dimer; 120 dimers comprise a particle. The surface proteins are shown in gray, with a middle gray S domain, a light gray preS2 domain, and a dark gray preS1 domain. For the topology of the surface proteins, see Figure 55.6. The virus particles also contain a cellular protein kinase (Pk) and cellular chaperones that are not shown here.*

and not from the plasma membrane. In contrast to other enveloped viruses the lipid content seems to be lower, resulting in a relatively high density of 1.16 g/ml in sucrose. Furthermore, the subunits of blood plasma-derived HBs particles are cross-linked by disulfide bonds and do not disassemble after the addition of detergent.

Within virions the surface proteins enclose the core which encapsidates the viral genome. The core particles interact with the internally localized preS domain of LHBs (Bruss 1997; Ponsel and Bruss 2003) (Figures 55.2 and 55.6d). The core protein consists of ca. 185 amino acids (HBV) with a basic carboxyterminus of four arginine-rich clusters. The core molecules form dimers in the cytosol (Zhou and Standring 1992), which are linked by disulfide bridges after release from the reducing environment in the cytosol (Jeng et al. 1991).

Capsid assembly occurs spontaneously. It is initiated by trimerization of the dimer (Zlotnick et al. 1999) and results in two populations of icosahedral core particles, either with a T = 3 or a T = 4 symmetry. They are composed of 180 and 240 core proteins respectively, and show diameters of 32 and 36 nm (Crowther et al. 1994; Kenney et al. 1995). The capsids do not form a closed shell but contain 2-nm holes that allow diffusion of nucleotides into the lumen. They show spikes on their surface, which have been successfully used as carrier sites for foreign epitopes in a highly immunogenic conformation (Pumpens and Grens 2001). Although capsid formation does not require any other viral component, the presence of RNA strongly enhances the assembly. This phenomenon is caused by the stabilizing interaction of RNA and the arginine clusters. Consequently, truncated core proteins lacking the carboxyterminus show a much slower assembly kinetic and are less stable than the wild-type. The localization of the carboxyterminus is, however, flexible. While being internally localized in RNA-containing core particles (Zlotnick et al. 1999) genome maturation results in an exposure on the capsid surface (Rabe et al. 2003).

In a patient's liver or in other eukaryotic cells, but not in bacteria, the assembly of the core particles is combined with the encapsidation of a cellular protein kinase. It is known that it phosphorylates serine residues within the carboxy-terminal part of the core protein (Gerlich et al. 1982). Reports on the trapped protein kinase are divergent (Barrasa et al. 2001; Daub et al. 2002, Duclos Vallee et al. 1998; Kau and Ting 1998; Kann and Gerlich 1994; Kann et al. 1993). Possibly, different kinases can replace each other regarding their function. In infected human liver, or artificial genome-expressing cell cultures, core particles encapsidate a complex of the pregenomic RNA and the viral DNA polymerase. The polymerase transcribes the pregenomic RNA into a negative DNA strand, which is used as the template for second strand DNA synthesis. The viral polymerase consists of four domains: (1) the priming

overexpressed and assemble either to subviral spheres of ca. 20 nm diameter or to filamentous structures, depending on the composition of the different surface proteins (Figure 55.2). In serum samples of highly viremic individuals, these particles can be found in up to 1 000-fold excess.

In contrast to the mammalian hepadnaviruses, the avian hepadnaviruses are not glycosylated and have only a large (36 kDa) and a small (18 kDa) surface protein and thus do not have division of the preS domain into preS1 and preS2 subdomains. Like the mammalian hepatitis B viruses, these proteins are overexpressed, resulting in the secretion of spherical particles of ca. 40–60 nm diameter.

Both the virion and the surface antigen particles are assembled at the endoplasmic reticulum (ER) and bud to the lumen of a post-ER intermediate compartment. Thus the lipid in the outer protein shell or the HBs particles is derived from an intracellular compartment

domain; (2) a so-called spacer or tether; (3) the reverse transcriptase domain, which catalyses RNA-dependent DNA synthesis; and (4) the RNase H domain, which degrades the RNA from the resulting DNA–DNA hybrid (for review, see Nassal and Schaller 1996). Because HBV DNA in infected hepatocytes remains unintegrated as an episomal minichromosome (Bock et al. 2001), the HBV polymerase is, in contrast to retro-viral polymerases, devoid of an integrase domain. Furthermore, no protease domain has been identified such as is found in retroviruses.

Genome structure and function

The HBV genome consists of a circular, partially double-stranded DNA in which the longer strand of negative polarity is ca. 3 200 nt long (Figure 55.3A). The 5′ end of this strand has a terminal redundancy of 8–10 nt. It is covalently bound to the primer domain of the viral polymerase. The polymerase presents the hydroxyl residue of tyrosine 96 (DHBV) or tyrosine 63 (HBV) as the acceptor for phosphodiester linkage to the first nucleotide of the negative DNA strand. The 5′ and 3′ end of this DNA strand are not covalently linked. The circular structure is caused by base pairing of the nega-tive with the positive DNA strand at the discontinuity around the two ends of the negative DNA strand. The positive DNA strand has a defined 5′ end ca. 230 nt (HBV) upstream of the 3′ end of the negative DNA strand. The 5′ end is linked to a capped RNA oligonu-cleotide, 18 nt long that acts as a primer for second strand DNA synthesis and represents the undegraded 5′ end of the pregenomic RNA (see section entitled Repli-cation, below, and Figure 55.3a). The length of the posi-tive DNA strand varies between 1 100 and 2 600 nt,

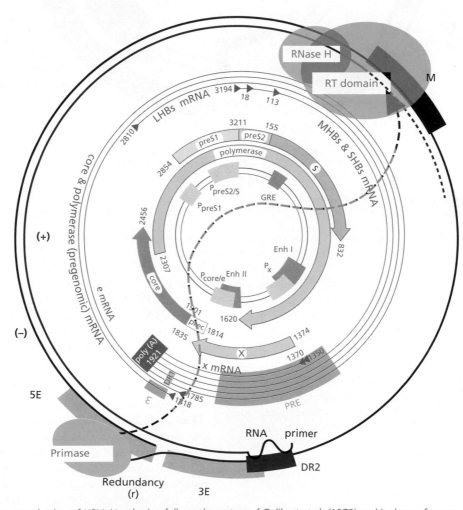

Figure 55.3 *Genome organization of HBV. Numbering follows the system of Galibert et al. (1979) and is shown for genotype A2 isolate 991 (GenBank association no. X51970.* **(a)** *Structure of virion DNA shown as the outer circle. The minus strand has a redundancy of 8–10 nt at the ends and is covalently linked to the primer (pr) domain of the polymerase. The active center of the reverse transcriptase domain (RT) is probably associated with the variable 3′ end of the incomplete plus strand, the RT domain is covalently linked with the primer domain via the tether domain. The plus strand starts at the 5′ end with a mRNA-derived cap and the 18 5′ terminal remaining bases of the RNA pregenome which are base-paired with the direct repeat DR2 to the minus strand. The circularization elements 5E, 3E, and M are also shown. (continued over)*

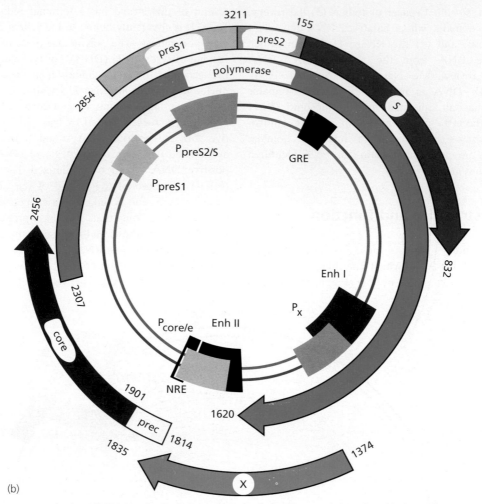

Figure 55.3 *Genome organization of HBV. Numbering follows the system of Galibert et al. (1979) and is shown for genotype A2 isolate 991 (GenBank association no. X51970. (Continued) (b) Open reading frames (ORFs) and some transcription regulating elements on the cccDNA. P: promoter, Enh: enhancer; GRE: glucocorticoid responsive element. Light gray promoters are liver-specific. ORFs start with the first conserved and translated start codons. Vertical lines within ORFs are internally used start codons. (Continued over)*

depending on how far the viral polymerase has proceeded. Therefore a single-stranded region of 600–2 100 nt is left and this gap can be partially filled in vitro by the viral polymerase after the addition of deoxynucleotides.

Cloning and sequencing of HBV DNA by many groups of workers confirmed the physical structure of the DNA. The genome of wild-type hepadnaviruses contains four conserved, partially overlapping, open reading frames (ORF) (Figure 55.3b), all on the negative DNA strand (Schlicht and Schaller 1989). Thus, the coding capacity of the 3 200 nt corresponds to 5 500 nt (had the ORFs been arranged in a linear manner). The ORFs encode:

- The core protein and an additional precore region which includes a signal peptide sequence; this additional precore peptide results in a secreted, proteolytically modified form of the core protein, called HBe (see section entitled Nonstructural proteins, below)
- The DNA polymerase

- The nested set of surface proteins
- A protein of unknown function, X protein (HBx), which was believed to be absent in the avian hepadnaviruses. Recent studies, however, describe the expression of an X-like protein from the DHBV genome via an unusual initiation site and the existence of an X-related gene in other avihepadnaviruses (Schuster et al. 2002).

The expression of the ORFs is controlled by at least four promoters, enhancers I and II (for review, see Tang and McLachlan 2001), glucocorticoid-responsive elements (GRE) increasing transcription, and a negative regulating element (NRE) that selectively inhibits the transcription from the core/precore promoter. Termination of transcription is encoded by a single polyadenylation signal so that all viral mRNAs share a common 3′ end.

On the level of the transcribed mRNAs, additional regulatory elements are found. Present on all mRNAs is the so-called post-transcriptional regulatory element (PRE), which suppresses splicing of the transcribed

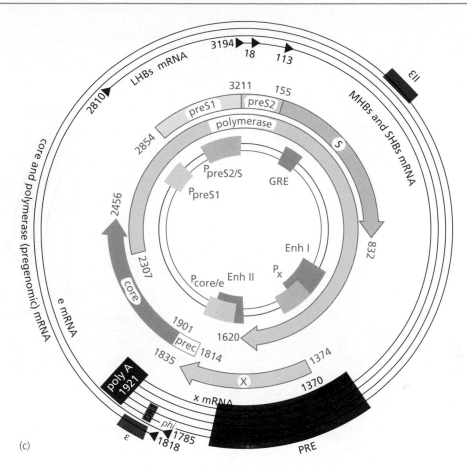

(c)

Figure 55.3 *Genome organization of HBV. Numbering follows the system of Galibert et al. (1979) and is shown for genotype A2 isolate 991 (GenBank association no. X51970. (Continued) (c) mRNAs of HBV. ε: encapsidation signal and polymerase binding site. DR1: direct repeat one PRE: post-transcriptional regulatory element preventing splicing and enabling transport to the cytoplasm.*

RNAs (Huang and Liang 1993). The pregenome contains signals to support reverse transcription and the formation of circularized DNA. This includes the ε signal, required for binding of the viral polymerase and subsequent initiation of reverse transcription, two direct repeats (DR) of 11 nt (orthohepadnavirus), which are termed DR1 and DR2. The minus-strand DNA, which is the product of reverse transcription of the RNA pregenome, comprises the M region, which supports the correct translocation of the polymerase to the site where subsequent plus-strand DNA synthesis is initiated. Circularization of the minus strand requires additional elements (Liu et al. 2004) as the terminal redundancy of the minus strand (r) and two flanking domains called 5E and 3E (Figure 55.3a) (see section entitled Replication, below).

Replication

OVERVIEW OF THE VIRAL LIFE CYCLE

Figure 55.4 outlines the essential steps in the viral life cycle. The mode of attachment and entry is not unequivocally identified. The uptake by clathrin-mediated endocytosis has been suggested for DHBV (Köck et al. 1996) (Figure 55.4). Recent data suggest actin-independence and microtubule-dependence of viral entry (Funk et al. 2004). These findings support the idea of endocytosis since endosomes are transported via microtubules towards the perinuclear region. Because hepadnaviruses multiply via RNA generated by the cellular RNA polymerase II, the DNA genome must be transported into the nucleus. Consequently, the DNA genome must escape from the endosome in a complex with viral proteins, which facilitate the transport towards the nuclear envelope. To pass the nuclear envelope, the genome must be transported through the nuclear pore complexes (NPC), which are the only sites for macromolecule exchange between the cytoplasm and the nucleus. At least inside the karyoplasm, the genome must be accessible to transcription factors and the polymerase II, which transcribes different sets of mRNAs.

For genome replication, one mRNA species of supergenomic length is used. This mRNA is translated into core protein and, in an overlapping reading frame, into the viral polymerase. This RNA can then specifically interact with the viral polymerase and cellular chaper-

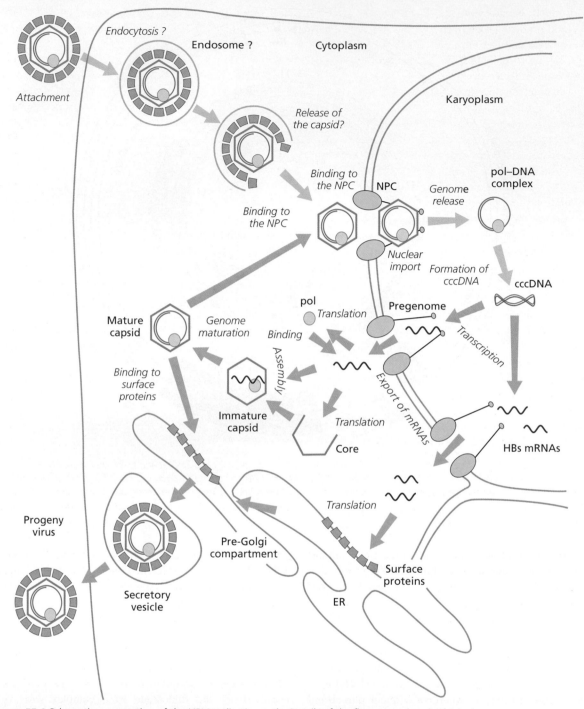

Figure 55.4 *Schematic presentation of the HBV replication cycle. Details of the figure are given in the text.*

ones. This complex is specifically encapsidated by the core protein into particles (Hu et al. 2002). Phosphorylation of at least some core protein subunits is required for the encapsidation (Gazina et al. 2000). Within the core particle, the encapsidated RNA serves as the template for reverse transcription and is therefore also called pregenomic RNA. The core particle containing the mature DNA genome can be either enveloped into the surface proteins and secreted as mature virus into the bloodstream or it can release the encapsidated DNA into the nucleus of the infected cell, leading to an amplification of the episomal viral DNA.

ATTACHMENT AND ENTRY

HBV infects naturally only humans and hominoidae, and is highly adapted to fully differentiated hepatocytes. Hepatocyte cultures are only susceptible for a very short time window, 1–3 days after explantation from the organ. Susceptibility can be prolonged and enhanced by addition of dimethyl sulfoxide and special hepatocyte media.

Primary duck hepatocytes are highly susceptible for DHBV and produce progeny virus after 2 days. Mammalian hepatocyte cultures are more difficult to obtain and less susceptible. Usually they require high virus input and produce little progeny virus with no spread from cell to cell. Permanent cell lines from hepatomas are usually not susceptible, but if transfected with double-stranded HBV DNA covering all genes, they express infectious HBV. Thus, the block in the susceptibility of permanent cell cultures comes at an early step in the viral life cycle before formation of covalently closed circular DNA (cccDNA). True infection requires species-, organ-, and differentiation-specific factors acting on attachment and uptake of the virus. Recently, a redifferentiated hepatoma cell line, Hepa RG, has been established which is after redifferentiation as susceptible as primary human hepatocytes (Gripon et al. 2002).

The scarcity of surgically obtained human liver and the low efficiency of the cell cultures have severely hampered studies on these early steps, but some limited data have been obtained for HBV. Additionally, studies with animal hepadnaviruses have been helpful. The preS1 protein sequence 10–36 (21–47 in HBV genotype A) is essential for binding of HBV to human hepatocyte membranes, and binding can be blocked by competing peptides or by antibodies against that sequence (Neurath et al. 1986; Pontisso et al. 1989). Such antibodies also block infection of primary human hepatocyte cultures (Maeng et al. 2000). Antibodies against SHBs in natural conformation also block infectivity, but a generally accepted role of SHBs in attachment has not been identified. Emergence of escape HBV mutants in infected anti-SHBs positive patients (Carman et al. 1997; Nainan et al. 2002) confirms the essential role of the SHBs antigen loop from amino acids 100–160 in vivo for viral spread. The woolly monkey hepadnavirus (Lanford et al. 1998) can infect human hepatocyte cultures, but much less efficiently than HBV. The determinant of the host range of this virus has been mapped to the region preS1 (1–40) that is also essential for attachment, with amino acids 5, 27, and 30 being most divergent (Chouteau et al. 2001).

In spite of their narrow host specificity, the human and the woolly monkey HBV, but not woodchuck HBV, quite efficiently infect primary hepatocyte cultures from the livers of *Tupaia belangeri* (Köck et al. 2001). These are small animals living in the tropical forests of South East Asia forming their own order (*Scandentia*) among the mammalians, unrelated to primates. They can be bred in large numbers in captivity and provide a more available source of fresh liver tissue than humans or primates. Using *Tupaia* hepatocytes for measuring infectivity of HBV, monoclonal antibodies against preS1 20–23 and against native SHBs have been found to be completely neutralizing while preS2 antibodies and a sequential SHBs antibody neutralized only partially (Glebe et al. 2003). With DHBV, both preS and S

antibodies have also been found to be neutralizing (Sunyach et al. 1999). As with human HBV, the preS sequence of DHBV is essential for binding and uptake and determines the host range (Ishikawa and Ganem 1995). Infectivity of HBV and DHBV for hepatocytes requires the myristoylation of the conserved glycin 2 of the preS domains (Bruss et al. 1996). Competing preS peptides are also more potent inhibitors if myristoylated (Urban and Gripon 2002). The preS sequence of DHBV binds to duck carboxypeptidase D that is an essential, but not sufficient, receptor for infection (Kuroki et al. 1995; Urban et al. 2000). For human HBV, numerous candidate receptors have been described, binding either to preS1, preS2, or SHBs but a connection to the infection process could up to now not be demonstrated.

The preS2 domain of HBV binds a modified form of natural human or primate serum albumin (Krone et al. 1990). The nature of the modification is unknown but it can be mimicked by treatment with glutaraldehyde. Such a modified human serum albumin mediates binding of preS2-containing HBsAg particles including HBV to human hepatocyte membranes (Pontisso et al. 1989), but it is not known whether this phenomenon contributes to infection. LHBs and SHBs are essential for both morphogenesis and infectivity of HBV or hepatitis delta virus (HDV), the envelope of which is derived from HBV. MHBs is nonessential for infectivity of HBV or HDV. Natural or artificial deletion mutants without the MHBs start codon are viable in patients and in cell cultures.

Recent work suggests a slow, actin-independent entry of DHBV, the details of which are not understood (Funk et al. 2004). The receptor for DHBV, carboxypeptidase D, shuttles between plasma membranes and the Golgi apparatus and may mediate uptake of DHBV into the cells (Breiner et al. 1998). The postulated second receptor mediating entry to the cytosol is still unknown. All hepadnaviruses at the amino end of the S domain or SHBs protein contain a short hydrophobic sequence that is similar to fusion peptides of many enveloped viruses. This sequence can indeed replace the fusion peptide in influenza virus hemagglutinin in the step of membrane fusion (Berting et al. 2000) and may play a similar role during entry of hepadnaviruses. In HBV-infected *Tupaia* hepatocyte cultures, HBV binding is very efficient, but the later steps seems to occur at low efficiency (Glebe et al. 2003).

At least in DHBV, the entire capsid is transported towards the nuclear envelope (Köck et al. 2003). Unpublished data after lipofection of HBV capsids reveal that this transport is indeed facilitated by using the cellular microtubule transport machinery (Rabe and Kann 2005) as was shown for other viruses (Whittaker et al. 2000).

NUCLEAR ENTRY AND FORMATION OF EPISOMAL VIRAL DNA

Liver cells are differentiated cells of which the vast majority are nondividing. As with other viruses replicating in the nuclei of arrested cells, the hepadnaviral genome has to travel through the cytoplasm towards the nuclear pores followed by passage through the pore. Furthermore, the conversion of the relaxed circular (rc) viral DNA to the cccDNA by cellular enzymes (Köck et al. 2003) requires its release from the capsid.

Most knowledge on the subsequent passage through the nuclear pores has been obtained by in vitro systems established for studying the nuclear import of cellular proteins. It has been shown that nucleocapsids bind to the NPC, following the 'classical' pathway of karyophilic proteins, which is mediated by the cellular proteins importin α and β (karyopherin α (and β). The exposure of a corresponding nuclear localization signal (NLS) on the surface of the nucleocapsids, which is bound by importin α, is dependent upon genome maturation and/ or phosphorylation of the core subunits (Kann et al. 1999). In contrast to herpes virus capsids and adenoviruses, which also migrate to the NPC, HBV capsids are small enough to pass the nuclear pore as entire particles (Panté and Kann 2002), as demonstrated after microinjection into *Xenopus* oocytes.

After release from the capsid within the nuclear basket (Rabe et al. 2003), the partially double-stranded DNA genome with its protein primer at the 5′ end of the negative DNA strand and its RNA primer at the 5′ end of the viral positive strand, must be converted by cellular DNA modifying enzymes to a cccDNA. In fact, formation of cccDNA is the first marker of successful infection, followed by replicative intermediates after 24 h. The central role of cccDNA for transcription of viral RNAs was confirmed by infecting chimpanzees with cloned, circular HBV DNA via intrahepatic injection (Will et al. 1985). The following steps for the generation of cccDNA are implied: (1) removal of the 5′ terminal redundancies from the negative strand and removal of the covalently bound polymerase; (2) removal of the RNA primer; (3) completion of the positive DNA strand; and (4) linkage of the 5′ and 3′ ends of each strand by DNA ligase. The positive DNA strand may be filled up by the viral polymerase (Köck et al. 2003), but cellular polymerases may be also required, because treatment of primary hepatocytes with ddG, an inhibitor of cellular DNA polymerases, resulted in suppression of cccDNA formation (Köck and Schlicht 1993).

TRANSCRIPTION AND TRANSLATION

The four promoters and two enhancers of HBV control expression of at least five overlapping RNAs of different sizes (see Figure 55.3c) by the cellular RNA polymerase II (for a review: Moolla et al. 2002). Like most eukaryotic mRNAs, the viral transcripts include a CAP structure at their 5′ terminus and are polyadenylated at their 3′ end. The genome contains only one polyadenylation signal TATAAA, which is conserved in all mammalian hepadnaviruses. The transcripts contain many potential

splice donor and acceptor sites, but they also contain a splice-suppressing sequence, homologous to the rev-responsive element (RRE) of human immunodeficiency virus (HIV). The corresponding sequence in hepatitis B viruses was termed PRE (Huang and Liang 1993). PRE acts context-dependently consistent with the observation that it has a secondary structure (Loeb et al. 2002). In contrast to the HIV-RRE however, the HBV RNA export is not sensitive to leptomycin B (Zang and Yen 1999), indicating that the nuclear export factor chromosome region maintenance (CRM)-1 is not involved whereas the corresponding WHV element is CRM-1 dependent (Popa et al. 2002). Probably, HBV-PRE acts like the constitutive transport element (CTE) found in the export of unspliced Mason–Pfizer monkey virus (MPMV) RNAs. CTE override the retention of intron-containing RNAs by a direct interaction with the export factor TAP, which is leptomycin insensitive. Poly-pyrimidine tract binding (PTB) protein has been reported to bind to PRE and to contribute to the nuclear export of HBV RNAs (Zang et al. 2001). HBV RNAs are post-transcriptionally down-regulated upon cytokine induction. The decrease of HBV mRNAs however is counteracted by a stabilization of the HBV transcripts mediated by the association to the auto-antigen La (Heise et al. 1999). La was shown to bind to a stem–loop structure located between nts 1275 and 1291 of HBV. It was reported that the turnover of HBV RNAs depends on structural features and less on the primary nucleotide sequence (Ehlers et al. 2004).

As in most eukaryotic mRNAs, the first reading frame is most efficiently translated. Thus, the different mRNAs are named after the first encoded ORF HBe-, HBc/pol-, preS1-, preS2/S-, and X-RNA. Among these RNAs, two sets can be discriminated: RNAs of subgenomic length, encoding X and the surface proteins; and RNAs longer than the genome (supergenomic RNAs), encoding HBe, core, and polymerase. Regulation of transcription from the HBV genome has been studied in great detail.

The HBx RNA of mammalian hepadnaviruses is ca. 700 nt long, and starts at two closely situated initiation sites (Schaller and Fischer 1991). The presence of multiple binding sites for liver-specific transcription factors (hepatonuclear factors (HNF) 3 and 4; C/EBP) in its promoter, which overlaps the enhancer I, makes it likely that the transcription of this RNA is regulated in a tissue-specific manner, but it can also be expressed in a large variety of nonhepatic cell lines.

The major transcript of the HBV genome of ca. 2.1 kb does not contain a clearly defined 5′ end, and is well transcribed in a large variety of hepatic and nonhepatic cell lines (Cattaneo and Will 1983). This subspecies of mRNA contains the preS2 and S regions with their start codons, resulting in the expression of MHBs when the first AUG is used. In most translation events, the second AUG is used, leading to the expression of the small surface protein, SHBs (Gallina et al. 1992). Its promoter is called preS2/S promoter and consists mainly of ubiquitously active SP1 binding sites (Raney et al. 1992), which explains the wide variety of cell lines and tissues in which the SHBs can be expressed.

In contrast to the above-mentioned transcripts, the LHBs-encoding mRNA of ca. 2.4 kb is transcribed in a liver-specific manner (Antonucci and Rutter 1989), requiring the presence of the liver-specific transcription factors HNF1 and 3 (Raney and McLachlan 1995). Because the expression of the encoded LHBs protein is essential for virus envelopment and secretion (Bruss and Ganem 1991), activation of the LHBs promoter seems to be an essential element in HBV–host cell restriction. In DHBV-transfected cells and DHBV-infected ducks, a common additional spliced mRNA is found with the start site of the pregenomic transcript, which seems to be essential for virus production (Obert et al. 1996). Because the resulting mRNA has the same length as the major LHBs mRNA, splicing of a 1.1 kb intron seems to be most probable. While splicing does not seem to be essential for HBV, various splice products have been identified in hepatocellular carcinoma cell lines (Rosmorduc et al. 1995) and in patients (Günther et al. 1996). A hepatitis B spliced protein (HBSP) composed of a fragment of pol and a new ORF seems to be often expressed and antibody against it may be associated with the generation of fibrosis (Soussan et al. 2003).

Two sets of supergenomic mRNAs exist, both of ca. 3.3 kb in length, being terminally redundant in ca. 150 nt. Owing to the redundancy of the RNAs, the polyadenylation signal, localized downstream of the AUG of the core ORF, must be ignored on the first passage of the transcription machinery. Apparently, this phenomenon is caused by the surrounding nucleotide sequences and by the length of the upstream region (Cherrington et al. 1992).

The transcription of these supergenomic RNAs is controlled by the core promoter and enhancer II which are liver specific owing to binding sites for nuclear hormone receptors, such as HNF4, retinoid X receptor, and peroxisome proliferator-activated receptor alpha (Tang and McLachlan 2001). The core/HBe promoter initiates the transcription of a subset of two classes of RNAs, which differ by ca. 30 nt at their 5′ end but have completely different biological functions. Only the longer mRNAs contain the AUG start codon of the preC region at their 5′ end, which is in frame with the AUG of the core reading frame. Therefore, these RNAs encode a primary translation product that differs from the core protein by 29 additional amino acids at the amino-terminal end. This additional domain, called preC, contains a hydrophobic sequence that serves as a signal sequence for secretion into the ER (see section entitled Nonstructural proteins, below). The resulting product is HBe antigen.

The genome replication is only supported by the other supergenomic transcript, which does not contain the preC AUG, but includes the initiation AUG at nt 1 900 for core protein (Ou et al. 1990). From this RNA, the overlapping pol ORF, beginning 407 nts downstream of the core AUG, is also translated, probably less efficiently. In contrast to retroviruses, which also have overlapping polymerase and nucleocapsid ORFs, expression of hepadnaviral polymerase occurs by de novo translational initiation and not by ribosomal frame shifting (Chang et al. 1990). The exact mechanism of pol translation remains unsolved because conflicting evidence has been reported for both an internal entry of the ribosomes at or near the pol AUG and for leaky scanning from the 5′ end of core/pol mRNA.

The ratio between pregenomic and 'preCore' HBe mRNA is variable and depends on the nucleotide sequence in the core promoter/enhancer. Particularly, mutations from A1762 to T and G1764 to A reduce HBeAg expression and enhance pregenome expression and thus replication (Buckwold et al. 1996). HNF 3β favors expression of HBe mRNA and inhibits pregenome transcription and replication (Banks et al. 2002).

In addition to cellular transcription factors, two virus encoded transcription factors regulate the gene expression of HBV. HBx protein is a promiscuous transactivator of many cellular genes and of the HBV genes (see below). The other transcription-activating element is located within the preS2 domain and acts only if located at the cytosolic side of the ER. This topology exists in LHBs protein and in carboxyterminally truncated forms of MHBs (Hildt et al. 1995). PreS2 activates the raf/MEK signal cascade that is essential for HBV replication (Stockl et al. 2003). HBx activates tyrosine kinases and calcium signaling which also activates HBV replication (Bouchard et al. 2003).

ASSEMBLY OF THE VIRAL NUCLEOCAPSID AND GENOME MATURATION

Expression of the viral nucleocapsid in *Escherichia coli* leads to core particles that, by electron microscopy, are indistinguishable from natural nucleocapsids found in infected liver (Kenney et al. 1995). (However, it should be considered that only the structure built by the first ca. 140 amino acids is depictable.) In these expression systems, devoid of any other viral protein, assembly is combined with nonspecific encapsidation of RNA. Specific encapsidation of the pregenomic RNA, as it occurs in vivo, is mediated by the epsilon (ε) signal and the viral polymerase (Bartenschlager et al. 1990; Hirsch et al. 1990). Mutations throughout the whole polymerase gene affect the ability for specific RNA encapsidation, suggesting a complex interaction between viral polymerase with pregenomic RNA and the core particle in which other proteins such as the cellular chaperone Hsp90 and co-chaperones may be involved (Hu and Seeger 1996; Beck and Nassal 2003).

The encapsidation signal ε of the pregenomic RNA was mapped within the preC region of DHBV and HBV

RNA (Nassal and Schaller 1996). Although ε is present in all HBV RNAs at the 3′ end and is redundant at the 5′ and 3′ ends of the supergenomic transcripts, only the 5′ terminal ε supports encapsidation (Junker-Niepmann et al. 1990). ε forms a base-paired stem–loop (see Figure 55.6a), conserved in its structure throughout all hepadnaviruses. Although ε seems to be sufficient for pregenome encapsidation by viral polymerase, additional sequence elements downstream increase the encapsidation efficiency (Hirsch et al. 1991; Calvert and Summers 1994). These elements may explain how the viral polymerase discriminates the 5′ terminal ε from the 3′ terminal ε in the super- and subgenomic RNAs. The nonreactivity of the HBe mRNA despite the 5′ terminal ε in encapsidation is caused by the translating ribosomes on the HBe RNA, which prevent the folding of ε or its interaction with the polymerase (Nassal et al. 1990). This indicates that only complete, translating 80S ribosomes are able to displace the ε-bound polymerase, because the pregenomic RNA must be scanned by the 40S ribosomal initiation complex for the initiation of core protein synthesis.

In addition to the polymerase and the pregenomic RNA, a protein kinase is encapsidated within core particles (Gerlich et al. 1982). This activity is associated with nucleocapsids, even when expressing the core gene alone in insect cells (Lanford and Notvall 1990). As mentioned above, the kinase is not unequivocally identified yet but it is known that it phosphorylates serine residues between the arginine clusters in the carboxy-terminal portion of the core protein (Lan et al. 1999).

Studies on the function of the protein kinase are difficult to perform since the carboxy-terminal part of the core protein is multifunctional. It comprises domains essential for RNA packaging and genome maturation (Nassal 1992). Hence, it is not surprising that point mutations of the protein kinase target sequences always resulted in a more or less complete inhibition of genome maturation. Using this approach, it has been shown that phosphorylation at serine 162 is required for specific encapsidation of the RNA pregenome (Gazina et al. 2000), mediated by the polymerase. However, phosphorylation in vitro inhibits interaction of nucleic acids and the core protein, implying that the majority of phosphorylation probably occurs after encapsidation of pregenomic RNA (Kann and Gerlich 1994).

The complex events that convert the linear RNA pregenome to the circular double-stranded DNA in the virion are outlined in Figure 55.5 (for review, see Ganem et al. 1994). Previous observations on the endogenous polymerase activity suggested that this enzyme is active only within nucleocapsids. However, DHBV RNA, which contains the ε signal, and the polymerase ORF, can be used in a cell-free translation system to express an active DHBV polymerase that can prime and elongate the first nucleotides of the negative-strand DNA (Wang and Seeger 1993). These data have

been confirmed by expression of the DHBV polymerase in *Escherichia coli*, which was able to initiate reverse transcription at a synthetic template after complementation with eukaryotic chaperones Hsc70 and Hsp40 (Beck and Nassal 2003). Noteworthy, these cell-free systems could only be established for the polymerase of DHBV and allow only the addition of some nucleotides; attempts to express the HBV polymerase in a similar manner failed.

The progress on DHBV research allowed the understanding of the initial events in hepadnaviral replication. The polymerase starts at the bulge of the ε signal (Figure 55.5a) and not, as originally concluded from primer extension experiments, within the 3′ terminal DR1. For the priming of the negative-strand DNA, the hydroxyl group of tyrosine 96 of the DHBV polymerase serves as the acceptor for the synthesis of a phosphodiester bridge with the first nucleotide. After the addition of the first 4 nt (DHBV, 3 nt in HBV) encoded by the bulge, the oligonucleotide polymerase complex dissociates from the bulge, and reanneals with a sequence complementary to the 3′ terminal DR1 (Figure 55.5b). These findings were confirmed for the HBV polymerase by expression in yeast. However, because there are many complementary sequences to the three or four initial bases of the negative DNA strand within the hepadnavirus genomes, additional factors must be involved. These include the primary and secondary structure of the surrounding RNA sequences of the DR1 as well as the distance between initiation site and DR1 that regulate the transfer of the polymerase nucleotide complex from ε to a sequence element φ at the 3′ terminal DR1 (Tang and McLachlan 2001). At DR1, reverse transcription, that means negative-strand DNA elongation, proceeds towards the 5′ end of the pregenome. The catalytic center for the polymerization reaction contains the typical YMDD motif as has been described for retroviruses. A further similarity is that the elongation of the negative DNA strand is combined with degradation of the RNA strand in the resulting DNA–RNA hybrid. Mapping of the 3′ end of the negative DNA strand showed that it nearly coincides with the 5′ end of the pregenomic RNA. Thus, the 3′ end of the negative DNA strand is obviously specified by 'run off', when the polymerase reaches the end of its RNA template, resulting in the terminal redundancy of the negative DNA strand of 8–10 nt (Figure 55.5c). Since the RNase H domain is separated from the polymerizing catalytic center in the polymerase, an RNA oligonucleotide of 17–18 bases does not become degraded. This oligonucleotide represents the 5′ end of the pregenome including the 5′ CAP. Together or concomitantly with the polymerase, the oligonucleotide translocates to the complementary region of DR2 on the minus-strand DNA. The translocation requires a folding of the minus strand mediated by a structural element within the S ORF termed the M region (Liu et al. 2003).

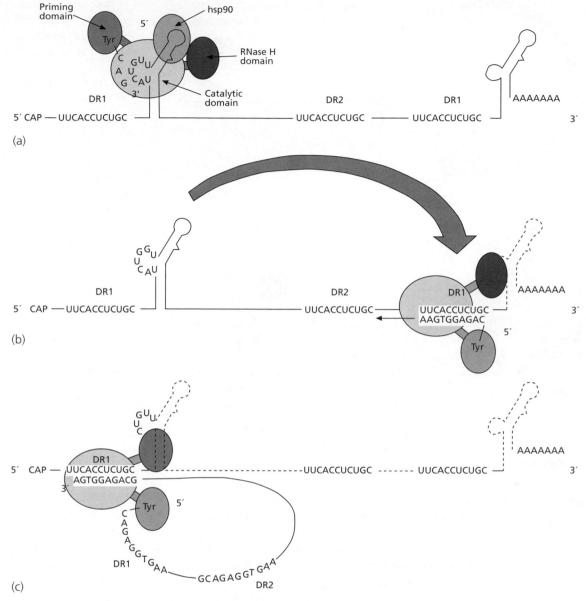

Figure 55.5 *Generation of the viral genome from the pregenomic RNA.* **(a)** *Binding of the viral polymerase and the cellular factor hsp90 to the encapsidation signal on the pregenomic RNA. Reverse transcription for the first 3 DNA nucleotides starts at the bulge of the stem–loop structure. The first nucleotide (C) is covalently linked to a hydroxyl group of a tyrosine within the priming domain of the polymerase.* **(b)** *Translocation (large arrow) of the polymerase–nucleotide complex to a complementary sequence on the DR1. Further negative DNA strand synthesis.* **(c)** *Completion of negative DNA strand synthesis. The degraded RNA template is depicted as a dotted line. The remaining undegraded RNA oligomer is shown in black. (continued over)*

At DR2, the polymerase uses the 3′ end of the RNA oligonucleotide as the primer for DNA synthesis, now accepting the single-stranded DNA of the minus strand as template. Since the polymerase is covalently bound to the 5′ end of the minus strand, this single strand must form a loop which narrows when the polymerase proceeds towards the 5′ end. Apparently, the distance between phosphodiester linked Tyr in the priming domain and the catalytic center of the polymerase allows that plus strand DNA synthesis reaches the 5′ end of the minus DNA strand template (Figure 55.5d, e). Because

the negative DNA strand is linear, second-strand synthesis could run off at the 5′ end of the template, but mature HBV genome in core particles is predominantly circular. Thus, the polymerase is able to bridge the gap between the 3′ and the 5′ end of the negative DNA strand. On the basis of mutational analysis, a melting of the 3′ end of the positive DNA strand and the 5′ end of the negative DNA strand (Figure 55.5f) was suggested. Due to the terminal redundancy r, the 3′ end of the positive DNA strand can anneal with the complementary 3′ end of the negative DNA strand (Figure 55.5g). Besides

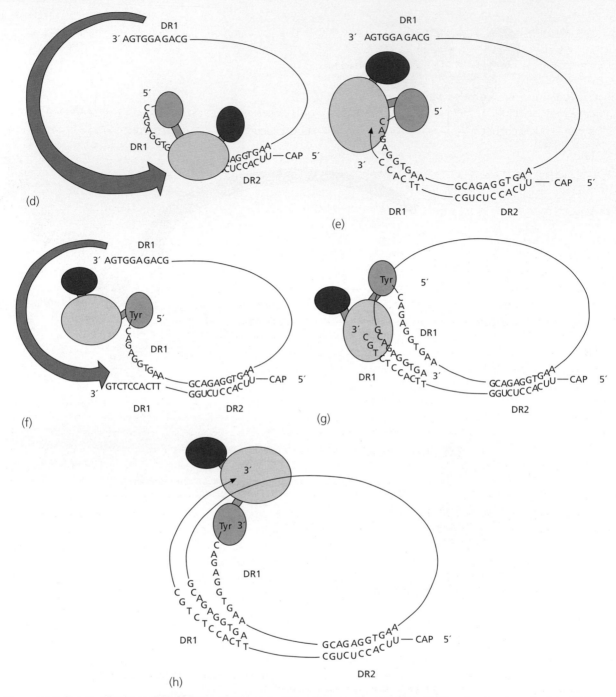

Figure 55.5 **(continued) Generation of the viral genome from the pregenomic RNA. (d)** *Translocation (arrow) of the RNA oligomer and the polymerase to a complementary sequence on the DR2.* **(e)** *Start of positive DNA strand synthesis, using the 3′ end of the RNA oligomer as a primer.* **(f)** *Melting of the 3′ end of the positive DNA strand and the 5′ end of the negative DNA strand. Translocation of the 3′ end of the negative DNA strand to the DR1 at the 3′ end of the positive DNA strand (arrow).* **(g)** *Annealing of the DR1 at the 3′ end of the negative DNA strand with the complementary sequence of DR1 at the 3′ end of the positive DNA strand (arrow).* **(h)** *Further positive DNA strand synthesis.*

r, however, there are additional requirements for circularization. This includes the adjacent regions termed 5E and 3E (Liu et al. 2003, 2004).

Annealing of the plus strand 3′ end and 5′ end of the minus strand reconstitute a continuous single-stranded DNA template for the polymerase. Thus, the polymerase should be able to synthesize a double-stranded

circular DNA with two nicks between the 5′ and 3′ end of both minus- and plus-strand DNA. The virion, however, contains a partially double-stranded DNA with the heterogeneous 3′ ends of the plus DNA strand leaving a single-stranded gap of ca. 800 nt. The reason for this phenomenon is unknown but one may hypothesize that the limited space within the capsid does not allow an ongoing synthesis since double-stranded DNA is less flexible than single-stranded DNA. A minority of virions contain a linear double-stranded DNA genome instead of the partially double-stranded circular DNA molecule. As shown for DHBV these virions are infectious. Within the nucleus the cccDNA is formed by circularisation of the linear DNA using nonhomologous recombination between the two ends (Yang and Summers, 1998).

TRAFFICKING OF PROGENY HEPADNAVIRAL CAPSIDS

Transport to the nucleus

Mature core particles may enter two different pathways, which are important for the viral life cycle. Because the HBV cccDNA in the nucleus is subject to slow degradation, the pool of intranuclear HBV genomes must be restored permanently to ensure viral persistence. The restoration of the pool is usually possible either by new infection of the hepatocyte with HBV, or by re-entry of viral DNA after release from the viral nucleocapsid. Amplification of cccDNA between 10 and 50 copies per cell occurs even in cultured hepatocytes that are not susceptible to DHBV and HBV infection, so it obviously does not require reinfection but nuclear entry of viral genomes from newly synthesized core particles in the cytoplasm. This 'short cut,' without secretion and reinfection, occurs predominantly at the beginning of infection. It leads to the establishment of chronic infection on the cellular level. In addition, this unusual strategy, which has only been described for pararetroviruses, avoids the appearance of the virus in the serum, and minimizes the risk of being neutralized by circulating antibodies. However, DHBV cores cannot spread from cell to cell but must be enveloped, secreted, and enter new cells (Funk et al. 2004).

The mechanism of how the viral genome is delivered to the nucleus has been studied in in vitro systems and seems to follow the same strategy as during initial infection. Apparently, the genome is transported within the core particles, which use the cellular microtubule transport system for reaching the perinuclear region, followed by an active nuclear import mediated by cellular nuclear import factors. For interaction with the import factors, the core proteins expose a 'classical' localization signal (NLS) on the capsid surface. The NLS is localized within the carboxy-terminal domain of the core proteins and within the lumen of the capsid after assembly. The exposure of the NLS on the capsid surface thus requires a structural change, which is caused by phosphorylation of the carboxy terminus (Rabe et al. 2003). The NLS is bound by the adapter protein importin α and subsequently by the cellular transport receptor importin β. Following the established pathway of nuclear import, importin β mediates the binding to the cytoplasmic fibers of the NPC and the transport through the pore into the nuclear basket (Panté and Kann 2002). Exclusively at this site, the core particles disintegrate and release the viral DNA into the karyoplasm (Rabe et al. 2003).

Envelopment and secretion

The second pathway for core particles is the envelopment into the surface proteins, followed by virus secretion. DHBV mutants defective for envelope proteins but competent for replication lead to intranuclear cccDNA accumulation up to 50 times the natural copy number. The expression of surface proteins results in envelopment of core particles and secretion of virus, and regulates amplification of cccDNA (Summers et al. 1990). After de novo infection of hepatocytes, transcription of HBs mRNA is a late event (Tuttleman et al. 1986). Thus, the regulation of DHBV cccDNA amplification via surface protein synthesis guarantees that a large pool of cccDNA has been generated in the infected cell before virus is exported.

In contrast to HDV, where only SHBs is required for assembly and secretion, assembly of HBV requires LHBs and SHBs (Bruss and Ganem 1991). Stepwise truncation of LHBs showed that only sequences proximal to amino acid 108 of preS are required for HBV assembly. A series of mutations determined that the highly conserved preS1 region between Arg103 and Ser124 at the transition to preS2 is essential (Bruss 1997). Using the same technique, envelopment-negative core mutants were identified. Although being spread throughout the primary amino acid sequence, these mutants clustered at two sites on the capsid surface. One cluster is localized in a ringlike groove around the tip of the spikes and the second cluster at the amino-terminal end of the flexible carboxy terminus of the core protein (Ponsel and Bruss 2003).

In the current model of HBV (Figure 55.6c,d; and see Figure 55.2), the preS domains in LHBs have a dual topology. The preS domain in part of the LHBs molecules is cytosolically retained by Hsc70 (Lambert and Prange 2003); the other part is exposed at the surface of HBV, allowing multiple functions of LHBs:

- Like matrix proteins of many other enveloped proteins, it mediates the budding of core particles together with their envelope proteins. For this task, a matrix protein must be fixed at the membrane, but its binding site for the viral capsid should be located on the cytosolic side.
- The preS1 domain is also the attachment site to the cell surface during infection. For this purpose the preS domain has to be accessible on the surface of the particle.

The mechanism by which the preS domain posttranslationally passes through the ER or post-ER membrane is unclear. Direct passage through the lipid bilayer without the involvement of signal recognition

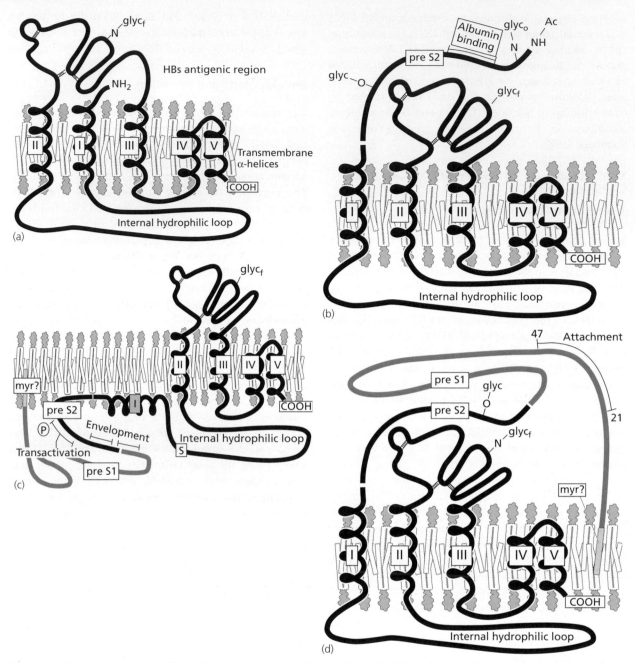

Figure 55.6 *Postulated topology of hepatitis B virus surface proteins.* **(a)** *SHBs;* **(b)** *MHBs;* **(c)** *LHBs with preS in the cytosol;* **(d)** *LHBs with the preS at the virus surface. In the nonassembled state, the bottom reflects the cytosolic side which represents, after encapsidation, the core particle of the inner part of the virus. The top of the figure represents nonassembled surface proteins in the lumen of the endoplasmic reticulum, after assembly and secretion the outside of the particle. The molecules of the membrane bilayer are depicted in gray and white. Predicted transmembrane helices are numbered I–V. ac: acetyl residue; N-glyco: obligatory complex N-linked glycan; N-glycf: facultative N-glycan; myr: myristylation site; O-glyc: O-linked glycan.*

particles (SRP) and secretion factors (sec) has been described for small amphipathic proteins, but the preS domain does not have this type of structure (Bruss et al. 1994). Incubation at low pH and at 37°C favors translocation of interior preS domains to the surface of virions (Bruss et al. 1994; Guo and Pugh 1997). The preS2 portion of preS carries a translocation motif that allows for energy-independent membrane passage (Oess and Hildt 2000) and may carry proteins into cells (Hafner

et al. 2003). However, there are no data that this motif is involved in the translocation of the preS domain itself.

The forces that drive the budding and assembly of HBV and HBs particles are not yet well understood. The carboxy-terminal part and parts of the two hydrophilic loops in the S domain can be deleted or substituted, but most of the cysteine residues in the internal loop are essential. The high sequence conservation in the four α-helices suggests a coil-to-coil interaction, which may contribute to the morphogenesis of virions and HBs particles (Berting et al. 1995).

The HBs particles mature in a pre-Golgi compartment. The *N*-linked glycosides of the HBs proteins at N146 of the S domain and N4 of preS2 are trimmed and modified to a complex biantennary oligosaccharide. *O*-linked glycan is linked to T37 of preS2, and an acetyl residue to the N-terminal methionine (Schmitt et al. 1999, 2004). Cultivation of HBV-expressing cells with inhibitors of glucosidase I (for example, *N*-butyldeoxy-nojirimycin) blocks the trimming and prevents the secretion of HBV (Block et al. 1994). MHBs is a specific target for this block of secretion (Lu et al. 1995).

HBsAg 20 nm spheres are constitutively secreted. However, HBs-filaments may be retained in the ER if they contain more LHBs than SHBs. The retention signal resides in the preS1 region (Gallina et al. 1995). MHBs does not significantly alter the secretion behavior if properly glycosylated.

Certain hepatocytes in HBsAg carriers seem to over-express LHBs, relative to SHBs, and contain a dilated ER, which gives them a ground glass appearance in light microscopy. Such cells probably do not contribute to HBV production and are often found in so-called healthy HBsAg carriers with low viremia (Dienes et al. 1990). Only cells that express core protein, polymerase, SHBs, and LHBs protein in a well-balanced mixture are able to assemble and secrete HBV.

Nonstructural proteins

In contrast to the positive-strand RNA viruses that do not use reverse transcription, retroviruses and the hepadnaviruses do not use a major part of their coding capacity for nonstructural proteins. However, LHBs and SHBs are not only essential structural components of the virion; they occur also as secreted antigens. Furthermore, MHBs is a nonessential structural protein of mammalian hepadnaviruses.

Two proteins that are not essential for replication in cell cultures are HBe protein and HBx protein. Neither HBe protein nor HBx protein have yet been identified as a structural component of the virion. They are therefore considered here as nonstructural proteins, although their presence in low amounts in virions cannot be excluded.

HBs PROTEINS

A peculiarity of all wild type hepadnaviruses is expression of the HBs proteins in large excess. Even in HBV carriers producing many virions, empty HBs particles are present in ca. 1 000-fold greater number than virions and may reach concentrations of up to 1 g/l, as major serum proteins such as IgM. In low viremic HBsAg carriers, HBsAg may be present in particle numbers up to 10^{12}/ml even though HBV DNA is barely detectable

by polymerase chain reaction (PCR). Thus, in a way, HBs proteins are nonstructural as well as structural proteins. HBsAg particles have a much longer half-life (>8 days) than virions, which disappear with a half-life of 1–3 days from the serum if replication is blocked (Chulanov et al. 2003). However, HBV-transfected hepatoma cells also produce an excess of HBs proteins. Thus, the excess of nonstructural HBs protein over virion-bound HBs protein is not only due to more rapid removal of virions from the circulation. The significance of this overexpression is not clear. It may contribute to an immune tolerance that is a precondition for highly productive persistent infection in an immunocompetent host. Furthermore the excess HBs proteins may block the HBV receptors of the host during late or persistent stages of infection and thereby allow the circulation of virions, which is a precondition for efficient transmissibility. The long delay of several weeks or even months between infection and the first appearance of virions and HBs protein is probably due to the slow replication of HBV, but may also be due in part to immediate readsorption to receptors not yet blocked. However, for DHBV intracellular down-regulation of the gp180 receptor by L-DHBs protein has been observed (Breiner et al. 2001).

The proportion of HBs proteins differs in the three morphological forms of HBs particles. Virions contain a high proportion of LHBs, HBs filaments intermediate amounts, but small amounts are present in 20 nm particles. The proportion of MHBs may be variable and is usually higher in HBs particles from high viremic carriers.

HBe PROTEIN

HBe protein was discovered by the analysis of HBsAg-positive sera from different donors by double diffusion in agar gels (Magnius and Espmark 1972). Some HBsAg carriers contained a precipitating antibody against a novel HBV antigen called e antigen (HBeAg). HBeAg was found predominantly in highly productive HBV carriers with a detectable endogenous HBV DNA polymerase, whereas anti-HBe was usually found in 'healthy' low viremic carriers. Sera from HBeAg-positive carriers typically have infectivity titers for chimpanzees of 10^8/ml or more and genome numbers of 10^9–10^{10}/ml, whereas anti-HBe- and HBsAg-positive sera have typically only ten infectious doses/ml (Shikata et al. 1977). The biochemical nature of HBe protein remained unclear until 1982, when recombinant HBc particles, devoid of any other viral component, were converted into HBeAg by treatment with protease and ionic detergents. Characterization of isolated HBe protein from the serum of HBV carriers revealed that it had an amino acid composition similar to that of HBc protein, but it had only ca. 15 kDa owing to a carboxy-terminal truncation at Val 149 of HBc.

It cannot be ruled out that a minor part of HBe protein in serum may be derived from degraded nucleocapsids or nonassembled HBc protein, but at least the major part of HBeAg, if not all, is generated by a biosynthetic pathway different from that of HBc protein. As mentioned in the section entitled Genome structure and function, above, HBV-containing cells express, besides the pregenomic RNA, a slightly longer RNA that contains not only the AUG for the HBc protein but also the AUG for the preC region 29 codons upstream. The preC sequence has the property of a signal peptide, which directs the nascent polypeptide to the membrane of the ER and causes its translocation to the ER lumen. The translocation is, however, incomplete, thus allowing the re-entry of part of the full-length HBe protein molecules with 25 kDa to the cytosol. This form of HBe protein may be transported to the nucleus because of its carboxy-terminal nuclear localization signal.

The major part of ER-associated HBe protein is cleaved at Ala19, thus generating a 22-kDa protein. During passage through the Golgi apparatus, a further protease cleaves HBe at Val149 or alternative sites downstream, generating proteins of 16–18 kDa. This cleavage is a precondition for release from the cell. HBe protein may oligomerize, but, in contrast to HBc, does not assemble to a closed particle. The tryptophan and cysteine residues in the remaining part of the preC peptide prevent assembly to corelike particles (Schlicht and Wasenauer 1991). The amount of HBeAg in the serum of HBV carriers by far exceeds the amount of HBc protein within circulating virions. Titers in enzyme immune assay (EIA) often reach 1:8 000, and detection by agar gel immune precipitation suggests amounts of several micrograms per milliliter. Thus, both major structural proteins HBs and HBc of the virion are accompanied by a large excess of slightly altered nonviral forms.

It is doubtful whether HBe protein has a direct function in the viral life cycle. The HBe mRNA does not support genome replication. HBe-negative mutated genomes of DHBV and WHV replicate in the natural hosts. Naturally occurring HBe-negative variants of HBV are present in many patients (see section Clinical and pathological aspects). It has even been found that preC-containing wild type genomes replicate less efficiently in transfected hepatoma cells than preC-negative genomes (Scaglioni et al. 1996).

The conservation of HBe protein in all known hepadnaviruses, in spite of its being nonessential, suggests that it provides an important advantage for the survival and spread of hepadnaviruses in their host population. A clue to the function of HBe protein may be the observation that newborn woodchucks infected with an HBe-negative mutant develop acute, but not chronic, infection as occurs with wild-type virus (Chen et al. 1992). It may be that HBe protein suppresses immune elimination of HBV, thus contributing to the development of a carrier state (Milich and Liang 2003). Furthermore, HBeAg is transferred in utero from a HBV carrier mother to the fetus (Wang and Zhang 2003).

HBx PROTEIN

HBV encodes a protein of 154 amino acids (141 in WHV and 138 in GSHV), the function of which is essentially unknown. The recent identification of a functional HBx protein in avian hepadnaviruses (Schuster et al. 2002) suggests that it is somehow essential during hepadnaviral replication in that it alters the host organism in a way that it is more permissive for viral replication. HBx is not essential for HBV production in transfected permanent cell lines (Yaginuma et al. 1987) or primary rat hepatocyte cultures (Blum et al. 1992). WHV genomes without a functional *HBx* gene do not replicate efficiently in woodchucks (Chen et al. 1993; Zoulim et al. 1994), but replicate sufficiently in vivo to induce immunity and may, thus, be considered as attenuated virus (Zhang et al. 2001). This observation suggests that HBx protein is not essential for low-level replication in vivo, but enhances infection (Xu et al. 2002). There may, however, also exist an effect of HBx on the immune system favoring tolerance against HBV, because HBV genomes with a truncated HBx variant have been observed preferably in immunodeficient patients (Repp et al. 1992). Evolution of such HBV genomes without a complete *HBx* gene in immunocompromised patients may indicate that HBx protein is not so necessary in patients without an efficient immune defense as in normal hosts. HBx protein may activate components of the specific and the innate immune system, for example, the nuclear factor of activated T cells NF-AT (Lara-Pezzi et al. 1998) or NF-κB (Su and Schneider 1997). HBV may enter lymphocytes and monocytes of HBV carriers and is weakly expressed. In these cells, HBx mRNA is expressed at highest levels compared to other HBV mRNAs (Stoll-Becker et al. 1997).

The genome position of the *HBx* gene and promoter next to HBV enhancer I is reminiscent of the genome position of the early 1A (*E1A*) gene of adenoviruses and of other immediate–early genes of DNA viruses. *E1A* is essential for adenovirus replication in most but not all cell types by *trans*-activating the early promoters of E2 and E4 in the adenovirus genomes. The *trans*-activating activity of HBx on HBV enhancer I and on various viral or cellular enhancers was first described in 1988 by Spandau and Lee and by Zahm et al. Numerous further studies (for example, Wu et al. 2002) confirmed the nonspecific promiscuous *trans*-activating activity of HBx (review by Murakami 2001), but usually the activation factor is low. HBx does not bind directly to DNA. If artificially expressed in the absence of other HBV genes, it is found most abundantly in the cytoplasm, but it is also present in the nucleus (Doria et al. 1995). Current evidence suggests that cytoplasmic HBx may act either via a tyrosine kinase signaling cascade and/or mitochondrial calcium channels (Bouchard et al. 2003) but other pathways also seem to exist (Hafner et al. 2003). However, the *trans*-activating activity seems to be maintained in some systems if a nuclear localization signal is added. Many potential nuclear binding partners of HBx protein have been identified in vitro: transcription factors (TF), ATF II, and CREB, the TATA-binding protein TFIID, TFIIB, RNA polymerase subunit RPB5, a novel X-associated protein XAP-1 which may be involved in DNA repair, the ubiquitous transcription factor Oct 1, tumor suppressor protein p53, DNA repair-associated transcription factor ERCC3, and single-stranded RNA. Furthermore, binding of HBx to XAP-C7, an α-subunit of the proteasome, or to XAP-P13, a subunit of the regulatory 26S complex of the proteasome, or to a liver-specific HBx-interacting protein XIP were reported. The highly divergent results of the in vitro binding studies allow, for the moment, only one conclusion: that HBx is very sticky. The association with the proteasome appears to be significant, because proteasome inhibitors may restore HBV replication activity of HBx-deficient mutants to wild-type levels (Zhang et al. 2004). A problem with all the *trans*-activation studies is that they depend on heavy transient overexpression of both HBx proteins and the target sequence. Moreover, they were carried out in culture systems that produce HBV without the presence of HBx and may thus be irrelevant in respect to the viral life cycle.

Many viral immediate–early transcription-activating factors, such as E1A of certain adenoviruses, or P6 and P7 of certain papillomavirus types, are also tumor proteins. They bind and inactivate tumor suppressor proteins such as Rb or p53. HBx was reported to bind and inactivate essential functions of p53. An Rb-inactivating factor of HBV has not yet been reported. HBx transforms the SV40TAg-immortalized fetal mouse hepatocyte line FMH 202 to overt malignancy if expressed in large amounts (Höhne et al. 1990). Similar results were obtained in p53-negative mouse cells (Oguey et al. 1996). Of several strains of mice transgenic for HBx protein, only one strain developed liver tumors; high expression of HBx in these mice was necessary. In one transgenic mouse line, an enhanced susceptibility against chemical carcinogens was noted (reviewed by Schaefer and Gerlich 1995). In human hepatocellular carcinoma (HCC) and cirrhotic liver HBx protein may be detected with selected anti-HBx antibodies in the cytoplasm of some but not all cells (Su et al. 1998). More recently, a very clear association of anti-HBx antibodies in the plasma and HBx antigen in the liver with the presence of HCC was found in contrast to findings in chronic hepatitis B patients (Hwang et al. 2003).

While immortalized cells may become malignant under high expression of HBx, primary cells seem to go into apoptosis (Terradillos et al. 1998; Schuster et al.

2000). HBx also enhances the apoptotic effect of tumor necrosis factor (TNF) alpha (Su and Schneider 1997). It appears that overexpressed HBx interacts with a variety of apoptosis-inducing or inhibiting factors, for example, c-FLIP (Kim and Seong 2003), mitochondrial membranes (Shirakata and Koike 2003), Bcl-2 (Terradillos et al. 2002), or the Fas-ligand (Yoo and Lee 2004). The oncogenic effect of HBx seems to reside in the amino terminal portion (Gottlob et al. 1998), whereas the proapoptotic and transcription-activating effect is in the carboxy-terminal portion (Schuster et al. 2000). HBx mutants present in HCCs abrogate the antiproliferative and transactivating effects of wt HBx and may, thus, maintain oncogenicity (Sirma et al. 1999). The proapoptotic function is conserved in the avihepadnaviruses (Schuster et al. 2002).

In natural infection, HBx mRNA is usually expressed in low levels. Furthermore, the half-life of HBx seems to be very low. Even if one postulates an oncogenic potential of HBx, this may explain why acutely infected patients and chronically infected HBV patients with high replication do not develop HCC. In WHV-infected woodchucks, WHxAg is localized in the cytoplasm of infected cells, but is rarely found in HCC (Jacob et al. 1997).

It is open to question whether HBx is not oncogenic at all in natural settings, or its expression is too low, or viral factors suppress the activity of HBx. With regard to the latter possibility, it has been observed that the core gene of HBV, if co-expressed, suppresses the *trans*-activating activities of the *HBx* gene on a variety of promoters. As with oncogenes from other viruses, *HBx* may be negatively controlled by viral genes the expression of which is stimulated by *HBx*. In HCC, *HBx* may be expressed from HBV DNA integrates, which often do not encode other complete HBV ORFs.

In summary, HBx probably has a role in liver-specific expression of HBV and a weak oncogenic potential that, however, can be effective only in combination with other oncogenesis-favoring events. The significance of the proaptotic effect is not understood.

Integration of HBV DNA and liver cancer

Integration of the viral genome into the host genome is not part of the hepadnaviral life cycle, in contrast to the retroviruses. Nevertheless, integration of HBV DNA fragments into the hepatocyte genome is a frequent event during HBV infection. Even if a full-length genome would be integrated the circular HBV genome is thereby disrupted and no longer able to express a viable pregenomic RNA. (Viable HBV DNA can be integrated for experimental purposes in the form of artificial linear constructs covering the sequence of the pregenome plus homologous or heterologous upstream transcription signals.) However, subgenomic mRNAs and viral proteins may be expressed from integrated HBV DNA fragments. Integration sites in the viral genome are very often around DR1 at one end and at variable sites at the other end. These integrates may express a carboxy-terminally truncated HBx protein fused to cellular sequences which still has *trans*-activating activity in experimental systems (Wollersheim et al. 1988). Furthermore, a cryptic polyadenylation site may be used that generates a polylysine tail at the carboxy-terminal end of a truncated HBx protein (Rakotomahanina et al. 1994).

The integrated HBV DNA is quite often composed of two, or even more, fragments that are linked together in a head-to-tail arrangement or in other complex rearrangements. Occasionally, such a rearranged DNA fragment may express truncated forms of preS/S proteins, in particular truncated MHBs and HBx. Such truncated LHBs or MHBs proteins have been found to *trans*-activate transcription factor AP1 and others, suggesting an additional growth-stimulating effect of these defective HBV proteins (Hildt et al. 1997). Such HBV DNA fragments induce malignant growth in cell cultures and nude mice (Luber et al. 1996).

With human HBV DNA, no clear preference for a defined integration site has been identified and it was noted that the integration site might be rearranged. It seems that integration of HBV DNA destabilizes the host genome. In two independent studies from Japan (Kawai et al. 2000; Okabe et al. 2000), a loss of heterozygosity was more often found in HBV-associated HCC than in nonviral or HCV-associated HCC. It has been suggested that oxidative stress – as may occur in inflammation – induces not only DNA-damage but also enhances HBV DNA integration (Dandri et al. 2002). A model has been proposed that topoisomerase I mediates the integration of HBV DNA around the DR1 site. A role of the integrated HBV DNA in the development of HCC is suggested by the fact that virtually all HCC-derived cell lines from HBV carriers contain one, or usually more, HBV DNA fragments and that the HCCs are usually of monoclonal origin. The model of insertional mutagenesis leading to deregulation of growth control genes has been verified for several human HCCs. One example is the fusion of a retinoic acid receptor β chain with 29 amino-terminal residues from preS1, which may lead to uncontrolled expression of this differentiation factor (Dejean et al. 1986). Another example is the insertion of preS2/S sequences of HBV into an intron of cyclin A, generating a preS2/2 fusion with cyclin A devoid of its amino-terminal degradation signals (Wang et al. 1990). This altered cyclin A has transforming properties in cell cultures. A third example is the activation of mevalonate kinase (Graef et al. 1994). More recently, a systematic search for HBV DNA integration sites revealed, in six of 21 isolates, insertion into cellular genes which are key regulators of cell proliferation and viability, among them the human telomerase reverse transcriptase gene (Gozuacik et al. 2001), which has also been found by others (Ferber et al. 2003). Further integration sites were reported next to the RNA-binding motif of Y chromosome gene which was found to be ectopically expressed in three of 10 HCCs from children (Tsuei et al. 2002). More typical are, however, integrations into Alu-type repeats, minisatellite-like, satellite III or a variable number of tandem repeat sequences, suggesting a preference of HBV DNA integration into sites where other multiple insertions have already occurred during evolution (Rogler and Chisari 1992).

Development of HCC is a regular event in woodchucks chronically infected with WHV. In HCCs of this animal, insertion of WHV DNA very often occurs upstream of a functional retrotransposon encoding cellular N-*myc*2. The viral enhancers activate the cellular N-myc2, which finally leads to the development of HCC (Flajolet et al. 1998). Insertion of hepadnaviral DNA into c-*myc* sequences was observed both in woodchucks and in ground squirrels. However, in human HCC c-*myc* or N-*myc* activation was found only occasionally (Buendia et al. 1993). Hepadnaviral DNA integration has also been found in HCC from ducks, but development of HCC in ducks seems to be exclusively correlated to exposure to aflatoxin B.

HBV genotypes, HBsAg subtypes, and HBV variants

The sequencing of numerous HBV isolates in the late 1970s and early 1980s has revealed a surprisingly high degree of conservation; even rodent hepadnaviruses are ca. 60 percent homologous to human HBV. Human HBV splits into eight identified genotypes, A to H, which diverge by 8–15 percent in the DNA sequence (Norder et al. 2004). Furthermore, genosubtypes with a typical predominant ethnical distribution have been defined: A1 in Africa, Brazil, and India, A2 in Europe and USA, B1 and B2 in Japan and China, B3 in Indonesia, B4 in Vietnam, C1 and C2 in Japan, Korea, and China, C3 in Oceania, C4 in Australian aborigines), D1–D3 in Europe, the Mediterranean, Middle East, and Central Asia, D4 in East Asia, E in West Africa and Madagascar, F1 and H in Central America, F2 in South America and Polynesia. The latter observation supports the debated theory of Thor Heyerdahl that a part of the Pacific Islands was settled from South America (Norder et al. 2004). Genotype G is rare and has no clear geographical pattern. HBV has also been found in apes, every species having its own genotype(s). Due to vertical and intrafamiliar transmission, the genotype usually reflects the ethnic origin even after several generations and not the actual geographical location. Americans or Canadians of East Asian origin usually have genotype B or C, Brazilians often genotype A1 originating from Africa.

Human and ape genotypes are phylogenetically equally distant (reviewed by Bartholomeusz and Schaefer 2004), but genotypes F and H branch off and are more distant. This suggests that there may have been a common ancestor to old world primates' hepadnaviruses and most human HBV genotypes whereas genotypes F and H may have been acquired in the new world. The next relative to human and ape hepadnaviruses has been isolated from woolly monkeys (a new world monkey) (Lanford et al. 1997). Since this virus is not viable in chimpanzees, it is considered an own species as is WHV (Mason et al. 2005). Avian hepadnaviruses are only distantly related to mammalian hepadnaviruses, despite their similar genomic organization and replication strategy.

The multiple functions of the viral nucleic acid sequences for the coding of overlapping genes, regulation of replication, transcription, and assembly of the virions prevent excessive variability. A hot spot of variability between virus species is the preS1 region, probably because of its role in host specificity and because the overlapping polymerase sequence functions in this region only as spacer.

Variability in the hydrophilic loop of the SHBs protein on the virion surface or on HBs particles, respectively, determines the serological HBsAg subtype. Besides the common antigenic determinant a, subtype-specific alleles d or y, and w1, w2, w3, w4, or r were described. Combinations of these alleles define nine HBsAg subtypes according to a workshop held in 1975 in Paris. Position 122 of SHBs is lysine for determinant d and arginine for determinant y. Position 160 is lysine for the four w alleles and arginine for r. Differentiation into w1 to w4 is mainly based on exchanges at position 127 (Norder et al. 1994). There is no clear correlation between genotype and HBsAg reactivity. Thus, HBV genomes should preferably be characterized by their genotype. Antigenic differences, defined by reactivity with monoclonal antibodies, also exist in the preS2 and preS1 regions. The predominant sequences of an HBV isolate are usually conserved within an infection chain from person to person, suggesting low variability. Obviously the existing genotypes of HBV are optimally adapted to replication in their host population. However, HBV turns out to be a quasi species at all stages of infection if a large number of cloned genomes is analyzed.

HBV variants can be generated by point mutations, small deletions or insertions, and by splicing events. The reverse transcription of HBV is very inaccurate and whereby all possible mutations may be created in a very short time. One can estimate that a highly viremic chronic carrier generates ca. 10^{13} new viral genomes per day. At an assumed error rate of 10^{-5}, 10^8 mutants per day are generated. While in the quasi-immunotolerant state one genome species is strongly favored, any kind of selection leads to a great variety of variants. Breakdown of immunotolerance is indicated by disappearance of

HBeAg and leads to a rapid accumulation of viable and nonviable mutants (Bozkaya et al. 1996). The main targets are

- the preS1/S2 junction leading to a loss of MHBs (Blackberg and Kidd-Ljunggren 2003)
- alterations in the binding sites for transcription factors in the core promoter and enhancer region (Erhardt et al. 2000) leading to less HBeAg production and stronger replication
- inactivation of the precore region, i.e. the HBeAg leader sequence (Chu et al. 2003)
- or deletions in the core protein (Günther et al. 1996).

The type of mutations leading to a HBeAg loss of production differs with the genotype (Chan et al. 1999; Tanaka et al. 2004). X-protein deletions are often found in immunosuppressed patients (Schlager et al. 2000). All these mutations supposedly develop under the host's own immune system as the only selective pressure. Active immunization with SHBs vaccine (Lu and Lorentz 2003) or passive immunization with anti-HBs (Carman et al. 1999) may select for escape mutations in the HBsAg antigen loop. Treatment with nucleoside or nucleotide analogues selects for mutations in the reverse transcriptase domain of the HBV DNA polymerase, which also become evident in the S domain (Locarnini 2003). Often, several types of selection come together leading to complex combinations of mutations. Typically, heavily mutated variants are more often found in late stage infection or HCC.

CLINICAL AND PATHOLOGICAL ASPECTS

Normal ('wild') types of *Hepadnavirus* species are not overtly cytopathogenic. Inflammatory liver disease is caused by the host immune response against viral antigens whereby cellular cytotoxic lymphocytes exert the strongest effect (Chisari and Ferrari 1995). Consequently, symptomatic liver disease is absent in persistently infected individuals whose immune system is either immature at birth or severely impaired. Some healthy adults may also develop persistent oligosymptomatic infection without an efficient immune response; possibly immunogenetic factors predispose for persistent infection.

Another type of oligosymptomatic infection occurs when the infectious dose is very low or the immune response is rapid and efficient, or both. In such cases, silent immunization results. Acute hepatitis occurs in most immunocompetent adults who are infected by the percutaneous route with highly infectious serum or blood. A variable, but usually small, proportion of such patients develops chronic disease after acute hepatitis B. Depending on the balance between viral replication and host defense, chronic disease may cease spontaneously or proceed over years or decades to liver cirrhosis or HCC,

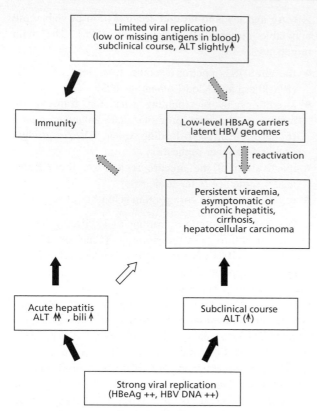

Figure 55.7 *Possible courses of hepatitis B virus infection. Black arrows show frequent courses, white arrows possible courses, and gray arrows rare or hypothetical events.*

or both. HCC usually develops in cirrhotic liver but may also appear independently of cirrhosis. In infections with high virus replication, extrahepatic manifestations (e.g. glomerulonephritis or periarteritis nodosa) due to circulating immune complexes may occur. Figure 55.7 illustrates the possible courses of HBV infection.

Clinical course of HBV infection

For more detailed descriptions and original literature, see textbooks on hepatology (e.g. Bircher et al. 1999) or on hepatitis viruses (e.g. Thomas 2000 or Lai and Locarnini 2002).

ACUTE HEPATITIS B

Diagnosis of acute hepatitis based merely on clinical symptoms is unreliable. Early nonspecific symptoms are malaise, poor appetite, nausea, and right upper quadrant abdominal pain which lasts for several days. In ca. 10 percent of patients with acute hepatitis B, a prolonged prodromal phase of up to 4 weeks occurs with serumlike sickness, including arthralgia or even frank arthritis, fever, and skin rash. In the more severe cases, after 3–6 days, fatigue and anorexia worsen and jaundice develops. Essential for the diagnosis is the determination of the alanine amino transferase (ALT) in the serum. In Germany, the upper limit of the normal range is 50 IU/l

for men and 35 IU/l for women (measured at 37°C). Clinical hepatitis is associated with values higher than 500 IU/l, reaching several thousand IU/l in severe cases (Thomas 2000). The level of ALT indicates the degree of hepatocyte damage. It increases sharply at the end of the prodromal phase and usually reaches peak values shortly before the appearance of jaundice caused by levels of high bilirubin in the serum. In less severe cases, bilirubin concentrations are below 50 µmol/l; in severe cases >340 µmol/l. In contrast to cholestatic jaundice, alkaline phosphatase is only moderately increased in the serum.

The time course of a typical acute hepatitis B is shown in Figure 55.8a. Clinical and biochemical data do not allow distinction between infections by the various hepatitis viruses. The most reliable serological marker for acute hepatitis B is IgM antibody against HBcAg (IgM anti-HBc). With the onset of symptoms, IgM anti-HBc appears and reaches peak values within a few days.

Many clinicians rely more on the detection of HBsAg in the serum. HBsAg appears during the incubation phase (Figure 55.8a), depending on the infective dose and the mode of exposure, several weeks or months after the infective event. It increases over several weeks, typically to peak levels of 10 000–100 000 PEI units/ml of HBsAg (PEI = Paul Ehrlich Institute, Germany). Decrease of HBsAg concentration starts with the onset of the prodromal phase and continues until complete recovery. Most patients remain HBsAg positive for several months.

In 2–10 percent of acute cases, HBsAg may have been eliminated so rapidly that it is already undetectable in the first available serum sample. To identify HBV as the etiological agent in these cases, it is essential to obtain a quantitative IgM anti-HBc result if no other cause for the hepatitis has been identified. Some EIAs for HBsAg may detect less well variants of HBsAg with altered *a* determinant, but these variants are rare in acute hepatitis B.

Persistence

Persistence of HBsAg for more than 6 months after onset in high concentrations (>100 PEI units/ml) means that (1) the acute hepatitis B evolved to chronicity (Figure 55.8b); or (2) a pre-existing chronic HBV infection was superimposed by an acute hepatitis of another etiology; or (3) the acute disease may actually be an exacerbation of chronic hepatitis B. Again, a high IgM anti-HBc during the early acute phase confirms recent acute HBV infection, whereas moderate amounts or absence indicate previous HBV infection.

Full recovery

Full recovery is assumed if the ALT reaches normal or close to normal levels and if HBsAg becomes negative

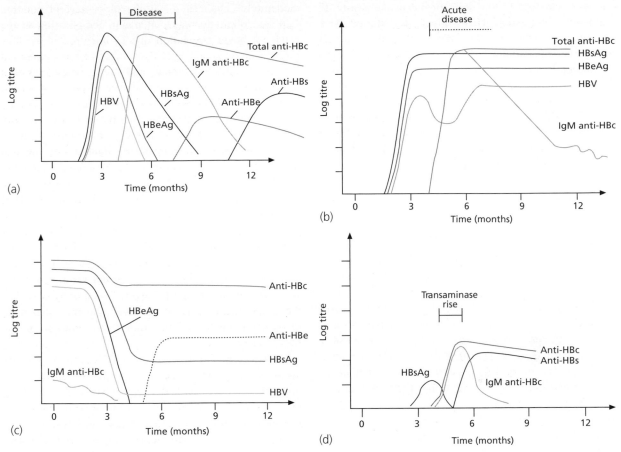

Figure 55.8 *Serological markers during the different courses of hepatitis B in arbitrary units:* **(a)** *acute hepatitis B, resolving;* **(b)** *acute hepatitis B, chronic evolution;* **(c)** *HBe seroconversion in chronic hepatitis B;* **(d)** *subclinical course of transient HBV infection.*

in EIA. This takes more than 6 months in some cases of protracted disease. Anti-HBs appears several weeks or even months after the disappearance of HBsAg. IgM anti-HBc falls to levels <100 PEI units, but may occasionally remain positive at low levels for several years. Anti-HBc of the IgG class may either persist lifelong or disappear after several years or decades.

HBV itself appears in the serum during the incubation period several weeks before HBsAg in amounts that allow its DNA to be detected by sensitive PCR techniques. Hybridization assays are not usually sensitive enough to detect HBV before HBsAg. Maximum concentration of 10^6–10^9 genomes/ml is reached before the onset of symptoms. About 40 percent of patients are already negative in hybridization assays (<10^6 genomes/ml) when the first serum sample is available.

Low-level persistence after recovery and reactivation

Cumulative evidence suggests that a major proportion of recovered patients retain intrahepatic HBV genomes. These continue to stimulate a cytotoxic T-cell response, which controls viral expression and replication (Rehermann et al. 1996). Occasionally, the cellular immune response is the only marker of the previous hepatitis B. Low level persistence may allow reactivation of HBV replication if the T-cell immunity breaks down, for example, after organ transplantation or during cancer therapy. Even a high anti-HBs level cannot reliably protect against reactivation because escape mutants may grow up. Cessation of immune suppression is extremely dangerous in that situation because memory T cells will proliferate and severely attack the infected liver (Westhoff et al. 2003). Thus, it is highly advisable to screen all patients before immunosuppression not only for overt (i.e. HBsAg positive), but also for occult HBV infection and to monitor for reactivation in positive patients.

Subclinical course and occult infections

The mild courses of transient HBV infection (Figure 55.8d) will usually go unnoticed unless sought after known exposure. For a few days, serology will show low amounts of HBV DNA, HBsAg, IgM anti-HBc, and a moderate transient rise of ALT to levels <500 IU/l for less than 4 weeks. Anti-HBc may appear at the peak of ALT, anti-HBs somewhat later. This inapparent course will often develop in healthy people who were exposed to low doses or mucocutaneously. In completely inapparent HBV infections without ALT elevation, markers of HBV may be difficult to detect and occasionally follow unexpected patterns. Anti-HBs may occur before anti-HBc or remain the only serological marker. In some transient infections, HBV DNA may be the only marker of infection. While these 'occult' HBV infections are irrelevant for the patient and his contact persons, HBV may be transmitted if such HBV infected persons donate blood or organs, particularly liver (Allain 2004).

Fulminant course

About 0.2 percent of clinically apparent cases of acute hepatitis B are so severe that the patients develop symptoms of hepatic failure within a few days and ensuing hepatic coma. This course is often fatal. Survivors recover completely and develop immunity to HBV characterized by anti-HBs and anti-HBc. Fulminant cases are often associated with coinfection by hepatitis delta virus (see Chapter 56, Hepatitis Delta virus) or possibly other hepatitis viruses. The significance of HBe-negative HBV variants for the development of fulminant hepatitis B is discussed controversially but they are found in ca. 50 percent of the cases.

Coinfection

Acute HBV-infection may occur together with hepatitis A virus (HAV), hepatitis C virus (HCV), HDV or HIV. None of the other hepatitis viruses aggravates the course of acute hepatitis, but HDV suppresses HBV viremia and enhances HBs antigenemia. HIV favors persistence of HBV. Pre-existent HCV may be transiently suppressed by HBV (Chulanov et al. 2003).

CHRONIC HEPATITIS B

Clinical signs of chronic hepatitis are usually mild and nonspecific. They include lack of energy, easy fatigability, and malaise. Myalgias, arthralgias, and skin rash may be present in cases with high virus replication due to circulating immune complexes. HBV-associated immune complex disease is an important cause of glomerulonephritis in tropical countries. The course of the disease is usually intermittent with acute exacerbations during which abdominal discomfort, nausea, weight loss, dark urine, jaundice, and mild fever may occur.

However, chronic HBV infection may go unnoticed until compensated or even decompensated cirrhosis of the liver is present. In this late phase of the disease the above-mentioned symptoms are enhanced and signs of hepatic encephalopathy may be present. Blood coagulation is decreased due to reduced synthesis of coagulation factors in the liver. Serum albumin is also decreased whereas IgG is increased, probably due to impaired degradation in the liver. The ALT levels are usually only

moderately enhanced to, at the most, several hundred IU/l and often fluctuate. A major complication is the collateral blood circulation due to impaired blood flow through the cirrhotic liver. Breakages of the esophageal varices are life-threatening, and are a result of portal hypertension. A further consequence of portal hypertension is the development of ascites in some cases.

It is important to distinguish between disease activity reflected by markers of viral replication, antiviral immune response, and hepatocyte damage, on the one hand, and symptoms caused by the lack of functional hepatocytes and the replacement of normal liver tissue by connective tissue on the other. Whereas the viral disease activity may come to an end either spontaneously or as a result of treatment, the conversion of normal liver tissue to cirrhotic tissue is irreversible. The liver status can be assessed only by histology, liver function tests, and determination of serum proteins synthesized or metabolized by the liver. Sonography describes the shape and density of the liver and may detect an increased diameter of the portal vein due to portal hypertension.

Most patients with persistent HBV infection are not aware of a previous acute hepatitis B episode. As pointed out above, HBV persistence very often develops in individuals who are immunologically immature or somehow impaired. Perinatal HBV infection virtually always results in persistence, unless HBe-negative variants are predominant. In the early years of life, symptoms are usually absent in HBV carriers despite high virus replication. The same is true for patients who acquired infection during significant immune deficiency. However, in otherwise healthy HBV carriers, a cytotoxic immune response will eventually develop and cause chronic disease. This cytotoxic immune response is directed primarily against the HBc protein, whereas the HBs protein seems to be a minor target in chronic hepatitis B. The HBc-specific T-cell response suppresses HBV replication and may even eliminate many HBV-expressing cells. As a result, an exacerbation of chronic hepatitis B may lead to a new form of persistent HBV infection, in which HBsAg is still present in the serum but the number of virions is much lower than in the previous phase of high viremia. HBeAg disappears and anti-HBe is often present in this phase. If HBV replication is constantly controlled by the immune system at low levels, the so-called healthy HBsAg carrier status is reached. Eventually, HBsAg may also disappear from the serum. In these cases, anti-HBc is often the only marker of HBV infection. This phase of low viral activity may be reached at all degrees of irreversible liver disease. Thus, a seemingly favorable serological constellation suggesting low viral replication does not necessarily mean insignificant liver disease.

During the high viremic HBeAg-positive phase, variability of the HBV epitope regions is low. In HBeAg-negative cases, however, considerable variability is observed. This variability may be generated by the immune elimination of the original strains.

A dangerous clinical situation occurs if a low viremic HBV carrier (with or without HBsAg or symptoms) is therapeutically immunosuppressed because of auto-immune disease, organ transplantation or anti-cancer therapy. In such cases, high HBV replication may reappear, but, as soon as the immune suppression is terminated, the existing memory cells induce a vigorous cytotoxic immune response that often results in fatal fulminant hepatitis B. In such cases, early pre-emptive therapy with an antiviral substance is indicated.

Coinfection of chronic hepatitis B patients with other hepatitis viruses and/or HIV is frequent. Intravenous drug users are often coinfected with HCV and/or HDV, male homosexuals often with HIV. Both HCV and HDV suppress replication of HBV, HCV often to the point that it becomes occult (Pontisso et al. 1993). In HIV coinfected patients, HBV may become the dominant pathogen under successful HIV therapy and requires an antiviral therapy, which is also effective against HBV (Rockstroh 2003). Superinfection of chronic hepatitis B patients with HAV does not lead to an aggravated course (Vento et al. 1998).

HEPATOCELLULAR CARCINOMA

HBV is the major cause of HCC in regions with high HBV prevalence. HCC usually develops after cirrhosis, but may also occur without cirrhosis. The involvement of HBV may not be recognized by testing for HBsAg in the serum, requiring the search for HBV DNA. In some cases in which the HCC contains integrated HBV DNA fragments no classic serological HBV marker may be present. However, in highly endemic areas of the world, people positive for HBsAg are 100 times more likely to develop HCC as compared to those who have anti-HBc and/or anti-HBs but no HBsAg (Beasley et al. 1981). An important cofactor is exposure to aflatoxin B (Ming et al. 2002). In low endemic areas the relative risk of HBsAg carriers to develop HCC is also increased. A British study found a 26-fold increased incidence of HCC in male HBsAg-positive blood donors compared to the male general population. The incidence was 33.5 per 100 000 persons year for male, but only 4.4 for female HBsAg carriers (Crook et al. 2003).

In some countries with intermediate HBV prevalence, HCV may be the major cause of HCC, but coinfection with HBV, HCV, and even HDV is quite common in HCC patients. In Italy, 45 percent of HCC patients have heavy alcohol intake, 36 percent HCV infection, and 22 percent HBV infection as risk factor for HCC (Donato et al. 1997). In Germany HBV is the leading risk factor for HCC (45 percent) followed by HCV (37 percent) and alcohol (Kubicka et al. 2000). While HBsAg persistence is associated with a highly increased risk for HCC, absence of HBsAg does not exclude development of an HBV-associated HCC (Yu et al. 1997; Tamori et al. 2003; Pollicino et al. 2004). It is believed that in addition to HBsAg, the level of HBV replication is positively correlated to the risk for HCC (Tang et al. 2004). The strong preponderance of HCC in male HBV carriers is positively correlated to the testosterone levels and to the structure of the androgen-receptor gene (Yu and Mertz 2001).

The development of HCC may be diagnosed early by quantitative measurement of α-fetoprotein (AFP) in the serum, but levels may be normal (<20 ng) before the HCC reaches a size of 3 cm. Levels above 1 000 ng/ml, or a sharp rise of AFP, indicate HCC. Abdominal imaging by ultrasound of HBsAg-positive patients, particularly those with liver cirrhosis, is advisable at intervals of 3–4 months.

Pathogenesis and immune response

The pathogenesis of HBV is based on the immune reaction. Virus replication itself is not overly pathogenic but subtle effects on hepatocyte function cannot be excluded. Transgenic mice expressing HBV or single HBV proteins are normal or almost normal. However, selective expression of LHBs in transgenic mice leads to storage of LHBs-containing filaments in the ER and pre-Golgi compartments. The LHBs-storing hepatocyte acquires a ground glass-like appearance. In mouse strains with very high expression of LHBs, hepatocytes become very sensitive to interferon-γ. Inflammatory liver disease and eventually HCC develop whereby the tumors no longer express LHBs (Rogler and Chisari 1992). LHBs containing ground glass hepatocytes are often found in healthy HBsAg, carriers but their diagnostic or pathogenetic significance in humans is not clear.

A potential pathogenic role has been suggested for HBx protein due to its apoptosis inducing properties, which may even protect against malignant transformation (Schuster et al. 2000). On the other hand, HBx has been reported to counteract p53-induced apoptosis (Wang et al. 2002) and to enhance malignancy of immortalized cells (Höhne et al. 1990; Oguey et al. 1996). HCCs usually contain variants of the *HBx* gene, which are less frequent in chronic hepatitis B patients (Yeh et al. 2000). Selective overexpression of HBx protein in a certain mouse strain has generated HCC late in life, but other mouse strains did not develop HCC. However, HBx-expressing mouse lineages were more susceptible to chemical carcinogens. Thus, HBx may be one oncogenic factor of HBV infection acting together with chronic inflammation (Nakamoto et al. 1998), insertional mutagenesis (Gozuacik et al. 2001), testosterone levels (Yu and Mertz 2001), or aflatoxin (Ming et al. 2002). Basal core promoter mutations 1762T and 1764A have been reported to be associated with HCC (Kuang et al. 2004; Kao et al. 2003), but this may be an indirect association because these mutations appear late in infection and lead to enhanced HBV replication (Blackberg and Kidd-Ljunggren 2003).

SHBs, HBc, and HBe proteins are not pathogenic when expressed in transgenic mice. SHBs and HBe protein are secreted whereas HBc protein is stored as HBc particles in the nucleus. Cytoplasmic HBc particles are rapidly degraded whereas nuclear HBc protein has a longer half-life. All these findings are in accordance with observations on human HBV infections. HBsAg, secreted HBeAg and nuclear HBcAg are not associated with disease per se.

There may be differences in pathogenicity and virulence between the various HBV genotypes. In Africa, Europe, and the USA genotypes A, D, and E predominate which lead less frequently to perinatal transmission, probably due to a shorter period of high level viremia in females. However, their horizontal transmission is frequent in early childhood (Dusheiko et al. 1985). In Asia, with genotypes B and C, perinatal transmission is frequent and seroconversion from anti-HBeAg to anti-HBe with a concomitant decrease in viremia occurs later. With genotype C, seroconversion to HBeAg occurs still later than in genotype B resulting in an even more progressive liver disease (Kao et al. 2004) and worse response to therapy.

HBeAg-negative variants are presumed to cause a more severe acute infection but less persistence. However, after persistence has been established by the HBeAg-positive virus, HBeAg negative variants can evolve and persist further.

Virtually all infected individuals develop anti-HBc antibodies. Development of IgM anti-HBc indicates significant ongoing HBV replication and is a serological marker of inflammatory disease. The appearance of anti-HBs usually shows that HBsAg production is low or absent. However, HBsAg and anti-HBs may co-exist and, rarely, HBs escape mutants are present. Anti-preS1 and anti-preS2 appear during recovery from acute hepatitis B earlier than anti-SHBs, and disappear earlier. In some cases, however, these antibodies may also contribute to the formation of circulating HBs immune complexes in chronic HBV carriers. Anti-HBx and anti-HBpol antibodies are detected in many but not all patients with acute or chronic hepatitis B, and are neither diagnostically nor pathogenetically important. HBs and HBe immune complexes contribute to extrahepatic manifestations of HBV, but are probably not a major pathogenic factor in viral hepatitis.

Administration of anti-SHBs in high doses protects against de novo infection with HBV. The administration of anti-SHBs to individuals already infected (for example, liver transplant recipients or some HBV-infected patients) favors outgrowth of HBs escape mutants. In vitro experiments with infection of cell cultures show that anti-preS2, and in particular anti-preS1, are also neutralizing antibodies, but their protective function in vivo is not well established.

The elimination of HBV-producing cells during acute hepatitis B is mediated mainly by a strong T-cell response to HBc/e and HBs proteins (Chisari and Ferrari 1995). Passive transfer of HBs-specific T-cell clones from immunized mice to HBs-transgenic mice induces acute hepatitis. The severity of the disease correlated directly with the dose of cytotoxic $CD8^+$ cells against HBs and the amount of HBs protein in the liver. It may result in fulminant hepatitis, as shown in animals with LHBs storage. The cytotoxic $CD8^+$ cells stimulate nonspecific inflammatory cells which form necroinflammatory foci, inducing necrosis of hepatocytes. However, these nonspecific cells are not necessary for HBV elimination (Sitia et al. 2002). The histological picture of this CD8+ cell-induced disease in transgenic mice is similar to that in acute or fulminant hepatitis B of humans. HBc/e- and HBs-specific $CD8^+$ cells have been isolated readily from the blood of patients with acute hepatitis B. In contrast, chronic hepatitis B patients have only low numbers of circulating or intrahepatic $CD8^+$ cells specific for HBs or HBc. This low number may explain the persistence of HBV and the continuous inflammation at moderate levels. Control of HBV replication in liver cells does not necessarily require the elimination of all HBV-expressing cells. Activated $CD8^+$ cells secrete interferon-γ and interleukin-2 which induce secretion of TNF-α. TNF-α reduces the stability of HBV mRNAs (Heise et al. 2001) and suppresses expression of HBV or its proteins, or both, without necessarily inducing cytolysis or apoptosis. In experimentally infected chimpanzees, $CD8^+$ cells induce the elimination of cccDNA even before cytotoxicity occurs, but final elimination of cccDNA is associated with hepatic turnover (Wieland et al. 2004a). A complete elimination of all cccDNA-containing cells is, however, not always achieved. $CD4^+$ lymphocytes against HBc/e are numerous in most patients with acute resolving hepatitis, but few are found during chronic hepatitis B. $CD4^+$ cells against HBs proteins are less abundant than those against HBc/e.

The mechanisms of how HBV escapes the immune system are not understood. Even in those individuals who resolve acute hepatitis B, HBV is able to replicate for weeks or even months without inducing an immune response. Evaluation of the gene expression pattern in acutely HBV-infected chimpanzees characterized HBV as a 'stealth virus' not visible to the innate immune system and with little influence on the host cells (Wieland et al. 2004b). Only after a period of several weeks of logarithmic expansion of HBV was the immune system activated, most likely via $CD4^+$ cells and interferon-γ. It is not known which factors finally activate the immune system after a long period of inertia.

HBV persistence seems to be caused by immune evasion and nonpathogenicity of the wild-type virus. It has been suggested that intrauterine transfer of maternal HBV antigens, particularly HBeAg, generates immune tolerance to HBV in the newborn, but most newborns of HBeAg-positive mothers respond very well to HBsAg vaccine. HBeAg in the serum may be involved in the suppression of a vigorous cytotoxic immune response against HBc protein, because newborns (both human and woodchuck) develop persistent infection only if the infecting HBV-positive serum is also HBeAg positive. However, HBeAg in cells also becomes a target for the inflammatory immune response (Milich and Liang 2003). Other potential factors supporting immune evasion are the high excess of secreted HBs proteins and the high resistance of SHBs protein to proteolytic degradation, which may impair antigen presentation.

Diagnosis

A survey of the significance of HBV parameters for different diagnostic problems is given in Table 55.1.

ACUTE HEPATITIS

According to the description in 'Acute hepatitis B', virtually all cases of acute hepatitis B show at the onset of symptoms easily detectable levels of anti-HBc. Thus, a test for anti-HBc clarifies whether a patient with hepatitis is infected with HBV. Lack of anti-HBc excludes HBV as the causative agent of a present acute hepatitis or of a subclinical transaminase rise (Table 55.1).

If anti-HBc is positive, a test for HBsAg and IgM anti-HBc should follow (Table 55.1). A negative or low IgM anti-HBc (<600 PEI units) excludes HBV as the cause of a clinically apparent acute hepatitis, but points to previous HBV infection, which may have resolved or be persistent. (Persistent infection is recognized by a positive HBsAg test, immunity by a positive anti-HBs.) During early or very late phases of the acute disease, IgM anti-HBc may have concentrations lower than 600 PEI units/ml. In mild HBV infections, IgM anti-HBc may also be lower (Gerlich et al. 1986).

HBsAg is at least positive in most hepatitis B-infected individuals transiently. It may be eliminated very rapidly in fulminant hepatitis with extremely strong immune elimination or in very mild infections with very low viral expression. Alternatively, HBsAg may be present, but undetectable, by the usual immune assays because of mutations in the major epitopes. Such cases can be diagnosed by the quantitative assay of IgM anti-HBc and by the test for HBV DNA using PCR. HBV infection of a patient may suggest, in addition, a risk of HDV, HCV, and HIV infection, and appropriate tests for these infections may be advisable.

The patient's disease status should be followed by determination of the ALT level until it is close to normal. An early favorable prognosis is possible if the HBeAg patient is negative already in the first serum sample, or HBV DNA negative in hybridization assays. These two parameters become negative in resolving cases within 4–6 weeks. Thus, a second assay of HBeAg or HBV DNA after 6 weeks, when they were initially positive, is advisable. Alternatively, the HBsAg quantity may be measured accurately by electroimmunodiffusion or a quantitative EIA. In resolving cases, HBsAg drops within 6 weeks by more than 60 percent. A definitive resolution may be assumed if HBsAg is negative and anti-HBs is positive but this may take up to one year. However, even in this condition, low-level viremia and intrahepatic persistence of HBV DNA has to be assumed in a major proportion of the convalescents.

CHRONIC HEPATITIS

Patients with symptoms of chronic hepatitis need a thorough examination of the liver, including liver function tests and, if possible, liver biopsy. The viral activity is not clearly correlated to disease activity or to the histological appearance of the liver, but HBsAg is virtually always detectable. In early phases of chronic infection, HBeAg is often present and HBV DNA detectable even by the insensitive hybridization assays. Quantities of ALT, HBV DNA, HBeAg, and IgM anti-HBc are often unstable, fluctuate or are occasionally even negative. HBeAg is sometimes absent, but HBV DNA is usually detectable however PCR may be required as a more sensitive technique for detection. The diagnostical parameters associated with persistent HBV infection are shown in Table 55.2.

A typical feature of late phase chronic HBV infection is the selection of variants with deletions or mutations leading to an altered expression of HBV or to altered gene products. Most frequent are mutations (stop codons, promoter inactivation, frame shifts) that abolish expression of HBeAg. Deletions also occur quite often in the B-cell epitope regions of HBcAg and preS. Deletions within the *HBx* gene are common in patients with impaired immune reactions and are often the only mutation in these people, but they are rare in HCC patients (Blackberg and Kidd-Ljunggren 2003).

INAPPARENT PERSISTENT HBV INFECTION

Infrequently, HBV infection is not recognized subjectively. Thus, HBV carriers are often detected accidentally – during blood donation, because of an occupational risk, before operations or during search for a

Table 55.1 *Serological parameters of HBV infection*

Serological parameters	
Ongoing or previous infection (prevalence)	Anti-HBc
Ongoing infection	HBsAg
Time of infection	IgM anti-HBc (quantitative)
Infectivity	HBV DNA (quantitative)
Natural immunity	Anti-HBc and anti-HBs
Immunity after vaccination	Anti-HBs (quantitative)

Table 55.2 *Three states of HBsAg carriership – typical parameters*

Parameters	Immune tolerance	Chronic disease	'Healthy' HBsAg carrier
Serum			
HBsAg µg/ml[a]	30–150	<30	<30
HBeAg PEI[b] – U/ml	2 000–10 000	<2 000 or absent	Negative, anti HBe[+]
HBV-g.e./ml[c]	10^9–10^{10}	10^6–10^9	$<10^6$
Anti-HBc	+ to ++	+++	+ to ++
IgM-antiHBc PEI units	<50	10–500	<10
ALT IU/ml 37°C	<120	>120, variable	<50
Liver			
HBcAg[+] cells	90–100%	Variable, low	Negative
HBsAg[+] cells	90–100%	Variable, low	Variable, frequent ground glass cells, LHBs[+]
Dynamics	Stable	Unstable	Stable
Interferon response	Transient or none	Often sustained	No treatment required

One IU HBV DNA in the WHO standard corresponds to ca. 5 g.e./ml.
a) 1 µg HBsAg = 1 000 PEI units or 2 000 WHO units. So-called ng units are often inaccurate.
b) PEI: Paul Ehrlich Institute for Sera and Vaccines, Langen, Germany.
c) g.e.: genome equivalents.

possible source of HBV infection. The most universal test to detect an ongoing or previous HBV infection is anti-HBc. However, anti-HBc may remain negative for up to 6 months post-infection, whereas HBsAg is positive much earlier. In some chronic HBV carriers who were infected perinatally, anti-HBc may remain negative lifelong although HBV replication is very strong. Anti-HBc may also be absent in reactivated HBV infections due to immune suppression or in conditions where antibody synthesis is generally suppressed. The earliest marker of HBV infection is HBV DNA in the serum if detected by a highly sensitive nucleic acid amplification technique (NAT) such as PCR.

If a person is identified as being positive for HBsAg, he or she should be tested for anti-HBc. Negative anti-HBc suggests an early phase of infection with a possible acute hepatitis B still to come, or a severe state of immune deficiency which, however, usually would have been known for other reasons. Absent IgM anti-HBc in the presence of IgG anti-HBc suggests low disease activity and a stable carrier state (Table 55.2). HBsAg carriers stay, by definition, HBsAg positive for more than 6 months. Positive HBeAg suggests high viremia and high infectivity, but some HBeAg-positive carriers have only moderate viremia ($<10^8$ genomes/ml) and are less infectious. Absence of HBeAg suggests low viremia ($<10^6$ HBV particles /ml) but does not exclude higher levels. A quantitative HBV DNA assay is therefore recommended. Most HBeAg-positive carriers and some HBeAg-negative carriers reach very high viremia levels of 10^9–10^{10} genome-containing HBV particles.

Chronically infected individuals may be divided into three groups, as shown in Table 55.2. The immunotolerant type is highly infectious but oligosymptomatic. The HBsAg carrier is also healthy but noninfectious (except for blood donation). A status between these two

extremes is usually associated with liver disease that, however, may be unrecognized. In this phase, disease activity is often fluctuating. Silent HBsAg carrierlike phases may change with flareups. Viremic HBV carriers often spontaneously reach the HBsAg carrier state after one or more episodes of recurrent liver disease. Unfortunately, this disease phase may be longlasting and result in liver cirrhosis or HCC. Thus, regular monitoring of ALT levels in persistently HBsAg-positive people is advisable until it is known whether a stable state is present. HBeAg and HBV DNA should also be regularly checked if positive.

NATURAL IMMUNITY

People who have been at risk for HBV may have acquired immunity by silent HBV infection. In order to detect natural immunity the person's blood should be tested for anti-HBc, and then, if positive, for anti-HBs. Naturally immune people should be anti-HBc and anti-HBs positive (see Table 55.1). It has, however, been noted that anti-HBs may occasionally disappear several years after an acute hepatitis B infection. Isolated anti-HBs without previous vaccination may be nonspecific and nonprotective, but asymptomatic transient HBV infection may also lead to low levels of anti-HBs without anti-HBc. Isolated anti-HBc may have different meanings:

- The person may be in the phase after disappearance of HBsAg but before the appearance of anti-HBs (so-called window period). In this case the titer should be high.
- It may be present long after previous HBV infection in which anti-HBs has already disappeared. In this case, the titer should be low.
- It may be a response to an HBV infection, in which HBsAg is mutated, bound in immune complexes or below the detection limit. Anti-HBe may be present.

- The anti-HBc test may react nonspecifically. Usually, the signal strength is low.

If distinction between the four situations is required, an HBV DNA assay by NAT may be helpful. If it is necessary to decide whether a person is immune, vaccination against HBV with one dose of vaccine is recommended and a quantitative test for anti-HBs should be done 1–2 weeks later. Situation (2) will lead to a rapid anamnestic response with a reappearance of anti-HBs at high titers. If this does not occur, vaccination should be continued by the regular schedule with two or three further doses. In situation (3), no anti-HBs may develop. For the discussion of vaccine-induced immunity see 'Active immunization'.

DETECTION OF HBV IN TISSUE SPECIMENS

Because of its ability to generate high viremia and antigenemia, HBV infection is usually easy to diagnose with the aid of serum samples. Liver biopsies are necessary to examine the degree of inflammation, necrosis, and fibrosis, and repeated biopsies give information on the progression of the disease. Because of the risk associated with biopsy, it should be done only if the clinical, biochemical, and virological data suggest severe, progressive disease. Once the biopsy is available, it may be stained for HBsAg, preS1 antigen, HBcAg, or HBV DNA. In HBsAg-positive patients, usually no more information can be derived from these stainings than from a complete quantitative HBV serology. The situation is different in HBsAg-negative patients with liver cirrhosis or HCC. Here, a liver biopsy or tumor tissue may allow detection of extracted HBV DNA by NAT and, if highly positive, by Southern blot. Distinct bands in a Southern blot prove mono- or oligoclonal outgrowth of hepatocytes with integrated HBV DNA and, thus, HBV-associated liver disease.

DIAGNOSTIC TESTS FOR HBV

HBsAg

HBsAg is detected qualitatively by solid-phase immune assays with unlabeled anti-HBs as the carrier and labeled anti-HBs for detection in the liquid phase. Originally, radioactive iodine 125 was used as label (radioimmune assay) but today enzymes (EIA) are preferred which generate a colored or fluorescent product. Chemoluminescence labeling is also used. The specificity and sensitivity is mostly determined by the quality of the anti-HBs reagent. Most commercially available assays use either as the solid phase or as label or for both just one monoclonal antibody against SHBs. While this is sufficient for most genotypes of wild-type HBV, mutants of the *SHBs* gene may escape detection in reactivated hepatitis B (Westhoff et al. 2003), in blood donors (Jongerius et al. 1998) or in the general population (Carman et al. 1997). Use of affinity-purified

polyvalent antibodies or several non-overlapping monoclonal antibodies, possibly also against preS epitopes, help to overcome this problem. Analytical sensitivity is also very important. An international standard is available for its validation which contains 33 IU/ml heat-inactivated SHBsAg of subtype adw2 and genotype A2. The detection limit should be below 0.1 IU/ml, but not all tests are so sensitive. Nonspecific reactions are usually rare (<0.1 percent) and may be verified by inhibition tests using polyvalent anti-HBs. Quantification may be achieved by using reference samples and appropriate dilutions of the sample which give a result in the proportionality range (<100 PEI units/ml) of the EIA. Results may be expressed either in PEI or in International Units /ml. One IU is 0.55 PEI-Unit. One PEI-Unit corresponds to 1 ng of fully native HBsAg. Unfortunately, many test kit producers use 'ng' units, which are calibrated with partially denatured HBsAg. Furthermore, test kits may react differently with various subtypes of HBsAg or with variants of HBsAg. A useful technique for quantifying HBsAg in the range of 1 000–100 000 PEI-units/ml is Laurell electrophoresis (Glebe and Gerlich 2004). This is the relevant range for quantitative assessment of acute and chronic hepatitis B.

Anti-HBc

Anti-HBc is usually determined by inhibition EIAs with recombinant HBcAg (expressed e.g. in *E. coli*) at the solid phase and labeled anti-HBc, the binding of which is inhibited by the anti-HBc within the samples. Sandwich assays with HBcAg at the solid phase and labeled HBcAg or labeled anti-IgG are also available. There are nonspecific inhibitors of HBcAg in human sera; nonspecific reactions may therefore be as frequent as 1 percent in the normal population. Repetition of the test using a test kit from a second producer usually yields a positive result if the reaction is specific, but a false-negative result in this second assay cannot be excluded. Divergent anti-HBc results in different tests are particularly frequent in individuals with a high risk of HBV exposure. Western blotting is not helpful and quantification of anti-HBc is not usually done. Chronic HBV carriers and acute hepatitis B patients may have end point titers up to 1:1 000 000 whereas immune people usually have titers below 1:1 000.

IgM anti-HBc

IgM anti-HBc is usually detected by the anti-μ capture EIA. This type of EIA binds via anti-μ antibodies IgM from the sample to the solid phase; thereafter labeled HBcAg is added. If the sample contains IgM anti-HBc, labeled HBcAg will be bound. Quantification is highly advisable. Results may be expressed in PEI units/ml or as an EIA index. Some commercial test kits employ very high cut-off values to give a positive result only with sera from acute hepatitis B, but all test kits react significantly stronger with sera from patients with active chronic hepatitis than the negative control giving values up to 600 PEI units/ml. Testing for IgM anti-HBc is advisable only if the screening for total anti-HBc was positive.

Anti-HBs

Anti-HBs is usually detected by a sandwich EIA with HBsAg at the solid phase and labeled HBsAg in the liquid phase. Some producers use natural purified HBsAg from HBV carrier plasma; others use recombinant HBsAg particles from yeast or from mammalian cells devoid of preS antigen. Thus, quantitative results obtained for one serum using various test kits may differ significantly. The detection limit is usually between 1 and 10 mIU/ml and saturation of the assay is reached at 100–1 000 mIU/ml. Sera may contain more than 100 000 mIU/ml after vaccination with HBsAg. Nonspecific results are possible, but they are rare. Coincident positivity of HBsAg and anti-HBs may occur in patients with chronic hepatitis B. The anti-HBs in these patients usually reacts with HBsAg subtypes not present in the HBV carrier. Normally, anti-HBs should be assayed only in anti-HBc-positive people or after vaccination.

HBeAg

HBeAg should be determined only in people with HBsAg. It is tested by EIA and may be quantified using PEI units. Detection limits of commercial assays are between 1 and 10 PEI units/ml and high viremia is usually associated with high HBeAg titers (>2 000 PEI units/ml). Anti-HBe is a less important marker of HBV infection. However, monitoring of chronic hepatitis B patients for seroconversion (Figure 55.8c) from HBeAg to anti-HBe is clinically relevant. Furthermore, assay of anti-HBe may help to interpret the significance of anti-HBc without HBsAg or anti-HBs.

HBV DNA

HBV DNA has become very important in the diagnosis of HBV infections and may be helpful for answering many questions:

- HBsAg positive anti-HBc negative samples need confirmation of specificity. A highly sensitive HBV DNA assay, preferable NAT, will react positively in almost all specifically positive samples.
- In anti-HBc positive but HBsAg and anti-HBs negative samples, HBV DNA can help to identify low level HBV carriers, or carriers with a mutated HBsAg which escaped detection.
- In very early phases of infection, inapparent transient or occult persistent HBV infection, HBV DNA may be the only detectable viral marker. Persistent low

level HBV infections are particularly frequent in HCV, HBV-coinfected persons.

For these applications an assay of the highest possible sensitivity is required. With todays techniques, usually few or even one DNA molecule in the tested sample volume are detectable. Thus, the sample volume is often the limiting factor. Unfortunately, some inapparent HBV infections show extremely low levels of viremia around 1 genome/ml (Kuhns et al. 2004). Nevertheless, HBV DNA assays should be employed whenever a serological pattern is inconsistent or of uncertain specificity. In-house NAT assays (if adequately validated) may be superior to commercially available assays because several target regions may be used. This can prevent false-negative results due to mutations in the primer or probe target regions.

In the 1990s, NAT was plagued by false-positive results due to cross contaminations between the amplificate and samples. The use of closed systems and/or degradation or amplicates has helped to avoid this problem during handling and extraction. However, cross contamination between samples is still a problem because sera may contain up to 10^{11} genome equivalents/ml. False-negative results due to polymerase inhibitors, false reagents, or wrong performance should be excluded by inclusion of an internal control or by spiking of a suspected false-negative sample with a known positive sample. False-negative results due to mutations in the target sequence of probes and primers remain a problem of unknown magnitude, but the existence of HBsAg true-positive, HBV DNA-negative samples give a hint to its existence. For diagnostic purposes only, NAT systems with detection of the amplificate by labeled probes should be used, because they are less prone to contamination by the amplificate. Techniques with in situ generation and measurement of the signal after each amplification step (real-time PCR) are preferable. The great advantage of these systems, besides their high contamination resistance and analytical sensitivity, is the ability to quantitate the complete range of concentrations from <100 to >10^{10} g.e./ml. The TaqMan system uses a fluorescent probe, which is degraded when being annealed to the amplificate and is thereby released from a fluorescence quencher. The fluorescence resonance energy transfer (FRET) technique uses two probes with two different fluorescence dyes. FRET can only occur and generate the signal when the probes bind next to each other to the amplificate. Due to the existence of a World Health Organization (WHO) approved International standard, both assays can be standardized. The WHO has preferred not to define the HBV DNA in g.e./ml or 'copies/ml' but in International Units, because different results were obtained with different methods of detection (Saldanha et al. 2001). These differences are most likely caused by variable losses during extraction, because the HBV

DNA carries the covalently bound HBV polymerase with it. This protein alters the extraction properties of the DNA, and it is the reason why for the standardization of HBV DNA assays HB-virion-derived DNA and not cloned DNA should be used. With adequate extraction and calibration one IU corresponds to ca. 5 g.e./ml of HBV genotype A2 (Heermann et al. 1999). One picogram HBV DNA is 280 000 g.e./ml.

Real-time PCR is superior to competitive PCR because it is more sensitive and does not reach an upper limit of quantification. Hybridization assays have been used for a long time to quantitate HBV DNA, but they are too insensitive (detection limit $>10^6$ g.e./ml) for therapy monitoring or assessment of infectivity. These are the main applications of HBV DNA quantitation.

HBV DNA genotyping or resistance testing can be done via hybridization of a NAT product with commercially available sets of probes, but sequencing of a NAT product covering the SHBs/RT region is a cost-effective and more informative in-house alternative.

Epidemiology

PREVALENCE

It is estimated that 50 percent of the world's population have had contact with HBV and about 10 percent of these (ca. 350 million) have developed persistent infection. HBV carriers have a high risk of developing liver cirrhosis and a 20 to 100-fold greater risk of developing HCC. Mortality from acute hepatitis B is low (<1 percent), but much higher from chronic hepatitis B. It is estimated that 1 million people per year die from the sequelae of chronic hepatitis B. Prevalence of anti-HBc, the best marker for current or previous infection, is highly variable in different geographic regions, ethnic or behavioral groups. Areas of low prevalence of anti-HBc positivity (<5 percent) are Northern Europe, North America, and parts of South America; areas with a particularly high prevalence (>50 percent) are sub-Saharan Africa, most parts of Asia and Oceania except India, where more than 10 percent of the adult population are HBsAg carriers. In Australia, New Zealand, and Alaska the native population is much more affected than the Caucasian immigrants. There are no hints that certain races are more susceptible to persistent infection. There may also be very large differences within a country; for example, southern Italy has a much higher prevalence than most northern areas. Lower socioeconomic status is often (but not always) connected with higher prevalence. In areas of low or moderate endemicity, prevalence increases gradually with age, being very low during childhood. In areas of high prevalence most individuals have acquired the infection before school age.

The prevalence pattern is changing due to lower incidence in young people. Vaccination has an efficacy of ca. 90 percent if performed optimally. Indeed in highly endemic countries like Taiwan or Oceania, which have implemented general vaccination in childhood, the prevalence of HBsAg has decreased by a factor of five from 14–20 percent to 3–5 percent (Lin et al. 2003; Wilson et al. 2000).

INCIDENCE

In many countries, hepatitis B is a notifiable disease and, thus, numbers on the annual incidence are available. In Germany, incidence of acute hepatitis B has continuously decreased from a high level in the seventies (>10 per 100 000 person years) to 1.7 per 100 000 person years, in 2002. Similar decreases are observed in other developed countries. Thus, acute hepatitis A and C are now more frequent than hepatitis B. In Germany, the peak incidence is found in males aged between 20–29 years pointing to i.v. drug use and male homosexuality as major risk factors. It is almost certain that acute hepatitis is under-reported. The true number of cases is probably two or three times higher. The true number of new HBV infections is even more difficult to determine, because most infections are subclinical, even those that finally lead to chronic hepatitis. On the basis of 6 percent prevalence of anti-HBc in the general population of Germany, even the general population must have had an incidence of 100–500 inapparent HBV infections per 100 000 person years before the 1980s. However, today's incidence is probably much lower.

MODES OF TRANSMISSION

Because of the extremely high infectivity titer of $>10^8$/ml serum, even the slightest trace of serum is dangerous, but other bodily secretions such as saliva, ejaculate, vaginal secretions or menstrual blood may also cause transmission, and titers of 10^6/ml may be present in these materials. HBsAg and HBV DNA have been detected in urine (Knutsson and Kidd-Ljunggren 2000), but there is no epidemiological evidence that the infection is transmitted by exposure to urine. Transmission is most efficient by intravenous injection, 100 times less efficient by the intramuscular or percutaneous route and least efficient by mucosal contact. Intact skin is impermeable to HBV but open wounds allow efficient entrance. Assuming an infectivity titer of 10^8/ml serum in an unrecognized HBV carrier, 1 nl of this serum (an invisible amount) would still contain 100 infectious doses, which would almost certainly cause infection if administered by a contaminated syringe or other medical device. Even dilution of this serum by $1:10^5$ (e.g. a blood spill of 0.1 ml has been washed away with 10 liters of water) would leave 1 ml of this liquid still infectious when administered percutaneously. Swallowing highly infectious blood or serum, blood splashes into the eyes, and contact with open wounds almost invariably lead to infection of susceptible individuals. Heterosexual contacts are a less effective but still relatively efficient way of transmission. Transmission has been very frequent between male homosexuals, depending on their sexual practices. The danger of transmission by intense kissing is unknown whereas bites transmit very efficiently. Experience suggests that the rate of transmission from HBV carriers to contacts is proportional to the genome titer, frequency and intensity of exposure. Genome titers $<10^6$/ml have been empirically found not to pose a risk to even the closest contact person unless contaminated syringes or similar devices are involved. HBsAg-positive mothers with a negative HBV DNA hybridization test ($<10^6$/ml) do not usually transmit HBV to their newborn babies (Ip et al. 1989). Thus, sources of infection are almost invariably (except for blood products) highly viremic HBV carriers. Even with very high titers, transmission to household contacts usually requires time and special situations; normal school or professional contact is not a risk. Transmissions occur more easily in nursery school or in injury-prone sports or jobs; for example, a young HBV carrier infected his co-pathfinders by hiking along the same thorny trail, and an HBV-positive butcher infected all his colleagues within a short time because of the many skin injuries they received during the course of their work. Nosocomial infections have been frequent in previous decades but today they occur only in rare cases of accidents or failures to follow hygiene. Transmission of HBV from patients to medical staff is a well-known risk, but the reverse is also well documented (Gunson et al. 2003). In recreational activities, devices for ear or nose piercing or tattooing have been sources of transmission, but the most significant are shared syringe and needles for intravenous drug use.

Control

Control of HBV includes counseling of HBV carriers, general hygiene, disinfection, blood screening, active and passive immunization, and treatment of persistent infection.

COUNSELING OF HBV CARRIERS

As pointed out under Modes of transmission above, even the slightest trace of highly infectious blood on a sharp item will transmit HBV if it penetrates the skin of a susceptible person. The job and the life style of a highly viremic HBV carrier must be analyzed as to whether their blood might contaminate sharp items that may percutaneously infect other people. The carrier should be informed that simple cleaning by wiping the blood away or washing with water will be insufficient to remove infectivity reliably. All highly viremic HBV carriers should be instructed to avoid injuries, to keep lost blood under control, and to disinfect items that are contaminated by their blood if they cannot be cleaned by regular washing.

Surgeons who have their hands and sharp instruments within the body of their patients cannot completely avoid small, often unnoticed, injuries. Thus, highly viremic carriers (HBeAg positive or HBV DNA hybridization positive ($>10^5$/ml)) should not operate or work as dentists. HBV transmission by HBeAg-negative and low-viremic ($<10^5$/ml) carriers has not yet been reported, except for one case (Corden et al. 2003). Operations performed by them should be safe if combined with wearing two pairs of gloves and an injury-avoiding technique. European recommendations added to this limit a safety margin and suggest that HBV carriers should have $<1\ 000$ g.e./ml when performing exposure prone procedures (Gunson et al. 2003). The main point is that all medical staff should be vaccinated and be tested at least once for HBsAg and for anti-HBs. No restrictions are necessary for noninvasive medical procedures.

Household contacts, close friends, and sexual partners should be vaccinated or (if appropriate) tested for anti-HBc and HBsAg, or both. Physicians should be informed before they do invasive procedures with the HBV carrier. To take appropriate precautions, it would be desirable that sexual partners and close social contacts should know that a person is a carrier of HBV; they may, however, fail to understand the nature of the risk and discriminate against the carrier. The HBeAg and HBV DNA status should be checked at least twice a year. The usefulness of antiviral therapy should be considered carefully, because an unsuccessful treatment might cause more harm than good.

HYGIENE

Human blood is almost ubiquitous in medical practice and laboratories, and HBV infections were once very frequent in the medical profession. Protection against the contamination with blood is now observed more strictly since the occurrence of HIV; this includes wearing gloves and facemasks and using safer equipment (for example, for blood taking) that causes fewer injuries.

Patients are now better protected by the use of disposable items, in particular syringes and needles, and by a generally higher awareness of hygiene. Breaking of hygiene rules during blood taking or injections still causes small outbreaks of HBV infection even in developed countries, and originates usually from an unrecognized highly viremic carrier. Nondisposable devices that cannot be autoclaved (e.g. endoscopes) can still pose a problem, if the available disinfection devices are not adequately used.

In dialysis centers, HBV carriers must have their own room with their own dialysis machine. Furthermore, dialysis patients should be vaccinated or – if nonresponders – monitored for HBsAg. Outbreaks of HBV have been observed in pediatric oncology wards despite good hygiene. Here patient-to-patient contact is common but HBV infections usually go unnoticed if the patients are not screened for HBsAg. Transmission from an operated highly viremic carrier to the next operated patient occurs occasionally even in these days and points to lack of hygiene. However, general screening of all patients, or at least of all those who undergo surgery, is considered to be cost-inefficient.

Isolation of patients with acute or chronic HBV infection is not essential if they are instructed as described above, behave responsibly, and do not lose blood in an uncontrolled fashion. However, HBV-carrying children should be supervised carefully.

DISINFECTION

Modern disinfectants should be validated with test organisms. In the European Community, a standard test is required in which a working dilution of a disinfectant must reduce the infectivity titer of poliovirus by a factor of $>10^4$ within 1 hour at room temperature. Because there is no feasible infectivity test for HBV, no disinfectant is formally validated for HBV even though it is one of the most important disinfection problems in medicine. The use of duck HBV as a model that can be titrated has been generally accepted, but its structural proteins (which are the targets) and its mode of transmission (almost exclusively vertical) are very different. A better model would be woodchuck HBV but the test system is not readily available. Inactivation of HBsAg or of the viral endogenous DNA polymerase is an inadequate substitute because their connection with infectivity is not established and a reduction by a factor of $>10^4$ has not been measured. The morphological alteration and disintegration test (MADT) using purified HBV particles and electron microscopy has been of some value. Disinfectants that inactivate simian virus 40 would also be expected to inactivate HBV, whereas adenovirus may be a more sensitive virus than HBV. Recently, agents that target viral DNA can be validated by PCR. Furthermore, neutralizing epitopes may be used as targets (Jursch et al. 2002) and finally cell cultures for infectivity testing of HBV have become available (Gripon et al. 2002; Gerlich et al. 2004).

SAFETY OF BLOOD PRODUCTS AND ORGAN DONATIONS

All blood or plasma donations must be tested as a minimum requirement by licensed highly sensitive tests for HBsAg; HBsAg-positive blood or plasma must not be used. However, in developing countries with very high HBV prevalence and very limited financial resources, HBsAg testing is often not done or is suboptimal. It has been estimated that in a highly endemic country like Ghana, the risk of children <10 years for acquiring HBV is 1:11 for unscreened and 1:360 for HBsAg screened blood (Allain et al. 2003). In Germany, the residual risk of HBV in a blood donation despite HBsAg screening is 1:100 000 to 1:500 000. While this risk is very low it is still 10 times higher than for HCV or HIV transmission. A similar situation exists in most developed countries. Additional measures like screening for HBV DNA and/or anti-HBc to reduce the small residual risk of HBV transmission are in most countries optional.

Donor blood may contain HBV despite HBsAg screening, because of:

- a mix-up in the blood bank
- a very early phase of HBV infection
- a late phase of HBV infection
- an escape mutant or a variant of HBV or
- immune complexing of HBsAg.

In cases (2) to (5) above, NAT may detect HBV DNA; in cases (3) to (5), anti-HBc should be also positive. Screening of every blood donation for HBV DNA by NAT has been introduced in sample pools by blood donation services of the German Red Cross (Roth et al. 2002) and in Japan (Minegishi et al. 2003). Screening for anti-HBc by EIA in low prevalence areas has also prevented a few cases of HBV infection in the recipients, but it caused a large loss of donors. In high prevalence areas, exclusion of anti-HBc positive persons is not feasible because most donors would be positive. To avoid loss of donors, anti-HBc-positive donors should be tested for anti-HBs and only anti-HBs-negative donors excluded. Anti-HBs-positive blood is thought to transfer protective antibody. HBV DNA-positive, HBsAg-negative blood with anti-HBs did not transmit HBV (Prince et al. 2001). Besides screening for HBV DNA, vaccination of non-yet immune donors against HBV would prevent transmission of fresh HBV-infections to recipients.

Anti-HBs in large plasma pools cannot exclude infectious HBV. In 1994, a clotting factor IX preparation transmitted HBV to at least 30 people, although the donors were screened for HBsAg the pool was anti-HBs positive and the transmitted HBV was not an escape mutant. The pool was, however, HBV DNA positive when tested by a highly sensitive NAT (detection limit 10 genomes/ml) and the product was suboptimally inactivated.

Since 1995, virtually all plasma protein products have been required to be treated with one or more validated virus inactivation steps, i.e. by heat at 60–70°C for 10–30 hours in the presence of protective factors. Experience suggests that low contamination by HBV ($<10^4$ infectious doses/ml) can be completely inactivated by such a heat treatment. High contamination can be prevented by donor screening for HBsAg and NAT testing of plasma pools. Treatment of plasma with solvent/detergent is probably effective against HBV as against other enveloped viruses. Recently, methods for chemical inactivation of cellular blood products have been developed and validated with DHBV infectivity and HBV DNA reaction in PCR (Aytay et al. 2004). HBV transmission by blood or blood products should be extremely rare exceptions today. However, if a new HBV infection occurs in a recipient, the producer of the product and the responsible public health institution should be notified and the source of infection identified.

For screening of organ and tissue donors, principally the same rules should be followed as for blood donors. However, livers from anti-HBc-positive donors will often reactivate HBV in the recipient and should be used only for HBV positive recipients or under protection with an antiviral substance and/or passive immunization.

Active immunization

All aspects of active and passive immunization have been described in detail by Ellis (1993). The first attempt to vaccinate against HBV used boiled HBsAg-containing serum as inactivated vaccine. More convincing success was obtained with HBsAg 20-nm particles purified from the plasma of HBV carriers. Residual infectivity of HBV and of other viruses potentially present in plasma was minimized by various inactivation procedures. The most frequently applied plasma-derived vaccine was treated with pepsin at pH 2, urea, and formalin. Other products were inactivated with higher doses of formalin or heating to 100°C. Plasma-derived HBsAg has been used in millions of recipients without any known transmission of viruses. Meanwhile, most countries use 'recombinant' HBsAg that has been expressed in transformed yeast cells. HBsAg expressed in mammalian cells is also used as a vaccine, but is more expensive and not generally available. Today, vaccines typically contain 10–20 μg purified 20-nm HBsAg particles as a standard dose, adsorbed to aluminium hydroxide as an adjuvant, and an antibacterial substance; some products are treated with formalin. Usually, three doses, the second 1 month after the first and the third at 6 months, are recommended for adults. For infants of HBsAg-negative mothers, combination with other vaccinations is recommended. The exact observance of the intervals is not essential, but long intervals between the second and the third dose favor development of high titers of anti-HBs. When rapid protection is required, or after exposure, a shortened schedule of 0, 1, and 2 months and a fourth dose after 6 or 12 months should be used. For infants, smaller doses (2.5–10 μg) are advisable, and for immunodeficient recipients, larger doses of 40 μg HBsAg. Vaccines with stronger adjuvants or HBs-encoding DNA are in clinical evaluation.

Indications for vaccination

The WHO has recommended the vaccination of all children worldwide during the first year of life. In areas where perinatal transmission is frequent, vaccination should start as soon as possible after birth. The same is true for children whose mothers are known to be HBsAg positive or who have not been tested for HBsAg. Post-exposure vaccination with four doses of 10 μg recombinant yeast-derived HBsAg (at 0, 1, 2, and 12 months) was reported to protect 95 percent of the babies born to HBsAg- and HBeAg-positive mothers. Most other studies on the prevention of perinatal HBV infection combined HBsAg vaccine with passive immunization (see 'Passive vaccination', below), but it is not clear whether immunoglobulins against HBV (HBIG) really improve the protection rate if highly efficacious active vaccines are used (for review, see West 1993). Studies without HBIG in South Africa (Hino et al. 2001) and in Oceania (Basuni et al. 2004) revealed a relatively low rate of vaccine failures and no selection of escape mutants whereas after passive/active immunizations escape mutants emerged (Nainan et al. 2002). Vaccination failure occurs more often in mothers with very high viremia ($>10^8$ g.e./ml). Thus, reduction of viremia to lower levels has been attempted with lamivudine therapy before delivery (Van Zonneveld et al. 2003).

In 2004, the majority of countries are following the WHO programme, but many countries with high prevalence have financial limitations and are not able to take part. Some countries with low prevalence do not consider early childhood vaccination to be necessary. In 2002, Germany had a vaccination coverage of 80 percent in early childhood and 60 percent in adolescents.

Among adults, vaccination is strongly recommended for people at risk. Everyone who is or will be in professional contact with blood from other persons, whether directly or indirectly, should be offered free vaccination against HBV by their employer or teaching institution. This includes not only medical and paramedical professions, but also people in the armed forces, the police, staff and inmates of prisons or other closed institutions, and social workers. Patients who need continuous invasive or infusion therapy should be vaccinated, as should relatives and close contacts of HBV carriers. Intravenous drug users should be offered free vaccination and also free access to syringes and needles. Travel to high-prevalence countries does not require hepatitis B vaccination unless close contact or a long stay is expected. Male homosexuals have a high risk of HBV infection and heterosexual promiscuity poses a greater risk than nonpromiscuous heterosexual activity. For many of these risk groups the combined vaccine containing HAV and HBs antigens is advisable.

Side-effects

The vaccine causes no local side effects except moderate pain at the injection site. Generalized nonspecific side effects are rare or mild. Recipients should be questioned about hypersensitivity to yeast components, formalin or the antibacterial substance, but such reactions are very rare. Induction of neurological autoimmune disorder has been suspected in some cases of being associated with hepatitis B vaccine, but several studies did not confirm this. It should be noted that HBsAg may be detected in the serum for a few days after vaccination, and thus for one week after vaccination no blood should be donated.

Pre- and post-testing

People to be vaccinated because of already existing high risk should be tested for anti-HBc before vaccination. Ethnic origin from a high prevalence area is also a risk. If anti-HBc is positive the serum sample should be tested further and the person vaccinated as described in 'Natural immunity,' above. If anti-HBc is negative, vaccination should be started following the schedule of the vaccine producers. If there is a high probability that HBV infection is already present, the person should be tested for HBsAg, even if negative for anti-HBc. An HBsAg-positive person should not be vaccinated, although accidental vaccination is not known to be harmful.

The immune response should be controlled by a quantitative anti-HBs test 4 weeks after the third dose in anyone who is at greater than average risk. Although T-cell responses and immunological memory may be more important than the anti-HBs itself, an easily detectable anti-HBs level is a marker of protection. The detection limit is 1–5 IU/l; 10 IU/l is considered to be a marker of protection. People with less or no anti-HBs should be revaccinated immediately with a further dose. Low responders with <100 IU/l should be revaccinated after one year, all others after 10 years if the special risk is still present, but the necessity of boosters is debated.

Children who have been vaccinated during the first year of life should be revaccinated at the onset of adolescence because then they are again at increased risk. Nonresponders after four doses may receive further doses if protection is urgently requested. Response rates are >90 percent in the healthy general population, but decrease strongly with age. Further risk factors for nonresponse are male gender, obesity, and smoking. Vaccines with preS antigen or other adjuvants may induce a better response but are not yet generally available at the time of writing.

Escape mutants

Post-exposure prophylaxis by active and passive vaccination is usually successful if given soon after injury (e.g. needle-sticks) with HBV-contaminated items. Active vaccination of newborns from HBeAg-positive mothers is also successful in up to 95 percent of cases. In ca. 5 percent of the children, HBsAg may appear in spite of vaccination or never be negative from the first day. Such infants may have already been infected in utero. In some children, HBsAg appears despite seemingly protective levels of anti-HBs. These children have escape variants, detectable by sequencing of the *SHBs* gene, with mutations in the major HBs epitopes between amino acids 120 and 150. Escape variants have been described with various genotypes except for genotype A. A frequent escape mutation is glycine 145 of the S protein to arginine (Nainan et al. 2002).

Although early experiments in chimpanzees suggested that immunization with one HBsAg subtype protected against all HBV genotypes, it should be noted that most recombinant vaccines have genotype A2 or HBsAg *adw2* respectively. It is possible that genotype-specific antibodies may contribute to protection.

Experiments in chimpanzees and in cell culture suggest that anti-preS1 and partially also anti-preS2 contribute to protection. Experiments with transgenic mice suggest that helper cell epitopes of the preS region may induce a better B-cell response against SHBs. The potentially better protection of humans by preS-containing vaccines has not yet been confirmed by field studies. However, induction of anti-HBs in many non-responders to the normal recombinant SHBs vaccine has been found with a vaccine containing preS1 and preS2 (Zuckerman et al. 2001). A similar vaccine induced a stronger and more rapid anti-HBs response than the conventional vaccine (Shapira et al. 2001).

PASSIVE VACCINATION

Normal immunoglobulin does not contain enough anti-HBs to be used for passive vaccination. A special immunoglobulin is produced from donors who are naturally immune and boosted with plasma-derived vaccine or from anti-HBc-negative donors who have particularly high titers after vaccination. 15 percent HBIG for intramuscular administration must contain 200 IU/ml; 5 percent HBIG for intravenous application must contain at least 50 IU/ml. Studies in the 1970s and 1980s showed that HBV infection was prevented in newborns from HBsAg- and HBeAg-positive mothers if HBIG was given within 24 h after birth. Active vaccination seems to be more effective and does not require complementation by passive immunization, but in many countries both active and passive vaccination are still required.

Passive immunization of HBeAg-positive liver transplant recipients usually fails unless combined with antiviral therapy, but in HBeAg-negative patients continuous levels of 100 IU/l of passively administered anti-HBs are able to prevent recurrence of liver disease. Passive immunization of the recipient prevents also viral reactivation in a transplanted anti-HBc positive donor liver (Roque-Afonso et al. 2002).

Passive immunization is recommended together with active immunization after proven accidental exposure of a nonimmune person. In these situations, the blood of the 'donor' should be rapidly tested for HBsAg and, if positive, the 'recipient' should be vaccinated passively and actively, after a blood sample has been taken for anti-HBc and anti-HBs testing.

TREATMENT

The treatment of acute hepatitis B can be directed against symptoms, but this is usually not necessary. Antiviral therapy of fulminant cases can be attempted but usually comes too late. The aim of antiviral or immunotherapy is to reduce persistent viral replication.

Immune modulators

Interferon-α and interferon-β have been used for the treatment of chronic hepatitis B. Success of interferon therapy depends very much on the status of the patient:. Patients with the so-called immunotolerant state (see Table 55.2) cannot usually be cured and should be monitored until they reach the state of chronic active disease, when the success rate of interferon therapy is much higher. Patients with a high probability of sustained response have typically $<10^9$ genomes/ml, low or absent HBeAg ($<2\,000$ PEI units), low HBsAg ($<30\,000$ PEI units/ml) and high ALT levels (>120 IU/l) (Burczynska et al. 1994; Erhardt et al. 2000). The higher the initial ALT levels are, the higher is the response rate in terms of low replication and HBeAg-negativity (Lok et al. 1998). Treatment is undertaken with quite high doses ($2.5–10$ MU/m^2 three times a week) if the patient tolerates the severe side effects such as flulike symptoms, depression, hair loss, leukopenia, and thrombopenia. Autoimmune antibodies should be monitored. Usually the HBV DNA concentration will fall within few weeks to levels $<10^6$ genomes/ml. Some patients do not respond at all, some may redevelop high levels of viremia even during therapy and others may become positive again soon after withdrawal of interferon. Six months of therapy are considered the minimum in responders before withdrawal is attempted. A relapse is not rare and a second course of interferon may be tried. Interferon may be harmful to patients with cirrhosis and is therefore not recommended in the terminal phases of chronic liver disease. In spite of its many disadvantages and relatively low efficacy, interferon has the advantage that in many cases it is able to induce seroconversion from HBeAg to anti-HBe and sustained cessation of viral replication, which is correlated with a very good clinical prognosis (Niederau et al. 1996).

Conjugation of interferon with polyethylene glycol (PEG) improves its pharmacological properties and has been used for therapy of chronic hepatitis B with at least as good success as standard interferon (Janssen et al. 2005). In this recent study, it was noted that genotypes A (47 percent) and B (44 percent) respond almost twice as well as genotypes C (28 percent) and D (25 percent). Combination with lamivudine did not improve the long-term response.

Immune therapy

Vaccination of chronic HBV carriers with licensed SHBs vaccines together with the application of interferon (Heintges et al. 2001) or with a MHBs-containing vaccine without interferon (Pol et al. 2001) increased the rate of HBV DNA negativation above rates in untreated controls but the effect was barely significant. Vaccination of chronic HBV patients with a preS1-, preS2-, and S-containing vaccine induced a Th2 response against these antigens but could not reduce the viremia (Jung et al. 2002). Hepadnaviral DNA vaccines or conventional protein vaccines alone or together with antivirals have been partially successful in the woodchuck (Menne et al. 2002) or duck model (Le Guerhier 2003), which warrants further studies. The successful use of a DNA vaccine in healthy humans to induce a protective Th1 and anti-HBs response is a further stimulus to follow this line (Roy et al. 2000). The optimal adjuvant and combination with antivirals has still to be found.

Antiviral substances

In the 1980s and early 1990s, only highly toxic nucleoside analogues were available. As a side-effect of HIV therapy, several nucleosidic inhibitors of reverse transcriptase were found to be active against HBV as well. Oral Lamivudine (3TC), at 100 mg per day, has been found to be very effective in reducing the viremia by several logs and to improve the HBV-associated liver disease. However, this drug and the other inhibitors of reverse transcription cannot block expression of the viral genes including the pregenome RNA and they cannot eliminate the pre-existing cccDNA of HBV. Lamivudine is able to suppress the release of mature HBV particles and infection of new target cells. Lamivudine induces an enhanced T-cell response against HBV antigen but this stimulation is transient and normally not sufficient to overcome persistent productive infection (Boni et al. 2003). Long-term therapy is necessary and well tolerated due to low toxicity. After 1 year of treatment most patients experience a clear improvement of ALT levels but more than half of them experience a relapse within 12 months after therapy. High pre-treatment levels of HBV DNA were predictive for a relapse after stop of therapy (Huang et al. 2003). Loss of HBeAg is a favorable prognostic marker for a sustained response to lamivudine. In one study (Dienstag et al. 1999), 32 percent of the patients seroconverted after 1 year on lamivudine, but usually the seroconversion rate is lower than with interferon and only twice above the control group, for example, in a study (Jonas et al. 2002) in HBeAg positive children. If HBeAg seroconversion has been reached and HBV DNA was undetectable by PCR, the favorable result is maintained in the majority (64 percent) of patients (Dienstag et al. 2003). The relapse rate can be further reduced by continuation of lamivudine therapy for 6 months (Ryu et al. 2003). Further extension was useful in one study (Chien et al. 2003) but not in another (Lee et al. 2003). One predictor of HBeAg seroconversion under therapy is a high pretreatment ALT level >5-fold the upper limit of normal (Perrillo et al. 2002), furthermore a rapid decrease of HBV DNA to levels $<10^4$/ml (Gauthier and Bourne 1999).

The limiting factor for a permanent therapy with lamivudine is the development of resistance. After 1 year of lamivudine, 23 percent of patients were resistant, after 5 years 65 percent. Resistance development was associated with hepatitis flares in most cases and in 5 percent with serious liver disease-related adverse events (Lok et al. 2003). Whether lamivudine should be stopped or continued once resistance has emerged is debated. The resistance occurs with mutations in the YMDD amino acid motif of the HBV reverse transcriptase domain of M204 to I or V or S (Stuyver et al. 2001). The mutant replicates less efficiently than the wild type, but compensatory additional mutations restore viability (Bock et al. 2002). The appearance of resistance severely impairs the long-term efficacy of lamivudine in cases of chronic hepatitis B, but this does not preclude its short-term usefulness. It is useful to suppress viremia in HBV patients before liver transplantation where reinfection is usually highly detrimental. However, lamivudine alone protects only a part of the patients and needs to be complemented at least for a short period of time with HBIG (Buti et al. 2003). Lamivudine is sufficient to suppress reactivation of HBV infection by an HBsAg-negative anti-HBc-positive donor liver or in anti-HBc-positive, HBsAg-negative recipients (Nery et al. 2003). Lamivudine also supports the establishment of adoptive immunity originating from an anti-HBs-positive liver donor in a HBV-positive recipient (Lo et al. 2003). Furthermore, it is useful to prevent reactivation of hepatitis in HBsAg-positive patients receiving various forms of immunosuppression or cancer therapy (Shibolet et al. 2002; Lau et al. 2003). In highly viremic pregnant women, lamivudine may suppress HBV to levels insufficient to infect the baby (Su et al. 2004). Lamivudine is also supportive in treatment of the HBV-induced immune complex disease polyarteritis nodosa (Guillevin et al. 2004).

If lamivudine resistance has developed, Adefovir – a nucleotide analogue and licensed drug – is in most cases effective (Perillo et al. 2004). Continuation of lamivudine together with Adefovir is not superior to Adefovir alone (Peters et al. 2004). Adefovir is active in HBeAg-positive (Marcellin et al. 2003) and HBeAg-negative chronic hepatitis B (Hadziyannis et al. 2003). The response rate is similar to that of lamivudine but resistance development is rare. Since Adefovir is nephrotoxic at higher doses than 10 mg/day, and expensive, therapy can start with lamivudine under close monitoring of viremia and continued with Adefovir if resistance arises.

Before licensing of Adefovir, Tenofovir, another inhibitor of reverse transcription, licensed for HIV, has been found even more effective (Dore et al. 2004) and should be considered in certain cases where both lamivudine and Adefovir have failed. Entecavir is also efficient against lamivudine-resistant HBV but further resistance can develop (Tenney and Levine 2004). Combination therapy, which is extremely valuable in HIV, has not yet been established for HBV. Combinations of Adefovir and lamivudine are not useful (Peters et al. 2004) combinations of lamivudine (Cooksley 2004; Janssen et al. 2005) or Adefovir (Marcellin and Lau 2004) with interferon were not superior to the single drugs.

Experimental drugs

Immunotherapy with various approaches has not reached advanced clinical studies. Even less developed are the various gene therapy approaches (Farrell 2000) including the most recent discovery of small interfering RNAs, which induce degradation of their target RNAs (McCaffrey et al. 2003). Inhibitory peptides which block viral attachment may also have potential (Glebe et al. 2005). In spite of modern drug design, high-throughput screening may still discover new drugs like the heteroaryl-pyrimidines, which inhibit maturation of HBV cores (Deres et al. 2003).

REFERENCES

Allain, J.P. 2004. Occult hepatitis B virus infection: implications in transfusion. *Vox Sang*, **86**, 83–91.

Allain, J.P., Candotti, D., et al. 2003. The risk of hepatitis B infection by transfusion in Kumasi, Ghana. *Blood*, **101**, 2419–25.

Antonucci, T.K. and Rutter, W.J. 1989. Hepatitis B virus (HBV) promoters are regulated by the HBV enhancer in a tissue specific manner. *J Virol*, **63**, 579–83.

Aytay, S., Ohagen, A., et al. 2004. Development of a sensitive PCR inhibition method to demonstrate HBV nucleic acid inactivation. *Transfusion*, **44**, 476–84.

Banks, K.E., Anderson, A.L., et al. 2002. Hepatocyte nuclear factor 3beta inhibits hepatitis B virus replication in vivo. *J Virol*, **76**, 12974–80.

Barrasa, M.I., Guo, J.T., et al. 2001. Does a cdc2 kinase-like recognition motif on the core protein of hepadnaviruses regulate assembly and disintegration of capsids? *J Virol*, **75**, 2024–8.

Bartenschlager, R., Junker-Niepmann, M. and Schaller, H. 1990. The P gene product of hepatitis B virus is required as a structural component for genomic RNA encapsidation. *J Virol*, **64**, 5324–32.

Bartholomeusz, A. and Schaefer, S. 2004. Hepatitis B virus genotypes: comparison of genotyping methods. *Rev Med Virol*, **14**, 3–16.

Basuni, A.A., Butterworth, L., et al. 2004. Prevalence of HBsAg mutants and impact of hepatitis B infant immunisation in four Pacific Island countries. *Vaccine*, **22**, 2791–9.

Beasley, R.P., Hwang, L.Y., et al. 1981. Hepatocellular carcinoma and hepatitis B virus. A prospective study of 22707 men in Taiwan. *Lancet*, **2**, 1129–33.

Beck, J. and Nassal, M. 2003. Efficient Hsp90-independent in vitro activation by Hsc70 and Hsp40 of duck hepatitis B virus reverse transcriptase, an assumed Hsp90 client protein. *J Biol Chem*, **278**, 36128–38.

Berting, A., Hahnen, J., et al. 1995. Computer-aided studies on the spatial structure of the small hepatitis B surface protein. *Intervirology*, **38**, 8–15.

Berting, A., Fischer, C., et al. 2000. Hemifusion activity of a chimeric influenza virus hemagglutinin with a putative fusion peptide from hepatitis B virus. *Virus Res*, **68**, 35–49.

Bircher, J., Benhamou, J.P., et al. (eds) 1999. *Oxford textbook of clinical hepatology*. New York, Oxford: Oxford University Press.

Blackberg, J. and Kidd-Ljunggren, K. 2003. Mutations within the hepatitis B virus genome among chronic hepatitis B patients with hepatocellular carcinoma. *J Med Virol*, **71**, 18–23.

Block, T.M., Lu, X., et al. 1994. Secretion of human hepatitis B virus is inhibited by the imino sugar N-butyldeoxynojirimycin. *Proc Natl Acad Sci USA*, **91**, 2235–9.

Blum, H.E., Zhang, Z.S., et al. 1992. Hepatitis B virus X protein is not central to the viral life cycle in vitro. *J Virol*, **66**, 1223–7.

Blumberg, B.S., Alter, H.J. and Visnich, S.A. 1965. A 'new' antigen in leukemia sera. *JAMA*, **191**, 541–6.

Blumberg, B.S., Gerstley, B.J., et al. 1967. A serum antigen (Australia antigen) in Down's syndrome, leukemia, and hepatitis. *Ann Intern Med*, **66**, 924–31.

Bock, C.T., Schwinn, S., et al. 2001. Structural organization of the hepatitis B virus minichromosome. *J Mol Biol*, **307**, 183–96.

Bock, C.T., Tillmann, H.L., et al. 2002. Selection of hepatitis B virus polymerase mutants with enhanced replication by lamivudine treatment after liver transplantation. *Gastroenterology*, **122**, 264–73.

Boni, C., Penna, A., et al. 2003. Transient restoration of anti-viral T cell responses induced by lamivudine therapy in chronic hepatitis B. *J Hepatol*, **39**, 595–605.

Bouchard, M.J., Puro, R.J., et al. 2003. Activation and inhibition of cellular calcium and tyrosine kinase signaling pathways identify targets of the HBx protein involved in hepatitis B virus replication. *J Virol*, **77**, 7713–19.

Bozkaya, H., Ayola, B. and Lok, A.S. 1996. High rate of mutations in the hepatitis B core gene during the immune clearance phase of chronic hepatitis B virus infection. *Hepatology*, **24**, 32–7.

Breiner, K.M., Urban, S. and Schaller, H. 1998. Carboxypeptidase D (gp180), a Golgi-resident protein, functions in the attachment and entry of avian hepatitis B viruses. *J Virol*, **72**, 8098–104.

Breiner, K.M., Urban, S., et al. 2001. Envelope protein-mediated down-regulation of hepatitis B virus receptor in infected hepatocytes. *J Virol*, **75**, 143–50.

Bruss, V. 1997. A short linear sequence in the pre-S domain of the large hepatitis B virus envelope protein required for virion formation. *J Virol*, **71**, 9350–7.

Bruss, V. and Ganem, D. 1991. The role of envelope proteins in hepatitis B virus assembly. *Proc Natl Acad Sci USA*, **88**, 1059–63.

Bruss, V., Lu, X., et al. 1994. Post-translational alterations in transmembrane topology of the hepatitis B virus large envelope protein. *EMBO J*, **13**, 2273–9.

Bruss, V., Hagelstein, J., et al. 1996. Myristylation of the large surface protein is required for hepatitis B virus in vitro infectivity. *Virology*, **218**, 396–9.

Buckwold, V.E., Xu, Z., et al. 1996. Effects of a naturally occurring mutation in the hepatitis B virus basal core promoter on precore gene expression and viral replication. *J Virol*, **70**, 5845–51.

Buendia, M.A., Paterlini, P., et al. 1993. Liver cancer. In: Zuckerman, A.J. and Thomas, H.C. (eds), *Viral hepatitis – scientific basis and management*. Edinburgh: Churchill Livingstone, 137–64.

Burczynska, B., Madalinski, K., et al. 1994. The value of quantitative measurement of HBeAg and HBsAg before interferon-α treatment of chronic hepatitis B in children. *J Hepatol*, **21**, 1097–102.

Buti, M., Mas, A., et al. 2003. A randomized study comparing lamivudine monotherapy after a short course of hepatitis B immune globulin (HBIg) and lamivudine with long-term lamivudine plus HBIg in the prevention of hepatitis B virus recurrence after liver transplantation. *J Hepatol*, **38**, 811–17.

Calvert, J. and Summers, J. 1994. Two regions of the avian hepadnavirus RNA pregenome are required in cis for encapsidation. *J Virol*, **68**, 2084–90.

Carman, W.F., Van Deursen, F.J., et al. 1997. The prevalence of surface antigen variants of hepatitis B virus in Papua New Guinea, South Africa and Sardinia. *Hepatology*, **26**, 1658–66.

Carman, W.F., Owsianka, A., et al. 1999. Antigenic characterization of pre- and post-liver transplant hepatitis B surface antigen sequences from patients treated with hepatitis B immune globulin. *J Hepatol*, **31**, 195–201.

Cattaneo, R. and Will, H. 1983. Signals regulating hepatitis B surface antigen transcription. *Nature*, **305**, 336–8.

Chan, H.L., Hussain, M. and Lok, A.S. 1999. Different hepatitis B virus genotypes are associated with different mutations in the core promoter and precore regions during hepatitis B e antigen seroconversion. *Hepatology*, **29**, 976–84.

Chang, L.J., Ganem, D. and Varmus, H.E. 1990. Mechanism of translation of the hepadnaviral polymerase (P) gene. *Proc Natl Acad Sci USA*, **87**, 5158–62.

Chen, H.S., Kew, M.C., et al. 1992. The precore gene of the woodchuck hepatitis virus genome is not essential for viral replication in the natural host. *J Virol*, **66**, 5682–4.

Chen, H.S., Kaneko, S., et al. 1993. The woodchuck hepatitis virus X gene is important for establishment of virus infection in woodchucks. *J Virol*, **66**, 1218–26.

Cherrington, J., Russnak, R. and Ganem, D. 1992. Upstream sequences and cap proximity in the regulation of polyadenylation in ground squirrel hepatitis virus. *J Virol*, **66**, 7589–96.

Chien, R.N., Yet, C.T., et al. 2003. Determinants for sustained HBeAg response to lamivudine therapy. *Hepatology*, **38**, 1267–73.

Chisari, F.V. and Ferrari, C. 1995. Hepatitis B virus immunopathogenesis. *Annu Rev Immunol*, **13**, 29–60.

Chouteau, P., Le Seyec, J., et al. 2001. A short N-proximal region in the large envelope protein harbors a determinant that contributes to the species specificity of human hepatitis B virus. *J Virol*, **75**, 11565–72.

Chu, C.J., Keeffe, E.B., et al. 2003. Hepatitis B virus genotypes in the United States: results of a nationwide study. *Gastroenterology*, **125**, 444–51.

Chulanov, V.P., Shipulin, G.A., et al. 2003. Kinetics of HBV DNA and HBsAg in acute hepatitis B patients with and without coinfection by other hepatitis viruses. *J Med Virol*, **69**, 313–23.

Cooksley, W.G. 2004. Treatment with interferons (including pegylated interferons) in patients with hepatitis B. *Semin Liver Dis*, **24**, Suppl 1, 45–53, Review.

Corden, S., Ballard, A.L., et al. 2003. HBV DNA levels and transmission of hepatitis B by health care workers. *J Clin Virol*, **27**, 52–8.

Crook, P.D., Jones, M.E. and Hall, A.J. 2003. Mortality of hepatitis B surface antigen-positive blood donors in England and Wales. *Int J Epidemiol*, **32**, 118–24.

Crowther, R.A., Kiselev, N.A., et al. 1994. Three-dimensional structure of hepatitis B virus core particles determined by electron cryomicroscopy. *Cell*, **77**, 943–50.

Dandri, M., Burda, M.R., et al. 2002. Increase in de novo HBV DNA integrations in response to oxidative DNA damage or inhibition of poly(ADP-ribosyl)ation. *Hepatology*, **35**, 217–23.

Dane, D.S., Cameron, C.H. and Briggs, M. 1970. Virus-like particles in serum of patients with Australia-antigen-associated hepatitis. *Lancet*, **1**, 695–8.

Daub, H., Blencke, S., et al. 2002. Identification of SRPK1 and SRPK2 as the major cellular protein kinases phosphorylating hepatitis B virus core protein. *J Virol*, **76**, 8124–37.

Dejean, A., Bougueleret, L., et al. 1986. Hepatitis B virus DNA integration in a sequence homologous to v-erb-A and steroid receptor genes in a hepatocellular carcinoma. *Nature (London)*, **322**, 70–2.

Deres, K., Schröder, C.H., et al. 2003. Inhibition of hepatitis B virus replication by drug-induced depletion of nucleocapsids. *Science*, **299**, 893–6.

Dienes, H.P., Gerlich, W.H., et al. 1990. Hepatic pre-S1 and pre-S2 expression pattern in viremic and non-viremic chronic hepatitis B. *Gastroenterology*, **98**, 1017–23.

Dienstag, J.L., Schiff, E.R., et al. 1999. Lamivudine as initial treatment for chronic hepatitis B in the United States. *N Engl J Med*, **341**, 1256–63.

Dienstag, J.L., Cianciara, J., et al. 2003. Durability of serologic response after lamivudine treatment of chronic hepatitis B. *Hepatology*, **37**, 748–55.

Donato, F., Tagger, A., et al. 1997. Hepatitis B and C virus infection, alcohol drinking, and hepatocellular carcinoma: a case-control study in Italy, Brescia HCC Study. *Hepatology*, **26**, 579–84.

Dore, G.J., Cooper, D.A., et al. 2004. Efficacy of tenofovir disoproxil fumarate in antiretroviral therapy-naive and -experienced patients coinfected with HIV-1 and hepatitis B virus. *J Infect Dis*, **189**, 1185–92.

Doria, M., Klein, N., et al. 1995. The hepatitis B virus HBx protein is a dual specificity cytoplasmic activator of Ras and nuclear activator of transcription factors. *EMBO J*, **14**, 4747–57.

Duclos-Vallee, J.C., Capel, F., et al. 1998. Phosphorylation of the hepatitis B virus core protein by glyceraldehyde-3-phosphate dehydrogenase protein kinase activity. *J Gen Virol*, **79**, 1665–70.

Dusheiko, G.M., Bowyer, S.M., et al. 1985. Replication of hepatitis B virus in adult carriers in an endemic area. *J Infect Dis*, **152**, 566–71.

Ehlers, I., Horke, S., et al. 2004. Functional characterization of the interaction between human La and hepatitis B virus RNA. *J Biol Chem*, **279**, 43437–47.

Ellis, R.W. 1993. *Hepatitis B vaccines in clinical practice*. New York: Marcel Dekker.

Erhardt, A., Reineke, U., et al. 2000. Mutations of the core promoter and response to interferon treatment in chronic replicative hepatitis B. *Hepatology*, **31**, 716–25.

Farrell, G.C. 2000. Clinical potential of emerging new agents in hepatitis B. *Drugs*, **60**, 701–10.

Ferber, M.J., Montoya, D.P., et al. 2003. Integrations of the hepatitis B virus (HBV) and human papillomavirus (HPV) into the human telomerase reverse transcriptase (hTERT) gene in liver and cervical cancers. *Oncogene*, **22**, 3813–20.

Findlay, G.M. and MacCallum, F.O. 1937. Note on acute hepatitis and yellow fever immunization. *Trans R Soc Trop Med Hyg*, **31**, 297–308.

Flajolet, M., Tiollais, P., et al. 1998. Woodchuck hepatitis virus enhancer I and enhancer II are both involved in N-myc2 activation in woodchuck liver tumors. *J Virol*, **72**, 6175–80.

Funk, A., Mhamdi, M., et al. 2004. Itinerary of hepatitis B viruses: delineation of restriction points critical for infectious entry. *J Virol*, **78**, 8289–300.

Galibert, F., Mandart, E., et al. 1979. Nucleotide sequence of the hepatitis B virus genome (subtype *ayw*) cloned in *E. coli*. *Nature (London)*, **281**, 646–50.

Gallina, A., De Koning, A., et al. 1992. Translational modulation in hepatitis B virus preS-S open reading frame expression. *J Gen Virol*, **73**, 139–48.

Gallina, A., Gazina, E. and Milanese, G. 1995. A C-terminal preS1 sequence is sufficient to retain hepatitis B virus L protein in 293 cells. *Virology*, **213**, 57–69.

Ganem, D., Pollack, J.R. and Tavis, J. 1994. Hepatitis B virus reverse transcriptase and its many roles in hepadnaviral genomic replication. *Infect Agents Dis*, **3**, 85–93.

Gauthier, J. and Bourne, E.J. 1999. Quantitation of hepatitis B viremia and emergence of YMDD variants in patients with chronic hepatitis B treated with lamivudine. *J Infect Dis*, **180**, 1757–62.

Gazina, E.V., Fielding, J.E., et al. 2000. Core protein phosphorylation modulates pregenomic RNA encapsidation to different extents in human and duck hepatitis B viruses. *J Virol*, **74**, 4721–8.

Gerlich, W.H., Goldmann, U., et al. 1982. Specificity and localization of the hepatitis B virus-associated protein kinase. *J Virol*, **42**, 761–6.

Gerlich, W.H., Uy, A., et al. 1986. Cutoff levels of immunoglobulin M antibody against viral core antigen for differentiation of acute, chronic and past hepatitis B virus infections. *J Clin Microbiol*, **24**, 288–93.

Gerlich, W.H., Wend, U. and Glebe, D. 2004. Quantitative assay of hepatitis B surface antigen in serum or plasma using Laurell electrophoresis. *Methods Mol Med*, **95**, 57–63.

Glebe, D. and Gerlich, W.H. 2004. Study of the endocytosis and intracellular localization of subviral particles of hepatitis B virus in primary hepatocytes. *Methods Mol Med*, **96**, 143–51.

Glebe, D., Aliakbari, M., et al. 2003. PreS1 antigen dependent infection of Tupaia hepatocyte cultures with human hepatitis B virus. *J Virol*, **77**, 9511–21.

Glebe D, Urban S, et al., 2005, Mapping of hepatitis B virus attachment site by infection-inhibiting preS1 lipopeptides using primary *Tupaia* hepatocytes.

Gottlob, K., Pagano, S., et al. 1998. Hepatitis B virus X protein transcription activation domains are neither required nor sufficient for cell transformation. *Cancer Res*, **58**, 3566–70.

Gozuacik, D., Murakami, Y., et al. 2001. Identification of human cancer-related genes by naturally occurring Hepatitis B Virus DNA tagging. *Oncogene*, **20**, 6233–40.

Graef, E., Caselmann, W.H., et al. 1994. Insertional activation of mevalonate kinase by hepatitis B virus DNA in a human hepatoma cell line. *Oncogene*, **9**, 81–7.

Gripon, P., Rumin, S., et al. 2002. Infection of a human hepatoma cell line by hepatitis B virus. *Proc Natl Acad Sci USA*, **99**, 15655–60.

Guillevin, L., Mahr, A., et al. 2004. Short-term corticosteroids then lamivudine and plasma exchanges to treat hepatitis B virus-related polyarteritis nodosa. *Arthritis Rheum*, **15**, 482–7.

Gunson, R.N., Shouval, D., et al. 2003. Hepatitis B virus (HBV) and hepatitis C virus (HCV) infections in health care workers (HCWs): guidelines for prevention of transmission of HBV and HCV from HCW to patients. *J Clin Virol*, **27**, 213–30.

Günther, S., Baginski, S., et al. 1996. Accumulation and persistence of hepatitis B virus core gene deletion mutants in renal transplant patients are associated with end-stage liver disease. *Hepatology*, **24**, 751–8.

Guo, J.T. and Pugh, J.C. 1997. Topology of the large envelope protein of duck hepatitis B virus suggests a mechanism for membrane translocation during particle morphogenesis. *J Virol*, **71**, 1107–14.

Hadziyannis, S.J., Tassopoulos, N.C., et al. 2003. Adefovir dipivoxil for the treatment of hepatitis B e antigen-negative chronic hepatitis B. *N Engl J Med*, **348**, 800–7.

Hafner, A., Brandenburg, B. and Hildt, E. 2003. Reconstitution of gene expression from a regulatory-protein-deficient hepatitis B virus genome by cell-permeable HBx protein. *EMBO Rep*, **4**, 767–73.

Heermann, K.H., Goldmann, U., et al. 1984. Large surface proteins of hepatitis B virus containing the pre-S sequence. *J Virol*, **52**, 396–402.

Heermann, K.H., Gerlich, W.H., et al. 1999. Quantitative determination of Hepatitis B Virus DNA in two international reference plasmas. *J Clin Microbiol*, **37**, 68–73.

Heintges, T., Petry, W., et al. 2001. Combination therapy of active HBsAg vaccination and interferon-alpha in interferon-alpha nonresponders with chronic hepatitis B. *Dig Dis Sci*, **46**, 901–6.

Heise, T., Guidotti, L.G. and Chisan, F.V. 1999. La autoantigen specifically recognises a predicted stem–loop in hepatitis B virus. *J Virol*, **73**, 5767–76.

Heise, T., Guidotti, L.G. and Chisan, F.V. 1999. La autoantigen specifically recognises a predicted stem-loop in hepatitis B virus RNA. *J Virol*, **73**, 5767–76.

Heise, T., Guidotti, L.G., et al. 2001. Characterization of nuclear RNases that cleave hepatitis B virus RNA near the La protein binding site. *J Virol*, **75**, 6874–83.

Hildt, E., Urban, S. and Hofschneider, P.H. 1995. Characterization of essential domains for the functionality of the MHBst transcriptional activator and identification of a minimal MHBst activator. *Oncogene*, **11**, 2055–66.

Hildt, E., Hofschneider, P.H. and Urban, S. 1997. The role of hepatitis B virus (HBV) in the development of hepatocellular carcinoma. *Semin Virology*, **7**, 333–47.

Hino, K., Katoh, Y., et al. 2001. The effect of introduction of universal childhood hepatitis B immunization in South Africa on the prevalence of serologically negative hepatitis B virus infection and the selection of immune escape variants. *Vaccine*, **19**, 3912–18.

Hirsch, R.C., Lavine, J.E., et al. 1990. Polymerase gene products of hepatitis B viruses are required for genomic RNA packaging as well as for reverse transcription. *Nature (London)*, **344**, 552–5.

Hirsch, R.C., Loeb, D.D., et al. 1991. *cis*-acting sequences required for encapsidation of duck hepatitis B virus pregenomic RNA. *J Virol*, **65**, 3309–16.

Höhne, M., Schaefer, S., et al. 1990. Malignant transformation of immortalized transgenic hepatocytes after transfection with hepatitis B virus DNA. *EMBO J*, **9**, 1137–45.

Hu, J. and Seeger, C. 1996. Hsp90 is required for the activity of a hepatitis B virus reverse transcriptase. *Proc Natl Acad Sci USA*, **93**, 1060–4.

Hu, J., Toft, D., et al. 2002. In vitro reconstitution of functional hepadnavirus reverse transcriptase with cellular chaperone proteins. *J Virol*, **76**, 269–79.

Huang, J. and Liang, T.J. 1993. A novel hepatitis B virus (HBV) genetic element with Rev response element-like properties that is essential for expression of HBV gene products. *Mol Cell Biol*, **13**, 7476–86.

Huang, Y.H., Wu, J.C., et al. 2003. Analysis of clinical, biochemical and viral factors associated with early relapse after lamivudine treatment for hepatitis B e antigen-negative chronic hepatitis B patients in Taiwan. *J Viral Hepat*, **10**, 277–84.

Hwang, G.Y., Lin, C.Y., et al. 2003. Detection of the hepatitis B virus X protein (HBx) antigen and anti-HBx antibodies in cases of human hepatocellular carcinoma. *J Clin Microbiol*, **41**, 5598–603.

Ip, H.M., Lelie, P.N., et al. 1989. Prevention of hepatitis B virus carrier state in infants according to maternal serum levels of HBV DNA. *Lancet*, **1**, 406–10.

Ishikawa, T. and Ganem, D. 1995. The pre-S domain of the large viral envelope protein determines host range in avian hepatitis B viruses. *Proc Natl Acad Sci USA*, **92**, 6259–63.

Jacob, J.R., Ascenzi, M.A., et al. 1997. Hepatic expression of the woodchuck hepatitis virus X-antigen during acute and chronic infection and detection of a woodchuck hepatitis virus X-antigen antibody response. *Hepatology*, **26**, 1607–15.

Janssen, H.H.A., von Zonnefeld, M., et al. 2005. Pegylated interferon alfa-2b alone or in combination with lamivudine for HBeAg-positive chronic hepatitis B: a randomised trial. *Lancet*, **365**, 123–9.

Jeng, K.S., Hu, C.P. and Chang, C. 1991. Different formation of disulfide linkages in the core antigen of extracellular and intracellular hepatitis B virus core particles. *J Virol*, **65**, 3924–7.

Jonas, M.M., Kelley, D.A., et al. 2002. Clinical trial of lamivudine in children with chronic hepatitis B. *N Engl J Med*, **346**, 1706–13.

Jongerius, J.M., Wester, M., et al. 1998. New hepatitis B virus mutant form in a blood donor that is undetectable in several hepatitis B surface antigen screening assays. *Transfusion*, **38**, 56–9.

Jung, M.C., Gruner, N., et al. 2002. Immunological monitoring during therapeutic vaccination as a prerequisite for the design of new effective therapies: induction of a vaccine-specific CD4+ T-cell proliferative response in chronic hepatitis B carriers. *Vaccine*, **20**, 3598–612.

Junker-Niepmann, M., Bartenschlager, R. and Schaller, H. 1990. A short cis-acting sequence is required for hepatitis B virus pregenome encapsidation and sufficient for packaging of foreign RNA. *EMBO J*, **9**, 3389–96.

Jursch, C.A., Gerlich, W.H., et al. 2002. Molecular approaches to validate disinfectants against hepatitis B virus. *Med Microbiol Immunol*, **190**, 189–97.

Kann, M. and Gerlich, W.H. 1994. Effect of core protein phosphorylation by protein kinase C on encapsidation of RNA within core particles of hepatitis B virus. *J Virol*, **68**, 7993–8000.

Kann, M., Thomassen, R. and Gerlich, W.H. 1993. Characterization of the endogenous protein kinase activity of the hepatitis B virus. *Arch Virol*, **8**, Suppl., 53–62.

Kann, M., Sodeik, B., et al. 1999. Phosphorylation-dependent binding of hepatitis B virus core particles to the nuclear pore complex. *J Cell Biol*, **145**, 45–55.

Kaplan, P.M., Greenman, R.L., et al. 1973. DNA polymerase associated with human hepatitis B antigen. *J Virol*, **12**, 995–1005.

Kao, J.H., Chen, P.J., et al. 2003. Basal core promoter mutations of hepatitis B virus increase the risk of hepatocellular carcinoma in hepatitis B carriers. *Gastroenterology*, **124**, 327–34.

Kao, J.H., Chen, P.J., et al. 2004. Hepatitis B virus genotypes and spontaneous hepatitis B e antigen seroconversion in Taiwanese hepatitis B carriers. *J Med Virol*, **72**, 363–9.

Kau, J.H. and Ting, L.P. 1998. Phosphorylation of the core protein of hepatitis B virus by a 46-kilodalton serine kinase. *J Virol*, **72**, 3796–803.

Kawai, H., Suda, T., et al. 2000. Quantitative evaluation of genomic instability as a possible predictor for development of hepatocellular carcinoma: comparison of loss of heterozygosity and replication error. *Hepatology*, **31**, 1246–50.

Kenney, J.M., von Bonsdorff, C.H., et al. 1995. Evolutionary conservation in the hepatitis B virus core structure: comparison of human and duck cores. *Structure*, **3**, 1009–19.

Kim, M.H. and Seong, B.L. 2003. Pro-apoptotic function of HBV X protein is mediated by interaction with c-FLIP and enhancement of death-inducing signal. *EMBO J*, **22**, 2104–16.

Knutsson, M. and Kidd-Ljunggren, K. 2000. Urine from chronic hepatitis B virus carriers: implications for infectivity. *J Med Virol*, **60**, 17–20.

Köck, J. and Schlicht, H.J. 1993. Analysis of the earliest steps of hepadnavirus replication: genome repair after infectious entry into hepatocytes does not depend on viral polymerase activity. *J Virol*, **67**, 4867–74.

Köck, J., Borst, E.M. and Schlicht, H.J. 1996. Uptake of duck hepatitis B virus into hepatocytes occurs by endocytosis but does not require passage of the virus through an acidic intracellular compartment. *J Virol*, **70**, 5827–31.

Köck, J., Nassal, M., et al. 2001. Efficient infection of primary *Tupaia* hepatocytes with purified human and woolly monkey hepatitis B virus. *J Virol*, **75**, 5084–9.

Köck, J., Kann, M., et al. 2003. Central role of a serine phosphorylation site within duck hepatitis B virus core protein for capsid trafficking and genome release. *J Biol Chem*, **278**, 28123–9.

Krone, B., Lenz, A., et al. 1990. Interaction between hepatitis B surface proteins and monomeric human serum albumin. *Hepatology*, **11**, 1050–6.

Kuang, S.Y., Jackson, P.E., et al. 2004. Specific mutations of hepatitis B virus in plasma predict liver cancer development. *Proc Natl Acad Sci USA*, **101**, 3575–80.

Kubicka, S., Rudolph, K.L., et al. 2000. Hepatocellular carcinoma in Germany: a retrospective epidemiological study from a low-endemic area. *Liver*, **20**, 312–18.

Kuhns, M.C., Kleinman, S.H., et al. 2004. Lack of correlation between HBsAg and HBV DNA levels in blood donors who test positive for HBsAg and anti-HBc: implications for future HBV screening policy. *Transfusion*, **44**, 1332–9.

Kuroki, K., Eng, F., et al. 1995. gp180, a host cell glycoprotein that binds duck hepatitis B virus particles, is encoded by a member of the carboxypeptidase gene family. *J Biol Chem*, **270**, 15022–8.

Lai, C.L. and Locarnini, S. (eds) 2002. *Hepatitis B virus: Vol 11 of human virus guides*. London: International Medical Press.

Lambert, C. and Prange, R. 2003. Chaperone action in the posttranslational topological reorientation of the hepatitis B virus large envelope protein: Implications for translocational regulation. *Proc Natl Acad Sci USA*, **100**, 5199–204.

Lan, Y.T., Li, J., et al. 1999. Roles of the three major phosphorylation sites of hepatitis B virus core protein in viral replication. *Virology*, **259**, 342–8.

Landers, T.A., Greenberg, H.B. and Robinson, W.S. 1977. Structure of hepatitis B Dane particle DNA and nature of the endogenous DNA polymerase reaction. *J Virol*, **23**, 368–76.

Lanford, R.E. and Notvall, L. 1990. Expression of hepatitis B virus core and precore antigens in insect cells and characterization of a core-associated kinase activity. *Virology*, **176**, 222–33.

Lanford, R.E., Chavez, D., et al. 1997. Isolation of a hepadnavirus from the woolly monkey, a New World primate. *Proc Natl Acad Sci USA*, **95**, 5757–61.

Lanford, R.E., Chavez, D., et al. 1998. Isolation of a hepadnavirus from the woolly monkey, a New World primate. *Proc Natl Acad Sci USA*, **95**, 5757–61.

Lara-Pezzi, E., Armesilla, A.L., et al. 1998. The hepatitis B virus X protein activates nuclear factor of activated T cells (NF-AT) by a cyclosporin A-sensitive pathway. *EMBO J*, **17**, 7066–77.

Lau, G.K., Yiu, H.H., et al. 2003. Early is superior to deferred preemptive lamivudine therapy for hepatitis B patients undergoing chemotherapy. *Gastroenterology*, **125**, 1742–9.

Lee, H.C., Suh, D.J., et al. 2003. Quantitative polymerase chain reaction assay for serum hepatitis B virus DNA as a predictive factor for post-treatment relapse after lamivudine induced hepatitis B e antigen loss or seroconversion. *Gut*, **52**, 1779–83.

Le Guerhier, F., Thermet, A., et al. 2003. Antiviral effect of adefovir in combination with a DNA vaccine in the duck hepatitis B virus infection model. *J Hepatol*, **38**, 328–34.

Lin, W.J., Li, J., et al. 2003. Suppression of hepatitis B virus core promoter by the nuclear orphan receptor TR4. *J Biol Chem*, **278**, 9353–60.

Liu, N., Tian, R. and Loeb, D.D. 2003. Base pairing among three cis-acting sequences contributes to template switching during hepadnavirus reverse transcription. *Proc Natl Acad Sci USA*, **100**, 1984–9.

Liu, N., Ji, L., et al. 2004. Cis-acting sequences that contribute to the synthesis of relaxed-circular DNA of human hepatitis B virus. *J Virol*, **78**, 642–9.

Lo, C.M., Fung, J.T., et al. 2003. Development of antibody to hepatitis B surface antigen after liver transplantation for chronic hepatitis B. *Hepatology*, **37**, 36–43.

Locarnini, S. 2003. Hepatitis B viral resistance: mechanisms and diagnosis. *J Hepatol*, **39**, Suppl 1, S124–32.

Loeb, D.D., Mack, A.A. and Tian, R. 2002. A secondary structure that contains the 5′ and 3′ splice sites suppresses splicing of duck hepatitis B virus pregenomic RNA. *J Virol*, **76**, 10195–202.

Lok, A.S., Ghany, M.G., et al. 1998. Predictive value of aminotransferase and hepatitis B virus DNA levels on response to interferon therapy for chronic hepatitis B. *J Viral Hepat*, **5**, 171–8.

Lok, A.S., Lai, C.L., et al. 2003. Long-term safety of lamivudine treatment in patients with chronic hepatitis B. *Gastroenterology*, **125**, 1714–22.

Lu, M. and Lorentz, T. 2003. De novo infection in a renal transplant recipient caused by novel mutants of hepatitis B virus despite the presence of protective anti-hepatitis B surface antibody. *J Infect Dis*, **187**, 1323–6.

Lu, X., Mehta, A., et al. 1995. Evidence that N-linked glycosylation is necessary for hepatitis B virus secretion. *Virology*, **213**, 660–5.

Luber, B., Arnold, N., et al. 1996. Hepatoma-derived integrated HBV DNA causes multi-stage transformation in vitro. *Oncogene*, **12**, 1597–608.

Lürmann, A. 1885. Eine Icterusepidemie. *Berl Klin Wochenschr*, **22**, 20–3.

Maeng, C.Y., Ryu, C.J., et al. 2000. Fine mapping of virus-neutralizing epitopes on hepatitis B virus PreS1. *Virology*, **270**, 9–16.

Magnius, L.O. and Espmark, J.A. 1972. A new antigen complex cooccurring with Australian antigen. *Acta Pathol Microbiol Scand*, **B80**, 335–7.

Marcellin, P. and Lau, G.K. 2004. Peginterferon alfa-2a alone, lamivudine alone, and the two in combination in patients with HBeAg-negative chronic hepatitis B. *N Engl J Med*, **351**, 1206–17.

Marcellin, P., Chang, T.T., et al. 2003. Adefovir dipivoxil for the treatment of hepatitis B e antigen-positive chronic hepatitis B. *N Engl J Med*, **348**, 808–16.

Mason, W.S., Burell, C.J., et al., 2005. Family *Hepadnaviridae*. In: Fauquet, C.M., Mayo, M.A. et al. *Virus taxonomy VIIIth report*, Elsevier/Academic Press, 373–84.

McCaffrey, A.P., Nakai, H., et al. 2003. Inhibition of hepatitis B virus in mice by RNA interference. *Nat Biotechnol*, **21**, 639–44.

Menne, S., Roneker, C.A., et al. 2002. Immunization with surface antigen vaccine alone and after treatment with 1-(2-fluoro-5-methyl-beta-L-arabinofuranosyl)-uracil (L-FMAU) breaks humoral and cell-mediated immune tolerance in chronic woodchuck hepatitis virus infection. *J Virol*, **76**, 5305–14.

Milich, D. and Liang, T.J. 2003. Exploring the biological basis of hepatitis B e antigen in hepatitis B virus infection. *Hepatology*, **38**, 1075–86.

Minegishi, K., Yoshikawa, A., et al. 2003. Superiority of minipool nucleic acid amplification technology for hepatitis B virus over chemiluminescence immunoassay for hepatitis B surface antigen screening. *Vox Sang*, **84**, 287–91.

Ming, L., Thorgeirsson, S.S., et al. 2002. Dominant role of hepatitis B virus and cofactor role of aflatoxin in hepatocarcinogenesis in Qidong, China. *Hepatology*, **36**, 1214–20.

Moolla, N., Kew, M., et al. 2002. Regulatory elements of hepatitis B virus transcription. *J Viral Hepat*, **9**, 323–31.

Murakami, S. 2001. Hepatitis B virus X protein: a multifunctional viral regulator. *J Gastroenterol*, **36**, 651–60.

Nainan, O.V., Khristova, M.L., et al. 2002. Genetic variation of hepatitis B surface antigen coding region among infants with chronic hepatitis B virus infection. *J Med Virol*, **68**, 319–27.

Nakamoto, Y., Guidotti, L.G., et al. 1998. Immune pathogenesis of hepatocellular carcinoma. *J Exp Med*, **188**, 341–50.

Nassal, M. 1992. The arginine-rich domain of the hepatitis B virus core protein is required for pregenome encapsidation and productive viral positive-strand DNA synthesis but not for virus assembly. *J Virol*, **66**, 4107–16.

Nassal, M. and Schaller, H. 1996. Hepatitis B virus replication – an update. *J Viral Hepatitis*, **3**, 217–26.

Nassal, M., Junker-Niepmann, M. and Schaller, H. 1990. Translational inactivation of RNA function: discrimination against a subset of genomic transcripts during HBV nucleocapsid assembly. *Cell*, **63**, 1357–63.

Nery, J.R., Nery-Avila, C., et al. 2003. Use of liver grafts from donors positive for antihepatitis B-core antibody (anti-HBc) in the era of prophylaxis with hepatitis-B immunoglobulin and lamivudine. *Transplantation*, **75**, 1179–86.

Neurath, A.R., Kent, S.B., et al. 1986. Identification and chemical synthesis of a host cell receptor binding site on hepatitis B virus. *Cell*, **46**, 429–36.

Niederau, C., Heintges, T., et al. 1996. Long-term follow-up of HBeAg-positive patients treated with interferon alfa for chronic hepatitis B. *N Engl J Med*, **334**, 1422–7.

Norder, H., Courouce, A.M. and Magnius, L.O. 1994. Complete genomes, phylogenetic relatedness, and structural proteins of six strains of the hepatitis B virus, four of which represent two new genotypes. *Virology*, **198**, 489–503.

Norder, H., Couroucé, A.M., et al. 2004. Genetic diversity of hepatitis B virus strains derived worldwide: genotypes, subgenotypes, and HBsAg subtypes. *Intervirology*, **47**, 286–309.

Obert, S., Zachmann Brand, B., et al. 1996. A splice hepadnavirus RNA that is essential for virus replication. *EMBO J*, **15**, 2565–74.

Oess, S. and Hildt, E. 2000. Novel cell permeable motif derived from the PreS2-domain of hepatitis-B virus surface antigens. *Gene Ther*, **7**, 750–8.

Oguey, D., Dumenco, L.L., et al. 1996. Analysis of the tumorigenicity of the X gene of hepatitis B virus in a nontransformed hepatocyte cell line and the effects of cotransfection with a murine p53 mutant equivalent to human codon 249. *Hepatology*, **24**, 1024–33.

Okabe, H., Ikai, I., et al. 2000. Comprehensive allelotype study of hepatocellular carcinoma: potential differences in pathways to hepatocellular carcinoma between hepatitis B virus-positive and -negative tumors. *Hepatology*, **31**, 1073–9.

Ou, J.H., Bao, H., et al. 1990. Preferred translation of human hepatitis B virus polymerase from core protein – but not from precore protein-specific transcript. *J Virol*, **64**, 4578–81.

Panté, N. and Kann, M. 2002. Nuclear pore complex is able to transport macromolecules with diameters of about 39 nm. *Mol Biol Cell*, **13**, 425–34.

Perrillo, R.P., Lai, C.L., et al. 2002. Predictors of HBeAg loss after lamivudine treatment for chronic hepatitis B. *Hepatology*, **36**, 186–94.

Perillo, R., Hann, H.W., et al. 2004. Adefovir dipivoxil added to ongoing lamivudine in chronic hepatitis B with YMDD mutant hepatitis B virus. *Gastroenterology*, **126**, 81–90.

Peters, M.G., Hann Hw, H., et al. 2004. Adefovir dipivoxil alone or in combination with lamivudine in patients with lamivudine-resistant chronic hepatitis B. *Gastroenterology*, **126**, 91–101.

Pol, S., Nalpas, B., et al. 2001. Efficacy and limitations of a specific immunotherapy in chronic hepatitis B. *J Hepatol*, **34**, 917–21.

Pollicino, T., Squadrito, G., et al. 2004. Hepatitis B virus maintains its pro-oncogenic properties in the case of occult HBV infection. *Gastroenterology*, **126**, 102–10.

Ponsel, D. and Bruss, V. 2003. Mapping of amino acid side chains on the surface of hepatitis B virus capsids required for envelopment and virion formation. *J Virol*, **77**, 416–22.

Pontisso, P., Ruvoletto, M.G., et al. 1989. Identification of an attachment site for human liver plasma membranes on hepatitis B virus particles. *Virology*, **173**, 522–30.

Pontisso, P., Ruvoletto, M.G., et al. 1993. Clinical and virological profiles in patients with multiple hepatitis virus infections. *Gastroenterology*, **105**, 1529–33.

Popa, I., Harris, M.E., et al. 2002. CRM1-dependent function of a cis-acting RNA export element. *Mol Cell Biol*, **22**, 2057–67.

Prince, A.M., Lee, D.H. and Brotman, B. 2001. Infectivity of blood from PCR-positive, HBsAg-negative, anti-HBs-positive cases of resolved hepatitis B infection. *Transfusion*, **41**, 329–32.

Pumpens, P. and Grens, E. 2001. HBV core particles as a carrier for B cell/T cell epitopes. *Intervirology*, **44**, 98–114.

Rabe, B., and Kann, M. 2005. Lipid-mediated entry of hepatitis B virus capsids in non-susceptible cells leads to highly efficient replication. *J Biol Chem*, in press.

Rabe, B., Vlachou, A., et al. 2003. Nuclear import of hepatitis B virus capsids and release of the viral genome. *Proc Natl Acad Sci USA*, **100**, 9849–54.

Rakotomahanina, C.K., Hilger, C., et al. 1994. Biological activities of a putative truncated hepatitis B virus X gene product fused to a polylysin stretch. *Oncogene*, **9**, 2613–21.

Raney, A.K. and McLachlan, A. 1995. Characterization of the hepatitis B virus large surface antigen promoter Sp1 binding site. *Virology*, **208**, 399–404.

Raney, A.K., Le, H.B. and McLachlan, A. 1992. Regulation of transcription from the hepatitis B virus major surface antigen promoter by the Sp1 transcription factor. *J Virol*, **66**, 6912–21.

Rehermann, B., Ferrari, C., et al. 1996. The hepatitis B virus persists for decades after patients' recovery from acute viral hepatitis despite active maintenance of a cytotoxic T-lymphocyte response. *Nat Med*, **2**, 1104–8.

Repp, R., Keller, C., et al. 1992. Detection of a hepatitis B virus variant with a truncated X gene and enhancer II. *Arch Virol*, **125**, 299–304.

Rockstroh, J.K. 2003. Management of hepatitis B and C in HIV co-infected patients. *J Acquir Immune Defic Syndr*, **34**, Suppl 1, S59–65.

Rogler, C.E. and Chisari, F.V. 1992. Cellular and molecular mechanisms of hepatocarcinogenesis. *Semin Liver Dis*, **12**, 265–78.

Roque-Afonso, A.M., Feray, C., et al. 2002. Antibodies to hepatitis B surface antigen prevent viral reactivation in recipients of liver grafts from anti-HBc positive donors. *Gut*, **50**, 95–9.

Rosmorduc, O., Petit, M.A., et al. 1995. In vivo and in vitro expression of defective hepatitis B virus particles generated by spliced hepatitis B virus RNA. *Hepatology*, **22**, 10–19.

Roth, W.K., Weber, M., et al. 2002. NAT for HBV and anti-HBc testing increase blood safety. *Transfusion*, **42**, 869–75.

Roy, M.J., Wu, M.S., et al. 2000. Induction of antigen-specific CD8+ T cells, T helper cells, and protective levels of antibody in humans by particle-mediated administration of a hepatitis B virus DNA vaccine. *Vaccine*, **19**, 764–78.

Ryu, S.H., Chung, Y.H., et al. 2003. Long-term additional lamivudine therapy enhances durability of lamivudine-induced HBeAg loss: a prospective study. *J Hepatol*, **39**, 614–19.

Saldanha, J., Gerlich, W., et al. 2001. An international collaborative study to establish a World Health Organization international standard for hepatitis B virus DNA nucleic acid amplification techniques. *Vox Sang*, **80**, 63–71.

Scaglioni, P.P., Melegari, M. and Wands, J.R. 1996. Biologic properties of hepatitis B viral genomes with mutations in the precore promoter and precore open reading frame. *Virology*, **233**, 374–81.

Schaefer, S. and Gerlich, W.H. 1995. In vitro transformation by hepatitis B virus DNA. *Intervirology*, **38**, 143–54.

Schaller, H. and Fischer, M. 1991. Hepatitis B virus. *Curr Top Microbiol Immunol*, **168**, 21–39.

Schlager, F., Schaefer, S., et al. 2000. Quantitative DNA fragment analysis for detecting low amounts of hepatitis B virus deletion mutants in highly viremic carriers. *Hepatology*, **32**, 1096–105.

Schlicht, H.F. and Schaller, H. 1989. Analysis of hepatitis B virus gene functions in tissue culture and in vivo. *Curr Top Microbiol Immunol*, **144**, 253–63.

Schlicht, H.J. and Wasenauer, G. 1991. The quaternary structure, antigenicity, and aggregational behavior of the secretory core protein of human hepatitis B virus are determined by its signal sequence. *J Virol*, **65**, 6817–25.

Schmitt, S., Glebe, D., et al. 1999. Analysis of the preS2 N- and O-linked glycans of the M surface protein from human hepatitis B virus. *J Biol Chem*, **274**, 11945–57.

Schmitt, S., Glebe, D., et al. 2004. Structure of preS2 N- and O-linked glycans in surface proteins from different genotypes of hepatitis B virus. *J Gen Virol*, **85**, 2045–53.

Schuster, R., Gerlich, W.H. and Schaefer, S. 2000. Induction of apoptosis by the transactivating domains of the hepatitis B virus X gene leads to suppression of oncogenic transformation of primary rat embryo fibroblasts. *Oncogene*, **19**, 1173–80.

Schuster, R., Hildt, E., et al. 2002. Conserved transactivating and pro-apoptotic functions of hepadnaviral X protein in ortho-and avihepadnaviruses. *Oncogene*, **21**, 6606–13.

Shapira, M.Y., Zeira, E., et al. 2001. Rapid seroprotection against hepatitis B following the first dose of a Pre-S1/Pre-S2/S vaccine. *J Hepatol*, **34**, 123–7.

Shibolet, O., Ilan, Y., et al. 2002. Lamivudine therapy for prevention of immunosuppressive-induced hepatitis B virus reactivation in hepatitis B surface antigen carriers. *Blood*, **100**, 391–6.

Shikata, T., Karasawa, T., et al. 1977. Hepatitis B e antigen and infectivity of hepatitis B virus. *J Infect Dis*, **136**, 571–6.

Shirakata, Y. and Koike, K. 2003. Hepatitis B virus X protein induces cell death by causing loss of mitochondrial membrane potential. *J Biol Chem*, **278**, 22071–8.

Sirma, H., Giannini, C., et al. 1999. Hepatitis B virus X mutants, present in hepatocellular carcinoma tissue abrogate both the antiproliferative and transactivation effects of HBx. *Oncogene*, **18**, 4848–59.

Sitia, G., Isogawa, M., et al. 2002. Depletion of neutrophils blocks the recruitment of antigen-nonspecific cells into the liver without affecting the antiviral activity of hepatitis B virus-specific cytotoxic T lymphocytes. *Proc Natl Acad Sci USA*, **99**, 13717–22.

Soussan, P., Tuveri, R., et al. 2003. The expression of hepatitis B spliced protein (HBSP) encoded by a spliced hepatitis B virus RNA is associated with viral replication and liver fibrosis. *J Hepatol*, **38**, 343–8.

Spandau, D.F. and Lee, C.H. 1988. Trans-activation of viral enhancers by the hepatitis B virus X protein. *J Virol*, **62**, 427–34.

Stockl, L., Berting, A., et al. 2003. Integrity of c-Raf-1/MEK signal transduction cascade is essential for hepatitis B virus gene expression. *Oncogene*, **22**, 2604–10.

Stoll-Becker, S., Repp, R., et al. 1997. Transcription of hepatitis B virus in peripheral blood mononuclear cells from persistently infected patients. *J Virol*, **71**, 5399–407.

Stuyver, L.J., Locarnini, S.A., et al. 2001. Nomenclature for antiviral-resistant human hepatitis B virus in the polymerase region. *Hepatology*, **33**, 751–7.

Su, F. and Schneider, R.J. 1997. Hepatitis B virus HBx protein sensitizes cells to apoptotic killing by tumor necrosis factor alpha. *Proc Natl Acad Sci USA*, **94**, 8744–9.

Su, G.G., Pan, K.H., et al. 2004. Efficacy and safety of lamivudine treatment for chronic hepatitis B in pregnancy. *World J Gastroenterol*, **10**, 910–12.

Su, Q., Schröder, C.H., et al. 1998. Expression of hepatitis B virus protein in HBV-infected human livers and hepatocellular carcinomas. *Hepatology*, **27**, 1109–20.

Summers, J. and Mason, W.S. 1982. Replication of the genome of a hepatitis B-like virus by reverse transcription of an RNA intermediate. *Cell*, **29**, 403–15.

Summers, J., Smith, P.M. and Horwich, A.L. 1990. Hepadnavirus envelope proteins regulate covalently closed circular DNA amplification. *J Virol*, **64**, 2819–24.

Sunyach, C., Rollier, C., et al. 1999. Residues critical for duck hepatitis B virus neutralization are involved in host cell interaction. *J Virol*, **73**, 2569–75.

Tamori, A., Nishiguchi, S., et al. 2003. HBV DNA integration and HBV-transcript expression in non-B, non-C hepatocellular carcinoma in Japan. *J Med Virol*, **71**, 492–8.

Tanaka, Y., Hasegawa, I., et al. 2004. A case-control study for differences among hepatitis B virus infections of genotypes A (suptypes Aa and Ae) and D. *Hepatology*, **40**, 747–55.

Tang, B., Kruger, W.D., et al. 2004. Hepatitis B viremia is associated with increased risk of hepatocellular carcinoma in chronic carriers. *J Med Virol*, **72**, 35–40.

Tang, H. and McLachlan, A. 2001. Transcriptional regulation of hepatitis B virus by nuclear hormone receptors is a critical determinant of viral tropism. *Proc Natl Acad Sci USA*, **98**, 1841–6.

Tenney, D.J. and Levine, S.M. 2004. Clinical emergence of entecavir-resistant hepatitis B virus requires additional substitutions in virus already resistant to Lamivudine. *Antimicrob Agents Chemother*, **48**, 3498–507.

Terradillos, O., Pollicino, T., et al. 1998. p53-independent apoptotic effects of the hepatitis B virus HBx protein in vivo and in vitro. *Oncogene*, **17**, 2115–23.

Terradillos, O., de La Coste, A., et al. 2002. The hepatitis B virus X protein abrogates Bcl-2-mediated protection against Fas apoptosis in the liver. *Oncogene*, **21**, 377–86.

Thomas, L. 2000. *Labor und Diagnose*, 5th edn. Frankfurt/Main: TH-Books.

Toh, H., Hayashida, H. and Miyata, T. 1983. Sequence homology between retroviral reverse transcriptase and putative polymerases of hepatitis B virus and cauliflower mosaic virus. *Nature (London)*, **305**, 827–9.

Tsuei, D.J., Chang, M.H., et al. 2002. Characterization of integration patterns and flanking cellular sequences of hepatitis B virus in childhood hepatocellular carcinomas. *J Med Virol*, **68**, 513–21.

Tuttleman, J.S., Pourcel, C. and Summers, J. 1986. Formation of the pool of covalently closed circular viral DNA in hepadnavirus-infected cells. *Cell*, **47**, 451–60.

Urban, S. and Gripon, P. 2002. Inhibition of duck hepatitis B virus infection by a myristoylated pre-S peptide of the large viral surface protein. *J Virol*, **76**, 1986–90.

Urban, S., Schwarz, C., et al. 2000. Receptor recognition by a hepatitis B virus reveals a novel mode of high affinity virus-receptor interaction. *EMBO J*, **19**, 1217–27.

Van Zonneveld, M., van Nunen, A.B., et al. 2003. Lamivudine treatment during pregnancy to prevent perinatal transmission of hepatitis B virus infection. *J Viral Hepat*, **10**, 294–7.

Vento, S., Garofano, T., et al. 1998. Fulminant hepatitis associated with hepatitis A virus superinfection in patients with chronic hepatitis C. *N Engl J Med*, **338**, 286–90.

Wang, G.H. and Seeger, C. 1993. Novel mechanism for reverse transcription in hepatitis B viruses. *J Virol*, **67**, 6507–12.

Wang, J., Chenivesse, X., et al. 1990. Hepatitis B virus integration in a cyclin A gene in a hepatocellular carcinoma. *Nature (London)*, **343**, 555–7.

Wang, J.T., Lee, C.Z., et al. 2002. Transfusion-transmitted HBV infection in an endemic area: the necessity of more sensitive screening for HBV carriers. *Transfusion*, **42**, 1592–7.

Wang, Z. and Zhang, J. 2003. Quantitative analysis of HBV DNA level and HBeAg titer in hepatitis B surface antigen positive mothers and their babies: HBeAg passage through the placenta and the rate of decay in babies. *J Med Virol*, **71**, 360–6.

West, D.J. 1993. Scope and design of hepatitis B vaccine clinical trials. In: Ellis, E.W. (ed.), *Hepatitis B virus in clinical practice*. New York, Basel, Hong Kong: Marcel Dekker, 159–78.

Westhoff, T.H., Jochimsen, F., et al. 2003. Fatal hepatitis B virus reactivation by an escape mutant following rituximab therapy. *Blood*, **102**, 1930.

Whittaker, G.R., Kann, M. and Helenius, A. 2000. Viral entry into the nucleus. *Annu Rev Cell Dev Biol*, **16**, 627–51.

Wieland, S.F., Spangenberg, H.C., et al. 2004. Expansion and contraction of the hepatitis B virus transcriptional template in infected chimpanzees. *Proc Natl Acad Sci USA*, **101**, 2129–34.

Wieland, S., Thimme, R., et al. 2004b. Genomic analysis of the host response to hepatitis B virus infection. *Proc Natl Acad Sci USA*, **101**, 6669–74.

Will, H., Cattaneo, R., et al. 1985. Infectious hepatitis B virus from cloned DNA of known nucleotide sequence. *Proc Natl Acad Sci USA*, **82**, 891–5.

Wilson, N., Ruff, T.A., et al. 2000. The effectiveness of the infant hepatitis B immunisation program in Fiji, Kiribati, Tonga and Vanuatu. *Vaccine*, **18**, 3059–66.

Wollersheim, M., Debelka, U. and Hofschneider, P.H. 1988. A transactivating function encoded in the hepatitis B virus X gene is conserved in the integrated state. *Oncogene*, **3**, 545–52.

Wu, C.G., Forgues, M., et al. 2002. SAGE transcript profiles of normal primary human hepatocytes expressing oncogenic hepatitis B virus X protein. *FASEB J*, **16**, 1665–7.

Xu, Z., Yen, T.S., et al. 2002. Enhancement of hepatitis B virus replication by its X protein in transgenic mice. *J Virol*, **76**, 2579–84.

Yaginuma, K., Shirakata, Y., et al. 1987. Hepatitis B virus (HBV) particles are produced in a cell culture system by transient expression of transfected HBV DNA. *Proc Natl Acad Sci USA*, **84**, 2678–82.

Yang, W. and Summers, J. 1998. Infection of ducklings with virus particles containing double-stranded duck hepatitis B virus DNAs illegitimate replication and reversion. *J Virol*, **72**, 8710–17.

Yeh, C.T., Shen, C.H., et al. 2000. Identification and characterization of a prevalent hepatitis B virus X protein mutant in Taiwanese patients with hepatocellular carcinoma. *Oncogene*, **19**, 5213–20.

Yoo, Y.G. and Lee, M.O. 2004. Hepatitis B virus X protein induces expression of Fas ligand gene through enhancing transcriptional activity of early growth response factor. *J Biol Chem*, **279**, 36242–9.

Yu, M.C., Yuan, J.M., et al. 1997. Presence of antibodies to the hepatitis B surface antigen is associated with an excess risk for hepatocellular carcinoma among non-Asian in Los Angeles County, California. *Hepatology*, **25**, 226–8.

Yu, X. and Mertz, J.E. 2001. Critical roles of nuclear receptor response elements in replication of hepatitis B virus. *J Virol*, **75**, 11354–64.

Zahm, P., Hofschneider, P.H. and Koshy, R. 1988. The HBV X-ORF encodes a transactivator: a potential factor in viral hepatocarcinogenesis. *Oncogene*, **3**, 169–77.

Zang, W.Q. and Yen, T.S. 1999. Distinct export pathway utilized by the hepatitis B virus posttranscriptional regulatory element. *Virology*, **259**, 299–304.

Zang, W.Q., Li, B., et al. 2001. Role of polypyrimidine tract binding protein in the function of the hepatitis B virus posttranscriptional regulatory element. *J Virol*, **75**, 10779–86.

Zhang, Z., Torii, N., et al. 2001. X-deficient woodchuck hepatitis virus mutants behave like attenuated viruses and induce protective immunity in vivo. *J Clin Invest*, **108**, 1523–31.

Zhang, Z., Protzer, U., et al. 2004. Inhibition of cellular proteasome activities enhances hepadnavirus replication in an HBx-dependent manner. *J Virol*, **78**, 4566–72.

Zhou, S. and Standring, D.N. 1992. Hepatitis B virus capsid particles are assembled from core-protein dimer precursors. *Proc Natl Acad Sci USA*, **89**, 10046–50.

Zlotnick, A., Johnson, J.M., et al. 1999. A theoretical model successfully identifies features of hepatitis B virus capsid assembly. *Biochemistry*, **38**, 14644–52.

Zoulim, F., Saputelli, J. and Seeger, C. 1994. Woodchuck hepatitis virus X protein is required for viral infection in vivo. *J Virol*, **68**, 2026–30.

Zuckerman, J.N., Zuckerman, A.J., et al. 2001. Evaluation of a new hepatitis B triple-antigen vaccine in inadequate responders to current vaccines. *Hepatology*, **34**, 798–802.

Hepatitis delta virus

JOHN M. TAYLOR

In 1977, the first clue to the existence of this virus came from a study of patients chronically infected with hepatitis B virus (HBV). A novel antigen, termed the delta antigen, was found in the hepatocyte nuclei of patient biopsies (Rizzetto et al. 1977). An initial interpretation was that the delta antigen might be a new variant of HBV. However, a more surprising explanation was subsequently obtained. By 1980, it was shown that this antigen was part of an infectious agent that could be transmitted to chimpanzees (Rizzetto et al. 1980). It is sometimes called the hepatitis delta agent, but more frequently hepatitis delta virus (HDV) or hepatitis D virus (HDV). Strictly speaking it is a subviral agent that is dependent upon HBV to provide the envelope proteins needed for the assembly of new virions. On one hand, this dependence of HDV replication on HBV means that many aspects of HDV and HBV biology overlap. On the other hand, the RNA genome of HDV and its strategy of replication have proven to have features unlike those of the helper HBV or any other infectious agent of animals.

PROPERTIES OF THE VIRUS

Classification

Currently, HDV is classified as the sole member of the genus *Deltavirus*. As mentioned above, it is a **satellite** of HBV, since its genome shows no obvious sequence relationship to that of HBV. The RNA genome of HDV and its mechanism of replication are unique relative to RNA viruses of animals, but, as discussed in the section on Plant viroid analogy below,

they show important similarities to certain infectious agents of plants.

Virion structure

In the serum of an HDV-infected individual, there are not only HDV particles but also the non-infectious, empty, surface antigen particles that are characteristic of HBV infection. The 42 nm diameter HBV may also be found, though surface antigen particles are always in at least 100-fold excess. The hepatitis B surface antigen particles, termed HBsAg, include both 22 nm diameter roughly spherical particles and elongated filaments. Several groups have tried to purify the HDV particles away from HBV and HBsAg particles. HDV was thus estimated to be around 38–43 nm in diameter (Bonino et al. 1984; He et al. 1989; Ryu et al. 1992). The envelope proteins of these particles include the same three found in HBV. Inside the HDV particle is the RNA genome and around 70 copies of the delta antigen (Ryu et al. 1993; Gudima et al. 2002). The size and shape of this HDV ribonucleoprotein structure may be more heterogeneous than initially claimed; it is certainly not like the more defined icosahedral core structures of HBV.

The single-stranded RNA genome of HDV is in several ways fundamentally different from other RNA viruses of animals (Lai 1995). At ca. 1 700 nt it is the smallest.

- The genome has a circular conformation whereas the other viral genomes are linear.
- The circle is able to fold on itself, with Watson and Crick base pairing of ca. 70 percent of the nucleotides, forming an unbranched rod-like structure.

- On the genome is a domain of about 85 nt, which acts as a self-cleaving ribozyme. When heated in vitro, in the presence of magnesium ions, this domain catalyzes a specific transesterification reaction. The reaction can also be reversed in vitro (Sharmeen et al. 1989), although there is evidence to suggest that in cultured cells, a host factor is needed to achieve ligation (Reid and Lazinski 2000). Recent studies have determined the structure of this ribozyme (Ferre-D'Amare et al. 1998) and the folding pathway followed to achieve this structure (Chadalavada et al. 2002).

Replication

As reviewed in Chapter 55, Hepatitis B, HBV is a hepatotropic virus but we still do not know the receptor(s) by which it enters hepatocytes. We do know, however, that antibodies against epitopes within the pre-S1 and pre-S2 domains of the HBV envelope proteins neutralize the virus. The same is true for HDV (Sureau et al. 1992). The replication of HDV in an infected animal is limited to the liver (Netter et al. 1994).

Inside infected cells there are not only HDV genomes but also complementary copies, called antigenomes. These have the same four properties mentioned for the genomes in the section on Virion structure above. In addition, the antigenomic RNA encodes, down one side of the rod-like structure, the 195 aa delta antigen. However, the antigenomic RNA, like the genomic RNA, is not translated. Translation of the delta antigen is considered dependent upon a third HDV RNA. This RNA is 5'-capped, 3'-polyadenylated, and cytoplasmic. Its size and sequence include the appropriate side of the antigenome; it is thus considered the mRNA for the delta antigen (Hsieh et al. 1990; Gudima et al. 1999). There is disagreement as to whether or not the mRNA transcription precedes that of antigenomic RNA or whether the two are separate and concurrent (Modahl and Lai 1998; Macnaughton et al. 2002). It has been estimated that an infected liver cell contains 300 000, 50 000, and 600 copies of the genome, antigenome, and mRNA, respectively (Chen et al. 1986). More recent quantitative studies indicate that during replication there is typically around 200 copies of the delta protein per molecule of genomic RNA (Gudima et al. 2002).

It is still not clear which host polymerase(s) carry out the HDV RNA synthesis. There is currently agreement that the host RNA polymerase II produces the transcripts of genomic RNA and mRNA (Modahl et al. 2000; Moraleda and Taylor 2001; Macnaughton et al. 2002). However, it has also been claimed that a different polymerase is needed to produce transcripts of antigenomic RNA (Modahl et al. 2000; Macnaughton et al. 2002).

Initially it was believed that during replication the majority of both genomic and HDV genomic RNAs were restricted to the nucleus (Taylor et al. 1987). More recent studies indicate that a significant fraction of the genomic RNA might by cytoplasmic (Gudima et al. 2002; Macnaughton and Lai 2002). There is even evidence that ribonucleoprotein complexes of HDV RNA and delta protein might undergo nuclear shuttling between the nucleus and the cytoplasm (Tavanez et al. 2002). Such complexes might also involve host proteins such as the splicing factor SC35 (Bichko and Taylor 1996), nucleolar proteins B23 and nucleolin (Lee et al. 1998; Huang et al. 2001), and the protein known as delta interacting protein A (Brazas and Ganem 1997).

During genome replication an ever-increasing fraction of the antigenomes undergo one or more post-transcriptional RNA-editing events. One such event is specific and essential for the life cycle. The adenosine located in the middle of the amber termination codon for the 195 aa delta antigen is deaminated by a host enzyme (Polson et al. 1996). Apparently only a small element of the rod-like folding structure of the antigenomic RNA is needed to define the target for this editing (Reid and Lazinski 2000). Transcription after editing leads to molecules of mRNA with the amber termination codon replaced by one for tryptophan. This altered mRNA encodes a somewhat longer protein, the 214-aa delta antigen. Both the small and large forms of the delta antigen are essential for HDV replication.

The small form of the delta antigen is required for genome replication (Kuo et al. 1989). The large delta antigen, which appears later in infection, does not support genome replication and, instead, can be a dominant-negative inhibitor of such replication (Chao et al. 1990). A more important property is that the large delta antigen is essential for the assembly of HDV ribonucleoprotein particles into new virions containing envelope proteins of the helper HBV (Chang et al. 1991). The large form becomes farnesylated at a site 4 aa from the new C terminus (Otto and Casey 1996). This modification is essential for virion formation (Glenn 1995; Glenn et al. 1998), presumably because it facilitates interactions with membranes and/or HBV envelope proteins. A monophosphorylated form of the large delta antigen has been detected, but only inside infected cells and not in serum particles (Bichko et al. 1997). Phosphorylated forms of the small delta protein have also been detected and may be needed for the support of genome replication (Mu et al. 2001).

The two forms of the delta antigen thus have quite distinct biological functions. At the same time, since they share a common 195 aa, they have some common properties (Hwang et al. 1995). These include:

- a domain involved in protein–protein dimerization and multimerization
- a bipartite signal which acts as a signal for localization to the nucleus

- a bipartite signal for protein–RNA interactions; the delta antigens have some specificity for recognizing HDV rodlike RNAs relative to other RNAs.

Both proteins are highly basic.

Experimental systems

The HBV envelope proteins are essential for virion formation, but replication of the HDV genome can be achieved in cells independent of the helper virus. Genome replication can be studied in established cell lines and even with in vitro systems.

Other than man, the only hosts that are known to allow complete replication of HDV are the chimpanzee and the woodchuck. The woodchuck hepatitis B virus (WHV) is a near relative of HBV, and it was found that HDV could replicate in woodchucks with WHV replacing HBV as helper (Ponzetto et al. 1984). Other hepadnaviruses, like duck hepatitis B virus (DHBV), are not able to support HDV replication; this may reflect the minimal ability of HDV to replicate in avian cells (Chang et al. 2000; Liu et al. 2001).

The only cultured animal cells that can be infected with HDV are primary hepatocytes. This is considered to reflect the need for the same receptors as used by the helper HBV. Thus, HDV with an HBV coat will infect human or chimpanzee hepatocytes (Sureau et al. 1991), and HDV that has been passaged in woodchucks, will infect woodchuck hepatocytes (Taylor et al. 1987). It is possible to implant human hepatocytes within the mouse and use these for HDV infection (Ohashi et al. 2000). Alternatively, injection of HDV into the mouse tail vein or peritoneal cavity can lead to infection of some mouse hepatocytes (Netter et al. 1993).

If one obviates the need for a receptor interaction by using techniques that directly fuse viral and cell membranes, then HDV can be introduced into established cell lines that are not necessarily of liver origin (Bichko et al. 1994). Under such conditions, HDV genome replication will occur. This can also be achieved by transfection of cells with HDV RNA or cDNA constructs. For RNA transfections, it is necessary that the small form of the delta antigen either is already present in the transfected cells or enters with the RNA. One interpretation is that HDV RNA will only migrate to the nucleus as a ribonucleoprotein complex with the delta antigen. In agreement with this idea, the initial requirement for a source of delta antigen can be met by providing a mRNA for this protein (Modahl and Lai 1998). Transfection can also be used to initiate HDV genome replication in mouse skeletal muscle (Polo et al. 1995a) and in mouse liver (Chang et al. 2001). Finally, using mice, made transgenic for HDV cDNA sequences, HDV genome replication can be detected in multiple tissues (Polo et al. 1995b).

If transfected cultured cells are also expressing the envelope proteins of the helper virus, then HDV virus-like particles are released. These will be infectious if not only the small but also the large envelope proteins of HBV are present; the large envelope protein contains the pre-S1, domain that is essential for HBV receptor interactions (Sureau et al. 1992).

Plant viroid analogy

Even though HDV is in many respects unique among RNA viruses of animals, it does seem to have some relatives in the plant world. Viroids, of which more than 25 have been described, are subviral agents of plants. Like HDV, they have small single-stranded RNA genomes that are circular in conformation and able to replicate via redirection of the host RNA polymerase II. In some cases they are known to contain both self-cleavage domains and the ability to self-ligate. However, unlike HDV, they are much smaller (only 240–375 nt), encode no proteins, and are not dependent in any way on a helper virus (Taylor 1999). In addition to the viroids there are also plant agents sometimes referred to as virusoids, which share similarities to HDV. However, the virusoids, unlike the viroids and HDV, replicate via an RNA polymerase provided by a helper virus (Taylor 1999).

CLINICAL AND PATHOLOGICAL ASPECTS

Transmission

Like HBV, HDV is a blood-borne pathogen. Cycles of HDV replication are dependent upon the envelope proteins produced by HBV; nevertheless, the modes of successful HDV transmission can be somewhat different from those of HBV. (Expression of envelope proteins via integrated copies of HBV DNA, might be able to support HDV replication cycles.) HDV is transmitted via contaminated needles among drug abusers and via blood products and transfusions. Sexual transmission is rare and so is perinatal transmission.

In natural situations, cycles of HDV replication fall into two classes: superinfections, where the patient is already infected with HBV, or co-infections, where the patient receives both HDV and the helper HBV at the same time. Superinfections are more likely than co-infections to lead to fulminant hepatitis. It has been hypothesized that since HDV replication may be aided by a more aggressive HBV replication, it could be the response of the host to the HBV replication that is the principal cause of pathogenesis (Casey et al. 1996). Some HDV infections pass through the acute phase and survive as a chronic infection. Such chronicity is also dependent upon a chronic HBV infection; thus, it should not be a surprise that HDV superinfections of patients already chronically infected with HBV are more likely, after the acute phase, to proceed onto chronicity.

A third mechanism of HDV infection was considered to arise in some patients with terminal HDV-associated cirrhosis that are given a liver transplantation from a virus-free donor. The interpretation was that hepatocytes of the new liver can first become infected by HDV alone; these would be nonproductive or latent infections, in which genome replication occurs but no particles are produced. Later, superinfection of such hepatocytes with HBV could lead to rescue and spread of the HDV (Rizzetto and Ponzetto 1995). Analogous latent infections were considered to be produced in experimental animals (Netter et al. 1994). More recently, the concept of latent infections, especially in humans, has been called into question because of evidence that at no time was HBV actually totally absent (Smedile et al. 1998).

Detection and clinical manifestations

There are several serum-based, commercially available, assays for HDV infection. The most widely used test is for antibodies (IgM and/or IgG) directed against the delta antigen. Tests that are more expensive are available for detection in serum of the delta antigen or the genomic RNA. Hybridization assays typically need more than 105 viral genomes per sample. By the use of reverse transcriptase to produce cDNA copies and the subsequent amplification of this cDNA with the polymerase chain reaction, as little as 10 molecules of the genome can be detected; however, sequence heterogeneity between isolates can render difficult the choice of appropriate oligonucleotide primers (Niro et al. 1997).

At one time, liver biopsy, with direct detection of delta antigen by immunohistochemistry, was considered the gold standard for detection of HDV infections (Rizzetto and Ponzetto 1995). However, in chronic infections, the number of infected hepatocytes and the level of replication per infected hepatocyte can be too low for easy detection. Not surprisingly, with more sophisticated in situ hybridization procedures, the sensitivity of detection can be increased. The possibility of adverse consequences of liver biopsy recommends against the use of this approach for routine purposes.

HDV infections may not always have a pathogenic effect. For example, on one Greek island there was an endemic chronic infection with both HBV and HDV, and yet infected individuals had no detectable signs of liver damage (Hadziyannis et al. 1993). By contrast, there have been local epidemics of HDV in the Amazon Basin of South America associated with a high incidence of fulminant hepatitis and death. It is possible that in such individuals there is an excessive HBV replication with associated immune response and liver damage and that the HDV, which after all depends upon HBV, replicates more efficiently (Casey et al. 1996). Early studies ascribed for such patients specific histological lesions, such as cytoplasmic eosinophilia, and microvesicular steatosis without an inflammatory infiltrate. Later studies argue against any direct involvement of HDV markers in such lesions. The lesions may reflect derangement in the secretory pathway of certain hepatocytes (Rizzetto and Ponzetto 1995) or the consequences of exposure to interferon presumably induced in response to the viral infection (Shimizu and Purcell 1989).

As recently reviewed (Gerin et al. 2001), the incubation period prior to an acute HDV infection is about 3–7 weeks. This is followed by a preicteric phase of about 1 week during which there can be various nonspecific symptoms, such as fatigue, lethargy, anorexia, and nausea. During this time the levels of virus in serum rise to a peak, and then fall, usually within a period of a few days. Peak titers of 10^{10}–10^{12} HDV particles per ml can be detected in the serum. Such titers are much higher than for HBV, which usually do not exceed 10^9–10^{10} particles per ml, but are similar to the titer of HBsAg 22 nm particles. Also detected in serum is an increase in biochemical markers of liver damage, such as alanine and aspartate aminotransferases. The appearance of jaundice defines the next phase, the icteric phase. Fatigue and nausea may persist. Serum bilirubin levels may become abnormal. Although the markers of HDV replication are decreasing, this phase may be the most severe clinical stage. At this point, a fulminant hepatitis may occur, but this is rare, though about ten times more frequent than for hepatitis induced by HBV alone, or by other hepatitis viruses. For most coinfections, the patient recovers over a period of weeks to months, and HDV infection is cleared. By contrast, with superinfections, the acute phase is usually followed by a chronic HDV infection. Such chronicity has a high chance of proceeding to cirrhosis and even hepatic failure. It has been previously thought that chronic HDV infections can progress not only to cirrhosis but also to hepatocellular carcinoma (Fattovich et al. 2000). One evaluation suggests that while chronic HDV infections frequently increase the risk of cirrhosis, they may only indirectly via HBV, increase the risk of hepatocellular carcinoma (Kew 1996).

Epidemiology and phylogenetics

HDV has been detected in many parts of the world, including Europe (Italy, Spain), Asia (China, Taiwan, Japan), the former USSR, and South America (Amazon Basin, Peru). The incidence in the USA is relatively low.

Chronic HBV infections are currently estimated at around 400 million worldwide. In 1993 it was estimated that there were around 25 million chronic cases of (both HBV and HDV) (Alter and Hadler 1993). However, worldwide the HDV levels are decreasing with the impact of HBV vaccination (which also protects against HDV), testing of blood prior to transfusions, and in some cases, altered patterns of intravenous drug usage. New cases of HDV are becoming rare and chronic HDV is being referred to as a 'vanishing disease' (Gaeta et al. 2000).

Primary sequence differences between isolates can be as much as 40 percent. Such sequence differences have been used to divide isolates into genotypes I–III. Genotype I contains the majority of isolates and it has been divided further into subgroups (Niro et al. 1997). Genotype II consists of several isolates from East Asia. Newer data suggest it is almost as widespread as genotype I (Ivaniushina et al. 2001). Genotype III includes only a small number of isolates from life-threatening infections in the Amazon Basin of South America. It is difficult to determine to what extent this pathogenesis is specific for the genotype of HDV relative to that due to the replication of the associated HBV, of genotype F (Casey et al. 1996; Gerin et al. 2001). Studies with transfected cells have shown that there are limitations in the ability of genomes of one genotype to be assisted in replication by the small delta proteins of other genotypes (Casey and Gerin 1998).

Pathogenicity and interactions with the helper virus

It has been reported that when the small form of the delta antigen is expressed in cultured cells there can be an associated cytopathic effect (Cole et al. 1991). In contrast to this, mice made transgenic for the expression of either the small or large forms of the delta antigen fail to show any associated pathology (Guilhot et al. 1994). Overall, it is agreed that there are no striking direct cytopathic effects of HDV (or HBV) replication (Gowans and Bonino 1993).

Nevertheless, HDV replication does have consequences for the infected cell. For example, mice experimentally infected with HDV showed that a small fraction of the hepatocytes became infected and were, within several days, somehow replaced, even in mice with a severe combined immunodeficiency (Netter et al. 1993). Also, some studies in tissue culture do support the interpretation that in cells replicating the HDV genome the rate of cell division is decreased (Bichko and Taylor 1996; Wang et al. 2001).

It has been noted that at the peak of an acute HDV infection, replication of the helper virus may be transiently suppressed (Gerin et al. 2001). However, in some cases this suppression can be as little as several-fold (Netter et al. 1994). It must be realized that there can also be evidence for 'interference' in patients infected with hepatitis C virus (HCV) superimposed on HBV and HDV (Jardi et al. 2001).

Treatment

Treatments with interferon-alpha are known to suppress particle production. However, the doses have to be very high and associated side effects are substantial. Moreover, when the patient is withdrawn from therapy, HDV production usually promptly resumes. The cure rate ascribable to such treatment, after subtraction of spontaneous cures, is probably <20 percent (Rizzetto and Ponzetto 1995; Lau et al. 1999).

A reasonable expectation was that suppression of HBV replication and assembly would indirectly suppress HDV replication. It was expected that some of the inhibitors, such as lamivudine, that act so potently on HBV replication should therefore inhibit HDV. Even the effects of interferon-alpha on HDV in large part might be indirect, via suppression of the HBV. However, from a study of four patients given 1 year of lamivudine therapy, it was observed that HDV RNA levels in the serum did not significantly decrease and liver damage continued (Lau et al. 1999).

Vaccination

In most cases, an HDV-specific vaccine is not needed since that for HBV is effective, indirectly. However, for individuals already chronically infected with HBV, an HDV vaccine might be of use. Several preliminary studies have used the delta antigen for vaccination, with variable success (Rizzetto and Ponzetto 1995).

REFERENCES

Alter, M. and Hadler, S.C. 1993. Delta hepatitis and infection in North America. *Prog Clin Biol Res*, **382**, 243–50.

Bichko, V.V. and Taylor, J.M. 1996. Redistribution of the delta antigens in cells replicating the genome of hepatitis delta virus. *J Virol*, **70**, 8064–70.

Bichko, V., Netter, H.J., et al. 1994. Introduction of hepatitis delta virus into animal cell lines via cationic liposomes. *J Virol*, **68**, 5247–52.

Bichko, V., Barik, S. and Taylor, J. 1997. Phosphorylation of the hepatitis delta virus antigens. *J Virol*, **71**, 512–18.

Bonino, F., Hoyer, W., et al. 1984. Delta hepatitis agent: structural and antigenic properties of the delta associated-particles. *Infect Immun*, **43**, 1000–5.

Brazas, R. and Ganem, D. 1997. Delta-interacting protein A and the origin of hepatitis delta antigen. *Science*, **276**, 825.

Casey, J.L. and Gerin, J.L. 1998. Genotype-specific complementation of hepatitis delta virus RNA replication by hepatitis delta antigen. *J Virol*, **72**, 2806–14.

Casey, J.L., Niro, G.A., et al. 1996. Hepatitis B virus/hepatitis D virus (HDV) coinfection in outbreaks of acute hepatitis in the Peruvian Amazon basin: the roles of HDV genotype III and HBV genotype F. *J Infect Dis*, **174**, 920–4.

Chadalavada, D.M., Senchak, S.E., et al. 2002. The folding pathway of the genomic hepatitis delta virus ribozyme is dominated by slow folding of the pseudoknots. *J Mol Biol*, **317**, 559–75.

Chang, F.L., Chen, P.J., et al. 1991. The large form of hepatitis δ antigen is crucial for the assembly of hepatitis δ virus. *Proc Natl Acad Sci U S A*, **88**, 8490–4.

Chang, J., Moraleda, G., et al. 2000. Limitations to the replication of hepatitis delta virus in avian cells. *J Virol*, **74**, 8861–6.

Chang, J., Sigal, L.J., et al. 2001. Replication of the human hepatitis delta virus genome is initiated in mouse hepatocytes following intravenous injection of naked DNA or RNA sequences. *J Virol*, **75**, 3469–73.

Chao, M., Hsieh, S.-Y., et al. 1990. Role of two forms of the hepatitis delta virus antigen: evidence for a mechanism of self-limiting genome replication. *J Virol*, **64**, 5066–9.

Chen, P.-J., Kalpana, G., et al. 1986. Structure and replication of the genome of hepatitis δ virus. *Proc Natl Acad Sci U S A*, **83**, 8774–8.

Cole, S., Gowans, E.J., et al. 1991. Direct evidence for cytotoxicity associated with expression of hepatitis delta virus antigen. *Hepatology*, **13**, 845–51.

Fattovich, G., Giustina, G., et al. 2000. Influence of hepatitis delta virus infection on morbidity and mortality in compensated cirrhosis type B. *Gut*, **46**, 420–6.

Ferre-D'Amare, A.R., Zhou, K., et al. 1998. Crystal structure of a hepatitis delta virus ribozyme. *Nature*, **395**, 567–74.

Gaeta, G.B., Stroffolini, T., et al. 2000. Chronic hepatitis D: a vanishing disease? An Italian multicenter study. *Hepatology*, **32**, 824–7.

Gerin, J.L., Casey, J.L., et al. 2001. Hepatitis delta virus. In: Knipe, D.M. and Howley, P.M. (eds), *Fields virology*, vol. 2. . Philadelphia: Lippincott Williams and Wilkins, 3037–50.

Glenn, J.S. 1995. Prenylation and virion morphogenesis. In: Dinter-Gottlieb, G. (ed.), *The unique hepatitis delta virus*. Austin, TX: R. G. Landes, Co., 83–94.

Glenn, J.S., Marsters, J.C. Jr, et al. 1998. Use of a prenylation inhibitor as a novel antiviral agent. *J Virol*, **72**, 9303–6.

Gowans, E.J. and Bonino, F. 1993. Hepatitis delta virus pathogenicity. *Prog Clin Biol Res*, **382**, 125–30.

Gudima, S., Dingle, K., et al. 1999. Characterization of the 5′-ends for polyadenylated RNAs synthesized during the replication of hepatitis delta virus. *J Virol*, **73**, 6533–9.

Gudima, S.O., Chang, J., et al. 2002. Parameters of human hepatitis delta virus replication: the quantity, quality, and intracellular distribution of viral proteins and RNA. *J Virol*, **76**, 3709–19.

Guilhot, S., Huang, S.-N., et al. 1994. Expression of hepatitis delta virus large and small antigens in transgenic mice. *J Virol*, **68**, 1052–8.

Hadziyannis, S.J., Dourakis, S.P., et al. 1993. Changing epidemiology and spreading modalities of hepatitis delta infection in Greece. *Prog Clin Biol Res*, **382**, 259–66.

He, L.-F., Ford, E., et al. 1989. The size of the hepatitis delta agent. *J Med Virol*, **27**, 31–3.

Hsieh, S.-Y., Chao, M., et al. 1990. Hepatitis delta virus genome replication: a polyadenylated mRNA for delta antigen. *J Virol*, **64**, 3192–8.

Huang, W.H., Yung, B.Y., et al. 2001. The nucleolar phosphoprotein B23 interacts with hepatitis delta antigens and modulates the hepatitis delta virus RNA replication. *J Biol Chem*, **276**, 25166–75.

Hwang, S.B., Jeng, K.-S., et al. 1995. Studies of functional roles of hepatitis delta antigen in delta virus RNA replication. In: Dinter-Gottlieb, G. (ed.), *The unique hepatitis delta virus*. Austin, TX: R. G. Landes, Co., 95–110.

Ivaniushina, V., Radjef, N., et al. 2001. Hepatitis delta virus genotypes I and II cocirculate in an endemic area of Yakutia, Russia. *J Gen Virol*, **82**, 2709–18.

Jardi, R., Rodriguez, F., et al. 2001. Role of hepatitis B, C and D viruses in dual and triple infection: influence of viral genotypes and hepatitis B precore and basal core promoter mutations on viral replicative interference. *Hepatology*, **34**, 404–10.

Kew, M.C. 1996. Hepatitis delta virus and hepatocellular carcinoma. *Viral Hepatitis Rev*, **2**, 285–90.

Kuo, M.Y.-P., Chao, M., et al. 1989. Initiation of replication of the human hepatitis delta virus genome from cloned DNA: role of delta antigen. *J Virol*, **63**, 1945–50.

Lai, M.M.C. 1995. The molecular biology of hepatitis delta virus. *Annu Rev Biochem*, **64**, 259–86.

Lau, D.T., Doo, E., et al. 1999. Lamivudine for chronic delta hepatitis. *Hepatology*, **30**, 546–9.

Lee, C.-H., Chang, S.C., et al. 1998. The nucleolin binding activity of hepatitis delta antigen is associated with nucleolus targeting. *J Biol Chem*, **273**, 7650–6.

Liu, Y.T., Brazas, R., et al. 2001. Efficient hepatitis delta virus RNA replication in avian cells requires a permissive factor(s) from mammalian cells. *J Virol*, **75**, 7489–93.

Macnaughton, T.B. and Lai, M.M. 2002. Genomic but not antigenomic hepatitis delta virus RNA is preferentially exported from the nucleus immediately after synthesis and processing. *J Virol*, **76**, 3928–35.

Macnaughton, T.B., Shi, S.T., et al. 2002. Rolling circle replication of hepatitis delta virus RNA is carried out by two different cellular RNA polymerases. *J Virol*, **76**, 3920–7.

Modahl, L.E. and Lai, M.M.C. 1998. Transcription of hepatitis delta antigen mRNA continues throughout hepatitis delta virus (HDV) replication: a new model of HDV RNA transcription and regulation. *J Virol*, **72**, 5449–56.

Modahl, L.E., Macnaughton, T.B., et al. 2000. RNA-dependent replication and transcription of hepatitis delta virus RNA involve distinct cellular RNA polymerases. *Mol Cell Biol*, **20**, 6030–9.

Moraleda, G. and Taylor, J. 2001. Host RNA polymerase requirements for transcription of the human hepatitis delta virus genome. *J Virol*, **75**, 10161–9.

Mu, J.J., Chen, D.S., et al. 2001. The conserved serine 177 in the delta antigen of hepatitis delta virus is one putative phosphorylation site and is required for efficient viral RNA replication. *J Virol*, **75**, 9087–95.

Netter, H.J., Kajino, K., et al. 1993. Experimental transmission of human hepatitis delta virus to the laboratory mouse. *J Virol*, **67**, 3357–62.

Netter, H.J., Gerin, J.L., et al. 1994. Apparent helper-independent infection of woodchucks by hepatitis delta virus and subsequent rescue with woodchuck hepatitis virus. *J Virol*, **68**, 5344–50.

Niro, G.A., Smedile, A., et al. 1997. The predominance of hepatitis delta virus genotype I among chronically infected Italian patients. *Hepatology*, **25**, 728–34.

Ohashi, K., Marion, P.L., et al. 2000. Sustained survival of human hepatocytes in mice: a model for in vivo infection with human hepatitis B and hepatitis delta viruses. *Nat Med*, **6**, 327–31.

Otto, J.C. and Casey, P.J. 1996. The hepatitis delta virus large antigen is farnesylated both in vitro and in animal cells. *J Biol Chem*, **271**, 4569–72.

Polo, J.M., Jeng, K.-S., et al. 1995a. Transgenic mice support replication of hepatitis delta virus RNA in multiple tissues, particularly in skeletal muscle. *J Virol*, **69**, 4880–7.

Polo, J.M., Lim, B., et al. 1995b. Replication of hepatitis delta virus RNA in mice after intramuscular injection of plasmid DNA. *J Virol*, **69**, 5203–7.

Polson, A.G., Bass, B.L., et al. 1996. RNA editing of hepatitis delta virus antigenome by dsRNA-adenosine deaminase. *Nature*, **380**, 454–6.

Ponzetto, A., Cote, P.J., et al. 1984. Transmission of the hepatitis B virus-associated δ agent to the eastern woodchuck. *Proc Natl Acad Sci U S A*, **81**, 2208–12.

Reid, C.E. and Lazinski, D.W. 2000. A host-specific function is required for ligation of a wide variety of ribozyme-processed RNAs. *Proc Natl Acad Sci U S A*, **97**, 424–9.

Rizzetto, M. and Ponzetto, A. 1995. Hepatitis delta virus infection: medical aspects. In: Dinter-Gottlieb, G. (ed.), *The unique hepatitis delta virus*. Austin, TX: R. G. Landes, Co., 125–39.

Rizzetto, M., Canese, M.G., et al. 1977. Immunofluorescence detection of a new antigen-antibody system associated to the hepatitis B virus in the liver and in the serum of HBsAg carriers. *Gut*, **18**, 997–1003.

Rizzetto, M., Canese, M.G., et al. 1980. Transmission of the hepatitis B virus-associated delta antigen to chimpanzees. *J Infect Dis*, **141**, 590–602.

Ryu, W.S., Bayer, M., et al. 1992. Assembly of hepatitis delta virus particles. *J Virol*, **66**, 2310–15.

Ryu, W.S., Netter, H.J., et al. 1993. Ribonucleoprotein complexes of hepatitis delta virus. *J Virol*, **67**, 3281–7.

Sharmeen, L., Kuo, M.Y., et al. 1989. Self-ligating RNA sequences on the antigenome of human hepatitis delta virus. *J Virol*, **63**, 1428–30.

Shimizu, Y.K. and Purcell, R.H. 1989. Cytoplasmic antigen of hepatocytes infected with non-A, non-B hepatitis or hepatitis delta virus: relationship to interferon. *Hepatology*, **10**, 764–8.

Smedile, A., Casey, J.L., et al. 1998. Hepatitis D viremia following orthotopic liver transplantation involves a typical HDV virion with a hepatitis B surface antigen envelope. *Hepatology*, **27**, 1723–9.

Sureau, C., Jacob, J.R., et al. 1991. Tissue culture system for infection with human hepatitis delta virus. *J Virol*, **65**, 3443–50.

Sureau, C., Moriarty, A.M., et al. 1992. Production of infectious hepatitis delta virus in vitro and neutralization with antibodies directed against hepatitis B virus pre-S antigens. *J Virol*, **66**, 1241–5.

Tavanez, J.P., Cunha, C., et al. 2002. Hepatitis delta virus ribonucleoproteins shuttle between the nucleus and the cytoplasm. *RNA*, **8**, 637–46.

Taylor, J., Mason, W., et al. 1987. Replication of human hepatitis delta virus in primary cultures of woodchuck hepatocytes. *J Virol*, **61**, 2891–5.

Taylor, J.M. 1999. Replication of human hepatitis delta virus: influence of studies on subviral plant pathogens. *Adv Vir Res*, **54**, 45–60.

Wang, D., Pearlberg, J., et al. 2001. Deleterious effects of hepatitis delta virus replication on host cell proliferation. *J Virol*, **75**, 3600–3604.

57

TT virus and other anelloviruses

MAURO BENDINELLI AND FABRIZIO MAGGI

TT virus (TTV) is one of several human viruses discovered in recent years, following the development of sensitive techniques for showing foreign nucleic acids in tissues. Soon after the discovery, it became clear that this novel virus was just one of a vast group of related, previously unrecognized viral agents, all of which were characterized by small, circular single-stranded DNA genomes with negative polarity. Presently, all these viruses are classified within a new genus, *Anellovirus*, that includes two species clearly distinct for their different genome sizes, TTV and TT minivirus (TTMV) [previously referred to as TTV-like minivirus (TLMV)].

Knowledge on TTV and related viruses has accumulated rapidly, but many fundamental aspects remain unresolved, particularly their significance for human health. In fact, anelloviruses have been found to be amazingly widespread, with abundant viral DNA detectable in the plasma of 80 percent or more of the general population worldwide, but in spite of this and the publication of more than 500 papers, no associated clinical disease has yet been identified. This unprecedented situation has actually led to the proposal that anelloviruses should be considered completely nonpathogenic and be regarded as the first recognized viral member of the normal commensal microflora (Mushahwar 2000). This view appears, however, somewhat premature considering all the many issues that still wait to be addressed (Bendinelli et al. 2001; Simmonds 2002).

DISCOVERY

TTV was first described in 1997 by Japanese workers who detected part of its genome whilst, in an attempt to identify additional agents of human hepatitis, were comparing by representational difference analysis, the nucleic acids contained in sequential blood samples of a patient (TT) with cryptogenetic post-transfusion hepatitis (Nishizawa et al. 1997). TTV discovery was soon followed by the detection, in diseased and healthy individuals, of numerous other viruses with genome properties clearly akin to those of TTV although often very divergent from it and from each other in sequence. The latter received specific names – SANBAN, YONBAN (meaning the third and the fourth, respectively, in Japanese), PMV, SENV, KAV – or were indicated with numbers (Hijikata et al. 1999; Hallett et al. 2000; Primi et al. 2000; Takahashi et al. 2000a; Tanaka et al. 2001) but are now classified as distinct genotypes of TTV. Furthermore, polymerase chain reaction (PCR) testing of certain blood donors for TTV produced shorter amplicons than expected, and further characterization revealed the existence of additional viruses also clearly related to TTV but with smaller genomes, namely TTMV (Takahashi et al. 2000b).

VIRIONS AND GENOMES

Physicochemical and immunoelectron microscopy studies have shown that the TTV particle has a density of 1.31–1.35 g/ml and is approximately spherical, 30–32 nm in diameter, and devoid of external lipids (Okamoto et al. 1998; Mushahwar et al. 1999; Itoh et al. 2000). Although most information on virion structure has been obtained with genotype 1, there are no indications that significant genotype-related differences might exist within TTV. TTMV, however, has a smaller size, as determined by filtration (Takahashi et al. 2000b). Like other non-enveloped viruses, both TTV and TTMV are unaffected by ether and chloroform and are believed to resist chemical and physical inactivating agents at least as effectively as parvoviruses and circoviruses (Todd et al. 2001).

Complete or near complete genome sequences, determined for a number of TTV and TTMV isolates, have revealed a high degree of divergence between the two viruses. The DNA of TTV is approximately 3 800 nt long (Erker et al. 1999; Kamahora et al. 2000; Muljono et al. 2001; Okamoto and Mayumi 2001; Hino 2002) whilst that of TTMV ranges around 2.8 kb. The general organization of the two genome types is, however, similar. Approximately one-third of their length has no coding functions (untranslated region (UTR)), but appears to control virus replication and expression through a number of regulatory sequences and secondary structures. Prominent among the latter is a stretch of approximately 100 nt with high guanine and cytosine content (GC region; Miyata et al. 1999). A number of such regulatory elements are highly conserved among TTV and TTMV isolates and are therefore exploited for designing universal primers (see below).

As deduced from the sequences, whilst no open reading frames (ORF) are present in the genomic DNA of either viruses, the antigenomes contain one large ORF (ORF1) and several partially or totally overlapping smaller ones (Kakkola et al. 2002; Yokoyama et al. 2002). ORF1 has a coding capacity of 770 and 675 amino acids in TTV and TTMV, respectively. The deduced encoded protein, which represents the putative capsid protein, contains an arginine-rich hydrophobic region at the N terminus, three hypervariable regions (HVR) (HVR-1, 2, and 3) located centrally, and variable numbers of potential glycosylation sites (Hijikata et al. 1999). The other ORFs are variously conserved amongst different genotypes. ORF2 encodes putative nonstructural proteins of approximately 120 and 100 amino acids in TTV and TTMV, respectively, which might have kinase activity in at least some genotypes. ORF3 seems to lead to two differently phosphorylated proteins, thus resembling gene *NS5A* of hepatitis C virus (HCV) (Asabe et al. 2001).

TAXONOMY AND NOMENCLATURE

At the time TTV was discovered, all known viruses of vertebrates with small circular, single-stranded DNA genomes were classified within the family *Circoviridae*, leading to the suggestion that the new virus should also be included in this family. Indeed, TTV has a high genome-relatedness to the *Chicken anemia virus* (CAV), a circovirus that causes damages to the poultry industry. However, the creation of a new virus family was also proposed (Mushahwar et al. 1999; Takahashi et al.

2000b; Okamoto and Mayumi 2001) to accommodate the considerable differences existing with other circoviruses [*Porcine circovirus* (PCV), *Beak and feather disease virus* (BFDV) of parrots], even though the latter have ambisense and not negative-strand genomes like CAV, TTV, and TTMV. More recently, following the advice of an appointed study group, the International Committee for the Taxonomy of Viruses (ICTV) has decided to classify TTV and TTMV as distinct species within a newly created, temporarily self-standing genus named *Anellovirus* (from *anellus*, Latin for ring). The ICTV has also decided to change the extended names of the two viruses in torque-teno-virus (TTV) (from the Latin words *torques* and *tenuis*, meaning necklace and thin, respectively) and torque-teno-minivirus (TTMV). This was suggested to conform to the rule that no official virus designation should be derived from people's names, without having to extensively modify the acronyms (Hino 2002).

Both TTV and TTMV show a remarkable degree of genetic heterogeneity. This diversity, which is especially high in the coding portion of the genomes (for example, amino acid divergence is as high as 68 percent in the ORF1 of isolates TA278 and SANBAN) has been exploited in order to group isolates. The criteria adopted for TTV are similar to the ones used for HCV: genotypes (identified by Arabic numbers) are defined by nucleotide divergences of 30 percent or greater, and subtypes (identified by small letters) by nucleotide divergences of between 15 percent and 29 percent. By such criteria, at least 40 genotypes of TTV, each (or most) subdivided in several subtypes, are presently known. In addition, genotypes have been clustered into five major TTV groups (designated 1–5), distinct from one another by nucleotide divergences of 50 percent or greater (Table 57.1). TTMV has been less investigated but existing data indicate that it may be even more diversified than TTV: comparison of full-length and ORF1 sequences has so far identified three clusters diverging by 40 percent or more at the nucleotide level (Table 57.1). Due to their considerable genetic distances, it is likely that in the future TTV genogroups will come to be regarded as distinct species. For both TTV and TTMV, the recognition of much greater diversity is expected with analysis of increasing numbers of sequences. It should also be noted that TTV-like viruses have been detected in several species of nonhuman primates, other mammals, and birds (Leary et al. 1999; Abe et al. 2000; Okamoto et al. 2002). From the limited amount of sequence data available, it would appear that primate viruses have undergone long-term co-evolution with their host species (Simmonds 2002).

INTERACTIONS WITH INFECTED CELLS

TTV and TTMV can been found in many tissues of the body and this, together with the demonstration of

Table 57.1 *Viruses recently classified in the genus* Anellovirus

Virus	Genogroup	No. of genotypes included	Representative isolates	Reference
TTV	1	6	TA278	Nishizawa et al. 1997
	2	6	PMV	Hallett et al. 2000
			KAV	Heller et al. 2001
	3	15	SANBAN	Hijikata et al. 1999
			SENV	Primi et al. 2000
	4	9	YONBAN	Takahashi et al. 2000a
			CT23	Peng et al. 2002
	5	4	JT33	Peng et al. 2002
TLMV	1	At least 4	CBD203	Takahashi et al. 2000b
			PB4TL	Biagini et al. 2001
	2	At least 2	CBD231	Takahashi et al. 2000b
	3	At least 2	NLC023	Biagini et al. 2001

replicative nucleic acid intermediates of TTV in several tissues, has suggested that both viruses might infect many different cell types (see below). However, the precise cell type(s) that support virus replication remain undetermined (Takahashi et al. 2002; Yu et al. 2002). In culture, only fresh human peripheral blood mononuclear cells have hitherto been found to permit TTV propagation (Maggi et al. 2001b; Mariscal et al. 2002).

Current understanding of TTV and TTMV replication mechanisms is scanty and mostly inferred from what is known about CAV. CAV grows in lymphoid cell lines and other cell types, is found in the nucleus, and appears to depend on cell proteins expressed during the S-phase for replication (Todd et al. 2001). TTV also appears to replicate in activated, but not resting, lymphoid cells (Maggi et al. 2001b; Mariscal et al. 2002). Viral DNA replication is believed to occur by the rolling circle mechanism. Such a mechanism, which is particularly well suited for replicating single-stranded DNA viruses, is indicated by the presence in the deduced ORF1 product of conserved Rep protein motifs typical of the many viruses that replicate in this manner (Hino 2002). It should be noted, however, that the great genetic diversity of TTV has also led to the theory that polymerases with low proofreading activity intervene (Umemura et al. 2001b). Indeed, the rates of nucleotide change reported for the HVR of TTV (up to 7.3×10^{-4} per site per year) are at least tenfold higher than in hepatitis B virus (HBV) and other DNA viruses and in a range similar to RNA viruses (Umemura et al. 2001b). Transcription profiles are poorly understood. Recently, TTV genome transcription and splicing has been found to produce three to four species of viral mRNA, transcribed from the negative strand and having different lengths but with common $5'$ and $3'$ terminals, in infected tissues (Okamoto et al. 2000a, 2001) and in experimental systems (Kamahora et al. 2000; Yokoyama et al. 2002).

Modes of virion assembly and release from producer cells are not known. In analogy with what is observed with other nonenveloped viruses, egress of progeny virions is likely to imply the destruction of infected cells. Genetic recombination between different genotypes appears to be a frequent event in TTV and TTMV (Worobey 2000; Biagini et al. 2001), indicating that the same cell can become infected with more than one genotype. Recombination is most often observed in the noncoding portion of the viral genome, most likely due to the high conservation of this region. As discussed below, individuals who harbor multiple genotypes are numerous, thus contributing to the explanation as to why recombination is a frequent occurrence. Available data exclude that TTV can persist as an episome or become integrated into cell DNA (Yu et al. 2002).

NATURAL HISTORY OF INFECTION

A well-documented property of both TTV and TTMV is that they readily establish chronic productive infections in many, if not all, exposed individuals. Apart from this, information about the infection course is still sketchy and almost exclusively limited to TTV. Whilst others appear likely (Okamoto and Mayumi 2001), three modes of TTV entry into the body have been clearly documented: inoculation of contaminated blood or blood-derived products (Simmonds et al. 1998; Bendinelli et al. 2001), transplacental infection (Morrica et al. 2000), and airborne infection (Maggi et al. 2003). In the latter study, 87 out of 100 young children hospitalized for acute respiratory infections were found to carry larger TTV loads in the nasal secretions than in blood and, in some, the same virus was demonstrable earlier in the nares than in the circulation, thus suggesting that the respiratory tract is a port of entry and also a site of primary virus amplification. This and other studies (Kobayashi et al. 1999; Matsumoto et al. 1999) have also shown that TTV becomes detectable in the blood within one or a few weeks after exposure, thus indicating that dissemination of infection throughout the body is rapid.

Self-limited TTV infections have been described (Lefrere et al. 1999; Matsumoto et al. 1999), and, according to a recent report (Ohto et al. 2002), their frequency depends on viral genotype; however, the possibility is not excluded that such findings reflect post-acute reductions of viremia levels under the detection threshold rather than true virus eradications. Large fluctuations of TTV viremia levels have been observed in a number of subjects over time (Ball et al. 1999; Matsumoto et al. 1999). In any case, prolonged, possibly lifelong, TTV persistence is by far the most frequent outcome (Lefrere et al. 1999; Matsumoto et al. 1999; Takayama et al. 1999). Plasma TTV loads vary extensively in chronically infected persons, ranging between 10^2 and more than 10^8 DNA copies per ml (Pistello et al. 2001). Similarly to what has been observed with other chronic plasma viremia-inducing viruses, TTV viremia is the result of the continuous shedding into, and clearance from, the bloodstream of large numbers of virions (Table 57.2).

Cerebrospinal fluid is usually virus-negative in infected individuals with an intact blood–brain barrier (Maggi et al. 2001a). All other anatomic sites tested have been found to harbor variably abundant TTV. These include liver, lung, pancreas, spleen, kidney, lymph nodes, skeletal muscles, thyroid gland, bone marrow, and circulating leukocytes. For some such tissues, namely liver, bone marrow, and circulating peripheral blood mononuclear cells, there are also molecular indicators (double-stranded viral DNA and viral mRNA) that TTV replicates locally (Okamoto et al. 1998, 2000a, b, c, 2001; Kikuchi et al. 2000; Suzuki et al. 2001). However, the possibility that these findings reflect circulating virus or ubiquitous virus-infected cells, such as lymphocytes and/or macrophages, cannot be excluded at present. That proliferating hematopoietic cells might be a major source of TTV is suggested by observations that baseline viremia decreased to undetectable levels in virus carriers treated with myelosuppressive drugs (Kanda et al. 1999). The possibility has also been suggested that different TTV genotypes differ in tropism and replicate preferentially in selected body compartments (Okamoto et al. 2001).

It is probable that the extraordinary ability of anelloviruses to persist and continuously release copious progeny into the systemic circulation is due to a complex combination of virus and host factors. That primary infections generally occur early in prenatal or postnatal life (see below) may be important for persistence by inducing partial immunotolerance. Also, if productive viral replication is indeed possible only in cycling cells (Maggi et al. 2001b; Mariscal et al. 2002), then only a fraction of potentially susceptible cells might be permissive at any given time, thus allowing even supposedly cytocidal agents, such as anelloviruses, to persist. On the other hand, it might well be that immune responses elicited by anelloviruses are not particularly vigorous and/or the immune effectors produced are incapable of controlling the infection with sufficient efficacy.

Immune responses have not been properly investigated as yet, at least partly due to lack of suitable viral antigens. A few attempts to produce recombinant TTV antigens have yielded confusing or negative results. Recently, an enzyme-linked immunosorbent assay using antigen extracted from the feces of a carrier has permitted the following of the antibody responses developed by two patients with post-transfusion TTV infections. Specific IgM and IgG were detected after 10–21 and 12–17 weeks, respectively (Tsuda et al. 2001), possibly indicating that humoral responses to TTV mount slowly. Furthermore, immunoprecipitation studies have shown that a variably large proportion of total TTV found in chronically infected patients has IgG bound to its surface (Nishizawa et al. 1999; Ott et al. 2000). It would be of interest to ascertain whether such immunocomplexed virus is still infectious for cells. The fact that mixed infections by multiple TTV strains are numerous (see below) indicates that antiviral immunity does not efficiently protect against superinfection by heterologous genotypes.

LABORATORY DIAGNOSIS

Reliable tissue culture and immunological methods for demonstrating TTV and TTMV or induced antibodies are lacking. Diagnosis of infection relies, therefore, solely on the detection of viral genomes in blood or other specimens. The PCR procedures most commonly used at present are listed in Table 57.3. Due to the great genetic diversity of both TTV and TTMV, the choice of the viral DNA segment targeted for amplification has an enormous impact on PCR assay sensitivity. For example, early tests for TTV, which targeted poorly conserved sequences in the ORF1 (Bendinelli et al. 2001), greatly underestimated the prevalence rates of infection since they almost exclusively detected genogroup 1 viruses. The UTR of both TTV and TTMV are now known to be most suitable for the design of primers capable of detecting all, or the majority of, the viral genotypes hitherto identified (Okamoto and Mayumi 2001). However, no method which has the potential to simultaneously detect all possible variants of both TTV and TTMV with a single test has yet been described. Quantitative real-time assays also exploit this region (Maggi et al. 2001c; Moen et al. 2002). On the other hand, the

Table **57.2** *Dynamics of chronic TTV viremia, relative to other viruses*

Virus	Mean virion half-life in plasma	New virions entering plasma per day	Reference
HBV	1.2 days	$>1.7 \times 10^{13}$	Whalley et al. 2001
HCV	2.7 hours	$>1.3 \times 10^{12}$	Neumann et al. 1998
HIV-1	< 1 hour	$>9.8 \times 10^9$	Ramratnam et al. 1999
TTV	6.5 hours	$>3.8 \times 10^{10}$	Maggi et al. 2001c

Table 57.3 *Methods currently in use for the diagnosis of TTV and TTMV*

Virus	Purpose	Type of test	Target region
TTV	Detection	Qualitative universal PCR	UTR
	Quantitation	Real-time universal PCR	UTR
	Typing	Group-specific PCR	ORF1 (genogroups 1–3)
			UTR (genogroups 4 and 5)
		Sequencing	ORF1 (all genogroups)
TTMV	Detection	Qualitative PCR	UTR
	Quantitation	Real-time PCR	UTR
	Typing	Sequencing	ORF1

genogroup-specific PCR assays that have been proposed for typing purposes as a practical alternative to sequencing methods are UTR- or ORF1-based, depending on the specific genotype targeted. Genogroup- or genotype-specific quantitative assays may also become valuable in future studies attempting to correlate definite viral types to disease (Maggi et al. 2003).

EPIDEMIOLOGY

The viruses discussed in this chapter are certainly among the most widespread viral agents of humans. The use of sensitive and broad-range PCR techniques has indeed shown that over two-thirds of the global population carries TTV in plasma and that active TTMV infection is possibly even more common (Biagini et al. 2000, 2001). Thus, almost everyone is infected with either TTV or TTMV or both. In fact, individuals who carry multiple genetic forms of the two viruses are more the rule than the exception (Umemura et al. 2001a). Significantly, a recent report has described the presence of as many as 15 different genotypes of TTMV in the blood of an immunocompromised subject (Vasconcelos et al. 2002). Prevalence rates are already very high during the first months of life and augment only moderately thereafter (Bendinelli et al. 2001; Maggi et al. 2003), but whether the proportion of individuals who carry multiple types of the two viruses varies with age remains to be established. Gender and socioeconomic conditions appear to be of little importance for spread of the infection. Geographical variations in total and genotype-specific prevalence rates would appear to exist (Gallian et al. 2000; Muljono et al. 2001; Umemura et al. 2001a); however, systematic studies conducted using uniform protocols that might permit really meaningful comparisons are lacking.

That anelloviruses can be transmitted via blood and blood products is obvious and has been repeatedly documented. However, their amazing diffusion in the general population implies the existence of much more frequent occasions of contagion, as also corroborated by frequent virus detection in saliva, nasal and genital secretions, tears, and feces. Intrauterine transmission is a clear possibility and has been repeatedly demonstrated with the detection of TTV in cord blood (Gerner et al.

2000; Inami et al. 2000; Matsubara et al. 2000; Fornai et al. 2001). Another route that has been clearly documented is through the respiratory tract (Maggi et al. 2003). Based on indirect evidence, fecal–oral spread is also very likely (Gallian et al. 2000; Lin et al. 2000; Tawara et al. 2000). The role in human epidemiology of the TTV-like viruses detected in other species, including pet and livestock animals, is unclear (Leary et al. 1999; Okamoto et al. 2002).

There are no available assays that permit the discrimination of whether viremia-negative subjects have skipped or have resolved the infection. Investigating this issue serologically is complicated by the poor definition of viral antigens and by the fact that virus in blood is frequently heavily immunocomplexed (Nishizawa et al. 1999; Ott et al. 2000; Tsuda et al. 2001; Kakkola et al. 2002).

ASSOCIATION WITH DISEASE

To date, there are no clinical manifestations that have been unequivocally linked to anelloviruses. As discussed in detail elsewhere (Bendinelli et al. 2001), early attempts to implicate TTV in those forms of liver disease that have a putative viral cause but are unrelated to known viruses have been frustrated, albeit it is still considered probable that, in some cases, TTV infection is associated with transient and mild elevations of liver enzyme levels (Nishizawa et al. 1997; Kanda et al. 1999; Tawara et al. 2000). Other cryptogenetic diseases that have been investigated include diabetes, cryoglobulinemia, psoriasis, rheumatoid arthritis, systemic lupus erythematosus, the Kawasaki syndrome, multiple sclerosis, and other neurological diseases. In all cases, results have excluded a TTV etiology or have been inconclusive.

As already mentioned, failure to identify associated diseases, together with the extraordinarily high prevalence rates of both TTV and TTMV active infections in the general population worldwide, has led to the hypothesis that these viruses might be completely nonpathogenic. However, at the time of writing it seems more appropriate to consider anelloviruses as 'orphans of disease,' similar to that previously done for many other viruses which in the early years after discovery could not be linked to any disease but were subsequently found to produce significant pathologies (e.g. echoviruses, reoviruses, Epstein–Barr virus, and others). Several aspects need investigating more thoroughly. For example, the possible clinical implications of primary infections, especially in infants, have been only marginally explored (Biagini et al. 2003; Maggi et al. 2003). Similarly, only recently is it becoming appreciated that only some types of TTV and TTMV might be pathogenic but their disease potentials might be blurred by many nonpathogenic types. Certain reports suggest that TTV genotypes 1a, 12, and 16 are especially damaging to the liver (Shibata et al. 2000; Umemura et al. 2001a) although others discount these findings (Yoshida et al. 2002). The possible consequences for the host's immune system of having to deal chronically with these viruses should also be attentively investigated, especially if proliferating lymphoid cells are confirmed to be a major site of virus infection. In this regard, recent findings have shown that among a large group of infants hospitalized for acute respiratory illnesses, the ones who exhibited higher plasma and nasal levels of TTV were also the ones who had more severe disease (Maggi et al. 2003). Furthermore, circulating loads of TTV are particularly high in patients with AIDS or other immunocompromising conditions (Christensen et al. 2000; Shibayama et al. 2001), possibly contributing to immune impairment. Accounts implicating TTV or TTMV in some renal ailments (Yokoyama et al. 2002) and in certain forms of anemia, neutropenia, and thrombocytopenia (Kikuchi et al. 2000; Simmonds 2002) are also worth further scrutiny.

CONTROL

As long as their clinical implications remain undefined, there will certainly be little attention paid on how the viruses discussed in this chapter might be controlled. Their epidemiologic features leave, however, little doubt that trying to prevent infections would be extremely difficult in the absence of specific multivalent vaccines. On the other hand, TTV has proven insensitive or only transiently sensitive to interferon in patients treated for other viral infections (Maggi et al. 1999, 2001c; Dai et al. 2002), albeit combined therapy with ribavirine seems more effective and selected viral genotypes more susceptible (Umemura et al. 2002). As expected, antiretroviral drugs have also shown no anti-TTV activity (Takamatsu et al. 2001). Thus, should it one day be regarded as clinically useful, treating established infections would most likely need the development of specific antivirals.

REFERENCES

Abe, K., Inami, T., et al. 2000. TT virus infection in nonhuman primates and characterization of the viral genome: identification of simian TT virus isolates. *J Virol*, **74**, 1549–53.

Asabe, S., Nishizawa, T., et al. 2001. Phosphorylation of serine-rich protein encoded by open reading frame 3 of the TT virus genome. *Biochem Biophys Res Commun*, **286**, 298–304.

Ball, J.K., Curran, R., et al. 1999. TT virus sequence heterogeneity in vivo: evidence for co-infection with multiple genetic types. *J Gen Virol*, **80**, 1759–68.

Bendinelli, M., Pistello, M., et al. 2001. Molecular properties, biology and clinical implications of TT virus, a recently identified widespread infectious agent of humans. *Clin Microbiol Rev*, **14**, 98–113.

Biagini, P., Gallian, P. and Touinssi, M. 2000. High prevalence of TT virus infection in French blood donors revealed by the use of three PCR systems. *Transfusion*, **40**, 590–5.

Biagini, P., Gallian, P., et al. 2001. Genetic analysis of full-length genomes and subgenomic sequences of TT virus-like mini virus human isolates. *J Gen Virol*, **82**, 379–83.

Biagini, P., Charrel, R.N., et al. 2003. Association of TT virus primary infection with rhinitis in newborn. *Clin Infect Dis*, **36**, 128.

Christensen, J.K., Eugen-Olsen, J., et al. 2000. Prevalence and prognostic significance of infection with TT virus in patients infected with human immunodeficiency virus. *J Infect Dis*, **181**, 1796–9.

Dai, C.Y., Yu, M.L., et al. 2002. The response of hepatitis C virus and TT virus to high dose and long duration interferon-alpha therapy in naive chronic hepatitis C patients. *Antivir Res*, **53**, 9–18.

Erker, J.C., Leary, T.P., et al. 1999. Analyses of TT virus full-length genomic sequences. *J Gen Virol*, **80**, 1743–50.

Fornai, C., Maggi, F., et al. 2001. High prevalence of TT virus (TTV) and TTV-like mini virus in cervical swabs. *J Clin Microbiol*, **39**, 2022–2024.

Gallian, P., Biagini, P., et al. 2000. TT virus: a study of molecular epidemiology and transmission of genotypes 1, 2 and 3. *J Clin Virol*, **17**, 43–9.

Gerner, P., Oettinger, R., et al. 2000. Mother-to-infant transmission of TT virus: prevalence, extent and mechanism of vertical transmission. *Pediatr Infect Dis J*, **19**, 1074–7.

Hallett, R.L., Clewley, J.P., et al. 2000. Characterization of a highly divergent TT virus genome. *J Gen Virol*, **81**, 2273–9.

Heller, F., Zachoval, R., et al. 2001. Isolate KAV: a new genotype of the TT-virus family. *Biochem Biophys Res Commun*, **289**, 937–41.

Hijikata, M., Takahashi, K. and Mishiro, S. 1999. Complete circular DNA genome of a TT virus variant (isolate name SANBAN) and 44 partial ORF2 sequences implicating a great degree of diversity beyond genotypes. *Virology*, **260**, 17–22.

Hino, S. 2002. TTV, a new human virus with single stranded circular DNA genome. *Rev Med Virol*, **12**, 151–8.

Inami, T., Konomi, N., et al. 2000. High prevalence of TT virus DNA in human saliva and semen. *J Clin Microbiol*, **38**, 2407–8.

Itoh, Y., Takahashi, M., et al. 2000. Visualization of TT virus particles recovered from the sera and feces of infected humans. *Biochem Biophys Res Commun*, **279**, 718–24.

Kakkola, L., Hedman, K., et al. 2002. Cloning and sequencing of TT virus genotype 6 and expression of antigenic open reading frame 2 proteins. *J Gen Virol*, **83**, 979–90.

Kamahora, T., Hino, S. and Miyata, H. 2000. Three spliced mRNAs of TT virus transcribed from a plasmid containing the entire genome in COS1 cells. *J Virol*, **74**, 9980–6.

Kanda, Y., Tanaka, Y., et al. 1999. TT virus in bone marrow transplant recipients. *Blood*, **93**, 2485–90.

Kikuchi, K., Miyakawa, H., et al. 2000. Indirect evidence of TTV replication in bone marrow cells, but not in hepatocytes, of a subacute hepatitis/aplastic anemia patient. *J Med Virol*, **61**, 165–70.

Kobayashi, M., Chayama, K., et al. 1999. Prevalence of TT virus before and after blood transfusion in patients with chronic liver disease treated surgically for hepatocellular carcinoma. *J Gastroenterol Hepatol*, **14**, 358–63.

Leary, T.P., Erker, J.C., et al. 1999. Improved detection systems for TT virus reveal high prevalence in humans, non-human primates and farm animals. *J Gen Virol*, **80**, 2115–20.

Lefrere, J.J., Roudot-Thoraval, F., et al. 1999. Natural history of the TT virus infection through follow-up of TTV DNA-positive multiple-transfused patients. *Blood*, **95**, 347–51.

Lin, C.L., Kyono, W., et al. 2000. Fecal excretion of a novel human circovirus, TT virus, in healthy children. *Clin Diagn Lab Immunol*, **7**, 960–3.

Maggi, F., Fornai, C., et al. 1999. High prevalence of TT virus viremia in Italian patients, regardless of age, clinical diagnosis, and previous interferon treatment. *J Infect Dis*, **180**, 838–42.

Maggi, F., Fornai, C., et al. 2001a. Low prevalence of TT virus in the cerebrospinal fluid of viremic patients with central nervous system disorders. *J Med Virol*, **65**, 418–22.

Maggi, F., Fornai, C., et al. 2001b. TT virus (TTV) loads associated with different peripheral blood cell types and evidence for TTV replication in activated mononuclear cells. *J Med Virol*, **64**, 190–4.

Maggi, F., Pistello, M., et al. 2001c. Dynamics of persistent TT virus infection, as determined in patients treated with alpha interferon for concomitant hepatitis C virus infection. *J Virol*, **75**, 11999–2004.

Maggi, F., Pifferi, M., et al. 2003. TT virus in the nasal secretions of children with acute respiratory diseases: relations to viremia and disease severity. *J Virol*, **77**, 2418–25.

Mariscal, L.F., Lopez-Alcorocho, J.M., et al. 2002. TT virus replicates in stimulated but not in nonstimulated peripheral blood mononuclear cells. *Virology*, **301**, 121–9.

Matsubara, H., Michitaka, K., et al. 2000. Existence of TT virus DNA in extracellular body fluids from normal healthy Japanese subjects. *Intervirology*, **43**, 16–19.

Matsumoto, A., Yeo, A.E.T., et al. 1999. Transfusion-associated TT virus infection and its relationship to liver disease. *Hepatology*, **30**, 283–8.

Miyata, H., Tsunoda, H., et al. 1999. Identification of a novel GC-rich 113-nucleotide region to complete the circular, single-stranded DNA genome of TT virus, the first human circovirus. *J Virol*, **73**, 3582–6.

Moen, E.M., Sleboda, J. and Grinde, B. 2002. Real-time PCR methods for independent quantitation of TTV and TLMV. *J Virol Methods*, **104**, 59–67.

Morrica, A., Maggi, F., et al. 2000. TT virus: evidence for transplacental transmission. *J Infect Dis*, **181**, 803–4.

Muljono, D.H., Nishizawa, T., et al. 2001. Molecular epidemiology of TT virus (TTV) and characterization of two novel TTV genotypes in Indonesia. *Arch Virol*, **146**, 1249–66.

Mushahwar, I.K. 2000. Recently discovered blood-borne viruses: are they hepatitis viruses or merely endosymbionts? *J Med Virol*, **62**, 399–404.

Mushahwar, I.K., Erker, J.C., et al. 1999. Molecular and biophysical characterization of TT virus: evidence for a new virus family infecting humans. *Proc Natl Acad Sci U S A*, **96**, 3177–82.

Neumann, A.U., Lam, N.P., et al. 1998. Hepatitis C viral dynamics in vivo and the antiviral efficacy of interferon-alpha therapy. *Science*, **282**, 103–7.

Nishizawa, T., Okamoto, H., et al. 1997. A novel DNA virus (TTV) associated with elevated transaminase levels in posttransfusion hepatitis of unknown etiology. *Biochem Biophys Res Commun*, **241**, 92–7.

Nishizawa, T., Okamoto, H., et al. 1999. Quasispecies of TT virus (TTV) with sequence divergence in hypervariable regions of the capsid protein in chronic TTV infection. *J Virol*, **73**, 9604–8.

Ohto, H., Ujiie, N., et al. 2002. TT virus infection during childhood. *Transfusion*, **42**, 892–8.

Okamoto, H. and Mayumi, M. 2001. TT virus: virological and genomic characteristics and disease associations. *J Gastroenterol*, **36**, 519–29.

Okamoto, H., Nishizawa, T., et al. 1998. Molecular cloning and characterization of a novel DNA virus (TTV) associated with posttransfusion hepatitis of unknown etiology. *Hepatol Res*, **10**, 1–16.

Okamoto, H., Nishizawa, T., et al. 2000a. TT virus mRNAs detected in the bone marrow cells from an infected individual. *Biochem Biophys Res Commun*, **279**, 700–7.

Okamoto, H., Takahashi, M., et al. 2000b. Replicative forms of TT virus DNA in bone marrow cells. *Biochem Biophys Res Commun*, **270**, 657–62.

Okamoto, H., Ukita, M., et al. 2000c. Circular double-stranded forms of TT virus DNA in the liver. *J Virol*, **74**, 5161–7.

Okamoto, H., Nishizawa, T., et al. 2001. Heterogeneous distribution of TT virus of distinct genotypes in multiple tissues from infected humans. *Virology*, **288**, 358–68.

Okamoto, H., Takahashi, M., et al. 2002. Genomic characterization of TT viruses (TTVs) in pigs, cats and dogs and their relatedness with species-specific TTVs in primates and tupaias. *J Gen Virol*, **83**, 1291–7.

Ott, C., Duret, L., et al. 2000. Use of a TT virus ORF1 recombinant protein to detect anti-TT virus antibodies in human sera. *J Gen Virol*, **81**, 2949–58.

Peng, Y.H., Nishizawa, T., et al. 2002. Analysis of the entire genomes of thirteen TT virus variants classifiable into the fourth and fifth genetic groups, isolated from viremic infants. *Arch Virol*, **147**, 21–41.

Pistello, M., Morrica, A., et al. 2001. TT virus levels in the plasma of infected individuals with different hepatic and extrahepatic pathologies. *J Med Virol*, **63**, 189–95.

Primi, D., Fiordalisi, G. et al. 2000. Identification of SENV genotypes. International patent number WO0028039 (http://ep.es-pacenet.com/).

Ramratnam, B., Bonhoeffer, S., et al. 1999. Rapid production and clearance of HIV-1 and hepatitis C virus assessed by large volume plasma apheresis. *Lancet*, **354**, 1782–5.

Shibata, M., Morizane, T., et al. 2000. TT virus infection in patients with fulminant hepatic failure. *Am J Gastroenterol*, **95**, 3602–6.

Shibayama, T., Masuda, G., et al. 2001. Inverse relationship between the titre of TT virus DNA and CD4 cell count in patients infected with HIV. *AIDS*, **15**, 563–70.

Simmonds, P. 2002. TT virus infection: a novel virus-host relationship. *J Med Microbiol*, **51**, 455–8.

Simmonds, P., Davidson, F., et al. 1998. Detection of a novel DNA virus (TTV) in blood donors and blood products. *Lancet*, **352**, 191–5.

Suzuki, F., Chayama, K., et al. 2001. Pathogenic significance and organic virus levels in patients infected with TT virus. *Intervirology*, **44**, 291–7.

Takahashi, K., Hijikata, M., et al. 2000a. Full or near full length nucleotide sequences of TT virus variants (types SANBAN and YONBAN) and the TT virus-like mini virus. *Intervirology*, **43**, 119–23.

Takahashi, K., Iwasa, Y., et al. 2000b. Identification of a new human DNA virus (TTV-like mini virus, TLMV) intermediately related to TT virus and chicken anemia virus. *Arch Virol*, **145**, 979–93.

Takahashi, M., Asabe, S., et al. 2002. TT virus is distributed in various leukocyte subpopulation at distinct levels, with the highest viral load in granulocytes. *Biochem Biophys Res Commun*, **290**, 242–8.

Takamatsu, J., Toyoda, H., et al. 2001. Effects of HAART on hepatitis C, hepatitis G and TT virus in multiply coinfected HIV-positive patients with haemophilia. *Haemophilia*, **7**, 575–81.

Takayama, S., Miura, T., et al. 1999. Prevalence and persistence of a novel DNA TT virus (TTV) infection in Japanese haemophiliacs. *Br J Haematol*, **104**, 626–9.

Tanaka, Y., Primi, D., et al. 2001. Genomic and molecular evolutionary analysis of a newly identified infectious agent (SEN virus) and its relationship to the TT virus family. *J Infect Dis*, **183**, 359–67.

Tawara, A., Akahane, Y., et al. 2000. Transmission of human TT virus of genotype 1a to chimpanzees with fecal supernatant or serum from patients with acute TTV infection. *Biochem Biophys Res Commun*, **278**, 470–6.

Todd, D., McNulty, M.S., et al. 2001. Animal circoviruses. *Adv Virus Res*, **57**, 1–70.

Tsuda, F., Takahashi, M., et al. 2001. IgM-class antibodies to TT virus (TTV) in patients with acute TTV infection. *Hepatol Res*, **19**, 1–11.

Umemura, T., Alter, H.J., et al. 2001a. Association between SEN virus infection and hepatitis C in Japan. *J Infect Dis*, **184**, 1246–51.

Umemura, T., Tanaka, Y., et al. 2001b. Observation of positive selection within hypervariable regions of a newly identified DNA virus (SEN virus). *FEBS Lett*, **510**, 171–4.

Umemura, T., Alter, H.J., et al. 2002. SEN virus: response to interferon alpha and influence on the severity and treatment response of coexistent hepatitis C. *Hepatology*, **35**, 953–9.

Vasconcelos, H.C.F., Cataldo, M. and Niel, C. 2002. Mixed infections of adults and children with multiple TTV-like mini virus isolates. *J Med Virol*, **68**, 291–8.

Whalley, S.A., Murray, J.M., et al. 2001. Kinetics of acute hepatitis B virus infection in humans. *J Exp Med*, **193**, 847–54.

Worobey, M. 2000. Extensive homologous recombination among widely divergent TT viruses. *J Virol*, **74**, 7666–70.

Yokoyama, H., Yasuda, J., et al. 2002. Pathological changes of renal epithelial cells in mice transgenic for the TT virus ORF1 gene. *J Gen Virol*, **83**, 141–50.

Yoshida, H., Kato, N., et al. 2002. Weak association between SEN virus viremia and liver disease. *J Clin Microbiol*, **40**, 3140–3145.

Yu, Q., Shiramizu, B., et al. 2002. TT virus: preferential distribution in CD19[+] peripheral blood mononuclear cells and lack of viral integration. *J Med Virol*, **66**, 276–84.

58

Retroviruses and associated diseases in humans

CHARLENE S. DEZZUTTI, WALID HENEINE, ROUMIANA S. BONEVA, AND
THOMAS M. FOLKS

INTRODUCTION AND GENERAL PROPERTIES OF THE *RETROVIRIDAE*

Retroviruses seem to have played a role in the evolution of human genetics, considering the large number of retroviral remnants within the human genome. Why, where, and how these viral residues occurred is a curious enigma of our genome. Did they arise from multiple infections, which over time devastated new evolving species of hominoids? Did such an occurrence result in survivors who either were infected with defective retroviruses or had modified their receptors to be resistant to primary infection? The answers may become apparent if, in several thousand years, remnants of human immunodeficiency virus (HIV) and human T-cell leukemia virus (HTLV) are found 'fixed' in the human genome.

Within the large family of retroviruses, lentiviruses, which include the HIVs, are unusual in that they possess complexities and degeneracies that differ from the biological properties of other, more stable, primate retroviruses, such as the deltaretroviruses and the spumaviruses. Nevertheless, these agents share the common feature of utilizing a reverse transcribing enzyme to replicate their genome. Retroviruses replicate in a unique manner. An enzyme carried by the viruses reverses the usual flow of genetic information (normally from DNA to RNA (messenger RNA) and then to protein) by causing the RNA genetic information to create a DNA (proviral) intermediate. This is a characteristic feature of all retroviruses. Viral genetic information in the DNA form is contained in this 'provirus,' which can be integrated into the genome of the host cell, where it may remain latent or nonexpressing for variable periods. Only when the provirus is activated, often by first messenger signals such as cytokines or antigens, are viral proteins and new viruses made. In the mature virion the genome is diploid, carried as a 60–70S dimer complex of two identical, positive-sense, single-stranded RNA copies, whereas reverse transcriptase (RT) is a meiotic event, resulting in a double-stranded haploid DNA provirus. The proviral genome structure of retroviruses is characterized by repeated sequences at either end of the genome, the long terminal repeats (LTR). These structures play an important role in viral expression because they contain promoter and enhancer elements. The genomes of all retroviruses that are able to replicate fully always include three genes coding for the three sets of structural proteins: those of the core proteins (gag), the envelope proteins (env) and the polymerase enzyme (pol). The genome arrangement LTR–gag–pol–env–LTR is common to all known retroviruses. A simplified retroviral life cycle is depicted in Figure 58.1.

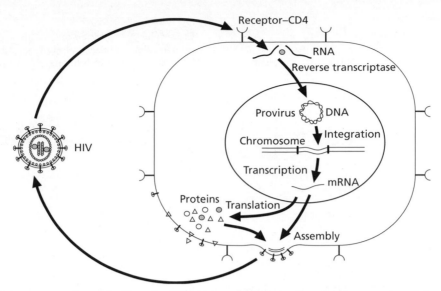

Figure 58.1 *Schematic representation of the life cycle of HIV. Virions attach to specific cell surface receptors. Following internalization and uncoating either via receptor-mediated endocytosis or by fusion at the plasma membrane, the reverse transcriptase in the core of the virion becomes activated and synthesizes a double-stranded DNA provirus. Circularized and linear forms of the provirus migrate to the nucleus and integrate in host chromosomal DNA. The integrated proviral genome may remain latent, but, if active, particularly in proliferating cells, it expresses positive-strand RNA. Full-length transcripts become packaged into progeny virions budding from the plasma membrane. Messenger RNA (mRNA) transcripts encode the structural and regulatory viral proteins, which can be recognized as antigens within infected cells.*

Among the viruses, retroviruses and the diseases they cause were some of the earliest to be described in detail (Weiss 1984). At the turn of the century, equine infectious anemia was one of the first animal infections recognized as having a viral etiology. Shortly afterwards, there were descriptions of filterable, transmissible agents associated with cancers among chickens that related both leukemias (avian leukosis, 1908) and solid tumours (Rous sarcoma, 1911) to infections with viruses. In 1936, breast cancer in mice was found to be transmitted by a virus in the animal's breast milk, and from the 1950s onwards leukemias in mice, cats, fish, apes, and other vertebrate hosts were found to be caused by retroviruses. Knowledge of these cancer-causing viruses has yielded important insights into the nature of neoplasia and catalyzed the search for similar agents as a cause of malignancy in humans. Despite the attraction of this idea, which implied the possibility of vaccines to prevent cancer, it was not until 1980 that the relationship between a retrovirus infection and human neoplasia was documented, leading to the eventual characterization of HTLV.

Recently, the family of *Retroviridae* has been reclassified into seven different genera (Table 58.1). Viruses from the genera *Lentivirus* and *Deltaretrovirus* are known to cause disease in humans while viruses from the genus *Spumavirus* have been shown to infect humans, but no disease associations yet have been found. The chapter presented here deals primarily with those non-HIV retroviruses that cause or are associated with human disease.

HUMAN T-LYMPHOTROPIC VIRUS TYPE 1 AND HUMAN T-LYMPHOTROPIC VIRUS TYPE 2

Morphology

Human T-lymphotropic virus type 1 (HTLV-1) was the first human retrovirus isolated in 1981 (Kalyanaraman et al. 1981; Poiesz et al. 1981). Shortly thereafter, Human T-lymphotropic virus type 2 (HTLV-2) was isolated from a person with hairy cell leukemia (Kalyanaraman et al. 1982). Both viruses are part of the *Orthoretrovirinae* subfamily. HTLV-1 and HTLV-2 are typical C-type retroviruses; they contain an electron-dense, centrally located nuclear core and they bud from the cell surface. Within the core are two positive-sense single-stranded RNA genomes. A unique feature about HTLV-1 and HTLV-2 is their inefficient ability to infect via cell-free virus. Rather, these viruses require cell-to-cell contact for productive infection. Despite this, electron microscopy has shown that chronically infected cells form normal viral particles that are assembled at the plasma membrane and released (Poiesz et al. 1980; Miyoshi et al. 1981; Ohtsuki et al. 1982). It is currently unknown why cell-free virus has reduced infectivity.

Genome organization

HTLV-1 and HTLV-2 are more than 9 kb in length and have similar genomic organization: *gag*, *pro/pol*, *env*, pX,

Table 58.1 Retroviridae *family*

Genus	Virus	Host	Growth in human cells in vitro	Mode of transmission to humans	Human disease or infection
Alpharetrovirus					
Avian leukosis virus	ALV	Birds			
Rous sarcoma virus	RSV	Birds			
Gammaretrovirus					
Moloney murine leukemia virus	MoMLV	Mice			
Feline leukemia virus	FeLV	Cats	Yes		
Porcine endogenous retrovirus	PoEV	Pigs	Yes	?[a]	?
Baboon endogenous virus	BaEV	Baboons	Yes	?[a]	?
Betaretrovirus					
Mouse mammary tumor virus	MMTV	Mice			
Mason–Pfizer monkey virus	MPMV	Monkeys	Yes	?	Infection
Deltaretrovirus					
Bovine leukemia virus	BLV	Cows			
Primate T-lymphotropic virus 1	HTLV-1	Humans	Yes	Mother to child, sexual transmission, blood	T-cell lymphoma, neurological disorders, HAM/TSP[b]
Primate T-lymphotropic virus 2	HTLV-2	Humans	Yes		
Epsilonretrovirus					
Walleye dermal sarcoma virus	WDSV	Fish			
Lentivirus					
Human immunodeficiency virus type 1	HIV-1	Humans	Yes	Mother to child, sexual transmission, blood	AIDS
Human immunodeficiency virus type 2	HIV-2	Humans	Yes		
Simian immunodeficiency virus	SIV	Monkeys	Yes	(biting, blood, other?)	Infection
Visna/maedi virus	VISNA	Sheep			
Equine infectious anemia virus	EIAV	Horses		(biting, blood, other?)	
Feline immunodeficiency virus	FIV	Cats	Yes		
Caprine arthritis encephalitis virus	CAEV	Goats			
Spumavirus					
Simian foamy virus	SFV$_{CPZ}$[c]	Nonhuman primate	Yes	(biting, blood, other?)	Infection

a) Risk of transmission to human from xenotransplantation.
b) TSP, tropical spastic paraparesis; HAM, HTLV-associated myelopathy.
c) No human species of *Spumavirus* (foamy) is known. Simian foamy viruses from a number of simian species have been isolated or sequences identified in humans (see section below on Zoonotic retroviral infections).

and are flanked by the LTRs (Figure 58.2). Further, they share approximately 65 percent of their nucleotide sequences. The *gag* gene encodes for a polypeptide precursor that contains the structural proteins, p19 (MA), p24 (CA), and p15 (NC). Sera from infected patients generally have antibodies that recognize p19 and p24. The *pro* gene encodes for the viral protease. Synthesis of the protease as part of the gag polyprotein

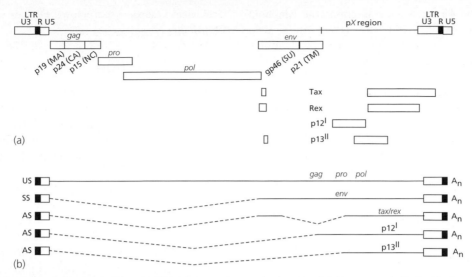

Figure 58.2 *Molecular genetic organization of HTLV.* **(a)** *Genomic organization. The 8.3-kb genome is flanked by long terminal repeats (LTR). Open reading frames are shown for the structural proteins, viral enzymes, and regulatory proteins.* **(b)** *RNA species. Unspliced, singly spliced, and multiply spliced RNA species are produced. Solid lines represent the exons and the dotted lines represent the intervening sequences.*

precursor is done by ribosomal frameshifting (Nam et al. 1988). The *pol* gene encodes the reverse transcriptase. The *env* gene encodes the transmembrane and external envelope glycoproteins, gp21 and gp46. The HTLV LTR is structured in a similar manner as other retroviral LTRs and contains three regions, U3, R, and U5. The U3 region contains transcriptional control sequences including the three imperfect 21 nt repeats that make up the Tax response element 1 (TRE-1), which is required for the *trans*-activation by Tax (see below) (Shimotohno et al. 1986). The U3 region also contains sequences for polyadenylation and termination of mRNAs. The R and U5 regions form the leader sequence encoded at the 5′ mRNAs. The R region is important for post-transcriptional control by Rex (see below).

As a complex retrovirus, HTLV-1 and HTLV-2 use alternative splicing and internal initiation codons to produce several regulatory and accessory proteins encoded by four open reading frames (ORF) located in the p*X* region of the viral genome between *env* and the 3′ LTR.

TAX (*TRANS*-ACTIVATING GENE)

The two originally described regulatory proteins, Tax and Rex, are generated from a doubly spliced, 2.1 kb mRNA encoded by ORF IV. The HTLV-1 *trans*-activator, Tax, is a 40 kDa protein. Tax contains a nuclear localization sequence that interacts with the cellular transcription factors, cyclic AMP-responsive element-binding protein (CREB) (Franklin and Nyborg 1995), nuclear factor-κB (NF-κB) (Sun and Ballard 1999), AP-1 (Jeang et al. 1991), and serum-response factor (SRF) (Fujii et al. 1992), and thus is a potent transcriptional activator not only from the viral promoter (Tax-responsive element), but also from enhancer elements of many cellular genes involved in host-cell proliferation.

These genes include the *IL-2*, *IL-2R*, *GM-CSF*, *Lck*, and others. On its own, Tax has been shown to immortalize T lymphocytes (Rosin et al. 1998) and transform rat fibroblasts (Tanaka et al. 1990). When HTLV-1 with mutations in the CREB region or the NF-κB region of Tax was introduced into primary T lymphocytes, the NF-κB mutant lost its ability to transform the cells, indicating that the NF-κB pathway may play a critical role in the transformation process (Robek and Ratner 1999). Collectively, these data suggest that Tax plays a direct role in the development of HTLV-1-associated leukemia, adult T-cell leukemia (ATL).

REX (REGULATOR OF VIRAL EXPRESSION)

Rex is a 27 kDa phosphoprotein encoded by the ORF IV. Rex has an essential role in viral replication and the regulation of viral structural genes by functioning as a post-transcriptional regulator that increases the expression of singly spliced and unspliced viral mRNAs (Hidaka et al. 1988). Rex binds to the mRNA through a *cis*-acting stem–loop structure, Rex responsive element, which is located within the R region of the viral LTR (Ballaun et al. 1991; Bar-Shira et al. 1991; Unge et al. 1991). For the production of infectious virus, Rex-mediated regulation is required to balance the spliced and unspliced mRNAs.

ADDITIONAL HTLV-1 ACCESSORY GENES

Additional gene products have recently been identified from the two other ORFs. ORF I encodes p12^{I}. p12^{I} is a highly hydrophobic protein that has been shown to localize to the endoplasmic reticulum with calcium-binding proteins (Ding et al. 2001). It has been shown that p12^{I} is necessary for optimal viral infectivity in nondividing lymphocytes (Collins et al. 1998; Albrecht et al. 2000) and activates NFAT-mediated transcription in lymphoid cells (Albrecht et al. 2002). Collectively these data suggest that $p12^I$ is important during early infection of T cells to facilitate cellular activation and viral replication. Much less is known about the ORF II product, $p13^{II}$. Recent reports have shown that $p13^{II}$ localizes to the mitochondria, altering the inner-membrane morphology and disrupting the inner-membrane potential (Ciminale et al. 1999; D'Agostino et al. 2002). These data suggest that $p13^{II}$ induces apoptosis of infected cells; however, this has not been observed, suggesting this viral protein may affect other mitochondrial functions.

Replication strategy

HTLV RECEPTOR

The identity of the HTLV-1 and HTLV-2 receptor(s) remains an enigma. It is unknown if both viruses share the same receptor, but mutual interference studies suggest that they may (Sommerfelt and Weiss 1990). Early work had proposed that the receptor may be located on human chromosome 17 (Sommerfelt et al. 1988; Gavalchin et al. 1995; Li et al. 1996); however, subsequent work failed to substantiate these results (Sutton and Littman 1996; Okuma et al. 1999; Jassal et al. 2001). Furthermore, this work has shown that the HTLV surface glycoprotein, gp46, can bind to cell lines derived from numerous species and cell types which implies broad expression of a common cellular antigen or possibly use of distinct cellular antigens for use as a receptor. It is currently unknown if one receptor or multiple receptors are required for HTLV binding and infection. Using an HTLV surface adhesion glycoprotein that binds to cell surface proteins important for HTLV-1-mediated entry, Nath et al. (Nath et al. 2003) showed binding to T cells, B cells, NK cells, and macrophage. Further, immune activation increased binding to $CD4^+$ and $CD8^+$ T cells, suggesting that the receptor(s) is up-regulated after activation of T cells (Manel et al. 2003a). Recent work has shown that treating susceptible cells with trypsin reduces infectivity, and entry was partially inhibited by ammonium chloride, suggesting that pH may play a role in entry (Trejo and Ratner 2000).

Cells infected with HTLV typically have metabolic alterations. Moreover, gammaretroviruses (Table 58.1) utilize receptors that belong to the multimembrane-spanning transporter family (Overbaugh et al. 2001). Together with this evidence and that presented above, Manel et al. (Manel et al. 2003b) showed that a ubiquitous glucose transporter, GLUT-1, was utilized as a receptor for HTLV-1 and HTLV-2. Interfering with the expression of GLUT-1, but not other similar proteins, reduced the binding of the HTLV-1 and HTLV-2 envelopes. In support of Igakura et al. (Igakura et al. 2003) data, the GLUT-1 expression is concentrated to the mobile membrane regions and should be involved in the 'virological synapse' (see below). Further work needs to confirm these results.

CELLULAR INFECTION

While the previous data suggest that HTLV has the potential to infect and replicate in a multitude of host species and cell types, in humans, HTLV-1 has shown a preferential tropism for $CD4^+$ T cells (Richardson et al. 1990). Recently, HTLV-1 was detected in $CD8^+$ T cells, and it was suggested that they might be a reservoir since there is low-level replication in these cells (Nagai et al. 2001). Like HTLV-1, HTLV-2 infects $CD4^+$ and $CD8^+$ T cells, but it has a broader cellular tropism in vivo as shown by detection of HTLV-2 genome in B cells, macrophage, and NK cells (Lal et al. 1995). However, the ability to replicate in non-T cells is poor as reflected in the lower proviral copy number in those non-T-cell types (Lal et al. 1995). It is currently unknown what factors in T cells, as opposed to other cell types, are required for optimal replication of HTLV-1 and HTLV-2.

HTLV rarely infects cells through cell-free virus as typified by the lack of HTLV transmission using serum/plasma as opposed to whole blood (Donegan et al. 1994). Direct cell-to-cell contact is required for efficient HTLV infection and results in syncytium formation between the infected cell and the uninfected cell. Cellular adhesion molecules that include ICAM-1, ICAM-3, and VCAM, have been shown to enhance syncytium formation (Hildreth et al. 1997; Daenke et al. 1999). It has been thought that the syncytium formation is involved in cell-to-cell infection, but until recently, how infection occurs has not been explained. Work by Igakura et al. (Igakura et al. 2003), showed that there is the formation of a 'virological synapse' that transfers HTLV between lymphocytes. These authors show that viral proteins and nucleic acids are polarized to the cell–cell junction within 40 minutes of cell contact. The polarization is accompanied by microtubule reorientation that transports Gag/nucleic acid complexes toward the cell–cell junction. The HTLV Env may have a role in the initiation of the virological synapse, but the formation of the synapse may be due to the up-regulation of certain adhesion molecules such as integrins (Dezzutti et al. 1995; Valentin et al. 1997; Yamamoto et al. 1997).

The kinetics of HTLV infection are thought to occur in a two-step process. Early after cell entry, there is a transient phase of RT followed by integration into the host's genome with subsequent persistent multiplication of infected cells. Integration is a requisite for expression of progeny virus and is responsible for persistence of the infection. In vitro studies have suggested that retroviruses may prefer to integrate into areas of the host genome that are transcriptionally active (Scherdin et al. 1990). It was also suggested that in persistently HTLV-infected cell lines, the provirus may integrate into GC-rich regions (Glukhova et al. 1999). However, in vivo work has shown that HTLV preferentially integrates into AT-rich regions and is not associated with transcriptionally active or GC-rich regions (Leclercq et al. 2000a, b).

Genetic diversity

As mentioned earlier, HTLV-1 and HTLV-2 share 65 percent genetic identity, and have minimal genetic variability (<10 percent) among different geographical isolates. The genetic stability of HTLV-1 and HTLV-2, despite long latency periods and high proviral load, is mainly attributed to clonal expansion of HTLV-harboring cells (Cavrois et al. 1996; Wattel et al. 1996). While the misincorporation rate of the HTLV RT is much lower than that of the HIV-1 RT (Mansky and Temin 1995; Mansky 2000), this is believed to play a lesser role in the genetic stability of these viruses. The LTR region has the lowest nucleotide homology, while the regulatory genes, *tax* and *rex*, have the highest nucleotide homology. The stability of the *env* gene may be due to its inability to tolerate mutations well. Pique et al. (Pique et al. 1990) performed insertion mutational analysis and showed that the majority of the mutations resulted in a nonfunctional envelope as shown by the lack of syncytia. These data suggest that the conformational constraints for processing and fusion abilities tend to limit the variability of the HTLV-1 envelope. Further, the utilization of the 'virological synapse' may allow HTLV-1 and perhaps HTLV-2 to escape the immune pressures that result in viral evolution.

While the overall genome of HTLV is highly conserved, nucleotide divergence in the LTR has been exploited to genotypically subtype both HTLV-1 and HTLV-2 (Slattery et al. 1999). There are four genetic subtypes of HTLV-1 based on the geographical origin of the virus: cosmopolitan (subtype A), Central African (subtype B), Australo-Melanesian (subtype C), and New Central African (subtype D) (Mahieux et al. 1997; Slattery et al. 1999). Likewise, HTLV-2 has four subtypes: IIa, IIb, IIc, and IId (Switzer et al. 1995; Slattery et al. 1999). Subtype IIa is commonly found among injecting drug users (IDU) worldwide, whereas subtype IIb is found primarily among Amerindians. This genetic heterogeneity within HTLV-1 and HTLV-2 has provided valuable information on geographical clustering and viral transmission (Switzer et al. 1995; Slattery et al. 1999).

Clinical and pathological aspects

Less than 5 percent of those persons infected with HTLV-1 develop the known diseases. Approximately 1–2 percent develops an aggressive T-cell malignancy known as ATL, and about 2–3 percent develop a chronic inflammatory disease called HTLV-1-associated myelopathy/tropical spastic paraparesis (HAM/TSP). Additional inflammatory diseases are also associated with HTLV-1 infection and they affect the skin (infective dermatitis), joints (HTLV-associated arthropathy), or the eye (uveitis). Rarely do persons concurrently develop ATL and HAM/TSP; however, there are documented cases of HAM/TSP with the other inflammatory diseases. It is currently unknown why there are distinct disease manifestations, but it may be due to the HTLV proviral load (Nagai et al. 1998; Manns et al. 1999b; Grant et al. 2002), the host immune response to HTLV (Jacobson et al. 1990), or the genetic background of the infected persons (Manns et al. 1998; Jeffery et al. 2000; Nishimura et al. 2000). For instance, studies calculating proviral load demonstrate that the proviral load is low among asymptomatic carriers compared to persons with HAM/TSP and ATL (Nagai et al. 1998; Manns et al. 1999b), suggesting that proviral load may be an indicator for future disease development.

ADULT T-CELL LEUKEMIA

An HTLV-1-infected person has an estimated 1 percent chance of developing adult T-cell leukemia (ATL) over their lifetime. Males are approximately 1.5 times more likely to develop ATL as females. ATL is diagnosed by seropositivity for HTLV-1, the presence of morphologically distinct $CD3^+/4^+/25^+$ lymphocytes with cleaved nuclei (flower cells)(Figure 58.3), and elevated serum lactate dehydrogenase activity. A comprehensive study on ATL published the outcome of 818 patients (Shimoyama 1991). That study characterized four clinically distinct subtypes of ATL. Smoldering ATL has the best prognosis with a mean survival time (MST) of >2 years and a projected 4-year survival of 62.8 percent. Smoldering ATL is characterized by skin and lung infiltration of leukemic cells and a normal leukocyte count with a low number of leukemic cells. Often it is hard to diagnose from the asymptomatic carrier since in both cases abnormal lymphocytes (flower cells) are detected in blood smears. However, only in ATL can clonal integration of HTLV-1 be detected by Southern blot. Chronic ATL has a MST of 24.3 months and a projected 4-year survival of 26.9 percent. In chronic ATL, there is a high leukocyte count, and it is associated with lymphadenopathy and hepatosplenomegaly. In both smoldering and chronic ATL, there is no association with hypercalcemia and no leukemic infiltration into the central nervous system, gastrointestinal tract, or bones. Lymphoma has a MST of 10.2 months with a projected 4-year survival of 5.7 percent. Acute ATL has a MST of 6 months and projected 4-year survival of 5 percent. These are both aggressive malignancies and are associated with massive lymphadenopathy, hepatosplenomegaly, lytic bone lesions, and multiple visceral lesions with skin and lung infiltration. Lymphoma and acute ATL patients are functionally immunosuppressed and

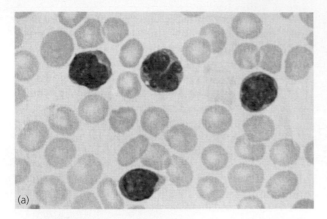

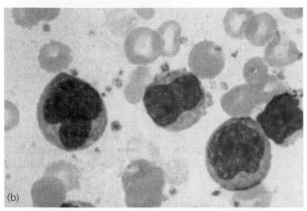

Figure 58.3 *Peripheral blood film of retrovirus infected patients.* **(a)** *Peripheral film of a patient with HTLV-I-associated adult T cell leukaemia/lymphoma (ATLL) showing lymphocytes with cleaved nuclei ×1000. (Courtesy of Professor D Gatovsky.)* **(b)** *Film of patient presenting with acute glandular fever illness during HIV seroconversion. Marked lymphocytosis with many abnormal immature-looking lymphocytes ×1500. (Courtesy of Dr C Ludlam.)*

may develop a variety of opportunistic infections. The difference between the lymphoma and acute types is whether or not the majority of leukemic cells is in the peripheral blood compartment. Lymphoma ATL has less than 1 percent leukemic cells present on a blood smear whereas acute ATL has a massive leukemic infiltrate in the peripheral blood.

HTLV-ASSOCIATED MYELOPATHY/TROPICAL SPASTIC PARAPARESIS

HTLV-1-infected persons have a lifetime risk of 0.25 percent for developing HTLV-associated myelopathy (HAM)/tropical spastic paraparesis (TSP) (Kaplan et al. 1990). Interestingly, females are three times as likely to develop HAM/TSP as are males. HAM/TSP is a slowly progressing myelopathy. The clinical features include the gradual onset of muscle weakness in the legs, hyperreflexia, clonus, extensor plantar responses, sensory disturbances, bowel and bladder dysfunction, impotence, and low back pain (Nagai and Jacobson 2001). However, unlike multiple sclerosis, HAM/TSP does not show periods of spontaneous improvement without treatment.

Diagnosis includes the presence of virus or HTLV-specific antibodies in the cerebrospinal fluid, brain, and spinal cord tissues. ATL flower cells are found in about half of HAM/TSP patients' peripheral blood and cerebrospinal fluid with a frequency of approximately 1 percent (Osame et al. 1987). Autopsy material from HAM/TSP patients shows loss of myelin and axons in the lateral, anterior, and posterior columns of the thoracic level of the spinal cord. This pathology is associated with an inflammatory infiltrate consisting of lymphocytes, predominately CD8[+] T cells, and foamy macrophages. The cytotoxic CD8[+] T cells are specific for HTLV-1 proteins, typically the pX gene products. It is thought that these HTLV-1-specific CD8[+] cytotoxic T lymphocytes are involved in the development of HAM/TSP by either directly lysing infected astrocytes (Kuroda et al. 1994; Lehky et al. 1995) or indirectly by secreting proinflammatory cytokines (Tendler et al. 1991; Kuroda and Matsui 1993).

OTHER INFLAMMATORY DISEASE ASSOCIATIONS

Other inflammatory disease associations include HTLV-associated uveitis (HU), HTLV-associated arthropathy (HAA), Sjögren's syndrome, and infective dermatitis (ID). HU, literally the inflammation of the uvea, is clinically characterized by the sudden onset of moderate or severe vitreous opacities with mild iritis and retinal vasculitis in one or both eyes (Mochizuki et al. 1996). Women are affected by HU twice as often as men. Patients with HU generally have a higher proviral load than asymptomatic HTLV-1 carriers, have viral particles and HTLV-1 provirus in their eyes, and accumulate HTLV-1-infected cells in their eyes (Ono et al. 1995; Sagawa et al. 1995). HU is self-limiting or responds well to treatment with topical or systemic corticosteroids; however, up to half of affected patients relapse. Generally, the visual prognosis is good after resolution (Takahashi et al. 2000).

HAA is indistinguishable from idiopathic rheumatoid arthritis with marked thickening of the synovial lining cells and lymphocytic infiltration of the sublining layer. The characteristic histopathological finding of an accumulation of HTLV-1 atypical lymphocytes in the synovial tissue and fluid as well as antibodies against HTLV-1 antigens in synovial fluid indicates that this is HAA (Sato et al. 1991). Epidemiologically, HTLV-1-infected persons are more likely to develop a polyarthropathy resembling rheumatoid arthritis than HTLV-1 negative persons (Motokawa et al. 1996). Furthermore, the arthropathy in the HTLV-1-infected persons was milder and onset was at a more advanced age compared to HTLV-1-negative persons with rheumatoid arthritis. The presence of HTLV-1 *Tax* is a common finding in synovial cells from persons with HAA. *Tax* expression is associated with increased inflammatory cytokine expression and synovial cell proliferation (Kitajima et al. 1991;

Miyasaka et al. 1991). Subsequent work with transgenic mice expressing the HTLV-1 *Tax* gene has shown the development of a polyarthropathy resembling rheumatoid arthritis (Iwakura et al. 1991, 1998) and it was associated with inflammatory cytokine expression (Iwakura et al. 1995).

Sjögren's syndrome is an autoimmune disorder characterized by a T-lymphocytic infiltration of salivary glands leading to ductal structure destruction (Eguchi et al. 1992; Ohyama et al. 1998). Epidemiologic reports have shown high seroprevalence of HTLV-1 among patients with Sjögren's syndrome in areas endemic for HTLV-1 (Eguchi et al. 1992; Terada et al. 1994). T-lymphocytic infiltrate in the salivary glands correlates to the clinical findings of Sjögren's syndrome (Nakamura et al. 2000). Furthermore, there is an accumulation of polyclonal HTLV-1-infected T cells expressing conserved T-cell receptor motifs in the salivary glands (Sasaki et al. 2000). The *Tax* gene sequence is detected in some salivary gland specimens, and expression of gene sequences homologous to HTLV-1 *Tax* may lead to the activation of autoreactive T cells in patients with Sjögren's syndrome (Sumida et al. 1994; Mariette et al. 2000).

ID is found commonly among children in the Caribbean and Japan. The average age at disease onset is 2 years with >50 percent of patients being female. Five major criteria are used for the diagnosis of ID (La Grenade et al. 1998) and include:

1 eczema of the scalp, axillae and groin, external ear and retroauricular areas, eyelid margins, paranasal skin, and/or neck
2 chronic watery nasal discharge without other signs of rhinitis and/or crusting of the anterior nares
3 chronic relapsing dermatitis with prompt response to appropriate therapy but prompt recurrence on withdrawal of antibiotics
4 usual onset in early childhood
5 HTLV-1 antibody seropositivity.

Skin lesions associated with ID become less severe with age, presumably due to the maturation of the immune system. Epidemiologic data indicate that ID is predictive of later ATL or HAM/TSP development (Hanchard et al. 1991; Tsukasaki et al. 1994; LaGrenade et al. 1995).

HTLV-2 ASSOCIATED DISEASES

Because of the genetic relatedness between HTLV-1 and HTLV-2, it was assumed that similar diseases would be associated with both viruses. However, no diseases have been definitively associated with HTLV-2. The estimated lifetime risk of disease development for HTLV-2-infected persons is unknown, but is less than that estimated for persons with HTLV-1 infection. A few reports have described forms of leukemia/lymphoma in HTLV-2-infected persons (Rosenblatt et al. 1986, 1987; Kaplan et al. 1991), but this is rare. There also has been a report

on a CD8$^+$ lymphocytosis associated with high HTLV-2 proviral copy numbers in intravenous drug users (Rosenblatt et al. 1990), but this has not been confirmed in other cohorts. Recently, HTLV-2 has been associated with a neurological disease resembling HAM/TSP (Jacobson et al. 1993; Murphy et al. 1997a; Silva et al. 2002) and ataxia (Harrington et al. 1993; Sheremata et al. 1993). These data suggest that HTLV-2-infected persons rarely develop disease; however, they should be followed up more closely for potential disease development.

IMMUNOSUPPRESSIVE NATURE OF HTLV-1 AND HTLV-2

While the majority of infected persons remain asymptomatic (>95 percent), recent studies report an increased incidence of infectious diseases (such as bronchitis and kidney and/or bladder infections) in HTLV-1- and HTLV-2-infected persons (Modahl et al. 1997; Murphy et al. 1997b, 1999) and an increased association with mortality, especially those persons with a high anti-HTLV-1 antibody titer (Arisawa et al. 1998). Higher rates of primary neoplasias have been reported in ATL patients, their siblings, and mothers as compared to HTLV-1-negative non-Hodgkin's lymphoma patients and their respective relatives in Japan (Kozuru et al. 1996). Clinical laboratory findings from asymptomatic HTLV-1 and HTLV-2-infected persons show altered blood chemistries and elevated absolute lymphocyte counts, but these findings were not significant enough to change their clinical evaluation or counseling of otherwise healthy HTLV-infected subjects (Glynn et al. 2000b). Some elderly HTLV-1-infected persons have anergic responses to purified protein derivative (PPD) (Suzuki et al. 1999). The inability to respond to PPD was found to be due in part to their inability to respond to IL-12. However, a more recent report showed that testing middle-aged HTLV-1- and HTLV-2-infected persons demonstrated no anergy to PPD, mumps, or *Candida albicans* antigens (Murphy et al. 2001). The wide spectrum of diseases indicates that further work is necessary to determine the full public health impact of HTLV infection in the general population.

Treatment

To date, therapy for ATL has had limited success. A combination of interferon-alpha (IFN-α) and zidovudine has been effective in a limited number of cases (Gill et al. 1995; Hermine et al. 1995). For persons with HAM/TSP, early disease can be alleviated by corticosteroids, and some relief is seen with zidovudine and danazol (Gout et al. 1991; Harrington et al. 1991). Lamivudine has been shown to decrease HTLV-1 proviral load, but has not been shown to clinically improve HAM/TSP patients who have established disease (Taylor et al. 1999). Despite a recent study showing that

HTLV-1 RT was equally susceptible to zidovudine, zalcitabine, didanosine, and stavudine, but resistant to lamivudine (Garcia-Lerma et al. 2001), lack of sustained clinical remission suggests that alternative treatments need to be found.

Long-term, high dose IFN-α therapy has been shown to reduce HTLV-1 proviral load and improve motor performance in six patients (Yamasaki et al. 1997). However, no randomized trials have been done to compare the effectiveness of these therapies for ATL or HAM/TSP treatment. Arsenic trioxide (As$_2$O$_3$), which causes apoptosis of HTLV-1-infected cell lines or fresh ATL cells from patients, has been proposed for the treatment of ATL (Ishitsuka et al. 1998). Its combination with IFN-α appears to have a high synergistic effect in vitro (Bazarbachi et al. 1999). The clinical application of IL-2R-directed therapy, using a humanized monoclonal antibody (or that antibody armed with radionuclides), provides a new perspective for the treatment of autoimmune disorders such as HAM/TSP and certain neoplastic diseases including ATL (Waldmann 1996). Antibodies directed toward both IL-15 and IL-2, or their receptors, inhibit almost completely the proliferation of peripheral blood mononuclear cells (PBMC) from HAM/TSP patients in vitro (Azimi et al. 1999). While these treatments show promise, they still need to be tested in a clinical setting.

Epidemiology

HTLV-1 and HTLV-2 share approximately 60 percent of their nucleotide sequences; yet they have distinct evolutionary and geographical distributions. HTLV-1 infects 15–20 million people worldwide, with endemic foci in southern Japan, the Caribbean, Melanesia, sub-Saharan Africa, and Central and South America (de The and Bomford 1993; Madeleine et al. 1993). The seroprevalence rate ranges from 3–6 percent in the Caribbean islands (Murphy et al. 1991) to approximately 27 percent in southern Japan (Mueller et al. 1996). HTLV-2 is endemic in Amerindian tribes throughout North and South America as well as pygmy tribes in Central Africa with seroprevalences ranging from 3 to 33 percent (Maloney et al. 1992; Hjelle et al. 1994). In the USA and Europe, the seroprevalence for both HTLV-1 and HTLV-2 among low-risk populations is less than 1 percent (Manns et al. 1999a). However, high-risk populations such as IDUs, who are predominately HTLV-2 infected, have a seroprevalence ranging from 0.4 to 20 percent (Kaplan and Khabbaz 1993).

HTLV-1 and HTLV-2 infections are spread through sexual, vertical, and parenteral transmission. Sexual transmission of HTLV-1 has been shown to primarily occur from male to female; however, female-to-male transmission does occur, albeit at a lower efficiency (Murphy et al. 1989; Stuver et al. 1993; Sullivan et al.

1993). Sexual transmission has been associated with older male partners, length of relationship, high anti-HTLV antibody titers, and high proviral load (Stuver et al. 1993; Kaplan et al. 1996). Less is known about the sexual acquisition of HTLV-2; however, in an HTLV-2 endemic area, there was a strong concordance of seropositivity between spouses (Vitek et al. 1995). The role of other sexually transmitted diseases in the spread of HTLV-1 or HTLV-2 is less clear. Persons engaging in high-risk sexual relationships have been shown to have a higher seroprevalence of HTLV-1 (Murphy et al. 1989; Wiktor et al. 1990; Nakashima et al. 1995). A history of having both ulcerative and nonulcerative sexually transmitted diseases has been associated with a higher prevalence of antibodies to HTLV-1, suggesting that they may affect HTLV-1 transmission (Murphy et al. 1989; Nakashima et al. 1995). Recently, cervicitis was shown to be associated with cervical shedding of HTLV-1 and thus may increase HTLV transmission (Zunt et al. 2002). More work is needed to fully address the role of sexually transmitted diseases in the sexual transmission of HTLV-1 and HTLV-2.

Vertical transmission, also known as mother-to-child transmission, primarily occurs through postnatal breastfeeding. HTLV-1 and HTLV-2-infected lymphocytes have been isolated from breast milk (Kinoshita et al. 1984; Heneine et al. 1992b). Mothers that have been shown to transmit HTLV to their children have higher viral antigen-producing capacity from isolated breast milk mononuclear cells as well as proviral load (Yoshinaga et al. 1995; Ureta-Vidal et al. 1999). Additional maternal factors that are important for transmission are high titer of HTLV antibodies (Hino et al. 1987; Hirata et al. 1992), and breastfeeding for more than 12 months (Takahashi et al. 1991; Wiktor et al. 1993; Hino et al. 1996). It was shown that reducing the length of breastfeeding significantly reduces the transmission of HTLV-1 (Takahashi et al. 1991; Wiktor et al. 1993). While the majority of vertical transmission occurs through breast milk, there is a minor population of children that becomes infected even if not breastfed. In utero transmission has been proposed as a secondary route for mother-to-child transmission. Several groups inconsistently found HTLV-1 proviral DNA in cord blood mononuclear cells from the HTLV-1-infected children, suggesting that in utero infection may not be a major route of transmission in children who were not breast-fed (Kawase et al. 1992; Katamine et al. 1994; Nyambi et al. 1996).

Transmission via saliva is considered possible but studies presenting direct evidence for this mode of transmission have not been published. HTLV-1 proviral DNA has been detected in saliva or mouthwashes from ATL (Taniguchi et al. 1993) and HAM/TSP patients (Soto-Ramirez et al. 1995; Achiron et al. 1996; Offen et al. 1998), and asymptomatic HTLV-infected carriers (Yamamoto et al. 1995; Achiron et al. 1996; Belec et al. 1996; Offen et al. 1998). Antibodies against HTLV-1 are also present in saliva (Archibald et al. 1987; Soto-Ramirez et al. 1995; Yamamoto et al. 1995). The association of the presence of viral RNA and local IgA in saliva has been thought to provide evidence that viral replication may occur in the oral cavity of HAM/TSP patients and some asymptomatic carriers (Soto-Ramirez et al. 1995). However, the neutralizing effect of saliva IgG on syncytium formation in vitro and the saliva's ability, even in the absence of antibodies, to inhibit cell-to-cell transmission of HTLV-1 in vitro demonstrate that transmission through the saliva, if it occurs at all, would be rare (Yamamoto et al. 1995).

Injecting drug use and sex with IDUs are the most important risk factors for HTLV-2 transmission (Kaplan and Khabbaz 1993). Because of the high risk of transfusion-related transmission of HTLV-1 and HTLV-2, screening of volunteer blood donors has been implemented in Japan, several Caribbean countries, various European countries, and the USA and Canada (Whyte 1997; Courouce et al. 1999; Glynn et al. 2000a). The effectiveness of these screening programs is manifested by reduced risk of transfusion-related transmission. In the USA, the incidence rates of seroconversion associated with HTLV in blood donors is estimated to be 1.59 per 100 000 persons per year (Glynn et al. 2000a), and the residual risk of transmitting HTLV infection by transfusing screened blood is estimated to be 1 in 641 000 (Schreiber et al. 1996).

Laboratory diagnosis

The most common assays used for screening persons detect antibodies in serum or plasma. However, such assays detect only past exposure to the viruses. Direct detection of HTLV-1 and HTLV-2 is achieved through the use of nucleic acid assays such as the polymerase chain reaction (PCR).

SEROLOGICAL DETECTION

The immunodominant regions of structural proteins and regulatory gene regions have been well characterized (Lal 1996) and are the basis for the development of diagnostic assays both for detection and differentiation of HTLV-1 and HTLV-2. Typically, an enzyme immunoassay (EIA) is used as the primary screening assay, and western blot (WB) is used as a confirmatory test. Particle agglutination assays, which are based on the agglutination of HTLV-1 lysate-coated gelatin particles by antibodies in a test specimen, are also used in various countries as screening assays.

The EIA is a colorimetric test that is both sensitive and simple to perform and generally now uses purified HTLV-1 and HTLV-2-infected cell lysates and/or HTLV-1 and HTLV-2 recombinant antigens or synthetic peptides. The addition of HTLV-2 antigens to test kits significantly improved the detection of antibodies to HTLV-2, compared with results using kits that contained only HTLV-1 antigens (Andersson et al. 1999; Liu et al. 1999; Poiesz et al. 2000). Comparative analysis of various commercial screening assays containing both HTLV-1 and HTLV-2 antigens indicates that sensitivity ranges from 98.9 to 100 percent for confirmed HTLV-1-positive specimens and 91.5 to 100 percent for confirmed HTLV-2 positive specimens. Specificity ranges from 90.2 to 100 percent for both infections (Andersson et al. 1999; Poiesz et al. 2000). These assays are used for both blood donor screening and as an aid in clinical diagnosis of HTLV-1 and HTLV-2 infection and related diseases. However, the EIAs cannot differentiate between infection with HTLV-1 and HTLV-2 because of the significant homology in structural proteins between the two viruses (Courouce et al. 1999). To serologically differentiate between these viruses, WB is used.

Although WB assays using purified viral lysates are highly sensitive for detecting p24^{gag} antibodies, they do not always detect antibodies to native envelope glycoproteins. Several approaches have addressed this issue in second-generation WB assays. In one, viral lysates have been spiked with recombinant p21e protein (p21e). Antibodies to p21e are detected more easily compared to those to gp46^{env}; however, some false-positive specimens have been identified by this test (Lal et al. 1992a; Busch et al. 1994; Kleinman et al. 1994). A second approach is a modified WB that contains type-specific gp46^{env} recombinant proteins from HTLV-1 and HTLV-2, as well as a truncated form of p21e (gd21) that reduces nonspecific reactivity (Varma et al. 1995) (Figure 58.3). This assay not only serves as a confirmatory serological test but also permits the differentiation of infection between HTLV-1 and HTLV-2 (Varma et al. 1995). The modified WB has improved specificity and is sensitive for most subtypes of HTLV-1 and HTLV-2 (Varma et al. 1995). Specimens with reactivity to p24^{gag} and p21e, but no reactivity to either rgp46^{I} or rgp46^{II}, are referred to as HTLV-positive untypeable. PCR analysis of these untypeable specimens has identified the presence of HTLV-specific sequences (Varma et al. 1995). In rare instances, specimens with confirmed HTLV infection have reactivity to p19^{gag} (in the absence of p24) and p21e (Cesaire et al. 1999; Rouet et al. 2001). Likewise, in some instances, antibody to p21e may represent an early antibody response during the 6-month seroconversion window period, and individuals with such reactivity should be retested in 6 months (Manns et al. 1992). It is the current policy of the US Public Health Service to recommend that the diagnostic criteria for WB tests require that a specimen demonstrating antibodies to p24^{gag} and to native gp46^{env} and/or recombinant p21e are considered seropositive for HTLV-1 or HTLV-2 (CDC and the U.S.P.H.S. Working Group 1993). Specimens reacting with any of the bands, but not satisfying the above criteria, are designated indeterminate. Specimens with no immunoreactivity to any bands are considered negative for antibodies to HTLV-1 and HTLV-2 (false-positive EIA specimens).

Both of the WB assays can give indeterminate results or show immunoreactivity to a single HTLV gene product, conditions which do not meet the criteria of seropositivity (Busch et al. 1994; Varma et al. 1995). Antibody to only Gag proteins (p24, p19) is the most common indeterminate pattern that is observed in EIA-reactive specimens, and extensive PCR analysis using primers to detect multiple gene regions have failed to detect HTLV-1 or HTLV-2 proviral sequences in these seroindeterminate persons thus indicating that these individuals are not likely to be infected with HTLV-1 or HTLV-2 (Lal et al. 1992b; Medrano et al. 1997; Cesaire et al. 1999; Rouet et al. 2001). Limited studies have also established that individuals with indeterminate WB profiles generally do not have risk factors for HTLV infection (Mauclere et al. 1997; Medrano et al. 1997; Cesaire et al. 1999; Rouet et al. 2001). Such indeterminate WB results appear to represent antibodies to different viral and cellular antigens that cross-react with HTLV proteins (Mahieux et al. 2000). However, recent data suggest that a small number of patients with chronic progressive neurological disease and HTLV-indeterminate WB patterns may be due to infection with a defective HTLV or have HTLV-1 in low copy numbers (Soldan et al. 1999; Waziri et al. 2000). The possibility that such indeterminate WB results may represent a novel retrovirus with partial homology to HTLV has also been explored; however, no amplification was observed using generic PCR primers that would amplify HTLV-related viruses (Vandamme et al. 1997; Busch et al. 2000).

NUCLEIC ACID DETECTION

Amplification of proviral DNA by PCR is the preferred method for determining infection status, testing the validity of serological assays, distinguishing between HTLV-1 and HTLV-2, and studying the in vivo tissue distribution. These qualitative and quantitative PCR techniques can be used to identify HTLV infections for subtyping purposes or for determining viral load.

Two quantitative PCR procedures have been successfully used on PBMCs to confirm and differentiate between HTLV-1 and HTLV-2 infections. The first uses HTLV consensus primers that allow amplification of both viruses; typing is achieved either by hybridizing the product to an HTLV-1-specific or HTLV-2-specific probe (Heneine et al. 1992a) (Figure 58.4) or by specific restriction digestion patterns (Tuke et al. 1992). A second approach employs type-specific primers and probes in separate amplifications (Heneine et al. 1992a). The PCR products can be detected with labeled internal probes by Southern blot hybridization. A solid-phase, nonradioactive, EIA-based detection system has been

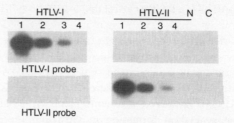

Figure 58.4 *Generic PCR amplification of HTLV-I and HTLV-II by SK110/SK111 and differentiation by type-specific probing. Numbers 1, 2, 3 and 4 refer to lysates of uninfected Hut-78 cells containing 1500, 150, 2 and 0 HTLV-I infected (MT-2) or HTLV-II (MO-T) cells, respectively. C, reagent cocktail control; N, Hut-78. The HTLV-I specific probe is SK112, and the HTLV-II probe is SK188.*

developed which seems highly sensitive and specific for detection and differentiation of both HTLV-1 and HTLV-2 (Dyster et al. 1994; Dezzutti et al. 1996).

Multiplex DNA PCR is a semiquantitative technique used for the simultaneous amplification, detection, and discrimination of different target sequences in one tube. In addition to primers for HTLV-1/HTLV-2 detection, primers for HIV-1/HIV-2 detection are also included. Primers for the *gag* region of HIV-1, *env* region of HIV-2, *pol* region of HTLV-1, and *Tax* of HTLV-2 are used to provide specific and sensitive coamplification of proviral sequences (Heredia et al. 1996; Vet et al. 1999). Multiplex PCR can detect fewer than ten proviral copies for each virus per sample and thus can provide an accurate measure of the number of copies of each proviral sequence that were originally present in the sample.

Additional quantitative nucleic acid assays have been developed to determine proviral DNA load. These assays include nested PCR with limiting dilution (Tosswill et al. 1998), quantitative competitive PCR (Albrecht et al. 1998), and real-time PCR (Kamihira et al. 2000; Miley et al. 2000). Primers have been designed for the *gag*, *tax*, or *pol* genes, and all are highly sensitive.

VIRUS ISOLATION, ANTIGEN DETECTION, AND REVERSE TRANSCRIPTASE ASSAYS

Viral isolation of HTLV-1 or HTLV-2 has been difficult due to the cell-associated nature of this virus. Nevertheless, cocultivation of HTLV-1- and HTLV-2-infected PBMCs with activated, allogeneic HTLV-negative PBMCs is used to obtain viral isolates. The culture supernatants are collected weekly, for up to 4 weeks, and the presence of p19^{gag} antigen in the supernatant is tested using an antigen-capture EIA. Alternatively, detection of viral replication in cultures supernatants is accomplished by detecting HTLV reverse transcriptase activity using an amplified reverse transcriptase (AMP-RT) assay (Yamamoto et al. 1996). This assay was shown to detect the presence of HTLV-1 and HTLV-2 in culture supernatants that were not detected by EIA.

ZOONOTIC RETROVIRUS INFECTIONS

The identification of isolated infections with either simian immunodeficiency virus (SIV) or simian foamy virus (SFV) in occupationally exposed workers suggested that occupational contact with nonhuman primates (NHP) may be associated with risks of transmission of simian retroviruses (Khabbaz et al. 1992, 1994; Schweizer et al. 1995, 1997). The recognition that human HIV-1 and HIV-2 infections originated from simian-to-human transmission of SIV has heightened concerns of cross-species transmission of animal retroviruses. Such transmissions could occur in various settings: occupational exposures to NHPs (e.g. in biomedical research), exposures to NHPs as pets or in zoological gardens, or in occasions when NHP organs have been used in xeno-transplantation. In addition to SIV and SFV, NHP are natural hosts to several exogenous retroviruses including simian T-lymphotropic viruses (STLV) and simian type D viruses (SRV) (Lowenstine and Lerche 1988).

Foamy viruses (FV), including SFV, belong to the *Spumavirus* genus in the family *Retroviridae*. FVs cause cytopathic effects with syncytium formation in vitro, but appear to be nonpathogenic in vivo. They establish persistent infections in many animal species, including nonhuman primates, cats, cows, and sea lions. SFVs infect more than 70 percent of captive nonhuman primates (Hooks and Gibbs 1975; Neumann-Haefelin et al. 1993; Schweizer et al. 1995; Meiering and Linial 2001), in which they appear to cause latent infection in almost all organs – spleen, liver, kidney, salivary gland, brain (Swack and Hsiung 1975) – and can be readily detected by PCR in PBMCs. Minimal viral replication appears to occur in the oral mucosa (Falcone et al. 1999).

Human infection with SFV

A foamy virus referred to as human foamy virus (HFV), now called prototype foamy virus (PFV), was isolated from a nasopharyngeal carcinoma specimen from a Kenyan man (Achong et al. 1971). Following its detection, seroepidemiologic studies in human populations have shown controversial results. Most studies did not find antibodies to PFV even in populations exposed to NHPs (Brown et al. 1978; Nemo et al. 1978; Schweizer et al. 1995). Some earlier serological studies reported seropositivity among certain populations from 6.9 percent among Pacific Islanders (Loh et al. 1980) to 17 percent in Kenyans (Achong and Epstein 1978) but later studies using confirmatory testing could not confirm PFV antibody presence even in sera highly reactive by enzyme-linked immunosorbent assay (ELISA) (Ali et al. 1996; Heneine et al. 2003). Most of the earlier studies did not always use adequate methods to control for false-positive results or additional confirmatory methods were not available at that time (Heneine et al. 2003).

The failure to find antibodies to PFV in sera from 250 persons, including 50 with nasopharyngeal carcinoma and Burkitt's lymphoma (Brown et al. 1978), the cross-reactivity of PFV with antibodies to SFV (Nemo et al. 1978), and sequence analyses all suggested that the PFV was most likely of chimpanzee origin (Herchenroder et al. 1994).

Recent studies, using WB for detection of antibodies and confirmatory testing for viral DNA, have documented seropositivity to SFV in 19 persons from Germany, the USA, and Canada (Schweizer et al. 1995, 1997; Heneine et al. 1998; Sandstrom et al. 2000; Brooks et al. 2002; Switzer et al. 2004). All of them have been occupationally exposed to nonhuman primates, their biological fluids, or to simian viruses in the laboratory. Sequence analysis confirmed that SFV infection has originated from baboons, chimpanzees, macaques, and African green monkeys (Heneine et al. 1998) (Figure 58.5). A study of Cameroonians who reported contact with nonhuman primates through hunting and butchering demonstrated SFV infection in natural settings (Wolfe et al. 2004). Ten of 1 099 (1 percent) persons had SFV WB positive results. Three WB-positive persons were also PCR-positive. Sequence analysis indicated that SFV was acquired from a mandrill, gorilla, and a DeBrazza guenon.

Characteristics of human infection with foamy viruses

Early studies raised questions about possible associations between PFV infection and a variety of human diseases (e.g. thyroiditis, amyotrophic lateral sclerosis, hemodialysis encephalopathy) (Cameron et al. 1978; Werner and Gelderblom 1979; Lagaye et al. 1992; Westphal et al. 1992; Stancek et al. 1995). Later studies, using more precise diagnostic methods, did not confirm such associations or endemic human infection (Heneine 1995; Schweizer et al. 1995, 1997; Ali et al. 1996; Rosener et al. 1996; Winkler et al. 2000).

Humans infected with SFV show persistent seropositivity by WB; testing of stored sera revealed that some persons have been seropositive for more than 20 years (Heneine et al. 1998; Switzer et al. 2004). The identification, by PCR, of two conserved SFV proviral DNA sequences in PBMCs confirms the persistent nature of the SFV infection (Heneine et al. 1998).

Although PFV can cause transient immunosuppression in experimentally infected mice and rabbits (Santillana-Hayat et al. 1993), currently there is no evidence that SFVs are pathogenic in their natural host (Weiss 1996; Linial 2000). Available data on the SFV-infected persons show that no obvious disease can be attributed to these infections at the time of their detec-

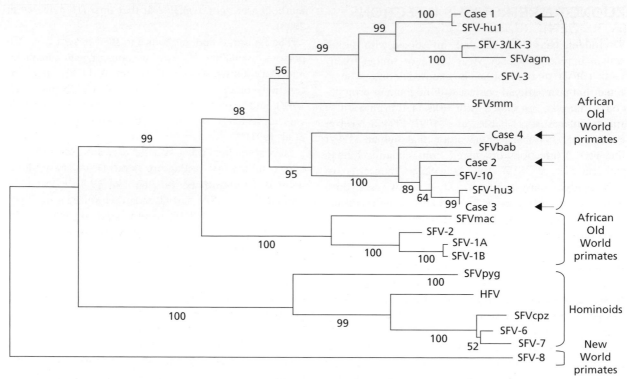

Figure 58.5 *NHP species origin of SFV infections in workers occupationally exposed to NHPs. Phylogenetic analysis by neighbor-joining of SFV pol sequences derived from peripheral blood lymphocytes of four case workers and from SFVhu1 and SFVh3, two SFV isolates obtained from case 1 and case 3, respectively. SFV sequences of different NHP species shown are SFVagm, SFVsmm, SFVbab, SFVmac, SFVpyg, obtained from African green monkey, sooty mangabey, baboon, and pygmy chimpanzee, respectively. SFVcpz and SFV-6 and SFV-7, from chimpanzees, SFV-8 from spider monkey (a New World monkey species). Numbers shown at branch nodes represent bootstrap percent values.*

tion (Schweizer et al. 1995, 1997; Heneine et al. 1998; Sandstrom et al. 2000; Brooks et al. 2002). Because FV are considered nonpathogenic and because they can infect a broad range of human cells and human cell lines in the laboratory (Meiering and Linial 2001), they are considered as potential candidates for gene transfer therapy (Bieniasz et al. 1997; Hill et al. 1999).

HTLV infections are an example that retroviruses may cause a disease in a small proportion of infected individuals and after a long latent period. To better characterize the course of SFV infection in humans, the US Centers for Disease Control and Prevention (CDC) has initiated a long-term follow-up of SFV-infected persons.

Human-to-human transmission

No evidence of male-to-female transmission in wives of six SFV-infected workers was found, suggesting that transmission of SFV among humans by sexual or less intimate contact may not occur easily (Schweizer et al. 1997; Heneine et al. 1998; Switzer et al. 2004). Four recipients of blood components from one SFV-infected donor were tested 1.9 to 7 years after transfusion and are not infected (Boneva et al. 2002). Although preliminary, these data suggest that secondary SFV transmis-

sion among humans appears unlikely and humans may be a dead-end host of the SFV infection – as is often the case with zoonoses. However, a larger number of SFV-infected persons and their contacts need to be followed for a longer period of time to confirm lack of human-to-human transmission and benign nature of the SFV infection in humans.

Other animal retroviruses

The observation that SFV appears to be readily transmissible to humans raises concerns that human contact with other domestic animals such as cats, all of which are known to harbor FV and other retroviruses (Tobaly-Tapiero et al. 2001), may be accompanied with risk of zoonosis. A study of persons occupationally exposed to cats by Butera et al. (Butera et al. 2000) found no evidence of infection with either feline foamy virus (FFV), feline leukemia virus (FeLV) or feline immunodeficiency virus (FIV) in 203 North American feline veterinary practitioners. Persons studied reported extensive duration of work with cats and multiple high-risk exposures. Similarly, Winkler et al. (1999) found no evidence of FFV zoonosis among Australian veterinarians, although exposure to felines were not clearly defined in that study.

XENOTRANSPLANTATION AND OTHER IATROGENIC RISKS OF INFECTION WITH ANIMAL RETROVIRUSES

Particular attention has been given to risks of transfer of animal retroviruses to humans through xenotransplantation – the use of live animal tissues or cells as xenografts. Interest in xenotransplantation has increased because of its potential to provide a solution for the chronic shortage of allotransplants or to provide porcine pancreatic islet cells for treatment of diabetes, or neuron cells for treatment of Parkinson's disease. Organs from NHPs have been used with some success in the past but currently pigs are the preferred source of animal xenografts. Both NHPs and pigs harbor endogenous retroviruses, which cannot be eliminated from source animals by pretransplant screening because their DNA is part of the cell's DNA. For example, porcine endogenous retroviruses (PoEV) and baboon endogenous viruses (BaEV) can infect human cells and have been extensively studied recently as potential causes of zoonotic infections in relation to xenotransplantation. SFV and BaEV sequences were detected in multiple tissue compartments of two human recipients of baboon livers (Allan et al. 1998). The presence of baboon mitochondrial DNA was also detected in these same tissues, suggesting that xenogeneic 'passenger leukocytes' harboring latent or active viral infections had migrated from the xenografts to distant sites within the human recipients. The persistence of SFV and BaEV in human recipients in the post-transplant period reveals the potential infectious risks associated with xenotransplantation (Allan et al. 1998). More than 200 persons exposed to various porcine xenografts have been tested for PoEV without evidence for infection (Herring et al. 2001). In one of the studies, about 23 percent of persons exposed to live porcine tissue had proviral sequences detected in quantities consistent with microchimerism but not infection (Paradis et al. 1999). PoEV has also been found as a contaminant of porcine factor VIII concentrates, which are used to treat hemophiliacs (Heneine et al. 2001); however, there was no evidence for PoEV infection in 88 recipients of this product (Heneine et al. 2001).

The identification of RT activity in chick-cell-derived vaccines including measles, mumps, and yellow fever vaccines has led to studies to identify the source of the RT activity and assess the risks it poses to vaccine recipients (Boni et al. 1996; Tsang et al. 1999). These investigations indicated that the RT activity in the measles, mumps, and rubella (MMR) vaccines and in yellow fever (YF) vaccines was found to be associated with viral particles containing RNA from the endogenous avian leukosis virus subgoup E (ALV-E) and the endogenous avian virus (EAV) (Weissmahr et al. 1997; Tsang et al. 1999; Johnson and Heneine 2001; Hussain et al. 2003). Both ALV-E and EAV originate from the chick embryonic fibroblasts used to propagate the measles and mumps vaccines, or from the chick embryos used for YF vaccine production. The detection of RT activity in all vaccine lots suggested that vaccine recipients might be universally exposed to these endogenous chicken retroviral particles. However, testing of MMR and YF vaccine recipients has thus far revealed no evidence of transmission of ALV-E or EAV to vaccine recipients. No antibody reactivity to either ALV-E or EAV was found in 206 US recipients of MMR vaccine and in 43 Brazilian recipients of YF vaccine (Hussain et al. 2001; Johnson and Heneine 2001). No ALV-E and EAV sequences were also detected by PCR in serum and peripheral blood lymphocyte samples from these vaccinees (Hussain et al. 2001; Johnson and Heneine 2001). While current data continue to support the use of chick-cell-derived MMR and YF vaccines, the presence of adventitious avian retroviral particles in these vaccines has raised questions about the suitability of primary chicken cell substrates for vaccine production.

Using retroviral vectors such as the Moloney murine leukemia virus for retrovirally mediated gene transfer has proven successful in treating certain genetic conditions. However, the recently reported lymphoproliferative disease in two of ten children treated for X-linked severe combined immunodeficiency demonstrates the risks that may be associated with retroviral integration and insertional mutagenesis (Hacein-Bey-Abina et al. 2003).

RETROVIRUSES, CANCER, AND DISEASES OF UNKNOWN ETIOLOGY

Interestingly, the literature is replete with studies showing the associations of cancer with retroviruses in animals. With the exception of the HTLV, humans are somewhat void of such associations. Our genome, on the other hand, contains remnants of retroviral elements (as endogenous retroviruses), suggesting that during our evolution we encountered and symbiotically associated with these viruses, which now provides a resistance to retroviral-mediated cancers. Retroviruses and/or retroviral components have been investigated for years as the putative agent in other diseases of unknown etiology. Numerous papers attempt to assign a retrovirus, its insertion, or gene product to the cause and association with many diseases such as multiple sclerosis, osteoarthritis, systemic lupus erythematosus, Sjögren's disease, Graves' disease, just to name a few. It has been neither the intent nor the aim of this chapter to refute those claims here, but rather to present the most scientifically accepted associations of retroviruses with human disease and infection. Retroviruses are constantly emerging and their ability to zoonotically transmit, recombine, mutate, and 'trap' other genes makes them a constant concern for the stewards of public health.

REFERENCES

Achiron, A., Pinhas-Hamiel, O., et al. 1996. Detection of proviral human T-cell lymphotrophic virus type I DNA in mouthwash samples of HAM/TSP patients and HTLV-I carriers. *Arch Virol*, **141**, 147–53.

Achong, B.G. and Epstein, M.A. 1978. Preliminary seroepidemiological studies on the human syncytial virus. *J Gen Virol*, **40**, 175–81.

Achong, B.G., Mansell, P.W., et al. 1971. An unusual virus in cultures from a human nasopharyngeal carcinoma. *J Natl Cancer Inst*, **46**, 299–307.

Albrecht, B., Collins, N.D., et al. 1998. Quantification of human T-cell lymphotropic virus type 1 proviral load by quantitative competitive polymerase chain reaction. *J Virol Methods*, **75**, 123–40.

Albrecht, B., Collins, N.D., et al. 2000. Human T-lymphotropic virus type 1 open reading frame I p12(I) is required for efficient viral infectivity in primary lymphocytes. *J Virol*, **74**, 9828–35.

Albrecht, B., D'Souza, C.D., et al. 2002. Activation of nuclear factor of activated T cells by human T- lymphotropic virus type 1 accessory protein p12(I). *J Virol*, **76**, 3493–501.

Ali, M., Taylor, G.P., et al. 1996. No evidence of antibody to human foamy virus in widespread human populations. *AIDS Res Hum Retroviruses*, **12**, 1473–83.

Allan, J.S., Broussard, S.R., et al. 1998. Amplification of simian retroviral sequences from human recipients of baboon liver transplants. *AIDS Res Hum Retroviruses*, **14**, 821–4.

Andersson, S., Thorstensson, R., et al. 1999. Comparative evaluation of 14 immunoassays for detection of antibodies to the human T-lymphotropic virus types I and II using panels of sera from Sweden and West Africa. *Transfusion*, **39**, 845–51.

Archibald, D., Essex, M., et al. 1987. Antibodies to HTLV-1 in saliva of seropositive individuals from Japan. *Viral Immunol*, **1**, 241–6.

Arisawa, K., Soda, M., et al. 1998. Human T-lymphotropic virus type-I infection, antibody titers and cause-specific mortality among atomic-bomb survivors. *Jpn J Cancer Res*, **89**, 797–805.

Azimi, N., Jacobson, S., et al. 1999. Involvement of IL-15 in the pathogenesis of human T lymphotropic virus type I-associated myelopathy/tropical spastic paraparesis: implications for therapy with a monoclonal antibody directed to the IL-2/15R beta receptor. *J Immunol*, **163**, 4064–72.

Ballaun, C., Farrington, G.K., et al. 1991. Functional analysis of human T-cell leukemia virus type I rex-response element: direct RNA binding of Rex protein correlates with in vivo activity. *J Virol*, **65**, 4408–13.

Bar-Shira, A., Panet, A. and Honigman, A. 1991. An RNA secondary structure juxtaposes two remote genetic signals for human T-cell leukemia virus type I RNA 3′-end processing. *J Virol*, **65**, 5165–73.

Bazarbachi, A., El-Sabban, M.E., et al. 1999. Arsenic trioxide and interferon-alpha synergize to induce cell cycle arrest and apoptosis in human T-cell lymphotropic virus type I- transformed cells. *Blood*, **93**, 278–83.

Belec, L., Jean Georges, A., et al. 1996. Human T-lymphotropic virus type I excretion and specific antibody response in paired saliva and cervicovaginal secretions. *AIDS Res Hum Retroviruses*, **12**, 157–67.

Bieniasz, P.D., Erlwein, O., et al. 1997. Gene transfer using replication-defective human foamy virus vectors. *Virology*, **235**, 65–72.

Boneva, R.S., Grindon, A.J., et al. 2002. Simian foamy virus infection in a blood donor. *Transfusion*, **42**, 886–91.

Boni, J., Pyra, H. and Schupbach, J. 1996. Sensitive detection and quantification of particle-associated reverse transcriptase in plasma of HIV-1-infected individuals by the product-enhanced reverse transcriptase (PERT) assay. *J Med Virol*, **49**, 23–8.

Brooks, J.I., Rud, E.W., et al. 2002. Cross-species retroviral transmission from macaques to human beings. *Lancet*, **360**, 387–8.

Brown, P., Nemo, G. and Gajdusek, D.C. 1978. Human foamy virus: further characterization, seroepidemiology, and relationship to chimpanzee foamy viruses. *J Infect Dis*, **137**, 421–7.

Busch, M.P., Laycock, M., et al. 1994. Accuracy of supplementary serologic testing for human T-lymphotropic virus types I and II in US blood donors. Retrovirus Epidemiology Donor Study. *Blood*, **83**, 1143–8.

Busch, M.P., Switzer, W.M., et al. 2000. Absence of evidence of infection with divergent primate T-lymphotropic viruses in United States blood donors who have seroindeterminate HTLV test results. *Transfusion*, **40**, 443–9.

Butera, S.T., Brown, J., et al. 2000. Survey of veterinary conference attendees for evidence of zoonotic infection by feline retroviruses. *J Am Vet Med Assoc*, **217**, 1475–9.

Cameron, K.R., Birchall, S.M. and Moses, M.A. 1978. Isolation of foamy virus from patient with dialysis encephalopathy. *Lancet*, **2**, 796.

Cavrois, M., Gessain, A., et al. 1996. Proliferation of HTLV-1 infected circulating cells in vivo in all asymptomatic carriers and patients with TSP/HAM. *Oncogene*, **12**, 2419–23.

CDC and the U.S.P.H.S. Working Group. 1993. Guidelines for counseling persons infected with human T-lymphotropic virus type I (HTLV-I) and type II (HTLV-II). *Ann Intern Med*, **118**, 448–54.

Cesaire, R., Bera, O., et al. 1999. Seroindeterminate patterns and seroconversions to human T-lymphotropic virus type I positivity in blood donors from Martinique, French West Indies. *Transfusion*, **39**, 1145–9.

Ciminale, V., Zotti, L., et al. 1999. Mitochondrial targeting of the p13II protein coded by the x-II ORF of human T-cell leukemia/lymphotropic virus type I (HTLV-I). *Oncogene*, **18**, 4505–14.

Collins, N.D., Newbound, G.C., et al. 1998. Selective ablation of human T-cell lymphotropic virus type 1 p12I reduces viral infectivity *in vivo*. *Blood*, **91**, 4701–7.

Courouce, A.M., Pillonel, J. and Saura, C. 1999. Screening of blood donations for HTLV-I/II. *Trans Med Rev*, **13**, 267–74.

Daenke, S., McCracken, S.A. and Booth, S. 1999. Human T-cell leukaemia/lymphoma virus type 1 syncytium formation is regulated in a cell-specific manner by ICAM-1, ICAM-3 and VCAM-1 and can be inhibited by antibodies to integrin beta2 or beta7. *J Gen Virol*, **80**, 1429–36.

D'Agostino, D.M., Ranzato, L., et al. 2002. Mitochondrial alterations induced by the p13II protein of human T-cell leukemia virus type 1. Critical role of arginine residues. *J Biol Chem*, **277**, 34424–33.

de The, G. and Bomford, R. 1993. An HTLV-I vaccine: why, how, for whom? *AIDS Res Hum Retroviruses*, **9**, 381–6.

Dezzutti, C.S., Rudolph, D.L. and Lal, R.B. 1995. Infection with human T-lymphotropic virus types I and II results in alterations of cellular receptors, including the up-modulation of T-cell counterreceptors CD40, CD54 and CD80 (B7-1). *Clin Diagn Lab Immunol*, **2**, 349–55.

Dezzutti, C.S., Patel, P.P., et al. 1996. Sensitivity and specificity of a DNA polymerase chain reaction nonisotopic-based detection method for the confirmation of infection with human T-lymphotropic virus types I and II. *Clin Diagn Virol*, **6**, 103–10.

Ding, W., Albrecht, B., et al. 2001. Endoplasmic reticulum and *cis*-Golgi localization of human T-lymphotropic virus type 1 p12(I): association with calreticulin and calnexin. *J Virol*, **75**, 7672–82.

Donegan, E., Lee, H., et al. 1994. Transfusion transmission of retroviruses: human T-lymphotropic virus types I and II compared with human immunodeficiency virus type 1. *Transfusion*, **34**, 478–83.

Dyster, L.M., Abbott, L., et al. 1994. Microplate-based DNA hybridization assays for detection of human retroviral gene sequences. *J Clin Microbiol*, **32**, 547–50.

Eguchi, K., Matsuoka, N., et al. 1992. Primary Sjogren's syndrome with antibodies to HTLV-I: clinical and laboratory features. *Ann Rheum Dis*, **51**, 769–76.

Falcone, V., Leupold, J., et al. 1999. Sites of simian foamy virus persistence in naturally infected African green monkeys: latent provirus is ubiquitous, whereas viral replication is restricted to the oral mucosa. *Virology*, **257**, 7–14.

Franklin, A.A. and Nyborg, J.K. 1995. Mechanisms of Tax regulation of human T cell leukemia virus type I gene expression. *J Biomed Sci*, **2**, 17–29.

Fujii, M., Tsuchiya, H., et al. 1992. Interaction of HTLV-1 Tax1 with p67SRF causes the aberrant induction of cellular immediate early genes through CArG boxes. *Genes Dev*, **6**, 2066–76.

Garcia-Lerma, J.G., Nidtha, S. and Heneine, W. 2001. Susceptibility of human T cell leukemia virus type 1 to reverse-transcriptase inhibitors: evidence for resistance to lamivudine. *J Infect Dis*, **184**, 507–10.

Gavalchin, J., Fan, N., et al. 1995. Regional localization of the putative cell surface receptor for HTLV-I to human chromosome 17q23.2-17q25.3. *Virology*, **212**, 196–203.

Gill, P.S., Harrington, W. Jr, et al. 1995. Treatment of adult T-cell leukemia-lymphoma with a combination of interferon alfa and zidovudine. *N Engl J Med*, **332**, 1744–8.

Glukhova, L.A., Zoubak, S.V., et al. 1999. Localization of HTLV-1 and HIV-1 proviral sequences in chromosomes of persistently infected cells. *Chromosome Res*, **7**, 177–83.

Glynn, S.A., Kleinman, S.H., et al. 2000a. Trends in incidence and prevalence of major transfusion-transmissible viral infections in US blood donors, 1991 to 1996. Retrovirus Epidemiology Donor Study (REDS). *JAMA*, **284**, 229–35.

Glynn, S.A., Murphy, E.L., et al. 2000b. Laboratory abnormalities in former blood donors seropositive for human T-lymphotropic virus types 1 and 2: a prospective analysis. *Arch Pathol Lab Med*, **124**, 550–5.

Gout, O., Gessain, A., et al. 1991. The effect of zidovudine on chronic myelopathy associated with HTLV-1. *J Neurol*, **238**, 108–9, [letter].

Grant, C., Barmak, K., et al. 2002. Human T cell leukemia virus type I and neurologic disease: events in bone marrow, peripheral blood, and central nervous system during normal immune surveillance and neuroinflammation. *J Cell Physiol*, **190**, 133–59.

Hacein-Bey-Abina, S., von Kalle, C., et al. 2003. LMO2-associated clonal T cell proliferation in two patients after gene therapy for SCID-X1. *Science*, **302**, 415–16.

Hanchard, B., LaGrenade, L., et al. 1991. Childhood infective dermatitis evolving into adult T-cell leukaemia after 17 years. *Lancet*, **338**, 1593–4.

Harrington, W.J. Jr, Sheremata, W.A., et al. 1991. Tropical spastic paraparesis/HTLV-1-associated myelopathy (TSP/HAM): treatment with an anabolic steroid danazol. *AIDS Res Hum Retroviruses*, **7**, 1031–4.

Harrington, W.J. Jr, Sheremata, W., et al. 1993. Spastic ataxia associated with human T-cell lymphotropic virus type II infection. *Ann Neurol*, **33**, 411–14.

Heneine, W. 1995. Absence of evidence for human spumaretrovirus sequences in patients with Graves' disease. *Biotechniques*, **18**, 244–8.

Heneine, W., Khabbaz, R.F., et al. 1992a. Sensitive and specific polymerase chain reaction assays for diagnosis of human T-cell lymphotropic virus type I (HTLV-I) and HTLV-II infections in HTLV-I/II-seropositive individuals. *J Clin Microbiol*, **30**, 1605–7.

Heneine, W., Woods, T., et al. 1992b. Detection of HTLV-II in breastmilk of HTLV-II infected mothers. *Lancet*, **340**, 1157–8, [letter].

Heneine, W., Switzer, W.M., et al. 1998. Identification of a human population infected with simian foamy viruses. *Nature Medicine*, **4**, 403–7.

Heneine, W., Switzer, W.M., et al. 2001. Evidence of porcine endogenous retroviruses in porcine factor VIII and evaluation of transmission to recipients with hemophilia. *J Infect Dis*, **183**, 648–52.

Heneine, W., Schweizer, M., et al. 2003. Human infection with foamy viruses. *Curr Top Microbiol Immunol*, **277**, 181–96.

Herchenroder, O., Renne, R., et al. 1994. Isolation, cloning, and sequencing of simian foamy viruses from chimpanzees (SFVcpz): high homology to human foamy virus (HFV). *Virology*, **201**, 187–99.

Heredia, A., Soriano, V., et al. 1996. Development of a multiplex PCR assay for the simultaneous detection and discrimination of HIV-1, HIV-2, HTLV-I and HTLV-II. *Clin Diagn Virol*, **7**, 85–92.

Hermine, O., Bouscary, D., et al. 1995. Brief report: treatment of adult T-cell leukemia-lymphoma with zidovudine and interferon alfa. *N Engl J Med*, **332**, 1749–51.

Herring, C., Cunningham, D.A., et al. 2001. Monitoring xenotransplant recipients for infection by PERV. *Clin Biochem*, **34**, 23–7.

Hidaka, M., Inoue, J., et al. 1988. Post-transcriptional regulator (rex) of HTLV-1 initiates expression of viral structural proteins but suppresses expression of regulatory proteins. *EMBO J*, **7**, 519–23.

Hildreth, J.E., Subramanium, A. and Hampton, R.A. 1997. Human T-cell lymphotropic virus type 1 (HTLV-1)-induced syncytium formation mediated by vascular cell adhesion molecule-1: evidence for involvement of cell adhesion molecules in HTLV-1 biology. *J Virol*, **71**, 1173–80.

Hill, C.L., Bieniasz, P.D. and McClure, M.O. 1999. Properties of human foamy virus relevant to its development as a vector for gene therapy. *J Gen Virol*, **80**, 2003–9.

Hino, S., Doi, H., et al. 1987. HTLV-I carrier mothers with high-titer antibody are at high risk as a source of infection. *Jpn J Cancer Res*, **78**, 1156–8.

Hino, S., Katamine, S., et al. 1996. Primary prevention of HTLV-I in Japan. *J Acquir Immune Defic Syndr Hum Retrovirol*, **13**, S199–203.

Hirata, M., Hayashi, J., et al. 1992. The effects of breastfeeding and presence of antibody to p40tax protein of human T cell lymphotropic virus type-I on mother to child transmission. *Int J Epidemiol*, **21**, 989–94.

Hjelle, B., Khabbaz, R.F., et al. 1994. Prevalence of human T cell lymphotropic virus type II in American Indian populations of the southwestern United States. *Am J Trop Med Hyg*, **51**, 11–15.

Hooks, J.J. and Gibbs, C.J. Jr 1975. The foamy viruses. *Bacteriol Rev*, **39**, 169–85.

Hussain, A.I., Shanmugam, V., et al. 2001. Lack of evidence of endogenous avian leukosis virus and endogenous avian retrovirus transmission to measles, mumps, and rubella vaccine recipients. *Emerg Infect Dis*, **7**, 66–72.

Hussain, A.I., Johnson, J.A., et al. 2003. Identification and characterization of avian retroviruses in chicken embryo-derived yellow fever vaccines: investigation of transmission to vaccine recipients. *J Virol*, **77**, 1105–11.

Igakura, T., Stinchcombe, J.C., et al. 2003. Spread of HTLV-I between lymphocytes by virus-induced polarization of the cytoskeleton. *Science*, **299**, 1713–16.

Ishitsuka, K., Hanada, S., et al. 1998. Arsenic trioxide inhibits growth of human T-cell leukaemia virus type I infected T-cell lines more effectively than retinoic acids. *Br J Haematol*, **103**, 721–8.

Iwakura, Y., Tosu, M., et al. 1991. Induction of inflammatory arthropathy resembling rheumatoid arthritis in mice transgenic for HTLV-I. *Science*, **253**, 1026–8.

Iwakura, Y., Saijo, S., et al. 1995. Autoimmunity induction by human T cell leukemia virus type 1 in transgenic mice that develop chronic inflammatory arthropathy resembling rheumatoid arthritis in humans. *J Immunol*, **155**, 1588–98.

Iwakura, Y., Itagaki, K., et al. 1998. The development of autoimmune inflammatory arthropathy in mice transgenic for the human T cell leukemia virus type-1 env-pX region is not dependent on H-2 haplotypes and modified by the expression levels of Fas antigen. *J Immunol*, **161**, 6592–8.

Jacobson, S., Shida, H., et al. 1990. Circulating CD8+ cytotoxic T lymphocytes specific for HTLV-I pX in patients with HTLV-I associated neurological disease. *Nature*, **348**, 245–8.

Jacobson, S., Lehky, T., et al. 1993. Isolation of HTLV-II from a patient with chronic, progressive neurological disease clinically indistinguishable from HTLV-I-associated myelopathy/tropical spastic paraparesis. *Ann Neurol*, **33**, 392–6.

Jassal, S.R., Pohler, R.G. and Brighty, D.W. 2001. Human T-cell leukemia virus type 1 receptor expression among syncytium-resistant cell lines revealed by a novel surface glycoprotein-immunoadhesin. *J Virol*, **75**, 8317–28.

Jeang, K.T., Chiu, R., et al. 1991. Induction of the HTLV-I LTR by Jun occurs through the Tax-responsive 21-bp elements. *Virology*, **181**, 218–27.

Jeffery, K.J., Siddiqui, A.A., et al. 2000. The influence of HLA class I alleles and heterozygosity on the outcome of human T cell lymphotropic virus type I infection. *J Immunol*, **165**, 7278–84.

Johnson, J.A. and Heneine, W. 2001. Characterization of endogenous avian leukosis viruses in chicken embryonic fibroblast substrates used in production of measles and mumps vaccines. *J Virol*, **75**, 3605–12.

Kalyanaraman, V.S., Sarngadharan, M.G., et al. 1981. Immunological properties of a type C retrovirus isolated from cultured human T-lymphoma cells and comparison to other mammalian retroviruses. *J Virol*, **38**, 906–15.

Kalyanaraman, V.S., Sarngadharan, M.G., et al. 1982. A new subtype of human T-cell leukemia virus (HTLV-II) associated with a T-cell variant of hairy cell leukemia. *Science*, **218**, 571–3.

Kamihira, S., Dateki, N., et al. 2000. Real-time polymerase chain reaction for quantification of HTLV-1 proviral load: application for analyzing aberrant integration of the proviral DNA in adult T-cell leukemia. *Int J Hematol*, **72**, 79–84.

Kaplan, J.E. and Khabbaz, R.F. 1993. The epidemiology of human T-lymphotropic virus types I and II. *Rev Med Virol*, **3**, 137–48.

Kaplan, J.E., Osame, M., et al. 1990. The risk of development of HTLV-I-associated myelopathy/tropical spastic paraparesis among persons infected with HTLV-I. *J Acquir Immune Defic Syndr*, **3**, 1096–101.

Kaplan, M.H., Hall, W.W., et al. 1991. Syndrome of severe skin disease, eosinophilia, and dermatopathic lymphadenopathy in patients with HTLV-II complicating human immunodeficiency virus infection. *Am J Med*, **91**, 300–9.

Kaplan, J.E., Khabbaz, R.F., et al. 1996. Male-to-female transmission of human T-cell lymphotropic virus types I and II: association with viral load. The Retrovirus Epidemiology Donor Study Group. *J Acquir Immune Defic Syndr*, **12**, 193–201.

Katamine, S., Moriuchi, R., et al. 1994. HTLV-I proviral DNA in umbilical cord blood of babies born to carrier mothers. *Lancet*, **343**, 1326–7.

Kawase, K., Katamine, S., et al. 1992. Maternal transmission of HTLV-1 other than through breast milk: discrepancy between the polymerase chain reaction positivity of cord blood samples for HTLV-1 and the subsequent seropositivity of individuals. *Jpn J Cancer Res*, **83**, 968–77.

Khabbaz, R.F., Rowe, T., et al. 1992. Simian immunodeficiency virus needlestick accident in a laboratory worker. *Lancet*, **340**, 271–3.

Khabbaz, R.F., Heneine, W., et al. 1994. Brief report: Infection of a laboratory worker with simian immunodeficiency virus. *N Engl J Med*, **330**, 172–7.

Kinoshita, K., Hino, S., et al. 1984. Demonstration of adult T-cell leukemia virus antigen in milk from three sero-positive mothers. *Gann*, **75**, 103–5.

Kitajima, I., Yamamoto, K., et al. 1991. Detection of human T cell lymphotropic virus type I proviral DNA and its gene expression in synovial cells in chronic inflammatory arthropathy. *J Clin Invest*, **88**, 1315–22.

Kleinman, S.H., Kaplan, J.E., et al. 1994. Evaluation of a p21e-spiked western blot (immunoblot) in confirming human T-cell lymphotropic virus type I or II infection in volunteer blood donors. The Retrovirus Epidemiology Donor Study Group. *J Clin Microbiol*, **32**, 603–7.

Kozuru, M., Uike, N., et al. 1996. High occurrence of primary malignant neoplasms in patients with adult T-cell leukemia/lymphoma, their siblings, and their mothers. *Cancer*, **78**, 1119–24.

Kuroda, Y. and Matsui, M. 1993. Cerebrospinal fluid interferon-gamma is increased in HTLV-I-associated myelopathy. *J Neuroimmunol*, **42**, 223–6.

Kuroda, Y., Matsui, M., et al. 1994. In situ demonstration of the HTLV-I genome in the spinal cord of a patient with HTLV-I-associated myelopathy. *Neurology*, **44**, 2295–9.

Lagaye, S., Ilyinskii, P.O., et al. 1992. Human spumaretrovirus-related sequences in the DNA of leukocytes from patients with Graves disease. *Intervirology*, **34**, 117–23.

La Grenade, L., Morgan, C., et al. 1995. Tropical spastic paraparesis occurring in HTLV-1 associated infective dermatitis. Report of two cases. *W Ind Med J*, **44**, 34–5.

La Grenade, L., Manns, A., et al. 1998. Clinical, pathologic, and immunologic features of human T-lymphotrophic virus type I-associated infective dermatitis in children. *Arch Dermatol*, **134**, 439–44.

Lal, R.B. 1996. Delineation of immunodominant epitopes of human T-lymphotropic virus types I and II and their usefulness in developing serologic assays for detection of antibodies to HTLV-I and HTLV-II. *J Acquir Immune Defic Syndr*, **13**, Suppl 1, S170–8.

Lal, R.B., Brodine, S., et al. 1992a. Sensitivity and specificity of a recombinant transmembrane glycoprotein (rgp21)-spiked western immunoblot for serological confirmation of human T-cell lymphotropic virus type I and type II infections. *J Clin Microbiol*, **30**, 296–9.

Lal, R.B., Rudolph, D.L., et al. 1992b. Failure to detect evidence of human T-lymphotropic virus (HTLV) type I and type II in blood donors with isolated gag antibodies to HTLV-I/II. *Blood*, **80**, 544–50.

Lal, R.B., Owen, S.M., et al. 1995. In vivo cellular tropism of human T-lymphotropic virus type II is not restricted to CD8+ cells. *Virology*, **210**, 441–7.

Leclercq, I., Mortreux, F., et al. 2000a. Host sequences flanking the human T-cell leukemia virus type 1 provirus in vivo. *J Virol*, **74**, 2305–12.

Leclercq, I., Mortreux, F., et al. 2000b. Basis of HTLV type 1 target site selection. *AIDS Res Hum Retroviruses*, **16**, 1653–9.

Lehky, T.J., Fox, C.H., et al. 1995. Detection of human T-lymphotropic virus type I (HTLV-I) tax RNA in the central nervous system of HTLV-I-associated myelopathy/tropical spastic paraparesis patients by in situ hybridization. *Ann Neurol*, **37**, 167–75.

Li, Q.X., Camerini, D., et al. 1996. Syncytium formation by recombinant HTLV-II envelope glycoprotein. *Virology*, **218**, 279–84.

Linial, M. 2000. Why aren't foamy viruses pathogenic? *Trends Microbiol*, **8**, 284–9.

Liu, H., Shah, M., et al. 1999. Sensitivity and specificity of human T-lymphotropic virus (HTLV) types I and II polymerase chain reaction and several serologic assays in screening a population with a high prevalence of HTLV-II. *Transfusion*, **39**, 1185–93.

Loh, P.C., Matsuura, F. and Mizumoto, C. 1980. Seroepidemiology of human syncytial virus: antibody prevalence in the Pacific. *Intervirology*, **13**, 87–90.

Lowenstine, L.J. and Lerche, N.W. 1988. Retrovirus infections of nonhuman primates: a review. *J Zoo Anim Med*, **19**, 168–87.

Madeleine, M.M., Wiktor, S.Z., et al. 1993. HTLV-I and HTLV-II world-wide distribution: reanalysis of 4,832 immunoblot results. *Int J Cancer*, **54**, 255–60.

Mahieux, R., Ibrahim, F., et al. 1997. Molecular epidemiology of 58 new African human T-cell leukemia virus type 1 (HTLV-1) strains: identification of a new and distinct HTLV-1 molecular subtype in Central Africa and in pygmies. *J Virol*, **71**, 1317–33.

Mahieux, R., Horal, P., et al. 2000. Human T-cell lymphotropic virus type I gag indeterminate Western blot patterns in Central Africa: relationship to *Plasmodium falciparum* infection. *J Clin Microbiol*, **38**, 4049–57.

Maloney, E.M., Biggar, R.J., et al. 1992. Endemic human T cell lymphotropic virus type II infection among isolated Brazilian Amerindians. *J Infect Dis*, **166**, 100–7.

Manel, N., Kinet, S., et al. 2003a. The HTLV receptor is an early T-cell activation marker whose expression requires de novo protein synthesis. *Blood*, **101**, 1913–18.

Manel, N., Kim, F.I., et al. 2003b. The ubiquitous glucose transporter GLUT-1 is a receptor for HTLV. *Cell*, **115**, 449–59.

Manns, A., Wilks, R.J., et al. 1992. A prospective study of transmission by transfusion of HTLV-I and risk factors associated with seroconversion. *Int J Cancer*, **51**, 886–91.

Manns, A., Hanchard, B., et al. 1998. Human leukocyte antigen class II alleles associated with human T-cell lymphotropic virus type I infection and adult T-cell leukemia/lymphoma in a Black population. *J Natl Cancer Inst*, **90**, 617–22.

Manns, A., Hisada, M. and La Grenade, L. 1999a. Human T-lymphotropic virus type I infection. *Lancet*, **353**, 1951–8.

Manns, A., Miley, W.J., et al. 1999b. Quantitative proviral DNA and antibody levels in the natural history of HTLV-I infection. *J Infect Dis*, **180**, 1487–93.

Mansky, L.M. 2000. In vivo analysis of human T-cell leukemia virus type 1 reverse transcription accuracy. *J Virol*, **74**, 9525–31.

Mansky, L.M. and Temin, H.M. 1995. Lower in vivo mutation rate of human immunodeficiency virus type 1 than that predicted from the fidelity of purified reverse transcriptase. *J Virol*, **69**, 5087–94.

Mariette, X., Agbalika, F., et al. 2000. Detection of the *tax* gene of HTLV-I in labial salivary glands from patients with Sjogren's syndrome and other diseases of the oral cavity. *Clin Exp Rheumatol*, **18**, 341–7.

Mauclere, P., Le Hesran, J.Y., et al. 1997. Demographic, ethnic, and geographic differences between human T cell lymphotropic virus (HTLV) type I-seropositive carriers and persons with HTLV-I Gag-indeterminate Western blots in Central Africa. *J Infect Dis*, **176**, 505–9.

Medrano, F.J., Soriano, V., et al. 1997. Significance of indeterminate reactivity to human T-cell lymphotropic virus in western blot analysis of individuals at risk. *Eur J Clin Microbiol Infect Dis*, **16**, 249–52.

Meiering, C.D. and Linial, M.L. 2001. Historical perspective of foamy virus epidemiology and infection. *Clin Microbiol Revs*, **14**, 165–76.

Miley, W.J., Suryanarayana, K., et al. 2000. Real-time polymerase chain reaction assay for cell-associated HTLV type I DNA viral load. *AIDS Res Hum Retroviruses*, **16**, 665–75.

Miyasaka, N., Higaki, M., et al. 1991. Production of interleukin-1 beta-like factor with synovial cell growth promoting activity from adult T-cell leukemia cells. *J Autoimmun*, **4**, 223–36.

Miyoshi, I., Kubonishi, I., et al. 1981. Type C virus particles in a cord T-cell line derived by co-cultivating normal human cord leukocytes and human leukaemic T cells. *Nature*, **294**, 770–1.

Mochizuki, M., Ono, A., et al. 1996. HTLV-I uveitis. *J Acquir Immune Defic Syndr*, **13**, Suppl 1, S50–6.

Modahl, L.E., Young, K.C., et al. 1997. Are HTLV-II-seropositive injection drug users at increased risk of bacterial pneumonia, abscess, and lymphadenopathy? *J Acquir Immune Defic Syndr Hum Retrovirol*, **16**, 169–75.

Motokawa, S., Hasunuma, T., et al. 1996. High prevalence of arthropathy in HTLV-I carriers on a Japanese island. *Ann Rheum Dis*, **55**, 193–5.

Mueller, N., Okayama, A., et al. 1996. Findings from the Miyazaki Cohort Study. *J Acquir Immune Defic Syndr*, **13**, Suppl 1, S2–7.

Murphy, E.L., Figueroa, J.P., et al. 1989. Sexual transmission of human T-lymphotropic virus type I (HTLV-I). *Ann Intern Med*, **111**, 555–60.

Murphy, E.L., Figueroa, J.P., et al. 1991. Human T-lymphotropic virus type I (HTLV-I) seroprevalence in Jamaica. I. Demographic determinants. *Amer J Epidemiol*, **133**, 1114–24.

Murphy, E.L., Fridey, J., et al. 1997a. HTLV-associated myelopathy in a cohort of HTLV-I and HTLV-II-infected blood donors. The REDS investigators. *Neurology*, **48**, 315–20.

Murphy, E.L., Glynn, S.A., et al. 1997b. Increased prevalence of infectious diseases and other adverse outcomes in human T lymphotropic virus types I- and II-infected blood donors. Retrovirus Epidemiology Donor Study (REDS) Study Group. *J Infect Dis*, **176**, 1468–75.

Murphy, E.L., Glynn, S.A., et al. 1999. Increased incidence of infectious diseases during prospective follow-up of human T-lymphotropic virus type II- and I-infected blood donors. Retrovirus Epidemiology Donor Study. *Arch Intern Med*, **159**, 1485–91.

Murphy, E.L., Wu, Y., et al. 2001. Delayed hypersensitivity skin testing to mumps and *Candida albicans* antigens is normal in middle-aged HTLV-I- and-II-infected U.S. cohorts. *AIDS Res Hum Retroviruses*, **17**, 1273–7.

Nagai, M. and Jacobson, S. 2001. Immunopathogenesis of human T cell lymphotropic virus type I-associated myelopathy. *Curr Opin Neurol*, **14**, 381–6.

Nagai, M., Usuku, K., et al. 1998. Analysis of HTLV-I proviral load in 202 HAM/TSP patients and 243 asymptomatic HTLV-I carriers: high proviral load strongly predisposes to HAM/TSP. *J Neurovirol*, **4**, 586–93.

Nagai, M., Brennan, M.B., et al. 2001. CD8$^+$ T cells are an in vivo reservoir for human T-cell lymphotropic virus type I. *Blood*, **98**, 1858–61.

Nakamura, H., Kawakami, A., et al. 2000. Relationship between Sjogren's syndrome and human T-lymphotropic virus type I infection: follow-up study of 83 patients. *J Lab Clin Med*, **135**, 139–44.

Nakashima, K., Kashiwagi, S., et al. 1995. Sexual transmission of human T-lymphotropic virus type I among female prostitutes and among patients with sexually transmitted diseases in Fukuoka, Kyushu, Japan. *Am J Epidemiol*, **141**, 305–11.

Nam, S.H., Kidokoro, M., et al. 1988. Processing of *gag* precursor polyprotein of human T-cell leukemia virus type I by virus-encoded protease. *J Virol*, **62**, 3718–28.

Nath, M.D., Ruscetti, F.W., et al. 2003. Regulation of the cell-surface expression of an HTLV-I binding protein in human T cells during immune activation. *Blood*, **101**, 3085–92.

Nemo, G.J., Brown, P.W., et al. 1978. Antigenic relationship of human foamy virus to the simian foamy viruses. *Infect Immun*, **20**, 69–72.

Neumann-Haefelin, D., Fleps, U., et al. 1993. Foamy viruses. *Intervirology*, **35**, 196–207.

Nishimura, M., Maeda, M., et al. 2000. Tumor necrosis factor, tumor necrosis factor receptors type 1 and 2, lymphotoxin-alpha and HLA-DRB1 gene polymorphisms in human T-cell lymphotropic virus type I associated myelopathy. *Hum Immunol*, **61**, 1262–9.

Nyambi, P.N., Ville, Y., et al. 1996. Mother-to-child transmission of human T-cell lymphotropic virus types I and II (HTLV-I/II) in Gabon: a prospective follow-up of 4 years. *J Acquir Immune Defic Syndr Hum Retrovirol*, **12**, 187–92.

Offen, D., Achiron, A., et al. 1998. HTLV-1 in mouthwash cells from a TSP/HAM patient and asymptomatic carriers. *Arch Virol*, **143**, 1029–34.

Ohtsuki, Y., Akagi, T., et al. 1982. Ultrastructural study on type C virus particles in a human cord T-cell line established by co-cultivation with adult T-cell leukemia cells. *Arch Virol*, **73**, 69–73.

Ohyama, Y., Nakamura, S., et al. 1998. Accumulation of human T lymphotropic virus type I-infected T cells in the salivary glands of patients with human T lymphotropic virus type I- associated Sjogren's syndrome. *Arthritis Rheum*, **41**, 1972–8.

Okuma, K., Nakamura, M., et al. 1999. Host range of human T-cell leukemia virus type I analyzed by a cell fusion-dependent reporter gene activation assay. *Virology*, **254**, 235–44.

Ono, A., Mochizuki, M., et al. 1995. Increased number of circulating HTLV-1 infected cells in peripheral blood mononuclear cells of HTLV-1 uveitis patients: a quantitative polymerase chain reaction study. *Br J Ophthalmol*, **79**, 270–6.

Osame, M., Matsumoto, M., et al. 1987. Chronic progressive myelopathy associated with elevated antibodies to human T-lymphotropic virus type I and adult T-cell leukemia-like cells. *Ann Neurol*, **21**, 117–22.

Overbaugh, J., Miller, A.D. and Eiden, M.V. 2001. Receptors and entry cofactors for retroviruses include single and multiple transmembrane-spanning proteins as well as newly described glycophosphatidyl inositol-anchored and secreted proteins. *Microbiol Mol Biol Rev*, **65**, 371–89.

Paradis, K., Langford, G., et al. 1999. Search for cross-species transmission of porcine endogenous retrovirus in patients treated with living pig tissue. The XEN 111 Study Group. *Science*, **285**, 1236–41.

Pique, C., Tursz, T. and Dokhelar, M.C. 1990. Mutations introduced along the HTLV-I envelope gene result in a non- functional protein: a basis for envelope conservation? *EMBO J*, **9**, 4243–8.

Poiesz, B.J., Ruscetti, F.W., et al. 1980. Detection and isolation of type C retrovirus particles from fresh and cultured lymphocytes of a patient with cutaneous T-cell lymphoma. *Proc Natl Acad Sci USA*, **77**, 7415–19.

Poiesz, B.J., Ruscetti, F.W., et al. 1981. Isolation of a new type C retrovirus (HTLV) in primary uncultured cells of a patient with Sezary T-cell leukaemia. *Nature*, **294**, 268–71.

Poiesz, B.J., Dube, S., et al. 2000. Comparative performances of an HTLV-I/II EIA and other serologic and PCR assays on samples from persons at risk for HTLV-II infection. *Transfusion*, **40**, 924–30.

Richardson, J.H., Edwards, A.J., et al. 1990. In vivo cellular tropism of human T-cell leukemia virus type 1. *J Virol*, **64**, 5682–7.

Robek, M.D. and Ratner, L. 1999. Immortalization of CD4+ and CD8+ T lymphocytes by human T-cell leukemia virus type 1 Tax mutants expressed in a functional molecular clone. *J Virol*, **73**, 4856–65.

Rosenblatt, J.D., Golde, D.W., et al. 1986. A second isolate of HTLV-II associated with atypical hairy-cell leukemia. *N Engl J Med*, **315**, 372–7.

Rosenblatt, J.D., Gasson, J.C., et al. 1987. Relationship between human T cell leukemia virus-II and atypical hairy cell leukemia: a serologic study of hairy cell leukemia patients. *Leukemia*, **1**, 397–401.

Rosenblatt, J.D., Plaeger-Marshall, S., et al. 1990. A clinical, hematologic, and immunologic analysis of 21 HTLV-II-infected intravenous drug users. *Blood*, **76**, 409–17.

Rosener, M., Hahn, H., et al. 1996. Absence of serological evidence for foamy virus infection in patients with amyotrophic lateral sclerosis. *J Med Virol*, **48**, 222–6.

Rosin, O., Koch, C., et al. 1998. A human T-cell leukemia virus Tax variant incapable of activating NF-kappaB retains its immortalizing potential for primary T-lymphocytes. *J Biol Chem*, **273**, 6698–703.

Rouet, F., Meertens, L., et al. 2001. Serological, epidemiological and molecular differences between human T-cell lymphotropic virus type 1 (HTLV-1)-seropositive healthy carriers and persons with HTLV-I Gag indeterminate Western blot patterns from the Caribbean. *J Clin Microbiol*, **39**, 1247–53.

Sagawa, K., Mochizuki, M., et al. 1995. Immunopathological mechanisms of human T cell lymphotropic virus type 1 (HTLV-I) uveitis. Detection of HTLV-I-infected T cells in the eye and their constitutive cytokine production. *J Clin Invest*, **95**, 852–8.

Sandstrom, P.A., Phan, K.O., et al. 2000. Simian foamy virus infection among zoo keepers. *Lancet*, **355**, 551–2.

Santillana-Hayat, M., Rozain, F., et al. 1993. Transient immunosuppressive effect induced in rabbits and mice by the human spumaretrovirus prototype HFV (human foamy virus). *Res Virol*, **144**, 389–96.

Sasaki, M., Nakamura, S., et al. 2000. Accumulation of common T cell clonotypes in the salivary glands of patients with human T lymphotropic virus type I-associated and idiopathic Sjogren's syndrome. *J Immunol*, **164**, 2823–31.

Sato, K., Maruyama, I., et al. 1991. Arthritis in patients infected with human T lymphotropic virus type I. Clinical and immunopathologic features. *Arthritis Rheum*, **34**, 714–21.

Scherdin, U., Rhodes, K. and Breindl, M. 1990. Transcriptionally active genome regions are preferred targets for retrovirus integration. *J Virol*, **64**, 907–12.

Schreiber, G.B., Busch, M.P., et al. 1996. The risk of transfusion-transmitted viral infections. The Retrovirus Epidemiology Donor Study. *N Engl J Med*, **334**, 1685–90.

Schweizer, M., Turek, R., et al. 1995. Markers of foamy virus infections in monkeys, apes, and accidentally infected humans: appropriate

testing fails to confirm suspected foamy virus prevalence in humans. *AIDS Res Hum Retroviruses*, **11**, 161–70.

Schweizer, M., Falcone, V., et al. 1997. Simian foamy virus isolated from an accidentally infected human individual. *J Virol*, **71**, 4821–4.

Sheremata, W.A., Harrington, W.J. Jr, et al. 1993. Association of '(tropical) ataxic neuropathy' with HTLV-II. *Virus Res*, **29**, 71–7.

Shimotohno, K., Takano, M., et al. 1986. Requirement of multiple copies of a 21-nucleotide sequence in the U3 regions of human T-cell leukemia virus type I and type II long terminal repeats for trans-acting activation of transcription. *Proc Natl Acad Sci U S A*, **83**, 8112–16.

Shimoyama, M. 1991. Diagnostic criteria and classification of clinical subtypes of adult T-cell leukaemia-lymphoma. A report from the Lymphoma Study Group (1984–87). *Br J Haematol*, **79**, 428–37.

Silva, E.A., Otsuki, K., et al. 2002. HTLV-II infection associated with a chronic neurodegenerative disease: clinical and molecular analysis. *J Med Virol*, **66**, 253–7.

Slattery, J.P., Franchini, G. and Gessain, A. 1999. Genomic evolution, patterns of global dissemination, and interspecies transmission of human and simian T-cell leukemia/lymphotropic viruses. *Genome Res*, **9**, 525–40.

Soldan, S.S., Graf, M.D., et al. 1999. HTLV-I/II seroindeterminate Western blot reactivity in a cohort of patients with neurological disease. *J Infect Dis*, **180**, 685–94.

Sommerfelt, M.A. and Weiss, R.A. 1990. Receptor interference groups of 20 retroviruses plating on human cells. *Virology*, **176**, 58–69.

Sommerfelt, M.A., Williams, B.P., et al. 1988. Human T cell leukemia viruses use a receptor determined by human chromosome 17. *Science*, **242**, 1557–9.

Soto-Ramirez, L.E., Garcia-Vallejo, F., et al. 1995. Human T-lymphotropic virus type I (HTLV-I)-specific antibodies and cell-free RNA in crevicular fluid-rich saliva from patients with tropical spastic paraparesis/HTLV-I-associated myelopathy. *Viral Immunol*, **8**, 141–50.

Stancek, D., Kosecka, G., et al. 1995. Links between prolonged exposure to xenobiotics, increased incidence of hepatopathies, immunological disturbances and exacerbation of latent Epstein–Barr virus infections. *Int J Immunopharmacol*, **17**, 321–8.

Stuver, S.O., Tachibana, N., et al. 1993. Heterosexual transmission of human T cell leukemia/lymphoma virus type I among married couples in southwestern Japan: an initial report from the Miyazaki Cohort Study. *J Infect Dis*, **167**, 57–65.

Sullivan, M.T., Williams, A.E., et al. 1993. Human T-lymphotropic virus (HTLV) types I and II infection in sexual contacts and family members of blood donors who are seropositive for HTLV type I or II. American Red Cross HTLV-I/II Collaborative Study Group. *Transfusion*, **33**, 585–90.

Sumida, T., Yonaha, F., et al. 1994. Expression of sequences homologous to HTLV-I *tax* gene in the labial salivary glands of Japanese patients with Sjogren's syndrome. *Arthritis Rheum*, **37**, 545–50.

Sun, S.C. and Ballard, D.W. 1999. Persistent activation of NF-kappaB by the tax transforming protein of HTLV-1: hijacking cellular IkappaB kinases. *Oncogene*, **18**, 6948–58.

Sutton, R.E. and Littman, D.R. 1996. Broad host range of human T-cell leukemia virus type 1 demonstrated with an improved pseudotyping system. *J Virol*, **70**, 7322–6.

Suzuki, M., Dezzutti, C.S., et al. 1999. Modulation of T-cell responses to a recall antigen in human T-cell leukemia virus type 1-infected individuals. *Clin Diagn Lab Immunol*, **6**, 713–17.

Swack, N.S. and Hsiung, G.D. 1975. Pathogenesis of simian foamy virus infection in natural and experimental hosts. *Infect Immun*, **12**, 470–4.

Switzer, W.M., Pieniazek, D., et al. 1995. Phylogenetic relationship and geographic distribution of multiple human T-cell lymphotropic virus type II subtypes. *J Virol*, **69**, 621–32.

Switzer, W.M., Bhullar, V., et al. 2004. Frequent simian foamy virus infection in persons occupationally exposed to nonhuman primates. *J Virol*, **78**, 2780–9.

Takahashi, K., Takezaki, T., et al. 1991. Inhibitory effect of maternal antibody on mother-to-child transmission of human T-lymphotropic virus type I. The Mother-to-Child Transmission Study Group. *Int J Cancer*, **49**, 673–7.

Takahashi, T., Takase, H., et al. 2000. Clinical features of human T-lymphotropic virus type 1 uveitis: a long-term follow-up. *Ocul Immunol Inflamm*, **8**, 235–41.

Tanaka, A., Takahashi, C., et al. 1990. Oncogenic transformation by the *tax* gene of human T-cell leukemia virus type I in vitro. *Proc Natl Acad Sci U S A*, **87**, 1071–5.

Taniguchi, S., Maekawa, N., et al. 1993. Detection of human T-cell lymphotropic virus type-1 proviral DNA in the saliva of an adult T-cell leukaemia/lymphoma patient using the polymerase chain reaction. *Br J Dermatol*, **129**, 637–41.

Taylor, G.P., Hall, S.E., et al. 1999. Effect of lamivudine on human T-cell leukemia virus type 1 (HTLV-1) DNA copy number, T-cell phenotype, and anti-tax cytotoxic T-cell frequency in patients with HTLV-1-associated myelopathy. *J Virol*, **73**, 10289–95.

Tendler, C.L., Greenberg, S.J., et al. 1991. Cytokine induction in HTLV-I associated myelopathy and adult T-cell leukemia: alternate molecular mechanisms underlying retroviral pathogenesis. *J Cell Biochem*, **46**, 302–11.

Terada, K., Katamine, S., et al. 1994. Prevalence of serum and salivary antibodies to HTLV-1 in Sjogren's syndrome. *Lancet*, **344**, 1116–19.

Tobaly-Tapiero, J., Bittoun, P., et al. 2001. Human foamy virus capsid formation requires an interaction domain in the N terminus of Gag. Isolation and characterization of an equine foamy virus. *J Virol*, **75**, 4367–75.

Tosswill, J.H., Taylor, G.P., et al. 1998. Quantification of proviral DNA load in human T-cell leukaemia virus type I infections. *J Virol Methods*, **75**, 21–6.

Trejo, S.R. and Ratner, L. 2000. The HTLV receptor is a widely expressed protein. *Virology*, **268**, 41–8.

Tsang, S.X., Switzer, W.M., et al. 1999. Evidence of avian leukosis virus subgroup E and endogenous avian virus in measles and mumps vaccines derived from chicken cells: investigation of transmission to vaccine recipients. *J Virol*, **73**, 5843–51.

Tsukasaki, K., Yamada, Y., et al. 1994. Infective dermatitis among patients with ATL in Japan. *Int J Cancer*, **57**, 293.

Tuke, P.W., Luton, P. and Garson, J.A. 1992. Differential diagnosis of HTLV-I and HTLV-II infections by restriction enzyme analysis of 'nested' PCR products. *J Virol Methods*, **40**, 163–73.

Unge, T., Solomin, L., et al. 1991. The Rex regulatory protein of human T-cell lymphotropic virus type I binds specifically to its target site within the viral RNA. *Proc Natl Acad Sci U S A*, **88**, 7145–9.

Ureta-Vidal, A., Angelin-Duclos, C., et al. 1999. Mother-to-child transmission of human T-cell-leukemia/lymphoma virus type I: implication of high antiviral antibody titer and high proviral load in carrier mothers. *Int J Cancer*, **82**, 832–6.

Valentin, H., Lemasson, I., et al. 1997. Transcriptional activation of the vascular cell adhesion molecule-1 gene in T lymphocytes expressing human T-cell leukemia virus type 1 Tax protein. *J Virol*, **71**, 8522–30.

Vandamme, A.M., Van Laethem, K., et al. 1997. Use of a generic polymerase chain reaction assay detecting human T- lymphotropic virus (HTLV) types I, II and divergent simian strains in the evaluation of individuals with indeterminate HTLV serology. *J Med Virol*, **52**, 1–7.

Varma, M., Rudolph, D.L., et al. 1995. Enhanced specificity of truncated transmembrane protein for serologic confirmation of human T-cell lymphotropic virus type 1 (HTLV-1) and HTLV-2 infections by Western blot (immunoblot) assay containing recombinant envelope glycoproteins. *J Clin Microbiol*, **33**, 3239–44.

Vet, J.A., Majithia, A.R., et al. 1999. Multiplex detection of four pathogenic retroviruses using molecular beacons. *Proc Nat Acad Sci U S A*, **96**, 6394–9.

Vitek, C.R., Gracia, F.I., et al. 1995. Evidence for sexual and mother-to-child transmission of human T lymphotropic virus type II among Guaymi Indians, Panama. *J Infect Dis*, **171**, 1022–6.

Waldmann, T.A. 1996. The promiscuous IL-2/IL-15 receptor: a target for immunotherapy of HTLV- I-associated disorders. *J Acquir Immune Defic Syndr Hum Retrovirol*, **13**, S179–85.

Wattel, E., Cavrois, M., et al. 1996. Clonal expansion of infected cells: a way of life for HTLV-I. *J Acquir Immune Defic Syndr Hum Retrovirol*, **13**, S92–9.

Waziri, A., Soldan, S.S., et al. 2000. Characterization and sequencing of prototypic human T-lymphotropic virus type 1 (HTLV-1) from an HTLV-1/2 seroindeterminate patient. *J Virol*, **74**, 2178–85.

Weiss, R.A. 1984. Human retroviruses in health and disease. *Princess Takamatsu Symposia*, **15**, 3–12.

Weiss, R.A. 1996. Reverse transcription. Foamy viruses bubble on. *Nature*, **380**, 201.

Weissmahr, R.N., Schupbach, J. and Boni, J. 1997. Reverse transcriptase activity in chicken embryo fibroblast culture supernatants is associated with particles containing endogenous avian retrovirus EAV-0 RNA. *J Virol*, **71**, 3005–12.

Werner, J. and Gelderblom, H. 1979. Isolation of foamy virus from patients with de Quervain thyroiditis. *Lancet*, **2**, 258–9.

Westphal, K.P., Kolde, G., et al. 1992. Diagnosis and treatment in a case of juvenile subacute necrotizing encephalopathy Leigh without cytochrome c oxidase deficiency. *Int J Clin Pharmacol Ther Toxicol*, **30**, 81–93.

Whyte, G.S. 1997. Is screening of Australian blood donors for HTLV-I necessary? *Med J Australia*, **166**, 478–81.

Wiktor, S.Z., Piot, P., et al. 1990. Human T cell lymphotropic virus type I (HTLV-I) among female prostitutes in Kinshasa, Zaire. *J Infect Dis*, **161**, 1073–7.

Wiktor, S.Z., Pate, E.J., et al. 1993. Mother-to-child transmission of human T-cell lymphotropic virus type I (HTLV-I) in Jamaica: association with antibodies to envelope glycoprotein (gp46) epitopes. *J Acquir Immune Defic Syndr*, **6**, 1162–7.

Winkler, I.G., Lochelt, M. and Flower, R.L. 1999. Epidemiology of feline foamy virus and feline immunodeficiency virus infections in domestic and feral cats: a seroepidemiological study. *J Clin Microbiol*, **37**, 2848–51.

Winkler, I.G., Flugel, R.M., et al. 2000. Antibody to human foamy virus not detected in individuals treated with blood products or in blood donors. *Vox Sang*, **79**, 118–19.

Wolfe, N.D., Switzer, W.M., et al. 2004. Naturally acquired simian retrovirus infections in central African hunters. *Lancet*, **363**, 932–7.

Yamamoto, A., Hara, H. and Kobayashi, T. 1997. Induction of the expression of gag protein in HTLV-I infected lymphocytes by anti-ICAM 1 antibody in vitro. *J Neurol Sci*, **151**, 121–6.

Yamamoto, S., Folks, T.M. and Heneine, W. 1996. Highly sensitive qualitative and quantitative detection of reverse transcriptase activity: optimization, validation, and comparative analysis with other detection systems. *J Virol Methods*, **61**, 135–43.

Yamamoto, T., Terada, K., et al. 1995. Inhibitory activity in saliva of cell-to-cell transmission of human T-cell lymphotropic virus type 1 in vitro: evaluation of saliva as an alternative source of transmission. *J Clin Microbiol*, **33**, 1510–15.

Yamasaki, K., Kira, J., et al. 1997. Long-term, high dose interferon-alpha treatment in HTLV-I-associated myelopathy/tropical spastic paraparesis: a combined clinical, virological and immunological study. *J Neurol Sci*, **147**, 135–44.

Yoshinaga, M., Yashiki, S., et al. 1995. A maternal risk factor for mother-to-child HTLV-I transmission: viral antigen-producing capacities in culture of peripheral blood and breast milk cells. *Jpn J Cancer Res*, **86**, 649–54.

Zunt, J.R., Dezzutti, C.S., et al. 2002. Cervical shedding of human T cell lymphotropic virus type I is associated with cervicitis. *J Infect Dis*, **186**, 1669–72.

Foamy viruses

AXEL RETHWILM

INTRODUCTION

The family of *Retroviridae* is taxonomically divided into two subfamilies: the *Orthoretrovirinae* and the *Spumaretrovirinae,* the latter are better known as foamy viruses (FV) (Table 59.1). The separation of the previously homogenous group of retroviruses into the two subfamilies by the International Committee of the Taxonomy of Viruses (ICTV) reflected the molecular biology of FVs and their replication pathway, which appears to be significantly different from all other retroviruses, and have common aspects with the replication strategy of hepadnaviruses (Linial 1999; Lecellier and Saïb 2000; Rethwilm 2003b; Flint et al. 2004). In this chapter, these findings will be reviewed and the general biology of FVs will be summarized.

NATURAL HISTORY AND GENERAL PROPERTIES OF FV

FVs have been known for more than 50 years. After long term cultivation of primary monkey cells a typical foamy cytopathic effect (CPE) emerged (Figure 59.1) that could be transferred in a cell-free manner to uninfected cell cultures (Enders and Peebles 1954; Rustigian et al. 1955; Lepine and Paccaud 1957; Paccaud 1957; Falke 1958; Plummer 1962). Following the detection of a reverse transcriptase activity in gradient-purified virions, FV were classified among the *Retroviridae* (Parks et al. 1971). Curiously the question of the

molecular basis of the FV-specific foamy degeneration of cells has not been addressed yet.

FVs have been found in the mammalian species which also naturally harbor lentiviruses, namely nonhuman primates (Hooks and Gibbs 1975; Swack 1981), felines (Lutz 1990; Pedersen 1990), bovines (Johnson et al. 1988; Amborski et al. 1989), equines (Tobaly-Tapiero et al. 2000), ovines (Flanagan 1992), and occasionally others (Hruska and Takemoto 1975; Rossignol et al. 1975; Kennedy-Stoskopf et al. 1986; Amborski et al. 1987; Meiering and Linial 2001; Saïb 2003). An overview is shown in Table 59.2. In particular, FVs from monkeys and great apes have been studied since the early years of FV research (Hooks and Gibbs 1975). It is a common experience that these simian foamy viruses (SFV) can influence studies on other simian (retro-) viruses, such as the immunodeficiency viruses, by reactivation from latency and destroying primary cell cultures (Voss et al. 1992; Feldmann et al. 1997).

Virus is shed in the saliva and can be easily isolated by throat swabs from infected monkeys and cats (Hooks and Gibbs 1975; Shroyer and Shalaby 1978; Alke et al. 2000). Transmission in monkeys is believed to occur by social contacts involving biting during juvenility (Meiering and Linial 2001; Falcone et al. 2003). After infection, the virus persists lifelong and can be isolated from many tissues (Hooks and Gibbs 1975; Falcone et al. 1999a; Falcone et al. 2003). Viral DNA at approximately one copy number per 10^2–10^3 cells can be found in most organs of perfused animals, although cellfree virus has not been detected in the plasma (Falcone et al. 1999a;

Table 59.1 *The ICTV nomenclature of the* Retroviridae

Subfamily	Genus	Example	Genome
Orthoretrovirinae	*Alpharetrovirus*	Avian leukosis virus (ALV)	Simple
	Betaretrovirus	Mouse mammary tumor virus (MMTV), Mason–Pfizer monkey virus (MPMV)	Simple
	Gammaretrovirus	Murine leukemia virus (MuLV)	Simple
	Deltaretrovirus	Bovine leukemia virus (BLV), Human T-cell leukemia virus (HTLV)	Complex
	Epsilonretrovirus	Walleye dermal sarcoma virus (WDSV)	Complex
	Lentivirus	Human immunodeficiency virus (HIV)	Complex
Spumaretrovirinae	Foamyviruses	Prototype foamy virus (PFV)	Complex

Falcone et al. 2003). The conservation of viral sequences over time is also suggestive of poor replication in vivo (Schweizer et al. 1999). Despite the prominent CPE FVs exhibit in adherent cell cultures, the in vivo infection is nonpathogenic (Linial 2000; Meiering and Linial 2001; Falcone et al. 2003). Continuous virus isolations by throat swabs and from peripheral blood lymphocytes

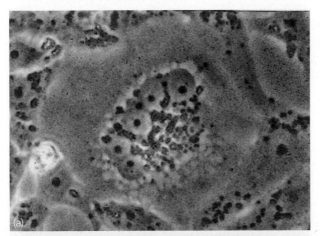

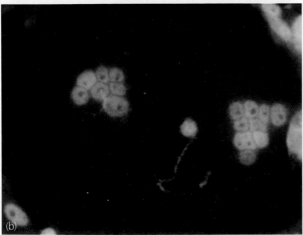

Figure 59.1 (a) *Micrograph of a typical FV cytopathic effect with the formation of multinucleated syncytia and vacuolation. SFVagm-infected Vero cell culture.* **(b)** *Nuclear staining in indirect immunofluorescence of SFVagm-infected cells with a SFVagm-positive monkey serum.*

(PBL) many years after primary infection indicate virus persistence (Hooks and Gibbs 1975; Hooks and Detrick-Hooks 1981; Meiering and Linial 2001; Falcone et al. 2003). More recently, the sequences of bovine foamy virus (BFV), feline foamy virus (FFV), and equine foamy virus (EFV) have also become available (Renshaw et al. 1991; Renshaw and Casey 1994a, 1994b; Helps and Harbour 1997; Winkler et al. 1997a; Tobaly-Tapiero et al. 2000; Hatama et al. 2001) and studies into the molecular biology, epidemiology, and persistence of FFV were performed (Winkler et al. 1998; Winkler et al. 1999; Alke et al. 2000; Hatama et al. 2001; Roy et al. 2003; Bodem et al. 2004).

In particular, the analysis of cats which were co-infected by FFV and feline immunodeficiency virus (FIV) did not reveal FFV-related diseases, which were triggered by FIV-induced immunosuppression (Zenger et al. 1993). Furthermore, the artificial immunosuppression in a limited number of SFV-infected monkeys by cyclosporin A resulted only in a higher rate of FV isolations by throat swabs, but not in disease that could be attributed to the virus (D. Neumann-Haefelin, personal communication). Similar results on virus isolation frequencies were obtained when analyzing cats co-infected with FFV and FIV (Bandecchi et al. 1992). The infection of laboratory animals, such as mice and rabbits, by FV of primate origin also leads to virus persistence in the absence of recognizable pathogenicity (Swack and Hsiung 1975; Hooks and Detrick-Hooks 1979; Brown et al. 1982; Santillana-Hayat et al. 1993; Saïb et al. 1997a; Schmidt et al. 1997b; Falcone et al. 2003).

Since human immunodeficiency virus (HIV) arose by trans-species transmissions from nonhuman primates to men (Hahn et al. 2000; Sharp et al. 2001; Peeters et al. 2002), much effort has been undertaken in identifying genuine human FV infections and a potential linkage with human diseases of a suspected infectious origin. In particular, neurological diseases were investigated after the discovery that mice transgenic for FV genes developed brain pathology (Bothe et al. 1991; Aguzzi et al. 1992; Aguzzi et al. 1993). Taking together the results from several studies, in which populations potentially at risk of contracting retroviral infections

Table 59.2 *Foamy virus isolates*[a]

Host species	Isolate	Key references
Macaque (*M. cyclopsis, M. mulatta, M. fascicularis*)	SFVmac	(Johnston 1961; Kupiec et al. 1991)
African green monkey (*C. aethiops*)	SFVagm	(Stiles et al. 1964)
Squirrel monkey (*S. sciureus*)	SFVsqu	(Johnston 1971)
Galago (*G. crass. panganiensis*)	SFVgal	(Johnston 1971)
Chimpanzee (*P. troglodytes* spp.)	SFVcpz	(Rogers et al. 1967; Hooks et al. 1972; Herchenröder et al. 1994)
Spider monkey (*Ateles* spp.)	SFVspm	(Hooks et al. 1973)
Capuchin (*Cebus* spp.)	SFVcap	(Hooks and Gibbs 1975)
Baboon (*P. cynocephalus*)	SFVbab	(Rhodes-Feuillette et al. 1979)
Orangutan (*P. pygmaeus*)	SFVora	(McClure et al. 1994; Verschoor et al. 2003)
Gorilla (*G. gorilla* sp.)	SFVgor	(Bieniasz et al. 1995a)
Marmoset (*C. jacchus*)	SFVmar	(Marczynska et al. 1981)
Felines	FFV	(Riggs et al. 1969; Helps and Harbour 1997; Winkler et al. 1997a)
Bovines	BFV	(Malmquist et al. 1969; Renshaw et al. 1991)
Equines	EFV	(Tobaly-Tapiero et al. 2000)

a) Modified from Meiering and Linial (2001); Falcone et al. (2003).

were screened for FV antibodies, humans do not appear to be a natural reservoir of FV (Hunsmann et al. 1990; Landay et al. 1991; Flügel et al. 1992; Folks et al. 1993; Heneine et al. 1994; Pyykkö et al. 1994; Schweizer et al. 1994; Simonsen et al. 1994; Heneine et al. 1995; Schweizer et al. 1995; Ali et al. 1996; Rösener et al. 1996).

However, additional studies identified a small population of FV-infected humans who were mostly people in contact with nonhuman primates, or material derived from them or African monkey hunters (Schweizer et al. 1997; Heneine et al. 1998; Sandstrom et al. 2000; Switzer et al. 2004; Wolfe et al. 2004). These trans-species infections were never caused by a hypothetical 'human' FV, but could always be traced back to a particular monkey virus (Heneine et al. 2003; Wolfe et al. 2004). Therefore, these isolates are called, for instance, SFVagm(hu) or SFVcpz(hu) to indicate that they were derived from humans zoonotically infected by SFV from African green monkey or chimpanzee, respectively. Virus isolations from FV-infected humans were unsuccessful from throat swabs and required PBL (Heneine et al. 1998; Heneine et al. 2003). Positive results twenty or more years after infection indicate lifelong persistence (Schweizer et al. 1997; Heneine et al. 2003; Switzer et al. 2004). As in their natural hosts, the infections of humans occur in the absence of any pathogenicity (Heneine et al. 2003). Furthermore, so far there is no indication that the virus is transmitted to other humans even by intimate contact or that FV other than those of primate origin can infect humans (Boneva et al. 2002; Heneine et al. 2003; Switzer et al. 2004). Thus humans are likely to represent a dead-end host to primate FV.

The absolute number of humans identified to be infected by SFV is small. A careful follow-up of these cases is required to ensure early recognition of a possible risk of a newly emerging pathogenic human retrovirus. However, given the very slow mutation rate of FV and their general apathogenicity, this scenario appears to be unlikely.

Curiously, the first FV that was molecularly cloned and is still the best-studied virus of this group was initially called 'human' FV, because it was reported to be derived from a human source (Achong et al. 1971; Rethwilm et al. 1987). Following sequencing of chimpanzee FVs, which revealed an almost identical nucleotide sequence (Herchenröder et al. 1994), and the large-scale sero-epidemiological studies with negative results mentioned above, the name 'human' FV was found to be inappropriate and misleading (Rethwilm 2003a). Instead, the name prototypic foamy virus (PFV) for this virus, which most likely is a chimpanzee FV, was coined (Rethwilm 2003a).

FV can infect a very large range of cell cultures (Hooks and Gibbs 1975; Hooks and Detrick-Hooks 1981). Pseudotyping experiments of vesicular stomatitis virus (VSV) with PFV envelope indicated that the unknown receptor must be ubiquitous, since even reptile cells could be infected (Hill et al. 1999). FVs make use of a pH-dependent endocytotic entrance pathway, which is vulnerable to various lysosomotropic agents (Picard-Maureau et al. 2003). Despite the ubiquitous presence of the receptor, not all cells support active virus replication. Reasons other than lack of receptor appear to be responsible for this (Meiering et al. 2001). In adherent cells, lytic infection results in cellfree virus titers of around 10^5–10^6 infectious units/ml (Yu and Linial 1993; Schmidt and Rethwilm 1995). Thus, any given cell produces only 0.1–1 cellfree progeny virus. However, the amount of cell-bound virus is approximately ten times higher (Neumann-Haefelin et al. 1983; Yu and Linial

1993). Of particular interest are cell lines of hematopoietic origin, because these cells often do not show the FV-typical giant cell CPE (Mikovits et al. 1996; Yu et al. 1996a). Yet these cells can be persistently infected and virus production is often low in the range of 10^2–10^3 infectious units/ml (Yu et al. 1996a). The virus–cell interaction in lymphoid cell lines may reflect the in vivo situation closer than fibroblastoid cells. In natural infection, lymphocytes probably disseminate the virus in the body. Active virus replication appears to be restricted to a few organs, like the oral mucosa (Falcone et al. 1999a; Falcone et al. 2003). Furthermore, gamma interferon (γ-IFN) secreted by activated lymphocytes is a potent suppressive factor of FVs that restricts virus replication in a species-specific manner (Falcone et al. 1999b). FV replication was shown to induce apoptosis (Ikeda et al. 1997; Mergia et al. 1997). However, this has not been further elucidated.

MOLECULAR BIOLOGY OF THE *SPUMARETROVIRINAE*

Morphology and composition of the FV particle

Electron microscopy studies revealed most of the details of the FV ultrastructure (Gelderblom and Frank 1987). Extracellular infectious particles are approximately 110 nm in diameter (Figure 59.2). They consist of an immature core of approximately 65 nm consisting of capsid (Gag) protein, which is either uncleaved or processed at the C-terminus where a 3 kD peptide is cleaved by the viral protease (see below). In primary FVs these two moieties are of 71 and 68 kD MW, which are present in around equimolar amounts in the viral particle (Hahn et al. 1994; Fischer et al. 1998). The capsid is surrounded by an envelope, in which the prominent viral glycoproteins (Env) are embedded in a trimeric arrangement (Wilk et al. 2000). In PFV the precursor of Env is of apparent 130 kD MW. Cellular proteases cleave this protein into three subunits, the 18-kDa leader peptide (gp18^{LP}), an around 80-kDa surface protein (gp80^{SU}), and the 48-kDa transmembrane subunit (gp48^{TM}). All three proteins are integral parts of the virion (Lindemann et al. 2001). At least in PFV another glycoprotein (gp170$^{Env-Bet}$) can be found at approximately 50 percent of the amount of gp130^{Env} (Giron et al. 1998; Lindemann and Rethwilm 1998). The gp170$^{Env-Bet}$ which is only loosely, if at all, associated with the virion appears not to be required for in vitro replication (Lindemann and Rethwilm 1998). It is generated from an alternatively spliced mRNA (Giron et al. 1998; Lindemann and Rethwilm 1998) which consists of the majority of the env open reading frame (ORF) fused to the bet ORF (see below). The polymerase (pol) ORF is expressed as a 127-kDa apparent MW precursor which is cleaved by the viral protease into the 85-kDa protease-reverse transcriptase/RNase H (PR-RT/RN) and the 41-kDa integrase (IN). All three proteins are found in virions (Netzer et al. 1993; Pfrepper et al. 1998). The molar ratio of Gag to Pol proteins approximates 15:1 (M. Cartellieri and A. Rethwilm, unpublished observation).

The genomes of FVs have been studied in detail for PFV and FFV (Moebes et al. 1997; Yu et al. 1999; Roy

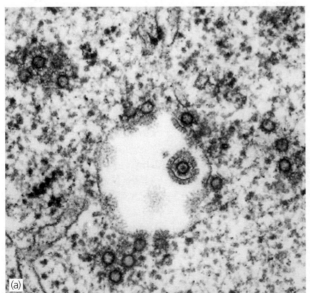
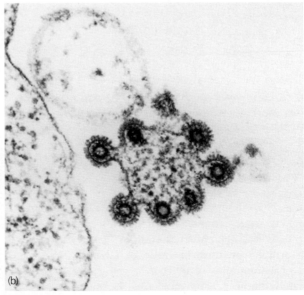

Figure 59.2 (a) *Electron micrograph of intracellular capsids, particles budding into intracellular compartments, and mature foamy virus.* **(b)** *Electron micrograph of budding foamy viruses revealing the prominent envelope glycoprotein spikes. The magnification in A and B is 96 000-fold. The pictures are a courtesy of Hanswalter Zentgraf (Heidelberg, Germany). (Continued over)*

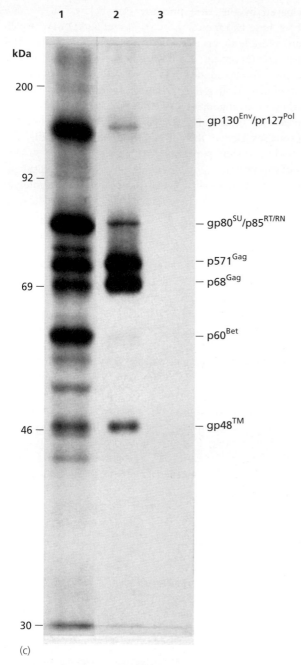

(c)

Figure 59.2 *(Continued)* **(c)** *Radioimmunprecipitation of metabolically labeled foamy virus proteins with positive monkey serum. Lane 1, intracellular virus proteins; lane 2, extracellular virion proteins; lane 3, lysate from uninfected cells reacted with positive serum. The molecular weight marker is indicated on the left and the main viral proteins on the right.*

et al. 2003). Interestingly, FVs contain a large amount of already reverse transcribed, mostly linear, cDNA (Yu et al. 1996a, 1999; Moebes et al. 1997; Roy et al. 2003). In orthoretroviruses, the ratio of DNA to RNA (late reverse transcripts of the *pol* or *gag* genes) is approximately one in 4×10^5 molecules. In spumaretroviruses, it was determined to be as high as one DNA in six RNA molecules (Yu et al. 1999; Roy et al. 2003). While some reports indicate that only the DNA form of the genome

is relevant for replication (Moebes et al. 1997; Yu et al. 1999; Roy et al. 2003), others point to a role of RNA as well (Delelis et al. 2003).

Genome organization and expression

FV genomes are large; the PFV genome (linear viral DNA) is 13.2 kb (Figure 59.3) and the FFV genome 11.7 kb long. The viral genes are flanked by long terminal repeats (LTR) (of 1770 bp in PFV), subdivided into U3 (1423-bp), R (194-bp), and U5 (153-bp) regions (Maurer et al. 1988; Schmidt et al. 1997a). Adjacent to the 5′ LTR a short untranslated sequence is positioned, which is followed by the canonical *gag*, *pol*, and *env* genes. The protease is encoded in the *pol* gene. Downstream of env and overlapping the 3′ LTR, two accessory ORFs can be found in all sequenced FVs. The first harbors the *tas* gene (for *t*ransactivator of *s*pumaretroviruses) and ORF-2 gives rise to Bet, an abundant protein of ill-defined function (see below).

After provirus integration an internal promoter (IP), which is located in the *env* gene upstream of the accessory ORFs gives rise to two major transcripts (Löchelt et al. 1993b; Campbell et al. 1994; Löchelt et al. 1994; Mergia 1994; Bodem et al. 1998a) which are often spliced in the 5′ untranslated region (Figure 59.3). To do this the IP has some weak basal activity (Löchelt et al. 1993a). The activity of the IP is essential for the remainder of the replication cycle (Löchelt et al. 1995). One of the IP transcripts leads to the Tas protein and the other to Bet (Löchelt et al. 1994). Bet is derived from a multispliced mRNA. The most significant splice uses a splice donor (SD) in ORF-1 and an ORF-2 splice acceptor (SA). Tas activates transcription from the IP and the 5′ LTR U3 promoter. The U3 promoter has no detectable activity in the absence of Tas (Keller et al. 1991). The Gag protein is translated from a (pre-)genome length transcript. Instead of being expressed as a Gag–Pol fusion protein, FV Pol uses its own mRNA for translation as an authentic protein (Bodem et al. 1996; Enssle et al. 1996; Löchelt and Flügel 1996; Yu et al. 1996a). This transcript is spliced from the major 5′ SD in U5 to an SA which is located in the *gag* gene (Figure 59.3). The *pol* gene-specific splicing event appears to be critical for viral replication (Jordan et al. 1996). The transcripts for the Env protein also make use of the major 5′ SD and a major (or one of the minor) SA sites at the 3′ end of the *pol* gene (Muranyi and Flügel 1991). Despite this complex splicing pattern, a post-transcriptional regulator of FV gene expression has not been detected (Baunach et al. 1993; Yu and Linial 1993; Lee et al. 1994; Adachi et al. 1995). However, an RNA element within the *pol* gene has been described to facilitate Gag protein expression of HIV (Wodrich et al. 2001). This result awaits further substantiation.

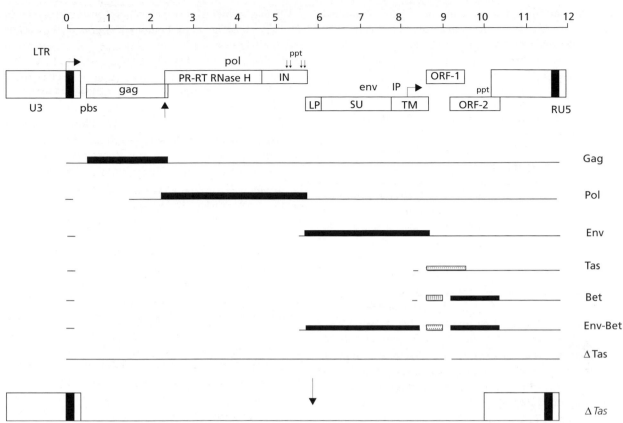

Figure 59.3 *Foamy virus genome organization (upper panel), main transcripts (middle panel), and ΔTas virus (bottom panel). Foamy virus genomes contain long terminal repeats (LTRs) at their ends, which are typically subdivided into U3, R, and U5 regions. First strand reverse transcription is initiated at the primer binding site (pbs). There are two polypurine tracts (ppt) for the initiation of second strand synthesis. RNA transcription initiates at the internal promoter (IP) or in the 5′ LTR. The canonical* gag, pol, end env *genes are indicated. Only one cleavage site for the viral protease has been identified in* gag *(arrow). The Pol precursor protein is expressed from a spliced mRNA and is also cleaved once between protease-reverse transcriptase and integrase. The Env precursor bears two cleavage sites for cellular proteases, one between the leader peptide (LP) and the surface (SU) domain and one between the latter and the transmembrane (TM) subunit. In addition, there are two further open reading frames (ORFs) downstream of* env. *ORF-1 gives rise to the Tas protein, which trans-activates transcription from the IP and the LTR promoter. Orf-1 transcripts are often spliced in the 5′ untranslated region (UTR) and can be generated from the IP or the 5′ LTR. This depends on the viral isolate. ORF-2 is expressed from a multispliced mRNA and gives rise to the Bet protein, which is highly expressed in infected cells, but of unknown function. Bet transcripts can also start from the IP or the main 5′ promoter. An Env–Bet fusion-protein is generated from the env mRNA that also uses the splice sites in the 5′ UTR of IP transcripts and splice sites in ORF-1 which lead to authentic Bet protein. These splicing events lead to an Env–ORF-2 fusion-protein in FFV. The function of Env–Bet (or Env–ORF-2) is ill-defined. The ΔTas transcript is of pregenomic length except for the small ORF-1 intron that has been spliced out. The ΔTas genome is transactivator-negative and helper virus-dependent (see text for details).*

Additional transcripts can be found in some FVs. Spliced tas and bet mRNAs originating in the 5′ LTR have been described for PFV, but not for FFV (Muranyi and Flügel 1991; Bodem et al. 1998a). The use of the *env* gene-located splice sites described above can give rise to a PFV Env-Bet fusion protein (Figure 59.3) from which the part of env coding for the membrane-spanning region of TM has been spliced out (Giron et al. 1998; Lindemann and Rethwilm 1998), or to an Env–ORF-2 fusion protein in FFV (Bodem et al. 1998a).

Aside from the (pre-)genomic transcript, a further transcript of almost (pre-)genomic length exists, from which only the small intron in the *tas* gene has been spliced out (Saïb et al. 1993). After reverse transcription this RNA leads to ΔTas virus (Saïb et al. 1993) which requires a helper virus for replication (see below).

Additional structural nucleic acid features include the primer binding side (pbs) 3′ of the 5′ LTR, which is specific for the t-RNA lysine[1,2] (Maurer et al. 1988), a dimer linkage site (Erlwein et al. 1997; Cain et al. 2001), the polypurine tract (ppt) 5′ of the 3′ LTR, and an internal stretch of purine-rich sequences which is located in the *pol* gene (Kupiec et al. 1988; Tobaly-Tapiero et al. 1991). The functional significance of this central ppt has not been completely determined yet, however, it is believed to have analogous functions to the ppt in HIV (Charneau and Clavel 1991; Charneau et al. 1992). Furthermore, RNA sequences involved in expression of structural proteins and in packaging the (pre-)genomic transcript and the Pol protein have been identified (Erlwein et al. 1998; Heinkelein et al. 1998, 2000b; Wu et al. 1998; Park and Mergia 2000; Russell et al. 2001; Heinkelein et al. 2002b). Full functional characterization of these sequences has not yet been carried out.

Antigens and function of individual proteins

CORE ANTIGEN (GAG)

Cleavage of the Gag precursor into matrix, capsid, and nucleocapsid subunits is a feature that is conserved among *Orthoretrovirinae* and is responsible for the maturation of the viruses. The process which can be viewed as condensation of the capsid after budding (Swanstrom and Wills 1997), does not occur in FVs (Figure 59.2). Instead, only a small peptide is chopped of the C-terminus of FV Gag by the viral protease. This cleavage is essential for virus replication (Enssle et al. 1997; Zemba et al. 1998) and capsids consisting only of the precursor tend not to close and to show an irregular morphology (Konvalinka et al. 1995; Fischer et al. 1998).

Viral capsids serve two antagonistic roles: on the one hand they must be stable enough to protect the nucleic acid from the hostile environment and, on the other, they must easily free this nucleic acid once uptake into a susceptible cell has occurred. Orthoretroviruses have solved this problem by using protease-mediated defined cleavages of their Gag proteins, which prepare the capsids for disassembly (Wills and Craven 1991; Boulanger and Jones 1996; Kräusslich and Welker 1996; Swanstrom and Wills 1997). Therefore, the question arises how spumaretroviruses meet this challenge. In one possible scenario, disassembly of capsids occurs by FV protease-mediated cleavages of Gag early following the viral uptake (Giron et al. 1997). The identification of further Gag cleavage sites in addition to the C-terminal p3 cleavage site by in vitro PR assays and the vulnerability of the virus by mutagenesis of these sites is consistent with this hypothesis (Pfrepper et al. 1999). However, in the respective study, other possible alterations on Gag morphogenesis have not been excluded. Furthermore, recent evidence indicates that the FV capsid structure is maintained in the first phase after infection (Petit et al. 2003).

FV Gag proteins also lack other conserved sequence motifs, such as the major homology region, or the nucleic acid-binding cysteine-histidine-boxes (Wills and Craven 1991; Swanstrom and Wills 1997). Instead, PFV Gag harbors three so-called glycine–arginine-rich (GR) boxes at the C terminus (Schliephake and Rethwilm 1994). The first of these boxes binds with equal affinity to RNA and DNA (Yu et al. 1996b), the second box harbors a nuclear localization signal which is responsible for primate FV Gag proteins being transiently transported into the nucleus of infected cells (Figure 59.1) (Schliephake and Rethwilm 1994), while no function has been assigned to the third box. Nuclear localization of Gag, however, does not seem to be essential for FV cell culture replication (Yu et al. 1996b). In sharp contrast to the lentiviruses FV Gag proteins are much less well conserved compared to Pol and Env proteins (Figure 59.4). It is, therefore, not surprising that even the GR-boxes of primate FV are not conserved in the equine, bovine, and feline isolates. Furthermore, FFV Gag has been shown not to have a nuclear phase (Bodem et al. 1998b).

FV capsids assemble in the cytoplasma (Baldwin and Linial 1998; Fischer et al. 1998). A coiled-coil domain in the N-terminal half of FV Gag has been identified as being required for Gag–Gag interactions (Tobaly-Tapiero et al. 2001). While orthoretroviral Gag proteins bear all the information required for particle budding from the plasma membrane (Wills and Craven 1991; Boulanger and Jones 1996), this is not the case in FVs where Gag depends on the presence of autologous Env to export the particles, either from the plasma membrane or from the endoplasmic reticulum (ER) (Baldwin and Linial 1998; Fischer et al. 1998; Pietschmann et al. 1999). However, the addition of a heterologous plasma membrane-targeting signal to the FV Gag N-terminus, together with the change of an arginine at position 50 to alanine, leads to Env-independent budding of Gag (Eastman and Linial 2001). The mutation of an arginine in a similar position of the *gag* gene of Mason–Pfizer virus, an orthoretrovirus that, like FVs, shows cytoplasmic capsid assembly (D-type morphology), has been reported previously to redirect capsid assembly to the plasma membrane (C-type morphology) (Rhee and Hunter 1990). Thus, like orthoretrovirus capsids, the FV Gag proteins show some flexibility in the intracellular location of particle assembly.

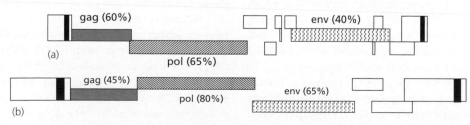

Figure 59.4 *Amino acids conservation among primate lentiviruses* **(a)** *and foamy viruses* **(b)**. *While in lentiviruses the Env protein is the most divergent structural viral protein, in primate FVs Gag is much more heterogenous than Env.*

RT ANTIGENS (POL)

FV Pol protein uses its own ATG start codon for expression from a spliced mRNA (Bodem et al. 1996; Jordan et al. 1996; Löchelt and Flügel 1996; Yu et al. 1996a). Sequences specifying protease, reverse transcriptase proper, RNase H, and integrase can be clearly identified on the basis of the conserved motifs of the active centers of the respective enzymes (Kögel et al. 1995a, 1995b). Unusually, the FV protease is not cleaved from the RT/RN (Pfrepper et al. 1998). The only consistent cleavage occurs between PR/RT/RN and IN (Pfrepper et al. 1998). A minor cleavage site has also been described between RT and RN of PFV (Pfrepper et al. 1998). Another peculiarity has been detected in the FFV PR. While the active center of retroviral proteases bears the strictly conserved DS/TG motif, FFV contains in this position a DSQ (Winkler et al. 1997a; Flügel and Pfrepper 2003). Nonetheless, the FFV PR containing this amino acid is enzymatically active (Flügel and Pfrepper 2003). The PFV Pol protein precursor, as well as its PR/RT/RN and IN subunits, were reported to be nuclear proteins when cells were transfected with eucaryotic expression constructs of the respective ORFs (Imrich et al. 2000). The functional significances of these findings have not been elucidated.

Since the Pol precursor protein of FVs is expressed independently from the Gag protein, FVs must have found a way of Pol incorporation into the particle in the absence of a Gag fusion partner. Interestingly, the presence of (pre-)genomic RNA is required in order to assemble Pol into viral capsids (Heinkelein et al. 2002b). In contrast to the hepadnaviruses, this RNA is incorporated in the absence of Pol into FV capsids (Baldwin and Linial 1998, 1999). Therefore, it is highly likely that in FVs (pre-)genomic RNA serves as a bridging molecule, which interacts with Gag on the one side and Pol on the other and, thereby, facilitates completion of particle assembly. The identification of separate sequences in the (pre-)genomic RNA for the interaction with Gag and Pol is consistent with this hypothesis (K. Peters, M. Heinkelein, and A. Rethwilm, unpublished results).

FV reverse transcriptase appears to be much more processive than orthoretroviral RT (Rinke et al. 2002). This is probably a prerequisite for FV reverse transcription prior to budding (see below).

ENVELOPE ANTIGENS (ENV)

The glycoproteins of FVs are another example of the highly divergent replication pathway that these viruses have developed. All orthoretroviral Env proteins are synthesized as precursors that are cleaved by cellular proteases into SU and TM subdomains which are part of the mature virion. TM is an MHC class I transmembrane protein (Einfeld 1996; Hunter 1997). It is anchored in the viral membrane and makes contacts to the SU subdomain (Swanstrom and Wills 1997). In murine leukaemia virus (MLV) and in Mason–Pfizer monkey virus, small peptides are cleaved from the cytoplasmic tail of TM to activate its fusogenic activity (Green et al. 1981; Henderson et al. 1984; Brody et al. 1992, 1994; Sommerfelt et al. 1992; Rein et al. 1994). However, this does not change the general organization of the glycoprotein complex. The orthoretroviral Env precursor bears a signal peptide sequence at the N-terminus that is responsible for ER translocation. This rather short sequence is cleaved from the remainder of the protein in the ER and degraded or further processed (Martoglio et al. 1997; Swanstrom and Wills 1997).

The signal or leader peptide of FV Env proteins is rather long and is also cleaved from the rest of the protein, however, in striking contrast to the situation in orthoretroviruses, the LP remains associated with the virion (Lindemann et al. 2001). Thus, FVs posses three glycosylated Env proteins (LP, SU, and TM), and two of these cross the viral membrane, LP at the N terminus and TM at the C terminus. Being initially synthesized as an MHC class III membrane protein (precursor), the mature Env consists of an MHC class II membrane protein (LP), the extraviral SU, and an MHC class I membrane protein (TM) (Lindemann et al. 2001). Furthermore, the LP points with its N-terminus to the viral capsid and makes contact to Gag (Lindemann et al. 2001; Wilk et al. 2001; Geiselhart et al. 2003). This is the reason for the specificity of the FV capsid–glycoprotein interaction and the molecular basis of the inability to pseudotype unmodified FV capsids with heterologous envelopes (Pietschmann et al. 1999). The mutation of only one conserved tryptophane residue in the cytoplasmic part of LP abrogates infectivity and the ability of Env to interact with Gag (Lindemann et al. 2001; Wilk et al. 2001), although the specific molecular way in which this interaction takes place is not yet known. Biophysical experiments point to contacts of LP with the Gag N terminus, which is believed to form a layer underneath the viral membrane akin to the matrix protein of orthoretrovirus Gag proteins (Wilk et al. 2001).

Not only is Env required to export FV capsids, Gag protein appears similarly to stimulate the quantitative release of Env from the plasma membrane (Pietschmann et al. 2000). The equine virus may represent an exception, because it was reported to bud exclusively from the plasma membrane (Tobaly-Tapiero et al. 2000; Lecellier et al. 2002a), while the other known FVs preferentially bud from intracellular membranes. Except in the case of EFV, an ER retrieval signal has been identified in the cytoplasmic tail of all FV TM proteins (Goepfert et al. 1995; Tobaly-Tapiero et al. 2000). This may, in the absence of Gag, hold back Env in intracellular compartments (Goepfert et al. 1997). However, additional elements in the membrane-spanning region of TM and the FV LP are at least equally important for this retrieval (Pietschmann et al. 2000; Lindemann et al. 2001).

Another interesting feature of FV Env is the ability to self-associate and form subviral particles (SVP). Such SVPs arise by self aggregation of hepatitis B virus (HBV) surface protein in HBV infection in numbers exceeding the infectious virus and are believed to deflect the anti-HBV immune response (Gerlich 1991). While the SVPs of HBV are abundantly shed from infected cells, the PFV SVPs are, probably due to the retention of Env in cytoplasmic compartments, less abundant (Shaw et al. 2003).

NONSTRUCTURAL PROTEINS

Tas

The FV Tas proteins are approximately 209–300 amino acids in length, depending on the specific virus isolate (Rethwilm 1995; Löchelt 2003). They act as transactivators of gene expression from the two FV promoters and are required for virus replication (Baunach et al. 1993; Rethwilm 1995; Löchelt 2003). Tas augments gene expression by direct binding to DNA motifs in the IP and the U3 region of the LTR (He et al. 1996; Zou and Luciw 1996; Kang et al. 1998; Kang and Cullen 1998; Bodem et al. 2004). Tas binds to the IP with higher affinity than to the U3 promoter and to the U3 promoter with higher avidity than to the IP (Kang et al. 1998; Löchelt 2003). Between FV promoters and Tas proteins from different species there is only little conservation and almost no cross-transactivation (Löchelt 2003; Bodem et al. 2004). Tas proteins have been dissected into several subdomains: at the N terminus a region is shared with the Bet protein. The variable length of this region is responsible for the length variability of Tas proteins from different species (Löchelt 2003). The promoter-targeting domain that shows a low degree of conservation between different Tas proteins and is responsible for recognition of the DNA target sites follows the domain shared with Bet (Löchelt 2003). Between this region and the C-terminal activation domain is located the nuclear localization signal (NLS), consisting of an accumulation of basic residues (Keller et al. 1991; Chang et al. 1995; Rethwilm 1995; Bodem et al. 1998b). The approximately 30 amino acids activation domain stimulates gene expression in a wide variety of lower and higher eukaryotic cells when targeted to a heterologous promoter via an unrelated DNA-binding motif (He et al. 1993).

The DNA-binding regions and the activation domains show no homology to known motifs. However, genetic evidence indicates that FV Tas proteins belong to the acidic class of transcriptional activators (Blair et al. 1994). FV Tas proteins are believed to interact with conserved components of the transcriptional machinery. In yeast cells the ADA2 transcriptional adapter molecule has been identified and shown to be required for activation by the PFV Tas activation domain (Blair et al. 1994). FV Tas proteins can also activate gene expression by binding to recognition sequences located elsewhere in the FV or in the host cellular genome (Campbell et al. 1996; Wagner et al. 2000; Kido et al. 2002).

Since the elements in the U3 region of the LTR, which are responsive to Tas, do not completely match with the DNA-binding sites (Mergia et al. 1992; Erlwein and Rethwilm 1993; Lee et al. 1993; Renne et al. 1993), it is likely that mechanisms in addition to direct binding of Tas are involved in the transcriptional regulation of FV promoters (He et al. 1996). Possibly, Tas has DNA-binding and protein–protein interaction capabilities. The cellular promyelocytic leukaemia protein (PML) complexes with and strongly inhibits PFV Tas function (Regad et al. 2001). PML is induced by IFN and this may explain the IFN-responsiveness of FVs. However, it was shown by others that on a cellular level PML is not involved in the establishment of viral latency (Meiering and Linial 2003). Viral latency appears to be the dominant form of persistence in the infected host (Falcone et al. 2003). Nuclear factor I (NFI) was identified as another element to repress FV gene expression (Kido et al. 2003). Its contribution to the state of viral latency remains to be determined.

Bet

Because Bet is a protein derived from an mRNA spliced from ORF-1 into ORF-2 (Figure 59.3), only one (Tas or Bet) of the two accessory FV proteins can be expressed at a time. In lytically infected cells there appears to be a strong preference to generate the Bet protein, while Tas is relatively rare (Baunach et al. 1993). The function of PFV Bet remains elusive, since the part of Bet (ORF-2) that is nonoverlapping with Tas (ORF-1) or with other sequences, such as the downstream ppt and 3′ LTR motifs required for integration, can be deleted or functionally ablated from infectious plasmids without adversely affecting their replication competence (Baunach et al. 1993; Yu and Linial 1993; Schmidt and Rethwilm 1995). Bet is mainly cytoplasmically located, however, a small portion of PFV Bet has been reported to enter the nucleus, as well as being shed from infected cells and taken up by other cells (Lecellier et al. 2002b). In FFV, Bet is required for the release of FFV particles in a cell-type dependent manner (Alke et al. 2001).

Using a reactivation system from viral latency by the addition of the phorbol ester PMA, it was shown that Bet counteracts IP activity (Meiering and Linial 2002). As outlined above, IP activity is the start of a series of events leading to progeny virus. It is possible that in latent infection the relative expression levels of Tas and Bet, even more than in lytic infection, shift in favour of Bet. Thus, the generation of Tas versus Bet is supposed to be the molecular switch that controls the outcome of an infection: lytic (little expression of

Tas, major expression of Bet) versus latent (no expression of Tas, exclusive expression of Bet) (Meiering and Linial 2002). However, the mechanisms controlling this switch remain to be determined. In addition, it is likely that Bet serves additional functions than controlling viral latency.

Interestingly, the overexpression of PFV Bet renders cells resistant to superinfection by the autologous virus (Saïb et al. 1995; Bock et al. 1998). Once delivered as plasmid DNA into the cells, establishment of the resistant phenotype was found to be unrelated to downregulation of viral uptake or the activity of viral promoters (Bock et al. 1998). It was, therefore, concluded that the block in replication most likely occurred between virus entry and provirus establishment (Bock et al. 1998). Any functional consequences of this for the viral replication cycle have not yet been analyzed.

Overview of the FV replication strategy

FVs appear to have acquired a unique replication strategy that has adopted aspects of the orthoretroviral and the hepadnaviral replication pathways (Nassal and Schaller 1993; Linial 1999; Lecellier and Saïb 2000; Rethwilm 2003b). An overview is presented in Figure 59.5. Although at first sight the FV genome organization looks like a typical complex retrovirus, the unique features cover any aspect of the replication strategy and the functions of individual proteins (Rethwilm 2003b). From provirus integration (Enssle et al. 1999; Juretzek et al. 2004), regulation of gene expression (Löchelt 2003), packaging of (pre-)genomic RNA and Pol proteins (Heinkelein et al. 2000b; Heinkelein et al. 2002b), capsid assembly (Linial and Eastman 2003), and cleavage by the viral protease (Flügel and Pfrepper 2003) to budding and Gag–Env interaction (Lindemann and Goepfert 2003), FV replication deviates from what are believed to be the standard rules of retrovirology (Vogt 1997).

Most striking is the generation of infectious full-length cDNA late in the replication cycle before budding of the particle (Yu et al. 1996a, 1999; Moebes et al. 1997; Roy et al. 2003). Aside from exiting the infected cell, this DNA can also recycle to the nucleus and integrate, resulting in the delivery of additional proviruses, at least in the absence of FV glycoprotein (Heinkelein et al. 2000a, 2003) (Figure 59.5). While this phenomenon is reminiscent of the life cycle of retrotransposons (Boeke and Stoye 1997), its significance for the FV replication cycle remains to be determined. The extent to which cDNA synthesis in the virus-producing cell is complete may depend on the actual cell type, which can explain why reverse transcription can also be detected early in the replication cycle (Delelis et al. 2003).

In addition, FVs generate a reverse-transcribed defective cDNA (the ΔTas genome in Figure 59.3) to an

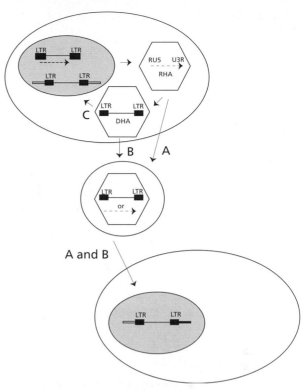

Figure 59.5 *Principal retroviral replication strategies. Orthoretroviruses make use of pathway A regardless of intracellular capsid assembly or assembly at the plasma membrane. Obligatory FV capsid assemble occurs in the cytoplasm. Furthermore, reverse transcription of the pregenomic RNA takes place at this stage and cDNA is exported (pathway B) or can recycle to the nucleus and integrate into the host cell genome to give rise to additional proviruses (pathway C). (Modified from Heinkelein et al. 2000a)*

extent that is likely to affect biological function (Saïb et al. 1993). The ΔTas is generated from an almost pregenomic length RNA, from which ORF-1 intron, normally used to generate Bet mRNA, has been spliced out (Figure 59.3). Thus, ΔTas are replication-defected. Depending on the number of ΔTas proviruses, which can express some Bet protein, cells become resistant to the infection by wildtype virus (Saïb et al. 1995). However, the exact relationship between wild-type and ΔTas genome, and whether this type of interference is taking place in vivo, is not known.

While orthoretroviruses are RNA viruses replicating through a DNA intermediate, where the step of reverse transcription occurs early in the replication cycle, FVs, like hepadnaviruses, are DNA viruses, which replicate through an RNA intermediate with a reverse transcription step late in the replication cycle. Unlike the hepadnaviruses, they require integration into the host cell genome for replication, similar to orthoretroviruses (Enssle et al. 1999; Meiering et al. 2000). This raises the question as to whether FVs may represent a functional or evolutionary link between these reverse transcribing virus families (Flint et al. 2004).

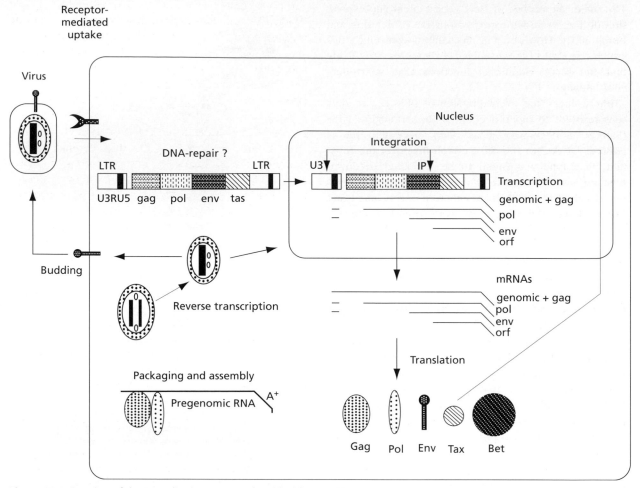

Figure 59.6 *Overview of the FV replication strategy. (Modified from Rethwilm 2003a)*

FV VECTORS

FV vectors based on PFV, SFV-1, and FFV have been developed over the last years (Mergia and Heinkelein 2003). Some of the vectors were replication-competent, taking advantage of the generally nonpathogenic nature of FV infection (Schmidt and Rethwilm 1995; Schwantes et al. 2002). These vectors may be used to deliver, for instance, suicide genes or genes for immunogenic proteins in vivo (Nestler et al. 1997; Schwantes et al. 2003). However, since the virus has no advantage from the additional genetic burden, these genes are usually lost quickly during replication, at least in vivo (Nestler et al. 1997; Schwantes et al. 2003).

More promising for future applications are replication-incompetent vectors based on FVs. There are several theoretical advantages of using FV vectors than MLV-derived vectors, which are the most widely and most successful retroviral vectors currently in use in clinical trials (Cavazzana-Calvo et al. 2004). First of all, the parental virus is nonpathogenic. As a consequence gene therapy with FV vectors should be safe, even in the unlikely event of generating replication-competent vector-derived retroviruses by recombination (Schenk et al.

1999; Bastone and Löchelt 2004). Furthermore, by separation of the packaging plasmids in three instead of two expression units (orthoretroviruses generate a Gag/Pol fusion protein) a further safety profile can be added to FV vectors (Heinkelein et al. 2002a; Trobridge et al. 2002a). Secondly, the genome of FVs is larger than that of MLV, possibly enabling the packaging of larger fragments of foreign DNA (Heinkelein et al. 2002a; Park et al. 2002; Trobridge et al. 2002a). Thirdly, FV can be concentrated without significant loss of infectivity, e.g. by centrifugation (Hill et al. 1999; Trobridge et al. 2002b). The receptor for FVs, although not currently known, is widespread, which allows targeting of a wide variety of cells (Mergia et al. 1996; Hill et al. 1999; Lindemann et al. 2000).

However, FVs do not infect resting cells (Bieniasz et al. 1995b; Trobridge and Russell 2004). The incoming capsid appears to be transported into the vicinity of the nucleus (Saïb et al. 1997b; Petit et al. 2003), but similar to MLV FVs appear to require the breakdown of the nuclear membrane for integration and subsequent gene expression (Hajihosseini et al. 1993). The difference from MLV is that, since FV reverse transcription has already taken place in the virus- or vector-producing cell, the form of the nucleic acid that is delivered into the target cell consists of DNA instead of RNA. Reverse transcription can be regarded as the most vulnerable step in retrovirus replication, and due to the greater stability of double-stranded DNA compared to single-stranded RNA, FVs may be ideal to target rarely cycling cells, such as hematopoietic progenitors.

In a variety of seminal experiments it has been shown that FV vectors can target CD34 antigen-positive human hematopoietic progenitors of different sources that are able to repopulate sublethally irradiated NOD/SCID mice with an efficiency comparable to vectors derived from lentiviruses and much superior to MLV vectors, provided that the target cells were not prestimulated (Hirata et al. 1996; Josephson et al. 2002; Leurs et al. 2003; Josephson et al. 2004). The transduction of hematopoietic stem cells was demonstrated by analysis of transgene expression and vector integration site determination in lymphoid and myeloid compartments after long-term engraftment (Josephson et al. 2002; Leurs et al. 2003; Josephson et al. 2004).

However, it must be noted that packaging cells for FV vectors, which would allow to better control for the quality of the vector preparations by standard means, are not yet available (Mergia and Heinkelein 2003). Furthermore, FV capsids do not currently allow the efficient pseudotyping by heterologous glycoproteins and the FV envelope glycoprotein complex exhibits considerable cell toxicity, which makes the handling of FV vectors painstaking. It remains to be seen whether the development of adenovirus–foamy virus hybrid vectors, which create a form of in vivo packaging cell line can overcome this problem (Picard-Maureau et al. 2004; Russell et al. 2004) or whether batches of FV vectors will have to be produced by the repeated transient transfection of cells.

Furthermore, the packaging signal on the (pre-)-genomic RNA and the mechanism of RNA, as well as Pol protein packaging have not yet been completely resolved (Heinkelein et al. 2000b, 2002b). It is known that at least two regions on the RNA are required for efficient packaging into particles (Erlwein et al. 1998; Heinkelein et al. 1998; Wu et al. 1998; Heinkelein et al. 2000b; Russell et al. 2001). One element resides in the 5′ leader region and extends into the *gag* gene, while the other element is located in the 3′ *pol* gene region. Thus, there is a need for a better understanding of the biochemical basis of RNA and Pol protein packaging and the mechanism of FV particle assembly to further improve current vectors and packaging constructs.

EPIDEMIOLOGY AND LABORATORY DIAGNOSIS

FV are highly prevalent in many monkey species from the Old and the New World (Hooks and Gibbs 1975; Hooks and Detrick-Hooks 1981; Swack 1981; Meiering

and Linial 2001; Falcone et al. 2003). Of these, only Old World FVs are characterized in greater detail. The rate of infection in the wild can be as high as 30 percent or above (Hooks and Gibbs 1975; Swack 1981; Meiering and Linial 2001). In captivity, infection rates may be anywhere between 70 percent and close to 100 percent (Hooks and Gibbs 1975; Hooks and Detrick-Hooks 1981; Swack 1981; Rösener et al. 1996; Meiering and Linial 2001; Falcone et al. 2003). Only a weak cross-neutralization was reported for SFVs originating from different species. Trans-species transmissions in captive monkeys and even dual infections with two different SFVs has been described (Hooks et al. 1972; Hooks and Gibbs 1975; Swack 1981; Meiering and Linial 2001).

As in monkeys, the FV prevalence in cats increases with age to an incidence of over 70–80 percent in domestic or feral animals over the age of nine (Bandecchi et al. 1992). Social contact is suspected to be the most likely mode of FFV transmission (Bandecchi et al. 1992). Two FFV serotypes which do not cross-neutralize and which have substantial differences in the env *SU* genes are documented (Winkler et al. 1998; Zemba et al. 2000). Because the Gag sequences are conserved, diagnostic tests rely on the detection of antibodies to this protein (Winkler et al. 1997b).

As already mentioned above, so far there is no indication of a naturally circulating human FV. However, since the detection of an SFV infection in a monkey caretaker (Schweizer et al. 1997), more extensive investigations led by the Centers for Disease Control and Prevention (CDC) in Atlanta, GA, USA on occupationally acquired FV infections were carried out (Heneine et al. 1998; Switzer et al. 2004). Altogether, approximately 5 percent of animal caretakers or laboratory personnel handling infected material were found to be sero- and PCR-positive (Brooks et al. 2002; Heneine et al. 2003; Switzer et al. 2004). Thus, the risk of occupational acquisition of an SFV infection appears to be much higher than that of contracting an infection with other nonhuman primate viruses (Brooks et al. 2002; Heneine et al. 2003; Switzer et al. 2004). No risk of attracting an FFV infection was found for veterinarians handling FV-infected cats (Butera et al. 2000).

Another population potentially at risk of FV infection are monkey hunters in the African bush. While an earlier investigation found no evidence of infection in a rather small sample (Goepfert et al. 1996), a more recent study identified 1 percent positives when screening over 1 000 human sera (Wolfe et al. 2004). Samples positive for FV antibodies were confirmed by nucleic acid detection and sequencing (Wolfe et al. 2004). Besides differences in the sample size, it should be noted that the methods of screening were also different in the two studies (Goepfert et al. 1996; Wolfe et al. 2004).

The method of choice to detect FV infections in humans consists of screening sera for antibody against a cocktail of antigens derived from the SFVs potentially being transmitted. An immunoblot coated with antigen derived from two SFVs (SFVagm and SFVcpz) has beenshown to react with serum samples, which are positive for a wide variety of different SFVs (Hussain et al. 2003). Antibody response in an immunoblot against the Gag antigens usually indicates positivity (Hahn et al. 1994; Hussain et al. 2003). The detection of an antibody response against the nonstructural Bet protein (Figure 59.2) corroborates serological diagnosis of infection (Hahn et al. 1994). Antiglycoprotein antibodies are only detected reliably by radio-immunoprecipitation (Netzer et al. 1990). In any case positive results in antibody tests should be confirmed by PCR diagnosis using primers from regions conserved in the FV genome, such as from the integrase gene (Schweizer and Neumann-Haefelin 1995; Khan et al. 1999). When the infecting virus is known and in culture, indirect immunofluorescence also reliably detect infection (Neumann-Haefelin et al. 1983). In this case a strong nuclear fluorescence should be visible, at least in some cells when dealing with FVs of primate origin (Figure 59.1).

Virus isolation can be done relatively easily from throat swabs of infected monkeys or cats using a wide variety of target cells, but preferably fibroblasts, to monitor the development of CPE (Hooks and Gibbs 1975; Swack 1981). Indicator cell lines bearing the *lacZ* gene under the control of different FV LTRs have been established for easy and quick monitoring of infection (Yu and Linial 1993; Bock et al. 1998; Roy et al. 2003). However, such cell lines are not available for all FVs. Virus isolation from humans requires particular conditions, such as the isolation from PBLs and potentially the addition of anti-interferon (Heneine et al. 1998; Falcone et al. 1999b).

The methods to diagnose FV infections are not generally in use and in the case of a suspected human SFV infection, one should refer to a more specialized and experienced laboratory. SFV-infected humans should not donate organs, blood or blood products (Allan et al. 1998; Boneva et al. 2002). Whenever possible, such individuals and their close contacts should be followed for the unlikely event of the emergence of a new retrovirus adapted to replicate efficiently in the human host (Peeters et al. 2002).

Zidovudine (AZT) is the only known antiretroviral drug that efficiently blocks FV replication (Rosenblum et al. 2001). In the event of reactivating latent FVs when culturing primary monkey cells, AZT at a concentration of 5–10 μm can be tried in order to block SFV replication.

Infections with foamy viruses are not of medical importance, but the study of their molecular biology has contributed much to our understanding of the ways retroviruses replicate and the use of foamy virus vectors may open a new field in somatic gene therapy.

ACKNOWLEDGMENTS

I am indebted to Myra O. McClure (London, UK) and Dirk Lindemann (Dresden, Germany) for their critical review of the manuscript.

REFERENCES

Achong, B.G., Mansell, P.W., et al. 1971. An unusual virus in cultures from a human nasopharyngeal carcinoma. *J Natl Cancer Inst*, **46**, 299–307.

Adachi, A., Sakai, H., et al. 1995. Functional analysis of human spumaretrovirus genome. *Virus Genes*, **11**, 15–20.

Aguzzi, A., Bothe, K., et al. 1992. Human foamy virus: an underestimated neuropathogen? *Brain Pathol*, **2**, 61–9.

Aguzzi, A., Wagner, E.F., et al. 1993. Human foamy virus proteins accumulate in neurons and induce multinucleated giant cells in the brain of transgenic mice. *Am J Pathol*, **142**, 1061–71.

Ali, M., Taylor, G.P., et al. 1996. No evidence of antibody to human foamy virus in widespread human populations. *AIDS Res Hum Retroviruses*, **12**, 1473–83.

Alke, A., Schwantes, A., et al. 2000. Characterization of the humoral immune response and virus replication in cats experimentally infected with feline foamy virus. *Virology*, **275**, 170–6.

Alke, A., Schwantes, A., et al. 2001. The bet gene of feline foamy virus is required for virus replication. *Virology*, **287**, 310–20.

Allan, J.S., Broussard, S.R., et al. 1998. Amplification of simian retroviral sequences from human recipients of baboon liver transplants. *AIDS Res Hum Retroviruses*, **14**, 821–4.

Amborski, G.F., Storz, J., et al. 1987. Isolation of a retrovirus from the American bison and its relation to bovine retroviruses. *J Wildl Dis*, **23**, 7–11.

Amborski, G.F., Lo, J.L. and Seger, C.L. 1989. Serological detection of multiple retroviral infections in cattle: bovine leukemia virus, bovine syncytial virus and bovine visna virus. *Vet Microbiol*, **20**, 247–53.

Baldwin, D.N. and Linial, M.L. 1998. The roles of Pol and Env in the assembly pathway of human foamy virus. *J Virol*, **72**, 3658–65.

Baldwin, D.N. and Linial, M.L. 1999. Proteolytic activity, the carboxy terminus of Gag, and the primer binding site are not required for Pol incorporation into foamy virus particles. *J Virol*, **73**, 6387–93.

Bandecchi, P., Matteucci, D., et al. 1992. Prevalence of feline immunodeficiency virus and other retroviral infections in sick cats in Italy. *Vet Immunol Immunopathol*, **31**, 337–45.

Bastone, P. and Löchelt, M. 2004. Kinetics and characteristics of replication-competent revertants derived from self-inactivating foamy virus vectors. *Gene Ther*, **11**, 465–73.

Baunach, G., Maurer, B., et al. 1993. Functional analysis of human foamy virus accessory reading frames. *J Virol*, **67**, 5411–18.

Bieniasz, P.D., Rethwilm, A., et al. 1995a. A comparative study of higher primate foamy viruses, including a new virus from a gorilla. *Virology*, **207**, 217–28.

Bieniasz, P.D., Weiss, R.A. and McClure, M.O. 1995b. Cell cycle dependence of foamy retrovirus infection. *J Virol*, **69**, 7295–9.

Blair, W.S., Bogerd, H. and Cullen, B.R. 1994. Genetic analysis indicates that the human foamy virus Bel-1 protein contains a transcription activation domain of the acidic class. *J Virol*, **68**, 3803–8.

Bock, M., Heinkelein, M., et al. 1998. Cells expressing the human foamy virus (HFV) accessory Bet protein are resistant to productive HFV superinfection. *Virology*, **250**, 194–204.

Bodem, J., Löchelt, M., et al. 1996. Characterization of the spliced pol transcript of feline foamy virus: the splice acceptor site of the pol transcript is located in gag of foamy viruses. *J Virol*, **70**, 9024–7.

Bodem, J., Löchelt, M., et al. 1998a. Detection of subgenomic cDNAs and mapping of feline foamy virus mRNAs reveals complex patterns of transcription. *Virology*, **244**, 417–26.

Bodem, J., Zemba, M. and Flügel, R.M. 1998b. Nuclear localization of the functional Bel 1 transactivator but not of the gag proteins of the feline foamy virus. *Virology*, **251**, 22–7.

Bodem, J., Kang, Y. and Flügel, R.M. 2004. Comparative functional characterization of the feline foamy virus transactivator reveals its species specificity. *Virology*, **318**, 32–6.

Boeke, J.D. and Stoye, J.P. 1997. Retrotransposons, endogenous retroviruses, and the evolution of retroelements. In: Coffin, J.M., Hughes, S.H. and Varmus, H.E. (eds), *Retroviruses*. Plainview, NY: Cold Spring Harbor Laboratory Press, 343–435.

Boneva, R.S., Grindon, A.J., et al. 2002. Simian foamy virus infection in a blood donor. *Transfusion*, **42**, 886–91.

Bothe, K., Aguzzi, A., et al. 1991. Progressive encephalopathy and myopathy in transgenic mice expressing human foamy virus genes. *Science*, **253**, 555–7.

Boulanger, P. and Jones, I. 1996. Use of heterologous expression systems to study retroviral morphogenesis. *Curr Top Microbiol Immunol*, **214**, 237–60.

Brody, B.A., Rhee, S.S., et al. 1992. A viral protease-mediated cleavage of the transmembrane glycoprotein of Mason–Pfizer monkey virus can be suppressed by mutations within the matrix protein. *Proc Natl Acad Sci USA*, **89**, 3443–7.

Brody, B.A., Rhee, S.S. and Hunter, E. 1994. Postassembly cleavage of a retroviral glycoprotein cytoplasmic domain removes a necessary incorporation signal and activates fusion activity. *J Virol*, **68**, 4620–7.

Brooks, J.I., Rud, E.W., et al. 2002. Cross-species retroviral transmission from macaques to human beings. *Lancet*, **360**, 387–8.

Brown, P., Moreau-Dubois, M.C. and Gajdusek, D.C. 1982. Persistent asymptomatic infection of the laboratory mouse by simian foamy virus type 6: a new model of retrovirus latency. *Arch Virol*, **71**, 229–34.

Butera, S.T., Brown, J., et al. 2000. Survey of veterinary conference attendees for evidence of zoonotic infection by feline retroviruses. *J Am Vet Med Assoc*, **217**, 1475–9.

Cain, D., Erlwein, O., et al. 2001. Palindromic sequence plays a critical role in human foamy virus dimerization. *J Virol*, **75**, 3731–9.

Campbell, M., Renshaw-Gegg, L., et al. 1994. Characterization of the internal promoter of simian foamy viruses. *J Virol*, **68**, 4811–20.

Campbell, M., Eng, C. and Luciw, P.A. 1996. The simian foamy virus type 1 transcriptional transactivator (Tas) binds and activates an enhancer element in the gag gene. *J Virol*, **70**, 6847–55.

Cavazzana-Calvo, M., Thrasher, A. and Mavillio, F. 2004. The future of gene therapy. *Nature*, **427**, 779–81.

Chang, J., Lee, K.J., et al. 1995. Human foamy virus Bel1 transactivator contains a bipartite nuclear localization determinant which is sensitive to protein context and triple multimerization domains. *J Virol*, **69**, 801–8.

Charneau, P. and Clavel, F. 1991. A single stranded gap in human immunodeficiency virus unintegrated linear DNA defined by central copy of the polypurine tract. *J Virol*, **65**, 2415–21.

Charneau, P., Alizon, M. and Clavel, F. 1992. A second origin of DNA plus-strand synthesis is required for optimal human immunodeficiency virus replication. *J Virol*, **66**, 2814–20.

Delelis, O., Saïb, A. and Sonigo, P. 2003. Biphasic DNA synthesis in spumaviruses. *J Virol*, **77**, 8141–6.

Eastman, S.W. and Linial, M.L. 2001. Identification of a conserved residue of foamy virus Gag required for intracellular capsid assembly. *J Virol*, **75**, 6857–64.

Einfeld, D. 1996. Maturation and assembly of retroviral glycoproteins. *Curr Top Microbiol Immunol*, **214**, 133–76.

Enders, J.F. and Peebles, T.C. 1954. Propagation in tissue cultures of cytopathogenic agents from patients with measles. *Proc Soc Exp Biol Med*, **86**, 277–86.

Enssle, J., Jordan, I., et al. 1996. Foamy virus reverse transcriptase is expressed independently from the Gag protein. *Proc Natl Acad Sci USA*, **93**, 4137–41.

Enssle, J., Fischer, N., et al. 1997. Carboxy-terminal cleavage of the human foamy virus Gag precursor molecule is an essential step in the viral life cycle. *J Virol*, **71**, 7312–17.

Enssle, J., Moebes, A., et al. 1999. An active foamy virus integrase is required for virus replication. *J Gen Virol*, **80**, 1445–52.

Erlwein, O. and Rethwilm, A. 1993. BEL-1 transactivator responsive sequences in the long terminal repeat of human foamy virus. *Virology*, **196**, 256–68.

Erlwein, O., Cain, D., et al. 1997. Identification of sites that act together to direct dimerization of human foamy virus RNA in vitro. *Virology*, **229**, 251–8.

Erlwein, O., Bieniasz, P.D. and McClure, M.O. 1998. Sequences in pol are required for transfer of human foamy virus-based vectors. *J Virol*, **72**, 5510–16.

Falcone, V., Leupold, J., et al. 1999a. Sites of simian foamy virus persistence in naturally infected African green monkeys: latent provirus is ubiquitous, whereas viral replication is restricted to the oral mucosa. *Virology*, **257**, 7–14.

Falcone, V., Schweizer, M., et al. 1999b. Gamma interferon is a major suppressive factor produced by activated human peripheral blood lymphocytes that is able to inhibit foamy virus-induced cytopathic effects. *J Virol*, **73**, 1724–8.

Falcone, V., Schweizer, M. and Neumann-Haefelin, D. 2003. Replication of primate foamy viruses in natural and experimental hosts. *Curr Top Microbiol Immunol*, **277**, 161–80.

Falke, D. 1958. Observation on the incidence of giant and foamy cells in normal monkey kidney cell cultures. *Zentralbl Bakteriol*, **170**, 377–87.

Feldmann, G., Fickenscher, H., et al. 1997. Generation of herpes virus saimiri-transformed T-cell lines from macaques is restricted by reactivation of simian spuma viruses. *Virology*, **229**, 106–12.

Fischer, N., Heinkelein, M., et al. 1998. Foamy virus particle formation. *J Virol*, **72**, 1610–15.

Flanagan, M. 1992. Isolation of a spumavirus from a sheep. *Aust Vet J*, **69**, 112–13.

Flint, S.J., Enquist, L.W., et al. 2004. *Principles of virology*, 2nd edn. Washington, DC: ASM Press.

Flügel, R.M. and Pfrepper, K.I. 2003. Proteolytic processing of foamy virus Gag and Pol proteins. *Curr Top Microbiol Immunol*, **277**, 63–88.

Flügel, R.M., Mahnke, C., et al. 1992. Absence of antibody to human spumaretrovirus in patients with chronic fatigue syndrome. *Clin Infect Dis*, **14**, 623–4.

Folks, T.M., Heneine, W., et al. 1993. Investigation of retroviral involvement in chronic fatigue syndrome. *CIBA Found Symp*, **173**, 160–6.

Geiselhart, V., Schwantes, A., et al. 2003. Features of the Env leader protein and the N-terminal Gag domain of feline foamy virus important for virus morphogenesis. *Virology*, **310**, 235–44.

Gelderblom, H. and Frank, H. 1987. *Spumavirinae*. In: Nermut, M.V. and Steven, A.C. (eds), *Animal virus structure*, Vol. 3. . Amsterdam: Elsevier, 305–12.

Gerlich, W. 1991. Hepatitis B surface proteins. *J Hepatol*, **13**, Suppl 4, S90–2.

Giron, M.L., Colas, S., et al. 1997. Expression and maturation of human foamy virus Gag precursor polypeptides. *J Virol*, **71**, 1635–9.

Giron, M.L., de The, H. and Saïb, A. 1998. An evolutionarily conserved splice generates a secreted env-Bet fusion protein during human foamy virus infection. *J Virol*, **72**, 4906–10.

Goepfert, P.A., Wang, G. and Mulligan, M.J. 1995. Identification of an ER retrieval signal in a retroviral glycoprotein. *Cell*, **82**, 543–4.

Goepfert, P.A., Ritter, G.D. Jr., et al. 1996. Analysis of West-African hunters for foamy virus infections. *AIDS Res Hum Retroviruses*, **12**, 1725–30.

Goepfert, P.A., Shaw, K.L., et al. 1997. A sorting motif localizes the foamy virus glycoprotein to the endoplasmic reticulum. *J Virol*, **71**, 778–84.

Green, N., Shinnick, T.M., et al. 1981. Sequence-specific antibodies show that maturation of Moloney leukemia virus envelope polyprotein involves removal of a COOH-terminal peptide. *Proc Natl Acad Sci USA*, **78**, 6023–7.

Hahn, H., Baunach, G., et al. 1994. Reactivity of primate sera to foamy virus Gag and Bet proteins. *J Gen Virol*, **75**, 2635–44.

Hahn, B.H., Shaw, G.M., Smith, X.X. and Smith, X.X. 2000. AIDS as a zoonosis: scientific and public health implications. *AIDS*, **287**, 607–14.

Hajihosseini, M., Iavachev, L. and Price, J. 1993. Evidence that retroviruses intregate into post-replication host DNA. *EMBO J*, **12**, 4969–74.

Hatama, S., Otake, K., et al. 2001. Isolation and sequencing of infectious clones of feline foamy virus and a human/feline foamy virus Env chimera. *J Gen Virol*, **82**, 2999–3004.

He, F., Sun, J.D., et al. 1993. Functional organization of the Bel-1 transactivator of human foamy virus. *J Virol*, **67**, 1896–904.

He, F., Blair, W.S., et al. 1996. The human foamy virus Bel-1 transcription factor is a sequence-specific DNA binding protein. *J Virol*, **70**, 3902–8.

Heinkelein, M., Schmidt, M., et al. 1998. Characterization of a cis-acting sequence in the Pol region required to transfer human foamy virus vectors. *J Virol*, **72**, 6307–14.

Heinkelein, M., Pietschmann, T., et al. 2000a. Efficient intracellular retrotransposition of an exogenous primate retrovirus genome. *EMBO J*, **19**, 3436–45.

Heinkelein, M., Thurow, J., et al. 2000b. Complex effects of deletions in the 5′ untranslated region of primate foamy virus on viral gene expression and RNA packaging. *J Virol*, **74**, 3141–8.

Heinkelein, M., Dressler, M., et al. 2002a. Improved primate foamy virus vectors and packaging constructs. *J Virol*, **76**, 3774–83.

Heinkelein, M., Leurs, C., et al. 2002b. Pregenomic RNA is required for efficient incorporation of pol polyprotein into foamy virus capsids. *J Virol*, **76**, 10069–73.

Heinkelein, M., Rammling, M., et al. 2003. Retrotransposition and cell-to-cell transfer of foamy viruses. *J Virol*, **77**, 11855–8.

Helps, C.R. and Harbour, D.A. 1997. Comparison of the complete sequence of feline spumavirus with those of the primate spumaviruses reveals a shorter gag gene. *J Gen Virol*, **78**, 2549–64.

Henderson, L.E., Sowder, R., et al. 1984. Quantitative separation of murine leukemia virus proteins by reversed-phase high pressure liquid chromatography reveals newly described gag and env cleavage products. *J Virol*, **52**, 492–500.

Heneine, W., Woods, T.C., et al. 1994. Lack of evidence for infection with known human and animal retroviruses in patients with chronic fatigue syndrome. *Clin Infect Dis*, **18**, 121–5.

Heneine, W., Musey, V.C., et al. 1995. Absence of evidence for human spumaretrovirus sequences in patients with Graves' disease. *J Acquir Immune Defic Syndr Hum Retrovirol*, **9**, 99–101.

Heneine, W., Switzer, W.M., et al. 1998. Identification of a human population infected with simian foamy viruses. *Nat Med*, **4**, 403–7.

Heneine, W., Schweizer, M., et al. 2003. Human infection with foamy viruses. *Curr Top Microbiol Immunol*, **277**, 181–96.

Herchenröder, O., Renne, R., et al. 1994. Isolation, cloning, and sequencing of simian foamy viruses from chimpanzees (SFVcpz): high homology to human foamy virus (HFV). *Virology*, **201**, 187–99.

Hill, C.L., Bieniasz, P.D. and McClure, M.O. 1999. Properties of human foamy virus relevant to its development as a vector for gene therapy. *J Gen Virol*, **80**, 2003–9.

Hirata, R.K., Miller, A.D., et al. 1996. Transduction of hematopoietic cells by foamy virus vectors. *Blood*, **88**, 3654–61.

Hooks, J.J. and Detrick-Hooks, B. 1979. Simian foamy virus-induced immunosuppression in rabbits. *J Gen Virol*, **44**, 383–90.

Hooks, J.J. and Detrick-Hooks, B. 1981. *Spumavirinae*: foamy virus group infections: comparative aspects and diagnosis. In: Kurstak, K. and Kurstak, C. (eds), *Comparative diagnosis of viral diseases*, Vol. 4. . New York: Academic Press, 599–618.

Hooks, J.J. and Gibbs, C.J. Jr. 1975. The foamy viruses. *Bacteriol Rev*, **39**, 169–85.

Hooks, J.J., Gibbs, C.J. Jr., et al. 1972. Characterization and distribution of two new foamy viruses isolated from chimpanzees. *Arch gesamte Virusforsch*, **38**, 38–55.

Hooks, J.J., Gibbs, C.J. Jr., et al. 1973. Isolation of a new simian foamy virus from a spider monkey brain culture. *Infect Immun*, **8**, 804–13.

Hruska, J.F. and Takemoto, K.K. 1975. Biochemical properties of a hamster syncytium-forming ('foamy') virus. *J Natl Cancer Inst*, **54**, 601–5.

Hunsmann, G., Flügel, R.M. and Walder, R. 1990. Retroviral antibodies in Indians. *Nature*, **345**, 120.

Hunter, E. 1997. Viral entry and receptors. In: Coffin, J.M., Hughes, S.H. and Varmus, H.E. (eds), *Retroviruses*. Plainview, NY: Cold Spring Harbor Labratory Press, 71–119.

Hussain, A.I., Shanmugam, V., et al. 2003. Screening for simian foamy virus infection by using a combined antigen Western blot assay: evidence for a wide distribution among Old World primates and identification of four new divergent viruses. *Virology*, **309**, 248–57.

Ikeda, Y., Itagaki, S., et al. 1997. Replication of feline syncytial virus in feline T-lymphoblastoid cells and induction of apoptosis in the cells. *Microbiol Immunol*, **41**, 431–5.

Imrich, H., Heinkelein, M., et al. 2000. Primate foamy virus Pol proteins are imported into the nucleus. *J Gen Virol*, **81**, 2941–7.

Johnson, R.H., de la Rosa, J., et al. 1988. Epidemiological studies of bovine spumavirus. *Vet Microbiol*, **16**, 25–33.

Johnston, P.B. 1961. A second immunologic type of simian foamy virus: monkey throat infections and unmasking by both types. *J Infect Dis*, **109**, 1–9.

Johnston, P.B. 1971. Taxonomic features of seven serotypes of simian and ape foamy viruses. *Infect Immun*, **3**, 793–9.

Jordan, I., Enssle, J., et al. 1996. Expression of human foamy virus reverse transcriptase involves a spliced pol mRNA. *Virology*, **224**, 314–19.

Josephson, N.C., Vassilopoulos, G., et al. 2002. Transduction of human NOD/SCID-repopulating cells with both lymphoid and myeloid potential by foamy virus vectors. *Proc Natl Acad Sci USA*, **99**, 8295–300.

Josephson, N.C., Trobridge, G. and Russell, D.W. 2004. Transduction of long-term and mobilized peripheral blood-derived NOD/SCID repopulating cells by foamy virus vectors. *Hum Gene Ther*, **15**, 87–92.

Juretzek, T., Holm, T., et al. 2004. Foamy virus integration. *J Virol*, **78**, 2472–7.

Kang, Y. and Cullen, B.R. 1998. Derivation and functional characterization of a consensus DNA binding sequence for the tas transcriptional activator of simian foamy virus type 1. *J Virol*, **72**, 5502–9.

Kang, Y., Blair, W.S. and Cullen, B.R. 1998. Identification and functional characterization of a high-affinity Bel-1 DNA binding site located in the human foamy virus internal promoter. *J Virol*, **72**, 504–11.

Keller, A., Partin, K.M., et al. 1991. Characterization of the transcriptional trans activator of human foamy retrovirus. *J Virol*, **65**, 2589–94.

Kennedy-Stoskopf, S., Stoskopf, M.K., et al. 1986. Isolation of a retrovirus and a herpesvirus from a captive California sea lion. *J Wildl Dis*, **22**, 156–64.

Khan, A.S., Sears, J.F., et al. 1999. Sensitive assays for isolation and detection of simian foamy retroviruses. *J Clin Microbiol*, **37**, 2678–86.

Kido, K., Doerks, A., et al. 2002. Identification and functional characterization of an intragenic DNA binding site for the spumaretroviral trans-activator in the human p57kip2 gene. *J Biol Chem*, **277**, 12032–9.

Kido, K., Bannert, H., et al. 2003. Bel1-mediated transactivation of the spumaretroviral internal promoter is repressed by nuclear factor I. *J Biol Chem*, **278**, 11836–42.

Kögel, D., Aboud, M. and Flügel, R.M. 1995a. Molecular biological characterization of the human foamy virus reverse transcriptase and ribonuclease H domains. *Virology*, **213**, 97–108.

Kögel, D., Aboud, M. and Flügel, R.M. 1995b. Mutational analysis of the reverse transcriptase and ribonuclease H domains of the human foamy virus. *Nucleic Acids Res*, **23**, 2621–5.

Konvalinka, J., Löchelt, M., et al. 1995. Active foamy virus proteinase is essential for virus infectivity but not for formation of a Pol polyprotein. *J Virol*, **69**, 7264–8.

Kräusslich, H.G. and Welker, R. 1996. Intracellular transport of retroviral capsid proteins. *Curr Top Microbiol Immunol*, **214**, 25–63.

Kupiec, J.J., Tobaly-Tapiero, J., et al. 1988. Evidence for a gapped linear duplex DNA intermediate in the replicative cycle of human and simian spumaviruses. *Nucleic Acids Res*, **16**, 9557–65.

Kupiec, J.J., Kay, A., et al. 1991. Sequence analysis of the simian foamy virus type 1 genome. *Gene*, **101**, 185–94.

Landay, A.L., Jessop, C., et al. 1991. Chronic fatigue syndrome: clinical condition associated with immune activation. *Lancet*, **338**, 707–12.

Lecellier, C.H. and Saïb, A. 2000. Foamy viruses: between retroviruses and pararetroviruses. *Virology*, **271**, 1–8.

Lecellier, C.H., Neves, M., et al. 2002a. Further characterization of equine foamy virus reveals unusual features among the foamy viruses. *J Virol*, **76**, 7220–7.

Lecellier, C.H., Vermeulen, W., et al. 2002b. Intra- and intercellular trafficking of the foamy virus auxiliary bet protein. *J Virol*, **76**, 3388–94.

Lee, A.H., Lee, H.Y. and Sung, Y.C. 1994. The gene expression of human foamy virus does not require a post-transcriptional transactivator. *Virology*, **204**, 409–13.

Lee, K.J., Lee, A.H. and Sung, Y.C. 1993. Multiple positive and negative cis-acting elements that mediate transactivation by bel1 in the long terminal repeat of human foamy virus. *J Virol*, **67**, 2317–26.

Lepine, P. and Paccaud, M. 1957. Contribution to the study of foamy virus. I. Study of FV I, FV II, FV III strains isolated from culture of renal cells of Cynocephalus. *Ann Inst Pasteur (Paris)*, **92**, 289–300.

Leurs, C., Jansen, M., et al. 2003. Comparison of three retroviral vector systems for transduction of nonobese diabetic/severe combined immunodeficiency mice repopulating human CD34+ cord blood cells. *Hum Gene Ther*, **14**, 509–19.

Lindemann, D. and Goepfert, P.A. 2003. The foamy virus envelope glycoproteins. *Curr Top Microbiol Immunol*, **277**, 111–29.

Lindemann, D. and Rethwilm, A. 1998. Characterization of a human foamy virus 170-kilodalton Env-Bet fusion protein generated by alternative splicing. *J Virol*, **72**, 4088–94.

Lindemann, D., Heinkelein, M. and Rethwilm, A. 2000. Aspects of foamy virus vectors: host range and replication-competent vectors. In: Cid-Arregui, A. and García-Carrancá, A. (eds), *Viral vectors basic science and gene therapy*. Natick, MA: Eaton Publishing, 515–22.

Lindemann, D., Pietschmann, T., et al. 2001. A particle-associated glycoprotein signal peptide essential for virus maturation and infectivity. *J Virol*, **75**, 5762–71.

Linial, M. 2000. Why aren't foamy viruses pathogenic? *Trends Microbiol*, **8**, 284–9.

Linial, M.L. 1999. Foamy viruses are unconventional retroviruses. *J Virol*, **73**, 1747–55.

Linial, M.L. and Eastman, S.W. 2003. Particle assembly and genome packaging. *Curr Top Microbiol Immunol*, **277**, 89–110.

Löchelt, M. 2003. Foamy virus transactivation and gene expression. *Curr Top Microbiol Immunol*, **277**, 27–61.

Löchelt, M. and Flügel, R.M. 1996. The human foamy virus pol gene is expressed as a Pro-Pol polyprotein and not as a Gag-Pol fusion protein. *J Virol*, **70**, 1033–40.

Löchelt, M., Aboud, M. and Flügel, R.M. 1993a. Increase in the basal transcriptional activity of the human foamy virus internal promoter by the homologous long terminal repeat promoter in cis. *Nucleic Acids Res*, **21**, 4226–30.

Löchelt, M., Muranyi, W. and Flügel, R.M. 1993b. Human foamy virus genome possesses an internal, Bel-1-dependent and functional promoter. *Proc Natl Acad Sci USA*, **90**, 7317–21.

Löchelt, M., Flügel, R.M. and Aboud, M. 1994. The human foamy virus internal promoter directs the expression of the functional Bel 1 transactivator and Bet protein early after infection. *J Virol*, **68**, 638–45.

Löchelt, M., Yu, S.F., et al. 1995. The human foamy virus internal promoter is required for efficient gene expression and infectivity. *Virology*, **206**, 601–10.

Lutz, H. 1990. Feline retroviruses: a brief review. *Vet Microbiol*, **23**, 131–46.

Malmquist, W.A., van der Maaten, M.J. and Boothe, A.D. 1969. Isolation, immunodiffusion, immunofluorescence, and electron microscopy of a syncytial virus of lymphosarcomatous and apparently normal cattle. *Cancer Res*, **29**, 188–200.

Martoglio, B., Graf, R. and Dobberstein, B. 1997. Signal peptide fragments of preprolactin and HIV-1 p-gp160 interact with calmodulin. *EMBO J*, **16**, 6636–45.

Marczynska, B., Jones, C.J. and Wolfe, L.G. 1981. Syncytium-forming virus of common marmosets (*Callithrix jacchus jacchus*). *Infect Immun*, **31**, 1261–9.

Maurer, B., Bannert, H., et al. 1988. Analysis of the primary structure of the long terminal repeat and the gag and pol genes of the human spumaretrovirus. *J Virol*, **62**, 1590–1.

McClure, M.O., Bieniasz, P.D., et al. 1994. Isolation of a new foamy retrovirus from orangutans. *J Virol*, **68**, 7124–30.

Meiering, C.D. and Linial, M.L. 2001. Historical perspective of foamy virus epidemiology and infection. *Clin Microbiol Rev*, **14**, 165–76.

Meiering, C.D. and Linial, M.L. 2002. Reactivation of a complex retrovirus is controlled by a molecular switch and is inhibited by a viral protein. *Proc Natl Acad Sci USA*, **99**, 15130–5.

Meiering, C.D. and Linial, M.L. 2003. The promyelocytic leukemia protein does not mediate foamy virus latency in vitro. *J Virol*, **77**, 2207–13.

Meiering, C.D., Comstock, K.E. and Linial, M.L. 2000. Multiple integrations of human foamy virus in persistently infected human erythroleukemia cells. *J Virol*, **74**, 1718–26.

Meiering, C.D., Rubio, C., et al. 2001. Cell-type-specific regulation of the two foamy virus promoters. *J Virol*, **75**, 6547–57.

Mergia, A. 1994. Simian foamy virus type 1 contains a second promoter located at the 3′ end of the env gene. *Virology*, **199**, 219–22.

Mergia, A. and Heinkelein, M. 2003. Foamy virus vectors. *Curr Top Microbiol Immunol*, **277**, 131–59.

Mergia, A., Pratt-Lowe, E., et al. 1992. cis-acting regulatory regions in the long terminal repeat of simian foamy virus type 1. *J Virol*, **66**, 251–7.

Mergia, A., Leung, N.J. and Blackwell, J. 1996. Cell tropism of the simian foamy virus type 1 (SFV-1). *J Med Primatol*, **25**, 2–7.

Mergia, A., Blackwell, J., et al. 1997. Simian foamy virus type 1 (SFV-1) induces apoptosis. *Virus Res*, **50**, 129–37.

Mikovits, J.A., Hoffman, P.M., et al. 1996. In vitro infection of primary and retrovirus-infected human leukocytes by human foamy virus. *J Virol*, **70**, 2774–80.

Moebes, A., Enssle, J., et al. 1997. Human foamy virus reverse transcription that occurs late in the viral replication cycle. *J Virol*, **71**, 7305–11.

Muranyi, W. and Flügel, R.M. 1991. Analysis of splicing patterns of human spumaretrovirus by polymerase chain reaction reveals complex RNA structures. *J Virol*, **65**, 727–35.

Nassal, M. and Schaller, H. 1993. Hepatitis B virus replication. *Trends Microbiol*, **1**, 221–8.

Nestler, U., Heinkelein, M., et al. 1997. Foamy virus vectors for suicide gene therapy. *Gene Ther*, **4**, 1270–7.

Netzer, K.O., Rethwilm, A., et al. 1990. Identification of the major immunogenic structural proteins of human foamy virus. *J Gen Virol*, **71**, 1237–41.

Netzer, K.O., Schliephake, A., et al. 1993. Identification of pol-related gene products of human foamy virus. *Virology*, **192**, 336–8.

Neumann-Haefelin, D., Rethwilm, A., et al. 1983. Characterization of a foamy virus isolated from *Cercopithecus aethiops* lymphoblastoid cells. *Med Microbiol Immunol (Berl)*, **172**, 75–86.

Paccaud, M. 1957. Study of foamy virus. II. Study of lesions in monkey and human kidney cells, monkey testicular cells and carcinomatous HeLa cells caused by foamy virus (strains FV I, FV II, and FV III). *Ann Inst Pasteur (Paris)*, **92**, 481–8.

Park, J. and Mergia, A. 2000. Mutational analysis of the 5′ leader region of simian foamy virus type 1. *Virology*, **274**, 203–12.

Park, J., Nadeau, P.E. and Mergia, A. 2002. A minimal genome simian foamy virus type 1 vector system with efficient gene transfer. *Virology*, **302**, 236–44.

Parks, W.P., Todaro, G.J., et al. 1971. RNA dependent DNA polymerase in primate syncytium-forming (foamy) viruses. *Nature*, **229**, 258–60.

Pedersen, N.C. 1990. Feline retrovirus infections. *Dev Biol Stand*, **72**, 149–55.

Peeters, M., Courgnaud, V., et al. 2002. Risk to human health from a plethora of simian immunodeficiency viruses in primate bushmeat. *Emerg Inf Dis*, **8**, 451–7.

Petit, C., Giron, M.L., et al. 2003. Targeting of incoming retroviral gag to the centrosome involves a direct interaction with the dynein light chain 8. *J Cell Sci*, **116**, 3433–42.

Pfrepper, K.I., Rackwitz, H.R., et al. 1998. Molecular characterization of proteolytic processing of the Pol proteins of human foamy virus reveals novel features of the viral protease. *J Virol*, **72**, 7648–52.

Pfrepper, K.I., Löchelt, M., et al. 1999. Molecular characterization of proteolytic processing of the Gag proteins of human spumavirus. *J Virol*, **73**, 7907–11.

Picard-Maureau, M., Jarmy, G., et al. 2003. Foamy virus envelope glycoprotein-mediated entry involves a pH-dependent fusion process. *J Virol*, **77**, 4722–30.

Picard-Maureau, M., Kreppel, F., et al. 2004. Foamy virus-adenovirus hybrid vectors. *Gene Ther*, **11**, 722–8.

Pietschmann, T., Heinkelein, M., et al. 1999. Foamy virus capsids require the cognate envelope protein for particle export. *J Virol*, **73**, 2613–21.

Pietschmann, T., Zentgraf, H., et al. 2000. An evolutionarily conserved positively charged amino acid in the putative membrane-spanning domain of the foamy virus envelope protein controls fusion activity. *J Virol*, **74**, 4474–82.

Plummer, G. 1962. Foamy virus of monkeys. *J Gen Microbiol*, **29**, 703–9.

Pyykkö, I., Vesanen, M., et al. 1994. Human spumaretrovirus in the etiology of sudden hearing loss. *Acta Otolaryngol*, **114**, 224.

Regad, T., Saïb, A., et al. 2001. PML mediates the interferon-induced antiviral state against a complex retrovirus via its association with the viral transactivator. *EMBO J*, **20**, 3495–505.

Rein, A., Mirro, J., et al. 1994. Function of the cytoplasmic domain of a retroviral transmembrane protein: p15E-p2E cleavage activates the membrane fusion capability of the murine leukemia virus Env protein. *J Virol*, **68**, 1773–81.

Renne, R., Mergia, A., et al. 1993. Regulatory elements in the long terminal repeat (LTR) of simian foamy virus type 3 (SFV-3). *Virology*, **192**, 365–9.

Renshaw, R.W. and Casey, J.W. 1994a. Analysis of the 5′ long terminal repeat of bovine syncytial virus. *Gene*, **141**, 221–4.

Renshaw, R.W. and Casey, J.W. 1994b. Transcriptional mapping of the 3′ end of the bovine syncytial virus genome. *J Virol*, **68**, 1021–8.

Renshaw, R.W., Gonda, M.A. and Casey, J.W. 1991. Structure and transcriptional status of bovine syncytial virus in cytopathic infections. *Gene*, **105**, 179–84.

Rethwilm, A. 1995. Regulation of foamy virus gene expression. *Curr Top Microbiol Immunol*, **193**, 1–24.

Rethwilm A. 2003a. Foreword. In *Foamy viruses*. vol. 277. Berlin: Springer.

Rethwilm, A. 2003b. The replication strategy of foamy viruses. *Curr Top Microbiol Immunol*, **277**, 1–26.

Rethwilm, A., Darai, G., et al. 1987. Molecular cloning of the genome of human spumaretrovirus. *Gene*, **59**, 19–28.

Rhee, S.S. and Hunter, E. 1990. A single amino acid substitution within the matrix protein of a type D retrovirus converts its morphogenesis to that of a type C retrovirus. *Cell*, **63**, 77–86.

Rhodes-Feuillette, A., Saal, F., et al. 1979. Isolation and characterization of a new simian foamy virus serotype from lymphocytes of a *Papio cynocephalus* baboon. *J Med Primatol*, **8**, 308–20.

Riggs, J.L., Oshiro, L.S., et al. 1969. Syncytium-forming agent isolated from domestic cats. *Nature*, **222**, 1190–1.

Rinke, C.S., Boyer, P.L., et al. 2002. Mutation of the catalytic domain of the foamy virus reverse transcriptase leads to loss of processivity and infectivity. *J Virol*, **76**, 7560–70.

Rogers, N.G., Basnight, M., et al. 1967. Latent viruses in chimpanzees with experimental kuru. *Nature*, **216**, 446–9.

Rosenblum, L.L., Patton, G., et al. 2001. Differential susceptibility of retroviruses to nucleoside analogues. *Antivir Chem Chemother*, **12**, 91–7.

Rösener, M., Hahn, H., et al. 1996. Absence of serological evidence for foamy virus infection in patients with amyotrophic lateral sclerosis. *J Med Virol*, **48**, 222–6.

Rossignol, J.M., Kress, M. and de Vaux Saint Cyr, C. 1975. Induction, by 5-bromo-2′-deoxyuridine, of a 'foamy' virus previously undetected in hamster cells transformed by SV40. *C R Acad Sci Hebd Seances Acad Sci D*, **281**, 1145–8.

Roy, J., Rudolph, W., et al. 2003. Feline foamy virus genome and replication strategy. *J Virol*, **77**, 11324–31.

Russell, R.A., Vassaux, G., et al. 2004. Transient foamy virus vector production by adenovirus vectors. *Gene Ther*, **11**, 310–16.

Russell, R.A., Zeng, Y., et al. 2001. The R region found in the human foamy virus long terminal repeat is critical for both Gag and Pol protein expression. *J Virol*, **75**, 6817–24.

Rustigian, R., Johnston, P. and Reihart, H. 1955. Infection of monkey kidney tissue cultures with virus-like agents. *Proc Soc Exp Biol Med*, **88**, 8–16.

Saïb, A. 2003. Non-primate foamy viruses. *Curr Top Microbiol Immunol*, **277**, 197–211.

Saïb, A., Peries, J. and de The, H. 1993. A defective human foamy provirus generated by pregenome splicing. *EMBO J*, **12**, 4439–44.

Saïb, A., Koken, M.H., et al. 1995. Involvement of a spliced and defective human foamy virus in the establishment of chronic infection. *J Virol*, **69**, 5261–8.

Saïb, A., Neves, M., et al. 1997a. Long-term persistent infection of domestic rabbits by the human foamy virus. *Virology*, **228**, 263–8.

Saïb, A., Puvion-Dutilleul, F., et al. 1997b. Nuclear targeting of incoming human foamy virus Gag proteins involves a centriolar step. *J Virol*, **71**, 1155–61.

Sandstrom, P.A., Phan, K.O., et al. 2000. Simian foamy virus infection among zoo keepers. *Lancet*, **355**, 551–2.

Santillana-Hayat, M., Rozain, F., et al. 1993. Transient immunosuppressive effect induced in rabbits and mice by the human spumaretrovirus prototype HFV (human foamy virus). *Res Virol*, **144**, 389–96.

Schenk, T., Enssle, J., et al. 1999. Replication of a foamy virus mutant with a constitutively active U3 promoter and deleted accessory genes. *J Gen Virol*, **80**, 1591–8.

Schliephake, A.W. and Rethwilm, A. 1994. Nuclear localization of foamy virus Gag precursor protein. *J Virol*, **68**, 4946–54.

Schmidt, M. and Rethwilm, A. 1995. Replicating foamy virus-based vectors directing high level expression of foreign genes. *Virology*, **210**, 167–78.

Schmidt, M., Herchenröder, O., et al. 1997a. Long terminal repeat U3 length polymorphism of human foamy virus. *Virology*, **230**, 167–78.

Schmidt, M., Niewiesk, S., et al. 1997b. Mouse model to study the replication of primate foamy viruses. *J Gen Virol*, **78**, 1929–33.

Schwantes, A., Ortlepp, I. and Löchelt, M. 2002. Construction and functional characterization of feline foamy virus-based retroviral vectors. *Virology*, **301**, 53–63.

Schwantes, A., Truyen, U., et al. 2003. Application of chimeric feline foamy virus-based retroviral vectors for the induction of antiviral immunity in cats. *J Virol*, **77**, 7830–42.

Schweizer, M. and Neumann-Haefelin, D. 1995. Phylogenetic analysis of primate foamy viruses by comparison of pol sequences. *Virology*, **207**, 577–82.

Schweizer, M., Turek, R., et al. 1994. Absence of foamy virus DNA in Graves' disease. *AIDS Res Hum Retroviruses*, **10**, 601–5.

Schweizer, M., Turek, R., et al. 1995. Markers of foamy virus infections in monkeys, apes, and accidentally infected humans: appropriate testing fails to confirm suspected foamy virus prevalence in humans. *AIDS Res Hum Retroviruses*, **11**, 161–70.

Schweizer, M., Falcone, V., et al. 1997. Simian foamy virus isolated from an accidentally infected human individual. *J Virol*, **71**, 4821–4.

Schweizer, M., Schleer, H., et al. 1999. Genetic stability of foamy viruses: long-term study in an African green monkey population. *J Virol*, **73**, 9256–65.

Sharp, P.M., Bailes, E., et al. 2001. The origins of acquired immune deficiency syndrome viruses: where and when? *Phil Trans R Soc Lond B*, **356**, 867–76.

Shaw, K.L., Lindemann, D., et al. 2003. Foamy virus envelope glycoprotein is sufficient for particle budding and release. *J Virol*, **77**, 2338–48.

Shroyer, E.L. and Shalaby, M.R. 1978. Isolation of feline syncytia-forming virus from orpharyngeal swab samples and buffy coat cells. *Am J Vet Res*, **39**, 555–60.

Simonsen, L., Heneine, W., et al. 1994. Absence of evidence for infection with the human spuma retrovirus in an outbreak of Meniere-like vertiginous illness in Wyoming, USA. *Acta Otolaryngol*, **114**, 223–4.

Sommerfelt, M.A., Petteway, S.R., et al. 1992. Effect of retroviral proteinase inhibitors on Mason–Pfizer monkey virus maturation and transmembrane glycoprotein cleavage. *J Virol*, **66**, 4220–7.

Stiles, G.E., Bittle, J.L. and Cabasso, V.J. 1964. Comparison of simian foamy virus strains including a new serological type. *Nature*, **201**, 1350–1.

Swack, N.S. 1981. Infections by foamy viruses. In: Beran, G.W. (ed.), *CRC handbook series in zoonoses: viral zoonoses*, vol. II. . Boca Raton, Florida, USA: CRC Press, 282–8.

Swack, N.S. and Hsiung, G.D. 1975. Pathogenesis of simian foamy virus infection in natural and experimental hosts. *Infect Immun*, **12**, 470–4.

Swanstrom, R. and Wills, J.W. 1997. Synthesis, assembly, and processing of viral proteins. In: Coffin, J.M., Hughes, S.H. and Varmus, H.E. (eds), *Retroviruses*. Plainview, NY: Cold Spring Harbor Labratory Press, 263–334.

Switzer, W.M., Bhullar, V., et al. 2004. Frequent simian foamy virus infection in persons occupationally exposed to nonhuman primates. *J Virol*, **78**, 2780–9.

Tobaly-Tapiero, J., Kupiec, J.J., et al. 1991. Further characterization of the gapped DNA intermediates of human spumavirus: evidence for a dual initiation of plus-strand DNA synthesis. *J Gen Virol*, **72**, 605–8.

Tobaly-Tapiero, J., Bittoun, P., et al. 2000. Isolation and characterization of an equine foamy virus. *J Virol*, **74**, 4064–73.

Tobaly-Tapiero, J., Bittoun, P., et al. 2001. Human foamy virus capsid formation requires an interaction domain in the N terminus of Gag. *J Virol*, **75**, 4367–75.

Trobridge, G., Josephson, N., et al. 2002a. Improved foamy virus vectors with minimal viral sequences. *Mol Ther*, **6**, 321–8.

Trobridge, G., Vassilopoulos, G., et al. 2002b. Gene transfer with foamy virus vectors. *Methods Enzymol*, **346**, 628–48.

Trobridge, G. and Russell, D.W. 2004. Cell cycle requirements for transduction by foamy virus vectors compared to those of oncovirus and lentivirus vectors. *J Virol*, **78**, 2327–35.

Verschoor, E.J., Langenhuijzen, S., et al. 2003. Structural and evolutionary analysis of an orangutan foamy virus. *J Virol*, **77**, 8584–7.

Vogt, P.K. 1997. Historical introduction to the general properties of retroviruses. In: Coffin, J.M., Hughes, S.H. and Varmus, H.E. (eds), *Retroviruses*. Plainview, NY: Cold Spring Harbor Laboratory Press, 1–25.

Voss, G., Nick, S., et al. 1992. Generation of macaque B lymphoblastoid cell lines with simian Epstein–Barr-like viruses: transformation procedure, characterization of the cell lines and occurrence of simian foamy virus. *J Virol Methods*, **39**, 185–95.

Wagner, A., Doerks, A., et al. 2000. Induction of cellular genes is mediated by the Bel1 transactivator in foamy virus-infected human cells. *J Virol*, **74**, 4441–7.

Wilk, T., de Haas, F., et al. 2000. The intact retroviral Env glycoprotein of human foamy virus is a trimer. *J Virol*, **74**, 2885–7.

Wilk, T., Geiselhart, V., et al. 2001. Specific interaction of a novel foamy virus Env leader protein with the N-terminal Gag domain. *J Virol*, **75**, 7995–8007.

Wills, J.W. and Craven, R.C. 1991. Form, function, and use of retroviral gag proteins. *AIDS*, **5**, 639–554.

Winkler, I., Bodem, J., et al. 1997a. Characterization of the genome of feline foamy virus and its proteins shows distinct features different from those of primate spumaviruses. *J Virol*, **71**, 6727–41.

Winkler, I.G., Löchelt, M., et al. 1997b. A rapid streptavidin-capture ELISA specific for the detection of antibodies to feline foamy virus. *J Immunol Methods*, **207**, 69–77.

Winkler, I.G., Flügel, R.M., et al. 1998. Detection and molecular characterisation of feline foamy virus serotypes in naturally infected cats. *Virology*, **247**, 144–51.

Winkler, I.G., Löchelt, M. and Flower, R.L. 1999. Epidemiology of feline foamy virus and feline immunodeficiency virus infections in domestic and feral cats: a seroepidemiological study. *J Clin Microbiol*, **37**, 2848–51.

Wodrich, H., Bohne, J., et al. 2001. A new RNA element located in the coding region of a murine endogenous retrovirus can functionally replace the Rev/Rev-responsive element system in human immunodeficiency virus type 1 Gag expression. *J Virol*, **75**, 10670–82.

Wolfe, N.D., Switzer, W.M., et al. 2004. Naturally acquired simian retrovirus infections in Central African hunters. *Lancet*, **363**, 932–7.

Wu, M., Chari, S., et al. 1998. cis-Acting sequences required for simian foamy virus type 1 vectors. *J Virol*, **72**, 3451–4.

Yu, S.F. and Linial, M.L. 1993. Analysis of the role of the bel and bet open reading frames of human foamy virus by using a new quantitative assay. *J Virol*, **67**, 6618–24.

Yu, S.F., Baldwin, D.N., et al. 1996a. Human foamy virus replication: a pathway distinct from that of retroviruses and hepadnaviruses. *Science*, **271**, 1579–82.

Yu, S.F., Edelmann, K., et al. 1996b. The carboxyl terminus of the human foamy virus Gag protein contains separable nucleic acid binding and nuclear transport domains. *J Virol*, **70**, 8255–62.

Yu, S.F., Sullivan, M.D. and Linial, M.L. 1999. Evidence that the human foamy virus genome is DNA. *J Virol*, **73**, 1565–72.

Zemba, M., Wilk, T., et al. 1998. The carboxy-terminal p3Gag domain of the human foamy virus Gag precursor is required for efficient virus infectivity. *Virology*, **247**, 7–13.

Zemba, M., Alke, A., et al. 2000. Construction of infectious feline foamy virus genomes: cat antisera do not cross-neutralize feline foamy virus chimera with serotype-specific Env sequences. *Virology*, **266**, 150–6.

Zenger, E., Brown, W.C., et al. 1993. Evaluation of cofactor effect of feline syncytium-forming virus on feline immunodeficiency virus infection. *Am J Vet Res*, **54**, 713–18.

Zou, J.X. and Luciw, P.A. 1996. The transcriptional transactivator of simian foamy virus 1 binds to a DNA target element in the viral internal promoter. *Proc Natl Acad Sci USA*, **93**, 326–30.

60

Human immunodeficiency virus

ULRICH SCHUBERT AND MYRA MCCLURE

INTRODUCTION

Since the beginning of the 1980s millions of people have been infected with human immunodeficiency virus (HIV) the causative agent of the acquired immune deficiency syndrome (AIDS), a multi-systemic, deadly, and so far incurable disease. HIV infections remain one of the most devastating diseases that humanity has ever faced. Unfortunately, there is little hope that an effective vaccine will be developed in the near future, nor are there other mechanisms available to stimulate the natural immunity against HIV. Current antiretroviral treatment is based on drugs that target either the viral reverse transcriptase (RT) or the protease (PR) or the viral envelope (gp41). A drawback to these treatments is that with HIV's high rate of mutation and replication, dynamic, drug-resistant mutants are evolving, particularly when anti-retroviral treatment suppresses virus replication to only marginal levels. Cellular genes have much lower mutation rates, and a potential solution to this problem is to target host cellular factors required for HIV replication. These include enzymes and interactive proteins that are essential for replication of HIV in host cells, which can be selectively manipulated without interfering with the vital functions of the organism.

GENOMIC ORGANIZATION AND REPLICATION CYCLE OF HIV

The *Retroviridae*, a family of viruses, which include the *Human immunodeficiency virus type 1* (HIV-1) and *Human immunodeficiency virus type 2* (HIV-2), belong to the gigantic group of eukaryotic retrotransposable elements (for review see Doolittle et al. 1990). Retroviruses are distinguished by their ability to reverse transcribe their RNA genomes into DNA intermediates by using the enzyme RT. The DNA form of the provirus genome is then integrated into a host cell chromosome by action of the viral enzyme integrase (Int). All retroviruses contain at least three major genes that encode the main virion structural components which are each synthesized as three polyproteins that produce either the inner virion interior (Gag, group specific antigen), the viral enzymes (Pol, *pol*ymerase), or the glycoproteins of the virion *env*elope (Env). In addition to virus structural proteins and viral enzymes, some retroviruses code for mostly small proteins with regulatory and auxiliary functions. While retroviruses share the same fundamental replication cycle and have the same basic genomic organization (e.g. the canonical *gag*, *pol*, and *env* genes) they do vary in the content of additional small regulatory genes and they have evolved different structures of their Gag proteins (for review see Coffin et al. 1997). The retroviral *gag* gene encodes the major structural protein and is entirely sufficient for virus particle formation (for review see Swanstrom and Wills 1997). According to the nomenclature defined by the International Committee on Taxonomy of Viruses (ICTV) convention (Hull 2001), orthoretroviruses contain RNA inside virus particles and are released from the plasma membrane. However, the assembly of orthoretroviruses follows two different strategies: Alpha-, gamma-, delta-, and lentiviruses (ICTV nomenclature) assemble on the inner leaflet of the plasma membrane and are released as immature virions. In contrast, beta-retroviruses and spumaviruses first assemble in the cytoplasm to form immature particles that are then transported to the plasma membrane where virus budding occurs.

Viruses of the genus *Lentivirus* including HIV-1, HIV-2, and *Simian immunodeficiency virus* (SIV), replicate preferentially in lymphocytes and in differentiated macrophages and cause long-lasting and mostly incurable chronic diseases. In contrast to gamma-retroviruses (ICTV nomenclature for oncoretroviruses) that require the breakdown of the nuclear membrane during mitosis for viral integration into host-cell chromosomes, lentiviruses are uniquely capable of infecting nondividing cells, preferentially nondividing macrophages and resting T-cells, as is the case for HIV-1 (Lewis and Emerman 1994).

As for other retroviruses, the HIV replication cycle begins with virus attachment and penetration through the plasma membrane. HIV binds to different cell-receptors, among them the differentiation antigen, CD4, acting as primary receptor, as well as different specific chemokine receptors that act as coreceptors after binding to CD4 (for review see Weiss 2002). The first retroviral receptor ever identified was the CD4 receptor on T-cells. It was established as the primary receptor for HIV-1 and HIV-2 and SIVs in 1984 (for review see Bour et al. 1995). However, the CD4 molecule alone is not adequate to allow Env-mediated membrane fusion and virus entry, as certain primary isolates of HIV-1 preferentially replicate in T-cell lines (T-cell-line trophic, 'TCL'-tropic), while others establish productive replication only in macrophage cultures ('M'-trophic). Thus, a second class of HIV receptors was predicted and finally identified as a member of the G protein-coupled seven transmembrane domain receptor superfamily acting as so called 'coreceptors' during HIV entry (for review see Berger et al. 1999). Coreceptors, in general, function as cellular receptors for α- and β-chemokines. Two types of coreceptors arbitrate the disparity in cell-type trophism:

the α-chemokine receptor CXCR4 (first described as 'fusin') that is typically present in T-cell lines, and the β-chemokine receptor CCR5 that is present on macrophages. In tissue culture, primary lymphocytes support replication of HIV, irrespective of its trophism. This phenomenon is demonstrated by the fact that cultures of activated peripheral blood mononuclear cells (PBMC) express both coreceptors, CXCR4 and CCR5. Notably, coreceptors symbolize an attractive target for anti-retroviral therapy. For example, the genetic heterogeneity in coreceptor alleles determines the vulnerability to HIV infection or disease progression. A well-characterized example is the identification of a truncated form of CCR5 (termed as the 'CCR5/d32' mutation) that in its homozygous form can protect individuals from HIV infection (Deng et al. 1996; Samson et al. 1996).

Following virus entry, the viral RNA genome is transcribed into double-stranded DNA, which as part of the preintegration complex (PIC) is transported to the nucleus where the proviral genome is integrated into chromosomes. Virus entry starts with the so-called 'uncoating' of the virus which is the fusion between the virus and host cell membrane followed by the release of the viral core into the cytoplasm. The virus core comprises all viral components that remain intact after the virus membrane is removed. Following membrane fusion, the reverse transcription complex (RTC) and the PIC is released from the virus core complex. While there is evidence that the CA molecules of the incoming virus are degraded via the ubiquitin proteasome system (UPS) (Schwartz et al. 1998), the three virus proteins Int, the matrix (MA), and the viral protein R (Vpr) molecules together with the provirus genome form the PIC. Although the PIC components comprise various nuclear import signals (for review see Sherman and Greene 2002), it is assumed that additional cellular and viral factors, including a central DNA flap, which is formed during reverse transcription (Zennou et al. 2000), facilitate the import of the PIC into the nucleus. It is worth noting that virus entry involves a number of consecutive and highly organized multistep events that might explain why approximately only one out of a thousand mature HIV-1 particles is capable of establishing a productive infection.

Further postentry events such as the reverse transcription of the viral genome, the nuclear import of the PIC, the integration of proviral DNA, the activation of HIV-1 LTR promoter driven retroviral gene expression, the export, the transport, and the splicing of viral RNA will not be described in detail in this review. Rather, late steps of the HIV-1 replication cycle, such as membrane targeting of Gag and Gag–Pol polyproteins, virus assembly, as well as budding and maturation will be explained in more detail. Following the early steps of the replication cycle and upon activation of integrated provirus, viral RNAs are processed and transported into the cytosol for translation of newly synthesized structural proteins that assemble at the plasma membrane into budding particles. The Gag polyprotein in HIV-1 and HIV-2 consists of different functional domains that mediate the recognition and binding of viral RNA, the membrane targeting of Gag and Gag–Pol polyproteins, virion assembly, and efficient particle release from the plasma membrane as the final step of virus budding (for review see Kräusslich and Welker 1996; Swanstrom and Wills 1997; Vogt 1997, 2000). The Gag polyprotein is the single viral protein sufficient and strictly required for virus particle assembly and budding, although further viral components such as the genomic RNA, the envelope, and the Gag–Pol precursor proteins are required for production of infectious progeny virions. The processing of the HIV-1 Gag polyprotein Pr55 by the viral PR generates the MA, CA, nucleocapsid (NC), and p6^{Gag} proteins (Swanstrom and Wills 1997). During proteolytic processing of HIV-1 Pr55^{Gag} two spacer peptides, p2 and p1, are also generated. The HIV-1 pol-encoded enzymes, PR, RT, and Int are proteolytically released from a large polyprotein precursor, Pr160^{GagPol}, the expression of which is the outcome from a rare frameshift event during Pr55^{Gag} translation (for review see Freed 2001). Similar to the Gag proteins, the Env glycoproteins are also synthesized from a polyprotein precursor protein. The resulting surface (SU) gp120 and transmembrane (TM) gp41 glycoproteins are produced by a cellular protease during trafficking of gp160 to the cell membrane. While gp120 harbors the domains that mediates virus binding to CD4 and coreceptors, the gp41 anchors the TM/SU complex in the virus membrane and includes the determinants that regulate fusion between cellular and virus membranes during virus entry. The N-terminus of the extra cellular ecto domain of gp41 harbors the hydrophobic domain, the so called 'fusion peptide' that in concert with two helical motifs of gp41 regulates membrane fusion by formation of a six-helix bundle (Weissenhorn et al. 1997). The highly polymorphic SU protein gp120 is organized into five conserved domains (C1 to C5), and five highly variable domains that in most of the known SU sequences are concentrated near loop structures and are stabilized by disulfide-bond formation.

In general, Gag proteins of different retroviruses exhibit a certain structural and functional similarity: MA mediates the plasma membrane targeting of the Gag polyprotein and lines the inner shell of the mature virus particle, CA regulates assembly of Gag and forms the core shell of the infectious virus, and NC regulates packaging and condensation of the viral genome. In addition to those canonical mature retrovirus proteins, other Gag domains have been described, such as the HIV-1 p6^{Gag} region that directs the incorporation of the regulatory protein Vpr into budding virions. Furthermore, p6^{Gag} harbors the late (L) domain required for efficient virus budding (Göttlinger et al. 1991).

HIV particles bud from the plasma membrane as immature noninfectious viruses consisting predominantly of uncleaved polyproteins. After virus release and in concert with PR activation which is autocatalytically released from the Gag–Pol polyprotein, processing of Gag and Gag–Pol polyproteins into its mature proteins and condensation of the inner core structure occurs resulting in the formation of mature infectious virus. Besides PR and Env, at least two other viral factors are known to promote efficient virus release: the HIV-1 specific accessory protein Vpu (Strebel et al. 1988) and the p6^{Gag} domain (Gottlinger et al. 1991). While Vpu supports virus release by an ion channel activity (Schubert et al. 1996b, c), p6^{Gag} contains the late assembly (L) domain that is required for efficient separation of assembled virions from the cell surface by a yet undefined mechanism that is further detailed below and involves the cellular UPS (Vogt 2000).

ROLE OF CELLULAR FACTORS IN HIV REPLICATION

From entry to release and maturation into infectious progeny virions, each individual step in the HIV replication cycle exploits cellular pathways. As for most other intracellular parasites, the replication of HIV is dependent on interaction with host cell factors, and some of these are specifically incorporated into progeny virions. Among the most abundant cellular proteins, and the first ever found in HIV-1 virions, is the peptidyl-prolyl isomerase (PPIase) cyclophilin A (CypA). This protein is specifically incorporated into HIV-1 virions, but not into virions of other lentiviruses, through an interaction with a proline-rich region that is conserved in the CA of all HIV-1 Gag polyproteins. In particular, Pro-222, which is conserved in the CA region of all HIV-1 Gag polyproteins appears to be important for the interaction of HIV-1 Gag with CypA (for review see Luban 1996). Earlier studies using two-hybrid screens found that HIV-1 Gag binds to most of the known members of the family of CyPs. CyPs were originally described as binding partners of cyclosporin A (CsA), an immunosuppressive cyclic undecapeptide used clinically to prevent allograft rejection. CsA binds with nanomolar affinity to CypA and this complex inhibits calcineurin, a calcium-dependent phosphatase that regulates gene expression of various cytokine genes in activated T-cells (for review see Ivery 2000). CyPs belong to the PPIases, a group of enzymes found in organisms ranging from prokaryotes to humans that catalyze the otherwise relatively slow cis/trans isomerization of peptidyl–prolyl bonds in vitro. A large body of evidence supports a function of CypA in formation of infectious HIV-1 viruses (for review see Ott 2002; Luban 1996). These studies were based either on mutation within gag or the use of competitive CypA inhibitors, such as CsA that interfere with the CypA–Gag interaction. A more conclusive proof that among the other 14 known members of mammalian CyPs, only CypA plays a functional role in supporting HIV-1 replication, was provided by selective genetic inactivation of the gene encoding CypA in human CD4[+] T-cells (Braaten and Luban 2001). The immunosuppressive activity of CsA is not correlated with anti-HIV activity as the non-immunosuppressive derivative NIM811 ([methyl-Ile[4]]-cyclosporin) represents an even more potent inhibitor of CypA-mediated HIV-1 replication than the parental CsA. Thus, CsA and related non-immunosuppressive derivatives form an interesting class of drugs that can modulate the interaction of CypA with other proteins.

Recent investigation of the conformational heterogeneity of the proline residues in the N terminus of the HIV-1 accessory protein Vpr suggested a functional interaction between Vpr and a host peptidyl–prolyl *cis/trans* isomerase (PPIase) that might regulate the *cis/trans* interconversion of the imidic bond within the conserved proline residues of Vpr in vivo (Bruns et al. 2003). The physical interaction between Vpr and the major host PPIase CypA involves the N-terminal region of Vpr and includes an essential role for proline in position 35 (Zander et al. 2003). The CypA inhibitor CsA, and non-immunosuppressive PPIase inhibitors, such as NIM811 and sanglifehrin A (SFA), block expression of Vpr without affecting pre- or post-translational events, such as transcription, intracellular transport or virus incorporation of Vpr. Similarly to CypA inhibition, Vpr expression is also reduced in HIV-1-infected CypA[−/−] knock-out T-cells. These studies provide the first evidence that, in addition to the interaction between CypA and HIV-1 capsid occurring during early steps in virus replication, CypA is also important for the de novo synthesis of Vpr and that in the absence of CypA activity, the Vpr-mediated cell cycle arrest is completely lost in HIV-1 infected T-cells.

Another example of host–virus interaction that has recently received much attention is the role of the UPS in virus budding. Efficient detachment of HIV-1 from the cell membrane is strictly dependent on the function of the L domain, a tetrapeptide motif (Pro–Thr/Ser–Ala–Pro (PT/SAP)) that encompass positions seven to ten of the p6[Gag] protein (for review see Freed 2002; Greene and Peterlin 2002). This process, which involves fission of the virus particle from the cell surface following envelopment and closing of the virus and cellular membrane, is commonly described as virus budding. L domain-deficient mutants of HIV-1 are characterized by late budding arrest, where virions remaining tethered to the plasma membrane by a thin membranous stalk that does not allow complete membrane fission (Göttlinger et al. 1991; Huang et al. 1995). Similar deficiencies in budding were reported for other retroviruses with L domain mutations within Gag polyproteins (for review see Freed 2002). Although the detailed molecular

mechanism(s) of how L domains regulate virus budding remain elusive, it is now generally believed that they function as a docking site for the cellular budding apparatus which normally is involved in the endocytotic recycling of cell surface-receptors (for review see Pornillos et al. 2002). Recent work provided an intriguing insight into the mechanism of how virus budding exploits a cellular machinery that is normally involved in vacuolar lysosomal protein sorting and multivesicular body (MVB) biogenesis (Martin-Serrano et al. 2003; von Schwedler et al. 2003). The recruitment of these cellular factors to the virus assembly site is facilitated by the interaction between the PTAP motif of p6[Gag] and at least one important factor which is the tumor susceptibility gene product (Tsg101) (Garrus et al. 2001; Martin-Serrano et al. 2001; Myers and Allen 2002; VerPlank et al. 2001), an E2 type ubiquitin ligase. Mechanistically, the interaction between Tsg101 and p6[Gag] is mediated by the N-terminal ubiquitin-binding domain, designated as ubiquitin E2 variant (UEV) sequence of Tsg101 that binds to the PTAP motif of p6[Gag] in a process that appears to be up-regulated when upstream lysine residues in p6[Gag] are mono-ubiquitinylated (Garrus et al. 2001; VerPlank et al. 2001; Pornillos et al. 2002; Demirov et al. 2002; Myers and Allen 2002). Recently, two additional binding partners of Tsg101 have been identified in virus budding: ALix/AIP1, a homologue of the yeast class E Vps protein Bro1 that binds to a C-terminal region of HIV-1 p6[Gag] and is also involved in L-domain function (Strack et al. 2003; von Schwedler et al. 2003), and Hrs, a regulator of MVB formation involving ESCRT recruitment to endosomes (Bache et al. 2003; Pornillos et al. 2002). The normal function of Tsg101 is to target multi-ubiquitinylated proteins into endosomal vesicles followed by MVB formation in a process that is similar to virus budding and involves the budding into the endosomal vesicles (Babst et al. 2000; Katzmann et al. 2002). Topologically, MVB generation is analogous to virus budding, since in both cases cytoplasmic material is extricated and enveloped by cellular membranes. Thus, it appears that HIV recruits the components of the MVB system to the budding machinery that follows two separate and cell-type-specific pathways: in T-cells HIV-1 buds primarily from the cell surface, while in monocytes/macrophages the virus buds into vacuoles of the MVB system (for review see Amara and Littman 2003). In general, there is mounting evidence that HIV-1 assembly and budding exploits the cellular protein sorting and trafficking pathway which itself is regulated by the UPS (for review see Schnell and Hicke 2003).

Another important example of the interaction of HIV-1 with host factors is the relationship between one HIV-1 accessory protein, the virus infectivity factor (Vif), and apolipoprotein B mRNA editing enzyme (APOBEC3G). APOBEC3G, also known as CEM15, is a member of cellular cytidine deaminase-editing enzyme family that represents another aspect of the so-called 'innate immune system' (for review see Vartanian et al. 2003; Rose et al. 2004; Navarro and Landau 2004; Schrofelbauer et al. 2004). The antiretroviral activity of APOBEC3G is based on its unique capability to hypermutate retroviruses, including HIV-1, with terminal consequences. This innate block in virus replication is counteracted by Vif, which in the virus producer cell binds to APOBEC3G, induces its polyubiquitination, and thus proteasomal degradation (Yu et al. 2003; Mangeat et al. 2003; Harris et al. 2003; Stopak et al. 2003). In this way Vif is precluding the presence of APOBEC3G in progeny virions. As a cytidine deaminase, APOBEC3G induces G to A hypermutation in proviral DNA and, thus, acts as an inhibitor of HIV-1 replication. Mechanistically, APOBEC3G causes changes of C to T in the viral DNA minus strand (Yu et al. 2004). This, in turn, leads to insertion of G in front of C, and A in front of T during DNA plus strand synthesis. The APOBEC3G induced hypermutation can interfere with HIV-1 replication in several ways: it may cause instability of the viral DNA, interference with plus-strand synthesis, or disturb functional gene expression from the proviral genome. The antiretroviral activity of APOBEC3G depends on its encapsidation into progeny virions, which is mediated through interaction with the NC region of the Gag polyprotein and/or with viral and nonviral RNAs (Alce and Popik 2004; Svarovskaia et al. 2004). It can be assumed that virion incorporation of APOBEC3G would maneuver the enzyme into close proximity with the reverse transcription complex.

Another example for host–virus interaction unraveled recently is the interaction between cellular and viral ion channel forming proteins, namely the HIV-1 specific virus protein u (Vpu) and the widely expressed acid-sensitive two-pore K^+ background channel TASK-1 (Hsu et al. 2004, for review see Strebel 2004). Most intriguingly, this interaction may be the consequence of a so called 'molecular piracy' as the N-terminal TM domain of TASK-1 shares striking similarity to that of Vpu. Further, the physical interaction between both TM domains may cause the intercalation of TASK-1 and Vpu into hetero-oligomeric channel complexes and, thus, may explain why TASK-1 suppresses Vpu-mediated virus release while Vpu abolishes TASK-1 channel conductance. This hypothesis was supported by the observation that sole expression of the homology sharing TM domain of TASK-1 can functionally complement the virus release function of Vpu. However, independent of whether Vpu itself acts as an ion channel or instead regulates the activity of a cellular ion channel, it remains an open question how the host cell membrane conductance controls late steps in virus budding.

A further accessory HIV protein was recently shown to interact specifically with a cellular factor: the HIV-1 Nef mimics an integrin receptor signal and thus recruits a nuclear transcription repressor host protein to the cell membrane (Witte et al. 2004). As detailed below, Nef is thought to obstruct T-cell activation by recruiting certain cellular factors into a so far undefined signaling complex to the cell membrane. Specifically, Nef directs the Polycomb Group (PcG) protein Eed, which represents a nuclear repressor of transcription, to the inner leaflet of the cell membrane. The Nef-mediated re-translocation of Eed causes activation of the Tat-dependent HIV-1 LTR promoter driven transcription, most likely because of the depletion of Eed repressor from the nucleus.

Further well-characterized examples for host virus protein interaction are the virus receptors (CD4 and chemokine receptors) which enable virus entry into specific host cells (Berger et al. 1999), the role of the chromatin-remodeling system (Yung et al. 2001) and the HMG I family proteins (Farnet and Bushman 1997) for proviral DNA integration, as well as the requirement of different factors of the endosomal protein trafficking and ubiquitinglation systems for virus release (for review see Perez and Nolan 2001; Vogt 2000; Luban 2001).

MOLECULAR STRUCTURE AND FUNCTION OF HIV REGULATOR PROTEINS

In addition to the canonical retroviral Gag, Pol, and Env proteins common to replication-competent retroviruses, HIV-1 and other lentiviruses encode further small proteins with either essential regulatory (Tat and Rev) or accessory (Vpu, Vif, Nef, and Vpr) functions that serve to accelerate viral replication. While Tat is critical for transcription driven by the HIV-1 LTR promoter, Rev is essential for transport of viral RNAs from the nucleus to the cytoplasm. The function of these essential regulatory HIV genes will not be discussed in this review. The focus will be on the accessory regulator proteins, with special emphasis on Vpr and Vpu. These proteins also called 'auxiliary,' since they are not essential for HIV-1 replication in certain cell lines, yet a growing number of in vivo studies report important roles of these HIV-1 gene products in the pathology and spread of HIV-1 (for review see Cohen et al. 1996).

THE LENTIVIRUS PROTEIN R (VPR)

The highly conserved 96-amino acid, 14-kDa viral protein R (Vpr), has received considerable attention and a number of biological functions have been attributed to its presence in various cellular and extra cellular compartments. The most intensively investigated biological functions of Vpr are those affecting the translocation of the PIC of the incoming virus from the cytoplasm to the nucleus, and the arrest in the G_2 phase of the cell cycle (for a recent comprehensive resume see Sherman and Greene 2002; Sherman et al. 2002; Bukrinsky and Adzhubei 1999). The nuclear targeting function of Vpr has been associated with HIV-1 infection of terminally differentiated macrophages. Regarding the second function of Vpr, that leads to G_2 cell cycle arrest in HIV-1-infected and/or Vpr-transfected human cells, it was suggested that this activity provides an intracellular milieu conducive to enhanced viral replication by increasing HIV-1 LTR-driven gene expression (Goh et al. 1998). This response has recently been linked with the capacity of Vpr to alter the structure of the nuclear lamina leading to transient, DNA-containing herniations of the nuclear envelope that intermittently rupture (de Noronha et al. 2001). Other studies suggest that the prolonged G_2 arrest induced by Vpr ultimately leads to apoptosis of the infected cell (Poon et al. 1998; Stewart et al. 2000). Conversely, early anti-apoptotic effects of Vpr have been described which are overlayed by its pro-apoptotic effects (Conti et al. 2000). These pro-apoptotic effects of Vpr may result from either effects on the integrity of the nuclear envelope or direct mitochondrial membrane permeabilization (Jacotot et al. 2001), perhaps involving Vpr-mediated formation of ion channels in cellular membranes (Piller et al. 1996).

Vpr is a virion-associated (Paxton et al. 1993), nucleocytoplasmic shuttling (Sherman et al. 2001) regulatory protein that is encoded by (and conserved among) primate lentiviruses, HIV-1, HIV-2, and the SIVs. Although dispensable for growth of HIV-1 in dividing cultured T cells, Vpr appears to play an important role in virus replication in vivo, since deletion of *vpr* and the related *vpx* genes in SIV severely compromises the pathogenic properties in experimentally infected rhesus macaques (Gibbs et al. 1995; Lang et al. 1993). Furthermore, HIV-2 and SIV also encode an additional Vpr-related protein, Vpx, that is believed to function synergistically with Vpr. The Vpr of HIV-1 is reported to exhibit numerous biological activities, including nuclear localization (based on the presence of at least two nuclear localization signals) (Heinzinger et al. 1994; Jenkins et al. 1998; Vodicka et al. 1998; Popov et al., 1998a, b; Sherman et al. 2000, 2001), ion channel formation (Piller et al. 1996), transcriptional activation of HIV-1 and heterologous promoters (Stark and Hay 1998; Felzien et al. 1998), co-activation of the glucocorticoid receptor (Kino et al. 1999), regulation of cell differentiation (Levy et al. 1993), induction of apoptosis (Stewart et al. 1997; Ayyavoo et al. 1997), cell cycle arrest (Levy et al. 1993; Rogel et al. 1995), and transduction through cell membranes (Henklein et al. 2000a). Although significant amounts of Vpr (approximately 0.15-fold molar ratio to viral core proteins, Müller et al. 2000) are packaged into budding HIV-1 particles in a process dependent on Vpr's interaction with the C-terminal p6^{gag} domain of the Gag polyprotein precursor Pr55 (Paxton et al. 1993), the biological role(s) of virion associated Vpr remains to be fully elucidated.

As the biologically relevant activity of the multifunctional Vpr has not yet been clarified, the molecular bases for many of its effects remain elusive. To date, structural studies of the full-length molecule have been hampered by the fact that this protein does not crystallize and the use of NMR techniques is complicated by the strong tendency for Vpr to undergo self-association. In addition, Vpr's structure depends critically on the solution conditions, and an unresolved apparent heterogeneity in the oligomeric composition of the polypeptide has been observed (Wecker et al. 2002; Henklein et al. 2000b). Many structural characterizations of Vpr have shown the important influence of environmental factors and indicate that in vivo folding of Vpr will probably require the presence of structure-stabilizing interacting factors (for review see Bukrinsky and Adzhubei 1999). The secondary structures in Vpr emerging from these analyses suggest the presence of an α-helix–turn–α-helix motif between residues 17 and 48 and an amphipathic α-helix located between amino acids 53–55 and 78–83 (Schüler et al. 1999). These helices are highly conserved and most likely play a key role in self-association and the interaction of Vpr with heterologous proteins (Felzien et al. 1998). Various investigations have shown that the C-terminal domain participates in a number of specific protein–protein and protein–nucleic acid interactions, such as that with NCp7 (de Rocquigny et al. 1997), Tat (Sawaya et al. 1999), RNA (de Rocquigny et al. 2000), and adenine nucleotide translocator of the mitochondrial pore (Jacotot et al. 2000).

STRUCTURE AND FUNCTION OF THE HIV-1 SPECIFIC VPU PROTEIN

The 81 amino acid Vpu is encoded exclusively by HIV-1 (Cohen et al. 1988; Strebel et al. 1988), with one exception, the HIV-1 related isolate SIV$_{cpz}$ that encodes a Vpu-like protein similar in length and predicted structure to the Vpu from HIV-1 isolates (Huet et al. 1990). The HIV-1 specific accessory gene *vpu* encodes an integral membrane phosphoprotein with various biological functions (for review see Bour and Strebel 2003): firstly, in the ER Vpu induces degradation of CD4 in a process involving the ubiquitin-proteasome pathway and CK-2 phosphorylation of its cytoplasmic tail (Vpu$_{CYTO}$) (Schubert et al. 1998; Margottin et al. 1998). In addition, there is evidence that Vpu interferes with the major histocompatibility complex (MHC) class I antigen presentation and regulates Fas-mediated apoptosis (Kerkau et al. 1997; Komoto et al. 2003; Akari et al. 2001). Secondly, Vpu augments virus release from a post-ER compartment by a cation-selective ion channel activity mediated by its transmembrane anchor (Vpu$_{TM}$) (Schubert et al., 1996a, and references therein). It was shown previously that Vpu can regulate cationic current when inserted into planar lipid bilayers and in *Xenopus* oocytes (Schubert et al. 1996a; Coady et al. 1998). However, the detailed mechanism how Vpu as a membrane conductance regulator supports virus budding remains elusive. The new insights are indicating that the virus release function of Vpu_{TM} involves the mutually destructive interaction between Vpu and the K^+ channel TASK-1 (Hsu et al. 2004, for review see Strebel 2004). Thus, it is now conceivable that Vpu affects membrane conductance through tuning the activity of host-cell ion channels (for review see Lamb and Pinto 1997).

Vpu is a class I oligomeric membrane-bound phosphoprotein (Maldarelli et al. 1993) composed of an amphipathic sequence of 81 amino acids comprising a hydrophobic N-terminal membrane anchor proximal to a polar C-terminal cytoplasmic domain. The latter contains a highly conserved region, from Glu-47 to Gly-58 that is present in all analyzed Vpu sequences. It also contains the phosphorylation sites for the casein kinase two (CK-2) that regulate Vpu's function in the ER (Schubert et al. 1994; Schubert and Strebel 1994). The structure and the orientation in the membrane of the N-terminal hydrophobic Vpu_{TM}, which is primarily associated with an ion-channel activity, either by itself (Schubert et al. 1996a) or in the context of full-length Vpu (Ewart et al. 1996), was first analyzed using the synthetic peptide Vpu^{1-39} (Wray et al. 1999). The tertiary U-shaped turn structure identified in solution, however, was inconsistent with the formation of ion-conducting membrane pores in planar lipid bilayers (Schubert et al. 1996a) since it is unlikely to be able to span the bilayer. Consequently, proton-decoupled ^{15}N cross-polarization solid-state NMR spectroscopy has been employed to investigate full-length Vpu and its isolated domains oriented in phospholipid bilayers using either synthetic discretely ^{15}N-labeled amino acids (Wray et al. 1999; Henklein et al. 2000b), or uniformly ^{15}N-labeled recombinant material (Marassi et al. 1999; Ma et al. 2002). Those solid state NMR data were consistent with a transmembrane alignment of a helical polypeptide, implying that the nascent helices in the folded solution structure reassemble to form a linear α-helix involving residues 6 to 29 that lies parallel to the bilayer normal with a tilt angle of $\leqslant 30°$ (Wray et al. 1999) and placing Trp^{22} near to and the Glu^{28}-Tyr-Arg-motif that is know to be important for helix termination, anchorage, and pore selectivity. Most recently, attention has focused on the ion channel activity of Vpu and its similarity to other viral ion channels (for review see Fischer and Sansom 2002). Molecular dynamic investigations of various Vpu fragments, combined with conductance measurements, provide evidence for water-filled five-helix bundles. In summary, the monomeric structure model of Vpu provides details of the topology and positions of secondary structure in the membrane bound state. However, more experimental and theoretical work is required to understand Vpu in its functional form in vivo where it exists as the phosphoprotein in multi-protein complexes involving CD4 and β-TrCp (Margottin et al. 1998), or in homo-oligomeric nonphosphorylated form required for its ion-channel activity in the cell membrane.

THE VIRAL INFECTIVITY FACTOR VIF

The 23-kDa phosphoprotein Vif represents a viral infectivity factor that is highly conserved among all lentiviruses with one exception, the equine infectious anemia virus (EIAV). Vif regulates virus infectivity in a cell-type-dependent fashion. Permissive cells like HeLa, Cos 293T, SupT1, CEM-SS, and Jurkat cells support HIV replication independently of Vif. In contrast, primary lymphocytes, macrophages, and certain cell lines that might express a specific cellular Vif interacting factor require Vif for production of fully infectious viruses (Strebel et al. 1987; Simon et al. 1998).

Until recently, the mechanism of how Vif supports formation of infectious virions was enigmatic. Contemporary findings, detailed above, support the intriguing hypothesis that at least one main function of Vif is to neutralize a natural host defense mechanism. This novel innate anti-HIV defense mechanism was recently revealed as the cellular cytidine deaminase APOBEC3G, which together with Vif is encapsidated into progeny virions (for review see Navarro and Landau 2004). Intriguing was the long known fact that Vif can act in *trans* when it is expressed in the virus producer, but not in the target cell, indicating that Vif must be situated at the virus assembly site (von Schwedler 1993). Consistent with this is the fact that relatively low levels of Vif molecules are detected in mature HIV-1 virions, yet its encapsidation is increased when unprocessed Gag or certain Gag mutants are expressed (Sova et al. 2001). Heterokaryon analysis of fusions between permissive and nonpermissive cells revealed that nonpermissive cells must contain a so far unknown, naturally occurring antiviral factor that is neutralized by Vif of the incoming virus (Simon et al. 1998a). This model of a post-entry function for Vif is further supported by the observation that Vif from diverse lentiviruses function in a species specific mode (Simon et al. 1998b). Several hypothesis have been put forward to explain the mechanism of Vif function: the activity of Vif might regulate reverse transcription and proviral DNA synthesis (Dornadula et al. 2000), Vif can support the formation of stable virus cores (Ohagen and Gabuzda 2000), or Vif might bind to viral RNA in order to support post-entry steps of virus replication (Khan et al. 2001). The discovery of the APOBEC3G–Vif interaction provides at least some explanation for these previous observations (Navarro and Landau 2004).

THE MULTIFUNCTIONAL NEF PROTEIN

Originally, the 27 kDa N-terminal myristoylated membrane-associated phosphoprotein Nef was described as a 'negative factor' that suppresses the HIV-LTR promoter activity (for review see Freed 2001; Frankel 1998; Steffens and Hope 2001; Marsh 1999). As one of the most intensively investigated HIV-1 accessory proteins, Nef has been shown to fulfill multiple functions during the viral replication cycle. However, the mechanism(s) of Nef has not yet been fully elucidated. In general, it is now widely accepted that, inconsistent with its originally 'negative' nomenclature, Nef plays an important stimulatory role in the replication and pathogenesis of HIV-1. The broad spectrum of Nef-associated activities so far described can be summarized in distinct classes: (i) modulation of cell activation and apoptosis, (ii) change in intracellular trafficking of cellular proteins, particularly of cell receptor proteins like CD4 and MHC class I, and (iii) increase of virus infectivity.

Well characterized and one of the earliest observation in the course of studying '*Nefology*' is the Nef-induced down-regulation of cell surface CD4 (Garcia and Miller 1991). This mechanism occurs on a post-translational level by augmentation of receptor internalization followed by lysosomal degradation, where Nef is binding to the adapter protein complex in clathrin-coated pits (Aiken et al. 1994). As there are at least two other mechanisms of HIV-1 receptor interference, induced by the envelope and Vpu proteins of HIV-1, it was speculated that intervention with the primary virus receptor, CD4, must be advantageous for HIV-1 replication. Indeed, excess of cell-surface CD4 was shown to interfere with encapsidation of Env and release of infectious HIV progeny viruses (Lama et al. 1999; Ross et al. 1999). Another influence on immune receptors is the Nef-mediated block in the transport of MHC-I antigen complexes to the cell surface, leading to the disturbance in the recognition of HIV-1 infected cells by cytotoxic T_{CD8} lymphocytes (CTL) (Collins et al. 1998; Schwartz et al. 1996, Le Gall et al. 2000). More recent studies described down-regulation of co-stimulatory protein CD28 induced by Nef (Swigut et al. 2001). As it appears, the mechanism(s) by which Nef blocks cell surface expression of CD4, MHC-I, and CD28 are independent and can be genetically separated (Le Gall et al. 2000; Piguet and Trono 2001; Piguet et al. 1999, 2000).

Nef is expressed relatively early in the HIV replication cycle, and there are reports that Nef is incorporated into budding virions where it can be cleaved by the viral protease. Nef is present during almost all steps of the viral lifecycle which might explain the multiple functions deployed by this accessory protein. Major attention has been focused towards the Nef-mediated modulation of the T-cell signal transduction and activation pathways (for review see Fackler and Baur 2002). Several lines of evidence supported the hypothesis that, by affecting the T cell receptor, Nef may support several aspects of the virus replication cycle, including regulation of apoptosis and immune evasion. Earlier studies in transgenic mice indicated Nef-dependent activation in T-cell signaling (Skowronski et al. 1993). Later studies indicate that Nef imitates T-cell receptor signalling motifs (Simmons et al. 2001). The Nef-induced T-cell activation requires the tyrosine kinase Zap70 and the zeta chain of the T-cell receptor (Xu et al. 1999). Further, Nef was shown to activate T-cells by binding to the Nef-associated kinase, also known as the p21-activated kinase 2 (PAK2) (Arora et al. 2000; Renkema et al. 2001). In addition to the activation of T-cells, Nef also induces cell death, although the mechanism and biological relevance of this Nef-function is less clear. It was also shown that expression of the death receptor Fas ligand (FasL) is activated by Nef and that this upregulation might increase killing of CTLs attacking HIV infected cells (Xu et al. 1997).

In terms of HIV related pathogenesis, it is becoming clear that the multifunctional Nef protein represents an attractive target for development of antiviral strategies, since this accessory protein has been explicitly characterized as a viral factor that increases the pathological potential and the replication of lentiviruses in vivo. For instance, virus isolates from so called long-term nonprogressing HIV-1 infected individuals maintain deletion in *nef* alleles (Rhodes et al. 2000). Consistent with the idea that Nef supports virus replication in vivo, Nef of SIV was shown to elevate virus replication and disease progression in SIV-infected rhesus macaques (Kestler et al. 1991).

DYNAMICS OF VIRAL REPLICATION

Before the direct quantification of plasma viral RNA was possible, estimates of viral dynamics were based on indirect parameters such as anti-HIV-1 antibody titer (Gaines et al. 1987), p24 antigenaemia (Paul et al. 1987), CD4 cell count (Goedert et al. 1987) and clinical progression. This lead to the belief that the natural course of HIV-1 infection included a 'latent stage' in which little or no viral replication occurred. It was not until 1989 that Ho et al. showed that viral replication and immune destruction was an on-going and active process. Thereafter, Pantaleo et al. (1993) and Embretson et al. (1993) demonstrated active viral replication during the 'latent' stage in tissues such as lymph nodes, tonsils and adenoids, and in cells such as T-helper cells and macrophages. The availability of drug regimes that could suppress all viral replication facilitated investigation of the dynamics of viral replication. Two groups (Ho et al. 1995; Wei et al. 1995) made use of viral load measurements to assay the rate of decline of plasma viremia in the presence of drug. They found that viral load fell exponentially within two weeks of starting therapy and that this decline was a combination of the clearance of free virus from the plasma and the removal of infected, productive cells. Both groups independently calculated the half-life of a virion in plasma to be 2–2.1 days, a higher replication rate than previously expected, and estimated viral production to be at least 10^8 or 10^9 virions per day.

Another study (Perelson et al. 1996) exploited the new potent antiretroviral therapy to demonstrate an exponential decrease in plasma viral load and to calculate the half-life of virion clearance to be 6 hours and the daily rate of virus production to be 10.3×10^9, greater than a one-log increase on previous estimations. It was calculated that 99 percent of plasma virus was released by recently infected cells. One year later, using a triple antiretroviral regime, Perelson and co-workers (1997) demonstrated that the therapy-induced viral decline was a two-stage event. This involved loss of plasma virus and virus from recently infected cells, followed by the loss of virus from long-lived infected cells such as tissue macrophages or dendritic cells, the half-life being approximately 1–4 weeks. A third stage was also predicted in which latently-infected cells required activation prior to virus production. Ho's prediction that HIV-1 could be eradicated from latently-infected cells with 3 years of Combined Antiretroviral Therapy (CART) (Ho 1997) was undermined by data showing that virus could still be detected from these latently infected cells after more than 2 years of CART, despite an undetectable plasma viremia (Wong et al. 1997b; Finzi et al. 1997; Chun et al. 1997).

The interplay between the immune response and virion production produces the viral load 'set point', which is prognostic of clinical outcome and disease progression in an infected individual (Mellors et al. 1996). It was proposed that lymphoid tissues trap virions early in infection, but as the lymphoid structure becomes damaged more virus is released to the circulating plasma. Calculations based on CD4 cell dynamics (Ho et al. 1995; Wei et al. 1995) estimated a daily turnover of between 1.8 and 2×10^9 cells, and led David Ho to propose the 'tap and sink' analogy for immune depletion. He hypothesized that the pool of CD4 cells was maintained as fast as it was destroyed during early infection but that, with time, the tap runs dry as new cells become fewer. Eventually the sink empties. Newer techniques using glucose-labeled CD4 cells have provided an insight into real-time CD4 cell dynamics and suggest that, in fact, HIV-1 infection affects the half-life of the CD4 cells, rather than their rate of production (Hellerstein et al. 1999). Hence, although the initial effect of CART is to increase the rate of CD4 cell production, the long-term aim is to increase the lifespan of cells.

ENZYME INFIDELITY AND GENETIC VARIATION

The *Lentiviridae* undergo extensive genetic variation. Variability results in part from RT infidelity combined with a lack of 3'-5' exonuclease activity, a proof-reading function common in mammalian polymerase enzymes which repairs incorrectly synthesized DNA. HIV-1 has one of the highest mutation rates of retrovirus RTs. In vitro studies on purified RT have estimated the error rate to be one base in every 3.4×10^5 (Preston et al. 1988; Roberts et al. 1988; Mansky and Temin 1995). When this mutation rate is considered in tandem with the estimated replication rate of ten billion new virions each day, the scope for diversity becomes apparent – every possible single point mutation is created daily in each infected individual. As a result, mutations that confer drug resistance may be present at undetectable levels prior to the commencement of anti-viral therapy. The majority of mutations are point mutations consisting of base-pair substitutions, although base insertions and deletions have been identified (Larder et al. 1999).

An alternative means by which variation may be introduced is via recombination. Each virion contains two RNA copies, both of which may contribute to a growing DNA strand during reverse transcription. Two viruses containing unique drug resistance mutations may create a single multidrug resistant virus by recombination (Moutouh et al. 1996). Following infection, the HIV-1 population develops into a 'quasi species' of genetic variants and as infection progresses, the homogeneity of the infecting population increases (McNearney et al. 1992). Viral variants may have different cell tropisms (e.g. brain and lymphoid tissue (Simmonds et al. 1991; Di Stefano et al. 1996) and co-receptor usage (Deng et al. 1996; Oberlin et al. 1996). Such genetic variation is inherent to the evolution of HIV-1 at an individual level, but also on a more global level, as illustrated by the presence of subtypes.

HIV-1 SUBTYPES

Analysis of viral sequences allows HIV-1 to be classified into three groups, representing the distinctive HIV-1 lineages, Main (M), Outlier (O) (Gurtler et al. 1994) and Non-M-Non-O (N) (Simon et al. 1998). The M group was initially subtyped following analyses of *gag* gene sequences from virus isolated in 15 countries (Louwagie et al. 1993), and has been further divided into individual subtypes (A–K) (Figure 60.1). Isolates containing RNA from more than one subtype are now appearing and have been termed circulating recombinant forms (CRF) (Carr et al. 1998), of which at least 14 have been identified (Robertson et al. 2000). The predominant example of a CRF is subtype AE, prevalent in Thailand. That these viruses might represent recombinants was confirmed from sequence analyses of *gag* and *env* genes (McCutchan et al. 1992; Louwagie et al. 1993), and from analyses of complete subtype AE genomes (Carr et al. 1996; Gao et al. 1996). However, the nonrecombinant subtype E 'source' isolate has yet to be identified, leading to uncertainty concerning the origins of

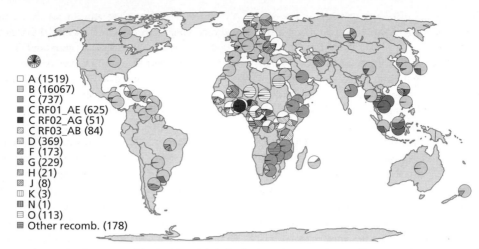

□ A (1519)
▦ B (16067)
▨ C (737)
■ C RF01_AE (625)
■ C RF02_AG (51)
▨ C RF03_AB (84)
▧ D (369)
▨ F (173)
▨ G (229)
▨ H (21)
▨ J (8)
▥ K (3)
▥ N (1)
▤ O (113)
▨ Other recomb. (178)

Figure 60.1 *HIV-1 subtype distribution worldwide. The global distribution of HIV-1 subtypes (from Los Alamos National Laboratory Database (2002) wwwII:hiv-web.lanl.gov/geography/index.html). Subtypes are represented by color, with the green subtype B predominating in Europe and the USA and the red, blue, and pink of subtypes A, C, and D, respectively, being prevalent in sub-Saharan Africa.*

subtype AE. Sub-subtypes are lineages closely related to particular subtypes, but not genetically distant enough to justify calling a new subtype. For example, subtype F comprises sub-subtype F1 and a newly found lineage sub-subtype F2 (Triques et al. 1999). A third F sub-subtype, F3, was later reclassified as subtype K (Triques et al. 2000). The subtypes of most HIV-1 strains can be determined by sequence analysis of any region of the genome as inter-subtype nucleotide sequence divergence may exceed 20, 15, and 25 percent for *gag*, *pol*, and *env*, respectively (Robertson et al. 2000).

HIV-1 subtypes show different geographical distributions. The majority of HIV-1 infections in Europe and North America are with subtype B, while in sub-Saharan Africa, subtypes A, C, and D predominate (Figure 60.1). Nevertheless, in the UK 25 percent of HIV-1 infections are estimated to be caused by non-B subtypes (Parry et al. 2001). In East Africa, subtypes A and D are most common, whereas in the south and south-east, subtype C predominates, although this subtype is also spreading eastwards (Koch et al. 2001). Cameroon is a source of Group O (Mauclere et al. 1997) and group N strains (Ayouba et al. 2000). Other continents display subtype variability. For example in India and south-east Asia subtype C is common (Bollinger et al. 1995) and in Thailand subtypes B and AE predominate (Gao et al. 1996; Ou et al. 1993).

In South America subtypes B, C, and F are found (Campodonico et al. 1996; Bongertz et al. 2000), and the developing epidemic in the former Soviet Union comprises subtypes A, B, C, G, and AB (Liitsola et al. 1998; Lukashov et al. 1995).

HIV-1 and HIV-2 show 50 percent genetic similarity (Korber et al. 1995) and demonstrate differing degrees of pathogenicity, transmissibility, and drug susceptibility (Marlink et al. 1994; Pauwels et al. 1990). Subtype variability may impact on issues as diverse as vaccine design,

detection, and quantification of HIV-1 infection, transmissibility, and pathogenicity.

THE CLINICAL IMPACT OF VIRAL DIVERSITY

Viral diversity impacts on the diagnosis of HIV-1 infection. The assay that is most widely applied to HIV-1 diagnosis is the enzyme-linked immunosorbent assay (ELISA). Until recently, ELISAs for the detection of antibodies to HIV-1 and HIV-2 were not equally sensitive for all subtypes. The earliest ELISAs failed to detect antibodies to group O and HIV-2, although incorporating antigens from these strains into newer assays overcame the problem (Schable et al. 1994). A recent study of the ability of six ELISAs to detect antibodies from all the major subtypes showed that the assays detected most HIV-1 group M variants (Koch et al. 2001) as well as group N (Masciotra et al. 2000).

Other clinical assays affected by viral diversity are those quantifying HIV infection. Viral load (VL) is the number of HIV-1 RNA copies per milliliter of plasma, and various techniques, based on differing technologies, are available for its quantification. The Roche Amplicor HIV-1 Monitor v1.5 assay (Roche Diagnostics, New Jersey, USA) (Mulder et al. 1994) uses reverse transcription and then PCR to amplify and quantify a region of the *gag* gene. The nucleic acid sequence-based amplification assay (NASBA) (Organon Teknika, Boxtel, The Netherlands) (Kievits et al., 1991; de Baar et al. 2001) directly amplifies RNA from *gag*. The HIV-1 Quantiplex branched DNA (bDNA) assay (Chiron Diagnostics, Emeryville, California, USA) (Pachl et al. 1995; Todd et al. 1995) uses sequential hybridization of probes targeting the *pol* gene to quantify viral RNA and the LCx quantitative assay (Abbott) uses RT-PCR amplification of *pol* (Swanson et al. 2000).

Each technique has a different sensitivity for viral load measurement, according to the subtype being tested (Alaeus et al. 1999; Holguin et al. 1999; Parekh et al. 1999; Clarke et al. 2000). This may preclude the comparison of viral loads from patients infected with different HIV-1 subtypes and, if different assays are used for consecutive readings in the same patient, any change in viral load may be difficult to interpret. For example, early versions of the Amplicor and NASBA assays detected HIV-1 subtypes A and H with lower degrees of sensitivity than other Group M subtypes (Coste et al. 1996), although comparisons of the more recent versions of these assays show that all subtypes are equally quantified (Swanson et al. 2001). As many viral load assays are PCR-based, polymorphic variability may compromise the binding of primers. Accordingly, assays can be improved by utilizing highly conserved regions of the genome, such as *pol* (Ernest et al. 2001) or by exploiting non-PCR amplification techniques, such as the bDNA assay (Parekh et al. 1999).

The influence of subtype on viral transmissibility has also been suggested by a number of studies, although data are limited. The difficulty with interpreting such studies is that there are many confounding factors. For example, coinfection with sexually transmitted pathogens such as *Neisseria gonorrhoeae* or herpes simplex virus also increase transmissibility (del Mar Pujades et al. 2002; Fawzi et al. 2001). There are data that suggest that subtype B isolates are less transmissible than non-B counterparts (Cameron et al. 1989; van Harmelen et al. 1997), and that the maternal transmission rate is lower in Tanzanian mothers infected with HIV-1 subtype D, than in those infected with A or C (Renjifo et al. 2001). Without larger controlled studies, such findings should be regarded with caution, particularly in the light of evidence to suggest that factors, such as viral load, significantly impact on virus transmission (Shaffer et al. 1999).

The degree of pathogenicity associated with HIV-1 infection is also multifactorial and, accordingly, attributing an effect to subtype is difficult. Some studies suggest that the rate of disease progression is similar, regardless of subtype (Alaeus et al. 1999; Weisman et al. 1999; Amornkul et al. 1999), whereas a study in Senegal suggested a survival advantage for those infected with subtype A HIV-1 (Kanki et al. 1999). More recently, in a study from Uganda, viruses with subtype D envelope were associated with faster disease progression (relative risk of death, 1.29; $P = 0.009$) and with a lower CD4 cell count ($P = 0.001$), compared with subtype A (Kaleebu et al. 2002).

SUBTYPE VARIABILITY AND THE PROSPECT OF A VACCINE

The lack of a vaccine for HIV-1 remains one of the major obstacles to controlling the epidemic. A number of approaches have led to clinical trials, including live vectors which express selected HIV-1 genes (Gupta et al. 2002; Corey et al. 1998; Ferrari et al. 1997), DNA vaccines (Caselli et al. 1999; Ayyavoo et al. 2000), live-attenuated *nef*-deleted virions (Khatissian et al. 2001; Wyand et al. 1999), and killed viral constructs (Moss et al. 2001). The high HIV-1 mutation rate and the development of quasi species facilitate the development of 'escape mutants' (Barouch et al. 2002) and restrict vaccine design. By using vaccines that utilize highly conserved regions of the HIV-1 genome, such as Tat and Rev, the impact of genetic variability is reduced and, accordingly, these vaccines have also been shown to be active against a range of subtypes (Goldstein et al. 2001), eliciting humoral and cellular responses (Caselli et al. 1999; Cafaro et al. 1999).

The extent of subtype effect on vaccine design remains unclear, especially as the majority of vaccines are designed to inhibit HIV-1 subtype B. Neutralizing antibodies are subtype-specific (Mascola et al. 1994), although broad cross-reactivity of neutralizing antibody activity to subtypes B and C has been reported (Bures et al. 2002; Dorrell et al. 1999). Cross-clade T-cell responses have been elicited. For example, an HIV-1 gp160-DNA construct encoding subtype B *env*, *tat*, and *rev* genes elicited specific and cross-reactive cell-mediated immune responses in mice (Arora and Seth 2001) and similar responses have been reported in human volunteers in Uganda (Cao et al. 2000; Van der Groen et al. 1998). Vaccines are being developed to express epitopes from a range of subtypes. For example, antibody responses to both subtypes AE and B have been reported using a vaccine that contains gp120 subunits from both (Berman et al. 1999). As many countries are affected by more than one subtype, it is likely that any effective vaccine will be required to induce broad responses (Agwale et al. 2002; Novitsky et al. 2001) and, accordingly, genetic libraries are being developed to document HIV-1 genetic variability with the aim of improving vaccine design (Mukai et al. 2002).

In 1991, antisera from human volunteers immunized with recombinant gp120 immunogens were examined for their capacity to neutralize field isolates of HIV-1 grown in primary peripheral blood mononuclear cells (PBMC) (McCormack et al. 2000; Beddows et al. 1999). None of the vaccine sera neutralized any primary HIV-1 isolates, even when homologous in sequence to the laboratory adapted isolates which could be neutralized by these sera. These data showed that the neutralization of primary isolates could not be achieved by sera raised to recombinant proteins, although these field isolates could be neutralized by human antisera from HIV+ subjects. Further work (Spenlehauer et al. 1998; Zhang et al. 2002) showed that the neutralization of laboratory HIV-1 strains is predominantly through a linear epitope of 33 amino acids at the tip of the third variable domain of gp120, called the V3 loop. The V3 loop is expressed on the surface of gp120 in cell-line adapted viruses, and is also present and highly immunogenic on the surface of the recombinant gp120 molecules. However, primary isolates of HIV-1 have a more cryptic V3 epitope, and antibodies to V3 do not neutralize these primary isolates if grown in primary cells. The molecular explanation for this phenomenon was published in 1996, with the characterization of the chemokine co-receptors for HIV entry. Primary isolates use CCR5 as the principal coreceptor, which is present on activated $CD4^+$ T cells; laboratory-adapted HIV-1 isolates grown in immortalized, transformed T-cell lines use CXCR4 as the coreceptor, which is responsible for the over-expression of V3 in these isolates (see earlier section for references).

Up to the present, September 2004, it has not been possible to engineer a recombinant envelope gp120 which induces antibodies that can neutralize primary HIV-1 isolates in PBMCs. It is highly likely that such an immunogen will require extensive investigation from structural biologists who may be able to engineer a gp120 molecule in its native trimeric conformation with the capacity to induce neutralizing antibodies against primary isolates. However, no such molecule is currently on the horizon.

Notwithstanding these negative neutralization experiments, the $rgp120_{MN}$ molecule was taken to two full phase III trials in the USA, Holland, and Thailand, by VaxGen. The first of these trials in >7000 HIV-negative subjects at risk of HIV-1 infection reported in March 2003 (www.vaxgen.com/pressrom/index.html 2003; Francis et al. 2003); there was no protection against infection, with equal numbers of infections in the active and placebo groups. The negative results of this VaxGen $rgp120_{MN}$ study have been bitterly disappointing for a world desperate for a prophylactic HIV vaccine, but extremely important for science. The results confirm the predictive value of laboratory-adapted and primary isolate neutralization data, and also support the predictive value of the macaque SHIV animal challenge model (Feinberg and Moore 2002; Moore and Burton 1999).

In the absence of natural immunity to HIV-1, and without an immunogen capable of inducing neutralization of all subtypes, attention turned to other correlates of protection from HIV-1. Immunologists studied children born to HIV-infected mothers, where only 30 percent become infected; long-term survivors of HIV-1 infection who might have beneficial immune responses; the primary immune response to HIV-1 where there is some evidence of immune-mediated viral suppression and the phenomenon of highly HIV-exposed but persistently HIV-sero-negative subjects (HEPS). These HEPS have been repeatedly described throughout the AIDS epidemic in all risk-groups. Rowland-Jones (1999), studying HEPS prostitute women in Nairobi, Kenya, demonstrated that absence of HIV-1 infection, despite repeated exposure to the virus, was associated with the presence of detectable HIV-specific, HLA class-I-restricted $CD8^+$ cytotoxic T-lymphocytes (CTL). When these women ceased regular commercial sex work, exposure to HIV lessened and they became more susceptible to infection. Her hypothesis was that exposure to HIV could, in some circumstances, lead to the induction of a protective cellular immunity.

This observation has subsequently led to a considerable amount of animal and human clinical research on the induction of HIV-specific cellular immunity through immunization. McMichael's group has shown that a priming immunization with DNA followed by boosting with a modified vaccinia virus (such as modified vaccinia Ankara, MVA) bearing the same genetic insert is a potent inducer of HIV-specific CTL (Mwau et al. 2004). In the macaque model, induction of SIV-specific CTL through DNA-MVA prime–boost immunization fails to protect against challenge with a pathogenic $SHIV_{89.6}$, but does lead to significant disease attenuation in the macaques (McMichael and Hanke 2003). There are now several clinical trials in humans at phase I/II of promising CTL-inducing immunogens; these include naked DNA, adenovirus, vaccinia, alphaviruses, peptides, and viruslike particles (VLP). However, the prospect of a prophylactic HIV vaccine which does not protect, but which might slow disease progression in vaccines would be extremely difficult to test in human trials, and would not fully address the world's urgent need for the prevention of HIV infection.

Should an effective HIV vaccine be developed, the immense genetic diversity of the HIV epidemic will place great evolutionary pressure on the virus to escape from vaccine-induced immunity. As with the emergence of point mutations conferring resistance to antiretroviral drugs, so vaccine-induced immunity is likely to promote naturally occurring mutants with lower susceptibility to vaccine induced cellular immunity. Phillips and co-authors (1991) first described the phenomenon of viral escape from a CTL epitope in 1991; the potential emergence of this phenomenon will need to be investigated in parallel to phase III vaccine trials in the future.

In 2004, there is no HIV vaccine. It is generally believed that a successful HIV vaccine will need to induce both HIV-specific cellular immunity as well as potent, broadly reactive primary isolate neutralizing antibodies. The reality of the research portfolio currently is that this prospect appears to be remote.

HIV THERAPY AND THE EMERGENCE OF RESISTANCE

In the two decades since the first antiretroviral was serendipitously identified, drugs to combat HIV infection have been developed at an increasing rate. These fall into well-defined categories (Table 60.1), according to which aspect of the virion lifecycle is being inhibited (Figure 60.2). CART, consisting of at least three antiretroviral drugs, is the current standard of care for

Table 60.1 *Drugs designed to inhibit HIV-1*

Site of action	Drug class	Drug
Reverse transcriptase	Nucleoside analogues	Zidovudine (AZT/ ZDV)
		Didanosine (ddl)
		Zalcitabine (ddC)
		Stavudine (D4T)
		Lamivudine (3TC)
		Abacavir (ABC)
		Emtricitibine (FTC)
	Nucleotide analogues	Adefovir Dipivoxil[a]
		Tenofovir PMPA
	Nonnucleoside analogues	Nevirapine (NEV)
		Delavirdine (DLV)
		Efavirenz (EFV)
Protease	Protease inhibitors	Saquinavir (hard and soft gel) (SQV)
		Ritonavir (RTN)
		Nelfinavir (NEL)
		Indinavir (IND)
		Amprenavir (AMP)
		Lopinavir
		Tipranavir[a]
		Atazanavir[a]
Integrase	Integrase inhibitors	S-1360[a]
Co-receptors	CCR5 inhibitor	SCH-C[a]
	CXCR4 inhibitor	AMD-3100[a]
Gp41	Fusion inhibitor	Envufutide (T-20)
		T-1249[a]

Drugs that contribute to the majority of CART regimes currently prescribed. Standard CART regimes include two nucleoside analogues in conjunction with either a protease inhibitor or a nonnucleoside analogue.
a) Still in research stages, under trial or not fully licensed at time of writing.

HIV-1-infected patients (Pozniak et al. 2003), and the availability of assays in simple kit form to quantify peripheral virus load has complemented drug development to optimize patient care (Nolte 1999).

Drugs designed to inhibit HIV-1 RT

NUCLEOSIDE REVERSE TRANSCRIPTASE INHIBITORS (NRTI)

The essential action of the NRTI class is to mimic the natural host nucleoside triphosphate molecules (dNTP), which depends on replacing the hydroxyl group at the 3′ position of the deoxyribose sugar ring in the natural dNTPs by an alternative moiety in the drug (Figure 60.3). For example, the azido group at the 3′ position in Zidovudine (ZDV) (3′-azido-3-deoxthymidine, an analogue of thymidine, also called AZT or Retrovir and produced by GlaxoSmithKline) promotes

the drug's chain-termination activity (Figure 60.3). This compound was initially designed as an anti-tumor agent and was found to inhibit the HIV-1 RT (Mitsuya et al. 1985). It competes in vitro with natural host nucleosides and is incorporated into the lengthening DNA strand by the viral RT, resulting in chain termination.

The NRTIs can be divided into the thymidine analogues: ZDV and Stavudine (2′,3′-didehydro-3′-deoxythymidine) or D4T, and non-thymidine analogues: Didanosine (2′,3′-dideoxyinosine), ddI; Zalcitabine (2′,3′-dideoxycytidine), ddC; Lamivudine ((-)-2′-deoxy-3′-thio-thiadine), 3TC; Emtricitibine ((-)B-l-3′-thio-2′-3′-dideoxy-5-fluorocytidine), FTC and Abacavir (IS, 4R)-4-[2-amino-6(cyclopropyl amino)-9H-purin-9-yl]-2-cyclopentene-1-methanol succinate), ABC). Since the former act predominantly in dividing cells and the latter in resting cells, combinations of the two groups are often coprescribed. An early clinical trial, designated the DELTA study (Delta Coordinating Committee 1996) which investigated whether two NRTIs in combination were more effective than AZT alone in delaying disease progression, demonstrated that combining AZT with ddI or ddC conferred a survival advantage over AZT monotherapy and heralded the concept of combination therapy.

Initial treatment with AZT monotherapy resulted in viral rebound and the discovery of a genotypic pattern of resistance, as mutations emerged initially at codons 41 and 215, then at 67, 70, 210, and 219. An alternative pathway leading to AZT resistance and broad cross-class resistance is the 'Q151M complex' (Shirasaka et al. 1995) associated with mutations at codons 62, 75, 77, and 116. These mutations seem to act via interference with the dNTP binding site (Shirasaka et al. 1995). This is seen more commonly when AZT is prescribed with ddI or ddC and confers 320-fold resistance to AZT and cross-resistance to ddI, ddC, D4T, Abacavir, and 3TC.

NUCLEOTIDE REVERSE TRANSCRIPTASE INHIBITORS (NTRTI)

The NtRTI require two intracellular phosphorylation events for activity. Two drugs originally from Gilead Sciences (Adefovir dipivoxil and Tenofovir (bis-POC PMPA)) are already monophosphorylated and, therefore, require only a single monophosphorylation for activation. Adefovir, although not licensed following problems with renal toxicity, had shown potent reductions in viral load after one year of monotherapy and appeared to have a favorable resistance profile compared to the NRTIs. It was also active against herpes simplex virus, cytomegalovirus, and hepatitis B virus (Xiong et al. 1997; Merta et al. 1990). Tenofovir which has similar activity without the toxicity, received FDA approval in the United States in 2001.

Although Adefovir has been withdrawn, it was active against viruses with the RT mutation in codon 184 and with AZT resistance (Miller et al. 1999; Gu et al. 1995).

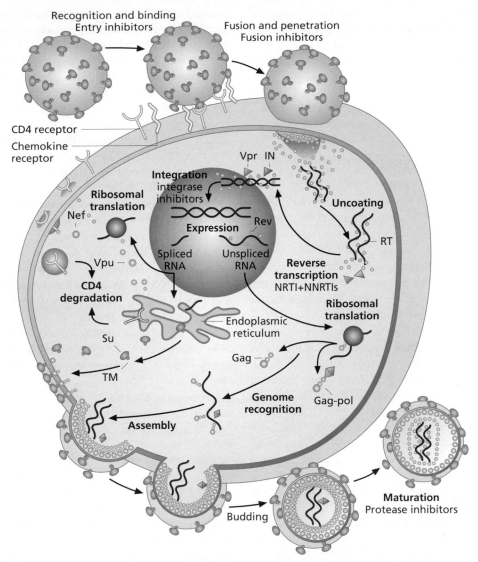

Figure 60.2 *The HIV-1 life cycle and site of action of antiretroviral drugs. Targets of drugs already approved for use by the FDA are shown in red. Others currently undergoing development and likely to be available for clinical trial in the near future are shown in blue. The HIV-1 core penetrates the host-cell post-entry via receptor-binding and fusion with the plasma membrane. Double-stranded proviral DNA resulting from the action of RT on the viral single-stranded RNA is translocated to the nucleus, where it is integrated into the host chromosomal DNA, courtesy of the viral integrase. Viral RNA is transcribed from the proviral DNA and viral proteins are translated from host cell ribosomes. New virions are assembled at the membrane from which they bud, maturing as they do so under the action of the viral protease. Redrawn from Pomerantz and Horn (2003) with permission.*

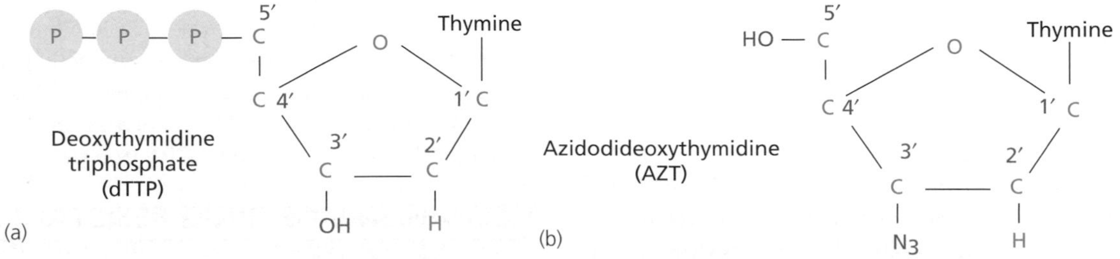

Figure 60.3 *Structure and mechanism of action of NRTIs. The structure of* **(a)** *the natural dNTP, deoxthymidine triphosphate (dTTP) and* **(b)** *azidodideoxythymidine (AZT, Zidovudine). The important difference is that the hydroxyl group attached to the carbon at position 3 of dTTP, which is vital to the DNA polymerase reaction, has been replaced by an azido group. Hence, when AZT is incorporated into the growing DNA strand, chain termination ensues.*

Mutations at codons 65 and 70 have been associated with resistance to Adefovir in vitro (Gu et al. 1995), and K70E has also been found in vivo (Mulato et al. 1998), although the significance of this is still undetermined. Interestingly, the activity of Adefovir against viruses containing the M184V mutation was 3–4-fold greater than against wild-type virus (Miller et al. 1999). Viruses containing the K65R and L210W mutation have reduced sensitivity to Tenofovir.

NONNUCLEOSIDE REVERSE TRANSCRIPTASE INHIBITORS (NNRTI)

The NNRTIs include Nevirapine, Efavirenz, Delavirdine, and the thiobenzimidazolone (TIBO) agents. These are noncompetitive inhibitors of RT (Spence et al. 1995) and bind to a specific site associated with codons 100–108 and 181–190 that provide the hydrophobic binding pocket within the polymerase domain of the p66 subunit of RT (Spence et al. 1995). These codons are also sites for key resistance mutations.

Although potent, the NNRTIs induce early resistance (Richman et al. 1994), often associated with mutations near codons 100 to 108 and 181 to 190, the locations of the drug-binding site. The Y181C mutation emerges rapidly in vitro, to cause 100-fold decrease in susceptibility to Nevirapine (Richman et al. 1991) and highly resistant strains have been identified in vivo within eight weeks of therapy (Richman et al. 1994; de Jong et al. 1997). Drug levels which exceed the IC_{50} of the resistant strains can be achieved in vivo using the higher dose of 400 mg, although with a higher incidence of side-effects (Havlir et al. 1995).

The K103N mutation seems to produce classwide resistance, including to newer drugs such as Efavirenz (DMP-266) (De Clercq 1998), although Efavirenz maintains some activity in the presence of the Y181C mutation (Jeffrey et al. 1998). The quinolone/quinoxaline class of NNRTIs, such as Nevirapine, also develop resistance through mutation at codon 190, but at the expense of enzymatic activity (Kleim et al. 1994). The major concern with NNRTIs is that only one mutation is required to induce resistance and, hence, they should be used in combination with other antiretroviral agents.

Drugs designed to inhibit HIV-1 protease

The viral protease acts to cleave and process the precursor proteins encoded by the *gag* and *gag–pol* genes. By inhibiting this posttranslational cleavage, the resultant virions are non-infectious. The RT inhibitors only block HIV-1 replication in acutely infected cells, whereas the protease inhibitors (PI) inhibit virus production from chronically infected cells, since they act at a late stage in the lifecycle (Lambert et al. 1992). The PIs inhibit the protease enzyme by acting as peptidomimetic competitive inhibitors at the enzymatic active site.

Therapy with PIs also appears to have a more suppressive effect on HIV-1 replication in lymph nodes than the RTIs (Gunthard et al. 1998a; Wong et al. 1997a).

Resistance and cross-resistance to PIs are well documented and at least 24 mutations have been identified in the 99 amino acid sequence (Figure 60.4). To provide prolonged efficacy, PIs need to be prescribed as part of a three-drug CART regime. Such regimes significantly reduce mortality and morbidity associated with HIV-1 infection (Palella et al. 1998) and, accordingly, have been given the acronym 'HAART,' for Highly Active Antiretroviral Therapy.

The interpretation of mutations associated with PI resistance is complex, especially with drugs such as Indinavir (Condra et al. 1996), when a large number of codons appear to be involved. Moreover, resistance is only one factor leading to drug failure. Others include the effects of bioavailability (Kupferschmidt et al. 1998; Vella and Floridia 1998; Perry and Noble 1998), cytochrome P450 metabolism (Wacher et al. 1998; Kupferschmidt et al. 1998), intolerance (Deeks et al. 1998; Sepkowitz et al. 1998; d'Arminio et al. 1998), and glycoprotein P transporter proteins (Kim et al. 1998; Wacher et al. 1998). Nevertheless, resistance remains a major cause of drug failure, and the issue of cross-resistance is becoming increasingly important, as failure on one PI may preclude the use of others (Condra et al. 1995).

A promising new class of antiretroviral agents are the 'Fusion inhibitors.' Two agents, T20 and T1249, bind to the HR1 domain of gp41 and disrupt the conformational change in this protein required for viral attachment and entry to the host cell (Kilby et al. 1998b; Lambert et al. 1999). As these drugs are peptides they cannot currently be given orally and, in addition, resistance has already been documented (Kilby et al. 1998b). Agents which bind to the co-receptors CCR5 (Simmons et al. 1997) and CXCR4 (Rusconi et al. 2000) or inhibit the -CD4 interaction (Jacobson et al. 2000) are also in development. For example, data on SCH-C, a CCR5 antagonist, have shown a 0.5 log_{10} reduction in viral load in a limited number of subjects over 10 days (Reynes et al. 2002). A CXCR4 antagonist termed AMD-3100 reduces viral load by 0.8 log_{10} RNA copies/ml (Schols et al. 2002), although antiviral potency has been questioned (Hendrix et al. 2002). The novel entry inhibitor BMS-806, is an antagonist of CD4-gp120 interactions and is still in preclinical development (Lin et al. 2002). It is active against multiple HIV-1 subtypes and against viruses displaying CXCR4 and CCR5 tropism.

MECHANISMS OF DRUG RESISTANCE

The infidelity of the retroviral RT results in a high mutation rate when viral genomic RNA is converted to DNA, as discussed. In the absence of complete viral inhibition, as might be associated with poor adherence,

MUTATIONS IN THE PROTEASE GENE ASSOCIATED WITH RESISTANCE

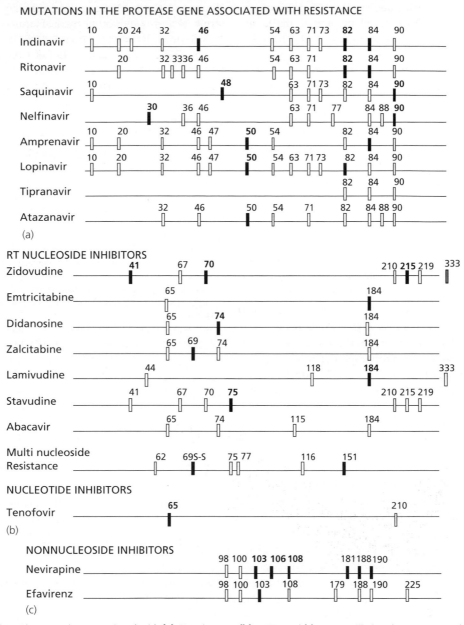

Figure 60.4 *Major point mutations associated with* (a) *PI resistance,* (b) *NRTI, and* (c) *NNRTI. Filled codons represent key mutations and white codons are secondary mutations.*

increased drug metabolism or drug sanctuary sites, there is increased opportunity for selection of drug-resistant mutants. According to the principles of natural selection, these variants soon become dominant and replicating viral RNA becomes detectable in the plasma. The recurrence of detectable plasma virus on therapy is often described as virological or therapeutic 'failure.' The point mutations in the *pol* gene that are commonly associated with drug resistance are detailed in Figure 60.4.

Although the genetic basis of HIV-1 drug resistance is well documented, the mechanisms underlying the loss of drug sensitivity are only now being understood. For the NRTI class of antiretroviral agents, there are two possible biochemical explanations for resistance. Either the retroviral RT develops increased ability to discriminate between natural dNTP molecules and inhibitors, or the enzyme acquires the ability to remove the chain-terminating inhibitors from the extending viral DNA in a process called 'pyrophosphorylysis' (Meyer et al. 1998; Boyer et al. 2001).

Certain mutations in HIV-1 RT decrease the activity of the nucleoside analogue by reducing its binding or altering the orientation of its binding so as to be unfavorable for incorporation. An example of such a mutation is the methionine to valine mutation at codon 184 of HIV-1 RT responsible for high-level resistance to 3TC and cross-resistance to other NRTIs (Tisdale et al. 1993). The beta-methyl group of the valine clashes sterically with the l-oxathiolane ring of 3TC, resulting in mal-positioning of 3TC-triphosphate and a markedly reduced incorporation of 3TC and other NRTIs into the viral cDNA.

The second mechanism, pyrophosphorylysis, is the opposite reaction to reverse transcription, resulting in the removal of chain-terminating inhibitors from the extending viral DNA (Meyer et al. 1998; Boyer et al. 2001). Some AZT resistance mutations enhance the ability of HIV-1 RT to excise AZT-monophosphate from the AZT-terminated cDNA, freeing up the 3' hydroxyl group (Figure 60.1) and allowing DNA polymerization to proceed. This excision reaction is catalyzed by ATP, and some AZT resistance mutations (e.g. 210W, 215Y/F) probably increase the binding affinity of ATP to the mutant enzyme. This enhanced excision capability of the mutant enzyme is not specific for AZT-monophosphate-terminated cDNA, and this helps to explain the cross-resistance observed between AZT and some other nucleoside analogues, such as D4T and Abacavir (Lennerstrand et al. 2001). Additionally, the 69SS mutation that confers multidrug resistance to the NRTI class also increases pyrophosphorylysis (Mas et al. 2000). Mutations such as M184V in RT, which confer resistance to 3TC, inhibit pyrophosphorylysis (Gotte et al. 2000). The M184V mutation alters the polymerase active site to interfere specifically with the ATP-mediated excision of AZT-MP from the end of the primer strand and, thereby, partially restores sensitivity to other NRTIs, such as AZT (Boyer et al. 2002).

The 20-year anniversary of the discovery of HIV-1 was celebrated in 2003. Within two decades research has changed the diagnosis of HIV infection in the western world from a certain death sentence to a manageable condition. However, viral latency (Wong et al. 1997b; Finzi et al. 1997), the recognition of tissue compartmentalization of replication which facilitates an evolutionary path independent of that taken by viruses in the periphery (Haggerty and Stevenson 1991; Zhu et al. 1996; Overbaugh et al. 1996; Zhang et al. 1998) and the persistence of low-level replication despite HAART (Dornadula et al. 1999; Dornadula et al. 2001), all conspire to undermine efforts to eradicate HIV-1 from infected hosts. Much remains to be understood of the way in which the virus responds in vivo to protect itself from annihilation, and further elucidation of the mechanism of replication will undoubtedly impact on the development of more novel and effective treatment regimens.

ACKNOWLEDGMENTS

We are thankful to the members of the laboratories at the Heinrich-Pette Institute (HPI), Hamburg, Germany and the Laboratory of Retrovirus Research at the Institute for Clinical and Molecular Virology, University of Erlangen-Nuremburg, and also Stefan Pöhlmann, Victor Wray, and Karin Metzner for comments on the manuscript. U.S. was supported by an Heisenberg grant from the German Research Council (DFG), and by DFG grants SFB-466-A11 and SFB 2003-A1, by grant IE-S08T06 from the German Human Genome Research, and by NIH/NIDDK RO1 grant DK59537-01.

REFERENCES

Agwale, S.M., Zeh, C., et al. 2002. Molecular surveillance of HIV-1 field strains in Nigeria in preparation for vaccine trials. *Vaccine*, **20**, 2131–9.

Aiken, C., Konner, J., et al. 1994. Nef induces CD4 endocytosis: requirement for a critical dileucine motif in the membrane-proximal CD4 cytoplasmic domain. *Cell*, **76**, 853-6, 4.

Akari, H., Bour, S., et al. 2001. The human immunodeficiency virus type 1 accessory protein Vpu induces apoptosis by suppressing the nuclear factor kappaB-dependent expression of antiapoptotic factors. *J Exp Med*, **194**, 1299–311.

Alaeus, A., Lidman, K., et al. 1999. Similar rate of disease progression among individuals infected with HIV-1 genetic subtypes A–D. *AIDS*, **13**, 901–7.

Alce, T.M. and Popik, W. 2004. APOBEC3G is incorporated into virus-like particles by a direct interaction with HIV-1 Gag nucleocapsid protein. *J Biol Chem*, **279**, 34083–6.

Amara, A. and Littman, D.R. 2003. After Hrs with HIV. *J Cell Biol*, **162**, 371-, 5.

Amornkul, P.N., Tansuphasawadikul, S., et al. 1999. Clinical disease associated with HIV-1 subtype B′ and E infection among 2104 patients in Thailand. *AIDS*, **13**, 1963–9.

Arora, A. and Seth, P. 2001. Immunization with HIV-1 subtype B gp160-DNA induces specific as well as cross reactive immune responses in mice. *Indian J Med Res*, **114**, 1–9.

Arora, V.K., Molina, R.P., et al. 2000. Lentivirus Nef specifically activates Pak2. *J Virol*, **74**, 11081–7.

Ayouba, A., Souquieres, S., et al. 2000. HIV-1 group N among HIV-1-seropositive individuals in Cameroon. *AIDS*, **14**, 2623–5.

Ayyavoo, V., Mahboubi, A., et al. 1997. HIV-1 Vpr suppresses immune activation and apoptosis through regulation of nuclear factor kappa B. *Nat Med*, **3**, 1117–23.

Ayyavoo, V., Kudchodkar, S., et al. 2000. Immunogenicity of a novel DNA vaccine cassette expressing multiple human immunodeficiency virus (HIV-1) accessory genes. *AIDS*, **14**, 1–9.

Babst, M., Odorizzi, G., et al. 2000. Mammalian tumor susceptibility gene 101 (TSG101) and the yeast homologue, Vps23p, both function in late endosomal trafficking. *Traffic*, **1**, 248–58.

Bache, K.G., Brech, A., et al. 2003. Hrs regulates multivesicular body formation via ESCRT recruitment to endosomes. *J Cell Biol*, **162**, 3, 435–42.

Barouch, D.H., Kunstman, J., et al. 2002. Eventual AIDS vaccine failure in a rhesus monkey by viral escape from cytotoxic T lymphocytes. *Nature*, **415**, 335–9.

Beddows, S., Lister, S., et al. 1999. Comparison of the antibody repertoire generated I healthy volunteers following immunization with a monomeric recombinant gp120 construct derived from a CCR5/CXCR4-using human immunodeficiency virus type 1 isolate with sera from naturally infected individuals. *J Virol*, **73**, 1740–5.

Berger, E.A., Murphy, P.M. and Farber, J.M. 1999. Chemokine receptors as HIV-1 coreceptors: roles in viral entry, tropism, and disease. *Annu Rev Immunol*, **17**, 657–700.

Berman, P.W., Huang, W., et al. 1999. Development of bivalent (B/E) vaccines able to neutralize CCR5-dependent viruses from the United States and Thailand. *Virology*, **265**, 1–9.

Bollinger, R.C., Tripathy, S.P. and Quinn, T.C. 1995. The human immunodeficiency virus epidemic in India. Current magnitude and future projections. *Medicine*, **74**, 97–106.

Bongertz, V. and Bou-Habib, D.C. 2000. HIV-1 diversity in Brazil: genetic, biologic, and immunologic characterization of HIV-1 strains in three potential HIV vaccine evaluation sites. Brazilian Network for HIV Isolation and Characterization. *J Acquir Immune Defic Syndr*, **23**, 184–93.

Bour, S. and Strebel, K. 2003. The HIV-1 Vpu protein: a multifunctional enhancer of viral particle release. *Microbes Infect*, **5**, 1029–39.

Bour, S., Geleziunas, R. and Wainberg, M.A. 1995. The human immunodeficiency virus type 1 (HIV-1) CD4 receptor and its central role in promotion of HIV-1 infection. *Microbiol Rev*, **59**, 63–93.

Boyer, P.L., Sarafianos, S.G., et al. 2001. Selective excision of AZTMP by drug-resistant human immunodeficiency virus reverse transcriptase. *J Virol*, **75**, 4832–42.

Boyer, P.L., Sarafianos, S.G., et al. 2002. The M184V mutation reduces the selective excision of zidovudine 5′-monophosphate (AZTMP) by the reverse transcriptase of human immunodeficiency virus type 1. *J Virol*, **76**, 3248–56.

Braaten, D. and Luban, J. 2001. Cyclophilin A regulates HIV-1 infectivity, as demonstrated by gene targeting in human T cells. *EMBO J*, **20**, 1300–9.

Bruns, K., Fossen, T., et al. 2003. Structural characterization of the HIV-1 Vpr N Terminus: Evidence OF *cis/trans*-proline isomerism. *J Biol Chem*, **278**, 43188–201.

Bukrinsky, M. and Adzhubei, A. 1999. Viral protein R of HIV-1. *Rev Med Virol*, **9**, 39–49.

Bures, R., Morris, L., et al. 2002. Regional clustering of shared neutralization determinants on primary isolates of clade C human immunodeficiency virus type 1 from South Africa. *J Virol*, **76**, 2233–44.

Cafaro, A., Caputo, A., et al. 1999. Control of SHIV-89.6P-infection of cynomolgus monkeys by HIV-1 Tat protein vaccine. *Nat Med*, **5**, 643–50.

Cameron, D.W., Simonsen, J.N., et al. 1989. Female to male transmission of human immunodeficiency virus type 1: risk factors for seroconversion in men. *Lancet*, **2**, 403–7.

Campodonico, M., Janssens, W., et al. 1996. HIV type 1 subtypes in Argentina and genetic heterogeneity of the V3 region. *AIDS Res Hum Retroviruses*, **12**, 79–81.

Cao, H., Mani, I., et al. 2000. Cellular immunity to human immunodeficiency virus type 1 (HIV-1) clades: relevance to HIV-1 vaccine trials in Uganda. *J Infect Dis*, **182**, 1350–6.

Carr, J.K., Salminen, M.O., et al. 1996. Full-length sequence and mosaic structure of a human immunodeficiency virus type 1 isolate from Thailand. *J Virol*, **70**, 5935–43.

Carr, J.K., Salminen, M.O., et al. 1998. Full genome sequences of human immunodeficiency virus type 1 subtypes G and A/G intersubtype recombinants. *Virology*, **247**, 22–31.

Caselli, E., Betti, M., et al. 1999. DNA immunization with HIV-1 tat mutated in the trans activation domain induces humoral and cellular immune responses against wild-type Tat. *J Immunol*, **162**, 5631–8.

Chun, T.W., Stuyver, L., et al. 1997. Presence of an inducible HIV-1 latent reservoir during highly active antiretroviral therapy. *Proc Natl Acad Sci USA*, **94**, 13193–7.

Clarke, J.R., Galpin, S., et al. 2000. Comparative quantification of diverse serotypes of HIV-1 in plasma from a diverse population of patients. *J Med Virol*, **62**, 445–9.

Coady, M.J., Daniel, N.G., et al. 1998. Effects of Vpu expression on Xenopus oocyte membrane conductance. *Virology*, **244**, 39–49.

Coffin, J., Hughes, S. and Varmus, H. 1997. *Retroviruses*. Plainview, NY: Cold Spring Harbor Press.

Cohen, E.A., Terwilliger, E.F., et al. 1988. Identification of a protein encoded by the vpu gene of HIV-1. *Nature*, **334**, 532–4.

Cohen, E.A., Subbramanian, R.A. and Gottlinger, H.G. 1996. Role of auxiliary proteins in retroviral morphogenesis. *Curr Top Microbiol Immunol*, **214**, 219–35.

Collins, K.L., Chen, B.K., et al. 1998. HIV-1 Nef protein protects infected primary cells against killing by cytotoxic T lymphocytes. *Nature*, **391**, 397–401.

Condra, J.H., Schleif, W.A., et al. 1995. In vivo emergence of HIV-1 variants resistant to multiple protease inhibitors. *Nature*, **374**, 569–71.

Condra, J.H., Holder, D.J., et al. 1996. Genetic correlates of in vivo viral resistance to indinavir, a human immunodeficiency virus type 1 protease inhibitor. *J Virol*, **70**, 8270–6.

Conti, L., Matarrese, P., et al. 2000. Dual role of the HIV-1 vpr protein in the modulation of the apoptotic response of T cells. *J Immunol*, **165**, 3293–300.

Corey, L., McElrath, M.J., et al. 1998. Cytotoxic T cell and neutralizing antibody responses to human immunodeficiency virus type 1 envelope with a combination vaccine regimen. AIDS Vaccine Evaluation Group. *J Infect Dis*, **177**, 301–9.

Coste, J., Montes, B., et al. 1996. Comparative evaluation of three assays for the quantitation of human immunodeficiency virus type 1 RNA in plasma. *J Med Virol*, **50**, 293–302.

d'Arminio, M.A., Testa, L., et al. 1998. Clinical outcome and predictive factors of failure of highly active antiretroviral therapy in antiretroviral-experienced patients in advanced stages of HIV-1 infection. *AIDS*, **12**, 1631–7.

de Baar, M.P., Timmermans, E.C., et al. 2001. One-tube real-time isothermal amplification assay to identify and distinguish human immunodeficiency virus type 1 subtypes A, B, and C and circulating recombinant forms AE and AG. *J Clin Microbiol*, **39**, 1895–902.

De Clercq, E. 1998. The role of non-nucleoside reverse transcriptase inhibitors (NNRTIs) in the therapy of HIV-1 infection. *Antiviral Res*, **38**, 153–79.

de Jong, M.D., Vella, S., et al. 1997. High-dose nevirapine in previously untreated human immunodeficiency virus type 1-infected persons does not result in sustained suppression of viral replication. *J Infect Dis*, **175**, 966–70.

Dean, M., Carrington, M., et al. 1996. Genetic restriction of HIV-1 infection and progression to AIDS by a deletion allele of the CKR5 structural gene. Hemophilia Growth and Development Study, Multicenter AIDS Cohort Study, Multicenter Hemophilia Cohort Study, San Francisco City Cohort, ALIVE Study. *Science*, **274**, 1069.

Deeks, S.G., Grant, R.M., et al. 1998. Activity of a ritonavir plus saquinavir-containing regimen in patients with virologic evidence of indinavir or ritonavir failure. *AIDS*, **12**, F97–102.

del Mar Pujades, R.M., Obasi, A., et al. 2002. Herpes simplex virus type 2 infection increases HIV incidence: a prospective study in rural Tanzania. *AIDS*, **16**, 451–62.

Demirov, D.G., Orenstein, J.M. and Freed, E.O. 2002. The late domain of human immunodeficiency virus type 1 p6 promotes virus release in a cell type-dependent manner. *J Virol*, **76**, 105–17.

Deng, H., Liu, R., et al. 1996. Identification of a major co-receptor for primary isolates of HIV-1. *Nature*, **381**, 661–6.

de Noronha, C.M., Sherman, M.P., et al. 2001. Dynamic disruptions in nuclear envelope architecture and integrity induced by HIV-1 Vpr. *Science*, **294**, 1105–8.

de Rocquigny, H., Petitjean, P., et al. 1997. The zinc fingers of HIV nucleocapsid protein NCp7 direct interactions with the viral regulatory protein Vpr. *J Biol Chem*, **272**, 30753–9.

de Rocquigny, H., Caneparo, A., et al. 2000. Interactions of the C-terminus of viral protein R with nucleic acids are modulated by its N-terminus. *Eur J Biochem*, **267**, 3654–60.

Di Stefano, M., Gray, F., et al. 1996. Analysis of ENV V3 sequences from HIV-1-infected brain indicates restrained virus expression throughout the disease. *J Med Virol*, **49**, 41–8.

Doolittle, R.F., Feng, D.F., et al. 1990. Retrovirus phylogeny and evolution. *Curr Top Microbiol Immunol*, **157**, 1–18.

Dornadula, G., Zhang, H., et al. 1999. Residual HIV-1 RNA in blood plasma of patients taking suppressive highly active antiretroviral therapy. *JAMA*, **282**, 1627–32.

Dornadula, G., Yang, S., et al. 2000. Partial rescue of the Vif-negative phenotype of mutant human immunodeficiency virus type 1 strains from nonpermissive cells by intravirion reverse transcription. *J Virol*, **74**, 2594–602.

Dornadula, G., Nunnari, G., et al. 2001. Human immunodeficiency virus type-1-infected persons with residual disease and virus reservoirs on suppressive highly active antiretroviral therapy can be stratified into relevant virologic and immunological subgroups. *J Infect Dis*, **183**, 1682–7.

Dorrell, L., Dong, T., et al. 1999. Distinct recognition of non-clade B human immunodeficiency virus type 1 epitopes by cytotoxic T lymphocytes generated from donors infected in Africa. *J Virol*, **73**, 1708–14.

Embretson, J., Zupancic, M., et al. 1993. Massive covert infection of helper T lymphocytes and macrophages by HIV during the incubation period of AIDS. *Nature*, **362**, 359–62.

Ernest, I., Alexandre, I., et al. 2001. Quantitative assay for group M (subtype A-H) and group O HIV-1 RNA detection in plasma. *J Virol Methods*, **93**, 1–14.

Ewart, G.D., Sutherland, T., et al. 1996. The Vpu protein of human immunodeficiency virus type 1 forms cation-selective ion channels. *J Virol*, **70**, 7108–15.

Fackler, O.T. and Baur, A.S. 2002. Live and let die: Nef functions beyond HIV replication. *Immunity*, **16**, 493–7.

Farnet, C.M. and Bushman, F.D. 1997. HIV-1 cDNA integration: requirement of HMG I(Y) protein for function of preintegration complexes in vitro. *Cell*, **88**, 483–92.

Fawzi, W., Msamanga, G., et al. 2001. Predictors of intrauterine and intrapartum transmission of HIV-1 among Tanzanian women. *AIDS*, **15**, 1157–65.

Feinberg, M.B. and Moore, J.P. 2002. AIDS vaccine models: challenging challenge viruses. *Nat Med*, **8**, 207–10.

Felzien, L.K., Woffendin, C., et al. 1998. HIV transcriptional activation by the accessory protein, VPR, is mediated by the p300 co-activator. *Proc Natl Acad Sci USA*, **95**, 5281–6.

Ferrari, G., Humphrey, W., et al. 1997. Clade B-based HIV-1 vaccines elicit cross-clade cytotoxic T lymphocyte reactivities in uninfected volunteers. *Proc Natl Acad Sci USA*, **94**, 1396–401.

Finzi, D., Hermankova, M., et al. 1997. Identification of a reservoir for HIV-1 in patients on highly active antiretroviral therapy. *Science*, **278**, 1295–300.

Fischer, W.B. and Sansom, M.S. 2002. Viral ion channels: structure and function. *Biochim Biophys Acta*, **1561**, 27–45.

Francis, D.P., Heyward, W.L., et al. 2003. Candidate HIV/AIDS vaccines: lessons learned from the world's first phase III efficacy trials. *AIDS*, **17**, 147–56.

Frankel, A.D. 1998. HIV-1: fifteen proteins and RNA. *Annu Rev Biochem*, **67**, 1–25.

Freed, E.O. 2001. HIV-1 replication. *Somat Cell Mol Genet*, **26**, 13–33.

Freed, E.O. 2002. Viral late domains. *J Virol*, **76**, 4679–87.

Gaines, H., von Sydow, M., et al. 1987. Antibody response in primary human immunodeficiency virus infection. *Lancet*, **854**, 1249–53.

Gao, F., Robertson, D.L., et al. 1996. The heterosexual human immunodeficiency virus type 1 epidemic in Thailand is caused by an intersubtype (A/E) recombinant of African origin. *J Virol*, **70**, 7013–29.

Garcia, J.V. and Miller, A.D. 1991. Serine phosphorylation-independent downregulation of cell-surface CD4 by nef. *Nature*, **350**, 6318, 508–11.

Garrus, J.E., von Schwedler, U.K., et al. 2001. Tsg101 and the vacuolar protein sorting pathway are essential for HIV-1 budding. *Cell*, **107**, 55–65.

Gibbs, J.S., Lackner, A.A., et al. 1995. Progression to AIDS in the absence of a gene for vpr or vpx. *J Virol*, **69**, 2378–83.

Goedert, J.J., Biggar, R.J., et al. 1987. Effect of T4 count and cofactors on the incidence of AIDS in homosexual men infected with human immunodeficiency virus. *JAMA*, **257**, 331–4.

Goh, W.C., Rogel, M.E., et al. 1998. HIV-1 Vpr increases viral expression by manipulation of the cell cycle: A mechanism for selection of Vpr *in vivo*. *Nat Med*, **4**, 65–71.

Goldstein, G., Tribbick, G. and Manson, K. 2001. Two B cell epitopes of HIV-1 Tat protein have limited antigenic polymorphism in geographically diverse HIV-1 strains. *Vaccine*, **19**, 1738–46.

Gotte, M., Arion, D., et al. 2000. The M184V mutation in the reverse transcriptase of human immunodeficiency virus type 1 impairs rescue of chain-terminated DNA synthesis. *J Virol*, **74**, 3579–85.

Göttlinger, H.G., Dorfman, T., et al. 1991. Effect of mutations affecting the p6 gag protein on human immunodeficiency virus particle release. *Proc Natl Acad Sci USA*, **88**, 3195–9.

Greene, W.C. and Peterlin, B.M. 2002. Charting HIV's remarkable voyage through the cell: Basic science as a passport to the future therapy. *Nat Med*, **8**, 673–80.

Gu, Z., Salomon, H., et al. 1995. K65R mutation of human immunodeficiency virus type 1 reverse transcriptase encodes cross-resistance to 9-(2-phosphonylmethoxyethyl)adenine. *Antimicrob Agents Chemother*, **39**, 1888–91.

Gunthard, H.F., Wong, J.K., et al. 1998a. Human immunodeficiency virus replication and genotypic resistance in blood and lymph nodes after a year of potent antiretroviral therapy. *J Virol*, **72**, 2422–8.

Gupta, K., Hudgens, M., et al. 2002. Safety and immunogenicity of a high-titered canarypox vaccine in combination with rgp120 in a diverse population of HIV-1-uninfected adults: AIDS Vaccine Evaluation Group Protocol 022A. *J Acquir Immune Defic Syndr*, **29**, 254–61.

Gurtler, L.G., Hauser, P.H., et al. 1994. A new subtype of human immunodeficiency virus type 1 (MVP-5180) from Cameroon. *J Virol*, **68**, 1581–8.

Haggerty, S. and Stevenson, M. 1991. Predominance of distinct viral genotypes in brain and lymph node compartments of HIV-1 infected individuals. *Viral Immunol*, **4**, 123–31.

Harris, R.S., Bishop, K.N., et al. 2003. DNA deamination mediates innate immunity to retroviral infection. *Cell*, **113**, 803–9.

Havlir, D., Cheeseman, S.H., et al. 1995. High-dose nevirapine: safety, pharmacokinetics, and antiviral effect in patients with human immunodeficiency virus infection. *J Infect Dis*, **171**, 537–45.

Heinzinger, N.K., Bukrinsky, M.I., et al. 1994. The Vpr protein of human immunodeficiency virus type 1 influences nuclear localization of viral nucleic acids in nondividing host cells. *Proc Natl Acad Sci USA*, **91**, 7311–15.

Hellerstein, M., Hanley, M.B., et al. 1999. Directly measured kinetics of circulating T lymphocytes in normal and HIV-1-infected humans. *Nat Med*, **5**, 83–9.

Hendrix, C., Collier, A., Lederman, M., et al. 2002. AMD-3100 CXCR4 Receptor Blocker Fails to Reduce HIV Viral Load by > 1 Log following 10-Day Continuous Infusion. *9th Conference on Retroviruses and Opportunistic Infections. 24–28 Feb 2002, Seattle, WA* Abstract 391.

Henklein, P., Bruns, K., et al. 2000a. Functional and structural characterization of synthetic Vpr from HIV-1 that transduces cells, localizes to the nucleus and induces G_2 cell cycle arrest. *J Biol Chem*, **275**, 32016–26.

Henklein, P., Kinder, R., et al. 2000b. Membrane interactions and alignment of structures within the HIV-1 Vpu cytoplasmic domain: effect of phosphorylation of serines 52 and 56. *FEBS Lett*, **482**, 220–4.

Ho, D.D. 1997. Perspectives series: host/pathogen interactions. Dynamics of HIV-1 replication in vivo. *J Clin Invest*, **99**, 2565–7.

Ho, D.D., Moudgil, T. and Alam, M. 1989. Quantitation of human immunodeficiency virus type 1 in the blood of infected persons. *N Engl J Med*, **321**, 1621–5.

Ho, D.D., Neumann, A.U., et al. 1995. Rapid turnover of plasma virions and CD4 lymphocytes in HIV-1 infection. *Nature*, **373**, 123–6.

Holguin, A., de Mendoza, C. and Soriano, V. 1999. Comparison of three different commercial methods for measuring plasma viraemia in patients infected with non-B HIV-1 subtypes. *Eur J Clin Microbiol Infect Dis*, **18**, 256–9.

Hsu, K., Seharaseyon, J., et al. 2004. Mutual functional destruction of HIV-1 Vpu and host TASK-1 channel. *Mol Cell*, **14**, 259–67.

Huang, M., Orenstein, J., et al. 1995. p6Gag is required for particle production from full-length human immunodeficiency virus type 1 molecular clones expressing protease. *J Virol*, **69**, 6810–18.

Huet, T., Cheynier, R., et al. 1990. Genetic organization of a chimpanzee lentivirus related to HIV-1. *Nature*, **345**, 356–9.

Hull, R. 2001. Classifying reverse transcribing elements. *Arch Virol*, **146**, 2255–61.

Ivery, M.T. 2000. Immunophilins: switched on protein binding domains? *Med Res Rev*, **20**, 452–84.

Jacobson, J.M., Lowy, I., et al. 2000. Single-dose safety, pharmacology, and antiviral activity of the human immunodeficiency virus (HIV) type 1 entry inhibitor PRO 542 in HIV-infected adults. *J Infect Dis*, **182**, 326–9.

Jacotot, E., Ravagnan, L., et al. 2000. The HIV-1 viral protein R induces apoptosis via a direct effect on the mitochondrial permeability transition pore. *J Exp Med*, **191**, 33–46.

Jacotot, E., Ferri, K.F., et al. 2001. Control of mitochondrial membrane permeabilization by adenine nucleotide translocator interacting with HIV-1 viral protein rR and Bcl-2. *J Exp Med*, **193**, 509–19.

Jeffrey, S., Baker, D. and Tritch, R. 1998. Resistance profile for Sustiva (Efavirenz, DMP266). *5th Conference on Retroviruses and Opportunistic Infections, Chicago, USA* Abstract 702.

Jenkins, Y., McEntee, M., et al. 1998. Characterization of HIV-1 vpr nuclear import: analysis of signals and pathways. *J Cell Biol*, **143**, 875–85.

Kaleebu, P., French, N., et al. 2002. Effect of human immunodeficiency virus (HIV) type 1 envelope subtypes A and D on disease progression in a large cohort of HIV-1-positive persons in Uganda. *J Infect Dis*, **185**, 1244–50.

Kanki, P.J., Hamel, D.J., et al. 1999. Human immunodeficiency virus type 1 subtypes differ in disease progression. *J Infect Dis*, **179**, 68–73.

Katzmann, D.J., Odorizzi, G. and Emr, S.D. 2002. Receptor downregulation and multivesicular-body sorting. *Nat Rev Mol Cell Biol*, **3**, 12, 893–905.

Kerkau, T., Bacik, I., et al. 1997. The human immunodeficiency virus type 1 (HIV-1) Vpu protein interferes with an early step in the biosynthesis of major histocompatibility complex (MHC) class I molecules. *J Exp Med*, **185**, 1295–305.

Kestler 3rd, H.W., Ringler, D.J., et al. 1991. Importance of the nef gene for maintenance of high virus loads and for development of AIDS. *Cell*, **65**, 651–62.

Khan, M.A., Aberham, C., et al. 2001. Human immunodeficiency virus type 1 Vif protein is packaged into the nucleoprotein complex through an interaction with viral genomic RNA. *J Virol*, **75**, 7252–65.

Khatissian, E., Monceaux, V., et al. 2001. Persistence of pathogenic challenge virus in macaques protected by simian immunodeficiency virus SIVmacDeltanef. *J Virol*, **75**, 1507–15.

Kievits, T., van Gemen, B., et al. 1991. NASBA isothermal enzymatic in vitro nucleic acid amplification optimized for the diagnosis of HIV-1 infection. *J Virol Methods*, **35**, 273–86.

Kilby, J.M., Hopkins, S., et al. 1998b. Potent suppression of HIV-1 replication in humans by T-20, a peptide inhibitor of gp41-mediated virus entry. *Nat Med*, **4**, 1302–7.

Kim, A.E., Dintaman, J.M., et al. 1998. Saquinavir, an HIV protease inhibitor, is transported by P-glycoprotein. *J Pharmacol Exp Ther*, **286**, 1439–45.

Kino, T., Gragerov, A., et al. 1999. The HIV-1 virion-associated protein vpr is a coactivator of the human glucocorticoid receptor. *J Exp Med*, **1**, 51–61.

Kleim, J.P., Bender, R., et al. 1994. Mutational analysis of residue 190 of human immunodeficiency virus type 1 reverse transcriptase. *Virology*, **200**, 696–701.

Koch, W.H., Sullivan, P.S., et al. 2001. Evaluation of United States-licensed human immunodeficiency virus immunoassays for detection of group M viral variants. *J Clin Microbiol*, **39**, 1017–20.

Komoto, S., Tsuji, S., et al. 2003. The vpu protein of human immunodeficiency virus type 1 plays a protective role against virus-induced apoptosis in primary CD4$^+$ T lymphocytes. *J Virol*, **77**, 10304–13.

Korber, B.T., Allen, E.E., et al. 1995. Heterogeneity of HIV-1 and HIV-2. *AIDS*, **9**, Suppl. A, S5–18.

Kräusslich, H.G. and Welker, R. 1996. Intracellular transport of retroviral capsid components. *Curr Top Microbiol Immunol*, **214**, 25–63.

Kupferschmidt, H.H., Fattinger, K.E., et al. 1998. Grapefruit juice enhances the bioavailability of the HIV protease inhibitor saquinavir in man. *Br J Clin Pharmacol*, **45**, 355–9.

Lama, J., Mangasarian, A. and Trono, D. 1999. Cell surface expression of CD4 reduces HIV-1 infectivity by blocking Env incorporation in a Nef and Vpu inhibitable manner. *Curr Biol*, **9**, 622–31.

Lamb, R.A. and Pinto, L.H. 1997. Do Vpu and Vpr of human immunodeficiency virus type 1 and NB of influenza B virus have ion channel activities in the viral life cycles? *Virology*, **229**, 1–11.

Lambert, D.M., Petteway-SR, J., et al. 1992. Human immunodeficiency virus type 1 protease inhibitors irreversibly block infectivity of purified virions from chronically infected cells. *Antimicrob Agents Chemother*, **36**, 982–8.

Lambert, D., Zhou, J. and Medinas, R. 1999. T1249, a second generation hybrid synthetic peptide inhibitor of HIV: isolates from T20-treated patients are sensitive to T1249. *3rd International Workshop on HIV Drug Resistance and Treatment Strategies. 23–26 June 1999, San Diego, USA* Abstract 10.

Lang, S.M., Weeger, M., et al. 1993. Importance of vpr for infection of rhesus monkeys with simian immunodeficiency virus. *J Virol*, **67**, 902–12.

Larder, B.A., Bloor, S., et al. 1999. A family of insertion mutations between codons 67 and 70 of human immunodeficiency virus type 1 reverse transcriptase confer multinucleoside analog resistance. *Antimicrob Agents Chemother*, **43**, 1961–7.

Le Gall, S., Buseyne, F., et al. 2000. Distinct trafficking pathways mediate Nef-induced and clathrin-dependent major histocompatibility complex class I down-regulation. *J Virol*, **74**, 9256–66.

Lennerstrand, J., Stammers, D.K. and Larder, B.A. 2001. Biochemical mechanism of human immunodeficiency virus type 1 reverse transcriptase resistance to stavudine. *Antimicrob Agents Chemother*, **45**, 2144–6.

Levy, D.N., Fernandes, L.S., et al. 1993. Induction of cell differentiation by human immunodeficiency virus 1 vpr. *Cell*, **72**, 541–50.

Lewis, P.F. and Emerman, M. 1994. Passage through mitosis is required for oncoretroviruses but not for the human immunodeficiency virus. *J Virol*, **68**, 510–16.

Liitsola, K., Tashkinova, I., et al. 1998. HIV-1 genetic subtype A/B recombinant strain causing an explosive epidemic in injecting drug users in Kaliningrad. *AIDS*, **12**, 1907–19.

Lin, P.F., Robinson, B.S., et al. 2002. Identification and Characterization of a Novel Inhibitor of HIV-1 Entry – I: Virology and Resistance. *9th Conference on Retroviruses and Opportunistic Infections. 24-28-4 Feb 2002, Seattle, WA* Abstract 9.

Louwagie, J., McCutchan, F.E., et al. 1993. Phylogenetic analysis of gag genes from 70 international HIV-1 isolates provides evidence for multiple genotypes. *AIDS*, **7**, 769–80.

Luban, J. 1996. Absconding with the chaperone: essential cyclophilin-Gag interaction in HIV-1 virions. *Cell*, **87**, 7, 1157–9.

Luban, J. 2001. HIV-1 and Ebola virus: the getaway driver nabbed. *Nat Med*, **12**, 1278–80.

Lukashov, V.V., Cornelissen, M.T., et al. 1995. Simultaneous introduction of distinct HIV-1 subtypes into different risk groups in Russia, Byelorussia and Lithuania. *AIDS*, **9**, 435–9.

Ma, C., Marassi, F.M., et al. 2002. Expression, purification, and activities of full-length and truncated versions of the integral membrane protein Vpu from HIV-1. *Protein Sci*, **11**, 546–57.

Maldarelli, F., Chen, M.Y., et al. 1993. Human immunodeficiency virus type 1 Vpu protein is an oligomeric type 1 integral membrane protein. *J Virol*, **67**, 5056–61.

Mangeat, B., Turelli, P., et al. 2003. Broad antiretroviral defence by human APOBEC3G through lethal editing of nascent reverse transcripts. *Nature*, **424**, 99–103.

Mansky, L.M. and Temin, H.M. 1995. Lower in vivo mutation rate of human immunodeficiency virus type 1 than that predicted from the fidelity of purified reverse transcriptase. *J Virol*, **69**, 5087–94.

Marassi, F.M., Ma, C., et al. 1999. Correlation of the structural and functional domains in the membrane protein Vpu from HIV-1. *Proc Natl Acad Sci USA*, **96**, 14336–41.

Margottin, F., Bour, S.P., et al. 1998. A novel human WD protein, h-beta TrCp, that interacts with HIV-1 Vpu connects CD4 to the ER degradation pathway through an F-box motif. *Mol Cell*, **1**, 565–74.

Marlink, R., Kanki, P., et al. 1994. Reduced rate of disease development after HIV-2 infection as compared to HIV-1. *Science*, **265**, 1587–90.

Marsh, J.W. 1999. The numerous effector functions of Nef. *Arch Biochem Biophys*, **365**, 192–8.

Martin-Serrano, J., Zang, T. and Bieniasz, P.D. 2001. HIV-1 and Ebola virus encode small peptide motifs that recruit Tsg101 to sites of particle assembly to facilitate egress. *Nat Med*, **7**, 1313–19.

Martin-Serrano, J., Zang, T. and Bieniasz, P.D. 2003. Role of ESCRT-I in retroviral budding. *J Virol*, **77**, 4794–804.

Mas, A., Parera, M., et al. 2000. Role of a dipeptide insertion between codons 69 and 70 of HIV-1 reverse transcriptase in the mechanism of AZT resistance. *EMBO J*, **19**, 5752–61.

Masciotra, S., Rudolph, D.L., et al. 2000. Serological detection of infection with diverse human and simian immunodeficiency viruses using consensus env peptides. *Clin Diagn Lab Immunol*, **7**, 706–9.

Mascola, J.R., Louwagie, J., et al. 1994. Two antigenically distinct subtypes of human immunodeficiency virus type 1: viral genotype predicts neutralization serotype. *J Infect Dis*, **169**, 48–54.

Mauclere, P., Loussert-Ajaka, I., et al. 1997. Serological and virological characterization of HIV-1 group O infection in Cameroon. *AIDS*, **11**, 445–53.

McCormack, S.T., Tilzey, A., et al. 2000. A phase I trial in HIV negative healthy volunteers evaluating the effect of potent adjuvants on immunogenecity of a recombinant gp120$_{W61D}$ derived from dual tropic R5X4 HIV-1$_{ACH320}$. *Vaccine*, **18**, 1166–77.

McCutchan, F.E., Hegerich, P.A., et al. 1992. Genetic variants of HIV-1 in Thailand. *AIDS Res Hum Retroviruses*, **8**, 1887–95.

McMichael, A.J. and Hanke, T. 2003. HIV vaccines 1983-2003. *Nat Med*, **9**, 874–80.

McNearney, T., Hornickova, Z., et al. 1992. Relationship of human immunodeficiency virus type 1 sequence heterogeneity to stage of disease. *Proc Natl Acad Sci*, **89**, 10247–51.

Mellors, J.W., Rinaldo-CR, J., et al. 1996. Prognosis in HIV-1 infection predicted by the quantity of virus in plasma. *Science*, **272**, 1167–70.

Merta, A., Votruba, I., et al. 1990. Inhibition of herpes simplex virus DNA polymerase by diphosphates of acyclic phosphonylmethoxyalkyl nucleotide analogues. *Antiviral Res*, **13**, 209–18.

Meyer, P.R., Matsuura, S.E., et al. 1998. Unblocking of chain-terminated primer by HIV-1 reverse transcriptase through a nucleotide-dependent mechanism. *Proc Natl Acad Sci USA*, **95**, 13471–6.

Miller, M.D., Anton, K.E., et al. 1999. Human immunodeficiency virus type 1 expressing the lamivudine- associated M184V mutation in reverse transcriptase shows increased susceptibility to adefovir and decreased replication capability in vitro. *J Infect Dis*, **179**, 92–100.

Mitsuya, H., Weinhold, K.J., et al. 1985. 3′-Azido-3′-deoxythymidine (BW A509U): an antiviral agent that inhibits the infectivity and cytopathic effect of human T-lymphotropic virus type III/ lymphadenopathy-associated virus in vitro. *Proc Natl Acad Sci USA*, **82**, 7096–100.

Moore, J.P. and Burton, D.R. 1999. HIV-1 neutralizing antibodies: how full is the bottle? *Nature Medicine*, **5**, 142–4.

Moss, R.B., Diveley, J., et al. 2001. Human immunodeficiency virus (HIV)-specific immune responses are generated with the simultaneous vaccination of a gp120-depleted, whole-killed HIV-1 immunogen with cytosine-phosphorothioate-guanine dinucleotide immunostimulatory sequences of DNA. *J Hum Virol*, **4**, 39–43.

Moutouh, L., Corbeil, J. and Richman, D.D. 1996. Recombination leads to the rapid emergence of HIV-1 dually resistant mutants under selective drug pressure. *Proc Natl Acad Sci USA*, **93**, 6106–11.

Mukai, T., Kurosu, T., et al. 2002. Construction and in vitro characterization of a molecularly cloned human immunodeficiency virus type 1 library. *Vaccine*, **20**, 1181–5.

Mulato, A.S., Lamy, P.D., et al. 1998. Genotypic and phenotypic characterization of human immunodeficiency virus type 1 variants isolated from AIDS patients after prolonged adefovir dipivoxil therapy. *Antimicrob Agents Chemother*, **42**, 1620–8.

Mulder, J., McKinney, N., et al. 1994. Rapid and simple PCR assay for quantitation of human immunodeficiency virus type 1 RNA in plasma: application to acute retroviral infection. *J Clin Microbiol*, **32**, 292–300.

Müller, B., Tessmer, U., et al. 2000. Human immunodeficiency virus type 1 Vpr protein is incorporated into the virion in significantly smaller amounts than gag and is phosphorylated in infected cells. *J Virol*, **74**, 9727–31.

Mwau, M., Cebere, I., et al. 2004. A human immunodeficiency virus 1 (HIV-1) clade A vaccine in clinical trials: stimulation of HIV-specific T-cell responses by DNA and recombinant modified vaccinia virus Ankara (MVA) vaccines in humans. *J Gen Virol*, **85**, 911–19.

Myers, E.L. and Allen, J.F. 2002. Tsg101, an inactive homologue of ubiquitin ligase e2, interacts specifically with human immunodeficiency virus type 2 gag polyprotein and results in increased levels of ubiquitinated gag. *J Virol*, **76**, 11226–35.

Navarro, F. and Landau, N.R. 2004. Recent insights into HIV-1 Vif. *Curr Opin Immunol*, **16**, 477–82.

Nolte, F.S. 1999. Impact of viral load testing on patient care. *Arch Pathol Lab Med*, **123**, 1011–14.

Novitsky, V., Rybak, N., et al. 2001. Identification of human immunodeficiency virus type 1 subtype C Gag-, Tat-, Rev- and Nef-specific elispot-based cytotoxic T-lymphocyte responses for AIDS vaccine design. *J Virol*, **75**, 9210–28.

Oberlin, E., Amara, A., et al. 1996. The CXC chemokine SDF-1 is the ligand for LESTR/fusin and prevents infection by T-cell-line-adapted HIV-1. *Nature*, **382**, 833–5.

Ohagen, A. and Gabuzda, D. 2000. Role of Vif in stability of the human immunodeficiency virus type 1 core. *J Virol*, **74**, 1105–11066.

Ott, D.E. 2002. Potential roles of cellular proteins in HIV-1. *Rev Med Virol*, **12**, 6, 359–74.

Ou, C.Y., Takebe, Y., et al. 1993. Independent introduction of two major HIV-1 genotypes into distinct high-risk populations in Thailand. *Lancet*, **341**, 1171–4.

Overbaugh, J., Anderson, R.J., et al. 1996. Distinct but related human immunodeficiency virus type 1 variant population in genital secretions and blood. *AIDS Res Hum Retroviruses*, **12**, 107–15.

Pachl, C., Todd, J.A., et al. 1995. Rapid and precise quantification of HIV-1 RNA in plasma using a branched DNA signal amplification assay. *J Acquir Immune Defic Syndr Hum Retrovirol*, **8**, 446–54.

Palella, F.J.J., Delaney, K.M., et al. 1998. Declining morbidity and mortality among patients with advanced human immunodeficiency virus infection. HIV Outpatient Study Investigators. *N Engl J Med*, **338**, 853–60.

Pantaleo, G., Graziosi, C., et al. 1993. HIV infection is active and progressive in lymphoid tissue during the clinically latent stage of disease. *Nature*, **362**, 355–8.

Parekh, B., Phillips, S., et al. 1999. Impact of HIV type 1 subtype variation on viral RNA quantitation. *AIDS Res Hum Retroviruses*, **15**, 133–42.

Parry, J.V., Murphy, G., et al. 2001. National surveillance of HIV-1 subtypes for England and Wales; design, methods and initial findings. *J Acquir Immune Defic Syndr*, **26**, 381–8.

Paul, D.A., Falk, L.A., et al. 1987. Correlation of serum HIV antigen and antibody with clinical status in HIV-infected patients. *J Med Virol*, **22**, 357–63.

Pauwels, R., Andries, K., et al. 1990. Potent and selective inhibition of HIV-1 replication in vitro by a novel series of TIBO derivatives. *Nature*, **343**, 470–4.

Paxton, W., Connor, R.I. and Landau, N.R. 1993. Incorporation of Vpr into human immunodeficiency virus type 1 virions: requirement for the p6 region of gag and mutational analysis. *Virology*, **67**, 7229–37.

Perelson, A.S., Neumann, A.U., et al. 1996. HIV-1 dynamics in vivo: virion clearance rate, infected cell life-span, and viral generation time. *Science*, **271**, 1582–6.

Perelson, A.S., Essunger, P., et al. 1997. Decay characteristics of HIV-1-infected compartments during combination therapy. *Nature*, **387**, 188–91.

Perez, O.D. and Nolan, G.P. 2001. Resistance is futile: assimilation of cellular machinery by HIV-1. *Immunity*, **15**, 687–90.

Perry, C.M. and Noble, S. 1998. Saquinavir soft-gel capsule formulation. A review of its use in patients with HIV infection. *Drugs*, **55**, 461–86.

Phillips, R.E., Rowland-Jones, S., et al. 1991. Human immunodeficiency virus genetic variation that can escape cytotoxic T cell recognition. *Nature*, **354**, 453–9.

Piguet, V. and Trono, D. 2001. Living in oblivion: HIV immune evasion. *Semin Immunol*, **13**, 1, 51–7.

Piguet, V., Schwartz, O., et al. 1999. The down regulation of CD4 and MHC-1 by primate lentiviruses: a paradigm for the modulation of cell surface receptors. *Immunol Rev*, **168**, 51–63.

Piguet, V., Wan, L., et al. 2000. HIV-1 Nef protein binds to the cellular protein PACS-1 to downregulate class I major histocompatibility complexes. *Nat Cell Biol*, **2**, 163–7.

Piller, S.C., Ewart, G.D., et al. 1996. Vpr protein of human immunodeficiency virus type 1 forms cation-selective channels in planar lipid bilayers. *Proc Natl Acad Sci USA*, **93**, 111–15.

Pomerantz, R.J. and Horn, D.L. 2003. Twenty years of therapy for HIV-1 infection. *Nature Med*, **9**, 867–73.

Poon, B., Grovit-Ferbas, K., et al. 1998. Cell cycle arrest by Vpr in HIV-1 virions and insensitivity to antiretroviral agents. *Science*, **281**, 266–9.

Popov, S., Rexach, M., et al. 1998a. Viral protein R regulates nuclear import of the HIV-1 pre-integration complex. *EMBO J*, **17**, 909–17.

Popov, S., Rexach, M., et al. 1998b. Viral protein R regulates docking of the HIV-1 preintegration complex to the nuclear pore complex. *J Biol Chem*, **273**, 13347–52.

Pornillos, O., Alam, S.L., et al. 2002a. Structure and functional interactions of the Tsg101 UEV domain. *EMBO J*, **21**, 2397–406.

Pornillos, O., Garrus, J.E. and Sundquist, W.I. 2002b. Mechanisms of enveloped RNA virus budding. *Trends Cell Biol*, **12**, 569–79.

Pozniak, A., Gazzard, B., et al. 2003. British HIV association (BHIVA) guidelines for the treatment of HIV-infected adults with antiretroviral therapy. *HIV Med*, **4**, Suppl. 1, 1–41.

Preston, B.D., Poiesz, B.J. and Loeb, L.A. 1988. Fidelity of HIV-1 reverse transcriptase. *Science*, **242**, 1168–71.

Renjifo, B., Fawzi, W., et al. 2001. Differences in perinatal transmission among human immunodeficiency virus type 1 genotypes. *J Hum Virol*, **4**, 16–25.

Renkema, G.H., Manninen, A. and Saksela, K. 2001. Human immunodeficiency virus type 1 Nef selectively associates with a catalytically active subpopulation of p21-activated kinase 2 (PAK2) independently of PAK2 binding to Nck or beta-PIX. *J Virol*, **75**, 2154–60.

Reynes, J., Rouzier, R., et al. 2002. SCH C: Safety and Antiviral Effects of a CCR5 Receptor Antagonist in HIV-1- Infected Subjects. *9th Conference on Retroviruses and Opportunistic Infections. 24–28 Feb 2002, Seattle, WA* Abstract 1.

Rhodes, D.I., Ashton, L., et al. 2000. Characterization of three nef-defective human immunodeficiency virus type 1 strains associated with long-term nonprogression. Australian Long-Term Nonprogressor Study Group. *J Virol*, **74**, 10581–8.

Richman, D.D., Shih, C.K., et al. 1991. Human immunodeficiency virus type 1 mutants resistant to nonnucleoside inhibitors of reverse transcriptase arise in tissue culture. *Proc Natl Acad Sci USA*, **88**, 11241–5.

Richman, D.D., Havlir, D., et al. 1994. Nevirapine resistance mutations of human immunodeficiency virus type 1 selected during therapy. *J Virol*, **68**, 1660–6.

Roberts, J.D., Bebenek, K. and Kunkel, T.A. 1988. The accuracy of reverse transcriptase from HIV-1. *Science*, **242**, 1171–3.

Robertson, D.L., Anderson, J.P., et al. 2000. HIV-1 nomenclature proposal. *Science*, **288**, 55–6.

Rogel, M.E., Wu, L.I. and Emerman, M. 1995. The human immunodeficiency virus type 1 vpr gene prevents cell proliferation during chronic infection. *J Virol*, **69**, 882–8.

Rose, K.M., Marin, M., et al. 2004. The viral infectivity factor (Vif) of HIV-1 unveiled. *Trends Mol Med*, **10**, 291–7.

Ross, T.M., Oran, A.E. and Cullen, B.R. 1999. Inhibition of HIV-1 progeny virion release by cell surface CD4 is relieved by expression of viral Nef protein. *Curr Biol*, **9**, 613–21.

Rowland-Jones, S.L. and Dong, T. 1999. Broadly cross-reactive HIV-specific cytotoxic T-lymphocytes in highly-exposed persistently seronegative donors. *Immunol Lett*, **66**, 9–14.

Rusconi, S., La Seta, C.S., et al. 2000. Combination of CCR5 and CXCR4 inhibitors in therapy of human immunodeficiency virus type 1 infection: in vitro studies of mixed virus infections. *J Virol*, **74**, 9328–32.

Samson, M., Libert, F., et al. 1996. Resistance to HIV-1 infection in caucasian individuals bearing mutant alleles of the CCR-5 chemokine receptor gene. *Nature*, **382**, 722–5.

Sawaya, B.E., Khalili, K., et al. 1999. Suppression of HIV-1 transcription and replication by a Vpr mutant. *Gene Ther*, **6**, 947–50.

Schable, C., Zekeng, L., et al. 1994. Sensitivity of United States HIV antibody tests for detection of HIV-1 group O infections. *Lancet*, **344**, 1333–4.

Schnell, J.D. and Hicke, L. 2003. Non-traditional functions of ubiquitin and ubiquitin-binding proteins. *J Biol Chem*, **278**, 35857–60.

Schols, D., Claes, S., et al. 2002. AMD-3100, a CXCR4 Antagonist, Reduced HIV Viral Load and X4 Virus Levels in Humans. *9th Conference on Retroviruses and Opportunistic Infections. 24–28 Feb 2002, Seattle, WA* Abstract 2.

Schrofelbauer, B., Yu, Q. and Landau, N.R. 2004. New insights into the role of Vif in HIV-1 replication. *AIDS Rev*, **6**, 34–9.

Schubert, U. and Strebel, K. 1994. Differential activities of the human immunodeficiency virus type-1 encoded Vpu protein are regulated by phosphorylation and occur in different cellular compartments. *J Virol*, **68**, 2260–71.

Schubert, U., Henklein, P., et al. 1994. The human immunodeficiency virus type 1 encoded Vpu protein is phosphorylated by casein kinase-2 (CK-2) at positions Ser52 and Ser56 within a predicted α-helix-turn-α-helix-motif. *J Mol Biol*, **236**, 16–25.

Schubert, U., Ferrer-Montiel, A.V., et al. 1996a. Identification of an ion channel activity of the Vpu transmembrane domain and its involvement in the regulation of virus release from HIV-1 infected cells. *FEBS Lett*, **398**, 12–18.

Schubert, U., Ferrer-Montiel, A.F., et al. 1996b. Identification of an ion channel activity of the Vpu transmembrane domain and its plausible involvement in the regulation of virus release from HIV-1-infected cells. *FEBS Letter*, **398**, 12-1, 8.

Schubert, U., Bour, S., et al. 1996c. The two biological activities of human immunodeficiency virus type 1 Vpu protein involve two separable structural domains. *J Virol*, **70**, 809–19.

Schubert, U., Anton, L.C., et al. 1998. CD4 glycoprotein degradation induced by human immunodeficiency virus type 1 Vpu protein requires the function of proteasomes and the ubiquitin-conjugating pathway. *J Virol*, **72**, 2280–8.

Schüler, W., Wecker, K., et al. 1999. NMR structure of the (52-96) C-terminal domain of the HIV-1 regulatory protein Vpr: molecular insights into its biological functions. *J Mol Biol*, **285**, 2105–17.

Schwartz, O., Marechal, V., et al. 1996. Endocytosis of major hstocompatibility complex class I molecules is induced by the HIV-1 Nef protein. *Nat Med*, **2**, 338–42.

Schwartz, O., Marechal, V., et al. 1998. Antiviral activity of the proteasome on incoming human immunodeficiency virus type 1. *J Virol*, **72**, 3845–50.

Sepkowitz, K.A., Rivera, P., et al. 1998. Postexposure prophylaxis for human immunodeficiency virus: frequency of initiation and completion of newly recommended regimen. *Infect Control Hosp Epidemiol*, **19**, 506–8.

Shaffer, N., Roongpisuthipong, A., et al. 1999. Maternal virus load and perinatal human immunodeficiency virus type 1 subtype E transmission, Thailand. Bangkok Collaborative Perinatal HIV Transmission Study Group. *J Infect Dis*, **179**, 590–9.

Sherman, M.P. and Greene, W.C. 2002. Slipping through the door: HIV entry into the nucleus. *Microbes Infect*, **4**, 67–73.

Sherman, M.P.D., de Noronha, C.M., et al. 2000. Human immunodeficiency virus type 1 Vpr contains two leucine-rich helices that mediate glucocorticoid receptor coactivation independently of its effects on G(2) cell cycle arrest. *J Virol*, **74**, 17, 8159–65.

Sherman, M.P., De Noronha, C.M., et al. 2001. Nucleocytoplasmic shuttling by human immunodeficiency virus type 1 Vpr. *J Virol*, **75**, 1522–32.

Sherman, M.P., Schubert, U., et al. 2002. HIV-1 Vpr displays natural protein-transducing properties: implications for viral pathogenesis. *Virology*, **302**, 95–105.

Shirasaka, T., Kavlick, M.F., et al. 1995. Emergence of human immunodeficiency virus type 1 variants with resistance to multiple dideoxynucleosides in patients receiving therapy with dideoxynucleosides. *Proc Natl Acad Sci USA*, **92**, 2398–402.

Simon, F., Mauclere, P., et al. 1998. Identification of a new human immunodeficiency virus type 1 distinct from group M and group O. *Nat Med*, **4**, 1032–103.

Simon, J.H., Gaddis, N.C., et al. 1998a. Evidence for a newly discovered cellular anti-HIV-1 phenotype. *Nat. Med*, **4**, 1397.

Simon, J.H., Miller, D.L., et al. 1998b. The regulation of primate immunodeficiency virus infectivity by Vif is cell species restricted: a role for Vif in determining virus host range and cross-species transmission. *EMBO J*, **17**, 1259–67.

Simmonds, P., Zhang, L.Q., et al. 1991. Discontinuous sequence change of human immunodeficiency virus (HIV) type 1 env sequence in plasma viral and lymphocyte-associated proviral populations in vivo: implications for models of HIV pathogenesis. *J Virol*, **65**, 6266–76.

Simmons, A., Aluvihare, V. and McMichael, A. 2001. Nef triggers a transcriptional program in T cells imitating single-signal T cell activation and inducing HIV virulence mediators. *Immunity*, **14**, 763–77.

Simmons, G., Clapham, P.R., et al. 1997. Potent inhibition of HIV-1 infectivity in macrophages and lymphocytes by a novel CCR5 antagonist. *Science*, **276**, 276–9.

Skowronski, J., Parks, D. and Mariane, R. 1993. Altered T cell activation and development in transgenic mice expressing the HIV-1 nef gene. *EMBO J*, **12**, 103–713.

Sova, P., Volsky, D.J., et al. 2001. Vif is largely absent from human immunodeficiency virus type 1 mature virions and associates mainly with viral particles containing unprocessed gag. *J Virol*, **12**, 5504–17.

Spence, R.A., Kati, W.M., et al. 1995. Mechanism of inhibition of HIV-1 reverse transcriptase by nonnucleoside inhibitors. *Science*, **267**, 988–93.

Spenlehauer, C., Saragosti, S., et al. 1998. Study of the V3 loop as a target epitope for antibodies involved in the neutralization of primary isolates versus T-cell-line-adapted strains of human immunodeficiency virus type 1. *J Virol*, **72**, 9855–64.

Stark, L.A. and Hay, R.T. 1998. Human immunodeficiency virus type 1 (HIV-1) viral protein R (Vpr) interacts with Lys-tRNA synthetase: implications for priming of HIV-1 reverse transcription. *J Virol*, **72**, 3037–44.

Steffens, C.M. and Hope, Th. 2001. Recent advances in the understanding of HIV accessory protein function. *AIDS*, **15**, Suppl., 21–6.

Stewart, S.A., Poon, B., et al. 1997. Human immunodeficiency virus type 1 Vpr induces apoptosis following cell cycle arrest. *J Virol*, **71**, 5579–92.

Stewart, S.A., Poon, B., et al. 2000. Human immunodeficiency virus type 1 vpr induces apoptosis through caspase activation. *J Virol*, **74**, 3105–11.

Stopak, K., de Noronha, C., et al. 2003. HIV-1 Vif blocks the antiviral activity of APOBEC3G by impairing both its translation and intracellular stability. *Mol Cell*, **12**, 591–601.

Strack, B., Calistri, A., et al. 2003. AIP1/ALIX is a binding partner for HIV-1 p6 and EIAV p9 functioning in virus budding. *Cell*, **114**, 689–99.

Strebel, K. 2004. HIV-1 Vpu: putting a channel to the TASK. *Mol Cell*, **14**, 150–2.

Strebel, K., Daugherty, D., et al. 1987. The HIV 'A' (sor) gene product is essential for virus infectivity. *Nature*, **328**, 728–30.

Strebel, K., Klimkait, T. and Martin, M.A. 1988. A novel gene of HIV-1, vpu, and its 16-kilodalton product. *Science*, **241**, 1221–3.

Svarovskaia, E.S., Xu, H., et al. 2004. Human APOBEC3G is incorporated into HIV-1 virions through interactions with viral and nonviral RNAs. *J Biol Chem*, **279**, 35822–8.

Swanson, P., Harris, B.J., et al. 2000. Quantification of HIV-1 group M (subtypes A-G) and group O by the LCx HIV RNA quantitative assay. *J Virol Methods*, **89**, 97–108.

Swanson, P., Soriano, V., et al. 2001. Comparative performance of three viral load assays on human immunodeficiency virus type 1 (HIV-1) isolates representing group M (subtypes A to G) and group O: LCx HIV RNA quantitative, AMPLICOR HIV-1 MONITOR version 1.5, and Quantiplex HIV-1 RNA version 3.0. *J Clin Microbiol*, **39**, 862–70.

Swanstrom, R. and Wills, J. 1997. Synthesis, assembly, and processing of viral proteins. In: Coffin, J., Hughes, S. and Varmus, H. (eds), *Retroviruses*. Plainview, NY: Cold Spring Harbor Press, 263–334.

Swigut, T., Shohdy, N. and Skowronski, J. 2001. Mechanism for down regulation of CD28 by Nef. *EMBO J*, **20**, 1593–604.

Tisdale, M., Kemp, S.D., et al. 1993. Rapid in vitro selection of human immunodeficiency virus type 1 resistant to 3′-thiacytidine inhibitors due to a mutation in the YMDD region of reverse transcriptase. *Proc Natl Acad Sci USA*, **90**, 5653–6.

Todd, J., Pachl, C., et al. 1995. Performance characteristics for the quantitation of plasma HIV-1 RNA using branched DNA signal amplification technology. *J Acquir Immune Defic Syndr Hum Retrovirol*, **10**, Suppl. 2, S35–44.

Triques, K., Bourgeois, A., et al. 1999. High diversity of HIV-1 subtype F strains in Central Africa. *Virology*, **259**, 99–109.

Triques, K., Bourgeois, A., et al. 2000. Near-full-length genome sequencing of divergent African HIV type 1 subtype F viruses leads to the identification of a new HIV type 1 subtype designated K. *AIDS Res Hum Retroviruses*, **16**, 139–51.

Van der Groen, G., Nyambi, P.N., et al. 1998. Genetic variation of HIV type 1: relevance of interclade variation to vaccine development. *AIDS Res Hum Retroviruses*, **14**, Suppl. 3, S211–21.

van Harmelen, J., Wood, R., et al. 1997. An association between HIV-1 subtypes and mode of transmission in Cape Town, South Africa. *AIDS*, **11**, 81–7.

Vartanian, J.P., Sommer, P. and Wain-Hobson, S. 2003. Death and the retrovirus. *Trends Mol Med*, **10**, 409–13.

VaxGen. VaxGen announces initial results of its Phase III AIDS vaccine trial. Press release Feb 24, 2003. http://www.vaxgen.com/pressroom/index.html

Vella, S. and Floridia, M. 1998. Saquinavir. Clinical pharmacology and efficacy. *Clin Pharmacokinet*, **34**, 189–201.

VerPlank, L., Bouamr, F., et al. 2001. Tsg101, a homologue of ubiquitin-conjugating (E2) enzymes, binds the L domain in HIV type 1 Pr55(Gag). *Proc Natl Acad Sci USA*, **98**, 7724–9.

Vodicka, M.A., Koepp, D.M., et al. 1998. HIV-1 Vpr interacts with the nuclear transport pathway to promote macrophage infection. *Genes Dev*, **12**, 175–85.

Vogt, V. 1997. Retroviral virions and genomes. In: Coffin, J., Hughes, S. and Varmus, H. (eds), *Retroviruses*. Plainview, NY: Cold Spring Harbor Press, 27–70.

Vogt, V.M. 2000. Ubiquitin in retrovirus assembly: actor or bystander? *Proc Natl Acad Sci USA*, **97**, 12945–7.

von Schwedler, U., Song, J., et al. 1993. Vif is crucial for human immunodeficiency virus type 1 proviral DNA synthesis in infected cells. *J Virol*, **67**, 4945–55.

von Schwedler, U.K., Stuchell, M., et al. 2003. The protein network of HIV budding. *Cell*, **114**, 2003, 701–13.

Wacher, V.J., Silverman, J.A., et al. 1998. Role of P-glycoprotein and cytochrome P450 3A in limiting oral absorption of peptides and peptidomimetics. *J Pharm Sci*, **87**, 1322–30.

Wecker, K., Morellet, N., et al. 2002. NMR structure of the HIV-1 regulatory protein Vpr in H20/trifluoroethanol. Comparison with the Vpr N-terminal (1-51) and C-terminal (52-96) domains. *Eur J Biochem*, **269**, 3779–88.

Wei, X., Ghosh, S.K., et al. 1995. Viral dynamics in human immunodeficiency virus type 1 infection. *Nature*, **373**, 117–22.

Weisman, Z., Kalinkovich, A., et al. 1999. Infection by different HIV-1 subtypes (B and C) results in a similar immune activation profile despite distinct immune backgrounds. *J Acquir Immune Defic Syndr*, **21**, 157–63.

Weiss, R.A. 2002. HIV receptors and cellular tropism. *IUBMB Life*, **53**, 4-5, 201–5.

Weissenhorn, W., Dessen, A., et al. 1997. Atomic structure of the ectodomain from HIV-1 gp41. *Nature*, **387**, 426–30.

Witte, V., Laffert, B., et al. 2004. HIV-1 Nef mimics an integrin receptor signal that recruits the polycomb group protein Eed to the plasma membrane. *Mol Cell*, **13**, 179–90.

Wong, J.K., Gunthard, H.F., et al. 1997a. Reduction of HIV-1 in blood and lymph nodes following potent antiretroviral therapy and the virologic correlates of treatment failure. *Proc Natl Acad Sci USA*, **94**, 12574–9.

Wong, J.K., Hezareh, M., et al. 1997b. Recovery of replication-competent HIV despite prolonged suppression of plasma viremia. *Science*, **278**, 1291–5.

Wray, V., Kinder, R., et al. 1999. Solution structure and orientation of the transmembrane anchor domain of the HIV-1-encoded virus protein U by high-resolution and solid-state NMR spectroscopy. *Biochemistry*, **38**, 5272–82.

Wyand, M.S., Manson, K., et al. 1999. Protection by live, attenuated simian immunodeficiency virus against heterologous challenge. *J Virol*, **73**, 8356–63.

Xiong, X., Flores, C., et al. 1997. In vitro characterization of the anti-human cytomegalovirus activity of PMEA (Adefovir). *Antiviral Res*, **36**, 131–7.

Yu, Q., Konig, R., et al. 2004. Single-strand specificity of APOBEC3G accounts for minus-strand deamination of the HIV genome. *Nat Struct Mol Biol*, **5**, 435–42.

Yu, X., Yu, Y., et al. 2003. Induction of APOBEC3G ubiquitination and degradation by an HIV-1 Vif-Cul5-SCF complex. *Science*, **302**, 1056–60.

Yung, E., Sorin, M., et al. 2001. Inhibition of HIV-1 virion production by a transdominant mutant of integrase interactor 1. *Nat Med*, **8**, 920–6.

Xu, X.N., Screaton, G.R., et al. 1997. Evasion of cytotoxic T lymphocyte (CTL) responses by nef-dependent induction of Fas ligand (CD95L) expression on simian immunodeficiency virus-infected cells. *J Exp Med*, **186**, 7–16.

Xu, X.N., Laffert, B., et al. 1999. Induction of Fas ligand expression by HIV involves the interaction of Nef with the T cell receptor zeta chain. *J Exp Med*, **189**, 1489–96.

Zander, K., Sherman, M.P., et al. 2003. Cyclophilin A Interacts with HIV-1 Vpr and Is required for its functional expression. *J Biol Chem*, **278**, 43202–13.

Zennou, V., Petit, C., et al. 2000. HIV-1 genome nuclear import is mediated by a central DNA flap. *Cell*, **101**, 173–85.

Zhang, H.D., Dornadula, G., et al. 1998. Human immunodeficiency virus type 1 in the semen of men receiving highly active antiretroviral therapy. *N Engl J Med*, **339**, 1803–9.

Zhang, P.F., Buoma, P., et al. 2002. A variable region 3 (V3) mutation determines a global neutralization phenotype and CD4-independent infectivity of a human immunodeficiency virus type 1 envelope associated with a broadly cross-reactive, primary virus-neutralizing antibody response. *J Virol*, **76**, 644–55.

Zhu, T., Wang, N., et al. 1996. Genetic characterization of human immunodeficiency virus type 1 in blood and genital secretions: evidence for viral compartmentalization and selection during sexual transmission. *J Virol*, **70**, 3098–107.

61

Prions of humans and animals

ADRIANO AGUZZI

PROPERTIES OF PRIONS

Introduction

Prion diseases, also termed transmissible spongiform encephalopathies (TSE), are inevitably fatal neurodegenerative conditions that affect humans and a wide variety of animals (Aguzzi et al. 2001c). Although prion diseases may present with certain morphological and pathophysiological features that parallel other progressive encephalopathies, such as Alzheimer's and Parkinson's disease (Aguzzi and Haass 2003; Aguzzi and Raeber 1998), they are unique in that they are transmissible. Homogenization of brain tissue from affected individuals and intracerebral inoculation into another individual of the same species will typically reproduce the disease. This important fact was recognized almost six decades ago in the case of scrapie (Cuille and Chelle 1939), a prototypic prion disease that affects sheep and goats.

The agent that elicits TSEs was termed prion by Stanley B. Prusiner, and defined as 'a small proteinaceous infectious particle which is resistant to inactivation by most procedures that modify nucleic acids' (Prusiner 1982). However, within the present chapter the term 'prion' will be used operationally to denote the infectious agent, without implying that it possesses particular chemical or structural characteristics.

Prions certainly differ from all other known infectious pathogens in several respects. First, prions do not appear to contain an informational nucleic acid genome longer than 50 bases that would code for their progeny. Second, the only known component of the prion is a modified protein that is encoded by a cellular gene. Third, the major, and possibly only, component of the prion is the scrapie isoform of the prion protein (PrP^{Sc} or PrP-res), which is a disease-associated conformer of the cellular isoform PrP^C (also termed PrP-sen).

A fundamental event in prion diseases is a conformational change that occurs during the conversion of PrP^C into PrP^{Sc}. PrP^C has been identified in all mammals and birds examined to date, as well as in the frog *Xenopus laevis* (Strumbo et al. 2001), and in fish (Oidtmann et al. 2003; Rivera-Milla et al. 2003). PrP^C is anchored to the external surface of cells by a glycolipid moiety (Stahl et al. 1987). The function of PrP^C is unknown. All attempts to identify post-translational chemical modifications that distinguish PrP^{Sc} from PrP^C have been unsuccessful to date (Stahl et al. 1993). PrP^C contains approximately 45 percent α-helix and two very short stretches of β-sheet (Riek et al. 1996). Conversion to PrP^{Sc} creates a protein that contains approximately 30 percent α-helix and 45 percent β-sheet. The mechanism by which PrP^C is converted into PrP^{Sc} remains unknown but PrP^C seems to bind to PrP^{Sc}, perhaps along with ancillary proteins, to form an intermediate complex during the formation of nascent PrP^{Sc} (Meier et al. 2003). Transgenic (Tg) mouse studies have provided genetic evidence that incoming prions in the inoculum interact preferentially with homotypic PrP^C during the propagation of prions (Prusiner et al., 1990; M. Scott et al. 1993).

The human prion diseases are referred to as kuru, Creutzfeldt–Jakob disease (CJD), variant CJD (vCJD), Gerstmann–Sträussler–Scheinker (GSS) disease, and fatal familial insomnia (FFI). The most common prion diseases of animals are scrapie of sheep and goats, bovine spongiform encephalopathy (BSE) or 'mad cow' disease, and chronic wasting disease (CWD) of deer and elk (Table 61.1). Kuru was the first of the human prion diseases to be transmitted to experimental animals, and it has often been suggested that kuru spread among the Fore people of Papua New Guinea by ritual cannibalism (Gajdusek et al. 1966; Gajdusek 1977). The experimental and presumed human-to-human transmission of kuru led to the belief that prion diseases are infectious disorders caused by unusual viruses similar to those causing scrapie in sheep and goats. Yet a paradox was presented by the occurrence of CJD in families, first reported more than 70 years ago (Kirschbaum 1924; Meggendorfer 1930), which appeared to be a genetic disease. The significance of familial CJD remained largely unappreciated until mutations in the protein coding region of the PrP gene on the short arm of chromosome 20 were discovered (Sparkes et al. 1986; Hsiao et al. 1989). The earlier finding that brain extracts from patients who had died of familial prion diseases inoculated into experimental animals often transmit disease posed a conundrum that was resolved with the genetic linkage of these diseases to mutations of the *PRNP* gene that encodes PrP^C (Masters et al. 1981a; Prusiner 1989a; Tateishi et al. 1992a). To date, all cases of familial prion disease were shown to cosegregate with *PRNP* missense or, in one case, nonsense mutations.

The most common form of prion disease in humans is sporadic CJD (sCJD). Its cause is unknown. Many attempts to show that the sporadic prion diseases are caused by infection have been unsuccessful (Malmgren et al. 1979; Brown et al. 1987; Harries Jones et al. 1988; Cousens et al., 1990). The discovery that inherited prion diseases are caused by germline mutation of the PrP gene raised the possibility that sporadic forms of these diseases might result from a somatic mutation (Prusiner 1989a). Alternatively, since PrP^{Sc} is formed from the cellular isoform of the prion protein, PrP^C, by a post-translational process (Borchelt et al. 1990), sporadic prion diseases may result from the spontaneous conversion of PrP^C into PrP^{Sc}.

CJD was reported to have a worldwide incidence of one case per 10^6 inhabitants annually (Masters and Richardson 1978). However, in countries that carry out active surveillance programs, reported CJD incidence is often higher (Aguzzi et al. 2000a), and in Switzerland it has reached $3.0/10^6$/year (Glatzel et al. 2002, 2003b), suggesting that many cases may go undetected. Less than 1 percent of CJD cases are infectious, and most of those seem to be iatrogenic. Between 10 and 15 percent of cases of prion disease are inherited, whilst the remaining cases are sporadic. Kuru was once the most common cause of death among New Guinea women in the Fore region of the Highlands (Gajdusek and Zigas 1957, 1959; Gajdusek et al. 1966) but has virtually disappeared with the cessation of ritualistic cannibalism (Alpers 1987; Mead et al. 2003). Most patients with CJD present primarily with dementia, but approximately 10 percent exhibit cerebellar dysfunction as the initial sign. People with either kuru or GSS usually present with ataxia, whereas those with FFI manifest insomnia and autonomic dysfunction (Hsiao and Prusiner 1990; Brown 1992; Medori et al. 1992b).

PrP^{CJD} has been found in the brains of most patients who died of prion disease. The term PrP^{CJD} is sometimes used when referring to the abnormal isoform of PrP in human brain. In this chapter, PrP^{Sc} is used interchangeably with PrP^{CJD}. PrP^{Sc} is always used after human CJD prions have been passaged into an experimental animal, because the nascent PrP^{Sc} molecules are produced from host PrP^C and the PrP^{CJD} in the inoculum serves only to initiate the process. In the brains of some patients with inherited prion diseases, as well as transgenic mice expressing mouse (Mo) PrP with the human GSS point mutation (Pro→Leu), detection of PrP^{Sc} by western blotting has been problematic despite clinical and neuropathological hallmarks of neurodegeneration (Hsiao et al. 1990, 1994), but histological techniques such as histoblotting (Taraboulos et al. 1992a) have often revealed protease-resistant PrP.

Experimental transmission of neurodegeneration from the brains of patients with inherited prion diseases to

Table 61.1 *Human prion diseases*

Disease	Etiology
Kuru	Infection
Creutzfeldt–Jakob disease:	
Iatrogenic	Infection
Sporadic	Unknown
Familial	*PRNP* mutation
Variant	Presumed BSE infection
Gerstmann–Sträussler–Scheinker disease	*PRNP* mutation
Fatal familial insomnia	*PRNP* mutation

inoculated rodents has been less frequent than with sporadic cases (Tateishi et al. 1992a). Whether this distinction between transmissible and nontransmissible inherited prion diseases will persist is unclear. Transgenic mice expressing a chimeric Hu/Mo PrP gene are highly susceptible to human prions from sporadic and iatrogenic CJD (iCJD) cases (Telling et al. 1994), and – somewhat unexpectedly – transgenic mice expressing a full-length bovine *Prnp* transgene appear to be the best model for transmission of human prions to date (Scott et al. 1999). There is hope that suitable transgenic mice may eventually make the use of apes and monkeys for the study of human prion diseases unnecessary. To date, this is not yet possible for several reasons:

- the molecular determinants that determine species barriers are not fully understood, and may encompass species-specific host factors additionally to PrP
- the peripheral pathophysiology of prion diseases may differ considerably between mice and humans.

Scrapie is the most common natural prion disease of animals. An investigation into the etiology of scrapie followed the vaccination of sheep for louping ill virus with formalin-treated extracts of ovine lymphoid tissue unknowingly contaminated with scrapie prions (Gordon 1946). Two years later, more than 1 500 sheep developed scrapie from this vaccine. In the late 1990s a similar incident led to widespread scrapie infection of Italian sheep herds. Although the transmissibility of experimental scrapie became well established, the spread of natural scrapie within and among flocks of sheep remained puzzling. Parry argued that host genes were responsible for the development of scrapie in sheep. He was convinced that natural scrapie is a genetic disease which could be eradicated by proper breeding protocols (Parry 1962; Parry and Livett 1973). He considered its transmission by inoculation to be of importance primarily for laboratory studies and communicable infection of little consequence in nature. Other investigators viewed natural scrapie as an infectious disease and argued that host genetics only modulates susceptibility to an endemic infectious agent (Dickinson et al. 1965).

Prion-infested offal is thought to be responsible for the epidemic of BSE (Wilesmith et al. 1992b). Prions in the offal from scrapie-infected sheep, or perhaps from rare cows affected by hypothetical 'sporadic BSE,' seem to have survived the rendering process that produced meat and bone meal (MBM). Whether the 'Ur-BSE prion' originated from sheep, or was autochtonous to cows, is a question that may not be solvable, and is of mainly academic and legal significance.

The MBM was fed to cattle as a nutritional supplement. After BSE was recognized, MBM produced from domestic animal offal was banned from further use. Since 1986, when BSE was first recognized, >180 000 cattle have died of BSE. More than 130 persons have

developed a 'new variant' of CJD (Chazot et al., 1996; http://www.doh.gov.uk/cjd/stats/aug02.htm, 2002; Will et al. 1996), which is likely to represent transmission of BSE to humans (Bruce et al. 1997; Collinge et al. 1996; Hill et al. 1997a).

As we learn about the molecular and genetic characteristics of prion proteins, our understanding of prions and their place in biology will undoubtedly undergo considerable change. Indeed, the discovery of PrP, the identification of pathogenic *PRNP* gene mutations, the differences in the structures of PrP^C and PrP^{Sc}, as well as studies of the process by which prions move from the site of infection to the brain, have already forced us to think about these diseases from viewpoints that had not been previously considered.

Development of the prion concept

HYPOTHESES ON THE NATURE OF THE SCRAPIE AGENT

The published literature contains a fascinating record of the structural hypotheses for the scrapie agent, proposed to explain the unusual features first of the disease and later those of the infectious agent. Among the earliest hypotheses was the notion that scrapie was a disease of muscle caused by the parasite *Sarcosporidia* (M'Fadyean, 1918; M'Gowan 1914). With the successful transmission of scrapie to animals, the hypothesis that scrapie is caused by a 'filtrable' virus became popular (Cuille and Chelle 1939; Wilson et al. 1950). With the findings of Tikvah Alper and her colleagues that scrapie infectivity resists inactivation by ultraviolet (UV) and ionizing irradiation (Alper et al. 1966, 1967), a myriad of hypotheses on the chemical nature of the scrapie agent emerged, including the quite prescient conjecture that it may consist of a self-replicating protein (Griffith 1967).

BIOASSAYS OF PRION INFECTIVITY

The experimental transmission of scrapie from sheep (Gordon 1946) to mice (Chandler 1961) gave investigators a more convenient laboratory model, which yielded considerable information on the nature of the unusual infectious pathogen that causes scrapie (Alper et al. 1966, 1967, 1978; Gibbons and Hunter 1967; Pattison and Jones 1967; Millson et al. 1971). Yet progress was slow because quantification of infectivity in a single sample required holding 60 mice for at least one year before accurate scoring could be accomplished (Chandler 1961).

Attempts to develop a more economical bioassay by relating the titre to incubation times in mice were unsuccessful (Eklund et al. 1963; Hunter and Millson 1964). However, some investigators used incubation times to characterize different 'strains' of scrapie agent, whilst others determined the kinetics of prion replication in rodents (Dickinson and Meikle, 1969; Kimberlin and Walker 1978a, 1979). Quantitative bioassays based on incubation times had been applied to the measurement of picorna and other viruses three decades earlier (Gard 1940). After scrapie incubation times were reported to be approximately 50 percent shorter in Syrian hamsters than in mice (Marsh and Kimberlin 1975), studies were undertaken to determine whether the incubation times in hamsters could be related to the titer of the inoculated sample. It was found that there was an excellent inverse correlation between the length of the incubation time and the logarithm of the dose of inoculated prions, and a more rapid and economical bioassay was developed (Prusiner et al. 1980a, 1982b). This improved bioassay for the scrapie agent in Syrian golden hamsters accelerated purification of the infectious particles by a factor of nearly 100. Still, the soaring costs of animal caretaking make it impossible for most institutions to carry out large-scale incubation-time-based prion titration studies. The recent development of a quantitative, highly sensitive cell-based bioassay by Klohn and Weissmann may foster a much-needed quantum leap in prion analytics (Klohn et al. 2003), which could prove crucial for many practical purposes, such as validation of prion decontamination procedures.

THE PRION CONCEPT

Once an effective protocol was developed for preparation of partially purified fractions of scrapie agent from hamster brain, it became possible to demonstrate that the procedures that modify or hydrolyze proteins produce a diminution in scrapie infectivity (Prusiner et al. 1981a, 1982b). At the same time, tests done in search of a scrapie-specific nucleic acid were unable to demonstrate any dependence of infectivity on a polynucleotide (Prusiner 1982; Riesner et al. 1993), in agreement with earlier studies reporting the extreme resistance of infectivity to UV irradiation at 254 nm (Alper et al. 1967).

On the basis of these findings, it seemed unlikely that the infectious pathogen capable of transmitting scrapie was a virus or a viroid. For this reason the term 'prion' was introduced to distinguish the proteinaceous infectious particles that cause scrapie, CJD, GSS, and kuru from both viroids and viruses (Prusiner 1982). Hypotheses for the structure of the infectious prion particle included:

- proteins surrounding a nucleic acid encoding them (a virus)
- proteins associated with a small polynucleotide
- proteins devoid of nucleic acid (Prusiner 1982).

Mechanisms postulated for the replication of infectious prion particles ranged from those used by viruses to the synthesis of polypeptides in the absence of nucleic acid template to post-translational modifications of cellular proteins. Subsequent discoveries have narrowed hypotheses for both prion structure and the mechanism of replication.

Considerable evidence has accumulated over the past decade supporting the prion hypothesis. But while the prion concept is now enjoying considerable acceptance, it should not go unmentioned that several core issues regarding prion replication are still entirely obscure (Chesebro 1998).

Discovery of the prion protein

Once the dependence of prion infectivity on protein was clear, the search for a scrapie-specific protein intensified. Although the insolubility of scrapie infectivity made purification problematic, this property was used by Prusiner along with its relative resistance to degradation by proteases to extend the degree of purification (Prusiner et al. 1980a, 1981b). In subcellular fractions from hamster brain enriched for scrapie infectivity, a protease-resistant polypeptide of 27–30 kDa (later designated PrP^{27-30}) was identified, which was absent from controls (Bolton et al. 1982; McKinley et al. 1983). Radioiodination of partially purified fractions revealed a protein unique to preparations from scrapie-infected brains (Bolton et al. 1982; Prusiner et al. 1982a).

Progress in the study of prions was greatly accelerated by the discovery of PrP and determination of its N-terminal sequence (Bolton et al. 1982; Prusiner et al. 1982a, 1984). Purification of PrP^{27-30} to near-homogeneity allowed determination of its NH_2-terminal amino acid sequence. Determination of a single, unique sequence for the NH_2 terminus of PrP^{27-30} permitted the synthesis of an isocoding mixture of oligonucleotides that was subsequently used to identify incomplete PrP cDNA clones from hamster (Oesch et al. 1985) and mouse (Chesebro et al. 1985). cDNA clones encoding the entire open reading frames (ORF) of Syrian hamster (SHa) and Mo PrP were subsequently recovered (Basler et al. 1986; Locht et al. 1986).

The experiments described above established that PrP is encoded by a chromosomal gene, and not by a nucleic acid within the infectious scrapie prion particle (Oesch et al. 1985; Basler et al. 1986). Levels of PrP mRNA remain unchanged throughout the course of scrapie infection – an unexpected observation which led to the identification of the normal PrP gene product, a protein of 33–35 kDa, designated PrP^C (Basler et al. 1986; Oesch et al. 1985). PrP^C is protease-sensitive and soluble in nondenaturing detergents, whereas PrP^{27-30} is the protease-resistant core of a 33–35 kDa disease-specific protein, designated PrP^{Sc}, which is insoluble in detergents (Meyer et al. 1986).

THE *PRNP* GENE LOCUS

The entire ORF of all known mammalian and avian *Prnp* genes is contained within a single exon (Figure 61.1) (Basler et al. 1986; Westaway et al. 1987; Hsiao et al. 1989; Gabriel et al. 1992). This feature of the PrP gene eliminates the possibility that PrP^{Sc} arises from alter-

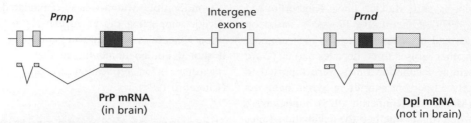

Figure 61.1 *Structure and organization of the chromosomal* Prnp *and* Prnd *genes. In all mammals examined the entire ORF is contained within a single exon. The 5'-untranslated region of the PrP mRNA is derived from either one or two additional exons (Basler et al. 1986; Puckett et al. 1991; Westaway et al. 1991, 1994a). Only one PrP mRNA has been detected. A prion protein homologue termed Dpl is encoded by the Prnd locus. PrP^{Sc} is thought to be derived from PrP^C by a post-translational process (Basler et al. 1986; Borchelt et al. 1990, 1992; Caughey et al. 1991b; Taraboulos et al. 1992b). The amino acid sequence of PrP^{Sc} is identical to that predicted from the translated sequence of the DNA encoding the PrP gene (Basler et al. 1986; Stahl et al. 1993), and no unique post-translational chemical modifications have been identified that might distinguish PrP^{Sc} from PrP^C. Thus, it seems likely that PrP^C undergoes a conformational change as it is converted to PrP^{Sc}. A second gene bearing remarkable structural homologies with* Prnp *was identified approximately 16 kb 3' of the* Prnp *locus, and was termed* Prnd. *The product of this locus is termed* Doppel.

native RNA splicing (Basler et al. 1986; Westaway et al. 1987, 1991), although mechanisms such as RNA editing or protein splicing remain a possibility (Blum et al. 1990; Kane et al. 1990). The two exons of the SHaPrP gene are separated by a 10 kb intron: exon 1 encodes a portion of the 5'-untranslated leader sequence whilst exon 2 encodes the ORF and the 3'-untranslated region (Basler et al. 1986). The murine and ovine PrP genes are composed of three exons; exon 3 is analogous to exon 2 of the hamster (Westaway et al. 1991, 1994a). The promoters of both the SHa and Mo PrP genes contain multiple copies of GC-rich repeats and are devoid of TATA boxes. These GC nonamers represent a motif that may function as a canonical binding site for the transcription factor Sp1.

PrP genes map to the short arm of human chromosome 20 and to the homologous region of mouse chromosome 2 (Sparkes et al. 1986). Hybridization studies demonstrated <0.002 *Prnp* gene sequences per ID_{50} unit in purified prion fractions, strongly suggesting that a nucleic acid encoding PrP^{Sc} cannot possibly constitute a component of the infectious prion particle (Oesch et al. 1985). This is a major feature that distinguishes prions from viruses, including retroviruses that carry cellular oncogenes and from satellite viruses that derive their coat proteins from other viruses previously infecting cells. Although *Prnp* mRNA is constitutively expressed in the brains of adult animals (Chesebro et al. 1985; Oesch et al. 1985), it is highly regulated during development (Manson et al. 1992; Sales et al. 2002). In the septum, levels of PrP mRNA and choline acetyltransferase increased in parallel during development (Mobley et al. 1988). In other brain regions, PrP gene expression occurred at an earlier age.

PrP amyloid

The discovery of PrP^{27–30} in fractions enriched for scrapie infectivity was accompanied by the identification of rod-shaped particles in the same fractions (Prusiner

et al. 1982a, 1983). The fine structure of these rod-shaped particles failed to reveal any regular substructure. Indeed, the irregular ultrastructure of the prion rods differentiates them from most viruses, which have regular, distinct structures (Williams 1954), and made them indistinguishable ultrastructurally from many purified amyloids (Cohen et al. 1982). This analogy was extended when the prion rods were found to display the tinctorial properties of amyloids (Prusiner et al. 1983). These findings were followed by the demonstration that amyloid plaques in the brains of humans and other animals with prion diseases contain PrP, as determined by immunoreactivity and amino acid sequencing (Bendheim et al. 1984; DeArmond et al. 1985; Kitamoto et al. 1986; Roberts et al. 1988; Tagliavini et al. 1991).

Solubilization of PrP^{27–30} into liposomes with retention of infectivity (Gabizon et al. 1987) suggests that large PrP polymers are not required for infectivity – although it is well possible that PrP^{Sc} oligomers may constitute nucleation centers pivotal to prion replication (Jarrett and Lansbury 1993; Lansbury 1994). In Tg(SHaPrP) mice inoculated with SHa prions, numerous amyloid plaques were found but none was observed if these mice were inoculated with mouse prions, indicating that amyloid formation is not an obligatory feature of prion diseases (Prusiner et al. 1990; Prusiner and DeArmond 1994). In agreement with these studies, PrP plaques are consistently found in some inherited prion diseases (Ghetti et al. 1989) but absent from others (Hsiao et al. 1991a).

Formation of PrP^{Sc}

Whether PrP^C is the substrate for PrP^{Sc} formation, or a restricted subset of PrP molecules are precursors for PrP^{Sc}, or whether reactive transition states exist (Weissmann 1991a), remains to be established. Several experimental results argue that PrP molecules destined to become PrP^{Sc} exit to the cell surface, as does PrP^C (Stahl et al. 1987) prior to its conversion into PrP^{Sc}

(Caughey and Raymond 1991; Borchelt et al. 1992; Taraboulos et al. 1992b).

Like other glycophosphatidylinositol (GPI)-anchored proteins, PrP^C seems to recirculate via a subcellular compartment bounded by cholesterol-rich, non-acidic, detergent-insoluble membranes denominated 'rafts' (Figure 61.2) (Keller et al. 1992; Anderson 1993; Shyng et al. 1994; Gorodinsky and Harris 1995; Taraboulos et al. 1995). Within the raft compartment, GPI-anchored PrP^C seems to be either converted into PrP^{Sc} or partially degraded (Taraboulos et al. 1995; Meier et al. 2003). After denaturation PrP^{Sc}, like PrP^C, can be released from the cell membranes by digestion with phosphatidyl-inositol-specific phospholipase C, suggesting that PrP^{Sc} is tethered only by the GPI anchor (Borchelt et al. 1993). In scrapie-infected cultured cells, PrP^{Sc} is trimmed at the N terminus to form PrP$^{27-30}$ in an acidic intra-cellular compartment (Caughey et al. 1991b; Taraboulos et al. 1992b). In contrast to cultured cells, the N-term-inal trimming of PrP^{Sc} is minimal in brain, where little PrP$^{27-30}$ is found (McKinley et al. 1991a). Deleting the GPI addition signal resulted in greatly diminished synth-esis of PrP^{Sc} (Rogers et al. 1993), and soluble dimeric PrP^C inhibits prion replication (Meier et al. 2003). In contrast to PrP^C, PrP^{Sc} accumulates primarily within cells, where it is deposited in cytoplasmic vesicles, many of which seem to be secondary lysosomes (Taraboulos et al. 1990b, 1992b; Caughey et al. 1991b; McKinley et al.

1991b; Borchelt et al. 1992). Studies of scrapie-infected brains suggest that PrP^{Sc} accumulates within either lyso-somes or late endosomes (Laszlo et al. 1992; Arnold et al. 1995).

Although most of the difference in the mass of PrP$^{27-30}$ predicted from the amino acid sequence and observed after post-translational modification is due to complex-type oligosaccharides (Endo et al. 1989; Haraguchi et al. 1989), these sugar chains are not required for PrP^{Sc} synthesis in scrapie-infected cultured cells, based on experiments with the asparagine-linked glycosylation inhibitor tunicamycin, and site-directed mutagenesis studies (Taraboulos et al. 1990a).

SEARCH FOR A CHEMICAL MODIFICATION OF PRP

The discovery that the entire ORF of the PrP gene is contained within a single exon, first in Syrian hamsters and later in humans and other animals, argued that PrP^{Sc} is not generated by alternative splicing (Basler et al. 1986; Gold-mann and Hunter 1988; Hsiao et al. 1989; Goldmann et al. 1991b; Westaway et al. 1994a, 1994b). This prompted a search for a post-translational chemical modification to explain the differences in the properties of these two PrP isoforms (Stahl et al. 1993). PrP^{Sc} was analyzed by mass spectrometry and gas phase sequencing in order to identify any amino acid substitutions or post-translational chemical modifications. The amino acid sequence was the same as

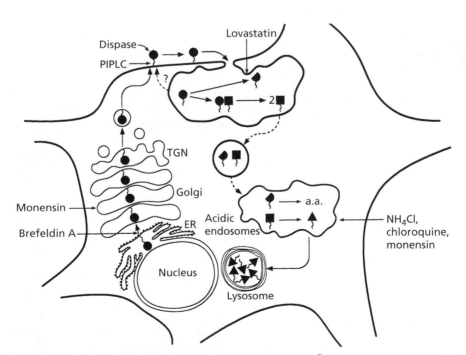

Figure 61.2 *Pathways of prion protein synthesis and degradation in cultured cells. PrP^{Sc} is denoted by squares; circles denote PrP^C. Before becoming protease-resistant, the PrP^{Sc} precursor transits through the plasma membrane and is sensitive to dispase or PIPLC added to the medium. PrP^{Sc} formation probably occurs in a compartment accessible from the plasma membrane, such as caveolae or early endosomes, both of which are non-acidic compartments. The synthesis of nascent PrP^{Sc} seems to require the interaction of PrP^C with existing PrP^{Sc}. In cultured cells, but not brain, the N terminus of PrP^{Sc} is trimmed to form PrP$^{27-30}$; PrP^{Sc} then accumulates primarily in secondary lysosomes. The inhibition of PrP^{Sc} synthesis by brefeldin A demonstrates that the endoplasmic reticulum (ER)–Golgi is not competent for its synthesis and that transport of PrP down the secretory pathway is required for the formation of PrP^{Sc}.*

that deduced from the translated ORF of the PrP gene, and no candidates for post-translational chemical modifications that might differentiate PrP^C from PrP^{Sc} were found (Stahl et al. 1993). These findings forced consideration of the possibility that conformation distinguishes the two PrP isoforms.

STRUCTURES OF PURIFIED PrP^C AND PrP^{SC}

Low-resolution structural studies indicated that PrP^C has a high α-helix content (ca. 40 percent) and little β-sheet (3 percent) (Pan et al. 1993). These findings were refined by Wüthrich and colleagues who determined the fine structure of PrP^C by nuclear magnetic resonance spectroscopy (Riek et al. 1996; Hornemann et al. 1997) (Figure 61.3a), and later also by crystallographic studies (Figure 61.3b) (Knaus et al. 2001). By contrast, the β-sheet content of PrP^{Sc} is ca. 40 percent and the α-helix ca. 30 percent as measured by Fourier-transformed infrared (FTIR) (Pan et al. 1993) and circular dichroism (CD) spectroscopy (Safar et al. 1993b) (Figure 61.4). No high-resolution structure is available for PrP^{Sc}, although interesting models have been conjectured on the basis of electron crystallography (Wille et al. 2002). That PrP^{27-30} has a high β-sheet content was inferred from the green-gold birefringence of the prion rods after staining with Congo red (Prusiner et al. 1983). Indeed, PrP^{27-30} polymerized into rod-shaped particles with ultrastructural appearance of amyloid (Figure 61.5) contains ca. 50 percent β-sheet and ca. 20 percent α-helix (Caughey et al. 1991a; Gasset et al. 1993; Safar et al. 1993a). In contrast to PrP^{27-30} which did polymerize into rod-shaped amyloids, neither purified PrP^C nor PrP^{Sc} formed aggregates detectable by electron microscopy (Figure 61.5) (McKinley et al. 1991a; Pan et al. 1993).

It is still possible that a hitherto undetected chemical modification of a small fraction of PrP^{Sc} initiates the conversion process into PrP^{Sc}. Limitations of the current analytical techniques for proteins prevent a stringent study of this question, and it is quite possible that PrP^{Sc} consists of inhomogeneous species, only some of which are capable of propagation. Because PrP^{Sc} seems to be the only component of the 'infectious' prion particle, it is likely that this conformational transition is a fundamental event in the propagation of prions. Accordingly, denaturation of PrP^{27-30} under conditions which reduced scrapie infectivity resulted in diminution of β-sheet content (Gasset et al. 1993; Safar et al. 1993b).

CONVERSION OF PrP^C INTO PrP^{SC}

Studies with Tg(SHaPrP) mice have provided genetic information about the process in which PrP^C is converted into PrP^{Sc} through the formation of a $PrP^C/$ PrP^{Sc} complex (Prusiner et al. 1990), even if such complex was not isolated physically. The level of PrP^C expression seems to be directly proportional to the rate of PrP^{Sc} formation and, thus, inversely related to the length of the incubation time. Formation of the $PrP^C/$ PrP^{Sc} complex was facilitated when the amino acid sequences of the two PrP isoforms were the same; SHaPrP differs from MoPrP at 16 positions out of 254. Differences in amino acid sequence delayed prion formation, resulting in a prolongation of the incubation time (Scott et al. 1989).

The protein-only hypothesis posits that the agent is devoid of nucleic acid and consists solely of an abnormal conformer of the cellular prion protein, PrP^C (Figure 61.6, p. 1355).

In vitro conversion of recombinant ^{35}S-labeled PrP^C to a PrP^{Sc}-like protease-resistant moiety was achieved by mixing with a 50-fold excess of PrP^{Sc} (Kocisko et al. 1994). The binding of PrP^C to PrP^{Sc} depends on the same residues (Kocisko et al. 1995) that render Tg(MH2M) mice susceptible to SHa prions (M. Scott et al. 1993) and seems to be strain-dependent (Bessen et al. 1995). However, evidence is still lacking that the converted material acquires infectious properties (Aguzzi and Heikenwalder 2003).

Propagation of prions

Initial transgenetic studies had shown that the 'species barrier' between mice and Syrian hamsters for the transmission of prions can be abolished by expression of a SHaPrP transgene in mice (Scott et al. 1989). Transgenic mice expressing human (Hu) PrP were then constructed. These Tg(HuPrP) mice inoculated with human prions failed to develop CNS dysfunction more frequently than nontransgenic controls (Telling et al. 1994). Faced with this apparent dichotomy, Scott constructed mice expressing a chimeric Hu/Mo PrP transgene designated MHu2M because earlier studies had shown that chimeric Syrian hamster/mouse (SHa/Mo) PrP transgenes supported transmission of either Mo or SHa prions (Scott et al., 1992; M. Scott et al. 1993). The Tg(MHu2M) mice expressing the chimeric transgene were highly susceptible to human prions, suggesting that Tg(HuPrP) mice have difficulty converting $HuPrP^C$ into PrP^{Sc} (Telling et al. 1994). Although MoPrP and HuPrP differ at 28 residues, only nine or perhaps fewer amino acids in the region between codons 96 and 167 feature in the species barrier in the transmission of human prions into mice, as demonstrated by the susceptibility of Tg(MHu2M) mice to human prions.

When Tg(HuPrP) mice were crossed with gene-targeted mice in which the MoPrP gene had been disrupted ($Prnp^{0/0}$) (Büeler et al. 1992), they were rendered susceptible to human prions. These findings suggested that Tg(HuPrP) mice were resistant to human prions because $MoPrP^C$ inhibited the conversion of $HuPrP^C$ into PrP^{Sc}: once $MoPrP^C$ was removed by gene ablation, the inhibition was abolished (Telling et al. 1995). Whereas earlier studies argued that PrP^C forms a complex with PrP^{Sc} during the formation of nascent

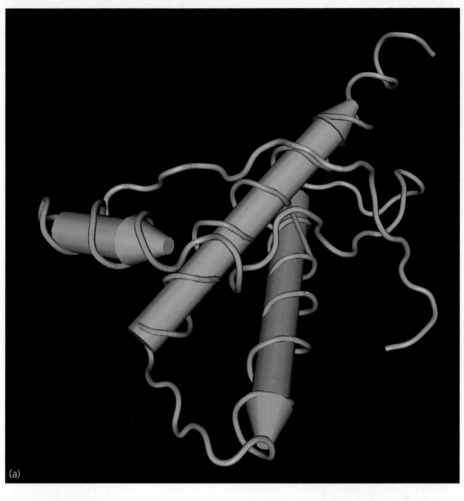

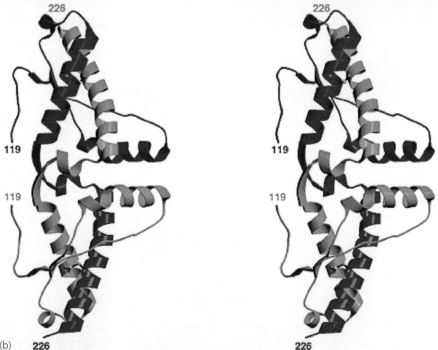

Figure 61.3 *The fine structure of the cellular prion protein, PrP^C.* **(a)** *Structure of the normal human prion protein, as submitted by R. Zahn, A. Liu, T. Luhrs and K. Wuthrich to the Molecular Modeling Database of the National Center for Biotechnology information (www.ncbi.nlm.nih.gov/Structure/mmdb/mmdbsrv.cgi?form=6&db=t&Dopt=s&uid=19138).* **(b)** *Crystal structure of a PrP dimer (reproduced from Knaus et al. 2001).*

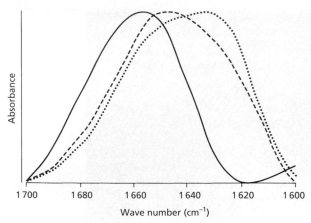

Figure 61.4 *Fourier transform infrared spectroscopy of prion proteins. The amide I′ band (1700–1600 cm⁻¹) of transmission FTIR spectra of PrP^C (solid line), PrP^Sc (dashed line) and PrP²⁷⁻³⁰ (dotted line). These proteins were suspended in a buffer in D_2O containing 0.15 M sodium chloride/10 mM sodium phosphate, pD 7.5 (uncorrected)/0.12 percent ZW. The spectra are scaled independently to be full scale on the ordinate axis (absorbance). (Reproduced from Pan et al. 1993)*

PrP^Sc (Prusiner et al. 1990), these findings suggested that PrP^C also binds to one (or more than one) additional macromolecule during the conversion process. Telling and colleagues called this second macromolecule 'protein X' with the proviso that a second binding site

on PrP^Sc might also function as protein X. However, 8 years after its initial postulation, no physical evidence for protein X has come forward, and Collinge and colleagues have observed exceptions to the genetic observations that had sparked the invention of protein X. Therefore, at present it is still possible that protein X is indeed a prion replication cofactor, but it is equally possible that it is nonexistent, that it exists but is not a protein, or that multiple host-encoded factors ('proteins X, Y, and Z') distinct from PrP may bind to PrP^Sc (Fischer et al. 2000; Maissen et al. 2001) and influence prion replication in vivo through a variety of direct and indirect mechanisms. On the basis of the available spectrum of data, one may speculate that the latter scenario is by far the most likely.

Transgenetics and gene targeting

Ablation of the PrP gene (*Prnp*^0/0) affected neither development nor behavior of the mice (Büeler et al. 1992; Manson et al. 1994a). In fact, *Prnp*^0/0 mice have remained healthy for more than 2 years. *Prnp*^0/0 mice are resistant to prions and do not propagate scrapie infectivity (Büeler et al. 1993; Prusiner et al. 1993; Sailer et al. 1994). *Prnp*^0/0 mice were sacrificed 5, 60, 120, and 315 days after inoculation with Rocky Mountain Laboratory prions passaged in CD-1 Swiss mice. Except for

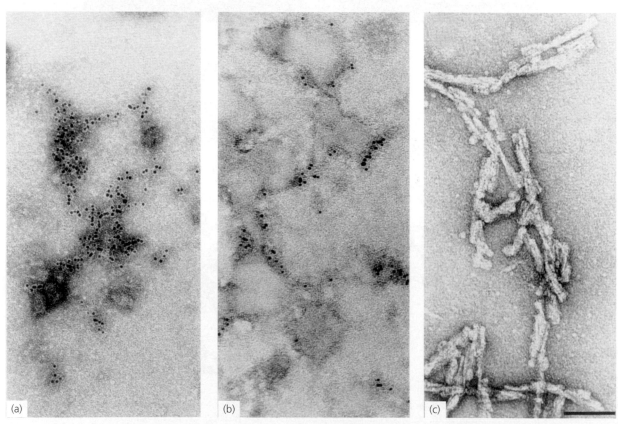

Figure 61.5 *Electron micrographs of negatively stained and immunogold-labeled prion proteins. (a) PrP^C. (b) PrP^Sc. (c) Prion rods composed of PrP²⁷⁻³⁰ were negatively stained with uranyl acetate. Bar, 100 nm. (Reproduced from Pan et al. 1993)*

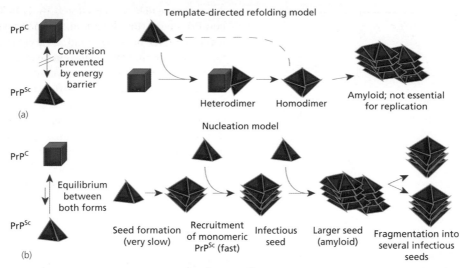

Figure 61.6 *Models for the conformational conversion of PrP^C into PrP^{Sc}. **(a)** The 'refolding' or template-assistance model postulates an interaction between exogenously introduced PrP^{Sc} and endogenous PrP^C, which is induced to transform itself into further PrP^{Sc}. A high-energy barrier may prevent spontaneous conversion of PrP^C into PrP^{Sc}. **(b)** The 'seeding' or nucleation-polymerization model proposes that PrP^C and PrP^{Sc} are in a reversible thermodynamic equilibrium. Only if several monomeric PrP^{Sc} molecules are mounted into a highly ordered seed, can further monomeric PrP^{Sc} be recruited and eventually aggregates to amyloid. Within such a crystallike seed, PrP^{Sc} becomes stabilized. Fragmentation of PrP^{Sc} aggregates increases the number of nuclei, which can recruit further PrP^{Sc} and thus results in apparent replication of the agent.*

residual infectivity from the inoculum detected at 5 days after inoculation, no infectivity was detected in the brains of *Prnp*$^{0/0}$ mice. *Prnp*$^{0/0}$ mice crossed with Tg(SHaPrP) mice were rendered susceptible to hamster prions but remained resistant to mouse prions (Büeler et al. 1993). Since the absence of PrP^C expression does not provoke disease, it is likely that scrapie and the other prion diseases result not from an inhibition of PrP^C function due to PrP^{Sc} but rather from interference with some as yet undefined cellular process (Hegde et al. 1998, 1999).

Mice heterozygous (*Prnp*$^{+/0}$) for ablation of the PrP gene had prolonged incubation times when inoculated with mouse prions (Figure 61.7) (Büeler et al. 1994; Manson et al. 1994b). The *Prnp*$^{+/0}$ mice developed signs of neurological dysfunction at 400–460 days after inoculation. Therefore, the amount of available PrP^C is rate-limiting for the development of disease – a finding with significant implications for prion therapy. These findings are in agreement with studies on Tg(SHaPrP) mice in which increased SHaPrP expression was accompanied by diminished incubation times (Prusiner et al. 1990), and reinforce the idea that the concentration of PrP^C in brain is rate-limiting for its conversion into PrP^{Sc}.

Because *Prnp*$^{0/0}$ mice do not express PrP^C, they can be easily immunized to produce α-PrP antibodies. *Prnp*$^{0/0}$ mice immunized with mouse or hamster prion rods produced α-PrP antisera that bound mouse, SHa, and human PrP (Prusiner et al. 1993; Brandner et al. 1996b). These findings contrast with earlier studies in which α-MoPrP antibodies could not be produced in mice, presumably because the mice had been rendered tolerant by the presence of MoPrP^C (Barry and Prusiner 1986; Kascsak

et al. 1987; Rogers et al. 1991). That *Prnp*$^{0/0}$ mice readily produce α-PrP antibodies is consistent with the hypothesis that the lack of an immune response in prion diseases is due to the fact that PrP^C and PrP^{Sc} share many epitopes. For reasons that are not understood, *Prnp*$^{0/0}$ mice have not proved useful to produce α-PrP antibodies that specifically recognize CD epitopes present on PrP^{Sc} but absent from PrP^C – although such experiments have now been attempted for more than a decade.

MODELING OF GSS IN TRANSGENIC MICE

The codon 102 point mutation found in GSS patients was introduced into the MoPrP gene and Tg(MoPrP-P101L)H mice were created expressing high (H) levels of the mutant transgene product. Two lines of Tg(MoPrP-P101L)H mice spontaneously developed CNS degeneration, characterized by clinical signs indistinguishable from experimental murine scrapie and neuropathology consisting of widespread spongiform morphology and astrocytic gliosis (Hsiao et al. 1990) and PrP amyloid plaques (Hsiao et al. 1994). Excitingly, transmission of brain homogenate from Tg(MoPrP-P101L)H mice to healthy mice expressing lower levels of the same transgene (denoted Tg196/*Prnp*$^{0/0}$) induced spongiform encephalopathy (Telling et al. 1996).

In other studies, modifying the expression of mutant and wild-type *Prnp* genes in transgenic mice permitted experimental manipulation of the pathogenesis of both inherited and infectious prion diseases. Although overexpression of the wtPrP-A transgene ca. eightfold was not deleterious to the mice, it did shorten scrapie incubation times to as little as 45 days after inoculation with mouse scrapie prions (Telling et al. 1996).

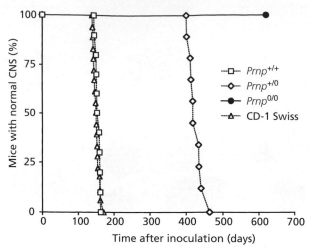

Figure 61.7 *Incubation times in PrP gene ablated* Prnp[+/0] *and* Prnp[0/0] *mice as well as wild-type* Prnp[+/+] *and CD-1 mice inoculated with RML mouse prions. The RML prions were heated and irradiated at 254 nm prior to intracerebral inoculation into CD-1 Swiss mice (open triangles),* Prnp[+/+] *mice (open squares),* Prnp[+/0] *mice (open diamonds) or* Prnp[0/0] *mice (solid circle).*

Prion diversity

The diversity of scrapie prions was first appreciated in goats inoculated with 'hyper' and 'drowsy' isolates (Pattison and Millson 1961b). Scrapie isolates or 'strains' from goats with a drowsy syndrome transmitted a similar syndrome to inoculated recipients, whereas those from goats with a 'hyper' or ataxic syndrome transmitted an ataxic form of scrapie to recipient goats. Subsequently, studies in mice demonstrated the existence of many scrapie 'strains' in which extracts prepared from the brains of mice inoculated with a particular preparation of prions produced a similar disease in inoculated recipients (Dickinson and Fraser 1979; Bruce and Dickinson 1987; Dickinson and Outram 1988). While the clinical signs of scrapie for different prion isolates in mice tended to be similar, the isolates could be distinguished by the incubation times, the distribution of CNS vacuolation that they produced, and whether or not amyloid plaques formed.

That such isolates could be propagated through multiple passages in mice suggested that the scrapie pathogen has a nucleic acid genome that is copied and passed on to nascent prions (Dickinson et al. 1968; Bruce and Dickinson 1987). But no evidence for scrapie-specific nucleic acid encoding information that specifies the incubation time and the distribution of neuropathological lesions has emerged from considerable efforts using a variety of experimental approaches. In striking contrast, mice expressing PrP transgenes have demonstrated that the level of PrP expression is inversely related to the incubation time (Prusiner et al. 1990). Furthermore, the distribution of CNS vacuolation and attendant gliosis are a consequence of pattern of PrP[Sc]

deposition which can be altered by both PrP genes and non-PrP genes (Prusiner et al. 1990). These observations taken together begin to build an argument for PrP[Sc] as the informational molecule in which prion 'strain'-specific information is encrypted. Deciphering the mechanism by which PrP[Sc] carries information for prion diversity and passes it onto the nascent prions is a challenging goal. Whether PrP[Sc] can adopt multiple conformations, each one of which produces prions exhibiting distinct incubation times and patterns of PrP[Sc] deposition, remains to be determined (Cohen et al. 1994). Preliminary immunochemical evidence suggests that PrP[Sc] of different strains may expose different epitopes (Safar et al. 1998), and may display different stability to chaotropic salts (Peretz et al. 2002) – which perhaps may provide indirect evidence for conformational differences, but may also indicate association with different 'third parties' of proteic or other nature.

PRION STRAINS AND VARIATIONS IN PATTERNS OF DISEASE

Scrapie was first transmitted to sheep and goats by intraocular inoculation (Cuille and Chelle 1939) and later by intracerebral, oral, subcutaneous, intramuscular, and intravenous injections of brain extracts from sheep developing scrapie. Incubation periods of 1–3 years were common, and often many of the inoculated animals failed to develop disease (Dickinson and Stamp 1969; Hadlow et al. 1980, 1982). Different breeds of sheep exhibited markedly different susceptibilities to scrapie prions inoculated subcutaneously, suggesting that the genetic background might influence host permissiveness (Gordon 1966).

The lengths of the incubation times have been used to distinguish prion strains inoculated into sheep, goats, mice, and hamsters. Dickinson and his colleagues developed a system for 'strain typing' by which mice with genetically determined short and long incubation times were used in combination with the F1 cross (Dickinson et al. 1968, 1984; Dickinson and Meikle 1971). For example, C57BL mice exhibited short incubation times of ca. 150 days when inoculated with either the ME7 or the Chandler isolates; VM mice inoculated with these same isolates had prolonged incubation times of ca. 300 days. The mouse gene controlling incubation times was labelled *Sinc* and long incubation times were said to be a dominant trait because of prolonged incubation times in F1 mice. Prion strains were categorized into two groups based on their incubation times:

1 those causing disease more rapidly in 'short' incubation time C57BL mice
2 those causing disease more rapidly in 'long' incubation time VM mice.

Noteworthy are the 22A and 87V prion strains that can be passaged in VM mice while maintaining their distinct characteristics.

MOLECULAR BASIS OF PRION STRAINS

The mechanism by which isolate-specific information is carried by prions remains enigmatic; indeed, explaining the molecular basis of prion diversity seems to be a formidable challenge. Some investigators are still contending that scrapie is caused by a viruslike particle containing a scrapie-specific nucleic acid that encodes the information expressed by each isolate (Bruce and Dickinson 1987). To date, no such polynucleotide has been identified, despite using a wide variety of techniques, including measurements of the nucleic acids in purified preparations. An alternative hypothesis has been suggested that PrP^{Sc} alone is capable of transmitting disease but the characteristics of PrP^{Sc} might be modified by a cellular nucleic acid (Weissmann 1991b). This accessory cellular polynucleotide is postulated to induce its own synthesis upon transmission from one host to another, but there is no experimental evidence to support its existence.

Two additional hypotheses not involving a nucleic acid have been offered to explain distinct prion isolates: a non-nucleic acid second component might create prion diversity, or post-translational modification of PrP^{Sc} might be responsible for the different properties of distinct prion isolates (Prusiner 1991). Whether the PrP^{Sc} modification is chemical or only conformational remains to be established, but no candidate chemical modifications have been identified (Stahl et al. 1993). Structural studies of GPI anchors of two SHa isolates have failed to reveal any differences; it is interesting that ca. 40 percent of the anchor glycans have sialic acid residues (Stahl et al. 1992). A portion of the PrP^C GPI anchors also have sialic acid residues; PrP is the first protein found to have sialic acid residues attached to GPI anchors.

Multiple prion isolates might be explained by distinct PrP^{Sc} conformers that act as templates for the folding of de novo synthesized PrP^{Sc} molecules during prion 'replication.' Although it is clear that passage history can be responsible for the prolongation of incubation time when prions are passed between mice expressing different PrP allotypes (Carlson et al. 1989) or between species (Prusiner et al. 1990), many scrapie strains show distinct incubation times in the same inbred host (Bruce et al. 1991).

PrP^{Sc} species associated with two hamster-adapted scrapie strains, hyper (HY) and drowsy (DY), proved to display characteristic clinical and histopathological properties as well as distinct biochemical patterns with respect to proteinase K digestion (Bessen and Marsh 1992, 1994) – which may be explainable by the presence of different conformations of PrP^{Sc}. Analogous findings have been made with other prion strains propagated in mice. In addition, PrP^{Sc} of certain strains differ in the ratio of diglycosylated to the monoglycosylated form. Based on the fragment size and the relative abundance

of individual bands, three distinct patterns (PrP^{Sc} types 1–3) were defined for sporadic and iCJD cases (Collinge et al. 1996; Parchi et al. 1996, 1999). By contrast, all cases of vCJD displayed a novel pattern, designated type 4 by Collinge, and type IIb by Parchi and Gambetti (Figure 61.8). Interestingly, brain extracts from BSE-infected cattle as well as BSE-inoculated macaques exhibited a type 4 pattern. Even more intriguingly, transmission of BSE or vCJD to mice produced mouse PrP^{Sc} with a type 4 pattern indistinguishable from the original inoculum (Hill et al. 1997a) – findings that impressively support the hypothesis that vCJD is the human counterpart to BSE. An additional tool, which may eventually serve to characterize prion strains, utilizes the differential affinity of certain antibodies for properly folded and denatured isoforms of PrP, thereby differentiating as many as eight different conformers (Safar et al. 1998). This provides further circumstantial evidence for the assumption that strain specificity is encrypted within the physical structure of PrP.

THE FUNCTION OF THE CELLULAR PRION PROTEIN

Despite considerable efforts, the physiological function of PrP^C is still unclear. A proposed role for PrP^C in synaptic function (Collinge et al. 1994) has been questioned by other investigators (Lledo et al. 1996) and a possible regulation of circadian rhythm by PrP^C has remained more-or-less anecdotal (Tobler et al. 1996). Hence, the only definite phenotype of $Prnp^{0/0}$ mice is their resistance to prion inoculation (Büeler et al. 1993). It seems, however, rather unlikely that a singular protein that is as highly conserved among species as PrP^C, from turtles to frogs, fish, and humans, has evolved for the sole reason of bestowing susceptibility to prion diseases.

If the function of PrP^C were completely unrelated to prion disease pathogenesis, PrP^C may be just one of many proteins whose function awaits clarification. Yet the function of PrP^C may very well have something to do, in a subtle way, with prion-induced damage. $Prnp$ ablation does not elicit disease, even when induced postnatally (Mallucci et al. 2002): hence prion pathology is unlikely to come about by simple loss of PrP^C function. If PrP^C transduces a signal (in analogy to many other GPI-linked proteins), or possesses some enzymatic activity, one could speculate that conversion to PrP^{Sc} may alter signal transduction strength, or substrate specificity, thereby conferring a toxic dominant function. In these scenarios, understanding the function of PrP^C may be instrumental to deciphering prion pathology, and perhaps even to devising therapeutical approaches.

Is PrP^C an enzyme? Glockshuber noted that PrP^C has similarities to membrane-anchored signal peptidases (Glockshuber et al. 1998), but his observation has not been substantiated by functional data. PrP^C can bind

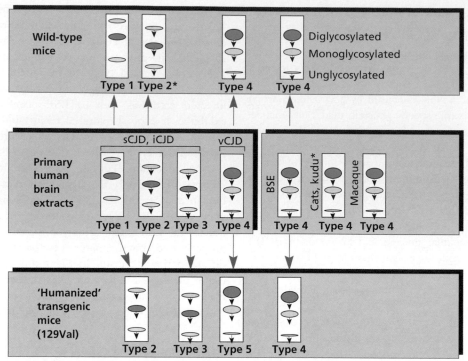

Figure 61.8 *Patterns of PrP glycosylation. Representation of the three glycosylated PrP^{Sc} moieties (un-, mono-, and diglycosylated PrP^{Sc}) in immunoblots of brain extracts after digest with proteinase K. Different inocula result in specific mobilities of the three PrP bands as well as different predominance of certain bands (middle panel). These characteristic patterns can be retained, or changed to other predictable patterns after passage in wild-type (upper panel) or humanized mice (PrP-deficient mice bearing a human PrP transgene, lower panel). Based on the fragment size and the relative abundance of individual bands, three distinct patterns (PrP^{Sc} types 1–3) were defined for sporadic and iatrogenic CJD cases. By contrast, all cases of vCJD displayed a novel pattern, designated as type 4 pattern.*

copper (Brown et al. 1997; Wadsworth et al. 1999), but reports of increased copper content of neurons lacking PrP^C have been questioned by contradictory findings (Waggoner et al. 2000). The speculation that PrP^C may be a superoxide dismutase (Brown et al., 1997; D.R. Brown et al. 1999) was perceived as particularly attractive in view of its multiple copper-binding sites. However, PrP^C does not make any measurable contribution to dismutase activity in vivo (Hutter et al. 2003; Waggoner et al. 2000). Interestingly, it was recently suggested that amino proximally truncated PrP^C may depress endogenous dismutase activity (Sakudo et al. 2003).

Perhaps PrP^C and PrP^{Sc} do not possess any intrinsic biological activity, yet they modify the function of other proteins. This supposition has prompted a search for PrP-interacting partners, and there is no dearth of PrP-binding proteins: the antiapoptotic protein Bcl-2 (Kurschner et al. 1995), caveolin (Gorodinsky and Harris 1995; Harmey et al. 1995), the laminin receptor precursor (Rieger et al. 1997), plasminogen (Fischer et al. 2000) and N-CAM (Schmitt-Ulms et al. 2001). None of these interactors, however, have yet revealed a functional pathway in which PrP^C would be involved in vivo. It was recently shown that PrP-deficient macrophages do not support bacterial 'swimming internalization' of the gram-negative bacterium, *Brucella abortus*

(Watarai et al. 2003) and that PrP^C interacts with a *Brucella* heat-shock protein, Hsp60. These intriguing findings raise the question of whether PrP^C is a part of a general Hsp60-dependent 'danger-sensing' mechanism (Aguzzi and Hardt 2003).

THE PRION DOPPELGANGER

After the advent of large-scale sequencing efforts and genome projects, it was realized that there is an ORF directly adjacent of *Prnp* that encodes a protein sharing significant homology with PrP^C (Moore et al. 1999). The novel gene, *Prnd*, is located 16 kb downstream of *Prnp* in the mouse genome, and encodes a protein of 179 residues, which was termed Dpl ('downstream of the *Prnp* locus' or 'Doppel,' German for 'double') (Moore et al. 1999; Weissmann and Aguzzi 1999; Behrens and Aguzzi 2002). The *Prnd* gene is evolutionarily conserved from humans to sheep and cattle, and shows roughly 25 percent identity with the carboxy-proximal two-thirds of PrP^C. Structural studies indicate that Dpl contains three α-helices, like PrP^C, and two disulfide bridges between the second and third helices (Lu et al. 2000; Silverman et al. 2000; Mo et al. 2001). Dpl mRNA is expressed at high levels in testis, less in other peripheral organs and, notably, at very low levels in brain of adult wild-type mice. However, significant *Prnd* mRNA transcripts were detected during embryogenesis and in the brains of newborn mice, arguing for a possible function of Dpl in brain development (Li et al. 2000).

To probe the function of Dpl, the *Prnd* gene was inactivated in embryonic stem (ES) cells (Behrens et al. 2001). Similarly to mice lacking PrP^C, mice devoid of Dpl survive to adulthood and do not show obvious phenotypical alterations, suggesting that Dpl is dispensable for embryogenesis and postnatal development (Behrens et al. 2002). The similarities between PrP^C and Dpl in primary amino acid sequence, structure, and subcellular localization suggest related biological functions: therefore a possible role of PrP^C and Dpl during development may be masked by functional redundancy. To address this question it will be necessary to generate mice lacking *Prnp* as well as *Prnd* and to study whether the lack of both PrP^C and Dpl will result in an exacerbation of the mutant phenotypes. These double-mutant mice may finally reveal the true physiological function of PrP^C and Dpl, and pave the way for the long-awaited understanding of these proteins.

ES cells carrying a homozygous null mutation of the *Prnd* locus, and a normal *Prnp* locus, were found to be capable of giving rise to all neural cell lineages when transplanted into host brains. The Dpl protein resembles an N-terminally truncated PrP^C protein lacking the octamer repeats. But the latter version of PrP^C is actually capable of supporting PrP^{Sc} propagation (Flechsig et al. 2000), suggesting that the Dpl protein may in principle be susceptible to conversion into 'Dpl^{Sc}.' However, presently there is no evidence whether upon scrapie inoculation Dpl can be converted into a misfolded β-strand-rich, protease-resistant conformation. After inoculation with scrapie prions, Dpl-deficient neural grafts showed spongiosis, gliosis, and unimpaired accumulation of PrP^{Sc} and infectivity similar to wild-type neuroectodermal grafts (Behrens et al. 2001). Therefore in neural grafts *Prnd* deficiency does not prevent prion pathogenesis. It is important to note, however, that this experimental approach does not rule out a role for Dpl in peripheral prion pathogenesis and in PrP^{Sc} transport to the brain. The latter possibility is worth studying, because *Prnd* is expressed in the spleen, a major peripheral reservoir of PrP^{Sc} and prion infectivity (Li et al. 2000).

Four polymorphisms in human *Prnd* were detected, but no strong association was found between any of these polymorphisms and human prion diseases (Mead et al., 2000; Peoc'h et al., 2000). These findings further argue against an important function of Dpl in neurons during prion disease, at least in genetically determined forms of these diseases.

Phenotypes of *Prnp*-deficient mice

Although this was not realized for several years, a Dpl-associated phenotype had been accidentally produced in knock-out mice lacking PrP^C. In the course of the 1990s, several mouse lines with targeted disruptions of *Prnp* were independently generated in various laboratories. All mutant mouse lines lacked significant portions of the *Prnp* ORF and did not produce PrP^C protein, but showed two strikingly different phenotypes. Zrch *Prnp*$^{0/0}$ and Edbg *Prnp*$^{-/-}$ (termed after the city of origin) showed only minor defects (Büeler et al. 1992; Collinge and Palmer 1994; Manson et al. 1994a; Tobler et al. 1996) whereas Ngsk *Prnp*$^{-/-}$, Zürich II and Rcm0 mice develop cerebellar Purkinje cell degeneration causing ataxia with advancing age (Sakaguchi et al. 1996; Moore et al. 1999; Rossi et al. 2001). This conundrum was solved when David Westaway and colleagues realized that in the brain of ataxic, but not of healthy *Prnp*-mutant mice, *Prnd* mRNA was up-regulated (Moore et al. 1999; Li et al. 2000). An intergenic splicing event places the Dpl locus under the control of the *Prnp* promoter, probably due to the deletion of the *Prnp* intron 2 sequence including its splicing acceptor (Moore et al. 1999). This intergenic splicing event could be detected at very low levels also in wild-type mice, but was greatly enhanced by the absence of the intron 2 splice acceptor (Moore et al. 1999). Whereas the *Prnp* promoter is strongly expressed in neuronal cells, the *Prnd* promoter is not (Moore et al. 1999; Li et al. 2000; Rossi et al. 2001) and therefore *Prnd* expression from the *Prnp* promoter results in overproduction of Dpl in the brain (Moore et al. 1999; Li et al. 2000; Rossi et al. 2001). Further experiments have demonstrated an inverse correlation between the mRNA levels of *Prnd* and the onset of ataxia. Disease progression was accelerated by increasing *Prnd* levels, supporting the notion that ectopic Dpl expression, but not functional loss of PrP^C, may be responsible for neuronal degeneration in ataxic *Prnp*-deficient mice (Rossi et al. 2001).

The function of the Doppel protein

Behrens and colleagues inactivated the *Prnd* gene. However, they have not been able to generate any progeny from intercrosses of *Prnd*$^{-/-}$ mice. Female *Prnd*$^{-/-}$ mice, when crossed to *Prnd*$^{-/-}$ or *Prnd*$^{+/-}$ mice, yielded litter sizes similar to those of wild-type. By contrast, male *Prnd*$^{-/-}$ mice were infertile. Their sexual activity was similar to that of controls, as shown by a normal number of copulation plugs. However, the number of spermatozoa in the cauda epididymis of *Prnd*$^{-/-}$ males was reduced, and motility of mutant sperm was decreased. Therefore, sterility of Dpl-mutant males is not due to behavioral abnormalities, but may be due to a spermatogenesis defect. Indeed, *Prnd*$^{-/-}$ sperm heads were severely malformed and lacked a discernible well-developed acrosome (Figure 61.9). As the acrosome is essential for sperm/egg interaction, this defect could explain the sterility of *Prnd*-deficient males.

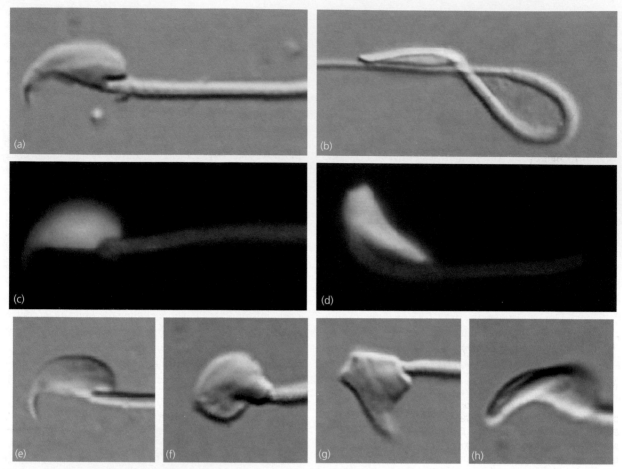

Figure 61.9 *Morphology of sperms in mice lacking the Doppel gene. Spermatozoa from Dpl-deficient mice are often heavily malformed. (a, b) Photographs of bright field images of spermatozoa isolated from wild-type* **(a)** *and* Prnd$^{-/-}$ *mice* **(b)**. **(c, d)** *Spermatozoa isolated from* Prnd$^{+/+}$ **(c)** *and* Prnd$^{-/-}$ *mice* **(d)** *were stained with mitotracker to detect mitochondria (in green) and with the DNA stain Hoechst (in blue). (e, h* *Photographs of bright-field images of sperm heads from* Prnd$^{+/+}$ **(e)** *and* Prnd$^{-/-}$ *mice* **(f–h)**

In vitro fertilization (IVF) experiments confirmed that spermatozoa isolated from *Prnd*$^{-/-}$ males were unable to fertilize wild-type oocytes. Spermatozoa of *Prnd*$^{-/-}$ males never penetrated the zona pellucida. However, if the zona pellucida was partially dissected and IVF was performed with sperm suspension from *Prnd*$^{-/-}$ males, fertility was partially rescued. These data indicate that *Prnd*$^{-/-}$ spermatozoa are capable of oocyte fertilization, albeit at a lower frequency than controls, but that they cannot overcome the barrier imposed by the zona pellucida (Figure 61.10).

A significant amount of PrP^C is expressed in mature spermatozoa. The PrP protein found in testes was truncated in its carboxy terminus in the vicinity of residue 200 (Shaked et al. 1999). A protective role for PrP against copper toxicity has been proposed: sperm cells originating from *Prnp*-ablated mice were found to be more susceptible to high copper concentrations than wild-type sperm. However, male *Prnp*$^{0/0}$ knockout mice are not sterile and produce normal litter sizes. PrP expressed in testes is clearly not capable of compensating for the absence of Dpl, suggesting

nonredundant functions for the two proteins. However, Dpl may mask a minor function of PrP^C in testes development or spermiogenesis; therefore, it will be very interesting to explore whether males lacking both PrP^C and Dpl might display a more severe defect than *Prnd*$^{-/-}$ single mutant mice. Also, it will be interesting to determine whether testicular expression of amino terminally truncated PrP^C restores the fertility of Dpl-deficient mice: if so, this would finally provide a long-sought experimental window into structure–function relationships affecting the physiology of PrP^C.

At present the molecular mechanism by which Dpl regulates acrosome development is unclear. Dpl may be present on the acrosomic vesicles through its GPI-anchor, and possibly participate in acrosome morphogenesis. Alternatively, Dpl may regulate acrosome function in a more indirect way. We have also observed that sperm isolated from *Prnd*$^{-/-}$ mice is greatly impaired in sperm/egg interaction and that *Prnd*$^{-/-}$ spermatozoa fail to trigger the acrosomal reaction. Oligosaccharides have been implicated in sperm binding

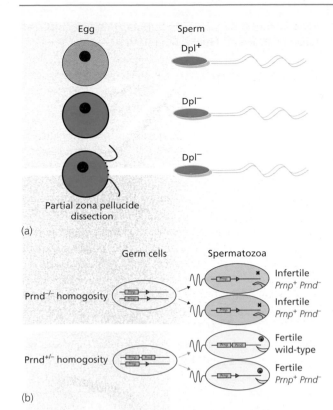

Figure 61.10 *A possible model for the function of the Doppel protein in fertilization.* **(a)** *Male sterility in mice that lack the Doppel protein appears to come about because Doppel-deficient sperms are incapable of fertilizing eggs. The process that appears to be disturbed relates to the acrosomal reaction and to the penetration of the zona pellucida. In fact, mechanical dissection of the zona pellucida restores, at least in part, fertility.* **(b)** *Interestingly, haploid spermatozoa lacking the Doppel gene (Prnd⁻) are perfectly fertile when generated in the context of a heterozygous Prnd⁺/⁻ mouse. Instead, Prnd⁻ sperms are infertile when generated in a Prnd⁻/⁻ mouse. This may be because sperms spend much of the maturation time in the form of syncytia, with maturing cells connected to each other by cytoplasmic bridges. This may allow sufficient amounts of Doppel protein to be transferred from Prnd⁺ to Prnd⁻ spermatids, and rescue fertility in trans.*

and signaling for the acrosome reaction, but the composition and structure of the essential carbohydrate moieties remain controversial (Wassarman et al. 2001). Dpl is a highly glycosylated protein located at the outside of the plasma membrane (Moore et al. 1999; Silverman et al. 2000); therefore, it is possible that Dpl present on the sperm plasma membrane is directly involved in sperm/egg interaction. With regard to the keen interest in the development of new methods of contraception (in particular those targeting the male), the phenotype of *Prnd⁻/⁻* mutant mice suggests that inhibition of Dpl function may provide a novel target for contraceptive intervention (Behrens and Aguzzi 2002).

In this context, it is interesting to mention that the laboratory of David Melton in Edinburgh has reported a slightly different phenotype of Dpl-deficient mice (communicated by D. Paisley and D. Melton). In

contrast to the mice generated in Zurich, Doppel-deficient homozygous males in Edinburgh appear to be able to fertilize eggs. In a series of IVFs, the Melton laboratory has reported that progression to the early cleavage divisions occurred, but was soon thereafter followed by death of the embryos at the preimplantation stage. Instead, there were no obvious malformations of sperms. Whether this discrepancy is related to a divergent genetic background of the mice utilized, whether it points to slightly different targeting strategies, or finally, whether it might uncover yet another surprising phenomenon in the genetics of prion-related genes, is – at the time of writing – wholly unclear.

CLINICAL AND PATHOLOGICAL ASPECTS OF PRION DISEASES

Scrapie

EXPERIMENTAL SCRAPIE

For decades, studies of experimental scrapie were performed exclusively with sheep and goats, which required incubation periods of 1–3 years. A crucial methodological advance in experimental studies of scrapie was created by the demonstration that scrapie could be transmitted to mice (Chandler 1961, 1963) which could be used for endpoint titrations of particular samples. In addition, pathogenesis experiments were performed directed at elucidating factors governing incubation times and neuropathological lesions (Eklund et al. 1967; Dickinson et al. 1968).

NATURAL SCRAPIE IN SHEEP AND GOATS

Even though scrapie was recognized as a distinct disorder of sheep with respect to its clinical manifestations as early as 1738, the disease remained an enigma, even with respect to its pathology, for more than two centuries (Parry 1983). Some veterinarians thought that scrapie was a disease of muscle caused by parasites, whilst others thought that it was a dystrophic process (M'Gowan 1914). An investigation into the etiology of scrapie followed the vaccination of sheep for louping-ill virus with formalin-treated extracts of ovine lymphoid tissue unknowingly contaminated with scrapie prions (Gordon 1946). Two years later, more than 1 500 sheep developed scrapie from this vaccine.

Scrapie of sheep and goats share with CWD of deer and elk a unique property among prion diseases: they seem to be readily communicable within flocks. Although the transmissibility of scrapie seems to be well established, the mechanism of the natural spread of scrapie among sheep is puzzling. The placenta has been implicated as one source of prions, accounting for the horizontal spread of scrapie within flocks (Pattison and Millson 1961a; Pattison 1964; Pattison et al. 1972;

Onodera et al. 1993). Whether this view is correct remains to be established. In Iceland, scrapie-infected flocks of sheep were destroyed and the pastures left vacant for several years; however, reintroduction of sheep from flocks known to be free of scrapie for many years eventually resulted in scrapie (Palsson 1979). The source of the scrapie prions that attacked the sheep from flocks without a history of scrapie is unknown. Transmission through mites has been advocated (Wisniewski et al. 1996), but its significance on the field remains somewhat anecdotal.

GENETICS OF SHEEP

Parry argued that host genes were responsible for the development of scrapie in sheep. He was convinced that natural scrapie is a genetic disease which could be eradicated by proper breeding protocols (Parry 1962, 1983). He considered its transmission by inoculation to be of importance primarily for laboratory studies and communicable infection of little consequence in nature. Other investigators viewed natural scrapie as an infectious disease, and argued that host genetics only modulates susceptibility to an endemic infectious agent (Dickinson et al. 1965). The incubation time gene for experimental scrapie in Cheviot sheep, called *Sip*, is said to be linked to a PrP gene (Hunter et al. 1989); however, the null hypothesis of nonlinkage has yet to be tested and this is important, especially in view of earlier studies which argue that susceptibility of sheep to scrapie is governed by a recessive gene (Parry 1962, 1983).

Polymorphisms at codons 136 and 171 of the PrP gene in sheep that produce amino acid substitutions have been studied with respect to the occurrence of scrapie in sheep (Clouscard et al. 1995). In Romanov and Ile-de-France breeds of sheep, a polymorphism in the PrP ORF was found at codon 136 (A→V) which correlates with scrapie (Laplanche et al. 1993b). Sheep homozygous or heterozygous for Val at codon 136 were susceptible to scrapie whereas those that were homozygous for Ala were resistant. Unexpectedly, only one of 74 scrapied autochthonous sheep had a Val at codon 136; these sheep were from three breeds denoted Lacaune, Manech, and Presalpes (Laplanche et al. 1993a).

In Suffolk sheep, a polymorphism in the PrP ORF was found at codon 171 (Q→R) (Goldmann et al. 1990a, 1990b). Studies of natural scrapie in the USA have shown that ca. 85 percent of the afflicted sheep are of the Suffolk breed. Only those Suffolk sheep homozygous for Gln (Q) at codon 171 had scrapie, although healthy controls with QQ, QR, and RR genotypes were found (Westaway et al. 1994b). These results argue that susceptibility in Suffolk sheep is governed by the PrP codon 171 polymorphism. Whether the PrP codon 171 or 136 polymorphisms in Cheviot sheep have the same profound influence on susceptibility to scrapie as has

been found for codon 171 in Suffolks is unknown (Goldmann et al. 1991a; Hunter et al. 1991).

Bovine spongiform encephalopathy

EPIDEMIC OF MAD COW DISEASE

In 1986, an epidemic of a previously unknown disease appeared in cattle in Great Britain (Wells et al. 1987): bovine spongiform encephalopathy (BSE) or 'mad cow' disease. BSE was shown to be a prion disease by demonstrating protease-resistant PrP in brains of ill cattle (Hope et al. 1988; Prusiner et al. 1993). Based mainly on epidemiological evidence, it has been proposed that BSE represents a massive common-source epidemic which has caused more than 180 000 cases to date (Weissmann and Aguzzi 1997). In Britain, cattle, particularly dairy cows, were routinely fed MBM as a nutritional supplement (Wilesmith et al. 1988, 1992a, b; Wilesmith and Wells 1991). The MBM was prepared by rendering the offal of sheep and cattle using a process that involved steam treatment and hydrocarbon solvent extraction. The extraction process produced a protein and fat-rich fractions; the protein or greaves fraction contained about 1 percent fat from which the MBM was prepared. In the late 1970s, the price of tallow prepared from the fat fraction fell, making it no longer profitable to use hydrocarbons in the rendering process. The resulting MBM contained about 14 percent fat: perhaps the high lipid content protected scrapie prions in the sheep offal from being completely inactivated by steam.

Since 1988, the practice of using dietary protein supplements for domestic animals derived from rendered sheep or cattle offal has been forbidden in the UK. Curiously, almost half of the BSE cases have occurred in herds where only a single affected animal has been found; several cases of BSE in a single herd are infrequent (Wilesmith et al. 1988; Dealler and Lacey 1990; Wilesmith and Wells 1991; Weissmann and Aguzzi 1997). In 1992, the BSE epidemic reached a peak, with over 35 000 cattle afflicted (Figure 61.11). In 1993, fewer than 32 000 cattle were diagnosed with BSE and in 1994 the number was approximately 22 000. In 2003, BSE had become a rare disease in British and European cattle, but regrettably (and quite unexplicably), it still had not completely disappeared.

TRANSMISSION OF BSE TO EXPERIMENTAL ANIMALS

Brain extracts from BSE cattle have transmitted disease to mice, cattle, sheep, and pigs after intracerebral inoculation (Fraser et al. 1988; Dawson et al. 1990a, b; Bruce et al. 1993). Transmissions to mice and sheep suggest that cattle preferentially propagate a single 'strain' of prions: seven BSE brains all produced similar incubation times as measured in each of three strains of inbred mice (Bruce et al. 1993). However, this notion was recently challenged on the basis of transgenetic studies (Asante et al. 2002). Incontrovertible evidence for the existence of several BSE strains, in the opinion of the author, has yet to be provided.

Of particular importance to the BSE epidemic is the recent transmission of BSE to the nonhuman primate marmoset after intracerebral inoculation followed by a prolonged incubation period (Baker et al. 1993). The potential parallels with kuru of humans, confined to the Fore region of New Guinea (Gajdusek et al. 1966; Gajdusek 1977), are worthy of consideration. Once the most common cause of death among women and children in that region, kuru has almost disappeared with the cessation of ritualistic cannibalism (Alpers 1987). Although it seems likely that kuru was transmitted orally, as proposed for BSE among cattle, some investigators argue that other routes of transmission were important because oral transmission of kuru prions to apes and monkeys has been difficult to demonstrate (Gajdusek 1977; Gibbs et al. 1980).

ORAL TRANSMISSION OF PRIONS

Besides BSE, four other animal diseases seem to have arisen from ingestion of prions. It has been suggested that an outbreak of transmissible mink encephalopathy in 1985 arose from the use for feed of a cow with a sporadic case of BSE (Will et al. 1996). The source of prions in CWD of mule, deer and elk is unclear (Williams and Young 1980, 1982). The prion-contaminated MBM thought to be the cause of BSE is also most likely the cause of feline spongiform encephalopathy (FSE) and exotic ungulate encephalopathy. FSE has been found in domestic cats throughout Europe, as well as in a puma and a cheetah (Willoughby et al. 1992). Three cases of FSE in domestic cats have been transmitted to laboratory mice and PrP^{Sc} has been identified in their brains by immunoblotting (Pearson et al. 1992). Whether FSE may have transmitted to a human (Zanusso et al. 1998) remains anectodal and unproven.

Prion disease has been found in the brains of the nyala, greater kudu, eland, gembok, and Arabian oryx in British zoos; all of these animals are exotic ungulates. Of eight greater kudu born into a herd maintained in a London zoo since 1987, five have developed prion disease. Except for the first case, none of the other four kudu was exposed to feeds containing ruminant-derived MBM (Kirkwood et al. 1993). Brain extracts prepared from a nyala and a greater kudu have been transmitted to mice (Kirkwood et al. 1990; Cunningham et al. 1993). PrP of the greater kudu differs from the bovine protein at four residues; Arabian oryx PrP differs from the sheep PrP at only one residue (Poidinger et al. 1993).

Chronic wasting disease of deer and elk

As the only prion disease of wildlife, CWD was initially reported in 1980 as a TSE in captive research deer in Colorado and Wyoming – the disease origin still remains completely obscure (Williams and Young 1980). Since 1980, free-ranging mule deer (*Odocoileus hemionus*), white-tailed deer (*Odocoileus virginanus)*, and Rocky Mountain elk (*Cervus elaphus nelsoni*) have been detected in the same region of Colorado and Wyoming (Spraker et al. 1997), but recently increased surveillance efforts across the USA and Canada have startlingly revealed CWD in adjacent states (Nebraska, New Mexico, and Utah) but also distant (Wisconsin, Illinois, Canada) from this original endemic region. Additionally, game-ranched elk have not escaped the disease, with CWD being first detected in 1997. The staggeringly high transmission apparent in captive deer (up to 90 percent infected in one facility, (Williams and Young 1992)) and in free-ranging deer (up to 15 percent, (Miller et al. 2000)), occurs by unknown mechanisms, but it is likely to be a horizontal route; saliva or feces could potentially harbor infectious prions and contaminate grazing areas.

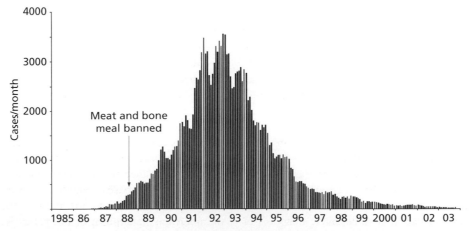

Figure 61.11 *Annual incidence of bovine spongiform encephalopathy in Great Britain. All cases were confirmed clinically and neuropathologically. (Statistics compiled by John Wilesmith, Central Veterinary Laboratory at Weybridge, United Kingdom)*

Clinical signs of CWD are remarkably subtle and nonspecific, characterized by lethargy, weight loss, flaccid hypotonic facial muscles, polydipsia/polyuria, excessive salivation, and behavioral changes, such as loss of fear of humans (Williams and Young 1980). Of the TSEs, histological brain lesions are most similar to BSE and scrapie, and include large single or septate intra-neuronal vacuoles prominent in the parasympathetic vagal nucleus of the medulla oblongata, and also evident in the thalamus, hypothalamus, pons, midbrain, and olfactory cortex (Williams and Young 1993; Spraker et al. 1997). Similar to scrapie, PrP^{CWD} is abundant in secondary lymphoid tissues, and can be detected in tonsil, Peyer's patches, and ileocecal lymph node by immunohistochemistry as early as 12 weeks after experimental oral CWD inoculation (Sigurdson et al. 1999).

The capacity for CWD transmission to other species is clearly an area of great concern. Unfortunately, very little is known about the risk for other wildlife species, domestic ruminants, or humans contracting the disease. Cattle have been inoculated intracerebrally with CWD, and by 2 years post-inoculation, three of 13 had developed a TSE (Hamir et al. 2001). No cattle which have been orally inoculated have shown clinical signs of a TSE at 63 months post-inoculation (M.W. Miller and E.S. Williams, unpublished findings). Thus, cattle appear to be highly resistant to CWD by a natural route of exposure. The ability of PrP^{CWD} to convert human PrP^c in vitro was determined to be inefficient, but similar to the efficiency of PrP^{BSE} or ovine PrP^{Sc} to convert human PrP^c (Raymond et al. 2000).

Human prion diseases

The human prion diseases are manifest as infectious, inherited, and sporadic disorders, and are often referred to as kuru, sCJD, familial CJD, vCJD, GSS syndrome, and FFI, depending upon the clinical, genetic, and neuropathological findings (Table 61.1).

DIAGNOSIS OF HUMAN PRION DISEASES

Human prion disease should be considered in any patient who develops a progressive subacute or chronic decline in cognitive or motor function. Typically adults between 40 and 70 (or more) years of age, patients often exhibit clinical features helpful in providing a premorbid diagnosis of prion disease, particularly sCJD (Roos et al. 1973; Brown et al. 1986a). There is as yet no specific diagnostic test for prion disease in the cerebrospinal fluid: the concentration of the proteins 14-3-3 (Hsich et al. 1996), S-100, and neuron-specific enolase is often increased, but these represent general markers of neuronal breakdown and do not allow for definite diagnosis of prion encephalopathy. A definitive diagnosis of human prion disease, which is invariably fatal, can often be made from the examination of brain tissue. Since

1992, knowledge of the molecular genetics of prion diseases has made it possible, using peripheral tissues, to diagnose inherited prion disease in living patients by sequencing the prion alleles.

A broad spectrum of neuropathological features in human prion diseases precludes a precise neuropathological definition. The classic neuropathological features of human prion disease include spongiform degeneration, gliosis, and neuronal loss in the absence of any significant inflammatory reaction (Budka et al. 1995). When present, amyloid plaques that stain with α-PrP antibodies are diagnostic.

The presence of protease-resistant PrP (PrP^{Sc} or PrP^{CJD}) in the infectious and sporadic forms, and in most of the inherited forms of these diseases, implicates prions in their pathogenesis. The absence of PrP^{CJD} in a biopsy specimen may simply reflect regional variations in the concentration of the protein (Serban et al. 1990). In some patients with inherited prion disease, PrP^{Sc} is barely detectable or undetectable (Little et al. 1986; Brown et al. 1992b; Manetto et al. 1992; Medori et al. 1992b); this situation seems to be mimicked in transgenic mice that express a mutant PrP gene and spontaneously develop neurological illness indistinguishable from experimental murine scrapie (Hsiao et al. 1990, 1994).

In humans and transgenic mice that have no detectable protease-resistant PrP but express mutant PrP, neurodegeneration may, at least in part, be caused by abnormal metabolism of mutant PrP (Hegde et al. 1998, 1999). Because molecular genetic analyses of PrP genes in patients with unusual dementing illnesses are readily performed, the diagnosis of inherited prion disease can often be established where there was little or no neuropathology (Collinge et al. 1990), atypical neurodegenerative disease (Collinge et al. 1990) or misdiagnosed neurodegenerative disease (Heston et al. 1966; Azzarelli et al. 1985), including Alzheimer's disease.

Since the prion is defined as the transmissible agent causing spongiform encephalopathies, horizontal transmission of neurodegeneration to experimental hosts should be considered the 'gold standard' of prion disease. However, transmission of inherited prion diseases from humans to experimental animals is frequently negative when using rodents, despite the presence of a pathogenic mutation in the PRNP gene (Tateishi et al. 1992b). New lines of transgenic mice with enhanced susceptibility to human or animal prions (Telling et al. 1994; Weissmann et al. 1998) are starting to enable transmission studies that were not practical in apes and monkeys (Brown et al. 1994b).

Stanley Prusiner advocates that the hallmark common to all prion diseases, whether sporadic, dominantly inherited or acquired by infection, is that they involve the aberrant metabolism of the prion protein (Prusiner 1991). The author of this chapter, however, contends that nontransmissible diseases involving aberrant states of PrP may differ significantly in their pathophysiology from TSE proper, and cautions that their classification can only be provisional given the current state of knowledge. The term 'prion' is used here in an operational meaning: it is not meant to be necessarily identical with PrP^{Sc}, but it simply denotes the infectious agent, whatever this agent exactly consists of (Aguzzi and Weissmann 1997). If one takes this viewpoint, PrP^{Sc} defined originally as the protease-resistant moiety associated with prion disease would be a mere surrogate marker for the prion. Even if this position may seem all too negativistic in view of the wealth of compelling evidence in favor of the protein-only hypothesis, we still do not understand the molecular details of prion replication.

Because protease resistance and infectivity of PrP^{Sc} may not necessarily be congruent, it is desirable to expand the range of reagents that will interact specifically with disease-associated prion protein, but not (or to a lesser degree) with its counterpart, PrP^{C}. One IgM monoclonal antibody termed 15B3 has been described a few years ago to fulfill the above conditions (Korth et al. 1997), but this antibody has not become generally available, and no follow-up studies have been published. Disappointingly, expression of the complementarity-determining regions of 15B3 in the context of a phage, as well as expression of its heavy chain variable region in transgenic mice, failed to reproduce the specificity of PrP^{Sc} binding (Heppner et al. 2001b).

The puzzling phenomenon was described that a prevalent constituent of blood serum, plasminogen, captures efficiently PrP^{Sc} but not PrP^{C} when immobilized onto the surface of magnetic beads (Fischer et al. 2000; Maissen et al. 2001). While the significance of this phenomenon in vivo has yet to be addressed, plasminogen binds to PrP^{Sc} from a variety of species and genotypes (Maissen et al. 2001), and the captured PrP^{Sc} retains the glycotype profile characteristic of the prion strain from which it was isolated (M. Maissen and A. Aguzzi, unpublished data).

In practical terms, however, a definitive diagnosis of human prion disease can be rapidly accomplished if PrP^{Sc} can be detected by western immunoblot analysis of brain homogenates in which samples are subjected to limited proteolysis to remove PrP^{C} before immunostaining (Bockman et al. 1985, 1987; Brown et al. 1986b; Serban et al. 1990). Because of regional variations in PrP^{Sc} concentration, methods using homogenates prepared from small brain regions may give false-negative results. Alternatively, PrP^{Sc} may be detected in situ in cryostat sections bound to nitrocellulose membranes followed by limited proteolysis to remove PrP^{C}, and guanidinium salt treatment to denature PrP^{Sc}, and thus enhance its accessibility to α-PrP antibodies (Taraboulos et al. 1992a). Denaturation of PrP^{Sc} in situ prior to immunostaining has also been accomplished by autoclaving fixed tissue sections (Kitamoto et al. 1992).

In the familial forms of the prion diseases, molecular genetic analyses of PRNP can be diagnostic and can be performed on DNA extracted from blood leukocytes antemortem. Unfortunately, such testing is of little value in the diagnosis of the sporadic or infectious forms of prion disease. Although the first missense PrP mutation was discovered when the two PrP alleles of a patient with GSS were cloned from a genomic library and sequenced (Hsiao et al. 1989), all subsequent novel missense and insertional mutations have been identified in PrP ORFs amplified by polymerase chain reaction (PCR) and sequenced. The 759 base pairs encoding the 253 amino acids of PrP reside in a single exon of the PrP gene, providing an ideal situation for the use of PCR. Amplified PrP ORFs can be screened for known mutations using one of several methods, the most reliable of which is automated sequencing. The list of disease-associated PRNP mutations is unlikely to be complete yet, and novel mutations may be found when the PrP ORF is sequenced. It is thinkable, but unproven, that mutations and/or polymorphisms in regulatory and intronic regions may contribute to CJD susceptibility.

When PrP amyloid plaques in brain are present, they are diagnostic for prion disease as noted above. Unfortunately, they are present in only ca. 10 percent of CJD cases but, by definition, in all cases of GSS. The amyloid plaques in CJD are compact (kuru plaques). Those in GSS are either multicentric (diffuse) or compact. The amyloid plaques in prion diseases contain PrP (Kitamoto et al. 1986; Roberts et al. 1986, 1988). The multicentric amyloid plaques that are pathognomonic for GSS may be difficult to distinguish from the neuritic plaques of Alzheimer's disease except by immunohistology (Ghetti et al. 1989; Nochlin et al. 1989; Ikeda et al. 1991). In the GSS kindreds, the diagnosis of Alzheimer's disease was excluded because the amyloid plaques failed to stain with β-amyloid antiserum, but stained with PrP antiserum. In subsequent studies, missense mutations were found in the PrP genes of these kindreds.

In summary, the diagnosis of prion disease may be made in patients on the basis of:

- the presence of PrP^{Sc}
- mutant PrP genotype or
- appropriate immunohistology,

and should not be excluded in patients with atypical neurodegenerative diseases until one, or preferably two, of these examinations have been performed.

Infectious prion diseases

IATROGENIC CREUTZFELDT–JAKOB DISEASE

Accidental transmission of CJD to humans seems to have occurred by corneal transplantation (Duffy et al. 1974), contaminated EEG electrode implantation (Bernoulli et al. 1977), and surgical operations using contaminated instruments or apparatus (Table 61.2) (Masters and Richardson 1978; Kondo and Kuroina 1981; Will and Matthews 1982; Davanipour et al. 1984). A cornea unknowingly removed from a donor with CJD was transplanted to an apparently healthy recipient who developed CJD after a prolonged incubation period. Corneas of animals have significant levels of prions (Buyukmihci et al. 1980), making this situation seem quite probable. The same improperly decontaminated EEG electrodes that caused CJD in two young patients with intractable epilepsy caused CJD in a chimpanzee 18 months after their experimental implantation (Bernoulli et al. 1979; Gibbs et al. 1994).

Surgical procedures may have resulted in accidental inoculation of patients with prions during their operations (Gajdusek 1977; Will and Matthews 1982; Brown et al. 1992c), presumably because some instrument or apparatus in the operating theatre became contaminated when a CJD patient underwent surgery. Although the epidemiology of these studies is highly suggestive, no proof for such episodes exists.

Since 1988, 11 cases have been recorded of CJD after implantation of dura mater grafts (Otto 1987; Thadani et al. 1988; Masullo et al. 1989; Nisbet et al. 1989; Miyashita et al. 1991; Willison et al. 1991; Brown et al., 1992c; Martinez Lage et al. 1993). All the grafts were thought to have been acquired from a single manufacturer whose preparative procedures were inadequate to inactivate human prions (Brown et al. 1992c). One case of CJD occurred after repair of an eardrum perforation with a pericardium graft (Tange et al. 1989). Thirty cases of CJD in physicians and healthcare workers have been reported (Berger and David 1993); however, no occupational link has been established (Ridley and Baker 1993). Whether any of these cases represents infectious prion diseases contracted during care of patients with CJD or processing specimens from these patients remains uncertain. It is interesting to note that surgical

operations of any kind appear to constitute a mild risk factor for subsequent CJD (Collins et al. 1999).

HUMAN GROWTH HORMONE THERAPY

The possibility of transmission of CJD from contaminated human grown hormone (HGH) preparations derived from human pituitaries has been raised by the occurrence of fatal cerebellar disorders with dementia in >80 patients ranging in age from 10 to over 60 years (Brown et al. 1985b; Buchanan et al. 1991; Fradkin et al. 1991; Brown 1992). Although one case of spontaneous CJD in a 20-year-old woman has been reported (Packer et al. 1980; Brown et al. 1985a; Gibbs et al. 1985), CJD in people under 40 years of age is extremely rare. These patients received injections of HGH every 2–4 days for 4–12 years (Gibbs et al., 1985; Koch et al., 1985; Powell Jackson et al. 1985; Tintner et al. 1986; Croxson et al. 1988; Marzewski et al. 1988; New et al. 1988; Anderson et al. 1990; Billette de Villemeur et al. 1991; Macario et al. 1991; Ellis et al., 1992). It is interesting that most of the patients presented with cerebellar syndromes that progressed over periods varying from 6 to 18 months. Some patients became demented during the terminal phases of their illnesses. This clinical course resembles kuru more than ataxic CJD in some respects (Prusiner et al. 1982c). Assuming that these patients developed CJD from injections of prion-contaminated HGH preparations, the possible incubation periods range from 4 to 30 years (Brown et al. 1992c). The longest incubation periods are similar to those (20–30 years) associated with recent cases of kuru (Gajdusek 1977; Prusiner et al. 1982c; Klitzman et al. 1984). Many patients received several common lots of HGH at various times during their prolonged therapies, but no single lot was administered to all the American patients. An aliquot of one lot of HGH has been reported to transmit CNS disease to a squirrel monkey after a prolonged incubation period (Gibbs et al. 1993). How many lots of the HGH might have been contaminated with prions is unknown.

CJD has an annual incidence of $1–1.5/10^6$ (Masters and Richardson 1978). Updated numbers can be found at the web site www.eurocjd.ed.ac.uk/euroindex.htm. About 1 percent of the population dies each year and most CJD patients die within one year of developing symptoms. Thus, one per 10^4 dead people may be infected with the CJD agent. Since 10 000 human pituitaries were typically processed in a single HGH preparation, the possibility of hormone preparations contaminated with CJD prions is not remote (Brown et al. 1985b). The concentration of CJD prions within infected human pituitaries is unknown; it is interesting that widespread degenerative changes have been observed in both the hypothalamus and pituitary of sheep with scrapie (Beck et al. 1964). The forebrains from scrapie-infected mice have been added to human pituitary suspensions to determine if prions and HGH co-purify (Lumley Jones

Table **61.2** *Transmission of prion diseases among humans (kuru and iatrogenic cases), as compiled from published reports and various national surveillance centers*

Diseases	No. of cases
Kuru (1957–82)	
Adult females	1 739
Adult males	248
Children and adolescents	597
Total	2 584
Iatrogenic Creutzfeldt–Jakob disease	
Electroencephalography electrodes	2
Corneal transplants	2
Human pituitary hormones	143
Dura mater grafts	114
Neurosurgical procedures	5
Total	266

et al. 1979). Bioassays in mice suggest that prions and HGH do not co-purify with currently used protocols (Taylor et al. 1985). Although these results seem reassuring, the relatively low titer of the murine scrapie prions used in these studies may not have provided an adequate test (Brown 1985). The extremely small size and charge heterogeneity exhibited by scrapie (Alper et al. 1966; Prusiner et al. 1978, 1980b, 1983; Bolton et al. 1985) and presumably CJD prions (Bendheim et al. 1985; Bockman et al. 1985) may complicate procedures designed to separate pituitary hormones from these slow infectious pathogens. Fortunately, the advent of recombinant protein production has rendered this problem obsolete – however, it is possible that a number of HGH-treated persons are incubating prions, and may pass it to others and/or develop iCJD in the future.

Molecular genetic studies have revealed that most patients developing iCJD after receiving pituitary-derived HGH are homozygous for either Met or Val at codon 129 of the PrP gene (Collinge et al. 1991; Brown et al. 1994a; Deslys et al. 1994). Homozygosity at the codon 129 polymorphism has also been shown to predispose individuals to sCJD (Palmer et al. 1991). It is interesting that valine homozygosity seems to be over-represented in these HGH cases compared to the general population.

Five cases of CJD have occurred in women receiving human pituitary gonadotropin (Cochius et al. 1990; Cochius et al. 1992; Healy and Evans 1993).

Inherited prion diseases

FAMILIAL PRION DISEASE

The recognition that ca. 10 percent of CJD cases are familial (Kirschbaum 1924; Meggendorfer 1930; Stender 1930; Davison and Rabiner 1940; Jacob et al. 1950; Friede and DeJong 1964; Rosenthal et al. 1976; Masters and Gajdusek 1979; Masters et al. 1981a, b) posed a perplexing problem once it was established that CJD is transmissible (Gibbs et al. 1968, 1969). Equally puzzling was the transmission of GSS to nonhuman primates (Gibbs et al. 1968, 1969; Masters et al. 1981a) and mice (Tateishi et al. 1979), because most cases of GSS are familial (Gerstmann et al. 1936). Like sheep scrapie, the relative contributions of genetic and infectious etiologies in the human prion diseases remained a conundrum until molecular clones of the PrP gene became available to probe the inherited aspects of these disorders.

PRP MUTATIONS AND GENETIC LINKAGE

The discovery of the PrP gene and its linkage to scrapie incubation times in mice (Carlson et al. 1986) raised the possibility that mutation might feature in the hereditary human prion diseases. A proline (P)→leucine (L) mutation at codon 102 was shown to be linked genetically to development of GSS with a logarithm of odds (LOD)

score exceeding 3 (Hsiao et al. 1989). This mutation may be due to the deamination of a methylated CpG in a germline PrP gene resulting in the substitution of a thymine (T) for cytosine (C). The P102L mutation has been found in ten different families in nine different countries, including the original GSS family (Doh-ura et al., 1989; Goldgaber et al. 1989; Goldhammer et al. 1993). Amyloid plaques isolated from patients with GSS (P102L) were composed of PrP molecules with an L at residue 102 based on protein sequencing of purified peptides (Kitamoto et al. 1991b). Patients with GSS who have a P→L substitution at PrP codon 105 have also been reported (Kitamoto et al. 1993a).

Some patients with a mutation at codon 117 have a dementing or telencephalic form of GSS (Doh-ura et al., 1989; Hsiao et al. 1991b), whereas others have an ataxic form of the disease (Mastrianni et al. 1995). In both forms of GSS (A117V), PrP amyloid plaques were found as well as spongiform degeneration. The factor or factors that determine the different phenotypes of this disease are unknown.

Patients with PrP mutations at codons 198 and 217 (Hsiao et al. 1992) were once thought to have familial Alzheimer's disease, but are now known to have prion diseases on the basis of PrP immunostaining of amyloid plaques and PrP gene mutations (Farlow et al. 1989; Ghetti et al. 1989; Nochlin et al. 1989; Giaccone et al. 1990). A genetic linkage study of this family produced a LOD score exceeding 6 (Dlouhy et al. 1992). Patients with the codon 198 mutation resulting in a phenylalanine (F)→serine (S) substitution (Hsiao et al. 1992) have numerous neurofibrillary tangles (NFT) that stain with antibodies to tau (τ) protein and have amyloid (Farlow et al. 1989; Ghetti et al. 1989; Nochlin et al. 1989; Giaccone et al. 1990) that are composed largely of a PrP fragment extending from residues 58 to 150 (Tagliavini et al. 1991). Because the F198S mutation is not contained within the major PrP peptide of the amyloid plaques, patients heterozygous at codon 129 were chosen to determine whether this peptide is derived from the mutant protein. Like the results of studies with GSS (P102L) (Kitamoto et al. 1991b) and GSS (Y145Stop) (Kitamoto et al. 1993b), protein sequencing revealed that the PrP peptides are derived exclusively from the mutant protein (Tagliavini et al. 1994). Similar results were found with PrP peptides from a patient of Swedish ancestry with the codon 217 mutation resulting in a glutamine (Q)→arginine (R) substitution (Hsiao et al. 1992). The neuropathology of patients with the codon 217 mutation was similar to that of patients with the codon 198 mutation (Ikeda et al. 1991).

One patient with a prolonged neurological illness spanning almost two decades who had PrP amyloid plaques and NFTs had an amber mutation of the PrP gene resulting in a stop codon at residue 145 (Kitamoto et al. 1993b; Kitamoto and Tateishi 1994). Staining of the plaques with α-PrP peptide antisera suggested that they might be composed exclusively of the truncated PrP molecules. That a PrP peptide ending at residue 145 polymerizes into amyloid filaments is to be expected since an earlier study noted above showed that the major PrP peptide in plaques from patients with the F198S mutation was an 11 kDa PrP peptide beginning at codon 58 and ending at ca. 150 (Tagliavini et al. 1991). A synthetic PrP peptide containing residues 90–145 was found to adopt an α-helical or β-sheet structure depending on the solvent as determined by two-dimensional magnetic resonance imaging, FTIR spectroscopy and fiber diffraction (Nguyen et al. 1995; Zhang et al. 1995).

An insert of 144 bp at codon 53 containing six octa-repeats has been described in patients with CJD from four families all residing in southern England (Owen et al. 1989, 1990b, 1991; Crow et al. 1990; Collinge et al. 1992; Poulter et al. 1992). This mutation must have arisen through a complex series of events, because the human PrP gene contains only five octarepeats, indicating that a single recombination event could not have created the insert. Genealogical investigations have revealed that all four families are related, arguing for a single founder born more than two centuries ago (Crow et al. 1990). The LOD score for this extended pedigree exceeds 11. Studies from several laboratories have demonstrated that two, four, five, six, seven, eight, or nine octarepeats in addition to the normal five are present in individuals with inherited CJD (Owen et al. 1989, 1990b, 1992; Goldfarb et al. 1991a; Brown 1993), whereas deletion of one octarepeat has been identified without the neurological disease (Laplanche et al., 1990; Vnencak Jones and Phillips 1992; Palmer et al., 1993).

For many years the unusually high incidence of CJD among Israeli Jews of Libyan origin was thought to be due to the consumption of lightly cooked sheep brain or eyeballs (Herzberg et al. 1974; Kahana et al. 1974, 1991). In reality, some Libyan and Tunisian Jews in families with CJD have a PrP gene point mutation at codon 200 resulting in a glutamate (E)→lysine (K) substitution (Goldfarb et al. 1990b; Hsiao et al. 1991a). One patient was homozygous for the E200K mutation but her clinical presentation was similar to that of heterozygotes (Hsiao et al. 1991a), arguing that familial prion diseases are true autosomal dominant disorders. The E200K mutation has also been found in Slovaks originating from Orava in north central Czechoslovakia (Goldfarb et al. 1990c), in a cluster of familial cases in Chile (Goldfarb et al. 1991b), and in a large German family living in the USA (Bertoni et al. 1992). It is likely that the E200K muta-tion has arisen independently multiple times through the deamidation of a methylated CpG as described above the codon 102 mutation (Hsiao et al. 1989, 1991a). In support of this hypothesis are records of Libyan and Tunisian Jews, indicating that they are descendants of Jews who settled on the island of Jerba off the southern coast of Tunisia around 500 BC and not from Sephardim (Udovitch and Valensi 1984).

Many families with CJD have been found to have a point mutation at codon 178, resulting in an aspartate (D)→asparagine (N) substitution (Fink et al. 1991; Goldfarb et al. 1991c, 1992a; Haltia et al. 1991; Brown et al. 1992a). In these patients as well as those with the E200K mutation, PrP amyloid plaques are rare; the neuropathological changes generally consist of wide-spread spongiform degeneration. A prion disease called fatal familial insomnia (FFI) was described in three Italian families with the D178N mutation (Lugaresi et al. 1986; Medori et al. 1992a). The neuropathology in these patients with FFI is restricted to selected nuclei of the thalamus. It is unclear whether all patients with the D178N mutation or only a subset present with sleep disturbances. It has been proposed that the allele with the D178N mutation encodes a methionine (M) at posi-tion 129 in FFI whereas a valine (V) is encoded at posi-tion 129 in familial CJD (Goldfarb et al. 1992b). The discovery that FFI is an inherited prion disease clearly widens the clinical spectrum of these disorders and raises the possibility that many other degenerative diseases of unknown etiology may be caused by prions (Johnson 1992; Medori et al. 1992b). The D178N muta-tion has been linked to the development of prion disease with a LOD score exceeding 5 (Petersen et al. 1992). Studies of PrP^{Sc} in FFI and familial CJD caused by the D178N mutation reveal that, after limited proteolysis, the molecular mass of the FFI PrP^{Sc} is ca. 2 kDa smaller (Monari et al. 1994). Whether this difference in protease resistance reflects distinct conformations of PrP^{Sc} that give rise to the different clinical and neuropathological manifestations of these inherited prion diseases remains to be established.

A valine (V)→isoleucine (I) mutation at PrP codon 210 produces CJD with classic symptoms and signs (Pocchiari et al. 1993; Ripoll et al. 1993). The V210I mutation is thought to be incompletely penetrant, like the E200K mutation was previously thought to be (Chapman et al. 1994; Spudich et al. 1995). It seems likely that, if a sufficiently large number of people with the V210I mutation could be analyzed, complete pene-trance that is age-dependent would be found.

Other point mutations at codons 208 and, possibly, 232 also segregate with inherited prion diseases (Kita-moto et al. 1993c; Kitamoto and Tateishi 1994; Mastrianni et al. 1995). The codon 208 mutation results in the substitution of arginine (R) for histidine (H). A patient with this mutation presented with a progressive dementia and widespread myoclonus was subsequently observed. The diagnosis of CJD was confirmed at autopsy. Patients with the codon 232 mutation present with dementia; this mutation is particularly notable, because it lies within the C-terminal signal sequence that is removed from PrP when the GPI anchor is attached (Stahl et al. 1992). Table 61.3 summarizes all mutations within the human *PRNP* gene that were found to cose-gregate with inherited prion disease.

Table 61.3 *Synopsis of all* PRNP *mutations and polymorphism, and their association with inherited prion diseases*

Presentation	Mutation in *PRNP*
Creutzfeldt–Jakob phenotype	D178N-129V, V180I, V180I-M232R, T183A, T188A, E196K, E200K, V203I, R208H, V210I, E211Q, M232R, 96 bpi, 120 bpi, 144 bpi, 168 bpi, 48 bpd
Gerstmann–Sträussler–Scheinker phenotype	P102L, P105L, A117V, G131V, F198S, D202N, Q212P, Q217R, M232T, 192 bpi
Fatal familial insomnia phenotype	D178N-129M
Vascular amyloid depositions	Y145STOP
Proven but unclassified prion disease	H187R, 216 bpi
Neuropsychiatric disorder, no proven prion disease	I138M, G142S, Q160s, T188K, T188R, M232R, P238S, 24 bpi, 48 bpi,
Polymorphisms, established influence on phenotype	M129V
Polymorphisms, suggested influence on phenotype	N171S, E219K
Silent polymorphisms	P68P, A117A, G124G, V161V, N173N, H177H, T188T, D202D, Q212Q, R228R, S230S

The wild-type human PrP gene contains five octarepeats [P(Q/H)GGG(G/–) WGQ] from codons 51–91. Deletion of a single octarepeat at codon 81 or 82 is not associated with prion disease (Laplanche et al. 1990; Puckett et al. 1991; Vnencak Jones and Phillips 1992); whether this deletion alters the phenotypic characteristics of a prion disease is unknown. There are common polymorphisms at codons 117 (Ala→Ala) and 129 (Met→Val); homozygosity for Met or Val at codon 129 seems to increase susceptibility to sCJD (Palmer et al. 1991). Octarepeat inserts of 16, 32, 40, 48, 56, 64, and 72 amino acids at codons 67, 75, or 83 are designated as bpi (base pair insertion). Point mutations are designated by the wild-type amino acid preceding the codon number and the mutant residue follows, e.g. P102L. These point mutations segregate with the inherited prion diseases and significant genetic linkage (underlined mutations) has been demonstrated where sufficient specimens from family members are available. The single letter codes for amino acids is as follows: A, Ala; D, Asp; E, Glu; F, Phe; I, Ile; K, Lys; L, Leu; M, Met; N, Asn; P, Pro; Q, Gln; R, Arg; S, Ser; T, Thr; V, Val; and Y, Tyr.

Along with the demonstration that PrP-deficient mice are resistant to prion infections, the linkage of *PRNP* mutations with hereditary prion disease provide a very solid piece of evidence in favor of Prusiner's protein-only hypothesis.

Variant Creutzfeldt–Jakob disease

The most recently recognized form of CJD in humans, new variant CJD (vCJD), was first described in 1996 and has been linked to BSE (Will and Zeidler 1996). vCJD represents a distinct clinicopathological entity that is characterized at onset by psychiatric abnormalities, sensory symptoms, and ataxia, and eventually leads to dementia along with other features usually observed in sCJD. What distinguishes vCJD from sporadic cases is that the age of patients is abnormally low (vCJD, 19–39 years; sCJD, 55–70 years) and duration of the illness is rather long (vCJD, 7.5–22 months; sCJD, 2.5–6.5 months). Moreover, vCJD displays a distinct pathology within the brain characterized by abundant 'florid plaques,' decorated by a daisy-like pattern of vacuolation. Most cases of vCJD have been observed in the United Kingdom (Will et al. 2000). For several years, it has been thought that prions are distributed much more broadly within the body of vCJD victims than of sCJD patients (Wadsworth et al. 2001). However, this view has recently been challenged by the finding of PrP^Sc in muscle and spleen of sCJD patients (Glatzel et al. 2003a).

What is the evidence that the agent causing vCJD may be identical with that of BSE when transmitted to humans? None of the arguments to date is conclusive,

yet each – and particularly when they are all considered together – is tantalizing. Much effort has gone into characterizing the 'strain properties' of the agent that affects cows and humans. Because the molecular substrate that underlies the nature of prion strains (which are heritable phenotypic traits that can be reproduced upon serial passage through experimental animals) is not known, strain-typing of prions has to rely on surrogate markers.

Two such markers have been particularly useful. One is the distribution of neuronal vacuoles in the brains of affected animals: for example, whereas some strains target the cortical cerebral ribbon, others mainly affect the midbrain (Fraser and Dickinson 1967). The BSE prion strain attacks the dorsal medulla and the superior colliculus (a part of the optical pathway) virulently and consistently (Bruce et al. 1997). Worryingly, BSE prions (extracted from the brains of affected cows) and vCJD prions derived from the brains of British patients produce the same lesional patterns when transmitted to panels of susceptible mice (Aguzzi 1996; Aguzzi and Weissmann 1996; Bruce et al. 1997).

The second marker for strain typing of prions comes from analyzing the biochemical properties of disease-associated PrP recovered from the brains of cattle and humans. Different steric conformations of PrP (which, according to the most popular hypothesis, account for the phenotypic strain properties) expose different sites to the action of proteolytic enzymes. These sites, in turn, can be identified by the different molecular masses of the resulting fragments. When used in conjunction with the ratio of diglycosylated to monoglycosylated PrP –

another parameter that seems to correlate with strain properties – these traits were again found to be indistinguishable between BSE and human vCJD prions (Collinge et al. 1996; Hill et al. 1997a). A third line of argument relating BSE and human vCJD concerns epidemiology of the disease. To date, the total number of definite or probable cases of vCJD is 136 in the UK (Table 61.4), but only a few cases in other countries including Ireland, France (Chazot et al. 1996), and Italy. Assuming that the quality of the epidemiologic surveillance is similar in these countries and in the rest of Europe (which has not reported cases of vCJD), the unavoidable conclusion is that the incidence of vCJD correlates with the prevalence of BSE.

One of the most powerful arguments is the study of pathogenesis in primates. In a classical experiment, Lasmezas and colleagues inoculated brain extracts from BSE-affected cows into cynomolgus macaques. After about 3 years, all inoculated primates (two adults and one infant) developed spongiform encephalopathy. The histopathological appearance of the disease was identical to that of vCJD and included characteristic 'florid plaques,' which have been recognized in every case of vCJD (Lasmezas et al. 1996b). These are spherical conglomerates of fibrillary birefringent material that stains positive with 'amyloidotropic' dyes such as Congo red. Characteristically, vCJD plaques are surrounded by a rim of microvacuolated brain tissue – a feature which they share with the deposits in sheep scrapie, but that is not seen in classical CJD, nor in any other human spongiform encephalopathy.

Impressive as all of these arguments may seem, however, each is phenomenological rather than causal. Distribution of histopathological lesions, as well as morphology of plaque deposits, is downstream of the molecular events responsible for prion strain specificity. Measurements of the 'glycotype ratio' may be more directly related to the essence of strains, but there is still no way to tell whether they might simply be surrogate markers. It would be desirable to measure the conformation of disease-associated PrP more directly. Some inroads have been made with a method that exploits the relative affinities of anti-PrP^C antibodies (Aguzzi 1998; Safar et al. 1998), but, to our knowledge, this possibility is restricted to differentiation of mouse and hamster PrPs, and has not yet been applied to investigating BSE and vCJD.

Given that a large fraction of the European population may have been exposed to BSE prions, yet only a minute minority developed vCJD, there can be hardly any doubt that additional genetic modifiers exist, other than *PRNP* polymorphisms. It was originally claimed that specific allelotypes of the major histocompatibility complex may represent such modifiers (Jackson et al. 2001), but this was not confirmed by later studies (Pepys et al. 2003).

So what will the numbers of vCJD victims be in the future? Terrible as the disease has been for patients, we

Table **61.4** *The Department of Health's latest information about the numbers of known cases of Creutzfeldt–Jakob disease*

Referral of suspect CJD			Deaths of definite and probable CJD					
Year	Referrals	Year	sporadic	Iatrogenic	Familial	GSS	vCJD[a]	Total deaths
1990	53	1990	28	5	0	0	–	33
1991	75	1991	32	1	3	0	–	36
1992	96	1992	45	2	5	1	–	53
1993	78	1993	37	4	3	2	–	46
1994	118	1994	53	1	4	3	–	61
1995	87	1995	35	4	2	3	3	47
1996	134	1996	40	4	2	4	10	60
1997	161	1997	60	6	4	1	10	81
1998	154	1998	63	3	4	1	18	89
1999	170	1999	62	6	2	0	15	85
2000	178	2000	49	1	2	1	28	81
2001	179	2001	56	3	2	2	20	83
2002	163	2002	72	0	4	1	17	94
2003[a]	107	2003[a]	35	4	1	0	15	55
Total	1 753	Total deaths	667	44	38	19	136	904

The Department of Health is issuing the latest information about the numbers of known cases of Creutzfeldt–Jakob disease. This includes cases of variant Creutzfeldt–Jakob disease (vCJD) – the form of the disease thought to be linked to BSE (as of September 2003). For updated information, see the following link: www.doh.gov.uk/cjd/cjd_stat.htm
Referrals: a simple count of all the cases which have been referred to the National CJD Surveillance Unit for further investigation. About half the cases referred in the past have turned out not to be CJD. Cases are notified to the Unit from neurologists, neuropathologists, neurophysiologists, general physicians, psychiatrists, EEG departments, etc.
Deaths: all columns show the number of deaths that have occurred in definite and probable cases of all types of CJD and GSS in the year shown.
Definite cases: the diagnosis was pathologically confirmed, in most cases by postmortem examination of brain tissue.
Probable vCJD cases: those who fulfill the 'probable' criteria and are either still alive, or have died and await postmortem pathological confirmation.
a) As at 1st September 2003.

have not yet seen a large-scale epidemic. Although many mathematical models have been generated (Ghani et al. 1998, 2000), the number of cases is still too small to predict future developments with any certainty. Since the year 2001, the incidence of vCJD in the UK appears to be stabilizing and may actually be even falling (Figure 61.12). One may argue that it is too early to draw any far-reaching conclusions, but each month passing without any dramatic rise in the number of cases increases the hope that perhaps the total number of vCJD victims will be limited (Valleron et al. 2001).

POSSIBLE TRANSMISSION OF ADDITIONAL PRION EPIZOOTICS TO HUMANS

There is no example of zoonotic transmission of prions from sheep and goat to humans: many epidemiologic studies have failed to implicate scrapie prions from sheep as a cause of CJD (Malmgren et al. 1979; Harries Jones et al. 1988; Cousens et al. 1990). However, there is uncertainty surrounding the danger of transmission to humans represented by CWD. Actually, even transmissibility of BSE to humans relies on circumstantial evidence. Epidemiology and biochemistry favor the link between BSE and vCJD, but are not really conclusive. The Koch postulates (which would unambiguously assign an infectious agent to a disease) have never been fulfilled, and experimental inoculation of humans was never performed. Also, accidental exposure to BSE infectivity of a sizable collective at a precisely defined time point has never occurred, or did not result in disease. For these reasons, speculations that variant Creutzfeldt–Jakob disease may not be due to BSE have never completely subsided.

Likewise, we do not know whether scrapie is just a veterinary problem that only affects sheep and goats, or whether it can cross species barriers and affect humans. Finally, it is unknown whether BSE, upon transmission to sheep, remains as dangerous for humans as cow-derived BSE, or whether it becomes attenuated and acquires the (allegedly) innocuous properties of bona fide sheep scrapie.

Another question relates to the possibility of chronic subclinical disease or a permanent 'carrier' status in cows as well as in humans. Evidence that such a carrier status may be produced by the passage of the infectious agent across species was first reported by Race and Chesebro (Aguzzi and Weissmann 1998; Race and Chesebro 1998), and has been confirmed by others (Hill et al. 2000) – at least for the passage between hamsters and mice. Immune deficiency can also lead to a similar situation in which prions replicate silently in the body, even when there is no species barrier (Frigg et al. 1999). So the problem of animal TSEs could be more widespread than is assumed, and may call for drastic measures in farming. Moreover, people carrying the infectious agent may transmit it horizontally (Aguzzi 2000), and the risks associated with this possibility can be met only if we know more about how the agent is transmitted and how prions reach the brain from peripheral sites.

PrP gene polymorphisms

POLYMORPHISMS AT CODONS 129 AND 219

At PrP codon 129, an amino acid polymorphism for M→V has been identified (Owen et al. 1990a). This polymorphism seems able to influence prion disease

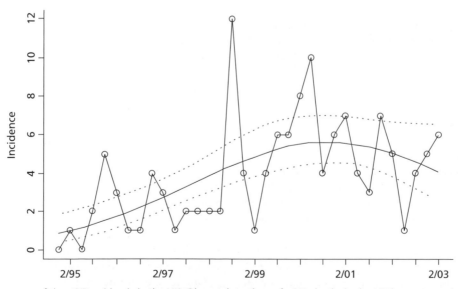

Figure 61.12 *The course of the vCJD epidemic in the UK. Observed numbers of vCJD deaths in the UK by a quarter (empty circles), and fitted quadratic trend (curved line) with 95 percent confidence interval for the trend (dotted line). The fitted trend shows a good fit to the data with a significant quadtratic term (P=0.002), which would indicate a departure from a constant exponential increase. This model estimates that the current quarterly incidence of deaths is 3.9 and shows that the epidemic reached a peak for deaths in about December 2000 (January 2000 to May 2003 with 95 percent confidence intervals). Regular updates are published by Mr N.J. Andrews (Communicable Disease Surveillance Centre, UK) at the web site: www.cjd.ed.ac.uk/vcjdq.htm*

expression, not only in inherited forms but also in iatrogenic and sporadic forms of prion disease. A second polymorphism resulting in an amino acid substitution at codon 219 (E→K) has been reported in the Japanese population, in which the K allele occurs with a frequency of 6 percent (Kitamoto and Tateishi 1994).

DOES HOMOZYGOSITY AT CODON 129 PREDISPOSE TO CJD?

Studies of caucasian patients with sporadic CJD have shown that most are homozygous for M or V at codon 129 (Palmer et al. 1991). This contrasts with the general population, in which frequencies for the codon 129 polymorphism in caucasians are 12 percent V/V, 37 percent M/M and 51 percent M/V (Collinge et al. 1991). By contrast, the frequency of the V allele in the Japanese population is much lower (Doh-ura et al. 1991; Miyazono et al. 1992) and heterozygosity at codon 129 (M/V) is more frequent (18 percent) in CJD patients than the general population, in whom the polymorphism frequencies are 0 percent V/V, 92 percent M/M and 8 percent M/V (Tateishi and Kitamoto 1993).

Although no specific mutations have been identified in the PrP gene of patients with sCJD (Goldfarb et al. 1990a), homozygosity at codon 129 in sCJD (Hardy 1991; Palmer et al. 1991) is consistent with the results of transgenic mouse studies. The finding that homozygosity at codon 129 predisposes to CJD supports a model of prion production that favors interactions between PrP molecules that are homologous in the H1 and H2 regions (Telling et al. 1995). However, there appears to be considerable evolutionary pressure for maintaining the prion gene. Protective polymorphisms in the human prion gene were heavily selected for, possibly because of evolutionary pressure from cannibalism-propagated prions (Mead et al. 2003). But if prion diseases were so frequent to skew the distribution of *Prnp* alleles, why were *Prnp*$^{-/-}$ individuals not selected for? This argues for an important, hitherto unidentified function of the cellular prion protein (Aguzzi and Hardt 2003).

BRAIN DAMAGE IN PRION DISEASES

An interesting question regards the molecular mechanism underlying neuropathological changes, in particular cell death, resulting from prion disease. Depletion of PrP^C is an unlikely cause, in view of the finding that abrogation of PrP does not cause scrapie-like neuropathological changes (Büeler et al. 1992), even when elicited postnatally (Mallucci et al. 2002). It is more likely that toxicity of PrP^{Sc} through some PrP^C-dependent process is responsible for neuronal dysfunction and death (Brandner et al. 1998, 1996a).

To address the question of neurotoxicity, brain tissue of *Prnp*$^{0/0}$ mice was exposed to a continuous source of PrP^{Sc}. Telencephalic tissue from transgenic mice overexpressing PrP (Fischer et al. 1996) was transplanted into the forebrain of *Prnp*$^{0/0}$ mice and the 'pseudochimeric' brains were inoculated with scrapie prions. All grafted and scrapie-inoculated mice remained free of scrapie symptoms for at least 70 weeks; this exceeded at least sevenfold the survival time of scrapie-infected donor mice (Brandner et al. 1996a). Therefore, the presence of a continuous source of PrP^{Sc} and of scrapie prions does not exert any clinically detectable adverse effects on a mouse devoid of PrP^C. On the other hand, the grafts develop characteristic histopathological features of scrapie after inoculation. The course of the disease in the graft is very similar to that observed in the brain of scrapie-inoculated wild-type mice (Brandner et al. 1998). Since grafts had extensive contact with the recipient brain, prions could navigate between the two compartments, as shown by the fact that inoculation of wild-type animals engrafted with PrP-expressing neuroectodermal tissue resulted in scrapie pathology in both graft and host tissue. Nonetheless, histopathological changes never extended into host tissue, even at the latest stages (>450 days), although PrP^{Sc} was detected in both grafts and recipient brain, and immunohistochemistry revealed PrP deposits in the hippocampus, and occasionally in the parietal cortex, of all animals (Brandner et al. 1996a). Thus, prions moved from the grafts to some regions of the PrP-deficient host brain without causing pathological changes or clinical disease. The distribution of PrP^{Sc} in the white matter tracts of the host brain suggests diffusion within the extracellular space (Jeffrey et al. 1994) rather than axonal transport.

These findings suggest that the expression of PrP^C by an infected cell, rather than the extracellular deposition of PrP^{Sc}, is one of the critical prerequisites for the development of scrapie pathology. Perhaps PrP^{Sc} is inherently nontoxic and PrP^{Sc} plaques found in spongiform encephalopathies are an epiphenomenon rather than a cause of neuronal damage. This hypothesis appears to be supported by the recent data (Ma and Lindquist 2002; Ma et al. 2002), indicating that exaggerated retrograde transport of the prion protein from the endoplasmatic reticulum into the cytosol, or functionally equivalent inhibition of proteasome function, might induce a self-propagating, extremely cytotoxic cellular form, which may ultimately be responsible for neuronal damage. These results are very novel and exciting, but they have been challenged (Roucou et al. 2003) and it is not clear whether they are universally valid (Drisaldi et al. 2003). Therefore it will be important to validate them by investigating whether the aggregated self-propagating material can also be transmitted between individual animals in a classic transmission experiment.

One may therefore propose that availability of PrP^C for some intracellular process elicited by the infectious agent, perhaps the formation of a toxic form of PrP (termed PrP* and discussed in Weissmann 1991a) other than PrP^{Sc} is responsible for spongiosis, gliosis, and neuronal death. This would be in agreement with the fact that in several instances, and especially in fatal familial insomnia, localized spongiform pathology is detectable although very little PrP^{Sc} is present (Aguzzi and Weissmann 1997).

PERIPHERAL PRION PATHOGENESIS

The fastest and most efficient method for inducing spongiform encephalopathy in the laboratory is intracerebral inoculation of brain homogenate. Inoculation of 1 000 000 ID$_{50}$ infectious units (defined as the amount of infectivity that will induce TSE with 50 percent likelihood in a given host) will yield disease in approximately 6 months; a remarkably strict inverse relationship can be observed between the logarithm of the inoculated dose and the incubation time (Prusiner et al., 1982b, Figure 61.13).

The above situation does not correspond to what typically happens in the field. There, acquisition of prion infectivity through any of several peripheral routes is the rule. However, prion diseases can also be initiated by feeding (Wells et al. 1987; Kimberlin and Wilesmith 1994; Anderson et al. 1996), by intravenous and intraperitoneal injection (Kimberlin and Walker 1978b) as

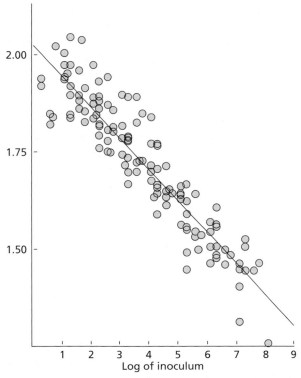

Figure 61.13 *Prion bioassay by the incubation time method. This figure is reproduced from an important study by Prusiner and colleagues that demonstrates an inverse logarithmic relationship between size of infectious inoculum and latency period of scrapie in experimental animals (Prusiner et al. 1982b). The relationship is so precise that incubation time can actually be used to back-calculate the prion titer of a test article, e.g. for inactivation studies. Measurement of prion titers by the incubation time method has become a standard procedure which can be used for both wild-type and transgenic animals.*

well as from the eye by conjunctival instillation (J.R. Scott et al. 1993), corneal grafts (Duffy et al. 1974) and intraocular injection (Fraser 1982). Two routes of infection have suggested for a long time that immune cells might be of importance for this phase of prion pathogenesis: oral challenge and administration by scarification (Aguzzi 2003). Therefore, these routes are discussed in some detail in the following paragraphs.

The pathway of orally administered prions

Upon oral challenge, an early rise in prion infectivity can be observed in the distal ileum of infected organisms. This is true for several animal species, but was most extensively investigated in the sheep (Wells et al. 1994; Vankeulen et al. 1996). There, Peyer's patches acquire strong immunopositivity for the prion protein. Immunohistochemical stains with antibodies to the prion protein typically reveal a robust signal in primary B-cell follicles and germinal centers, which roughly colocalizes with the complement receptor, CD35, in a wide variety of secondary lymphoid organs including appendix and tonsils (Hill et al. 1997b). Although conventional light microscopy does not allow differentiating between PrP^C and PrP^{Sc}, western blot analysis has not left any doubt about the fact that Peyer's patches do accumulate the disease-associated form of the prion protein.

The latter is true also in the mouse model of scrapie, which is being used as a convenient experimental paradigm by many laboratories including ours. Administration of mouse-adapted scrapie prions (Rocky Mountain Laboratory (RML) strain, originally derived from the Chandler sheep scrapie isolate) induces a surge in intestinal prion infectivity as early as a few days after inoculation (Prinz et al. 2003c). All of the above evidence conjures the suggestion that Peyer's patches may represent a portal of entry for orally administered prions on their journey from the luminal aspect of the gastroenteric tube to the central nervous system. However, the question as to whether the same applies for BSE-affected cattle has been answered less unambiguously.

In a monumental study of BSE pathogenesis in cattle carried out at the UK Veterinary Laboratory Agency, cows of various ages were fed with 100 g, 10 g, 1 g, or 100 mg of brain homogenate derived from BSE-sick cows (Bradley 2000). A large variety of tissues was taken at various points in time, homogenized, and transmitted intracerebrally to indicator organisms in order to assess their prion content. This study was designed to be performed over a time frame of more than a decade and is still under way at the time of writing: it has uncovered a transient surge in infectivity in the distal ileum of cows at approximately 6 months post-infection. Infectivity then subsides, but it appears to return to the terminal ileum at the end stages of disease, perhaps by means of some sort of retrograde transport (Wells et al. 1998). Although this was not formally confirmed, it appears likely that Peyer's patches are the sites of prion accumulation in the gastrointestinal tract of cattle challenged orally with prions.

Oral prion susceptibility correlates with number but not structure of Peyer's patches

Recruitment of activated B lymphocytes to Peyer's patches requires $\alpha_4\beta_7$ integrin as an essential homing receptor: Peyer's patches of mice that lack β_7 integrin are normal in number, but are atrophic and almost entirely devoid of B cells (Wagner et al. 1996). Therefore, it seemed interesting to investigate the susceptibility to orally administered prions of $\beta_7^{-/-}$ mice. Surprisingly, minimal infectious dose and disease incubation after oral exposure to logarithmic dilutions of prion inoculum were similar in $\beta_7^{-/-}$ and wild-type mice (Prinz et al. 2003c). Despite their atrophy, Peyer's patches of both $\beta_7^{-/-}$ and wild-type mice contained 3–4 $\log LD_{50}/g$ prion infectivity at 125 or more days after challenge.

Why does reduced mucosal lymphocyte trafficking not impair, as expected, the susceptibility to orally initiated prion disease? One possible reason may relate to the fact that, despite marked reduction of B cells, M cells were still present in $\beta_7^{-/-}$ mice. In contrast, mice deficient in both tumor necrosis factor (TNF) and lymphotoxin (LT)-α (TNF-$\alpha^{-/-} \times$ LT-$\alpha^{-/-}$) or in lymphocytes (RAG-1$^{-/-}$, μMT), in which numbers of Peyer's patches are reduced in number, were highly resistant to oral challenge, and their intestines were virtually devoid of prion infectivity at all times after challenge. Therefore, lymphoreticular requirements for enteric and for intraperitoneal uptake of prions differ from each other and that susceptibility to prion infection following oral challenge correlates with the number of Peyer's patches, but is independent of the number of intestinal mucosa-associated lymphocytes (Prinz et al. 2003c).

Transepithelial enteric passage of prions: a role for membranous epithelial cells (M cells)?

The requirements for transepithelial passage of prions are of obvious interest to prion pathogenesis. Membranous epithelial cells (M cells) are key sites of antigen sampling for the mucosal-associated lymphoid system (MALT) and have been recognized as major ports of entry for enteric pathogens in the gut via transepithelial transport (Neutra et al. 1996). Interestingly, maturation of M cells is dependent on signals transmitted by intraepithelial B cells. The group of Jean-Pierre Kraehenbuhl (Lausanne) has developed efficient in vitro systems, in which epithelial cells can

be instructed to undergo differentiation to cells that resemble M cells by morphological and functional–physiological criteria. Therefore, it became feasible to investigate whether M cells are a plausible site of prion entry in a coculture model (Kerneis et al. 1997). Colon carcinoma cells (line CaCo-2) were seeded on the upper face of transwell filters and cultured until confluency was reached. Next, B-lymphoblastoid cells Raji B cells were added onto the lower side of the filters. Lymphoid cells migrated through the pores of the filter and settled within the epithelial monolayer (Figure 61.14), inducing differentiation of some CaCo-2 cells into M cells. Successful conversion was monitored by measuring transport of fluorescein-conjugated latex beads in cocultures that exhibited a high transepithelial resistance and were therefore tight. Active transepithelial transport of beads, but not passive leakage, was blocked at 4°C. Scrapie prions were administered to the apical compartment of cocultures that combined integrity and active transport of beads. After 24 hours, infectivity was determined within the basolateral compartment by bioassay with *tga20* mice, which overexpress a *Prnp* transgene and develop scrapie rapidly after infection (Fischer et al. 1996). Upon challenge with 5 $\log LD_{50}$ scrapie prions, prions were consistently recovered in the basolateral compartment of co-cultures containing M cells, suggesting transepithelial prion transport (Figure 61.14). Even at low prion doses (3 $\log LD_{50}$), infectivity was found in at least one M cell-containing co-culture. By contrast, there was hardly any prion transport in CaCo-2 cultures without M cells (Heppner et al. 2001a).

These findings indicate that M cell differentiation is necessary and sufficient for active transepithelial prion transport in vitro. M cell-dependent uptake of foreign antigens or particles is known to be followed by rapid transcytosis directly to the intraepithelial pocket, where key players of the immune system, e.g. macrophages, dendritic cells, and lymphocytes (Neutra et al. 1996), are located. Therefore, prions may exploit M cell-dependent transcytosis to gain access to the immune system (Aguzzi and Heppner 2000). While these findings suggest that M cells are a plausible candidate for the mucosal portal of prion infection, it still remains to be established whether the pathway delineated above does, indeed, represent the first portal of entry of orally administered prions into the body. This will necessitate in vivo experimentation, for example by ablation of M cells through suicide transgenetic strategies, or by M cell-specific expression of *Prnp* transgenes.

Uptake of prion through the skin

Even less well understood, yet possibly much more efficient than oral administration of prions, is challenge by scarification. Application of one droplet of scrapie inoculum to skin abrasions and subsequent delivery of

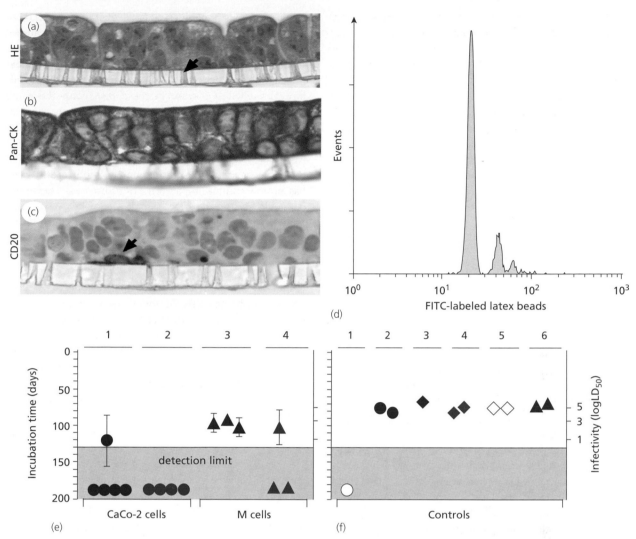

Figure 61.14 *Transepithelial transport of prions via M-cells. Filter membranes with 3 μm pores were overlaid with epithelial cells (colon carcinoma, line CaCo-2). Human B-lymphoblastoid Raji cells were then cultured on the back side of the membrane. (a) Morphology of co-cultures on filters, visualized by hematoxylin and eosin (HE) stains. (b) Immunohistochemical stain for cytokeratins (pan-CK) visualizing human CaCo-2 epithelial cells and (c) for the B-cell marker CD20, displaying B cells that have successfully migrated through the pores of the filter (arrow). (d) Flow cytometric analysis demonstrating active (i.e. temperature-dependent) transport of FITC-conjugated latex beads from the apical to the basolateral chamber compartment upon integration of B cells within pouches of the epithelial CaCo-2 cell layer, and differentiation of M cells. Intactness of co-cultures was assessed by measuring transepithelial resistance at $37^\circ C$, which was typically >200 Ωcm^2. The presence of additional peaks corresponds to aggregates of several latex beads. (e) Recovery of prion infectivity upon challenge with different prion inocula [5 (black) or 3 (red) $logLD_{50}$ input infectious units] was only visible in co-cultures containing M cells (triangles, lanes 3, 4). No prion transport was observed in CaCo-2 cultures (circles, lanes 1, 2) without M cells, except in one case in which traces of infectivity were present. Controls: mock inoculum (lane 1), CaCo-2 culture (Ca) after slight mechanical manipulation resulting in a transepithelial resistance <50 Ωcm^2 (lane 2). Prion infectivity dilutions as indicated before (positive control, lanes 3, 4) and after incubating with either CaCo-2 (lane 5) or M cell containing (M) cultures (lane 6). Each symbol represents the mean incubation time in days (ordinate) of four tga20 indicator mice until terminal disease.*

sweeping strokes until blood is leaking has been shown to be a highly efficacious method of inducing prion disease (Carp 1982; Taylor et al. 1996). It is thinkable that dendritic cells in the skin may become loaded with the infectious agent by this method, and in fact recent work has implicated dendritic cells as potential vectors of prions in oral (Huang et al. 2002) and in hemato-genous spread (Aucouturier et al. 2001) of the agent. It is equally possible (and perhaps more probable), however, that scarification induces direct neural entry of

prions into skin nerve terminals. The latter hypothesis has not yet been studied in much detail, but it would help explain the remarkable speed with which central nervous system pathogenesis follows inoculation by this route: dermal inoculation of scarified mice yields typical latency periods of the disease that are similar to those obtained by intracerebral inoculation. The possibility of direct neural spread of the agent has been brought up also by a series of elegant experiments in the laboratories of Oldstone and Chesebro: transgenic mice that lack the endogenous prion gene but express a *Prnp* transgene exclusively in nervous tissue (under transcriptional control of the neuron-specific enolase regulatory elements) can be efficiently infected by the oral route despite lack of prion protein expression in lymphoid organs (Race et al. 1995). Of course, these experiments do not exclude that dendritic or other mobile cells may participate in neuroinvasion even if they do not express endogenous PrP^C. Rapid neuroinvasion was reported following intralingual inoculation, and may also exploit a direct intraneural pathway (Bartz et al. 2003).

LYMPHOCYTES AND PRION PATHOGENESIS

More than a decade ago the normal prion protein was found to be consistently expressed, albeit at moderate levels, in circulating lymphocytes (Cashman et al. 1990). Subsequently, it was clearly shown in a wealth of experimental paradigms that innate or acquired deficiency of lymphocytes would impair peripheral prion pathogenesis, whereas no aspects of pathogenesis were affected by the presence or absence of lymphocytes upon direct transmission of prions to the central nervous system (Kitamoto et al. 1991a; Lasmezas et al. 1996a). Klein and colleagues pinpointed the lymphocyte requirement to B cells (Aguzzi 1997; Klein et al. 1997): at first sight this was very surprising, since there had been no suggestions that any aspect of humoral immunity would be involved in prion diseases. In the same study, it was shown that T-cell deficiency brought about by ablation of the T-cell receptor (TCR)-α chain did not affect prion pathogenesis (Table 61.5).

TCR-α-deficient mice, however, still contain TCR-γδ T lymphocytes. Although the latter represent a subpopulation of T cells, the experiments described did not allow excluding a role for TCR-γδ T lymphocytes. Therefore, we challenged also TCR-β/δ-deficient mice with prions. Incubation times after intracerebral and intraperitoneal inoculation of limiting or saturating doses of prions, however, elicited disease in these mice with the same kinetics as in wild-type mice (M. Klein and A. Aguzzi, unpublished data). Also, accumulation of PrP^{Sc} and development of histopathological changes in the brain were indistinguishable in these two strains of mice. We therefore conclude that the complete absence of T cells has no measurable impact on prion diseases. Therefore, it is unlikely that the T-cell infiltrates which have been reported to occur in the central nervous system during the course of prion infections (Betmouni et al. 1996; Betmouni and Perry 1999; Perry et al. 2002) represent more than an epiphenomenon.

In 1996–97, when the results of the studies described above were being collected, there was no precise mechanistic model for the role of B cells in prion pathogenesis. It had become rather clear, on the other hand, that lymphocytes alone could not account for the entirety of prion pathogenesis, and an additional sessile compartment had to be involved: adoptive transfer of *Prnp*$^{+/+}$ bone marrow to *Prnp*$^{0/0}$ recipient mice did not suffice to restore infectability of *Prnp*-expressing brain grafts, indicating that neuroinvasion was still defective (Blättler et al. 1997).

In an immediately subsequent series of bone marrow transfer experiments, it emerged that peripheral prion pathogenesis required the physical presence of B cells, yet intraperitoneal infection occurred efficiently even in B-cell-deficient hosts that had been transferred with B cell from *Prnp* knock-out mice (Klein et al. 1998).

Table 61.5 *Susceptibility of various strains of immunodeficient mice to intracerebrally or intraperitoneally administered prions (Klein et al. 1997)*

Defect	Genotype	Intracerebral route		Intraperitoneal route	
		Scrapie	Time to terminal disease	Scrapie	Time to terminal disease
T	CD4$^{0/0}$	7/7	159±11	8/8	191±1
T	CD8$^{0/0}$	6/6	157±15	6/6	202±5
T	β$_2$-μ$^{0/0}$	8/8	162±11	7/7	211±6
T	Perforin$^{-/-}$	3/4	171±2	4/4	204±3
T and B	SCID	7/8	160±11	6/8	226±15
T and B	RAG 2$^{0/0}$	7/7	167±2	0/7	healthy (>504)
T and B	RAG 1$^{0/0}$	3/3	175±2	0/5	healthy (>58)
T and B	AGR$^{0/0}$	6/6	184±10	0/7	healthy (>425)
B	μMT	8/8	181±6	0/8	healthy (>510)
IgG	t11μmt	5/5	170±3	4/4	223±2
FDC	TNFR1$^{0/0}$	7/7	165±3	9/9	216±4
Controls	129Sv	4/4	167±9	4/4	193±3
	C57BL/6	4/4	166±2	4/4	206±2

We measured the latency of scrapie (days from inoculation to terminal disease) upon delivery of a standard prion inoculum. All mice developed spongiform encephalopathy after intracerebral inoculation. By contrast, all mice that carried a defect in B-cell differentiation stayed healthy after intraperitoneal inoculation of RML scrapie prions. Intriguingly, in this and in several subsequent studies, TNFRI$^{-/-}$ developed disease with the same kinetics as wild-type mice, although there are no morphologically detectable follicular dendritic cells in the spleens of TNFRI$^{-/-}$ mice.

Therefore, the presence of B cells – but not expression of the cellular prion protein by these cells – is indispensable for pathogenesis upon intraperitoneal infection in the mouse scrapie model (Aguzzi et al. 2001a).

The above results have been reproduced and confirmed several times over the years by many laboratories in various experimental paradigms: the requirement for B cells in particular appears to be very stringent in most instances investigated. However, it has emerged that not all strains of prions induce identical patterns of peripheral pathogenesis, even when propagated in the same, isogenic strain of host organism. One quite intriguing exception to the B-cell requirement appears to have been recently identified: Manuelidis and colleagues have reported efficient peripheral infection of B-cell-deficient mice with a mouse-adapted strain of human CJD prions (Shlomchik et al. 2001). Despite its somewhat selective interpretation of previously published reports, this study is interesting in that it identifies the unique situation of a prion strain that induces a highly anomalous peripheral pathogenesis.

Straining the lymphocytes

Another interesting discrepancy that remains to be addressed concerns the actual nature of the cells that replicate and accumulate prions in lymphoid organs. In the RML paradigm, four series of rigorously controlled experiments over 5 years (Aguzzi et al. 2000b; Kaeser et al. 2001; Klein et al. 2001; Prinz et al. 2002) unambiguously reproduced the original observation by Thomas Blättler and colleagues that transfer of wild-type ($Prnp^{+/+}$) bone marrow cells (or fetal liver cells) to PrP-deficient ($Prnp^{0/0}$) mice restored accumulation and replication of prions in spleen (Blättler et al. 1997). By contrast, Karen Brown and colleagues reported a diametrically opposite outcome of similar experiments when mice were inoculated with prions of the ME7 strain (K.L. Brown et al. 1999). Since trivial experimental artifacts appear to have been excluded, it is enticing to speculate that this discrepancy may identify yet another significant difference in the cellular tropism of different prion strains.

It is important to note that the Blättler results do not necessarily indicate that lymphocytes are the primary splenic repository of prions: in fact, other experiments suggest that this is quite unlikely. Instead, bone marrow transplantation may

- transfer an ill-defined population with the capability to replenish splenic stroma and to replicate prions, or
- less probably, donor-derived PrP^C expressing hematopoietic cells may confer prion replication capability to recipient stroma by virtue of 'GPI painting,' i.e. the post-translational cell-to-cell transfer of glycophosphoinositol linked extracellular membrane proteins (Kooyman et al. 1998).

Some evidence might be accrued for either possibility: stromal splenic follicular dendritic cells have been described by some authors to possibly derive from hematopoietic precursors, particularly when donors and recipients were young (Szakal et al. 1995; Kapasi et al. 1998). Conversely, instances have been described in which transfer of GPI-linked proteins occurs in vivo with surprisingly high efficiency (Kooyman et al. 1995). Most recently, GPI painting has been described specifically for the cellular prion protein (Liu et al. 2002).

While it has been known for a long time that specific strains of prions may preferentially affect specific subsets of neurons, the Blättler/Brown paradox may uncover an analogous phenomenon in peripheral prion pathogenesis. The latter question may be much more important than it may appear at face value, and its clarification may warrant the investment of significant resources, since the molecular and cellular basis of peripheral tropism of prion strains is likely to be directly linked to the potential danger of BSE in sheep (Bruce et al. 2002; Glatzel and Aguzzi 2001; Kao et al. 2002), as well the potential presence of vCJD prions in human blood (Aguzzi 2000).

PRION HIDEOUTS IN LYMPHOID ORGANS

As mentioned above, prion infectivity rises very rapidly (in a matter of days) in the spleen of intraperitoneally infected mice. Although B lymphocytes are crucial for neuroinvasion, a series of prion titrations in $Prnp$-expressing and $Prnp$-ablated mice, as well as reciprocal bone marrow chimeras thereof, has virtually ruled out the hypothesis that the bulk of infectivity might be contained in lymphocytes. Instead, all evidence points to the fact that most splenic prion infectivity resides in a 'stromal' fraction. Therefore, lymphocytes may be important for trafficking prions within lymphoid organs, but they do not appear to represent a major hideout for the infectious agent. Follicular dendritic cells (FDC) are a prime candidate prion reservoir, since they express large amounts of cellular prion protein, and PrP accumulations tend to co-localize with FDCs in light and electron microscopical analyses of prion-infected spleens. More recently, elegant immunoelectron microscopic studies have evidenced that strong PrP immunoreactivity is situated in the immediate neighborhood of iccosomes (Jeffrey et al. 2000).

A definitive assessment of the contribution of FDCs to prion pathogenesis continues to be problematic since the histogenesis and the molecular characteristics of these cells are ill-defined. In particular, there is a dearth of molecular markers for FDCs. FDCs express S-100 proteins, as well as the complement receptors 2 (CD35) and 4 (identical to the marker FDC-M2). All of these markers, however, are also expressed by additional cell types, even within lymphoid organs (Bofill et al. 2000). The FDC-M1 marker recognized by hybridoma clone 4C11 appears to be more specific, but it stains also tingeable body macrophages, which are most likely of hematopoietic origin. In addition, the antigen recognized by 4C11 has not been molecularly characterized.

Identification of FDC-specific genes would be extremely important and useful to this effect, since it would allow for transgenic studies of FDC histogenesis using fluorescent marker proteins. Other studies on the immediate wish list that would depend on FDC-specific transcription might include:

- transgenetic expression of *Prnp*-restricted to FDCs
- lineage ablation experiments by expressing conditional suicide genes – such as diphtheria toxin receptor or herpes simplex virus thymidine kinase – in FDCs.

Gene deletion experiments in mice have shown that signaling by both TNF and lymphotoxins is required for FDC development (Fu et al. 1997; Koni et al. 1997; Endres et al. 1999). Membrane-bound LT-α/β (LT-α$_1$/β$_2$ or LT-α$_2$/β$_1$) heterotrimers signal through the LT-β receptor (LT-βR) (Ware et al. 1995), thereby activating a signaling pathway required for the development and maintenance of secondary lymphoid organs (Mackay et al. 1997; Matsumoto et al. 1997). Membrane LT-α/β heterotrimers are mainly expressed by activated lymphocytes (Browning et al. 1993, 1995). Maintenance of pre-existing FDCs in a differentiated state requires continuous interaction with B lymphocytes expressing surface LT-α/β (Gonzalez et al. 1998). Inhibition of the LT-α/β pathway in mice by treatment with LT-βR-immuno-

globulin fusion protein (LT-βR-IgFcγ) (Crowe et al. 1994) leads to the disappearance of mature, functional FDCs (defined as cells that express markers such as FDC-M1, FDC-M2, or CD35) within one day, both in spleen and in lymph nodes (Mackay et al. 1997; Mackay and Browning 1998). Prolonged administration of LT-βR-IgFcγ leads to disruption of B-cell follicles.

All of the above prompted a study of the effect of selective ablation of functional FDCs on the pathogenesis of scrapie in mice. FDC depletion was maintained by weekly administration of LT-βR-IgFcγ for 8 weeks. Histological examination of spleen sections revealed that FDC networks had disappeared 1 week after treatment (Figure 61.15), as expected (Montrasio et al. 2000).

In mice, following peripheral inoculation, infectivity in the spleen rises within days and reaches a plateau after a few weeks (Bruce 1985; Büeler et al. 1993; Rubenstein et al. 1991). Even after intracerebral inoculation, spleens of C57BL/6 animals contain infectivity already 4 days post-infection (Büeler et al. 1993). However, western blot analysis (Figure 61.16) revealed that 8 weeks after inoculation spleens of control mice showed strong bands of protease-resistant PrP, whereas mice injected weekly with LT-βR-IgFcγ, starting either 1 week before or 1 week after inoculation, showed no detectable signal (less than one-fiftieth of the controls).

Prion infectivity in three spleens for each time point was assayed by intracerebral inoculation into indicator mice (Fischer et al. 1996). In spleens of mice treated with LT-βR-IgFcγ 1 week before intraperitoneal inoculation,

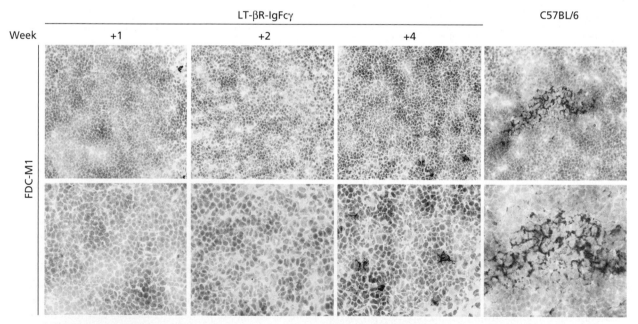

Figure 61.15 *Depletion of follicular dendritic cells by pharmacological inhibition of lymphotoxin signaling. Time course of FDC depletion in spleen of LT-βR-IgFcγ-treated mice. Left to right: spleen histology at 1 week, 2 weeks, and 4 weeks after administration of lymphotoxin antagonist. Right hand column shows administration of human immunoglobulin for control. Frozen sections of treated (left) and control mice (right) immunostained with follicular dendritic cell specific antibody FDC-M1 at different times points after injection of LT-βR-IgFcγ (original magnifications: upper row 8×25; lower row 8×63). Germinal centers FDC networks were depleted 1 week after treatment as described (Mackay and Browning 1998; Montrasio et al. 2000). Some FDC-M1 positive cells, which may represent residual FDCs or tingeable body macrophages, were still detectable in the spleens of treated mice.*

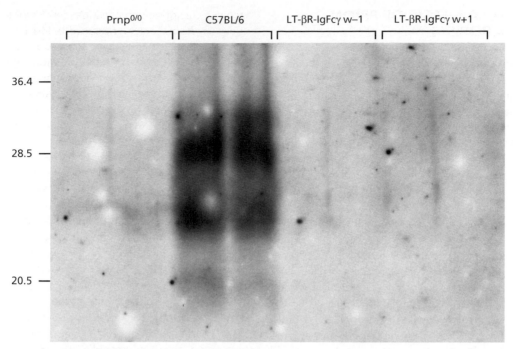

Figure 61.16 *Inhibition of lymphotoxin signalling blocks prion replication in lymphoid organs. Accumulation of PrP[Sc] in spleens of LT-βR-IgFcγ-treated mice 8 weeks after inoculation. Immunoblot analysis of spleen extracts (200 μg total protein) from LT-βR-IgFcγ-treated and control mice sacrificed 8 weeks after inoculation. All spleen samples were treated with proteinase K. Mice analyzed (left to right): Prnp[0/0]; untreated, LT-βR-IgFcγ-treated C57BL/6 mice either 1 week before (LT-βR-IgFcγ w−1) or after (LT-βR-IgFcγ w+1) prion inoculation. Spleens of two mice for each group were analyzed. Immunoreactive PrP was detected using a rabbit antiserum against mouse-derived PrP (1B3) (Farquhar et al. 1994) and enhanced chemiluminescence. The position of the molecular mass standards (in kDa) is indicated on the left side of the fluorogram. The three diagnostic bands of PrP[Sc] are only recognized in untreated mice. LT-βR-IgFcγ treatment led to complete disappearance of the signal (reduction >50-fold).*

no infectivity could be detected after 3 or 8 weeks (<1.0 logID$_{50\text{\p}}$units/ml 10 percent homogenate). Traces of infectivity, possibly representing residual inoculum, were present in the 1-week samples. In mice treated with LT-βR-IgFcγ 1 week after inoculation, the titers were about 2.2 and 4.1 logID$_{50}$ units/ml 10 percent homogenate at 3 weeks and at borderline detectability at 8 weeks after infection, suggesting that some prion accumulation took place in the first weeks after inoculation but was reversed under treatment with LT-βR-IgFcγ by 8 weeks. Spleens of scrapie-inoculated control mice treated with unspecific pooled human immunoglobulins (huIgG) 1 week after inoculation had 4.5 and 5.5 logID$_{50}$ units/ml 10 percent homogenate 8 weeks after intraperitoneal inoculation.

To assess whether prolonged depletion of mature FDCs would perturb the progression of the disease, C57BL/6 mice were subjected to weekly administration of the fusion protein up to 8 weeks post-inoculation and observed for more than 340 days. Mice receiving LT-βR-IgFcγ starting 1 week after inoculation developed the disease with about 25 days delay as compared to control mice. Whenever FDC depletion was initiated 1 week before inoculation, the effect on incubation time was even more pronounced: Two out of three mice developed scrapie symptoms 60 days later than huIgG-treated controls and one mouse survived >340 days (Montrasio

et al. 2000). Double-color immunofluorescence analysis of spleen sections of terminally sick animals revealed that the FDC networks were reconstituted after interruption of LT-βR-IgFcγ administration at 8 weeks and that PrP[C] and/or PrP[Sc] colocalized with FDCs. Immunoblot analysis showed that PrP[Sc] accumulation was restored upon reappearance of FDCs in the spleens of terminal sick LT-βR-IgFcγ-treated mice.

These results show that follicular dendritic cells are essential for the deposition of PrP[Sc] and generation of infectivity in the spleen and suggest that they participate in the process of neuroinvasion. Therefore, the requirement for B cells for these processes might be explained by their essential role in the maturation of FDCs. PrP knock-out mice expressing PrP transgenes only in B cells do not sustain prion replication in the spleen or elsewhere, suggesting that prions associated with splenic B cells (Raeber et al. 1999a) may be acquired from FDCs. Finally, these results suggest that strategies aimed at depleting FDCs might be envisaged for post-exposure prophylaxis (Aguzzi and Collinge 1997) of prion infections initiated at extracerebral sites. The distance between follicular dendritic cells and sympathetic nerve terminals in lymphoid organs appears to control the velocity of neuroinvasion, since juxtaposition of FDCs and sympathetic nerve terminals increases the velocity of neuroinvasion (Prinz et al. 2003a).

THE CELLULAR BASIS OF PRION LYMPHOTROPISM

As discussed above, inhibition of the LT-β signaling pathway with a soluble receptor depletes FDCs (Mackay and Browning 1998) and abolishes prion replication in spleens, thereby prolonging the latency of scrapie after intraperitoneal challenge (Montrasio et al. 2000). This suggests that B-cell-deficient μMT mice (Kitamura et al. 1991) may be resistant to intraperitoneal prion inoculation (Klein et al. 1997) because of impaired FDC maturation (Klein et al. 1998; Montrasio et al. 2000). However, additional experimentation appears to indicate that PrP^C-expressing hematopoietic cells are required in addition to FDCs for efficient lymphoreticular prion propagation (Blättler et al. 1997; Kaeser et al. 2001). This apparent discrepancy called for additional studies of the molecular requirements for prion replication competence in lymphoid stroma. Therefore peripheral prion pathogenesis was studied in mice lacking TNF-α, LTα/β, or their receptors. After intracerebral inoculation, all treated mice developed clinical symptoms of scrapie with incubation times, attack rates, and histopathological characteristics similar to those of wild-type mice, indicating that TNF/LT signaling is not relevant to cerebral prion pathogenesis. Upon intraperitoneal prion challenge, mice defective in LT signaling (LT-α$^{-/-}$, LTβ$^{-/-}$, LT-βR$^{-/-}$, or LT-α$^{-/-}$TNF-α$^{-/-}$) proved virtually non-infectible with ≤5 logLD$_{50}$ scrapie infectivity, and establishment of subclinical disease (Frigg et al. 1999) was prevented. By contrast, TNFR1$^{-/-}$ mice were almost fully susceptible to all inoculum sizes, and TNF-α$^{-/-}$ mice showed dose-dependent susceptibility. TNFR2$^{-/-}$ mice had intact FDCs and germinal centers, and were fully susceptible to scrapie. Unexpectedly, all examined lymph nodes of TNFR1$^{-/-}$ and TNF-α$^{-/-}$ mice had consistently high infectivity titers (Prinz et al. 2002). Even inguinal lymph nodes, which are distant from the injection site and do not drain the peritoneum, contained infectivity titers equal to all other lymph nodes. Therefore, TNF deficiency prevents lymphoreticular prion accumulation in spleen but not in lymph nodes.

Why is susceptibility to peripheral prion challenge preserved in the absence of TNFR1 or TNF-α$^{-/-}$, while deletion of LT signaling components confers high resistance to peripheral prion infection? After all, each of these defects (except TNFR2$^{-/-}$) abolishes FDCs. For one thing, prion pathogenesis in the lymphoreticular system appears to be compartmentalized, with lymph nodes (rather than spleen) being important reservoirs of prion infectivity during disease. Second, prion replication appears to take place in lymph nodes even in the absence of mature FDCs.

Bone marrow chimeric mice were generated in order to determine whether hematopoietic components are involved in prion propagation in TNFR1$^{-/-}$ lymph nodes. In Prnp$^{0/0}$ mice grafted with TNFR1$^{-/-}$ hematopoietic cells, high infectivity loads were detectable in lymph nodes but not spleens, indicating that TNFR1-deficient, PrP^C-expressing hematopoietic cells may support prion propagation within lymph nodes (Prinz et al. 2002). These findings are in line with previous studies, which showed that chimeras of PrP-deficient hosts with PrP-expressing hematopoietic cells can accumulate prions chronically (Blättler et al. 1997; Kaeser et al. 2001). The PrP signal colocalized with a subset of macrophages in TNFR1$^{-/-}$ lymph nodes. Since marginal zone macrophages are in close contact to FDCs and also interact with marginal zone B cells, this cell type is certainly a candidate supporter in prion uptake and replication. On the other hand, it has been reported that in short-time infection experiments depletion of macrophages appears to enhance the amount of recoverable infectivity, implying that macrophages may degrade prions rather than transport them (Beringue et al. 2000). The finding that a cell type other than mature FDCs is involved in prion replication and accumulation within lymph nodes may be relevant to the development of post-exposure prophylaxis strategies.

SYMPATHETIC NERVES: A NEUROIMMUNE LINK?

In the last several years, a model has emerged that predicts prion neuroinvasion to consist of two distinct phases (Aguzzi et al. 2001c). The details of the first phase are discussed above: widespread colonization of lymphoreticular organs is achieved by mechanisms that depend on B lymphocytes (Klein et al. 1997, 1998), follicular dendritic cells (Montrasio et al. 2000), and complement factors (Klein et al. 2001). The second phase has long been suspected to involve peripheral nerves, and possibly the autonomic nervous system, and may depend on expression of PrP^C by these nerves (Glatzel and Aguzzi 2000). Glatzel and colleagues have been attempting to test the requirement for expression of PrP^C in peripheral nerves for several years, and have developed a gene transfer protocol to spinal ganglia aimed at resolving this question (Glatzel et al. 2000); however, they were never able to recover infectivity in spinal cords of Prnp$^{0/0}$ mice whose spinal nerves had been transduced by Prnp-expressing adenoviruses (M. Glatzel and A. Aguzzi, unpublished results). Also, fast axonal transport does not appear to be involved in prion neuroinvasion, since mice that are severely impaired in this transport mechanism experience prion pathogenesis with kinetics similar to that of wild-type mice (Künzi et al. 2002).

There is substantial evidence suggesting that prion transfer from the lymphoid system to the CNS occurs along peripheral nerves in a PrP^C-dependent fashion

(Blättler et al. 1997; Glatzel and Aguzzi 2000; Race et al. 2000). Studies focusing on the temporal and spatial dynamics of neuroinvasion have suggested that the autonomic nervous system might be responsible for transport from lymphoid organs to the CNS (Clarke and Kimberlin 1984; Cole and Kimberlin 1985; Beekes et al. 1998; McBride and Beekes 1999).

The innervation pattern of lymphoid organs is mainly sympathetic (Felten and Felten 1988). Glatzel and colleagues have shown that denervation by injection of the drug 6-hydroxydopamine (6-OHDA), as well as 'immunosympathectomy' by injection of antibodies against nerve growth factor (NGF) leads to a rather dramatic decrease in the density of sympathetic innervation of lymphoid organs (Figure 61.17), and significantly delayed the development of scrapie (Glatzel et al. 2001) (Figure 61.18). Sympathectomy appears to delay the transport of prions from lymphatic organs to the thoracic spinal cord, which is the entry site of sympathetic nerves to the CNS. Transgenic mice overexpressing NGF under control of the K14 promoter, whose spleens are hyperinnervated, developed scrapie significantly earlier than nontransgenic control mice. No alteration in lymphocyte subpopulations was detected in spleens at any time point investigated. In particular, no significant differences in content of FDCs were detected between treated and untreated mice, which negates the possibility that the observed protection may be due to modulation of FDC microanatomy.

While the sympathetic nervous system may represent a major component of the second phase of prion neuroinvasion, many details remain to be elucidated. It is not known whether prions can be transferred directly from FDCs to sympathetic endings, or whether additional cell types are involved. The latter possibility is particularly enticing, since FDCs have not been shown to entertain physical contact with sympathetic nervous system terminals.

Moreover, it is unclear how prions are actually transported within peripheral nerves. Axonal and non-axonal transport mechanisms may be involved, and non-neuronal cells (such as Schwann cells) may play a role. Within the framework of the protein-only hypothesis, one may hypothesize a 'domino' mechanism, by which incoming PrP^{Sc} converts resident PrP^C on the axolemmal surface, thereby propagating spatially the infection. While speculative, this model is attractive since it may accommodate the finding that the velocity of neural prion spread is extremely slow (Kimberlin et al. 1983) and may not follow the canonical mechanisms of fast axonal transport. Indeed, recent studies may favor a non-axonal transport mechanism that results in periaxonal deposition of PrP^{Sc} (Hainfellner and Budka 1999; Glatzel and Aguzzi 2000).

The fact that denervated mice eventually developed scrapie may be due to an alternative, low-efficiency route of entry that may become uncovered by the absence of sympathetic fibers, or because of incomplete sympathectomy. Entry through the vagal nerve has been proposed in studies of the dynamics of vacuolation

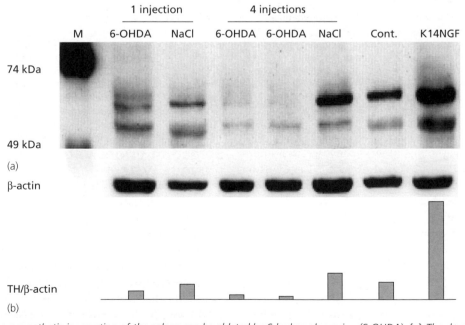

(a)

(b)

Figure 61.17 *The sympathetic innervation of the spleen can be ablated by 6-hydroxydopamine (6-OHDA).* **(a)** *The density of sympathetic innervation correlates with the concentration of tyrosine hydroxylase, which was measured by western blot analysis in spleens of adult 6-OHDA-treated mice, K14NGF transgenic mice, and controls. The two main tyrosine hydroxylase bands are visible at ca. 55 kDa. While there is a certain increase in sympathetic innervation with age, it is obvious that 6-OHDA treatment depletes, and the K14NGF transgene increases sympathetic innervation.* **(b)** *Quantification of tyrosine hydroxylase content by chemiluminescence scanning. The bars represent the ratio between signal intensity of the tyrosine hydroxylase band and that of the corresponding β-actin bands (arbitrary units).*

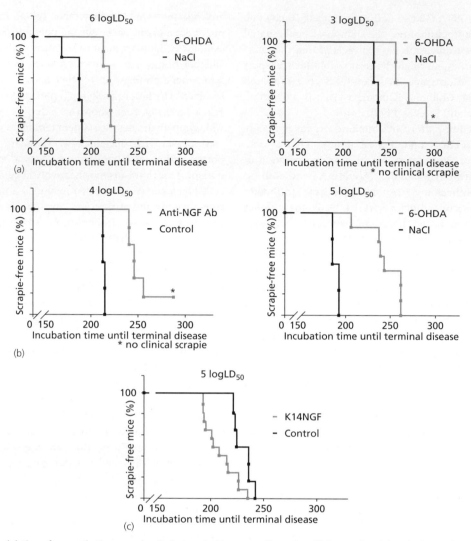

Figure 61.18 *Modulation of sympathetic nerve density in lymphoid organs affects the efficiency of peripheral prion pathogenesis. Survival plots displaying the incubation time (days) until development of terminal scrapie in C57BL/6 mice inoculated intraperitoneally with prions (a–c) and of tga20 indicator mice inoculated intracerebrally with spinal cord and spleen samples (d). Mice injected with 6-OHDA in their adulthood (a), as well as mice injected neonatally with anti-NGF antibodies or with 6-OHDA (b) developed terminal scrapie significantly later than their respective controls. Instead K14NGFmice, which have hyperinnervated spleens, developed terminal scrapie earlier than matched wild-type siblings of the same genetic background (c). The size of inoculum is expressed in infectious units (logLD_{50}).*

following oral and intraperitoneal challenge with prions (Baldauf et al. 1997; Beekes et al. 1998). There was no evidence for transport along the vagal nerve in sympathectomized mice, since vagal nuclei were affected similarly to other regions of the brainstem unrelated to the vagal system. This supports the hypothesis that delayed neuroinvasion in denervated mice may occur because of residual innervation of lymphoreticular organs.

The surprising finding that infectious titers in hyperinnervated spleens are at least two logs higher and show enhanced PrP^{Sc} accumulations compared to control mice suggests that sympathetic nerves, besides being involved in the transport of prions, may also accumulate and replicate prions in lymphatic organs (Clarke and Kimberlin 1984). Obviously, this finding has implications related to the permanence and possibly eradication of prions in subclinically infected hosts.

Spread of prions within the central nervous system

Ocular administration of prions has proved particularly useful to study neural spread of the agent, since the retina is a part of the central nervous system and intraocular injection does not produce direct physical trauma to the brain, which may disrupt the blood–brain barrier and impair other aspects of brain physiology. The assumption that spread of prions occurs axonally rests mainly on the demonstration of diachronic spongiform changes along the retinal pathway following intraocular infection (Fraser 1982).

To investigate whether spread of prions within the CNS is dependent on PrP^C expression in the visual pathway, PrP-producing neural grafts were used as sensitive indicators of the presence of prion infectivity in the brain of an otherwise PrP-less host. Following inoculation with prions into the eye of grafted $Prnp^{0/0}$ mice, none of the grafts showed signs of scrapie. Therefore, it was concluded that infectivity administered to the eye of PrP-deficient hosts cannot induce scrapie in a PrP-expressing brain graft (Brandner et al. 1996b).

Engraftment of $Prnp^{0/0}$ mice with PrP^C-producing tissue might lead to an immune response to PrP which, in turn, was shown to be in principle capable of neutralizing infectivity (Heppner et al. 2001b). In order to definitively rule out the possibility that prion transport was disabled by a neutralizing immune response, $Prnp^{0/0}$ mice were rendered tolerant by expressing PrP^C under the control of the *lck* promoter. These mice overexpress PrP on T lymphocytes, but are resistant to scrapie and do not replicate prions in brain, spleen, and thymus after intraperitoneal inoculation with scrapie prions (Raeber et al. 1999b). Engraftment of these mice with PrP-overexpressing neuroectoderm did not lead to the development of antibodies to PrP after intracerebral or intraocular inoculation, presumably due to clonal deletion of PrP-immunoreactive T lymphocytes. As before, intraocular inoculation with prions did not provoke scrapie in the graft, supporting the conclusion that lack of PrP^C, rather than immune response to PrP, prevented prion spread (Brandner et al. 1996b). Therefore, PrP^C appears to be necessary for the spread of prions along the retinal projections and within the intact CNS.

These results indicate that intracerebral spread of prions is based on a PrP^C-paved chain of cells, perhaps because they are capable of supporting prion replication. When such a chain is interrupted by interposed cells that lack PrP^C, as in the case described here, no propagation of prions to the target tissue can occur. Perhaps prions require PrP^C for propagation across synapses: PrP^C is present in the synaptic region (Fournier et al. 1995) and certain synaptic properties are altered in $Prnp^{0/0}$ mice (Collinge et al. 1994; Whittington et al. 1995). Perhaps transport of prions within (or on the surface of) neuronal processes is PrP^C-dependent. Within the framework of the protein-only hypothesis (Griffith 1967; Prusiner 1989b), these findings may be accommodated by a 'domino-stone' model in which spreading of scrapie prions in the CNS occurs per continuitatem through conversion of PrP^C by adjacent PrP^{Sc} (Aguzzi 1997).

INNATE IMMUNITY AND ANTIPRION DEFENSE

Macrophages and Toll-like receptors

Cells of the monocyte/macrophage lineage typically represent the first line of defense against an extremely broad variety of pathogens. In the case of prions, it might be conceivable that macrophages protect against prions. However, it would be equally conceivable that macrophages, by virtue of their phagocytic properties and of their intrinsic mobility, may function as Trojan horses that transport prion infectivity between sites of replication within the body. This interesting question has not yet been fully resolved.

In a short-term prion infection paradigm, Beringue and colleagues administered dichloromethylene disphosphonate encapsulated into liposomes to mice: this eliminates for a short period of time all spleen macrophages. Accumulation of newly synthesized PrP^{Sc} was accelerated, suggesting that macrophages participate in the clearance of prions, rather than being involved in PrP^{Sc} synthesis (Beringue et al. 2000).

On the basis of the results presented above, Beringue and colleagues have suggested that activation or targeting of macrophages may represent a therapeutic pathway to explore in TSE infection. This suggestion was taken up by Sethi and Kretzschmar, who recently reported that activation of Toll-like receptors (TLR), which function as general stimulators of innate immunity by driving expression of various sets of the immune regulatory molecules, can effect post-exposure prophylaxis in an experimental model of intraperitoneal scrapie infection (Sethi et al. 2002). In this experimental paradigm, administration of prions intraperitoneally elicited disease after approximately 180 days, whereas the administration of CpG oligodeoxynucleotides 7 hours after prion inoculation and daily for 20 days led to disease-free intervals of 'more than 330 days' – although it appears that all inoculated mice died of scrapie shortly thereafter (communicated by H. Kretzschmar at the TSE conference in Edinburgh in September, 2002).

This finding is very surprising, since most available evidence indicates that general activation of the immune system would typically sensitize mice to prions, rather than protect them. The mechanism by which activation of TLRs can result in post-exposure prophylaxis is wholly unclear at present, particularly in view of the fact that mice lacking MyD88 (Adachi et al. 1998), which is an essential mediator of TLR signaling, develop prion disease with exactly the same sensitivity and kinetics as wild-type mice (Prinz et al. 2003b). Moreover, repeated administration of CpG oligonucleotides (ODN) was shown to produce a profound depletion of follicular dendritic cells, which are prominent peripheral prion reservoirs (Heikenwälder et al. 2004). This finding suggests that the alleged protective effect of CpG-ODN administration relies on indiscriminate destruction of immune organs rather than any specific anti-prion effect.

The complement system

Another prominent component at the crossroads between innate and adaptive immunity is represented by the complement system. Opsonization by complement system components also appears to be relevant to prion pathogenesis: mice genetically engineered to lack complement factors (Klein et al. 2001), or mice depleted of the C3 complement component by administration of cobra venom (Mabbott et al. 2001), exhibit a remarkable resistance to peripheral prion inoculation. This phenomenon may, once again, be related to the pathophysiology of FDCs, which typically function as antigen traps. Trapping mechanisms essentially consist of capture of immune complexes by Fcγ receptors, and binding of opsonized antigens (linked covalently to C3d and C4b complement adducts) to the CD21/CD35 complement receptors.

Capture mediated by Fcγ receptors does not appear to be very important in prion disease: for one thing, knockout mice lacking Fcγ receptors (Takai et al. 1994, 1996; Hazenbos et al. 1996; Park et al. 1998) are just as susceptible to intraperitoneally administered scrapie as wild-type mice. Furthermore, introduction into μMT mice of a generic immunoglobulin μ chain fully restored prion neuroinvasion irrespective of whether this heavy chain allowed for secretion of immunoglobulins, or only for production of membrane-bound immunoglobulins. We therefore conclude that circulating immunoglobulins are certainly not crucial to prion replication in lymphoid organs and to neuroinvasion.

A second mechanism exploited by FDCs for antigen trapping involves covalent linking of proteolytic fragments of the complement components C3 and C4 (Szakal and Hanna 1968; Carroll 1998). The CD21/CD35 complement receptors on FDCs bind C3b, iC3b, C3d, and C4b through short consensus repeats in their extracellular domain. Ablation of C3, or of its receptor CD21/CD35, as well as C1q (alone or combined with BF/C2$^{-/-}$), delayed neuroinvasion significantly after intraperitoneal inoculation when a limiting dose of prions was administered. These effects suggest that opsonization of the infectious agent may enhance its accessibility to germinal centers by facilitating docking to FDCs.

Very large prion inocula ($>10^6$ infectious units) appear to override the requirement for a functional complement receptor in prion pathogenesis. This is similar to systemic viral infections and coreceptor-dependent retention within the follicular compartment, whose necessity can be overridden by very high affinity antigens (Fischer et al. 1998) or adjuvants (Wu et al. 2000). Additional retention mechanisms for prions may therefore exist in FDCs, which are not complement-dependent, or which may depend on hitherto unidentified complement receptors.

ADAPTIVE IMMUNITY AND PRE-EXPOSURE PROPHYLAXIS AGAINST PRIONS

For many conventional viral agents, vaccination is the most effective method of infection control. But is it at all possible to induce protective immunity in vivo against prions? Prions are extremely sturdy and their resistance against sterilization is proverbial. Preincubation with anti-PrP antisera was reported to reduce the prion titer of infectious hamster brain homogenates by up to 2 log units (Gabizon et al. 1988) and an anti-PrP antibody was found to inhibit formation of PrP^{Sc} in a cell-free system (Horiuchi and Caughey 1999). Also, antibodies (Klein et al. 2001) and F(ab) fragments raised against certain domains of PrP (Peretz et al. 2001) can suppress prion replication in cultured cells. However, it is difficult to induce humoral immune responses against PrP^C and PrP^{Sc}. This is most likely due to tolerance of the mammalian immune system to PrP^C, which is an endogenous protein expressed rather ubiquitously. Ablation of the *Prnp* gene (Büeler et al. 1992), which encodes PrP^C, renders mice highly susceptible to immunization with prions (Brandner et al. 1996b), and many of the best available monoclonal antibodies to the prion protein have been generated in *Prnp*$^{0/0}$ mice (Prusiner et al. 1993). However, *Prnp*$^{0/0}$ mice are unsuitable for testing vaccination regimens since they do not support prion pathogenesis (Büeler et al. 1993).

It was therefore asked whether genes encoding high-affinity anti-PrP antibodies (originally generated in *Prnp*$^{0/0}$ mice) may be utilized to reprogram B-cell responses of prion-susceptible mice that express PrP^C. Indeed, the introduction of the epitope-interacting region of heavy chain of 6H4, a high-affinity anti-PrP monoclonal antibody (Korth et al. 1997), into the germline of mice sufficed to produce high-titer anti-PrP^C immunity. The 6H4μ heavy chain transgene induced similar anti-PrP^C titers in *Prnp*$^{0/0}$, *Prnp*$^{0/+}$ and *Prnp*$^{+/+}$ mice, indicating that deletion of autoreactive B cells does not prevent anti-PrP immunity. The buildup of anti-PrP^C titers, however, was more sluggish in the presence of endogenous PrP^C, suggesting that some clonal deletion is actually occurring.

How can these observations be interpreted? The total anti-PrP^C titer results from pairing of one transgenic μ heavy chain with a large repertoire of endogenous κ and λ chains: some pairings may lead to reactive moieties, while others may be anergic (Figure 61.19a). Maybe the B-cell clones with the highest affinity to PrP^C are being eliminated by the immune tolerization machinery, and only clones with medium affinity are retained (Figure 61.19a). This would explain the delay in titer buildup in the presence of PrP^C, and would be in agreement with our affinity measurements – indicating that the total molar avidity of 6H4μ serum is approximately 100-fold lower that that of the original 6H4 antibody from which the transgene was derived (Figure 61.19b). But most intriguingly, expression of the 6H4μ heavy chain sufficed to block peripheral prion pathogenesis upon intraperitoneal inoculation of the prion agent (Heppner et al. 2001a).

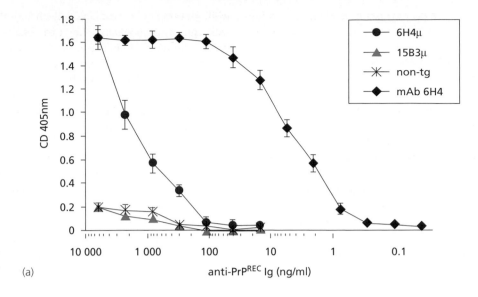

(a)

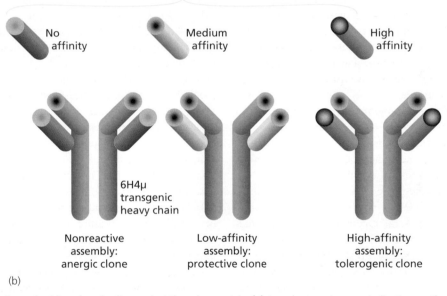

(b)

Figure 61.19 *Affinity and avidity of antibodies against the prion protein.* **(a)** *In order to gain some indication on the relative avidity of the immune response against PrP^C in 6H4 transgenic mice, we compared the binding of serum from transgenic mice to a dilution series of the 6H4 original monoclonal antibody. When normalized against the immunoglobulin concentration, taking into account that the anti-PrP^C antibodies 6H4 transgenic mice are pentameric, we found that the total avidity of the transgenic serum is approximately 2 log units lower than that of the monoclonal antibody from which the transgene was derived. A possible explanation for this phenomenon is depicted in* **(b)**. *While the heavy chain is kept constant in the transgene, it may pair with a large repertoire of endogenous light chains. Some of the pairs will yield very high affinity antibodies, others will have low affinity, but the majority may have no affinity at all for the prion protein. It is possible that some degree of clonal deletion occurs, and that combinations with the highest affinity are eliminated.*

PrP^C is a normal protein expressed by most tissues of the body. Therefore an anti-PrP immune response may conceivably induce an autoimmune disease, and defeat any realistic prospect for prion vaccination. We did not observe any blatant autoimmune disease as a consequence of anti-prion immunization – unless PrP^C was artificially transgenically expressed at nonphysiological, extremely high levels.

The strategy outlined above delivers proof-of-principle that a protective humoral response against prions can be mounted by the mammalian immune system, and suggests that B cells are not intrinsically tolerant to PrP^C. If the latter is generally true, lack of immunity to prions may be due to T-helper tolerance. The latter problem is not trivial, but may perhaps be overcome by presenting PrP^C to the immune system along with highly active adjuvants. These findings, therefore, encourage a reassessment of the possible value of active and passive immunization (Westaway and Carlson 2002), and perhaps of reprogramming B-cell repertoires by μ-chain transfer, in prophylaxis or in therapy of prion diseases.

Prion immunization and its reduction to practice

As described above, monoclonal antibodies and F(ab) fragments recognizing PrP were shown to prevent de novo scrapie infection, and to abolish PrP^{Sc} as well as prion infectivity in chronically scrapie-infected neuro-blastoma cells (Enari et al. 2001). Furthermore, transgenic expression of anti-PrP antibodies in mice arrested peripheral scrapie pathogenesis (Heppner et al. 2001b). In line with these results, White and colleagues confirmed the efficiency of anti-PrP antibodies in preventing prion disease by injecting such antibodies into wild-type mice upon peripheral prion challenge (White et al. 2003).

The prionostatic efficacy of anti-PrP antibodies is highest in extraneural compartments: transgenic 6H4μ mice expressing anti-PrP-specific IgM molecules were not protected when prions were administered intracerebrally (Aguzzi and Heppner, unpublished observations), and passive transfer of PrP-specific IgG immunoglobulins (White et al. 2003) was inefficient when started after the onset of clinical signs. This may be due to the limited influx of immunoglobulins into the central nervous system (CNS) and to the high prion load of clinically symptomatic animals.

By providing stable, sustained titers, active immunization may obviate to some of the problems listed above. However, host tolerance to endogenous PrP^{C} remains a major obstacle to devising active immunization regimens. Nevertheless, several recent studies suggest that the induction of anti-PrP antibodies in wild-type mice is, in principle, feasible (Souan et al. 2001; Koller et al. 2002; Sigurdsson et al. 2002; Arbel et al. 2003; Schwarz et al. 2003; Rossett et al. 2004). While anti-PrP immunoglobulin titers could be measured in most of these studies, the titers were rather low. Accordingly, the biological efficacy of these immunization series, if evaluated at all, was limited.

A systematic exploration of the efficacy of active immunization strategies against PrP (Heikenwälder et al. 2004) found that it was exceedingly difficult to elicit antibody titers to native cell-bound PrP^{C} as displayed on the cell surface of PrP^{C}-overexpressing splenocytes (Raeber et al. 1999b). This suggests that host tolerance to endogenous PrP^{C} is non-permissive to generating high-affinity anti-PrP B-cell clones, or leads to deletion or anergy of the cognate T-cell clones. Expression of PrP^{C} within the thymus did not prevent humoral immune responses to recombinant bacterially expressed PrP completely. However, extrathymic and extraneural PrP^{C} – even if expressed in very small amounts – blocked all immune responses to both PrP^{C} and bacterially expressed PrP. One must conclude, therefore, that while antibodies recognizing cell-surface PrP^{C} interfere with prion pathogenesis in two independent paradigms, humoral immune responses may not be of much value if their affinity does not extend to bona fide eukaryotic PrP^{C} as displayed on cell surfaces.

PROGRESS IN THE DIAGNOSIS OF PRION DISEASES

As with any other disease, early diagnosis would significantly advance the chances of success of any possible intervention approaches. Unfortunately, the situation in prion diagnosis continues to be rather primitive. Presymptomatic diagnosis is virtually impossible, and the earliest possible diagnosis is based on clinical signs and symptoms. Hence, prion infection is typically diagnosed after the disease has considerably progressed.

A significant advance in prion diagnostics was accomplished in 1997 by the discovery that protease-resistant PrP^{Sc} can be detected in tonsillar tissue of vCJD patients (Hill et al. 1997b). It was hence proposed that tonsil biopsy may be the method of choice for diagnosis of vCJD (Hill et al. 1999). Furthermore, there have been reports of individual cases showing detection of PrP^{Sc} at preclinical stages of the disease in tonsil (Schreuder et al. 1996) as well as in the appendix (Hilton et al. 1998), indicating that lymphoid tissue biopsy may represent a potential test for asymptomatic individuals. These observations triggered large screenings of human populations for subclinical vCJD prevalence, using appendectomy and tonsillectomy speciments (Glatzel et al. 2003b). PrP^{Sc}-positive lymphoid tissue were long considered to be a vCJD-specific feature which would not apply to any other forms of human prion diseases (Hill et al. 1999). However, a recent survey of peripheral tissues of patients with sCJD has identified PrP^{Sc} in as many as one-third of skeletal muscle and spleen samples (Glatzel et al. 2003a). In addition, PrP^{Sc} was found in the olfactory epithelium of patients suffering from sCJD (Zanusso et al. 2003). These unexpected findings raise the hope that minimally invasive diagnostic procedures may take the place of brain biopsy in intravital CJD diagnostics.

The sensitivity of PrP^{Sc} detection was significantly improved by the sodium phosphotungstic (NaPTA) precipitation method (Safar et al. 1998). By concentrating PrP^{Sc} prior to western blot analysis, this procedure improves the sensitivity of diagnostic assays by as much as four orders of magnitude (Wadsworth et al. 2001). An interesting development was brought about by the conformation-dependent immunoassay (CDI), in which conformational differences of PrP isoforms are mapped by quantitating the relative binding of antibodies to denatured and native protein (Safar et al. 1998). Rather than relying on protease resistance, the CDI measures a variety of misfolded PrP isoforms, which may increase its sensitivity (Safar et al. 2002; Bellon et al. 2003).

Be that as it may, all techniques described above suffer from the fact that PrP^{Sc} continues to represent a surrogate marker for prion infectivity – since:

- PrP^{Sc} has not been incontrovertibly shown to be congruent with the prion
- several manipulations in vitro and in vivo can render PrP^C protease-resistant without bestowing infectivity on it.

Therefore, determination of prion infectivity by bioassay remains the golden standard: as in Pasteur's age, the concentration of the infectious agent is determined by inoculating serial dilutions of the test material into experimental animals, and the dilution at which 50 percent of the animals contract the disease (termed ID$_{50}$) is determined. Naturally, this system is riddled with inconveniences: scores of animals need to be sacrificed, and the incubation times are lengthy (transgenetic overexpression of PrP^C can help, but only to some extent). Also the method tends to be breathtakingly inaccurate: the inoculation schemes used in most studies typically suffer from standard errors of ± 1 order of magnitude!

A radical improvement of this situation is likely to be brought about by the use of prion-susceptible cell lines (Bosque and Prusiner 2000). The determination of prion infectivity endpoints combines the sensitivity and intrinsic biological validity of the bioassay (i.e. direct measurement of the infectivity) with the speed and convenience of an in vitro methodology amenable to medium-throughput automation (Klohn et al. 2003).

PERSPECTIVES IN PRION IMMUNOLOGY

Until approximately 10 years ago, it was thought that prion diseases are completely independent of the immune system. The lack of overt inflammation in spongiform lesions lent support to this viewpoint. It is fascinating to note that this view has been turned completely upside down, and it is now obvious that the relationships between the infectious agent and various components of the immune system are intimate, complex, and multifaceted. While several crucial questions are still open, notably regarding the true portal of entry of BSE prions into the human body, and the mechanism by which they cause vCJD, a fascinating multitude of unexpected findings has been reported, some of them in extraordinary detail.

In the long run, one would hope that this accrued knowledge will be put into useful practice. To that effect, it is encouraging to note that a sizable number of the steps in prion transport which have been discussed above appears to be rate-limiting. Because of that, these steps lend themselves as a target for interventions, which may be therapeutic or prophylactic (Aguzzi et al. 2001b).

A number of substances appear capable of influencing the outcome of a contact of mammalian organisms with prions: a non-exhaustive list includes compounds as diverse as Congo red (Caughey and Race 1992), amphotericin B (Pocchiari et al. 1987), anthracyclin derivatives (Tagliavini et al. 1997), sulfated polyanions (Caughey and Raymond 1993), pentosan polysulfate (Farquhar et al. 1999), soluble lymphotoxin-β receptors (Montrasio et al. 2000), porphyrins (Priola et al. 2000), branched polyamines (Supattapone et al. 2001), and β-sheet breaker peptides (Soto et al. 2000). However, it is sobering that none of the substances have yet made it to any validated clinical use: quinacrine appears to represent the most recent unfulfilled promise (Collins et al. 2002). On the other hand, the tremendous interest in this field has attracted researchers from various neighboring disciplines, including immunology, genetics, and pharmacology, and therefore it is to be hoped that rational and efficient methods for managing prion infections will be developed in the future.

CONCLUDING REMARKS

Do prions exist in lower organisms?

In *Saccharomyces cerevisiae*, ure2 and [URE3] mutants were described that can grow on ureidosuccinate under conditions of nitrogen repression such as glutamic acid and ammonia (Lacroute 1971). Mutants of *URE2* exhibit mendelian inheritance, whereas [URE3] is cytoplasmically inherited (Wickner 1994). The [URE3] phenotype can be induced by UV irradiation and by overexpression of ure2p, the gene product of ure2; deletion of ure2 abolishes [URE3]. The function of ure2p is unknown but it has substantial homology with glutathione-S-transferase; attempts to demonstrate this enzymic activity with purified ure2p have been unsuccessful (Coschigano and Magasanik 1991). Whether the [URE3] protein is a post-translationally modified form of ure2p which acts upon unmodified ure2p to produce more of itself remains to be established.

Another yeast prion is the [PSI] phenotype (Wickner 1994). [PSI] is a non-mendelian inherited trait that can be induced by overexpression of *Sup35* (Cox et al. 1988; Chernoff et al. 1993). The production of [PSI] has recently been shown to require the molecular chaperone Hsp104, suggesting that this protein functions in producing an altered form of *Sup35* (Chernoff et al. 1995). Both [PSI] and [URE3] can be cured by exposure of the yeast to 3 mm GdnHCl. The mechanism responsible for abolishing [PSI] and [URE3] with a low concentration of GdnHCl is unknown. In the filamentous fungus *Podospora anserina*, the *het-s* locus controls the vegetative incompatibility; conversion from the S^s to the s state seems to be a post-translational, autocatalytic process (Deleu et al. 1993). If any of the examples above cited can be shown to function in a manner similar to prions in animals, many new, more rapid and economical approaches to prion diseases should be forthcoming.

Unresolved problems in prion science

The study of prions has taken several unexpected directions over the past few years. The discovery that prion diseases in humans are uniquely both genetic and infectious has greatly strengthened and extended the prion concept. However, the areas that are still obscure do not relate only to the details: some of these concern the core of the prion concept (Chesebro 1998). In my opinion, there are five large groups of questions regarding the basic science of prion replication and of development of TSE diseases that deserve to be addressed with a vigorous research effort:

- Which are the molecular mechanisms of prion replication? How does the disease-associated prion protein, PrP^{Sc}, achieve the conversion of its cellular sibling, PrP^{C}, into a likeness of itself? Which other proteins assist this process? Can we inhibit this process? If so, how?
- What is the essence of prion strains, which are operationally defined as variants of the infectious agent capable of retaining stable phenotypic traits upon serial passage in syngeneic hosts? The existence of strains is very well known in virology, but it was not predicted to exist in the case of an agent that propagates epigenetically.
- How do prions reach the brain after having entered the body? Which molecules and which cell types are involved in this process of neuroinvasion? Which inhibitory strategies are likely to succeed?
- The mechanisms of neurodegeneration in spongiform encephalopathies are not understood. Which are the pathogenetic cascades that are activated upon accumulation of disease-associated prion protein, and ultimately lead to brain damage?
- What is the physiological function of the highly conserved, normal prion protein, PrP^{C}? The *Prnp* gene encoding PrP^{C} was indentified in 1985 (Oesch et al 1985; Basler et al. 1986), *Prnp* knock-out mice were described in 1992 (Büeler et al., 1992), and some PrP^{C}-interacting proteins have been identified (Oesch et al. 1990; Rieger et al. 1997; Yehiely et al. 1997; Zanata et al. 2002). Yet the function of PrP^{C} remains unknown.

GLOSSARY OF PRION TERMINOLOGY

Prion Agent of transmissible spongiform encephalopathy (TSE), with unconventional properties. The term does not have structural implications other than that a protein is an essential component.

'Protein-only' hypothesis Maintains that the prion is devoid of informational nucleic acid, and that the essential pathogenic component is protein (or glycoprotein). Genetic evidence indicates that the protein is an abnormal form of PrP (perhaps identical with PrP^{Sc}). The association with other 'non-informational' molecules (such as lipids, glycosaminoglycans, or perhaps even short nucleic acids) is not excluded.

PrP^{C} The naturally occurring form of the mature *Prnp* gene product. Its presence in a given cell type is necessary, but not sufficient, for replication of the prion.

PrP^{Sc} An 'abnormal' form of the mature *Prnp* gene product found in tissue of TSE sufferers, defined as being partly resistant to digestion by proteinase K under standardized conditions. It is believed to differ from PrP^{C} only (or mainly) conformationally, and is often considered to be the transmissible agent or prion.

These definitions (Aguzzi and Weissmann 1997) describe our terminology which is, however, not agreed on by convention and is not necessarily used by others.

ACKNOWLEDGMENTS

I am indebted to Stanley B. Prusiner for allowing me to use an earlier version of this chapter as the basis for the first half of the present manuscript. This article is dedicated to the present and past members of my laboratory, whose enthusiastic commitment led to the work described here. Special thanks to Petra Schwarz for maintaining our prion-infected mouse colony in an impeccable shape, and to Susanne Tiefenthaler and Jacqueline Wiedler for excellent assistance. Christina Sigurdson provided crucial help with the chapter on CWD. The work of my laboratory is supported by the Canton of Zurich, the Faculty of Medicine at the University of Zurich, the Swiss Federal Offices of Education and Science, of Health, and of Animal Health, the Swiss National Foundation, the National Center for Competence in Research on neural plasticity and repair, the Migros foundation, the Coop Foundation, the U.K. Department for Environment, Food, & Rural Affairs, the US Department of Defense (National Prion Research Program), and the Stammbach Foundation. Individual members of the Aguzzi lab have been directly supported by the EMBO Fellowship Programme (Isabelle Arrighi), HFSP and Bonizzi-Theler Foundation (Frank Heppner, Mark Zabel), DFG (Michael Klein, Marco Prinz, Kirsten Mertz, Frank Baumann), the Koetser Foundation (Nicolas Genoud), the FAN Society for the Support of Young Academic Scientists (Mathias Heikenwälder, Christoph Huber), the SBF Foundation (Christoph Huber), the Catello family (Mathias Heikenwälder), the Federal Office of Health (Manuela

Maissen), the Center of Neuroscience Zurich and the UBS Bank (Magdalini Polymenidou), the Roche Foundation (Mark Zabel), the UK Biotechnology and Biological Sciences Research Council (Gino Miele), and the Career Development Awards of the University of Zurich (Markus Glatzel, Erich Brunner).

REFERENCES

Adachi, O., Kawai, T., et al. 1998. Targeted disruption of the MyD88 gene results in loss of IL-1- and IL-18-mediated function. *Immunity*, **9**, 143–50.

Aguzzi, A. 1996. Between cows and monkeys. *Nature*, **381**, 734.

Aguzzi, A. 1997. Neuro-immune connection in spread of prions in the body? *Lancet*, **349**, 742–3.

Aguzzi, A. 1998. Protein conformation dictates prion strain. *Nat Med*, **4**, 1125–6.

Aguzzi, A. 2000. Prion diseases, blood and the immune system: concerns and reality. *Haematologica*, **85**, 3–10.

Aguzzi, A. 2003. Prions and the immune system: a journey through gut, spleen, and nerves. *Adv Immunol*, **81**, 123–7.

Aguzzi, A. and Collinge, J. 1997. Post-exposure prophylaxis after accidental prion inoculation. *Lancet*, **350**, 1519–20.

Aguzzi, A. and Haass, C. 2003. Games played by rogue proteins in prion and Alzheimer's disease. *Science*, **302**, 814–18.

Aguzzi, A. and Hardt, W.D. 2003. Dangerous liaisons between a microbe and the prion protein. *J Exp Med*, **198**, 1–4.

Aguzzi, A. and Heikenwalder, M. 2003. Prion diseases: Cannibals and garbage piles. *Nature*, **423**, 127–9.

Aguzzi, A. and Heppner, F.L. 2000. Pathogenesis of prion diseases: a progress report. *Cell Death Differ*, **7**, 889–902.

Aguzzi, A. and Raeber, A.J. 1998. Transgenic models of neurodegeneration. Neurodegeneration: of (transgenic) mice and men. *Brain Pathol*, **8**, 695–7.

Aguzzi, A. and Weissmann, C. 1996. Spongiform encephalopathies: a suspicious signature. *Nature*, **383**, 666–7.

Aguzzi, A. and Weissmann, C. 1997. Prion research: the next frontiers. *Nature*, **389**, 795–8.

Aguzzi, A. and Weissmann, C. 1998. Spongiform encephalopathies. The prion's perplexing persistence. *Nature*, **392**, 763–4.

Aguzzi, A., Hegyi, I. et al. 2000a. Rapport des activitées 1996–1999. Hôpital universitaire de Zurich, Département de pathologie, Institut de neuropathologie. Centre nationale de référence pour les prionoses (NRPE).

Aguzzi, A., Klein, M.A., et al. 2000b. Prions: pathogenesis and reverse genetics. *Ann N Y Acad Sci*, **920**, 140–57.

Aguzzi, A., Brandner, S., et al. 2001a. Spongiform encephalopathies: insights from transgenic models. *Adv Virus Res*, **56**, 313–52.

Aguzzi, A., Glatzel, M., et al. 2001b. Interventional strategies against prion diseases. *Nat Rev Neurosci*, **2**, 745–9.

Aguzzi, A., Montrasio, F. and Kaeser, P.S. 2001c. Prions: health scare and biological challenge. *Nat Rev Mol Cell Biol*, **2**, 118–26.

Alper, T., Haig, D.A. and Clarke, M.C. 1966. The exceptionally small size of the scrapie agent. *Biochem Biophys Res Commun*, **22**, 278–84.

Alper, T., Cramp, W.A., et al. 1967. Does the agent of scrapie replicate without nucleic acid? *Nature*, **214**, 764–6.

Alper, T., Haig, D.A. and Clarke, M.C. 1978. The scrapie agent: evidence against its dependence for replication on intrinsic nucleic acid. *J Gen Virol*, **41**, 503–16.

Alpers, M. 1987. Epidemiology and clinical aspects of kuru. In: Prusiner, S.B. and McKinley, M.P. (eds), *Prions – novel infectious pathogens causing scrapie and Creutzfeldt–Jakob disease*. Orlando: Academic Press, 451–65.

Anderson, J.R., Allen, C.M.C. and Weller, R.O. 1990. Creutzfeldt–Jakob disease following human pituitary-derived growth hormone administration. *Br Neuropathol Soc Proc*, **16**, 543.

Anderson, R.G.W. 1993. Caveolae: where incoming and outgoing messengers meet. *Proc Natl Acad Sci U S A*, **90**, 10909–13.

Anderson, R.M., Donnelly, C.A., et al. 1996. Transmission dynamics and epidemiology of BSE in British cattle. *Nature*, **382**, 779–88.

Arbel, M., Lavie, V. and Solomon, B. 2003. Generation of antibodies against prion protein in wild-type mice via helix 1 peptide immunization. *J Neuroimmunol*, **144**, 38–45.

Arnold, J.E., Tipler, C., et al. 1995. The abnormal isoform of the prion protein accumulates in late-endosome-like organelles in scrapie-infected mouse brain. *J Pathol*, **176**, 403–11.

Asante, E.A., Linehan, J.M., et al. 2002. BSE prions propagate as either variant CJD-like or sporadic CJD-like prion strains in transgenic mice expressing human prion protein. *EMBO J*, **21**, 6358–66.

Aucouturier, P., Geissmann, F., et al. 2001. Infected splenic dendritic cells are sufficient for prion transmission to the CNS in mouse scrapie. *J Clin Invest*, **108**, 703–8.

Azzarelli, B., Muller, J., et al. 1985. Cerebellar plaques in familial Alzheimer's disease (Gerstmann–Straussler–Scheinker variant?). *Acta Neuropathol Berl*, **65**, 235–46.

Baker, H.F., Ridley, R.M., et al. 1993. Evidence for the experimental transmission of cerebral beta-amyloidosis to primates. *Int J Exp Pathol*, **74**, 441–54.

Baldauf, E., Beekes, M. and Diringer, H. 1997. Evidence for an alternative direct route of access for the scrapie agent to the brain bypassing the spinal cord. *J Gen Virol*, **78**, 1187–97.

Barry, R.A. and Prusiner, S.B. 1986. Monoclonal antibodies to the cellular and scrapie prion proteins. *J Infect Dis*, **154**, 518–21.

Bartz, J.C., Kincaid, A.E. and Bessen, R.A. 2003. Rapid prion neuroinvasion following tongue infection. *J Virol*, **77**, 583–91.

Basler, K., Oesch, B., et al. 1986. Scrapie and cellular PrP isoforms are encoded by the same chromosomal gene. *Cell*, **46**, 417–28.

Beck, E., Daniel, P.M. and Parry, H.B. 1964. Degeneration of the cerebellar and hypothalamo-neurohypophysial systems in sheep with scrapie; and its relationship to human system degenerations. *Brain*, **87**, 153–76.

Beekes, M., McBride, P.A. and Baldauf, E. 1998. Cerebral targeting indicates vagal spread of infection in hamsters fed with scrapie. *J Gen Virol*, **79**, 601–7.

Behrens, A. and Aguzzi, A. 2002. Small is not beautiful: antagonizing functions for the prion protein PrP^c and its homologue Dpl. *Trends Neurosci*, **25**, 150–4.

Behrens, A., Brandner, S., et al. 2001. Normal neurogenesis and scrapie pathogenesis in neural grafts lacking the prion protein homologue Doppel. *EMBO Rep*, **2**, 347–52.

Behrens, A., Genoud, N., et al. 2002. Absence of the prion protein homologue Doppel causes male sterility. *EMBO J*, **21**, 3652–8.

Bellon, A., Seyfert-Brandt, W., et al. 2003. Improved conformation-dependent immunoassay: suitability for human prion detection with enhanced sensitivity. *J Gen Virol*, **84**, 1921–5.

Bendheim, P.E., Barry, R.A., et al. 1984. Antibodies to a scrapie prion protein. *Nature*, **310**, 418–21.

Bendheim, P.E., Bockman, J.M., et al. 1985. Scrapie and Creutzfeldt–Jakob disease prion proteins share physical properties and antigenic determinants. *Proc Natl Acad Sci U S A*, **82**, 997–1001.

Berger, J.R. and David, N.J. 1993. Creutzfeldt–Jakob disease in a physician: a review of the disorder in health care workers. *Neurology*, **43**, 205–6.

Beringue, V., Demoy, M., et al. 2000. Role of spleen macrophages in the clearance of scrapie agent early in pathogenesis. *J Pathol*, **190**, 495–502.

Bernoulli, C., Siegfried, J., et al. 1977. Danger of accidental person-to-person transmission of Creutzfeldt–Jakob disease by surgery. *Lancet*, **1**, 478–9, [letter].

Bernoulli, C.C., Masters, C.L., et al. 1979. Early clinical features of Creutzfeldt–Jakob disease (subacute spongiform encephalopathy). In: Prusiner, S.B. and Hadlow, W.J. (eds), *Slow transmissible diseases of the nervous system*. New York: Academic Press, 229–51.

Bertoni, J.M., Brown, P., et al. 1992. Familial Creutzfeldt-Jakob disease (codon 200 mutation) with supranuclear palsy. *JAMA*, **268**, 2413–15.

Bessen, R.A. and Marsh, R.F. 1992. Biochemical and physical properties of the prion protein from two strains of the transmissible mink encephalopathy agent. *J Virol*, **66**, 2096–101.

Bessen, R.A. and Marsh, R.F. 1994. Distinct PrP properties suggest the molecular basis of strain variation in transmissible mink encephalopathy. *J Virol*, **68**, 7859–68.

Bessen, R.A., Kocisko, D.A., et al. 1995. Non-genetic propagation of strain-specific properties of scrapie prion protein. *Nature*, **375**, 698–700.

Betmouni, S. and Perry, V.H. 1999. The acute inflammatory response in CNS following injection of prion brain homogenate or normal brain homogenate. *Neuropathol Appl Neurobiol*, **25**, 20–8.

Betmouni, S., Perry, V.H. and Gordon, J.L. 1996. Evidence for an early inflammatory response in the central nervous system of mice with scrapie. *Neuroscience*, **74**, 1–5.

Billette de Villemeur, T.B., Beauvais, P., et al. 1991. Creutzfeldt–Jakob disease in children treated with growth hormone. *Lancet*, **337**, 864–5, [letter].

Blättler, T., Brandner, S., et al. 1997. PrP-expressing tissue required for transfer of scrapie infectivity from spleen to brain. *Nature*, **389**, 69–73.

Blum, B., Bakalara, N. and Simpson, L. 1990. A model for RNA editing in kinetoplastid mitochondria: 'guide' RNA molecules transcribed from maxicircle DNA provide the edited information. *Cell*, **60**, 189–98.

Bockman, J.M., Kingsbury, D.T., et al. 1985. Creutzfeldt–Jakob disease prion proteins in human brains. *N Engl J Med*, **312**, 73–8.

Bockman, J.M., Prusiner, S.B., et al. 1987. Immunoblotting of Creutzfeldt–Jakob disease prion proteins: host species-specific epitopes. *Ann Neurol*, **21**, 589–95.

Bofill, M., Akbar, A.N. and Amlot, P.L. 2000. Follicular dendritic cells share a membrane-bound protein with fibroblasts. *J Pathol*, **191**, 217–26.

Bolton, D.C., McKinley, M.P. and Prusiner, S.B. 1982. Identification of a protein that purifies with the scrapie prion. *Science*, **218**, 1309–11.

Bolton, D.C., Meyer, R.K. and Prusiner, S.B. 1985. Scrapie PrP 27-30 is a sialoglycoprotein. *J Virol*, **53**, 596–606.

Borchelt, D.R., Scott, M., et al. 1990. Scrapie and cellular prion proteins differ in their kinetics of synthesis and topology in cultured cells. *J Cell Biol*, **110**, 743–52.

Borchelt, D.R., Taraboulos, A. and Prusiner, S.B. 1992. Evidence for synthesis of scrapie prion proteins in the endocytic pathway. *J Biol Chem*, **267**, 16188–99.

Borchelt, D.R., Rogers, M., et al. 1993. Release of the cellular prion protein from cultured cells after loss of its glycoinositol phospholipid anchor. *Glycobiology*, **3**, 319–29.

Bosque, P.J. and Prusiner, S.B. 2000. Cultured cell sublines highly susceptible to prion infection. *J Virol*, **74**, 4377–86.

Bradley, R. 2000. Veterinary research at the Central Veterinary Laboratory, Weybridge, with special reference to scrapie and bovine spongiform encephalopathy. *Rev Sci Tech*, **19**, 819–30.

Brandner, S., Isenmann, S., et al. 1996a. Normal host prion protein necessary for scrapie-induced neurotoxicity. *Nature*, **379**, 339–43.

Brandner, S., Raeber, A., et al. 1996b. Normal host prion protein (PrPC) is required for scrapie spread within the central nervous system. *Proc Natl Acad Sci U S A*, **93**, 13148–51.

Brandner, S., Isenmann, S., et al. 1998. Identification of the end stage of scrapie using infected neural grafts. *Brain Pathol*, **8**, 19–27.

Brown, D.R., Qin, K., et al. 1997. The cellular prion protein binds copper in vivo. *Nature*, **390**, 684–7.

Brown, D.R., Wong, B.S., et al. 1999. Normal prion protein has an activity like that of superoxide dismutase. *Biochem J*, **344**, 1–5, [published erratum appears in *Biochem J* 2000; **345**, 767].

Brown, K.L., Stewart, K., et al. 1999. Scrapie replication in lymphoid tissues depends on prion protein-expressing follicular dendritic cells. *Nat Med*, **5**, 1308–12.

Brown, P. 1985. Virus sterility for human growth hormone. *Lancet*, **2**, 729–30, [letter].

Brown, P. 1992. The phenotypic expression of different mutations in transmissible human spongiform encephalopathy. *Rev Neurol Paris*, **148**, 317–27.

Brown, P. 1993. Infectious cerebral amyloidosis: clinical spectrum risks and remedies. In: Brown, F. (ed.), *Developments in biological standardization*. Basel: Karger, 91–101.

Brown, P., Cathala, F., et al. 1985a. Epidemiologic implications of Creutzfeldt–Jakob disease in a 19-year-old girl. *Eur J Epidemiol*, **1**, 42–7.

Brown, P., Gajdusek, D.C., et al. 1985b. Potential epidemic of Creutzfeldt–Jakob disease from human growth hormone therapy. *N Engl J Med*, **313**, 728–31.

Brown, P., Cathala, F., et al. 1986a. Creutzfeldt–Jakob disease: clinical analysis of a consecutive series of 230 neuropathologically verified cases. *Ann Neurol*, **20**, 597–602.

Brown, P., Coker Vann, M., et al. 1986b. Diagnosis of Creutzfeldt–Jakob disease by Western blot identification of marker protein in human brain tissue. *N Engl J Med*, **314**, 547–51.

Brown, P., Cathala, F., et al. 1987. The epidemiology of Creutzfeldt–Jakob disease: conclusion of a 15-year investigation in France and review of the world literature. *Neurology*, **37**, 895–904.

Brown, P., Goldfarb, L.G., et al. 1992a. Phenotypic characteristics of familial Creutzfeldt–Jakob disease associated with the codon 178Asn PRNP mutation. *Ann Neurol*, **31**, 282–5.

Brown, P., Goldfarb, L.G., et al. 1992b. Atypical Creutzfeldt–Jakob disease in an American family with an insert mutation in the PRNP amyloid precursor gene. *Neurology*, **42**, 422–7.

Brown, P., Preece, M.A. and Will, R.G. 1992c. 'Friendly fire' in medicine: hormones, homografts, and Creutzfeldt–Jakob disease. *Lancet*, **340**, 24–7.

Brown, P., Cervenakova, L., et al. 1994a. Iatrogenic Creutzfeldt–Jakob disease: an example of the interplay between ancient genes and modern medicine. *Neurology*, **44**, 291–3.

Brown, P., Gibbs, C.J. Jr, et al. 1994b. Human spongiform encephalopathy: the National Institutes of Health series of 300 cases of experimentally transmitted disease. *Ann Neurol*, **35**, 513–29.

Browning, J.L., Ngam-ek, A., et al. 1993. Lymphotoxin beta, a novel member of the TNF family that forms a heteromeric complex with lymphotoxin on the cell surface. *Cell*, **72**, 847–56.

Browning, J.L., Dougas, I., et al. 1995. Characterization of surface lymphotoxin forms. Use of specific monoclonal antibodies and soluble receptors. *J Immunol*, **154**, 33–46.

Bruce, M., Chree, A. et al. 1993. Transmissions of BSE, scrapie and related diseases to mice. *Proceedings of the IXth International Congress of Virology*, Glasgow, 93.

Bruce, M.E. 1985. Agent replication dynamics in a long incubation period model of mouse scrapie. *J Gen Virol*, **66**, 2517–22.

Bruce, M.E. and Dickinson, A.G. 1987. Biological evidence that scrapie agent has an independent genome. *J Gen Virol*, **68**, 79–89.

Bruce, M.E., McConnell, I., et al. 1991. The disease characteristics of different strains of scrapie in Sinc congenic mouse lines: implications for the nature of the agent and host control of pathogenesis. *J Gen Virol*, **72**, 595–603.

Bruce, M.E., Will, R.G., et al. 1997. Transmissions to mice indicate that 'new variant' CJD is caused by the BSE agent. *Nature*, **389**, 498–501.

Bruce, M.E., Boyle, A., et al. 2002. Strain characterization of natural sheep scrapie and comparison with BSE. *J Gen Virol*, **83**, 695–704.

Buchanan, C.R., Preece, M.A. and Milner, R.D. 1991. Mortality, neoplasia and Creutzfeldt–Jakob disease in patients treated with human pituitary growth hormone in the United Kingdom. *BMJ*, **302**, 824–8.

Budka, H., Aguzzi, A., et al. 1995. Neuropathological diagnostic criteria for Creutzfeldt–Jakob disease (CJD) and other human spongiform encephalopathies (prion diseases). *Brain Pathol*, **5**, 459–66.

Büeler, H.R., Fischer, M., et al. 1992. Normal development and behaviour of mice lacking the neuronal cell-surface PrP protein. *Nature*, **356**, 577–82.

Büeler, H.R., Aguzzi, A., et al. 1993. Mice devoid of PrP are resistant to scrapie. *Cell*, **73**, 1339–47.

Büeler, H., Raeber, A., et al. 1994. High prion and PrPSc levels but delayed onset of disease in scrapie-inoculated mice heterozygous for a disrupted PrP gene. *Mol Med*, **1**, 19–30.

Buyukmihci, N., Rorvik, M. and Marsh, R.F. 1980. Replication of the scrapie agent in ocular neural tissues. *Proc Natl Acad Sci U S A*, **77**, 1169–71.

Carlson, G.A., Kingsbury, D.T., et al. 1986. Linkage of prion protein and scrapie incubation time genes. *Cell*, **46**, 503–11.

Carlson, G.A., Westaway, D., et al. 1989. Primary structure of prion protein may modify scrapie isolate properties. *Proc Natl Acad Sci U S A*, **86**, 7475–9.

Carp, R.I. 1982. Transmission of scrapie by oral route: effect of gingival scarification. *Lancet*, **1**, 170–1, [letter].

Carroll, M.C. 1998. CD21/CD35 in B cell activation. *Semin Immunol*, **10**, 279–86.

Cashman, N.R., Loertscher, R., et al. 1990. Cellular isoform of the scrapie agent protein participates in lymphocyte activation. *Cell*, **61**, 185–92.

Caughey, B. and Race, R.E. 1992. Potent inhibition of scrapie-associated PrP accumulation by congo red. *J Neurochem*, **59**, 768–71.

Caughey, B. and Raymond, G.J. 1991. The scrapie-associated form of PrP is made from a cell surface precursor that is both protease- and phospholipase-sensitive. *J Biol Chem*, **266**, 18217–23.

Caughey, B. and Raymond, G.J. 1993. Sulfated polyanion inhibition of scrapie-associated PrP accumulation in cultured cells. *J Virol*, **67**, 643–50.

Caughey, B.W., Dong, A., et al. 1991a. Secondary structure analysis of the scrapie-associated protein PrP 27-30 in water by infrared spectroscopy. *Biochemistry*, **30**, 7672–80, [published erratum appears in *Biochemistry* 1991; **30**, 10600].

Caughey, B., Raymond, G.J., et al. 1991b. N-terminal truncation of the scrapie-associated form of PrP by lysosomal protease(s): implications regarding the site of conversion of PrP to the protease-resistant state. *J Virol*, **65**, 6597–603.

Chandler, R.L. 1961. Encephalopathy in mice produced by inoculation with scrapie brain material. *Lancet*, **1**, 1378–9.

Chandler, R.L. 1963. Experimental scrapie in the mouse. *Res Vet Sci*, **4**, 276–85.

Chapman, J., Ben Israel, J., et al. 1994. The risk of developing Creutzfeldt–Jakob disease in subjects with the PRNP gene codon 200 point mutation. *Neurology*, **44**, 1683–6.

Chazot, G., Broussolle, E., et al. 1996. New variant of Creutzfeldt–Jakob disease in a 26-year-old French man. *Lancet*, **347**, 1181, [letter].

Chernoff, Y.O., Derkach, I.L. and Inge-Vechtomov, S.G. 1993. Multicopy SUP35 gene induces de-novo appearance of psi-like factors in the yeast *Saccharomyces cerevisiae*. *Curr Genet*, **24**, 268–70.

Chernoff, Y.O., Lindquist, S.L., et al. 1995. Role of the chaperone protein Hsp104 in propagation of the yeast prion-like factor [psi+]. *Science*, **268**, 880–4.

Chesebro, B. 1998. BSE and prions: uncertainties about the agent. *Science*, **279**, 42–3.

Chesebro, B., Race, R., et al. 1985. Identification of scrapie prion protein-specific mRNA in scrapie-infected and uninfected brain. *Nature*, **315**, 331–3.

Clarke, M.C. and Kimberlin, R.H. 1984. Pathogenesis of mouse scrapie: distribution of agent in the pulp and stroma of infected spleens. *Vet Microbiol*, **9**, 215–25.

Clouscard, C., Beaudry, P., et al. 1995. Different allelic effects of the codons 136 and 171 of the prion protein gene in sheep with natural scrapie. *J Gen Virol*, **76**, 2097–101.

Cochius, J.I., Burns, R.J., et al. 1990. Creutzfeldt–Jakob disease in a recipient of human pituitary-derived gonadotrophin. *Aust N Z J Med*, **20**, 592–3.

Cochius, J.I., Hyman, N. and Esiri, M.M. 1992. Creutzfeldt–Jakob disease in a recipient of human pituitary-derived gonadotrophin: a second case. *J Neurol Neurosurg Psychiatry*, **55**, 1094–5.

Cohen, A.S., Shirahama, T. and Skinner, M. 1982. Electron microscopy of amyloid. In: Harris, J.R. (ed.), *Electron microscopy of proteins*. New York: Academic Press, 165–206.

Cohen, F.E., Pan, K.M., et al. 1994. Structural clues to prion replication. *Science*, **264**, 530–1.

Cole, S. and Kimberlin, R.H. 1985. Pathogenesis of mouse scrapie: dynamics of vacuolation in brain and spinal cord after intraperitoneal infection. *Neuropathol Appl Neurobiol*, **11**, 213–27.

Collinge, J. and Palmer, M.S. 1994. Human prion diseases. *Baillières Clin Neurol*, **3**, 241–7.

Collinge, J., Owen, F., et al. 1990. Prion dementia without characteristic pathology. *Lancet*, **336**, 7–9.

Collinge, J., Palmer, M.S. and Dryden, A.J. 1991. Genetic predisposition to iatrogenic Creutzfeldt–Jakob disease. *Lancet*, **337**, 1441–2.

Collinge, J., Brown, J., et al. 1992. Inherited prion disease with 144 base pair gene insertion. 2. Clinical and pathological features. *Brain*, **115**, 687–710.

Collinge, J., Whittington, M.A., et al. 1994. Prion protein is necessary for normal synaptic function. *Nature*, **370**, 295–7.

Collinge, J., Sidle, K.C., et al. 1996. Molecular analysis of prion strain variation and the aetiology of 'new variant' CJD. *Nature*, **383**, 685–90.

Collins, S., Law, M.G., et al. 1999. Surgical treatment and risk of sporadic Creutzfeldt-Jakob disease: a case-control study. *Lancet*, **353**, 693–7.

Collins, S.J., Lewis, V., et al. 2002. Quinacrine does not prolong survival in a murine Creutzfeldt–Jakob disease model. *Ann Neurol*, **52**, 503–6.

Coschigano, P.W. and Magasanik, B. 1991. The *URE2* gene product of *Saccharomyces cerevisiae* plays an important role in the cellular response to the nitrogen source and has homology to glutathione *S*-transferases. *Mol Cell Biol*, **11**, 822–32.

Cousens, S.N., Harries Jones, R., et al. 1990. Geographical distribution of cases of Creutzfeldt–Jakob disease in England and Wales 1970–84. *J Neurol Neurosurg Psychiatry*, **53**, 459–65.

Cox, B.S., Tuite, M.F. and McLaughlin, C.S. 1988. The psi factor of yeast: a problem in inheritance. *Yeast*, **4**, 159–78.

Crow, T. J., Collinge, J. et al. 1990. Mutations in the prion gene in human transmissible dementia. *Seminar on Molecular Approaches to Research in Spongoform Encephalopathies in Man*, Medical Research Council, London.

Crowe, P.D., VanArsdale, T.L., et al. 1994. A lymphotoxin-beta-specific receptor. *Science*, **264**, 707–10.

Croxson, M., Brown, P., et al. 1988. A new case of Creutzfeldt–Jakob disease associated with human growth hormone therapy in New Zealand. *Neurology*, **38**, 1128–30.

Cuille, J. and Chelle, P.L. 1939. Experimental transmission of trembling to the goat. *C R Seances Acad Sci*, **208**, 1058–160.

Cunningham, A.A., Wells, G.A., et al. 1993. Transmissible spongiform encephalopathy in greater kudu (*Tragelaphus strepsiceros*). *Vet Rec*, **132**, 68.

Davanipour, Z., Goodman, L., et al. 1984. Possible modes of transmission of Creutzfeldt–Jakob disease. *N Engl J Med*, **311**, 1582–3, [letter].

Davison, C. and Rabiner, A.M. 1940. Spastic pseudosclerosis (disseminated encephalomyelopathy; corticopallidospinal degeneration). Familial and nonfamilial incidence (a clinico-pathologic study). *Arch Neurol Psychiatry*, **44**, 578–98.

Dawson, M., Wells, G.A. and Parker, B.N. 1990a. Preliminary evidence of the experimental transmissibility of bovine spongiform encephalopathy to cattle. *Vet Rec*, **126**, 112–13.

Dawson, M., Wells, G.A., et al. 1990b. Primary parenteral transmission of bovine spongiform encephalopathy to the pig. *Vet Rec*, **127**, 338, [letter].

Dealler, S.F. and Lacey, R.W. 1990. Transmissible sponigform encephalopathies: the threat of BSE to man. *Food Microbiol*, **7**, 253–79.

DeArmond, S.J., McKinley, M.P., et al. 1985. Identification of prion amyloid filaments in scrapie-infected brain. *Cell*, **41**, 221–35.

Deleu, C., Clave, C. and Begueret, J. 1993. A single amino acid difference is sufficient to elicit vegetative incompatibility in the fungus *Podospora anserina*. *Genetics*, **135**, 45–52.

Deslys, J.P., Marce, D. and Dormont, D. 1994. Similar genetic susceptibility in iatrogenic and sporadic Creutzfeldt–Jakob disease. *J Gen Virol*, **75**, 23–7.

Dickinson, A.G. and Fraser, H. 1979. An assessment of the genetics of scrapie in sheep and mice. In: Prusiner, S.B. and Hadlow, W.J. (eds), *Slow transmissible diseases of the nervous system*. New York: Academic Press, 367–86.

Dickinson, A.G. and Meikle, V.M. 1969. A comparison of some biological characteristics of the mouse-passaged scrapie agents, 22A and ME7. *Genet Res*, **13**, 213–25.

Dickinson, A.G. and Meikle, V.M. 1971. Host-genotype and agent effects in scrapie incubation: change in allelic interaction with different strains of agent. *Mol Gen Genet*, **112**, 73–9.

Dickinson, A.G. and Outram, G.W. 1988. Genetic aspects of unconventional virus infections: the basis of the virino hypothesis. *Ciba Found Symp*, **135**, 63–83.

Dickinson, A.G. and Stamp, J.T. 1969. Experimental scrapie in Cheviot and Suffolk sheep. *J Comp Pathol*, **79**, 23–6.

Dickinson, A.G., Young, G.B., et al. 1965. An analysis of natural scrapie in Suffolk sheep. *Heredity Edinburgh*, **20**, 485–503.

Dickinson, A.G., Meikle, V.M. and Fraser, H. 1968. Identification of a gene which controls the incubation period of some strains of scrapie agent in mice. *J Comp Pathol*, **78**, 293–9.

Dickinson, A.G., Bruce, M.E. et al. 1984. Scrapie strain differences: the implications of stability and mutation. *Proceedings of Workshop on Slow Transmissible Diseases*, Japanese Ministry of Health and Welfare, Tokyo, 105–18.

Dlouhy, S.R., Hsiao, K., et al. 1992. Linkage of the Indiana kindred of Gerstmann–Straussler–Scheinker disease to the prion protein gene. *Nat Genet*, **1**, 64–7.

Doh-ura, K., Tateishi, J., et al. 1989. Pro-leu change at position 102 of prion protein is the most common but not the sole mutation related to Gerstmann–Straussler syndrome. *Biochem Biophys Res Commun*, **163**, 974–9.

Doh-ura, K., Kitamoto, T., et al. 1991. CJD discrepancy. *Nature*, **353**, 801–2.

Drisaldi, B., Stewart, R.S., et al. 2003. Mutant PrP is delayed in its exit from the endoplasmic reticulum, but neither wild-type nor mutant PrP undergoes retrotranslocation prior to proteasomal degradation. *J Biol Chem*, **278**, 21732–43.

Duffy, P., Wolf, J., et al. 1974. Possible person-to-person transmission of Creutzfeldt–Jakob disease. *N Engl J Med*, **290**, 692–3.

Eklund, C.M., Hadlow, W.J. and Kennedy, R.C. 1963. Some properties of the scrapie agent and its behavior in mice. *Proc Soc Exp Biol Med*, **112**, 974–9.

Eklund, C.M., Kennedy, R.C. and Hadlow, W.J. 1967. Pathogenesis of scrapie virus infection in the mouse. *J Infect Dis*, **117**, 15–22.

Ellis, C.J., Katifi, H. and Weller, R.O. 1992. A further British case of growth hormone induced Creutzfeldt–Jakob disease. *J Neurol Neurosurg Psychiatry*, **55**, 1200–2.

Enari, M., Flechsig, E. and Weissmann, C. 2001. Scrapie prion protein accumulation by scrapie-infected neuroblastoma cells abrogated by exposure to a prion protein antibody. *Proc Natl Acad Sci USA*, **98**, 9295–9.

Endo, T., Groth, D., et al. 1989. Diversity of oligosaccharide structures linked to asparagines of the scrapie prion protein. *Biochemistry*, **28**, 8380–8.

Endres, R., Alimzhanov, M.B., et al. 1999. Mature follicular dendritic cell networks depend on expression of lymphotoxin beta receptor by radioresistant stromal cells and of lymphotoxin beta and tumor necrosis factor by B cells. *J Exp Med*, **189**, 159–68.

Farlow, M.R., Yee, R.D., et al. 1989. Gerstmann–Straussler–Scheinker disease. I. Extending the clinical spectrum. *Neurology*, **39**, 1446–52.

Farquhar, C., Dickinson, A. and Bruce, M. 1999. Prophylactic potential of pentosan polysulphate in transmissible spongiform encephalopathies. *Lancet*, **353**, 117, [letter].

Farquhar, C.F., Dornan, J., et al. 1994. Effect of Sinc genotype, agent isolate and route of infection on the accumulation of protease-resistant PrP in non-central nervous system tissues during the development of murine scrapie. *J Gen Virol*, **75**, 495–504.

Felten, D.L. and Felten, S.Y. 1988. Sympathetic noradrenergic innervation of immune organs. *Brain Behav Immun*, **2**, 293–300.

Fink, J.K., Warren, J.T. Jr, et al. 1991. Allele-specific sequencing confirms novel prion gene polymorphism in Creutzfeldt–Jakob disease. *Neurology*, **41**, 1647–50.

Fischer, M., Rülicke, T., et al. 1996. Prion protein (PrP) with amino-proximal deletions restoring susceptibility of PrP knockout mice to scrapie. *EMBO J*, **15**, 1255–64.

Fischer, M.B., Goerg, S., et al. 1998. Dependence of germinal center B cells on expression of CD21/CD35 for survival. *Science*, **280**, 582–5.

Fischer, M.B., Roeckl, C., et al. 2000. Binding of disease-associated prion protein to plasminogen. *Nature*, **408**, 479–83.

Flechsig, E., Shmerling, D., et al. 2000. Prion protein devoid of the octapeptide repeat region restores susceptibility to scrapie in PrP knockout mice. *Neuron*, **27**, 399–408.

Fournier, J.G., Escaig Haye, F., et al. 1995. Ultrastructural localization of cellular prion protein (PrPc) in synaptic boutons of normal hamster hippocampus. *C R Acad Sci III*, **318**, 339–44.

Fradkin, J.E., Schonberger, L.B., et al. 1991. Creutzfeldt–Jakob disease in pituitary growth hormone recipients in the United States. *JAMA*, **265**, 880–4.

Fraser, H. 1982. Neuronal spread of scrapie agent and targeting of lesions within the retino-tectal pathway. *Nature*, **295**, 149–50.

Fraser, H. and Dickinson, A.G. 1967. Distribution of experimentally induced scrapie lesions in the brain. *Nature*, **216**, 1310–11.

Fraser, H., McConnell, I., et al. 1988. Transmission of bovine spongiform encephalopathy to mice. *Vet Rec*, **123**, 472.

Friede, R.L. and DeJong, R.N. 1964. Neuronal enzymatic failure in Creutzfeldt–Jakob disease. A familial study. *Arch Neurol*, **10**, 181–95.

Frigg, R., Klein, M.A., et al. 1999. Scrapie pathogenesis in subclinically infected B-cell-deficient mice. *J Virol*, **73**, 9584–8.

Fu, Y.X., Huang, G., et al. 1997. Independent signals regulate development of primary and secondary follicle structure in spleen and mesenteric lymph node. *Proc Natl Acad Sci U S A*, **94**, 5739–43.

Gabizon, R., McKinley, M.P. and Prusiner, S.B. 1987. Purified prion proteins and scrapie infectivity copartition into liposomes. *Proc Natl Acad Sci U S A*, **84**, 4017–21.

Gabizon, R., McKinley, M.P., et al. 1988. Immunoaffinity purification and neutralization of scrapie prion infectivity. *Proc Natl Acad Sci U S A*, **85**, 6617–21.

Gabriel, J.M., Oesch, B., et al. 1992. Molecular cloning of a candidate chicken prion protein. *Proc Natl Acad Sci U S A*, **89**, 9097–101.

Gajdusek, D.C. 1977. Unconventional viruses and the origin and disappearance of kuru. *Science*, **197**, 943–60.

Gajdusek, D.C. and Zigas, V. 1957. Degenerative disease of the central nervous system in New Guinea – the endemic occurrence of 'kuru' in the native population. *N Engl J Med*, **257**, 974–8.

Gajdusek, D. and Zigas, V. 1959. Clinical, pathological and epidemiological study of an acute progressive degenerative disease of the central nervous system among natives of the eastern highlands of New Guinea. *Am J Med*, **26**, 442–69.

Gajdusek, D.C., Gibbs, C.J. and Alpers, M. 1966. Experimental transmission of a Kuru-like syndrome to chimpanzees. *Nature*, **209**, 794–6.

Gard, S. 1940. Encephalomyelitis of mice. II. A method for the measurement of virus activity. *J Exp Med*, **72**, 69–77.

Gasset, M., Baldwin, M.A., et al. 1993. Perturbation of the secondary structure of the scrapie prion protein under conditions that alter infectivity. *Proc Natl Acad Sci U S A*, **90**, 1–5.

Gerstmann, J., Sträussler, E. and Scheinker, I. 1936. Über eine eigenartige hereditär-familiäre Erkrankung des Zentralnervensystems. Zugleich ein Beitrag zur Frage des vorzeitigen lokalen Alterns. *Z Neurol*, **154**, 736–62.

Ghani, A.C., Ferguson, N.M., et al. 1998. Estimation of the number of people incubating variant CJD. *Lancet*, **352**, 1353–4, [letter].

Ghani, A.C., Donnelly, C.A., et al. 2000. Assessment of the prevalence of vCJD through testing tonsils and appendices for abnormal prion protein. *Proc R Soc Lond B Biol Sci*, **267**, 23–9.

Ghetti, B., Tagliavini, F., et al. 1989. Gerstmann–Straussler–Scheinker disease. II. Neurofibrillary tangles and plaques with PrP-amyloid coexist in an affected family. *Neurology*, **39**, 1453–61.

Giaccone, G., Tagliavini, F., et al. 1990. Neurofibrillary tangles of the Indiana kindred of Gerstmann–Straussler–Scheinker disease share antigenic determinants with those of Alzheimer disease. *Brain Res*, **530**, 325–9.

Gibbons, R.A. and Hunter, G.D. 1967. Nature of the scrapie agent. *Nature*, **215**, 1041–3.

Gibbs, C.J. Jr, Gajdusek, D.C., et al. 1968. Creutzfeldt–Jakob disease (spongiform encephalopathy): transmission to the chimpanzee. *Science*, **161**, 388–9.

Gibbs, C.J. Jr, Gajdusek, D.C. and Alpers, M.P. 1969. Attempts to transmit subacute and chronic neurological diseases to animals. *Int Arch Allergy Appl Immunol*, **36**, Suppl, 519–52.

Gibbs, C.J. Jr, Amyx, H.L., et al. 1980. Oral transmission of kuru, Creutzfeldt–Jakob disease, and scrapie to nonhuman primates. *J Infect Dis*, **142**, 205–8.

Gibbs, C.J. Jr, Joy, A., et al. 1985. Clinical and pathological features and laboratory confirmation of Creutzfeldt–Jakob disease in a recipient of pituitary-derived human growth hormone. *N Engl J Med*, **313**, 734–8.

Gibbs, C.J. Jr, Asher, D.M., et al. 1993. Creutzfeldt–Jakob disease infectivity of growth hormone derived from human pituitary glands. *N Engl J Med*, **328**, 358–9.

Gibbs, C.J. Jr, Asher, D.M., et al. 1994. Transmission of Creutzfeldt–Jakob disease to a chimpanzee by electrodes contaminated during neurosurgery. *J Neurol Neurosurg Psychiatry*, **57**, 757–8.

Glatzel, M. and Aguzzi, A. 2000. PrP(C) expression in the peripheral nervous system is a determinant of prion neuroinvasion. *J Gen Virol*, **81**, 2813–21.

Glatzel, M. and Aguzzi, A. 2001. The shifting biology of prions. *Brain Res Brain Res Rev*, **36**, 241–8.

Glatzel, M., Flechsig, E., et al. 2000. Adenoviral and adeno-associated viral transfer of genes to the peripheral nervous system. *Proc Natl Acad Sci U S A*, **97**, 442–7.

Glatzel, M., Heppner, F.L., et al. 2001. Sympathetic innervation of lymphoreticular organs is rate limiting for prion neuroinvasion. *Neuron*, **31**, 25–34.

Glatzel, M., Rogivue, C., et al. 2002. Incidence of Creutzfeldt–Jakob disease in Switzerland. *Lancet*, **360**, 139–41.

Glatzel, M., Abela, E., et al. 2003a. Extraneural pathological prion protein in sporadic Creutzfeldt–Jakob disease. *N Engl J Med*, **349**, 1812–20.

Glatzel, M., Ott, P.M., et al. 2003b. Human prion diseases: epidemiology and integrated risk assessment. *Lancet Neurol*, **2**, 757–63.

Glockshuber, R., Hornemann, S., et al. 1998. Prion protein structural features indicate possible relations to signal peptidases. *FEBS Lett*, **426**, 291–6, [published erratum appears in *FEBS Lett* 1998; **431**, 130].

Goldfarb, L.G., Brown, P., et al. 1990a. Creutzfeldt–Jakob disease and kuru patients lack a mutation consistently found in the Gerstmann–Straussler–Scheinker syndrome. *Exp Neurol*, **108**, 247–50.

Goldfarb, L.G., Korczyn, A.D., et al. 1990b. Mutation in codon 200 of scrapie amyloid precursor gene linked to Creutzfeldt–Jakob disease in Sephardic Jews of Libyan and non-Libyan origin. *Lancet*, **336**, 637–8, [letter].

Goldfarb, L.G., Mitrova, E., et al. 1990c. Mutation in codon 200 of scrapie amyloid protein gene in two clusters of Creutzfeldt–Jakob disease in Slovakia. *Lancet*, **336**, 514–15, [letter].

Goldfarb, L.G., Brown, P., et al. 1991a. Transmissible familial Creutzfeldt–Jakob disease associated with five, seven, and eight extra octapeptide coding repeats in the *PRNP* gene. *Proc Natl Acad Sci U S A*, **88**, 10926–30.

Goldfarb, L.G., Brown, P., et al. 1991b. Creutzfeldt–Jacob disease associated with the PRNP codon 200[Lys] mutation: an analysis of 45 families. *Eur J Epidemiol*, **7**, 477–86.

Goldfarb, L.G., Haltia, M., et al. 1991c. New mutation in scrapie amyloid precursor gene (at codon 178) in Finnish Creutzfeldt–Jakob kindred. *Lancet*, **337**, 425, [letter].

Goldfarb, L.G., Brown, P., et al. 1992a. Creutzfeldt–Jakob disease cosegregates with the codon 178[Asn] *PRNP* mutation in families of European origin. *Ann Neurol*, **31**, 274–81.

Goldfarb, L.G., Petersen, R.B., et al. 1992b. Fatal familial insomnia and familial Creutzfeldt–Jakob disease: disease phenotype determined by a DNA polymorphism. *Science*, **258**, 806–8.

Goldgaber, D., Goldfarb, L.G., et al. 1989. Mutations in familial Creutzfeldt–Jakob disease and Gerstmann–Straussler–Scheinker's syndrome. *Exp Neurol*, **106**, 204–6.

Goldhammer, Y., Gabizon, R., et al. 1993. An Israeli family with Gerstmann–Straussler–Scheinker disease manifesting the codon 102 mutation in the prion protein gene. *Neurology*, **43**, 2718–19.

Goldmann, W. and Hunter, N. 1988. The PrP gene in natural scrapie. *Alzheimer Dis Assoc Disord (Abstr suppl)*, **2**, 330.

Goldmann, W., Hunter, N., et al. 1990a. The PrP gene of the sheep, a natural host of scrapie. *VIIIth International Congress of Virology*, Berlin, 284 [Abstr].

Goldmann, W., Hunter, N., et al. 1990b. Two alleles of a neural protein gene linked to scrapie in sheep. *Proc Natl Acad Sci U S A*, **87**, 2476–80.

Goldmann, W., Hunter, N., et al. 1991a. Different scrapie-associated fibril proteins (PrP) are encoded by lines of sheep selected for different alleles of the *Sip* gene. *J Gen Virol*, **72**, 2411–17.

Goldmann, W., Hunter, N., et al. 1991b. Different forms of the bovine PrP gene have five or six copies of a short, G-C-rich element within the protein-coding exon. *J Gen Virol*, **72**, 201–4.

Gonzalez, M., Mackay, F., et al. 1998. The sequential role of lymphotoxin and B cells in the development of splenic follicles. *J Exp Med*, **187**, 997–1007.

Gordon, W.S. 1946. Advances in veterinary research. *Vet Res*, **58**, 516–20.

Gordon, W.S. 1966. Variation in susceptibility of sheep to scrapie and genetic implications. *Report of Scrapie Seminar*, US Department of Agriculture, Washington, DC, 53–67.

Gorodinsky, A. and Harris, D.A. 1995. Glycolipid-anchored proteins in neuroblastoma cells form detergent-resistant complexes without caveolin. *J Cell Biol*, **129**, 619–27.

Griffith, J.S. 1967. Self-replication and scrapie. *Nature*, **215**, 1043–4.

Hadlow, W.J., Kennedy, R.C., et al. 1980. Virologic and neurohistologic findings in dairy goats affected with natural scrapie. *Vet Pathol*, **17**, 187–99.

Hadlow, W.J., Kennedy, R.C. and Race, R.E. 1982. Natural infection of Suffolk sheep with scrapie virus. *J Infect Dis*, **146**, 657–64.

Hainfellner, J.A. and Budka, H. 1999. Disease associated prion protein may deposit in the peripheral nervous system in human transmissible spongiform encephalopathies. *Acta Neuropathol (Berl)*, **98**, 458–60.

Haltia, M., Kovanen, J., et al. 1991. Familial Creutzfeldt–Jakob disease in Finland: epidemiological, clinical, pathological and molecular genetic studies. *Eur J Epidemiol*, **7**, 494–500.

Hamir, A.N., Cutlip, R.C., et al. 2001. Preliminary findings on the experimental transmission of chronic wasting disease agent of mule deer to cattle. *J Vet Diagn Invest*, **13**, 91–6.

Haraguchi, T., Fisher, S., et al. 1989. Asparagine-linked glycosylation of the scrapie and cellular prion proteins. *Arch Biochem Biophys*, **274**, 1–13.

Hardy, J. 1991. Prion dimers: a deadly duo? *Trends Neurosci*, **14**, 423–4.

Harmey, J.H., Doyle, D., et al. 1995. The cellular isoform of the prion protein, PrPc, is associated with caveolae in mouse neuroblastoma (N2a) cells. *Biochem Biophys Res Commun*, **210**, 753–9.

Harries Jones, R., Knight, R., et al. 1988. Creutzfeldt–Jakob disease in England and Wales, 1980-1984: a case-control study of potential risk factors. *J Neurol Neurosurg Psychiatry*, **51**, 1113–19.

Hazenbos, W.L., Gessner, J.E., et al. 1996. Impaired IgG-dependent anaphylaxis and Arthus reaction in Fc gamma RIII (CD16) deficient mice. *Immunity*, **5**, 181–8.

Healy, D.L. and Evans, J. 1993. Creutzfeldt–Jakob disease after pituitary gonadotrophins. *BMJ*, **307**, 517–18, [editorial].

Hegde, R.S., Mastrianni, J.A., et al. 1998. A transmembrane form of the prion protein in neurodegenerative disease. *Science*, **279**, 827–34.

Hegde, R.S., Tremblay, P., et al. 1999. Transmissible and genetic prion diseases share a common pathway of neurodegeneration. *Nature*, **402**, 822–6.

Heikenwälder, M., Polymenidou, M., et al. 2004. Lymphoid follicle destruction and immunosuppression after repeated CPG oligodeoxynucleotide administration. *Nature Medicine*, **10**, 187–92.

Heppner, F.L., Christ, A.D., et al. 2001a. Transepithelial prion transport by M cells. *Nat Med*, **7**, 976–7.

Heppner, F.L., Musahl, C., et al. 2001b. Prevention of scrapie pathogenesis by transgenic expression of anti-prion protein antibodies. *Science*, **294**, 178–82.

Herzberg, L., Herzberg, B.N., et al. 1974. Letter: Creutzfeldt–Jakob disease: hypothesis for high incidence in Libyan Jews in Israel. *Science*, **186**, 848.

Heston, L.L., Lowther, D.L. and Leventhal, C.M. 1966. Alzheimer's disease. A family study. *Arch Neurol*, **15**, 225–33.

Hill, A.F., Desbruslais, M., et al. 1997a. The same prion strain causes vCJD and BSE. *Nature*, **389**, 448–50, [letter].

Hill, A.F., Zeidler, M., et al. 1997b. Diagnosis of new variant Creutzfeldt–Jakob disease by tonsil biopsy. *Lancet*, **349**, 99.

Hill, A.F., Butterworth, R.J., et al. 1999. Investigation of variant Creutzfeldt–Jakob disease and other human prion diseases with tonsil biopsy samples. *Lancet*, **353**, 183–9.

Hill, A.F., Joiner, S., et al. 2000. Species-barrier-independent prion replication in apparently resistant species. *Proc Natl Acad Sci U S A*, **29**, 10248–53.

Hilton, D.A., Fathers, E., et al. 1998. Prion immunoreactivity in appendix before clinical onset of variant Creutzfeldt–Jakob disease. *Lancet*, **352**, 703–4, [letter].

Hope, J., Reekie, L.J., et al. 1988. Fibrils from brains of cows with new cattle disease contain scrapie-associated protein. *Nature*, **336**, 390–2.

Horiuchi, M. and Caughey, B. 1999. Specific binding of normal prion protein to the scrapie form via a localized domain initiates its conversion to the protease-resistant state. *EMBO J*, **18**, 3193–203.

Hornemann, S., Korth, C., et al. 1997. Recombinant full-length murine prion protein, mPrP(23-231): purification and spectroscopic characterization. *FEBS Lett*, **413**, 277–81.

Hsiao, K. and Prusiner, S.B. 1990. Inherited human prion diseases. *Neurology*, **40**, 1820–7.

Hsiao, K., Baker, H.F., et al. 1989. Linkage of a prion protein missense variant to Gerstmann–Straussler syndrome. *Nature*, **338**, 342–5.

Hsiao, K.K., Scott, M., et al. 1990. Spontaneous neurodegeneration in transgenic mice with mutant prion protein. *Science*, **250**, 1587–90.

Hsiao, K., Meiner, Z., et al. 1991a. Mutation of the prion protein in Libyan Jews with Creutzfeldt–Jakob disease. *N Engl J Med*, **324**, 1091–7.

Hsiao, K.K., Cass, C., et al. 1991b. A prion protein variant in a family with the telencephalic form of Gerstmann–Straussler–Scheinker syndrome. *Neurology*, **41**, 681–4.

Hsiao, K., Dlouhy, S.R., et al. 1992. Mutant prion proteins in Gerstmann–Straussler–Scheinker disease with neurofibrillary tangles. *Nat Genet*, **1**, 68–71.

Hsiao, K.K., Groth, D., et al. 1994. Serial transmission in rodents of neurodegeneration from transgenic mice expressing mutant prion protein. *Proc Natl Acad Sci U S A*, **91**, 9126–30.

Hsich, G., Kinney, K., et al. 1996. The 14-3-3 brain protein in cerebrospinal fluid as a marker for transmissible spongiform encephalopathies. *N Engl J Med*, **335**, 924–30.

http://www.doh.gov.uk/cjd/stats/aug02.htm (2002). Monthly Creutzfeldt–Jakob disease statistics. (Department of Health).

Huang, F.P., Farquhar, C.F., et al. 2002. Migrating intestinal dendritic cells transport PrP(Sc) from the gut. *J Gen Virol*, **83**, 267–71.

Hunter, G.D. and Millson, G.C. 1964. Studies on the heat stability and chromatographic behaviour of the scrapie agent. *J Gen Microbiol*, **37**, 251–8.

Hunter, N., Foster, J.D., et al. 1989. Linkage of the gene for the scrapie-associated fibril protein (PrP) to the *Sip* gene in Cheviot sheep. *Vet Rec*, **124**, 364–6.

Hunter, N., Foster, J.D., et al. 1991. Restriction fragment length polymorphisms of the scrapie-associated fibril protein (PrP) gene and their association with susceptibility to natural scrapie in British sheep. *J Gen Virol*, **72**, 1287–92.

Hutter, G., Heppner, F.L. and Aguzzi, A. 2003. No superoxide dismutase activity of cellular prion protein in vivo. *Biol Chem*, **384**, 1279–85.

Ikeda, S., Yanagisawa, N., et al. 1991. A variant of Gerstmann–Sträussler–Scheinker disease with β-protein epitopes and dystrophic neurites in the peripheral regions of PrP-immunoreactive amyloid plaques. In: Natvig, J.B., Forre, O., et al. (eds), *Amyloid and amyloidosis 1990*. Dordrecht: Kluwer Academic, 737–40.

Jackson, G.S., Beck, J.A., et al. 2001. HLA-DQ7 antigen and resistance to variant CJD. *Nature*, **414**, 269–70.

Jacob, H., Pyrkosch, W. and Strube, H. 1950. Die erbliche Form der Creutzfeldt-Jakobschen Krankheit. *Arch Psychiatr Zeitschr Neurol*, **184**, 653–74.

Jarrett, J.T. and Lansbury, P.T. Jr 1993. Seeding 'one-dimensional crystallization' of amyloid: a pathogenic mechanism in Alzheimer's disease and scrapie? *Cell*, **73**, 1055–8.

Jeffrey, M., Goodsir, C.M., et al. 1994. Correlative light and electron microscopy studies of PrP localisation in 87V scrapie. *Brain Res*, **656**, 329–43.

Jeffrey, M., McGovern, G., et al. 2000. Sites of prion protein accumulation in scrapie-infected mouse spleen revealed by immuno-electron microscopy. *J Pathol*, **191**, 323–32.

Johnson, R.T. 1992. Prion disease. *N Engl J Med*, **326**, 486–7, [editorial; comment].

Kaeser, P.S., Klein, M.A., et al. 2001. Efficient lymphoreticular prion propagation requires prp(c) in stromal and hematopoietic cells. *J Virol*, **75**, 7097–106.

Kahana, E., Alter, M., et al. 1974. Creutzfeldt–Jakob disease: focus among Libyan Jews in Israel. *Science*, **183**, 90–1.

Kahana, E., Zilber, N. and Abraham, M. 1991. Do Creutzfeldt-Jakob disease patients of Jewish Libyan origin have unique clinical features? *Neurology*, **41**, 1390–2.

Kane, P.M., Yamashiro, C.T., et al. 1990. Protein splicing converts the yeast *TFP1* gene product to the 69-kD subunit of the vacuolar H+-adenosine triphosphatase. *Science*, **250**, 651–7.

Kao, R.R., Gravenor, M.B., et al. 2002. The potential size and duration of an epidemic of bovine spongiform encephalopathy in British sheep. *Science*, **295**, 332–5.

Kapasi, Z.F., Qin, D., et al. 1998. Follicular dendritic cell (FDC) precursors in primary lymphoid tissues. *J Immunol*, **160**, 1078–84.

Kascsak, R.J., Rubenstein, R., et al. 1987. Mouse polyclonal and monoclonal antibody to scrapie-associated fibril proteins. *J Virol*, **61**, 3688–93.

Keller, G.A., Siegel, M.W. and Caras, I.W. 1992. Endocytosis of glycophospholipid-anchored and transmembrane forms of CD4 by different endocytic pathways. *EMBO J*, **11**, 863–74.

Kerneis, S., Bogdanova, A., et al. 1997. Conversion by Peyer's patch lymphocytes of human enterocytes into M cells that transport bacteria. *Science*, **277**, 949–52.

Kimberlin, R.H. and Walker, C.A. 1978a. Evidence that the transmission of one source of scrapie agent to hamsters involves separation of agent strains from a mixture. *J Gen Virol*, **39**, 487–96.

Kimberlin, R.H. and Walker, C.A. 1978b. Pathogenesis of mouse scrapie: effect of route of inoculation on infectivity titres and dose-response curves. *J Comp Pathol*, **88**, 39–47.

Kimberlin, R.H. and Walker, C.A. 1979. Pathogenesis of scrapie: agent multiplication in brain at the first and second passage of hamster scrapie in mice. *J Gen Virol*, **42**, 107–17.

Kimberlin, R.H. and Wilesmith, J.W. 1994. Bovine spongiform encephalopathy. Epidemiology, low dose exposure and risks. *Ann N Y Acad Sci*, **724**, 210–20.

Kimberlin, R.H., Hall, S.M. and Walker, C.A. 1983. Pathogenesis of mouse scrapie. Evidence for direct neural spread of infection to the CNS after injection of sciatic nerve. *J Neurol Sci*, **61**, 315–25.

Kirkwood, J.K., Wells, G.A., et al. 1990. Spongiform encephalopathy in an arabian oryx (*Oryx leucoryx*) and a greater kudu (*Tragelaphus strepsiceros*). *Vet Rec*, **127**, 418–20.

Kirkwood, J.K., Cunningham, A.A., et al. 1993. Spongiform encephalopathy in a herd of greater kudu (*Tragelaphus strepsiceros*): epidemiological observations. *Vet Rec*, **133**, 360–4.

Kirschbaum, W.R. 1924. Zwei eigenartige Erkrankungen des Zentralnervensystems nach Art der spastischen Pseudosklerose (Jakob). *Z Ges Neurol Psychiatr*, **92**, 175–220.

Kitamoto, T. and Tateishi, J. 1994. Human prion diseases with variant prion protein. *Philos Trans R Soc Lond B Biol Sci*, **343**, 391–8.

Kitamoto, T., Tateishi, J., et al. 1986. Amyloid plaques in Creutzfeldt–Jakob disease stain with prion protein antibodies. *Ann Neurol*, **20**, 204–8.

Kitamoto, T., Muramoto, T., et al. 1991a. Abnormal isoform of prion protein accumulates in follicular dendritic cells in mice with Creutzfeldt–Jakob disease. *J Virol*, **65**, 6292–5.

Kitamoto, T., Yamaguchi, K., et al. 1991b. A prion protein missense variant is integrated in kuru plaque cores in patients with Gerstmann–Straussler syndrome. *Neurology*, **41**, 306–10.

Kitamoto, T., Shin, R.W., et al. 1992. Abnormal isoform of prion proteins accumulates in the synaptic structures of the central nervous system in patients with Creutzfeldt–Jakob disease. *Am J Pathol*, **140**, 1285–94.

Kitamoto, T., Amano, N., et al. 1993a. A new inherited prion disease (*PrP-P105L* mutation) showing spastic paraparesis. *Ann Neurol*, **34**, 808–13.

Kitamoto, T., Iizuka, R. and Tateishi, J. 1993b. An amber mutation of prion protein in Gerstmann–Straussler syndrome with mutant PrP plaques. *Biochem Biophys Res Commun*, **192**, 525–31.

Kitamoto, T., Ohta, M., et al. 1993c. Novel missense variants of prion protein in Creutzfeldt–Jakob disease or Gerstmann–Straussler syndrome. *Biochem Biophys Res Commun*, **191**, 709–14.

Kitamura, D., Roes, J., et al. 1991. A B cell-deficient mouse by targeted disruption of the membrane exon of the immunoglobulin mu chain gene. *Nature*, **350**, 423–6.

Klein, M.A., Frigg, R., et al. 1997. A crucial role for B cells in neuroinvasive scrapie. *Nature*, **390**, 687–90.

Klein, M.A., Frigg, R., et al. 1998. PrP expression in B lymphocytes is not required for prion neuroinvasion. *Nat Med*, **4**, 1429–33.

Klein, M.A., Kaeser, P.S., et al. 2001. Complement facilitates early prion pathogenesis. *Nat Med*, **7**, 488–92.

Klitzman, R.L., Alpers, M.P. and Gajdusek, D.C. 1984. The natural incubation period of kuru and the episodes of transmission in three clusters of patients. *Neuroepidemiology*, **3**, 3–20.

Klohn, P.C., Stoltze, L., et al. 2003. A quantitative, highly sensitive cell-based infectivity assay for mouse scrapie prions. *Proc Natl Acad Sci U S A*, **100**, 11666–71.

Knaus, K.J., Morillas, M., et al. 2001. Crystal structure of the human prion protein reveals a mechanism for oligomerization. *Nat Struct Biol*, **8**, 770–4.

Koch, T.K., Berg, B.O., et al. 1985. Creutzfeldt–Jakob disease in a young adult with idiopathic hypopituitarism. Possible relation to the administration of cadaveric human growth hormone. *N Engl J Med*, **313**, 731–3.

Kocisko, D.A., Come, J.H., et al. 1994. Cell-free formation of protease-resistant prion protein. *Nature*, **370**, 471–4.

Kocisko, D.A., Priola, S.A., et al. 1995. Species specificity in the cell-free conversion of prion protein to protease-resistant forms: a model for the scrapie species barrier. *Proc Natl Acad Sci U S A*, **92**, 3923–7.

Koller, M.F., Grau, T. and Christen, P. 2002. Induction of antibodies against murine full-length prion protein in wild-type mice. *J Neuroimmunol*, **132**, 113–16.

Kondo, K. and Kuroina, Y. 1981. A case-control study of Creutzfeldt–Jakob disease: association with physical injuries. *Ann Neurol*, **11**, 377–81.

Koni, P.A., Sacca, R., et al. 1997. Distinct roles in lymphoid organogenesis for lymphotoxins alpha and beta revealed in lymphotoxin beta-deficient mice. *Immunity*, **6**, 491–500.

Kooyman, D.L., Byrne, G.W., et al. 1995. In vivo transfer of GPI-linked complement restriction factors from erythrocytes to the endothelium. *Science*, **269**, 89–92.

Kooyman, D.L., Byrne, G.W. and Logan, J.S. 1998. Glycosyl phosphatidylinositol anchor. *Exp Nephrol*, **6**, 148–51.

Korth, C., Stierli, B., et al. 1997. Prion (PrPSc)-specific epitope defined by a monoclonal antibody. *Nature*, **390**, 74–7.

Künzi, V., Glatzel, M., et al. 2002. Unhampered prion neuroinvasion despite impaired fast axonal transport in transgenic mice overexpressing four-repeat tau. *J Neurosci*, **22**, 7471–7.

Kurschner, C., Morgan, J.I., et al. 1995. The cellular prion protein (PrP) selectively binds to Bcl-2 in the yeast two-hybrid system: identification of candidate proteins binding to prion protein. *Brain Res Mol Brain Res*, **30**, 165–8.

Lacroute, F. 1971. Non-Mendelian mutation allowing ureidosuccinic acid uptake in yeast. *J Bacteriol*, **106**, 519–22.

Lansbury, P.T. 1994. Mechanism of scrapie replication. *Science*, **265**, 1510.

Laplanche, J.L., Chatelain, J., et al. 1990. Deletion in prion protein gene in a Moroccan family. *Nucleic Acids Res*, **18**, 6745.

Laplanche, J.L., Chatelain, J., et al. 1993a. French autochthonous scrapied sheep without the 136Val PrP polymorphism. *Mamm Genome*, **4**, 463–4.

Laplanche, J.L., Chatelain, J., et al. 1993b. PrP polymorphisms associated with natural scrapie discovered by denaturing gradient gel electrophoresis. *Genomics*, **15**, 30–7.

Lasmezas, C.I., Cesbron, J.Y., et al. 1996a. Immune system-dependent and -independent replication of the scrapie agent. *J Virol*, **70**, 1292–5.

Lasmezas, C.I., Deslys, J.P., et al. 1996b. BSE transmission to macaques. *Nature*, **381**, 743–4.

Laszlo, L., Lowe, J., et al. 1992. Lysosomes as key organelles in the pathogenesis of prion encephalopathies. *J Pathol*, **166**, 333–41.

Li, A., Sakaguchi, S., et al. 2000. Physiological expression of the gene for PrP-like protein, PrPLP/Dpl, by brain endothelial cells and its ectopic expression in neurons of PrP- deficient mice ataxic due to purkinje cell degeneration. *Am J Pathol*, **157**, 1447–52.

Little, B.W., Brown, P.W., et al. 1986. Familial myoclonic dementia masquerading as Creutzfeldt–Jakob disease. *Ann Neurol*, **20**, 231–9.

Liu, T., Li, R., et al. 2002. Intercellular transfer of the cellular prion protein. *J Biol Chem*, **277**, 47671–8.

Lledo, P.M., Tremblay, P., et al. 1996. Mice deficient for prion protein exhibit normal neuronal excitability and synaptic transmission in the hippocampus. *Proc Natl Acad Sci U S A*, **93**, 2403–7.

Locht, C., Chesebro, B., et al. 1986. Molecular cloning and complete sequence of prion protein cDNA from mouse brain infected with the scrapie agent. *Proc Natl Acad Sci U S A*, **83**, 6372–6.

Lu, K., Wang, W., et al. 2000. Expression and structural characterization of the recombinant human doppel protein. *Biochemistry*, **39**, 13575–83.

Lugaresi, E., Medori, R., et al. 1986. Fatal familial insomnia and dysautonomia with selective degeneration of thalamic nuclei. *N Engl J Med*, **315**, 997–1003.

Lumley Jones, R., Benker, G., et al. 1979. Large-scale preparation of highly purified pyrogen-free human growth hormone for clinical use. *Br J Endocrinol*, **82**, 77–86.

Ma, J. and Lindquist, S. 2002. Conversion of PrP to a self-perpetuating PrPSc-like conformation in the cytosol. *Science*, **298**, 1785–8.

Ma, J., Wollmann, R. and Lindquist, S. 2002. Neurotoxicity and neurodegeneration when PrP accumulates in the cytosol. *Science*, **298**, 1781–5.

Mabbott, N.A., Bruce, M.E., et al. 2001. Temporary depletion of complement component C3 or genetic deficiency of C1q significantly delays onset of scrapie. *Nat Med*, **7**, 485–7.

Macario, M.E., Vaisman, M., et al. 1991. Pituitary growth hormone and Creutzfeldt–Jakob disease. *BMJ*, **302**, 1149.

Mackay, F. and Browning, J.L. 1998. Turning off follicular dendritic cells. *Nature*, **395**, 26–7.

Mackay, F., Majeau, G.R., et al. 1997. Lymphotoxin but not tumor necrosis factor functions to maintain splenic architecture and humoral responsiveness in adult mice. *Eur J Immunol*, **27**, 2033–42.

Maissen, M., Roeckl, C., et al. 2001. Plasminogen binds to disease-associated prion protein of multiple species. *Lancet*, **357**, 2026–8.

Mallucci, G.R., Ratte, S., et al. 2002. Post-natal knockout of prion protein alters hippocampal CA1 properties, but does not result in neurodegeneration. *EMBO J*, **21**, 202–10.

Malmgren, R., Kurland, L., et al. 1979. The epidemiology of Creutzfeldt–Jakob disease. In: Prusiner, S.B. and Hadlow, W.J. (eds), *Slow transmissible diseases of the nervous system*. New York: Academic Press, 93–112.

Manetto, V., Medori, R., et al. 1992. Fatal familial insomnia: clinical and pathologic study of five new cases. *Neurology*, **42**, 312–19.

Manson, J., West, J.D., et al. 1992. The prion protein gene: a role in mouse embryogenesis? *Development*, **115**, 117–22.

Manson, J.C., Clarke, A.R., et al. 1994a. 129/Ola mice carrying a null mutation in PrP that abolishes mRNA production are developmentally normal. *Mol Neurobiol*, **8**, 121–7.

Manson, J.C., Clarke, A.R., et al. 1994b. PrP gene dosage determines the timing but not the final intensity or distribution of lesions in scrapie pathology. *Neurodegeneration*, **3**, 331–40.

Marsh, R.F. and Kimberlin, R.H. 1975. Comparison of scrapie and transmissible mink encephalopathy in hamsters. II. Clinical signs, pathology, and pathogenesis. *J Infect Dis*, **131**, 104–10.

Martinez Lage, J.F., Sola, J., et al. 1993. Pediatric Creutzfeldt–Jakob disease: probable transmission by a dural graft. *Childs Nerv Syst*, **9**, 239–42.

Marzewski, D.J., Towfighi, J., et al. 1988. Creutzfeldt–Jakob disease following pituitary-derived human growth hormone therapy: a new American case. *Neurology*, **38**, 1131–3.

Masters, C.L. and Gajdusek, D.C. 1979. Familial Creutzfeldt–Jakob disease and other familial dementias: an inquiry into possible models of virus-induced familial diseases. In: Prusiner, S.B. and Hadlow, W.J. (eds), *Slow transmissible diseases of the nervous system*. New York: Academic Press, 143–94.

Masters, C.L. and Richardson, E.P. 1978. Subacute spongiform encephalopathy (Creutzfeldt–Jakob disease). The nature and progression of spongiform change. *Brain*, **101**, 333–44.

Masters, C.L., Gajdusek, D.C. and Gibbs, C.J. 1981a. Creutzfeldt–Jakob disease virus isolations from the Gerstmann–Sträussler syndrome with an analysis of the various forms of amyloid plaque deposition in the virus-induced spongiform encephalopathies. *Brain*, **104**, 559–588.

Masters, C.L., Gajdusek, D.C. and Gibbs, C.J. 1981b. The familial occurrence of Creutzfeldt–Jakob disease and Alzheimer's disease. *Brain*, **104**, 535–58.

Mastrianni, J.A., Curtis, M.T., et al. 1995. Prion disease (PrP-A117V) presenting with ataxia instead of dementia. *Neurology*, **45**, 2042–50.

Masullo, C., Pocchiari, M., et al. 1989. Transmission of Creutzfeldt–Jakob disease by dural cadaveric graft. *J Neurosurg*, **71**, 954–5.

Matsumoto, M., Fu, Y.X., et al. 1997. Distinct roles of lymphotoxin alpha and the type I tumor necrosis factor (TNF) receptor in the establishment of follicular dendritic cells from non-bone marrow-derived cells. *J Exp Med*, **186**, 1997–2004.

McBride, P.A. and Beekes, M. 1999. Pathological PrP is abundant in sympathetic and sensory ganglia of hamsters fed with scrapie. *Neurosci Lett*, **265**, 135–8.

McKinley, M.P., Bolton, D.C. and Prusiner, S.B. 1983. A protease-resistant protein is a structural component of the scrapie prion. *Cell*, **35**, 57–62.

McKinley, M.P., Meyer, R.K., et al. 1991a. Scrapie prion rod formation in vitro requires both detergent extraction and limited proteolysis. *J Virol*, **65**, 1340–51.

McKinley, M.P., Taraboulos, A., et al. 1991b. Ultrastructural localization of scrapie prion proteins in cytoplasmic vesicles of infected cultured cells. *Lab Invest*, **65**, 622–30.

Mead, S., Beck, J., et al. 2000. Examination of the human prion protein-like gene doppel for genetic susceptibility to sporadic and variant Creutzfeldt–Jakob disease. *Neurosci Lett*, **290**, 117–20.

Mead, S., Stumpf, M.P., et al. 2003. Balancing selection at the prion protein gene consistent with prehistoric kurulike epidemics. *Science*, **300**, 640–3.

Medori, R., Montagna, P., et al. 1992a. Fatal familial insomnia: a second kindred with mutation of prion protein gene at codon 178. *Neurology*, **42**, 669–70.

Medori, R., Tritschler, H.J., et al. 1992b. Fatal familial insomnia, a prion disease with a mutation at codon 178 of the prion protein gene. *N Engl J Med*, **326**, 444–9.

Meggendorfer, F. 1930. Klinische und genealogische Beobachtungen bei einem Fall von spastischer Pseudosklerose Jakobs. *Z Ges Neurol Psychiatr*, **128**, 337–41.

Meier, P., Genoud, N., et al. 2003. Soluble dimeric prion protein binds PrP(Sc) in vivo and antagonizes prion disease. *Cell*, **113**, 49–60.

Meyer, R.K., McKinley, M.P., et al. 1986. Separation and properties of cellular and scrapie prion proteins. *Proc Natl Acad Sci USA*, **83**, 2310–14.

M'Fadyean, J.M. 1918. Scrapie. *J Comp Pathol*, **31**, 102–31.

M'Gowan, J.P. 1914. *Investigation into the disease of sheep called 'scrapie'*. Edinburgh: William Blackwood.

Miller, M.W., Williams, E.S., et al. 2000. Epizootiology of chronic wasting disease in free-ranging cervids in Colorado and Wyoming. *J Wildl Dis*, **36**, 676–90.

Millson, G.C., Hunter, G.D. and Kimberlin, R.H. 1971. An experimental examination of the scrapie agent in cell membrane mixtures. II. The association of scrapie activity with membrane fractions. *J Comp Pathol*, **81**, 255–65.

Miyashita, K., Inuzuka, T., et al. 1991. Creutzfeldt–Jakob disease in a patient with a cadaveric dural graft. *Neurology*, **41**, 940–1.

Miyazono, M., Kitamoto, T., et al. 1992. Creutzfeldt–Jakob disease with codon 129 polymorphism (valine): a comparative study of patients with codon 102 point mutation or without mutations. *Acta Neuropathol Berl*, **84**, 349–54.

Mo, H., Moore, R.C., et al. 2001. Two different neurodegenerative diseases caused by proteins with similar structures. *Proc Natl Acad Sci USA*, **98**, 2352–7.

Mobley, W.C., Neve, R.L., et al. 1988. Nerve growth factor increases mRNA levels for the prion protein and the beta-amyloid protein precursor in developing hamster brain. *Proc Natl Acad Sci USA*, **85**, 9811–15.

Monari, L., Chen, S.G., et al. 1994. Fatal familial insomnia and familial Creutzfeldt–Jakob disease: different prion proteins determined by a DNA polymorphism. *Proc Natl Acad Sci U S A*, **91**, 2839–42.

Montrasio, F., Frigg, R., et al. 2000. Impaired prion replication in spleens of mice lacking functional follicular dendritic cells. *Science*, **288**, 1257–9.

Moore, R.C., Lee, I.Y., et al. 1999. Ataxia in prion protein (PrP)-deficient mice is associated with upregulation of the novel PrP-like protein doppel. *J Mol Biol*, **292**, 797–817.

Neutra, M.R., Frey, A. and Kraehenbuhl, J.P. 1996. Epithelial M cells: gateways for mucosal infection and immunization. *Cell*, **86**, 345–8.

New, M.I., Brown, P., et al. 1988. Preclinical Creutzfeldt–Jakob disease discovered at autopsy in a human growth hormone recipient. *Neurology*, **38**, 1133–4.

Nguyen, J.T., Inouye, H., et al. 1995. X-ray diffraction of scrapie prion rods and PrP peptides. *J Mol Biol*, **252**, 412–22.

Nisbet, T.J., MacDonaldson, I. and Bishara, S.N. 1989. Creutzfeldt–Jakob disease in a second patient who recieved a cadaveric dura mater graft. *JAMA*, **261**, 1118.

Nochlin, D., Sumi, S.M., et al. 1989. Familial dementia with PrP-positive amyloid plaques: a variant of Gerstmann–Straussler syndrome. *Neurology*, **39**, 910–18.

Oesch, B., Westaway, D., et al. 1985. A cellular gene encodes scrapie PrP 27-30 protein. *Cell*, **40**, 735–46.

Oesch, B., Teplow, D.B., et al. 1990. Identification of cellular proteins binding to the scrapie prion protein. *Biochemistry*, **29**, 5848–55.

Oidtmann, B., Simon, D., et al. 2003. Identification of cDNAs from Japanese pufferfish (*Fugu rubripes*) and Atlantic salmon (*Salmo salar*) coding for homologues to tetrapod prion proteins. *FEBS Lett*, **538**, 96–100.

Onodera, T., Ikeda, T., et al. 1993. Isolation of scrapie agent from the placenta of sheep with natural scrapie in Japan. *Microbiol Immunol*, **37**, 311–16.

Otto, D. 1987. Jacob–Creutzfeldt disease associated with cadaveric dura. *J Neurosurg*, **67**, 149.

Owen, F., Poulter, M., et al. 1989. Insertion in prion protein gene in familial Creutzfeldt–Jakob disease. *Lancet*, **1**, 51–2, [letter].

Owen, F., Poulter, M., et al. 1990a. Codon 129 changes in the prion protein gene in Caucasians. *Am J Hum Genet*, **46**, 1215–16.

Owen, F., Poulter, M., et al. 1990b. An in-frame insertion in the prion protein gene in familial Creutzfeldt–Jakob disease. *Brain Res Mol Brain Res*, **7**, 273–6.

Owen, F., Poulter, M., et al. 1991. Insertions in the prion protein gene in atypical dementias. *Exp Neurol*, **112**, 240–2.

Owen, F., Poulter, M., et al. 1992. A dementing illness associated with a novel insertion in the prion protein gene. *Brain Res Mol Brain Res*, **13**, 155–7.

Packer, R.J., Cornblath, D.R., et al. 1980. Creutzfeldt–Jakob disease in a 20-year-old woman. *Neurology*, **30**, 492–6.

Palmer, M.S., Dryden, A.J., et al. 1991. Homozygous prion protein genotype predisposes to sporadic Creutzfeldt–Jakob disease. *Nature*, **352**, 340–2.

Palmer, M.S., Mahal, S.P., et al. 1993. Deletions in the prion protein gene are not associated with CJD. *Hum Mol Genet*, **2**, 541–4.

Palsson, P.A. 1979. Rida (scrapie) in Iceland and its epidemiology. In: Prusiner, S.B. and Hadlow, W.J. (eds), *Slow transmissible diseases of the nervous system*. New York: Academic Press, 357–66.

Pan, K.M., Baldwin, M., et al. 1993. Conversion of alpha-helices into beta-sheets features in the formation of the scrapie prion proteins. *Proc Natl Acad Sci U S A*, **90**, 10962–6.

Parchi, P., Castellani, R., et al. 1996. Molecular basis of phenotypic variability in sporadic Creutzfeldt–Jakob disease. *Ann Neurol*, **39**, 767–78.

Parchi, P., Giese, A., et al. 1999. Classification of sporadic Creutzfeldt–Jakob disease based on molecular and phenotypic analysis of 300 subjects. *Ann Neurol*, **46**, 224–33.

Park, S.Y., Ueda, S., et al. 1998. Resistance of Fc receptor- deficient mice to fatal glomerulonephritis. *J Clin Invest*, **102**, 1229–38.

Parry, H.B. 1962. Scrapie: a transmissible and hereditary disease of sheep. *Heredity*, **17**, 75–105.

Parry, H.B. 1983. *Scrapie disease in sheep*. New York: Academic Press.

Parry, H.B. and Livett, B.G. 1973. A new hypothalamic pathway to the median eminence containing neurophysin and its hypertrophy in sheep with natural scrapie. *Nature*, **242**, 63–5.

Pattison, I.H. 1964. The spread of Scrapie by contact between affected and healthy sheep, goats or mice. *Vet Rec*, **76**, 333–6.

Pattison, I.H. and Jones, K.M. 1967. The possible nature of the transmissible agent of scrapie. *Vet Rec*, **80**, 2–9.

Pattison, I.H. and Millson, G.C. 1961a. Experimental transmission of scrapie to goats and sheep by the oral route. *J Comp Pathol*, **71**, 171–6.

Pattison, I.H. and Millson, G.C. 1961b. Scrapie produced experimentally in goats with special reference to the clinical syndrome. *J Comp Pathol*, **71**, 101–8.

Pattison, I.H., Hoare, M.N., et al. 1972. Spread of scrapie to sheep and goats by oral dosing with foetal membranes from scrapie-affected sheep. *Vet Rec*, **90**, 465–8.

Pearson, G.R., Wyatt, J.M., et al. 1992. Feline spongiform encephalopathy: fibril and PrP studies. *Vet Rec*, **131**, 307–10.

Peoc'h, K., Guerin, C., et al. 2000. First report of polymorphisms in the prion-like protein gene (*PRND*): implications for human prion diseases. *Neurosci Lett*, **286**, 144–8.

Pepys, M.B., Bybee, A., et al. 2003. MHC typing in variant Creutzfeldt–Jakob disease. *Lancet*, **361**, 487–9.

Peretz, D., Williamson, R.A., et al. 2001. Antibodies inhibit prion propagation and clear cell cultures of prion infectivity. *Nature*, **412**, 739–43.

Peretz, D., Williamson, R.A., et al. 2002. A change in the conformation of prions accompanies the emergence of a new prion strain. *Neuron*, **34**, 921–32.

Perry, V.H., Cunningham, C. and Boche, D. 2002. Atypical inflammation in the central nervous system in prion disease. *Curr Opin Neurol*, **15**, 349–54.

Petersen, R.B., Tabaton, M., et al. 1992. Analysis of the prion protein gene in thalamic dementia. *Neurology*, **42**, 1859–63.

Pocchiari, M., Schmittinger, S. and Masullo, C. 1987. Amphotericin B delays the incubation period of scrapie in intracerebrally inoculated hamsters. *J Gen Virol*, **68**, 219–23.

Pocchiari, M., Salvatore, M., et al. 1993. A new point mutation of the prion protein gene in familial and sporadic cases of Creutzfeldt–Jakob disease. *Ann Neurol*, **34**, 802–7.

Poidinger, M., Kirkwood, J. and Almond, W. 1993. Sequence analysis of the PrP protein from two species of antelope susceptible to transmissible spongiform encephalopathy. *Arch Virol*, **131**, 193–9.

Poulter, M., Baker, H.F., et al. 1992. Inherited prion disease with 144 base pair gene insertion. 1. Genealogical and molecular studies. *Brain*, **115**, 675–85.

Powell Jackson, J., Weller, R.O., et al. 1985. Creutzfeldt–Jakob disease after administration of human growth hormone. *Lancet*, **2**, 244–6.

Prinz, M., Montrasio, F., et al. 2002. Lymph nodal prion replication and neuroinvasion in mice devoid of follicular dendritic cells. *Proc Natl Acad Sci U S A*, **99**, 919–24.

Prinz, M., Heikenwalder, M., et al. 2003a. Positioning of follicular dendritic cells within the spleen controls prion neuroinvasion. *Nature*, **425**, 957–62.

Prinz, M., Heikenwalder, M., et al. 2003b. Prion pathogenesis in the absence of Toll-like receptor signalling. *EMBO Rep*, **4**, 195–9.

Prinz, M., Huber, G., et al. 2003c. Oral prion infection requires normal numbers of Peyer's patches but not of enteric lymphocytes. *Am J Pathol*, **162**, 1103–11.

Priola, S.A., Raines, A. and Caughey, W.S. 2000. Porphyrin and phthalocyanine antiscrapie compounds [see comments]. *Science*, **287**, 1503–6.

Prusiner, S.B. 1982. Novel proteinaceous infectious particles cause scrapie. *Science*, **216**, 136–44.

Prusiner, S.B. 1989a. Creutzfeldt–Jakob disease and scrapie prions. *Alzheimer Dis Assoc Disord*, **3**, 52–78.

Prusiner, S.B. 1989b. Scrapie prions. *Annu Rev Microbiol*, **43**, 345–74.

Prusiner, S.B. 1991. Molecular biology of prion diseases. *Science*, **252**, 1515–22.

Prusiner, S.B. and DeArmond, S.J. 1994. Prion diseases and neurodegeneration. *Annu Rev Neurosci*, **17**, 311–39.

Prusiner, S.B., Hadlow, W.J., et al. 1978. Partial purification and evidence for multiple molecular forms of the scrapie agent. *Biochemistry*, **17**, 4993–9.

Prusiner, S.B., Groth, D.F., et al. 1980a. Molecular properties, partial purification, and assay by incubation period measurements of the hamster scrapie agent. *Biochemistry*, **19**, 4883–91.

Prusiner, S.B., Groth, D.F., et al. 1980b. Gel electrophoresis and glass permeation chromatography of the hamster scrapie agent after enzymatic digestion and detergent extraction. *Biochemistry*, **19**, 4892–4898.

Prusiner, S.B., Cochran, S.P., et al. 1981a. Determination of scrapie agent titer from incubation period measurements in hamsters. *Adv Exp Med Biol*, **134**, 385–99.

Prusiner, S.B., McKinley, M.P., et al. 1981b. Scrapie agent contains a hydrophobic protein. *Proc Natl Acad Sci U S A*, **78**, 6675–9.

Prusiner, S.B., Bolton, D.C., et al. 1982a. Further purification and characterization of scrapie prions. *Biochemistry*, **21**, 6942–50.

Prusiner, S.B., Cochran, S.P., et al. 1982b. Measurement of the scrapie agent using an incubation time interval assay. *Ann Neurol*, **11**, 353–8.

Prusiner, S.B., Gajdusek, C. and Alpers, M.P. 1982c. Kuru with incubation periods exceeding two decades. *Ann Neurol*, **12**, 1–9.

Prusiner, S.B., McKinley, M.P., et al. 1983. Scrapie prions aggregate to form amyloid-like birefringent rods. *Cell*, **35**, 349–58.

Prusiner, S.B., Groth, D.F., et al. 1984. Purification and structural studies of a major scrapie prion protein. *Cell*, **38**, 127–34.

Prusiner, S.B., Scott, M., et al. 1990. Transgenetic studies implicate interactions between homologous PrP isoforms in scrapie prion replication. *Cell*, **63**, 673–86.

Prusiner, S.B., Groth, D., et al. 1993. Ablation of the prion protein (PrP) gene in mice prevents scrapie and facilitates production of anti-PrP antibodies. *Proc Natl Acad Sci U S A*, **90**, 10608–12.

Puckett, C., Concannon, P., et al. 1991. Genomic structure of the human prion protein gene. *Am J Hum Genet*, **49**, 320–9.

Race, R. and Chesebro, B. 1998. Scrapie infectivity found in resistant species. *Nature*, **392**, 770.

Race, R., Oldstone, M. and Chesebro, B. 2000. Entry versus blockade of brain infection following oral or intraperitoneal scrapie administration: role of prion protein expression in peripheral nerves and spleen. *J Virol*, **74**, 828–33.

Race, R.E., Priola, S.A., et al. 1995. Neuron-specific expression of a hamster prion protein minigene in transgenic mice induces susceptibility to hamster scrapie agent. *Neuron*, **15**, 1183–91.

Raeber, A.J., Klein, M.A., et al. 1999a. PrP-dependent association of prions with splenic but not circulating lymphocytes of scrapie-infected mice. *EMBO J*, **18**, 2702–6.

Raeber, A.J., Sailer, A., et al. 1999b. Ectopic expression of prion protein (PrP) in T lymphocytes or hepatocytes of PrP knockout mice is insufficient to sustain prion replication. *Proc Natl Acad Sci U S A*, **96**, 3987–92.

Raymond, G.J., Bossers, A., et al. 2000. Evidence of a molecular barrier limiting susceptibility of humans, cattle and sheep to chronic wasting disease. *EMBO J*, **19**, 4425–30.

Ridley, R.M. and Baker, H.F. 1993. Occupational risk of Creutzfeldt–Jakob disease. *Lancet*, **341**, 641–2.

Rieger, R., Edenhofer, F., et al. 1997. The human 37-kDa laminin receptor precursor interacts with the prion protein in eukaryotic cells. *Nat Med*, **3**, 1383–8.

Riek, R., Hornemann, S., et al. 1996. NMR structure of the mouse prion protein domain PrP(121-321). *Nature*, **382**, 180–2.

Riesner, D., Kellings, K., et al. 1993. Prions and nucleic acids: search for 'residual' nucleic acids and screening for mutations in the PrP-gene. *Dev Biol Stand*, **80**, 173–81.

Ripoll, L., Laplanche, J.-L., et al. 1993. A new point mutation in the prion protein gene at codon 210 in Creutzfeldt–Jakob disease. *Neurology*, **43**, 1934–8.

Rivera-Milla, E., Stuermer, C.A. and Malaga-Trillo, E. 2003. An evolutionary basis for scrapie disease: identification of a fish prion mRNA. *Trends Genet*, **19**, 72–5.

Roberts, G.W., Lofthouse, R., et al. 1986. Prion-protein immunoreactivity in human transmissible dementias. *N Engl J Med*, **315**, 1231–3, [letter].

Roberts, G.W., Lofthouse, R., et al. 1988. CNS amyloid proteins in neurodegenerative diseases. *Neurology*, **38**, 1534–40.

Rogers, M., Serban, D., et al. 1991. Epitope mapping of the Syrian hamster prion protein utilizing chimeric and mutant genes in a vaccinia virus expression system. *J Immunol*, **147**, 3568–74.

Rogers, M., Yehiely, F., et al. 1993. Conversion of truncated and elongated prion proteins into the scrapie isoform in cultured cells. *Proc Natl Acad Sci U S A*, **90**, 3182–6.

Roos, R., Gajdusek, D.C. and Gibbs, C.J. Jr 1973. The clinical characteristics of transmissible Creutzfeldt–Jakob disease. *Brain*, **96**, 1–20.

Rosenthal, N.P., Keesey, J., et al. 1976. Familial neurological disease associated with spongiform encephalopathy. *Arch Neurol*, **33**, 252–9.

Rossett, M.B., Ballerina, C., et al. 2004. Breaking immune tolerance to the prion protein using prion protein peptides plus oligodeoxynucleotide-CpG in mice. *J Immunol*, **172**, 5168–74.

Rossi, D., Cozzio, A., et al. 2001. Onset of ataxia and Purkinje cell loss in PrP null mice inversely correlated with Dpl level in brain. *EMBO J*, **20**, 1–9.

Roucou, X., Guo, Q., et al. 2003. Cytosolic prion protein is not toxic and protects against Bax-mediated cell death in human primary neurons. *J Biol Chem*, **278**, 40877–81.

Rubenstein, R., Merz, P.A., et al. 1991. Scrapie-infected spleens: analysis of infectivity, scrapie-associated fibrils, and protease-resistant proteins. *J Infect Dis*, **164**, 29–35.

Safar, J., Roller, P.P., et al. 1993a. Conformational transitions, dissociation, and unfolding of scrapie amyloid (prion) protein. *J Biol Chem*, **268**, 20276–84.

Safar, J., Roller, P.P., et al. 1993b. Thermal stability and conformational transitions of scrapie amyloid (prion) protein correlate with infectivity. *Protein Sci*, **2**, 2206–16.

Safar, J., Wille, H., et al. 1998. Eight prion strains have PrP(Sc) molecules with different conformations. *Nat Med*, **4**, 1157–65.

Safar, J.G., Scott, M., et al. 2002. Measuring prions causing bovine spongiform encephalopathy or chronic wasting disease by immunoassays and transgenic mice. *Nat Biotechnol*, **20**, 1147–50.

Sailer, A., Büeler, H., et al. 1994. No propagation of prions in mice devoid of PrP. *Cell*, **77**, 967–8.

Sakaguchi, S., Katamine, S., et al. 1996. Loss of cerebellar Purkinje cells in aged mice homozygous for a disrupted PrP gene. *Nature*, **380**, 528–31.

Sakudo, A., Lee, D.C., et al. 2003. Impairment of superoxide dismutase activation by N-terminally truncated prion protein (PrP) in PrP-deficient neuronal cell line. *Biochem Biophys Res Commun*, **308**, 660–7.

Sales, N., Hassig, R., et al. 2002. Developmental expression of the cellular prion protein in elongating axons. *Eur J Neurosci*, **15**, 1163–77.

Schmitt-Ulms, G., Legname, G., et al. 2001. Binding of neural cell adhesion molecules (N-CAMs) to the cellular prion protein. *J Mol Biol*, **314**, 1209–25.

Schreuder, B.E.C., Vankeulen, L.J.M., et al. 1996. Preclinical test for prion diseases. *Nature*, **381**, 563.

Schwarz, A., Kratke, O., et al. 2003. Immunization with a synthetic prion protein-derived peptide prolongs survival times of mice orally exposed to the scrapie agent. *Neurosci Lett*, **350**, 187–9.

Scott, J.R., Foster, J.D. and Fraser, H. 1993. Conjunctival instillation of scrapie in mice can produce disease. *Vet Microbiol*, **34**, 305–9.

Scott, M., Foster, D., et al. 1989. Transgenic mice expressing hamster prion protein produce species- specific scrapie infectivity and amyloid plaques. *Cell*, **59**, 847–57.

Scott, M., Groth, D., et al. 1993. Propagation of prions with artificial properties in transgenic mice expressing chimeric PrP genes. *Cell*, **73**, 979–88.

Scott, M.R., Kohler, R., et al. 1992. Chimeric prion protein expression in cultured cells and transgenic mice. *Protein Sci*, **1**, 986–97.

Scott, M.R., Will, R., et al. 1999. Compelling transgenetic evidence for transmission of bovine spongiform encephalopathy prions to humans. *Proc Natl Acad Sci U S A*, **96**, 15137–42.

Serban, D., Taraboulos, A., et al. 1990. Rapid detection of Creutzfeldt–Jakob disease and scrapie prion proteins. *Neurology*, **40**, 110–17.

Sethi, S., Lipford, G., et al. 2002. Postexposure prophylaxis against prion disease with a stimulator of innate immunity. *Lancet*, **360**, 229–30.

Shaked, Y., Rosenmann, H., et al. 1999. A C-terminal-truncated PrP isoform is present in mature sperm. *J Biol Chem*, **274**, 32153–8.

Shlomchik, M.J., Radebold, K., et al. 2001. Neuroinvasion by a Creutzfeldt–Jakob disease agent in the absence of B cells and follicular dendritic cells. *Proc Natl Acad Sci U S A*, **98**, 9289–94.

Shyng, S.L., Heuser, J.E. and Harris, D.A. 1994. A glycolipid-anchored prion protein is endocytosed via clathrin-coated pits. *J Cell Biol*, **125**, 1239–50.

Sigurdson, C.J., Williams, E.S., et al. 1999. Oral transmission and early lymphoid tropism of chronic wasting disease PrPres in mule deer fawns (*Odocoileus hemionus*). *J Gen Virol*, **80**, 2757–64.

Sigurdsson, E.M., Brown, D.R., et al. 2002. Immunization delays the onset of prion disease in mice. *Am J Pathol*, **161**, 13–17.

Silverman, G.L., Qin, K., et al. 2000. Doppel is an *N*-glycosylated, glycosylphosphatidylinositol-anchored protein. Expression in testis and ectopic production in the brains of Prnp$^{0/0}$ mice predisposed to Purkinje cell loss. *J Biol Chem*, **275**, 26834–41.

Soto, C., Kascsak, R.J., et al. 2000. Reversion of prion protein conformational changes by synthetic beta-sheet breaker peptides. *Lancet*, **355**, 192–7.

Souan, L., Tal, Y., et al. 2001. Modulation of proteinase-K resistant prion protein by prion peptide immunization. *Eur J Immunol*, **31**, 2338–46.

Sparkes, R.S., Simon, M., et al. 1986. Assignment of the human and mouse prion protein genes to homologous chromosomes. *Proc Natl Acad Sci U S A*, **83**, 7358–62.

Spraker, T.R., Miller, M.W., et al. 1997. Spongiform encephalopathy in free-ranging mule deer (*Odocoileus hemionus*), white-tailed deer (*Odocoileus virginianus*) and Rocky Mountain elk (*Cervus elaphus nelsoni*) in northcentral Colorado. *J Wildl Dis*, **33**, 1–6.

Spudich, S., Mastrianni, J.A., et al. 1995. Complete penetrance of Creutzfeldt–Jakob disease in Libyan Jews carrying the E200K mutation in the prion protein gene. *Mol Med*, **1**, 607–13.

Stahl, N., Borchelt, D.R., et al. 1987. Scrapie prion protein contains a phosphatidylinositol glycolipid. *Cell*, **51**, 229–40.

Stahl, N., Baldwin, M.A., et al. 1992. Glycosylinositol phospholipid anchors of the scrapie and cellular prion proteins contain sialic acid. *Biochemistry*, **31**, 5043–53.

Stahl, N., Baldwin, M.A., et al. 1993. Structural studies of the scrapie prion protein using mass spectrometry and amino acid sequencing. *Biochemistry*, **32**, 1991–2002.

Stender, A. 1930. Weitere Beiträge zum Kapitel 'Spastische Pseudosklerose Jakobs'. *Z Neurol Psychiatr*, **128**, 528–43.

Strumbo, B., Ronchi, S., et al. 2001. Molecular cloning of the cDNA coding for *Xenopus laevis* prion protein. *FEBS Lett*, **508**, 170–4.

Supattapone, S., Wille, H., et al. 2001. Branched polyamines cure prion-infected neuroblastoma cells. *J Virol*, **75**, 3453–61.

Szakal, A.K. and Hanna, M.G. Jr 1968. The ultrastructure of antigen localization and viruslike particles in mouse spleen germinal centers. *Exp Mol Pathol*, **8**, 75–89.

Szakal, A.K., Kapasi, Z.F., et al. 1995. Multiple lines of evidence favoring a bone marrow derivation of follicular dendritic cells (FDCs). *Adv Exp Med Biol*, **378**, 267–72.

Tagliavini, F., Prelli, F., et al. 1991. Amyloid protein of Gerstmann–Straussler–Scheinker disease (Indiana kindred) is an 11 kd fragment of prion protein with an N-terminal glycine at codon 58. *EMBO J*, **10**, 513–19.

Tagliavini, F., Prelli, F., et al. 1994. Amyloid fibrils in Gerstmann–Straussler–Scheinker disease (Indiana and Swedish kindreds) express only PrP peptides encoded by the mutant allele. *Cell*, **79**, 695–703.

Tagliavini, F., McArthur, R.A., et al. 1997. Effectiveness of anthracycline against experimental prion disease in Syrian hamsters. *Science*, **276**, 1119–22.

Takai, T., Li, M., et al. 1994. FcR gamma chain deletion results in pleiotrophic effector cell defects. *Cell*, **76**, 519–29.

Takai, T., Ono, M., et al. 1996. Augmented humoral and anaphylactic responses in Fc gamma RII-deficient mice. *Nature*, **379**, 346–9.

Tange, R.A., Troost, D. and Limburg, M. 1989. Progressive fatal dementia (Creutzfeldt–Jakob disease) in a patient who received homograft tissue for tympanic membrane closure. *Eur Arch Otorhinolaryngol*, **247**, 199–201.

Taraboulos, A., Rogers, M., et al. 1990a. Acquisition of protease resistance by prion proteins in scrapie-infected cells does not require asparagine-linked glycosylation. *Proc Natl Acad Sci U S A*, **87**, 8262–6.

Taraboulos, A., Serban, D. and Prusiner, S.B. 1990b. Scrapie prion proteins accumulate in the cytoplasm of persistently infected cultured cells. *J Cell Biol*, **110**, 2117–32.

Taraboulos, A., Jendroska, K., et al. 1992a. Regional mapping of prion proteins in brain. *Proc Natl Acad Sci U S A*, **89**, 7620–4.

Taraboulos, A., Raeber, A.J., et al. 1992b. Synthesis and trafficking of prion proteins in cultured cells. *Mol Biol Cell*, **3**, 851–63.

Taraboulos, A., Scott, M., et al. 1995. Cholesterol depletion and modification of COOH-terminal targeting sequence of the prion protein inhibit formation of the scrapie isoform. *J Cell Biol*, **129**, 121–32.

Tateishi, J. and Kitamoto, T. 1993. Developments in diagnosis for prion diseases. *Br Med Bull*, **49**, 971–9.

Tateishi, J., Ohta, M., et al. 1979. Transmission of chronic spongiform encephalopathy with kuru plaques from humans to small rodents. *Ann Neurol*, **5**, 581–4.

Tateishi, J., Doh-ura, K., et al. 1992a. Prion protein gene analysis and transmission studies of Creutzfeldt–Jakob disease. In: Prusiner, S.B., Collinge, J., et al. (eds), *Prion diseases of humans and animals*. London: Ellis Horwood, 129–34.

Tateishi, J., Kitamoto, T., et al. 1992b. Creutzfeldt–Jakob disease with amyloid angiopathy: diagnosis by immunological analyses and transmission experiments. *Acta Neuropathol Berl*, **83**, 559–63.

Taylor, D.M., Dickinson, A.G., et al. 1985. Preparation of growth hormone free from contamination with unconventional slow viruses. *Lancet*, **2**, 260–2.

Taylor, D.M., McConnell, I. and Fraser, H. 1996. Scrapie infection can be established readily through skin scarification in immunocompetent but not immunodeficient mice. *J Gen Virol*, **77**, 1595–9.

Telling, G.C., Scott, M., et al. 1994. Transmission of Creutzfeldt–Jakob disease from humans to transgenic mice expressing chimeric human-mouse prion protein. *Proc Natl Acad Sci USA*, **91**, 9936–40.

Telling, G.C., Scott, M., et al. 1995. Prion propagation in mice expressing human and chimeric PrP transgenes implicates the interaction of cellular PrP with another protein. *Cell*, **83**, 79–90.

Telling, G.C., Haga, T., et al. 1996. Interactions between wild-type and mutant prion proteins modulate neurodegeneration in transgenic mice. *Genes Dev*, **10**, 1736–50.

Thadani, V., Penar, P.L., et al. 1988. Creutzfeldt–Jakob disease probably acquired from a cadaveric dura mater graft. Case report. *J Neurosurg*, **69**, 766–9.

Tintner, R., Brown, P., et al. 1986. Neuropathologic verification of Creutzfeldt–Jakob disease in the exhumed American recipient of human pituitary growth hormone: epidemiologic and pathogenetic implications. *Neurology*, **36**, 932–6.

Tobler, I., Gaus, S.E., et al. 1996. Altered circadian activity rhythms and sleep in mice devoid of prion protein. *Nature*, **380**, 639–42.

Udovitch, A.L. and Valensi, L. 1984. *The last Arab Jews: the communities of Jerba, Tunisia*. London: Harwood Academic.

Valleron, A.J., Boelle, P.Y., et al. 2001. Estimation of epidemic size and incubation time based on age characteristics of vCJD in the United Kingdom. *Science*, **294**, 1726–8.

Vankeulen, L.J.M., Schreuder, B.E.C., et al. 1996. Immunohistochemical detection of prion protein in lymphoid tissues of sheep with natural scrapie. *J Clin Microbiol*, **34**, 1228–31.

Vnencak Jones, C.L. and Phillips, J.A. 1992. Identification of heterogeneous PrP gene deletions in controls by detection of allele-specific heteroduplexes (DASH). *Am J Hum Genet*, **50**, 871–2.

Wadsworth, J.D., Hill, A.F., et al. 1999. Strain-specific prion-protein conformation determined by metal ions. *Nat Cell Biol*, **1**, 55–9.

Wadsworth, J.D.F., Joiner, S., et al. 2001. Tissue distribution of protease resistant prion protein in variant CJD using a highly sensitive immuno-blotting assay. *Lancet*, **358**, 171–80.

Waggoner, D.J., Drisaldi, B., et al. 2000. Brain copper content and cuproenzyme activity do not vary with prion protein expression level. *J Biol Chem*, **275**, 7455–8.

Wagner, N., Lohler, J., et al. 1996. Critical role for beta7 integrins in formation of the gut-associated lymphoid tissue. *Nature*, **382**, 366–70.

Ware, C.F., VanArsdale, T.L., et al. 1995. The ligands and receptors of the lymphotoxin system. *Curr Top Microbiol Immunol*, **198**, 175–218.

Wassarman, P.M., Jovine, L. and Litscher, E.S. 2001. A profile of fertilization in mammals. *Nat Cell Biol*, **3**, E59–64.

Watarai, M., Kim, S., et al. 2003. Cellular prion protein promotes *Brucella* infection into macrophages. *J Exp Med*, **198**, 5–17.

Weissmann, C. 1991a. Spongiform encephalopathies. The prion's progress. *Nature*, **349**, 569–71.

Weissmann, C. 1991b. A 'unified theory' of prion propagation. *Nature*, **352**, 679–83.

Weissmann, C. and Aguzzi, A. 1997. Bovine spongiform encephalopathy and early onset variant Creutzfeldt–Jakob disease. *Curr Opin Neurobiol*, **7**, 695–700.

Weissmann, C. and Aguzzi, A. 1999. Perspectives: neurobiology. PrP's double causes trouble. *Science*, **286**, 914–15.

Weissmann, C., Fischer, M., et al. 1998. The use of transgenic mice in the investigation of transmissible spongiform encephalopathies. *Rev Sci Tech*, **17**, 278–90.

Wells, G.A., Scott, A.C., et al. 1987. A novel progressive spongiform encephalopathy in cattle. *Vet Rec*, **121**, 419–20.

Wells, G.A., Dawson, M., et al. 1994. Infectivity in the ileum of cattle challenged orally with bovine spongiform encephalopathy. *Vet Rec*, **135**, 40–1.

Wells, G.A., Hawkins, S.A., et al. 1998. Preliminary observations on the pathogenesis of experimental bovine spongiform encephalopathy (BSE): an update. *Vet Rec*, **142**, 103–6.

Westaway, D. and Carlson, G.A. 2002. Mammalian prion proteins: enigma, variation and vaccination. *Trends Biochem Sci*, **27**, 301–7.

Westaway, D., Goodman, P.A., et al. 1987. Distinct prion proteins in short and long scrapie incubation period mice. *Cell*, **51**, 651–62.

Westaway, D., Mirenda, C.A., et al. 1991. Paradoxical shortening of scrapie incubation times by expression of prion protein transgenes derived from long incubation period mice. *Neuron*, **7**, 59–68.

Westaway, D., Cooper, C., et al. 1994a. Structure and polymorphism of the mouse prion protein gene. *Proc Natl Acad Sci U S A*, **91**, 6418–22.

Westaway, D., Zuliani, V., et al. 1994b. Homozygosity for prion protein alleles encoding glutamine-171 renders sheep susceptible to natural scrapie. *Genes Dev*, **8**, 959–69.

White, A.R., Enever, P., et al. 2003. Monoclonal antibodies inhibit prion replication and delay the development of prion disease. *Nature*, **422**, 80–3.

Whittington, M.A., Sidle, K.C., et al. 1995. Rescue of neurophysiological phenotype seen in PrP null mice by transgene encoding human prion protein. *Nat Genet*, **9**, 197–201.

Wickner, R.B. 1994. [URE3] as an altered URE2 protein: evidence for a prion analog in *Saccharomyces cerevisiae*. *Science*, **264**, 566–9.

Wilesmith, J.W. and Wells, G.A. 1991. Bovine spongiform encephalopathy. *Curr Top Microbiol Immunol*, **172**, 21–38.

Wilesmith, J.W., Wells, G.A., et al. 1988. Bovine spongiform encephalopathy: epidemiological studies. *Vet Rec*, **123**, 638–44.

Wilesmith, J.W., Hoinville, L.J., et al. 1992a. Bovine spongiform encephalopathy: aspects of the clinical picture and analyses of possible changes 1986–1990. *Vet Rec*, **130**, 197–201.

Wilesmith, J.W., Ryan, J.B., et al. 1992b. Bovine spongiform encephalopathy: epidemiological features 1985 to 1990. *Vet Rec*, **130**, 90–4.

Will, R. and Zeidler, M. 1996. Diagnosing Creutzfeldt–Jakob disease – case identification depends on neurological and neuropathological assessment. *BMJ*, **313**, 833–4.

Will, R.G. and Matthews, W.B. 1982. Evidence for case-to-case transmission of Creutzfeldt–Jakob disease. *J Neurol Neurosurg Psychiatry*, **45**, 235–8.

Will, R.G., Ironside, J.W., et al. 1996. A new variant of Creutzfeldt–Jakob disease in the UK. *Lancet*, **347**, 921–5.

Will, R.G., Zeidler, M., et al. 2000. Diagnosis of new variant Creutzfeldt–Jakob disease. *Ann Neurol*, **47**, 575–82.

Wille, H., Michelitsch, M.D., et al. 2002. Structural studies of the scrapie prion protein by electron crystallography. *Proc Natl Acad Sci USA*, **99**, 3563–8.

Williams, E.S. and Young, S. 1980. Chronic wasting disease of captive mule deer: a spongiform encephalopathy. *J Wildl Dis*, **16**, 89–98.

Williams, E.S. and Young, S. 1982. Spongiform encephalopathy of Rocky Mountain elk. *J Wildl Dis*, **18**, 465–71.

Williams, E.S. and Young, S. 1992. Spongiform encephalopathies in Cervidae. *Rev Sci Tech*, **11**, 551–67.

Williams, E.S. and Young, S. 1993. Neuropathology of chronic wasting disease of mule deer (*Odocoileus hemionus*) and elk (*Cervus elaphus nelsoni*). *Vet Pathol*, **30**, 36–45.

Williams, R.C. 1954. Electron microscopy of viruses. *Adv Virus Res*, **2**, 183–239.

Willison, H.J., Gale, A.N. and McLaughlin, J.E. 1991. Creutzfeldt-Jacob disease following cadaveric dura mater graft. *J Neurol Neurosurg Psychiatry*, **54**, 940, [letter].

Willoughby, K., Kelly, D.F., et al. 1992. Spongiform encephalopathy in a captive puma (*Felis concolor*). *Vet Rec*, **131**, 431–4.

Wilson, D.R., Anderson, R.D. and Smith, W. 1950. Studies in scrapie. *J Comp Pathol*, **60**, 267–82.

Wisniewski, H.M., Sigurdarson, S., et al. 1996. Mites as vectors for scrapie. *Lancet*, **347**, 1114, [letter].

Wu, X., Jiang, N., et al. 2000. Impaired affinity maturation in Cr2-/- mice is rescued by adjuvants without improvement in germinal center development. *J Immunol*, **165**, 3119–27.

Yehiely, F., Bamborough, P., et al. 1997. Identification of candidate proteins binding to prion protein. Erratum in *Neurobiol Dis*, **3**, 339–55. *Neurobiol Dis*, **10**, 67–8.

Zanata, S.M., Lopes, M.H., et al. 2002. Stress-inducible protein 1 is a cell surface ligand for cellular prion that triggers neuroprotection. *EMBO J*, **21**, 3307–16.

Zanusso, G., Nardelli, E., et al. 1998. Simultaneous occurrence of spongiform encephalopathy in a man and his cat in Italy. *Lancet*, **352**, 1116–17, [letter].

Zanusso, G., Ferrari, S., et al. 2003. Detection of pathologic prion protein in the olfactory epithelium in sporadic Creutzfeldt–Jakob disease. *N Engl J Med*, **348**, 711–19.

Zhang, H., Kaneko, K., et al. 1995. Conformational transitions in peptides containing two putative alpha-helices of the prion protein. *J Mol Biol*, **250**, 514–26..

PART III

SYNDROMES CAUSED BY A RANGE OF VIRUSES

62

Infections of the central nervous system

JÜRGEN SCHNEIDER-SCHAULIES, SIBYLLE SCHNEIDER-SCHAULIES, AND
VOLKER TER MEULEN

INTRODUCTION

Viral infections of the central nervous system (CNS) represent clinically important, often life-threatening complications of systemic viral infections. Except for rabies, they do not result per se from a pathogen-specific tropism for neural tissue, as most viruses associated with CNS disorders frequently infect humans without involving this organ. Some of these viruses cause clinically significant diseases only when invasion of the CNS takes place, for example certain entero- or arthropod-borne viruses. Other agents, such as herpes simplex or mumps viruses, usually induce a mild illness, which may follow a more severe course when the CNS is infected. The establishment of a CNS viral infection depends not only on the biological properties of the invading agent but also on the breakdown of the host defense mechanisms that normally protect CNS cells from infection. Moreover, the degree of damage to CNS tissues is influenced by several special features that set the CNS apart from other tissues. Brain cells are not unusual in their fine structure, but they are unique in the high degree of cell differentiation and the interaction between cell types, as revealed by the synapses between neurons and the relationship between myelin sheath and axons. These peculiarities, together with the existence of a blood–brain barrier (BBB) in the absence of lymphatic tissue in the CNS, play a major role in the development of neurological disease.

Virological, immunological, and molecular biological studies have provided important information on the etiology and pathogenesis of many acute and chronic disorders of the CNS associated with viral infections of animals and humans. In addition, information obtained from in vitro studies of infected neural cells in culture has helped our understanding of the processes involved in a wide range of virus-induced neurological diseases. Although many unresolved problems still remain, great progress has been made in molecular virology and neuroimmunology. Many sensitive techniques have been developed that allow a better characterization of the virus–cell and virus–host interactions occurring in CNS infections.

Rather than give a complete account of all virus infections of the CNS, this chapter is intended to give an overview of the most common human viral CNS disorders and to promote insights that may emerge by comparing this aspect of human diseases. The single viral agents and their corresponding (peripheral) diseases are dealt with separately in specific chapters.

INTERACTIONS OF VIRUSES WITH THE HUMAN CNS

Pathways of virus spread to the nervous system

Successful infection of the CNS by virus depends on a number of factors, and it is the direct interplay between the host's immune system in controlling or attenuating infection on the one hand, and the neurotropism and neurovirulence of the infecting virus on the other, that has profound consequences for the host. Virus invasion of the CNS can be established via any of the commonly recognized routes for infection: vector-borne, fecal–oral, direct contact and aerosol.

VECTOR-BORNE

The most common route of infection associated with severe disorders of the CNS is via the bite of an infected arthropod vector which delivers virus inoculum through the dead keratinized layer of the skin into the dermis or bloodstream. Viruses belonging to the families *Alphaviridae*, *Bunyaviridae*, and *Flaviviridae* are usually transmitted to humans through the bite of an infected mosquito or tick, after the virus has replicated to high titers in the salivary glands of the insect. A number of the arthropod-borne viruses (arboviruses) are highly pathogenic and the CNS is often involved. Of the viruses commonly associated with CNS disease, Japanese encephalitis virus, a Flavivirus, is the most important, with thousands of reported infections each year and an associated case fatality rate of about 10 percent (see section on Japanese encephalitis). Infection with arboviruses is limited geographically and seasonally to conditions that support the virus vector.

FECAL–ORAL

The fecal–oral route has long been established as an important mode of transmission of numerous enteroviruses, and classically with epidemics of poliomyelitis. Enteric viruses, which replicate primarily in the alimentary tract, are shed in fecal matter, which in turn may contaminate food and water supplies, particularly in areas of poor sanitation. These viruses are able to resist and survive gastric acidity. Enteric viruses are responsible for large epidemics of disease which, unlike the arboviruses mentioned above, are not restricted geographically. In Europe enteroviruses are the leading cause of CNS disturbances, although 90 percent of these infections are clinically inapparent. Of the remainder, symptoms may range from paralytic poliomyelitis to nonparalytic meningitis, as well as the more rare encephalitides.

DIRECT CONTACT

Direct contact (sexual, prenatal, or by mechanical means, e.g. by needle, bite), as a mode of transmission for a number of viruses that cause CNS disease, is by nature a particularly emotive subject. Infection by direct contact involves the transfer of virus-infected cells or body fluids. These viruses include human immunodeficiency virus (HIV), herpes simplex virus (HSV), rabies virus, and *Cytomegalovirus* (CMV). More rarely, infection of the (CNS) with rabies virus or CMV has been reported following corneal tissue grafts. Vertical transfer of virus from mother to fetus, commonly HSV, CMV, rubella, human T-lymphotropic virus type I (HTLV-I) and HIV, may lead to severe CNS disease in newborns. In addition, breastfeeding by infected mothers is associated with HTLV-I, HIV and CMV infections in newborns.

AEROSOL

Establishment of CNS infection via the respiratory tract is not widely recognized as a common event. The exception to this generalization is mumps virus, when, during epidemics of parotitis, about 0.1–10 percent of infected individuals develop quite severe meningitis. Infection of the CNS by rabies virus has been documented following the inhalation of virus-laden aerosols by visitors to bat caves, where the virus is maintained in the bat population, or in laboratory workers exposed to high concentrations of virus. Aerosols may also be associated with the transmission of other potentially neurotropic pathogens, such as measles virus and varicella-zoster virus.

Regardless of the site of entry, for successful infection of the host by a virus a period of replication at this initial site is required, and the virus must also evade the local immune response. The possible exception to the above concerns arthropod-borne viruses, which are often inoculated directly into the bloodstream and initial replication is usually established in lymphatic tissue. Replication of virus at the site of entry or in lymphatic tissue increases the viral load and allows the establishment of viremia. Once in the bloodstream, virus is able to disseminate throughout the host and infection of susceptible secondary organs and tissues can take place. The ability of the immune system to terminate virus infection rapidly before significant viremia levels are reached largely dictates the outcome of a number of potential viral diseases of the CNS. Two main routes for the invasion of the CNS by virus are recognized: hematogenous and neural.

Entry into the CNS

THE HEMATOGENOUS ROUTE

The bloodstream, with its extensive network of vessels serving every part of the body, forms the perfect dissemination vehicle for invading viruses. The extent to which tissues and organs become exposed to virus depends on the length of time that a high viral load is maintained in the bloodstream and the efficiency with which the immune system can clear virus. Whether infection will be established by the virus depends on a number of factors, including the presence of specific cellular receptors for that virus. Before virus can enter the CNS, the so-called blood–brain barrier must be circumvented (Zhang 1999). The BBB comprises endothelial cells of the cerebral microvasculature, pericytes, astrocyte foot processes, and the basal lamina, which together are a formidable barrier (Pardridge 1999; Miller 1999). However, the CNS is accessible to activated lymphocytes and macrophages which, if infected with virus, afford access to this normally protected environment (Persidsky 1999). Circumvention of the BBB by the transport of virus within infected cells is thought to be highly significant for CNS infection with mumps and measles viruses (Wolinsky et al. 1976; Fournier et al. 1985) and HIV (Haase 1986). Direct measles virus infection of the endothelial cells of the BBB is commonly found in patients suffering from subacute sclerosing panencephalitis (SSPE) (Allen et al. 1996). The choroid plexus is widely believed to be an important portal of entry for bloodborne virus to the CNS. This is based largely on the fine structure analysis of the choroid plexus itself, in which fenestrated endothelium and a sparse basement membrane combine to form a more permeable region. The choroid plexus is a major target of replication or transport of mumps and arboviruses, which subsequently infect ependymal cells lining the ventricles and finally the underlying brain tissue.

THE NEURAL ROUTE

A number of viruses establish CNS infection by directly infecting nerves of the CNS. Viruses such as HSV, poliovirus, and rabies (Sabin 1956; Martin and Dolvio 1983; Iwasaki et al. 1985) infect peripheral nerve endings and, by retrograde axonal transport, spread through the CNS. Entry into neurons is believed to occur via receptor-mediated endocytosis, after which virus is transported in vesicles. The exact mechanism of transport of virus within nerves remains to be established, although movement is known to occur via fast axonal transport (Kristensson 1982), which involves the passage of viral material in vesicles along microtubules. Viral replication occurs once virus particles reach the neuronal cell body and newly synthesized virion components accumulate at postsynaptic sites. The site of inoculation can influence the ultimate distribution of lesions in the CNS, especially for viruses that spread along neural routes. For example, HSV infection of the genitourinary tract establishes latency of virus in the sacral ganglia, whereas infection with HSV orally establishes latency in the trigeminal ganglia. At the time of primary infection, HSV is transported from the mucous membrane by retrograde axonal transport, whereas during periods of reactivation virus is transported to the periphery by anterograde flow. Once the CNS has been invaded, advancement of infection by many neurotropic viruses occurs through cell-to-cell spread (trans-synaptic transport).

The factors influencing the release of virus from presynaptic nerve terminals and the uptake of progeny at postsynaptic terminals are unknown. It is important to note that direct infection of peripheral nerve endings by virus may also take place during the viremic phase of an infection. For example, during the high-titer viremia found in clinically apparent infections of humans with the *Flavivirus* Japanese encephalitis virus (JEV), the possibility that neurons of the olfactory bulb will be infected is enhanced. Retrograde transport of virus within specialized neurons is then possible. The olfactory mucosa itself offers a unique pathway for the spread of viruses into the CNS, where the apical processes of receptor cells penetrate beyond the surface of the epithelium as olfactory rods. However, olfactory uptake and spread is not a common route of virus infection of the CNS (Johnston 1994). Once in the CNS, the cellular tropism and neurovirulence of virus and its ability to avoid the immune response will largely determine the outcome of disease.

Tropism and neurovirulence

CELLULAR RECEPTORS AND HOST FACTORS

The ability of a virus to infect specific cell populations of the CNS defines its neurotropism, which is influenced either by host cell expression of receptors or by genes important for viral replication. In general, the distribution of specific cellular receptors for viruses within a host governs the susceptibility of tissue(s) or organs to virus infection. In recent years, many cell surface proteins have been identified as viral receptors that normally serve various physiological functions (Schneider-Schaulies 2000; Schweighardt and Atwood 2001) (Table 62.1).

Besides the viral receptor the virus attachment protein itself plays a central role in the initial interaction of the virus with its target cell. Numerous virus–cell attachment proteins have been identified by analysis of genetic recombinants, genetic reassortants, and mutant viruses (Kennedy 1990). This approach has been used, for example, to define the neurotropism of serotype 3 reovirus, which has been mapped to the *S1* gene that encodes the σ1 protein (Tyler 1991). Similarly, neutralization escape mutants of rabies virus, with a single amino acid substitution in the envelope glycoprotein G that serves in viral cell attachment, revealed a lower virulence than the parent virus (Tyler 1990). A more detailed molecular view of a ligand in virus receptor–molecular interactions was obtained with the X-ray crystallographic analysis of the poliovirus virion. The analysis revealed that a series of peaks in the VP1 capsid proteins surrounded by a broad valley composed of VP1 and VP3 forms the receptor-binding pocket (Almond 1991). It is thought that other picornaviruses may have cell attachment proteins of similar topology. An exception to this is foot-and-mouth disease virus (FMDV), an aphthovirus, for which the virus attachment protein

Table 62.1 *Examples of viruses associated with CNS disease and their receptors*

Virus (family)	Receptor	References
Flaviviridae		
Tick-borne encephalitis virus (TBEV)	Heparan sulfate	Mandl et al. 2001
Lentiviridae		
HIV-1, 2	CD4	Dalgleish et al. 1984; Klatzmann et al. 1984
HIV-1	Galactosylceramide	Harouse et al. 1991
	Chemokine receptors	Berger et al. 1999
Herpesviridae		
CMV	Heparan sulfate	Compton et al. 1993
HSV	Heparan sulfate, HveA, -B, -C	WuDunn and Spear 1989; Montgomery et al. 1996; Geraghty et al. 1998
Human herpesvirus-6	CD46	Santoro et al. 1999
Paramyxoviridae		
Measles virus	Membrane cofactor protein (CD46) Signaling lymphocytic activation molecule (CD150)	Dörig et al. 1993; Naniche et al. 1993; Tatsuo et al. 2000
Picornaviridae		
Polioviruses	PVR (CD155) (immunoglobulin-like)	Koike et al. 1990; Mendelsohn et al. 1989
Echovirus 1, 8	VLA-2 (α-chain, integrin)	Bergelson et al. 1992; Bergelson and Finberg 1993
Echovirus 22	$\alpha_v\beta_3$ (integrin)	Roivainen et al. 1991
Echovirus 7 (6, 11, 12, 20, 21?)	Decay-accelerating factor (CD55)	Bergelson et al. 1994
Rhabdoviridae		
Rabies virus	Acetylcholine receptor (α_{-1}) Neural cell adhesion molecule (NCAM) Nerve growth factor receptor (NGFR)	Lentz 1990; Thoulouze et al. 1998; Tuffereau et al. 1998

(VAP) is exposed on VP1 (Mason et al. 1994). Mutations occurring in the VAP may be responsible for altered tropism of the virus, or even defective virus that is no longer able to bind to its receptor. This may be manifested by attenuation of virus infectivity, and is thought to be important in relation to the immunogenicity of vaccines.

In further attempts to unravel which factors govern the neurovirulence of poliovirus, a combination of nucleotide sequencing and gene cloning identified the genetic differences between wildtype and live attenuated vaccine strains (Almond 1991). Of the changes detected, the most significant were localized in the 5′ nontranslated region (NTR) at positions 480, 481, and 472 of poliovirus serotypes 1, 2, and 3, respectively. These mutations were associated with the ability of the virus to replicate in the brains of mice or neuroblastoma cells in culture (La Monica et al. 1987). A more detailed investigation of both the structure and the related function of mutated 5′ NTR regions of poliovirus revealed that attenuating mutations in vaccine strains act through the disruption of a stem–loop structure in the region of nucleotide positions 470–540. Computer-generated analysis has hinted that the greater the disruption of the system structure, the greater the temperature sensitivity

and the degree of attenuation. Further analysis of the intracellular protein interactions associated with this poliovirus stem–loop structure may provide an explanation of why motor neurons are the specific targets of these viruses.

In addition to viral factors, host factors also influence viral tropism and virulence and modulate the viral pathogenesis of CNS infections. In this context, a lack of enzymatic activity required for maturational cleavage of viral proteins, or completion of the virus replicating cycles, will lead to incomplete infection of target cells, thereby limiting tropism and spread of the virus. On the other hand, this may facilitate the establishment of a persistent infection, as has been demonstrated in the case of SSPE (Billeter et al. 1994). Moreover, it has been observed that many neurotropic viruses more readily invade the CNS of the young, owing to an immature immune response, reduced capacity to produce interferon, and dependence of the susceptibility of viral infection on the stage of cell differentiation, as well as the age-specific nature and distribution of receptor proteins (Coyle 1991). Bias of infection for a particular gender has also been noted. The CNS disorder tropical spastic paraparesis/HTLV-I associated myelopathy (TSP/HAM), for which HTLV-I is the proposed etiological agent, has a prevalence in females, with a female:male ratio of 1.6:1.

Neurovirulence and viral gene expression

Neurovirulence is the capacity of a virus to multiply and to extend infection after it has invaded the nervous system. This property, together with the effectiveness of the host immune response, determines the degree of tissue damage. Point mutations in envelope proteins of several viruses have been shown to influence neurovirulence in animal models. Some examples are Sindbis virus (Lee et al. 2002), murine coronavirus (Philips et al. 2002), measles virus (Moeller et al. 2001), and yellow fever virus/Japanese encephalitis virus chimera (Arroyo et al. 2001).

Many viruses contain nontranscribed genetic elements, referred to as promoters or enhancers, that regulate the transcription of specific genes. It is interesting that virus enhancers may exhibit cell or tissue specificity, and possibly species specificity, thus promoting or limiting virus infection. Important roles for viral enhancer elements in determining cell type-specific gene expression have also been described for picornaviruses. In the poliovirus-induced pathogenesis the internal ribosomal entry site (IRES) plays an important role for neurovirulence (Ohka and Nomoto 2001).

The available data suggest that, in general, the outer capsid or envelope glycoproteins of neurotropic viruses are probably important determinants of virulence. This assumption is based, for instance, on the observation that amino acid sequence changes – of proteins, or genetic reassortments between virulent and avirulent strains of a given neurotropic virus – can lead to an attenuated infection. On the other hand, not all changes in viral genes result in attenuation, as mutations causing reversions to neurovirulence have been seen in poliovirus isolates from vaccine recipients (Almond 1987). Moreover, when one region of a viral protein is linked to neurotropism and neurovirulence, changes in that protein could have dramatic effects on the resulting infections, as documented in studies of Theiler's murine encephalomyelitis virus infections (Nash 1991). Usually not only one gene contributes to the neurovirulence of a virus, as found for example for Theiler's virus, in which mutations of the envelope proteins, as well as the polymerase, influence the outcome of the disease (Reddi and Lipton, 2002; van Eyll and Michiels 2000). Taken together, the interplay of host and viral factors determines the tropism and virulence of viruses that infect the CNS.

Virus–cell interactions in the CNS

The interaction of infectious viruses with susceptible cells leads in general to cell destruction, and is largely determined by the genetic constitution of the host cell and by the type of viral agent. This destruction can occur following cytolysis, persistent or even latent infection, cell transformation, or be caused by infection-independent mechanisms. After infectious virus has reached the CNS, disease develops only if viral spread is accomplished and sufficient numbers of susceptible cells are infected, resulting in brain dysfunction. In this respect, a number of unique features of the CNS are noteworthy. First, the CNS contains a highly differentiated cell population, with complex functionally integrated cell-to-cell connections and highly specialized cytoplasmic membranes. This probably results in the great variability in virus receptor sites and their density on cells. Second, CNS tissue is unique in its high metabolic rate and a low regenerative capacity. Although persistent infection by a noncytopathic virus in cells of tissue with a low energy requirement and a high rate of regeneration may be tolerated, in CNS tissue such infections may interfere with normal cell functions, especially when neurons are affected. Third, the brain's relative isolation from the immune system is another feature that plays an important role in the establishment and pathogenesis of CNS infections.

ACUTE INFECTIONS

Acute infections lead to cell death and the release of progeny virus. Cell destruction is induced by the products of the viral genome or their effect on the regulatory mechanism of the cell. For some viruses, such as herpes and polio viruses, the molecular events during a lytic infection have been well described for tissue culture systems, and it may be inferred that similar processes occur during CNS infections. One of the most severe acute viral infections of the CNS is caused by herpes simplex virus (HSV), which results mainly from the primary infection. Productive replication in brain tissue leads to cell destruction, which in its extent and pathology depends on the neuroinvasiveness and neurovirulence of the virus and on the effectiveness of the host defense mechanisms. Extensive molecular biological studies have defined several regions on the viral genome as specific contributors to these processes (Stevens 1993). Among the HSV genes, 37 seem not to be necessary for HSV replication in tissue culture, and are referred to as 'supplemental essential genes.' They may be linked to the properties of neuroinvasiveness and neurovirulence by allowing the virus to invade the CNS, to replicate in a variety of different brain cells, and to spread efficiently from cell to cell. Another destructive disease of nervous tissue occurs after poliovirus infection (Melnick 1990). Following primary replication of poliovirus in the tonsils, the lymph nodes of the neck, and Peyer's patches in the small intestine, the virus spreads along the axons of peripheral nerves, and may invade the spinal cord and brain. Here, neuronal tissue can be damaged or completely destroyed as a consequence of intracellular replication. The anterior and, in severe cases, the posterior horn cells of the spinal cord are most prominently involved, resulting in a flaccid paralysis (see Chapter 40, Picornaviruses).

PERSISTENT INFECTIONS

Within the group of viruses that can establish persistent infections, a variety of virus–cell and virus–host interactions exist that lead to a number of different disease processes:

- Latent viral infections are characterized by long periods of pretended viral absence followed by intermittent episodes of viral replication and the formation of infectious virus (recurrence). This may either remain clinically silent or result in clinical disease (recrudescence). During latency, the virus remains within the host in a quiescent form.
- In chronic viral infections virus can be reproducibly and continuously recovered from the host, with or without the development of clinical disease. Disease may be caused by the replication of virus or by immunopathological mechanisms.
- In slow virus infections, a long incubation period of months to years is followed by a slow, progressive disease course that is usually fatal. The concentration of virus in the CNS increases until disease becomes clinically apparent.

The establishment and maintenance of persistent infections in the CNS may be governed by viral factors or host cell factors, or both, depending on the individual virus–host-cell relationships. As a general mechanism, virus-induced apoptosis may be an important pathogenic mechanism of CNS damage. On the other hand, virus-mediated inhibition of the apoptotic pathway has been linked to the establishment of persistent infections in brain cells (Levine et al. 1991). In the human nervous system, only the latent and the slow virus type of infection are found. The classic latent infection is caused by HSV types 1 and 2. HSV is transmitted from human to human by skin or mucous membrane contact, and is able to remain latent in the nervous system for the lifetime of the host. Its occurrence is not restricted to sensory neurons, and it has also been detected in neurons of peripheral nerve ganglia, the adrenal medulla, the retina and the CNS (Stevens 1993). The establishment of the latent phase is controlled and executed by the neuron rather than by the virus itself, and HSV gene expression is almost completely abolished except for the expression of a set of so-called latency-associated transcripts (LAT)(Taylor et al. 2002). No infectious virus can be isolated during latency. Although the underlying molecular events that trigger viral reactivation are still unknown, clinical observations indicate that recurrence is associated with physical or emotional stress, immune suppression, UV light, or nerve damage. HSV in latently infected neurons is refractive to the immune system and cannot be cleared from those cells. The role of the immune system in controlling HSV infection is not entirely clear, because recurrences can be observed even in the presence of an apparently normal cell-mediated and humoral immune response. Although there seems to be no impact on nerve function during silent periods of latency, reactivation of HSV leads to the destruction of infected neurons.

The best-studied slow virus disease of humans associated with a conventional virus is subacute sclerosing panencephalitis SSPE (ter Meulen et al. 1983). The disease develops after the establishment of a persistent measles virus infection in brain cells months to years after acute measles. How and when the virus reaches the CNS, and the mechanisms that trigger the disease, remain unknown. In brain material obtained post mortem, the accumulation of viral nucleocapsids in virtually any CNS cell population, together with a general failure to reisolate infectious virus, points to the presence of a defective viral replication cycle (see below). In general, gene functions required for intracellular amplification of the viral genome are functionally maintained, whereas those associated with viral maturation and budding are highly restricted. This allows the virus to survive and replicate intracellularly while evading immune surveillance. In fact, an exceedingly high humoral immune response against measles virus proteins, except for the matrix (M) protein, in both serum and CSF of patients with SSPE is pathognomonic.

Infection-independent mechanisms

Experimental evidence suggests that some viruses may trigger apoptosis in neural cells, thereby leading to rapid destruction of the host cell before the virus is efficiently replicated (Levine et al. 1991). Viral invasion of the CNS may not always lead to infection of susceptible cells, but it may trigger pathological changes in the absence of viral spread. This is particularly important in parainfectious conditions, such as acute measles encephalitis, in which the presence of the infectious agent cannot be unequivocally demonstrated, or HIV, in which the infected CNS cells can support only minimal viral replication. As is apparent from tissue culture studies and animal experiments, HIV gene products such as gp120, tat, and nef, as well as soluble factors and nitric oxide released from virus-infected microglial cells, may contribute to the pathogenesis of HIV brain infections (Patrick et al. 2002). This occurs by the induction of neuronal damage and the functional impairment of both neuronal and macroglial cells that, per se, seem not to be susceptible to viral infection.

Viral impact on specific neural cell functions

The interaction of a virus with the CNS may cause severe dysfunction of the infected cell, even if only restricted areas of the CNS are involved. In rat astrocytoma cells persistently infected with measles virus, a strong reduction in the cAMP response to catecholamines was observed, the density of β-adrenergic receptors was decreased by 50 percent and their G protein coupling was affected (Halbach and Koschel 1979; Koschel and Münzel 1980). The endothelin-1-induced Ca^{2+} signal was absent in the same cells, 95 percent of the binding sites for endothelin-1 being lost (Tas and Koschel 1991).

A further example of the direct disturbance of brain cell functions is infection with rabies virus (RV). This virus causes a nonlytic infection of brain cells that rapidly eads to the death of the infected individual. In contrast to the limited cytopathology, death seems to result from interference of the virus with neuronal cell functions in vital centers of the brain that regulate sleep, body temperature, and respiration (Tsiang 1993). The uptake and release of γ-aminobutyric acid (GABA) was reduced by 45 percent in the cortical neurons of rabies-infected embryonic rats (Ladogana et al. 1994), and binding of 5-hydroxytryptamine to serotonin receptor subtypes was reduced by 50 percent in infected rat brains (Ceccaldi et al. 1993). It is conceivable that disturbances of specialized receptor sytems for neurotransmitter and neurohormone turnover, as well as for the generation of chemical signals and electrical potentials, might be the main cause of death in this viral infection, rather than cytopathic effects or immunopathogenesis.

Induction of cytokine and chemokine expression in the brain

Cytokines are produced in response to viral infection in the CNS and are secreted either from infected brain cells or from mononuclear cell infiltrates. Virus-induced cytokine patterns in CSF and in brain tissue of both humans and experimentally infected animals have been intensively studied. Although individual variations may be observed between different virus infections, there seems to be a common set of cytokines induced in the CNS, as in the periphery. These include type I (IFN-α/β) and type II (IFN-γ) interferons, the proinflammatory cytokines interleukin (IL)-1 and tumor necrosis factor (TNF)-α, IL-6, and, generally in lower amounts, IL-2 (Maudsley et al. 1989; Plata-Salaman 1991). For example, in the CSF of SSPE patients elevated levels of IFN-α/β are observed, and brain cells staining for IFN-γ and TNF-α have been detected in autopsy material (Neumann 2001; Joncas et al. 1976; Cosby et al. 1989; Hofman et al. 1991). In the brains of HIV-1 infected patients, where CD4+ microglial cells are the major cell population supporting viral replication, these cells are the source of intrathecal synthesis of IL-1, IL-6, granulocyte–macrophage colony-stimulating factor (GM-CSF), and TNF-α (Merrill and Chen 1991). In addition to the cytokines, a set of infection-induced chemokines attracts inflammatory mononuclear cells across the BBB. Besides lymphoid cells and endothelial cells, as neural cells microglia and astrocytes are the main producers of chemokines such as macrophage inflammatory proteins (MIP-1α, 1β, and 2), macrophage chemotactic proteins (MCP-1, -2, -3), interferon-γ-inducible protein (IP-10), IL-8, growth-related oncogene (GRO α and β), and regulated upon activation of normal T cell expressed and secreted (RANTES). Together with cytokines, which induce or enhance the expression of adhesion molecules on endothelial cells of the BBB, these chemokines promote the migration of monocytes, lymphocytes, eosinophils, and basophils across the BBB into the brain (Persidsky 1999). Viral infection of the CNS parenchyma strongly stimulates local chemokine expression. In simian immunodeficiency virus (SIV)-induced neuropathogenesis in primates the chemokines MIP-1α, MIP-1β, RANTES, MCP-3, and IP-10 play a major role in recruiting inflammatory cell infiltrates (Sasseville et al. 1996). In tissue culture it has been shown that the HIV transactivator tat stimulates the expression of MCP-1 by astroctyes. In addition, this chemokine was detected in the brains and CSF of patients with HIV-associated dementia (Conant et al. 1998).

The multiple effects of cytokines in the CNS may be beneficial in stimulating immunological surveillance and intracellular viral resistance (mainly type I and II IFNs and TNF-α) (Schijns et al. 1991; Shankar et al. 1992). This occurs by recruitment and activation of cells of the immune system as well as by induction of MHC molecules (Campbell 1991; Neumann 2001; Plata-Salaman 1991) or antiviral proteins such as MxA, RNA-dependent protein kinase R (PKR), or 2′,5′-A synthetase in brain cells that directly interfere with intracellular viral replication (Staeheli 1990). Triggering of immune responses and inflammatory reactions by proinflammatory cytokines such as IL-1 and TNF-α, together with the induction of neurotoxins (Giulian et al. 1990) and reactive oxygen intermediates (Nathan 1992), may, however, also contribute directly to the immunopathology observed in most viral CNS conditions. Proinflammatory cytokines such as IL-1 or TNF-α produced by immune cells or by CNS cells in response to infection may be essential to the process of neuronal destruction (Quagliarello et al. 1991; Selmaj 1992), as indicated by the meningitis and BBB damage that followed injection of these cytokines into rat brains. Moreover, it has been shown for experimental allergic encephalitis that neurospecific T cells recruit activated inflammatory cells through the action of TNF-α and IFN-γ (Ruddle et al. 1990). In addition, these cytokines can prime macrophages for the production of inducible reactive oxygen and nitrogen intermediates (Ding et al. 1988), which are thought to play an important role in cytotoxicity (Nathan 1992).

Direct analysis of cytokine expression in human CNS diseases is often difficult to perform, because the production of cytokines may be localized, the levels may be very low, and cytokines normally are rather unstable once secreted. Moreover, the role of cytokines in the development of viral CNS infection and in viral neuro-pathogenesis cannot be studied in humans for obvious reasons, and so suitable animal models must be used. For example, experimentally induced CNS infections with borna disease virus (BDV) in rats represent a recent example of an animal model to study the role of cytokines in neurological disorders (Bode 1995; Rott and Becht 1995; Stitz et al. 1995; Briese et al. 1999). Induction of IL-1α, IL-2, IL-6, TNF-α, and IFN-γ mRNA synthesis has been found in rat brains 2 weeks after intranasal infection, and IL-2 as well as IFN-γmRNA expression correlated well with the appearance of CD4$^+$ and CD8$^+$ lymphocytes during the early stages of BDV infection (Shankar et al. 1992). Moreover, mRNA levels for inducible nitric oxide synthetase (iNOS) were upregulated (Koprowski et al. 1993). It is interesting that the levels of iNOS mRNA correlated not only with the degree of neurological involvement and CNS inflammation but also with the levels of TNF-α, IL-1, and IL-6 mRNA (Selmaj 1992), potential mediators of iNOS expression (Nathan 1992). In the chronic phase of BDV infection of the CNS, levels of IL-1, IL-6, and TNF-α decreased dramatically, whereas mRNA levels for IFN-γ were greatly elevated, probably indicating that IFN-γ may act to reduce inflammation and to improve neurological signs during the transition phase from acute to chronic disease. In fact, IFN-γ has a pronounced synergistic effect in the TNF- and IL-1-mediated induction of manganese superoxide dismutase, which has been linked to the protection of uninfected cells from reactive oxygen toxicity during immune responses (Harris et al. 1991). To date, BDV has not been identified as a clear etiological agent of any known human disease (Carbone 2001).

MHC expression in the brain and its relation to viral infection

An effective immunological response to viral infections of the CNS is undoubtedly hampered by the relative lack of MHC and costimulatory molecule expression in this tissue. MHC class I expression is believed to be virtually absent from the surface of neurons, whereas MHC class II expression is confined to microglia and pericytes at the BBB (Pardridge 1999). Not only is MHC class I 'passively' absent, but surface contact with neurons also suppresses its expression on the surface of microglial cells (Hoek et al. 2000). In tissue culture, astrocytes and endothelial cells

have also been found to express MHC class II after induction. Much attention has been focused on the ability of certain cytokines, such as IFN-γ and TNF-α, to induce or upregulate MHC class I and II, and adhesion molecules such as ICAM-1 on glial cells (Frohman et al. 1989). However, the presence of these factors in the CNS indicates that an inflammatory process had already been initiated, which is not likely to occur soon after a virus has entered the CNS. In support of this notion, infection-dependent upregulation of MHC class I expression on a variety of cell types (reviewed in Maudsley et al. 1989), and also MHC class II induction on otherwise negative cells (including astrocytes), has been described (Massa et al. 1986, 1987). Interestingly, infected neurons can be an intrathecal source of IFN-γ and express MHC class I after inhibition of their electrical activity, either experimentally or after infection (Neumann et al. 1997).

Although it is certain that induction or augmentation of immunoregulatory surface molecules on the surface of brain cells is a prerequisite for an efficient immune response, their role in neuropathogenesis is unclear. For instance, MHC class II expression was readily inducible in the SJL and CBA mouse strains, which are susceptible to experimentally induced CNS infections with Theiler's virus, but not in the resistant BALB/c mice (Nash et al. 1985). In contrast, BN rats, which live well with experimental *Coronavirus* JHM or MV infections, showed a constitutive high MHC class II expression in the brain, whereas in Lewis rats, in which MHC class II expression occurs as a consequence of the viral infection, immuno-pathological (autoimmune) processes are observed in a significant proportion of animals. This illustrates that the early presence of immunoregulatory molecules in the brain may provide protection, whereas the same process could lead to pathology and disease when MHC molecules are expressed several days or weeks later (Sedgwick and Dörries 1991). Induction of MHC molecules on neural cells is, however, not sufficient to result in elimination of virus, as illustrated by observations in brain tissue from patients with progressive multifocal leukoencephalopathy (PML), a slow papovavirus infection predominantly involving oligodendrocytes. Here, both MHC class I and II are expressed in the lesions, yet viral clearance does not occur, probably because no reactive T cells are generated by the immunosuppressed patient. This may allow the establishment of persistence and ultimately chronic viral infection with progressive disease (Achim and Wiley 1992).

The immune response to viral infections in the CNS

PASSAGE OF EFFECTOR LYMPHOCYTES INTO THE CNS

The BBB is the sentinel in the development of an inflammatory response in the CNS. Adhesion of lymphocytes and their subsequent migration through the capillary endothelium is essential for the development of an inflammatory reaction. Adhesion molecules expressed on the brain capillary endothelium act as important ligands to receptors on the surface of lymphocytes, and mediate both adhesion and subsequent migration (Cross 1992) (Figure 62.1). Two families of molecules on the endothelium are well known in the initiation of adhesion. The initial binding seems to be mediated by those belonging to the selectin (CD62) family (E-selectin, L-selectin, and P-selectin). The second family comprises the Ig superfamily of adhesion molecules such as ICAM-1 (CD54) and VCAM-1 (CD106), which bind to integrin molecules on lymphocytes (Springer 1994; Risau et al. 1998; Pardridge 1999).

Migration is mediated by the secretion of chemoattractant molecules released by the endothelium, as well as by astrocytes and microglial cells (Ransohoff et al. 1993; Persidsky 1999; Zhang 1999). Because adhesion to the capillary endothelium is an important step before cell

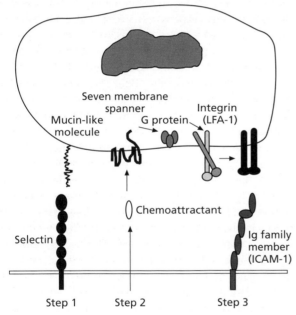

Figure 62.1 *Sequential steps in the traffic of leukocyte adhesion to the vascular endothelium. Selectins (CD62) on the surface of vascular endothelial cells initially interact with carbohydrate residues, often displayed on mucin-like molecules on flowing leukocytes to mediate a labile adhesion (Step 1). This interaction brings leukocytes into close proximity with chemoattractants (released from the endothelial cells lining the vessel wall) which bind to receptors that span the membrane seven times on the surface of leukocytes. Binding of chemoattractants to their receptors subsequently triggers the activation of G proteins, which then transduce signals to activate integrin adhesiveness (e.g. by activating leukocyte function antigen 1, LFA-1) (Step 2). The interaction of the latter with surface proteins of the Ig superfamily (expressed on the endothelial cells, such as intercellular adhesion molecule 1, ICAM-1) mediates strong adhesion, leading to an arrest of the rolling leukocyte (Step 3). Following directional cues from chemoattractants, and using integrins for traction, leukocytes then cross the endothelial lining of the blood–brain barrier and enter the CNS.*

migration, it follows that factors influencing the expression of the receptor molecules on the capillary endothelium or on the lymphocyte surface are likely to influence the extent and severity of the inflammatory response. Proinflammatory cytokines such as IL-1, TNF-α, and IFN-γ increase the expression of the Ig superfamily of adhesion receptors. In fact, ICAM-1 and -2 and VCAM-1 are expressed on CNS microvessels in experimental allergic encephalomyelitis (EAE), and its expression coincides with inflammatory cell infiltration (Engelhardt 1998; Cannella et al. 1991). Furthermore, in the human brain, ICAM-1 is expressed on vessels in viral encephalitic lesions (Sobel et al. 1990). Studies in vitro have shown that antibodies to proinflammatory cytokines, or cytokines that have an antagonistic effect, such as transforming growth factor-β_2 (TGF-β_2), alter the adhesion of lymphocytes to the capillary endothelium (Fabry et al. 1995). The anti-inflammatory properties of TGF-β have been exploited in the amelioration of two distinct T cell-mediated EAEs (Racke et al. 1991, 1993), and it can interfere with the adhesion of lymphocytes to endothelial cells, possibly inhibiting the entry of effector cells into the CNS (Cai et al. 1991; Gamble and Vadas 1991). In support of this suggestion, TGF-β treatment in EAE does not influence the appearance of sensitized cells in peripheral blood and lymph nodes, but does prevent the accumulation of T cells in the brain and spinal cord. This suggests that the protective effect of TGF-β is exerted at the level of the target organ, the CNS, its vascular endothelium, or both (Santambrogio et al. 1993). It has been shown that T cells require prior activation to cross the BBB (Hickey et al. 1991). However, once the BBB was breached, no activation-dependent differences in the homing pattern of T lymphocytes were observed (Trotter and Steinman 1985).

THE HUMORAL IMMUNE RESPONSE IN THE CNS

The control of virus infection depends on the efficient generation of both humoral and cell-mediated immune responses. Antibodies, which attack predominantly extracellular virus particles released from infected cells, are required to limit the spread of some viruses in the host. For example, it seems that the humoral immune reaction is essential in controlling poliovirus infections. For infections with other viruses, such as varicella-zoster, *Cytomegalovirus*, or measles virus, T-cell responses may be more important than antibody. In this context it is important to remember that the immune response to viral infections of the CNS is initiated in peripheral lymphoid tissue, with subsequent entry of activated (end-differentiated) T cells into the meninges, brain parenchyma, and cerebrospinal fluid (Sedgwick et al. 1991a, 1991b).

Inhibition of virus entry into the brain and blockade of intracerebral viral spread

Specific antibodies are the main tool of the infected host in preventing extracellular viral spread from primary sites of infection to other organs during viremia (Sissons and Oldstone 1985). Virtually all viral CNS infections are preceded by primary peripheral infection, and so it is obvious that virus neutralization and opsonization during viremia comprise one of the most efficient defense reactions preventing viral entry into the CNS. Agammaglobulinemic patients suffer more frequently from persistent CNS infections than do fully immunocompetent hosts (Smith et al. 1992), and peripheral virus-specific antibodies usually prevent neuroinvasion in perinatal viral hosts that do not display full immune competence. For example, lethal encephalomyelitis experimentally induced by the murine *Coronavirus* JHM (JHMV) in newborn or suckling rats is prevented by nursing the babies from JHMV-immunized mothers (Wege et al. 1983), and teratogenic effects induced by lymphocytic choriomeningitis virus (LCMV) in neonates are not observed when they are nursed by immunized mothers or injected with LCMV-specific neutralizing monoclonal antibodies (Baldridge and Buchmeier 1992; Baldridge et al. 1993). Moreover, experimental virus infections of the CNS in immunocompetent hosts usually remain subclinical, provided high titers of virus-neutralizing antibodies are mounted (Jubelt et al. 1991; Rima et al. 1991).

Nevertheless, in some instances viruses escape extracerebral neutralization and invade the CNS. If retrograde transport occurs along the axons of peripheral nerves, the virus is inaccessible for an immune system. Neither virus-specific antibodies nor cytotoxic T lymphocytes (CTL) can prevent the axonal transport of the virus to the CNS, particularly because nerve cells are thought to be unable to upregulate MHC class I molecules (Momburg et al. 1986). Using leukocytes as 'Trojan horses' is another way to escape neutralization by antibodies, although this hypothesis has so far not been supported by direct experimental evidence. Viral infection of peripheral recirculating monocytes may enhance invasion of the perivascular space in the CNS, because, in contrast to ramified microglia, the perivascular type of this cell is frequently exchanged by peripheral monocytes (Sedgwick et al. 1991a, 1991b, 1993).

Once in its target cell, the virus continues replicating and spreading in the CNS until immune effector cells are recruited into the brain parenchyma. Plasma cells of the B-lymphocyte lineage home to virus-infected sites in the tissue (Dörries et al. 1991), where they secrete virus-specific antibodies (Schwender et al. 1991), and cytotoxic T lymphocytes provide an early virus-specific defense mechanism in the brain parenchyma. Although the latter may efficiently lyse virus-infected cells, the formation of secondary virus-infected foci in the tissue by extracellular spread of the virus is prevented only when virus-specific antibodies are secreted intracerebrally in close proximity to infected sites. This has been confirmed in several animal models of virus-induced encephalitis. In addition to extracellular spread, virus-specific antibodies

may inhibit dissemination from cell to cell, for example by interfering with cell fusion (Dietzschold et al. 1992). Moreover, antiviral antibodies may be directly involved in attenuating intracellular viral replication in vivo and in vitro. This concept, known as antibody-induced antigenic modulation (Fujinami and Oldstone 1980), has been established for MV infections in brain cells and mice with severe combined immunodeficiency (SCID) infected with Sindbis virus (Levine et al. 1991).

Although it is generally assumed that the protective effect of a virus-neutralizing antibody in the CNS is mainly due to binding of its Fab part to viral epitopes necessary for infection of the target cell, the Fc part of the antibody molecule may also contribute. A monoclonal antibody specific for the yellow fever virus (YFV) nonstructural protein NS1 protects mice from encephalitis only when given as an intact molecule, but not as a F(ab)2 fragment, which normally neutralizes YFV efficiently in vitro. Moreover, only monoclonal antibodies of the IgG_{2a} subclass efficiently prevented acute encephalitis in this virus system, indicating that only binding of a distinct IgG subclass to NS1 allows recognition by FcR expressing cells. Similar observations have been made for Semliki Forest virus (SFV) infection of mice, in which IgG_{2a} is the dominant subclass in the CSF, as well as for LCMV-induced encephalitis, which can be prevented with an IgG_{2a} monoclonal antibody (Baldridge and Buchmeier 1992). In rabies virus-infected mice, however, protection from lethal disease is achieved by both IgG_1 and IgG_{2a} subclasses (Dietzschold et al. 1992).

Successful action of the humoral immune response requires very rapid migration of virus-specific plasma cells into the brain parenchyma. This is usually achieved if viral CNS infection occurs concomitantly with the acute peripheral infection and pre-existing plasma cells can immediately enter the brain tissue. When viral CNS infection occurs late after primary infection, the immune response has to be initiated in local secondary lymphatics, such as the cervical lymph nodes. The period until humoral effector systems reach the brain parenchyma may be determined by the genetic background of the host, as documented for *Coronavirus* JHM-induced encephalomyelitis in two genetically different rat strains (Schwender et al. 1991).

The effect of a late or a rather unspecific recruitment of humoral immunity to the CNS facilitates viral spread within the CNS. Consequently, large infected areas will result in a vigorous infiltration of virus-specific T cells, leading to enhancement of neurological disease. This intimate relation between virus-specific humoral response and T cell-mediated immunopathology was shown in acute LCMV-induced encephalitis of mice. In this model, mice injected with neutralizing antibodies before and shortly after viral infection were protected from lethal encephalitis, and CTL responses were diminished compared with unprotected mice (Wright and Buchmeier 1991).

Enhancement of viral pathogenesis by humoral effector systems

Humoral immunity is not generally thought to contribute to the pathology of viral CNS infection. Nevertheless, there are theoretical considerations and experimental data obtained in vitro that do not strictly rule out disease-enhancing properties of humoral immune responses. As in the periphery, intrathecal antibody synthesis could help to augment viral pathogenesis by antibody-dependent enhancement (ADE): i.e. antibody-complexed viral particles can be taken up by cells either by binding to Fc receptors (FcR) or, in the case of activation of the complement cascade, by attachment via the C3 receptor. In both cases, cells of the monocyte/macrophage lineage, such as microglial cells, are prime targets for ADE in the CNS (Aloisi 2001; Homsy et al. 1989) In addition, the engagement of FcR triggers activation of macrophages or microglia, which may lead to unspecific tissue destruction. Binding of immune complexes to the FcR can stimulate the release of toxic substances, causing the destruction of healthy cells surrounding the infected areas. This assumption is supported by the observation in vitro of macrophage-dependent oligodendroglia cell degeneration in mixed glial cell cultures when they are treated with immune complexes formed by canine distemper virus (CDV) and CDV-specific antibodies (Botteron et al. 1992).

The presence of virus-specific antibodies in the CNS opens one pathway allowing a complement-dependent immunological effector mechanism to operate: the antibody-activated cytolytic action of complement (Speth et al. 2001). Activation of the complement cascade in the CSF has been demonstrated in patients suffering from HIV-1 infection (Reboul et al. 1989). Opsonized virions will bind to cellular complement receptors, an interaction which can amplify the infection of cells with HIV-1 rather than induce lysis of the virus (Stoiber et al. 2001). There is, however, no evidence for antibody-mediated tissue destruction in the CNS of AIDS patients (Lenhardt and Wiley 1989). Although not proven, there is some reason to suggest that complement-mediated lysis could contribute to the pathogenesis of SSPE, caused by a persistent measles virus infection of the human CNS. One of the cellular receptors for measles virus, CD46, was found to be absent in CNS lesions of SSPE patients, whereas it is present on a fraction of cells in uninfected regions of the brain (McQuaid and Cosby 2001; Ogata et al. 1997). Because the normal function of CD46 is to protect cells from autologous lysis by activated complement (Liszweski et al. 1991), the sera and CSF of SSPE patients reveal high complement activity (Oldstone et al. 1975), and CD46 down-regulation enhances the complement-mediated lysis of cells in tissue culture (Schnorr et al. 1995), it is tempting to speculate that this mechanism may contribute to the pathology of SSPE.

Viral persistence and virus-specific antibodies

Incomplete elimination of virus from the CNS may result in persistent infection that is usually accompanied by a long-lasting intrathecal antibody synthesis with specificity for viral proteins (Rammohan et al. 1983; Tyor et al. 1992). Over time there is selection of high-avidity antiviral antibodies, and the respective clones are preferentially recruited to the CNS. In this case, isoelectric focusing of CSF specimens will show a restricted 'oligoclonal pattern' of antibody clones, compared to the polyclonal distribution detectable in paired serum specimens. The presence of these oligoclonal bands can therefore be used as a diagnostic marker in viral infections of the CNS (Felgenhauer and Reiber 1992).

In addition to intrathecal virus-specific antibody synthesis being a reliable indicator of viral infection of the CNS, the long-lasting presence of antiviral antibodies at high titers may contribute to the selection of virus variants. In fact, changes in neural cell tropism have been shown for neurotropic JHMV grown in the presence of virus-neutralizing monoclonal antibodies (Buchmeier et al. 1984).

THE CELL-MEDIATED IMMUNE RESPONSE

T cell-mediated immune protection is usually mediated by cell destruction. Because a timely T-cell immune response encounters a small number of infected cells, the disease should be limited in most acute viral encephalitides, and the benefits will outweigh the harmful effects of the cell-mediated immune response. Paradoxically, the host's immune response to viral infection, which is usually protective outside the CNS, can be destructive when operating within this isolated compartment with such a low regenerative capacity. Cell lysis and toxic cytokines may themselves cause pathological changes while helping to clear virus, particularly during a long-lasting persistent infection.

The role of CD4⁺ and CD8⁺ T cells

Although both $CD4^+$ and $CD8^+$ T cells can be relatively easily isolated and grown in culture from the CSF of patients with viral encephalitis and meningoencephalitis, their relative contributions to antiviral defense are uncertain. As is apparent in some animal models, the presence and function of $CD4^+$ cells are more important than $CD8^+$ T cells in viral CNS infections. This is in contrast to the situation in peripheral tissues in which, for example, during acute and chronic viral hepatitis cytotoxic MHC class I-restricted $CD8^+$ T cells attack virus-infected hepatocytes and thus mediate protection as well as cell destruction (Almond et al. 1991).

Although there is still some controversy, results obtained in the Theiler's virus model in mice indicate that the ability to generate $CD8^+$ T cells is not essential for viral clearance. In both C57BL/10 mice, which develop an acute encephalitis followed by subsequent clearance of virus from the CNS, and SJL mice, which experience a persistent viral infection with demyelination lesions, there are CD8[+] CTLs in the CNS (Lindsley et al. 1991). Furthermore, β2-microglobulin-deficient transgenic mice that lack MHC class I and, therefore, functional CD8[+] cells, develop persistent encephalitis with extensive demyelination. However, neither antibody titers nor viral persistence was significantly affected (Pullen et al. 1993).

Consistent with these findings, CD4[+] cells proved indispensable in achieving viral clearance from the CNS of rats after transfer into animals experimentally infected with MV, whereas CD8[+] cells were not vital for recovery from the acute infection. It must be remembered, however, that in different species different virus-specific immune effector cells are generated in the control of viral infections in the periphery; even within a single species there is no unique T-cell subset used for antiviral defense. In many murine virus infections, including HSV, influenza A virus, LCMV, and mouse poxvirus, CD8[+] CTLs are important in combating infection (Moskophidis et al. 1987; Nash et al. 1987; Ahmed et al. 1988; Askonas et al. 1988). However, the clearance of murine hepatitis virus from the brain by CD8[+] T cells depends on CD4[+] help (Williamson and Stohlman 1990), and in the protective immunity to retroviruses both CD8[+] and CD4[+] T cells were only partially effective, whereas the combination of both led to full protection (Hom et al. 1991). In contrast, recovery from acute murine CMV infection can proceed in the absence of the CD8[+] subset, and it is mediated by CD4[+] T cells that develop a compensatory protective activity absent from normal mice (Jonjic et al. 1990). CD4[+] T cells seem to be required for the maintenance of spontaneous recovery from friend murine leukemia virus-induced leukemia (Robertson et al. 1992). These examples illustrate that there is no general assignment of a determinative role in vivo to either T-lymphocyte subset in the recovery from viral infections. It seems, however, that in the CNS antiviral cell-mediated activity is largely dependent on CD4[+] T cells.

Mechanisms of T cell-mediated antiviral activity in the brain

The mechanism of the antiviral activity of CD4[+] T cells in vivo has not been completely elucidated. A detailed characterization in vitro revealed that all protective T-cell lines produce large amounts of IL-2, IFN-γ, and TNF-α, but not IL-4 or IL-6, defining them as Th1 cells (Liebert and Finke 1995). If cytokines secreted by Th1 cells are important, two requirements should be met: virus-primed T cells have to invade the CNS and home in on sites of infection; and blocking cytokine function should abolish protection. Adoptive transfer experiments in MV-infected rats as well as in mice, using a genetic marker, revealed that MV-specific CD4[+] T cells from a donor animal enter the brain of the host. These cells accumulated in infected areas, where they represented

≤5 percent of all infiltrating T cells in immunocompetent animals. Furthermore, the neutralization of IFN-γ by the administration of antibodies rendered all mice susceptible to MV-induced acute encephalitis, suggesting that cytokines may indeed play an important role in the immune surveillance of the CNS. The mechanism of cytokine activity may be to assist in recruiting effector cells into the CNS (see also under Virus cell interaction in the CNS). The main source of IFN-γ and TNF-α in MV infection of the murine CNS seems to be CD4[+] T cells.

In the Theiler's murine encephalomyelitis virus (TMEV) encephalitis model in mice, susceptibility to infection is associated with MHC and maps to the class I locus H-2D, which is highly upregulated in the CNS, in contrast to the H-2K locus (Nash et al. 1987). In susceptible strains CD8[+] T cells apparently fail to recognize viral antigens in the context of MHC class I, so the virus persists and eventually causes disease. After depletion of CD8[+] T cells in vivo, virus clearance is delayed and demyelinating disease develops, indicating that CD8[+] T cells are not involved in demyelination and are not vital for recovery from acute infection. In contrast, depletion of CD8[+] cells after the acute phase does reduce disease. Observations made in β2-microglobulin-deficient transgenic mice, however, suggest that CD8[+] T cells may play a role in clearing viral persistence from glial cells (Pullen et al. 1993). Depletion studies of CD4[+] cells in the TMEV model suggest that the major role of CD4[+] T cells in picornavirus infections is probably to control the early stages of infection by providing B-cell help and thus enable the production of neutralizing antibody (Virelizier 1989). TMEV-specific proliferation of CD4[+] MHC class II-restricted T cells was found in both resistant and susceptible strains (Clatch et al. 1987).

There is a strong correlation in a number of susceptible strains between demyelination and a CD4[+] T cell-mediated DTH response, and one DTH T-cell epitope in susceptible mice has been mapped to the VP2 protein (Geretry et al. 1994). The incidence of demyelinating disease was reduced following suppression of MHC II restricted CD4[+] T-cell function after viremia. After TMEV infection and initial T-cell infiltration into the CNS, MHC class II induction on astrocytes is a key step in allowing local antigen presentation and amplification of immunopathological responses within the CNS, and hence the development of demyelinating disease (Borrow and Nash 1992). A bystander effect caused by the induction of mononuclear cell infiltration, and activation of macrophages, which in turn can lead to damage on myelin sheaths, is probably responsible for the observed immunopathology.

Virus-induced cell-mediated autoimmune reactions against brain antigens

Another possibility involves T cells reactive against brain cell antigens, which could be induced during the course of infection and may exacerbate current pathology or initiate new lesions. There are several possibilities of how a virus could induce strong cell-mediated immunity (CMI) responses to brain antigen:

- When enveloped viruses multiply in living cells, they may incorporate host antigens into their envelope. In this context these antigens might then be recognized by the host and thus elicit an immune reaction.
- Viruses with a tropism for lymphocytes and macrophages might be involved in the destruction of lymphocyte subpopulations or the generation/expansion of autoreactive lymphocyte clones.
- Immune responses raised against certain viral antigens may cross-react with normal host cell antigens and lead to autoimmunity by molecular mimicry (Oldstone 1989; Fujinami and Oldstone 1985). Synthetic peptides derived from common viruses (based on motifs required for MHC class II binding and T-cell receptor recognition) can activate human T-cell lines specific for MBP (Wucherpfennig and Strominger 1995).

The frequency of induction of T cells reactive against brain antigens, and their role in the pathology of human viral CNS infections, are unclear. One study suggests that a significant proliferative response of isolated peripheral lymphocytes occurs against myelin basic protein (MBP) in patients with acute measles encephalomyelitis (Johnston et al. 1984). Moreover, MBP was detected in the CSF of such patients as a consequence of myelin breakdown. MBP-specific lymphoproliferative responses have also been seen after postinfectious encephalomyelitis following rubella virus, varicella-zoster virus, and respiratory infection, and in patients with postexposure rabies immunization (Johnston and Griffin 1986). The latter disorder is probably the human equivalent of EAE, because these patients received rabies vaccine prepared in brain tissue. Continuing the analogy to EAE, it is not surprising that an MBP-specific lymphoproliferative response in these virus infections is considered to be of pathogenic importance. In experimental CNS infections autoimmune T cells do not seem to be involved in the induction of demyelination in Theiler's virus in mice, as tolerance induced to myelin antigens blocked the induction of EAE but did not affect the development of demyelinating disease (Kennedy et al. 1990). However, in rats infected with JHMV or MV, MBP-reactive CD4$^+$ T cells were detected that could transfer EAE to naive uninfected animals (Watanabe et al. 1983; Liebert et al. 1988). These observations support the hypothesis that viruses could be involved in the initiation of autoimmune processes.

Consequences of antiviral mechanisms in the CNS

In summary, immune responses generated in the periphery encounter great difficulties when combating CNS virus infections. If neurons are infected, elimination of the cells may not be of any advantage to the host as the immune response, although beneficial in the periphery, would inflict enormous damage when attacking cells that lack the capacity to regenerate. Hence, rapid elimination of infected cells is necessary to prevent virus amplification. In contrast, the development of a delayed immune response may allow the virus to spread in the CNS and, even if ultimately effective against the virus, may be destructive to the host. Thus, precautions are built into the system to prevent potentially damaging and disease-inducing immune responses during persistent infections in which the virus, at least temporarily, does not destroy its host cell.

The fine regulation of intracerebral immune surveillance has yet to be elucidated. However, it is clear that a delicate balance is normally maintained between the morphological and functional integrity of the CNS and the ability of the immune system to combat virus and eliminate infected cells. At present the evidence indicates that:

- The immune response to viral infections of the CNS is initiated in peripheral lymphoid tissues, followed by entry of activated end-differentiated T and B cells into the CSF, meninges, and brain parenchyma.
- During viral infections different sets of cytokines and chemokines are induced.
- Together with interferon-induced proteins, these factors contribute to the establishment of persistent infections, which may depend on downregulation of replication of certain viruses by lack of certain factors, or the restriction of viral gene expression, or both.
- During viral infections, MHC class I or II antigens are expressed extensively on microglial cells which present viral antigen produced by infected cells, and also on astrocytes oligodendrocytes, and damaged neurons.
- Full development of the inflammatory response requires virus-specific T cells; natural killer (NK) cells, γ/δ T cells, mononuclear phagocytes, B cells, and plasma cells participate in a bystander response.
- In many viral systems T cells are required for viral elimination, but clearance of virus may also depend on the timely presence of virus-specific antibodies.
- Immunopathology and autoimmunity may result from inopportune or inefficient T-cell responses generated after the viral agent has succeeded in establishing a persistent infection in brain cells as a result of immune-mediated damage during attempted viral clearance.

VIRUSES AND ASSOCIATED CNS DISORDERS IN HUMANS

As mentioned previously, except for rabies virus, human pathogenic viruses do not per se reveal a tropism for the

CNS, but rather cause CNS diseases in the course of an infection in the periphery. A summary of the relative frequencies of the ability of human pathogenic viruses to cause CNS diseases is given in Table 62.2. For example, CNS involvement is quite frequent with mumps virus infections, whereas the proportion of patients with measles developing CNS complications is generally small. The same applies to EBV infections, which are ubiquitous and normally clinically inapparent, CNS complications being observed only rarely. The following sections thus focus on viral infections of the CNS that are of major clinical interest and which have been investigated in more detail.

Polyomaviruses

Progressive multifocal leukoencephalopathy (PML) is a demyelinating disease of the CNS resulting from infection of oligodendrocytes with JC virus (JCV), a *Polyomavirus* (Richards 1988, Dörries 2000) (see Chapter 24 Polyomaviruses). Until the AIDS epidemic, experience with this disease was limited. Once regarded by most neurologists as a clinical curiosity, PML has now been recognized as an AIDS-associated disorder and the HIV-encoded transactivator Tat has been found to be an activator of the JCL promoter (Remenick et al. 1991). Current estimates suggest that 1–4 percent of all HIV-infected people will develop PML (Berger et al. 1987; Berger and Major 1999). In AIDS patients, as in those with other underlying diseases, PML usually progresses inexorably to death within a mean of 4 months. More than 80 percent succumb within 1 year of diagnosis. However, on rare occasions individuals with PML experience both clinical and radiographic recovery, including full neurological recovery, in the absence of specific therapeutic intervention.

The spread of JCV is thought to occur via the respiratory route (Shah 1990). To date, no disease has been convincingly associated with the acute infection. Usually, asymptomatic persistent infections with JCV (and the closely related BK virus) are established; consequently, 80–90 percent of the healthy adult population have IgG antibodies against JCV (Padgett and Walker 1983). Kidney, CNS, and in some cases peripheral blood mononuclear cells, have been identified as sites of persistent

infection (Houff et al. 1988; Arthur et al. 1989; Elsner and Dörries 1992; Dörries et al. 1994). It is not yet entirely clear how these persistent infections are established and maintained. Although heterogeneity within the JCV control regions in brain isolates could be defined, these changes could be linked neither to the persistent phenotype of the infection nor to the efficiency and frequency of reactivation (Elsner and Dörries 1992). On the other hand, it has been suggested that the cell type specificity of JCV in vitro and in vivo is controlled by host and viral transcription factors that actively regulate JCV gene expression by interacting with the viral control region (Feigenbaum et al. 1987; Chowdhury et al. 1990; Lynch and Frisque 1991; Ranganathan and Khalili 1993). Reactivation of viral replication leading to PML is almost exclusively confined to immunosuppressed individuals (Walker and Frisque 1986), strongly suggesting that the host's immune system plays a major role in controlling viral replication in persistence. However, there is no evidence as to how the immune response controls virus persistence and prevents reactivation. Because only a minority of patients with underlying cellular immunodeficiency ultimately develop PML, it is possible that the presence of JCV and immunosuppression alone is not sufficient for its development.

The AIDS epidemic has dramatically altered the epidemiology of PML (Holman et al. 1991). Instead of affecting chiefly elderly people, PML has become a disease of the young and middle-aged affected with AIDS. It is interesting that this disease rarely occurs in immunosuppressed children with HIV infection (Berger et al. 1992), perhaps as a result of the smaller percentage of children infected with JCV. The high prevalence of antibodies in the adult population and the rarity of PML in children supports the contention that PML results from reactivation of JCV in individuals who have become immunosuppressed. Until the early 1980s (before the AIDS epidemic), the vast majority of patients with PML had lymphoproliferative disorders leading to immunosuppression, such as Hodgkin's disease, chronic lymphocytic leukemia and lymphosarcoma, tuberculosis, lupus erythematosus, or sarcoidosis (Brooks and Walker 1984). In contrast, AIDS has been estimated to be the underlying disease behind PML in 55–85 percent of all current cases in which PML was reported within 1 year

Table 62.2 *Viruses causing acute meningoencephalitis and acute encephalitis in humans*

Frequent	Infrequent	Rare
Herpes simplex virus 1 and 2	Varicella-zoster virus	Adenovirus
Mumps	Measles	Epstein–Barr virus
Enteroviruses	Rubella	Reovirus
Arboviruses	Influenza virus A and B	Parainfluenza virus 1–3
Rabies	Cytomegalovirus	Respiratory syncytial virus
		Human parvovirus
		Lymphocytic choriomeningitis virus

after the initial diagnosis of AIDS (Gullota et al. 1992; Kaye et al. 1992; Major et al. 1992).

The clinical hallmark of PML is the presence of focal neurological changes associated with radiographic evidence of white matter lesions, depending on the location of the CNS infection. Cardinal features of PML, apparent on clinical examination, include an insidiously progressive psychomotor slowing, impaired memory, and apathy. The most common presentations include weakness, visual deficits, and cognitive abnormalities, which occur in approximately one-third of patients (Brooks and Walker 1984). Weakness is typically a hemiparesis, but monoparesis, hemiplegia, and quadriparesis may be observed as the disease progresses. Other motor disturbances include limb and trunk ataxia, resulting most often from cerebellar involvement. Nearly one-third of patients have cerebellar signs at the time of diagnosis (von Einsiedel et al. 1993). Extrapyramidal disease is rare at onset, but bradykinesia and rigidity may be detected in a substantial minority of patients with advanced disease. Dystonia and severe dysarthria have also been observed as a consequence of lesions in the basal ganglia. Neuro-ophthalmic symptoms occur in 50 percent of patients and are the presenting manifestation in 30–45 percent. The most common visual deficits are homonymous hemianopia or quadrantanopia due to lesions of the optic tracts. The spectrum of cognitive changes observed is quite broad. Unlike the slowly evolving global dementia of the HIV-associated dementia complex, the mental impairments of PML often advance more rapidly and typically occur in conjunction with focal neurological deficits.

Neuropathologically, the cardinal feature of PML is demyelination, i.e. the loss of oligodendroglial cells and myelin sheaths (Figure 62.2). Demyelination is typically multifocal, but on rare occasions may also be unifocal. Although these lesions may develop in any location in the white matter, they have a predilection for the parieto-occipital regions. Not infrequently, lesions involve the cerebellum, brainstem and, less commonly, the spinal cord (Bauer et al. 1969; Kuchelmeister et al. 1993; von Einsiedel et al. 1993).

Other histopathological hallmarks of PML include hyperchromatic, enlarged oligodendroglial nuclei, and enlarged bizarre astrocytes with lobulated hyperchromatic nuclei (Figure 62.2). The abnormal astrocytes may undergo mitosis and have quite a malignant appearance. In situ hybridization for JCV DNA allows the detection of virions in the nuclei of infected oligodendroglial cells. Virions are detected less frequently in reactive astrocytes, and only rarely in macrophages engaged in removing the affected oligodendrocytes (Mazlo and

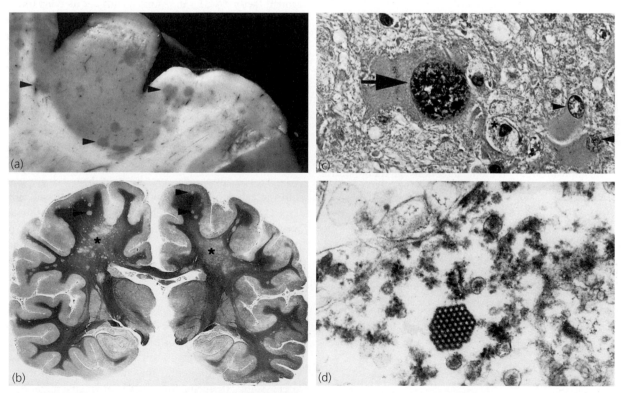

Figure 62.2 (a) *Close-up of the cortex of a patient who died from PML. Several small foci of demyelination are situated mainly at the border between the gray and the white matter.* **(b)** *Whole mount of the cerebrum of the same patient, stained with a myelinotropic dye. Again, there are several round areas of demyelination, as well as larger polycyclical (several circular confluent) regions of confluent foci in the central white matter.* **(c)** *Swollen, grotesquely deformed oligodendrocyte with a very large nucleus (×400). For comparison, see the two reactive astrocytes at the right of the picture (arrowed).* **(d)** *Electron micrograph showing papovaviruses within the affected oligodendrocytes. (Courtesy of Dr Adriano Aguzzi.)*

Tariska 1992). The subcellular distribution of virions, particularly in cells usually not involved in papovavirus infection (the nucleus and cytoplasm of neurons), has been reported in two cases (Boldorini et al. 1993). Although neuropathological findings do not reveal fundamental differences between cases of AIDS and non-AIDS PML, the former more frequently present with extensive lesions of a particularly destructive, necrotizing character.

The application of quantitative PCR to CSF samples enables premortem diagnosis with less invasive procedures than brain biopsy (Dörries 2000). Confirmation of PML requires the demonstration of typical histopathological changes and the detection of JCV in brain samples obtained from biopsies or at autopsy using conventional techniques, including electron microscopy, virus isolation, immunocytochemistry, and in situ hybridization. Recently, it was found that the newly approved cidofovir diphosphate, a structural analog of deoxycytidine trisphosphate, is not only a potent inhibitor of human herpes and papillomaviruses, but also a selective anti-polyomavirus agent.

Alphaherpesviruses

Of the numerous herpesviruses so far characterized, eight have been isolated from humans (see Chapters 25, 26, 27, 28, and 29). Among these, three members of the subfamily *Alphaherpesvirinae*, herpes simplex virus-1 and -2, and varicella-zoster virus (VZV), have been identified as etiological agents in the pathogenesis of human disease processes in both the peripheral and the central nervous system. HSV is responsible for the viral encephalitis with the highest fatality rate. Alphaherpesviruses have a variable host range and short replication cycles and spread rapidly in infected cell cultures, resulting in complete cell destruction. Paradoxically, they can establish latent, lifelong infections in their natural hosts, including those with natural or vaccine-induced immunity. These latent infections occur primarily, but not exclusively, in neural tissue of sensory and autonomic nerve ganglia and the CNS.

Human herpesviruses -6, -7, and -8 have been isolated from human peripheral blood mononuclear cells (PBMC) in recent years. Their association with human CNS diseases has not yet been fully defined, although a pathogenic role of HHV-6 has been suggested for multiple sclerosis (Challoner et al. 1995; Gutierrez and Vergara 2002).

HERPES SIMPLEX VIRUS

Following infection, HSV-1 and HSV-2 replicate at the mucocutaneous surface before entering nerve axons. Virus then moves centripetally via retrograde fast axonal transport to cell bodies of neurons in sensory and autonomic nerve ganglia, and in some cases to the CNS

(Figure 62.3). Following retrograde transport, the virus replicates in the sensory ganglia that innervate the site of infection. In experimental work in animals there is evidence of lytic virus infection in neurons and accessory cells, and virus can be recovered from ganglionic homogenates. Once replication in the sensory ganglia is complete, antiviral drugs cannot eliminate the virus if it enters its latent state. In acutely infected ganglia two types of virus–neuron interaction can occur, resulting in either lytic or latent infection. Cellular factors involved in repressing immediate early gene expression may be paramount in this. After acute ganglionic infection subsides, virus persists in neurons, probably for the lifetime of the host. Infectious virus cannot be recovered from ganglionic homogenates during the latent phase of infection, but can be isolated from ganglionic explant cultures. Periodically, latent virus is reactivated either spontaneously or by a variety of stimuli. During this reactivation process, virus (or perhaps subviral particles) is transported centrifugally via the nerve cell axon to the original peripheral infection site, where replication can then recur.

The exact role of the cell in establishing latent HSV-1 infections is still unclear, because of the small number of latently infected cells present in vivo as well as the difficulty of establishing authentic in vitro latency systems. The dependence of latency on the presence of nerve growth factor (NGF) in primary cultures of sympathetic and sensory neurons has been described (Wilcox and Johnson 1988; Wilcox et al. 1990). Moreover, neurons in culture express factors that inhibit the expression of HSV-1 immediate–early genes (Ash 1986; Kemp et al. 1990; Wheatley et al. 1991; Lillycrop et al. 1993) and therefore arrest HSV-1 replication at an early stage, before irreversible cell damage.

Some molecular aspects of HSV latency and reactivation have been described (for review see Millhouse and Wigdahl 2000). The genome persists as a circularized or a linear concatenated structure that is not integrated into the cellular DNA in human and mouse tissue. The viral DNA is not extensively methylated, and estimates suggest that 20–30 copies of the viral genome may be present in individual cells. A set of RNAs, predominantly stable introns of 1.5 and 2 kb length, is produced in latently infected neurons, where they are the only viral transcripts detectable (latency-associated transcripts (LAT)) (Figure 62.4). They extend from a region in IR_L (large internal repeat region) without an assigned coding role into an oppositely orientated coding region. Mutations in the region encoding LATs have been reported as affecting entry into or reactivation from the latent state. It seems that LAT elements have been conserved in evolution, thus strongly suggesting that there are important functions that may include the silencing of genes such as *ICP0*, an activator of the viral replication, or the expression of proteins contributing to reactivation. Recently, an anti-apoptotic function of the

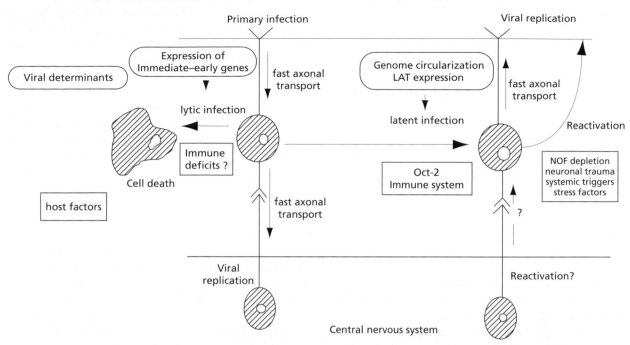

Figure 62.3 *Schematic representation of mechanisms of HSV-1 replication in the nervous system. After primary infection at peripheral tissues, the virion travels via fast axonal transport to peripheral sensory ganglia (PSG). Under conditions favoring viral replication (e.g. immune disruption), expression of HSV-1 immediate–early genes, followed by a complete viral replication cycle, will ensue, leading to neuronal cell death. Again by fast axonal transport, the virus may seed the CNS, causing an acute lytic infection (primary HSV-1 encephalitis). By contrast, in the presence of an effective immune system, viral replication will be prevented in PSG and probably CNS neurons (due at least in part to host cell factors such as neuronal-specific Oct-2 transcription factor). This may lead to either an abortive (not reactivatable) or a latent infection that is characterized by the circularization of the viral genomic DNA and a marked restriction of viral gene expression where no immediate–early genes, but only latency-associated transcripts (LATs), are expressed. Under specific systemic (e.g. menstruation) and local triggering conditions, the latent genome can reactivate in PSG, travel to the periphery, and replicate there. The ability of reactivated HSV-1 to invade the CNS is uncertain, as is reactivation from latent infections established in the CNS. NGF, neuronal growth factor.*

LATs has been described which promotes neuronal survival (Perng et al. 2001).

Primary CNS infection with HSV

Infection with HSV-1, generally limited to the oropharynx, can be transmitted by respiratory droplets or through direct contact of a susceptible individual with infected secretions. Thus, initial replication of virus occurs in the oropharyngeal mucosa. The trigeminal ganglia become colonized and harbor latent virus. HSV-2 infection is usually the consequence of transmission via a genital route. In these circumstances, virus replicates in the vaginal tract or on penile skin and eventually seeds the sacral ganglia. After recovery from the primary infection only a small percentage of individuals experience recurrent infections. HSV encephalitis is mainly associated with HSV-1 infection, whereas ascending myelitis or meningitis is linked mainly to HSV-2 (Shyu et al. 1993). Of these clinical entities, encephalitis is the most common and most severe HSV infection of the CNS. The clinical course is variable,

depending on the location as well as the acuteness of the infection.

HSV infections of the newborn can be aquired in utero, intrapartum (75–80 percent of all cases), or postnatally. The clinical presentation of infection reflects the site and extent of viral replication. Neonatal HSV infection is almost invariably symptomatic and frequently lethal. Intrauterine infection is apparent at birth and is characterized by severe manifestations, such as microcephaly or hydrocephaly. Intrapartum or postnatally acquired HSV infections may lead to encephalitis or disseminated infection that involves multiple organs, including acute brain infections. In infants with disseminated infections the virus probably seeds the brain by a blood-borne route, resulting in multiple areas of cortical hemorrhagic necrosis. In contrast, infants who present only with encephalitis probably develop brain disease as a consequence of retrograde axonal transmission of virus to the CNS. Clinical manifestations of encephalitis with or without associated disseminated disease include seizures (both focal and generalized), lethargy, irritability, tremors, poor feeding, temperature instability, a

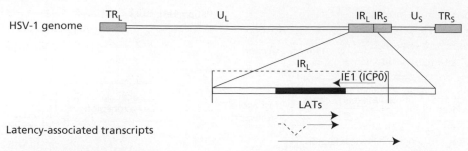

Figure 62.4 *The HSV-1 genome is a linear DNA molecule containing unique long (U_L) and short (U_S) regions bounded by the terminal and internal repeat regions (TR and IR, respectively). The region encoding the major species of latency-associated transcripts (LATs) that are expressed during viral latency is located within the IR_L region (as indicated by the black bar in the enlarged section). As also indicated, some LATs extend from the LAT locus into the IR_S region. The major LAT species expressed partly overlap with viral genes encoded in the opposite direction on the genome, as exemplified for the immediate–early 1 gene (IE1 or ICP0). LATs may interfere with the expression of these genes because they are antisense to their mRNAs, leading to the formation of dsRNA molecules.*

bulging fontanelle, and pyramidal tract signs. Cultures of CSF yield virus in 25–40 percent of cases. Likely findings on CSF examination include pleocytosis and proteinosis, which increase with progressive disease. Death occurs in 50 percent of untreated infants with localized CNS disease, and is usually related to brainstem involvement. With rare exceptions, survivors are left with neurological impairment.

Clinical manifestations of HSV encephalitis in older children and adults reflect the areas of pathology in the brain. These include primarily a focal encephalitis associated with fever, altered consciousness, bizarre behavior, disordered mentation, and localized neurological signs. These clinical findings are generally associated with neurodiagnostic evidence of localized temporal lobe disease. Histopathological findings include widespread areas of hemorrhagic necrosis, mirroring the area of infection, with oligodendrocytic involvement, gliosis and, frequently, astrocytosis late in the disease course (Figure 62.5). Primary HSV-2 infections can, independent of gender, be associated with fever, dysuria, localized inguinal adenopathy, and malaise. The severity of primary infection and its association with complications is statistically higher in women than in men, for unknown reasons. Systemic complaints are common in both sexes, approaching 70 percent of all cases. The most common complications include aseptic meningitis (approximately 20 percent). Following primary genital herpetic infection, sacral radiculomyelitis (which can lead to neuralgias) and meningoencephalitis can also occur. The relationship between HSV infections of the brain and chronic degenerative disease and psychiatric disorders requires further investigation.

Latent infection by HSV

Despite the wide range of anti-HSV immune responses to the initial infection, the nonreplicating latent virus can persist in the ganglia for the lifetime of the patient. Whether latency per se causes any neurological injury is

unknown, but it is well recognized that latent HSV is the source of virus responsible for recurrent infections in the peripheral nervous system. It is assumed that latent virus is reactivated to a replication-competent form and transported via sensory nerves to cutaneous or ocular sites, where further replication results in recurrent HSV infections. The pathological changes induced by the replication of HSV are similar in both primary and recurrent infection.

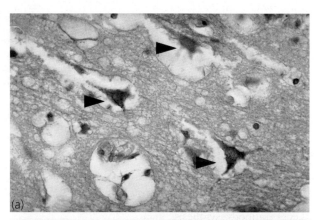

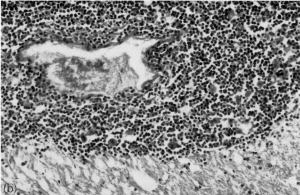

Figure 62.5 *Herpes simplex type 1 encephalitis.* **(a)** *Strongly positive intraneuronal staining with anti-HSV-1 immunostain (arrowed) (×400).* **(b)** *Massive accumulation of inflammatory cells (predominantly lymphocytes) in the neighborhood of small vessels ('cuffing') (×50). (Courtesy of Dr Adriano Aguzzi.)*

HSV encephalitis in immunocompetent individuals is about 1 million times less frequent than the peripheral disease. The source of virus behind HSV-1 encephalitis in immunocompetent individuals is unclear, as the ability of HSV-1 to reactivate in the CNS seems to be extremely limited. Despite the presence of HSV-1 nucleic acid in the human brain (Fraser et al. 1981; Steiner and Kennedy 1995), there is no convincing evidence of recurrent encephalitis induced by HSV-1, and attempts to reactivate it from explanted CNS tissue have generally failed. On rare occasions reactivated virus may be transported from the trigeminal ganglia to the cerebral cortex, resulting in HSV encephalitis. However, not all cases of HSV encephalitis are caused by the strain responsible for cold sores in an individual. Therefore, it is assumed that, in about half of patients, HSV encephalitis occurs as a primary infection (Whitley 1990). Moreover, even with a history of a prior HSV-1 infection, a second primary infection with another HSV-1 strain may be responsible for the encephalitis.

Diagnosis and treatment of HSV encephalitis

The severity of HSV-associated CNS complications warrants the application of rapid and specific diagnostic approaches in order to achieve effective treatment. Seroconversion or an increase in serum antibody titer are not diagnostic of CNS infection. Serological diagnosis requires proof of intrathecal synthesis of virus-specific antibodies, which is evident only when the quantity of specific antibodies in the CNS cannot be explained by transport of antibodies from the periphery across the BBB into the CNS. Classically, CNS HSV IgG antibody is distinguished from peripheral blood-derived HSV antibody appearing in the CSF by the calculation of an antibody index (CSF HSV IgG:serum HSV IgG/CSF albumin:serum albumin); HSV antibody index values >1.5 are considered indicative of intrathecal Ig synthesis. Several approaches are available to determine intrathecal antibody synthesis, including techniques such as enzyme linked immunosorbent assay (ELISA), isoelectric focusing (IEF) or Western blotting using protein antigens (virus purified, or expressed as recombinant proteins) (Klapper and Cleator 1992). For the detection of viral antigens or nucleic acids, brain biopsies stained with virus-specific antibodies or hybridized with virus-specific probes have been used successfully (with a sensitivity of 80–85 percent and a specificity of 100 percent). More recently, PCR-based analysis of CSF samples has been widely used as a less invasive, highly sensitive method more appropriate for clinical application for the diagnosis of HSV encephalitis, particularly in the acute phase of disease in the absence of virus-specific antibodies and in suspicious relapses (Calvario et al. 2002).

The currently accepted antiviral treatment is acyclovir, and new therapeutic drugs, i.e. penciclovir and oral prodrugs, valacyclovir, and Famciclovir (Naesens and De Clercq 2001), potent therapeutic antiviral drugs that specifically interfere with HSV polymerase function and are highly effective in reducing both mortality and morbidity. In fact, the early and systemic application of aciclovir has reduced the mortality of HSV encephalitis from 70 to 20 percent of affected patients.

The use of steroid treatment in HSV encephalitis is a matter of controversy. As brain edema is believed to represent the major cause of mortality associated with herpes encephalitis, reduction of intracranial pressure is another important consideration in the overall treatment.

VARICELLA-ZOSTER CNS COMPLICATIONS

As the name implies, varicella-zoster virus (VZV) causes two distinct clinical symptoms: chickenpox and shingles (for review see Wood 2000). Chickenpox (varicella) is a ubiquitous, highly contagious disease that spreads rapidly in a susceptible population, and is seen predominantly in childhood as the manifestation of primary infection with this virus. In contrast, shingles (herpes zoster) is the manifestation of a recurrent VZV infection. It usually occurs in the elderly or in immunocompromised individuals, and is characterized by a painful vesicular eruption, generally limited to a single dermatome. A live attenuated vaccine against VZV infection is available (Takahashi et al. 1974; Black et al. 1999).

As with HSV, a primary infection with VZV is thought to pass centripetally from skin and mucosal lesions to the corresponding sensory ganglia via contiguous sensory nerve endings and sensory nerve fibers. At the same time, some seeding of ganglia might also occur through direct spread of the virus owing to a varicella-associated viremia. Once in the ganglion, the virus sets up a latent infection in the neuronal cells without replicating or damaging them.

Immune responses to VZV may play a role in maintaining the latent state, and certainly seem to be responsible for preventing clinically apparent reactivation. Reactivation of VZV occurs only rarely, usually once in an individual's lifetime. The main factors that trigger reactivation include generalized immunosuppression, such as HIV infection, or certain cancers (e.g. Hodgkin's disease), suggesting that alteration in the host immunity to VZV may allow the development of zoster. Accumulating evidence points to CMI as the principal factor in the appearance of zoster. Zoster is seen most frequently in cases where CMI is lost (e.g. in bone marrow transplantation), and is accompanied by acute inflammation of the corresponding sensory nerve and ganglion. Acute lymphocytic inflammation, focal hemorrhage and neuronal destruction have also been described. In addition, the sensory nerve shows degeneration and demyelination, both peripherally and centrally, and the presence of viral antigen in neuronal and satellite cells and within the corresponding sensory nerves has been described.

VZV latency and reactivation are quite different from HSV latency and reactivation (reviewed by Hay and Ruyechan 1994). In contrast to HSV, VZV seems able to establish ganglionic latency in nonneural cells (satellite cells that surround the neurons) and to express several lytic cycle viral genes while latent; these genes probably represent very early events in viral multiplication. LAT-like molecules have not been described in these infections, and VZV has no genomic region directly corresponding to LAT. The proposed block at the molecular level, however, may be quite weak, allowing small amounts of virus to be produced on a regular basis.

CNS involvement in varicella is seen in about one case per 1 000. It occurs most often in children aged 5–14 years. The pathogenesis of the neurological complications of varicella is not well understood. Direct invasion of the CNS is seen in some cases, particularly with disseminated visceral infection, whereas other CNS manifestations seem to be immune mediated in origin. Involvement of the ganglia and nerves precedes the development of cutaneous lesions. Similar changes are often observed in adjacent ganglia. The inflammatory and degenerative changes can be traced peripherally to the cutaneous lesions and centrally into the adjacent segments of the spinal cord or brainstem. The myelitis is generally unilateral and predominantly involves the posterior horns. Degeneration with neuronal necrosis and neuronophagia may also involve the posterior columns and the gray matter. A mild lymphocytic meningitis is frequently present and is most intense in the involved area. Anterior nerve root degeneration can be associated with a motor neuron radiculitis. VZV can be isolated from CSF and nerve tissue, which suggests that these changes represent direct viral invasion. CNS involvement is responsible for 20 percent of admissions to hospital. The most common presentation is acute cerebellitis, which appears towards the end of the first or the beginning of the second week after the onset of the rash and is usually transient. A more serious form of encephalitis occurring earlier during the course of varicella is a progressive encephalopathy with loss of conciousness and convulsions. If the brain swelling cannot be reduced the patient may assume a decorticate position. Less common neurological presentations seen in varicella include meningoencephalitis, transverse myelitis, peripheral neuritis, and Reye's syndrome.

In contrast to neuralgia, the most common and important clinical manifestation of herpes zoster encephalitis is a rare complication. Typically, the rash involves the cranial or upper cervical nerves, and little is known about its pathogenesis. Lesions of disseminated herpes zoster are identical to those of fatal varicella. In zoster meningoencephalitis there are lesions ranging from mononuclear infiltration of the meninges to necrotizing encephalitis with axonal degeneration, macrophage infiltration, and characteristic intranuclear inclusions and viral particles in the glial cells.

Enteroviruses

The genus *Enterovirus* belongs to the family *Picornaviridae* (see Chapter 40, Picornaviruses). It contains a number of viruses that give rise to infections of the CNS, notably polioviruses, enteroviruses, coxsackie, and echoviruses. Epidemics of poliovirus, for instance, were once a worldwide scourge, but with widespread vaccination and the eradication program since 1988 the number of annual cases could be reduced from approximately 350 000 to 497 in 2001, mostly in Africa and Asia. Of the 853 confirmed polio cases in 2002, 651 occured in India. Aseptic meningitis due to other enteroviruses is now the most frequent neurological infection of viral origin. It may occur sporadically or in epidemic form, with significant morbidity and, depending on specific host factors, mortality. Enteroviruses multiply in the lymphoid tissue of the alimentary tract and cause a wide range of syndromes. The extent to which enteroviruses are responsible for CNS disease is very difficult to gauge because of both underreporting and the subclinical nature of infection in approximately 90 percent of cases. Children are the main targets of enterovirus infection, and also serve as a mode for virus dissemination. In general, gender does not seem to predispose to a certain type of disease, although cases of childhood paralytic poliomyelitis are twice as common in males as in females.

POLIOMYELITIS

Natural infection with poliovirus occurs via the oral route, whereupon virus replicates in the tonsils, the lymphatic tissue which drains the neck, Peyer's patches, and the small intestine. Whether infection of lymphoid tissue such as the tonsils is achieved after initial replication of virus in the gut and subsequent viremia, or during the initial infection following ingestion, is a topic of debate. It is generally held that, for successful invasion of the CNS by poliovirus, a viremic phase is required, although some evidence suggests that direct infection of the CNS can take place via nerve endings in the gut.

Once poliovirus has gained access to the CNS the outcome of disease can be devastating, and is based largely on the highly cytopathic nature of poliovirus replication. The majority of infections (90–95 percent) are, however, silent, although virus may be recovered in the stools or from throat swabs of infected persons. Abortive infections (4–8 percent) include self-limiting forms of poliovirus infection and may present as an upper respiratory tract infection, gastroenteritis, or an influenza-like illness. Nonparalytic poliomyelitis (1–2 percent) presents initially as an abortive infection that is followed by invasion of the CNS by virus. Accompanying the assault on the CNS by virus are symptoms of aseptic meningitis with back pain and muscle spasms.

Paralytic poliomyelitis/polio encephalitis (0.1–2 percent), such as nonparalytic poliomyelitis, will generally present as an abortive infection during the prodromal stages, although there is often no evidence of an early phase of infection. The illness may be biphasic (often seen in children), with meningeal irritation and, finally, the onset of asymmetric flaccid paralysis (when whole muscle groups are involved) or paresis (when muscle group involvement is somewhat limited). Poliomyelitis can be divided into three basic types (spinal, bulbar, and bulbospinal), depending on the site of nerve cell involvement. Bulbar paralysis is more common in children and generally does not involve the limbs, whereas adults presenting with bulbar poliomyelitis typically have limb paralysis.

The gross pathology of poliovirus infection has been widely studied (Bodian and Horstmann 1965). Classically, there is extensive damage to the large anterior horn cells of the spinal cord. When paralysis is associated with poliomyelitis the cervical and lumbar areas (which serve limbs) are particularly affected. In fatal cases of poliomyelitis there may also be involvement of the brainstem motor nuclei, as seen in bulbar poliomyelitis, or of nerve cells of the motor cortex or thalamus and hypothalamus. After infection of cells of the CNS by poliovirus, the earliest histological change is vascular engorgement, rapidly followed by perivascular infiltration. The infiltrate comprises mainly lymphocytes and, to some degree, polymorphonuclear neutrophils, plasma cells and microglia. Cell damage is largely due to cytolytic replication of poliovirus within cells. Infected nerves swell and undergo satellitosis before being phagocytosed by mononuclear cells. Viral destruction of cells results in degeneration of axons and axon sheaths, followed by atrophy of the affected area and astrocytic scarring. Flaccid paralysis accompanies these changes, followed by a widespread atrophy of muscle no longer innervated by affected nerves. Death is often due to respiratory failure as a result of respiratory paralysis or secondary complications (e.g. bacterial pneumonia). People affected by paralytic poliomyelitis may develop new muscle weakness and prominent midday fatigue 25–30 years later as part of the postpolio syndrome (PPS) (Munsat 1991; Stone 1994; Dalakas 2002). The basis for the muscle weakness is an ongoing motor neuron deterioration related to the extensive motor unit remodeling during recovery from poliomyelitis, leading to postpoliomyelitis progressive muscular atrophy, whereas the basis for midday fatigue may be related to the abnormal presence of cytokines, possibly owing to persistence of poliovirus in the CNS.

ENTEROVIRUS

Of the numerous serotypes of enteroviruses that are recognized, two deserve special recognition with respect to disease involvement of the CNS: enterovirus serotypes 70 and 71 (for review, see Yin-Murphy 1994).

Both are transmitted by the fecal–oral route, although ocular infections with enterovirus 70 may be mediated by facecloths and bath towels, etc. Although enterovirus 70 has a marked predilection for epithelial cells of the conjunctiva, the fact that patients may exhibit signs of CNS involvement suggests neurotropism. However, enterovirus 70 has yet to be isolated from the CSF or CNS of infected patients.

The three forms of CNS disease caused by enterovirus 70 are the spinal form, the cranial form, and a combination of the two. The spinal form is by far the most commonly encountered and is characterized by an asymmetrical flaccid paralysis or paresis, with one or more limbs involved. Paralysis is the manifestation of infection of the anterior horn cells of the spinal cord by enterovirus 70. Atrophy of the affected muscle groups resembles poliomyelitis. In the cranial form, acute motor cranial nerve palsy is seen which may involve single nerves or groups of nerves. In the spinal cord there is marked degeneration of anterior horn cells and neuroglial cell proliferation. Immunofluorescence staining for enterovirus 70 antigen reveals the presence of virus in the microglial or neuronal cells, or both.

Although expression of clinical disease of the CNS by enterovirus 70 is somewhat rare, enterovirus 71 has caused epidemics of aseptic meningitis and encephalitis (Minn 2002). Originally described in California, the virus has been associated with neurological disease on a worldwide scale. The major clinical manifestation is that of aseptic meningitis, which may often be concomitant with encephalitis, bulbospinal disturbances, and polyneuritis. Children under 5 years of age are particularly susceptible to the most severe forms of enterovirus 71-associated neurological disease, including aseptic meningitis, brainstem and/or cerebellar encephalitis, and acute flaccid paralysis. Because the majority of patients are hospitalized for possible bacterial infection, a rapid test such as RT-PCR for the diagnosis of enteroviral meningitis may reduce hospitalizations and unnecessary treatments (Stellrecht et al. 2002). Studies in primates with strains of virus isolated from patients with CNS disease show degeneration and necrosis of the neurons and neuronophagia by polymorphonuclear and mononuclear cells. Analysis of the CNS reveals predominantly perivascular cuffing in the lumbar and cervical cord, with minor involvement of specific areas of the brain (including the medulla oblongata and midbrain).

COXSACKIE VIRUSES

Coxsackie viruses A and B also enter the host primarily via the oral route and follow essentially the same path as poliovirus, with replication in the Peyer's patches of the alimentary tract. Most infections are clinically silent, although some individuals exhibit greater susceptibility than others (a male:female infection ratio of 1.5:2.0 is observed for clinical disease). The reasons for this discrepancy remain elusive. Nervous system involvement has been documented for coxsackie viruses A7 and A9, and for B1–B6, which induce an aseptic meningitis and poliovirus-like paralysis. coxsackie virus B may also cause chronic meningitis and/or encephalitis in immunocompromised persons. Encephalitis, ataxia, and paralysis of the cranial nerves are rare. Both coxsackie viruses A and B are responsible for aseptic meningitis, although echoviruses (see below) are more frequently involved. Pathological changes with encephalitic and poliomyelitis cases in laboratory animals include brown fat necrosis and myocarditis, which is widespread in animals infected with coxsackie B virus (for review see Whitton 2002).

ECHOVIRUSES

Echoviruses have been associated with a number of syndromes, including aseptic meningitis, encephalitis, paralysis, ataxia, and Guillain–Barré syndrome, to list those affecting the CNS. Humans are the only recognized host for echoviruses, and several epidemics of disease have been attributed to them. Assigning a particular serotype to a specific syndrome has not been possible, although Guillain–Barré syndrome has been linked to infection with echovirus 9. In addition, echovirus 4 has been isolated from patients with bilateral limb paralysis. Similar syndromes have been noted for adults and children infected with echovirus serotypes 6, 9, 14, 17, 19, and 30. Primary infection results in replication of virus in the alimentary tract, after which other organs are seeded following an initial viremia. The nature of the secondary target is largely random. Occasional peripheral neuropathies have been documented following expression of the virus in the CNS. Initial clinical symptoms of CNS invasion by echoviruses can mimic bulbospinal poliomyelitis, although the major clinical manifestation is that of lymphocytic meningitis. Neonatal infection with echoviruses may lead to encephalitis with white matter sclerosis. In general, infection of newborns and younger children with echovirus is more severe than in older people.

Flaviviruses

There are currently about 70 registered flaviviruses (see Chapter 46, Flaviviruses), of which about 50 percent are associated with human disease (Heinz et al. 2000). Of those that cause significant CNS disease, Japanese encephalitis virus (JEV), which causes epidemics over much of Asia, carries the highest mortality rate of any flavivirus. In epidemics, mortality rates range from 10 to 20 percent in most outbreaks to >30 percent (Umenai et al. 1985; Bu' Lock 1986). tick-borne encephalitis virus (TBEV) has long been recognized as a public health problem in eastern Europe. In Russia, the virus caused high mortality in the 1930s, prompting a great effort to isolate the causative agent and to produce a vaccine

(Silber and Soloviev 1946). A number of subtypes of TBE have been defined in different geographical locations, including eastern subtypes such as Sofyn, the agent of Russian spring–summer encephalitis (RSSE) (Silber and Soloviev 1946), and western subtypes, such as Hypr (Blaskovic et al. 1967) and Neudörfl (Ackerman et al. 1986). Mosquito-borne JEV continues to threaten large populations, even though massive vaccination campaigns have been undertaken. Vaccination may, however, be undermined to a large degree by the high antigenic variation in different subtypes of JEV. Other mosquito-borne flaviviruses that tend to involve the CNS include St. Louis encephalitis (SLEV) and Murray Valley encephalitis (MVEV). SLE became a serious public health problem in the USA in the 1960s and continues to cause concern during sporadic outbreaks (Kokernot et al. 1969). MVE causes epidemics in Australia, disease occurring intermittently in areas that have experienced periods of high rainfall. Epidemics in the southern hemisphere are usually recorded from January to March and coincide with high population levels of the mosquito vector. Recently, the emergence of JEV and West Nile virus (WNV) in new geographic areas several thousand kilometres from their known habitats has caused considerable concern. JEV appeared in the Australian zoogeographic region in 1995 about 3 000 km from its nearest known focus in Bali, and WNV jumped from the Middle East to the United States in 1999 (Mackenzie et al. 2002b; Roehrig et al. 2002). The JEV group of the genus *Flavivirus* comprises several viruses, including *Japanese encephalitis*, *West Nile*, *St. Louis encephalitis*, and *Murray Valley viruses*.

JAPANESE ENCEPHALITIS VIRUS

Japanese encephalitis (JE) occurs in epidemic form in temperate areas of Asia, the northern parts of tropical southeast Asia, and northern parts of Australia. With respect to number of cases (30 000–50 000 annually) and associated morbidity and mortality, JE is the most important of the arbovirus encephalitides, which is transmitted to humans via the bite of an infected mosquito (*Culex* spp.) and the case fatality rate of which is up to 35 percent (Solomon and Vaughn 2002). JEV has a major mammalian amplifying host in the pig, and indeed most epidemic activity is driven by mosquito–pig transmission cycles.

After humans become infected, virus is thought to replicate in the skin and is transported to local lymph nodes, probably in migrating dendritic cells.

How JEV invades the CNS is unknown. After a variable incubation period of 6–16 days the disease may be asymptomatic or fulminant in course. Death may be rapid, occurring 10 days after onset in some cases. For patients who develop encephalitis, the disease pattern begins with headache, cough, coryza, nausea, vomiting, and gastroenteritis, proceeding to the onset of high fever and alterations in sensory perception (including confusion or delirium, which may result in coma). Other patients present with aseptic meningitis and have no encephalitic features. Seizures are uncommon in adults, but are often (20 percent or more) seen in children. Facial motor weakness is often observed and upper motor neuron paralysis and paresis are common. Neurological sequelae are common (up to 70 percent) in survivors of symptomatic JEV infection, and are particularly severe in children. Such sequelae include convulsive disorders, motor abnormalities, impaired intellect, and emotional disturbances.

The areas of the brain infected by JEV include the cerebral cortex, the cerebellum, and the spinal cord. The highest concentration of infected neurons is in the thalamus and brainstem. Once in the CNS JEV virus replicates very efficiently in neurons, and it is the destruction of these cells by virus that is directly related to the manifestation of encephalitis. The brain and meninges of JE patients show edema, congestion, and focal hemorrhages. Microscopically, there is degeneration and necrosis of neurons, with accompanying neuronophagia in the cerebral cortex, cerebellum, and spinal cord. There is marked destruction of Purkinje cells in the cerebellum, as well as perivascular cuffing and inflammatory infiltrates in surrounding neural tissue. JE antigen is usually not detected in glial cells.

Vaccination against JEV ideally should be routinely practiced in all areas where the virus causes human disease (Monath 2002). For a laboratory confirmation of JE, rapid diagnostic kits based on ELISA techniques are available. There is currently no specific antiviral treatment.

WEST NILE VIRUS

Although mosquitos are the vector for WNV, birds are instrumental in its spread, acting both as a viral reservoir and in geographical spread. Geographically, WNV infections have been described in Egypt (1951–1975), Israel (1951–1980), France, Spain, Africa, India, Pakistan, since 1996 in Romania, and since 1999 in the eastern states of the USA (Murgue et al. 2002; Roehrig et al., 2002).

After an incubation period of 2–6 days patients develop a sudden onset of high fever with chills, malaise, headache, backache, arthralgia, myalgia, and retro-orbital pain, which is made worse by eye movement (Solomon and Vaughn 2002). Other nonspecific features are common. A rash appears from the second to the fifth day of illness in about 50 percent of patients, and is more common in young children. Neurological manifestations of WNV infection are similar to those of JEV infection, including aseptic meningitis, encephalitis, myelitis, or combinations of the three. After 1–7 days of a febrile prodrome, with headache, weakness, and gastrointestinal symptoms, patients become drowsy, confused, and disorientated. Although in most cases the prodrome is nonspecific, up to 16 percent of patients

may have features suggestive of WN fever, including eye pain, facial congestion, pharyngeal or conjunctival hyperemia, lymphadenopathy, arthralgia, or cutaneous eruptions. In some patients the illness is biphasic, with two fever peaks. Focal neurological signs include upper motor neuron weakness, lower cranial nerve palsies, tremor, and ataxia. WNV infection may also cause a flaccid paralysis of the limbs and respiratory muscles, which may require ventilation. Urinary incontinence or retention may also occur. The case fatality rate for patients with symptoms of the CNS due to WNV infection is 5–10 percent. Whereas younger patients are more likely to present with WN fever or aseptic meningitis, older patients are more likely to develop encephalitis and to die.

WNV infections are most frequently diagnosed by assessment of the antibody response in an IgM antibody capture ELISA. There is currently no specific antiviral treatment.

ST. LOUIS ENCEPHALITIS VIRUS

St. Louis encephalitis virus is a mosquito-borne *Flavivirus* that occurs in both endemic and epidemic forms in the USA and represents the most important arbovirus disease of North America. The virus is transmitted by *Culex* spp.

Clinically, infection with SLEV can range from inapparent infections to fulminant encephalitis and death. Patients usually present with or progress rapidly to one of three established syndromes: febrile headache, aseptic meningitis, or encephalitis. The febrile headache is often accompanied by vomiting and nausea. Analysis of the CSF may reveal pleocytosis. There are no apparent signs of meningeal involvement or neurological abnormalities. Aseptic meningitis presents as an acute febrile illness with signs of meningeal irritation and pleocytosis in the CSF. Encephalitis attributed to SLEV infection also includes meningoencephalitis and encephalomyelitis. Alterations in the state of consciousness or localized neurological abnormalities, or both, may be seen. Brinker and co-workers (Brinker et al. 1979) analyzed data from 18 reports of patients with SLE. It is estimated that 70–80 percent of patients suffer from headache, nuchal rigidity, and an altered level of consciousness. Almost 50 percent display tremors, pathological reflexes, and confusion. Some 20–30 percent of patients exhibit multiple cranial nerve abnormalities, hypoactive deep tendon reflexes, positive Babinski signs, or myalgia. More significantly, 11–20 percent of those infected have VIIth cranial nerve lesions, lower motor neuron lesions, hyperactive deep tendon reflexes, or myoclonus, and progress to coma. Up to 10 percent exhibit convulsions, paresis, photophobia, nystagmus, or ataxia. There is a striking increase in case fatality rates for SLEV infection, depending on age. A fatality rate of approximately 2 percent is observed for young adults, rising to 22 percent for the elderly. Of those infected with SLEV, approximately 50 percent with fatal disease die within 1 week after the onset of symptoms.

MURRAY VALLEY ENCEPHALITIS

Murray Valley encephalitis virus is the major *Flavivirus* in Australia and Papua New Guinea (Mackenzie et al. 2002a).

Antigenically, it is closely related to both JE and SLE viruses. In a number of respects the clinical presentation of patients suffering from MVE is similar to that of JE infection. Clinically, the disease begins with a prodrome of fever, headache, photophobia, myalgia, nausea, and vomiting. There are often early signs of CNS involvement that include drowsiness, speech difficulties, disorientation, and ataxia. Patients who do not progress to coma generally have a favorable prognosis, but may display sequelae including tremors, incontinence, stiffened limbs and neck, and speech impediments. Patients who enter coma often develop respiratory paralysis, necessitating mechanical aid for breathing. Fatalities are usually the result of secondary infection or extensive brain destruction, accompanied by decerebrate rigidity.

TICK-BORNE ENCEPHALITIS

The tick-borne encephalitis (TBE) complex of the family *Flaviviridae* comprises 14 antigenically related viruses, eight of which are significant human pathogens (Heinz et al. 2000). The two most important are Russian spring–summer encephalitis (RSSE) and Central European encephalitis (CEE). These differ in pathogenicity, the former being associated with much higher rates of morbidity and mortality.

RSSE is characterized by a gradual onset following 10–14 days' incubation after the transmission of virus from the bite of an infected tick. The patient suffers a prodromal phase of severe headache, nausea, photophobia, weakness, fever, and chills. The body temperature may rise as high as 41°C and the fever lasts 5–7 days. These symptoms are followed by neck stiffness, sensory changes, visual disturbances, and variable neurological dysfunction, including paresis, paralysis, sensory loss, and convulsions (Silber and Soloviev 1946). The more severe cases can develop central paralysis or involve the brainstem or spinal cord, which may lead to bulbospinal or spinal paralysis. In fatal cases death occurs within the first week after onset, with case fatality rates of approximately 30 percent (Gresikova and Beran 1981). Disease is more severe in children than in adults. Recovery from infection is protracted, with neurological sequelae in 30–69 percent of survivors, manifested by residual flaccid paralysis of the shoulders and arms. These sequelae probably reflect permanent damage to neurons.

In comparison to RSSE, infection with CEE subtypes of virus is much milder, with a number of abortive infections. Classically, CEE is a biphasic illness with a prodromal period resembling influenza that either resolves completely or is followed by the sudden onset of encephalitis. Onset of illness is often rapid, with fever, severe headache, photophobia, nuchal rigidity, nausea, and vomiting. Patients who present with brainstem involvement or have ascending paralysis generally have a poor prognosis. Although case fatality rates range between 1 and 5 percent, 20 percent of survivors suffer minor neuropsychiatric sequelae (Radsel-Medvescek et al. 1980). It is interesting that a small percentage of patients who recover from CEE have a progressive chronic encephalitis with remissions and relapses (Silber and Soloviev 1946).

Clinical signs are swelling, congestion, and petechial hemorrhages in the brain, similar to other flavivirus encephalitides. There is also meningeal and perivascular inflammation, with neuronal degeneration and necrosis, neuronophagia, and glial nodule formation in the cerebellar cortex, brainstem, basal ganglia, and spinal cord. Far Eastern subtypes have a tropism for neurons of the gray matter of the medulla oblongata and upper cervical cord. The predominance of lower motor neuron paralysis of the upper extremities, observed in many cases of encephalitis, may be explained by the vulnerability of the anterior horn cells of the cervical cord to virus infection.

Retroviruses

In this section, two neurotropic human pathogenic retroviruses, HIV and human T-lymphotropic virus (also known as human T-cell leukemia virus-1 (HTLV-1)), that cause distinct syndromes affecting the CNS are considered (see also Chapters 58, Retroviruses and associated diseases in humans and 60, Human immunodeficiency virus), Both viruses have a prolonged incubation period (average of 8–10 years for HIV, and up to 40 years for HTLV-I-associated myelopathy). Some similarities exist between modes of transmission via the transfer of body fluids containing free virus or, more often, infected cells. HIV and HTLV-I both have a primary tropism for lymphocytes.

HIV-ASSOCIATED DEMENTIA

Exactly how HIV gains access to the CNS is unknown. In early acute infections HIV can be detected as free virus in the CSF of patients with no apparent neurological disturbances. Crossing of the BBB is believed to occur through passage of the virus in infected peripheral blood macrophages or activated T cells (Gartner 2000; Patrick et al. 2002). In the brain, HIV infects mainly microglial cells. Additional evidence points to possible infection of brain capillary endothelial cells, which are CD4-negative, but chemokine receptor and SIGNR-positive (Mukhtar et al. 2002; Soilleux et al. 2002). Furthermore, galactosylceramide (GalC) has been proposed to fulfil a receptor function in brain-derived cells (Harouse et al. 1991). Differences in tropism between strains of HIV could be demonstrated. In general, macrophage-tropic strains replicate more efficiently in cells of neural origin than strains of a T-cell tropic nature.

AIDS itself is often characterized by a high prevalence of marked and extensive neurological disturbances. In numerical terms, it is suggested that as many as 80 percent of AIDS patients will have neuropathological abnormalities at postmortem, and that as many as half of these will have suffered neurological disturbances prior to death. Transient neurological disturbances can also be detected at the time of seroconversion, and may include aseptic meningitis (characterized by headache, fever, and cellular pleocytosis of the CSF), acute encephalopathy, and myelopathy. All these disturbances are usually self-limiting during early infection. As HIV infection progresses to AIDS a new spectrum of neurological complications may emerge, which are globally described as the AIDS dementia complex or HIV-associated dementia (HAD) (Cortegis 1994). The primary stages of HAD show mild impairment of memory, as well as loss of concentration and the ability to process information. Symptoms may then progress to severe cognitive dysfunction and possibly paralysis. Morphologically, features associated with HAD include either a diffuse leukoencephalopathy with severe reduction in myelin, or areas of discrete demyelination and multinucleated giant cells (Figure 62.6). Clinically, HAD is suspected in AIDS patients presenting with memory loss, disturbances in concentration, depression, and motor complaints. Specific afflictions associated with HAD include peripheral neuropathy, cerebral tumors, and vascular lesions. Peripheral neuropathies are often observed in severely immunosuppressed patients who present with painful paraesthesiae. These are due to axonal degeneration of small myelinated and unmyelinated fibers as a result of exposure to toxic factors (see below). It is interesting to note that the inflammatory neuropathies, including demyelinating polyneuropathy, are identical in clinical course to Guillain–Barré syndrome or chronic inflammatory demyelinating polyneuropathy (Cornblath et al. 1987; Tyor et al. 1995). In the latter condition the nerves show perivascular lymphocytic and monocytic infiltrates, believed to be mediated by T cells and macrophages. Cerebrovascular

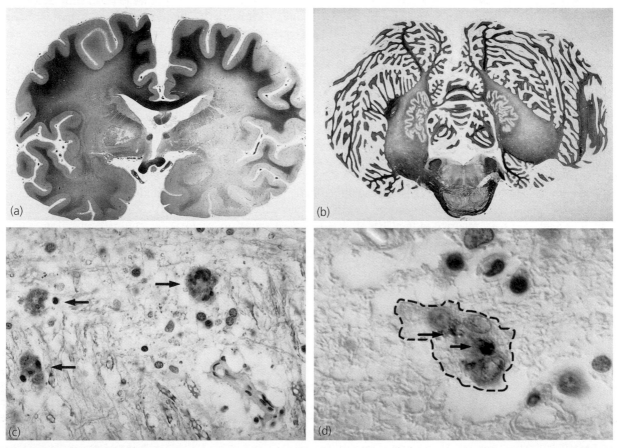

Figure 62.6 *HIV encephalopathy.* **(a)** *Whole mount of a brain slice, stained with a myelinotropic dye (Luxol fast blue). The hallmark of HIV leukoencephalopathy is diffuse reduction of myelin stain in the central white matter.* **(b)** *Whole mount of the cerebellum of the same patient. Leukoencephalopathy is evident in the deep cerebellar white matter.* **(c)** *High-power micrograph of HIV leukoencephalopathy, showing loss of myelin and typical multinucleated giant cells (arrows) (×200).* **(d)** *Immunostaining of a multinucleated giant cell for the HIV protein p24, showing granular immunoreactivity (arrows) (×400). (Courtesy of Dr Adriano Aguzzi.)*

complications such as vasculitis and hemorrhages are often found in areas of cerebral tumor or demyelination. Hemorrhages may occur as a result of alterations in coagulation (Snider et al. 1983).

Mechanism of CNS disturbances in neuro-AIDS

Despite the observation that HAD is associated with HIV infection of microglia/macrophages, the number of HIV-infected cells and the amount of viral antigen in the CNS do not correlate well with measures of cognitive decline (Glass et al. 1995). Direct viral infection of susceptible cells of the CNS may induce syncytia formation, producing multinucleated giant cells. Multinucleated giant cells are usually formed by macrophages or microglial cells and are considered a hallmark of subacute encephalitis in HIV-infected brains and spinal cord, but not in peripheral nerves (Cornblath et al. 1987) (Figure 62.6). As only a restricted number of cells of the CNS are susceptible to infection by HIV, secondary mechanisms of cellular injury are paramount in producing neurological disturbances in AIDS patients.

The release of neurotoxic soluble factors by cells in response to viral assault or to binding of virus proteins is an important facet of the disease process of HIV.

Infection of monocytes or macrophages by HIV is known to stimulate the synthesis and release of a number of cytokines, including chemokines, IL-1β, TNF-α, interferons, and nitric oxide (NO) (Garden 2002; Ryan et al. 2002; Wang et al. 2002). Possibly the most notable change associated with HIV dementia with AIDS is the upregulation of TNF-α. TNF-α levels were higher in patients with advanced dementia and those with multinucleated giant cells or diffuse myelin pallor (Wilt et al. 1995). The release of cytokines makes the BBB more permeable to inflammatory cells, which may then infiltrate the CNS to establish additional neurological sequelae. Although significant levels of quinolinic acid have been reported in the CNS of HIV-1 seropositive patients, whether there is a direct causal relationship with the observed neurological findings remains questionable. Induction of TGF-β by macrophages and astrocytes has also been linked to CNS disorders (Wahl et al. 1991). Studies examining levels of specific chemokines in patients with HAD have shown that β-chemokines (RANTES and MIP-1α) are elevated in the CSF of patients, but higher levels were associated with the preservation of cognitive function (Letendre et al. 1999). Microglia also release excitatory amino acids and related substances that most likely contribute to the neuronal disfunction in HAD, including glutamate, quinolinate, L-cysteine, and the amine Ntox (Garden 2002). These substances can induce N-methyl-D-aspartate (NMDA) receptor-mediated neuronal apoptosis.

Autoimmunity is also thought to be important in the process of HIV-induced neurological disease, and may be based on the partial identity between viral antigens and antigenic determinants on cells (i.e. molecular mimicry). An autoimmune process was proposed following the observation that small demyelinated regions of the brain seem similar to those in post-infectious encephalomyelitis or experimental allergic encephalitis (Kumar et al. 1989). AIDS patients with peripheral neuropathy have autoantibodies to an unidentified protein on the surface of neurons. In addition, fluorescence studies have shown antibody attached to the perineurium in tissues from AIDS patients. AIDS patients suffering from peripheral neuropathy who undergo subsequent plasmapheresis obtain relief of symptoms similar to that observed in the autoimmune conditions of Guillain–Barré syndrome and thrombocytopenic purpura. Autoantibodies to peripheral nerves are associated with peripheral neuropathy. A likely target in the nervous system is the myelin sheath of nerves. Antibody levels to myelin basic protein have been described in CSF of AIDS patients that correlate directly with the severity of dementia (Liuzzi et al. 1994). Cross-reactivity of anti-gp41 antibodies with certain proteins of astrocytes could compromise the function of these cells. Moreover, cross-reaction of anti-V3 antibody with human brain proteins may also be an important part of the pathogenic process. Further brain-reactive proteins in the sera of infected patients may lead to immune complex disease.

A number of HIV products (e.g. gp120) are toxic to cultured human brain cells in vitro. NMDA antagonists have been shown to reduce toxic effects attributed to gp120 interaction (Lipton et al. 1991). The same viral protein can also affect the permeability of the cell membrane, leading to ion influx/efflux and loss of electrical potential. Inhibitors of the p38 MAP kinase have been shown to abrogate neuronal apoptosis due to HIV gp120 exposure or α-chemokine (SDF-1) toxicity (Kaul and Lipton 1999). The HIV proteins gp41 and Tat have been shown to be toxic for cultured cells: Tat exhibits some homology with a neurotoxin and induces cellular aggregation and fascicle formation in primary rat cortical brain cells (Garry and Koch 1992). In addition, Tat may induce differentiation of these cells (Kolson et al. 1993). The clinical relevance of these findings, however, remains unclear. When discussing HIV infection, it is also important to consider that neurotropic effects may reflect infection with an additional agent. A number of studies have shown the presence of viruses such as *Cytomegalovirus* (Figure 62.7), or polyomaviruses in the CNS of AIDS patients, and have led to the suggestion that secondary infections are the primary cause of neurological disturbances.

HTLV-I ASSOCIATED MYELOPATHY/TROPICAL SPASTIC PARAPARESIS

Human T-lymphotropic virus type I infects 10–20 million people worldwide, and is endemic in southern Japan, the

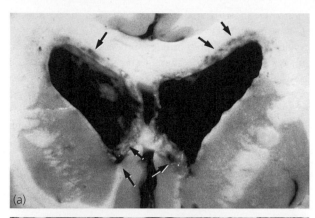

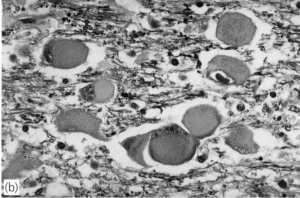

Figure 62.7 Cytomegalovirus *encephalitis in an AIDS patient.* **(a)** *Typical CMV-induced damage with areas of necrosis and microhemorrhage located in subependymal positions (arrows).* **(b)** *Focus of CMV encephalitis within the corpus callosum (x400). Characteristic cytomegalic cells with large inclusion bodies representing viral products. (Courtesy of Dr Adriano Aguzzi.)*

Caribbean, Central and South America, the Middle East, Melanesia, and equatorial regions of Africa.

HTLV-I was established as an etiologic agent of acute T-cell leukemia (ATL). A correlation between tumor cells and a monoclonal or oligoclonal pattern of viral genome integration, infection of lymphocytes in vitro resulting in immortalized T cells, and the establishment of HTLV-I oncogenic animal model systems has been reported (Cann and Chen 1990). In 1985 it was discovered that a number of HTLV-I-seropositive patients in the Caribbean and Japan were suffering from a chronic myelopathy. Since then, increasing evidence has accumulated linking HTLV-I infection with what is now termed HTLV-I-associated myelopathy (HAM) or tropical spastic paraparesis (TSP), collectively known as HAM/TSP, which is developed by 0.25–3 percent of virus carriers (Jacobson 2002).

HAM/TSP presents as a clinical disease very distinct from ATL. The disorder is characterized by weakness and spasticity of the extremities, hyperreflexia, peripheral sensory loss, and chronic inflammation. The development of HAM/TSP correlates with the presence of lesions in the white matter of the spinal cord, including demyelination and axonal changes. In the subacute

disease there is progressive paralysis of the lower extremities and associated impotence, incontinence, and sensory symptoms, paradoxically often with minimal sensory findings on examination. Lesions are localized primarily in the thoracic spinal cord, with little, if any, cerebral involvement. In cases of late disease, hyalinization of vessels with necrosis and demyelination of the spinal cord, particularly in the throracic region, is observed. Because many patients are infected through breastfeeding from infected mothers or via sexual transmission, the virus is thought to be transmitted by infected lymphocytes. The incubation period is particularly long, with onset often in the fourth or fifth decade of life.

Gross examination of the brain reveals no apparent abnormalities, although the majority of cases exhibit severe loss of myelin and atrophy of the spinal cord, and some thickening of the meninges. These clinical findings are associated with HAM/TSP patients with a long history of illness, whereas in cases with a clinical history of 1 year or less the spinal cord often seems normal (Fukura et al. 1989). The major finding in HAM/TSP cases is a chronic inflammatory process, with perivascular infiltrates involving the gray and, more often, the white matter of the spinal cord. Numerous inflammatory cells, including $CD4^+$ and $CD8^+$ T cells, B cells, and foamy macrophages, are present in damaged areas of the spinal cord parenchyma (Wu et al. 1993). Later in the disease, immunohistochemical analysis of the affected lesions shows the predominance of $CD8^+$ T cells (Umehara et al. 1993). HTLV-I sequence analysis of PBMCs of HAM/TSP patients demonstrates a pattern of polyclonal integration, in contrast to an oligoclonal or monoclonal pattern associated with ATL patients. Most HAM/TSP patients have higher titers of anti-HTLV-I antibodies than do asymptomatic HTLV-I patients. The amount of proviral DNA in HAM/TSP patients correlates with the number of CTL. HTLV-I-specific sequences have been localized to astrocytes in affected areas of the CNS (Lehky et al. 1995). An autoimmune basis for HAM/TSP has been proposed after the isolation of circulating MHC class I-restricted CTLs from HAM/TSP patients. The CTLs show specific activity against a nine amino acid peptide of the HTLV-I tax protein, and are restricted to the HLA-A201 haplotype (Elovaara et al. 1993; Koenig et al. 1993). The presence of HTLV-I-specific CTL correlates with the production of several cytokines and chemokines, such as IFN-γ, TNF-α, IL-2, MIP-1α/β, and matrix metalloproteinases (Biddison et al. 1997; Kubota et al. 1998; Giraudon et al. 2000). In HLA-A201 patients the increased HTLV-I proviral DNA loads in CSF in comparison to PBMC were propotional to the frequency of tax-specific $CD8^+$ T cells. This observation supports the hypothesis that the HTLV-I proviral load may drive the increased virus-specific immune responses that have been suggested to be immunopathogenic in HAM/TSP (Soldan 2001). The data led to the following immunopathogenesis model of HAM/TSP: processing and presentation of HTLV-I-specific peptides in association with high proviral loads and viral protein expression in CD4$^+$ and CD8$^+$ T cells may lead to the activation and expansion of antigen-specific T-cell responses in the CNS. Numbers of inflammatory CD8$^+$ T cells in the spinal cord lesions of HAM/TSP patients tend to increase with disease progression, and together with inflammatory cytokines and chemokines, immunopathogenesis may be enhanced.

To help in understanding the disease process involved in HAM/TSP, an animal model using Wistar–King–Aptekman (WKA) rats has been developed in which the characteristics and distribution of lesions in the rat CNS are similar to those observed in human cases (Ishiguro et al. 1992; Kasai et al. 1999). After an icubation period of approximately 15 months the rats develop a chronic progressive myelopathy with paraparesis of the hind limbs. HTLV-I proviral DNA was localized in some microglia/macrophages in spinal cord lesions. In addition, provirus was evident not only in ED-1-negative lymphoid cells, but also in ED-1-positive macrophages from lymph nodes. These infected microglia/macrophages may relate to cause the myeloneuropathy through neurotoxic cytokine synthesis. The expression of the antiapoptotic gene bcl-2 was strongly downregulated in oligodendrocytes of infected rats. This may increase the susceptibility to TNF-α-induced apoptosis of oligodendrocytes and result in the development of the characteristic disease (Jiang et al. 2000).

Paramyxoviruses

The two paramyxoviruses frequently liable to cause CNS diseases are mumps and measles viruses, both members of the subfamily *Paramyxovirinae* (see Chapters 33, 34, and 35).

MUMPS VIRUS INFECTIONS OF THE CNS

Mumps is a highly communicable and generally self-limited infection caused by mumps virus (MuV). It occurs in epidemics among susceptible school-aged children and is characterized clinically by nonsuppurative salivary gland enlargement. Although parotitis is the most obvious manifestation, mumps is clearly a systemic infection that can involve virtually all organs, including the CNS. Indeed, CNS involvement during acute mumps infection occurs with such high frequency that it should be considered a primary manifestation, rather than a complication. The spectrum of CNS infections caused by mumps virus ranges from aseptic meningitis, which is very common but usually mild, to fulminant encephalitis, which is very rare but potentially fatal. The term 'mumps meningoencephalitis' is often used to designate overlap syndromes that have features of both these typical forms. Mumps vaccine has successfully been used

by many countries, and high coverage has shown a rapid decline in mumps morbidity (Galazka et al. 1999).

Mumps is a highly contagious infection that is transmitted from human to human (the only known natural host) by droplets. Infected individuals may transmit the virus for about 10–16 days. During the incubation period (which averages 18 days), primary viral replication takes place in epithelial cells of the upper respiratory tract, followed by spread of the virus to regional lymph nodes and subsequent viremia, with systemic dissemination.

Symptomatic CNS involvement occurs in 10–20 percent of cases (Russell and Donald 1958; Galazka et al. 1999). The vast majority of cases of CNS MuV infections are uncomplicated aseptic meningitis, whereas symptomatic encephalitis occurs in >0.1 percent of cases (Klemola et al. 1965; Levitt et al. 1970). The incidence of CNS inflammation as evidenced by pleocytosis in the CSF (observed in only 60 percent of cases) is actually much higher than the incidence of clinical meningoencephalitis (Bang and Bang 1943).

Although differences in neurotropism among MuV isolates have been demonstrated in animal models, there is no direct evidence that cases of human mumps encephalitis are caused by virus strains with enhanced neurotropism or virulence.

Patients with symptomatic mumps CNS infection most often present with fever, vomiting, and headache. Other frequent findings include nuchal rigidity, lethargy, and abdominal pain (possibly from pancreatitis). Defervescence is usually the first sign of clinical recovery, which is normally complete within 7–10 days. Patients with simple mumps aseptic meningitis have signs of meningeal irritation, however, with normal cortical function. Cases of mumps encephalitis present with seizures, markedly depressed levels of consciousness, and focal neurological signs. Typical findings also include psychiatric disturbances, lethargy, and stupor. CNS symptoms appear about 5 days after the onset of parotitis, although they may accompany or even precede the development of salivary gland enlargement. No association between the parotitis and the frequency or severity of CNS manifestations has been established. Other neurological manifestations of mumps include myelitis and polyneuropathy.

Confirmation of CNS involvement in patients with mumps is based on examination of the CSF. CSF findings do not differ significantly between mumps patients with meningitis and those with encephalitis. MuV can be isolated from CSF in 30–50 percent of patients with CSF pleocytosis (Björvatn and Wolontis 1971; Wolontis and Björvatn 1973). The spinal fluid opening pressure is normal. Infiltrating cells are predominantly lymphocytes, but significant amounts of polymorphonuclear leukocytes may be seen in the early stages of infection. CSF pleocytosis resolves slowly, and complete normalization of the spinal fluid may require several weeks (Azimi et al. 1975). No correlation has been established between the magnitude of the CSF pleocytosis and the severity of clinical illness.

MuV spreads readily to the CNS, either as free plasma virus or within infected mononuclear cells (Fleischer and Kreth 1982). Initially, viral replication occurs in choroidal epithelial cells, with shedding of progeny virus into the CSF (Herndon et al. 1974). The development of mumps encephalitis probably results from a direct extension of the virus from ependymal cells into neurons within the brain parenchyma, as has been demonstrated in experimentally induced mumps encephalitis in hamsters (Wolinsky et al. 1974). Because of the low case:fatality ratio, autopsy reports describing the pathological findings in mumps meningoencephalitis are rare and variable (reviewed in Gnann 1991). Histological changes are seen in the white matter of the cerebral hemispheres and cerebellum, and in the white and gray matter of the brainstem and spinal cord. The most commonly recorded features are diffuse edema of the brain, limited mononuclear cell infiltration of the meninges, perivascular infiltration with mononuclear cells, glial cell proliferation, focal areas of neuronal cell destruction, and localized demyelination. A few cases of purported chronic mumps encephalitis have been described, but available data are insufficient to support a role for mumps virus in chronic CNS infection (Ito et al. 1991).

MEASLES VIRUS INFECTIONS OF THE CNS

Measles virus (MV) is a highly contagious agent that leads to a well-defined acute disease in unvaccinated individuals, followed by seroconversion and a lifelong immunity against reinfection. As hallmarks of acute measles, a transient, marked lymphopenia and immunosuppression are observed which favor the establishment and fatal outcome of opportunistic infections, and are the main reasons for the annual death toll of approximately 1 million children worldwide, particularly in developing countries (Clements and Cutts 1995; Schneider-Schaulies and ter Meulen 2002). Before the advent of vaccination, approximately 8 million deaths were due to measles annually. Vaccination protects not only from complications such as otitis media, pneumonia, and diarrhea, but also from acute and subacute encephalitis (Duclos and Ward 1998). Patients with a history of acute measles develop a lifelong immunity.

MV infections have also been linked etiologically to the establishment of CNS disease processes that include an early acute measles encephalitis and two late complications: subacute sclerosing panencephalitis and measles inclusion body encephalitis (MIBE). Moreover, some studies have suggested a pathogenic role of MV for other disease processes, including multiple sclerosis (ter Meulen and Katz 1997), chronic liver disease (Robertson et al. 1987; Andjaparidze et al. 1989), Paget's disease (Basle et al. 1986), otosclerosis

(McKenna and Mills 1989) and, more recently, Crohn's disease (Wakefield et al. 1993). However, none of these diseases has been linked unequivocally to measles virus.

Acute measles encephalitis

CNS involvement in the course of measles is fairly common, as EEG and CSF changes are found in half of all patients with acute measles (Gibbs et al. 1959; Reinicke et al. 1974). Acute encephalitis is observed in 0.5–1 per 1 000 cases (Katz 1995). In general, about 15 percent of cases are fatal, and 20–40 percent of those who recover are left with lasting neurological sequelae. Encephalitis usually develops within about 8 days after the onset of measles. Occasionally, it may also occur during the prodromal stage. Measles encephalitis is characterized by a resurgence of fever, headache, seizures, cerebellar ataxia, and coma. As is commonly seen in postinfectious encephalitis induced by other viruses, demyelination, perivascular cuffing, gliosis, and the appearance of fat-laden macrophages near the blood vessel walls are detectable histopathologically. Petechial hemorrhages may be present, and in some cases inclusion bodies have been observed in brain cells. CSF findings in measles encephalitis usually consist of mild pleocytosis and the absence of MV-specific antibodies. Long-term sequelae include selective brain damage, with retardation, recurrent convulsive seizures, hemiplegia, and paraplegia. It is not entirely clear what pathogenic role MV plays in the development of acute measles encephalitis. MV has been occasionally recovered from CSF samples (McLean et al. 1966) and brain tissue of patients (ter Meulen et al. 1972; Ogura et al. 1997), including the detection of MV-specific nucleic acids by PCR techniques (Nakayama et al. 1995). Because there is no evidence that MV is regularly present in the nervous system, and because there is an aberrant immune reaction to brain antigens, acute measles encephalitis is considered an autoimmune disease (Griffin 1995).

Measles inclusion body encephalitis

MIBE has been recognized only recently and is confined to immunosuppressed children with, for example, leukemia undergoing axial irradiation therapy. The incubation period ranges from weeks to several months. The condition commences with convulsions, myoclonic jerks as seen in SSPE. The seizures are often focal and localized to one site; other findings include hemiplegia, coma, or stupor. However, the disease course is more rapid than that of SSPE, and proceeds to death within weeks or a few months. Characteristically, no or only low titers of MV-specific antibodies are mounted in the serum and CSF of patients.

Subacute sclerosing panencephalitis

SSPE is a rare, fatal, slowly progressive degenerative disease of the CNS. It is generally seen in children and young adults aged 5–15 years after acute measles, with an incidence of approximately 1 in 100 000 cases – after infection with wildtype virus, and not after vaccination (Duclos and Ward 1998). Boys are more likely than girls to develop SSPE, and half the patients have contracted measles before the age of 2 years. No unusual features of acute measles have ever been demonstrated. The course of SSPE is variable and usually starts with a generalized intellectual deterioration, which may last for weeks or months, until definite neurological signs or motor dysfunctions such as dyspraxia, generalized convulsions, aphasia, visual disturbances, and mild repetitive simultaneous myoclonic jerks appear. Viral invasion of the retina leads, in 75 percent of cases, to a chorioretinitis, often affecting the macular area, followed by blindness. Finally, the disease proceeds to progressive cerebral degeneration, leading to coma and inevitable death. The illness generally lasts for 1–3 years, but more rapid forms have been described. Neuropathological findings include a diffuse encephalitis affecting both the gray and the white matter, characterized by perivascular cuffing and diffuse lymphocytic infiltrations. Gliosis is usually observed. Neurons, oligodendroglial cells, fibrous astrocytes, and endothelial cells contain large aggregates of intranuclear inclusion bodies that contain MV nucleocapsid structures, visible on immunohistological examination (Allen et al. 1996). Giant cell formation or membrane changes consistent with virus maturation have not been detected.

Characteristic EEG changes are usually the first diagnostic hint and are regarded as characteristic and even pathognomonic for SSPE. They consist of periodic high-amplitude slow-wave complexes that are synchronous with myoclonic jerks recurring at 3.5–20-second intervals. These periodic complexes (Radermecker) are remarkably stereotypical in an individual patient, in that their form remains identical in any given lead. They are bilateral, usually synchronous, and symmetrical. Moreover, they usually consist of two or more δ waves and are biphasic, triphasic, or polyphasic in appearance. This EEG pattern, however, is variable within the course of the disease and from one patient to another, and may disappear as the disease progresses. Other important pathognomonic findings are the very high titers of measles antibodies in serum – except those against the M protein – and a pronounced increase in the γ-globulin in the CSF. In the CSF, the humoral immune response is oligoclonally restricted, as revealed by isoelectric focusing (Dörries and ter Meulen 1984). This indicates that antibodies are synthesized intrathecally by a restricted number of plasma cells that have invaded the CNS.

VIRUS–HOST INTERACTIONS

Acute MV infections are characterized by the marked tropism of the virus for PBMCs, including lymphocytes, monocytes/macrophages, and dendritic cells (Borrow and Oldstone 1995; Ohgimoto et al. 2001). The virus is present in a highly cell-associated form and is efficiently spread via infected PBMCs, in which both viral nucleic acid and proteins can easily be detected and from which infectious virus can be recovered. Subsequently, endothelial cells and underlying tissue in various organs are infected. Infected PBMCs have been proposed as potential carriers, but have not been positively identified. Exactly how and when the virus reaches the brain in SSPE is not known. Some PCR-based studies described MV-specific nucleic acids in autopsy brain material obtained from patients with no history of measles-associated CNS illness (Katayama et al. 1995), suggesting that persistent MV infections of the brain may be more frequent than initially thought and may stay clinically inapparent throughout life. It is also not known which cellular receptors mediate the infection of neural cells, as the known receptors – CD150 for wildtype and vaccine MV (Tatsuo et al. 2000; Erlenhoefer et al. 2001) and CD46 only for vaccine strains (Dörig et al. 1993; Naniche et al. 1993) – owing to their cell type-specific expression, are not sufficient to explain the CNS infection (Ogata et al. 1997; McQuaid and Cosby 2002). Virus spread in the brain occurs directly from cell to cell, most likely involving local microfusion events (summarized in Schneider-Schaulies et al. 2001).

No specific defects of cell-mediated immunity have been detected in SSPE, yet in both CNS diseases, SSPE and MIBE, large amounts of MV nucleocapsid structures are present within infected cells (ter Meulen et al. 1983). However, rescue of infectious virus in tissue culture is rarely possible (Ogura et al. 1997), indicating that the viral replication cycle is defective. As with other persistent infections, MV gene expression is markedly restricted during persistence. Viral envelope proteins are generally expressed at extremely low levels, whereas internal proteins required for intracellular viral reproduction (N, P) can be detected easily. As characterized mainly in autopsy material, this is generally achieved by particular restrictions of the viral envelope-specific mRNAs (M, F, and H), and by mutations within the envelope-specific genes that interfere with a functional expression of the corresponding proteins (reviewed in Billeter et al. 1994) (summarized in Figure 62.8). It is significant for the pathogenesis that mutations introduced into the envelope gene reading frames are of two types: point mutations, caused by the naturally high infidelity of the viral polymerase during transcription/replication, and clustered hypermutations, ascribed to a cellular unwinding/modifying enzyme complex. Functional alterations or complete abolition of the MV envelope proteins seem to readily explain why the formation of infectious virus particles, viral budding, and the formation of giant cells are not encountered in persistent MV CNS infections (Cathomen et al. 1998). Moreover, important antigenic structures are mainly lacking on the surface of infected cells, which thus escape detection by the MV-specific humoral immune response.

Although it is not understood what triggers the development of a MV CNS disease, some progress has been made in understanding which factors lead to and maintain the establishment of a persistent MV infection in brain cells. Increasing evidence suggests that MV that infects brain cells is primarily nondefective, and that host factors initially attenuate viral gene expression on both transcriptional and translational levels (reviewed by Schneider-Schaulies et al. 1994). In addition, MV-specific double-stranded RNA intermediates, as formed accidentally during viral transcription and replication, serve as targets for a cellular enzyme (dsRNA adenosine deaminase activity (DRADA)) present in large amounts in brain cells in vitro. This enzyme introduces up to 50 percent of nucleotide transitions within a given double-stranded target RNA, thus profoundly altering the coding sequences (Billeter et al. 1994) (Figure 62.9, p. 1435). There is still, however, some controversy about whether mutations within the viral genome are a prerequisite for the establishment of persistent MV infection in brain cells, whether mutant viruses have a selective advantage in replication and spread in the brain, or if mutations are important for the long-term maintenance of MV persistence. The last possibility is weakened by the high variability of the mutations encountered in individual patients with SSPE and MIBE, and also by the finding that, at least in an animal model, persistent MV CNS infections have been established in the absence of detectable mutations. In summary, the IFN response and its possible lack in neurons, a steep viral expression gradient, the accumulation of point and hypermutations within envelope genes, the antibody-induced antigenic modulation, and the observed cell-to-cell spread of nucleocapsids support the persistent brain infection, with failure of the immune response to eliminate the virus (for review see Schneider-Schaulies et al. 1995).

In newborn rodents the hamster neurotropic strain HNT, or the rat brain-adapted MV strain CAM/RB, spread efficiently, causing an age-dependent lethal acute encephalitis or subacute encephalitis (for review see Liebert and Finke 1995). Resistance and susceptibility to MV-induced encephalitis correlate with the MHC haplotype of the respective inbred strain. In resistent mouse strains depletion of the CD4$^+$ T cell subset by mAb led to a breakdown of resistance, whereas depletion of CD8$^+$ T cells had no effect. A breakdown of resistance is also observed after neutralization of IFN-γ, leading to the generation of a Th2 response. Further investigation of this measles encephalitis model revealed that CD4$^+$ T cells are able to protect either alone (resistant mice), through cooperation with CD8$^+$ T cells (intermediate susceptible), or after immunization as secondary T cells (susceptible mice), and CD8$^+$ T cells are able to protect alone after immunization if they are cytolytic (Weidinger et al. 2000). As found earlier in nontransgenic mice, IFN-γ has also a critical role in the protection of CD46-transgenic mice against MV encephalitis (Patterson et al. 2002). Interestingly, this protection functions in a noncytolytic manner without neuronal loss.

CONCLUSIONS AND OUTLOOK

The observation that viruses can induce slowly progressive neurological diseases with diverse pathologies has led to speculations that other neurological diseases of unknown cause may have a viral etiology, the prime candidate being multiple sclerosis. This potential, together with epidemiological, neuropathological, immunological, and clinical findings, has encouraged extensive virological studies in pursuit of relevant infectious agents. Although several claims have been made for viruses isolated from multiple sclerosis patients, no infectious agent has yet been linked to the disease. Other diseases, such as amyotrophic lateral sclerosis, continuous focal epilepsy, or Alzheimer's disease, also reveal certain features that would be compatible with a viral infection. Recently, borna disease virus, which has been linked to a variety of neurological diseases in several animal hosts, has also been associated with certain psychiatric disorders in humans, such as schizophrenia and manic depression. No direct evidence is yet available to support the possibility that viruses cause these diseases, but their involvement cannot be ruled out.

A better understanding of the pathogenesis of viral CNS infections is a prerequisite to obtaining new and more effective means of prevention. However, each virus has different protection requirements. On the other hand, neurotropic virus infections also offer interesting possibilities for studying the structure and function of the nervous system, as in studies using neurotropic rabies or HSV for tracing neural pathways (Kruypers and Ugolini 1990). Moreover, neurotropic viruses are also used as vehicles to bring foreign genes to the CNS. Gene therapy approaches have been used in animal experiments to reduce tumor growth in brain tissue (Tapscott et al. 1994). It is therefore conceivable that a controlled viral infection of the CNS might be used for the selective expression of, for example, pharmacological agents or neurotransmitters in order to influence functional aspects of the CNS. Thus, studies of viral infections of the CNS offer new perspectives, leading to a better understanding of the pathogenesis of disease.

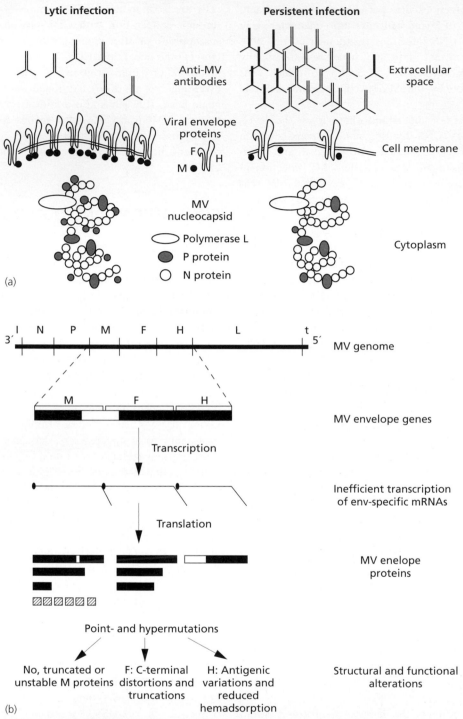

Figure 62.8 *Mechanisms of Measles virus persistence in the human CNS.* **(a)** *During acute infection the viral ribonucleocapsid particle (RNP) consisting of the genomic RNA encapsidated by the N protein and the transcriptase complex (L and P proteins) is amplified intracellularly. Concomitantly, the viral glycoproteins F and H (expressed as complexes) are expressed at the surface of the infected cell, with the M protein underlying their integration sites. In persistent infections the RNP structures are easily detected in large amounts in the cytoplasm (and the nucleus) of the infected brain cell. The expression of both the glycoproteins and the M protein is generally low or even absent. Pathognomonic for SSPE, a humoral hyperimmune reaction to viral antigens (mainly to N and H protein) is observed both in CSF and in serum.* **(b)** *The structural genes of MV are encoded in a linear arrangement along the MV genome: I represents the leader, t the trailer region that contains the viral promoter sequences and encapsidation sites. In persistent infections, the expression of the MV envelope genes M, F, and H (shown enlarged, the white region indicates a 1-kb noncoding region separating the M and F reading frames) is greatly reduced by different mechanisms: (1) the frequency of the corresponding mRNAs is very low, and (2) their reading frames are more or less affected by mutations that lead to complete abolition or truncated or distorted expression of the corresponding gene product. Most mutations have been encountered within the M gene, and all F proteins characterized so far have truncated C termini. Both point mutations (introduced by the viral polymerase) and hypermutations (clustered transitions most probably introduced by a cellular enzyme complex; see Figure 62.9) have been described.*

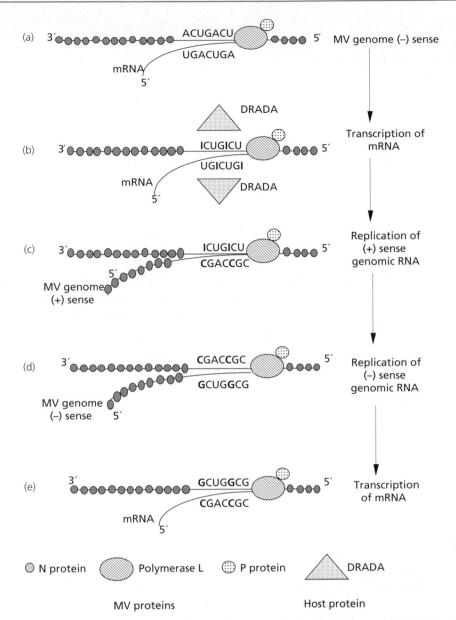

Figure 62.9 *DRADA (dsRNA adenosine deaminase activity): a cellular enzyme altering viral sequences. DRADA, initially detected and described in vitro in extracts of frog oocytes, is able to introduce clustered transitions into dsRNA structures both in vivo and in vitro. Increasing evidence suggests that unencapsidated viral dsRNAs (step a), accidentally formed during transcription/replication of negative-strand RNA viruses, may serve as targets for this cellular enzyme activity (step b) that deaminates adenosine (A) to inosine (I) residues. During replication of the positive-strand genome a cytidine (C) residue will be introduced instead of the expected uridine (U) into the positive-strand intermediate (step c); upon replication of this altered (+) genome, G will be introduced into the (–) genomic RNA (step d), which will in turn lead to the introduction of C into the mRNA (step e), replacing the initial U (step a). Although DRADA is mainly found in the nucleus, some activity has been consistently detected in the cytoplasm, in particular of neural cells.*

ACKNOWLEDGMENTS

The work in the authors' laboratory was supported by the Deutsche Forschungsgemeinschaft and the Bundesministerium für Forschung und Technologie.

REFERENCES

Achim, C.L. and Wiley, C.A. 1992. Expression of major histocompatibility complex antigens in the brains of patients with progressive multifocal leukoencephalopathy. *J Neuropathol Exp Neurol*, **51**, 257–63.

Ackerman, R., Kruger, K., et al. 1986. Spread of early summer meningoencephalitis in the Federal Republic of Germany. *Dtsch Med Wochenschr*, **111**, 927–33.

Ahmed, R., Butler, L.D. and Bhatti, L. 1988. T4⁺ T helper cell function in vivo: differential requirement for induction of antiviral cytotoxic T cell and antibody response. *J Virol*, **62**, 2102–6.

Allen, I.V., McQuaid, S., et al. 1996. The significance of measles virus antigen and genome distribution in the CNS in SSPE for mechanisms of viral spread and demyelination. *J Neuropathol Exp Neurol*, **55**, 471–80.

Almond, J.W. 1987. The attenuation of poliovirus neurovirulence. *Annu Rev Microbiol*, **41**, 153–80.

Almond, J.W. 1991. Poliovirus neurovirulence. *Semin Neurosci*, **3**, 101–8.

Almond, P.S., Bumgardner, G.L., et al. 1991. Immunogenicity of class I⁺ class II⁻ hepatocytes. *Transplant Proc*, **23**, 108–9.

Aloisi, F. 2001. Immune function of microglia. *Glia*, **36**, 165–79.

Andjaparidze, O.G., Chaplygina, N.M., et al. 1989. Detection of measles virus genome in blood leucocytes of patients with certain autoimmune diseases. *Arch Virol*, **105**, 287–91.

Arroyo, J., Guirakhoo, F., et al. 2001. Molecular basis for attenuation of neurovirulence of a yellow fever virus/Japanese encephalitis virus chimera vaccine (ChimeriVax-JE). *J Virol*, **75**, 934–42.

Arthur, R.R., Dagostin, S. and Shah, K. 1989. Detection of BK virus and JC virus in urine and brain tissue by the polymerase chain reaction. *J Clin Microbiol*, **27**, 1174–9.

Ash, R.J. 1986. Butyrate-induced reversal of herpes simplex virus restriction in neuroblastoma cells. *Virology*, **155**, 584–92.

Askonas, B.A., Taylor, P.M. and Esquivel, F. 1988. Cytotoxic T cells in influenza infection. *Ann NY Acad Sci*, **532**, 230–44.

Azimi, P.H., Shaban, S., et al. 1975. Mumps meningoencephalitis: prolonged abnormality of cerebrospinal fluid. *JAMA*, **234**, 1161–2.

Baldridge, J.R. and Buchmeier, M.J. 1992. Mechanisms of antibody-mediated protection against lymphocytic choriomeningitis virus infection: mother-to-baby transfer of humoral protection. *J Virol*, **66**, 4252–7.

Baldridge, J.R., Pearce, B.D., et al. 1993. Teratogenic effects of neonatal arenavirus infection on the developing rat cerebellum are abrogated by passive immunotherapy. *Virology*, **197**, 669–77.

Bang, H.O. and Bang, J. 1943. Involvement of the central nervous system in mumps. *Acta Med Scand*, **113**, 487–505.

Basle, M.F., Fournier, J.G. and Rozenblatt, S. 1986. Measles virus RNA detected in Paget's disease bone tissue by in situ hybridisation. *J Gen Virol*, **67**, 907–13.

Bauer, W., Chamberlin, W. and Horenstein, S. 1969. Spinal demyelination in progressive multifocal leucoencephalopathy. *Neurology*, **19**, 287–94.

Bergelson, J.M. and Finberg, R.W. 1993. Integrins as receptors for virus attachment and cell entry. *Trends Microbiol*, **1**, 287–9.

Bergelson, J.M., Shepley, M.P., et al. 1992. Identification of the integrin VLA-2 as a receptor for echovirus 1. *Science*, **255**, 1718–20.

Bergelson, J.M., Chan, M., et al. 1994. Decay accelerating factor (CD55), a glycosylphosphatidyl-anchored complement regulatory protein, is a receptor for several echoviruses. *Proc Natl Acad Sci USA*, **91**, 6245–50.

Berger, E.A., Murphy, P.M. and Farber, J.M. 1999. Chemokine receptors as HIV-1 coreceptors: roles in viral entry, tropism, and disease. *Annu Rev Immunol*, **17**, 657–700.

Berger, J.R. and Major, E.O. 1999. Progressive multifocal leukoencephalopathy. *Semin Neurol*, **19**, 193–200.

Berger, J.R., Kaszovitz, B., et al. 1987. Progressive multifocal leukoencephalopathy associated with human immunodeficiency virus infection. A review of the literature with a report of sixteen cases. *Ann Intern Med*, **107**, 78–87.

Berger, J.R., Scott, S., et al. 1992. Progressive multifocal leukoencephalopathy in HIV-infected children. *AIDS*, **2**, 837–41.

Biddison, W.E., Kubota, R., et al. 1997. Human T cell leukemia virus type I (HTLV-I)- specific CD8+ CTL clones from patients with HTLV-I-associated neurologic disease secrete proinflammtory cytokines, chemokines, and matrix metalloproteinase. *J Immunol*, **159**, 2018–25.

Billeter, M.A., Cattaneo, R., et al. 1994. Generation and properties of measles virus mutations typically associated with subacute sclerosing panencephalitis. *Ann NY Acad Sci*, **724**, 367–77.

Björvatn, B. and Wolontis, S. 1971. Mumps meningoencephalitis in Stockholm November 1964–July 1971. *Scand J Infect Dis*, **5**, 253–60.

Black, S., Shinefield, H., et al. 1999. Postmarketing evaluation of the safety and effectiveness of varicella vaccine. *Pediatr Infect Dis J*, **18**, 1041–6.

Blaskovic, D., Pucekova, G. and Kubinyi, L. 1967. An epidemiological study of tick-borne encephalitis in the Tribec region: 1956–63. *Bull WHO*, **36**, 89–94.

Bode, L. 1995. Human infections with Borna disease virus and potential pathogenic implications. *Curr Top Microbiol Immunol*, **190**, 103–30.

Bodian, D. and Horstmann, D.M. 1965. Polioviruses. In: Horsfall, F.L. and Tamm, I. (eds), *Viral and rickettsial infections of man*, 4th edn. Philadelphia: JB Lippincott, 430–73.

Boldorini, R., Cristina, S., et al. 1993. Ultrastructural studies in the lytic phase of progressive multifocal leukoencephalopathy in AIDS patients. *Ultrastruct Pathol*, **17**, 599–609.

Borrow, P. and Nash, A.A. 1992. Susceptibility to Theiler's virus-induced demyelinating disease correlates with astrocyte class II induction and antigen presentation. *Immunology*, **76**, 133–9.

Borrow, P. and Oldstone, M.B.A. 1995. Measles virus–mononuclear cell interactions. *Curr Top Microbiol Immunol*, **191**, 85–100.

Botteron, C., Zurbriggen, A., et al. 1992. Canine distemper virus-immune complexes induce bystander degeneration of oligodendrocytes. *Acta Neuropathol (Berlin)*, **83**, 402–7.

Briese, T., Hornig, M. and Lipkin, W.I. 1999. Bornavirus immunopathogenesis in rodents: models for human neurological diseases. *J Neurovirol*, **5**, 604–12.

Brinker, K.R., Paulson, G., et al. 1979. St Louis encephalitis in Ohio, September 1975: clinical and EEG in 18 cases. *Arch Intern Med*, **139**, 561–6.

Brooks, B.R. and Walker, D.L. 1984. Progressive multifocal leukoencephalopathy. *Neurol Clin*, **2**, 299–313.

Buchmeier, M., Lewicki, H., et al. 1984. Murine hepatitis virus-4 (strain JHM) induced neurologic disease is modulated in vivo by monoclonal antibody. *Virology*, **132**, 261–70.

Bu'Lock, F.A. 1986. Japanese B encephalitis in India: a growing problem. *QJ Med*, **60**, 825–36.

Cai, J.P., Falanga, V. and Chin, Y.H. 1991. TGF-β regulates the adhesive interactions between mononuclear cells and microvascular endothelium. *J Invest Dermatol*, **97**, 169–78.

Calvario, A., Bozzi, A., et al. 2002. Herpes consensus PCR test: a useful diagnostic approach to the screening of viral diseases of the central nervous system. *J Clin Virol*, **25**, 45–51.

Campbell, I.L. 1991. Cytokines in viral diseases. *Curr Opin Immunol*, **3**, 486–91.

Cann, A.J. and Chen, I.S.Y. 1990. Human T-cell leukemia virus types I and II. In: Fields, B.N., Knipe, D.M., et al. (eds), *Fields' virology*, 2nd edn. New York: Raven Press, 1501–28.

Cannella, B., Cross, A.H. and Raine, C.S. 1991. Adhesion-related molecules in the CNS: upregulation correlates with inflammatory cell influx during relapsing EAE. *Lab Invest*, **65**, 23–33.

Carbone, K.M. 2001. Borna disease virus and human disease. *Clin Microbiol Rev*, **14**, 513–27.

Cathomen, T., Mrkic, B., et al. 1998. A matrix-less measles virus is infectious and elicits extensive cell fusion: consequences for propagation in the brain. *EMBO J*, **17**, 3899–908.

Ceccaldi, P.E., Fillion, M.P., et al. 1993. Rabies virus selectively alters 5-HT1 receptor subtypes in rat brain. *Eur J Pharmacol*, **245**, 129–38.

Challoner, P.B., Smith, K.T., et al. 1995. Plaque-associated expression of human herpesvirus 6 in multiple sclerosis. *Proc Natl Acad Sci USA*, **92**, 7440–4.

Chowdhury, M., Taylor, J.P., et al. 1990. Regulation of the human neurotropic virus promoter by JCV-T antigen and HIV-1 tat protein. *Oncogene*, **5**, 1737–42.

Clatch, R.J., Lipton, H.L. and Miller, S.D. 1987. Class II restricted T cell responses in Theiler's murine encephalomyelitis virus (TMEV)-induced demyelinating disease. II. Survey of host immune responses and central nervous system virus titers in inbred mouse strains. *Microb Pathog*, **3**, 327–37.

Clements, C.J. and Cutts, F.T. 1995. The epidemiology of measles: thirty years of vaccination. *Curr Topic Microbiol Immunol*, **191**, 13–33.

Compton, T., Nowlin, D.M. and Cooper, N.R. 1993. Initiation of human cytomegalovirus infection requires initial interaction with cell surface heparan sulphate. *Virology*, **193**, 834–42.

Conant, K., Garsino-Demo, A., et al. 1998. Induction of monocyte chemoattractant protein-1 in HIV-1 Tat-stimulated astrocytes and elevation in AIDS dementia. *Proc Natl Acad Sci USA*, **95**, 3117–21.

Cornblath, D.R., McArthur, J.C., et al. 1987. Inflammatory demyelinating peripheral neuropathies associated with human T-cell lymphotropic virus type III infection. *Ann Neurol*, **21**, 32–40.

Cortegis, P. 1994. AIDS dementia complex: a review. *J AIDS*, **7**, 38–48.

Cosby, S.L., Macquaid, S., et al. 1989. Examination of eight cases of multiple sclerosis and 56 neurological and nonneurological controls for genomic sequences of measles virus. *J Gen Virol*, **70**, 2027–36.

Coyle, P. 1991. Viral infections in the developing nervous system. *Semin Neurosci*, **3**, 157–63.

Cross, A.H. 1992. Immune cells traffic control and central nervous system. *Semin Neurosci*, **4**, 312–19.

Dalakas, M.C. 2002. Pro-inflammatory cytokines and motor neuron dysfunction: is there a connection in post-polio syndrome? *J Neurol Sci*, **205**, 5–8.

Dalgleish, A.G., Beveriev, P.C.L., et al. 1984. The CD4 (T4) antigen is an essential component of the receptor for the AIDS retrovirus. *Nature (Lond)*, **312**, 763–7.

Dietzschold, B., Kao, M., et al. 1992. Delineation of putative mechanisms involved in antibody-mediated clearance of rabies virus from the central nervous system. *Proc Natl Acad Sci USA*, **89**, 7252–6.

Ding, A.H., Nathan, C.F. and Stuehr, D.J. 1988. Release of reactive nitrogen and oxygen intermediates from mouse peritoneal macrophages: comparison of activating cytokines and evidence for independent production. *J Immunol*, **141**, 2407–12.

Dörig, R.E., Marcil, A., et al. 1993. The human CD46 molecule is a receptor for measles virus (Edmonston strain). *Cell*, **75**, 295–305.

Dörries, K. 2000. Human polyomaviruses. In: Zuckermann, A.J., Banatvala, J.E. and Pattison, J.R. (eds), *Principles and practice of clinical virology*, 4th edn. Chichester: John Wiley & Sons, 619–43, Chapter 23.

Dörries, R. and ter Meulen, V. 1984. Detection and identification of virus-specific oligoclonal IgG in unconcentrated cerebrospinal fluid by immunoblot technique. *J Neuroimmunol*, **7**, 77–89.

Dörries, R., Schwender, S., et al. 1991. Population dynamics of lymphocyte subsets in the central nervous system of rats with different susceptibility to coronavirus-induced demyelinating encephalitis. *Immunology*, **74**, 539–45.

Dörries, K., Vogel, E., et al. 1994. Infection of human polyomavirus JC and BK in peripheral blood leukocytes from immunocompetent individuals. *Virology*, **198**, 59–70.

Duclos, P. and Ward, B.J. 1998. Measles vaccines. A review of adverse events. *Drug Exp*, **6**, 435–54.

Elovaara, I., Koenig, S., et al. 1993. High human T-cell lymphotropic virus type I (HTLV-I) specific precursor cytotoxic T-lymphocyte frequencies in patients with HTLV-I associated neurological disease. *J Exp Med*, **177**, 1567–73.

Elsner, C. and Dörries, K. 1992. Evidence of human polyomavirus BK and JC infection in normal brain tissue. *Virology*, **191**, 72–80.

Engelhardt, B. 1998. The role of alpha 4-integrin in T lymphocyte migration into the inflamed and noninflamed central nervous system. *Curr Topic Microbiol Immunol*, **231**, 51–64.

Erlenhoefer, C., Wurzer, W., et al. 2001. CD150 (SLAM) is a receptor for measles virus, but not involved in viral contact-mediated proliferation inhibition. *J Virol*, **75**, 4499–505.

Fabry, Z., Topham, D.J., et al. 1995. TGF-β2 decreases migration of lymphocytes in vitro and homing of cells into the CNS in vivo. *J Immunol*, **155**, 325–32.

Feigenbaum, L., Khalili, K., et al. 1987. Regulation of the host range of human papovavirus JCV. *Proc Natl Acad Sci USA*, **84**, 3695–8.

Felgenhauer, K. and Reiber, H. 1992. The diagnostic significance of antibody specificity indices in multiple sclerosis and herpes virus induced diseases of the nervous system. *Clin Invest*, **70**, 28–37.

Fleischer, B. and Kreth, H.W. 1982. Mumps virus replication in human lymphoid cell lines and in peripheral blood lymphocytes: preference for T cells. *Infect Immun*, **35**, 25–31.

Fournier, J.G., Tardieu, M., et al. 1985. Detection of measles virus RNA in lymphocytes from peripheral blood and brain in perivascular infiltrates of patients with subacute sclerosing panencephalitis. *N Engl J Med*, **313**, 910–15.

Fraser, N.W., Lawrence, N.C., et al. 1981. Herpes simplex virus type 1 DNA in human brain tissue. *Proc Natl Acad Sci USA*, **78**, 6461–5.

Frohman, E.M., Frohman, T.C., et al. 1989. The induction of intercellular adhesion molecule 1 (ICAM-1) expression on human fetal astrocytes by interferon-gamma, tumor necrosis factor alpha, lymphotoxin and interleukin-1: relevance to intracerebral antigen presentation. *J Neuroimmunol*, **23**, 117–24.

Fujinami, R.S. and Oldstone, M.B.A. 1980. Alterations in expression of measles virus polypeptides by antibody: molecular events in antibody-induced antigenic modulation. *J Immunol*, **125**, 78–85.

Fujinami, R.S. and Oldstone, M.B.A. 1985. Amino acid homology and immune responses between the encephalitogenic site of myelin basic protein and virus: a mechanism for autoimmunity. *Science*, **230**, 1043–5.

Fukura, H., Tashiro, K., et al. 1989. CT and MRI findings in HAM: a report on five cases. *Progr CT*, **11**, 69–73.

Galazka, A.M., Robertson, S.E. and Kraigher, A. 1999. Mumps and mumps vaccine: a global review. *Bull WHO*, **77**, 3–14.

Gamble, J.R. and Vadas, M.A. 1991. Endothelial cell adhesiveness for human T lymphocytes is inhibited by TGF-β1. *J Immunol*, **146**, 1149–56.

Garden, G.A. 2002. Microglia in human immunodeficiency virus-associated neurodegeneration. *Glia*, **40**, 240–51.

Garry, R.F. and Koch, G. 1992. Tat contains a sequence related to snake neurotoxins. *AIDS*, **6**, 1541–2.

Gartner, S. 2000. HIV infection and dementia. *Science*, **287**, 602–4.

Geraghty, R.J., Krummenacher, C., et al. 1998. Entry of alpha herpesviruses mediated by poliovirus receptor-related protein 1 and poliovirus receptor. *Science*, **280**, 1618–20.

Geretry, S.J., Karpus, W.J., et al. 1994. Class II-restricted T cell responses in Theiler's murine encephalomyelitis virus-induced demyelinating disease. *J Immunol*, **152**, 908–24.

Gibbs, F.A., Gibbs, L., et al. 1959. Electroencephalographic abnormality in 'uncomplicated' childhood diseases. *JAMA*, **171**, 1050–5.

Giraudon, P., Szymocha, R., et al. 2000. T lymphocytes activated by persistent viral infection differentially modify the expression of metalloproteinases and their endogenous inhibitors, TIMPs, in human astrocytes: relevance to HTLV-I- induced neurological disease. *J Immunol*, **164**, 2718–27.

Giulian, D., Vaca, K. and Noonan, C.A. 1990. Secretion of neurotoxins by mononuclear phagocytes infected with HIV-1. *Science*, **250**, 1593–6.

Glass, J.D., Fedor, H., et al. 1995. Immunocytochemical quantitation of human immunodeficiency virus in the brain: correlations with dementia. *Ann Neurol*, **38**, 755–62.

Gnann, J.W. 1991. Meningitis and encephalitis caused by mumps virus. In: Scheld, W.M., Whitley, R.J. and Durack, D.T. (eds), *Infections of the central nervous system*. New York: Raven Press, 113–26.

Gresikova, M. and Beran, G.W. 1981. Tick-borne encephalitis. In: Beran, G.W. (ed.), *Viral zoonoses vol I: CRC Handbook Series in Zoonoses, section B*. Boca Raton: CRC Press, 201–8.

Griffin, D.E. 1995. Immune responses during measles virus infections. *Curr Topic Microbiol Immunol*, **191**, 117–34.

Gullota, F., Masini, T., et al. 1992. Progressive multifocal leukoencephalopathy in gliomas in an HIV-negative patient. *Pathol Res Pract*, **188**, 964–72.

Gutierrez, J. and Vergara, M.J. 2002. Multiple sclerosis and human herpesvirus 6. *Infection*, **30**, 145–9.

Haase, A.T. 1986. Pathogenesis of lentivirus infections. *Nature (Lond)*, **332**, 130–6.

Halbach, M. and Koschel, K. 1979. Impairment of hormone dependent signal transfer by chronic SSPE virus infection. *J Gen Virol*, **42**, 615–19.

Harouse, J.M., Bhat, S., et al. 1991. Inhibition of entry of HIV-1 in neural cell lines by antibodies against galactosyl ceramide. *Science*, **253**, 320–3.

Harris, C.A., Derbin, K.S., et al. 1991. Manganese superoxide dismutase is induced by IFN-γ in multiple cell types: synergistic induction of IFN-γ and tumor necrosis factor of IL-1. *J Immunol*, **147**, 149–54.

Hay, J. and Ruyechan, T. 1994. Varizella-zoster virus – a different kind of herpesvirus latency? *Semin Virol*, **5**, 241–7.

Heinz, F.X., Collett, M.S., et al. 2000. Flaviviridae. In: Van Regenmortel, M.H.V., Fauquet , C.M., et al. (eds), *Virus taxonomy, classification and nomenclature of viruses: 7th report of the International Committee for the Taxonomy of Viruses*. San Diego: Academic Press, 859–78.

Herndon, R.M., Johnston, R.T., et al. 1974. Ependymitis in mumps virus meningitis. *Arch Neurol*, **30**, 475–9.

Hickey, W.F., Hsu, B.L. and Kimura, H. 1991. T-lymphocyte entry into the CNS. *J Neurosci Res*, **28**, 254–63.

Hoek, R.M., Ruuls, S.R., et al. 2000. Down-regulation of the macrophage lineage through interaction with OX2 (CD200). *Science*, **290**, 1768–71.

Hofman, F.M., Hinton, D.R., et al. 1991. Lymphokines and immunoregulatory molecules in subacute sclerosing panencephalitis. *Clin Immunol Immunopathol*, **58**, 331–42.

Holman, R.C., Janssen, R.S., et al. 1991. Epidemiology of progressive multifocal leukoencephalopathy in the United States: analysis of national mortality and AIDS surveillance data. *Neurology*, **41**, 1733–6.

Hom, R.C., Finberg, R.W., et al. 1991. Protective cellular retroviral immunity requires both CD4+ and CD8+ T cells. *J Virol*, **65**, 220–4.

Homsy, J., Meyer, M., et al. 1989. The Fc and not CD4 receptor mediates antibody enhancement of HIV infection in human cells. *Science*, **244**, 1357–60.

Houff, S.A., Major, E.O., et al. 1988. Involvement of JC virus-infected mononuclear cells from the bone marrow and spleen in the pathogenesis of progressive multifocal leukoencephalopathy. *N Engl J Med*, **318**, 301–5.

Ishiguro, N., Abe, M., et al. 1992. A rat model of HTLV-I infection. Humoral antibody response, provirus integration and HAM/TSP-like myelopathy in seronegative HTLV-I carrier rats. *J Exp Med*, **176**, 981–9.

Ito, M., Go, T., et al. 1991. Chronic mumps virus encephalitis. *Pediatr Neurol*, **7**, 467–70.

Iwasaki, Y., Liu, D., et al. 1985. On the replication and spread of rabies virus in the human central nervous system. *J Neuropathol Exp Neurol*, **44**, 185–95.

Jacobson, S. 2002. Immunopathogenesis of human T cell lymphotropic virus type I-associated neurologic disease. *J Infect Dis*, **186**, 187–92.

Jiang, X., Ikeda, H., et al. 2000. A rat model for human T lymphotropic virus type I-associated myelopathy. Down-regulation of bcl-2 expression and increase in sensitivity to TNF-a of the spinal oligodendrocytes. *J Neuroimmunol*, **106**, 105–13.

Johnston, R.T. 1994. Nervous system viruses. In: Webster, R.G. and Granoff, A. (eds), *Encyclopedia of virology*, Vol. II. London: Academic Press, 907–14.

Johnston, R.T., Griffin, D.E., et al. 1984. Measles encephalomyelitis: clinical and immunological studies. *N Engl J Med*, **310**, 137–41.

Johnston, R.T. and Griffin, D.E. 1986. Virus-induced autoimmune demyelinating disease of the CNS. In: Notkins, A.L. and Oldstone, M.B.A. (eds), *Concepts in viral pathogenesis*, Vol. II. New York: Springer Verlag, 203–9.

Joncas, J.H., Robillard, L.R., et al. 1976. Interferon in serum and cerebrospinal fluid in subacute sclerosing panencephalitis. *Can Med Assoc J*, **115**, 309–15.

Jonjic, S., Pavic, I., et al. 1990. Efficacious control of cytomegalovirus infection after long-term depletion of CD8+ T lymphocytes. *J Virol*, **64**, 5457–64.

Jubelt, B., Ropka, S.L., et al. 1991. Susceptibility and resistance to poliovirus-induced paralysis of inbred mouse strains. *J Virol*, **65**, 1035–40.

Kasai, T., Ikeda, H., et al. 1999. A rat model of human T lymphotropic virus type I (HTLV-I) infection: in situ detection of HTLV-I provirus DNA in microglia/macrophages in affected spinal cords of rats with HTLV-I-induced chronic progressive myeloneuropathy. *Acta Neuropathol*, **97**, 107–12.

Katayama, Y., Hotta, H., et al. 1995. Detection of measles virus nucleoprotein mRNA from autopsied brain tissues. *Arch Virol*, **76**, 3201–4.

Katz, M. 1995. Clinical spectrum of measles. *Curr Topic Microbiol Immunol*, **191**, 1–12.

Kaul, M. and Lipton, S.A. 1999. Chemokines and and activated macrophages in HIV gp120-induced neuronal apoptosis. *Proc Natl Acad Sci USA*, **96**, 8212–16.

Kaye, B.R., Neuwelt, C.M., et al. 1992. Central nervous system systemic lupus erythematosus mimicking progressive multifocal leukoencephalopathy. *Ann Rheum Dis*, **51**, 1152–6.

Kemp, L.M., Dent, C.L. and Latchman, D.S. 1990. Octamer motif mediates transcriptional repression of HSV immediate early genes and octamer-containing cellular promoters in neuronal cells. *Neuron*, **4**, 215–22.

Kennedy, M.K., Tan, L.J., et al. 1990. Inhibition of murine relapsing experimental autoimmune encephalomyelitis by immune tolerance to proteolipid protein and its encephalitogenic peptides. *J Immunol*, **144**, 909–15.

Kennedy, P.G.E. 1990. The use of molecular techniques in studying viral pathogenesis in the nervous system. *Trends Neurosci*, **13**, 424–31.

Klapper, P.E. and Cleator, G.M. 1992. The diagnosis of herpes encephalitis. *Rev Med Microbiol*, **3**, 151–8.

Klatzmann, D., Champagne, E., et al. 1984. T lymphocyte T4 molecule behaves as the receptor for human retrovirus LAV. *Nature (Lond)*, **312**, 767–78.

Klemola, E., Kaarinen, L., et al. 1965. Studies on viral encephalitis. *Acta Med Scand*, **177**, 707–16.

Koenig, S., Woods, R.M., et al. 1993. Characterization of MHC class I restricted cytotoxic T cell responses to tax in HTLV-1 infected patients with neurologic disease. *J Immunol*, **151**, 3874–83.

Koike, S., Horie, H., et al. 1990. The poliovirus receptor protein is produced both as membrane bound and secreted forms. *EMBO J*, **9**, 3217–24.

Kokernot, R.H., Hayes, J., et al. 1969. St Louis encephalitis in the USA. *Am J Trop Med Hyg*, **18**, 750–71.

Kolson, D.L., Buchhalter, J., et al. 1993. HIV-1 Tat alters normal organization of neurons and astrocytes in primary rodent brain cell cultures. *AIDS Res Hum Retrovir*, **9**, 677–85.

Koprowski, H., Zeng, Y.M., et al. 1993. In vivo expression of inducible nitric oxid synthetase in experimentally induced neurological disease. *Proc Natl Acad Sci USA*, **90**, 3024–7.

Koschel, K. and Münzel, P. 1980. Persistent paramyxovirus infections and behaviour of α-adrenergic receptors in C6 rat glioma cells. *J Gen Virol*, **47**, 513–17.

Kristensson, K. 1982. Implications of axoplasmic transport for the spread of virus infections in the nervous system. In: Weiss, D.G. and Gorio, A. (eds), *Axoplasmic transport in physiology and pathology*. New York: Springer Verlag, 153–8.

Kruypers, H.G.J.M. and Ugolini, G. 1990. Viruses as transneuronal tracers. *Trends Neurosci*, **13**, 71–5.

Kubota, R., Kawanishi, T., et al. 1998. Demonstration of human T cell lymphotropic virus type I (HTLV-I) tax-specific CD8+ lymphocytes directly in peripheral blood of HTLV-I-associated myelopathy/tropical spastic paraparesis patients by intracellular cytokine detection. *J Immunol*, **161**, 482–8.

Kuchelmeister, K., Gullotta, F. and Bergmann, M. 1993. Progressive multifocal leukoencephalopathy (PML) in the acquired immune deficiency syndrome (AIDS). A neuropathological autopsy study of 21 cases. *Pathol Res Pract*, **189**, 163–73.

Kumar, M., Resnick, L., et al. 1989. Brain reactive antibodies and the AIDS dementia complex. *J AIDS*, **2**, 469–71.

Ladogana, A., Bouzamondo, E., et al. 1994. Modification of tritiated gamma-amino-n-butyric acid transport in rabies virus-infected primary cortical cultures. *J Gen Virol*, **75**, 623–7.

La Monica, N., Almond, J.W. and Racaniello, V.R. 1987. A mouse model for poliovirus neurovirulence identifies mutations that attenuate the virus for humans. *J Virol*, **61**, 2917–20.

Lee, P., Knight, R., et al. 2002. A single mutation in the E2 glycoprotein important for neurovirulence influences binding of sindbis virus to neuroblastoma cells. *J Virol*, **76**, 6302–10.

Lehky, T.J., Fox, C.H., et al. 1995. Detection of human T-lymphotropic virus type I (HTLV-I) tax RNA in the central nervous sytem of HTLV-I-associated myelopathy/tropical spastic paraparesis patients by in situ hybridization. *Ann J Neurovirol Neurol*, **37**, 167–75.

Lenhardt, T.M. and Wiley, C.A. 1989. Absence of humorally mediated damage within the central nervous system of AIDS patients. *Neurology*, **39**, 278–80.

Lentz, T.L. 1990. The recognition event between virus and host cell receptor: a target for antiviral agents. *J Gen Virol*, **71**, 751–66.

Letendre, S.L., Lanier, E.R., et al. 1999. Cerebrospinal fluid beta chemokine concentrations in neurocognitively impaired individuals infected with human immunodeficiency virus type 1. *J Infect Dis*, **180**, 310–19.

Levine, B., Hardwick, J.M., et al. 1991. Antibody-mediated clearance of alphavirus infection from neurons. *Science*, **254**, 856–60.

Levitt, L.P., Rich, T.A., et al. 1970. Central nervous system mumps. *Neurology*, **20**, 829–34.

Liebert, U.G. and Finke, D. 1995. Measles virus infections in rodents. *Curr Topic Microbiol Immunol*, **191**, 149–66.

Liebert, U.G., Linington, C. and ter Meulen, V. 1988. Induction of autoimmune reactions to myelin basic protein in measles virus encephalitis in Lewis rats. *J Neuroimmunol*, **17**, 103–18.

Lillycrop, K.A., Estridge, J.K. and Latchman, D.S. 1993. The octamer binding protein Oct-2 inhibits transactivation of the herpes simplex virus immediate–early genes by the virion protein Vmw65. *Virology*, **196**, 888–91.

Lindsley, M.D., Thiemann, R. and Rodriguez, M. 1991. Cytotoxic T cells isolated from the central nervous systems of mice infected with Theiler's virus. *J Virol*, **65**, 6612–20.

Lipton, S.A., Sucher, N.J., et al. 1991. Synergistic effects of HIV coat protein and NMDA receptor-mediated neurotoxicity. *Neuron*, **7**, 111–18.

Liszewski, M.K., Post, T.W. and Atkinson, J.P. 1991. Membrane cofactor protein (MCP or CD46): newest member of the regulators of complement activation gene cluster. *Annu Rev Immunol*, **9**, 431–55.

Liuzzi, G.M., Mastroianni, C.M., et al. 1994. Myelin degrading activity in the CSF of HIV-1 infected patients with neurological diseases. *Neuroreport*, **6**, 157–60.

Lynch, K.J. and Frisque, R.J. 1991. Factors contributing to the restricted DNA replicating activity of JC virus. *Virology*, **180**, 306–17.

Mackenzie, J.S., Barrett, A.D.T. and Deubel, V. 2002a. The Japanese encephalitis serological group of flaviviruses: a brief introduction to the group. *Curr Topic Microbiol Immunol*, **267**, 1–10.

Mackenzie, J.S., Johansen, C.A., et al. 2002b. Japanese encephalitis as an emerging virus: the emergence and spread of Japanese encephalitis virus in Australia. *Curr Topic Microbiol Immunol*, **267**, 49–73.

Major, E.O., Amemiya, K., et al. 1992. Pathogenesis and molecular biology of progressive multifocal leukoencephalopathy, the JC virus induced demyelinating disease of the human brain. *Clin Microbiol Rev*, **5**, 49–73.

Mandl, C.W., Kroschewski, H., et al. 2001. Adaptation of tick-borne encephalitis virus to BHK-21 cells results in the formation of multiple

heparan sulfate binding sites in the envelope protein and attenuation in vivo. *J Virol*, **75**, 5627–37.

Martin, X. and Dolvio, M. 1983. Neuronal and transneuronal tracing in the trigeminal system of the rat using the herpes virus suis. *Brain Res*, **273**, 253–76.

Mason, P.W., Rieder, E. and Baxt, B. 1994. RGD sequence of foot and mouth disease virus is essential for infecting cells via the natural receptor but can be by-passed by an antibody-dependent enhancement pathway. *Proc Natl Acad Sci USA*, **91**, 1932–6.

Massa, P.T., Dörries, R. and ter Meulen, V. 1986. Viral antigens induce Ia antigen expression on astrocytes. *Nature (Lond)*, **320**, 543–6.

Massa, P.T., Schimpl, A., et al. 1987. Tumor necrosis factor amplifies measles virus-mediated Ia induction on astrocytes. *Proc Natl Acad Sci USA*, **84**, 7242–5.

Maudsley, D.J., Morris, A.G. and Tomkins, P.T. 1989. Regulation by interferon of the immune responses to viruses via the major histocompatibility complex antigens. In: Dimmock, N.J. and Minor, P.D. (eds), *Immune responses, virus infections and disease*. Oxford: IRL Press, 15–32.

Mazlo, M. and Tariska, I. 1992. Progressive multifocal leukoencephalopathy: ultrastructural findings in two brain biopsies. *Acta Neuropathol (Berlin)*, **56**, 323–39.

McKenna, M.J. and Mills, B.G. 1989. Immunohistochemical evidence of measles virus antigen in active otosclerosis. *Otolaryngol Head Neck Surg*, **101**, 415–18.

McLean, D.M., Best, J.M., et al. 1966. Viral infection of Toronto children during 1965. II. Measles encephalitis and other complications. *Can Med Assoc J*, **94**, 905–10.

McQuaid, S. and Cosby, S.L. 2002. An immunohistochemical study of the distribution of the measles virus receptors, CD46 and SLAM, in normal human tissues and subacute sclerosing panencephalitis. *Lab Invest*, **82**, 403–9.

Melnick, J.L. 1990. Enteroviruses, polioviruses, Coxsackieviruses, echoviruses and newer enteroviruses. In: Fields, B.N., Knipe, D.M., et al. (eds), *Fields' virology*, 2nd edn. New York: Raven Press, 549–604.

Mendelsohn, C.L., Wimmer, E. and Racaniello, V. 1989. Cellular receptor for poliovirus: molecular cloning, nucleotide sequence, and expression of a new member of the immunoglobulin superfamily. *Cell*, **56**, 855–65.

Merrill, J.E. and Chen, I.S.Y. 1991. HIV-1, macrophages, glial cells, and cytokines in AIDS nervous system disease. *FASEB J*, **5**, 2391–7.

Miller, D.W. 1999. Immunobiology of the blood–brain barrier. *J Neurovirol*, **5**, 57–578.

Millhouse, S. and Wigdahl, B. 2000. Molecular circuitry regulating herpes simplex virus type 1 latency in neurons. *J Neurovirol*, **6**, 6–24.

Minn, P.C. 2002. An overview of the evolution of enterovirus 71 and its clinical and public health significance. *FEMS Microbiol Rev*, **26**, 91–107.

Momburg, F., Koch, N., et al. 1986. In vivo induction of H-2K/D antigens by recombinant interferon-γ. *Eur J Immunol*, **16**, 551–7.

Moeller, K., Duffy, I., et al. 2001. Recombinant measles viruses expressing altered hemagglutinin (H) genes: functional separation of mutations determining H antibody escape from neurovirulence. *J Virol*, **75**, 7612–20.

Monath, T.P. 2002. Japanese encephalitis vaccines: current vaccines and future prospects. *Curr Topic Microbiol Immunol*, **267**, 105–38.

Montgomery, R.I., Warner, M.S., et al. 1996. Herpes simplex virus-1 entry into cells is mediated by a novel member of the TNF/NGF receptor family. *Cell*, **87**, 427–36.

Moskophidis, D., Cobbold, P., et al. 1987. Mechanism of recovery from acute virus infection: treatment of lymphocytic choriomeningitis virus-infected mice with monoclonal antibodies reveals that Lyt-2+ T lymphocytes mediate clearance of virus and regulate the antiviral antibody response. *J Virol*, **61**, 1867–74.

Mukhtar, M., Harley, S., et al. 2002. Primary isolated brain microvascular endothelial cells express diverse HIV/SIV-associated chemokine coreceptors and DC-SIGN and L-SIGN. *Virology*, **25**, 78–88.

Munsat, T.L. 1991. Poliomyelitis – new problems with an old disease. *N Engl J Med*, **324**, 1206–7.

Murgue, B., Zeller, H. and Deubel, V. 2002. The ecology and epidemiology of wets Nile virus in Africa, Europe and Asia. *Curr Topic Microbiol Immunol*, **267**, 196–221.

Naesens, L. and De Clercq, E. 2001. Recent developments in herpesvirus therapy. *Herpes*, **8**, 12–16.

Nakayama, T., Mori, T., et al. 1995. Detection of measles virus genome directly from clinical samples by reverse transcriptase–polymerase chain reaction and genetic variability. *Virus Res*, **35**, 1–16.

Naniche, D., Varior-Krishnan, G., et al. 1993. Human membrane cofactor protein (CD46) acts as a cellular receptor for measles virus. *J Virol*, **67**, 6025–32.

Nash, A.A. 1991. Virological and pathological processes involved in Theiler's virus infection of the central nervous system. *Semin Neurosci*, **3**, 109–16.

Nash, A.A., Leung, K.N. and Wildy, P. 1985. The T cell-mediated immune response of mice to herpes simplex virus. In: Roizman, B. and Lopez, C. (eds), *The herpesviruses*, 4th edn. New York: Plenum Press, 87–102.

Nash, A.A., Jayasuriya, A., et al. 1987. Different roles for L3T4$^+$ and Lyt 2$^+$ T cell subsets in the control of an acute herpes simplex virus infection of the skin and nervous system. *J Gen Virol*, **68**, 825–33.

Nathan, C. 1992. Nitric oxide as a secretory product of mammalian cells. *FASEB J*, **6**, 3051–64.

Neumann, H. 2001. Control of glial immune function by neurons. *Glia*, **36**, 191–9.

Neumann, H., Schmidt, H., et al. 1997. Major histocompatibility complex (MHC) class I gene expression in single neurons of the central nervous system: differential regulation by interferon (IFN)-γ and tumor necrosis factor (TNF)-α. *J Exp Med*, **185**, 305–16.

Ogata, A., Czub, S., et al. 1997. Absence of measles virus receptor (CD46) in lesions of subacute sclerosing panencephalitis (SSPE) brains. *Acta Neuropathol*, **94**, 444–9.

Ogura, H., Ayata, M., et al. 1997. Efficient isolation of subacute sclerosing panencephalitis virus from patient brains by reference to magnetic resonance and computed tomographic images. *J Neurovirol*, **3**, 304–9.

Ohgimoto, S., Ohgimoto, K., et al. 2001. The hemagglutinin protein is an important determinant for measles virus tropism for dendritic cells in vitro and immunosuppression in vivo. *J Gen Virol*, **82**, 1835–44.

Ohka, S. and Nomoto, A. 2001. The molecular basis of poliovirus neurovirulence. *Dev Biol*, **105**, 51–8.

Oldstone, M.B.A. 1989. Molecular mimicry as a mechanism for the cause and a probe uncovering etiologic agent(s) of autoimmune disease. *Curr Topic Microbiol Immunol*, **145**, 127–35.

Oldstone, M.B.A., Bokisch, V.A., et al. 1975. Subacute sclerosing panencephalitis: destruction of human brain cells by antibody and complement in an autologous system. *Clin Immunol Immunopathol*, **4**, 52–8.

Padgett, B.L. and Walker, D.L. 1983. Virologic and serologic studies of progressive multifocal leukoencephalopathy. *Prog Clin Biol Res*, **105**, 107–17.

Pardridge, W.M. 1999. Blood–brain barrier biology and methodology. *J Neurovirol*, **5**, 556–69.

Patrick, M.K., Johnston, J.B. and Power, C. 2002. Lentiviral neuropathogenesis: Comparative neuroinvasion, neurotropism, neurovirulence and host neurosusceptibility. *J Virol*, **76**, 7923–31.

Patterson, C.E., Lawrence, D.M., et al. 2002. Immune-mediated protection from measles virus-induced central nervous system disease is noncytolytic and gamma interferon dependent. *J Virol*, **76**, 4497–506.

Perng, G.C., Jones, C., et al. 2000. Virus-induced neuronal apoptosis blocked by the herpes simplex virus latency-associated transcript. *Science*, **287**, 1500–3.

Persidsky, Y. 1999. Model systems for studies of leukocyte migration across the blood–brain barrier. *J Neurovirol*, **5**, 579–90.

Philips, J.J., Chua, M.M., et al. 2002. Murine coronavirus spike glycoprotein mediates degree of viral spread, inflammation, and virus-induced immunopathology in the central nervous system. *Virology*, **15**, 109–20.

Plata-Salaman, C.R. 1991. Imunoregulators in the central nervous system. *Neurosci Biobehav Rev*, **15**, 185–215.

Pullen, L.C., Miller, S.D., et al. 1993. Class I-deficient resistant mice intracerebrally inoculated with Theiler's virus show an increased T cell response to viral antigens and susceptibility to demyelination. *Eur J Immunol*, **23**, 2287–93.

Quagliarello, V.J., Wispelwey, B., et al. 1991. Recombinant human IL-1 induced meningitis and blood-brain barrier injury in the rat. *J Clin Invest*, **87**, 1360–6.

Racke, M.K., Dhib-Jalbut, S., et al. 1991. Prevention and treatment of chronic relapsing EAE by transforming growth factor 1. *J Immunol*, **146**, 3012–19.

Racke, M.K., Sriram, S., et al. 1993. Long-term treatment of chronic relapsing EAE by transforming growth factor 2. *J Neuroimmunol*, **46**, 175–83.

Radsel-Medvescek, A., Marolt-Gomiscek, M., et al. 1980. Late sequelae after tick-borne meningoencephalitis in patients treated at the Hospital for Infectious Diseases, University Medical Centre of Ljubljana, during the period 1974–1975. *Zentralbl Bakteriol*, Suppl. 9, 281–4.

Rammohan, K.W., McFarland, H.F., et al. 1983. Antibody-mediated modification of encephalitis induced by hamster neurotropic measles virus. *J Infect Dis*, **147**, 546–50.

Ranganathan, P.N. and Khalili, K. 1993. The transcriptional enhancer element, kappa B, regulates promoter activity of the human neurotropic virus JCV in cells derived from the CNS. *Nucleic Acid Res*, **21**, 1959–64.

Ransohoff, R.M., Hamilton, T.A., et al. 1993. Astrocyte expression of MRNA encoding cytokines IP-10 and JE/MCP-1 in experimental autoimmune encephalomyelitis. *FASEB J*, **7**, 592–9.

Reboul, J., Schuller, E., et al. 1989. Immunoglobulins and complement components in 37 patients infected by HIV-1 virus: comparison of general (systemic) and intrathecal immunity. *J Neurol Sci*, **89**, 243–52.

Reddi, H.V. and Lipton, H.L. 2002. Heparan sulfate mediates infection of high-neurovirulence Theiler's viruses. *J Virol*, **76**, 8400–7.

Reinicke, V., Mordhorst, C.A. and Ingerslev, N. 1974. Central nervous system affection in connection with ordinary measles. *Scand J Infect Dis*, **6**, 131.

Remenick, J., Radonovich, M.F. and Brady, J.N. 1991. Human immunodeficiency virus Tat transactivation: induction of a tissue-specific enhancer in a nonpermissive cell line. *J Virol*, **65**, 5641–6.

Richards, E.P. 1988. Progressive multifocal leukoencephalopathy 30 years later. *N Engl J Med*, **318**, 315–16.

Rima, B.K., Duffy, N., et al. 1991. Correlation between humoral immune responses and presence of virus in the CNS in dogs experimentally infected with canine distemper virus. *Arch Virol*, **121**, 1–8.

Risau, W., Esser, S. and Engelhardt, B. 1998. Differentiation of blood–brain barrier endothelial cells. *Pathol Biol*, **46**, 171–5.

Robertson, D.A.F., Zhang, S.L., et al. 1987. Persistent measles virus genome in autoimmune chronic active hepatitis. *Lancet*, **2**, 9–11.

Robertson, M.N., Spangrude, G.J., et al. 1992. Role and specificity of T-cell subsets in spontaneous recovery from Friend virus-induced leukemia in mice. *J Virol*, **66**, 3271–7.

Roehrig, J.T., Layton, M., et al. 2002. The emergence of West Nile virus in north America: ecology, epidemiology, and surveillance. *Curr Topics Microbiol Immunol*, **267**, 223–40.

Roivainen, M., Hyypia, T., et al. 1991. RGD-dependent entry of coxsackievirus A9 into host cells and its bypass after cleavage of VP1 protein by intestinal proteases. *J Virol*, **65**, 4735–43.

Rott, R. and Becht, H. 1995. Natural and experimental Borna disease in animals. *Curr Topic Microbiol Immunol*, **190**, 17–30.

Ruddle, N.H., Bergman, C.M., et al. 1990. An antibody to lymphotoxin and tumor necrosis factor prevents transfer of experimental allergic encephalomyelitis. *J Exp Med*, **172**, 1193–200.

Russell, R.R. and Donald, J.C. 1958. The neurological complications of mumps. *Br Med J*, **2**, 27–30.

Ryan, L.A., Cotter, R.L., et al. 2002. Macrophages, chemokines and neuronal injury in HIV-1-associated dementia. *Cell Mol Biol*, **48**, 137–50.

Sabin, A.B. 1956. Pathogenesis of poliomyelitis. Reappraisal in the light of new data. *Science*, **123**, 1151–7.

Santambrogio, L., Hochwald, G.M., et al. 1993. Studies on the mechanism by which TGF-β protects against EAE. *J Immunol*, **151**, 1116–23.

Santoro, F., Kennedy, P.E., et al. 1999. CD46 is a cellular receptor for human herpesvirus 6. *Cell*, **99**, 817–27.

Sasseville, V.G., Smith, M.M., et al. 1996. Chemokine expression in simian immunodeficiency virus-induced AIDS encephalitis. *Am J Pathol*, **149**, 1459–67.

Schijns, V.E.C.J. and Van der Neut, R. 1991. Tumour necrosis factor α, interferon-γ and interferon-β exert antiviral activity in nervous tissue cells. *J Gen Virol*, **72**, 809–15.

Schneider-Schaulies, J. 2000. Cellular receptors for viruses: links to tropism and pathogenesis. *J Gen Virol*, **81**, 1413–29.

Schneider-Schaulies, J., ter Meulen, V. and Schneider-Schaulies, S. 2001. Measles virus interactions with cellular receptors: consequences for viral pathogenesis. *J Neurovirol*, **7**, 391–9.

Schneider-Schaulies, S., Schnorr, J.J., et al. 1994. The role of host factors in measles virus persistence. *Semin Virol*, **5**, 273–80.

Schneider-Schaulies, S., Schneider-Schaulies, J., et al. 1995. Measles virus gene expression in neural cells. *Curr Topic Microbiol Immunol*, **191**, 101–16.

Schneider-Schaulies, S. and ter Meulen, V. 2002. Modulation of immune functions by measles virus. *Springer Semin Immunopathol*, **24**, 127–48.

Schnorr, J.J., Dunster, L.M., et al. 1995. Measles virus-induced down-regulation of CD46 is associated with enhanced sensitivity to complement-mediated lysis of infected cells. *Eur J Immunol*, **25**, 976–84.

Schweighardt, B. and Atwood, W.J. 2001. Virus receptors in the human central nervous system. *J Neurovirol*, **7**, 187–95.

Schwender, S., Imrich, H. and Dörries, R. 1991. The pathogenic role of virus-specific antibody-secreting cells in the central nervous system of rats with different susceptibility to coronavirus-induced demyelinating encephalitis. *Immunology*, **74**, 533–8.

Sedgwick, J.D. and Dörries, R. 1991. The immune system response to viral infection of the CNS. *Semin Neurosci*, **3**, 93–100.

Sedgwick, J., Schwender, S., et al. 1991a. Isolation and direct characterization of resident microglia cells from the normal and inflamed central nervous system. *Proc Natl Acad Sci USA*, **88**, 7438–42.

Sedgwick, J.D., Mössner, R., et al. 1991b. MHC-expressing nonhematopoietic astroglial cells prime only CD8+ T lymphocytes: astroglial cells as perpetuators but not initiators of CD4+ T cell responses in the central nervous system. *J Exp Med*, **173**, 1235–46.

Sedgwick, J.D., Schwender, S., et al. 1993. Resident macrophages (ramified microglia) of the adult brown Norway rat central nervous system are constitutively major histocompatibility complex class II positive. *J Exp Med*, **177**, 1145–52.

Selmaj, K.W. 1992. The role of cytokines in inflammatory conditions of the central nervous system. *Semin Neurosci*, **4**, 221–9.

Shah, K.V. 1990. Polyomaviruses. In: Fields, B.N., Knipe, D.M., et al. (eds), *Fields' virology*, 2nd edn. New York: Raven Press, 1609–23.

Shankar, V., Kao, M., et al. 1992. Kinetics of virus spread and changes in levels of several cytokine mRNAs in the brain after intranasal infection of rats with Borna disease virus. *J Virol*, **66**, 992–8.

Shyu, W.C., Lin, J.C., et al. 1993. Recurrent ascending myelitis: an unusual presentation of herpes simplex virus type 2 infection. *Ann Neurol*, **34**, 625–7.

Silber L.A., Soloviev V.D. 1946. *American review of Soviet medicine*, Special Supplement. New York: American-Soviet Medical Society, 1–50.

Sissons, J.G.P. and Oldstone, M.B.A. 1985. Host response to viral infections. In: Fields, B.N. and Knipe, J.M. (eds), *Fields' virology*. New York: Raven Press, 265–79.

Smith, T.W., De Girolami, U. and Hickey, W.F. 1992. Neuropathology of immunosuppression. *Brain Pathol*, **2**, 183–94.

Snider, W.D. and Simpson, D.M. 1983. Primary lymphoma of the nervous system associated with acquired immune-deficiency syndrome. *N Engl J Med*, **308**, 45.

Sobel, R.A., Mitchell, M.E. and Fondren, G. 1990. Intercellular adhesion molecule-1 (ICMA-1) in cellular immune reaction in the human CNS. *Am J Pathol*, **136**, 1309–16.

Soilleux, E.J., Morris, L.S., et al. 2002. Expression of human immunodeficiency virus (HIV)-binding lectin DC-SIGNR: consequences for HIV infection and immunity. *Hum Pathol*, **33**, 652–9.

Soldan, S. 2001. Immune response to HTLV-I and HTLV-II. In: Walker, G.P.B. (ed.), *Retroviral immunology: immune responses and restoration*. Totowa, NJ: Humana Press, 159–90.

Solomon, T. and Vaughn, D.W. 2002. Pathogenesis and clinical features of Japanese encephalitis and West Nile virus infections. *Curr Topic Microbiol Immunol*, **267**, 171–94.

Speth, C., Dierich, M.P. and Gasque, P. 2001. Neuroinvasion by pathogens: a key role of the complement system. *Mol Immunol*, **38**, 669–79.

Springer, T.A. 1994. Traffic signals for lymphocyte recirculation and leukocyte emigration: the multistep paradigm. *Cell*, **76**, 301–3.

Staeheli, P. 1990. Interferon-induced proteins and the antiviral state. *Adv Virus Res*, **38**, 147–200.

Steiner, I. and Kennedy, P.G.E. 1995. Herpes simplex virus latent infection in the nervous system. *J Neurovirol*, **1**, 19–29.

Stellrecht, K.A., Harding, I., et al. 2002. The impact of an enteroviral RT-PCR assay on the diagnosis of aseptic meningitis and patient management. *J Clin Virol*, **25**, S19–26.

Stevens, J.G. 1993. HSV-1 neuroinvasiveness. *Intervirology*, **35**, 152–63.

Stitz, L., Dietzschold, B. and Carbone, K.M. 1995. Immunopathogenesis of Borna disease. *Curr Topic Microbiol Immunol*, **190**, 75–92.

Stoiber, H., Kacani, L., et al. 2001. The supportive role of complement in HIV pathogenesis. *Immunol Rev*, **180**, 168–76.

Stone, R. 1994. Post-polio syndrome: remembrance of viruses past. *Science*, **264**, 909.

Takahashi, M., Otsuka, T., et al. 1974. Live vaccine used to prevent the spread of varicella in children in hospital. *Lancet*, **2**, 1288–90.

Tapscott, S.J., Miller, A.D., et al. 1994. Gene therapy of rat 9L gliosarcoma tumors by transduction with selectable genes does not require drug selection. *Proc Natl Acad Sci USA*, **91**, 8185–9.

Tas, P.W. and Koschel, K. 1991. Loss of the endothelin signal pathway in C6 rat glioma cells persistently infected with measles virus. *Proc Natl Acad Sci USA*, **88**, 6736–9.

Tatsuo, H., Ono, N., et al. 2000. SLAM (CDw150) is a cellular receptor for measles virus. *Nature*, **406**, 893–7.

Taylor, T.J., Brockman, M.A., et al. 2002. Herpes simplex virus. *Front Biosci*, **1**, 752–64.

ter Meulen, V. and Katz, M. 1997. The proposed viral etiology of multiple sclerosis and related demyelinating diseases. In: Raine, C.S., McFarland, H. and Tourtellotte, W.W. (eds), *Multiple sclerosis: clinical and pathogenetic basis*. London: Chapman & Hall, 287–305.

ter Meulen, V., Kackell, Y., et al. 1972. Isolation of infectious measles virus in measles encephalitis. *Lancet*, **2**, 1172–5.

ter Meulen, V., Stephenson, J.R. and Kreth, H.W. 1983. Subacute sclerosing panencephalitis. In: Fraenkel-Conrat, H. and Wagner, R.R. (eds), *Comprehensive virology*. New York: Plenum Press, 105–59.

Thoulouze, M.I., Lafage, M., et al. 1998. The neural cell adhesion molecule is a receptor for rabies virus. *J Virol*, **72**, 7181–90.

Trotter, J. and Steinman, L. 1985. Homing of Lyt-2$^+$ and Lyt-2$^-$ T cell subsets and B lymphocytes to the CNS of mice with EAE. *J Immunol*, **132**, 2919–25.

Tsiang, H. 1993. Pathophysiology of rabies virus infection of the nervous system. *Adv Virus Res*, **42**, 375–411.

Tuffereau, C., Benejeau, J., et al. 1998. Low-affinity nerve growth factor receptor (P75 NTR) can serve as a receptor for rabies virus. *EMBO J*, **17**, 7250–9.

Tyler, K.L. 1990. Pathogenesis of viral infections. In: Fields, B.N., Knipe, D.M., et al. (eds), *Fields' virology*, 2nd edn. New York: Raven Press, 191–240.

Tyler, K.L. 1991. Pathogenesis of reovirus infections of the central nervous system. *Semin Neurosci*, **3**, 117–24.

Tyor, W.R., Wesselingh, S., et al. 1992. Long term intraparenchymal Ig secretion after acute viral encephalitis in mice. *J Immunol*, **149**, 4016–20.

Tyor, W.R., Wesselingh, S., et al. 1995. Unifying hypothesis for the pathogenesis of HIV-associated dementia complex, vacuolar myelopathy and sensory neuropathy. *J AIDS*, **9**, 379–88.

Umehara, F., Izumo, S., et al. 1993. Immunocytochemical analysis of the cellular infiltrate in the spinal cord lesions in HTLV-I-associated myelopathy. *J Neuropathol Exp Neurol*, **52**, 424–30.

Umenai, T., Krzyskov, R., et al. 1985. Japanese encephalitis: current worldwide status. *Bull WHO*, **63**, 625–31.

van Eyll, O. and Michiels, T. 2000. Influence of the Theiler's virus L* protein on macrophage infection, viral persistence, and neurovirulence. *J Virol*, **74**, 9071–7.

Virelizier, J.L. 1989. Cellular activation and human immunodeficiency virus infection. *Curr Opin Immunol*, **2**, 409–13.

von Einsiedel, R.W., Fife, T.D., et al. 1993. Progressive multifocal leukoencephalopathy in AIDS: a clinicopathologic study and review of the literature. *J Neurol*, **240**, 391–406.

Wahl, S.M., Allen, J.B., et al. 1991. Macrophage and astrocyte-derived transforming growth factor as a mediator of central nervous system dysfunction in acquired immune deficiency syndrome. *J Exp Med*, **173**, 981–91.

Wakefield, A.J., Pittilo, R.M., et al. 1993. Evidence of persistent measles virus infection in Crohn's disease. *J Med Virol*, **39**, 345–53.

Walker, D.L. and Frisque, R.J. 1986. The biology and molecular biology of JC virus. In: Salzman, N.P. (ed.), *The Papovaviridae*. London: Plenum Press, 327–77.

Wang, J., Asensie, V.C., et al. 2002. Cytokines and chemokines as mediators of protection and injury in the central nervous system assessed in transgenic mice. *Curr Topic Microbiol Immunol*, **265**, 23–48.

Watanabe, R., Wege, H. and ter Meulen, V. 1983. Adoptive transfer of EAE-like lesions from rats with coronavirus induced demyelinating encephalomyelitis. *Nature (Lond)*, **305**, 150–3.

Wege, H., Watanabe, R., et al. 1983. Coronavirus JHM-induced demyelinating encephalomyelitis in rats: influence of immunity on the course of disease. *Prog Brain Res*, **59**, 221–31.

Weidinger, G., Czub, S., et al. 2000. Role of CD4+ and CD8+ T cells in the prevention of measles virus-induced encephalitis in mice. *J Gen Virol*, **81**, 2707–13.

Wheatley, S.C., Dent, C.L., et al. 1991. A cellular factor binding to the TAATGARAT DNA sequence prevents the expression of the HSV-1 immediate-early genes following infection of nonpermissive cell lines derived from dorsal root ganglion neurons. *Exp Cell Res*, **194**, 78–82.

Whitley, R.J. 1990. Herpes simplex viruses. In: Fields, B.N., Knipe, B.M., et al. (eds), *Fields' virology*, 2nd edn. New York: Raven Press, 1843–86.

Whitton, J.L. 2002. Immunopathology during coxsackievirus infection. *Springer Semin Immunopathol*, **24**, 201–13.

Wilcox, C.L. and Johnson, E.M. 1988. Characterisation of nerve growth factor-dependent herpes simplex virus latency in neurons in vitro. *J Virol*, **62**, 393–9.

Wilcox, C.L., Smith, R.L., et al. 1990. Nerve growth factor dependence of herpes simplex virus latency in peripheral sympathetic and sensory neurons. *J Neurosci*, **10**, 1268–75.

Williamson, J. and Stohlman, S. 1990. Effective clearance of mouse hepatitis virus from the central nervous system both requires CD4$^+$ and CD8$^+$ T cells. *J Virol*, **64**, 4589–92.

Wilt, S.G., Milward, E., et al. 1995. In vitro evidence for a dual role of tumour necrosis factor-alpha in human immunodeficiency virus type 1 encephalopathy. *Ann Neurol*, **37**, 381–94.

Wolinsky, J.S., Baringer, J.R., et al. 1974. Ultrastructure of mumps virus replication in newborn hamster central nervous system. *Lab Invest*, **31**, 402–12.

Wolinsky, J.S., Klassen, T. and Baringer, J.R. 1976. Persistence of neuroadapted mumps virus in brains of newborn hamsters after intraperitoneal inoculation. *J Infect Dis*, **133**, 260–7.

Wolontis, S. and Björvatn, B. 1973. Mumps meningoencephalitis in Stockholm: November 1964–July 1971. II. Isolation attempts from the cerebrospinal fluid in a hospitalised group. *Scand J Infect Dis*, **2**, 261–71.

Wood, M.J. 2000. History of varicella zoster virus. *Herpes*, **7**, 60–5.

Wright, K.E. and Buchmeier, M.J. 1991. Antiviral antibodies attenuate T-cell-mediated immunopathology following acute lymphocytic choriomeningitis virus infection. *J Virol*, **65**, 3001–6.

Wu, E., Dickson, D.W., et al. 1993. Neuronoaxonal dystrophy in HTLV-I associated myelopathy/tropical spastic paraparesis: neuropathologic and neuroimmunologic correlations. *Acta Neuropathol*, **86**, 224–35.

Wucherpfennig, K.W. and Strominger, J.L. 1995. Molecular mimicry of T cell mediated autoimmunity: viral peptides activate human T cell lines specific for myelin basic protein. *Cell*, **80**, 695–705.

WuDunn, D. and Spear, P.G. 1989. Initial interaction of herpes simplex virus with cells is binding to heparansulfate. *J Virol*, **63**, 52–60.

Yin-Murphy, M. 1994. Enteroviruses. In: Webster, R.G. and Granoff, A. (eds), *Encyclopedia of virology*. London: Academic Press, 378–91.

Zhang, J.R. 1999. Molecular and cellular mechanisms for microbial entry into the CNS. *J Neurovirol*, **5**, 591–603.

63

Viral infections of the fetus and neonate, other than rubella

GISELA ENDERS

INTRODUCTION

General factors in transmission of infection

The virus infections that may be transmitted from the mother during gestation or perinatally to the fetus or neonate are listed in Table 63.1. The importance of the various infections depends both on the frequency of maternal infection in the epidemiological situations prevailing in different geographic areas and on the frequency and seriousness of the infections in the embryo, the fetus, and the neonate. In this chapter, the various infections with known consequences for the fetus and infant are discussed more in order of importance than on a taxonomic basis. Details of the viruses themselves are given in their respective chapters in this volume. Virus infections in pregnancy with possible or suspected consequences for the fetus and infant (measles virus, mumps virus, Epstein–Barr virus, influenza a virus, human herpesvirus 6, human herpesvirus 7, and human herpesvirus 8, molluscum contagiosum virus, hantavirus, denguevirus, adenovirus, human respiratory syncytial virus, West Nile virus, TT virus, SEN virus) cannot be discussed on account of shortage of space. Full description of infections in pregnancy is published elsewhere (Enders 2005).

Transmission of a virus to the products of conception may occur within the uterus (congenital or prenatal infection), and during delivery or shortly thereafter (perinatal infection) (Table 63.2). Some viruses are transmitted only when the mother has an acute primary infection in pregnancy, others from chronically infected mothers. All such infections can be transmitted if maternal primary infection occurs shortly before delivery.

In pregnancy, the immune response is modified by a shift towards a Th2-type profile, which is associated with immunological tolerance (Reinhard et al. 1998). It has been hypothesized that this allows protection of the fetal allograft but may also influence the immune defense against microorganisms (Wegmann et al. 1993). However, data from animals and humans fit the Th1/Th2 concept, but newer results (e.g. the role of NK cells) suggest that the Th1/Th2 paradigm in pregnancy is an oversimplification and the situation is more complex (Chaouat et al. 2004).

In certain viral infections, though with some exceptions, the presence of antibodies in the female before conception protects both her and the fetus against infection and disease. In the presence of certain vaccine-acquired antibodies (e.g. rubella, measles, mumps, varicella) silent reinfection of the mother may occur, but usually without causing infection or disease of the fetus. Antibodies to viruses that establish latent or chronic infection

Table **63.1** *Virus infections in pregnancy with known consequences for the fetus and infant*

| Virus | Consequences for the fetus and infant | |
	Congenital infection	Perinatal infection
Rubella virus	+	−
Cytomegalovirus	+	+
Varicella-zoster virus	+	+
Herpes simplex viruses 1, 2	+/−	+
Parvovirus B19	+	−
Human immunodeficiency viruses 1, 2	+/−	+
Hepatitis virus A (*Picornavirus*)	+/−	+/−
Hepatitis viruses B, C, D, G	+/−	+
Hepatitis virus E	+	+
Enteroviruses: coxsackie/ echoviruses (*Picornavirus*)	+/−	+
Lymphocytic choriomeningitis virus	+	−
Genital human papillomaviruses	+/−	+
Hemorrhagic fever viruses[a, b]	+	+
Vaccinia virus[b]	+	−

+, common; +/−, less common; −, none.
a) Imported or in the respective geographic area.
b) Not described in detail.

(e.g. herpesviruses, human immunodeficiency viruses) before conception cannot prevent reactivation or recurrence, with consequent risks of fetal or neonatal infection.

The consequences of maternal infection for the embryo, fetus, or neonate are mainly determined by the gestational age and additional factors, such as the type of virus and its pathogenicity for the developing fetus. In the first few weeks of gestation many organisms may infect the pregnant woman and may lead to death and resorption of the embryo. Therefore the incidence of such infections is not known. The effect of embryonic or fetal infection may be apparent as early as the 6th to 8th week of gestation (WG) (WG 6–8). Infection acquired in utero may result in resorption of the embryo, abortion (until WG 20); intrauterine death (after WG 21);

stillbirth (after WG 37); intrauterine growth retardation; prematurity (defined as the birth of a viable infant before the 37th week of gestation); malformation and other systemic abnormalities, and the sequelae of chronic postnatal infection. Signs of disease may be absent at birth, but serious sequelae may become apparent months or years later. Structural defects may occur following early maternal infection at the time of organogenesis (WG 3–8), for example caused by rubella. Maternal infection after WG 9 may lead to systemic abnormalities due to inhibition of organ development. Neonatal disease may also be caused by late intrauterine or perinatal infection.

The total rate of pregnancy loss after implantation due to all causes amounts to 31 percent (Wilcox et al. 1988). In cases with later implantation (>8–10 days after ovulation) the risk of early pregnancy loss markedly increases (Wilcox et al. 1999). Among the factors – mostly of unknown nature – that can affect the outcome of pregnancy, only 5–10 percent are attributable to maternal microbial infections and, of these, approximately 2 percent lead to congenital malformation or systemic abnormalities. These low rates are due to the existence of complex mechanisms of protection. The placenta is a powerful barrier with a wide variety of macrophages and lymphocytes. It allows the transit of maternal IgG, while preventing a large number of infective agents from reaching the embryo or the fetus. Furthermore, cellular immunity develops by the 12th week of gestation when antigen-presenting cells are detectable and the expression of MHC class I and II molecules by a variety of fetal tissues is evident (Lewis and Wilson 2001).

Diagnostic procedures

For the laboratory diagnosis of maternal, intrauterine, and perinatally acquired infections, new techniques for detecting both viruses and their antibodies have become available. The traditional methods for detecting viruses and viral antigens have been replaced or supplemented by detection of specific nucleic acid by various molecular biological techniques, such as the polymerase chain

Table **63.2** *Transmission of viral infections to embryo, fetus, and neonate*

Transmission	Mode	Time of gestation	Infections
Transovarian	Infected sperm	Early	Seldom: CMV, HIV-1
Intrauterine	Hematogenous transplacental	1st to 39th week	Rubella virus, CMV, parvovirus B19, VZV, coxsackie and echoviruses, HIV-1,[a] HBV,[a] HCV[a]
	Local extension from foci of infection (e.g. ovaries)		
	Ascending from vaginal tract	Late, after rupture of membranes	CMV, HSV, HIV-1
Perinatal	Infected birth canal	Delivery	CMV, HSV, HIV-1, HBV, HCV, HPV
Early postnatal	Breast milk/environment	After birth	CMV, HSV, HBV, HIV-1, HCV?

CMV, cytomegalovirus; HBV, hepatitis B virus; HCV, hepatitis C virus; HIV, human immunodeficiency virus; HPV, human papillomaviruses; HSV, herpes simplex virus; VZV, varicella-zoster virus.
a) Possible, but rare.

reaction (PCR). For serology, basic and newly developed supplementary tests are now available. Whether the virological or serological route for diagnosis is pursued depends on the particular agent and on the availability of sensitive and specific assays for detecting it.

Unless stated otherwise, the techniques for diagnosing the various viral infections are the same as those used in nonpregnant people and are described in the relevant chapters in this volume.

Direct tests on the fetus commenced in 1983 (Daffos et al. 1983); the methods include ultrasound screening at low and high levels, detection of fetal infection by identification of the agent in chorionic villi biopsies, amniotic fluid, and fetal blood (Table 63.3) and by tests for specific IgM/IgA antibodies and cellular immunity in fetal blood. Methods for ensuring the purity of fetal blood samples are essential, and nonspecific biological, biochemical, and immunological factors reflecting fetal functions are also applied (Forestier et al. 1988). The optimal time for chorionic villi sampling (CVS) is at about WG 11, when the risk of spontaneous abortion is lowest. In case of positive results, CVS has the advantage of early decision on further management of the pregnancy, however there is a risk of false-positive results due to contamination with maternal blood still containing the infectious agent. The added risk of fetal complications after amniocentesis is 0.2–1 percent (Hanson et al. 1990; Blackwell et al. 2002; Scott et al. 2002) and the risk linked to fetal blood sampling by experienced teams is 0.5–1 percent in healthy fetuses (Maxwell et al. 1991).

Invasive prenatal diagnosis has been applied to pregnancies complicated by infections with, for example, rubella virus, cytomegalovirus, parvovirus B19, varicella-zoster virus, *Toxoplasma gondii* and *Borrelia burgdorferi* infections (Enders and Jonatha 1987; Daffos et al. 1988; Enders 1994; Hohlfeld et al. 1994; Tercanli

et al. 1996; Enders and Miller 2000; Enders et al. 2001, 2004). Prenatal diagnosis has proved helpful in rescuing many unaffected fetuses from being lost by termination of pregnancy.

To interpret the results obtained by tests on the fetus (Table 63.3), the pathogenicity of the agent for mother and fetus, the time of maternal infection during gestation, and the specificity and sensitivity of the various methods must be considered. The ultrasound findings at high level are of major importance when deciding to continue or terminate a pregnancy. The predictive value of tests on the fetus can be fully estimated only by follow-up investigations: in cases of therapeutic abortion by detection of the virus or other agent in fetal tissue; or, if pregnancy continues, by tests for agents and specific antibodies in the infant.

In pediatric diagnosis, congenital infection can be assumed if either virus or IgM antibodies are detected in samples collected shortly after birth; perinatal or early postnatal infection is diagnosed if tests for virus and IgM antibody were negative soon after birth, but positive in samples obtained 3–4 weeks later (Tables 63.4 and 63.5).

It should be remembered that, even though clinically apparent congenital virus infections are infrequent, there are some important ones whose risk can now be reduced by preventive measures (vaccination in childhood and before pregnancy, safe sexual behavior before and during pregnancy, hygienic measures, and for certain infections passive prophylaxis in case of contact or therapy). Great progress has been made in achieving a correct laboratory diagnosis followed by intervention, such as prenatal diagnosis, therapy in utero, e.g. red cell intrauterine transfusion or therapeutic abortion if appropriate. The need and value of the formerly so-called TORCH or STORCH screening (Editorial 1990), now known under the acronym TORCHES-CLAP (*Toxoplasma gondii*, rubella virus, cytomegalovirus,

Table 63.3 *Prenatal diagnosis of fetal infection*

Week of gestation	Investigation	Sample	Object of detection
⩾11	Biopsy	Chorionic villi	Virus: by nucleic acid (PCR), antigen, culture
18–23	Amniocentesis	Amniotic fluid	Virus: by nucleic acid (PCR), antigen, culture
17–39	Ultrasonography of high level		Anatomical abnormalities
22–23	Cordocentesis and amniocentesis	Fetal blood (ensure purity of sample)	Specific IgM
			Total IgM (mg/dl)
			Other nonspecific biological, biochemical markers
		Fetal blood/amniotic fluid	Virus: by nucleic acid (PCR), antigen, culture
⩾24	If ultrasound is abnormal, investigation as for weeks 22–23		

PCR, polymerase chain reaction.

Table 63.4 *Virological differentiation between congenital and perinatal infections*

| Type of infection | Transmission | Viral Infection | | |
		At birth	Neonate	Infant
Congenital	Intrauterine	+	+	+/−
Perinatal/early postnatal	Extrauterine	−	+/−	+

Adapted from Griffiths (1990). +, positive; +/−, positive or negative; −, negative.

Herpes simplex virus, enteroviruses, syphilis (*Treponema pallidum*), chickenpox (varicella-zoster virus), Lyme disease (*Borrelia burgdorferi*), acquired immune deficiency syndrome (AIDS) (human immunodeficiency virus), parvovirus B19, not to mention hepatitis B virus, hepatitis C virus, hepatitis D virus, hepatitis G virus, hepatitis E virus, papillomavirus, and lymphocytic choriomeningitis virus) should be re-evaluated from time to time (Sutherland 1993; Klein and Remington 2001). This appears necessary with respect to changing epidemiology due to increasing vaccination and progress in preventing certain infections important for pregnancy. Moreover, globalization provides opportunities for the emergence/re-emergence of infectious diseases. The role of newly recognized viral pathogens in pregnancy, imported or in the respective geographic area, has to be elucidated.

CYTOMEGALOVIRUS

Cytomegalovirus (CMV), a gammaherpesvirus, is the most frequent viral cause of congenital infection in humans, with symptomatic disease at birth, and short- and long-term sequelae. CMV establishes latency and persists so for life, periodically reactivating from this latent state. In immunocompetent persons, including pregnant women, primary CMV infection is usually asymptomatic and only a small portion (<10 percent) presents with clinical symptoms such as mononucleosis-like illness. Primary maternal CMV infection is the major risk for congenital disease. Recurrent infection, which quantitatively accounts for most of the congenital infections in highly immune populations worldwide is always asymptomatic and clinical manifestations in the infected fetus or newborn infant are rare.

Infection in pregnancy

EPIDEMIOLOGY OF MATERNAL CMV INFECTION

CMV antibody prevalence differs in various populations according to socioeconomic factors, race, geographic location, and lifestyle. In the USA and western Europe, the antibody prevalence rates in women aged 20–40 years from the higher socioeconomic group ranges from <40–60 percent (mean 45 percent) compared to 85 percent in the lower socioeconomic group. In developing countries more than 90 percent of young women are positive for CMV antibodies (Yow et al. 1988; Istas et al. 1995; Enders et al. 2003).

CMV is not very contagious and requires close or intimate contact with infectious secretions. No data have indicated CMV transmission through respiratory droplets. Infections in adolescent women (aged 14–20) are acquired mainly by sexual/oral contact with saliva, genital secretions, and semen (Shen et al. 1994), particularly in those of lower socioeconomic groups who change sex partners frequently (Istas et al. 1995; Coonrod et al. 1998). Women aged ≥25 years in the middle and upper socioeconomic classes may acquire infection predominantly by close contact with asymptomatic infants and toddlers excreting CMV in saliva and urine (Stagno and Cloud 1994; Sobaszek et al. 2000).

Primary infection, as well as recurrent or secondary infection, can lead to vertical transmission and congenital infection. The annual rate of primary infection in susceptible pregnant women ranges in British, American, Swedish, and German studies generally from 0.4 to 4.1 percent (Ades 1992; Stagno et al. 1986; Enders et al. 2003). As shown in the US study primary infection is lower (2 percent) in the higher income group as compared to the lower income group with 6 percent (Stagno et al. 1986). Furthermore, it was documented that the annual seroconversion rate increased with the

Table 63.5 *Serological differentiation between congenital and perinatal infections*

| Type of infection | Transmission | Virus-specific antibodies | | |
		At birth	Neonate <4 weeks	Infant >4 weeks to 1 year
Congenital	Intrauterine	IgM+/−	IgM+	IgM−
		IgG+	IgG+	IgG+
Perinatal/early postnatal	Extrauterine	IgM−	IgM+/−	IgM+
		IgG+	IgG+	IgG+
None	None	IgM−	IgM−	IgM−
		IgG+	IgG+	IgG−

Adapted from Griffiths (1990). +, positive; +/−, positive or negative; −, negative.

number of pregnancies from about 2 to 3 percent in the first pregnancy to 4 to 7 percent between the second and third pregnancy (Stagno et al. 1986; Yow et al. 1988). It also became evident that seronegative mothers whose children acquired the infection in daycare centers have a 30 percent annual risk for seroconversion. On average these mothers acquired the infection within 4.2 months (range 3–7 months) after their children became infected (Adler 1988). The route of transmission among children in group daycare is caused by horizontal transmission from child to child. This is supported by analysis of the restriction enzyme digestion patterns of CMV-DNA of the virus isolates of the infected children (Adler 1988). The highest risk is posed by toddlers in their second year of life. These children are an important potential source for infection of susceptible parents or caregivers. The risk for seroconversion among seronegative caregivers ($n = 202$) was 11 percent per year in contrast to seronegative women employed in a local hospital ($n = 229$) with 2.0 percent (Adler 1992). Over all, approximately 25 percent of serious congenital infections occurring each year in the USA can be attributed to exposure in daycare centers.

PRIMARY INFECTION AND EFFECTS ON THE FETUS

Primary infection is defined as first contact with the virus. Characteristic symptoms (lymphadenitis with fever and hepatic dysfunction) occur in only 6.5 percent and suspicious symptoms (lymphadenitis with flulike symptoms) in about 19.4 percent (Daiminger et al. 2004). Therefore diagnosis of infection and immune status relies on laboratory tests. The association between primary CMV infection and fetal loss is not clear. In one early study, the number of spontaneous abortions after primary infection in early gestation was higher (4/26; 15 percent) than in the control group (16/744; 2 percent) (Griffiths and Baboonian 1984). A further low numbered study could not confirm an association between primary infection in early gestation and abortion (Yow et al. 1988). Although some studies published in the 1990s detected CMV DNA in abortive or placental tissue, up to now no correlation between active CMV infection and fetal loss was found, supporting the fact that CMV is not a major abortion-related factor (Spano et al. 2002).

Primary infection in pregnancy, regardless of socioeconomic status, accounts for 24–75 percent (mean 40 percent) of congenital infection (Stagno et al. 1986). These data were confirmed by newer studies on prenatal diagnosis in which intrauterine transmission rates varied between 23.5 and 68 percent (Revello et al. 1995; Ruellan-Eugene et al. 1996; Bodus et al. 1999; Lazzarotto et al. 2000; Liesnard et al. 2000; Azam et al. 2001; Enders et al. 2001).

Most studies reported a constant transmission rate throughout pregnancy following maternal primary infection, but some workers found a higher rate in late pregnancy. However all authors agree that the risk for congenital disease is strongly connected with infection in the first 12 weeks of pregnancy (Stagno et al. 1986; Enders et al. 2001; Daiminger et al. 2004). The risk of fetal damage following preconceptional maternal infection (8 to 2 weeks before last menstrual period) appears to be low, but more data are needed to confirm this observation (Revello et al. 2002; Daiminger et al. 2004). In this respect, the study of Fowler et al. (2004) is of interest, reporting that maternal infection up to 2 years before renewed pregnancy may still pose a risk for congenital infection (Plotkin 2004).

RECURRENT INFECTION AND EFFECTS ON THE FETUS

Recurrent (or secondary) infections are defined as either reactivation of endogenous virus or reinfection with a new strain. The most frequent mechanism for recurrent infection during pregnancy seems to be reactivation of latent virus. However, reinfection by CMV strains other than the original infecting strain, particularly in women with multiple sexual partners, has been demonstrated by restriction enzyme analysis (Chou 1990) and indirectly by measuring antibody specificity of glycoprotein H against CMV laboratory strains and isolates (Boppana et al. 2001).

Recurrent infections occur in the presence of both humoral and cellular immunity, but in the absence of a viremic phase. In contrast to primary infection the transmission rate is very low and amounts to only 1 percent (Fowler et al. 2003), however quantitatively recurrent infections account for most of the subclinical infections worldwide (Stagno et al. 1986; Fowler et al. 2003; Griffiths and Baboonian 1984). It is generally recognized by the presence of specific IgG antibodies before conception or by the presence of IgG antibodies in the first 12 weeks of gestation in the absence of IgM antibodies and by detection of congenital infection in the offspring (Fowler et al. 1992).

Recurrent infection occurs most frequently in the late second and third trimester, when a marked transient depression of CMV-specific cellular immunity was observed (Gehrz et al. 1981; Baboonian et al. 1989). With advancing gestational age the rate of viral shedding from the uterine cervix and urine increases (Shen et al. 1993) suggesting that productive CMV infection in nonpregnant women and in women during early gestation is under the control of the cellular immune system. In relation to CMV and pregnancy it is interesting that the rate of viral shedding from urinary or genital secretions of seropositive pregnant women is inversely related to age. For genital secretion, in one study, the high level of 15 percent at the age of 11–14 years falls to undetectable levels in women aged 31 years and older. For urinary excretion, the rate falls from a peak of 8 percent in the younger age group to zero in women

>26 years old. No excretion occurred from either site in postmenopausal women (Knox et al. 1979). Less well investigated is the influence of age in males on CMV excretion in semen (Shen et al. 1994). The relationship between maternal age and congenital infection and disease for maternal primary and recurrent infection in different populations is not yet well defined.

Between 1970 and 1973, it became evident that congenital infection can occur in consecutive pregnancies. In three independent studies, the first infant was severely affected or died and the second born in each case was subclinically infected. Thereafter, several case reports on congenital infection with disease in infants of seropositive mothers with and without immunosuppression have been published (Stagno 2001). Some recent publications indicate that symptomatic infection at birth in infants born to immune mothers may be more frequent than previously recognized (Ahlfors et al. 1999; Boppana et al. 1999; Casteels et al. 1999). However, it should be remembered that, in immune mothers, the rate of vertical transmission is about 1 percent, the rate of defects at birth in newborns less than 1 percent and the risk of late sequelae 5–8 percent (unilateral hearing loss approximately 5 percent or microcephaly 2 percent).

PATHOGENESIS OF FETAL INFECTION

In primary maternal infection, it is assumed that intrauterine infection results from maternal viremia with subsequent placental infection and hematogenous dissemination to the fetus. It is still undefined whether cell-free or leukocyte-associated virus is required for the spread from the mother to the fetus through the placenta. In detail, infected leukocytes may transmit the infection to uterine microvascular endothelial cells which are in direct contact with the cytotrophoblasts of anchoring villi with subsequent infection of underlying tissues of villous cores including fibroblasts, fetal macrophages, and endothelial cells (Sinzger et al. 1993; Gabrielli et al. 2001). Alternatively infected maternal leukocytes may directly spread the infection to the villous stroma through breaches of the syncytiotrophoblast layer (Hemmings et al. 1998). As a further hypothesis, transportation of antibody-coated CMV virions by transcytosis through the intact syncytiotrophoblast has been discussed (Fisher et al. 2000).

Following direct infection of placental and chorionic tissue, the virus may also spread to amniotic cells that are then ingested by the fetus. In this case the virus replicates in the oropharynx and is then carried through the fetal blood circulation to target tissues such as the kidney. The renal tubular epithelium seems to be a major site of replication. By either mechanism of intrauterine infection the fetus would excrete CMV via urine into amniotic fluid, which seems therefore to be the optimal specimen for prenatal diagnosis of CMV fetal infection.

Other modes of intrauterine transmission may include transovarian infection by infected semen (Shen et al. 1994) and in late pregnancy, by ascending infection from the vagina after premature rupture of the membranes (Ohyama et al. 1992).

The pathogenesis of fetal infection in twin pregnancies is not yet systematically evaluated with respect, for example, to type (primary or recurrent) and time of maternal infection. From the literature it appears, that in the case of monozygotic/monoamniotic pregnancies both fetuses are infected, whereas in dizygotic/diamniotic pregnancies one or both fetuses can be infected. The infected fetuses show various degrees of symptoms at birth. Gabrielli et al. (2003) presented the possibility of horizontal (fetus-to-fetus) transmission for a dichoriotic, diamniotic twin pregnancy with fused placentas. They found that only one fetus was infected at WG 21, whereas both fetuses were infected at birth. Altogether, because intrauterine transmission occurs in only 30–40 percent of pregnant women with primary infection, a mechanism that is not understood but is generally referred to as placental barrier must operate to prevent fetal infection.

In recurrent infection, the mode of CMV transmission in immune mothers is not well known. It is unclear how the virus evades the immune system under these circumstances. Latent CMV reactivates from sites that are less accessible to virologic examination, like placental tissue, ovaries, endometrium, or cervix (Mocarski et al. 1990; Reddehase et al. 1994). Reactivation of CMV especially from macrophages during local immunosuppression in the uterus may be a possible mechanism (Revello and Gerna 2004). As shown by dot-blot hybridization of PCR products CMV DNA was detected in 30 percent of placentas of seropositive mothers, localized mostly to the villi, the extravillous trophoblasts, and decidual cells. The frequency of CMV DNA detection in placentas increased from 18.2 percent for deliveries in the second trimester to 32.9 percent in the third trimester (Kumazaki et al. 2002). This is compatible with the increasing rate for cervical and urinary shedding with advancing gestational age.

In the fetus, the fetal cellular and humoral immune responses to infection are reduced compared to that of the adult (Lewis and Wilson 2001). Cellular immunity such as CMV-specific CD8 cells could be detected in congenitally infected fetuses as soon as WG 22, but may not be fully functional as shown by IFN-γ secretion (Elbou Ould et al. 2004). Humoral immune responses are triggered by immunoglobulin-secreting plasma cells, which are detectable by the 15th week of gestation (Toivanen et al. 1969; Gathings et al. 1981).

CONGENITAL DISEASE

Congenital CMV infection, affecting worldwide approximately 0.2–2 percent of all live-born infants (in the USA, mean approximately 1 percent), is one of the leading causes of mental deficiencies. Up to one in ten newborns has signs at birth commonly associated with congenital CMV disease and about half of these have the classic stigmata of cytomegalic inclusion disease (CID). Another 5 percent present with milder or atypical involvement (e.g. hydrocephalus, hemolytic anemia, pneumonitis, and inguinal hernia) and approximately 90 percent are born with subclinical, but chronic, infection (Demmler 1994). Table 63.6 presents the clinical manifestations of congenital CMV disease in the newborn period. Most of the data come from the USA National Congenital CMV Disease Registry, the worldwide greatest analysis of congenital disease (*n* = 786 babies in the 11th year of investigation) (Demmler 2002).

Congenital CMV infection is the leading nongenetic cause of sensorineural hearing loss (SNHL) in childhood, causing 20–30 percent of all deafness cases (Barbi et al. 2003). By universal otoacoustic emission (OAE) screening of neonates as practiced, for example, in the USA, only about half of all SNHL caused by congenital CMV can be detected and late onset hearing loss, which generally occurs up to 6 years of age will pass unnoticed (Fowler et al. 1999). Ocular disease, which manifests principally by chorioretinitis, is detected more frequently in infants symptomatic at birth (Table 63.6). Because 23 percent of infants with chorioretinitis have either progression of lesions or delayed onset after the first year of life, serial eye examinations are recommended (Anderson et al. 1996; Coats et al. 2000). SNHL usually passes unnoticed for the first 1–2 months of life, as does the less common chorioretinitis. Among the most infected infants mortality ranges between 10 and 12 percent mainly in the neonatal period. More than 90 percent of the survivors have major long-term sequelae. The severity of neurologic impairment is highly variable. In infants with symptomatic infection, normal cranial computer tomographic scan (CT) and normal head circumference proved to be a predictor of favorable cognitive and neurologic outcome (Noyola et al. 2001). However, in symptomatically infected infants presenting with abnormal CT (about 70 percent) and microcephaly, subsequent neurologic abnormalities and mental retardation (IQ <70) may be expected in 90 and 56 percent, respectively (Boppana et al. 1997). Still no factors are identified for predicting progression of hearing loss. Table 63.7 compares the sequelae in congenital CMV infection in infants symptomatic and asymptomatic at birth. Asymptomatically infected infants have a 10 to 15 percent risk of abnormal development, such as SNHL, chorioretinitis, and microcephaly with varying degrees of mental retardation and neuromuscular defects. Except for SNHL, which may be detected even at school age, these sequelae usually present during the first 2 years of life (Table 63.7).

Encouraging aspects are that infants with asymptomatic infection at birth seem to have no differences in IQ and other neuropsychological tests compared with a healthy control collective (Temple et al. 2000; Kashden et al. 1998; Demmler 2004). Furthermore, children with congenital CMV infection, including those with systemic signs at birth, are unlikely to be at increased risk of subsequent neurodevelopmental or intellectual impairment if they show normal development at 12 months of age (Ivarsson et al. 1997).

Table 63.6 *Clinical manifestations and abnormalities in the newborn period with congenital CMV infection*

Abnormalities	Percentage (approx.)
Prematurity (<38 weeks)	34
Small for gestational age	47
Petechiae and purpura	54
Jaundice	36
Hepatomegaly	47
Splenomegaly	44
Pneumonia	11
Thrombocytopenia	54
Hemolytic anemia	13
Elevated liver enzyme values	46
Neurological findings	
One or more of the following	72
Microcephaly	40
Intracranial calcification	43
Lethargy/poor feeding	25
Convulsions	7
Hearing impairment	41
Chorioretinitis	11
Death in the first 6 weeks	12

Table 63.7 *Sequelae in children with congenital cytomegalovirus infection*

Sequelae	Symptomatic at birth (%)	Asymptomatic at birth (%)
Sensorineural hearing loss	41–58	7.4
Bilateral hearing loss	37	2.7
Speech difficulties	27	1.7
Chorioretinitis with/without optic atrophy	20	2.5–3.9
Visual impairment	22	1.2
IQ <70	55	3.7
Microcephaly with convulsions or paresis/paralysis	52	2.7
Microcephaly	37	1.8
Convulsions	23	0.9
Paresis/paralysis	13	0
Death after the newborn period	6	0.3

According to/adapted from: Stagno (2001); Anderson et al. (1996); Coats et al. (2000); Dahle et al. (2000).

PERINATAL AND EARLY POSTNATAL INFECTION

Perinatal infection is acquired by passage through the infected birth canal and early postnatal infection mainly by infected breast milk of a CMV-IgG-positive mother as a result of primary or recurrent infection. The source of both types of infection is due to local reactivation of the virus in the cervical and mammary gland.

The correct rate of perinatal infection is more difficult to determine because it can only be assumed in vaginally delivered infants of seropositive mothers with detection of virus in their cervicovaginal secretion at the time of delivery and in throat or ear swabs of the newborns. In an earlier study of this kind, the rate of perinatal infection was found to be 57 percent; in a similar more recent study restricted to preterm infants it was 22 percent (Hamprecht et al. 2001).

The CMV excretion rate in breast milk of seropositive mothers using highly sensitive diagnostic methods for detection of CMV such as DNA with PCR amounts to 88–96 percent (Mosca et al. 2001; Hamprecht et al. 2001). Instead of the less sensitive virus culture detection of CMV pp65 late mRNA was used to indicate replicating virus. Viral shedding in breast milk was seen as early as 2–3 weeks after delivery, peaks in activity by 3–6 weeks, and ending in most individuals by 8–10 weeks (Hamprecht et al. 2001; Numazaki et al. 2001). It is known that there is a considerable variability in perinatal and early postnatal CMV transmission throughout the world, which is due to maternal factors such as age, practice of breast-feeding and socioeconomic, geographic, and ethnic background.

Breast-feeding in premature infants is beneficial. However, breast-feeding of a high-risk group of preterm infants may be associated with symptomatic CMV infection (Hamprecht et al. 2001; Maschmann et al. 2001). This is shown in a 3-year prospective study of 176 preterm infants weighing <1 500 g (<32nd week of gestation) with a high infection rate of 38 percent (33/87 infants). The mean incubation period between positive DNA detection in breast milk and virus or viral DNA detection in the infant was 42 days (range 28–69 days). Half (16 of 33) of the infected infants had symptoms compatible with CMV disease: hepatomegaly, neutropenia, thrombocytopenia, and four infants had sepsis-like deterioration in the early phase of CMV infection. All infants recovered and thus far, no negative effect on neurodevelopment or hearing was found at follow-up of 22 CMV-infected preterm infants at 2–4.5 years of age and matched controls. Besides the relatively favorable outcome of infected preterm infants by breast-feeding, prevention of CMV infection through contaminated breast milk was and still is a challenge. The aim is removing CMV from breast milk without destroying nutritional–immunological factors (Forsgren 2004).

Perinatal and early postnatal CMV infection are as chronic as congenital infection with virus shed into urine up to 6 years (mean 3.9 years) and into saliva up to 2–4 years with the highest quantity excreted during the first 6 months of life. However, the quantity of virus excreted is less than in infants with symptomatic congenital infection.

Transfusion-acquired early postnatal CMV infection and disease is hardly observed due to the use of CMV antibody-negative blood available through more sensitive screening methods and improved pathogen inactivation methods (Roback 2002).

Diagnosis

DIAGNOSIS IN PREGNANCY

Primary CMV infection in pregnancy is usually detected by chance, as primary infection is generally asymptomatic or may cause nonspecific symptoms.

With the basic serological tests, primary infection can best be detected by seroconversion or rising IgG and IgM antibody titers to high level within 2–4 weeks of onset. Medium- to low-level IgM antibodies can be detected in less recent primary infection, as well as in persistent (chronic) and recurrent infection. This makes IgM an insufficient marker for diagnosing and timing primary infection, particularly since the various commercial IgM tests greatly differ in sensitivity and specificity (Landini 1993; Daiminger et al. 1999). Therefore, sera with positive IgM results should be retested in supplementary assays such as the IgG avidity enzyme immunoassay (EIA) (Eggers et al. 2000), the microneutralization assay (Eggers et al. 1998), and the gB/gH recombinant immunoblot (Eggers et al. 2001). Thus, primary maternal infection may be diagnosed with a single serum sample up to WG 20 by negative or low values in the IgG avidity assay and the microneutralization test (Enders et al. 2003, personal communication).

The cellular immune response determined by CMV-specific lymphoproliferative or cytotoxic assays in women with recent primary CMV infection is not routinely assessed, for example, for the prediction of intrauterine transmission. The first study of this kind (Stern et al. 1986) revealed that newborns of women with a good lymphocyte response were not infected ($n = 8$), whereas mothers whose lymphocytes did not respond delivered infected babies (4/6). In a later study there was a fair, but not complete correlation between a strong lymphocyte response and birth of noninfected infants (Fernando et al. 1993).

The detection of virus shedding in cervical secretion and urine in pregnant women is of little value for distinguishing primary from recurrent maternal infection, because CMV may be excreted intermittently in primary as well as recurrent infection.

Breast milk of lactating seropositive mothers of preterm infants may be investigated for presence of CMV DNA by PCR. However, negative results are of minor value for deciding whether or not to breast feed as excretion may be delayed or often intermittent.

Altogether there is presently no serologic or immunologic test that can predict, for example, protection against intrauterine infection and disease in the fetus (Weinberg 2002).

DIAGNOSIS IN THE FETUS

Prenatal invasive diagnosis of fetal CMV infection is increasingly used in pregnant women with serological suspicion of acute or recent primary infection and in those with abnormal findings by ultrasound examination, whose CMV antibody status is mostly unknown. A variety of sonographic findings has been reported from a number of authors: ascites, fetal growth retardation, cerebral ventriculomegaly, microcephaly, hydrocephalus internus, and oligohydramnion are the most common features. A wide range of brain abnormalities (e.g. intracranial calcification) and hyperechogenic fetal bowel has also been documented in addition to cardiomegaly, hepato- and splenomegaly, hydrops fetalis, or placentomegaly as reviewed by Crino (Crino 1999; Enders et al. 2001). In one study, more than two fetal abnormalities were recorded in 46 percent (27/58) and only one sign in 22 percent (13/58). Fetal abnormalities were first observed between WG 18 and 22 in 40 percent and beyond WG 23 to 32 in 60.3 percent at which time termination of pregnancy is a difficult option (Enders et al. 2001 and update 2001–2004). For detection of fetal intracranial abnormalities transvaginal sonography in WG 22–37 (mean gestational age of 27.5 weeks) provided additional information for all fetuses and fetal magnetic resonance imaging (MRI) in one of two cases (Malinger et al. 2003). In counseling the parents it is necessary to mention not only what can be seen of the characteristic manifestations of congenital infection but also what cannot be seen, like hearing defects or chorioretinitis.

Prenatal diagnosis relies on the detection of viral DNA by PCR and infectious virus by the rapid shell vial culture in amniotic fluid and on the detection of DNA and CMV-specific IgM antibodies in fetal blood (Table 63.3). Detection of CMV in chorionic villi was more rarely attempted. Amniotic fluid is the preferred specimen not only because of the relatively low technical risk of fetal loss with amniocentesis in undamaged fetuses (0.2–1 percent) but also because CMV is excreted into fetal urine, which accumulates in amniotic fluid as pregnancy proceeds. For avoiding false-negative results, amniotic fluid should be obtained after WG 21. In all instances an interval of at least 6 weeks between presumed onset of maternal infection and invasive procedure is recommended (Revello et al. 1995; Bodus et al. 1999; Liesnard et al. 2000; Enders et al. 2001; Gouarin et al. 2001).

In fetal blood obtained after WG 20 CMV DNA detection by PCR was found to be more sensitive (92.6 percent) than detection of IgM antibodies with a sensitivity of approximately 50–80 percent, especially in fetuses with overt infection (Enders et al. 2001 and update 2001–2004; Lipitz et al. 1997; Hagay et al. 1996; Revello et al. 1995; Liesnard et al. 2000).

In one study, the predictive value of prenatal diagnosis on fetal infection, as estimated by the outcome of pregnancy, for positive results (obtained with at least two detection methods) was 100 percent (74/74) and for negative results 96.1 percent (149/155) (Enders et al., 2001 and update 2001–2004). Generally, isolated positive PCR results in only one sample must be considered with caution. Therefore additional cell culture-based methods (shell vial assay or isolation in cell culture) or alternative DNA and RNA detection methods (e.g. nucleic acid sequence based amplification (NASBA), quantitative PCR), PCR in another sample, for example, fetal blood, or in addition a second sampling may be performed for a safe prediction of fetal infection.

The following virological markers may be useful for the prognosis of fetal outcome: viral load in amniotic fluid (Lazzarotto et al. 2000; Guerra et al. 2000; Enders et al. 2001; Gouarin et al. 2002) or fetal blood (Revello et al. 1999b) and presence of CMV-specific IgM antibodies in fetal blood (Revello et al. 1999b; Enders et al. 2001). Also nonspecific biological, biochemical, and immunological markers for fetal function (Azam et al. 2001; Forestier et al. 1988) may provide supportive evidence of congenital disease.

The present experience suggests that prenatal diagnosis carried out with well-controlled serological and virological techniques and ultrasound screening at high level saves a considerable number of pregnancies, since fetal infection can be excluded in about 75 percent of primary maternal infections in pregnancy (Enders et al. 2001 and update 2001–2004, personal communication).

DIAGNOSIS IN INFANTS

The diagnosis of suspected congenital infection in newborns is confirmed by detection of virus in saliva, urine, blood, and by detection of IgM antibodies in cord blood or blood of the neonate.

All the different CMV genotypes (four gB and four gN variants) can be vertically transmitted and produce congenital disease. However, up to now, it seems that the 'potential of infectivity' and ability to produce severe disease is not related to a single polymorphic gene alone (Barbi et al. 2001; Pignatelli et al. 2003).

The virus detection is carried out today mainly by detection of CMV DNA by PCR using commercial and 'in-house' tests of various sensitivities and by detection of infectious virus in the shell vial culture or less frequently in conventional cell culture. Virological tests must be initiated within 2 weeks after birth to distinguish congenital from perinatal or early postnatally acquired infection. It is of interest that higher CMV DNA levels are detected in serum (Nelson et al. 1995) and peripheral leukocytes (Revello et al. 1999a) of symptomatic infants than in asymptomatic infants and that in the former the mean duration of leuko-DNAemia was longer (156 ± 50 versus 40 ± 8 days).

More recently a simple and reliable diagnosis of congenital infection can be accomplished by demonstration of CMV DNA in dried blood spots (DBS) on Guthrie cards (Barbi et al. 2000). The DBS test could be used as an alternative to viral culture. The main benefit comes from the fact that congenital infection may retrospectively be diagnosed beyond the neonatal period or to link morbid conditions like SNHL or white matter abnormalities in brain MRI to congenital infection. However the sensitivity of the DBS test, especially when used retrospectively has to be further investigated.

Antibody testing for detecting prenatal infection is less informative. After birth, approximately 70 percent of symptomatic newborns are IgM antibody positive in contrast to only 30 percent of asymptomatic infected neonates; IgM antibodies are usually detectable for 3–4 months in declining levels (Revello et al. 1999a; Enders et al. 2001). IgG antibodies measured in the cord blood or in the blood of the newborn are mostly of maternal origin. An initial decrease of IgG antibody is followed by an IgG antibody increase and lifelong persistence at medium to low titers. The presence of IgG antibody in asymptomatic infants ⩾8 months of age can be due to congenital or perinatal/early postnatal infection (see also Table 63.5). In this respect the IgG avidity test is helpful in identification of the type of infection (G. Enders, personal communication).

Management

MANAGEMENT IN PREGNANCY

Preventing primary CMV infection by hygienic measures and altering their lifestyle is difficult to achieve and only effective in women who want to become pregnant or are pregnant as they may be highly motivated to follow hygienic guidelines (Adler et al. 1996).

Seronegative pregnant women with significant exposure to CMV at home or at work should be serologically controlled in 2–3-weekly intervals up to 12 weeks after first exposure and at delivery to demonstrate that no infection has occurred (Enders 2003).

For passive prophylaxis, several intravenous hyper-immunoglobulin preparations (CMVIG) with known neutralizing antibody titers are available. They may be used for forensic aspects in seronegative pregnant women with close occupational contact to newborns, infants, or toddlers known to excrete CMV with the goal of preventing maternal infection. From our own experience, passive prophylaxis is less important or needed than observing correct hygienic measures. Antenatal care

directives for CMV seronegative pregnant caregivers differ from country to country from reinforcement of hygienic measures to (for example, in Germany) removal from the workplace for the whole of the pregnancy or restriction to work with infants more than 3 years of age.

In cases of suspected primary infection in the first and second trimester of pregnancy, ultrasound screening at high level and prenatal diagnosis for assessing fetal infection is recommended up to WG 23. This is a better option than the often unnecessary immediate termination of pregnancy.

Treatment of pregnant women with suspected primary CMV infection with the antiviral drugs ganciclovir, foscarnet, and recently valganciclovir (all of which cross the placenta) is not recommended due to their potential teratogenic and embryonic toxicity according to animal studies. Thus far, ganciclovir was applied only in single pregnancies in which the mother had preceding organ transplantation or suffered from severe disease. Whether CMV-infected fetuses benefit from intravascular administration of ganciclovir or CMVIG preparations cannot be finally assessed since only a few case reports with diverse outcome have been published (Revello et al. 1993; Negishi et al. 1998; Nigro et al. 1999; Matsuda et al. 2004, G. Enders personal communication). New drugs for treatment of CMV, e.g. non-DNA polymerase inhibitors, are in development and some of them will hopefully enter clinical trials for safety and efficiency in the near future (Emery and Hassan-Walker 2002).

Delivery: cesarean section is not recommended in case of presumed maternal primary and fetal congenital CMV infection – unless the fetus is highly damaged.

Breast-feeding of seropositive mothers in uninfected and congenital infected newborns is not contraindicated. Recommendations for breast-feeding of very low birth weight (VLBW) preterm infants (WG <32, body weight <1 500 g) born to IgG-seropositive mothers vary from country to country between breast-feeding after counseling the parents for possible risks and feeding breast milk following various virus inactivation methods (Holder pasteurization or a new procedure for gentle virus inactivation up to corrected WG 34). Other intervention strategies for seronegative women are avoidance of iatrogenic transmission in in vitro fertilization (IVF) programs by using screened semen or screened blood products for seronegative pregnant women in case of emergency or seronegative donors in organ transplantation.

MANAGEMENT OF THE NEONATE

In infants of mothers with suspected CMV infection in pregnancy, screening for CMV congenital infection should be performed by detection of virus in urine or saliva within 14 days after birth or by DBS test on Guthrie cards followed by auditory screening of infected infants up to school age, so that affected infants can receive intervention (e.g. cochlea implants) as promptly as possible (Fowler et al. 1999).

An increasing number of neonates with hearing defects will now be identified due to the more universally practised auditory screening in industrialized countries by otoacustic emissions or auditory brain stem response. It should be remembered that about half of all cases with sensorineural hearing loss caused by CMV will be missed due to the late onset of hearing loss in formerly asymptomatic newborns.

In infants with congenital disease at birth antiviral therapy is an option and its aim is the suppression of virus replication in order to prevent the progression of auditory, visual, and mental impairment and the occurrence of further or late manifestations. From a number of studies it is known that there is a reduction of virus load during therapy, but no complete virus elimination. After cessation of therapy, virus shedding usually returns to preceding or even higher levels especially when treatment was suspended too early (Barbi et al. 1996). According to several studies – using different treatment regimes – i.v. ganciclovir is fairly well tolerated even in preterm infants. Acute symptoms (pneumonia, hepatitis, chorioretinitis) seem to resolve by early treatment (Hocker et al. 1990; Stronati et al. 1995; Nigro et al. 1994; Liberek et al. 2002; Barampouti et al. 2002). In the USA, a large-randomized controlled multicenter clinical trial (with and without 6 mg/kg i.v. twice a day for 6 weeks) was performed in infants with congenital disease at birth and central nervous system (CNS) involvement and showed very promising results with respect to safety and antiviral effects (phase I (Trang et al. 1993); phase II (Whitley et al. 1997)). The results from phase III indicate that i.v. ganciclovir therapy in symptomatically infected neonates prevented hearing deterioration at 6 months and might prevent it thereafter (⩾1 year) (Kimberlin et al. 2003).

The availability of oral therapy (oral ganciclovir and most recently valganciclovir) would be a great advance in long-term maintenance therapy usually following the initial i.v. treatment. Thus far, there are only few pharmacokinetic studies on oral ganciclovir application in infants (Michaels et al. 2003). In infants dosage should be related to body surface or body weight and controlled by drug monitoring in blood plasma. The effect of oral valganciclovir with a ten times higher bioavailability than oral ganciclovir is still under investigation. Preliminary results in seven infants show that valganciclovir is well tolerated, effective in a transient reduction of the viral load, and effective in resolving acute symptoms (G. Enders, personal communication).

There is good agreement that asymptomatic congenitally infected infants should not be treated with ganciclovir so far, but should be closely surveilled for onset of late manifestations, which may then justify treatment. Early after birth, e.g. via breast milk, infected preterm infants with symptomatic disease seem to benefit from early therapy in preventing severe disease (G. Enders, personal communication).

The overall effectiveness of ganciclovir i.v. treatment is difficult to judge from the multicenter study and from the increasing number of observational studies, due to the erratic natural course of the congenital disease.

With regard to childhood vaccination, it has been observed that the recently used sixfold vaccine combination (DTPa, hepatitis B, poliovirus 1, 2, 3, HiB), measles, mumps, and rubella (MMR), and lately varicella is well tolerated in asymptomatic and symptomatic congenitally infected infants producing satisfactory antibody levels against the various vaccine components (G. Enders, personal communication).

FUTURE MEASURES AND PUBLIC HEALTH ASPECTS

Opinions vary on the value and cost-effectiveness of screening programs for CMV. Universal antenatal CMV antibody screening is not officially recommended or has not been introduced into any prenatal programs in industrialized countries (Revello and Gerna 2002; Enders et al. 2003). Such programs have shown to be helpful for the guidance of pregnant seronegative women in commonsense measures for preventing the acquisition of primary infection and for reassuring IgG-positive/IgM-negative women that they are protected against primary infection. In case of recurrent infection there is only a low risk of the birth of a child with congenital disease. However, to such women a closer surveillance in the following pregnancy by serology and ultrasonography (WG 21–24) should be recommended.

For active prophylaxis, several vaccines are under investigation (Pass and Burke 2002) and currently four of them have reached clinical trials: Towne live-attenuated virus, subunit glycoprotein B (gB/MF59) (Mitchell et al. 2002), canary pox, and an improved Towne (chimeric CMV) vaccine. Further vaccines consisting of plasmid DNA, dense bodies, or synthetic peptides are in development (Plotkin 2001). To be effective, these vaccines should induce persisting titers of serum-neutralizing and mucosal antibodies comparable to those found after natural infection. Induction of cellular immunity (cytotoxic lymphocyte response of importance for protection) would also be beneficial, but will not be achieved with subunit vaccines alone. Potential vaccine recipients would be young boys and girls before puberty. Encouraging aspects come from a study by Griffiths (Griffiths et al. 2001) showing by a mathematic modeling approach that in developed countries a vaccine applied to 1-year old infants with only modest efficiency (60 percent protective effect against primary infection) would nevertheless be sufficient in eradication of CMV from the population.

The public health impact of congenital CMV infection is enormous, especially when the late sequelae of congenital CMV infection are more definitely associated with CMV congenital infection (Istas et al. 1995), which is presently the case (2004). The annual costs of supporting children with congenital CMV in the USA approaches two billion US dollars (Griffiths 2002; Prober and Enright 2003).

VARICELLA-ZOSTER VIRUS

Varicella-zoster virus (VZV) is an alphaherpesvirus that causes two main clinical syndromes: primary infection gives rise to varicella (chickenpox) and recurrent infection to herpes zoster (shingles). Varicella is highly contagious, whereas herpes zoster is less so. Chickenpox in pregnancy may be associated with severe maternal disease, spontaneous abortion, and infrequently, during the first two trimesters, with congenital varicella syndrome (CVS). Maternal varicella around term carries the risk of serious neonatal disease. Zoster at any time during pregnancy does not result in congenital anomalies or neonatal disease.

Infection in pregnancy

INCIDENCE

Varicella in pregnancy is relatively uncommon because in densely populated areas of the northern hemisphere, approximately 95 percent women of childbearing age are seropositive. However, this figure may be smaller in some populations (e.g. black women in the USA and in countries of the southern hemisphere) (Gray et al. 1990; Dworkin 1996; Seward et al. 2000). Reliable data on the incidence of varicella in pregnancy are not available, but extrapolation from the consultation rates for chickenpox in adults aged 15–44 years in the UK suggest an infection risk of approximately 2–3 per 1 000 with an average mortality rate of 1/1 million pregnancies (Department of Health 1996a; Fairley and Miller 1996). In Germany, the seroprevalence to varicella was studied annually from 1984 to 1997 in more than 26 000 pregnant women aged 20–40 years; the seronegative rate was about 5–6 percent, with no significant change over the period (Enders 1984; Enders and Miller 1994; Enders and Miller 2000, and update 2004). Based on the suggested infection risk of 2 per 1 000 in the UK in all adults aged 15–44 years, the frequency of varicella in pregnancy was calculated to be 8 000 in the USA, 1 600 cases per year in Germany, and 1 400 in England and Wales (Department of Health 1996a; Enders and Miller 2000). Asymptomatic reinfection is possible and second attacks of varicella have also been reported (Martin et al. 1994, Enders et al. personal communication). An upward shift of incidence to adults aged 15–44 years has been recognized in England (Miller et al. 1993a) and in the USA (Gray et al. 1990; Choo et al. 1995). Zoster in pregnancy may have an annual incidence of 2 per 1 000, similar to that in nonpregnant adults aged 15–40 years (Miller et al. 1993b; Schmader 2001). There is no evidence that the incidence in adults has changed over the last few decades.

ADVERSE EFFECTS IN PREGNANCY

Anecdotal evidence suggests that varicella is more severe in pregnant women than in other adults, particularly the risk of varicella pneumonia. However, there are no reliable population-based prospective studies to confirm this impression (Nathwani et al. 1998). Among 1 721 pregnant women with varicella followed up prospectively by the author between 1980 and 1999, no cases of pneumonia nor deaths were recorded (Enders and Miller 1994, 2000). However, outside this study, we investigated three very severe cases of VZV pneumonia between WG 22 and 33 (1992–1997). All three women survived and two of the three infants were born healthy and uninfected. In the third pregnancy, intrauterine death and spontaneous abortion occurred in WG 23. This indicates that varicella pneumonia associated with pregnancy is rare, although mortality data from the UK suggest that the risk of fatal varicella appears to be five-fold higher in pregnant than in nonpregnant immunocompetent adults (Miller et al. 1993b).

VZV pneumonia is the most common serious maternal complication in pregnancy (Haake et al. 1990; Katz et al. 1995). It usually develops within 1 week of the rash. The predominant signs and symptoms are fever, cough, dyspnea, and tachypnea. The outcome is unpredictable and there may be rapid progress to hypoxia and respiratory failure. Pneumonia is regarded as a medical emergency requiring prompt diagnosis and treatment. Studies reporting the outcome of varicella pneumonia in pregnancy show an excess of cases in the third trimester, suggesting that the risk to the mother may be greatest towards term. For example, 28 of 34 cases reported in 1989 and 1991 occurred in the third trimester (Esmonde et al. 1989; Smego and Asperilla 1991). Of the nine deaths reported as due to varicella in pregnancy in England and Wales between 1985 and 1998, seven occurred between 27 and 32 weeks of gestation.

In pregnancies complicated by varicella, spontaneous abortion, stillbirth, and prematurity do not seem to be significantly increased (Paryani and Arvin 1986; Balducci et al. 1992). In a prospective study of a total of 1 721 VZV-complicated pregnancies, the incidence of fetal loss due to spontaneous abortion during the first 20 weeks was 2.9 percent ($n = 49$) and of intrauterine death after the 20th week 0.6 percent ($n = 11$) of 1 612 live-born infants (Enders and Miller 1994, 2000). In pregnancies complicated by localized zoster rarely has dissemination been reported in immune-competent women.

Effects on the fetus

CONGENITAL VARICELLA SYNDROME

The risk of congenital varicella syndrome is an important concern. Since its first description by Laforet and Lynch (1947) more than 112 such cases have been reported in the English and German medical literature (Sauerbrei and Wutzler 2003). A causal association with maternal infection has been confirmed in only a few cases in live-born infants by isolation of VZV or detection of viral DNA from skin lesions at birth and in some more cases in tissues following therapeutic abortion or intrauterine death (e.g. Da Silva et al. 1990; Scharf et al. 1990; Puchhammer-Stöckl et al. 1994; Sauerbrei et al. 1996; Sauerbrei 1998; Hartung et al. 1999; Schulze-Oechtering et al. 2004).

CLINICAL MANIFESTATIONS

The clinical manifestations of CVS range from severe multisystem involvement, resulting in death in the neonatal period, to dermatomal skin scarring, limb hypoplasia, or both as the only defects. Table 63.8 shows the clinical features of CVS and their relative frequencies of 48 well-documented cases from the world literature, as well as the 13 prospective and the 12 retrospective cases investigated by Enders and Miller (2000).

PATHOGENESIS OF CVS

The precise mechanism of infection with VZV in utero is unknown. It is generally accepted that transplacental transmission of VZV may take place during the viremic phase, resulting in congenital infection (Trlifojova et al. 1986). The pattern of defects in CVS, particularly the limb hypoplasia and scarring, suggests that they are due to intrauterine zoster. The extremely short period between reactivation and fetal infection may be the

result of an inadequate cell-mediated immune response in early gestation (Higa et al. 1987).

The clinical consequences of congenital VZV infections depend on the stage of pregnancy at which maternal infection occurs (Table 63.9).

Intrauterine varicella infection can, however, occur without clinical sequelae at any stage of pregnancy, the proportion rising from 5–10 percent in the first and second trimester to 25 percent towards WG 36 and reaching approximately 50 percent when maternal varicella occurs 1–4 weeks before delivery (Miller et al. 1989). It seems possible that fetal infection early in pregnancy may result in clinical manifestations with healing of lesions before birth. Localized zoster in pregnancy could theoretically result in fetal infection, if the dermatomes involved were T10 to L1, as sensory nerves to the uterus originate from these segments; but no such cases have yet been documented (Miller et al. 1993b; Enders and Miller 2000).

The risk of zoster in infancy and childhood following maternal varicella in the second and third trimesters is 0.6 percent (4/618) and 1.6 percent (7/431), respectively, and the overall risk 1 percent (Enders and Miller, 1994, 2000, and update 2004). In the prenatal diagnosis study of Mouly et al. (1997) the rate of localized early herpes zoster in infants born to mothers with varicella before the 24th week of pregnancy was 3.8 percent (3/78).

RISK OF CONGENITAL VARICELLA SYNDROME

Several workers undertook prospective studies to estimate the risk of CVS following maternal varicella infection at various stages of pregnancy (Enders 1984; Paryani and Arvin 1986; Balducci et al. 1992; Jones et al. 1994; Pastuszak et al. 1994). In the largest reported prospective study (Enders and Miller, 1994, 2000, and update 2004), including 1 795 pregnant women with acute varicella with known outcome the overall risk during the first 20 weeks of gestation is 1.4 percent, the highest (3.0 percent) being observed between weeks 13 and 20. The latest gestational age at which CVS occurred was WG 19, which is consistent with the findings in one retrospective report (Alkalay et al. 1987). In a recent prospective study in 2002, involving 347 pregnant women with primary VZV infection only one case

Table 63.8 *Congenital varicella syndrome*

Main signs	Number of infants (%)	
	$n = 48^a$	$n = 25^b$
Skin: dermatomal cicatricial skin lesions, contractures	39	18
Skeleton: Limb hypoplasia associated with reduction deformaties	21	18
Eye: microphthalmia, chorioretinitis, cataract, Horner syndrome	26	11
CNS: microcephaly, brain atrophy, paralysis, convulsions, encephalitis, mental retardation	26	14
Other organ defects (e.g. gastrointestinal, genitourinary)	5	5
Multiorgan involvement (e.g. hemorrhagic rash and dystrophy)	ND	6
Death postpartum and later	ND	9
Female	ND	13
Male	ND	12

ND, no data.
a) From world literature.
b) Enders and Miller (1994, 2000); 13 prospective and 12 retrospective cases.

Table 63.9 *Clinical manifestations of congenital varicella infection following chickenpox in pregnancy*

Stage of maternal infection	Sequelae
First and second trimester	Congenital varicella syndrome
Second and third trimester	Herpes zoster in infancy or childhood
Perinatal	Disseminated neonatal varicella

From Miller et al. (1993b).

of CVS with typical skin scars and left retinal macular lesion occurred, however, after maternal varicella at WG 24 (Harger et al. 2002). In zoster in pregnancy involving 504 women with localized zoster there was no serological evidence of intrauterine infection and no congenital varicella syndrome (CVS) symptoms in the infants (Enders and Miller 1994, 2000, Enders update 2004). Various congenital defects have been reported after maternal zoster (Webster and Smith 1977; Higa et al. 1987), but only one infant with characteristic limb hypoplasia and skin scarring has been described following disseminated maternal zoster at WG 12 with presumed maternal viremia (Higa et al. 1987).

Based on the estimate of risk, together with the incidence of chickenpox in pregnancy and the annual rate of births, the number of CVS cases, which could be expected to occur each year is 44 in the USA, eight in England/Wales (UK), and nine in Germany (Enders and Miller 2000). The incidence of the CVS in Australia has been reported as 1–2 of 100 000 pregnancies per year which is 2.3 cases per year (Forrest et al. 2000). This confirms the low frequency of CVS.

The possibility of reinfection with adverse consequences for the fetus, has been raised (Martin et al. 1994). In our investigation on asymptomatic reinfection in 347 seropositive pregnant women with close exposure a significant rise of IgG antibodies was detected in 203 women and a rise of IgG and IgM antibodies in 144 women. In one case of reinfection at WG 37 varicella-like symptoms were noted together with a very high rise of IgG and IgM antibodies. Reinfection could be recognized by the already high avidity index in the first low-level IgG serum sample. Pregnancy outcome was documented in about 70 percent of the cases. In the newborns, no abnormal serology nor defects or illness consistent with CVS or neonatal varicella were observed (Enders, personal communication).

Re-exposure to VZV also induces a VZV-specific cellular immune response with an expansion of antigen-specific $CD4^+$ T cells and changes in cytotoxic $CD8^+$ T cells and NK cells. This T-cell response of VZV-specific $CD4^+$ memory T cells largely resembles the primary immune response to VZV (Vossen et al. 2004).

Neonatal varicella

Severe neonatal disease is generally attributed to intrauterine infection and lack of maternal antibody. If the mother's rashes appears more than 6 days before delivery, the infant invariably has maternal antibodies. When it is <6 days before delivery, only some infants have significant titers of antibody, whereas those born <3 days after onset of maternal rash, or infants whose mothers develop varicella after delivery are VZV IgG-negative. Infants at greatest risk of severe or fatal illness are those whose mothers' rashes appears 5 days before

to 2 days after delivery (Gershon 1975; Miller et al. 1989). The interval between the onset of rash in the mother and infant is usually 12–13 days, but may be as brief as 2 days, suggesting transplacental infection. In one retrospective series, the clinical attack rate was estimated to be 17 percent (Meyers 1974) and the fatality rate 30 percent (Gershon 1975). According to a more recent large prospective study the commonly cited fatality rate of 30 percent seems to be an overestimate due to selective reporting of fatal outcomes (Miller et al. 1989). The annual incidence of neonatal varicella is only known from Australia, which is 5.8 per 100 000 live births or one in 17 000 pregnancies. Of interest is that all these 44 infants recovered without reported sequelae (Forrest et al. 2000).

A severe outcome of neonatal varicella is not limited to transplacentally acquired infection, but occasionally occurs in early postnatally acquired infection (minimum incubation period 8 days after birth) despite the use of varicella immunoglobulin (VZIG) even at high dosage.

Most of the concern surrounding neonatal varicella relates to infants whose mothers develop varicella. But it should be borne in mind that maternal immunity to varicella does not always protect the neonate exposed postnatally at home. There have been occasional reports of varicella in neonates of mothers with a past history of chickenpox (Bendig et al. 1998; Baba et al. 1982). All the cases (two and five) were of moderate severity or mild. Miller et al. (1989) followed up 36 infants who had a home exposure to varicella during the first 4 weeks of life. Six infants (17 percent) were infected, three with symptoms (mild to severe) and three without clinical features. Clearly, passively acquired VZV antibody provides incomplete protection, particularly under conditions of close exposure. Following neonatal varicella reactivation is not uncommon giving rise to zoster within a few months or years of the primary infection. Further zoster episodes have not been reported in these children, suggesting that good cell-mediated immunity develops after reactivation.

Despite the potential for horizontal transmission of VZV from zoster cases, neonates do not seem to be at risk of infection if maternal zoster occurs around the time of delivery (Miller et al. 1993b; Enders and Miller 2000). The reason for this is the lower infectivity of zoster compared to chickenpox; furthermore, if the onset of maternal zoster is ≥ 4 days before delivery, the infant passively acquires antibody from the mother, whose own pre-existing immunity is reinforced as a result of her recent reactivation.

Diagnosis

DIAGNOSIS IN PREGNANCY

In typical cases of varicella and zoster a clinical diagnosis is usually sufficient. In pregnancy VZV infection should be verified serologically. To detect specific IgG, IgM, and IgA antibodies, the enzyme-linked immunosorbent assay (ELISA) with whole virus has become the most widely used method, and for a very rapid determination of the immune status in case of exposure the latex agglutination (LA) test is also employed. Results with both tests correlate well with cell-mediated immunity as determined by lymphoproliferative assays (Weinberg et al. 1996). It should be known that in the majority of adults (e.g. pregnant women) following primary infection VZV IgG antibodies are detected before VZV IgM antibodies due to strong cross-reaction with herpes simplex virus type 1 (Enders and Miller 2000). More recently the IgG avidity test – which is investigated for its diagnostic value since 1990 (Thomas et al. 1990) – proved in our in-house version very useful for assuring protection against VZV disease in persons with low-level IgG antibodies, for diagnosing recent infection in the absence of IgM antibodies and for differentiation of asymptomatic or symptomatic reinfection from primary infection (G. Enders, personal communication).

Virus detection is unnecessary in uncomplicated varicella, but is used in cases complicated by pneumonia or encephalitis to guide antiviral therapy and in prenatal diagnosis. Rapid diagnosis can be achieved in smears of vesicle fluid or respiratory secretion by immunofluorescence applying monoclonal antibodies for identification. Virus detection with the conventional methods such as cell culture is only successful with varicella or zoster vesicular fluid containing free virus, whereas cell-associated virus can, apart from the rapid diagnosis, be demonstrated by detection of VZV DNA. Initially VZV DNA has been detected in amniotic fluid and fetal blood by dot-blot hybridization (Gottard et al. 1991), but now detection by single round and nested PCR is the method of choice. However, positive results with n-PCR only must be judged with caution.

DIAGNOSIS IN THE FETUS

Invasive prenatal diagnosis (PD) to exclude fetal infection with VZV is feasible, but not generally recommended. PD should only be performed in women with varicella up to WG 21–22, since the risk of CVS is limited to this period. In cases where VZV DNA is detected in the amniotic fluid and the ultrasonographic scan is considered normal, the majority of infants have no clinical manifestation at birth (Mouly et al. 1997; G. Enders personal communication 1996–2004). Amniotic fluid taken at WG 18–21 and >4–6 weeks after the onset of maternal varicella is technically easy to obtain and yields the best results. In case of varicella infection and genetic indication for prenatal diagnosis the latter could be done earlier, but not before all vesicles have disappeared in order to avoid iatrogenic infection of the fetus. High-level ultrasound screening is recommended between WG 19 and 23. If the findings are abnormal,

both amniotic fluid and fetal blood should be tested for VZV DNA. Tests for fetal VZV-specific IgM are not helpful, because VZV IgM antibodies are usually not detected in fetal blood. Skeletal defects may be evident by ultrasound earlier, but cerebral or ocular abnormalities are seldom recognized before WG 22–23. They may not become evident until much later in pregnancy, when therapeutic abortion is not an option. The combined use of ultrasound and magnetic resonance imaging (MRI) may document earlier the extent of tissue damage, particularly involvement of the CNS (Verstraelen et al. 2003). These findings are substantiated by the author's own prospective series on invasive prenatal diagnosis of 195 women with acute varicella up to WG 24 between 1991 and July 2004. In nine cases, detection of VZV DNA in amniotic fluid and fetal blood was associated with suspicious finding for CVS by high-level ultrasound and in some cases by additional MRI between WG 20 and 27. Following termination of pregnancy in six cases, VZV DNA could also be demonstrated by PCR in fetal blood and various types of fetal tissues and also in fluids and tissues in three cases who died shortly after birth (Enders and Miller 2000; G. Enders personal communication 2000–2004).

DIAGNOSIS IN INFANCY

The criteria for the diagnosis of fetal varicella syndrome in the infant include maternal symptomatic varicella infection during early pregnancy, presence of dermatomal cicatrial skin lesions, limb hypoplasia, and some of the other signs and symptoms associated with CVS recognizable at birth (see Table 63.8). Laboratory confirmation of intrauterine VZV infection is more important in cases with less typical CVS features. Concerning the immunological evidence of in utero VZV infection, IgM antibody detection, and detection of cellular immune response are unreliable markers, because IgM antibodies are only exceptionally detected with the presently used commercial ELISA IgM tests even in infants with CVS. Also the detection of a positive cellular immune response over the age of 1 month by the standard lymphocyte proliferation (^{3}H-thymidine) test has been rarely accomplished (Paryani and Arvin 1986). Attempts with the newly developed interferon-γ ELISPOT assay have not been made thus far (Smith et al. 2001). Detecting persistent VZV IgG antibodies in the infant seems to be more indicative of congenital VZV as shown in CVS cases assessed prospectively and retrospectively since 1980–2003 (Enders and Miller 1994, 2000). An even later criterion of intrauterine VZV infection is the occurrence of zoster in early infancy. Therefore, attempts to detect VZV DNA by PCR in body fluids or skin biopsies and EDTA blood should be undertaken. Positive results are limited (Mehraein et al. 1991; Puchhammer-Stöckl et al. 1994; Schulze-Oechtering et al. 2004). In contrast, DNA detection in tissues of various organs obtained postmortem is the method of choice in cases of early death and the demonstration of miliary calcified necrosis by histopathological techniques may further support intrauterine varicella infection (Hartung et al. 1999).

Management

MANAGEMENT IN PREGNANCY

Passive prophylaxis with varicella-zoster immunoglobulin

The value of passive prophylaxis is difficult to assess because of the differences in quality of the various varicella-zoster-immunoglobulin (VZIG) preparations used worldwide. This concerns IgG antibody concentration and the test used for establishing the international units (IU). Passive antibody prophylaxis with a standardized preparation of VZIG for intramuscular application is available in the USA (CDC 1996), in the UK, France, Scandinavian countries, and Australia for exposed susceptible pregnant women to prevent or attenuate varicella.

The English preparations have a relatively low IgG antibody concentration (700 IU per adult dose) and administration of VZIG is recommended within 4–10 days of a close (e.g. home) exposure. Their effect is to attenuate disease rather than to prevent infection (Miller et al. 1993b).

In Germany, two preparations of VZV immunoglobulins with defined antibody concentrations are available for passive prophylaxis, one for intramuscular and the other for intravenous administration, with an IgG antibody concentration of approximately 2 000 IU per adult dose. The dosage for example for a 70-kg woman is 20 ml Varicellon i.m. (2 000 IU) or 70 ml Varitect i.v. (1 750 IU). It should be given within 24–72 (96) hours after exposure. According to the experience of Enders and Miller (2000) in 212 seronegative pregnancies, even if VZIG is given in the recommended dosage and within 24–72 (96) hours of exposure, infection is prevented in only 54 percent. Of the remaining cases VZIG administration results in subclinical infection (5 percent) or in modified to normal disease (41 percent). When VZIG is given 4–5 days after exposure, there is still a mitigating effect in 20 percent of patients.

In the UK and Germany, postexposure prophylaxis with VZIG is recommended only for seronegative pregnant women with significant exposure to an acute case of varicella (e.g. household contact, face-to-face contact, contact indoors with a case of chickenpox for >1 h). As a consequence of the findings in the largest prospective study (Enders and Miller 1994), that no case of CVS occurred in maternal varicella after WG 20, VZIG is no longer recommended for women exposed after WG 21. However, VZIG prophylaxis for women exposed later in

pregnancy is officially recommended, also in Germany by the RKI, to reduce the risk of rare maternal complications of varicella such as pneumonia. In the UK, however, VZIG is only issued for women exposed after WG 20 if national supplies permit (Department of Health 1996b). These recommendations differ from the US recommendation, which includes all susceptible pregnant women with close contact throughout pregnancy.

It is clear that seropositive women do not need VZIG. They can be assured that they are protected against clinical disease but not completely against reinfection. In the case of exposure to zoster, passive prophylaxis is only recommended for seronegative women up to WG 21 intimately exposed to persons with extensive zoster lesions.

Whether VZIG has any benefit in preventing intrauterine infection and of CVS is not known. A certain benefit of VZIG administration during pregnancy in case of contact is deduced from the prospective studies of Enders et al. (Enders and Miller 1994 and 2000 with update). There were no CVS cases in 108 pregnancies in which maternal varicella occurred despite VZIG prophylaxis and no persistent IgG antibodies could be detected at the age of 7 months in eight infants tested.

One other study (Pastuszak et al. 1994) indicates that in order to prove such a benefit a prospective study would be needed, which includes the following: a large cohort of VZV-seronegative women with confirmed close contact to VZV who all receive the same in neutralizing units of a standardized preparation of VZIG.

Besides postexposure prophylaxis with VZIG, oral acyclovir (ACV) given at the 9th day of incubation or within 24 h after onset of exanthema (5 × 800 mg/day for 5 days) and vaccination with live-varicella vaccine within 72 h after contact may be effective. In the UK and Australia in contrast to Germany, oral ACV is offered to persons presenting within 24 h of onset of rash and given for 5 days; pregnant women over 20 weeks of gestation with varicella are treated with this regimen. However, the use of oral ACV during the incubation period or vaccination in early pregnancy is not established.

The recommendations in the UK and Germany for postexposure prophylaxis to varicella in early and late pregnancy are summarized in Table 63.10.

The medical advice for acute varicella at various stages in pregnancy is summarized in Table 63.11.

Management of exposure to zoster and zoster in pregnancy is presented in Table 63.12.

Active prophylaxis with vaccine

In the USA, universal vaccination of children, adolescents, and young adults including all nonpregnant women

Table 63.10 *Recent exposure to varicella in pregnancy – high contagiousness*

VZV exposure in pregnancy

Ask for previous varicella:
If yes: no testing
If no or doubtful
↓

Quick antibody test (ELISA, LA test)
AB positive: previous infection
AB low or equivocal: repeat test in 2–3 weeks
AB negative: susceptible

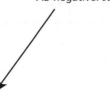

First and second trimester: risk for CVS	**End of third trimester around delivery: risk for severe neonatal varicella**
VZIG: until WG 21 within 24–72 (96 h) after exposure[a]	No VZIG after WG 37, because it may shift onset of exanthem to delivery, better to induce labor
New: >20 WG: ACV oral within 24 h after onset of exanthem	
Check after 2–3 weeks for preventive effect	Check antibody status in 2–3 weeks

AB, varicella-zoster antibodies; ACV, acyclovir; CVS, congenital varicella syndrome; ELISA, enzyme-linked immunosorbent assay; LA test, latex agglutination test; VZIG, varicella immunoglobulin; WG, week of gestation.
a) Personal recommendations by G. Enders; official German recommendations also include women exposed beyond 21 WG.

of childbearing age with no history of varicella has been recommended since 1996 (CDC 1996). The effectiveness of this universal childhood vaccination in the USA is indicated by a significant decline of varicella cases in the total population and, in particular, in the vaccinated age group of 1–4 years. Also the rate of hospitalization in all age groups has decreased within the first 3 years since the beginning of routine childhood vaccination. Furthermore, a reduction in pediatric hospitalizations for VZV-related invasive group A streptococcal infections

Table 63.11 *Acute varicella throughout pregnancy*

Management for acute varicella throughout pregnancy	
First and second trimester	
1. Counsel	Risk of CVS is low
2. Mention	Prenatal diagnosis possible in case of acute varicella in WG 1–20, ~4 weeks after onset of varicella: VZV-DNA detection with PCR/n-PCR in amniotic fluid (WG >18–21) Advocate: Ultrasound control of high level (MRI) in WG 19–24, if abnormal: PCR/n-PCR in amniotic fluid and fetal blood in WG 23/24; IgM antibodies not detected
3. Observe	VZV pneumoniae occurring mainly late second and third trimester: advice immediate i.v. acyclovir therapy at any stage of pregnancy and intensive medical support
Third trimester	
More than 6 days prior to delivery →	No VZIG
4–5 days prior to delivery →	If birth cannot be delayed: VZIG to mother Instead of VZIG – new: ACV oral within 24 h of onset of rash (5 × 800 mg/day for 5 days) not yet practisized VZIG to neonate and ACV i.v. before or at onset of prodromal signs
2–4 days after delivery →	VZIG to neonate
	No isolation of mother/child (rooming-in). Breast-feeding possible, in case of florid exanthem, pump off breast milk. Observe neonate ⩾12 days in hospital and until age of 28 days at home

ACV, acyclovir; CVS, congenital varicella syndrome; n-PCR, nested polymerase chain reaction; VZIG, varicella immunoglobulin; VZV, varicella zoster virus; WG, week of gestation.

Table 63.12 *Exposure to zoster and zoster in pregnancy – low contagiousness, no risk for CVS or perinatal infection*

Management for exposure to zoster and zoster in pregnancy		
Recent exposure to zoster lesion		
Determination of VZV IgG antibody status:		
VZV IgG antibody positive	→	no VZIG
VZV IgG antibody negative	→	VZIG only if close contact until WG ±21
Onset of zoster		
1st–3rd trimester	→	No VZIG
(1st), 2nd, 3rd trimester	→	Acyclovir if severe manifestations, i.v., oral
±4 days prior to delivery	→	No VZIG to newborn
		Cover maternal zoster lesions
		Breast-feeding: yes, if no vesicles in area of nipples; otherwise pump off breast milk
3–4 days after delivery	→	VZIG for newborn 0.5 ml/kg weight, since maternal antibody level is still low

CVS, congenital varicella syndrome; VZIG, varicella immunoglobulin; VZV, varicella-zoster virus; WG, week of gestation.

parallel to the increase of vaccination rates has been observed. In most European countries, the universal childhood vaccination is still controversial. In July 2004, Germany, however, introduced the US childhood vaccination program encouraged by the favorable US experience (Wagenpfeil et al. 2004). It is hoped that the shift in the proportion of cases to older persons will be minimized by catch-up vaccination of adolescents and adults. Selective vaccination is recommended for seronegative risk-patients, their family contacts, healthcare workers, women who want to become pregnant, and also adolescents at the age of 12–15 years without varicella history. Children aged 1–12 years generally receive one dose of vaccine, whereas from 13 years on two doses of vaccine with an interval of 6 weeks are recommended.

Pregnancy is a contraindication for administration of live-attenuated varicella vaccine. However, the virulence of the vaccine virus is less than wild-type VZV, so the risk to the fetus, if any, is even lower and therefore inadvertent administration is no reason for termination of pregnancy. As a precaution, however, nonpregnant women who are vaccinated should avoid becoming pregnant for 1 month following each injection. A varicella vaccine in the pregnancy registry in the USA has been established, similar to that for rubella vaccine. Between 1995 and 2000, 362 women were inadvertently exposed to varicella during pregnancy or within 3 months of conception. In this group 58, of 92 seronegative women received their first dose of vaccine (Varivax) during the first or second trimester. No cases of congenital varicella syndrome were identified in 56 live-births (Shields et al. 2001). With respect to transmitting vaccine virus from vaccinees, there is one report in which the vaccinated child transmitted vaccine virus to its pregnant mother (Long 1997). Despite this observation recommendation of the German Vaccine Commission (STIKO) does not consider pregnancy of the mother as a contraindication

to the vaccination of her own child (Robert Koch Institut 2004).

Furthermore, postpartum vaccination of varicella-susceptible women need not be delayed because of breast-feeding. In a study of 217 postvaccination breast milk specimens, varicella DNA was not detected by PCR. In addition, none of the breast-fed infants became seropositive (Bohlke et al. 2003).

Antiviral therapy

For antiviral chemotherapy of VZV infection, acyclovir (which has an excellent safety record), valacyclovir, brivudin, and famciclovir are available.

The efficacy of intravenous acyclovir in the treatment of chickenpox in immunocompromised people is well established. By oral application, valacyclovir, brivudin, and famciclovir have a higher bioavailability than ACV. All these drugs in intravenous and oral form are not licensed for use in pregnancy. However, in varicella complicated by, for example, pneumonia or signs of dissemination, early treatment with intravenous acyclovir at any stage of pregnancy is essential and life-saving (Haake et al. 1990; Smego and Asperilla 1991). The prospective follow-up of a total of 1 207 women treated by oral and intravenous application during the first, second, and third trimester with ACV did not show an increase in the number of birth defects when compared with those expected in the general population, or any consistent pattern of defects. Similar data have been reported on the outcome of 94 pregnancies in which oral valacyclovir had been given (Enders and Miller 2000). The use of oral ACV following exposure as a postprophylactic measure has already been discussed. For cases of CVS antiviral therapy is recommended, particularly, in those in which VZV DNA in fluids and lesions is detected (ACV 30–60 mg/kg/day i.v., divided into three single doses).

MANAGEMENT OF THE NEONATE

For neonates whose mothers have varicella around the time of delivery, prophylaxis with VZIG is recommended to prevent neonatal infection or to modify the disease. In the USA and Germany, prophylaxis is only recommended for neonates whose mothers develop varicella between 5 days before, to 2 days after, delivery (CDC 1996); while in the UK prophylaxis is recommended for any infant whose mother develops varicella in the 14-day period centered on delivery (Department of Health 1996b). In the UK, VZIG is also recommended for infants with nonmaternal postnatal exposure during the first 7 days of life and who lack VZV antibodies. In the USA and UK, susceptible infants can be identified by testing a stored antenatal blood sample from mothers with a negative history of chickenpox. In the USA and Germany, prophylaxis for postnatal exposure is restricted to premature infants. However, all preterm infants less than 28 weeks or infants weighing less than 1 000 g exposed to acute cases should be given VZIG (0.5 ml/kg i.m.) regardless of a positive maternal history of varicella (Deutsche Gesellschaft für pädiatrische Infektiologie 2003) and regardless of low-level IgG antibodies in the infant.

If severe varicella develops in the infant despite treatment with VZIG, high-dose intravenous acyclovir should be given (Reynolds et al. 1999). Fatal outcomes have been reported despite VZIG prophylaxis and treatment with ACV (Holland et al. 1986; King et al. 1986). All were in infants whose mothers developed varicella within the period 4 days before, to 2 days after, delivery. Early treatment with intravenous ACV of infected neonates in this high-risk period is therefore recommended (Nathwani et al. 1998; Reynolds et al. 1999). Prophylactic use of intravenous ACV in this group has also been advocated (Sills et al. 1987), but there is no evidence of efficacy. For limitation of the existing symptoms and further symptoms by interrupting possibly still ongoing virus replication, ACV therapy is carried out.

At present, there is no convincing information about whether mothers who develop varicella in the high-risk period around the time of delivery should breastfeed or be isolated from their infants. Not unexpectedly, VZV DNA has been detected by PCR in breast milk (Yoshida et al. 1992), but whether VZV was transmitted to the newborn via breast milk could not be determined because the mother was breast-feeding in the 24 h prior to rash onset. Furthermore, neonates whose mothers have varicella shortly before delivery may have already been infected transplacentally at the time of birth.

For those infants whose mothers develop varicella in the puerperium, transmission during the infectious period before rash onset is likely. Therefore isolation of the infant from the mother is questioned (Trompeter et al. 1986; Stephenson 1993).

Management of nosocomial exposure

Despite the concern raised when varicella exposure occurs in an antenatal clinic or neonatal intensive care unit, documented nosocomial transmissions in these groups are rare. This is probably due to the low intensity of exposure, particularly in neonatal units. Furthermore, the majority (approximately 90–95 percent) of the neonates, also premature and low birth weight infants, have low or medium maternal antibody titers which may be protective. The index case is often a healthcare worker or visitor and control measures may require extensive VZV antibody testing of patients and staff contacts. To avoid unnecessary use of VZIG for the newborn only neonates of seronegative mothers should receive VZIG.

Newborns with CVS have to be isolated from other neonates although there is no report of an infection transmitted by the respiratory route or by intimate contact. Asymptomatic newborns whose mothers develop varicella 5 days before to 2 days after delivery do not need to be isolated from other babies.

For more than 20 years it has been stipulated that medical and healthcare workers should know their immunity status and since the availability of live vaccine in 1995, vaccination of susceptible healthcare workers is recommended.

Recommendations for limiting nosocomial spread of varicella are listed in Table 63.13.

HERPES SIMPLEX VIRUS TYPES 1 AND 2

Maternal herpes simplex virus (HSV), primary and recurrent genital infection, which is frequently asymptomatic, may cause neonatal herpes. Although infrequent, neonatal herpes is a devastating disease with a high rate of morbidity and mortality despite early and appropriate therapy. Because its incidence is significantly higher in the USA than elsewhere, special efforts are being made in that country to establish a reliable and cost-effective strategy for prevention.

Infection in pregnancy

EPIDEMIOLOGY OF MATERNAL HSV INFECTION

In the past, approximately 90 percent of herpetic genital infections were caused by HSV-2, but more recently HSV-1 has been implicated as the cause of up to 40 percent of cases of primary genital herpes in seronegative adults. However, the reactivation rate for genital HSV-2 is at least twice as high as for HSV-1, and so too are the risks of transmission by sexual intercourse and of neonatal herpes infection (Forsgren 1992; Koelle et al. 1992; Corey et al. 1996). This was confirmed in a recent study in the UK. The prevalence of HSV-1 antibodies among attenders of a sexually transmitted disease

Table 63.13 *Limitation of nosocomial varicella transmission*

Group	Action
For hospital staff	
Test for VZV IgG antibody	In personnel before working in maternity/newborn wards and wards for immunosuppressed patients
In case of exposure, test for IgG antibody if immunity status is unknown	Seropositive staff: remain on ward
	Seronegative staff: removal from work 8–21 days after exposure to a case of varicella or immediate vaccination with live vaccine
	Vaccinees: develop IgG antibody in low titer within 10–12 days. Should avoid close association with susceptible high-risk individuals if they develop some vesicles
For pregnant women	
Exposed to cases with acute varicella shortly before and after delivery	Determine IgG antibody titer
	Mother antibody-positive → no VZIG to neonate
	Mother antibody-negative → VZIG to neonate
For infants in neonatal care	
In case of exposure in the first 7 days of life	Determine IgG antibody titer
	Infants VZV-IgG positive → no VZIG[a]
	Infants VZV-IgG negative → VZIG
Newborn with CVS	Isolation mother and baby (rooming-in), contagiousness low

VZIG, varicella immune globulin; VZV, varicella-zoster virus.
a) Except premature neonates born before 25 weeks gestational age and/or with birth weight of less than 1 000 g.

(STD) clinic was 60 percent and among the blood donors 46 percent ($n = 1\,494$). The increasing genital herpes infection due to HSV-1 was strongly associated with early age of first sexual intercourse (Cowan et al. 2002).

Seroprevalence studies with HSV type-specific antigens have demonstrated rates of HSV-1 infection of approximately 30 percent in people aged 20–40 years in higher socioeconomic groups and approximately 80 percent in those of lower socioeconomic groups (Corey and Spear 1986a, 1986b; Johnson et al. 1989). Thus people with higher living standards now acquire HSV-1 infection less frequently in childhood than they did in the past. The consequent lack of partial cross-protection may be one of the reasons for the higher frequency and severity of primary HSV-2 and HSV-1 genital infection (Koutsky et al. 1990; Bernstein 1991).

Most surveys of seroprevalence have shown a relatively low but increasing rate of HSV-2 infection during the last decade in the general adult population in the developed world; for example, in the USA from 16 percent in 1976–1980 to approximately 22 percent in 1989–1991 (Johnson et al. 1989, 1994). HSV-2 seroprevalence in women of childbearing age in the USA varied from 10 to 35 percent in white women and from 35 to 60 percent in black women (Johnson et al. 1989; Arvin and Prober 1990). In other surveys, the HSV-2 seroprevalences in pregnant women in various countries ranged between 10 and 33 percent, and in most of the HSV-2-seropositive women, a large proportion (55–87 percent) had asymptomatic infections (Slomka 1996). This finding led to alterations to the preventive strategies previously suggested (Prober et al. 1988; Randolph et al. 1993). A global review of type-specific HSV sero-epidemiologic surveys shows that HSV-2 prevalence is higher in Africa and the Americas (South America), lower in western and southern Europe than in northern Europe and north America, and lowest in Asia (Smith and Robinson 2002).

CLASSIFICATION OF GENITAL HERPES INFECTION

Genital herpes infections are defined as primary first episode, nonprimary first episode, or recurrent infections. Primary first episode infections are those with seroconversion for either type 1 or type 2; in nonprimary first episode infection, seroconversion occurs to one type in the presence of antibody to the other type; and in recurrent – also called reactivated – infection, homologous antibodies to the type in question are already present.

Primary infection

Initial genital infection due to herpes may be either asymptomatic or associated with severe symptoms. With symptomatic primary infection, lesions may occur on the vulva, vagina, or cervix, or on all three between 2 and 14 days following exposure to infectious virus. These lesions are larger in number and size than those observed in patients with recurrent disease and patients who have had prior infection with HSV-1.

When systemic symptoms (malaise, myalgia, and fever) occur (low risk), they are most commonly restricted to presumed primary herpetic infections. These symptoms reflect the viremia that occurs more likely with primary infection. Subclinical cervical and vulvar shedding occur at a rate of approximately 2.3 percent in women with HSV-2 infection and 0.65 percent in women with HSV-1 infection (ACOG, 2000a).

Nonprimary first episode

Prior infection with HSV-1 does not fully protect a patient from initial infection with HSV-2 in the genital tract. There are fewer systemic manifestations, less pain, a briefer duration of viral shedding, and a more rapid resolution of the clinical lesions in the nonprimary infection. These episodes are usually thought to be the result of an initial HSV-2 infection in the presence of partially protective HSV-1 antibodies.

Recurrent infection

Shedding of the virus from the genital tract without symptoms or signs of clinical lesions (subclinical shedding) is episodic and lasts an average of 1.5 days (ACOG 2000b). The clinical signs of genital herpes are present in approximately 25–30 percent of infected women (Table 63.14).

EFFECT ON PREGNANCY

The form of genital infection at the time of delivery is of major importance, whereas primary or recurrent oropharyngeal type 1 infections are of little significance. Severe disease after primary oropharyngeal or genital infection in pregnancy is rare. The first case of disseminated HSV infection in pregnancy was reported by Flewett et al. (1969). Since then 25 cases have been described in the English language literature (Kang and Graves 1999; Frederick et al. 2002), which occurred between WG 22 and 38 with an average gestational age of 36 weeks. Both HSV serotypes have been implicated with type 2 more prevalent accounting for 63 percent of cases. HSV hepatitis presents as anicteric hepatic dysfunction with highly elevated transaminases, fever, and abdominal tenderness. Symptoms of central nervous system involvement ranging from lethargy to seizures and coma may be observed in 50 percent of cases. Maternal mortality from 24 reported cases is 39 percent. Three of those received ACV therapy and six were not or inadequately treated. Early diagnosis and early initia-

Table 63.14 *Classification of genital herpes simplex infection and viral shedding*

Infection	Clinical characteristics
Primary first-episode infection: HSV-2 (HSV-1)	Seroconversion for either type 1 or 2
	Characteristic genital lesions, sometimes with systemic illness
	Low risk of disseminated severe disease
	Virus shedding in the cervix (ca. 3 weeks) and in high concentration, often continuing after clinical healing
Nonprimary first-episode infection: HSV-2, (HSV-1)	Seroconversion to one type in the presence of antibody to the other type
	Significant to moderate local symptoms, but little systemic illness
	Virus shedding often similar to that in primary infection
Recurrent infection: HSV-2 (HSV-1)	Homologous pre-existing antibody
	Usually minor or no local symptoms
	Viral shedding in low concentration during the very early phase for 2–5 days

(HSV-1), less common.

tion of antiviral therapy with i.v. acyclovir plays a major role in improving survival. Only three patients (20 percent) on antiviral acyclovir died and these three received antivirals late in their clinical course, whereas the mortality rate in patients without antiviral therapy was 67 percent. The overall perinatal mortality, excluding terminated gestations, was 39 percent, but evidence of HSV infections by virus detection in the tissues of these infants was very limited. The review of the reported cases shows that fever and anicteric hepatitis in the third trimester should prompt an investigation for disseminated herpes simplex infection and early treatment with acyclovir will reduce maternal and fetal mortality and morbidity.

Primary genital infections with HSV-2 up to midgestation have been associated with an increased rate of abortion (Nahmias et al. 1971). However, these findings were not confirmed in another study of 94 women with seroconversion during pregnancy (Brown et al. 1997). In the second or third trimester, intrauterine growth retardation and prematurity can occur (Brown et al. 1987). Furthermore, maternal primary, and less often nonprimary first episode infection during the first or second trimester, may lead to congenital infection with severe disease evident at birth (Hutto et al. 1987; Hoppen et al. 2001).

RISK FACTORS IN MOTHER–INFANT TRANSMISSION

Most infants with neonatal herpes acquire infection by passage through an infected birth canal. Mothers with a known history of genital herpes and those with unrecognized genital herpes infection (approximately 70 percent) are at risk of transmitting HSV to their infants. For the intrapartum route of transmission, the risk of neonatal infection depends on the form of maternal genital infection and is directly related to viral shedding into the cervicovaginal secretion at the onset of labor.

Brown and colleagues (Brown et al. 1991) made a prospective study of the very important group of women who are asymptomatic at onset of labor. Viral shedding in the genital tract at the beginning of labor occurred in 56 of 15 923 women (0.35 percent). Of these, 51 shed HSV-2 and five HSV-1. Serological tests revealed that 35 percent of the women with HSV shedding at the onset of labor had recently acquired primary infection or first episode genital infection. Vertical transmission occurred in 12.5 percent in women with positive HSV cultures and in 0.02 percent of those with negative cultures, indicating that viral shedding is not always detectable. Neonatal herpes developed in 33 percent of the babies born to women with recent primary or first episode genital infections, but in only 3 percent of those born to mothers with recurrent asymptomatic infection. The incidence of neonatal herpes in this study population was one per 2 000 live births. In a new prospective study of Brown et al. (2003) the outcome of 58 632 pregnancies with an incidence of neonatal herpes of 1:3 200 per live births. One of the novel finding in this study was that the neonatal HSV infection rate was reduced by cesarean delivery (1.2 percent) versus vaginal delivery (7.7 percent). Only one woman with subclinical nonprimary first-episode HSV-2 infection infected her child after undergoing a cesarean delivery because of failure to progress 19 h after rupture of the membranes. Another novel finding was the high efficiency of transmission of HSV-1 (45 percent) from mother to infant, both from primary infection and reactivation of genital HSV-1, among women with genital shedding.

The results of this study indicate that the risk of virus transmission to vaginally delivered infants is approximately 44 percent (3/3 with HSV-1; 1/6 with HSV-2) in women with primary infection 23 percent (0/1 with HSV-1; 4/16 with HSV-2) in those with nonprimary first-episode HSV genital infection shortly (<2 weeks) before delivery, 1.3 percent (2/11 with HSV-1; 0/140 with HSV-2) in women with recurrent lesions and <3 percent in those with recurrent asymptomatic infection (Brown et al. 2003).

ADDITIONAL RISK FACTORS IN MOTHER–INFANT TRANSMISSION

Additional risk factors for virus transmission and neonatal disease are prolonged ruptured or leaky membranes (>6 h before delivery), increasing the risk of intrauterine infection by the ascending route. Fetal scalp electrode monitoring, forceps delivery, or vacuum extraction may provide portals of virus entry in the newborn (Brown et al. 1991; Malm et al. 1991; Forsgren 1992). Other risk factors for neonatal HSV not statistically proven were younger maternal age (Brown et al. 2003).

Effects on the neonate

INCIDENCE OF NEONATAL DISEASE

Neonatal herpes in the USA occurs at an estimated annual rate of one per 3 500–5 000 deliveries, but may be as high as one per 2 000 in certain population groups with high HSV-2 seroprevalence (e.g. Whitley 1994). For unknown reasons, the annual incidence is much lower in some other countries, for example, the UK (1/40 000–60 000) and Sweden (1/15 000), even though the seroprevalences of HSV-1 and HSV-2 in European countries are comparable with those in the USA. In general, a larger proportion of neonatal infections in these countries, as well as in Germany (where no incidence rates are available) has been predominantly caused between 1993 and 1994 by HSV-2 than HSV-1, thereafter up to now by HSV-1 (1995–2004). A nationwide survey in Japan also indicated that twice as many neonatal infections are due to HSV-1 (Morishima et al. 1996). Similar observations have been reported from the Netherlands, where 73 percent of neonatal herpes cases (2.4 cases per 100 000 neonates) are caused by HSV-1 with a seroprevalence rate for HSV-1 of 61–75 percent and for HSV-2 of 11–35 percent in three different cities (Amsterdam, Nijmegen, Rotterdam) (Gaytant et al. 2002).

PATHOGENESIS OF NEONATAL INFECTION

Of the reported neonatal herpes cases in the USA, approximately 4 percent are acquired in utero, 86 percent intrapartum, and 10 percent postnatally (Whitley 1993; Arvin and Whitley 2001).

Transmission of infection in utero occurs transplacentally in <2 percent of cases, most probably in early to mid-gestation, because physical signs are present at birth and include some unusual stigmata (e.g. hydrocephalus, chorioretinitis); a further 2–3 percent arise late in gestation by the ascending route. In intrapartum transmission, the higher infection rate in infants born to mothers with primary or primary first-episode genital herpes shortly before delivery, causing most cases of neonatal herpes, is related both to viral shedding in high concentration and to the absence of maternal neutralizing antibodies (see, for example, Yeager et al. 1980; Brown et al. 1991; Whitley 1994). This is in contrast to recurrent infection, in which virus is shed for a shorter period in low amounts and maternal antibodies against the infecting type are passed to the newborn. Postnatal infections are acquired from maternal sources (oral, genital, and breast lesions), or close contact with people with herpetic lesions (e.g. of the mouth or fingers), or by nosocomial spread from other infected babies.

IMMUNE RESPONSE IN THE INFECTED NEWBORN

In infected newborns the cellular immune response is suppressed and delayed as indicated by an absent or delayed T-lymphocyte proliferative response and decreased interferon-α and -γ production in response to herpes simplex antigen (see, for example, Kahlon and Whitley 1988; Cederblad et al. 1989). The IgG antibody response is initially not recognizable because, in the first 6–8 weeks, it cannot be distinguished from maternal antibody. Specific IgM antibodies develop within the first 2–3 weeks of illness and remain detectable for approximately 6–8 weeks. Specific IgG antibodies persist at medium to low titers for life. Transplacentally transferred neutralizing and antibody-dependent cell-mediated cytotoxic (ADCC) antibodies modify the severity of neonatal disease (Kohl et al. 1989).

CLINICAL MANIFESTATIONS

Neonatal herpes is almost invariably overt and frequently lethal. The most severely affected infants are those with in utero infection acquired early in pregnancy (<2 percent) with physical signs apparent at birth. Lesions include skin vesicles or scarring, chorioretinitis, microcephaly, and hydrocephaly (Hutto et al. 1987). So far, more than 30 such cases have been identified but the estimated incidence (one per 200 000 live births) is low. Infants with intrauterine infections acquired late by the ascending route (2–3 percent) usually present only with skin or eye lesions at birth, without multiorgan involvement (Baldwin and Whitley 1989; Whitley 1993; Arvin and Whitley 2001). Yet, there are also reports on disseminated neonatal herpes caused by late maternal ascending infection (Vasileiadis et al. 2003).

In a scheme based on large prospective studies, neonatal herpes cases are classified according to the three general patterns of infection, each occurring in about one third of cases (Forsgren 1992; Whitley 1994; Harrison 1995; Arvin and Whitley 2001) (Table 63.15).

In general, neonatal disease caused by HSV-1 seemed to have a better prognosis than that caused by HSV-2 (Forsgren 1992). However, in the national Japanese survey on neonatal herpes, although similar patterns of disease were evident, the type of virus had no significant effects on mortality, morbidity, and response to treatment (Morishima et al. 1996). This was also shown by Enders et al. (unpublished).

Diagnosis

DIAGNOSIS IN PREGNANCY

Maternal infection with typical mucocutaneous lesions in the oropharynx and the genital tract is easily diagnosed but less typical, minor genital lesions need laboratory confirmation.

PCR is the most sensitive method for detecting both HSV-1 and HSV-2, and can be used at the onset of labor for a rapid decision on the mode of delivery (Schalasta et al. 2000), high levels of HSV DNA in the maternal secretion increasing the probability of transmission to the infant. Assessment of the type-specific antibodies to both HSV-1 and HSV-2 in late pregnancy is essential for identifying mothers at risk of infecting their infants during delivery. The risk is highest in women with primary or nonprimary first-episode infection who seroconvert during pregnancy. ELISA and immunofluorescence tests with nontype-specific antigens detect seroconversion for IgG and IgM antibodies in primary oropharyngeal and genital infections and rises in specific IgG in genital first episodes; in recurrent infections (symptomatic or asymptomatic), there is no rise in specific IgG level and IgM is not detectable. The more cumbersome neutralization test, although not routinely used, is employed for determining the amount of protective antibodies in maternal and newborn blood.

None of the conventional tests, however, can accurately distinguish between type 1- and type 2-specific antibodies. This is possible only with assays (e.g. immunoblot, immunodot, gG2 indirect ELISA) employing recombinant expressed or native purified glycoprotein G antigen (gG-1 for HSV-1, gG-2 for HSV-2) (Svennerholm et al.

Table 63.15 *Classification, pattern, and outcome of neonatal HSV disease*

Disease	Onset of signs after birth	Mortality		Prognosis in survivors
		No therapy	With therapy	
Disseminated CNS, lung, liver, adrenals, SEM	6–12 days[a]	>80%	>50%	40% develop normally
CNS encephalitis/meningitis in 37–48% without SEM	16–18 days	>50%	15%	In ca. 56% neurological and ophthalmological impairment and recurrent skin lesions
SEM skin/eye/mouth	7–10 days	ND	0%	In ≥20% neurological impairment, recurrent skin lesions

ND, no data.
a) Onset at 12 days is less frequent.

1984; Johnson et al. 1989; Forsgren 1992; Slomka 1996; Enders et al. 1998; Ashley 2002). HSV-2 type-specific IgM antibodies may also be detected more easily by such assays (Ho et al. 1993). However, certain problems with immunoblot versus ELISA tests with regard to low values have to be recognized (Cherpes et al. 2003). It should be noted that the interval between onset of a primary or first episode genital infection to the detection of type-specific antibodies may range from 2 to 3 weeks for HSV-1 and from 2 to 4 weeks for HSV-2 (Ashley et al. 1988; Ho et al. 1993). The influence of immediate ACV therapy on prolonging seroconversion has to be considered (Ashley and Corey 1984).

DIAGNOSIS IN NEONATE AND INFANT

Cases with skin vesicles are easily recognized; neonatal herpes should also be considered in the differential diagnosis of severe generalized disease or of encephalitis within the first 6 weeks of life.

The most direct means of laboratory diagnosis is viral detection, especially by PCR, which is particularly useful for tests on cerebrospinal fluid (CSF). Serology is of little help in the first weeks of life. Testing the maternal serum together with acute phase and later sera of the infant is essential. A presumptive retrospective diagnosis of a child damaged by HSV-2 is obtained by demonstrating persistent IgG antibodies to HSV-2 or by isolating the virus from recurrent vesicles, because HSV-2 infections are rare before the onset of sexual activity (Malm et al. 1991).

Management in pregnancy and of the neonate

At the first antenatal visit, a careful history should be taken of genital infections in the woman herself and her sexual partner, together with visual inspection of her genital tract both at this visit and at the onset of labor. If lesions are seen, swabs should be taken for virus detection, but a decision on cesarean section rests mainly on the presence of visible lesions. If serological tests are used, seroconversion to HSV-2 antibody-positive during pregnancy may be an indication for rapid virus detection by PCR and possible treatment; this approach might reduce the need for cesarean section.

Cesarean sections, considered at present as the only effective means of preventing neonatal herpes infection, are performed on up to 70 percent of women in the USA with a history of genital herpes, because of possible fetal infection and of medicolegal considerations. It is recommended generally for women with visible cervicovaginal lesions at onset of labor, irrespective of the antibody status or viral shedding, and is best performed before rupture of the membranes. The procedure will, however, not always prevent neonatal herpes, even if performed before rupture of the membranes, and

especially not after they have been ruptured for more than 4 h (Stone et al. 1989; Randolph et al. 1993).

Prenatal diagnosis is not recommended because the fetus is rarely transplacentally infected until midgestation. Termination of pregnancy in women with disseminated disease is not an option.

For immunoprophylaxis, specific immunoglobulins, humanized murine and human monoclonal antibodies, and hyperimmunoglobulin with high neutralizing activity (but never commercially available) have been developed for administration to neonates lacking maternal antibodies. Vaccines for prevention and treatment, particularly of HSV-2 genital infections, have also been developed and a candidate subunit vaccine is still on trial (Stanberry et al. 2002; Whitley and Roizman 2002).

Acyclovir or its derivatives are the mainstay of antiviral therapy for both topical and systemic application. Although this drug is not licensed for use in pregnancy, no association has so far been identified between its use in pregnancy and adverse effects in mother or child (Kroon and Whitley 1995). This was shown by a large registry of acyclovir use in pregnancy for both HSV and varicella pneumonia which was established in the USA (1984–1998). Up until its closure in 1998, no evidence of any increase in adverse fetal effects related to drug exposure in any trimester, in comparison with the general population, was reported (Enders and Miller 2000).

In maternal primary disseminated infection, early intravenous treatment with acyclovir (i.v. 10 mg/kg every 8 h for 10–14 days) at any stage of pregnancy is recommended. Oral treatment with acyclovir (400 mg three times daily for 14 days) is considered beneficial for women with recognized primary or non-primary first-episode genital infection in the later stages of pregnancy. This is also the case in maternal primary oral infection (e.g. gingivostomatitis) shortly before term, at delivery, or in the neonatal period and in primary genital herpes in the neonatal period. To suppress viral shedding during labor in women with recurrent lesions in late pregnancy, prophylactic oral use (400 mg three times daily) approximately 10 days before delivery (Stray-Pedersen 1990; Haddad et al. 1993) is still controversial for various reasons, such as potential renal toxicity for the fetus, occasional virus shedding despite suppressive treatment (Katz et al. 1995), and the question of its value. The need for suppressive therapy in the above-mentioned target group is limited, because there is only a low prospective risk to babies born to women with recurrent lesions, in contrast to those born to mothers with unrecognized primary and non-primary first-episode genital infections (Kroon and Whitley 1995; Arvin and Whitley 2001). Hence a recently published double-blind, randomized, placebo-controlled trial of acyclovir in late pregnancy shows that acyclovir significantly reduced, but did not eliminate, herpes simplex virus lesions in the genital tract and detection of HSV

DNA by PCR in genital secretion in late pregnancy (Watts et al. 2003).

The prophylactic administration of acyclovir to vaginally delivered asymptomatic newborns at risk of infection depends mainly on the form of maternal infection and the virus load in the maternal secretion. Follow up for clinical and laboratory signs of infection is recommended up to 4 weeks after delivery (e.g. Forsgren 1992; Whitley 1994; Arvin and Whitley 2001). Opinions on administration of acyclovir to exposed vaginally delivered infants who have no signs of infection are controversial. However, prophylactic treatment should be considered for infants of mothers with high-risk markers for primary or primary first-episode genital infection.

B19 VIRUS (PARVOVIRUS B19)

The *B19 virus* (B19), belonging to the genus *Erythrovirus*, family *Parvoviridae*, was discovered in the plasma of healthy blood donors in 1975, and recognized in 1983 as the cause of erythema infectiosum. In 1984, its causative role in hydrops fetalis and fetal death became evident and in 1993 blood group P antigen (glycolipide-globoside) was identified as the cellular receptor for parvovirus B19 (Brown et al. 1993). Since 1995, parvovirus B19 has become associated with a wide spectrum of hematological and nonhematological complications.

Recently, a second human erythrovirus, the V9 isolate, was detected in the serum and bone marrow of a child with transient aplastic anemia (Nguyen et al. 1999; Servant et al. 2002). The prevalence of V9 and its association with clinical disease and significance for pregnancy remains to be evaluated.

Postnatal infection

Postnatal infection of parvovirus B19 is acquired through aerosol droplets by the respiratory route by close person-to-person contact, but may also occur through blood-derived products administered parenterally. Transmission via respiratory secretions is greatest during viremia and before clinical signs are apparent, complicating efforts to control transmission. The incubation time ranges between 8 and 18 days (Anderson et al. 1985; Joseph 1986), the contagious period lasts from 5 to 7 days before, and until 2 to 4 days after, onset of symptoms. First-phase illness appears approximately 8 days after infection and second-phase illness with typical symptoms about 17/18 days. All immunocompetent people with or without characteristic symptoms develop antibodies to parvovirus B19 and presumably lasting immunity that protect them against infection with the virus in the future. The seroprevalence rate in childbearing age, in adults and in pregnancy ranges from 30 to 60 percent in individual countries and with regional differences (Cohen and Buckley 1988; Enders and Biber 1990; Kelly et al. 2000).

Infections in temperate climates are common in late winter, spring, and the early summer months. Rates of infection may rise to an epidemic level every 3–4 years. During epidemic periods, women of childbearing age show an annual seroconversion rate of 13 percent compared with 1.5 percent in endemic periods (Koch and Adler 1989; Valeur-Jensen et al. 1999; Jensen et al. 2000). During outbreaks, secondary spread to seronegative contacts is very common. The infection rate in susceptible children and adults is up to 50 percent within families and approximately 20 percent for care workers and teachers in primary school being highest for those in contact with younger and greater numbers of infected children (Gillespie et al. 1990). During school outbreaks, 10–60 percent of students may get fifth disease (CDC 2000). A serological study on the occupational risk in employees of hospital and elementary schools during an endemic period revealed that those persons in daily contact with school-age children had a fivefold increased annual occupational risk for infection (Adler et al. 1993).

In pregnancy, approximately 60 percent of infections are asymptomatic or clinically uncharacteristic, for example, without the typical slapped-cheek rash and the lacy red rash on the trunk and limbs, but often associated with joint swelling which lasts usually for 1–2 weeks, and more rarely for several months. Most frequently affected are the joints of the hands, wrists, and knees (Woolf et al. 1989; Enders and Biber 1990).

Effects on the fetus

PATHOGENESIS OF FETAL INFECTION

The main cellular receptor for B19 virus (the blood group P antigen, a glycolipid-globoside), is expressed on mature erythrocytes and erythroid progenitor cells. Abundant productive infection with cell lysis has only been demonstrated in the nucleated, rapidly dividing erythroid progenitors (burst-forming units erythroid (BFU-E) and colony-forming units erythroid (CFU-E)) in bone marrow and fetal liver (Morey and Fleming 1992). The inhibition of fetal erythropoiesis occurs mainly in the late pronormoblast stage in which intranuclear inclusions (Lantern cells) are commonly detected. Direct toxic cell injury, as well as B19-induced apoptosis and cell cycle arrest may be involved in the pathogenesis of erythroid aplasia (Chisaka et al. 2003). The damage of the erythroid progenitor cells, e.g. in the bone marrow, spleen, and liver during the time of a rapidly expanding red-cell volume combined with a shortened fetal red-cell life span of 45–70 days produces a profound aplastic crisis in the fetus with a resultant anemia culminating in cardiovascular decompensation, hydrops, ascites, and fetal death.

P antigen is also presented on nonerythroid cells, for example, megakaryocytes, endothelial cells, placental villous trophoblast cells, and cardiac myocytes. However, none of these cells are fully permissive for B19 replication. Various reasons for the nonpermissiveness are discussed and include incomplete virus replication (Liu et al. 1992), the need for a second receptor for viral entry (Weigel-Kelley et al. 2003) or a viral phospholipase A2 which appears to be necessary for B19 infectivity (Zadori et al. 2001; Heegaard and Brown 2002). Nevertheless, B19 was found to infect fetal myocardial cells and was associated with fetal myocarditis (Soulie 1995; von Kaisenberg et al. 2001). Hence, not only anemia but also myocarditis may be implicated in the pathogenesis of hydrops fetalis.

The presence of the globoside receptor on trophoblast cells may play a role in transmission of the virus across the placenta. It was observed that the immunoreactivity for globoside was strongest in the villous trophoblast cells of first trimester placentas with diminished reactivity in second trimester placentas and a near lack of staining for the antigen in those of third trimester. The observed change found in globoside immunoreactivity correlates well with the fact that fetal outcome is worse when maternal infection occurs during the first or second trimester as compared with an infection occurring near term (Jordan and DeLoia 1999). Furthermore, an enhanced apoptotic activity within placental villous trophoblast cells in pregnancies complicated by B19 infection was described. Damage to the protective trophoblast layer may compromise the integrity of the placenta, and cause fetal loss not necessarily associated with fetal infection (Jordan and Butchko 2002).

FETAL COMPLICATIONS

The virus may cross the placenta at any time during pregnancy and infection is possible as early as 6 weeks of gestation (Nunoue et al. 2002). The overall transplacental transmission rate was estimated to be 33 percent based on an adverse outcome, parvovirus B19 IgM in cord or neonatal blood, and on the persistence of specific IgG antibodies (Miller et al. 1998; Public Health Laboratory Service Working Party on Fifth Disease 1990) and others have reported similar rates (Gratacós et al. 1995; Koch et al. 1998).

The major risks are spontaneous abortion, stillbirth, and hydrops fetalis (HF). The interval between onset of maternal infection and fetal complications may range from 2 to 17 weeks (Miller et al. 1998), 2–6 weeks (Yaegashi et al. 1998), and 2–20 weeks (Nunoue et al. 2002).

Fetal loss

The rates of fetal loss varied in some small numbered prospective studies between 1.66 percent (one of 60 infected mothers) (Gratacós et al. 1995), 5 percent

(2/39) (Rodis et al. 1990), 15 percent (7/48) Yaegashi et al. 1999), and 0 percent (0/52) (Harger et al. 1998). In two prospective studies from the UK, 427 pregnant women with acute B19 virus infection were investigated (Public Health Laboratory Service Working Party on Fifth Disease 1990; Miller et al. 1998). The excess rate of fetal loss was confined to the first 20 weeks of gestation and averaged 9 percent. In our prospective study, 1 018 pregnant women with B19 infection were enrolled and the excess rate of fetal loss was also confined to the first 20 WG, but slightly smaller (5.6 percent). The median interval between maternal infection and diagnosis of fetal death was 2 weeks (Enders et al. 2004). Although the majority of B19 infections associated with fetal death occur in the first 20 WG, intrauterine death in late pregnancy without signs of fetal hydrops has been reported by different authors (Skjöldebrand-Sparre et al. 2000; Tolfvenstam et al. 2001; Norbeck et al. 2002). According to our observations and to the findings of other studies (e.g. Miller et al. 1998), there seems to be no such association.

Nonimmune hydrops fetalis

In 1984, the first case of hydrops fetalis associated with confirmed parvovirus B19 infection was reported by Brown et al. (1984). The risk of fetal hydrops in the two English studies (Public Health Laboratory Service Working Party on Fifth Disease 1990; Miller et al. 1998) was diagnosed to be 2.9 percent. In our investigation, hydrops fetalis was diagnosed in 3.9 percent (40/1018) throughout pregnancy with a maximum of 7.1 percent (23/322) when maternal infection occurred between WG 13 and 20. The rate was lower than 1 percent when maternal B19 infection occurred after WG 32. The median interval between maternal infection and diagnosis of hydrops was 21 days. In the rates of hydrops, there were no significant differences between asymptomatic and symptomatic maternal infection (Enders et al. 2004). It should be noted that hydrops can resolve spontaneously without apparent ill-effects on the infant (Morey et al. 1991; Pryde et al. 1992, Sheikh et al. 1992; Zerbini et al. 1993; Tercanli et al. 1996). In the large study of Rodis et al. (1998a) with 539 cases of parvovirus B19 induced hydrops 34 percent resolved spontaneously.

DISEASES POSSIBLY DUE TO FETAL PARVOVIRUS B19 INFECTION

In addition to the fetal complications described above, B19 virus infection has been suspected to lead, if the fetus survives, to specific and permanent organ defects. Most of those findings have been made in aborted fetuses with B19 infection and involvement of myocardial cells (Porter et al. 1988), eye anomalies, and damage to other tissues (Weiland et al. 1987) or with bilateral cleft lip and palate, micrognathia, and webbed joints (Tiessen et al. 1994). Systematic studies, however, have failed to substantiate congenital malformations caused by parvovirus B19.

Brown and colleagues (1994) described three cases with chronic anemia closely resembling congenital red cell aplasia (Diamond–Blackfan anemia). In all three, the sera lacked B19 DNA, but viral DNA was found in bone marrow. In one instance hepatic disease was associated with intrauterine B19 infection in a premature newborn (Metzman et al. 1989). Furthermore, a case of 'prune belly' after maternal B19 infection and hydrops fetalis has been reported (Walther et al. 1994). There is a more important preliminary report on three live-born infants with severe nervous system anomalies following serologically confirmed maternal B19 infection (Conry et al. 1993), but a follow-up on these children is missing. One report concerns fetal B19 infection and meconium peritonitis (Schild et al. 1998) and another one fetal parvovirus B19 myocarditis with terminal cardiac heart failure and perinatal heart transplantation (von Kaisenberg et al. 2001).

IMMEDIATE AND LONG-TERM OUTCOME OF B19 INFECTION IN PREGNANCY

In the study of Miller et al. (1998), no abnormalities attributable to parvovirus B19 infection were found at birth in surviving infants and no late effects were diagnosed at 7–10 years. The congenital infection rate was estimated with 22 percent based on the detection of IgG antibodies in children at least 1 year of age. It was concluded that the maximum possible risk of congenital abnormality is under 1 percent and the long-term development will be normal (Miller et al. 1998). In another study, the favorable long-term outcome in 108 children exposed in utero to maternal parvovirus B19 infection at the median age of 4 years (range from 6 months to 7 years) was described (Rodis et al. 1998b). Our observations on the outcome of live-born infants of mothers with serological proven B19 infection at birth and at age 8 to 24 months also indicate that there are no parvovirus B19 attributable immediate or long-term clinical consequences (G. Enders, unpublished 2004).

Diagnosis

DIAGNOSIS IN PREGNANCY

B19 virus infection should be excluded in pregnant women who are contacts to patients with erythema infectiosum. In pregnant women with exanthems, lymphadenopathy, or arthralgia, B19 infection as well as rubella must be considered. Anamnestic data about type and time of contact are helpful. In pregnant women with suspected hydrops fetalis or fetal anemia on sonography, parvovirus B19 infection should be confirmed or excluded.

Detection of specific IgM with or without IgG antibodies indicates acute B19 infection. This should be confirmed by testing a second serum. IgG antibodies in the absence of IgM antibodies indicate previous infection ($\geq$4 months) or protection (Searle et al. 1997; Ferguson et al. 1997). However, depending on the serological assay used, IgM antibodies may decline to undetectable levels within 4–6 weeks. The significance of detecting NS1-specific IgG has been continuously discussed and contested since it was suggested that this antibody was suggested to be associated with an altered course of disease (von Poblotzki et al. 1995). Conversely, others have found no evidence of NS1 IgG antibodies representing a marker of persistent infection or contributing to pathogenesis. Most of the studies find that, irrespective of the underlying disease, NS1-specific IgG antibodies appear late in infection (>6 weeks), and the NS1 antibody test may, therefore, be used to exclude very recent infections in patients with an otherwise unclear serology (Hemauer et al. 2000; Searle et al. 1998). Neither raised levels of alpha-1 fetoprotein (AFP) nor human chorionic gonadotropin (hCG) levels in maternal serum have been found to be regular prognostic markers for fetal complications in pregnant women with parvovirus B19 infection (Saller et al. 1993; Komischke et al. 1997). However, both markers are frequently elevated when fetal complications were already evident.

Maternal B19 infection can be confirmed by detection of B19 DNA using PCR when diagnostic interpretation of serological results is difficult. Large amounts of B19 DNA are present in the blood shortly before and after onset of symptoms and can persist at low titers for 2–6 months or even longer (Musiani et al. 1995; G. Enders et al. unpublished). This, however, also depends on the sensitivity of the PCR employed with refined PCR-based techniques such as automated sample preparation and real-time quantitative PCR with a detection limit of 234 IU/ml (Schorling et al. 2004).

DIAGNOSIS IN THE FETUS

Fetal infection is suspected most frequently when hydrops is diagnosed by ultrasonography after a serologically confirmed B19 virus infection in the mother or at routine scan without knowledge of maternal serology. The most reliable way to diagnose fetal infection is to detect B19 DNA by PCR in amniotic fluid, body effusions, or fetal blood. The severity of hydrops fetalis has been graded according to the degree of fetal anemia or ascites (Fairley et al. 1995; Schild et al. 1999). Mild hydrops is not usually associated with significant anemia (Hb 7.2–11.5 g/dl), and may resolve spontaneously over time (category I). Moderate hydrops fetalis is associated with Hb values of 5.7–7.2 g/dl (category II). In cases with generalized hydrops, fetal Hb values range between 1.9 and 5.4 g/dl (category III). Without very early intervention, most cases end in intrauterine death (Tercanli et al. 1996). In prenatal diagnostic centers more recently,

Doppler sonography is employed to recognize fetal anemia by measuring the peak systolic velocity (PSV) in the middle cerebral artery (MCA) (Delle Chiaie et al. 2001; Cosmi et al. 2002). According to the work of Cosmi et al., it seems to be a reliable predictor of parvovirus-induced fetal anemia.

In the case of pathologic PSV values, fetal blood sampling should be considered to determine fetal Hb and reticulocyte count, as well as to confirm B19 infection by detecting viral DNA, IgM antibodies, or both. To detect B19 DNA in fetal blood by PCR, it is important that heparin is not used for moistening the needle employed for cordocentesis, because this anticoagulant may inhibit *Taq* polymerase by binding to DNA (Beutler et al. 1990; Schwarz et al. 1992) and can cause false-negative results. Fetal parvovirus B19-IgM antibodies are a less reliable marker for fetal infection than the detection of B19 DNA in fetal blood or amniotic fluid (Schild et al. 1999). This is confirmed by our results performing the laboratory investigation of fetal specimens obtained at prenatal diagnosis in 349 B19-affected pregnancies (G. Enders, personal observation). In addition, B19 can be identified by histopathology, immunohistochemistry, and in situ hybridization in fetal tissues (Wright et al. 1996).

Management in pregnancy and of the neonate

When acute infection is diagnosed in pregnancy, weekly ultrasound monitoring at low level up to 8–12 weeks after onset of maternal infection is recommended to detect signs of fetal infection such as increased volume of amniotic fluid, skin or placental edema, ascites, and pleural and pericardial effusions early in the course of disease. In such cases the patient should be referred immediately to a prenatal tertiary diagnostic center for further tests and, if necessary, for intrauterine therapy (Schild et al. 1999).

In case of late maternal B19 infection after the 32nd week of pregnancy, fetal complications are less likely. If such an exceptional case occurs near term, the induction of labor or cesarean section may be performed. After delivery, no special precautions (e.g. isolation mother/child) are needed and breastfeeding is not contra-indicated. No observations have been reported that late intrauterine or perinatally infected newborns pose an occupational risk to medical personnel or care workers.

TREATMENT OF THE HYDROPIC FETUS

Intrauterine transfusion as a new therapy regimen in B19-infected hydropic fetuses was first reported from Germany (Schwarz et al. 1988; Schwarz et al. 1990). Initially, this treatment was controversial, since the case of intrauterine transfusion rests against the spontaneous resolution of fetal hydrops. However, the findings in a study conducted in the UK during the epidemic year of

1993/1994 indicated that timely intrauterine transfusion of fetuses with severe hydrops fetalis reduces the risk of fetal death. In this study, the surviving fetuses had no abnormalities related to B19 infection (Fairley et al. 1995). In the meantime, an increasing number of studies on invasive prenatal diagnostics and intrauterine transfusion in fetuses mainly with hydrops fetalis and their favorable immediate and long-term outcomes were reported worldwide (e.g. Rodis et al. 1998a; Schild et al. 1999; Eis-Hübinger et al. 1998; Swain et al. 1999; Forestier et al. 1999; Grab et al. 2002). From all these studies there is little evidence of damage to fetuses infected with parvovirus B19, treated by intrauterine transfusion, and born alive. This is important for the justification of intrauterine treatment of infected fetuses.

PROPHYLAXIS AND THERAPY

Screening in pregnancy for B19 virus antibodies is not recommended and exclusion from work of pregnant women in, for example, childcare centers and elementary schools during the highest risk period between the 9th and 24th week of pregnancy may be considered, but is not officially recommended (Crowcroft et al. 1999). Efforts to prevent contact with infected individuals are of very limited effect, since people are contagious before they develop the rash (CDC 2000).

Passive prophylaxis with immunoglobulin may be effective, since all immunoglobulin preparations for i.v./i.m. application tested contain parvovirus B19-IgG antibodies which can be measured in international units per milliliter and neutralizing antibodies detectable by using a reverse-transcriptase polymerase chain reaction (Ballou et al. 2003). Postexposure prophylaxis with immunoglobulins in pregnancy is presently not recommended; however, pre-exposure prophylaxis has been proven to be beneficial in patients with chronic parvovirus infection and in nosocomial outbreaks in hospitals.

Antiviral drugs are not available for treatment and a parvovirus B19 vaccine is presently not licensed for use. A recombinant human parvovirus B19 vaccine has been developed and is composed of the VP1 and VP2 capsid proteins and formulated with a special adjuvant has recently been evaluated in a randomized, double-blind phase 1 trial in healthy B19-seronegative adults. The vaccine seems to be safe and immunogenic, since all volunteers developed neutralizing antibody titers that peaked after the third immunization and were sustained thus far through 1 year (Ballou et al. 2003).

It is now evident from all the available information that approximately 94 percent of parvovirus B19-affected pregnancies have a normal outcome, that the risk of fetal damage is low and no malformations were observed, and that in case of moderate to severe fetal anemia intrauterine transfusion(s) reduce the risk of fetal death. Therefore a pregnancy does not need to be terminated when B19 infection occurs. Even so, although studies on immediate and long-term outcome of surviving infants following maternal infection in pregnancy have increased recently, further such studies are needed.

HUMAN IMMUNODEFICIENCY VIRUS

AIDS is caused by the lentiviruses human immunodeficiency virus 1 and human immunodeficiency virus 2 (HIV-1 and HIV-2). At the end of 2003, more than 40 million people were living worldwide with human immunodeficiency virus (HIV), including about 19 million women (estimated by UNAIDS); 700 000 children under the age of 15 years are infected annually, most of them by mother-to-child transmission. Prenatal care is an important means of detecting HIV infection in pregnancy. Progress in diagnosis, therapy, and interventional measures has drastically reduced the risk of vertical transmission in industrialized countries.

Effects on pregnancy

Pregnancy does not seem to accelerate progression of HIV-1 disease as demonstrated in studies from the USA and Europe (Burns et al. 1998; Weisser et al. 1998; Saada et al. 2000). Data from developing countries suggest a weak association between pregnancy and an adverse maternal outcome related to HIV infection (French and Brocklehurst 1998). Furthermore, a greater frequency of spontaneous abortion, preterm birth, low birth weight, intrauterine growth retardation, stillbirth, and infant death was shown among HIV-infected women (Brocklehurst and French 1998).

Mother–infant transmission

The main factor associated with increased risk of vertical transmission is the maternal plasma HIV-1 RNA level (e.g. Cooper et al. 2002). In former studies a critical threshold for transmission was estimated to be 100 000 RNA copies/ml of plasma (Fang et al. 1995), but later studies could not confirm this threshold (European Collaborative Study 1999). A lower copy number decreases the risk of transmission significantly (Ioannidis et al. 2001), whereas in pregnant women with undetectable virus copies the transmission rate might be reduced completely (Mofenson et al. 1999). Further factors associated with increased risk of vertical transmission as low maternal $CD4^+$ cell counts, advanced clinical HIV disease, increased levels of beta-2-microglobulin and race/ethnicity are also assumed to reflect the viral load (Cunningham et al. 2004). Other factors are, for example, co-existing sexually transmitted diseases, drug abuse, low vitamin A, chorioamnionitis, rupture of the membranes >4 h before birth regardless of the mode of delivery, and premature delivery (e.g. Minkoff et al. 1995; Landesman et al. 1996). Also immunological

factors contribute to the risk of vertical transmission. A mother–child HLA class I concordance, several HLA-B alleles, maternal SDF1 chemokine receptor ligand polymorphism, and infant homozygosity in a mutation of the regulatory region of chemokine receptor 5 gene increase the risk of perinatal HIV-1 transmission (Polycarpou et al. 2002; Winchester et al. 2004; John et al. 2000; Kostrikis et al. 1999), whereas the presence of maternal neutralizing antibodies decreases the risk (Scarlatti et al. 1993). Also some MHC class II alleles of the infant are associated with reduced or enhanced risk of vertical HIV infection (Winchester et al. 1995).

ROUTES OF TRANSMISSION

Mother-to-child transmission may occur in utero, intrapartum, or by breast-feeding. Intrauterine infection in early pregnancy seems possible, but is more likely to occur shortly before delivery. It is usually assumed to occur by hematogenous spread across the placenta. However, it may also spread from pelvic organs in which replication is occurring, and in late pregnancy by ascending infection from the vagina after rupture of the membranes.

Intrapartum transmission causes a substantial proportion of the cases of vertical transmission (Chouquet et al. 1999). Possible mechanisms include transfusion of the mother's blood to the fetus during labor contractions, infection after the rupture of membranes, and direct contact of the fetus with infected secretions or blood from the maternal genital tract.

The mainly postnatal route of HIV transmission is by breast-feeding. Breast-feeding is associated with an additional 15 to 20 percent risk of HIV transmission (Nduati et al. 2000). Modifying infant feeding practices with early cessation of breast-feeding at 4–6 months or inactivation of HIV in breast milk reduces the risk of postnatal transmission (Rollins et al. 2004).

RATES OF PERINATAL TRANSMISSION

Transmission rates for HIV-1 range today from <2 up to 40 percent depending on geographic areas, socioeconomic conditions, therapeutic and obstetrical interventions. With optimal management of the mother and the newborn, a transmission rate below 2 percent can be achieved (Buchholz et al. 2002).

HIV-2 infections in pregnant women are still rarely reported. However, in the few studies the perinatal transmission rates range form 0 to 4 percent (Adjorlolo-Johnson et al. 1994; De Cock et al. 1994). The much lower rate of transmission of HIV-2 compared with HIV-1 is possibly due to a 37-fold lower maternal RNA level in HIV-2-infected women (O'Donovan et al. 2000).

Effect on infant

Two patterns of disease have been described for infants vertically infected with HIV-1. In one, infection progresses rapidly to AIDS within the first year of life in approximately 25 percent. In the remainder it progresses more slowly and, of these, approximately 25 percent remain asymptomatic until pre-adolescence (Grubman et al. 1995). In two European prospective studies an estimated one-fifth of infected children will have been diagnosed with AIDS or have died by 12 months of age, rising to a third by 6 years of age (Blanche et al. 1997). In a study from Malawi, the mortality rate of HIV-infected children up to the age of 3 years was 45 percent, the major causes of death were wasting and respiratory conditions (Taha et al. 1999).

The more rapid progression of disease in vertically infected infants compared with adults is explained by the relative immaturity of the immune system, the infectious dose, the route of infection, and infections with opportunistic organisms. In children infected with HIV-1, the wide range of clinical manifestations includes features of severe immunodeficiency, nonspecific symptoms and AIDS-related diseases. The prospects for survival of children with opportunistic infections, neurological disease, and lymphoma are worse than for those with lymphocytic interstitial pneumonitis or bacterial infections.

Diagnosis

DIAGNOSIS IN PREGNANCY

Prenatal HIV testing offers the best opportunity for the prevention of perinatal HIV infection. Voluntary HIV screening in pregnancy has been implemented in the USA, Canada, and western European countries in gynecological, prenatal, and other obstetric clinics. For instance in Germany, HIV testing has been included since 1987 in routine prenatal care if the pregnant woman gives her consent. Over recent years, substantial increasing prenatal testing rates have been observed in the USA and Canada. Data from the USA indicate that in 2000, 93 percent of HIV-infected women knew their HIV status before delivery. However, an estimated 280–370 perinatal HIV transmissions continue to occur in the USA each year (CDC 2002a). In western countries, pregnant women remain at low risk of acquiring HIV infection. In Germany, from 1987 to 2004, the seroprevalence of HIV has been surveyed in 325 000 pregnant women resulting in a HIV prevalence of 0.03 percent (G. Enders 2004, unpublished results).

HIV screening in pregnancy is performed with sensitive antibody detecting enzyme immunoassays (EIA). Newer assays include the detection of p24 antigen which improves the diagnosis of a primary HIV infection when p24 antigen is present, but antibodies are not yet synthesized. Reactive HIV screening assays have to be confirmed serologically, for example, with western blot or immunofluorescence assays. For the management of HIV-1-infected women, the viral load in the blood is determined by quantifying RNA and the cellular immune status by counting the $CD4^+$ T cells.

DIAGNOSIS IN THE FETUS

Tests on the fetus of an HIV-infected woman are not recommended, because most vertical transmissions of HIV occur intrapartum and only occasionally during late pregnancy. Furthermore, as in the case of hepatitis C virus (HCV) or hepatitis B virus (HBV) infections, contamination with maternal blood during amnio- or cordocentesis may transmit the virus to the fetus (Enders and Braun 2000; Geipel et al. 2001). An invasive prenatal diagnostic, for example, for the detection of chromosomal anomalies should be performed only when strictly indicated and with antiretroviral therapy/prophylaxis (Buchholz et al. 2002; Maiques et al. 2003).

DIAGNOSIS IN NEONATAL AND INFANT

Early diagnosis of HIV infection in infants born to an HIV-positive mother is not recommended by conventional serological tests, because IgG antibodies reflect maternal serology and IgM antibody determination lacks sensitivity and specificity (Schupbach et al. 1994). Although tests for HIV-specific IgA antibodies are less sensitive compared with virological tests especially for early diagnosis of HIV infection in the first 3 months of life, they may be useful in countries without facilities for viral culture or PCR detection (Livingston et al. 1995). In general, HIV infection can be definitively diagnosed in most infected infants by the age of 1 month and in virtually all infected infants by the age of 6 months by using viral diagnostic assays. A positive virological test (i.e. detection of HIV by culture or polymerase chain reaction) indicates possible HIV infection and should be confirmed by a repeat virological test on a second specimen as soon as possible. Pediatric HIV testing is recommended by the age of 48 h, at age 1–2 months, and at age 3–6 months. At birth only about 40 percent of infected children had positive viral assays. Then the sensitivity increases rapidly during the first week, with over 90 percent of infected children testing positive by the age of 1 month (Peckham and Gibb 1995). HIV DNA and/or RNA PCR is the preferred virological method; HIV culture has a sensitivity similar to that of HIV PCR, but HIV culture is more complex, expensive, and time-consuming to perform compared to HIV PCR. The use of HIV p24 antigen testing alone is not recommended for diagnosis, because the sensitivity and specificity of this assay is less compared with other HIV virological tests. HIV infection is diagnosed by two positive HIV virological tests performed on separate blood samples. HIV infection can be reasonably excluded among children with one negative virological test at the age of 1–4 month, and one at age ⩾4 months. Definitively excluded is the HIV infection at the age of 18 months, if HIV IgG antibody is negative in the absence of hypogammaglobulinemia and if the child has neither clinical symptoms of HIV infection nor negative HIV virological assays (CDC 1998a).

Previously cases of HIV clearance in children were described in several studies (e.g. Newell et al. 1996). Later investigations of 42 suspected transient HIV-1-infected children could not confirm a cleared HIV infection in any of these cases (Frenkel et al. 1998). Most cases suggest mislabeling of specimens or contamination in the laboratory, therefore rare cases of HIV clearance may be possible but have to be proven carefully.

Management

MANAGEMENT IN PREGNANCY

The great progress over the past few years for treatment of HIV infection has also dramatically influenced the management of HIV-infected pregnant women (European Collaborative Study 2001; Friese 2003).

Prevention

Most HIV infections are acquired sexually, the risk of transmission is associated with the viral load in genital secretions which can be different from the viral load in the peripheral blood (Robert Koch Institut 2003). The optimal preventive measure is sexual contact only with a partner known to be uninfected and the avoidance of unprotected sexual intercourse. Despite extensive worldwide research activities, a successful HIV preventive vaccine is not yet available (Stratov et al. 2004). After occupational exposure (e.g. accidental needlestick of healthcare workers), an antiretroviral postexposure therapy reduces the risk of HIV transmission (Cardo et al. 1997). For HIV exposures relating to sexual or drug injection, the post-exposure therapy can be offered under strict indication when the probability of HIV infection is high, therapy can be initiated promptly and adherence to the regime is likely. This therapy should never be considered as a routinely used form of primary HIV prevention (Robert Koch Institut 2002a).

Chemotherapy

In 1996, the ACTG 076 trial demonstrated a reduction of the vertical transmission after administration of zidovudine monotherapy throughout pregnancy and to the newborn for the first 6 weeks of life (Sperling et al. 1996). Shorter courses of therapy and treatment with other drugs, e.g. nevirapine or zidovudine/lamivudine also reduced the rate of vertical transmission. Studies with highly active antiretroviral therapy (HAART) resulted in the lowest transmission rates (Cooper et al. 2002). When combination therapy is administered during pregnancy, zidovudine should be included whenever possible. Maternal indication for therapy is based on the clinical, immunological, or virological status as published

in current guidelines for the treatment of nonpregnant women (e.g. NIH 2004). To reduce the risk of vertical transmission, antiretroviral therapy is recommended even for pregnant women with a HIV-1 viral load below 1 000 copies/ml (Ioannidis et al. 2001). The possible risks of teratogenic drug effects of antiretroviral therapy during the first trimester of pregnancy are so far unknown. Exposure to maternal antiretroviral therapy was not associated with prevalence or pattern of congenital abnormalities, but was associated with reversible anemia in the newborn. However, treatment with some drugs, e.g. efavirenz, should be avoided because teratogenic effects occurred among animal species. The data on the teratogenic potential of antiretroviral agents are limited, currently approved agents and selected information regarding their use in pregnancy are available (US Department of Health and Human Services 2002). New antiretroviral agents, e.g. the 36-amino-acid peptide enfuvirtide, which prevents the fusion of the virus with the cell membrane, may improve the therapy response even in pretreated patients (Lazzarin et al. 2003).

Mode of delivery

Cesarean section before onset of labor or rupture of membranes effectively reduces the rate of transmission (European Mode of Delivery Collaboration 1999). In a meta-analysis of 15 prospective cohort studies, the elective cesarean section decreased the risk by approximately 50 percent as compared with other modes of delivery and independently of the effects of treatment with zidovudine (International Perinatal HIV Group 1999). In women with viral loads below 1 000 copies/ml, a benefit of cesarean section has not yet been demonstrated (Minkoff 2001), but generally cesarean section is recommended when possible.

MANAGEMENT OF THE NEONATE

Among the infants of HIV-infected women, no malformations or an increase in birth defects relating to HIV infection was observed (Brocklehurst and French 1998). Breast-feeding is not recommended in countries where appropriate milk substitutes are available. The risk of HIV transmission through breast-feeding is greatest in early infancy (before 6 months of age), and persists as long as breast-feeding continues (Nduati et al. 2000). In developing countries, however, breast-feeding is encouraged because artificial feeding in a poor hygienic environment greatly increases morbidity and mortality from diarrheal diseases and respiratory infections (Van de Perre 1995). In these countries, a threefold higher mortality rate in HIV-infected mothers who breast-fed their infants was reported compared with those who fed their infants with formula (Nduati et al. 2000). However, these limited results did not warrant any change in current policies on breast-feeding nor on infant feeding by HIV-infected women (World Health Organization

2001). After delivery, zidovudine is administered in general to the newborn for up to 6 weeks according to PATCG protocol 076. In developing countries the single dose nevirapine given to pregnant women in labor and to neonates shortly after birth effectively reduced the rate of perinatal HIV transmission and appears to be one of the most cost-effective options for the prevention of perinatal HIV transmission (Jackson et al. 2003). Management of infants and children is rapidly evolving and becoming increasingly complex, for example, considering possible early and late side-effects. Therefore the management of these children should be directed to a specialist wherever possible.

HEPATITIS VIRUSES

The list of hepatitis viruses continues to expand. Of those so far identified, types B, C, and E are of known significance in pregnancy and for the newborn (Table 63.16).

Hepatitis A virus

Hepatitis A virus (HAV) (enterovirus 72) is acquired by the fecal–oral route, and has an incubation period of approximately 4 weeks.

INFECTION IN PREGNANCY AND IN NEONATES

Hepatitis A virus has no apparent adverse effect on the outcome of pregnancy. Transmission during birth (e.g. by exposure to maternal feces or by breastfeeding) is very rare (e.g. Zhuang 1989; CDC 1990; Ye 1990; Zhang et al. 1990; ACOG 1998). In one investigation, neonatal infection was diagnosed in an infant born to a mother with hepatitis A 10 days after premature labor, the evidence indicating that he was infected by his mother before or during birth. In another case, vertical transmission of HAV resulted in a symptomatic neonatal disease. After a trip to India, the mother developed symptomatic hepatitis A infection during the 4th month of pregnancy (Fagan et al. 1999). HAV may spread within the neonatal intensive care unit, causing asymptomatic infection in neonates, and symptomatic or asymptomatic infection in staff members as a result of lapses in infection control precautions (Watson et al. 1993). Neonates, even when infected parenterally by transfusion with hepatitis A-contaminated blood (a rare event) rarely have biochemical evidence of hepatitis (Azimi et al. 1986). They are, however, a potential source of infection for nonimmune staff members, as the virus is excreted in the stools of infected neonates and infants for up to 5 months (Rosenblum et al. 1991). This is much longer than in older children, except those in whom icteric hepatitis relapses, as has been reported in 3–20 percent of children (Sjogren et al. 1987).

CONTROL MEASURES

Infection can be controlled by adopting simple hygienic measures and by the sanitary disposal of excreta. Strict isolation of cases is not effective, as fecal shedding of the virus peaks during the prodromal phase. For pre- and postexposure prophylaxis, human normal immunoglobulin preparations (HNIG) are in use and may be given to neonates born within 2 weeks of maternal illness, to neonates in an intensive care unit if a case occurs on the ward, and to nonimmune staff members (Zhang et al. 1990). Inactivated vaccines are effective, and will replace immunoglobulin for pre-exposure prophylaxis; they seem also to be useful for post-exposure prophylaxis as documented in a randomized study (Sagliocca et al. 1999). Neither HNIG nor inactivated hepatitis A vaccines are contraindicated in pregnancy.

Hepatitis B virus

Hepatitis B virus (HBV), a hepadnavirus, is transmitted primarily by the parenteral route, by blood, by sexual contact through contaminated secretions from acutely infected patients or carriers, and by vertical transmission. Perinatal infection and infection during the first year of life have important consequences because 90 percent of these infants become chronic carriers, compared with only approximately 5–10 percent of those infected after the age of 12 years. Such chronicity increases the risk of cirrhosis and hepatocellular carcinoma. Since the commencement of the hepatitis B vaccination approximately 20 years ago, the prevalence of chronic HBV infections has been reduced substantially among populations whose infection rates were previously high. CDC estimates that perinatal HBV infections in the USA declined 75 percent during the period 1987–2000 (CDC 2002b).

INFECTION IN PREGNANCY

The annual incidence of acute hepatitis B cases in pregnant women is not known because pregnancy status is not recorded in most countries. Pregnancy does not appear to influence the severity or mortality rates of acute HBV infections in countries under good living conditions (e.g. Shalev and Bassan 1982). No teratogenic effects have been associated with maternal HBV infection.

MOTHER–CHILD TRANSMISSION

About 90 percent of vertical transmission occurs as a consequence of intrapartum exposure to contaminated blood and genital secretions. In approximately 10 percent infection results from hematogenous transplacental transmission.

The main risk factors for intrauterine HBV infection are maternal serum HBeAg positivity (Wang and Zhu

Table 63.16 *Effects of hepatitis A–G infection on pregnancy, on the fetus, and the newborn*

Hepatitis	Increased morbidity/ mortality after acute infection	Increased incidence of abortion or IUD	Congenital defects	Vertical transmission			Postnatal disease[d]	
				Intrauterine	Perinatal	Early postnatal infection	Early	Late
A (HAV)	No	Controversial	No	Possible[c]	No	Possible[b]	No	No
B (HBV)	No	No	No	Possible[b]	Yes	Yes	No	Yes
C (HCV)	No	No	No	Possible[b]	Yes	Possible	No	Yes
D (HDV) co-superinfection with HBV	No	No	No	Possible[b]	Yes, only in HBsAg and HDV RNA positive mothers	N/A	No	N/A
E (HEV)	Yes mortality ±20% 3rd trimester	Yes ±12%	No	Yes	Yes	N/A	Yes with increased mortality	N/A
G (HGV)	No[a]	No[a]	No[a]	Possible	No	Possible	No[a]	N/A

IUD, intrauterine death; N/A, data not yet available.

a) Provisional.
b) Possible, but rare.
c) One case reported.
d) Following congenital infection.

2000), a history of threatened preterm labor, HBV in the placenta especially in the villous capillary endothelial cells (Xu et al. 2001, 2002), a high HBV viremia level in pregnant women (Zhang et al. 1998) which is particularly elevated in women acutely infected in the third trimester, and transplacental leakage of maternal blood to the fetus (Lin et al. 1987; Ohto et al. 1987). As reported by Xu et al. (2002), the intrauterine infection rate increased linearly and significantly with maternal HBV DNA concentration. Results of the pathology study showed that HBV infection rates decrease gradually from the maternal side to the fetal side in the placental cell layers.

Recently, it has been found that breast-feeding of infants of chronic HBV carriers poses no additional risk for transmission of the hepatitis B virus (Hill et al. 2002). The early postnatal HBV infections result from close contact between infant and the infected parent(s). In hyperendemic areas, most HBV-related complications occur during adulthood, but nearly half of the primary infected persons becoming chronic HBV carriers have acquired their infection during the perinatal period through the transmission from hepatitis B e antigen (HBeAg)-positive mothers. The other half is from horizontal transmission mainly through intrafamilial spread or injection using unsterilized needles (Chang 1998).

RATE OF TRANSMISSION

The transmission rate from asymptomatic carrier mothers who are positive only for HBsAg is approximately 10–20 percent in the absence of immune prophylaxis. Mothers positive for both HBsAg and HBeAg, and thus highly infectious, transmit the virus in 80–90 percent of cases (see, for example, Stevens et al. 1979). For predicting persisting infection in infants and a possible failure of neonatal hepatitis B passive/active vaccination in earlier studies, the HBV DNA viral load in the maternal serum of the HBeAg-positive mothers seemed to be the most important factor (e.g. Burk et al. 1994; Del Canho et al. 1994). In a more recent case–control study conducted to find out why some infants born full-term to HBeAg-seropositive mothers became infected despite full passive-active immunoprophylaxis, allelic base changes in maternal HBV genotype were determined as risk factors (Ngui et al. 1998).

OUTCOMES OF PERINATAL AND POSTNATAL INFECTION

Most infants born to carrier mothers are HBsAg-negative at birth and, without immunoprophylaxis, seroconvert in the first 3 months after delivery. Perinatally and postnatally infected newborns and infants are asymptomatic. Fulminant hepatitis secondary to perinatal HBV infection has been reported in infants aged 2–6 months, particularly if the mother is anti-HBe-positive and the infecting virus has undergone mutations in the pre-core region of its DNA (see for example,

Carman et al. 1990; Omata et al. 1991; Terazawa et al. 1991; Waters et al. 1992; Schödel 1994; von Weizsäcker et al. 1995; Hsu et al. 1999; Ogata et al. 1999; Zuckerman 2000). A recent publication, however, indicates that HBV genomic heterogeneity is not primarily involved either in the initiation of infection nor the failure of neonatal HBV immunoprophylaxis (Cacciola et al. 2002). The risk of chronicity in perinatally and early postnatally infected infants and the rate of progression to liver disease or hepatocellular carcinoma are currently under observation. In earlier studies of almost 350 Chinese and Italian children followed from 1 to 10 years, no progression of liver disease was noted, although almost 50 percent had histological findings of chronic active hepatitis or cirrhosis at presentation (Bortolotti et al. 1986; Lok and Lai 1988). Some more recent observations (Chang 1998) confirm that children with chronic hepatitis B virus infection are mostly asymptomatic. They are generally active and growing well with very rare exceptions. Even with acute exacerbation of liver function and active inflammation, jaundice, or growth failure is uncommon. However, hepatocellular carcinoma may also follow perinatal or childhood HBV infection (Hsu et al. 1987). This is demonstrated in a Japanese long-term follow-up study of 3 to 22 years (mean, 11 years) in 52 adolescents with perinatally acquired HBV infection where hepatocellular carcinoma has been diagnosed in two cases (a 21-year-old and a 16-year-old). All children carrying hepatitis B surface antigen should be observed carefully to monitor the possible development of hepatocellular carcinoma, especially in the anti-HBe-positive phase after spontaneous seroconversion or even after interferon treatment (Fujisawa et al. 2000). It is known that hepatitis B pathology is a dynamic process between the virus, the infected cell, and the host's immune response. In this context, more studies are needed to clear the function of the soluble core gene product (HBeAg) of hepatitis B virus. It has been proposed that transplacentally passed HBeAg might induce fetal immunotolerance to HBeAg (Milich et al. 1990; Wang and Zhu 2000).

DIAGNOSIS IN PREGNANCY

Screening in pregnancy for HBsAg detects both acutely infected and asymptomatic carrier women whose babies are at risk of perinatal infection. Since the beginning of the late 1980s, in most European countries, universal antenatal screening is carried out and is advocated in the USA and in Canada (CDC 1991; ACOG 1993) because selective screening has been of low efficiency (Boxall 1995). Antenatal screening is usually done early in pregnancy together with screening tests for blood group and syphilis (Grosheide et al. 1995). In Germany, selective HBsAg screening was introduced in 1987, but since 1994 has formed part of the obligatory prenatal care program. Testing is performed in the third trimester with the same blood sample as provided for the second obligatory indirect Coombs' test (Kassenärztliche Bundesvereinigung 1994).

The screening procedures in pregnancy are as follows. If the test for HBsAg is negative, no further testing is done unless there is a clinical indication of hepatitis or suspicion of behavioral risk factors (then testing anti-HBc is carried out). If the HBsAg result is positive, anti-HBc IgM testing and, if this test is positive, quantification of HBV DNA may also be carried out. For results notification requirement to healthy authorities exists. The HBsAg result is documented in the prenatal care notes and, if positive, the obstetrician is advised to administer active/passive hepatitis B immunization to the neonate within 12 h after birth. If antenatal HBsAg screening is not documented, it will be done at delivery. In Germany, universal antenatal HBsAg screening was estimated to be cost-effective over a wide range of assumption (Kassenärztliche Bundesvereinigung 1994). Tests for anti-HBc only in the case of negative results for HBsAg have not been included in the German strategy of antenatal screening. Although an anti-HBc prevalence of 8.71 percent was calculated in the middle-aged adult German population, 1.40 percent of the individuals had anti-HBc, only 7.7 percent of them or 0.1 percent of the whole population were DNA positive in the absence of HBsAg indicating infectiousness (Jilg et al. 2001). However, some countries, e.g. Switzerland, include anti-HBc testing in the antenatal screening algorithm. As a consequence, newborns of the solely anti-HBc-positive mothers also obtain active-passive hepatitis B immune prophylaxis shortly after delivery (personal communication, Professor Zimmermann, Universitätsspital Zürich, Department für Frauenheilkunde und Geburtshilfe, Switzerland).

MANAGEMENT IN PREGNANCY

Preventive measures are designed to prevent transmission by transfusion, transplantation, syringe-borne infection, frequent changes of sex partner, and nosocomial infection between patients. Pregnant women in sexual or household contact with HBV-infected individuals should be offered active/passive immunization after their HBsAg, anti-HBc, and anti-HBs seronegativity is established. The specific antiviral drugs lamivudine, adefovir, entecavir, and pegylated interferon-α are not recommended for pregnant women (Balfour 1999; Anonymous 2002; Schalm et al. 2002). During pregnancy, acute HBV infection is treated by supportive measures as in nonpregnant patients.

Invasive prenatal diagnosis in the second and third trimester is not indicated since transmission occurs primarily during delivery. If genetic reasons are the indication for prenatal diagnosis, a potential risk of iatrogenic infection of the fetus in viremic mothers has to be considered (Enders and Braun 2000; Delamare et al. 1999).

Termination of pregnancy is contraindicated.

Cesarean section is not usually recommended, but may be performed in women with high serum levels of HBV DNA and HBeAg and with acute infection in late pregnancy (Schalm and Pit-Grosheide 1989; Del Canho et al. 1994; Wang et al. 2002).

MANAGEMENT OF NEONATES

In the USA, all newborns are vaccinated at birth regardless of the maternal HBsAg status, with anti-HBs testing of infants at age of 7 months born to HBsAg-positive mothers (Committee on Infectious Diseases 1994). The detailed vaccination procedure is given by the Advisory Committee on Immunization (www.cdc.gov/nip/acip). In most western European countries (term and preterm) babies of mothers with positive HBsAg test or unknown HBsAg status are immunized within 12 hours after birth simultaneously with hepatitis B immunoglobulin (HBIG) and a hepatitis B low-dose vaccine, and again with hepatitis B vaccine only at 1 and 6 months of age; 1 month later, a test for anti-HBs is recommended (Robert Koch Institut 2002b). Infants of mothers with negative HBsAg status are vaccinated within the routine infant program starting at age of 2 months (Robert Koch Institut 2002b).

Perinatal immune prophylaxis has been effective in western populations, protecting 93–95 percent of infants 1 month after the third dose (antibody levels ⩾10 mIU/ml). This was confirmed by a recent study carried out in a population at high risk of infection by examining 522 children in southern Italy born to HBsAg-positive mothers 5–14 years after postpartum immunization. Four hundred of 505 (79.2 percent) children had protective anti-HBsAg titers ⩾10 mIU/ml. Thus, HBV vaccination of children born to HBsAg carrier mothers seems to provide immediate and long-term protection against HBV infection. There was no evidence that the emergence of HBV escape mutants secondary to the immune pressure against wild-type HBV is of concern (Mele et al. 2001). In areas with low HBV endemicity, for vaccination of infants low-dose vaccine (5 μg) is used, whereas in areas with high HBV endemicity, normal dose of vaccine (10 μg) seems to be more effective in perinatal and infant vaccination (Lee 1995; Milne et al. 1995).

In 1991, recognizing the difficulty of vaccinating high-risk adults and the substantial burden of HBV-related disease acquired from infections in childhood, a comprehensive strategy to eliminate HBV transmission in the USA was recommended (CDC 1991, 1995, 2002b). It includes universal childhood vaccination, antenatal screening, vaccination of all nonvaccinated young adults, and vaccination of groups at risk because of their occupation, behavior, contacts, travel, etc. This strategy was taken up by the majority of western countries, including Germany (Robert Koch Institut 1995) and various Asian (Ruff et al. 1995) and African countries.

For elimination of HBV transmission, it is important to sustain high vaccine-coverage rates among infants, children, adolescents, and adults at increased risk for HBV infection. However, if the efforts to vaccinate the latter group are not greatly expanded, complete elimination of HBV transmission might take another 20 years to achieve (CDC 2002b; Robert Koch Institut 2002b).

Hepatitis C virus

Hepatitis C virus (HCV), with >6 genotypes and >70 subtypes, is the etiological agent of most cases of non-A, non-B post-transfusion and sporadic hepatitis (Simmonds 1995; Maertens and Stuyver 1997). Acute HCV infections are asymptomatic in 75 percent of cases and in the remainder symptoms are mild, but >50 percent of infected adults develop chronic liver disease. Information on the perinatal implications of HCV is still constantly expanding. Based on observational data of more than 77 studies carried out in approximately 18 countries, vertical transmission has been confirmed to occur generally at a low rate (1–5 percent) and is favored mainly by a high maternal virus load in the blood. Maternal risk factors such as coinfection with HIV increase the vertical transmission rate to more than 20 percent (Roberts and Yeung 2002).

INFECTION IN PREGNANCY

The important risk factors for infection in pregnancy are intravenous drug abuse, sexual contact with intravenous drug users, high promiscuity, and infection with other sexually transmitted diseases. Other risk factors are previous transfusions, transplantation, and administration of blood products.

In pregnant women at normal risk, antibody prevalence is 0.7–2.5 percent, being higher than in blood donors (approximately 0.2–0.5 percent) in the same geographical area (Bohman et al. 1992; Marranconi et al. 1994; Pipan et al. 1996). In a UK study, the HCV seroprevalence in mothers born in the UK was 0.13–0.15 percent and 0.81 percent in mothers born elsewhere in Europe (Ades et al. 2000). In pregnant women from high-risk populations, antibody prevalence rates are >2.5 percent, irrespective of the geographic region.

It appears that pregnancy has no impact on the viral load and the clinical course of acute hepatitis C or the activity of chronic infection (Reth et al. 1995). In addition, abortions or intrauterine deaths are not increased in acute or chronic HCV infection (Dinsmoor 2001).

MOTHER–INFANT TRANSMISSION

Routes of transmission

Hepatitis C can be transmitted in utero and during parturition. Intrauterine transmission is suggested in some reports because viral RNA was detected in cord or neonatal blood (e.g. Kurauchi et al. 1993; Kojima and Yamanaka 1994), but not always in follow-up sera of the infants. As in HBV infection, intrauterine transmission may occur late in pregnancy due to placental leakage in cases of threatened abortion and preterm labor (e.g. Lin et al. 1987). The major route, however, is intrapartum transmission, which probably occurs by contact with contaminated blood. This route is verified by detection of viral RNA in nonbreast-fed infants >1 month old (e.g. Resti et al. 1995; Zanetti et al. 1995). Several studies of mother–infant pairs with follow-up of the infants show that the risk of vertical transmission is higher in mothers with acute infection in late pregnancy (Kuroki et al. 1991; Lynch-Salamon and Combs 1992) or chronic hepatitis (Degos et al. 1991); in high-risk mothers co-infected with HIV-1, but not with HBV; and particularly if a high level of HCV RNA is present in maternal blood, with (Zanetti et al. 1995) or without (e.g. Ohto et al. 1994; Tajiri et al. 2001) behavioral risk cofactors.

There is no evidence of transmission by breast milk in asymptomatic carrier mothers, but it cannot be fully excluded in symptomatic mothers (Kumar and Shahul 1998; Mast 2004).

Rates of vertical transmission and infection

In low risk groups   In prospective studies of the world literature from 1994 to 2001 on vertical HCV transmission in low-risk, HIV-negative mothers a mean transmission rate of 5.5 percent (range, 0–11.1 percent) was reported (Ohto et al. 1994; Moriya et al. 1995; Giacchino et al. 1995; Meisel et al. 1995; Pipan et al. 1996; Kumar et al. 1997; Resti et al. 1998; Xiong et al. 1998; Conte et al. 2000; Ceci et al. 2001; Tajiri et al. 2001; Lima et al. 2004). All these studies indicate that infants are infected only by HCV-RNA-positive mothers, particularly those with a high viral load. One investigation reports that vertical transmission of HCV can occur irrespective of the maternal viral load (Pipan et al. 1996).

Older studies from 1990–1992 on vertical transmission in anti-HCV-positive and HIV-1-negative mothers indicate that, on the basis of antibody persistence the infection rate in infants followed up for 10–12 months was 4.5 percent (4/88) (Lynch and Ghidini 1993). In one of these older studies, in which both HCV RNA detection and antibody persistence were used as markers of infection of infants, RNA was found not only in infants who seroconverted or who had persisting antibody, but also in those who became and remained antibody negative (Thaler et al. 1991). This puzzling observation was also made in later studies (e.g. Giacchino et al. 1995; Paccagnini et al. 1995) and may indicate false-positive PCR results or seroreversion with clearance of infection, as has been found in a few infants born to HIV-1-positive mothers (Newell et al. 1996).

In high risk groups   Several studies tried to establish the rate of vertical transmission of HCV in mothers of high-risk groups with and without HIV-1 coinfection. In studies (1995–2002) from various countries, vertical transmission rates in children born to HCV-RNA-positive mothers with HIV infection ranged from 44 to 8 percent, whereas the transmission rate in children born to HCV-RNA-positive mothers without HIV infection range from 10 to 0 percent (Zanetti et al. 1995; Zuccotti et al. 1995; Paccagnini et al. 1995; Tovo et al. 1997; Mazza et al. 1998; Thomas et al. 1998; Papaevanegelou 1998; Zanetti et al. 1998; Gibb et al. 2000; Resti et al. 2002).

The investigations of Zanetti and colleagues (1995, 1998) and Zuccotti and co-workers (1995) show clearly a higher maternal HCV RNA positivity in HIV-1 coinfected mothers than in those with HCV RNA alone, and a higher rate of vertical transmission in the group positive for HIV-1 and HCV RNA. The study of Paccagnini et al. (1995) further indicates that HCV and HIV transmission, alone or in combination, can occur in infants born to coinfected mothers.

Some authors (Kudesia et al. 1995; Fischler et al. 1996; Spencer et al. 1997) recorded no vertical transmission in HCV-infected pregnant women engaged in injection drug use (IDU). In contrast to these studies, Resti et al. (1998) have shown that intravenous drug use itself and post-transfusional hepatitis is an important risk factor for transmission of hepatitis C virus (Resti et al. 1998). In their more recent study Resti et al. (2002) have postulated that transmission occurs mainly in those women who are former or current injection drug users and not in HIV-coinfected women. However, it has been questioned why transmission would be associated with a history of IDU in women who do not currently engage in IDU (Armstrong et al. 2003). Furthermore, Yeung et al. (2001) have examined the results of prior studies

and have confirmed that transmission is more strongly associated with HIV coinfection than with IDU.

The outcomes of HCV-infected children in four studies of maternal low risk groups and in five studies of maternal high risk groups are summarized in Table 63.17. Nearly all the infected infants showed signs of liver involvement during the follow-up period. Increased, but fluctuating, values of alanine aminotransferase (ALT) were usually detected as well as histological evidence of liver disease. Tests for HCV RNA were repeatedly positive in all children aged $\geqslant 6$ months; HCV antibodies persisted beyond 14 months of age in 12 infants; there was temporary seroreversion in nine infants and loss of HCV antibodies in six infants aged 6–9 months despite persistence of HCV RNA.

These studies in high- and low-risk groups which have already been discussed above and some further studies reflect various courses of the infection in apparently vertically infected infants (especially in the first year of life), e.g. transient viremia without real infection, acute self-limited clinically inapparent infection, or clearance of HCV-RNA (Bortolotti et al. 1997; Sasaki et al. 1997; Ketzinel-Gilad et al. 2000). Long-term observations are needed to clarify if chronic hepatitis in infants will spontaneously resolve or progress to chronic liver disease.

Although transmission via breast milk has been suggested in one study (Gürakan et al. 1994), the majority of studies that have examined transmission rates with breastfeeding have not noted any significant increase in transmission in infants who were breast-fed, compared with those who were bottle-fed (Kumar and Shahul 1998; Lin et al. 1995; Zanetti et al. 1995; Zimmermann et al. 1995; Tovo et al. 1997; Resti et al. 2002; European Paediatric Hepatitis C Virus Network

Table 63.17 Outcome of hepatitis C-infected infants born to mothers of low and high risk groups

Study	Country	Risk group	HCV RNA pos.	Anti-HCV pos.	Abnormal ALT value
Ohto et al. (1994)	Japan	Low	3	2/3	3/3
Giacchino et al. (1995)	Italy	Low	2	2/2	2/2[a]
Ceci et al. (2001)	Italy	Low	2	2/2	2/2
Tajiri et al. (2001)	Japan	Low	9	9/9	9/9
Zanetti et al. (1995)	Italy	High	8[b]	6/8	8/8
Paccagnini et al. (1995)	Italy	High	14[c]	11/14	10[d]/14
Spencer et al. (1997)	Australia	High	6[e]	6/6	6/6
Mazza et al. (1998)	Italy	High	6	6/6	6/6
Zanetti et al. (1998)	Italy	High	17	15/17	16/17

ALT, alanine aminotransferase; HCV, hepatitis C.
a) Histological signs of liver disease: 2/2.
b) Three HIV co-infected.
c) Four HIV co-infected.
d) Histological signs of liver disease: 4/10.
e) Two of six infants initially HCV RNA-positive were negative at age of 30 months.

2001). In recent studies, the authors were unable to find HCV RNA in any breast milk samples tested (Kage et al. 1997; Polywka et al. 1997).

According to the knowledge that vertical HCV transmission occurs like HIV transmission around the time of delivery, the effect of the mode of delivery on transmission was of interest. Of the various studies (Paccagnini et al. 1995; Spencer et al. 1997; Tovo et al. 1997; Resti et al. 1998; Thomas et al. 1998; Conte et al. 2000; European Paediatric Hepatitis C Virus Network 2001) only two reported significantly lower transmission rates with elective cesarean section. One study reported that in mothers with high viral load, vaginal delivery resulted in a vertical transmission rate of 44 percent (7/16) (Okamoto et al. 2000). In contrast, the eight patients with a high viral load who underwent elective cesarean section (prior to labor) did not transmit HCV to their ten neonates. In the study of Gibb et al. (2000) in 441 HCV-infected women in the UK, there were no cases of neonatal HCV following elective cesarean delivery in 31 patients. This transmission rate was significantly lower than that for vaginal delivery and emergency cesarean section combined. Unfortunately, data on maternal HCV RNA levels were not available for the patients in this study.

A viral factor which influence the risk of mother-to-infant transmission may be the HCV genotype (e.g. Zuccotti et al. 1995), but this could not be substantiated in a number of further investigations (e.g. Mazza et al. 1998).

At present, the guidelines from the American Academy of Pediatrics, the Centers for Disease Control and Prevention (CDC), and the American College of Obstetricians and Gynecologists (ACOG) do not prohibit breast-feeding in infants of HCV-positive mothers (CDC 1998b; American Academy of Pediatrics 1998; ACOG 2000c). It is likely that most of the individual studies done thus far lack the statistical power to detect differences in transmission following interventions such as cesarean section or formula feeding. The current guidelines from the CDC and ACOG recommend cesarean section only for obstetric indications in patients who are infected with hepatitis C (CDC 1998b).

It might be of interest that mothers who have already delivered an HCV-infected child can be advised that this event does not increase the probability of infecting the second child (Resti et al. 2000).

The contribution of vertical transmission to community-acquired HCV infection in western populations seems to be low (e.g. Alter et al. 1992; Goto et al. 1994; Yoshii et al. 1999), but may be important among children living in areas of high HCV prevalence (Chang et al. 1994).

DIAGNOSIS IN PREGNANCY

Laboratory tests for HCV infection in pregnancy are the same as for nonpregnant people. With regard to vertical transmission, a maternal viral load of more than 10^{6-7} IU/ml is considered high, 10^{4-6} as moderate and $<10^4$ as low or negative values. Commercially available qualitative and quantitative HCV RNA assays provide good sensitive, specific, and reproducible results today.

DIAGNOSIS IN INFANCY

Infants born to anti-HCV-positive and, particularly, to HCV-RNA-positive mothers should be tested at birth, at 6–8 weeks and at the age of 10–12 months for HCV RNA and, facultatively, for anti-HCV persistence. Liver function tests should be performed on HCV-RNA-positive infants at 2–3-monthly intervals and also on infants with antibodies persisting beyond 12 months of age.

MANAGEMENT IN PREGNANCY

Screening tests

Universal screening of pregnant women with anti-HCV antibodies is not recommended (CDC 1991). Selective screening should be performed in women with behavioral risk factors, with known positive HIV or HBsAg status, in those with signs of hepatitis or with a history of transfusion or transplantation and in nonpregnant and pregnant women with an HCV-positive partner. In cases of anti-HCV positivity, PCR for HCV RNA should be performed; if positive, the viral load should be determined toward the end of pregnancy.

Avoiding infection

The possibility of sexual transmission exists, predominantly in cases of high promiscuity. In contrast to previous findings, HCV RNA has been detected recently in seminal plasma by using highly sensitive PCR techniques (Hsu et al. 1991; Terada et al. 1992; Levy et al. 2000; Bourlet et al. 2003).

Although the risk of virus transmission is low, the presence of HCV RNA in seminal plasma suggest a possible risk of sexual transmission. It is noteworthy that French legislation has introduced a screening for HCV RNA in seminal fluids of HCV-infected men who are involved in programs of assisted reproductive techniques (Bourlet et al. 2003).

At present there is no contraindication to pregnancy for HCV-positive women or for anti-HCV-negative women with an HCV-positive partner.

Invasive prenatal diagnosis in the second and third trimester is not indicated since transmission occurs primarily during delivery and since, for example, genetic reasons for prenatal diagnosis, a potential risk of iatrogenic infection of the fetus in viremic mothers has to be considered (Enders and Braun 2000; Delamare et al. 1999).

Termination of pregnancy is not indicated.

Passive/active prophylaxis and therapy

The efficacy of passive prophylaxis for HCV by intravenous immunoglobulin seems limited (e.g. Krawczynski et al. 1996), and a vaccine is not yet available (Choo et al. 1994; Zanetti et al. 2003). Treatment with IFN-α or pegylated IFN-α alone or in combination with ribavirin (Di Bisceglie et al. 1995; Collier and Chapman 2001) is not indicated in pregnancy (McDonnell and Lucey 1995). However, more recently some reports suggest continuing pregnancy if they were exposed inadvertently at the beginning of pregnancy to interferon (Hiratsuka et al. 2000; Trotter and Zygmunt 2001; Ozaslan et al. 2002), but less so in case of therapy with ribavirin (Mishkin and Deschenes 2001; Hegenbarth et al. 2001).

Mode of delivery

If the viral load in the maternal serum is high, elective cesarean section has been suggested, to reduce the rate of vertical transmission (Paccagnini et al. 1995; Gibb et al. 2000), but should rather be reserved for cases acquiring acute infection during the second and third trimester (Lin et al. 1996). After delivery no special precautions (e.g. isolation) are needed.

Breast-feeding

Breast-feeding by HCV-positive mothers is not contraindicated, because of the generally low risk of early postnatal transmission, unless they have a high viral load in the serum. In this case, breast milk may be quickly assessed for HCV RNA before routine breast-feeding is recommended (Pipan et al. 1996).

MANAGEMENT OF THE NEONATE

Prolonged follow-up of infants (up to 24 months) born to anti-HCV and HCV-RNA-positive mothers is of great importance. Treatment of chronic hepatitis C in infants and children is usually started not before the age of more than 2 years. Treatment with interferon-α alone yielded poor results, but the combination therapy of interferon-α 2b with ribavirin is an important advance (Wirth et al. 2002).

Hepatitis D virus

Hepatitis D virus (HDV) is also known as delta agent. HDV is a defective single-stranded RNA virus that requires the helper function of HBV for viral replication since the envelope of HDV consists of HbsAg and a unique internal antigen, the delta antigen. HDV is transmitted principally by blood and blood products, but also by sexual contact or injecting drug use. There is considerable regional variation in its prevalence. The prevalence of HDV is generally low among both asymptomatic HBV carriers and among patients with chronic HBV-related liver disease in countries with low prevalence of chronic HBV infection. In countries with moderate and high levels of chronic HBV prevalence, the prevalence of HDV infection is highly variable (CDC 2001a). Vertical transmission is rare.

INFECTION IN PREGNANCY AND IN THE NEONATE

A study in northern Italy demonstrated an incidence of anti-HDV antibody among HBsAg-positive pregnant patients lower than that in a group of HBsAg-positive patients with chronic liver disease (7 versus 20 percent) (Zanetti et al. 1982). Exacerbation of HDV infection during pregnancy has not been reported. Vertical transmission seems possible either during late pregnancy or intrapartum (Ramia and Bahakim 1988; Riongeard et al. 1992). Perinatal infection has been described in an infant born to a mother positive for both HBeAg and anti-HDV, but in none whose mothers were anti-HBe-positive (Smedile et al. 1981). Prevalence rates of HDV as estimated by HDAg or anti-HDV antibody in hepatitis B-infected children range from 1.6 percent in Taiwan to 12.5 percent in parts of Italy, China, and the Balkans, and up to 25 percent in the Amazon basin in Brazil (e.g. Chen et al. 1990; Torres and Mondolfi 1991).

PROPHYLAXIS

Measures to control the spread of HBV are also effective in preventing transmission of HDV infection to the infant. Administration of HBIG and HBV vaccine within 12–24 h after birth to newborns of HBsAg-positive mothers seems to prevent both HBV and HDV infection (Silverman et al. 1991). Zanetti and colleagues (1982) reported serological evidence of HDV infection only in newborns who did not receive HBV immunoprophylaxis.

Hepatitis E virus

Hepatitis E virus (HEV) a currently unclassified probably zoonotic RNA-virus (HEV-like viruses) is transmitted enterically and is responsible for waterborne epidemics and for sporadic outbreaks in tropical and subtropical countries (Mast and Alter 1993; Emerson and Purcell 2003).

In contrast to hepatitis A, HEV affects mainly young adults (15–40 years old) and has considerable implications in pregnancy. The death rate due to hepatitis E in the general population is 0.5–3 percent, in pregnant women as high as 15–25 percent (Mast and Krawczynski 1996).

INFECTION IN PREGNANCY AND IN THE NEONATE

During epidemics, the incidence of HEV infection in pregnant women is nine times higher than in nonpregnant women or in men (Khuroo et al. 1981; Khuroo and Kamili 2003). Both in epidemic and in sporadic outbreaks, HEV causes fulminant hepatitis and maternal death, especially among women in the third trimester (Nanda et al. 1995). Mortality in pregnant women is as high as 25 percent compared with the overall mortality of 0.5–3 percent (Krawczynski 1993; Purdy and Krawczynski 1994; Kumar et al. 2004). The reasons remain unknown, but it seems unlikely that HEV is the sole cause of liver failure in pregnant women (Fagan et al. 1994).

According to the early observations of Khuroo and co-workers (1981), even mild HEV infection during pregnancy seems to cause a high rate of abortion and intrauterine death and increased perinatal mortality in babies born to women with fulminant hepatitis. Another report suggests that, unlike other hepatitis viruses, HEV often causes intrauterine infection, as well as substantial perinatal morbidity and mortality (Khuroo et al. 1995) and a more recent report suggests significant vertical transmission of HEV among HEV-RNA-positive mothers with appreciable perinatal morbidity and mortality (Kumar et al. 2001, 2004). Excluding mothers with acute hepatic disease, breast-feeding appears to be safe in HEV seropositive mothers (Kumar et al. 2001).

PROPHYLAXIS

Fecally contaminated drinking water is the most common vehicle of transmission. Hygienic precautions (e.g. adequate heating of drinking water and food) are necessary in areas where HEV is endemic. Immunoglobulin prepared from plasma collected in industrialized countries does not prevent HEV infection, immunoglobulin prepared from donors in endemic areas is of unknown efficacy (CDC 2001b). Until now, no effective antiviral drugs exist. A recombinant capsid vaccine is under evaluation in Nepal with adult volunteers receiving three doses of HEV vaccine or placebo over 6 months (Purcell et al. 2003).

Hepatitis G virus

An additional agent that may be responsible for as yet unexplained liver disease was discovered in 1995–1996 by molecular amplification and named hepatitis G virus (HGV) also known as GB virus C (Simons et al. 1995; Linnen et al. 1996). At present, HGV infection is mainly detected by reverse-transcriptase polymerase chain reaction (RT-PCR), but serological assays are now also in use. The clinical importance of this agent is as yet unclear. No causal relationship between HGV and hepatitis has been established (Alter 1996; Alter et al. 1997). Mother-to-infant transmission has been demonstrated without evidence of disease manifestations.

INFECTION IN PREGNANCY AND IN THE NEONATE

Few data are yet available on vertical mother-to-child transmission and infection of the infant. Feucht and

colleagues (1996) studied mothers belonging to a behavioral-risk group; 61 mother–infant pairs were investigated. In six of 30 mothers coinfected with HCV and three of 17 coinfected with HIV-1, HGV viremia was detected by RT-PCR. Vertical transmission of HGV occurred in three of the nine infants, but co-transmission with HIV-1 or HCV could not be demonstrated. The rate of vertical transmission for HIV-1 was 11.8 percent (2/17) and for HCV 6.7 percent (2/30), corresponding with the reported vertical transmission rates of these viruses.

During follow-up of all 61 infants for vertical transmission of HGV, HCV, and HIV-1 every 3 months for >1 year, none of the three HGV-infected infants or the two with HCV infection became icteric or showed other biochemical or clinical signs of hepatitis.

In another report on vertical transmission of HGV, three HGV-positive pregnant women (one coinfected with HCV, but all three negative for HIV-1) and their three infants were studied. All three women had elective cesarean delivery because of obstetric indications, and their infants were not infected with HGV or HCV during the 12 months of observation. These negative results may indicate that mother-to-infant transmission does not occur in women from low-risk populations or that cesarean delivery minimizes infection because there is less microtransfusion from mother to fetus compared with other modes of delivery (Lin et al. 1996). Viazov et al. demonstrated a mother-to-infant transmission of 56 percent. During follow-up studies, none of the GBV-C/HGV-infected infants had elevated levels of ALT or clinical signs of liver disease. Prospective epidemiological and clinical studies are further needed to determine the long-term outcome of this infection (Viazov et al. 1997).

ENTEROVIRUSES

There is no convincing evidence that maternal infection in early pregnancy with any of the picornaviruses is associated with teratogenic defects. Maternal poliomyelitis caused by wild-type poliovirus is now largely of historical interest. In the prevaccination era, poliovirus infections in pregnancy could result in abortion, stillbirth, and, rarely, in neonatal disease. Transplacental transmission of the virus to the fetus was demonstrated especially in maternal poliomyelitis in late pregnancy, but seldom in early pregnancy (Bates 1955; Carter 1956).

Coxsackie virus and ECHO viruses

Maternal enterovirus infections with various coxsackie and ECHO viruses may be followed by spontaneous abortion, intrauterine death, placentitis, and multiorgan fetal infection, as demonstrated in various prospective studies (Basso et al. 1990; Garcia et al. 1991; Frisk and

Diderholm 1992; Dommergues et al. 1994). In our investigations, during the past 14 years on the untoward effects of coxsackie/ECHO virus in pregnancy, involving 288 women with serologically suspected or virologically proven coxsackie/ECHO virus infections during pregnancy, fetal loss of 6.5 percent, but no teratogenic defects in the newborns were reported. In addition, no enterovirus RNA (virus culture was not attempted) could be detected in amniotic fluid of 30 women with symptomatic infection, who underwent prenatal diagnosis (18–24 WG) (G. Enders 2004, unpublished). A recent case report shows that a late intrauterine enterovirus infection (coxsackie virus B3) could be diagnosed antenatally in amniotic fluid by virus culture, but surprisingly not by enterovirus RNA detection (Ouellet et al. 2004). Late intrauterine, intrapartum, or early postnatally acquired infections are of importance for the newborns.

CONGENITAL AND PERINATAL INFECTION

Clinical manifestations in the neonate or infant often include sepsis, meningoencephalitis, hepatitis, myocarditis, and coagulation disorders (Kulhanjian 1992; Bendig et al. 2003). Meningitis is a common manifestation of neonatal enterovirus infection, and enteroviruses seem to be responsible as often as bacteria for meningitis in the first month of life (Shattuck and Chonmaitree 1992). Onset 1–2 days after birth suggests intrauterine or intrapartum transmission and disease is severe in approximately 80 percent of cases. Onset 5–6 days after birth suggests that the infant has acquired infection by contact with infected mothers, siblings, or an infected neonate in the maternity unit. The course of illness is less severe in such cases (Simoes and Abzug 1993).

More recently it was described, that in utero coxsackie virus infection of the placenta was associated with the development of severe respiratory failure and central nervous system sequelae in the newborn (Euscher et al. 2001). This underscores the importance of detailed pathologic and viral examination of the placenta in cases of systemic illness in the newborn. Data on the long-term prognosis of neonates with enteroviral meningitis are still incomplete and contradictory. Children <2 years of age with enteroviral meningitis do not have long-term sequelae (Rorabough et al. 1992). Encephalitis occasionally occurs and in young infants may have neurological sequelae. Furthermore, it was reported that varicella-like congenital skin lesions in the newborn may be one of the leading manifestations of intrauterine infection with coxsackie B viruses (e.g. CVB3) (Sauerbrei et al. 2000).

MANAGEMENT IN PREGNANCY AND OF THE NEONATE

Enterovirus infections in early pregnancy occasionally cause abortion but are not teratogenic, and the mother should be reassured accordingly. Prenatal diagnosis

should be considered in the differential diagnosis of nonimmune *hydrops fetalis* with pericardial effusion and fetal tachycardia, particularly in women with suspicion of recent enterovirus infection. Acute symptomatic or asymptomatic infections towards the end of pregnancy carry the risk of intrauterine infection causing severe neonatal disease. In case of known infection of the mother, the child should be isolated at delivery and the baby should be fed with expressed maternal breast milk. The use of intravenous immunoglobulin up to the age of 14 days as a preventive measure for neonates exposed to infected infants did not confer significant benefit (Abzug et al. 1993). Pleconaril may be used as an emergency medication (Ouellet et al. 2004). In hospitals, adequate hygienic measures must be observed because of the ready spread of these viruses in neonatal units.

LYMPHOCYTIC CHORIOMENINGITIS VIRUS

Lymphocytic choriomeningitis virus (LCMV) is a rodent-borne *Arenavirus*. The infected animals may be asymptomatic, but may excrete the virus for months. The illness in infected people is influenza-like and accompanied by fever, headache, nausea, and myalgia lasting 5–10 days; a small proportion develop meningitis or choriomeningitis, which in adults usually resolves without sequelae.

LCM virus infection is an often undiagnosed cause of congenital disease with features similar to those of cytomegalovirus or *Toxoplasma gondii*. Infection with LCMV in the first trimester of pregnancy may cause abortion (Ackermann et al. 1975; Biggar et al. 1975; Deibel et al. 1975), and infection of the fetus can result in congenital hydrocephalus, chorioretinitis, severe hyperbilirubinemia, and myopia (Sheinbergas 1975; Sheinbergas 1976; Enders et al. 1999). Although the number of published studies on intrauterine and perinatal infections is limited, the incidence of serious sequelae in infants seems to be high (Barton et al. 1995; Enders et al. 1999; Barton and Mets 2001).

Because healthy mice and hamsters shed LCMV chronically, pregnant women should avoid direct contact with these animals and their excreta.

HUMAN PAPILLOMAVIRUSES

Juvenile laryngeal papillomatosis (JLP) is associated most often with human papillomavirus (HPV) types 6 and 11; it is an uncommon but potentially serious problem, which is best treated by prevention if possible.

Infection in pregnancy

Growth of HPV warts is stimulated by several factors, including pregnancy. Some of the lesions may grow markedly during pregnancy, only to recede postpartum.

This phenomenon is thought to be related to hormonal influences or to changes in local cellular immunity. Rarely, the lesions become so large as to obstruct the birth canal and extensive formation of HPV condylomata may lead to premature rupture of the membranes, chorioamnionitis, and intrapartum infection of the fetus (Young et al. 1973).

Effects on the fetus and the neonate

Overall, the risk of perinatal transmission seems to be low, and it is still unclear how frequent it progresses to clinical lesions (Watts et al. 1996; Syrjanen and Puranen 2000). Nevertheless, transmission from mother to fetus and to the newborn may occur both in clinically apparent and subclinical maternal infection, and may lead to intrauterine infections, perinatal infections, or both. Approximately 50 percent of children with JLP are born to mothers with genital HPV (Quick et al. 1980; Nikolaidis et al. 1985), and HPV types 6 and 11, which are the most common in anogenital tract infections (Ferenczy 1989), are identified in >80 percent of JLP cases. Gastric and nasopharyngeal aspirates of babies born to mothers with genital tract HPV have been reported to contain HPV DNA (Ferenczy 1989; Sedlacek et al. 1989). The possibility of perinatal transmission is supported by the detection of DNA from HPV types 6, 11, 16, and 18 in foreskin specimens from neonates (Roman and Fife 1986).

Association with JLP

The long latent period from birth to development of JLP (>7 years) and the observation that HPV types found in newborns often differs from those detected in their mothers make association with intrauterine or perinatal infection difficult. Postnatally acquired infection from a variety of sources may account for numerous cases of JLP. For example, HPV may be transmitted on fomites after contact with individuals with warts (Patsner et al. 1990) and sexual abuse may also result in postnatal infection (Fleming et al. 1987). Recent data from Scandinavia indicate that despite the increasing rate of genital HPV infections in pregnant women, the incidence of JLP remains very low (Lindbergh and Elbrond 1990).

Diagnosis

The HPV infection may be latent without evident warts or manifest with warts. The diagnostic methodology extends from gynecological examinations, PAP smear tests, and colposcopy to the direct detection of the viral nucleic acids with molecular biology techniques such as PCR or hybrid capture (Arena et al. 2002). HPV antibodies are detectable in children of infected mothers,

but there is generally no correlation between seropositivity and the detection of DNA in either the oral or the genital mucosa (Syrjanen and Puranen 2000; Burd 2003). Women under treatment for cytologically and virologically proven HPV infection should be examined at intervals until lesions and HPV DNA are no longer detectable. Testing their partners is recommended.

Management

The treatment of pregnant women with HPV-induced genital warts should be started as early as possible and directed at elimination of the virus near term to diminish risk of the infant's acquiring HPV infection by passage through an infected birth canal. Laser vaporization is proposed as an effective invasive technique for treatment of warts in pregnant women (Arena et al. 2001). As noninvasive methods, topically applicable immune modifiers have been reported. Prophylactic cesarean section in pregnant women with genital HPV infection is not advocated except in the rare event of large condylomata obstructing the birth canal.

Preventive and therapeutic vaccines, usually composed of recombinant viruslike particles directed against HPV, are under development (Hines et al. 1995; Borysiewicz et al. 1996). Beside this more classical technology, a new strategy based on genetic immunization with naked HPV DNA is now evaluated (Moniz et al. 2003; Burd 2003; Roden et al. 2004).

REFERENCES

Abzug, M., Keyserling, H., et al. 1993. Intravenous immune globulin treatment of neonatal enterovirus infection. *Pediatr Res*, **33**, 287A.

Ackermann, R., Stammler, A., and Armbruster, B. 1975. Isolierung von Virus der Lymphozytären Choriomeningitis aus Abrasionsmaterial nach Kontakt der Schwangeren mit einem Syrischen Goldhamster (*Mesocricetusauratus*). *Infection*, 47–9.

ACOG. 1993. Guidelines for hepatitis B virus screening and vaccination during pregnancy. *Int J Gynecol Obstet*, **40**, 172–4.

ACOG. 1998. ACOG Educational Bulletin. Viral hepatitis in pregnancy. Number 248, July 1998 (replaces No. 174, November 1992). American College of Obstetricians and Gynecologists. *Int J Gynaecol Obstet*, **63**, 195–202.

ACOG. 2000a. ACOG Practice Bulletin. Management of herpes in pregnancy. Number 8, October 1999. Clinical management guidelines for obstetrician-gynecologists. *Int J Gynaecol Obstet*, **68**, 165–73.

ACOG. 2000b. ACOG Practice Bulletin. Medical management of endometriosis. Number 11, December 1999 (replaces Technical Bulletin Number 184, September 1993). Clinical management guidelines for obstetrician-gynecologists. *Int J Gynaecol Obstet*, **71**, 183–96.

ACOG. 2000c. ACOG Educational Bulletin. Breastfeeding: maternal and infant aspects. Number 258. Washington, DC: American College of Obstetricians and Gynecologists.

Ades, A.E. 1992. Methods for estimating the incidence of primary infection in pregnancy: a reappraisal of toxoplasmosis and cytomegalovirus data. *Epidemiol Infect*, **108**, 367–75.

Ades, A.E., Parker, S., et al. 2000. HCV prevalence in pregnant women in the UK. *Epidemiol Infect*, **125**, 399–405.

Adjorlolo-Johnson, G., De Cock, K.M., et al. 1994. Prospective comparison of mother-to-child transmission of HIV-1 and HIV-2 in Abidjan, Ivory Coast. *J Am Med Assoc*, **272**, 462–6.

Adler, S.P. 1988. Molecular epidemiology of cytomegalovirus: viral transmission among children attending a day care center, their parents, and caretakers. *J Pediat*, **112**, 366–72.

Adler, S.P. 1992. Cytomegalovirus and pregnancy. *Curr Opin Obstet Gynecol*, **4**, 670–5.

Adler, S.P., Manganello, A.-M.A., et al. 1993. Risk of human parvovirus B19 infections among school and hospital employees during endemic periods. *J Infect Dis*, **168**, 361–8.

Adler, S.P., Finney, J.W., et al. 1996. Prevention of child-to-mother transmission of cytomegalovirus by changing behaviors: a randomized controlled trial. *Pediatr Infect Dis J*, **15**, 240–6.

Ahlfors, K., Ivarsson, S.A. and Harris, S. 1999. Report on a long-term study of maternal and congenital cytomegalovirus infection in Sweden. Review of prospective studies available in the literature. *Scand J Infect Dis*, **31**, 443–57.

Alkalay, A.L., Pomerance, J.J. and Rimoin, D.L. 1987. Fetal varicella syndrome. *J Pediatr*, **111**, 320–3.

Alter, H.J. 1996. The cloning and clinical implications of HGV and HGBV-C. *N Engl J Med*, **334**, 1536–7.

Alter, H.J., Nakatsuji, Y., et al. 1997. The incidence of transfusion-associated hepatitis G virus infection and its relation to liver disease. *N Engl J Med*, **336**, 747–54.

Alter, M.J., Margolis, H.S., et al. 1992. The natural history of community acquired hepatitis C in the United States. *N Engl J Med*, **327**, 1899–905.

American Academy of Pediatrics, Committee on Infectious Disease. 1998. Hepatitis C virus infection. *Pediatrics*, **101**, 481–5.

Anderson, K.S., Amos, C.S., et al. 1996. Ocular abnormalities in congenital cytomegalovirus infection. *J Am Optom Assoc*, **67**, 273–278.

Anderson, M.J., Higgins, P.G., et al. 1985. Experimental parvoviral infection in humans. *J Infect Dis*, **152**, 257–65.

Anonymous. 2002. Adefovir (Hepsera) for chronic hepatitis B infection. *Med Lett Drugs Ther*, **44**, 105–6.

Arena, S., Marconi, M., et al. 2001. Pregnancy and condyloma. Evaluation about therapeutic effectiveness of laser CO_2 on 115 pregnant women. *Minerva Ginecol*, **53**, 389–96.

Arena, S., Marconi, M., et al. 2002. HPV and pregnancy: diagnostic methods, transmission and evaluation. *Minerva Ginecol*, **54**, 225–37.

Armstrong, G.L., Perz, J.F. and Alter, M.J. 2003. Comment on: Perinatal hepatitis C virus transmission – role of human immunodeficiency virus infection and injection drug use. *J Infect Dis: 872, author reply*, **187**, 872, author reply 872–4.

Arvin, A.M. and Prober, C.G. 1990. Herpes simplex virus infections. *Pediatr Infect Dis J*, **9**, 764–7.

Arvin, A.M. and Whitley, R.J. 2001. Herpes simplex virus infections. In: Remington, J.S. and Klein, J.O. (eds), *Infectious diseases of the fetus and newborn infant*, 5th edn. Philadelphia: W.B. Saunders, 425–46.

Ashley, R.L. 2002. Performance and use of HSV type-specific serology test kits. *Herpes*, **9**, 38–45.

Ashley, R.L. and Corey, L. 1984. Effect of acyclovir treatment of primary genital herpes on the antibody response to herpes simplex virus. *J Clin Invest*, **73**, 681–8.

Ashley, R.L., Militoni, J., et al. 1988. Comparison of Western blot (immunoblot) and glycoprotein G-specific immunodot enzyme assay for detecting antibodies to herpes simplex virus type 1 & 2 in human sera. *J Clin Microbiol*, **26**, 662–7.

Azam, A., Vial, Y., et al. 2001. Prenatal diagnosis of congenital cytomegalovirus infection. *Obstet Gynecol*, **97**, 443–8.

Azimi, P.H., Roberto, R.R., et al. 1986. Transfusion-acquired hepatitis A in a premature infant with secondary spread in an intensive care nursery. *Am J Dis Child*, **140**, 23–7.

Baba, K., Yabuuchi, H., et al. 1982. Immunologic and epidemiologic aspects of varicella infection acquired during infancy and early childhood. *J Pediatr*, **100**, 881–5.

Baboonian, C., Grundy, J.E., et al. 1989. Effect of pregnancy plasma upon in vitro parameters of cell mediated immunity. *FEMS Microbiol Immunol*, **1**, 189–97.

Balducci, J., Rodis, J.F., et al. 1992. Pregnancy outcome following first-trimester varicella infection. *Obstet Gynecol*, **79**, 5–6.

Baldwin, S. and Whitley, R.J. 1989. Intrauterine herpes simples virus infection. *Teratology*, **39**, 1–10.

Balfour, H.H. 1999. Antiviral drugs. *N Engl J Med*, **340**, 1255–68.

Ballou, W.R., Reed, J.L., et al. 2003. Safety and immunogenicity of a recombinant parvovirus B19 vaccine formulated with MF59C.1. *J Infect Dis*, **187**, 675–8.

Barampouti, F., Rajan, M. and Aclimandos, W. 2002. Should active CMV retinitis in non-immunocompromised newborn babies be treated? *Br J Ophthalmol*, **86**, 248–9.

Barbi, M., Binda, S., et al. 1996. Cytomegalovirus in peripheral blood leukocytes of infants with congenital or postnatal infection. *Pediatr Infect Dis J*, **15**, 898–903.

Barbi, M., Binda, S., et al. 2000. Cytomegalovirus DNA detection in Guthrie cards: a powerful tool for diagnosing congenital infection. *J Clin Virol*, **17**, 159–65.

Barbi, M., Binda, S., et al. 2001. CMV gB genotypes and outcome of vertical transmission: study on dried blood spots of congenitally infected babies. *J Clin Virol*, **21**, 75–9.

Barbi, M., Binda, S., et al. 2003. A wider role for congenital cytomegalovirus infection in sensorineural hearing loss. *Pediatr Infect Dis J*, **22**, 39–42.

Barton, L.L., Peters, C.J., et al. 1995. Lymphocytic choriomeningitis virus: an unrecognized teratogenic pathogen. *Emerg Infect*, **1**, 152–3.

Barton, L.L. and Mets, M.B. 2001. Congenital lymphocytic choriomeningitis virus infection: decade of rediscovery. *Clin Infect Dis*, **33**, 370–4.

Basso, N.G., Fonseca, M.E., et al. 1990. Enterovirus isolation from foetal and placental tissues. *Acta Virol (Praha)*, **34**, 49–57.

Bates, T. 1955. Poliomyelitis in pregnancy, fetus and newborn. *Am J Dis Child*, **90**, 189.

Bendig, J.W.A., Meurisse, E.V., et al. 1998. Neonatal varicella despite maternal immunity. *Lancet*, **352**, 1985–6.

Bendig, J.W., Franklin, O.M., et al. 2003. Coxsackievirus B3 sequences in the blood of a neonate with congenital mycarditits, plus serological evidence of maternal infection. *J Med Virol*, **70**, 606–9.

Bernstein, D.I. 1991. Effects of prior HSV-1 infection on genital HSV-2 infection. *Prog Med Virol*, **38**, 109–27.

Beutler, E., Gelbart, T. and Kuhl, W. 1990. Interference of heparin with the polymerase chain reaction. *BioTechniques*, **9**, 166.

Biggar, R.J., Woodall, J.P., et al. 1975. Lymphocytic choriomeningitis virus outbreak associated with pet hamsters. *J Am Med Assoc*, **232**, 494–500.

Blackwell, S.C., Abundis, M.G., et al. 2002. Five-year experience with midtrimester amniocentesis performed by a single group of obstetricians-gynecologists at a community hospital. *Am J Obstet Gynecol*, **186**, 1130–2.

Blanche, S., Newell, M.L., et al. 1997. Morbidity and mortality in European children vertically infected by HIV-1. The French Pediatric HIV Infection Study Group and European Collaborative Study. *J Acq Imm Def Syn Hum Retrovir*, **14**, 442–50.

Bodus, M., Hubinont, C., et al. 1999. Prenatal diagnosis of human cytomegalovirus by culture and polymerase chain reaction: 98 pregnancies leading to congenital infection. *Prenat Diagn*, **19**, 314–17.

Bohlke, K., Galil, K., et al. 2003. Postpartum varicella vaccination: is the vaccine virus excreted in breast milk? *Obstet Gynecol*, **102**, 970–7.

Bohman, V.R., Stettler, R.W., et al. 1992. Seroprevalence and risk factors for hepatitis C virus antibody in pregnant women. *Obstet Gynecol*, **80**, 609–13.

Boppana, S.B., Fowler, K.B., et al. 1997. Neuroradiographic findings in the newborn period and long-term outcome in children with symptomatic congenital cytomegalovirus infection. *Pediatrics*, **99**, 409–14.

Boppana, S.B., Fowler, K.B., et al. 1999. Symptomatic congenital cytomegalovirus infection in infants born to mothers with preexisting immunity to cytomegalovirus. *Pediatrics*, **104**, 55–60.

Boppana, S.B., Rivera, L.B., et al. 2001. Intrauterine transmission of cytomegalovirus to infants of women with preconceptional immunity. *N Engl J Med*, **344**, 1366–71.

Bortolotti, F., Calzia, R., et al. 1986. Liver cirrhosis associated with chronic hepatitis B virus infection in childhood. *J Pediatr*, **198**, 224–7.

Bortolotti, F., Resti, M., et al. 1997. Hepatitis C virus infection and related liver disease in children of mothers with antibodies to the virus. *J Pediatr*, **130**, 990–3.

Borysiewicz, L.K., Fiander, A., et al. 1996. A recombinant vaccinia virus encoding human papillomavirus types 16 and 18, E6 and E7 proteins as immunotherapy for cervical cancer. *Lancet*, **347**, 1523–7.

Bourlet, T., Levy, R., et al. 2003. Multicenter quality control for the detection of hepatitis C RNA in seminal plasma specimens. *J Clin Microbiol*, **41**, 789–93.

Boxall, E.H. 1995. Antenatal screening for carriers of hepatitis B virus. *Br Med J*, **311**, 1178–9.

Brocklehurst, P. and French, R. 1998. The association between maternal HIV infection and perinatal outcome: a systematic review of the literature and meta-analysis. *Br J Obstet Gynaecol*, **105**, 836–48.

Brown, K.E., Anderson, S.M. and Young, N.S. 1993. Erythrocyte P antigen: cellular receptor for B19 parvovirus. *Science*, **262**, 114–17.

Brown, K.E., Green, S.W., et al. 1994. Congenital anaemia after transplacental B19 parvovirus infection. *Lancet*, **343**, 895–6.

Brown, T., Anand, A., et al. 1984. Intrauterine parvovirus infection associated with hydrops fetalis. *Lancet*, **2**, 1033–4.

Brown, Z.A., Vontver, L.A., et al. 1987. Effects on infants of a first episode of genital herpes during pregnancy. *N Engl J Med*, **317**, 1246–51.

Brown, Z.A., Benedetti, L., et al. 1991. Neonatal herpes simplex virus infection in relation to asymptomatic maternal infection at the time of labor. *N Engl J Med*, **324**, 1247–52.

Brown, Z.A., Selke, S., et al. 1997. The acquisition of herpes simplex virus during pregnancy. *N Engl J Med*, **337**, 509–15.

Brown, Z.A., Wald, A., et al. 2003. Effect of serologic status and cesarean delivery on transmission rates of herpes simplex virus form mother to infant. *J Am Med Assoc*, **289**, 203–9.

Buchholz, B., Marcus, U., et al. 2002. German-Austrian recommendations for HIV-therapy in pregnancy – common declaration of the German AIDS-society (DAIG), the Austrian AIDS-society (OEAG) as well as the Robert-Koch Institute Berlin (RKI), the German Association of Physicians specialized in HIV care (DAGNAE), the German Society of Pediatric and Youth Medicine (DGKJ), the German AIDS Pediatric Association (PAAD), the German Society of Obstetrics and Gynecology (DGGG), the National Reference Center for Retroviruses (NRZ), German AIDS Assistance (DAH). *Eur J Med Res*, **7**, 417–33.

Burd, E.M. 2003. Human papillomavirus and cervical cancer. *Clin Microbiol Rev*, **16**, 1–17.

Burk, R.D., Hwang, L., et al. 1994. Outcome of perinatal hepatitis B virus exposure is dependent on maternal virus load. *J Infect Dis*, **170**, 1418–23.

Burns, D.N., Landesman, S., et al. 1998. The influence of pregnancy on human immunodeficiency virus type 1 infection: antepartum and postpartum changes in human immunodeficiency virus type 1 viral load. *Am J Obstet Gynecol*, **178**, 355–9.

Cacciola, I., Cerenzia, G., et al. 2002. Genomic heterogeneity of hepatitis B virus (HBV) and outcome of perinatal HBV infection. *J Hepatol*, **36**, 426–32.

Cardo, D.M., Culver, D.H., et al. 1997. A case-control study of HIV seroconversion in health care workers after percutaneous exposure. Centers for Disease Control and Prevention Needlestick Surveillance Group. *N Engl J Med*, **337**, 1485–90.

Carman, W.F., Fagan, E.A., et al. 1990. Association of a pre-core variant of HBV with fulminant hepatitis. *Hepatology*, **14**, 219–22.

Carter, H.M. 1956. Congenital poliomyelitis. *Obstet Gynecol*, **8**, 373.

Casteels, A., Naessens, A., et al. 1999. Neonatal screening for congenital cytomegalovirus infections. *J Perinat Med*, **27**, 116–21.

CDC. 1990. Protection against viral hepatitis. Recommendations of the immunization practices advisory committee (ACIP). *Morb Mort Wkly Rep*, **39**, 1–26.

CDC. 1991. Hepatitis B virus: a comprehensive strategy for eliminating transmission in the United States through universal childhood vaccination: recommendations of the Immunization Practices Advisory Committee (ACIP). *Morb Mort Wkly Rep*, **40**, 1–19.

CDC. 1995. Update. Recommendations to prevent hepatitis B virus transmission – United States. *Morb Mort Wkly Rep*, **44**, 574–5.

CDC. 1996. Prevention of varicella. *Morb Mort Wkly Rep*, **45**, 1–36.

CDC. 1998a. Guidelines for the use of antiretroviral agents in pediatric HIV infection. *Morb Mort Wkly Rep*, **47**, 1–31.

CDC. 1998b. Recommendations for prevention and control of hepatitis C virus infection and HCV-related chronic disease. *Morb Mort Wkly Rep*, **47**, 1–39.

CDC. 2000. Parvovirus B19 infection (fifth disease), www.cdc.gov/ncidod/diseases/parvovirus/B19.htm.

CDC. 2001a. Hepatitis D (delta) virus, www.cdc.gov/ncidod/diseases/hepatitis/slideset/hep_d/slide_1.htm.

CDC. 2001b. Hepatitis E, www.cdc.gov/ncidod/diseases/hepatitis/slideset/hep_e/slide_1.htm.

CDC. 2002a. HIV testing among pregnant women – United States and Canada, 1998–2001. *Morb Mort Wkly Rep*, **51**, 1013–6.

CDC. 2002b. Hepatitis B vaccination – United States, 1982–2002. *Morb Mort Wkly Rep*, **51**, 549–2.

Ceci, O., Margiotta, M., et al. 2001. Vertical transmission of hepatitis C virus in a cohort of 2,447 HIV-seronegative pregnant women: a 24-month prospective study. *J Pediatr Gastroenterol Nutr*, **33**, 570–5.

Cederblad, B., Riesenfeld, T. and Alm, G.A. 1989. Deficient herpes simplex virus-induced interferon alpha production by blood leukocytes of preterm and term newborn infants. *Pediatr Res*, **27**, 7–10, published erratum appears in *Pediatr Res*, 1990, **27**, 507.

Chang, M.H. 1998. Chronic hepatitis virus infection in children. *J Gastroenterol Hepatol*, **13**, 541–8.

Chang, T.-T., Liou, T.-C., et al. 1994. Intrafamilial transmission of hepatitis C virus: the important role of inapparent transmission. *J Med Virol*, **42**, 91–6.

Chaouat, G., Ledee-Bataille, N., et al. 2004. Th1/Th2 paradigm in pregnancy: paradigm lost? Cytokines in pregnancy/early abortion: re-examining the Th1/Th2 paradigm. *Int Arch Allergy Immunol*, **134**, 93–119.

Chen, G.H., Zhang, M.D. and Huang, W. 1990. Hepatitis delta virus superinfection in Guangzhou area. *Chin Med J (Engl)*, **103**, 451–4.

Cherpes, T.L., Ashley, R.L., et al. 2003. Longitudinal reliability of focus glycoprotein G-based type-specific enzyme immunoassays for detection of herpes simplex virus types 1 and 2 in women. *J Clin Microbiol*, **41**, 671–4.

Chisaka, H., Morita, E., et al. 2003. Parvovirus B19 and the pathogenesis of anemia. *Rev Med Virol*, **13**, 347–59.

Choo, P.W., Donahue, J.G., et al. 1995. The epidemiology of varicella and its complications. *J Infect Dis*, **172**, 706–12.

Choo, Q.L., Kuo, G., et al. 1994. Vaccination of chimpanzees against infection by the hepatitis C virus. *Proc Natl Acad Sci USA*, **91**, 1294–8.

Chou, S. 1990. Differentiation of cytomegalovirus strains by restriction analysis of DNA sequences amplified from clinical specimens. *J Infect Dis*, **162**, 738–42.

Chouquet, C., Richardson, S., et al. 1999. Timing of human immunodeficiency virus type 1 (HIV-1) transmission from mother to child: Bayesian estimation using a mixture. *Stat Med*, **18**, 815–33.

Coats, D.K., Demmler, G.J., et al. 2000. Ophthalmologic findings in children with congenital cytomegalovirus infection. *J AAPOS*, **4**, 110–16.

Cohen, B.J. and Buckley, M.M. 1988. The prevalence of antibody to human parvovirus B19 in England and Wales. *J Med Microbiol*, **25**, 151–3.

Collier, J. and Chapman, R. 2001. Combination therapy with interferon-alpha and ribavirin for hepatitis C: practical treatment issues. *BioDrugs*, **15**, 225–38.

Committee on Infectious Diseases. 1994. Update on timing of hepatitis B vaccination for premature infants and for children with lapsed immunization. *Pediatrics*, **94**, 403–4.

Conry, J.A., Török, T. and Andrews, P.I. 1993. Perinatal encephalopathy secondary to in utero human parvovirus B19 (HPV) infection. *Neurology*, **43**, A346, Abstract 736S.

Conte, D., Fraquelli, M., et al. 2000. Prevalence and clinical course of chronic hepatitis C virus (HCV) infection and rate of HCV vertical transmission in a cohort of 15,250 pregnant women. *Hepatology*, **31**, 751–5.

Coonrod, D., Collier, A.C., et al. 1998. Association between cytomegalovirus seroconversion and upper genital tract infection among women attending a sexually transmitted disease clinic: a prospective study. *J Infect Dis*, **177**, 1188–93.

Cooper, E.R., Charurat, M., et al. 2002. Combination antiretroviral strategies for the treatment of pregnant HIV-1-infected women and prevention of perinatal HIV-1 transmission. *J Acq Imm Def Syn*, **29**, 484–94.

Corey, L. and Spear, P.G. 1986a. Infections with herpes viruses II. *N Engl J Med*, **314**, 749–57.

Corey, L. and Spear, P.G. 1986b. Infections with herpes simplex viruses I. *N Engl J Med*, **314**, 686–91.

Corey, L., Wald, A. and Hobson, A.C. 1996. Reactivation of herpes simplex virus type 2. *21st Herpesvirus Workshop, Chicago, July 27–August 2 1996*. 263.

Cosmi, E., Mari, G., et al. 2002. Noninvasive diagnosis by Doppler ultrasonography of fetal anemia resulting from parvovirus infeciton. *Am J Obstet Gynecol*, **187**, 1290–3.

Cowan, F.M., Copas, A., et al. 2002. Herpes simplex virus type 1 infection: a sexually transmitted infection of adolescence? *Sex Transm Infect*, **78**, 346–8.

Crino, J.P. 1999. Ultrasound and fetal diagnosis of perinatal infection. *Clin Obstet Gynecol*, **42**, 71–80.

Crowcroft, N.S., Roth, C.E., et al. 1999. Guidance for control of parvovirus B19 infection in healthcare settings and the community. *J Pub Hlth Med*, **21**, 439–46.

Cunningham, C.K., Balasubramanian, R., et al. 2004. The impact of race/ethnicity on mother-to-child transmission in the United States in pediatric AIDS clinical trials group protocol 316. *J Acq Imm Def Syn*, **36**, 3, 800–7.

Da Silva, O., Hammerberg, O. and Chance, G.W. 1990. Fetal varicella syndrome. *Pediatr Infect Dis J*, **9**, 854–5.

Daffos, F., Capella-Pavlovsky, M. and Forestier, F. 1983. Fetal blood sampling via the umbilical cord using a needle guided by ultrasound. Report of 66 cases. *Prenat Diagn*, **3**, 271–7.

Daffos, F., Forestier, F., et al. 1988. Prenatal management of 746 pregnancies at risk for congenital toxoplasmosis. *N Engl J Med*, **118**, 271–5.

Dahle, A.J., Fowler, K.B., et al. 2000. Longitudinal investigation of hearing disorders in children with congenital cytomegalovirus. *J Am Acad Audiol*, **11**, 283–90.

Daiminger, A., Bäder, U., et al. 1999. Evaluation of two novel enzyme immunoassays using recombinant antigens to detect cytomegalovirus-specific immunoglobulin M in sera from pregnant women. *J Clin Virol*, **13**, 161–71.

Daiminger, A., Bäder, U. and Enders, G. 2004. Pre- and periconceptional primary cytomegalovirus infection: risk of vertical transmission and congenital disease. *Br J Obstet Gynaecol*, **112**, 166–72.

De Cock, K.M., Zadi, F., et al. 1994. Retrospective study of maternal HIV-1 and HIV-2 infections and child survival in Abidjan, Cote d'Ivoire. *Br Med J*, **308**, 441–3.

Degos, F., Maisonneuve, P., et al. 1991. Neonatal transmission of HCV from mother with chronic hepatitis. *Lancet*, **338**, 758.

Deibel, R., Woodall, J.P., et al. 1975. Lymphocytic choriomeningitis virus in man. Serological evidence of association with pet hamsters. *J Am Med Assoc*, **232**, 501–4.

Del Canho, R., Grosheide, P.M., et al. 1994. Failure of neonatal hepatitis B vaccination, the role of HBV-DNA levels in hepatitis B carrier mothers and HLA antigen. *J Hepatol*, **20**, 483–6.

Delamare, C., Carbonne, B., et al. 1999. Detection of hepatitis C virus RNA (HCV RNA) in amniotic fluid: a prospective study. *J Hepatol*, **31**, 416–20.

Delle Chiaie, L., Buck, G., et al. 2001. Prediction of fetal anemia with Doppler measurement of the middle cerebral artery peak systolic velocity in pregnancies complicated by maternal blood group alloimmunization or parvovirus B19 infection. *Ultrasound Obstet Gynecol*, **18**, 232–6.

Demmler, G.J. 1994. Cytomegalovirus. In: Gonik, B. (ed.), *Viral diseases in pregnancy*. New York, Berlin, Heidelberg: Springer-Verlag, 69–91.

Demmler, G.J. 2002. Congenital CMV disease, www.bcm.tmc.edu/pdi/infect/cmv/cu6-1-02.htm

Demmler, G.J. 2004. CMV updates, spring 2004, www.bcm.tmc.edu/pdi/infect/cmv

Department of Health. 1996a. *Report on confidential enquiries into maternal deaths in the United Kingdom. 1985–87, 1988–90, 1991–93, 1994–96*. London: HMSO.

Department of Health. 1996b. *Immunisation against infectious disease*. Salisbury D.M. and Begg N. (eds). London: HMSO.

Deutsche Gesellschaft für pädiatrische Infektiologie. 2003. *Handbuch: Infektionen bei Kindern und Jugendlichen*, 4th edn. Munich: Futuramed Verlag.

Di Bisceglie, A.M., Conjeevaram, H.S., et al. 1995. Ribavirin as therapy for chronic hepatitis C. *Ann Intern Med*, **123**, 897–903.

Dinsmoor, M.J. 2001. Hepatitis C in pregnancy. *Curr Womens Health Rep*, **1**, 27–30.

Dommergues, M., Petitjean, J., et al. 1994. Fetal enteroviral infection with cerebral ventriculomegaly and cardiomyopathy. *Fetal Diagn Ther*, **9**, 77–8.

Dworkin, R.H. 1996. Racial differences in herpes zoster and age at onset of varicella. *J Infect Dis*, **174**, 239–40.

Editorial. 1990. TORCH syndrome and TORCH screening. *Lancet*, **335**, 1559–61.

Eggers, M., Metzger, C. and Enders, G. 1998. Differentiation between acute primary and recurrent human cytomegalovirus infection in pregnancy, using a microneutralization assay. *J Med Virol*, **56**, 351–8.

Eggers, M., Bäder, U. and Enders, G. 2000. Combination of microneutralization and avidity assays: improved diagnosis of recent primary human cytomegalovirus infection in single serum sample of second trimester pregnancy. *J Med Virol*, **60**, 324–30.

Eggers, M., Radsak, K., et al. 2001. Use of recombinant glycoprotein antigen gB and gH for diagnosis of primary human cytomegalovirus infection during pregnancy. *J Med Virol*, **63**, 135–42.

Eis-Hübinger, A.M., Dieck, D., et al. 1998. Parvovirus B19 infection in pregnancy. *Intervirology*, **41**, 178–84.

Elbou Ould, M.A., Luton, D., et al. 2004. Cellular immune response of fetuses to cytomegalovirus. *Pediatr Res*, **55**, 280–6.

Emerson, S.U. and Purcell, R.H. 2003. Hepatitis E virus. *Rev Med Virol*, **13**, 145–54.

Emery, V.C. and Hassan-Walker, A.F. 2002. Focus on new drugs in development against human cytomegalovirus. *Drugs*, **62**, 1853–8.

Enders, G. 1984. Varicella-zoster virus infection in pregnancy. In: Melnick, J.L. (ed.), *Progress in medical virology*. Basel: Karger, 166–96.

Enders, G. 1994. Pränatale Diagnostik: Meilensteine auf dem Gebiet der pränatalen Infektionsdiagnostik und der vorgeburtlichen Medizin. *Abbott Times*, **4**, 8–16.

Enders, G. 2003. Infektionsgefährdung: Mutterschutz im Krankenhaus, Arbeitsmedizin, Sozialmedizin. *Umweltmedizin*, **38**, 324–35.

Enders, G. 2005. *Infektionen und Impfungen in der Schwangerschaft*, 3rd edn. Munich: Urban & Fischer.

Enders, G. and Biber, M. 1990. Parvovirus B19 infections in pregnancy. *Behring Inst Mitt*, **85**, 74–8.

Enders, G. and Braun, R. 2000. Pre- and peripartum transmission of hepatitis C virus. *Internist (Berl)*, **41**, 676–8.

Enders, G. and Jonatha, W. 1987. Prenatal diagnosis of intrauterine rubella. *Infection*, **15**, 162–7.

Enders, G. and Miller, E. 1994. Consequences of varicella and herpes zoster in pregnancy: prospective study of 1739 cases. *Lancet*, **343**, 1548–51.

Enders, G. and Miller, E. 2000. Varicella and herpes zoster in pregnancy and the newborn. In: Arvin, A.M. and Gershon, A.A. (eds), *Varicella-zoster virus: virology and clinical management*. Cambridge: Cambridge University Press, 317–47.

Enders, G., Risse, B., et al. 1998. Seroprevalence study of herpes simplex virus type 2 among pregnant women in Germany using a type-specific enzyme immunoassay. *Eur J Clin Microbiol Infect Dis*, **17**, 870–2.

Enders, G., Varho-Gobel, M., et al. 1999. Congenital lymphocytic choriomeningitis virus infection: an underdiagnosed disease. *Pediatr Infect Dis J*, **18**, 652–5.

Enders, G., Bäder, U., et al. 2001. Prenatal diagnosis of congenital cytomegalovirus infection in 189 pregnancies with known outcome. *Prenat Diagn*, **21**, 362–77.

Enders, G., Bäder, U., et al. 2003. Zytomegalievirus (CMV) Durchseuchung und Häufigkeit von CMV-Primärinfektionen bei schwangeren Frauen in Deutschland. *Bundesgesundheitsbl Gesundheitsforsch Gesundheitsschutz*, **46**, 426–32.

Enders, M., Weidner, A., et al. 2004. Fetal morbidity and mortality after acute human parvovirus B19 infection in pregnancy: prospective evaluation of 1018 cases. *J Prenat Diagn*, **7**, 513.

Esmonde, T.F., Herdman, G. and Anderson, G. 1989. Chickenpox pneumonia. An association with pregnancy. *Thorax*, **44**, 812–15.

European Collaborative Study. 1999. Maternal viral load and vertical transmission of HIV-1: an important factor but not the only one. The European Collaborative Study. *AIDS*, **13**, 1377–85.

European Collaborative Study. 2001. HIV-infected pregnant women and vertical transmission in Europe since 1986. *AIDS*, **15**, 761–70.

European Mode of Delivery Collaboration. 1999. Elective caesarean-section versus vaginal delivery in prevention of vertical HIV-1 transmission: a randomised clinical trial. *Lancet*, **353**, 1035–9.

European Paediatric Hepatitis C Virus Network. 2001. Effects of mode of delivery and infant feeding on the risk of mother-to-child transmission of hepatitis C virus. *Br J Obstet Gynaecol*, **108**, 371–7.

Euscher, E., Davis, J., et al. 2001. Coxsackie virus infection of the placenta associated with neurodevelopmental delays in the newborn. *Obstet Gynecol*, **98**, 1019–26.

Fagan, E.A., Menon, T., et al. 1994. Equivocal serological diagnosis of sporadic fulminant hepatitis E in pregnant Indians. *Lancet*, **344**, 342–3.

Fagan, E.A., Hadzic, N., et al. 1999. Symptomatic neonatal hepatitis A disease from a virus variant acquired in utero. *Pediatr Infect Dis J*, **18**, 389–91.

Fairley, C.K. and Miller, E. 1996. Varicella-zoster virus – a changing scene? *J Infect Dis*, **174**, Suppl. 3, 31409.

Fairley, C.K., Smoleniec, J.S., et al. 1995. Observational study of effect of intrauterine transfusions on outcome of fetal hydrops after parvovirus B19 infection. *Lancet*, **346**, 1335–7.

Fang, G., Burger, H., et al. 1995. Maternal plasma human immunodeficiency virus type 1 RNA level: a determinant and projected threshold for mother-to-child transmission. *Proc Natl Acad Sci USA*, **92**, 12100–4.

Ferenczy, A. 1989. HPV-associated lesions in pregnancy and their clinical implications. *Clin Obstet Gynecol*, **32**, 191–9.

Ferguson, M., Walker, D. and Cohen, B. 1997. Report of a collaborative study to establish the international standard for parvovirus B19 serum IgG. *Biologicals*, **25**, 283–8.

Fernando, S., Pearce, J.M. and Booth, J.C. 1993. Lymphocyte responses and virus excretion as risk factors for intrauterine infection with cytomegalovirus. *J Med Virol*, **41**, 108–13.

Feucht, H.H., Zöllner, B., et al. 1996. Vertical transmission of hepatitis G. *Lancet*, **347**, 615–16.

Fisher, S., Genbacev, O., et al. 2000. Human cytomegalovirus infection of placental cytotrophoblasts in vitro and in utero: implications for transmission and pathogenesis. *J Virol*, **74**, 6808–20.

Fischler, B., Lindh, G., et al. 1996. Vertical transmission of hepatitis C virus infection. *Scand J Infect Dis*, **28**, 353–6.

Fleming, K.A., Venning, V. and Evans, M. 1987. DNA typing of genital warts and diagnosis of sexual abuse of children. *Lancet*, **2**, 454.

Flewett, T.H., Parker, G.F. and Philip, W.M. 1969. Acute hepatitis due to herpes simplex virus in an adult. *J Clin Path*, **22**, 60.

Forestier, F., Cox, W., et al. 1988. The assessment of fetal blood samples. *Am J Obstet Gynecol*, **158**, 1184–8.

Forestier, F., Tissot, J.D., et al. 1999. Haematological parameters of parvovirus B19 infection in 13 fetuses with hydrops foetalis. *Br J Haematol*, **104**, 925–7.

Forrest, J.M., Mego, S. and Burgess, M.A. 2000. Congenital and neonatal varicella in Australia. *J Paediatr Child Health*, **36**, 108–13.

Forsgren, M. 1992. Herpes simplex virus infection in the perinatal period. *Rev Med Microbiol*, **3**, 129–36.

Forsgren, M. 2004. Cytomegalovirus in breast milk: reassessment of pasteurization and freeze-thawing. *Paediatr Res*, **56**, 526–8.

Fowler, K.B., Stagno, S., et al. 1992. The outcome of congenital cytomegalovirus infection in relation to maternal antibody status. *N Engl J Med*, **326**, 663–7.

Fowler, K.B., Dahle, A.J., et al. 1999. Newborn hearing screening: Will children with hearing loss caused by congenital cytomegalovirus infection be missed? *J Pediatr*, **135**, 60–4.

Fowler, K.B., Stagno, S. and Pass, R.F. 2003. Maternal immunity and prevention of congenital cytomegalovirus infection. *J Am Med Assoc*, **289**, 1008–11.

Fowler, K.B., Stagno, S. and Pass, R.F. 2004. Interval between births and risk of congenital cytomegalovirus infection. *Clin Infect Dis*, **38**, 1035–7.

Frederick, D.M., Bland, D. and Gollin, Y. 2002. Fatal disseminated herpes simplex virus infection in a previously healthy pregnant woman. *J Reprod Med*, **47**, 591–6.

French, R. and Brocklehurst, P. 1998. The effect of pregnancy on survival in women infected with HIV: a systematic review of the literature and meta-analysis. *Br J Obstet Gynaecol*, **105**, 827–35.

Frenkel, L.M., Mullins, J.I., et al. 1998. Genetic evaluation of suspected cases of transient HIV-1 infection of infants. *Science*, **280**, 1073–7.

Friese, K. 2003. Human-Immundefizien-Virus Typ 1 und 2. In: Friese, K., Schäfer, A. and Hof, H. (eds), *Infektionskrankheiten in Gynäkologie und Geburtshilfe*. Berlin, Heidelberg: Springer-Verlag, 121–48.

Frisk, G. and Diderholm, H. 1992. Increased frequency of coxsackie B virus IgM in women with spontaneous abortion. *J Infect*, **24**, 141–5.

Fujisawa, T., Komatsu, H., et al. 2000. Long-term outcome of chronic hepatitis B in adolescents or young adults in follow-up from childhood. *J Pediatr Gasteroenterol Nutr*, **30**, 201–6.

Gabrielli, L., Losi, L., et al. 2001. Complete replication of human cytomegalovirus in explants of first trimester human placenta. *J Med Virol*, **64**, 499–504.

Gabrielli, L., Lazzarotto, T., et al. 2003. Horizontal in utero acquisition of cytomegalovirus infection in a twin pregnancy. *J Clin Microbiol*, **41**, 1329–31.

Garcia, A.G., Basso, N.G., et al. 1991. Enterovirus associated placental morphology: a light, virological, electron microscopic and immunohistologic study. *Placenta*, **12**, 533–47.

Gathings, W.E., Kubagawa, H. and Cooper, M.D. 1981. A distinctive pattern of B cell immaturity in perinatal humans. *Immunol Rev*, **5**, 107–26.

Gaytant, M.A., Steegers, E.A., et al. 2002. Seroprevalences of herpes simplex virus type 1 and type 2 among pregnant women in the Netherlands. *Sex Transm Dis*, **29**, 710–14.

Gehrz, R.C., Christianson, W.R., et al. 1981. Cytomegalovirus-specific humoral and cellular immune response in human pregnancy. *J Infect Dis*, **143**, 391–5.

Geipel, A., Gembruch, U., et al. 2001. Fetales Infektionsrisiko bei invasiver Pränataldiagnostik. Bei Frauen mit nachgewiesener HIV-, HBV-, HCV- oder CMV-Infektion. *Gynkologe*, **34**, 453–7.

Gershon, A.A. 1975. Varicella in mother and infant: problems old and new. In: Krugman, S. and Gershon, A.A. (eds), *Infections in the fetus and newborn infant*. New York: Alan R Liss, 79–95.

Giacchino, R., Picciotto, A., et al. 1995. Vertical transmission of hepatitis C. *Lancet*, **345**, 1122–3.

Gibb, D.M., Goodall, R.L., et al. 2000. Mother-to-child transmission of hepatitis C virus: evidence for preventable peripartum transmission. *Lancet*, **356**, 904–7.

Gillespie, S.M., Carter, M.L., et al. 1990. Occupational risk of human parvovirus B19 infection for school and day-care personnel during an outbreak of erythema infectiosum. *J Am Med Assoc*, **263**, 2061–5.

Goto, M., Fujiyama, S., et al. 1994. Intrafamilial transmission of hepatitis C virus. *J Gastroenterol Hepatol*, **9**, 13–18.

Gottard, H., Rabensteiner, A., et al. 1991. Nachweis des Varizellenvirus mit der DNA-Sonde im fetalen Blut und im Fruchtwasser. *Geburtsh Frauenheilk*, **51**, 63–4.

Gouarin, S., Palmer, P., et al. 2001. Congenital HCMV infection: a collaborative and comparative study of virus detection in amniotic fluid by culture and by PCR. *J Clin Virol*, **21**, 47–55.

Gouarin, S., Gault, E., et al. 2002. Real-time PCR quantification of human cytomegalovirus DNA in amniotic fluid samples from mothers with primary infection. *J Clin Microbiol*, **40**, 1767–72.

Grab, D., Kittelberger, M., et al. 2002. Kindliche Entwicklung nach maternaler Ringelrötelninfektion in der Schwangerschaft. *Gyne*, **7**, 299–303.

Gratacós, E., Torres, P.J., et al. 1995. The incidence of human parvovirus B19 infection during pregnancy and its impact on perinatal outcome. *J Infect Dis*, **171**, 1360–3.

Gray, G.C., Palinkas, L.A. and Kelley, P.W. 1990. Increasing incidence of varicella hospitalizations in the United States Army and Navy personnel: are today's teenagers more susceptible? Should recruits be vaccinated? *Pediatrics*, **86**, 867–73.

Griffiths, P.D. 1990. Virus infections of the fetus and neonate, other than rubella. In: Collier L.H. and Timbury, M.C. (eds), *Topley & Wilson's principles of bacteriology, virology and immunity*, 8th edn, *Virology*, Vol. 4. London: Edward Arnold, 533–45.

Griffiths, P.D. 2002. Strategies to prevent CMV infection in the neonate. *Semin Neonatol*, **7**, 293–9.

Griffiths, P.D. and Baboonian, C. 1984. A prospective study of primary cytomegalovirus infection during pregnancy: final report. *Br J Obstet Gynaecol*, **91**, 307–15.

Griffiths, P.D., McLean, A., et al. 2001. Encouraging prospects for immunization against primary cytomegalovirus infection. *Vaccine*, **19**, 1356–62.

Grosheide, P.M., Wladimiroff, J.W., et al. 1995. Proposal for routine antenatal screening at 14 weeks for hepatitis B surface antigen. *Br Med J*, **311**, 1197–9.

Grubman, S., Gross, E., et al. 1995. Older children and adolescents living with perinatally acquired human immunodeficiency virus infection. *Pediatrics*, **95**, 657–63.

Guerra, B., Lazzarotto, T., et al. 2000. Prenatal diagnosis of symptomatic congenital cytomegalovirus infection. *Am J Obstet Gynecol*, **183**, 476–82.

Gürakan, B., Oran, O. and Yigit, S. 1994. Vertical transmission of hepatitis C virus. *N Engl J Med*, **331**, 399.

Haake, D.A., Zakowski, P.C., et al. 1990. Early treatment of acyclovir for varicella pneumonia in otherwise healthy adults: retrospective controlled study and review. *Rev Infect Dis*, **112**, 788–98.

Haddad, J., Langer, B., et al. 1993. Oral acyclovir and recurrent genital herpes during late pregnancy. *Obstet Gynecol*, **82**, 102–4.

Hagay, Z.J., Biran, G., et al. 1996. Congenital cytomegalovirus infection: a long-standing problem still seeking a solution. *Am J Obstet Gynecol*, **174**, 241–5.

Hamprecht, K., Maschmann, J., et al. 2001. Epidemiology of transmission of cytomegalovirus from mother to preterm infant by breastfeeding. *Lancet*, **357**, 513–18.

Hanson, F.W., Happ, R.L., et al. 1990. Ultrasonography guided early amniocentesis in singleton pregnancies. *Am J Obstet Gynecol*, **162**, 1376–81.

Harger, J.H., Adler, S.P., et al. 1998. Prospective evaluation of 618 pregnant women exposed to parvovirus B19: risks and symptoms. *Obstet Gynecol*, **91**, 413–20.

Harger, J.H., Ernest, J.M., et al. 2002. Frequency of congenital varicella syndrome in a prospective cohort of 347 pregnant women. *Obstet Gynecol*, **100**, 260–5.

Harrison, C.J. 1995. Neonatal herpes simplex virus (HSV) infections. *Nebr Med J*, **10**, 311–15.

Hartung, J., Enders, G., et al. 1999. Prenatal diagnosis of congenital varicella syndrome and detection of varicella-zoster virus in the fetus: a case report. *Prenat Diagn*, **19**, 163–6.

Heegaard, E.D. and Brown, K.E. 2002. Human parvovirus B19. *Clin Microbiol Rev*, **15**, 485–505.

Hegenbarth, K., Maurer, U., et al. 2001. No evidence for mutagenic effects of ribavirin: report of two normal pregnancies. *Am J Gastroenterol*, **96**, 2286–7.

Hemauer, A., Gigler, A., et al. 2000. Seroprevalence of parvovirus B19 NS1-specific IgG in B19-infected and uninfected individuals and in infected pregnant women. *J Med Virol*, **60**, 48–55.

Hemmings, D.G., Kilani, R., et al. 1998. Permissive cytomegalovirus infection of primary villous term and first trimester trophoblasts. *J Virol*, **72**, 4970–9.

Higa, K., Dan, K. and Manabe, H. 1987. Varicella-zoster virus infections during pregnancy: hypothesis concerning the mechanisms of congenital malformations. *Obstet Gynecol*, **69**, 214–22.

Hill, J.B., Sheffield, J.S., et al. 2002. Risk of hepatitis B transmission in breast-fed infants of chronic hepatitis B carriers. *Obstet Gynecol*, **99**, 1049–52.

Hines, J.F., Ghim, S., et al. 1995. Prospects for a vaccine against human papillomavirus. *Obstet Gynecol*, **86**, 860–6.

Hiratsuka, M., Minakami, H., et al. 2000. Administration of interferon-alpha during pregnancy: effects on fetus. *J Perinat Med*, **28**, 372–6.

Ho, D.W.T., Field, P.R., et al. 1993. Detection of immunoglobulin M antibodies to glycoprotein G-2 by western blot (immunoblot) for diagnosis of initial herpes simplex virus type 2 genital infections. *J Clin Microbiol*, **31**, 3157–64.

Hocker, J.R., Cook, L.N., et al. 1990. Ganciclovir therapy of congenital cytomegalovirus pneumonia. *Pediatr Infect Dis J*, **9**, 743–5.

Hohlfeld, P., Daffos, F., et al. 1994. Prenatal diagnosis of congenital toxoplasmosis with a polymerase chain reaction test on amniotic fluid. *N Engl J Med*, **331**, 695–9.

Holland, P., Isaacs, D. and Moxon, E.R. 1986. Fatal neonatal varicella infection. *Lancet*, **2**, 1156.

Hoppen, T., Eis Hübinger, A.M., et al. 2001. Intrauterine herpes simplex virus infection. *Klin Padiatr*, **213**, 63–8.

Hsu, H.C., Wu, M.Z., et al. 1987. Childhood hepatocellular carcinoma develops exclusively in hepatitis B surface antigen carriers in three decades in Taiwan: a report of 51 cases strongly associated with rapid development of liver cirrhosis. *J Hepatol*, **5**, 260–7.

Hsu, H.H., Wright, T.L., et al. 1991. Failure to detect hepatitis C virus genome in human secretions with polymerase chain reaction. *Hepatology*, **14**, 763–7.

Hsu, H.Y., Chang, M.H., et al. 1999. Changes of hepatitis B surface antigen variants in carrier children before and after universal vaccination in Taiwan. *Hepatology*, **30**, 1312–17.

Hutto, C., Arvin, A.M., et al. 1987. Intrauterine herpes simplex virus infections. *J Pediatr*, **110**, 97–101.

International Perinatal HIV Group. 1999. The mode of delivery and the risk of vertical transmission of human immunodeficiency virus type 1 – a meta-analysis of 15 prospective cohort studies. *N Engl J Med*, **340**, 977–87.

Ioannidis, J.P., Abrams, E.J., et al. 2001. Perinatal transmission of human immunodeficiency virus type 1 by pregnant women with RNA virus loads <1000 copies/ml. *J Infect Dis*, **183**, 539–45.

Istas, A.S., Demmler, G.J., et al. 1995. Surveillance for congenital cytomegalovirus disease: a report from the National Congenital Cytomegalovirus Disease Registry. *Clin Infect Dis*, **20**, 665–70.

Ivarsson, S.-A., Lernmark, B. and Svanberg, L. 1997. Ten-year clinical, developmental, and intellectual follow-up of children with congenital cytomegalovirus infection without neurologic symptoms at one year of age. *Pediatrics*, **99**, 800–3.

Jackson, J.B., Musoke, P., et al. 2003. Intrapartum and neonatal single-dose nevirapine compared with zidovudine for prevention of mother-to-child transmission of HIV-1 in Kampala, Uganda: 18-month follow-up of the HIVNET 012 randomised trial. *Lancet*, **362**, 859–68.

Jensen, I.P., Thorsen, P., et al. 2000. An epidemic of parvovirus B19 in a population of 3,596 pregnant women: a study of sociodemographic and medical risk factors. *Br J Obstet Gynaecol*, **107**, 637–43.

Jilg, W., Hottentrager, B., et al. 2001. Prevalence of markers of hepatitis B in the adult German population. *J Med Virol*, **63**, 96–102.

John, G.C., Rousseau, C., et al. 2000. Maternal SDF1 3'A polymorphism is associated with increased perinatal human immunodeficiency virus type 1 transmission. *J Virol*, **74**, 5736–9.

Johnson, R.E., Nahmias, A.J., et al. 1989. Seroepidemiologic survey of the prevalence of herpes simplex virus type 2 infection in the United States. *N Engl J Med*, **321**, 7–12.

Johnson, R.E., Lee, F., et al. 1994. US genital herpes trends during the first decade of AIDS: prevalences increased in young whites and elevated in blacks. *Sex Transm Dis*, **21**, 109.

Jones, K.L., Johnson, K.A. and Chambers, C.D. 1994. Offspring of women infected with varicella during pregnancy: a prospective study. *Teratology*, **49**, 29–32.

Jordan, J.A. and Butchko, A.R. 2002. Apoptotic activity in villous trophoblast cells during B19 infection correlates with clinical outcome: assessment by the caspase-related M30 Cytodeath antibody. *Placenta*, **23**, 547–53.

Jordan, J.A. and DeLoia, J.A. 1999. Globoside expression within the human placenta. *Placenta*, **20**, 103–8.

Joseph, P.R. 1986. Incubation period of fifth disease. *Lancet*, **13**, 1390–1, letter to the editor.

Kage, M., Ogasawara, S., et al. 1997. Hepatitis C virus RNA present in saliva but absent in breast-milk of the hepatitis C carrier mother. *J Gastroenterol Hepatol*, **12**, 518–21.

Kahlon, J. and Whitley, R.J. 1988. Antibody response of the newborn after herpes simplex virus infection. *J Infect Dis*, **158**, 925.

Kang, A.H. and Graves, C.R. 1999. Herpes simplex hepatitis in pregnancy: a case report and review of the literature. *Obstet Gynecol Surv*, **54**, 463–8.

Kashden, J., Frison, S., et al. 1998. Intellectual assessment of children with asymptomatic congenital cytomegalovirus infection. *J Dev Behav Pediatr*, **19**, 254–9.

Kassenärztliche Bundesvereinigung. 1994. Generelles Screening auf Hepatitis B in der Schwangerschaft. *Dtsch Ärztebl*, **91**, A2778–9.

Katz, V.L., Kuller, J.A., et al. 1995. Varicella during pregnancy. Maternal and fetal effects. *West J Med*, **163**, 446–50.

Kelly, H.A., Siebert, D., et al. 2000. The age-specific prevalence of human parvovirus immunity in Victoria, Australia compared with other parts of the world. *Epidemiol Infect*, **124**, 449–57.

Ketzinel-Gilad, M., Colodner, S.L., et al. 2000. Transient transmission of hepatitis C virus from mothers to newborns. *Eur J Clin Microbiol Infect Dis*, **19**, 267–74.

Khuroo, M.S. and Kamili, S. 2003. Aetiology, clinical course and outcome of sporadic acute viral hepatitis in pregnancy. *J Viral Hepat*, **10**, 61–9.

Khuroo, M.S., Teli, M.R., et al. 1981. Incidence and severity of viral hepatitis in pregnancy. *Am J Med*, **70**, 252–5.

Khuroo, M.S., Kamili, S. and Jameel, S. 1995. Vertical transmission of hepatitis E virus. *Lancet*, **345**, 1025–6.

Kimberlin, D.W., Lin, C.Y., et al. 2003. Effect of ganciclovir therapy on hearing in symptomatic congenital cytomegalovirus disease involving the central nervous system: a randomised controlled trial. *J Pediatr*, **143**, 16–25.

King, S.M., Gorensek, M., et al. 1986. Fatal varicella-zoster infection in a newborn treated with varicella-zoster immunoglobulin. *Pediatr Infect Dis*, **5**, 588–9.

Klein, J.O. and Remington, J.S. 2001. Current concepts of infections of the fetus and newborn infant. In: Remington, J.S. and Klein, J.O. (eds), *Infectious diseases of the fetus and newborn infant*. Philadelphia: W.B. Saunders, 1–23.

Knox, G.E., Pass, R.F., et al. 1979. Comparative prevalence of subclinical cytomegalovirus and herpes simplex virus infections in the genital and urinary tracts of low income, urban women. *J Infect Dis*, **140**, 419–22.

Koch, W.C. and Adler, S.P. 1989. Human parvovirus B19 infections in women of childbearing age and within families. *Pediatr Infect Dis J*, **8**, 83–7.

Koch, W.C., Harger, J.H., et al. 1998. Serologic and virologic evidence for frequent intrauterine transmission of human parvovirus B19 with a primary maternal infection during pregnancy. *Pediatr Infect Dis J*, **17**, 489–94.

Koelle, D.M., Benedetti, J.K., et al. 1992. Asymptomatic reactivation of herpes simplex virus in women after the first episode of genital herpes. *Ann Intern Med*, **116**, 433–7.

Kohl, S., West, M.S., et al. 1989. Neonatal antibody-dependent cellular cytotoxic antibody levels are associated with the clinical presentation of neonatal herpes simplex virus infection. *J Infect Dis*, **160**, 770.

Kojima, T. and Yamanaka, T. 1994. Transmission routes of hepatitis C virus: analysis of anti-HCV-positive pregnant women and their family members. *Nippon Sanka Fujinka Gakkai Zasshi*, **46**, 573–80.

Komischke, K., Searle, K. and Enders, G. 1997. Maternal serum alpha-fetoprotein and human chorionic gonadotropin in pregnant women with acute parvovirus B19 infection with and without fetal complications. *Prenat Diagn*, **17**, 1039–46.

Kostrikis, L.G., Neumann, A.U., et al. 1999. A polymorphism in the regulatory region of the CC-chemokine receptor 5 gene influences perinatal transmission of human immunodeficiency virus type 1 to African-American infants. *J Virol*, **73**, 10264–71.

Koutsky, L.A., Ashley, R.L., et al. 1990. The frequency of unrecognised type 2 herpes simplex virus infection among women. Implications for the control of genital herpes. *Sex Transm Dis*, **17**, 90–4.

Krawczynski, K. 1993. Hepatitis E. *Hepatology*, **17**, 932–41.

Krawczynski, K., Alter, M.J., et al. 1996. Effect of immune globulin on the prevention of experimental hepatitis C virus infection. *J Infect Dis*, **173**, 822–8.

Kroon, S. and Whitley, R. 1995. *Management strategies in herpes: can we improve management of perinatal HSV infections?* Worthing: PPS Europe.

Kudesia, G., Ball, G. and Irving, W. 1995. Vertical transmission of hepatitis C. *Lancet*, **345**, 1122.

Kulhanjian, J. 1992. Fever, hepatitis and coagulopathy in a newborn infant. *Pediatr Infect Dis J*, **11**, 1069–72.

Kumar, R.M., Frossad, P.M. and Hughes, P.F. 1997. Seroprevalence and mother-to-infant transmission of hepatitis C in asymptomatic Egyptian women. *Eur J Obstet Gynecol Reprod Biol*, **75**, 177–82.

Kumar, R.M. and Shahul, S. 1998. Role of breast-feeding in transmission of hepatitis C virus to infants of HCV-infected mothers. *J Hepatol*, **29**, 191–7.

Kumar, R.M., Uduman, S., et al. 2001. Sero-prevalence and mother-to-infant transmission of hepatitis E virus among pregnant women in the United Arab Emirates. *Eur J Obstet Gynecol Reprod Biol*, **100**, 9–15.

Kumar, A., Beniwal, M., et al. 2004. Hepatitis E in pregnancy. *Int J Gynaecol Obstet*, **85**, 240–4.

Kumazaki, K., Ozono, K., et al. 2002. Detection of cytomegalovirus DNA in human placenta. *J Med Virol*, **68**, 363–9.

Kurauchi, O., Furui, T., et al. 1993. Studies on transmission of hepatitis C virus from mother to child in the perinatal period. *Arch Obstet Gynecol*, **253**, 121–6.

Kuroki, T., Nishiguchi, S., et al. 1991. Mother-to-child transmission of hepatitis C virus. *J Infect Dis*, **164**, 427–8.

Laforet, E.G. and Lynch, C.L. 1947. Multiple congenital defects following maternal varicella: report of a case. *N Engl J Med*, **236**, 534–7.

Landesman, S.H., Kalish, L.A., et al. 1996. Obstetrical factors and the transmission of human immunodeficiency virus type 1 from mother to child. *N Engl J Med*, **334**, 1617–23.

Landini, M.P. 1993. New approaches and perspectives in cytomegalovirus diagnosis. In: Melnick, J.L. (ed.), *Progress in medical virology*. Basel: Karger, 157–77.

Lazzarin, A., Clotet, B., et al. 2003. Efficacy of enfuvirtide in patients with drug-resistant HIV-1 in Europe and Australia. *N Engl J Med*, **348**, 2186–95.

Lazzarotto, T., Varani, S., et al. 2000. Prenatal indicators of congenital cytomegalovirus infection. *J Pediatr*, **137**, 90–5.

Lee, S.S. 1995. Hepatitis B vaccination strategy for newborn babies. *Lancet*, **346**, 900–1.

Levy, R., Tardy, J.C., et al. 2000. Transmission risk of hepatitis C virus in assisted reproductive techniques. *Hum Reprod*, **15**, 810–16.

Lewis, D.B. and Wilson, C.B. 2001. Developmental immunology and role of host defences in fetal and neonatal susceptibility to infection. In: Remington, J.S. and Klein, J.O. (eds), *Infectious diseases of the fetus and newborn infant*, 5th edn. Philadelphia: W.B. Saunders, 25–138.

Liberek, A., Rytlewska, M., et al. 2002. Cytomegalovirus disease in neonates and infants – clinical presentation, diagnostic and therapeutic problems – own experience. *Med Sci Monit*, **8**, CR815–20.

Liesnard, C., Donner, C., et al. 2000. Prenatal diagnosis of congenital cytomegalovirus infection: prospective study of 237 pregnancies at risk. *Obstet Gynecol*, **95**, 881–8.

Lima, M.P., Pedro, R.J. and Rocha, M.D. 2004. Mother-to-infant transmission of hepatitis C virus (HCV) in Brazil. *J Trop Pediatr*, **50**, 236–8.

Lin, H.H., Lee, T.Y., et al. 1987. Transplacental leakage of HBeAg-positive maternal blood as the most likely route in causing intrauterine infection with hepatitis B virus. *J Pediatr*, **111**, 877–81.

Lin, H.H., Kao, J.H., et al. 1995. Absence of infection in breast-fed infants born to hepatitis C virus-infected mothers. *J Pediatr*, **126**, 589–91.

Lin, H.H., Kao, J.H., et al. 1996. Least microtransfusion from mother to fetus in elective cesarean delivery. *Obstet Gynecol*, **87**, 244–8.

Lindbergh, H. and Elbrond, O. 1990. Laryngeal papillomas: the epidemiology in a Danish subpopulation 1965–84. *Clin Otolaryngol*, **15**, 125–31.

Linnen, J., Wages, J., et al. 1996. Molecular cloning and disease association of hepatitis G virus: a transfusion-transmissible agent. *Science*, **271**, 505–8.

Lipitz, S., Yagel, S., et al. 1997. Prenatal diagnosis of fetal primary cytomegalovirus infection. *Obstet Gynecol*, **89**, 763–7.

Liu, J.M., Green, S.W., et al. 1992. A block in full-length transcript maturation in cells nonpermissive for B19 parvovirus. *J Virol*, **66**, 4686–92.

Livingston, R.A., Hutton, N., et al. 1995. Human immunodeficiency virus-specific IgA in infants born to human immunodeficiency virus-seropositive women. *Arch Pediatr Adolesc*, **149**, 503–7.

Lok, A.S.F. and Lai, C.L. 1988. A longitudinal follow-up of asymptomatic hepatitis B surface antigen positive Chinese children. *Hepatology*, **8**, 1130–3.

Long, S.S. 1997. Toddler-to-mother transmission of varicella-vaccine virus: how bad is that? *J Pediatrics*, **131**, 10–12.

Lynch, L. and Ghidini, A. 1993. Perinatal infections. *Curr Opin Obstet Gynecol*, **5**, 24–32.

Lynch-Salamon, D.I. and Combs, C.A. 1992. Hepatitis C in obstetrics and gynecology. *Obstet Gynecol*, **79**, 621–9.

Maertens, G. and Stuyver, L. 1997. Genotypes and genetic variation of hepatitis C virus. In: Zuckerman, A.J. and Harrison, T.J. (eds), *Molecular medicine of viral hepatitis*. Chichester: John Wiley & Sons, 183–233.

Maiques, V., Garcia-Tejedor, A., et al. 2003. HIV detection in amniotic fluid samples. Amniocentesis can be performed in HIV pregnant women? *Eur J Obstet Gynecol Reprod Biol*, **108**, 137–41.

Malinger, G., Lev, D., et al. 2003. Fetal cytomegalovirus infection of the brain: the spectrum of sonographic findings. *Am J Neuroradiol*, **24**, 28–32.

Malm, G., Forsgren, M., et al. 1991. A follow-up study of children with neonatal herpes simplex virus infections with particular regard to nervous disturbances. *Acta Pediatr Scand*, **80**, 226–34.

Marranconi, F., Fabris, P., et al. 1994. Prevalence of anti-HCV and risk factors for hepatitis C virus infection in healthy pregnant women. *Infection*, **22**, 333–7.

Martin, K.A., Junker, A.K., et al. 1994. Occurrence of chickenpox during pregnancy in women seropositive for varicella-zoster virus. *J Infect Dis*, **170**, 991–5.

Maschmann, J., Hamprecht, K., et al. 2001. Cytomegalovirus infection of extremely low-birth weight infants via breast milk. *Clin Infect Dis*, **33**, 1998–2003.

Mast, E.E. 2004. Mother-to-infant hepatitis C virus transmission and breastfeeding. *Adv Exp Med Biol*, **554**, 211–16.

Mast, E.E. and Alter, M.J. 1993. Epidemiology of viral hepatitis: an overview. *Semin Virol*, **4**, 274–83.

Mast, E.E. and Krawczynski, K. 1996. Hepatitis E: an overview. *Annu Rev Med*, **47**, 257–66.

Matsuda, H., Kawakami, Y., et al. 2004. Intrauterine therapy for a cytomegalovirus-infected symptomatic fetus. *Br J Obstet Gynaecol*, **111**, 756–7.

Maxwell, D.J., Johnson, P., et al. 1991. Fetal blood sampling and pregnancy loss in relation to indication. *Br J Obstet Gynaecol*, **98**, 892–7.

Mazza, C., Ravaggi, A., et al. 1998. Prospective study of mother-to-infant transmission of hepatitis C virus (HCV) infection. Study Group for Vertical Transmission. *J Med Virol*, **54**, 12–19.

McDonnell, M. and Lucey, M.R. 1995. Hepatitis C infection. *Curr Opin Infect Dis*, **8**, 384–90.

Mehraein, Y., Rehder, H., et al. 1991. Die Diagnostik fetaler Virusinfektionen durch In-situ-Hybridisierung. *Geburtsh Frauenheilk*, **51**, 984–9.

Meisel, H., Reip, A., et al. 1995. Transmission of hepatitis C virus to children and husbands by women infected with contaminated anti-D immunoglobulin. *Lancet*, **345**, 1209–11.

Mele, A., Tancredi, F., et al. 2001. Effectiveness of hepatitis B vaccination in babies born to hepatitis B surface antigen-positive mothers in Italy. *J Infect Dis*, **184**, 905–8.

Metzman, R., Anand, A., et al. 1989. Hepatic disease associated with intrauterine parvovirus B19 infection in a newborn premature infant. *J Pediatr Gastroenter Nutr*, **9**, 112–14.

Meyers, J.D. 1974. Congenital varicella in term infants: risk reconsidered. *J Infect Dis*, **129**, 215–17.

Michaels, M.G., Greenberg, D.P., et al. 2003. Treatment of children with congenital cytomegalovirus infection with ganciclovir. *Pediatr Inf Dis J*, **22**, 504–8.

Milich, D.R., Jones, J.E., et al. 1990. Is a function of the secreted hepatitis B e antigen to induce immunologic tolerance in utero. *Proc Natl Acad Sci USA*, **87**, 6599–03.

Miller, E., Cradock-Watson, J. and Ridehalgh, M. 1989. Outcome in newborn babies given anti-varicella-zoster immunoglobulin after perinatal maternal infection with varicella-zoster virus. *Lancet*, **2**, 371–3.

Miller, E., Vurdien, J.E. and Farrington, P. 1993a. Shift in age in chickenpox. *Lancet*, **341**, 308–9.

Miller, E., Marshall, R. and Vurdien, J.E. 1993b. Epidemiology, outcome and control of varicella-zoster virus infection. *Rev Med Microbiol*, **4**, 222–30.

Miller, E., Fairley, C.K., et al. 1998. Immediate and long term outcome of human parvovirus B19 infection in pregnancy. *Br J Obstet Gynaecol*, **105**, 174–8.

Milne, A., Rodgers, E. and Hopkirk, N. 1995. Hepatitis B vaccination of babies in Melanesia. *Lancet*, **346**, 318.

Minkoff, H. 2001. Prevention of mother-to-child transmission of HIV. *Clin Obstet Gynecol*, **44**, 210–25.

Minkoff, H., Burns, D.N., et al. 1995. The relationship of the duration of ruptured membranes to vertical transmission of human immunodeficiency virus. *Am J Obstet Gynecol*, **173**, 585–9.

Mishkin, D. and Deschenes, M. 2001. Conception soon after discontinuing interferon/ribavirin therapy: a successful outcome. *Am J Gastroenterol*, **96**, 2285–6.

Mitchell, D.K., Holmes, S.J., et al. 2002. Immunogenicity of a recombinant human cytomegalovirus gB vaccine in seronegative toddlers. *Pediatr infect Dis J*, **21**, 133–8.

Mocarski, E.S., Abenes, G.B., et al. 1990. Molecular genetic analysis of cytomegalovirus gene regulation in growth, persistence and latency. *Curr Top Microbiol Immunol*, **154**, 46–74.

Mofenson, L.M., Lambert, J.S., et al. 1999. Risk factors for perinatal transmission of human immunodeficiency virus type 1 in women treated with zidovudine. Pediatric AIDS Clinical Trials Group Study 185 Team. *N Engl J Med*, **341**, 385–93.

Moniz, O.M., Ling, M., et al. 2003. HPV DNA vaccines. *Front Biosci*, **8**, D55–68.

Morey, A.L. and Fleming, K.A. 1992. Immunophenotyping of fetal haemopoietic cells permissive for human parvovirus B19 replication in vitro. *Br J Haematol*, **82**, 302–9.

Morey, A.L., Nicolini, U., et al. 1991. Parvovirus B19 infection and transient fetal hydrops. *Lancet*, **337**, 496.

Morishima, T., Morita, M. et al. 1996. Clinical survey on neonatal herpes simplex virus (HSV) infection in Japan. *21st Herpesvirus Workshop*, July 27–August 2, 401.

Moriya, T., Sasaki, F., et al. 1995. Transmission of hepatitis C virus from mothers to infants: its frequency and risk factors revisited. *Biomed Pharmacother*, **49**, 59–64.

Mosca, F., Pugni, L., et al. 2001. Transmission of cytomegalovirus. *Lancet*, **357**, 1800.

Mouly, F., Mirlesse, V., et al. 1997. Prenatal diagnosis of fetal varicella zoster virus infection with polymerase chain reaction of amniotic fluid in 107 cases. *Am J Obstet Gynecol*, **177**, 894–8.

Musiani, M., Zerbini, M., et al. 1995. Parvovirus B19 clearance from peripheral blood after acute infection. *J Infect Dis*, **172**, 1360–3.

Nahmias, A.J., Josey, W.E., et al. 1971. Perinatal risk associated with maternal genital herpes simplex virus infection. *Am J Obstet Gynecol*, **110**, 825.

Nanda, S.K., Ansari, I.H., et al. 1995. Protracted viremia during acute sporadic hepatitis E virus infection. *Gastroenterology*, **108**, 225–30.

Nathwani, D., Maclean, A., et al. 1998. Varicella infections in pregnancy and the newborn. *J Infect*, **36**, 59–71.

Nduati, R., John, G., et al. 2000. Effect of breastfeeding and formula feeding on transmission of HIV-1: a randomized clinical trial. *J Am Med Assoc*, **283**, 1167–74.

Negishi, H., Yamada, H., et al. 1998. Intraperitoneal administration of cytomegalovirus hyperimmunoglobulin to the cytomegalovirus-infected fetus. *J Perinatol*, **18**, 466–9.

Nelson, C.T., Istas, A.S., et al. 1995. PCR detection of cytomegalovirus DNA in serum as a diagnostic test for congenital cytomegalovirus infection. *J Clin Microbiol*, **33**, 3317–18.

Newell, M.L., Dunn, D., et al. 1996. Detection of virus in vertically exposed HIV-antibody negative children. *Lancet*, **347**, 213–15.

Ngui, S.L., Andrews, N.J., et al. 1998. Failed postnatal immunoprophylaxis for hepatitis B: characteristics of maternal hepatitis B virus as risk factors. *Clin Infect Dis*, **27**, 100–6.

Nguyen, Q.T., Sifer, C., et al. 1999. Novel human erythrovirus associated with transient aplastic anemia. *J Clin Microbiol*, **37**, 2483–7.

Nigro, G., Scholz, H. and Bartmann, U. 1994. Ganciclovir therapy for symptomatic congenital cytomegalovirus infection: a two-regimen experience. *J Pediatr*, **124**, 318–22.

Nigro, G., La Torre, R., et al. 1999. Hyperimmunoglobulin therapy for a twin fetus with cytomegalovirus infection and growth restriction. *Am J Obstet Gynecol*, **180**, 1222–6.

NIH. 2004. Recommendations for use of antiretroviral drugs in pregnant HIV-1-infected women for maternal health and interventions to reduce perinatal HIV-1 transmission in the United States. *Public Health Service Task Force*, assessed 23 June 2004, www.aidsinfo.nih.gov

Nikolaidis, E.T., Trost, D.C., et al. 1985. The relationship of histologic and clinical factors in laryngeal papillomatosis. *Arch Pathol Lab Med*, **109**, 24–9.

Norbeck, O., Papadogiannakis, N., et al. 2002. Revised clinical presentation of parvovirus B19-associated intrauterine fetal death. *Clin Infect Dis*, **35**, 1032–8.

Noyola, D.E., Demmler, G.J., et al. 2001. Early predictors of neurodevelopmental outcome in symptomatic congenital cytomegalovirus infection. *J Pediatr*, **138**, 325–31.

Numazaki, K., Chiba, S. and Asanuma, H. 2001. Transmission of cytomegalovirus. *Lancet*, **357**, 1799.

Nunoue, T., Kusuhara, K. and Hara, T. 2002. Human fetal infection with parvovirus B19: maternal infection time in gestation, viral persistence and fetal prognosis. *Pediatr Infect Dis J*, **21**, 1133–6.

O'Donovan, D., Ariyoshi, K., et al. 2000. Maternal plasma viral RNA levels determine marked differences in mother-to-child transmission rates of HIV-1 and HIV-2 in the Gambia. MRC/Gambia Government/ University College London Medical School working group on mother–child transmission of HIV. *AIDS*, **14**, 441–8.

Ogata, N., Cote, P.J., et al. 1999. Licensed recombinant hepatitis B vaccines protect against infection with the prototype surface gene mutants of hepatitis B virus. *Hepatology*, **30**, 779–86.

Ohto, H., Lin, H.H., et al. 1987. Intrauterine transmission of hepatitis B virus is closely related to placental leakage. *J Med Virol*, **21**, 1–6.

Ohto, H., Terazawa, S., et al. 1994. Transmission of hepatitis C virus from mothers to infants. *N Engl J Med*, **330**, 744–50.

Ohyama, M., Motegi, Y., et al. 1992. Ascending placentofetal infection caused by cytomegalovirus. *Br J Obstet Gynaecol*, **99**, 770.

Okamoto, M., Nagata, I., et al. 2000. Prospective reevaluation of risk factors in mother-to-child transmission of hepatitis C virus: high virus load, vaginal delivery, and negative anti-NS4 antibody. *J Infect Dis*, **182**, 1511–14.

Omata, M., Ehata, T., et al. 1991. Mutations in the precore region of hepatitis B virus DNA in patients with fulminant and severe hepatitis. *N Engl J Med*, **324**, 1699–704.

Ouellet, A., Sherlock, R., et al. 2004. Antenatal diagnosis of intrauterine infection with coxsackievirus B3 associated with live birth. *Infect Dis Obstet Gynecol*, **12**, 23–6.

Ozaslan, E., Yilmaz, R., et al. 2002. Interferon therapy for acute hepatitis C during pregnancy. *Ann Pharmacother*, **36**, 1715–18.

Paccagnini, S., Principi, N., et al. 1995. Perinatal transmission and manifestation of hepatitis C virus infection in a high risk population. *Pediatr Infect Dis J*, **14**, 195–9.

Papaevangelou, V., Pollack, H., et al. 1998. Increased transmission of vertical hepatitis C virus (HCV) infection to human immunodeficiency virus (HIV)-infected infants of HIV- and HCV-coinfected women. *J Infect Dis*, **178**, 1047–52.

Paryani, S.G. and Arvin, A.M. 1986. Intrauterine infection with varicella-zoster virus after maternal varicella. *N Engl J Med*, **314**, 1542–6.

Pass, R.F. and Burke, R.L. 2002. Development of cytomegalovirus vaccines: Prospects for prevention of congenital CMV infection. *Semin Pediatr Infect Dis*, **13**, 196–204.

Pastuszak, A.L., Levy, M., et al. 1994. Outcome after maternal varicella infection in the first 20 weeks of pregnancy. *N Engl J Med*, **330**, 901–5.

Patsner, B., Baker, D.A. and Orr, J.W.J. 1990. Human papillomavirus genital tract infections during pregnancy. *Clin Obstet Gynecol*, **33**, 258–67.

Peckham, C.S. and Gibb, D. 1995. Mother-to-child transmission of the human immunodeficiency virus. *N Engl J Med*, **333**, 298–302.

Pignatelli, S., Dal Monte, P., et al. 2003. Intrauterine cytomegalovirus infection and glycoprotein N (gN) genotypes. *J Clin Virol*, **28**, 38–43.

Pipan, C., Amici, S., et al. 1996. Vertical transmission of hepatitis C virus in low-risk pregnant women. *Eur J Clin Microbiol Infect Dis*, **15**, 116–20.

Plotkin, S.A. 2001. Vaccination against cytomegalovirus. *Arch Virol Suppl*, **17**, 121–34.

Plotkin, S.A. 2004. Congenital cytomegalovirus infection and its prevention. *Clin Infect Dis*, **38**, 1038–9.

Polycarpou, A., Ntais, C., et al. 2002. Association between maternal and infant class I and II HLA alleles and of their concordance with the risk of perinatal HIV type 1 transmission. *AIDS Res Hum Retrovir*, **18**, 741–6.

Polywka, S., Feucht, H., et al. 1997. Hepatitis C virus infection in pregnancy and the risk of mother-to-child transmission. *Eur J Clin Microbiol Infect Dis*, **16**, 121–4.

Porter, H.J., Quantrill, A.M. and Fleming, K.A. 1988. B19 parvovirus infection in myocardial cells. *Lancet*, **1**, 535–6.

Prober, C.G. and Enright, A.M. 2003. Congenital cytomegalovirus (CMV) infections: hats off to Alabama. *J Pediatr*, **143**, 4–6.

Prober, C.G., Hensleigh, P.A., et al. 1988. Use of routine viral cultures at delivery to identify neonates exposed to herpes simplex virus. *N Engl J Med*, **318**, 887–91.

Pryde, P.G., Nugent, C.E., et al. 1992. Spontaneous resolution of nonimmune hydrops fetalis secondary to human parvovirus B19 infection. *Obstet Gynecol*, **79**, 859–61.

Public Health Laboratory Service Working Party of Fifth Disease. 1990. Prospective study of human parvovirus (B19) infection in pregnancy. *Br Med J*, **300**, 1166–70.

Puchhammer-Stöckl, E., Kunz, C., et al. 1994. Detection of varicella-zoster virus (VZV) DNA in fetal tissue by polymerase chain reaction. *J Perinat Med*, **22**, 65–9.

Purcell, R.H., Nguyen, H., et al. 2003. Pre-clinical immunogenicity and efficacy trial of a recombinant hepatitis E vaccine. *Vaccine*, **21**, 2607–15.

Purdy, M.A. and Krawczynski, K. 1994. Hepatitis E. *Gastroenterol Clin North Am*, **23**, 537–46.

Quick, C.A., Watts, S.L., et al. 1980. Relationship between condylomata and laryngeal papillomata: clinical and molecular virological evidence. *Ann Otol Rhinol Laryngol*, **89**, 467–71.

Ramia, S. and Bahakim, H. 1988. Perinatal transmission of hepatitis B virus-associated hepatitis D virus. *Ann Inst Pasteur Virol*, **139**, 285–90.

Randolph, A.G., Washington, A.E. and Prober, C.G. 1993. Caesarean delivery for women presenting with genital herpes lesions. *J Am Med Assoc*, **270**, 77–82.

Reddehase, M.J., Balthesen, M., et al. 1994. The conditions of primary infection define the load of latent viral genome in organs and the risk of recurrent cytomegalovirus disease. *J Exp Med*, **179**, 185–93.

Reinhard, G., Noll, A., et al. 1998. Shift in the Th1/Th2 balance during human pregnancy correlate with apoptotic changes. *Biochem Biophys Res Commun*, **245**, 933–8.

Resti, M., Azzari, C., et al. 1995. Mother-to-infant transmission of hepatitis C virus. *Acta Paediatr*, **84**, 251–5.

Resti, M., Azzari, C., et al. 1998. Mother to child transmission of hepatitis C virus: prospective study of risk factors and timing of infection in children born to women seronegative for HIV-1. Tuscany Study Group on Hepatitis C Virus Infection. *Br Med J*, **317**, 437–41.

Resti, M., Bortolotti, F., et al. 2000. Transmission of hepatitis C virus from infected mother to offspring during subsequent pregnancies. *J Pediatr Gastroenterol Nutr*, **30**, 491–3.

Resti, M., Azzari, C., et al. 2002. Italian Study Group on Mother-to-Infant Hepatitis C Virus Transmission. Maternal drug use is a preeminent risk factor for mother-to-child hepatitis C virus transmission: results from a multicenter study of 1372 mother–infant pairs. *J Infect Dis*, **185**, 567–72.

Reth, P., Sola, R., et al. 1995. The effect of pregnancy on the course of chronic hepatitis C. *Gastroenterol Hepatol*, **18**, 162, letter, in Spanish.

Revello, M.G. and Gerna, G. 2002. Diagnosis and management of human cytomegalovirus infection in the mother, fetus, and newborn infant. *Clin Microbiol Rev*, **15**, 680–715.

Revello, M.G. and Gerna, G. 2004. Pathogenesis and prenatal diagnosis of human cytomegalovirus infection. *J Clin Virol*, **29**, 71–83.

Revello, M.G., Percivalle, E., et al. 1993. Prenatal treatment of congenital human cytomegalovirus infection by fetal intravascular administration of ganciclovir. *Clin Diagn Virol*, **1**, 61–7.

Revello, M.G., Baldanti, F., et al. 1995. Polymerase chain reaction for prenatal diagnosis of congenital human cytomegalovirus infection. *J Med Virol*, **47**, 462–6.

Revello, M.G., Zavattoni, M., et al. 1999a. Diagnostic and prognostic value of human cytomegalovirus load and IgM antibody in blood of congenitally infected newborns. *J Clin Virol*, **14**, 57–66.

Revello, M.G., Zavattoni, M., et al. 1999b. Prenatal diagnostic and prognostic value of human cytomegalovirus load and IgM antibody response in blood of congenitally infected fetuses. *J Infect Dis*, **180**, 1320–3.

Revello, M.G., Zavattoni, M., et al. 2002. Diagnosis and outcome of preconceptional and periconceptional primary human cytomegalovirus infections. *J Infect Dis*, **186**, 553–7.

Reynolds, L., Struik, S. and Nadel, S. 1999. Neonatal varicella: varicella-zoster immunoglobulin (VZIG) does not prevent disease. *Arch Dis Child Fetal Neonatal Ed*, **81**, F69–70.

Riongeard, P., Sankale, J.L., et al. 1992. Infection due to hepatitis delta virus in Africa: report from Senegal and review. *Clin Infect Dis*, **14**, 510–14.

Roback, J.D. 2002. CMV and blood transfusions. *Rev Med Virol*, **12**, 211–19.

Robert Koch Institut. 1995. Impfempfehlungen der Ständigen Impfkommission am Robert-Koch-Institut (STIKO). *Inf Fo*, **4**, i–xii.

Robert Koch Institut. 2002a. Postexpositionelle Prophylaxe der HIV-Infektion. Deutsch-Österreichische Empfehlungen Aktualisierung Mai 2002. Gemeinsame Erklärung der Deutschen AIDS-Gesellschaft (DAIG) und der Österreichischen AIDS-Gesellschaft (ÖAG), www.rki.de/infekt/aids_std/expo/hiv.htm

Robert Koch Institut. 2002b. Impfempfehlungen der Ständigen Impfkommission (STIKO) am Robert-Koch-Institut/Stand: Juli 2002. *Epidemiol Bull*, **28**, 227–42.

Robert Koch Institut. 2003. HIV-Infektionen/AIDS: 10. Retroviruskonferenz in Boston – epidemiologische Aspekte. *Epidemiol Bull*, **15**, 111–15.

Robert Koch Institut. 2004. Empfehlungen der Ständigen Impfkommission (STIKO) am Robert Koch-Institut/Stand Juli 2004. *Epidemiol Bull*, **30**, 235–50.

Roberts, E.A. and Yeung, L. 2002. Maternal–infant transmission of hepatitis C virus infection. *Hepatology*, **36**, 106–13.

Roden, R.B., Ling, M. and Wu, T.C. 2004. Vaccination to prevent and treat cervical cancer. *Hum Pathol*, **35**, 971–82.

Rodis, J.F., Quinn, D.L., et al. 1990. Management and outcomes of pregnancies complicated by human B19 parvovirus infection: a prospective study. *Am J Obstet Gynecol*, **163**, 1168–71.

Rodis, J.F., Borgida, A.F., et al. 1998a. Management of parvovirus infection in pregnancy and outcomes of hydrops: a survey of members of the Society of Perinatal Obstetricians. *Am J Obstet Gynecol*, **179**, 985–8.

Rodis, J.F., Rodner, C., et al. 1998b. Long-term outcome of children following maternal human parvovirus B19 infection. *Obstet Gynecol*, **91**, 125–8.

Rollins, N., Meda, N., et al. 2004. Preventing postnatal transmission of HIV-1 through breast-feeding: modifying infant feeding practices. *J Acq Imm Def Syn*, **35**, 188–95.

Roman, A. and Fife, K. 1986. Human papillomavirus DNA associated foreskins of normal newborns. *J Infect Dis*, **153**, 855–61.

Rorabough, M., Berlin, L., et al. 1992. Absence of neurodevelopmental sequelae from aseptic meningitis. *Pediatr Res*, **31**, 177A.

Rosenblum, L.S., Villarino, M.E., et al. 1991. An outbreak in a neonatal intensive care unit: risk factors for transmission and evidence of prolonged viral excretion among preterm infants. *J Infect Dis*, **164**, 476–82.

Ruellan-Eugene, G., Barjot, P., et al. 1996. Evaluation of virological procedures to detect fetal cytomegalovirus infection: avidity of IgG antibodies, virus detection in amniotic fluid and maternal serum. *J Med Virol*, **50**, 9–15.

Ruff, T.A., Gertig, D.M., et al. 1995. Lombok hepatitis B model immunization project: toward universal infant hepatitis B immunization in Indonesia. *J Infect Dis*, **171**, 290–6.

Saada, M., Le Chenadec, J., et al. 2000. Pregnancy and progression to AIDS: results of the French prospective cohorts. Serogest und Seroco Study Groups. *AIDS*, **14**, 2355–60.

Sagliocca, L., Amoroso, P., et al. 1999. Efficacy of hepatitis A vaccine in prevention of secondary hepatitis A infection: a randomised trial. *Lancet*, **353**, 1136–9.

Saller, D.N., Rogers, B.B. and Canick, J.A. 1993. Maternal serum biochemical markers in pregnancies with fetal parvovirus B19 infection. *Prenat Diagn*, **13**, 467–71.

Sasaki, N., Matsui, A., et al. 1997. Loss of circulating hepatitis C virus in children who developed a persistent carrier state after mother-to-baby transmission. *Pediatr Res*, **42**, 263–7.

Sauerbrei, A. 1998. Varicella-zoster virus infections in pregnancy. *Intervirology*, **41**, 191–6.

Sauerbrei, A. and Wutzler, P. 2003. Fetales Varizellensyndrom. *Monatsschr Kinderheilkd*, **151**, 209–13.

Sauerbrei, A., Müller, D., et al. 1996. Detection of varicella zoster virus in congenital varicella syndrome: a case report. *Obstet Gynecol*, **88**, 687–9.

Sauerbrei, A., Gluck, B., et al. 2000. Congenital skin lesions caused by intrauterine infection with coxsackievirus B3. *Infection*, **28**, 326–8.

Scarlatti, G., Albert, J., et al. 1993. Mother-to-child transmission of human immunodeficiency virus type 1: correlation with neutralizing antibodies against primary isolates. *J Infect Dis*, **168**, 207–10.

Schalasta, G., Arents, A., et al. 2000. Fast and type-specific analysis of herpes simplex virus types 1 and 2 by rapid PCR and fluorescence melting-curve-analysis. *Infection*, **28**, 85–91.

Schalm, S.W. and Pit-Grosheide, P. 1989. Prevention of hepatitis B transmission at birth. *Lancet*, **1**, 44.

Schalm, S., De Man, R., et al. 2002. Combination and newer therapies for chronic hepatitis B. *J Gastroenterol Hepatol*, **17**, Suppl. 3, S338–41.

Scharf, A., Scherr, O., et al. 1990. Virus detection in the fetal tissue of a premature delivery with congenital varicella syndrome. A case report. *J Perinat Med*, **18**, 317–22.

Schild, R.L., Plath, H., et al. 1998. Fetal parvovirus B19 infection and meconium peritonitis. *Fetal Diagn Ther*, **13**, 15–18.

Schild, R.L., Bald, R., et al. 1999. Intrauterine management of fetal parvovirus B19 infection. *Ultrasound Obstet Gynecol*, **13**, 161–6.

Schmader, K. 2001. Herpes zoster in older adults. *Clin Infect Dis*, **32**, 1481–6.

Schödel, F. 1994. Emerging viral mutants in hepatitis B. *Lancet*, **343**, 355.

Schorling, S., Schalasta, G., et al. 2004. Quantification of parvovirus B19 DNA using COBAS AmpliPrep automated sample preparation and LightCycler real-time PCR. *J Mol Diagn*, **6**, 37–41.

Schulze-Oechtering, F., Roth, B., et al. 2004. Kongenitales Varizellensyndrom – besteht eine Infektionsgefahr für die Umgebung. *Z Geburtsh Neonatol*, **208**, 25–8.

Schupbach, J., Tomasik, Z., et al. 1994. IgG, IgM, and IgA response to HIV in infants born to HIV-1 infected mothers. Swiss Neonatal HIV Study Group. *J Acq Imm Def Syn*, **7**, 421–7.

Schwarz, T.F., Roggendorf, M., et al. 1988. Human parvovirus B19 infection in pregnancy. *Lancet*, **2**, 566–7.

Schwarz, T.F., Nerlich, A. and Roggendorf, M. 1990. Parvovirus B19 infection in pregnancy. *Behring Inst Mitt*, **85**, 69–77.

Schwarz, T.F., Jäger, G., et al. 1992. Diagnosis of human parvovirus B19 infections by polymerase chain reaction. *Scand J Infect Dis*, **24**, 691–6.

Scott, F., Peters, H., et al. 2002. The loss for invasive prenatal testing in a specialised obstetric ultrasound practice. *Aust NZ J Obstet Gynaecol*, **42**, 55–8.

Searle, K., Guilliard, C. and Enders, G. 1997. Parvovirus B19 diagnosis in pregnant women – quantification of IgG antibody levels (IU/ml) with reference to the international parvovirus B19 standard serum. *Infection*, **25**, 32–4.

Searle, K., Schalasta, G. and Enders, G. 1998. Development of antibodies to the nonstructural protein NS1 of parvovirus B19 during acute symptomatic and subclinical infection in pregnancy: implications for pathogenesis doubtful. *J Med Virol*, **56**, 192–8.

Sedlacek, T.V., Lindheim, S., et al. 1989. Mechanism for human papillomavirus transmission at birth. *Am J Obstet Gynecol*, **161**, 55–9.

Servant, A., Laperche, S., et al. 2002. Genetic diversity within human erythroviruses: identification of three genotypes. *J Virol*, **76**, 9124–34.

Seward, J., Galil, K. and Wharton, M. 2000. Epidemiology of varicella. In: Arvin, A.M. and Gershon, A.A. (eds), *Varicella-zoster virus: virology and clinical management*. Cambridge: Cambridge University Press, 187–205.

Shalev, E. and Bassan, H.M. 1982. Viral hepatitis during pregnancy in Israel. *Int J Gynaecol Obstet*, **20**, 73–8.

Shattuck, K. and Chonmaitree, T. 1992. The changing spectrum of neonatal meningitis over a fifteen-year period. *Clin Pediatr (Phila)*, **31**, 130–6.

Sheikh, A.U., Ernest, J.M. and O'Shea, M. 1992. Long-term outcome in fetal hydrops from parvovirus B19 infection. *Am J Obstet Gynecol*, **167**, 337–41.

Sheinbergas, M.M. 1975. Antibody to lymphocytic choriomeningitis virus in children with congenital hydrocephalus. *Acta Virol (Praha)*, **19**, 165–6.

Sheinbergas, M.M. 1976. Hydrocephalus due to prenatal infection with the lymphocytic choriomeningitis virus. *Infection*, **4**, 185–91.

Shen, C.Y., Chang, S.F., et al. 1993. Cytomegalovirus excretion in pregnant and nonpregnant women. *J Clin Microbiol*, **31**, 1635–6.

Shen, C.Y., Chang, S.F., et al. 1994. Cytomegalovirus is present in semen from a population of men seeking fertility evaluation. *J Infect Dis*, **169**, 222–3.

Shields, K.E., Galil, K., et al. 2001. Varicella vaccine exposure during pregnancy: data from the first 5 years of the pregnancy registry. *Obstet Gynecol*, **98**, 14–19.

Sills, J.A., Galloway, A., et al. 1987. Acyclovir in prophylaxis and perinatal varicella. *Lancet*, **1**, 161.

Silverman, N.S., Darby, M.J., et al. 1991. Hepatitis B prevalence in an unregistered prenatal population. *J Am Med Assoc*, **266**, 282–5.

Simmonds, P. 1995. Variability of hepatitis C virus. *Hepatology*, **21**, 570–83.

Simoes, E.A.F. and Abzug, M.J. 1993. Enteroviruses: issues in poliomyelitis immunization and perinatal enterovirus infections. *Curr Opin Infect Dis*, **6**, 547–52.

Simons, J.N., Leary, T.P., et al. 1995. Isolation of novel virus-like sequences associated with human hepatitis. *Nature Med*, **1**, 564–9.

Sinzger, C., Müntefering, H., et al. 1993. Cell types infected in human cytomegalovirus placentitis identified by immunohistochemical double staining. *Virchows Arch A Pathol Anat Histopathol*, **423**, 249–56.

Sjogren, M.H., Tanno, H., et al. 1987. Hepatitis A virus in stool during clinical relapse. *Ann Intern Med*, **106**, 221–6.

Skjöldebrand-Sparre, L., Tolfvenstam, T., et al. 2000. Parvovirus B19 infection: association with third-trimester intrauterine fetal death, 2000. *Br J Obstet Gynaecol*, **107**, 476–80.

Slomka, M.J. 1996. Seroepidemiology and control of genital herpes: the value of type specific antibodies to herpes simplex virus. *CDR Rev*, **6**, R41–5.

Smedile, A., Dentico, P., et al. 1981. Infection with HBV associated delta agent in HBsAg carriers. *Gastroenterology*, **81**, 992–7.

Smego, R.A. and Asperilla, M.O. 1991. Use of acyclovir for varicella pneumonia during pregnancy. *Obstet Gynecol*, **78**, 1112–16.

Smith, J.G., Liu, X., et al. 2001. Development and validation of a gamma interferon ELISPOT assay for quantitation of cellular immune responses to varicella-zoster virus. *Clin Diagn Lab Immunol*, **8**, 871–9.

Smith, J.S. and Robinson, N.J. 2002. Age-specific prevalence of infection with herpes simplex virus type 2 and 1: a global review. *J Infect Dis*, **186**, Suppl. 1, S3–S28.

Sobaszek, A., Fantoni-Quinton, S., et al. 2000. Prevalence of cytomegalovirus infection among health care workers in pediatric and immunosuppressed adult units. *J Occup Environ Med*, **42**, 1109–14.

Soulie, J.C. 1995. Cardiac involvement in fetal parvovirus B19 infection. *Pathol Biol (Paris)*, **43**, 416–19.

Spano, L., Vargas, P., et al. 2002. Cytomegalovirus in human abortion in Espirito Santo, Brazil. *J Clin Virol*, **2**, 173.

Spencer, J.D., Latt, N., et al. 1997. Transmission of hepatitis C virus to infants of human immunodeficiency virus-negative intravenous drug-using mothers: rate of infection and assessment of risk factors for transmission. *J Viral Hepat*, **4**, 395–409.

Sperling, R.S., Shapiro, D.E., et al. 1996. Maternal viral load, zidovudine treatment, and the risk of transmission of human immunodeficiency virus type 1 from mother to infant. Pediatric AIDS Clinical Trials Group Protocol 076 Study Group. *N Engl J Med*, **335**, 1621–9.

Stagno, S. 2001. Cytomegalovirus. In: Remington, J.S. and Klein, J.O. (eds), *Infectious diseases of the fetus and newborn infant*, 5th edn. Philadelphia: W.B. Saunders, 389–425.

Stagno, S. and Cloud, G.A. 1994. Working parents: the impact of day care and breast-feeding on cytomegalovirus infections in offspring. *Proc Natl Acad Sci USA*, **91**, 2384–9.

Stagno, S., Pass, R.F., et al. 1986. Primary cytomegalovirus infection in pregnancy: incidence, transmission to fetus and clinical outcome. *J Am Med Assoc*, **256**, 1904–8.

Stanberry, L.R., Spruance, S.L., et al. 2002. Glycoprotein-D-adjuvant vaccine to prevent genital herpes. *N Engl J Med*, **347**, 1703–5.

Stephenson, T. 1993. Chickenpox in pregnancy. *Br Med J*, **306**, 1753.

Stern, H., Hannington, G., et al. 1986. An early marker of fetal infection after primary cytomegalovirus infection in pregnancy. *Br Med J*, **292**, 718–20.

Stevens, C.E., Neurath, R.A., et al. 1979. HBeAg and anti-HBe detection by radioimmunoassay: correlation with vertical transmission of hepatitis B virus in Taiwan. *J Med Virol*, **3**, 237–41.

Stone, K.M., Brooks, C.A., et al. 1989. National surveillance for neonatal herpes simplex virus infections. *Sex Transm Dis*, **16**, 152–6.

Stratov, I., DeRose, R., et al. 2004. Vaccines and vaccine strategies against HIV. *Curr Drug Targets*, **5**, 71–88.

Stray-Pedersen, B. 1990. Acyclovir in late pregnancy. *Lancet*, **2**, 756.

Stronati, M., Revello, M.G., et al. 1995. Ganciclovir therapy of congenital human cytomegalovirus hepatitis. *Acta Pediatr*, **84**, 340–1.

Sutherland, S. 1993. *Torch screening reassessed*, 2nd edn. London: Public Health Laboratory Service.

Svennerholm, B., Olofsson, S., et al. 1984. Herpes simplex virus type-selective enzyme linked immunosorbent assay with helix pomatia lectin-purified antigens. *J Clin Microbiol*, **19**, 235–9.

Syrjanen, S. and Puranen, M. 2000. Human papillomavirus infections in children: the potential role of maternal transmission. *Crit Rev Oral Biol Med*, **11**, 259–74.

Swain, S., Cameron, A.D., et al. 1999. Prenatal diagnosis and management of nonimmune hydrops fetalis. *Aust NZ J Obstet Gynaecol*, **39**, 285–90.

Taha, T.E., Kumwenda, N.I., et al. 1999. Mortality after the first year of life among human immunodeficiency virus type 1-infected and uninfected children. *Pediatr Infect Dis J*, **18**, 689–94.

Tajiri, H., Miyoshi, Y., et al. 2001. Prospective study of mother-to-infant transmission of hepatitis C virus. *Pediatr Infect Dis J*, **20**, 10–14.

Temple, R.O., Pass, R.F. and Boll, T.J. 2000. Neuropsychological functioning in patients with asymptomatic congenital cytomegalovirus infection. *J Dev Behav Pediatr*, **21**, 417–22.

Terada, S., Kawanishi, K. and Katayama, K. 1992. Minimal hepatitis C infectivity in semen. *Ann Intern Med*, **117**, 171–2.

Terazawa, S., Kojima, M., et al. 1991. Hepatitis B virus mutants with precore-region defects in two babies with fulminant hepatitis and mothers positive for antibody to hepatitis B antigen. *Pediatr Res*, **29**, 5–9.

Tercanli, S., Enders, G. and Holzgreve, W. 1996. Aktuelles Management bei mütterlichen Infektionen mit Röteln, Toxoplasmose, Zytomegalie, Varizellen und Parvovirus B19 in der Schwangerschaft. *Gynäkologe*, **29**, 144–63.

Thaler, M.M., Park, C.K., et al. 1991. Vertical transmission of hepatitis C virus. *Lancet*, **338**, 17–18.

Thomas, D.L., Villano, S.A., et al. 1998. Perinatal transmission of hepatitis C virus from human immunodeficiency virus type 1-infected mothers. Women and Infants Transmission Study. *J Infect Dis*, **177**, 1480–8.

Thomas, H.I.J., Morgan-Capner, P. and Meurisse, E.V. 1990. Studies on the avidity of IgG1 subclass antibody specific for varicella-zoster virus. *Serodiagn Immunother Infect Dis*, **4**, 371–7.

Tiessen, R.G., van Elsacker-Niele, A.M., et al. 1994. A fetus with a parvovirus B19 infection and congenital anomalies. *Prenat Diagn*, **14**, 173–6.

Toivanen, P., Rossi, T. and Hirvonen, T. 1969. Immunoglobulins in human fetal sera at different stages of gestation. *Experientia*, **25**, 527–8.

Tolfvenstam, T., Papadogiannakis, N., et al. 2001. Frequency of human parvovirus B19 infection in intrauterine fetal death. *Lancet*, **357**, 1494–7.

Torres, J.R. and Mondolfi, A. 1991. Protracted outbreak of severe delta hepatitis: experience in an isolated Amerindian population of the Upper Orinoco basin. *Rev Infect Dis*, **13**, 52–5.

Tovo, P.A., Palomba, E., et al. 1997. Increased risk of maternal–infant hepatitis C virus transmission for women coinfected with HIV type 1. Italian Study Group for HCV Infection in Children. *Clin Infect Dis*, **25**, 1121–4.

Trang, J.M., Kidd, L., et al. 1993. Linear single-dose pharmacokinetics of ganciclovir in newborns with congenital cytomegalovirus infections. *Clin Pharmacol Ther*, **53**, 15–21.

Trlifojova, J., Brenda, R. and Benes, C. 1986. Effect of maternal varicella-zoster virus infection on the outcome of pregnancy and the analysis of transplacental virus transmission. *Acta Virol (Praha)*, **30**, 249–55.

Trompeter, R.S., Bradley, J.M. and Griffiths, P.D. 1986. Varicella-zoster in the newborn. *Lancet*, **1**, 744.

Trotter, J.F. and Zygmunt, A.J. 2001. Conception and pregnancy during interferon-alpha therapy for chronic hepatitis C. *J Clin Gastroenterol*, **32**, 76–8.

US Department of Health and Human Services. 2002. Safety and toxicity of individual antiretroviral agents ind pregnancy. 23 May 2002, www.aidsinfo.nih.gov/guidelines/perinatal/STMay23.pdf

Valeur-Jensen, A.K., Pedersen, C.B., et al. 1999. Risk factors for parvovirus B19 infection in pregnancy. *J Am Med Assoc*, **281**, 1099–105.

Van de Perre, P. 1995. Postnatal transmission of human immunodeficiency virus type 1: the breast-feeding dilemma. *Am J Obstet Gynecol*, **173**, 483–7.

Vasileiadis, G.T., Roukema, H.W., et al. 2003. Intrauterine herpes simplex infection. *Am J Perinatol*, **20**, 55–8.

Verstraelen, H., Vanzieleghem, B., et al. 2003. Prenatal ultrasound and magnetic resonance imaging in fetal varicella syndrome: correlation with pathology findings. *Pren Diag*, **23**, 705–9.

Viazov, S., Riffelmann, M., et al. 1997. Transmission of GBV-C/HGV from drug-addicted mothers to their babies. *J Hepatol*, **27**, 85–90.

von Kaisenberg, C.S., Bender, G., et al. 2001. A case of fetal parvovirus B19 myocarditis, terminal cardiac heart failure, and perinatal heart transplantation. *Fetal Diagn Ther*, **16**, 427–32.

von Poblotzki, A., Gigler, A., et al. 1995. Antibodies to parvovirus B19 NS-1 protein in infected individuals. *J Gen Virol*, **76**, 519–27.

von Weizsäcker, F., Pult, I., et al. 1995. Selective transmission of variant genomes from mother to infant in neonatal fulminant hepatitis B. *Hepatology*, **21**, 8–13.

Vossen, M.T.M., Gent, M.R., et al. 2004. Development of virus-specific CD4+ T cells on reexposure to varicella-zoster virus. *J Infect Dis*, **190**, 72–82.

Wagenpfeil, S., Neiss, A., et al. 2004. Empirical data on the varicella situation in Germany for vaccination decisions. *Clin Microbiol Infect*, **10**, 425–30.

Walther, J.U., Gloning, K.P. and Schwarz, T.F. 1994. Prune belly nach Hydrops fetalis bei mütterlicher Parvovirus-B19-Infektion. *Monatsschr Kinderheilkd*, **142**, 592–5.

Wang, J.S. and Zhu, Q.R. 2000. Infection of the fetus with hepatitis B e antigen via the placenta. *Lancet*, **355**, 989.

Wang, J., Zhu, Q., et al. 2002. Effect of delivery mode on maternal-infant transmission of hepatitis B virus by immunoprophylaxis. *Chin Med J*, **115**, 1510–12.

Waters, J.A., Kennedy, M., et al. 1992. Loss of common A determinant of hepatitis B surface antigen by a vaccine-induced escape mutant. *J Clin Invest*, **90**, 2543–7.

Watson, J.C., Fleming, D.W., et al. 1993. Vertical transmission of hepatitis A resulting in an outbreak in a neonatal intensive care unit. *J Infect Dis*, **167**, 567–71.

Watts, D.H., Koutsky, L.A., et al. 1996. Risk of perinatal transmission of human papillomavirus (HPV) is low: results from a prospective cohort study. *Am J Obstet Gynecol*, **174**, 319.

Watts, D.H., Brown, Z.A., et al. 2003. A double-blind, randomized, placebo-controlled trial of acyclovir in late pregnancy for the reduction of herpes simplex virus shedding and cesarean delivery. *Am J Obstet Gynecol*, **188**, 836–43.

Webster, M.H. and Smith, C.S. 1977. Congenital abnormalities and maternal herpes zoster. *Br Med J*, **2**, 1193.

Wegmann, T.G., Lin, H., et al. 1993. Bidirectional cytokine interactions in the maternal–fetal relationship: is successful pregnancy a TH2 phenomenon? *Immunol Today*, **14**, 353–6.

Weigel-Kelley, K.A., Yoder, M.C. and Srivastava, A. 2003. Alpha5beta1 integrin as a cellular coreceptor for human parvovirus B19: requirement of functional activation of beta1 integrin for viral entry. *Blood*, **102**, 3927–33.

Weiland, H.T., Vermey-Keers, C., et al. 1987. Parvovirus B19 associated with fetal abnormality. *Lancet*, **1**, 682–3, letter.

Weinberg, A. 2002. The role of immune reconstitution in cytomegalovirus infection. *Biodrugs*, **16**, 89–95.

Weinberg, A., Hayward, A.R., et al. 1996. Comparison of two methods for detecting varicella-zoster virus antibody with varicella-zoster virus cell-mediated immunity. *J Clin Microbiol*, **34**, 445–6.

Weisser, M., Rudin, C., et al. 1998. Does pregnancy influence the course of HIV infection? Evidence from two large Swiss cohort studies. *J Acq Imm Def Syn Hum Retrovir*, **17**, 404–10.

Whitley, R.J. 1993. Neonatal herpes simplex virus infections. *J Med Virol*, **1**, 13–21.

Whitley, R.J. 1994. Herpes simplex virus infections of women and their offspring: implications for a developed society. *Proc Natl Acad Sci USA*, **91**, 2441–7.

Whitley, R.J. and Roizman, B. 2002. Herpes simplex viruses: is a vaccine tenable? *J Clin Invest*, **110**, 145–51.

Whitley, R.J., Cloud, G., et al. 1997. Ganciclovir treatment of symptomatic congenital cytomegalovirus infection: results of a phase II study. *J Infect Dis*, **175**, 1080–6.

Wilcox, A.J., Weinberg, C.R., et al. 1988. Incidence of early loss of pregnancy. *N Engl J Med*, **319**, 189–94.

Wilcox, A.J., Baird, D.D. and Weinberg, C.R. 1999. Time of implantation of the conceptus and loss of pregnancy. *New Engl J Med*, **340**, 1796–9.

Winchester, R., Chen, Y., et al. 1995. Major histocompatibility complex class II DR alleles DRB1*1501 and those encoding HLA-DR13 are preferentially associated with a diminution in maternally transmitted human immunodeficiency virus 1 infection in different ethnic groups: determination by an automated sequence-based typing method. *Proc Natl Acad Sci USA*, **92**, 12374–8.

Winchester, R., Pitt, J., et al. 2004. Mother-to-child transmission of HIV-1: strong association with certain maternal HLA-B alleles independent of viral load implicates innate immune mechanisms. *J Acq Imm Def Syn*, **36**, 659–70.

Wirth, S., Lang, T., et al. 2002. Recombinant alfa-interferon plus ribavirin therapy in children and adolescent with chronic hepatitis C. *Hepatology*, **36**, 1280–4.

Woolf, A.D., Campion, G.V., et al. 1989. Clinical manifestations of human parvovirus B19 in adults. *Arch Intern Med*, **149**, 1153–6.

World Health Organization. 2001. Effect of breastfeeding on mortality among HIV-infected women. WHO statement, 7 June 2001, www.who.int/reproductive-health/RTIs/MTCT/WHO_statement_on_breast_feeding_June_2001.html

Wright, C., Hinchliffe, S.A. and Taylor, C. 1996. Fetal pathology in intrauterine death due to parvovirus B19 infection. *Br J Obstet Gynaecol*, **103**, 133–6.

Xiong, S.K., Okajima, Y., et al. 1998. Vertical transmission of hepatitis C virus: risk factors and infantile prognosis. *J Obstet Gynaecol Res*, **24**, 57–61.

Xu, D.Z., Yan, Y.P., et al. 2001. Role of placental tissue in the intrauterine transmission of hepatitis B virus. *Am J Obstet Gynecol*, **185**, 981–7.

Xu, D.Z., Yan, Y.P., et al. 2002. Risk factors and mechanism of transplacental transmission of hepatitis B virus: a case-control study. *J Med Virol*, **67**, 20–6.

Yaegashi, N., Niinuma, T., et al. 1998. The incidence of, and factors leading to, parvovirus B19-related hydrops fetalis following maternal infection; report of 10 cases and meta-analysis. *J Infect*, **37**, 28–35.

Yaegashi, N., Niinuma, T., et al. 1999. Serologic study of human parvovirus B19 infection in pregnancy in Japan. *J Infection*, **38**, 30–5.

Ye, J.Y. 1990. Outcome of pregnancy complicated by hepatitis A in the urban districts of Shanghai. *Chung-Hua Fu Chan Ko Tsa Chih*, **25**, 219–21.

Yeager, A.S., Arvin, A.M., et al. 1980. Relationship of antibody to outcome in neonatal herpes simplex virus infections. *Infect Immun*, **29**, 532–8.

Yeung, L.T., King, S.M., et al. 2001. Mother-to-infant transmission of hepatitis C virus. *Hepatology*, **34**, 223–9.

Yoshida, M., Yamagami, N., et al. 1992. Case report detection of varicella-zoster virus DNA in maternal breast milk. *J Med Virol*, **38**, 108–10.

Yoshii, E., Shinzawa, H., et al. 1999. Molecular epidemiology of hepatitis C virus infection in an area endemic for community-acquired acute hepatitis C. *Tohoku J Exp Med*, **188**, 311–16.

Young, R.L., Acosta, A. and Kaufman, R.H. 1973. The treatment of large condylomata acuminata complicating pregnancy. *Obstet Gynecol*, **41**, 65–73.

Yow, M.D., Williamson, D.W., et al. 1988. Epidemiologic characteristics of cytomegalovirus infection in mothers and their infants. *Am J Obstet Gynecol*, **158**, 1189–95.

Zadori, Z., Szelei, J., et al. 2001. A viral phospholipase A_2 is required for parvovirus infectivity. *Dev Cell*, **1**, 291–302.

Zanetti, R.A., Gerroni, P., et al. 1982. Perinatal transmission of the hepatitis B virus and of the HBV-associated delta agent from mothers to offspring in northern Italy. *J Med Virol*, **9**, 139–48.

Zanetti, A.R., Tanzi, E., et al. 1995. Mother-to-infant transmission of hepatitis C virus. *Lancet*, **345**, 289–91.

Zanetti, A.R., Tanzi, E., et al. 1998. A prospective study on mother-to-infant transmission of hepatitis C virus. *Intervirology*, **41**, 208–12.

Zanetti, A.R., Romano, L. and Bianchi, S. 2003. Primary prevention of hepatitis C virus infection. *Vaccine*, **21**, 692–5.

Zerbini, M., Musiani, M., et al. 1993. Symptomatic parvovirus B19 infection of one fetus in a twin pregnancy. *J Clin Infect Dis*, **17**, 262–3.

Zhang, R.L., Zeng, J.S. and Zhang, H.Z. 1990. Survey of 34 pregnant women with hepatitis A and their neonates. *Chin Med J (Engl)*, **103**, 552–5.

Zhang, S.L., Han, X.B., et al. 1998. Relationship between HBV viremial level of pregnant women and intrauterine infection, nested PCR for detection of HBV DNA. *World J Gastroenterol*, **4**, 61–3.

Zhuang, Y.L. 1989. Acute hepatitis A in pregnancy: a report of 43 cases. *Chung-Hua Fu Chan Ko Tsa Chih*, **24**, 136–8.

Zimmermann, R., Perucchini, D., et al. 1995. Hepatitis C virus in breast milk. *Lancet*, **345**, 928, letter.

Zuccotti, G.V., Ribero, M.L., et al. 1995. Effect of hepatitis C genotype on mother-to-infant transmission of virus. *J Pediatr*, **127**, 278–80.

Zuckerman, A.J. 2000. Effect of hepatitis B virus mutants on efficacy of vaccination. *Lancet*, **355**, 1382–4.

64

Virus infections in immunocompromised patients

ANTHONY SIMMONS

Perturbations of immunity can influence the pathogenesis of viral infections in several ways. Prominent among these is increased frequency or severity of disease, exemplified par excellence by the debilitating manifestations of many herpesvirus infections in immunocompromised hosts. However, not all viral infections are exacerbated by immunosuppression and the acute stages of some diseases, such as hepatitis B, may be unusually mild. This is presumably because immunologically mediated lysis of infected cells contributes more than virally induced cell damage to the pathogenesis of some diseases in normal hosts.

Diagnosis of viral infections in immunocompromised patients can be difficult. Total and differential leukocyte counts tend to be unhelpful, clinical signs and symptoms of infection are often atypical, and symptoms produced by the host's immune response (e.g. the rash of measles) may be absent. Serology has little role in diagnosis because patients with dysfunctional immunity do not usually mount appropriate immune responses rapidly enough to influence decisions about management. The mainstay of diagnosis is detection of virus in appropriate clinical specimens: rapid procedures, such as direct antigen detection, nucleic acid detection and culture amplified enzyme immunoassays, have increased the usefulness of laboratory diagnosis enormously (Simmons 1996). In some situations (e.g. post-transplantation), regular surveillance cultures may be helpful: virus shedding may precede the onset of symptoms, and initiation of therapy as soon as virus is detected may prevent extensive tissue damage.

The AIDS pandemic has created an explosive increase in the number of profoundly immunocompromised people worldwide. The clinical manifestations of viral infections in human immunodeficiency virus (HIV)-infected individuals often differ significantly from the signs and symptoms caused by the same viruses in patients with other types of immune deficiency. Accordingly, a significant part of this chapter is devoted specifically to patients infected with HIV.

HIV-INFECTED ADULTS

The progressive decline in immunological function associated with HIV infection is usually monitored by measuring the absolute CD4$^+$ T-cell count. In general, significant opportunistic viral infections (Table 64.1) are not seen until CD4$^+$ T cells fall below 200/mm^3 and the most severe problems are associated with CD4$^+$ T-cell counts of <100/mm^3. Herpesviruses, particularly cytomegalovirus (CMV) and herpes simplex viruses types 1 and 2 (HSV-1 and HSV-2), are common causes of serious disease in profoundly immunosuppressed HIV-infected individuals and therefore herpesviruses receive particular attention here. Infections caused by papillomaviruses and enteric viruses are also given special consideration. Importantly, in locations where highly active antiretroviral therapy (HAART) is available, the prevalence in patients with AIDS of severe complications caused by viruses has been reduced considerably. Where appropriate, the discussion includes diagnosis and treatment of first-episode disease, prophylaxis against recurrence and, finally, measures to prevent acquisition of infection in previously unexposed individuals.

Table 64.1 *Opportunistic viral infections in HIV-infected patients*

Virus	Prominent clinical manifestations	References
Adenovirus	Gastroenteritis	Khoo et al. 1995
Retrovirus	Gastroenteritis	Grohmann et al. 1993
BK virus	Nephropathy, encephalitis	Vallbracht et al. 1993
Herpesviruses		
Cytomegalovirus	Retinitis, gastrointestinal disease, encephalitis, adrenalitis	Drew 1988; Peters et al. 1991
Epstein–Barr virus	Oral hairy leukoplakia, lymphoma	Andersson 1991
Herpes simplex virus type 1	Mucocutaneous lesions, keratoconjunctivitis	Stewart et al. 1995
Herpes simplex virus type 2	Genital and perianal ulceration	Stewart et al. 1995
Human herpesvirus 6	Pneumonitis, disseminated infection	Knox and Carrigan 1994
Human herpesvirus 8	Kaposi's sarcoma?	Chang et al. 1994
Varicella-zoster virus	Retinitis, recurrent dermatomal zoster, disseminated zoster, pneumonia, prolonged varicella	Buchbinder et al. 1992; Kelly et al. 1994
Hepatitis B virus	Increased rate of chronic infection	Hadler et al. 1991
Human papillomavirus	Recurrent and persistent anogenital warts, premalignant and malignant tumors, oral lesions	Palefsky 1991
Human parvovirus B19	Persistent anemia, red cell aplasia	Frickhofen et al. 1990
Influenza virus	Increased severity of illness	Safrin et al. 1990
JC virus	Progressive multifocal leukoencephalopathy	Berger et al. 1987
Measles virus	Encephalitis, pneumonia	Mustafa et al. 1993
Molluscum contagiosum virus	Disseminated cutaneous lesions	Epstein 1992
Parainfluenza virus	Exacerbation of respiratory symptoms	Hague et al. 1992
Picobirnavirus	Gastroenteritis	Grohmann et al. 1993
Respiratory syncytial virus	Increased mortality, prolonged viral shedding	Chandwani et al. 1990

Herpesvirus infections

Several genetically distinct herpesviruses have been isolated from humans. Some, namely HSV-1 and HSV-2, varicella-zoster virus (VZV), Epstein–Barr virus (EBV) and CMV have been recognized for decades. By contrast, human herpesviruses types 6 and 7 (HHV-6 and HHV-7) are relatively recent discoveries and the latest addition to the list, referred to here as *Human herpesvirus 8* HHV-8, is of particular interest in the present context because it is found in Kaposi's sarcoma (KS) cells (Chang et al. 1994).

Most well-characterized herpesviruses establish latent infections from which disease can periodically reactivate. In some cases, there are prolonged periods of asymptomatic virus shedding. Human herpesvirus (HHV) infections are generally acquired in early childhood and therefore most of the clinical problems associated with herpesviruses in adults are the result of reactivations. With the exception of varicella and herpes zoster, primary and recurrent HHV infections are often clinically unapparent and transmission of infection commonly occurs during periods of asymptomatic virus shedding.

The herpesviruses that cause greatest morbidity among HIV-infected people are HSV, CMV, VZV, and EBV. Occasional disease has been associated with

HHV-6 and HHV-8 is thought to have a causal relationship with KS.

HERPESVIRUSES AS COFACTORS IN PROGRESSION OF HIV-RELATED DISEASE

Aside from their direct clinical impact, it has been suggested that herpesviruses could be cofactors in the development of AIDS, i.e. herpesviruses might accelerate progression toward immunodeficiency and death by influencing the pathogenesis of HIV infection at the molecular or cellular level. Epidemiologic data supporting this hypothesis are limited. A study of HIV-infected hemophiliacs suggested more rapid progression to AIDS in CMV-seropositive compared with CMV-seronegative patients (Webster et al. 1989), but this result could not be confirmed in a similar study elsewhere (Rabkin et al. 1993). Probably the best way to address the hypothesis is to study the effect of herpesvirus-specific antiviral drugs on HIV progression. There have been several clinical trials in which patients have been treated prophylactically with the anti-herpes compound aciclovir, in addition to zidovudine. Two groups (Cooper et al. 1993; Youle et al. 1994) showed, independently, that combination therapy increased survival time compared with zidovudine alone. However, neither study showed a decrease in deaths related to any of the known human herpesviruses and the explanation for the apparent benefit of combination therapy remains obscure.

Although the proposal that herpesviruses promote the development of AIDS is in the realms of speculation, several molecular mechanisms can be envisaged by which HIV replication, or reactivation of latent provirus, could be enhanced.

For instance; all HHVs encode proteins called trans-activators, which up-regulate viral gene expression during replication. Some herpesvirus transactivators are 'promiscuous,' i.e. they can upregulate expression not only of herpesvirus genes but also of genes belonging to other viruses or host cells. In vitro, several herpesvirus transactivators have been shown to interact with the HIV long terminal repeat, which is the main region of the HIV genome responsible for controlling gene expression. Thus, co-infection of a cell with a herpesvirus and HIV could, in principle, result in enhanced HIV replication. Alternatively, reactivation of latent HIV might be stimulated by superinfection with a herpesvirus. The best candidates for herpesviruses that might enhance HIV replication are CMV and HHV-6 because these viruses are commonly found in the same tissues as HIV in autopsy specimens (Emery et al. 1999). Therefore, coinfection of, for example, lymphocytes with HIV and either CMV or HHV-6 is a theoretical possibility. Furthermore, HHV-6 infection has been shown to transactivate the HIV *tat* gene in vitro (Garzino-Demo et al. 1996).

Promiscuous transactivation of various cellular genes could also, in principle, promote the spread of HIV. For example, virus induced up-regulation of CD4, the main cell surface receptor for HIV, might facilitate the spread of HIV from cell to cell. Similarly, up-regulation of cell surface Fc receptors, a property of most herpesviruses, could enable antibody-coated HIV particles to enter CD4$^+$ cell types, thereby expanding the pool of HIV-infected cells.

Coinfection of a cell with more than one type of virus raises the possibility of phenotypic mixing and the formulation of virus pseudotypes. This phenomenon is well established in vitro and can be manipulated to the extent that HIV genomes can be packaged into the capsids of vesicular stomatitis viruses. Formation of pseudotypes comprising HIV genomes packaged into particles containing herpesvirus glycoproteins has not been documented in vivo, but nevertheless, pseudotype formation remains a theoretical way in which HIV genomes could gain entry into a wide variety of other-wise resistant cell types.

HERPES SIMPLEX VIRUSES TYPES 1 AND 2

Herpes simplex is one of the commonest infections of humans. HSV-2 is transmitted almost exclusively by sexual contact; consequently, HSV-2 seropositivity is rare before the onset of sexual activity. The epide-miology of HSV-1 is more diverse; infection is commonly acquired during infancy or childhood from infected oral secretions, but sexual transmission of HSV-1 is becoming increasingly common. HSV latently infects primary sensory neurons innervating the portal of entry, creating a reservoir of infection that can periodically give rise to recrudescent disease. The generally early acquisition of HSV means that most episodes of herpes simplex seen in the clinic are recrudescences.

In the context of HIV infection, HSV causes a wide spectrum of disease, including genital herpes, perioral and facial herpes, perianal lesions, proctitis, conjunctivitis and keratitis, aseptic meningoencephalitis, herpetic Whitlow, autonomic nervous system dysfunction and acute necrotizing retinitis. In profoundly immuno-compromised patients, with CD4$^+$ T-cell counts of <100/mm^3, extensive and chronic mucocutaneous ulceration is a frequently encountered and troublesome clinical problem, particularly in the genital and perianal regions (Safrin et al. 1991). In the absence of a normal inflammatory response, the lesions tend to respond slowly or poorly to antiviral therapy and they are often indolent or atypical in appearance.

In addition to prolonged mucocutaneous ulceration, there are several other severe manifestations of HSV infections in AIDS patients that merit further consideration. HSV may invade the esophagus or other parts of the gastrointestinal tract, giving rise to symptoms that reflect the region of the gut that is infected. Disseminated infection is rare but life-threatening. Many organs may be involved, including the lungs, liver, and adrenals. Prolonged ulcerative lesions and visceral disease are AIDS-defining illnesses.

There is evidence to suggest that genital ulceration facilitates sexual transmission of HIV and, in industrialized nations, the commonest cause of genital ulceration is HSV. By extrapolation, it has been proposed that genital herpes promotes the spread of HIV and there is some evidence that indirectly supports this contention (Holmberg et al. 1988; Stamm et al. 1988; Keet et al. 1990; Hook et al. 1992; Gwanzura et al. 1998).

Prevention of exposure

Strictly speaking, strategies designed to prevent exposure to HSV apply only to those rare individuals who are HSV-seronegative. However, first episode genital infections caused by HSV-2 in people previously exposed only orally to HSV-1 may be symptomatic; i.e. prior HSV-1 infection is, at best, only partially cross-protective against HSV-2 (Xu et al. 2002). Furthermore, in HIV-infected people, exogenous reinfection of the genital tract with different strains of HSV-2 is a possibility. With these considerations in mind, it is recommended that all HIV-infected people use latex condoms during every sexual contact. Condom usage is essential irrespective of whether the sexual partner has noticeable herpetic lesions, because HSV is frequently shed from the genital tract asymptomatically.

Treatment and suppression of symptoms

HSV replication is inhibited by aciclovir, its pro-drug valaciclovir, and famciclovir. Aciclovir is available in oral and intravenous formulations; the appropriate route of administration and dose depend on the severity of lesions and the degree of immunological impairment. Primary genital herpes can be managed with oral aciclovir or valaciclovir unless immune function is profoundly impaired or lesions are unusually severe, in which case intravenous aciclovir is required. Recurrent genital herpes in patients with early HIV infection generally resolves spontaneously. In this group of patients, the approach to management is the same as for immunocompetent people: symptomatic relief of mild, infrequent outbreaks or, in selected patients who experience clear prodromal symptoms, episodic valaciclovir (Bodsworth et al. 1997) or famciclovir. Continuous administration of valaciclovir should be considered for patients with frequent episodes (Patel et al. 1997) or when lesions tend to heal slowly. In advanced HIV infection, when immune suppression is profound, herpetic lesions often require prolonged therapy with high doses of an antiviral compound; treatment failure is not uncommon, even when the drug is administered intravenously (Whitley and Gnann 1992). In this patient population, emergence of aciclovir-resistant viral strains, which are also resistant to the related nucleoside analogue ganciclovir is an increasingly recognized problem (Chatis and Crumpacker 1992). There are few avenues available for the treatment of recalcitrant lesions caused by aciclovir-resistant virus, the main option being intravenous foscarnet or perhaps cidofovir (Kopp et al. 2002).

Aciclovir resistance

Aciclovir is a nucleoside analogue which, when phosphorylated, inhibits DNA replication. The drug is phosphorylated by an HSV-encoded enzyme, thymidine kinase (TK), hence it is active only in HSV-infected cells. Emergence of HSV strains resistant to aciclovir is rare in immunocompetent hosts, even after long-term suppressive therapy. The situation is different in immunocompromised hosts, particularly patients with advanced HIV infection, in whom aciclovir resistance is a significant clinical problem.

HSV becomes resistant to aciclovir by way of viral TK mutations that decrease the ability of the virus to phosphorylate the drug. Such mutations can also affect the ability of TK to phosphorylate nucleosides required for virus replication. However, TK-altered HSV strains are able to grow in most cell types, because cellular kinases substitute for viral TK. Consequently, aciclovir-resistant viruses may cause aggressive mucocutaneous lesions, However, non-dividing cells, notably neurons, express unusually low amounts of endogenous kinases and, in these cells, replication of aciclovir-resistant HSV strains is, fortuitously, inhibited. This has important practical consequences: HSV must replicate in neurons in order to reactivate from latency and, therefore, the latency/ reactivation cycle is interrupted for aciclovir-resistant viruses. The subtle influence of viral TK on the pathogenesis of herpes simplex may explain, in part, why aciclovir resistance is largely confined to patients treated over long periods for recalcitrant cutaneous lesions.

VARICELLA-ZOSTER VIRUS

Varicella is a common disease of childhood that is generally benign in immunocompetent hosts. In industrialized nations, seropositivity to VZV is >90 percent by the age of 15 years and therefore varicella is uncommon in adults. In the USA varicella vaccination is commonplace, further enhancing immunity among the young. This is fortunate, because the clinical impact of varicella in adults with impaired cellular immunity is high. Clinical manifestations include extensive, often hemorrhagic, cutaneous lesions and pneumonitis.

VZV establishes latency in sensory ganglia in much the same way as herpes simplex, although it has been suggested that the virus may be dormant in satellite glia rather than in neurons (Croen et al. 1988). However, despite controversy about the cell specificity of latent VZV for over a decade, it is now widely accepted that the virus is latent mainly in neurons, with only a small proportion of glia infected (Kennedy 2002). Recurrent VZV infection (herpes zoster, or shingles) is characterized by a blistering dermatomal rash and pain. HIV infection has a substantial impact on the incidence of VZV recurrence. HIV-infected adults are nine times more likely than the general population to develop herpes zoster (Holmberg et al. 1995) and the annual incidence of the disease is seven times higher in HIV-infected adults than in the general population. HIV-positive homosexual men are 17 times more likely to develop zoster than demographically matched HIV-negative subjects (Buchbinder et al. 1992).

The clinical manifestations of recurrent VZV infections in HIV-infected patients depend on the degree of immunological impairment. In the early stages of HIV infection, the signs and symptoms resemble herpes zoster in immunologically normal hosts. By contrast, repeated episodes of severe, prolonged, and sometimes atypical disease (Nikkels et al. 1999) are characteristic of advanced HIV infection. A few patients develop VZV retinitis, which has a particularly poor prognosis if the $CD4^+$ T-cell count is <50/mm^3. In some cases, atypical herpes zoster may require laboratory tests for confirmation of the diagnosis, in which case material from a recently erupted lesion should be sent for virus culture, rapid antigen detection or, if available, culture amplified enzyme immunoassay. Antemortem diagnosis of herpes zoster is particularly difficult when atypical manifestations of the disease, such as retinitis, meningoencephalitis, optic neuritis, and visceral involvement, occur in the absence of cutaneous lesions.

Prophylaxis and treatment

Most adults with no history of chickenpox have antibodies to VZV, and serological tests are useful for determining whether an HIV-infected patient is truly at risk of acquiring primary VZV infection. Seronegative patients should avoid contact with varicella- and herpes zoster; if contact is documented, they should receive varicella-zoster immunoglobulin (VZIG) within 96 hours of exposure. In addition, household contacts should be vaccinated against VZV if they have no history of chickenpox or are known to be seronegative provided they themselves do not have advanced HIV infection. The prophylactic effect of varicella vaccine, administered to susceptible HIV-infected people before CD4$^+$ T cells become depleted, has yet to be fully evaluated. However, varicella is not a cofactor for progression to AIDS (Aronson et al. 1992) and is a generally benign illness early in the course of HIV. As a consequence, varicella vaccine (Oka strain) should be considered for non-immunocompromised HIV-positive children.

Most cases of herpes zoster respond well to valaciclovir, famciclovir, or high-dose oral aciclovir. Disseminated, recurrent, or unusually severe cases should be treated intravenously. Aciclovir-resistant VZV strains have been isolated from severely immunocompromised people on long-term suppressive therapy (Lyall et al. 1994). The usual cause of resistance is mutation of the viral TK gene; aciclovir-resistant VZV remains sensitive to intravenous foscarnet (Balfour et al. 1994).

CYTOMEGALOVIRUS

CMV infection is extremely common among men who have sex with men (MSM) and intravenous drug users (IVDU) and in these populations it is generally acquired before HIV. Therefore primary CMV infections are rare among HIV-infected MSM and IVDU. Other HIV-infected people should be informed that CMV is shed in body fluids including semen, saliva, and cervical secretions and advised to use latex condoms during sexual contact. Reactivation of CMV does not cause illness in immunocompetent adults. By contrast, when cellular immunity is impaired, reactivation has many potential clinical manifestations, including retinitis, esophagitis, colitis, pneumonitis, and CNS disease. The spectrum of disease caused by recurrent CMV infection is significantly different in HIV-infected people compared with transplant recipients. For instance, necrotizing retinitis and CNS disease, common complications of CMV infec-

tion in advanced AIDS (Drew 1988; Jacobson and Mills 1988), are very unusual in the transplant setting. Conversely, CMV pneumonitis is unusual in HIV-infected adults but is not uncommon in transplant recipients.

CMV is frequently present in body fluids of AIDS patients and it is often difficult to establish a causal relationship between CMV and disease. Detection of CMV in affected organs provides circumstantial evidence that disease is CMV-related, but this approach frequently fails. CMV is often detected in bronchoalveolar lavage specimens from AIDS patients but this alone is not predictive of CMV pneumonitis; histological examination of cells or tissue for characteristic cytomegaly is required to establish the diagnosis.

Prevention, pre-emptive therapy, and treatment

HAART has had a profound impact on the previously high incidence of CMV disease in HIV-infected persons. However, not all patients are able or ready to take HAART and in some cases HAART may have failed. CMV remains therefore a significant problem. Unfortunately, immunization is not an option currently available for protection against primary CMV infection in the immunocompromised but general prophylactic measures are appropriate, including counseling about the risks of sexual transmission and the increased risk of CMV acquisition in the child care setting. In the latter situation, good hygienic practices including hand washing can reduce the risk of acquisition. In reality, measures to prevent exposure apply to only a small proportion of HIV-infected adults but it is essential that patients understand that CMV is present in genital secretions. Finally, if CMV-seronegative patients require transfusion, blood products should be obtained from CMV-seronegative donors.

Many adults are already infected with CMV when HIV infection is diagnosed and reconstituting immunity with HAART is the most effective way of preventing CMV disease from developing in seropositive persons. Ways to predict and prevent development of CMV disease (primary prophylaxis) are being explored, allowing pre-emptive therapy to be commenced before irreversible damage has been done. CMV viremia per se is no more predictive of CMV disease than CD4$^+$ T-cell counts (Salmon-Ceron et al. 2000); most patients who develop CMV disease have <200 CD4$^+$ T cells/mm^3, and the risk increases as the CD4$^+$ T-cell count falls. The greatest risk is in patients with <50 CD4$^+$ T cells/mm^3, in whom the median time to development of retinitis is 6 months. Anti-CMV drugs are generally too toxic for continuous administration to profoundly immuno-compromised persons (CD4$^+$ T-cell count <50/mm^3) and therefore true prophylaxis in AIDS patients awaits the development of safer, orally active compounds. Oral ganciclovir has been investigated for primary prophylaxis of CMV in AIDS but neutropenia, anemia, cost, and lack of proven efficacy have made its use a generally unpopular option.

The mainstays of treatment for established disease are intravenous ganciclovir, foscarnet, cidofovir, and fomivirsen, given intravitreally for retinitis. These drugs are toxic and treatment is not curative, so it is usual to reduce the dosage to maintenance levels after an initial period of induction. Without maintenance, relapse is inevitable; even on maintenance, relapse is common, necessitating periods of reinduction.

EPSTEIN–BARR VIRUS

HIV infection promotes the development of a variety of EBV-related diseases. Oral hairy leukoplakia is an EBV-associated hyperkeratotic disease of the tongue that is very common in HIV-infected patients but very rare otherwise. It responds to aciclovir but relapses if therapy is stopped. Lymphomas occur with greatly increased frequency in HIV-positive individuals, and a high proportion of the tumors, which tend to be monoclonal, contain cells expressing EBV antigens. Despite intensive chemotherapy, the prognosis is poor, especially in patients with low CD4$^+$ T-cell counts.

HUMAN HERPESVIRUSES 6 AND 7

HHV-6 and HHV-7 are ubiquitous, closely related betaherpesviruses, and most humans are infected with these agents in early childhood. Primary infection may be asymptomatic or cause roseola infantum. It is probable that both viruses establish latent infections in lymphoid tissues; in immunocompromised people, latent infection may reactivate and disseminate. HHV-6 is also known to be resident in the brain. In AIDS patients, HHV-6 has been detected in a wide variety of tissues postmortem and may cause fatal pneumonitis (Knox and Carrigan 1994). Further work is required to clarify its clinical impact.

HUMAN HERPESVIRUS 8 (KAPOSI'S SARCOMA-ASSOCIATED HERPESVIRUS)

HHV-8 is found in KS but not in normal skin. It is also associated with primary effusion lymphomas and some cases of multicentric Castelman's disease. On the basis of nucleotide sequence analysis, this agent is a gamma-2 herpesvirus, related to herpesvirus saimiri of squirrel monkeys and newly identified viruses of chimps and gorillas (Lacoste et al. 2000). Several lines of evidence suggest that HHV-8 plays an etiologic role in KS. First, antibodies against the virus are found in the sera of virtually all KS patients. Second, HHV-8 encodes several homologs of human proteins that could modulate cellular behavior, including a variety of cytokines (IL-6, MIPs, IRFs), cyclin D and a G-protein-coupled receptor (GPCR). Retinoblastoma protein and p53 are inhibited by viral cyclin D and the latency-associated nuclear antigen respectively and mice transgenic for GPCR have Kaposi-like regions in the skin. Finally, HHV-8 viral load in lymphocytes (Campbell et al. 2000) and skin lesions (Boivin et al. 2000) have been shown to increase with increasing disease burden.

Prevention and treatment

There is evidence to suggest that acquisition of HHV-8 after being infected with HIV may be associated with accelerated progression to KS, making prophylaxis against HHV-8 a priority. Counseling can be based on the three known routes of transmission, which are kissing (virus in saliva), sexual (virus in semen), bloodborne, and mother to child (Plancoulaine et al. 2000). Avoidance of deep kissing with persons with KS is currently accepted as advisable to reduce the risk of oral transmission. There is no evidence to support the supposition that latex condoms reduce the transmission of HHV-8 but their use is advisable for protection against not only HHV-8 but many other sexually transmissible infections. Owing to the lack of routine serological tests for HHV-8, screening of blood has not been possible and finally, there are no current recommendations for preventing mother-to-child transmission.

The prevalence of KS is lower among AIDS patients treated for retinitis with either ganciclovir or foscarnet, both of which inhibit HHV-8 replication in vitro, suggesting that these compounds might be useful for prevention or treatment of KS. However, the efficacies of antiviral therapies for HHV-8 infection have not been established and this remains a research priority. Finally, restoration of immune function with HAART, where it is available, has greatly reduced the prevalence of KS.

Human papillomavirus infections

Of the 70 or so known Human papillomavirus (HPV) infections, more than 25 have been detected in the genital region. Some HPVs, notably types 16 and 18, are associated with precancerous intraepithelial neoplasias of the cervix, vagina, vulva, penis, and anus. HIV-induced immune dysfunction increases the prevalence of detectable genital HPV infection and HPV-associated intraepithelial neoplasia (Northfelt and Palefsky 1992), as does iatrogenic immunosuppression (Penn 1986). However, the association between HIV and HPV is not explicable solely on the basis of immunosuppression, because HPV DNA is detectable with increased frequency in the genital tracts of women with early HIV infection, before there is a measurable decline in the CD4$^+$ T-cell count. Both direct interaction between HIV and HPV and the common risk factors for their acquisition may contribute to the association between HIV infection and HPV-related disease.

In HIV-infected women, cervical intraepithelial neoplasia (CIN) recurs more frequently than expected after treatment (Maiman et al. 1990), and recurrence is related to severity of immunosuppression. Although CIN does not seem to progress unusually rapidly to invasive cancer, the latter is an AIDS-defining condition according to the Centers for Disease Control and Prevention guidelines. It is recommended that women have a pelvic examination and Papanicolaou (Pap) smear twice during the first year after HIV diagnosis and once per year thereafter. The usefulness of cytological screening of HPV-positive MSM for early detection of anal high-grade intraepithelial neoplasia is currently unclear (Piketty et al. 2003).

Hepatitis C

HIV infection and hepatitis C share some common risk factors (primarily injecting drug use and hemophilia) and therefore it is prudent to screen all HIV-positive patients for hepatitis C virus (HCV). This is important for helping in the interpretation of abnormal liver function tests and also because in patients with HIV infection the course of hepatitis C may be accelerated (Thomas et al. 1996). The safety of treatment for hepatitis C in HIV-infected patients is currently under investigation.

Enteric infections

Diarrhea is very common among HIV-infected patients. Potential viral causes include astroviruses, adenoviruses, picobirnavirus, and caliciviruses (Grohmann et al. 1993), on the basis that they are detected more frequently in patients with diarrhea than in patients without diarrhea. CMV is also associated with gastrointestinal disease in HIV-infected adults (Laughon et al. 1988).

PICOBIRNAVIRUSES

Picobirnaviruses are small, bisegmented, double-stranded RNA viruses that have been detected in a wide variety of vertebrates, including pigs, in which they are associated with diarrhea (Gatti et al. 1989). They can be grown in mammalian cell cultures, suggesting that they are vertebrate viruses rather than viruses of other intestinal organisms such as protozoa. It is not known with certainty whether picobirnaviruses cause diarrhea in humans (Glass et al. 2001) but their detection in a significant proportion of fecal specimens from HIV-infected patients with diarrhea raises this possibility (Giordano et al. 1998, 1999). Development of serological tests might help to determine the prevalence of picobirnavirus infections in the human population.

ENTERIC ADENOVIRUSES

Reported rates of faecal carriage of adenoviruses among patients with advanced HIV infection are very high (Cunningham et al. 1988). Adenovirus infections of the gastrointestinal tract are frequently asymptomatic, and

when symptoms are noted they are often mild. In immunocompetent people, adenoviruses associated with diarrhea (Liste et al. 2000; Pollok 2001; Trevino et al. 2001) usually belong to subgenera A, C, or F, but in HIV-antibody-positive patients at least one report suggests that the most predominant fecal isolates belong to subgenus D (Khoo et al. 1995). There is some suggestion that prolonged infections in patients with CD4$^+$ T-cell counts <200/mm^3 may allow antigenic drift and genetic recombination between different serotypes (Hierholzer et al. 1988).

JC polyoma virus and progressive multifocal leukoencephalopathy

Progressive multifocal leukoencephalopathy (PML) is a neurological disease caused by JC polyoma virus (JCV). It is characterized by multiple foci of demyelination throughout the CNS. PML has a global distribution and, in patients who do not have AIDS, it is most common in people over the age of 50. The disease is seen in patients with a wide variety of disorders associated with impaired immune function but very rarely in immunocompetent hosts. JCV is found in the nuclei of oligodendrocytes in affected areas of the brain, and viral DNA is present in the cerebrospinal fluid (Gibson et al. 1993). The clinical features of PML are gradual deterioration of cerebral function, progressing to dementia, blindness, paralysis, and eventual coma and death, usually within 6 months of onset.

No treatment is curative and currently, the best initial approach to therapy for PML is improving the underlying immunodeficiency. Addition of cidofovir to HAART has been reported to improve clinical outcome in PML patients and reduce JCV DNA load in cerebrospinal fluid, indicating control of JCV replication (De Luca et al. 2000).

HIV-INFECTED CHILDREN

The impact of opportunistic viral infections on HIV-infected children has yet to be fully determined. However, as in adults, herpesviruses are a major problem.

Herpesvirus infections

There are marked differences in the clinical manifestations of herpesvirus infections in HIV-infected children compared with adults. In part, the differences depend on whether HIV infection precedes primary infections with herpesviruses.

HERPES SIMPLEX VIRUSES

In children, herpes simplex is almost always limited to the oropharynx. Esophagitis is rare, as is dissemination or invasion of the CNS. Furthermore, there is no evidence suggesting that neonatal herpes is more common among the offspring of HIV-infected mothers. The diagnostic method of choice is detection of virus or viral antigens in material collected from newly erupted lesions. Treatment follows guidelines similar to those applied to herpes simplex in adults: oral or intravenous aciclovir according to the severity of disease and suppressive therapy with oral aciclovir for frequently recurrent episodes.

VARICELLA-ZOSTER VIRUS

A small number of cases of varicella in HIV-positive children have been reported in the literature, including a recent outbreak at a summer camp for infected children. Some cases run an uneventful course whereas others may be prolonged or complicated by sepsis, pneumonia, or cerebral vasculitis/aneurism. Recurrent varicella- and herpes zoster have been documented. The severity of complications seems to be inversely related to the CD4$^+$ T-cell count (Jura et al. 1989). Diagnosis is usually possible on clinical grounds. Atypical disease may require laboratory confirmation by detection of VZV in material collected from a freshly erupted vesicle.

Prophylaxis and treatment

Serological tests may be required to identify children who are susceptible to primary infection with VZV. Seronegative children should avoid contact with chickenpox and herpes zoster; when exposure is documented, VZIG may be useful. However, even when VZIG is given within 96 hours of exposure, protection is not guaranteed (Srugo et al. 1993). Varicella vaccine has recently been reported to be beneficial and safe in mildly immunocompromised HIV-infected children (ACIP 1999).

Aciclovir is effective in the treatment of varicella in HIV-infected children (Jura et al. 1989). Intravenous therapy is recommended, particularly for children with poor immune function.

CYTOMEGALOVIRUS

CMV infection is very common among infants whose mothers are HIV-antibody-positive. Furthermore, maternal HIV infection seems to increase the prevalence of congenital CMV. CMV-related disease is an important AIDS indicator event in HIV-infected children, and dissemination of CMV in children with advanced HIV infection carries a high mortality. There is evidence to suggest that HIV-related disease develops up to three times more rapidly in CMV-infected infants compared with uninfected infants. Therefore prophylaxis is a desirable but currently unattainable goal.

There are differences in the clinical manifestations of CMV infection in HIV-infected children and adults that most probably represent the different outcomes of primary and recurrent infections, respectively. Pneumonitis and hepatitis, the commonest diseases caused by CMV in HIV-infected children, are probably the result of primary infection. By contrast, CMV retinitis, which is common in adults and rare in children, is thought to follow reactivation of latent virus in the immune host.

Diagnosis of CMV disease is notoriously difficult, owing to the high prevalence of asymptomatic infection by the age of 2 years. Detection of CMV in urine is common and not indicative of CMV disease. Detection of CMV in the diseased organ [by culture, viral antigen detection, culture amplified antigen detection or polymerase chain reaction (PCR)] is currently the best diagnostic approach but the predictive value of a positive result is not absolute.

Prophylaxis and treatment

Ganciclovir, foscarnet, and cidofovir have all been used to treat CMV disease in children. Toxicity is less of a problem in children compared with adults but the drugs must be given intravenously, creating problems with compliance. Realistically, neither drug is suitable for prophylactic use.

EPSTEIN–BARR VIRUS

EBV DNA has been detected in the lungs of HIV-infected patients with lymphoid interstitial pneumonitis (LIP). LIP is rare in HIV-infected adults but is one of the commonest complications of HIV infection in infants under the age of 2 years. Clinical manifestations of LIP include lymphadenopathy, parotitis, bronchospasm, tachypnea, and sleep apnea. Serum immunoglobulin levels may be unusually high, with an associated hyperviscosity syndrome. Chest infections may complicate the disease and therefore immunization against bacterial pathogens is recommended. Diagnosis rests on sequential clinical assessments and chest X-ray changes over a period of 2 months, together with lung biopsy if necessary. Further work is merited to determine whether EBV, the host response to it, or other viruses, plays an etiologic role in LIP because, if this is the case, specific therapy may be possible. Corticosteroids and zidovudine have been reported to be useful in the management of the disease.

Respiratory syncytial virus infections

Pneumonitis, rather than bronchiolitis or wheezing, seems to be a prominent clinical manifestation of respiratory syncytial virus (RSV) in HIV-infected children (Chandwani et al. 1990). Bronchiolitis is thought to be the result of immune-mediated damage to the lung, which might explain its rarity in immunocompromised hosts. In infants with low CD4$^+$ T-cell counts, RSV pneumonia may be life-threatening as a result of secondary bacterial infection (Chandwani et al. 1990). Pre-emptive antibacterial therapy may therefore be worthwhile in severely immunocompromised children who fail to respond promptly to ribavirin.

IMMUNE DEFICIENCIES NOT CAUSED BY HIV

Malignant tumors, cytotoxic chemotherapy or radiotherapy, and congenital disorders may all profoundly compromise the immune system, predisposing patients to unusually severe or prolonged infections with a wide range of viruses.

Herpesvirus infections

It has been known for a long time that herpesviruses are important opportunistic pathogens in patients with disorders of cellular immunity. The potential manifestations of infection are diverse and sometimes life-threatening.

HERPES SIMPLEX

The frequency and severity of recurrent episodes of herpes simplex are increased in patients with dysfunctional immunity, particularly allograft recipients (Naraqi et al. 1977; Rand et al. 1977; Meyers et al. 1980), those with malignancy or those receiving anti-tumor chemotherapy (Muller et al. 1972) and patients with Wiskott–Aldrich syndrome (St Geme et al. 1965). In allograft recipients, herpes simplex most commonly presents in the second week after transplantation.

Shedding of HSV may be asymptomatic or may present as vesicles or ulcers. Lesions may be widespread and persistent, and may involve the esophagus or rectum, causing pain and gastrointestinal disturbances. Ulcers may become indolent and, in immobile patients, perianal ulcers may be confused with pressure sores. Major manifestations of visceral infection are pneumonia and hepatitis.

Virus detection is the mainstay of laboratory diagnosis. In the case of a superficial infection, the specimen required is material collected from the base of the lesion. To diagnose HSV pneumonia, bronchoalveolar lavage fluid or, preferably, a lung biopsy specimen is necessary. Virus culture is probably the most sensitive diagnostic procedure in routine use but it can take up to 7 days before a characteristic cytopathic effect (CPE) develops. More rapid procedures include direct detection of viral antigens and culture-amplified enzyme immunoassays, in which inoculated cell cultures are tested for the presence of viral antigens after 24–48 hours, in order to prevent the development of cytopathology.

Prophylaxis and treatment

To control reactivation of HSV caused by iatrogenic immunosuppression, bone marrow recipients are often given aciclovir prophylactically, commencing at the start of induction chemotherapy. However, some transplant units believe it is more cost effective to treat episodes as they arise.

Intravenous aciclovir is recommended for the treatment of all HSV disease in profoundly immunocompromised patients, irrespective of whether the infection is localized or disseminated at the time of diagnosis. Oral aciclovir or valaciclovir may be appropriate for localized herpes simplex in patients who are not severely immunocompromised, with the caveat that intestinal absorption of the drug may be reduced by irradiation of the gut or systemic chemotherapy.

VARICELLA

Varicella is an aggressive and potentially fatal disease in people with severe cellular immune defects. The rash may be florid or hemorrhagic, and visceral manifestations include hepatitis, pneumonitis, and encephalitis. Most cases of varicella can be diagnosed on clinical grounds but, occasionally, virus culture or antigen detection tests are required, particularly to distinguish the disease from disseminated herpes simplex.

Treatment and prophylaxis

Intravenous aciclovir is of proven efficacy for the treatment of visceral disease caused by VZV in children with malignant disease (Schulmann 1985). The drug is beneficial in immunocompromised children presenting at the time of emergence of rash (Nyerges et al. 1988) and treatment should begin as soon as possible after rash eruption to be effective in reducing the incidence of visceral complications.

For prevention of varicella, live-attenuated varicella vaccine (Oka strain) is safe and effective when given to children with leukemia (in remission) or other malignancies, provided that anticancer chemotherapy is suspended from 1 week before to 1 week after vaccination. Passive immunization with VZIG is useful for seronegative people known to have been exposed to varicella. VZIG is potentially beneficial when given within 96 hours of exposure but protection is not a certainty (Kavaliotis et al. 1998).

HERPES ZOSTER

Herpes zoster (recrudescent VZV infection) is common in VZV-seropositive immunocompromised children and adults and, unlike zoster in immunocompetent people, episodes may be recurrent. After bone marrow transplantation, 30 percent of patients develop herpes zoster within a year, with a peak incidence in the fourth month (Locksley et al. 1985). The disease is also common in renal transplant recipients (Naraqi et al. 1977) and in patients with Hodgkin's disease (Schulmann 1985).

Infection may be confined to a single dermatome or may involve overlapping or noncontiguous dermatomes. Cutaneous dissemination of infection is not uncommon and, in severely immunocompromised patients, life-threatening visceral dissemination may occur.

Treatment and prophylaxis

Oral aciclovir, valaciclovir, or famciclovir may be used to treat localized herpes zoster in patients who are not severely immunocompromised (e.g. those on maintenance chemotherapy). Treatment should be commenced as soon as possible after eruption of the rash. In profoundly immunocompromised patients and in patients with signs of disseminated disease, intravenous aciclovir is currently the treatment of choice.

At the present time it is not feasible or cost effective to prevent herpes zoster in immunocompromised patients by continuous administration of antiviral compounds. This situation might change in the future if safe and inexpensive oral compounds with high activity against VZV become available. There is interest in determining whether herpes zoster can be prevented in immunocompetent adults by vaccination with the Oka strain of VZV. If this approach proves to be effective, it may be applicable to some immunocompromised patients, given that vaccination of leukemic children during periods of remission safely protects them against varicella.

CYTOMEGALOVIRUS INFECTIONS

CMV infection is usually asymptomatic in the immunocompetent host. Primary infection is acquired at any time throughout life; by 40 years of age, 50–70 percent of the general population are infected, with the lower prevalence correlated with higher socioeconomic class. Primary infection or reinfection of an immune host may be acquired as a result of transfusion of CMV-seropositive blood or blood products, or receipt of a kidney from a seropositive donor. However, reactivation of latent virus is the cause of most CMV infections in immunocompromised hosts. CMV is a major cause of morbidity and mortality in allograft recipients (Peterson et al. 1980; Meyers et al. 1982). Characteristically, reactivation is detected in the second and third months after bone marrow transplantation.

CMV causes a wide range of clinical syndromes in people with dysfunctional immunity, prominent among which are hepatitis, gastrointestinal disease, and pneumonitis. The last is thought to be immunologically mediated (Grundy et al. 1987) and responds poorly to specific antiviral therapy. In bone marrow recipients, graft-versus-host disease is a risk factor for development of CMV pneumonitis. Reactivation of CMV may be manifest as fever without localizing signs of infection, creating considerable difficulty in diagnosis. Surveillance cultures of urine, saliva, and blood, taken twice weekly,

are useful in this respect, because virological evidence of active infection precedes disease. In addition, quantification of CMV load in whole blood or plasma has been shown to be a useful predictor of CMV disease in solid organ transplant recipients.

Diagnosis of CMV disease requires detection of virus in material from the affected organ. For diagnosis of CMV pneumonitis, a transbronchial biopsy is a suitable specimen. Detection of virus in buffy coat cells may be a useful adjunct to diagnosis when material cannot be obtained from the affected organ. In order to be useful in patient management, virus detection must be rapid. On average, 16 days are required to identify CMV in conventional cell cultures, making virus culture impractical when decisions have to be made about therapy. Rapid diagnosis depends on direct immunohistochemical detection of viral antigen in biopsy material (Volpi et al. 1983) or culture amplified antigen detection methods. The latter approach is both rapid and sensitive and is based on the principle that a few cells in an inoculated monolayer express immediate early CMV antigens, which can be detected, for instance, by enzyme immunoassay, within 24–48 hours of infection.

Quantification of CMV in plasma or leukocytes by PCR is a rapid and potentially useful diagnostic tool in solid organ transplant recipients (Ferreira-Gonzalez et al. 1999).

EPSTEIN–BARR VIRUS INFECTIONS

Primary EBV infection is very common in early childhood and adolescence, and more than 90 percent of the adult population is EBV-seropositive. EBV replicates in B lymphocytes and pharyngeal epithelial cells and the virus is transmitted in saliva. In the normal host, lytic infection is kept under control by cytotoxic T lymphocytes (CTL) with specificity for virally encoded antigens. After recovery from primary infection, EBV persists in a latent form in B lymphocytes. In renal allograft recipients and other profoundly immunocompromised patients, lytic infection is not adequately controlled, leading to frequently recurrent or persistent virus shedding and an unusually high virus load in the blood. In one report, EBV was detected in throat washings from more than 80 percent of seropositive renal transplant patients (Chang et al. 1978).

There has been considerable debate as to whether EBV can persist in epithelial cells in addition to lymphoid tissue. Current evidence suggests that lymphocytes are the only true reservoir of EBV in vivo. Carriage of EBV is lost following ablation of lymphoid tissue in EBV-seropositive patients undergoing bone marrow transplantation (Gratama et al. 1990). Furthermore, the characteristic pattern of viral gene expression associated with latency is not evident in epithelial cells at sites of oral hairy leukoplakia (Sandvej et al. 1992).

Primary EBV infections may be asymptomatic or cause infectious mononucleosis (IM). The clinical features of reactivated infection are poorly character-ized: fever and hepatitis have been implicated as poten-tial manifestations of recrudescent disease but undoubt-edly most reactivations must be asymptomatic. Primary and recurrent infections are associated with B-cell lymphomas in transplant recipients (Hanto et al. 1982; Ho et al. 1985), and EBV nuclear antigen and EBV DNA can be detected in the tumor cells. The incidence of lymphomas in transplant patients has increased substantially with the use of more aggressive immuno-suppressive regimens, and recipients of bone marrow, heart, and liver grafts are most at risk. Rapidly progres-sive lymphomas that develop early after transplantation are most commonly the result of primary rather than recurrent EBV infections, acquired either from the graft or from transfused blood. Lymphoma tends to be a late complication of recurrent EBV infection. Post-transplant lymphomas are resistant to standard antitumor chemo-therapies, and aciclovir is not beneficial.

All post-transplantation lymphomas contain EBV DNA. The higher the virus load in the blood, the greater is the risk of developing lymphoma (Riddler et al. 1994; Savoie et al. 1994), consistent with the hypothesis that failure to control lytic infection predis-poses to the outgrowth of malignant cells. Tumors are often multifocal and particularly affect the gastro-intestinal tract, liver, and CNS. They may progress from a polyclonal to a monoclonal phenotype, presumably representing dominance by the most rapidly growing cell in the original tumor. Different tumors in the same patient commonly have different clonal origins.

The lymphoma cells have several properties in common with EBV-transformed lymphoblastoid cell lines, suggesting that EBV may be the only factor underlying tumor development in vivo. Chromosomal translocations of the Burkitt's lymphoma type and c-myc rearrange-ments have been reported but are rare. Tumors may regress with improved immune function (Starzl et al. 1984), suggesting that they remain sensitive to attack by EBV-specific CTLs. The possibility of treating post-transplant lymphomas by adoptive transfer of CTL is being explored.

X-linked lymphoproliferative syndrome

X-linked lymphoproliferative syndrome (XLPS) is a rare form of immunodeficiency that selectively predisposes affected males to life-threatening EBV-related disease (Purtilo et al. 1975). About 75 percent of those affected die within a few weeks of primary EBV infection. The remainder has a greatly increased risk of developing lymphomas or hypogammaglobulinemia.

Many patients with XLPS fail to control the initial proliferation of EBV-transformed B cells associated with acute IM, despite the presence of reactive T cells. This may result in a disease resembling immunoblastic lymphoma in transplant patients. Infiltration of organs by lymphocytes is a common cause of death in these individuals. Alternatively, the initial proliferation of B cells and reactive T cells may abate, to be followed by widespread infiltration and destruction of lymphoid tissues and bone marrow by phagocytic cells (Sullivan and Woda 1989). This type of pathology is indistinguish-able from the virus-associated hemophagocytic syndrome.

The genetic defect responsible for XLPS is closely linked to two X-chromosome markers, DXS42 and 37. Several phenotypic defects have been identified in XLPS patients and carriers, including failure to develop anti-bodies to EBV nuclear antigens. IgM to IgG switching is defective and the ability of T cells to produce interferon-gamma (IFN-γ) is reduced. It has been postulated that patients with XLPS have a critical defect in their ability to support the activity of EBV-specific CTLs.

Papillomavirus infections

Warts are common in patients with dysfunctional cellular immunity, including those with leukemia or lymphoma and renal transplant recipients (Koranda et al. 1974). Most infections probably represent reactivations of latent virus.

EPIDERMODYSPLASIA VERRUCIFORMIS

Epidermodysplasia verruciformis (EV) is a rare disease that is first manifest in infancy or childhood by the development of multiple warts that do not regress spon-taneously. Patients with EV have a poorly understood immunological defect that predisposes them, apparently quite specifically, to papillomavirus disease. There is often a family history of the disease but its pattern of inheritance is not clear. Parental consanguinity is common, suggesting that the trait is recessive.

A mixture of typical flat warts and reddish-brown plaques is characteristic. The lesions are caused by a wide variety of papillomavirus types, most of which rarely cause warts in the general population. Some of the warts, particularly those in areas of the body exposed to the sun, progress to intraepithelial or inva-sive squamous carcinomas (Jablonska and Majewski 1994).

Enteric viruses

Many viruses have been associated with gastroenteritis. In immunocompetent hosts, illness is usually mild and shedding of virus in the feces is transient. By contrast, enteric viruses cause significant morbidity in immuno-compromised patients. Rotaviruses, adenoviruses, astro-viruses, caliciviruses, and small round viruses have all been associated with severe or persistent diarrhea in patients with perturbed immune function (Chrystie et al. 1982; Pedley et al. 1984; Oishi et al. 1991; Cox et al.

1994; Romberg 1994), bone marrow recipients being particularly at risk. A nosocomial outbreak of rotavirus infection, with severe diarrhea, has been documented in renal transplant recipients (Peigue-Lafeuille et al. 1991). Although enteroviruses are not usually associated with gastrointestinal disease, coxsackie A viruses have been implicated as causes of diarrhea in the contexts of hypo-gammaglobulinemia (Johnson et al. 1982) and bone marrow transplantation (Townsend et al. 1982).

ENTEROVIRAL MENINGOENCEPHALITIS

Severe and persistent enterovirus infections are seen in patients with congenital hypogammaglobulinemia, despite regular immunoglobulin replacement therapy. This finding is unusual in that hypogammaglobulinemic patients respond normally to other viral infections. The most frequent complication is chronic, often fatal, meningoencephalitis. Patients may present with neck stiffness, headache, lethargy, weakness or seizures, with or without fever. These features are often associated with a dermatomyositis-like syndrome, characterized by edema of the extremities, sometimes with an erythematous or violaceous rash overlying groups of muscles. Echovirus types 2, 3, 5, 9, 11, 17, 19, 24, 25, 30, and 33, and coxsackie virus B3 have been isolated from the cerebrospinal fluid or brain tissue, and occasionally from muscle, in these patients (Mease et al. 1981: Cooper et al. 1983). Respiratory illness caused by enteroviruses has also been described, and evidence of disseminated infection has been found in fatal cases.

Measles

Dysfunctional cellular immunity predisposes to persistence of measles virus with potentially lethal consequences. Two complications, namely giant cell pneumonia and measles inclusion body encephalitis (MIBE), are recognized, neither of which is seen in immunocompetent hosts. Giant cell pneumonia usually presents 2–3 weeks after exposure to measles. The characteristic measles rash may be absent, in which case the diagnosis may remain obscure until postmortem. Laboratory approaches to diagnosis include detection of virus or viral antigens in nasopharyngeal fluid, bronchoalveolar lavage fluid or lung tissue, and demonstration of multi-nucleated giant cells with characteristic inclusion bodies in histological sections of lung.

MIBE usually arises within 6 months of exposure to measles virus and is occasionally accompanied by giant cell pneumonia or retinopathy. The disease may be rapidly progressive and has a poor prognosis; rapid deterioration leads to death within a few weeks of onset. The underlying pathology is one of gliosis. Intracytoplasmic and intranuclear inclusion bodies are present in glial cells and neurons, and inflammatory cell infiltration of the brain is minimal. Defective measles virus has been detected in the brains of MIBE patients and it is possible that the disease is an accelerated version of subacute sclerosing panencephalitis (Ohuchi et al. 1987).

Measles vaccine contains live attenuated virus and is not generally recommended for administration to immunocompromised patients. The current vaccination program for normal children reduces the number of susceptible patients among those who subsequently develop dysfunctional immunity, and may reduce the chance of exposure in non-immune individuals. Measles in previously vaccinated hosts has, however, been reported. Administration of normal human immunoglobulin after exposure to measles virus has some beneficial effect, but may not prevent complications, particularly MIBE (Kay and Rankin 1984). There is as yet no specific antiviral therapy with proven efficacy for the treatment of measles or its complications in immunocompromised hosts, but sporadic case reports suggest that aerosolized ribavirin might be of some benefit to patients with pneumonitis.

Polyomavirus infections

BK virus (BKV) and JCV are human polyomaviruses which, according to serological studies, are ubiquitous. It was thought that active, persistent infections were rare in immunocompetent hosts, but recent data suggest that urinary excretion of JCV is common in older people and pregnant women.

About half of renal transplant recipients have serological or other evidence of prior exposure to *Polyomavirus* (Hogan et al. 1980; Gardner et al. 1984), in keeping with the high seropositivity rate in the general population. BKV and JCV are commonly detected in the urine of transplant patients, suggesting that immunosuppression allows latent infections to reactivate. Primary and reactivated infections are usually asymptomatic, although ureteric stenosis has been reported and there may be an association with impaired graft function. Infections are frequent in the second month after renal transplantation, but late infections, occurring several months or even years later, are not unusual.

Urinary excretion of BKV and JCV is also common after bone marrow transplantation (O'Reilly et al. 1981) and has been reported in association with leukemia, lymphoma, solid tumors and Wiskott–Aldrich syndrome. Infection is generally asymptomatic, although deterioration in renal and hepatic function has been observed; BK viruria following bone marrow transplantation may be associated with hemorrhagic cystitis (Rice et al. 1985).

Polyomavirus infections of the urinary tract may be diagnosed by electron microscopy or by demonstrating characteristic intranuclear inclusions in exfoliated urinary epithelial cells. The presence of Polyomavirus antigens within these cells can be confirmed by immunofluorescence. BKV can be isolated in cell cultures, such as human embryo lung fibroblasts.

A minority of non-AIDS immunocompromised patients infected with JCV may develop PML. The factors predisposing to PML are unclear and virus has been detected in the brains of normal individuals. It has been suggested that JCV may adapt itself for growth in the nervous system during the course of infection. In support of this hypothesis, structural alterations in the archetypal regulatory region of the JCV genome have been found in JCV DNA from PML brains. Structural variations in the regulatory region have also been reported among viral DNAs from different organs in the same infected patient (Loeber and Dorries 1988). However, the issue of virus adaptation to different tissues is controversial because different organs have been shown to be infected with the same JCV subtype and PML isolates can be the same subtype as urinary isolates (Myers et al. 1989).

Diagnosis of PML is based on the characteristic clinical picture, and should be confirmed by brain biopsy. The histological appearances are typical and polyomavirus particles can be demonstrated by electron microscopy. Immunofluorescence microscopy of acetone-fixed brain tissue may reveal the presence of polyomavirus antigens. Virus may also be isolated in primary cultures of human fetal glial cells.

No agent has proven efficacy for the treatment of polyomavirus infections; reduction of immunosuppressive therapy, when practicable is, however, beneficial.

REFERENCES

ACIP. 1999. Prevention of varicella. Update recommendations of the Advisory Committee on Immunization Practices (ACIP). *MMWR Recomm Rep*, **48**, 1–5.

Andersson, J.P. 1991. Clinical aspects of Epstein–Barr virus infection. *Scand J Infect Dis*, **80**, Suppl, 94–104.

Aronson, J.E., McSherry, G., et al. 1992. Varicella does not appear to be a cofactor for human immunodeficiency virus infection in children. *Pediatr Infect Dis J*, **11**, 1004–8.

Balfour, H.H. Jr, Benson, C., et al. 1994. Management of acyclovir-resistant herpes simplex and varicella-zoster virus infections. *J Acquir Immune Defic Syndr*, **7**, 254–60.

Berger, J.R., Kaszovita, B., et al. 1987. Progressive multifocal leuko-encephalopathy associated with human immunodeficiency virus infection. *Ann Intern Med*, **107**, 78–87.

Bodsworth, N.J., Crooks, R.J., et al. 1997. Valaciclovir versus aciclovir in patient initiated treatment of recurrent genital herpes: a randomised, double blind clinical trial. International Valaciclovir HSV Study Group. *Genitourin Med*, **73**, 110–16.

Boivin, G., Gaudreau, A., et al. 2000. Evaluation of the human herpesvirus 8 DNA load in blood and Kaposi's sarcoma skin lesions from AIDS patients on highly active antiretroviral therapy. *AIDS*, **14**, 1907–10.

Buchbinder, S.P., Katz, M.H., et al. 1992. Herpes zoster and human immunodeficiency virus infection. *J Infect Dis*, **166**, 1153–6.

Campbell, T.B., Borok, M., et al. 2000. Relationship of human herpesvirus 8 peripheral blood virus load and Kaposi's sarcoma clinical stage. *AIDS*, **14**, 2109–16.

Chandwani, S., Borkowsky, W., et al. 1990. Respiratory syncytial virus infection in human immunodeficiency virus-infected children. *J Pediatr*, **117**, 251–4.

Chang, R.S., Lewis, J.P., et al. 1978. Oropharyngeal excretion of Epstein–Barr virus by patients with lymphoproliferative disorders and by recipients of renal homografts. *Ann Intern Med*, **88**, 34–40.

Chang, Y., Cesarman, E., et al. 1994. Identification of herpesvirus-like DNA sequences in AIDS-associated Kaposi's sarcoma. *Science*, **266**, 1865–9.

Chatis, P.A. and Crumpacker, C.S. 1992. Resistance of herpesviruses to antiviral drugs. *Antimicrob Agents Chemother*, **36**, 1589–95.

Chrystie, I.L., Booth, I.W., et al. 1982. Multiple faecal virus excretion in immunodeficiency. *Lancet*, **1**, 282.

Cooper, D.A., Pehrson, P.O., et al. 1993. The efficacy and safety of zidovudine alone or as cotherapy with acyclovir for the treatment of patients with AIDS and AIDS-related complex: a double-blind randomized trial. European-Australian Collaborative Group. *AIDS*, **7**, 197–207.

Cooper, J.B., Pratt, W.R., et al. 1983. Coxsackievirus B3 producing fatal meningoencephalitis in a patient with X-linked agammaglobulinemia. *Am J Dis Child*, **137**, 82–3.

Cox, G.J., Matsui, S.M., et al. 1994. Etiology and outcome of diarrhea after marrow transplantation: a prospective study. *Gastroenterology*, **107**, 1398–407.

Croen, K.D., Ostrove, J.M., et al. 1988. Patterns of gene expression and sites of latency in human nerve ganglia are different for varicella-zoster and herpes simplex viruses. *Proc Natl Acad Sci U S A*, **85**, 9773–7.

Cunningham, A.L., Grohman, G.S., et al. 1988. Gastrointestinal viral infections in homosexual men who were symptomatic and seropositive for human immunodeficiency virus. *J Infect Dis*, **158**, 386–91.

De Luca, A., Giancola, M.L., et al. 2000. Cidofovir added to HAART improves virological and clinical outcome in AIDS-associated progressive multifocal leukoencephalopathy. *AIDS*, **14**, F117–21.

Drew, W.L. 1988. Cytomegalovirus infection in patients with AIDS. *J Infect Dis*, **158**, 449–56.

Emery, V.C., Atkins, M.C., et al. 1999. Interactions between beta-herpesviruses and human immunodeficiency virus in vivo: evidence for increased human immunodeficiency viral load in the presence of human herpesvirus 6. *J Med Virol*, **57**, 278–82.

Epstein, W.L. 1992. Molluscum contagiosum. *Semin Dermatol*, **11**, 184–9.

Ferreira-Gonzalez, A., Fisher, R.A., et al. 1999. Clinical utility of a quantitative polymerase chain reaction for diagnosis of cytomegalovirus disease in solid organ transplant patients. *Transplantation*, **68**, 991–6.

Frickhofen, N., Abkowitz, J.L., et al. 1990. Persistent B19 parvovirus infection in a patient infected with human immunodeficiency virus infection type (HIV-1): a treatable cause of anaemia in AIDS. *Ann Intern Med 113*, **1**, 926–33.

Gardner, S.D., MacKenzie, E.F., et al. 1984. Prospective study of the human polyomaviruses BK and JC and cytomegalovirus in renal transplant recipients. *J Clin Pathol*, **37**, 578–86.

Garzino-Demo, A., Chen, M., et al. 1996. Enhancement of TAT-induced transactivation of the HIV-1 LTR by two genomic fragments of HHV-6. *J Med Virol*, **50**, 20–4.

Gatti, M.S., de Castro, A.F., et al. 1989. Viruses with bisegmented double-stranded RNA in pig faeces. *Res Vet Sci*, **47**, 397–8.

Gibson, P.E., Knowles, W.A., et al. 1993. Detection of JC virus DNA in the cerebrospinal fluid of patients with progressive multifocal leukoencephalopathy. *J Med Virol*, **39**, 278–81.

Giordano, M.O., Martinez, L.C., et al. 1998. Detection of picobirnavirus in HIV-infected patients with diarrhea in Argentina. *J Acquir Immune Defic Syndr Hum Retrovirol*, **18**, 380–3.

Giordano, M.O., Martinez, L.C., et al. 1999. Diarrhea and enteric emerging viruses in HIV-infected patients. *AIDS Res Hum Retroviruses*, **15**, 1427–32.

Glass, R.I., Bresee, J., et al. 2001. Gastroenteritis viruses: an overview. *Novartis Found Symp*, **238**, 5–19.

Gratama, J.W., Oosterveer, M.A., et al. 1990. Serological and molecular studies of Epstein–Barr virus infection in allogeneic marrow graft recipients. *Transplantation*, **49**, 725–30.

Grohmann, G.S., Glass, R.I., et al. 1993. Enteric viruses and diarrhea in HIV-infected patients.. *N Engl J Med*, **329**, 14–20.

Grundy, J.E., Shanley, J.D., et al. 1987. Is cytomegalovirus interstitial pneumonitis in transplant recipients an immunopathological condition? *Lancet*, **2**, 996–9.

Gwanzura, L., McFarland, W., et al. 1998. Association between human immunodeficiency virus and herpes simplex virus type 2 seropositivity among male factory workers in Zimbabwe. *J Infect Dis*, **177**, 481–4.

Hadler, S.C., Judson, F.N., et al. 1991. Outcome of hepatitis B virus infection in homosexual men and its relation to prior human immunodeficiency virus infection. *J Infect Dis*, **163**, 454–9.

Hague, R.A., Burns, S.E., et al. 1992. Virus infections of the respiratory tract in HIV-infected children. *J Infect*, **24**, 31–6.

Hanto, D.W., Frizzera, G., et al. 1982. Epstein–Barr virus-induced B-cell lymphoma after renal transplantation: acyclovir therapy and transition from polyclonal to monoclonal B-cell proliferation. *N Engl J Med*, **306**, 913–18.

Hierholzer, J.C., Adrian, T., et al. 1988. Analysis of antigenically intermediate strains of subgenus B and D adenoviruses from AIDS patients. *Arch Virol*, **103**, 99–115.

Ho, M., Miller, G., et al. 1985. Epstein–Barr virus infections and DNA hybridization studies in posttransplantation lymphoma and lymphoproliferative lesions: the role of primary infection. *J Infect Dis*, **152**, 876–86.

Hogan, T.F., Borden, E.C., et al. 1980. Human polyomavirus infections with JC virus and BK virus in renal transplant patients. *Ann Intern Med*, **92**, 373–8.

Holmberg, S.D., Stewart, J.A., et al. 1988. Prior herpes simplex virus type 2 infection as a risk factor for HIV infection. *JAMA*, **259**, 1048–50.

Holmberg, S.D., Buchbinder, S.P., et al. 1995. The spectrum of medical conditions and symptoms before acquired immunodeficiency syndrome in homosexual and bisexual men infected with the human immunodeficiency virus. *Am J Epidemiol*, **141**, 395–404.

Hook, E.W. III, Cannon, R.O., et al. 1992. Herpes simplex virus infection as a risk factor for human immunodeficiency virus infection in heterosexuals. *J Infect Dis*, **165**, 251–5.

Jablonska, S. and Majewski, S. 1994. Epidermodysplasia verruciformis. In: zur Hausen, H. (ed.), *Human pathogenic papillomaviruses*. Heidelberg: Springer-Verlag, 157–75.

Jacobson, M.A. and Mills, J. 1988. Serious cytomegalovirus disease in the acquired immunodeficiency syndrome (AIDS). Clinical findings, diagnosis, and treatment. *Ann Intern Med*, **108**, 585–94.

Johnson, J.P., Yolken, R.H., et al. 1982. Prolonged excretion of group A coxsackievirus in an infant with agammaglobulinemia. *J Infect Dis*, **146**, 712.

Jura, E., Chadwick, E.G., et al. 1989. Varicella-zoster virus infections in children infected with human immunodeficiency virus. *Pediatr Infect Dis J*, **8**, 586–90.

Kavaliotis, J., Loukou, I., et al. 1998. Outbreak of varicella in a pediatric oncology unit. *Med Pediatr Oncol*, **31**, 166–9.

Kay, H.E. and Rankin, A. 1984. Immunoglobulin prophylaxis of measles in acute lymphoblastic leukaemia. *Lancet*, **1**, 901–2.

Keet, I.P., Lee, F.K., et al. 1990. Herpes simplex virus type 2 and other genital ulcerative infections as a risk factor for HIV-1 acquisition. *Genitourin Med*, **66**, 330–3.

Kelly, R., Mancao, M., et al. 1994. Varicella in children with perinatally acquired human immunodeficiency virus infection. *J Pediatr*, **124**, 271–3.

Kennedy, P.G. 2002. Key issues in varicella-zoster virus latency. *J Neurovirol*, **8**, Suppl 2, 80–4.

Khoo, S.H., Bailey, A.S., et al. 1995. Adenovirus infections in human immunodeficiency virus-positive patients: clinical features and molecular epidemiology. *J Infect Dis*, **172**, 629–37.

Knox, K.K. and Carrigan, D.R. 1994. Disseminated active HHV-6 infections in patients with AIDS. *Lancet*, **343**, 577–8.

Kopp, T., Geusau, A., et al. 2002. Successful treatment of an aciclovir-resistant herpes simplex type 2 infection with cidofovir in an AIDS patient. *Br J Dermatol*, **147**, 134–8.

Koranda, F.C., Dehmel, E.M., et al. 1974. Cutaneous complications in immunosuppressed renal homograft recipients. *JAMA*, **229**, 419–24.

Lacoste, V., Mauclere, P., et al. 2000. KSHV-like herpesviruses in chimps and gorillas. *Nature*, **407**, 151–2.

Laughon, B.E., Druckman, D.A., et al. 1988. Prevalence of enteric pathogens in homosexual men with and without acquired immunodeficiency syndrome. *Gastroenterology*, **94**, 984–93.

Liste, M.B., Natera, I., et al. 2000. Enteric virus infections and diarrhea in healthy and human immunodeficiency virus-infected children. *J Clin Microbiol*, **38**, 2873–7.

Locksley, R.M., Flournoy, N., et al. 1985. Infection with varicella-zoster virus after marrow transplantation. *J Infect Dis*, **152**, 1172–81.

Loeber, G. and Dorries, K. 1988. DNA rearrangements in organ-specific variants of polyomavirus JC strain GS. *J Virol*, **62**, 1730–5.

Lyall, E.G.H., Ogilvie, M.M., et al. 1994. Acyclovir resistant varicella-zoster and HIV infection. *Arch Dis Child*, **70**, 133–5.

Maiman, M., Fruchter, R.G., et al. 1990. Human immunodeficiency virus infection and cervical neoplasia. *Gynecol Oncol*, **38**, 377–82.

Mease, P.J., Ochs, H.D., et al. 1981. Successful treatment of echovirus meningoencephalitis and myositis-fasciitis with intravenous immune globulin therapy in a patient with X-linked agammaglobulinemia. *N Engl J Med*, **304**, 1278–81.

Meyers, J.D., Flournoy, N., et al. 1980. Infection with herpes simplex virus and cell-mediated immunity after marrow transplant. *J Infect Dis*, **142**, 338–46.

Meyers, J.D., Flournoy, N., et al. 1982. Nonbacterial pneumonia after allogeneic marrow transplantation: a review of ten years' experience. *Rev Infect Dis*, **4**, 1119–32.

Muller, S.A., Herrmann, E.C. Jr, et al. 1972. Herpes simplex infections in hematologic malignancies. *Am J Med*, **52**, 102–14.

Mustafa, M.M., Weitman, S.D., et al. 1993. Subacute measles encephalitis in the young immunocompromised host: report of two cases diagnosed by polymerase chain reaction and treated with ribavirin, and review of the literature. *Clin Infect Dis*, **16**, 654–60.

Myers, C., Frisque, R.J., et al. 1989. Direct isolation and characterization of JC virus from urine samples of renal and bone marrow transplant patients. *J Virol*, **63**, 4445–9.

Naraqi, S., Jackson, G.G., et al. 1977. Prospective study of prevalence, incidence, and source of herpesvirus infections in patients with renal allografts. *J Infect Dis*, **136**, 531–40.

Nikkels, A.F., Snoeck, R., et al. 1999. Chronic verrucous varicella zoster virus skin lesions: clinical, histological, molecular and therapeutic aspects. *Clin Exp Dermatol*, **24**, 346–53.

Northfelt, D.W. and Palefsky, J.M. 1992. Human papillomavirus-associated anogenital neoplasia in persons with HIV infection. *AIDS Clin Rev*, 241–59.

Nyerges, G., Meszner, Z., et al. 1988. Acyclovir prevents dissemination of varicella in immunocompromised children. *J Infect Dis*, **157**, 309–13.

Ohuchi, M., Ohuchi, R., et al. 1987. Characterization of the measles virus isolated from the brain of a patient with immunosuppressive measles encephalitis. *J Infect Dis*, **156**, 436–41.

Oishi, I., Kimura, T., et al. 1991. Serial observations of chronic rotavirus infection in an immunodeficient child. *Microbiol Immunol*, **35**, 953–61.

O'Reilly, R.J., Lee, F.K., et al. 1981. Papovavirus excretion following marrow transplantation: incidence and association with hepatic dysfunction. *Transplant Proc*, **13**, 262–6.

Palefsky, J. 1991. Human papillomavirus infection among HIV-infected individuals: implications for development of malignant tumors. *Hematol Oncol Clin North Am*, **5**, 357–70.

Patel, R., Bodsworth, N.J., et al. 1997. Valaciclovir for the suppression of recurrent genital HSV infection: a placebo controlled study of once daily therapy. International Valaciclovir HSV Study Group. *Genitourin Med*, **73**, 105–9.

Pedley, S., Hundley, F., et al. 1984. The genomes of rotaviruses isolated from chronically infected immunodeficient children. *J Gen Virol*, **65**, Pt 7, 1141–50.

Peigue-Lafeuille, H., Henquell, C., et al. 1991. Nosocomial rotavirus infections in adult renal transplant recipients. *J Hosp Infect*, **18**, 67–70.

Penn, I. 1986. Cancers of the anogenital region in renal transplant recipients. Analysis of 65 cases. *Cancer*, **58**, 611–16.

Peters, B.S., Beck, E.J., et al. 1991. Cytomegalovirus infection in AIDS. Patterns of disease, response to therapy and trends in survival. *J Infect*, **23**, 129–37.

Peterson, P.K., Balfour, H.H. Jr, et al. 1980. Cytomegalovirus disease in renal allograft recipients: a prospective study of the clinical features, risk factors and impact on renal transplantation. *Medicine (Baltimore)*, **59**, 283–300.

Piketty, C., Darragh, T.M., et al. 2003. High prevalence of anal human papillomavirus infection and anal cancer precursors among HIV-infected persons in the absence of anal intercourse. *Ann Intern Med*, **138**, 453–9.

Plancoulaine, S., Abel, L., et al. 2000. Human herpesvirus 8 transmission from mother to child and between siblings in an endemic population. *Lancet*, **356**, 1062–5.

Pollok, R.C. 2001. Viruses causing diarrhoea in AIDS. *Novartis Found Symp*, **238**, 276–83.

Purtilo, D.T., Cassel, C.K., et al. 1975. X-linked recessive progressive combined variable immunodeficiency (Duncan's disease). *Lancet*, **1**, 935–40.

Rabkin, C.S., Hatzakis, A., et al. 1993. Cytomegalovirus infection and risk of AIDS in human immunodeficiency virus-infected hemophilia patients. National Cancer Institute Multicenter Hemophilia Cohort Study Group. *J Infect Dis*, **168**, 1260–3.

Rand, K.H., Rasmussen, L.E., et al. 1977. Cellular immunity and herpesvirus infections in cardiac-transplant patients. *N Engl J Med*, **296**, 1372–7.

Rice, S.J., Bishop, J.A., et al. 1985. BK virus as cause of haemorrhagic cystitis after bone marrow transplantation. *Lancet*, **2**, 844–5.

Riddler, S.A., Breinig, M.C., et al. 1994. Increased levels of circulating Epstein–Barr virus (EBV)-infected lymphocytes and decreased EBV nuclear antigen antibody responses are associated with the development of posttransplant lymphoproliferative disease in solid-organ transplant recipients. *Blood*, **84**, 972–84.

Romberg, W.M. 1994. Die Epilepsie des Erzherzog Carl von Osterreich (1771–1847). *Wurzbg Medizinhist Mitt*, **12**, 245–53.

Safrin, S., Ashley, R., et al. 1991. Clinical and serologic features of herpes simplex virus infection in patients with AIDS. *AIDS*, **5**, 1107–10.

Salmon-Ceron, D., Mazeron, M.C., et al. 2000. Plasma cytomegalovirus DNA, pp65 antigenaemia and a low CD4 cell count remain risk factors for cytomegalovirus disease in patients receiving highly active antiretroviral therapy. *AIDS*, **14**, 1041–9.

Sandvej, K., Krenacs, L., et al. 1992. Epstein–Barr virus latent and replicative gene expression in oral hairy leukoplakia. *Histopathology*, **20**, 387–95.

Savoie, A., Perpete, C., et al. 1994. Direct correlation between the load of Epstein–Barr virus-infected lymphocytes in the peripheral blood of pediatric transplant patients and risk of lymphoproliferative disease. *Blood*, **83**, 2715–22.

Schulmann, S. 1985. Acyclovir treatment of disseminated varicella in childhood malignant neoplasms. *Am J Dis Child*, **139**, 137–40.

Simmons, A. 1996. Rapid diagnosis of viral infections. In: Collee, J., Fraser, A., et al. (eds), *Practical medical microbiology*, 14th edn. London: Churchill Livingstone, 655–73.

Srugo, J., Israele, V., et al. 1993. Clinical manifestations of varicella-zoster virus infections in human immunodeficiency virus-infected children.. *Am J Dis Child*, **147**, 742–5.

St Geme, J., Prince, J., et al. 1965. Impaired cellular resistance to herpes simplex virus in Wiskott–Aldrich syndrome. *N Engl J Med*, **273**, 229–34.

Stamm, W.E., Handsfield, H.H., et al. 1988. The association between genital ulcer disease and acquisition of HIV infection in homosexual men. *JAMA*, **260**, 1429–33.

Starzl, T.E., Nalesnik, M.A., et al. 1984. Reversibility of lymphomas and lymphoproliferative lesions developing under cyclosporin-steroid therapy. *Lancet*, **1**, 583–7.

Stewart, J.A., Reef, S.E., et al. 1995. Herpesvirus infections in persons infected with human immunodeficiency virus. *Clin Infect Dis*, **21**, Suppl 1, 114–20.

Sullivan, J.L. and Woda, B.A. 1989. X-linked lymphoproliferative syndrome. *Immunodefic Rev*, **1**, 325–47.

Thomas, D.L., Shih, J.W., et al. 1996. Effect of human immunodeficiency virus on hepatitis C virus infection among injecting drug users. *J Infect Dis*, **174**, 690–5.

Townsend, T.R., Bolyard, E.A., et al. 1982. Outbreak of Coxsackie A1 gastroenteritis: a complication of bone-marrow transplantation. *Lancet*, **1**, 820–3.

Trevino, M., Prieto, E., et al. 2001. [Diarrhea caused by adenovirus and astrovirus in hospitalized immunodeficient patients]. *Enferm Infecc Microbiol Clin*, **19**, 7–10.

Vallbracht, A., Löhler, J., et al. 1993. Disseminated BK type polyomavirus infection in an AIDS patient with central nervous system disease. *Am J Pathol*, **143**, 29–39.

Volpi, A., Whitley, R.J., et al. 1983. Rapid diagnosis of pneumonia due to cytomegalovirus with specific monoclonal antibodies. *J Infect Dis*, **147**, 1119–20.

Webster, A., Lee, C.A., et al. 1989. Cytomegalovirus infection and progression towards AIDS in haemophiliacs with human immunodeficiency virus infection. *Lancet*, **2**, 63–6.

Whitley, R.J. and Gnann, J.W. Jr 1992. Acyclovir: a decade later. *N Engl J Med*, **327**, 782–9.

Xu, F., Schillinger, J.A., et al. 2002. Seroprevalence and coinfection with herpes simplex virus type 1 and type 2 in the United States, 1988–1994. *J Infect Dis*, **185**, 1019–24.

Youle, M.S., Gazzard, B.G., et al. 1994. Effects of high-dose oral acyclovir on herpesvirus disease and survival in patients with advanced HIV disease: a double-blind, placebo-controlled study. European-Australian Acyclovir Study Group. *AIDS*, **8**, 641–9.

PART IV

PRINCIPLES OF DIAGNOSIS AND CONTROL

Safety in the virology laboratory

GRAHAM LLOYD AND MICHAEL P. KILEY

INTRODUCTION

Both the emergence and re-emergence of new virological agents and the perceived threats associated with bioterrorism are requiring scientists, engineers, and biosafety professionals to design safe working environments and ensure the protection of the community. In addition, disease eradication programs, such as the World Health Organization (2003) plan for the elimination of wild polioviruses, calls for the establishment of limited holdings and inventories of the agent, possibly raising future containment requirements. Most current safety legislation is based on the principles laid down in a variety of government regulations, which may differ slightly from country to country. Examples of such regulations include the Health and Safety at Work Act 1974 and Heath and Safety Control of Substances Hazardous to Health 2002 (Health and Safety Executive 2002) in the UK, the occupational safety and health laws in the USA, European Directive 1993, and Labour Canada regulations, all of which place a duty of care on employers in relation to the safety of their employees and others. International and national legislation increasingly demand employees to co-operate with employers and place a duty on them to avoid putting themselves, colleagues, or others at potential risk. Therefore, overall safety in the virology, or any other, laboratory is the responsibility of all laboratory workers.

People in a supervisory or managerial position are responsible and increasingly accountable for the health, safety, and welfare of all staff and visitors in laboratories under their jurisdiction (Health and Safety Executive, 2000). The emphasis in this chapter, though, is the unique subset of safety issues resulting from the operation of a microbiology laboratory using pathogenic or potentially pathogenic agents. The ability to perform accurate risk assessments (job hazard analysis), based on our understanding of science, is of key importance.

In his review of laboratory-acquired infections, Pike (1979) concluded 'the knowledge, the techniques, and the equipment to prevent most laboratory infections are available.' Over the last decade safety-related technology has advanced significantly, developing biosafety systems that provide a safer working environment. Despite these advances, laboratory accidents still occur at a disturbing rate; unfortunately, as in the past, the most common cause of such accidents is human error. New, sophisticated biosafety systems and improved training methods are still necessary to cope with the increased challenges raised by the emergence and re-emergence of significant pathogenic viruses such as arenaviruses, dengue viruses, Ebola virus, hantavirus, the new hepatitis viruses, severe acute respiratory syndrome (SARS), influenza strains (H5N1), and human immunodeficiency virus (HIV). The fundamental concepts on which to construct a laboratory safety program must therefore ensure minimal risk to both laboratory workers and the community. These concepts include both the proper use and maintenance of new safety equipment and, especially, a greater appreciation of good laboratory practice and proper risk assessment.

A safety program must be based on a sound understanding of the microbiological properties of the agent to be manipulated; a microbiological risk assessment programme (Advisory Committee on Dangerous Pathogens 1996); an understanding of the protective potential of scientific equipment and facilities; comprehensive personnel training and development appropriate to the studies to be undertaken; and use of guidelines and protocols, with the understanding that both must be flexible and dynamic. Any understanding of the properties of a micro-organism must include its virulence, means of spread, tropism, infectious dose, and environmental stability. For a safety program to be effective, it must have the support of laboratory workers and managers. Laboratory management have the ultimate responsibility of providing a safe working environment as described above.

This chapter discusses the typical components of a prudent virology laboratory safety programme. Topics include facilities, containment criteria, work practices, biohazard surveillance, waste management, and training. It must be repeated, though, that the cornerstone of any worthwhile safety program is accurate risk assessment and management that is based on full understanding of the infectious and pathogenic potential of the agents under investigation.

Information on laboratory safety and biosafety may be found in a variety of national and international guidelines or codes of practice (National Institute of Health 1987 (Japan); Ministry of Health 1988 (Sweden); Association Française de Normalisation 1990; Standards Australia/Standards New Zealand 2002, US Department of Health and Human Services 1999 (being updated); World Health Organization 2004; UK Advisory Committee on Dangerous Pathogens 1995a, b, 2001; Health Canada 2004.

HISTORICAL PERSPECTIVE – LABORATORY-ACQUIRED INFECTIONS

The risk of infection is higher in virology laboratories than in the general population, although the risk of exposure to infectious agents is somewhat less than among other groups of healthcare workers.

To determine the essential components of a laboratory safety program, it is first necessary to assess the 'risk' of infection associated with working in a virus laboratory. Pike (1979) compiled the best collection of data to date dealing with accidental infections of laboratory workers with pathogenic micro-organisms. The analysis was based on global data relating to laboratory-acquired infections recorded from the beginning of the

century. Although much of the data covers the period before the age of chemotherapy and biosafety cabinets, it still gives some idea of the potential risk to people working in laboratories. The study concluded that most of the reported infections occurred mainly in research rather than clinical laboratories. However, the data did not provide any information about the changing pattern of laboratory techniques or the relative importance of different groups of infectious agents responsible for the infections.

Examination of these data, as well as analyzing more recent anecdotal and unpublished information, has demonstrated a major shift away from bacteria and rickettsiae as the chief causes of laboratory-acquired infections. Most such infections reported since the 1970s have been of viral origin especially in research environments working with high threat or newly emerged viruses (see Table 65.1). The trend is generally a decrease in aerosol infections and an increase in bloodborne diseases associated with technique failures and work associated with animal studies.

The overall decrease in aerosol infections in the laboratory is probably due to the development and introduction of engineering controls (i.e. microbiological safety cabinets); increased awareness of the routes of infection and of the need for safe working practices in the laboratory. The increasing availability of antiviral drugs, as well as the increase in the number of vaccines available, has also played a role in the decrease in illness due to laboratory infections. Despite these general trends, though, laboratory-acquired infections still occur regularly; however, because of the lack of a worldwide reporting system and the absence of adequate medical surveillance, their true extent may never be known. In some countries, for example the UK (Health and Safety Executive 1986), microbiological accidents must be reported.

Table 65.1 lists some of the ongoing concerns relating to laboratory-acquired infections in virology laboratories reported since 1970. Unfortunately, these are merely examples that emphasize the need for a strong and continuing biosafety program in all virus laboratories. The Subcommittee of Arbovirus Laboratory Safety (1980) collated a number of reports relating to arbovirus incidents involving laboratory workers: Crimean-Congo hemorrhagic fever virus (eight cases, one death); Chikungunya virus (39 cases); Japanese encephalitis virus (22 cases); Argentinian hemorrhagic fever virus (21 cases); Kyasanur Forest disease virus (133 cases); Marburg virus (31 cases, five deaths); Rift Valley fever virus (47 cases); West Nile virus (18 cases); western equine encephalitis virus (seven cases, two deaths); yellow fever virus (38 cases, eight deaths); and numerous others.

The use of vaccinia virus in laboratories has increased in recent years, partly as a consequence of international concerns about the potential use of variola virus (smallpox) as a bioterrorist weapon. Although the vaccine is considered safe, it can produce mild to

Table 65.1 *Examples of laboratory acquired viral infections*

Agent	References	Country/Date	Laboratory type	Exposure details
Marburg virus	Martini et al. (1969)	Germany 1968 Yugoslavia 1968	Tissue culture	Direct
Lassa virus	Leifer et al. (1970)	USA 1969	Research	Direct
Ebola virus	Emond et al. (1977)	UK 1976	Research	Needlestick while inoculating guinea pigs
Hantaan virus	Lloyd and Jones (1986)	UK 1976	Research	Aerosol
Junin virus	Weissenbacher et al. (1978)	Argentina 1978	Research	Aerosol (?)
Hantaan virus	Desmyter et al. (1983)	Belgium 1983	Animal house	Aerosol
Dengue virus	(Kiley, unpublished)	USA 1988	Research	Direct
Marburg virus	International Society for Infectious Disease (2001)	Russian Federation 1990	Research	Direct
Sabià virus	Ryder and Gordsman (1995)	USA 1994	Research	Aerosol, centrifugation incident
Herpes 'B' virus	Centers for Disease Control and Prevention (1998)	USA 1998	Research	Fatal mucocutaneous exposure
West Nile virus	Campbell and Lanciotti (2002)	USA 2002	Animal house	Scalpel injury during bird necropsy
West Nile virus	Cambell and Lanciotti (2002)	USA 2002		Needlestick while harvesting mouse brains
Severe acute respiratory syndrome (SARS)	World Health Organization (2004a)	Singapore 2002	Research	PhD student working on WNV at BSL3, sample also contained SARs. CoV exposure not identified
Severe acute respiratory syndrome (SARS)	Taiwan Department of Health (2003)	Taiwan 2003	Research	Researcher working on SARS in P4 laboratory. Source of infection unknown
Severe acute respiratory syndrome (SARS)	World Health Organization, (2004)	China 2004	Research	2 research workers (7 associated, 1 fatal) in BSL3 laboratory, exposure incident/s not identified
Ebola virus	(International Society for Infectious Disease 2004a)	USA 2004	Research	Needlestick
Ebola virus	(International Society for Infectious Disease 2004b)	Russian Federation 2004	Research	Needlestick during guinea pig inoculation at BSL4, fatal

moderate disease in vaccines and can be disseminated to their close contacts (Fenner et al. 1988; Spencer and Lightfoot 2001; Centers for Disease Control and Prevention 2002) or through auto-inoculation causing vaccinia keratouveitis (Lee et al. 1994). There have been 18 previously reported cases of laboratory-related vaccinia infection, of which at least three were accidental infections of laboratory workers with recombinant vaccinia (Jones et al. 1986; Openshaw et al. 1991; Mempel et al. 2003) and through the manipulation of vaccinia virus-infected cells (Moussatche et al. 2003). This re-emphasizes the potential risks of human infection associated with the increasing volume of recombinant work.

It should be noted that most of the incidents could have been prevented by the use of common, readily available, biosafety practices and validated training schemes. An example of this was seen during the investigation into the cause of several laboratory-acquired dengue virus infections which occurred over a brief period in the late 1980s. It was determined that each infection was due to entry of the virus through a skin abrasion or wound and that these infections could have been prevented by the use of common safety practices such as covering exposed skin or by wearing gloves and greater appreciation of infectious disease transmission.

COMPONENTS OF A BIOSAFETY PROGRAM

Rules and regulations about the use, management, and disposal of hazardous and carcinogenic chemicals in the laboratory have been in place for some time. The US Fire Protection Agency, US Occupational Safety and Health Administration (OSHA) regulations, UK Health and Safety Executive, and Labour Canada are agencies that enforce the regulations which are backed by law. Before 1989, the criteria for working safely with biological materials consisted of a series of guidelines and recommendations issued by such organizations as the US Centers for Disease Control and Prevention (CDC) and the National Institutes of Health (NIH), the UK Public Health Laboratory Service (PHLS) or professional groups. The Canadian MRC/HWC guidelines were published in 1990.

The recent concern for laboratory safety was generated by the appearance of HIV, as well as the continuing problem of hepatitis B infections among healthcare workers. In addition potential infections from emergent and re-emergent pathogens have led to the adoption of regulations to reduce occupational exposure to bloodborne pathogens. These regulations have taken various forms, such as the UK Management of Health and Safety at Work Regulations 1992, Control of Substances Hazardous to Health Regulations (COSHH) 2002, Categorisation of Biological Agents According to Hazard and Categories of Containment 1995 and 2000, Workplace (Health, Safety and Welfare) Regulations 1992, Safe Working and the Prevention of Infection in Clinical Laboratories 2003; the European Directives to Member States, relating to the protection and exposure of workers to biological agents 1990; the US OSHA Bloodborne Pathogens Standard (29 CFR part 1910.1030); and the Canadian WHIMIS Biosafety Guidelines. They include most of the information in earlier guidelines with recommendations that stress the importance of employee training and education, the use of safety equipment and the duty of care to be provided by an employer ensuring a safe working environment. Although the new regulations cover many areas relating to laboratory safety, they should be viewed only as a starting point. A comprehensive laboratory safety program relating to work with biological agents should ensure that:

- Senior management actively support and resource it.
- Full and proper risk assessment policies and procedures are in place, and take into account the agent (virulence, transmissibility, routes of infection); the work being considered; and the codes of practice needed to prevent exposure.
- Laboratories, their equipment, and other facilities are properly maintained for the safe conduct of the work.

- Laboratories undergo regular safety audits to ensure compliance with agreed protocols and the identification of new hazards.
- Laboratory workers are provided with suitable safety information, safety instruction, and training as part of their continuing professional development.
- An effective infection control program, including monitoring of exposure, health surveillance, and listing of employees working with class 3 and 4 organisms, is developed and implemented.

All staff, regardless of their position, have a duty to protect themselves, their colleagues, and the community from any hazard arising from their work.

Developing a laboratory safety program

Each safety program, while having similar objectives, will vary according to the type of institution involved and any unique features present in the local regulations. Factors to be considered include the scope of the work being undertaken, the level of technical expertise of laboratory staff, the availability of personal protective equipment (laboratory coats and gowns, gloves, eye protection, respiratory protective equipment, ear defenders), and laboratory hardware designed to ensure a safe work environment. Of equal importance is engineering support to ensure the proper installation and maintenance of biosafety cabinets and fume hoods, eye washes, and the proper air balance. Equally important is the establishment of a continually defined program of facility and equipment validation undertaken after the maintenance program that ensures equipment safety standards are being maintained. It is also crucial that staff understand, and use, the correct procedures for operating laboratory equipment.

MICROBIOLOGICAL RISK ASSESSMENT AND INFECTION CONTROL

The exact incidence of occupational infection among laboratory workers is unknown. A number of published reports detail individual or small group outbreaks of laboratory-acquired infections, retrospective studies, and anecdotal information but there has been no report that has succeeded in determining the population at risk for any of these incidents. The overall mortality of reported cases is approximately 4 percent, but this number is probably very high considering the unknown denominator and the great number of unreported illnesses.

All virology laboratories should provide safe working conditions for all staff. In order to accomplish this goal it is essential to understand and determine the possible risks involved in the manipulation and propagation of viruses (including genetically manipulated viruses), the propagation of viruses in cell cultures, and undertaking viral immunoassays. In addition, the potential hazards of chemicals and radiological products used must be taken into account during the risk assessment to reduce exposure to nonmicrobiological hazards.

It is increasingly recognized that a structured microbiological risk assessment (MRA) is necessary to identify and characterize microbiological hazards associated with laboratory working practices. Such formal risk assessments underpin current legislation in the UK (Advisory Committee on Dangerous Pathogens 1996, Health and Safety Executive 1986); Europe (EC Directive 89/391 2000); Canada (Workplace Hazardous Materials Information System (WHIMIS), 1987), and the USA (OSHA). Although such legislation requires employees to make suitable assessments of risk, they do not offer any formal guidelines on conducting risk analysis. Several agencies have begun to produce risk assessment guidelines on specific viruses: for example, HIV ((UK) Department of Health 1990); hepatitis ((UK) Public Health Service 1992); and bovine spongiform encephalitis ((UK) Health and Safety Executive 1996). For the process to be meaningful, it is important that formal risk analysis be undertaken on laboratory work practices, including the following:

● Risk assessment that identifies the source(s) of the hazard(s) and quantifies the risk of each hazard within the conditions examined.
● Identification of the gravity of the risk, to guide the management of that risk.
● A formal record of the assessment and recommendation of working practice that is communicated to all staff.
● A regular review and corrective action process.
● A corrective action plan.

For any risk assessment to be acceptable, some attempt at measurement or quantification of the risk(s) must be made. This relies on available experimental data, case and epidemiological information, and population studies including mathematical modeling, all of which relate to different aspects of risk.

It is important when establishing an infection control/ medical surveillance program that the institution's authorities understand the relative risks that their employees face. This requires information about infectious agents and other potential sources of risk that are likely to be found at their institution. Laboratories should be especially alert if dealing with large numbers and wide varieties of clinical, environmental, or veterinary materials received for laboratory diagnosis or research.

Knowledge of infectious disease processes is the cornerstone of an infection control program. People must be identified whose duties include routine and anticipated tasks involving or potentially involving exposure to infectious material. Particular duties must be evaluated for their 'infectious potential.' It is the job that is rated and not the individual, although anyone who is highly susceptible to infection should be excluded from duties that are not a risk to the normal population. Especially vulnerable are people whose immune system has been compromised, for whatever reason. The infectious potential of any job is usually determined by asking a series of questions about the work involved. For example, does the individual routinely come in contact with virus-containing blood or blood products? Does the individual routinely handle incoming shipments of potentially infectious material? What is the level of experimental animal handling? Other information required may include the type of laboratory equipment that is used, the nature of the materials used, and whether test samples are inactivated.

Once it has been determined that a worker is at risk, a written infection control plan for that position must be considered. This plan should contain an exposure determination (the criteria used to evaluate the position), a schedule, and method for meeting any relevant safety standards and the content of any training to be undertaken. A well-structured and recorded training programme is vitally important to overall laboratory safety. Training should include familiarization with the nature of laboratory pathogens, and proper and safe use of laboratory equipment. A laboratory safety manual (or code of laboratory practice) must be developed and made available to all employees and should include all approved laboratory protocols, as well as a list of duties and responsibilities. One of the responsibilities of any laboratory worker should be to report any incident that might have the potential for an occupational exposure, according to a defined incidence policy.

Any infection control policy should include medical surveillance. This should incorporate a medical evaluation including an occupational/medical history and a physical examination covering conditions that a physician feels might interfere with a worker's ability to use personal protective equipment. It is also essential to ensure that all workers are adequately immunized.

A major goal of an effective medical surveillance policy is to educate workers of the need, and indeed the requirement, to report an occupational exposure. Employees should also have the right to a confidential medical evaluation and follow-up after reporting such an incident. Elements of such a follow-up include documentation of the events surrounding the exposure, the source (if known), and the route of exposure. For incidents involving possible exposure to HIV or Lassa virus, a quick decision may be necessary as to whether to begin azidothymidine (AZT) or other treatment regimen, or ribavirin treatment. It is therefore prudent to have an established policy covering the various possibilities within any establishment handling viruses. Continuing follow-up, including counseling and illness reporting, should also be part of the program.

A surveillance policy designed for reporting illnesses away from the work site should also be developed.

A typical plan should include employees carrying an information card that will notify treating physicians that the patient may be at risk of certain diseases because of his or her occupation. The card would also contain a means for contacting the employee's institution if it is deemed necessary, such as a physician noting symptoms compatible with a disease related to that person's work. The system is important for two reasons:

1 It is essential for an employer to know if more than one employee has contracted a similar disease, because this may be an indication of a common occupational source.
2 Maintenance of a good reporting system helps to determine any source of infection. Experience has taught us that examination of most laboratory accident reports seldom pinpoints the source of occupationally acquired illnesses.

It is evident that a good infection control/medical surveillance program requires well designed and clearly written procedures and policies. It is also essential that the policy be made known to all employees at their induction and any modifications circulated as part of a continuing process of awareness. Results of investigations of laboratory incidents, with a guarantee of anonymity, should be widely published for educational purposes. Laboratory workers should be made to appreciate the ultimate goal and benefit of policy and not be made to fear it.

All workers in microbiology laboratories should provide a baseline serum sample; consideration should be given to establishing a system whereby employees are tested at quarterly intervals for evidence of infection by any agents used in the laboratory, the purpose being to detect silent infections. Although this policy has not been adopted in all parts of the world, knowledge of such subclinical infections can lead to examination of safety procedures, which may result in changes that will eliminate the potential for infections with clinical, and therefore possibly political, consequences. A major laboratory has recently been able to detect silent infections with a virus with known pathogenic relatives that were being studied there. Procedural and protocol changes have eliminated the potential for what could have been a very serious incident.

Definition of hazard groups

The classification of microbial pathogens is based on the inherent hazard of the organism. The corresponding minimum levels of containment set out in Tables 65.2 and 65.3 are intended to compensate for microbial risks encountered when working with pathogens as defined in the various hazard groups. 'Hazard' is taken as expressing the level of danger associated with the nature of the organism and 'risk' as the probability that in some circumstances the dangers will be manifested as an infection. The more inherently infectious the microbe, the higher the risk. In reality there are different levels of risk arising from work with viruses, depending on such factors as the immune status of the individual, the dose, the route, and the site of infection.

Categorizing any virus into the currently recognized four hazard groups depends on whether the organism is:

- infectious for people
- hazardous to laboratory workers
- transmissible to the community; and
- susceptible to effective prophylaxis or treatment.

All pathogenic viruses (and other microorganisms) are assigned to one of the higher hazard groups according to the infective hazard they pose for healthy workers (Table 65.3). The categorization does not allow for any additional risks that an organism can present to people who may be more severely affected for other reasons, such as pre-existing disease, compromised immunity, pregnancy, or the effects of medication.

The hazard group assigned to a particular organism indicates the minimum level of containment under which it must be handled. It should be noted that viruses listed under one category may require a containment level different from that normally assigned. The decision may be influenced by the techniques used (animal infection, virus concentration procedures, or production of an aerosol). It should also be noted that some organisms are subject to monitoring by national departments of agriculture and fisheries.

STANDARD MICROBIOLOGICAL CODE OF SAFETY PRACTICES

The importance of establishing good laboratory practices cannot be overstated. Previous investigations of laboratory accidents indicate that failures in good laboratory practice are frequently the direct cause of accidents. Information derived from the investigation of laboratory accidents, practical experience obtained from working in microbiological laboratories and the application of informed risk assessment have contributed to the development of a list of good working practices.

- Management practice should ensure that all laboratory personnel are competent and understand the biological and other hazards found in a laboratory, and are fully trained to the biohazard level required before undertaking any work.
- The laboratory director should be the individual responsible for granting or limiting access to the laboratory. In general, people who are at increased risk of infection or for whom infection may be particularly dangerous should be excluded from the laboratory. Some other situations, such as a pregnancy, will have to be considered on an individual basis. Children under the age of 16 years should not

Table 65.2 *Comparative categorization of biological agents and categories of containment*

Country/Organization	Biological hazard classification	Facility designation
Australia	Biosecurity level 1	Biosecurity level 1
	Biosecurity level 2	Biosecurity level 2
	Biosecurity level 2(E)	Biosecurity level 2(E)
	Biosecurity level 3	Biosecurity level 3
	Biosecurity level 3(E)	Biosecurity level 3(E)
	Biosecurity level 3(Z)	Biosecurity level 3(Z)
	Biosecurity level 4	Biosecurity level 4
Canada	Risk group 1	Containment level 1
	Risk group 2	Containment level 2
	Risk group 3	Containment level 3
	Risk group 4	Containment level 4
European Directive	Group 1	Containment level 1
	Group 2	Containment level 2
	Group 3	Containment level 3
	Group 4	Containment level 4
UK	Hazard group 1	Laboratory containment 1
	Hazard group 2	Laboratory containment 2
	Hazard group 3	Laboratory containment 3
	Hazard group 4	Laboratory containment 4
USA	Class 1	Biosafety 1
	Class 2	Biosafety 2
	Class 3	Biosafety 3
	Class 4	Biosafety 4
	Class 5[a]	Biosafety 3 or 4[b]
WHO	Risk group 1	Basic biosafety level 1
	Risk group 2	Basic biosafety level 2
	Risk group 3	Containment biosafety level 3
	Risk group 4	Maximum containment 4

E, exotic; Z, zoonotic.
a) Non-indigenous pathogens.
b) Facility use dependent upon virus and work involved.

be allowed in the laboratory. Animals not involved in laboratory procedures should never be allowed in the laboratory.

- A laboratory code of practice should be available, read, and signed before a new member of staff commences work.
- Laboratories should have a designated biological safety officer and/or a safety committee whose

responsibilities include ensuring that all work is carried out in accordance with established safety practices.

- Laboratories must be kept clean, neat, and orderly, and all materials or equipment not pertinent to the work should be kept to the minimum.
- Access to the laboratory must be strictly limited to authorized personnel especially biosafety level

Table 65.3 *Summary of agent hazard category and associated basis risk assessment*

Hazard group	Agent risk categorization
1	Biological agent unlikely to cause human disease
2	Biological agent that may cause disease and which may be a hazard to laboratory workers, but is unlikely to spread to community. Laboratory exposure rarely produces infection and effective prophylaxis or treatment is usually available. Examples: herpes viruses, paramyxoviruses, picornaviruses, adenoviruses
3	Biological agent can cause severe human disease, and presents a serious hazard to employees. It may present a threat of community spread. Usually an effective prophylaxis or treatment available. Examples include hepatitis B virus (HBV), hantaviruses, Japanese B encephalitis, Rift Valley fever virus, yellow fever virus, rabies virus
4	Biological agent causes severe human infections, serious threat to employees, high risk of community spread, no effective prophylaxis or treatment available. Examples Lassa virus, Ebola virus, smallpox virus, Crimean-Congo hemorrhagic fever virus, Russian spring–summer encephalitis virus

3 (BL3) and 4 laboratories. The laboratory door should remain closed and an international biohazard sign should be prominently displayed on the door, indicating that the room contains potentially infectious material. When an infectious agent (or agents) used in the laboratory requires special provisions for entry (e.g. vaccination), the relevant information must be included in the sign, together with the name of the individual responsible for the laboratory.

- A disinfection policy should be available, regularly reviewed, and displayed.
- Work surfaces should be decontaminated daily, and immediately following any spill involving potentially infectious material.
- All procedures should minimize the production of aerosols. This usually requires the development of standard operating practice and risk assessments for all laboratory procedures, and the timely review of these procedures to ensure that they are abreast of current technology and take advantage of the latest innovations in safety.
- Procedures that have the potential for producing an infectious aerosol should be undertaken within a biosafety cabinet. It is essential that all people who use such cabinets understand the principles of their operation.
- Laboratory coats, gowns, smocks, or uniforms should be worn in the laboratory, and removed before leaving the laboratory for other areas. Although a regular laboratory coat is sufficient for most clinical/diagnostic laboratory situations, a rear-closing, solid-front gown is required when practicing BL3 procedures.
- Face and eye protection or other such devices must be worn when it is necessary to protect from splashes, impacting objects, harmful substances, especially if the work is carried out on the open bench.
- Gloves must be worn for all procedures that might involve contact between broken skin or mucous membranes and potentially infectious material, toxins, or infected animals. This usually means wearing gloves for most laboratory work, including drawing blood. Gloves used in the laboratory are generally made of latex or a vinyl compound (usually polvinylchloride (PVC)), and there seems to be no difference in barrier effectiveness between gloves made of either material. When choosing gloves, consideration should be given to the toxic products (e.g. vinyl chloride and hydrochloric acid) produced when PVC gloves are incinerated.
- Mechanical pipetting devices should be used; mouth pipetting should never be permitted. Modern mechanical pipetting devices are available for almost any laboratory situation.
- Eating, drinking, smoking, application of cosmetics, or storage of food should be strictly prohibited in laboratory work areas.

- Staff must wash their hands immediately after handling any infectious materials or animals and when leaving the laboratory. For this purpose sinks, preferably with foot or elbow controls and located near the exit door, should be provided in each laboratory. Because of the number of times hands are washed it is probably best to use a mild soap with a lanolin base; although these soaps are not disinfectants, their use should remove most surface microbes from the skin.
- All contaminated or infectious liquid or solid materials must be decontaminated before disposal or cleaning for reuse. Contaminated materials that are autoclaved or incinerated at a site away from the laboratory must be packaged and labeled properly for transport and have the outside of the container disinfected chemically.
- Accidents and incidents should be immediately reported to and recorded by the person responsible for the work and to the proper safety and occupational health authorities.
- Appropriate medical surveillance and treatment should be provided.
- Hypodermic needles, syringes and needles, and scalpels, collectively referred as 'sharps,' are the main source of accidents. It is therefore especially important that laboratory workers, as well as others, use and dispose of these items with extreme caution. Needles and syringes should be restricted to parenteral injection and aspiration of fluids from laboratory animals. Only needle-locking syringes or disposable syringe–needle units should be used. Needles should not be recapped or removed by hand; attempts to perform these procedures are a major cause of needlestick injuries. Whenever a person's free hand is near a syringe and there is a needle in the other hand, the potential for an accident is very high. Several recent needlestick injuries have occurred when used syringes, capped or uncapped, were placed in the pocket of a laboratory coat and either the individual wearing the coat or a colleague was subsequently stuck. Hypodermic needles and syringes should not be used as substitutes for pipetting devices in the manipulation of infectious fluids. Once used, needles should be promptly placed in a puncture-proof container and decontaminated, preferably by incineration or autoclaving, before disposal.
- Any soiled 'sharp,' except nondisposable items, should be placed in a sharps disposal container. The sharps container itself must be of rigid construction and leak-proof. The top opening should be large enough so that the used sharps can be dropped into the container without the need to overfill it. These containers should have a top that closes easily and tightly when it is full, and they should be placed at convenient locations throughout the laboratory. When full, a container should be decontaminated by

autoclaving and then it and its contents should be incinerated.

- In modern laboratories instrumentation is a potential source of laboratory accidents. These accidents may involve chemical or electrical hazards or the possibility of infection with a biological agent. Centrifuges – ultra, high speed, or clinical – are always a potential source of aerosols. Care should be taken to load and unload centrifuge tubes containing infectious or harmful material in a biosafety cabinet. It is also prudent to use sealed tubes or safety heads while centrifuging such dangerous material. Automated analyzers are another potential source of danger in the laboratory. Blood or serum samples are often introduced into the instrument under pressure, which can increase the potential for aerosolization. The level of containment of such equipment will depend on the risk assessment and the infectious nature of the material.
- A program for insect and rodent control should be in place.
- If an autoclave is not present in the laboratory, all potentially infectious material for decontamination must be taken out of the laboratory in containers that preclude both aerosolization and leakage of the contents.

BIOSAFETY LABORATORIES

The design or refurbishment of virology laboratories increasingly has to respond to an increasingly national and global regulatory environment, and advances in scientific, technical, and industrial biosafety capabilities (Advisory Committee on Dangerous Pathogens 2001; Health Canada 2004; US Department of Health and Human Services 1999; World Health Organization 2004). Primary and secondary containment practices are increasingly more complex and their introduction varies throughout the world. There is a need to establish a common system for the implementation of common standards for future design and operation of virology laboratories that ensures worker and public confidence in biocontainment and biosafety strategies employed. Laboratory operation should also introduce a detailed record system for the monitoring and revalidation of facilities, equipment, and plant which should become more detailed the higher the biosafety level (BSL) category.

Working with potentially infectious viruses in the microbiological laboratory requires an appreciation both of work practices and of the facilities needed to make such laboratories a safe environment. Guidelines on the safe handling of pathogens have evolved over the past decade and have reached the point where there is general agreement on the basic principles of biosafety in the laboratory (Table 65.4). Four biosafety levels have been described (BL1–BL4), which comprise combinations of laboratory practices and procedures, safety equipment, and laboratory facilities appropriate for the operations performed and the hazard posed by the infectious agent. Essentially, the numerical designation of a safety level increases with an increase in the risks involved in working with an agent.

The levels of containment are intended to reflect the risks encountered when working with biological agents as categorized in the various hazard groups. All laboratories in which there is likely to be exposure to human

Table 65.4 *General summary of relation between hazard groups and biosafety level, work practices, and containment level*

Hazard group	Biosafety level (BL)	Working practices and procedures (use)	Primary engineering control requirements
1	BL1	Standard microbiological practices (SMP)	No special engineering requirements; containment achieved by adherence to standard laboratory practice
2	BL2	BL1 work practice, plus: Limit access. Limit aerosols. Biohazard signs. Laboratory code of practice. Protective personal equipment (PPE): gloves, laboratory coats, face protection as needed. Infectious waste decontaminated	Procedures that produce potentially infectious aerosols performed in a biological safety cabinet (BSC). On-site autoclave required
3	BL3	BL2 work practice, plus: All virus material contained. Restricted access. PPE: gloves, protective laboratory clothing, respiratory protection as needed	Inward airflow. Air-lock facility. Exhaust air discharged from laboratory via HEPA filtration (optional). On-site/integrated autoclave required
4	BL4 (maximum containment)	BL3 work practice, plus Change of clothing before entry. Shower on exit. All waste autoclaved before leaving facility. Regular engineering and biosafety maintenance	HEPA-filtered supply and exhaust air. Work undertaken in BSC class III cabinets or BSC II using an air-supplied positive full-body pressure suit in an air-tight laboratory. Integrated laboratory required. All waste decontaminated

pathogens (whether or not they are to be propagated or concentrated) require a minimum of BL2 containment. When there is a likelihood or strong indication that material (specimens or samples) contains BL3 or BL4 agents, additional controls are necessary.

Many national guidelines list the essential laboratory procedures that are basic to good laboratory practice (Table 65.5). It must be emphasized that good microbiological practice is fundamental to laboratory safety and cannot be replaced by specialized equipment or safety barriers, which can only supplement it.

It should be noted that although these classifications may be reasonable for clinical and research laboratories, they are not applicable to many industrial, food science, and agricultural laboratories.

Rules associated with animal facilities parallel those for laboratories. Additional considerations should be given to the requirements of individual species that take into account behavior, husbandry requirements, housing standards, zoonoses, parasites, and size (Advisory Committee on Dangerous Pathogens 1997; Richmond and Quimby 1999).

Biosafety level 1

BL1 practices, safety equipment, and laboratory facilities require no special engineering features for work with organisms that present no danger to humans. Examples of laboratories that may be operated at this level include undergraduate training and teaching laboratories. In these laboratories work is undertaken with well-characterized agents that are most unlikely to cause disease in normal healthy adult humans. Many agents not normally able to produce disease in healthy individuals may produce severe illness in elderly people, the immunodeficient, or the immunosuppressed, and can cause allergic or toxogenic responses, so appropriate precautions must be taken. Also, vaccine strains that, because they are attenuated in virulence, do not usually produce disease in healthy individuals may produce severe disease in some individuals. The latter two categories of organisms should be manipulated under BL2 conditions.

Work is generally conducted on the bench, and specialized containment equipment is not normally

Table 65.5 *Exposure controls: summary of minimum containment requirements for laboratories and animal rooms*

Containment requirements	Containment levels			
	1	2	3	4
Laboratory site: separated from other activities in the building	No	No	Yes	Yes
Facility: sealable	No	No	Yes	Yes
Ventilation				
Workplace maintained at air pressure negative to atmosphere	Opt	Opt	Yes	Yes
Through safety cabinet	No	Opt	Opt	No
Mechanical: direct	No	Opt	Opt	No
Mechanical: independent	No	No	Opt	Yes
Supply and extract air HEPA filtered	No	No	Yes, on extract	Yes on input and double on extract
Airlock	No	No	Yes	Yes
Airlock: with shower	No	No	No/Opt	Yes
Effluent treatment	No	No	Yes	Yes
Autoclave site				
On site	No	No	No	No
En suite	No	Yes	Yes	Yes
In laboratory: free-standing	No	No	Opt	No
In laboratory: double-ended	No	No	Rec	Yes
Microbiological safety cabinet/enclosure	No	Opt	Yes	Yes
Biosafety cabinet	NR	I	I/III	III I/II[a]
Facility to contain own equipment	NR	No	Yes as far as reasonably practical	Yes
Safe storage of biological material		Yes	Yes, secure storage	Yes, secure storage
Efficient vector control, e.g. rodents and insects		Yes, for animal containment	Yes, for animal containment	Yes

NR, not required; Opt, optional; Rec, recommended.
a) Class I and II biological safety cabinets permitted with use of positive-pressure suits.

required. Laboratory personnel should have specific training in the procedures undertaken within the laboratory and be supervised by experienced senior staff. The following laboratory facilities and basic work practices apply to viruses assigned to BL1.

LABORATORY FACILITIES

In the interests of safety, floors should be slip resistant, seamless, be impermeable to liquids, and resistant to most if not all chemicals. Laboratories should be designed so that the floors, walls, and ceilings are easy to clean. Benchtops should be impervious to water and resistant to acids, alkalis, organic solvents, and moderate heat. Laboratory furniture should be of similar resistant materials and be arranged so as not to obstruct workers while performing their duties. Equipment should be placed where it is easily accessible for cleaning and, if it is likely to produce an aerosol, in the safest possible location. Attention should be paid to door swings because a door opening in the wrong direction has the potential to knock items from someone's hands. Equipment must not be placed near thermostats, because it may interfere with temperature control. Floors should be nonskid, to reduce the likelihood of slipping. Hand-washing facilities must be provided, preferably near the point of exit.

Biosafety level 2

Conditions described for BL2 are usually applicable to clinical, diagnostic, research, and teaching facilities in which work is done with a wide variety of microorganisms that cause human disease and may be a hazard to laboratory workers but unlikely to spread to the community. Laboratory exposure rarely produces infection, and effective prophylaxis or treatment is usually available. Many of the agents that require BL2 containment are already present in the community, and community vaccination programs for them are routine.

Hepatitis A virus, herpes simplex types 1 and 2, measles virus, Epstein–Barr virus, and certain viral vaccines are among those that can be manipulated at the BL2 level. Generally the agents that are assigned to this level cause bloodborne diseases and do not have a history of infection via the respiratory route. It is not surprising, then, that the usual routes of laboratory-acquired infections with agents in this group are auto-inoculation, ingestion, and mucous membrane exposure to the infectious agent. Procedures with agents assigned to this level that have a high probability of aerosol production should be conducted in primary containment equipment (e.g. Class 2 biosafety cabinet) or similar devices.

The competence expected of laboratory workers is greater than that of a newly qualified graduate. Personnel at this level need to be familiar with the institution's safety policy, to have received training in the handling of the viruses and be supervised by a competent senior member of staff.

LABORATORY DESIGN

The laboratory requiring BL2 containment is generally similar in construction and design to a BL1 facility. It also incorporates criteria for microbiological practices in association with additional primary and secondary containment facilities (Figure 65.1).

The equipment is selected according to the following principles:

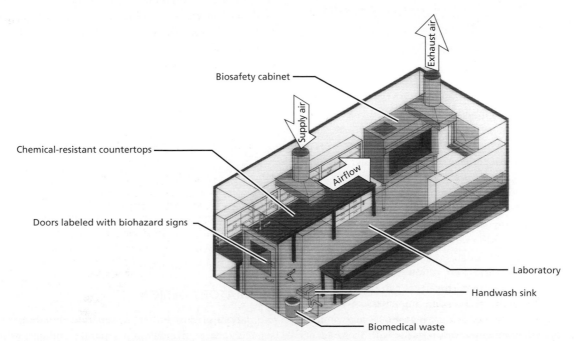

Figure 65.1 *A schematic of a generic BL2 laboratory design (courtesy of Smith Carter, architects, engineers, planners, interior designers).*

- Designed to prevent or limit exposure of the operator to infectious material.
- Constructed of materials that are resistant to corrosion and meet structural requirements.
- Installed to aid operation, maintenance, cleaning, decontamination, and safety testing.
- Complies with safety specifications.

Laboratories that anticipate working with potentially infectious material should use a biosafety cabinet, isolator, or other suitable containment. Standard laboratory working practice is undertaken at this level, with additional features that reflect the higher containment level (see Tables 65.3, 65.4, and 65.5). Procedures with the potential for creating infectious aerosols should be conducted within a biosafety containment cabinet. These include grinding, blending, vigorous shaking or mixing, sonic disruption, and opening containers of infectious materials. Intranasal inoculation of animals and harvesting infectious tissues from animals or eggs should also be done in a biosafety cabinet or equivalent. Any work with high concentrations of infectious agents should be carried out in a containment cabinet. The reduction of aerosols is also a consideration when working with many of the analytical machines found in any virology laboratory. Special precautions should be taken with machines such as cell sorters and when loading analytical machines where the sample may be under pressure and more likely to produce an aerosol. In many cases a splash-guard may suffice.

There may be occasions when agents routinely manipulated at BL2 may require BL3 containment, or at least BL3 practices. This usually occurs when the procedures produce concentrations significantly exceeding the physiological concentration of the agent in nature. A higher biosafety level should also be considered for studies involving animals.

Biosafety level 3

All the laboratory design features and working practices required for BL2 are applicable to BL3, with special emphasis on some of them. The work practices, safety equipment and facilities for BL3 apply when working with indigenous or exotic agents and when aerosol infection is a significant possibility resulting in disease that may have serious, or even lethal, consequences. Agents for which BL3 safeguards are routinely recommended include *Hantavirus* (Hantaan virus, Seoul virus, Sin Nombre virus) and St. Louis encephalitis virus. Two of the more exotic agents that require BL3 containment are Rift Valley fever virus and yellow fever virus, hemorrhagic fever viruses from Africa that can be worked with at this level provided workers are immunized.

Although auto-inoculation, ingestion, and mucous membrane contamination are hazards with these agents, the major concern is aerosol infection. The requirements for BL3 are more stringent than those for BL2 and are aimed at controlling aerosol production and possible spread into the community.

The laboratory staff must understand the safety procedures, as well as the risks involved in working with the agents used in their laboratory. Training, including the use of specialized equipment, should be done by competent scientists who have experience of working with the viruses contained at this level.

LABORATORY DESIGN

The laboratory has engineering and design features and physical containment equipment additional to those found at BL2 (see Tables 65.4 and 65.5). Principal differences from BL2 requirements are that the laboratory must be separated from other laboratory space by an anteroom and that personnel access is strictly controlled. The laboratory must be maintained at an air pressure negative to the atmosphere (maintain a verifiable inward directional air flow) and extracted air must be high efficiency particulate air (HEPA)-filtered (in some countries) and discharged to the outside so that it is dispersed clear of adjacent buildings or air intakes (Figure 65.2). Additional aerosol protection when working with animals is afforded by a variety of newly designed flexible-film isolators (Figure 65.3).

LABORATORY PRACTICES

All work involving infectious material is undertaken within biosafety cabinets by staff wearing full frontal gowns, gloves, and eye protection. Alternatively, some laboratories prefer to use class III cabinets. Contaminated solid materials that are to be decontaminated at a site away from the laboratory are sealed in a leak-proof container before being removed to an autoclave and then incineration. Contaminated liquids are autoclaved or disinfected in the laboratory area. An autoclave should be available in the laboratory or laboratory suite.

Biosafety level 4

This containment level is to be used when working with viruses that cause severe human disease (some with a high mortality rate), and present a serious hazard to laboratory workers for which there is no vaccine or generally no reliable treatment. A variety of agents causing hemorrhagic fevers, including Lassa virus, Marburg virus, Ebola virus, Crimean-Congo hemorrhagic fever virus, and related viruses, are those most commonly studied at BL4.

LABORATORY DESIGN

The laboratory is either a separate building or an isolated zone equivalent to a separate building within a building. Mainly because of their high construction and

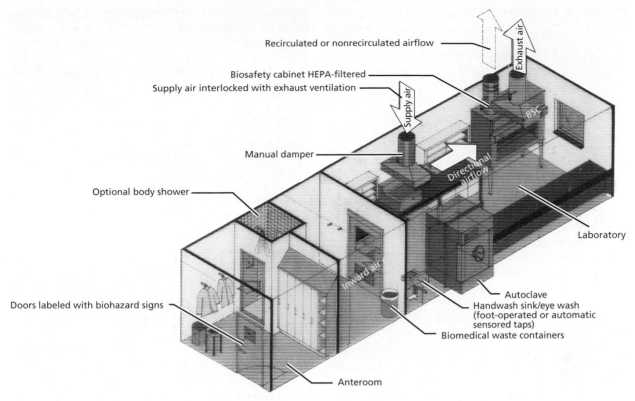

Figure 65.2 *A schematic of a generic BL3 laboratory design (courtesy of Smith Carter, architects, engineers, planners, interior designers).*

operational costs, there are fewer than ten BL4 laboratories in the world.

There are two operational designs that provide efficient primary containment. The first and oldest system is based on protecting the worker from exposure by containing the agent within a series of interconnecting airtight class III biosafety cabinets (Figure 65.4).

Each cabinet is equipped with its own HEPA-filtered air supply and extracts exhaust air via HEPA filters in series, and can be independently sealed and fumigated without interference with the rest of the system. All equipment (refrigerators, freezers, microscopes, centrifuges, and incubators) is built as an integral part of the system. All staff has a complete change of clothing and shower after each day's work. All work is conducted through glove ports. The cabinet system is connected to a double-ended high-containment autoclave, through which all liquid and solid waste is decontaminated before being removed for incineration. A chemical 'dunk tank' or formaldeclave is located at the other end of the system, through which suitably packaged material can be taken in or out of the system. The whole system is incorporated within a laboratory providing environmental protection and operating an interlocking HEPA-filtered supply and exhaust air system.

The alternative system, 'the suit laboratory' isolates the workers from the laboratory environment by means of fully encapsulating suits supplied with air from outside the laboratory (Figure 65.5). By the use of special construction techniques (impermeable surfaces and welded ductwork) the laboratory facility provides the biosafety barrier that ensures the protection of the exterior environment. Work with infectious material is carried out within class II biosafety cabinets. Air from the room and biosafety cabinets is removed via HEPA filtration, the HEPA filters are also an integral component of the supply air ductwork. A special chemical shower must be provided to decontaminate the surface of the suit before the worker leaves the area. A double-doored autoclave is provided for decontaminating waste materials to be removed from the suit area. When necessary, appropriate material may be removed from the laboratory, without heat treatment, by proper packaging and removal through the chemical shower or a dunk tank.

Laboratory practices

Basic work practices are undertaken in the same manner in both systems. Because of the complexity of the work, a detailed code of practice should be developed and form part of an individualized training program. On entering, staff should put on a complete change of clothing; before leaving, they must shower before putting on their own clothing. Entry and exit of personnel and supplies must only be through an airlock or pass-through system. All fluid effluents from the facility, including shower water, must be rendered safe before final release.

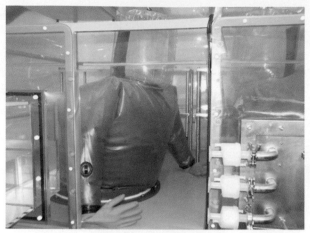

Figure 65.3 *Flexible-film isolator design for animal containment level 3 and 4 work (courtesy of Health Protection Agency, UK).*

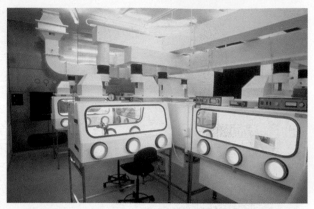

Figure 65.4 *Cabinet-line BL4 laboratory (courtesy of Health Protection Agency, UK).*

A regular, rigorous, preventative maintenance program for the engineering controls, air flow, autoclave, safety cabinets, etc., should be developed to ensure continued integration of the facilities and suitability of the safety procedures. Within the UK the Health and Safety Commission institute regular safety inspections of the facilities, safety management, and procedures.

LABORATORY WASTE

The general principle involved in the treatment of laboratory waste is that all infectious or potentially infectious laboratory waste must be rendered noninfectious before leaving the laboratory. An alternative is to develop a system whereby infectious material can be safely delivered to an off-site disposal facility. A robust disinfection and waste policy is regarded as an operational necessity at this level.

In general, local regulations cover the disposal of infectious waste. There are different interpretations of what constitutes 'infectious waste,' so this must be considered when developing a waste management program. A program designed to minimize the production of regulated waste will reap cost savings because disposal of regulated waste is far more costly.

PACKING AND SHIPPING OF INFECTIOUS MATERIALS

The safe shipment of infectious substances or diagnostic specimens within or between countries is important for everyone involved with the process, basic guidance being provided by the World Health Organization (1997). Although no reports of illness have been attributed to the transportation of such materials, there are numerous areas of conflicting guidelines throughout the world. Because these packages have the potential for harboring

infectious agents and move in public places during their journey, their transportation is strictly regulated. Postal and transport authorities have always been aware of the potential hazards to their employees of infectious material transported and handled by them.

In many countries such material is sent through the mail, and local regulations apply; guidelines are often issued (e.g. the *Post Office Guide* in the UK and the *Postal Service Manual* in the USA). The USPS requirements for the mailing of 'diseased tissue, blood, serum, and cultures of pathogenic microorganisms' are listed in their Postal Service Manuals.

The US Department of Transportation, the UK's Health and Safety Executive, and Canada's Transport Canada have major responsibility for safe transportation and provide the authorization for the movement of hazardous materials within their respective countries and to foreign countries. The importation of infectious agents that are predominately pathogenic to animals also needs to take into account various national regulations and permit requirements (UK: Importation of Animal Pathogens Order 1980, 1998; Canada: Animal Disease Protection Act; USA: USDA, APHIS 9 CFR Parts 94 and 95). Workers sending infectious material to other laboratories should ensure that these laboratories have the facilities to work with the agent. This applies particularly to the transfer of viruses in hazard groups 3 and 4. In response to the anthrax attacks in the USA during 2001, the USA (2002 42 CFR Part 73) and UK (Home Office 2001) introduced antiterrorism legislation which made laboratories and their personnel accountable and responsible for possessing, working with, and transferring high-threat pathogens known as 'selected agents.'

An agreement between the Universal Postal Union (UPU), the International Air Transport Association (IATA), and the International Civil Aviation Organization (ICAO) led to new regulations for overseas mail in the 1990s. These are currently being modified and due for publication in 2004/5. The IATA/ICAO guidelines and procedures also should be considered because they were designed to facilitate the safe shipment of

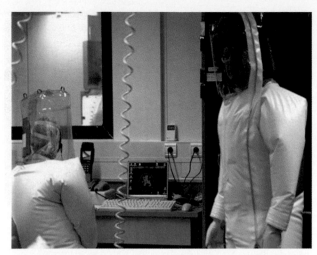

Figure 65.5 *BL4 suit laboratory (courtesy of Lyon CL4 facility, France).*

infectious substances while ensuring the safety of the transport personnel and the general public. The regulations define the terms 'diagnostic specimen,' 'biological product' and 'etiological agent,' and give minimum packaging requirements and volume limits for each.

The regulations define a diagnostic specimen as 'any human or animal material including, but not limited to, excreta, secretions, blood and its components, tissue, and tissue fluids, being shipped for the purposes of diagnosis (excluding live infected animals).' These must be transported under ICAO/IATA packing instruction 602. Infectious substances are 'substances containing viable microorganisms or toxins known or suspected to cause diseases in animals or humans (including HIV)' and are transported according to ICAO/IATA packing instruction 650.

With regard to packaging, all guidelines indicate that no one may knowingly transport or cause to be transported, directly or indirectly, any diagnostic specimens or biological product which they reasonably believe may contain an etiological agent unless such material is packaged to withstand leakage of contents, shocks, pressure changes, and other conditions incident to ordinary handling in transportation. The major decision to be made, then, when determining the transport requirements for any sample is whether it contains an etiological agent. It is prudent to be conservative in this matter and assume that each specimen may contain an agent unless it is certain that it does not.

The current packaging requirement is for triple packaging. A securely closed, watertight primary container is enclosed in a second, durable watertight container, with enough material in the space between them to absorb all the contents of the primary container in the event of leakage. Each set of primary and secondary containers is then enclosed in an outer shipping container constructed of fiberboard, cardboard, wood, or other material of equivalent strength. An etiological agent/biomedical

material sticker is required for the outer mailing package. Any packaging requiring solid carbon dioxide (dry ice) should ensure that it permits the release of carbon dioxide gas to prevent the build-up of pressure.

Although on 1 January 1995, IATA (a voluntary organization of air carriers) issued requirements for packaging, and has established a certification procedure for packaging companies who wish to provide packages to ship 'infectious material' on aircraft, the issues of updated guidelines is expected in 2004/5. Certification of packaging will continue to be a requirement. With the increased concern surrounding the transport of infectious material internationally and nationally, individuals should recognize that the importation and export of infectious materials requires the approval of a number of government departments and biosafety and biosecurity agencies.

SUMMARY

An increasing variety of publications already covers the many topics involved in general safety, laboratory safety, and biosafety. In this chapter we have tried to make virologists aware of the range of guidelines and regulations that affect work in a virology laboratory. We have also attempted to present the issue of biosafety from the view of the scientist. It is increasingly recognized that virological scientific programs need to be conducted in an efficient, safe, and secure manner. Because it is the scientists who should have the best knowledge of the nature of the agents under investigation, including factors such as pathogenic potential, they should play a pivotal role in the development of continuing biosafety policy.

The biosafety professionals have knowledge of the guidelines and regulations that apply to the operation of a virology laboratory. They also have knowledge of the latest in validated biosafety technology and practices that have been developed around the world. In addition, occupational safety and health professionals generally have information in such areas as transportation of specimens and requirements for importation of agents, which can help the laboratory function more efficiently. Increasingly it is recognized that scientists need to be responsible and accountable for the agents they work with and provide both the public and regulatory agencies evidence-based information that work is conducted within appropriately designed containment systems.

With the current expansion of high containment laboratories throughout the world it is essential that international cooperation and consensus is established in facility design, commissioning, operation, and maintenance in accordance with our understanding of infectious disease processes. Equally the establishment of well-managed biosafety training programs address the 'duty of care' required. The operational integrity of these facilities will be dependent upon the establishment of good working relationships between scientists, specialist engineers, and biosafety professionals being established. This will ensure that the primary mission of the laboratory, the research, developmental and detection programs, can be conducted efficiently, safely, and securely.

REFERENCES

Advisory Committee on Dangerous Pathogens (UK). 1995a. *Categorisation of biological agents according to hazard and categories of containment.* 4th edn. London: HMSO.

Advisory Committee on Dangerous Pathogens (UK). 1995b. *Protection against blood-borne infections at work – HIV and hepatitis.* London: HMSO.

Advisory Committee on Dangerous Pathogens (UK). 1996. *Microbiological risk assessment: an interim report.* London: HMSO.

Advisory Committee on Dangerous Pathogens (UK). 1997. *Working safely with research animals: management of infection risks.* London: HMSO.

Advisory Committee on Dangerous Pathogens (UK). 2000. *Second supplement to Categorisation of biological agents according to hazard and categories of containment.* London: HMSO.

Advisory Committee on Dangerous Pathogens (UK). 2001. *The management, design and operation of microbiological containment laboratories.* London: HMSO.

Association Française de Normalisation. 1990. *Liste des espèces microbiennes communement reconnues comme pathogènes pour l'homme* [List of microbial species known to be pathogenic for man]. Paris: AFNOR.

Department of Health (UK). 1990. *Guidance for clinical health care workers: protection against infection with HIV and hepatitis viruses.* London: HMSO.

Department of Health (Taiwan). 2003. *A SARS confirmed case infected in research laboratory in Taiwan.* http/sars.doh.gov.tw/news/200312701.html

Cambell, G. and Lanciotti, M.D. 2002. Laboratory-acquired West Nile virus infections – United States. *Morb Mortal Wkly Rep*, **51**, 1133–5.

Centers for Disease Control and Prevention. 1998. Fatal cercopithecine herpesvirus 1 (B virus) infection following a mucocutaneous exposure and interim recommendations for worker protection. *Morb Mortal Wkly Rep*, **47**, 1073–6, 1083.

Centers for Disease Control and Prevention. 2002. *Smallpox response plan and guidelines (version 3.0).* URL: http//www.bt.cdc.gov/agent/smallpox/response-plan/index.asp

Desmyter, J., LeDuc, J.W., et al. 1983. Laboratory rat associated outbreak of haemorrhagic fever with renal syndrome due to hantaan-like virus. *Lancet*, **2**, 1445–8.

EC Directive. 1993. *Biological agents directive.* 93/88/EEC.

EC Directive 54. 2000. *Protection of workers from risks related to exposure to biological agents at Work*, 89/391/EEC.

Emond, R.T.D., Evans, B., et al. 1977. A case of Ebola virus infection. *Br Med J*, **2**, 541–4.

Fenner, F., Henderson, D.A., et al. 1988. *Smallpox and its eradication.* Geneva: World Health Organization.

Health and Safety Executive (UK). 1986. *A guide to the reporting of injuries, diseases and dangerous occurrences regulations (RIDDOR).* London: HMSO.

Health and Safety Executive (UK). 1996. *BSE (bovine spongiform encephalopathy): background and general occupational guidance.* London: HMSO.

Health and Safety Executive (UK). 2000. *Management of health, safety and welfare. Mangement of Health and Safety at Work Regulations 1999. Approved code of practice and guidance L21*, (2nd edn). London: HMSO.

Health and Safety Executive (UK). 2002. *The control of substances hazardous to health regulations (2002). Approved code of practice and guidance L5*, 4th edn. London: HMSO.

Health Canada. 2004. *Laboratory biosafety guidelines*, 3rd edn. Ottawa: Laboratory Centre for Disease Control, Health Protection Branch.

Home Office (UK). 2001. *The anti-terrorism, crime and security Act 2001 (Commencement No. 40 Order 2002*: SI 202/1279. London: The Stationery Office.

International Society for Infectious Diseases. 2001. Marburg virus, laboratory infection in Russia, htttp://www.promedmail.org. ProMed archive No 20010208.0248.

International Society for Infectious Diseases. 2004a. Ebola, virus, laboratory accident – USA (Maryland). htttp://www.promedmail.org. ProMed archive No. 20040220.0550.

International Society for Infectious Diseases. 2004b. Ebola, lab accident death – Russia (Siberia), htttp://www.promedmail.org. ProMed archive No. 20040823.2350.

Jones, L., Ristow, S., et al. 1986. Accidental human vaccination with vaccinia virus expressing nucleoprotein gene. *Nature*, **319**, 543.

Labour Canada. 1987. *Workplace hazardous materials information system (WHIMIS).* Canada Labour Code, Bill C-70, Ottawa.

Lee, S.F., Buller, R., et al. 1994. Vaccinia keratouveitis manifesting as a masquerade syndrome. *Am J Ophthalmol*, **117**, 480–7.

Leifer, E., Gocke, D.J. and Bourne, H. 1970. Lassa fever. A new virus disease of man from West Africa. II. Report of a laboratory acquired infection. *Am J Trop Med Hyg*, **19**, 677–9.

Lloyd, G. and Jones, N. 1986. Infections of laboratory workers with Hantaan virus acquired from immunocytomas propagated in laboratory rats. *J Infect*, **12**, 117–25.

Martini, G.A., Knauff, H.G., et al. 1969. A hitherto unknown infectious disease contracted from monkeys. *German Med Mth*, **8**, 457–69.

Mempel, M., Isa, G., et al. 2003. Laboratory-acquired infection with recombinant vaccinia virus containing an immunomodulating construct. *J Invest Dermatol*, **120**, 356–8.

Ministry of Health (Sweden). 1988. *Arbetarskyddsstyrelsens kungörelse med foreskrifter om mikroorganismer samt allmana rad om tillämpningen av foreskrifterna.* [Statement of the Workers' Protection Board containing regulations on micro-organisms, with general advice on their application]. Stockholm: Ministry of Health.

Moussatche, N., Tuyama, M., et al. 2003. Accidental infection of laboratory worker with vaccinia virus. *Emerg Inf Dis*, **9**, 1–6.

Openshaw, P.J.M., Alwan, W.H., et al. 1991. Accidental infection of laboratory worker with recombinant vaccinia virus. *Lancet*, **338**, 459.

National Institutes of Health. 1987. *Regulations on the safety control of laboratories handling pathogenic agents.* Tokyo: National Institute of Health.

Pike, R.M. 1979. Laboratory-associated infections: incidence, fatalities, causes and prevention. *Annu Rev Microbiol*, **33**, 41–66.

Public Health Laboratory Service. 1992. Exposure to hepatitis B virus: guidance on post-exposure prophylaxis. *Commun Dis Rep*, **2**, 9.

Richmond, J.Y. and Quimby, F. 1999. Considerations for working safely with infectious disease agents in research animal. In: Zak, O. and Sande, M.A. (eds), *Handbook of animal models of infection.* London: Academic Press.

Ryder, R.W. and Gordsman, E.J. 1995. Laboratory acquired Sabià virus infection. *N Engl J Med*, **333**, 1716, letter.

Spencer, R.C. and Lightfoot, N.F. 2001. Preparedness and response to bioterrorism. *J Infect*, **43**, 104–10.

Standards Australia/Standards New Zealand. 2002. *Safety in laboratories – microbiological aspects and containment facilities.* Sydney, NSW: Standards Australia International (Standard AS/NZS 2243.3.2002).

Subcommittee on Arbovirus Laboratory Safety. 1980. Laboratory safety for arboviruses and certain other viruses of vertebrates. *Am J Trop Med Hyg*, **29**, 1359–81.

UK Department Environment, Food and Rural Affairs. 1980. *Importation of animal pathogens order 1980.* London: HMSO.

UK Department Environment, Food and Rural Affairs. 1998. *Specific animal pathogens order*. London: HMSO.

US Department of Health and Human Services. 1999. *Biosafety in microbiological and biomedical laboratories*, HHS Publication No (CDC) 93-8395, 4th edn. Washington, DC: Centers for Disease Control and National Institutes of Health.

US Department of Health and Human Services. 2002. *Possession, use, and transfer of selected agents and toxins; Interim Final rule, Part IV 42 Part 73*.

Weissenbacher, M.C., Grela, M.E., et al. 1978. Inapparent infections with Junin virus among laboratory workers. *J Infect Dis*, **137**, 309–13.

World Health Organization. 1997. *Guidelines for the safety transport of infectious substances and diagnostic specimens*. Geneva: WHO.

World Health Organization. 2003. *WHO global eradication plan for laboratory containment of wild poliovirus*, 2nd edn. Geneva: Department of Vaccines and Biologicals, WHO.

World Health Organization. 2004. *Laboratory biosafety manual*, 3rd edn (revised). Geneva: WHO.

World Health Organization. 2004a. *New case of laboratory-confirmed SARS in China*. http://www.who.int/csr/don/2004-01-31/en/

World Health Organization. 2004b. *Severe case in Singapore linked to accidental laboratory contamination*. http://www.who.int/csr/don/2004-09-24/en/

FURTHER READING

Furr, A.K. 2000. *CRC handbook of laboratory safety*, 5th edn. Boca Raton, FL: CRC Press.

Health and Safety Commission. 1994. *Management of health and safety in the health services: Information for directors and managers*. London: HMSO.

Health and Safety Commission. 2002a. *Control of substances hazardous to health regulations. Approved code of practice*. London: HMSO.

Health and Safety Commission. 2002b. *Management of health and safety at work regulations 1999. Approved code of practice and guidance*, L21, 2nd edn. London: HMSO.

Health and Safety Executive. 1992. *Workplace (health, safety and welfare) regulations 1992. Approved code of practice*. London: HMSO.

Health Services Advisory Committee. 2003. *Safe working and the prevention of infection in clinical laboratories*. London: HMSO.

Lee, H.V. and Johnson, K.M. 1982. Laboratory acquired infections with Hantaan virus the etiologic agent of Korean haemorrhagic fever. *J Infect Dis*, **146**, 645–51.

National Research Council USA, 1989, *Biosafety in the laboratory. Prudent practices for the handling and disposal of infectious materials*. Washington, DC: National Academy Press.

66

The laboratory diagnosis of viral infections

STEVEN SPECTER AND MAURO BENDINELLI

During the past three decades the diagnostic virology laboratory has emerged as an important adjunct to patient care. This is a result of several factors, including enhanced technology that has allowed for more accurate, useful and rapid detection of viruses, improvements in patient management resulting from increased understanding of viral pathophysiology, and the development of a growing arsenal of antiviral chemotherapeutic agents. Molecular biology and antigen detection techniques have emerged as the methods of choice for rapid viral detection in many cases. This often allows detection and quantitation of virus in a matter of a few hours, resulting in direct application of collected results to patient healthcare. The viral diagnostic laboratory now has a vast array of methods to assist in diagnosis, including cytology, cell culture, antigen detection, electron microscopy, nucleic acid detection, measurement of antibodies, and, most recently, antiviral susceptibility testing. These techniques are facilitated by the development of specific reagents, test kits, and automated instruments, many of which are commercially available, as well as published algorithms for how to test for specific viral agents.

In an age when administrators are examining all costs, the performance of viral testing is often driven by outcomes assessment. The laboratory is now able to provide data that lead to cost savings related to:

- number of hospital days saved due to rapid and accurate diagnosis

- decrease in unnecessary antibiotic use
- improved hospital infection control
- application of specific antiviral therapy or other patient management issues.

These all have become valid reasons for performing testing, in addition to the age-old standards of collecting epidemiologic information and screening the blood supply.

Thus, this chapter strives to assess the methods currently in use for their importance in achieving viral diagnoses, with little comment on the actual manner in which these tests are performed. For this reason many of the historically important procedures may only receive passing mention.

PRINCIPLES OF DIAGNOSIS

In the course of virus infection it is possible to detect virus, viral antigens, nucleic acids, or antibodies to the virus as a means of identification of the etiologic agent. A good understanding of viral pathophysiology and host response is needed in order to determine the most appropriate specimen(s) to collect and the best type of testing to perform. During the viral incubation period, which can last from 1 day to months or even years depending on the virus, virus or viral subunits are the best targets for detection methods. This is also a period when virus may be found in blood or other body fluids in some infections. By the time signs or symptoms of disease become apparent, virus is usually present in the target tissues but may be more readily isolated or otherwise detected from other tissues. For example, enteroviruses are more easily detected in stool than in the cerebrospinal fluid (CSF) in infections of the central nervous system (CNS). Collection of a serum sample early in infection is also important since the rise in antibody titers in later specimen(s) is often a useful way to identify a cause of infection. For serological identification of virus it is necessary to either test for IgM antibodies as an indicator of recent infection or to look for a significant titer rise. This must be at least a two-dilution increase to limit the possibility that technical error is a factor (most commonly a fourfold rise, since use of twofold dilutions is mostly performed). For persistent infections or late infection it may be difficult to isolate virus; thus, detection of viral antigen or nucleic acids may be easier than virus.

Specimens

Collection and submission to the laboratory of an appropriate sample is a vital factor in successful diagnosis. Ideally one should know exactly what is necessary to collect and submit specimens to a particular laboratory to optimize results (Smith 2000) (Table 66.1). This is best accomplished by contacting the laboratory to which the specimen will be submitted for direction.

Specimens should be collected and submitted to the laboratory as rapidly as possible after the recognition of

a clinical problem. Failure to get the laboratory a good specimen is the greatest contributor to improper results. The suspected etiology(ies) should help guide the choice of specimen site(s). Not all specimens are directly related to the clinical presentation and knowledge of the most appropriate specimen(s) for each condition as well as the laboratory that is going to be used are important. It is best to err on the side of too much sample, if the amount of material needed is in question, as most laboratories do not complain about too much material as compared to too little. Of similar importance is the submission of vital supportive data on the label of the container for the specimen including patient name, identification number, specimen source, date and time of collection, and ordering physician. Each specimen should be accompanied by a requisition form with identical information as the specimen label plus other useful information such as clinical diagnosis and suspected virus(es).

Another important factor for successful laboratory diagnosis is transport of the specimen to the laboratory. A number of commercial media are available to preserve specimens during transport including Culturettes, Micro Test Multi-Microbe (M4-3), Virocult, Viral Transport Medium (VTM) and ViraTrans. While these all-purpose transport media are usually sufficient for the transport of most specimens, occasionally a specific specimen type may require special medium (Johnson 1990).

DETECTION OF VIRIONS OR THEIR COMPONENTS

Cytopathology

One of the oldest and most rapid methods of detecting viruses is to directly examine stained clinical material using light microscopy. Cytological alterations that are pathognomonic for specific viruses can be readily visualized in virus-infected tissues and cells (Table 66.2). More often, the examination of material by microscopy may only raise a suspicion of viral infection or may limit detection to a viral family, requiring more specific methods for viral identification. Nevertheless, these rapid examinations may quickly rule in or out viral infection. Cytological staining using Giemsa (Tzanck preparation), Papanicalaou (Pap) or Wright stain, while rapid, has relatively low sensitivity when compared with modern methods of antigen or nucleic acid detection. Inability to distinguish herpes simplex virus (HSV) from varicella-zoster virus (VZV) somewhat limits the utility of Tzanck preparations.

The most commonly used viral cytology procedure is the Pap stain of cervical scrapings to detect premalignant lesions. Since its implementation nearly 50 years ago, Pap staining has helped to dramatically decrease the incidence of cervical cancer. The most common

Table 66.1 *Specimens useful for viral studies*

Specimen type	Disease category (examples)
Nasopharyngeal wash or aspirate	Respiratory tract infection Certain exanthems CNS infections (especially enteroviruses)
Throat wash or swab	Respiratory tract infection
Sputum	Respiratory infection (HSV, CMV)
Bronchoalveolar lavage	Lower respiratory infection (CMV, influenza virus, parainfluenza virus)
Rectal swab or stool (5 mg)	Gastroenteritis and enterovirus infections
Cerebrospinal fluid	Meningitis, encephalitis
Brain biopsy	Meningitis, encephalitis (HSV, *Rabies virus*)
Blood	CMV, HIV, HBV, HCV
Vesicle fluid or lesion scraping	HSV, VZV, HPV
Endocervical swab	Genital infections (HPV, HSV)
Swab (eye)	Ocular infections (adenovirus, HSV)
Urine	CMV, BK virus, mumps virus
Serum	Antibody studies (most viruses)

Table 66.2 *Cytopathology of viral infections*

Virus	Clinical presentation	Inclusion bodies/Cytologic finding
Adenovirus	Hemorrhagic cystitis	Intranuclear, basophilic
	Pneumonia, upper respiratory tract infection	Intranuclear, eosinophilic (early); basophilic (late)
	Acute keratoconjunctivitis	Intranuclear, eosinophilic (early); basophilic (late)
BK polyoma virus	Urinary tract	Intranuclear, mucoid (early); cytoplasmic, dense, full, basophilic (late)
CMV	Urinary tract	Intranuclear, basophilic surrounded by halo (owl eye)
		Intracytoplasmic, eosinophilic
	Pneumonia	Cytomegaly, small intracytoplasmic, eosinophilic
HSV	Tracheobronchitis	Large ground-glass nucleus (early); intranuclear, eosinophilic (late); multinuclear cells
	Local cystitis, generalized infection	Large ground-glass nucleus (early); intranuclear, eosinophilic (late)
	Herpes genitalis	Multinuclear cells
HPV	Cervical dysplasia, condyloma accuminatum	Enlarged nucleus (hyperchromatic), intranuclear, basophilic (rare)
		Koilocytes (perivascular cytoplasmic clearing and vacuolar degeneration)
Measles virus	Nasal secretions in prodrome	Lymphocytic nuclei in mulberry-like clusters
	Pneumonia	Intranuclear and intracytoplasmic, eosinophilic; multinucleated giant cells
	Exanthem	Intracytoplasmic; multinucleated giant cells
Molluscum contagiosum virus	Genital lesions	Intracytoplasmic, large, dense staining, nucleus displaced bean-shaped squamous cells
	Papule on eyelid or conjunctiva	Intracytoplasmic, basophilic, dense; nucleus displaced
Parainfluenza virus	Bronchiolitis, pneumonia	Intracytoplasmic, eosinophilic; cytomegaly; single or multiple nuclei
RSV	Tracheobronchitis, pneumonia	Intracytoplasmic, basophilic, large multinucleated cells
VZV	Chickenpox, shingles	Intranuclear, eosinophilic, multinucleated cells

abnormal findings using the Pap test are atypical squamous cells of undetermined significance (ASCUS) and atypical glandular cells of undetermined significance (AGUS), which are associated with human papillomavirus (HPV) infection. In follow-up, HPV DNA testing can be useful for identifying women who are more likely to have underlying high-grade squamous intraepithelial lesions (Solomon et al. 2001). The management of patients with equivocal Pap tests is a clinically debated topic and has led to the re-evaluation of the need for this test and development of new clinical paradigms, which may soon preclude the common use of this procedure in favor of molecular tests for HPV. Smith and Yassin (2000) have written a chapter elsewhere that details many of the uses for cytology in viral diagnosis.

Electron microscopy

Electron microscopy (EM) can be used to directly examine specimens for the presence of viral particles. Most commonly, negative-staining methods are used to directly visualize viruses. EM is particularly helpful when trying to detect non-cultivatable or fastidious viruses, although high concentrations are required (Chrystie 1996; Petric and Szymanski 2000). It is rapid and relatively inexpensive, provided an electron microscope is available to the laboratory. In recent times, the emergence of new viral agents has emphasized the value of EM, notably for Ebola virus, hantaviruses, and other agents causing viral hemorrhagic fevers. It has also been suggested that EM could play an important part in early identification of an etiologic agent in a biological warfare or bioterrorist attack. The major limitations of EM are the high cost of the microscope, the expertise needed, and the frequent lack of precise identification of the virus detected, as well as low sensitivity and specificity. Successful detection requires the presence of 10^5 or greater particles/ml. EM is effective for identification of virus morphologically by family, which may be sufficient clinically in many cases, and can be enhanced by the use of antibodies (immune EM), which permits identification of specific viruses.

The rapidity of EM and ability to visualize the actual virus particle are the major advantages of this technique.

Negative staining of liquid specimens can be accomplished in under an hour and specimens that need concentrating by ultracentrifugation, agar diffusion, or pseudoreplica methods can be done in about 2 hours. In solid tissues the specimens would require thin sectioning and this would result in a 2-day process to accommodate the steps of fixation, staining, embedding, and then sectioning. EM is particularly useful for gastrointestinal infections, as virions are often in high concentration. Other specimens, such as urine or CSF, usually require concentration.

Detection and quantitation of viral antigens

Immunological methods are highly effective for detection of viral antigens. They offer a high degree of sensitivity and specificity, are rapid, and the costs are reasonable. Availability of commercial reagents facilitates the detection of many agents. Virtually all methods use antibodies that are tagged with a fluorochrome, enzyme, or radiolabel. Radioimmunoassay is used to a much lesser extent today due to issues of exposure to radioisotopes and the high cost of disposal of radioactivity.

IMMUNOFLUORESCENCE

The direct staining of clinical specimens using monoclonal or polyclonal antibodies bound to fluorescent dye is extensively used in many laboratories for the detection of a wide variety of viral antigens. This may be accomplished using either direct or indirect techniques. In direct immunofluorescence (IF), a single fluorochrome-labeled antibody is used. Indirect IF uses two antibodies, one specific for the antigen under scrutiny and a second fluorochrome-labeled antibody to the immunoglobulin (species specific) used as the first antibody. Indirect IF offers a few advantages, including increased sensitivity and one reagent (the second antibody) that can be used for testing for many viruses. There are many uses for IF including direct staining of smears, cells present in body fluids, tissues, and applications of flow cytometry or cell sorting (McSharry 2000; Schutzbank and McGuire 2000; Madeley and Peiris 2002).

IF has several distinct advantages: it is rapid, simple to perform, and does not require live virus. Results in some cases can be obtained in 1–2 hours, thus impacting on patient management, need for hospitalization, length of hospital stay, and mortality. Specimen requirements are simpler than those for viral culture since maintenance of live virus is not needed. In addition, the visualization of results allows for determination of specificity, examination of the appropriateness of the specimen, and specimen quality. The quality of a specimen is a critically important factor in viral diagnosis and has come under greater scrutiny by regulatory agencies in recent years. Determining that specimens contain sufficient numbers of cells, proper cell types, etc., can be very important in reflecting on the predictive value of the test result.

The IF methods also have their limitations: they require special microscopes, which can be expensive, specially trained microscopists who can interpret results accurately, and reagents that are specific for a particular virus. Thus, multiple smears would be needed to test for several viruses and a new virus would not be detected. It is therefore advisable to use IF in combination with culture methods for detection of viruses. Diagnosis is dependent on the quality of specimens as with all tests, so it is important that uniform, well-made smears be submitted for IF testing.

ENZYME IMMUNOASSAYS

Enzyme immunoassays (EIA) can be performed to detect either antigens or antibodies in clinical specimens. This versatility has resulted in widespread use of EIA in diagnostic virology. Most commonly these assays are performed using a solid-phase format, referred to as enzyme-linked immunosorbent assay (ELISA), with the particular target reagent bound to plastics in a microtiter well (Leland 2000). Many reagents are commercially available for detection of viruses and this form of testing is routine in many laboratories. EIAs are generally highly specific, have high sensitivity, and can be performed rapidly, within minutes to hours. Some solid-phase assays have been adapted to a disposable membrane format for use in physicians' offices, notably for influenza and respiratory syncytial virus (RSV). Also, EIA can be used for the detection of antigens in tissues using immunoperoxidase staining (Docherty et al. 2000).

There are some limitations to EIA, including lack of availability of reagents for some viruses, lack of cost-effectiveness for viruses that have a large number of serotypes (e.g. rhinoviruses) that are not cross reactive, and less sensitivity compared to molecular techniques.

RADIOIMMUNOASSAYS

Radioimmunoassays (RIA) have generally fallen out of use for most viral assays due to the expense of disposal and the potential of radiation exposure, and have generally been replaced by EIA. RIA rivals EIA in specificity and sensitivity and could be used for the same antigens as EIA if desired. Details on use of RIA in viral diagnosis can be found elsewhere (Mushahwar and Brawner 2000).

Detection and quantitation of viral nucleic acids

Recent years have witnessed an exponential growth in the use of diagnostic methods based on the search for viral nucleic acids in clinical samples. The advantages of this approach are, in fact, several-fold (Table 66.3). In particular, rapid turnaround times for all viruses, including the ones that are fastidious or noncultivable (Table 66.4) and do not accumulate sufficient amounts of antigenic material in the host's tissues, or express unusual, not readily detected antigens (Ireland et al. 2000) to be detectable with current immunoassays, and relative ease of automation represent important features in the clinical virology setting since they permit significant improvements in the management of viral diseases without weighing unbearably on work loads. The common denominator of all genome-based methods is the use of stretches of nucleic acids (oligonucleotides, cDNA, RNA) that are complementary to, and thus capable of hybridizing with, segments of the viral genome being targeted. It follows that, although the many, variably sophisticated methods that have been designed around this basic principle vary greatly, choosing the correct segment of viral genome to be targeted is always very critical. In fact, because genome detection methods are extremely sensitive to sequence variation, selected sequences should be as conserved as possible in order for the method to detect and quantify all the possible variants of the virus with equal efficiency. This may sometimes be hard to achieve, as exemplified by the difficulties encountered in developing diagnostic methods that reveal with sufficient efficiency all the lentiviruses that may cause AIDS, including all subtypes of group M human immunodeficiency virus type 1 (HIV-1), group O HIV-1, and human immunodeficiency virus type 2 (HIV-2).

For several years, the only practical means for revealing the presence of viral genetic material in clinical samples was by nucleic acid hybridization techniques, which, however, were limited in sensitivity or required radioactive reagents. The hybridization-based assays that were designed for the diagnostic laboratory routine were therefore relatively few and found limited application. The advent of amplification techniques, which increase the copy numbers of selected segments of nucleic acids (nucleic acid amplification) or the signals generated by these when coupled to appropriate detectors or probes (signal amplification) has permitted the development of assays with exquisitely high levels of sensitivity and tremendously expanded the diagnostic potential of viral genome detection. Indeed, currently the detection of viral genomes is considered to be the most accurate indicator of infection for several viruses. Consequently, a large share of the virological tests carried out in an average diagnostic laboratory is presently based on this approach, albeit the high cost of many commercial reagents often remains a critical issue.

HYBRIDIZATION TESTS

In certain viral infections, selected clinical specimens can contain enough viral genetic material to be detectable directly, i.e. without the need for amplification technologies. In these cases, genome detection may be successfully carried out by reacting the specimens with nucleic acid probes of appropriate specificity and checking whether these have bound to target viral DNA or RNA. Technical variations are numerous. Examining thin-tissue sections or smears (in situ hybridization) may provide clinically useful histological information in addition to virus detection, but requires too much expertise and is too cumbersome for routine use. Thus, hybridization tests are usually performed on extracted nucleic acids in solution or, more frequently, immobilized on a solid support (e.g. dot-(spot)-blot hybridization). In the latter instance, extracted nucleic acid can be digested with restriction enzymes and electrophoresed (e.g. Southern-blot hybridization), thus allowing for much more specificity. The probes can be either DNA or RNA, may vary extensively in length, covering the entire viral genome or segments of it, and can be labeled with a variety of signal-generating systems (biotin, digoxigenin, etc.), although only ^{32}P and other radioactive tracers guarantee maximum sensitivity. Some hybridization tests also provide a semi-quantitative estimate of sample content in viral nucleic acids.

In past years, hybridization tests have found large practical application for detection of certain viruses,

Table 66.3 *Advantages and limits of genome detection methods in the laboratory diagnosis of viral infection*

Advantages	Limits
High sensitivity and specificity	Risk of cross-contamination
Detection of fastidious or noncultivable viruses	Risk of cross-reactions with nonrelevant nucleic acids
Virus detection also in clinical samples from which virus isolation can be difficult (patients treated with antivirals, CSF, etc.)	Risk of false negatives and false positives due to inhibitors or degradation of primes, probes, and templates
Quantitation of viral load	Viral phenotype not analyzable
Ease of automation	Comparatively high cost of commercial methods
High throughput	Detection of clinically irrelevant viruses
Rapid turnaround time	
Specimen deterioration less critical than for virus isolation	

Table 66.4 *Slow, difficult or impossible to isolate in tissue culture from clinical specimens*

Human virus
Coronaviruses
Enteric adenoviruses (serotypes 40 and 41)
Epstein–Barr virus (EBV)
GB virus-C (GBV-C)
Hepatitis A virus (HAV)
Hepatitis B virus (HBV)
Hepatitis C virus (HCV)
Hepatitis delta virus (HDV)
Hepatitis E virus (HEV)
Human herpesvirus 8 (HHV-8)
Human immunodeficiency virus (HIV)
Human metapneumovirus
Human papillomavirus (HPV)
Human parvovirus
Human polyomaviruses BK virus and JC virus
Human T-lymphotropic virus (HTLV)
Norwalk virus and other caliciviruses
Rotaviruses
Selected enteroviruses (most coxsackie A viruses)
Torque-teno-virus (TTV)

such as HPV in anogenital specimens and hepatitis B virus (HBV), hepatitis delta virus (HDV), and parvovirus B19 in plasma, but have now been almost completely replaced by more sensitive amplification-based techniques. As examples, the lower limit of sensitivity of commercial hybridization assays for HBV and parvovirus B19 detection in plasma ranged around 10^5–10^7 genome copies/ml whereas current amplification methods consistently yield a positive result with only a few hundred copies (Bendinelli et al. 2000; Heegaard and Brown 2002).

AMPLIFICATION METHODS

In the large majority of viral infections, no matter whether acute or chronic, the amount of genetic material of viral origin present in patient tissues is below the detection threshold of even the most sensitive among the direct hybridization tests discussed above. This explains the great success of many amplification methods that have been introduced in diagnostic virology in the last decade. In fact, these are capable of specifically and reproducibly detecting 10–100 viral genomes, thus performing at levels that were previously achievable only by the isolation of viruses capable of growing with great efficiency in tissue culture. Another important reason is that several amplification-based methods have permitted the development of quantitative assays, which precisely determine the number of viral genomes (viral load) in plasma and other specimens. This, in conjunction with the recent recognition that viral load determinations reflect and reliably measure active infection, has led to widespread use of quantita-

tive assays for monitoring the levels of virus in the plasma of patients infected with chronic viremia inducing viruses, such as HIV, HBV, hepatitis C virus (HCV), and human cytomegalovirus (CMV). Viral loads are in fact now considered important parameters for treatment decision-making. Thanks to expanded availability of suitable reagents coupled with improved understanding of other technical issues, viral load assays have rapidly become increasingly reliable and user friendly and have acquired an important role in the clinical management of the above infections, contributing significantly to improved patient care.

Signal amplification methods

In essence, these methods are evolved formats of the hybridization tests discussed above, which have been designed to increase manifold – and make easily measurable – the strength of the signals generated by DNA or RNA probes that have formed hybrids with template viral nucleic acids. Several stratagems have been conceived for this purpose and exploit different technologies representing the basis for a number of widely used commercial kits. These include EIA technologies using monoclonal antibodies to specific nucleic acid hybrids, chemiluminescent technologies using triggerable substrates, and the recently developed branched-chain DNA (bDNA) technology. The latter consists of an intricate network of simultaneous hybridization events between multiple sets of oligonucleotide probes (capture probes, extender and amplifier secondary probes, labeled tertiary probes), some of which contain unnatural bases to optimize their complementarity performance characteristics. Since the intensity of amplified signals is proportional to the number of template sequences present in the specimens being tested, these assays are valuable not only for detecting but also for quantitating viral nucleic acids over a wide range of concentrations. For example, the HIV bDNA assays currently on the market can detect as few as 50 viral genomes per ml plasma. However, in general signal amplification assays tend to be somewhat less sensitive than methods based on nucleic acid amplification. On the other hand, they are less prone to technical problems generated by carryover contamination (see below).

Nucleic acid amplification methods

These methods are based on the use of enzymatic machineries that replicate nucleic acids under controlled conditions in vitro, increasing their copy number to a point where detection is possible by conventional or nonconventional techniques. The template amplified can be either viral DNA or RNA (target amplification) or, less frequently, the detectors that have interacted with viral nucleic acids (probe amplification). The polymerase chain reaction (PCR) developed by Mullis and colleagues at the Cetus Corporation in the late 1980s (Mullis et al. 1986) is the conceptual progenitor of all methods in this category and still represents a widely exploited technology in a variety of nested, non-nested, monoplex, multiplex, and quantitative configurations, that in many instances have become standard laboratory practice. For amplification of RNA viruses, PCR-based methods require that target RNA is first converted into cDNA by a reverse transcriptase (RT) or by a bifunctional enzyme having both RT and polymerase activities [reverse transcriptase polymerase chain reaction (RT-PCR)]. However, several other methods have been developed that achieve viral nucleic acid amplification by using different principles and enzymatic systems. These include nucleic acid sequence-based amplification (NASBA), transcription-mediated amplification (TMA), and strand displacement amplification (SDA), which use a variety of enzyme combinations and amplification schemes. An example of probe amplification methods are the ligase chain reaction (LCR), the cycling probe technology (CPT), and the cleavase invader assay. Some such techniques require that the reaction mixtures undergo cycles of defined temperature changes, thus needing specific instrumentation, while others are isothermal and need no special instruments (Table 66.5).

Nucleic acid amplification methods are at high risk of carryover contamination, the source being mainly the sequences amplified (amplicons) in previous runs, which readily become dispersed in the environment and generate false-positive results, but also other specimens. Control of cross-contamination requires the implementation of rigorous physical precautions, the description of which is beyond the scope of this chapter, as well as the need to include in each assay appropriate numbers of negative control samples interspersed with test samples. It is also important to note that the enzymatic reactions at the basis of nucleic acid amplification assays are variably prone to inhibition by a multiplicity of substances, including heme, heparin, urine, calcium alginate, polysaccharides, and polyamines. The latter problem is usually overcome by the use of extensive nucleic acid

Table 66.5 *Nucleic acid amplification methods used in the laboratory diagnosis of viral infections*

Method	Template amplified	Thermal cycling required
PCR	Target DNA	Yes
RT-PCR	Target RNA	Yes
NASBA	Target RNA	No
TMA	Target RNA	No
SDA	Target DNA	No
LCR	Detector DNA	Yes
CPT	Detector chimeric DNA-RNA	No
Cleavase invader	Detector DNA	No

purification procedures or of systems that specifically capture the target template.

Microarrays

Microarrays are amplification/hybridization methods miniaturized in such a way as to make it possible to assay, in a single run, specimens against a large number (thousands) of probes and consist of slides or microchips that carry microspots of cDNA or oligonucleotides bound to their surface. In perspective, this technology is expected to allow not only the search of many different viruses in a single test but also the simultaneous recognition of clinically and epidemiologically useful characteristics of detected virus (genotype, susceptibility to drugs, etc.) that at present need to be investigated separately (see below) as well as cellular gene alterations characteristic of a specific type of pathology. Although offering much promise, microarrays have yet to find wide application in the diagnosis of viral infections.

Real-time methods

The term real-time refers to methods in which the two major phases of amplification technologies, i.e. amplification and amplified product detection, occur simultaneously in a single, closed tube or well. These methods require intercalating dyes, probes, or molecular beacons labeled in such a way that the signal emitted changes concomitant with amplicon formation and dedicated instruments with precision optics that reveal such change as soon as it has occurred. They considerably shorten assay times, have an extremely high throughput and minimize cross-contamination problems (Mackay et al. 2002).

Commercial kits and automation

Virus detection and quantitation using commercial assays in kit format and with an increasing level of standardization and automation have gradually invaded most diagnostic laboratories. In fact, the performance characteristics of well standardized commercial assays having built-in carryover protection systems are generally superior to those of the in-house-developed PCR and NASBA assays (many of the other methods are too complex to be developed independently in the user laboratory), that are, however, still in use for testing clinical samples for the presence of uncommon viruses and for cost containment. Commercial kits often come with automated or semiautomated platforms. Automated steps may include sample preparation, nucleic acid extraction, amplification reaction, reading both sample and appropriate control values, data processing, and report generation. Automation can dramatically decrease laboratory-to-laboratory differences as well as labor requirements. The automation level of real-time techniques is often quite high. Rapid point-of-care viral genome detection methods may also become available in the future, possibly as a spinoff of the portable amplification systems that are being developed for screening the environment for pathogens considered potential biological weapons. A note of caution regarding these advances is that a loss of the technical skills needed for handling and characterizing viruses is also anticipated.

DETECTION OF VIRAL INFECTIVITY

Animal inoculation

The use of animals to grow viruses for laboratory identification has virtually disappeared from the diagnostic laboratory. This has resulted more from the development of sensitive techniques to detect viruses, as well as the health risks and the costs involved in handling the animals. It is likely that animal inoculation will be limited to specialized laboratories who might investigate suspected new pathogens for which other techniques have not yet been developed. A detailed description of animal inoculation is provided in Landry and Hsiung (2000).

Virus isolation in embryonated eggs

Similar to the use of animal inoculation, use of embryonated eggs has yielded to cell culture and direct detection methods for viral diagnosis. The embryonated hen's egg, however, was a very useful vessel for growing viruses, which could be cultivated on the chorioallantoic membrane or in the allantoic or amniotic sacs. Eggs are still used for the large-scale production of some viruses in vaccine production processes (e.g. influenza viruses).

Eggs used for virus isolation must be obtained from a facility that raises them in specific pathogen-free conditions and dedicated equipment is required. Eggs are incubated at 37°C in a humidified atmosphere (40–70 percent) and rotated several times every day to ensure the health of the developing embryo. Eggs are examined by candling, a visual inspection process using a light box with a hole at the top, to make certain that the embryos are developing properly. A detailed description of inoculation and evaluation procedures is described by Landry and Hsiung (2000).

Virus isolation in cell culture

Work in the 1930s pioneered the use of cell culture for the propagation of viruses. Since that time the numbers and types of cultured cells have expanded tremendously and variations of standard uses of cell culture have enhanced the ability to detect and identify viruses (Landry and Hsiung 2000). As a result of these changes, viruses can be isolated more rapidly and in many cases viral identification also results.

STANDARD CELL CULTURE

Three types of culture are routinely used to isolate viruses: primary cells, diploid cell lines, and heteroploid cell lines. Cells may be used as monolayers or cell suspensions to isolate viruses. Lymphocytes for cultivation of HIV and certain herpesviruses, such as Epstein–Barr virus (EBV), human herpesvirus 6 (HHV-6), and human herpesvirus 7 (HHV-7), have been especially useful in suspension culture. Each cell type has distinct characteristics that make it susceptible to a limited number of viruses (Table 66.6). Thus, it is often important to use in parallel several cell types in order to cover the array of viruses that might be associated with pathology in a particular illness or organ system. For example, respiratory tract infection during the traditional season for such infections might include human diploid fibroblasts as well as HEp-2 cells, primary monkey kidney cells, and A549 cells, which can support growth of almost all of the common causes of respiratory tract infections and can help differentiate among them (Landry and Hsiung 2000). In addition to susceptibility, sensitivity and the speed with which cells begin to show infection are factors to be considered in selecting cell lines. Other important factors to consider in setting up a cell culture laboratory are:

- whether or not to prepare and maintain cell lines in-house or purchase them commercially, which must be based on cost and availability
- what are the common specimens encountered so that appropriate numbers of the most needed cells are readily available (this may be seasonally adjusted)
- what is the availability of experienced skilled technologists.

Cell cultures must be carefully maintained and replaced regularly to ensure that cells will be capable of replicating virus when needed, as older cultures often have reduced susceptibility and contaminated cultures cannot yield useful results. This includes visual inspection prior to inoculation and addition of antibiotics and antifungal agents to specimens in the initial processing steps. Typically, tubes for standard cell culture are 16×125 mm screw-cap tubes and they are held at 35°C. When inoculated, cultures may be maintained in stationary position or in roller tubes and incubated at the same temperature except for certain viruses (e.g. rhinoviruses that are incubated at slightly lower temperatures). Tubes are usually kept at a slight angle (5–7°C). Cells are observed daily for evidence of infection.

DETECTION OF VIRAL PRESENCE

Classically, detection of viral infection is dependent upon light microscopy of unstained cells for visualization of evidence of cytopathology. Cytopathic effect (CPE) is the term used for morphological changes noted as a result of viral replication in the cell culture. The CPE of

Table 66.6 *Cell lines sensitive to common viral agents*

Cell line	Viruses
A549 cells	Adenovirus, HSV
HeLa cells	HSV
HEp-2 cells	Adenovirus, HSV, RSV
Human embryonic kidney	Adenovirus, BK virus, HSV
Human diploid fibroblasts	CMV, HSV, VZV, enteroviruses, rhinoviruses
Madin–Darby canine kidney (MDCK)	Influenza viruses
NCI-H929	Adenovirus, enteroviruses, MuV, measles virus, parainfluenza viruses, RSV
Primary monkey kidney cells	Enteroviruses, influenza viruses
Primary rabbit kidney cells	HSV
Engineered cell lines	
BHK-21 (baby hamster kidney-inducible β-galactosidase gene with HSV-inducible promotor)	HSV
Super E-mix (CaCo-2 and BGMK-high expression of decay accelerating factor)	Enteroviruses
Mixed cell cultures	
E-mix A (RD and NCI H292)	Enteroviruses
E-mix B (BGMK and A549)	Enteroviruses
Super E-mix (CaCo-2 and BGMK) high expression of decay accelerating factor)	Enteroviruses
H and V mix (CV-1 and MRC5)	CMV, HSV, VZV
R-mix (A549 and ML)	Adenoviruses, influenza A and B viruses, parainfluenza viruses, RSV

cells may be described as clumping, destruction, granulation, rounding or vacuolation, giant cell or syncytia formation, or refractile cells. A presumptive identification of the etiologic agent may often be made, with a high degree of accuracy, based on the type of CPE in the cell line(s) used, specimen source, and information on the clinical presentation. It is important to examine cells at least once every 2 days and to maintain sham-inoculated controls for each cell line inoculated. The presence of adventitious agents in cells, especially simian viruses in primary monkey cells, is not uncommon.

In some circumstances, viruses will not cause a visible CPE and it is necessary to resort to other methods to detect their presence. Mumps virus (MuV) will not normally cause CPE but addition of guinea pig red blood cells (RBC) to infected primary monkey kidney cells will result in adherence of the RBC to the cells (hemadsorption), thus demonstrating the presence of infection. This results from a viral glycoprotein (hemagglutinin) being inserted into the cell membrane as part of the viral replicative cycle. Alternatively, viruses that do not cause CPE following infection may be detected using an interference assay. In this regard, rubella virus (RUBV) isolation may be detected by interference with echovirus 11 to replicate and cause cell destruction of African green monkey kidney cells.

Whilst all the assays described will isolate virus and may provide presumptive evidence, they do not provide definitive evidence of the identification of the etiologic agent. Identification can be achieved by using specific antiviral antibodies, most effectively monoclonal antibodies, in conjunction with cell culture. This can be achieved by using antibodies labeled with a fluorochrome (IF) or an enzyme (EIA) as described above.

Enhanced cell culture

Over the past few decades several advances have been introduced that have allowed for more rapid, sensitive and cost-effective use of cell culture. The first of these involved low-speed centrifugation of cell cultures to enhance the infectivity of viruses. Subsequently, the use of labeled antibodies for early detection of viral antigen allowed for greatly decreased time to detection as compared to awaiting development of CPE. Thereafter, cell culture has been enhanced by the identification of genetic regulatory elements that are specific to particular viruses, allowing for cell lines to be engineered to yield highly specific detection of a virus. More recently, the admixture of different cell types into a single culture vessel has allowed for a broader array of viruses to be identified in a single tube.

CYTOSPINNING (SHELL VIALS)

The use of the shell vial assay was adapted for detection of CMV as reported by Gleaves et al. (1984). The assay used MRC-5 cells (human diploid fibroblasts) grown on a coverslip in a vial, infected with a specimen, and submitted to low-speed centrifugation followed by overnight incubation. Labeled antibody to an early antigen of CMV is used to stain cells after 24 or 48 hours and often yields a positive result a week or more sooner than waiting for the development of CPE. When used in combination with standard cell culture, the shell vial assay can result in more rapid detection and increases the overall rate of detection for CMV. The success of this assay for CMV has stimulated development of shell vial assays for other viruses and testing can now be done for adenovirus, enteroviruses, respiratory viruses, HSV and VZV. Depending on the virus suspected, an increased number of shell vials was inoculated, the time of incubation was extended and the variety of cell lines used was increased (Olsen et al. 1993). In the case of detection for a variety of viruses, such as respiratory viruses, a cocktail of antibodies can be used to determine if infection is present. The antibodies are used in such a way that the staining pattern is suggestive of a particular virus. Subsequent testing of a second shell vial containing the positive specimen using a monospecific antibody can then identify the etiologic agent.

ENGINEERED CELL LINES

Principles of histochemistry, genetic engineering, and cell culture were combined to enhance the development of a rapid, specific method for detection of HSV by Stabell and Olivo (Olivo 1996). They used BHK-21 (baby hamster kidney) cells that had been stably transformed with a β-galactosidase from *Escherichia coli* attached to an HSV-inducible promoter. When these cells are infected with either herpes simplex virus 1 (HSV-1) or herpes simplex virus 2 (HSV-2), the β-galactosidase is induced and then an X-gal colorimetric substrate is added, infected cells turn blue, while other viruses do not induce the enzyme and cells remain colorless. This method has been incorporated into a commercial kit that has been marketed as the enzyme-linked virus-inducible system (ELVIS) (Olivo 1996). When compared to standard isolation in cell culture that takes considerably longer at times, this test was highly sensitive and specific for both herpes simplex viruses. There are advantages to this method including its rapidity, use of relatively inexpensive substrate as compared to antibodies, and the ability to use cells to look for both the color change and CPE. The method is adaptable for other viruses, both DNA and RNA viruses, and a format for antiviral susceptibility testing for HSV (Olivo 1996) may further broaden the usefulness of this approach.

MIXED CELL CULTURES

The most recent significant development in virus isolation methodology is the use of a mixture of cells in a shell vial format. The choice of cells has been focused on the ability to isolate and identify viruses that have a common pathological presentation, such as enteroviruses or respiratory viruses. The cell mixture allows for a broader range of viruses to be isolated in a single culture. The mixtures have been designated by the cell types included in the culture and the specimen type submitted. R-mix uses a combination of A549 cells and mink lung cells and is useful for the detection of adenoviruses, influenza viruses, parainfluenza viruses, and RSV (Huang et al. 2000; St George et al. 2002). There are three combinations used for enteroviruses, designated E-mix A (RD and NCI-H292) and E-mix B (BGMK and A549) and Super E-mix (CaCo-2 and BGMK cells that have been genetically engineered to express a receptor for enteroviruses), which will also detect some additional viruses (Buck et al. 2002; Huang et al. 2002). The choice would depend on specimen type and clinical diagnosis since enteroviruses are seen in a variety of disease entities. In addition, there are H and V mix cells for the detection of herpesviruses (CMV, HSV, and VZV) that use CV-1 and MRC-5 cells (Huang et al. 2000). Preliminary results using these cell mixtures indicate that they perform similarly to or better than conventional cell culture or single-cell shell vial cultures and are more cost effective. By contrast, these cell mixtures do not appear to be as sensitive as PCR in comparison testing.

CHARACTERIZATION OF DETECTED VIRUSES

Viruses detected in clinical specimens by one or more of the methods discussed above generally need to be further investigated in order to achieve their precise identification (typing). In addition, they may need to undergo supplemental analyses that can provide clinically useful information, including antiviral drug susceptibility testing.

Typing

A precise identification of detected viruses is often necessary because viral agents belonging to different species or types within a same family or genus may vary greatly in pathogenic potential, and most virus detection methods do not allow such differentiation. Typing is also essential for epidemiologic surveillance purposes. Criteria that may be of guidance in typing a virus detected in a clinical specimen are numerous, including nature of the specimen, epidemiologic data, virion morphology and physical–chemical properties, electrophoretic pattern of segmented viral genomes, presence or absence of a lipid envelope, range of infectable cell types or animals, type of CPE or pathological manifestations produced, ability to agglutinate the RBC of different animal species, etc. However, generally such elements only provide presumptive evidence that permits one to narrow, sometimes substantially, the number of type-specific tests the laboratory will eventually need to perform. For example, assessing the hemagglutination properties of an adenovirus isolated in tissue culture may assign it to one of the subgenera A–F but does not obviate the need for further typing. In fact, ultimate identification is based on an accurate definition of their antigenic makeup (serotyping) and/or nucleotide sequence analysis (genotyping) of detected viruses, the choice between the two being mainly dictated by how detection has occurred.

SEROTYPING

Viruses demonstrated by isolation in tissue culture, embryonated eggs, or experimental animals, or revealed by antigen detection methods are generally typed serologically. This is achieved by investigating how selected biological properties of the isolate behave when this is probed with type-specific immune sera. Although neutralization remains the most reliable means of serotype classification due to its exquisite specificity, it is technically demanding and labor-intensive. Also, it may be complicated by the poor neutralizability of certain fresh isolates by antisera raised against prototype viral strains or by the concomitant presence of more than one virus in the sample. In the case of viruses for which a profusion of different serotypes exist, performing the neutralization tests with pooled antisera represents a considerable help since it reduces the number of immune sera that need to be individually used in final identification. For example, serotyping of enteroviruses can be facilitated by the use of standardized antiserum pools provided by international agencies.

Additional frequently used methods for serotyping are inhibition of hemagglutination or hemadsorption and examination of virus-infected cells by IF or other immunostaining techniques. Finally, especially when the virus is difficult to cultivate, dissection of intertypic antigenic differences can be carried out with enzyme immunoassays, immune EM (which relies on the antibody-mediated agglutination of viral particles), immunochromatography, and other serological tests.

GENOTYPING

Although applicable to any virus, genotyping is most frequently used for the ones that have been demonstrated by nucleic acid detection and consists in analyzing segments of the viral genome that present unequivocally distinct type-specific nucleotide sequences. Genome regions suitable for typing can be the same used for virus detection as in the case of HCV genotyping (Zein 2000; Nolte 2001). However, because detection methods often target highly conserved genomic segments, genotyping frequently requires the prior amplification of additional carefully selected segments of the viral genome. For example, while human T-lymphotropic virus (HTLV) detection by PCR in Ficoll-purified peripheral blood mononuclear cells (PBMC) is usually carried out with primer sets targeted

to the *tax* gene, differentiation of human T-lymphotropic virus type 1 (HTLV-1) and human T-lymphotropic virus type 2 (HTLV-2) is achieved by amplifying positive samples in a region of the *pol* gene (Schüpbach and Gallo 2000). Amplified segments are then sequenced, and obtained sequences compared to those existing in data banks with the help of special computer algorithms. Alternatively, the viral genotype can be deduced from the patterns generated by the amplicons when sized or examined for restriction fragment length polymorphism (RFLP), electrophoretic mobility following duplex formation with reference amplicons (heteroduplex mobility assay), denaturation at different temperatures (melting curve analysis; Whiley et al. 2001), or binding to carefully chosen genotype-specific oligonucleotide detectors immobilized on solid supports, such as membrane strips (line probe assay). The latter method has been exploited in several commercial kits since it is technically the least demanding. However, sequencing is regarded as the 'gold standard' since it permits pairwise comparisons, calculation of genetic identities on the basis of percent homology, and performance of phylogenetic investigations that may be useful for documenting epidemiologic links and other purposes. In addition, if the tracts of viral genome analyzed are sufficiently long, sequencing has the potential of revealing viral hybrids that may form as a result of recombinational events between viruses belonging to different genotypes. For some viruses, recombinants are a common occurrence. For example, recombinants of HIV-1 not only are frequently found in multiply exposed patients but also have the ability to be transmitted from patient to patient (circulating recombinant forms; Thomson et al. 2002).

As an alternative molecular strategy to classification, proposed, for example, for differentiating among orthopoxviruses (Ropp et al. 1999) and HCV genotype identification (Schröter et al. 2002), group- or type-specific PCR assays can be constructed which provide a positive result only when a specific viral group or type is present in the clinical specimen. Of note, this strategy has the potential to give a definitive diagnosis based on a single assay without the need for additional testing but is practicable only when the number of possible genotypes is minimal. Examples are the detection of the polyomaviruses BK virus and JC virus in urine (Biel et al. 2000) and of coxsackie virus A16, a frequent cause of hand-foot-and-mouth disease (Bendig et al. 2001).

Differentiating between wild-type and attenuated vaccine virus strains

This differentiation is necessary whenever a virus suspected to be responsible for a clinical form is detected in a patient who has recently been immunized against the same virus by means of an attenuated vaccine or has been in contact with vaccinees. The assays involved are generally conducted in reference laboratories and may be phenotypic and/or genotypic. For example, discrimination between vaccine and wild-type strains of poliovirus can be based on in vitro growth behavior at different temperatures, intratypic serodifferentiation using strain-specific antibodies, RFLP patterns, or sequencing of PCR products. Molecular methods have found application also for discriminating the vaccine strains of the measles virus (Bellini and Rota 1998) and varicella virus (Loparev et al. 2000) from their wild-type counterparts.

ANTIVIRAL DRUG-SUSCEPTIBILITY TESTING

Patient treatment with antiviral agents frequently – if not invariably, especially if therapy is sufficiently prolonged – determines the emergence of virus mutants that show a decreased susceptibility to the drug(s) used and often also to other drugs having mechanisms of action similar to the ones in use. Because this usually leads to reduced patient response to therapy, revealed by rising viral loads and/or clinical deterioration, monitoring patients for the appearance of drug-resistant mutants is gradually becoming routine in clinical practice for evaluating whether and how antiviral regimens have to be modified. This is in turn impacting on diagnostic virology laboratories to an increasing extent. Currently, viruses obtained from antiviral naive patients are generally drug sensitive. However, as with antibacterial drugs, increased availability and use of powerful antiviral agents is likely in the future to lead to the circulation in the community of viruses that present baseline drug susceptibility characteristics that diverge to a variable extent from naive viruses. This development, which already has been observed with HIV-1 (Boden et al. 1999), is bound to extend the need for drug-susceptibility testing of viruses prior to initiation of treatment.

Phenotypic drug-resistance assays

Ideally, for better reflecting what is happening in patients, drug-resistance profiles should be based on the phenotype characteristics of detected viruses. This implies that the virus is isolated in tissue culture, grown at sufficiently high titers, titrated, and finally tested for the ability to replicate in the presence of graded concentrations of each of the drugs of interest. Thus, conventional phenotypic assays are laborious and, with the almost sole exception of HSV-susceptibility testing, take weeks to be completed. In addition, concerns exist that in vitro passage may result in the selection of an altered virus population having drug-susceptibility characteristics different from the one in the patient. In the case of HIV-1, an effort to circumvent these shortcomings has been the development of recombinant virus-based phenotypic assays, in which the relevant genes are directly PCR amplified from the patient and inserted into engineered HIV-1 clones from which such genes have been deleted, and the resulting chimeras subjected to phenotype analysis. It should be noted, however, that even the latter assays do not resolve the other major pitfall of phenotypic resistance tests, namely that attempts to standardize protocols and interpretation guidelines have met with limited success, due to the many technical and interpretational variables that may influence assay results. These include assay format (plaque reduction, dye uptake, yield reduction, flow cytometry, etc.), virus dose, type of cell substrate, viral strains adopted as drug-susceptible and resistant controls, duration of incubation, readout (CPE, accumulation of viral components, infectivity, etc.), and endpoint (50 versus 90 or 99 percent inhibition).

Genotypic drug-resistance assays

Due to the problems inherent to phenotypic assays, for certain viruses (HIV-1, HBV, CMV, influenza), these have been largely replaced by tests that analyze the genome of detected viruses. The procedure most often used consists in amplifying and sequencing the entire genetic region(s) known to control drug susceptibility. Alternatively, if the mutations involved are limited in number or only the most common need to be detected, PCR amplification can be confined to short genome segments, and the resulting amplicons examined by restriction enzyme digestion, melting curve analysis, or line probe assays, as well as by automatic or hybridization sequencing. Genotypic assays are much faster and less labor intensive than phenotypic assays but may miss resistant mutants that are still in the minority in the patient's total viral population. A further limitation stems from the fact that the multiple effects of individual mutations can make it extremely difficult to infer how different combinations of mutations, generated, for example, as a result of multidrug therapies, can impact on actual viral phenotype (level of resistance, cross-resistance, multidrug resistance, etc.). Of note, for HIV-1, an interesting solution has been to scrutinize the nucleotide sequences against constantly updated databases that embrace large numbers of data correlating HIV-1 genotype to phenotype (virtual phenotype). For a recent review of genotypic testing for HIV-1 drug resistance see Shafer (2002).

Viral parameters of poorly defined clinical utility

As discussed in the above sections, viral load and drug-susceptibility determinations have become an integral part in the management of several viral diseases. In recent years, however, there have been numerous efforts to identify further virological parameters that may help at formulating precise prognoses and effective antiviral treatments. One avenue has consisted in attempts to correlate disease severity with variably subtle differences that may exist among different strains of a given virus or may evolve as a result of virus–host or virus–drug(s) interplay. For example, in HIV-1 the features considered have included genetic complexity, tropism for lymphocytes or macrophages, co-receptor usage, cytopathicity, syncytium-inducing ability, sensitivity to antibody-mediated neutralization, and replicative capacity. In particular, the latter parameter has received attention especially following the introduction of highly active antiretroviral therapy (HAART) due to the observation that certain drug-resistant HIV-1 isolates with mutated enzymes exhibit impaired replication rates (Brenner et al. 2002), leading to controversy regarding whether failing drugs should be stopped or rather continued in order not to remove the force that provides selective advantage to such unfit mutants (Deeks et al. 2001).

Similar studies have also involved several hepatitis viruses, although the range of parameters considered has been more restricted due to failure of these viruses to grow in vitro. HCV quasi-species composition has received particular attention in the hope that the swarm of viral variants found in patients may provide a recapitulation of the selective forces that have impacted and are impacting on the virus and of virus ability to evolve and resist host's defense mechanisms (Maggi et al. 1997). Although the findings in chronically infected patients have been inconclusive (Farci et al. 2002), recent evidence suggests that, when studied in the viral hypervariable region 1 at the time of seroconversion, quasispecies composition can predict the outcome of acute HCV infection (Farci et al. 2000).

A second approach has been trying to find correlations between disease progression and status of the infecting viruses in patients tissues. An early example was the correlation that was established between HBV replication activity and HBeAg detection in plasma (Bendinelli et al. 2000). More recently, suggestions have been put forward that detection of CMV DNA in plasma and not only in the peripheral blood leukocytes of bone marrow transplant recipients correlates with increased likelihood of progression to clinical disease (Boeckh et al. 1997) and that detecting viral mRNA, particularly late rather than early transcripts, in the tissues of transplanted patients is an indication of persistent infections reactivation (Lam et al. 1998; Gerna et al. 1999; Blok et al. 2000; Van den Bosch et al. 2001). Also, determining the physical state (integrated versus episomal) of HPV DNA in genital samples has been proposed as a measure of the risk of oncogenic progression (Kalantari et al. 2001).

To date, however, the overall practical product of these studies has been disappointing, since few, if any, of the parameters proposed have reached general acceptance and none has found extensive application in everyday clinical and laboratory practice. It should also be noted that, at least as currently performed, many of the parameters considered are too laborious for most clinical virology laboratories and are susceptible to artifacts. As an example, viral quasispecies analysis implies the amplification of selected regions of the viral genome followed by cloning or separation by gel mobility of the resulting amplicons and sequencing of the different variants (Gomez et al. 1999) or, as suggested in a recent report, mass spectroscopy of the peptides encoded by such amplicons (Ayers et al. 2002). Similarly, discriminating between viral genomic DNA and the cDNA formed as a result of mRNA reverse transcription and amplification can be extremely arduous. It is therefore to be expected that, even if eventually validated, many of the proposed parameters will remain in the realm of clinical research for a long time.

ANALYSIS OF THE HOST'S IMMUNE RESPONSE TO THE INFECTING VIRUS

Cell-mediated immune responses

Early attempts to exploit cell-mediated immune (CMI) responses, in particular delayed hypersensitivity skin tests, for the diagnosis of viral infections led to the conclusion that they could at most have some utility in epidemiologic surveys. The measurement of CMI responses has had a resurgence in the past two decades as a tool for monitoring patients who are virus infected or at risk of becoming infected. This is related to our recognition of the pathogenetic significance of cellular immune function and cytokines in viral infections. HIV infection and AIDS are perhaps the circumstances where this is most thoroughly used but other states of immunocompromise, notably bone marrow transplantation, have seen benefits from such testing. Testing of CMI function has included measurement of a variety of functional and nonfunctional parameters (Table 66.7), including circulating lymphocyte subset counts, cytotoxic T lymphocytes (CTL) and natural killer cell activities, response to specific antigens and to polyclonal lymphocyte phytomitogens, and cytokine production and profiles. Mawle (1996) has written a useful review that details many of the assays used to measure cellular immunity.

The determination of total T lymphocytes as well as the number of helper ($CD4^+$) and cytotoxic ($CD8^+$) T cells has achieved its greatest importance in HIV-infected individuals as this is used for staging of disease, evidence of progression to AIDS, and as an indication of

Table 66.7 *Cell-mediated immunity used for clinical virology*

Cell numbers	Cell functions	Cytokines
CD4, CD8, CD4:CD8 ratios	Cytotoxic T cells	T helper cell populations
NK cells	NK cells	Th1 – IL-2, IFN-γ Th2 – IL-4, IL-1

efficacy of antiviral therapy. Absolute cell numbers as well as CD4:CD8 cell ratios are used for these purposes. The availability of monoclonal antibodies to measure these cell numbers has made this testing easy to perform in virtually any laboratory; however, it is more precisely accomplished using flow cytometry.

Testing of cellular cytotoxicity is usually performed using a radioactivity label release (^{51}Cr) assay. This testing requires a step to separate and collect PBMCs and then test them under conditions that are optimal for measuring virus-specific CTL. This testing has been used in evaluating AIDS patients and individuals with herpesvirus infections but is still not routinely used in the clinical laboratory.

Nonspecific or antigen-specific blastogenic responses as a measure of immune competence provide insight into CMI function, either generally or regarding a specific disease. More recently there has been an association of subsets of helper T cells with immune status, such that production of specific cytokines is associated with a predominance of CMI [Th1 cells, which produce interferon-gamma (IFN-γ) and interleukin (IL)-2] or antibody responses (Th2 cells, which produce IL-4, IL-5 and IL-10). Th1 responses are considered to favor a better prognosis in HIV infection and many virus infections, whereas Th2 responses would be considered to be important in other types of infections.

Antibody responses

Although at present somewhat overshadowed by the recent success story of molecular methods, serological tests for antiviral antibodies (serodiagnosis) have had and still have an important position in the diagnosis of viral infections. The reasons are several-fold. First, certain serological tests (in particular, detection of antiviral IgM) represent a rapid means for identifying several acute viral infections. Second, the technologies most frequently used are within reach of most laboratories since they do not demand the expertise and the equipment that are instead essential for most other virological procedures. Third, serology is theoretically valuable for establishing an etiologic diagnosis in all viral diseases, regardless of whether the etiologic virus is easily demonstrable by direct means or not. Fourth, serological tests are generally inexpensive in labor and reagents. Fifth, the market offers a vast selection of high-quality serological reagents, many of which are available in kit format and are suitable for automation. Finally and possibly most importantly, if the implicated virus is one of the many that tend to persist for prolonged periods of time or indefinitely in their hosts, serodiagnosis represents the only means, together with viral load determination when available, by which it can be demonstrated that a primary infection or a reactivation of a chronic infection is ongoing at the time of disease. When clinical, anamnestic, and epidemiologic

data are compatible, this represents strong evidence that the disease under scrutiny is indeed caused by that virus.

Classically, the procedures exploitable for serodiagnosis include virus neutralization (which for decades has been the standard against which the other test systems were evaluated), complement fixation (CF), hemagglutination inhibition (HI), passive agglutination of latex particles or RBC, immunoblotting, indirect IF, and RIA. These methods are still in use for some viruses (e.g. neutralization for poliovirus and CF for uncommon agents for which no other assay is available), or for selected purposes (e.g. immunoblots for confirmation of HIV or HCV seropositivity assessed with other methods). However, currently, the scene is dominated by solid-phase EIAs, that have become enormously popular in diagnostic virology as well as in other fields due to their sensitivity (comparable to RIA), speed, ability to measure antibodies of different isotypes, use of nonhazardous reagents, and aptitude to be automated. The antigens used are purified viral preparations and, increasingly, recombinant or synthetic peptides. It is, however, possible that in the future, other practical methods will be adapted for viral serology. For example, flow-cytometry-based serological methods are being advocated for their ability to detect antibodies to more that one virus in a single assay (Álvarez-Barrientos et al. 2000).

For viruses that constantly cause chronic infections (HIV-1 and HIV-2, HTLV-1 and HTLV-2) or are very uncommon (rabies in unvaccinated individuals), the interpretation of serological data is unique since the detection of antibodies of any isotype virtually always denotes infection. For all other viruses, demonstration of ongoing infection by serology requires that the antiviral antibody response is shown to have been elicited (boosted in the case of virus reactivations) recently. This is a consequence of the long duration of most antiviral antibodies, often with little or no reduction in total titer for many years or lifelong, particularly if they have been generated by systemic infections. Thus, mere seropositivity reveals that the individual has been exposed to the tested virus but is not informative of whether this has occurred recently or more or less remotely or even as the result of artificial immunization. In a sense, seronegativity may be more informative because it excludes the infection or indicates that antibody production has not yet started.

Demonstration that an antiviral antibody response has been triggered recently can be achieved with one or more of the approaches below.

TITRATION OF PAIRED SERUM SAMPLES

Two serum samples, one collected as early after disease onset as possible (acute-phase serum) and the second at least 1 week later (convalescent-phase serum), are titrated for antiviral antibodies simultaneously and in the same run. Although seroconversion is rarely observed especially in systemic diseases with an incubation period of weeks, this approach often permits the observation of a significant rise (fourfold or greater) in total or IgG antibody titer between the first and the second serum. Major pitfalls of this procedure are:

- if the acute-phase serum is drawn too late, antibodies may be already reaching peak levels and a significant rise in titer can be missed
- the result of testing is very often retrospective and, therefore, of little use for patient care.

DETERMINATION OF ANTIVIRAL IGM IN SERUM

This approach is currently the most widely used. Typically, during acute primary virus infections virus-specific IgM antibodies appear in serum between 5 and 10 days after initiation of infection, reach peak concentrations at 2–4 weeks, and then usually decline to undetectable levels at 2–4 months, although they may last considerably longer in some infections. In the course of persistent infections, IgM antibodies are usually negative, although they can briefly reappear during episodes of intense reactivations of virus replication. Thus, detecting IgM to a given virus, with or without the corresponding IgG, even in a single serum sample obtained during the acute phase of illness, denotes current or very recent primary infection or reactivation of a persistent infection by that virus. By contrast, the presence of virus-specific IgG but not IgM signifies past infection. Examples of acute viral infections in which specific IgM tests are particularly useful for diagnosis include hepatitis A, rubella, measles, CMV and EBV infections. Also, because IgM as well as IgA do not cross the placental barrier, detecting antibodies of these classes in a newborn is strongly diagnostic for a congenital infection.

The development of sensitive, specific, and reproducible tests for antiviral IgM that can be used on a routine basis has taken considerable effort, mainly due to the possible presence of IgM rheumatoid factors (RF) which, by binding to the Fc portion of IgG, can generate false positives and/or abundant IgG which can compete for antigen binding and produce false negatives. Methods used in the past have relied on IgM physicochemical separation or inactivation by reducing agents and on IgG removal with certain bacterial cell wall proteins (*Staphylococcus aureus* protein A, streptococcal protein G) or other means. However, the ones presently employed are almost exclusively variations around the use of highly selective class-specific anti-IgM antibodies to detect and/or to capture the IgM. The commercial kits that utilize the latter technology are numerous, varied for the use of different solid-phase supports, have different indicator labels to signal IgM–anti-IgM complex formation, and different inbuilt systems for RF and IgG removal (not needed for capture assays), and are generally dependable.

MEASUREMENT OF ANTIBODIES AGAINST DIFFERENT VIRAL EPITOPES

The various subsets of antibodies generated in response to an infecting virus and directed to diverse epitopes of the structural and nonstructural viral proteins may present consistent and marked differences in the kinetics of appearance, decline, and disappearance that are utilizable for staging the infection. This approach has wide application in HBV and EBV serology, where measuring separately the antibodies directed to different antigens has considerable clinical utility. As an example, Table 66.8 provides a key to the interpretation of the serological profiles to EBV that are most frequently encountered.

DETERMINATION OF ANTIVIRAL IGA IN SERUM

Appearance, level, and duration of serum IgA are less predictable than either IgG or IgM. In general, however, IgA antibodies are made acutely, like IgM antibodies although they tend to last longer. Albeit no IgA assay is widely used in routine diagnostic testing, detection of virus-specific serum IgA has been suggested to have practical utility in several situations. These include identification of HIV-1 infections in newborns (Moodley et al. 1997), rapid diagnosis of influenza (Voeten et al.

Table 66.8 *Interpretation of serological test results for EBV infection*

Anti-VCA[a] IgM	Total anti-VCA	Total anti-EBNA[b]	Total anti-EA[c]	Interpretation
−	−	−	−	No infection
+	±	−	±	Acute primary infection
+	+	+	−	Recent infection
−	+	−	+	Recent infection in immunocompromised
+	+	+	+	Resolution of acute primary infection or reactivation
−	+	+	+	Past infection or reactivation
−	+	+	−	Past infection

a) VCA, viral capsid antigen.
b) EBNA, EBV nuclear antigen.
c) EA, early antigen.

1998) and dengue fever (Talarmin et al. 1998), and diagnosis of EBV-associated nasopharyngeal carcinoma (Hsu et al. 2001).

DETERMINATION OF ANTIVIRAL ANTIBODY AVIDITY

This approach exploits the fact that the strength of antibody binding to antigens increases with time after initiation of immune responses. The parameter used (avidity index) is the ratio of the antibody titers obtained in a standard serological assay (generally EIA) with and without treating the formed antigen–antibody complexes with an appropriate concentration of a protein denaturant, such as urea or guanidine, before addition of the secondary antibody. The test has been successfully used in the diagnosis of a number of viruses, including several herpesviruses, hantaviruses, encephalitis viruses, HCV, and measles virus. In pregnant women, it has been found valuable, together with other assays, for measuring the risk of transmitting CMV infection to the fetus (Lazzarotto et al. 2001).

ANTIBODY IN ALTERNATIVE SPECIMENS

Due to the blood–brain barrier, normally the CSF is devoid of IgM and has an IgG content 250–500-fold lower than serum. Thus, in the absence of concomitant signs of barrier damage, finding specific IgM or increased CSF/serum ratios of specific IgG is indicative of intrathecal antibody synthesis resulting from CNS infection. For alphaviruses, bunyaviruses, and flaviviruses, the presence of specific IgG in the CSF is highly suspicious, although only the presence of specific IgM is truly diagnostic. For more common viruses, CSF antibody analysis provides diagnostic hints only if evidence of intrathecal synthesis is obtained. Currently, it is almost always preferred to examine the CSF for viral nucleic acids.

Studies have also advocated the testing of urine and oral, ocular, or genital fluids for antiviral antibodies as easily obtainable, noninvasive alternatives to serum or plasma or as a means for obtaining additional informa-tion in selected clinical conditions. In general, these specimens have proven valuable for epidemiologic purposes but are not commonly used for diagnosis. Methods need to be developed specifically or validated for use with each type of specimen and some are commercially available. For maximum sensitivity, assays may be designed to recognize IgA as well as IgG and IgM antibodies (Zmuda et al. 2001).

CAUTIONARY NOTE

Serodiagnosis of viral infections can be complicated by a number of factors (Table 66.9), thus calling for considerable judgment in the interpretation of results. Whenever possible, serological diagnoses should be confirmed with virus detection methods.

QUALITY ASSURANCE/QUALITY CONTROL

Quality assurance affects all aspects of the diagnostic laboratory through a comprehensive program that strives toward constant improvement (Warford 2000). Oversight of services related to the virology laboratory includes specimen handling (collection, transport, storage, and testing), monitoring of procedures, reporting of results and their interpretation. The importance of laboratory participation in this process is well documented (Nutting et al. 1996). Laboratories in the USA are currently highly regulated under the Clinical Laboratory Improvement Act, instituted in 1992, which provides strict standards for quality improvement. These regulations address personnel qualifications, assessment of competence and defined responsibilities, written and approved procedures, quality control for test reagents and equipment (includes maintenance), test method verification and validation, proficiency testing of all analytes and staff members, analysis and improvement of all laboratory services, and a well-documented reference section for accreditation requirements, methods,

Table 66.9 *Considerations for interpreting serological data for diagnosis of viral infections*

Considerations
Superficial infections may elicit no or very weak systemic antibody responses
Antibody production may be delayed or absent in newborns, elderly, and immunocompromised individuals
IgM antibodies may persist for protracted periods after primary infections or may be stimulated in reactivation of latent viruses
False-positive IgM tests are a common occurrence in certain lymphoproliferative disorders
Reinfections and reactivations may not produce significant rises in total and IgG antibodies
Antibodies may cross-react within certain virus groups (e.g. alphaviruses, herpesviruses, parainfluenza viruses)
Passively acquired IgG antibodies are common finding in newborns and in individuals recently treated with blood transfusions or immunoglobulins
Antibody appearance in the CSF may be delayed by 2–4 weeks
Defects in the blood–brain barrier produced by any nonviral neurological disease can cause leakage of serum antibodies into the CSF

and quality assurance literature. Five major areas have been identified where quality assurance is mandated:

1 documentation of competency testing, staff duties and training
2 a well-maintained procedures manual that conforms to National Committee for Clinical Laboratory Standards (NCCLS) formatting
3 proficiency testing
4 quality control
5 a specimen log complete that includes test requisitions (Warford 2000).

The goal of these quality assurance efforts should be the constant improvement of laboratory services to the benefit of patient care. In other countries, regulations are more or less detailed and enforced but there is no doubt that a stringent quality control surveillance is of great help in keeping good patient care standards.

A comprehensive program for quality control that is well documented and regularly reviewed must include all procedures performed in the diagnostic virology laboratory. When appropriate, corrective actions must be taken in a timely manner and must be documented in writing. Quality control is documented by daily checking of all materials and equipment with weekly review by a supervisor. Excellent quality control practices are essential to establish the reliability of clinical laboratories and for the provision of good patient care; this is dependent on attention to all details for all aspects of the laboratory. A particularly important issue for the clinical virology laboratory is prevention of contamination, which is critical to successful performance of both molecular diagnostic techniques and cell culture. Nearly all issues related to quality control measures and scheduling are covered in documents prepared by the NCCLS and can be found at their website (www.nccls.org).

FROM LABORATORY FINDINGS TO DIAGNOSIS

Demonstration of a virus by cell cultures or EM is virtually always a definitive indication that virus is present in a disease state. Whilst this usually is suggestive of an etiologic role for the particular virus, this is not always the case. Results may be complicated by mixed infections with more than one organism or an organism might be isolated that does not have a pathogenic role. Recently, it has been discovered that many respiratory tract infections result from infection with human metapneumovirus. In several cases this virus and other human respiratory pathogens have been detected concurrently and it is not yet clear whether one or both viruses contribute to disease pathology. Alternatively, certain small round viruses can be routinely visualized in the gastrointestinal tract but association with any pathology has been far more difficult to establish. The same can presently be said of TT virus and related

anelloviruses, which are found, often at high titers, in the circulation of many diseased and healthy individuals, with no apparent relation to disease.

Presence of virus as determined by detection of viral nucleic acid is indicative of current or recent viral infection but does not necessarily reflect that live virus is present nor that the virus is responsible for the ongoing clinical manifestations. There has been extensive evaluation of the detection of quantities of nucleic acid to determine viral load and its relationship to disease state, progression, and the efficacy of antiviral therapy (Johanson et al. 2001). It is clear that viral load determination in plasma is very important in infections by CMV, HCV, HBV, and HIV.

Serological tests are more complex to interpret but have the potential of demonstrating that the virus is sustaining a primary or reactivated infection at the time clinical symptoms are present (see above).

In all cases, detection of virus, viral antigens, or viral nucleic acid is preferable to antibody detection as an indicator of current or recent viral infection. In many cases, direct testing for virus rather than antiviral antibody can provide rapid diagnosis that can be vital in affecting the management of the patient or patient contacts. Improved technology, automation, and reagents have allowed rapid, cost-effective viral detection, which has contributed significantly to better patient care.

Thus, the viral diagnostic laboratory has become a most important adjunct to patient care. The physician can be provided data on rapid, sensitive, and accurate testing that can identify a virus, indicate its genotype, phenotype, and/or serotype as is appropriate. In this regard, in an increasing number of cases the physician can select an antiviral agent and can even tailor drug combinations to avoid specific patterns of antiviral resistance. It is exciting to recognize the advances we have witnessed over these past 30 years in viral diagnosis and therapy, and to project to the future when even more effective tools can be expected to impact on the ability of physicians to help their patients.

REFERENCES

Álvarez-Barrientos, A., Arroyo, J., et al. 2000. Applications of flow cytometry to clinical microbiology. *Clin Microbiol Rev*, **13**, 167–95.

Ayers, M., Siu, K., et al. 2002. Characterization of hepatitis C virus quasispecies by matrix-assisted laser desorption ionization-time of flight (mass spectroscopy) mutation detection. *J Clin Microbiol*, **40**, 3455–62.

Bellini, W.J. and Rota, P.A. 1998. Genetic diversity of wild-type measles viruses: implications for global measles elimination programs. *Emerg Infect Dis*, **4**, 1–7.

Bendig, J.W.A., O'Brien, P.S. and Muir, P. 2001. Serotype-specific detection of coxsackievirus A 16 in clinical specimens by reverse transcription-nested PCR. *J Clin Microbiol*, **39**, 3690–2.

Bendinelli, M., Pistello, M., et al. 2000. Blood-borne hepatitis viruses: hepatitis B, C, D, and G viruses and TT virus. In: Specter, S.,

Hodinka, R.L. and Young, S.A. (eds), *Clinical virology manual*, 3rd edn. Washington, DC: ASM Press, 306–37.

Biel, S.S., Held, T.K., et al. 2000. Rapid quantification and differentiation of human polyomavirus DNA in undiluted urine from patients after bone marrow transplantation. *J Clin Microbiol*, **38**, 3689–95.

Blok, M.J., Lautenschlager, I., et al. 2000. Diagnostic implications of human cytomegalovirus immediate early-1 and pp67 mRNA detection in whole-blood samples from liver transplant patients using nucleic acid sequence-based amplification. *J Clin Microbiol*, **38**, 4485–91.

Boden, D., Hurley, A., et al. 1999. HIV-1 drug resistance in newly infected individuals. *JAMA*, **282**, 1135–41.

Boeckh, M., Gallez-Hawkins, G.M., et al. 1997. Plasma polymerase chain reaction for cytomegalovirus DNA after allogeneic marrow transplantation: comparison with polymerase chain reaction using peripheral blood leukocytes, pp65 antigenemia, and viral culture. *Transplantation*, **64**, 108–13.

Brenner, B.G., Routy, J.P., et al. 2002. Persistence and fitness of multidrug-resistant human immunodeficiency virus type 1 acquired in primary infection. *J Virol*, **76**, 1753–61.

Buck, G.E., Wiesemann, M. and Stewart, L. 2002. Comparison of mixed cell culture containing genetically engineered BGMK and CaCo-2 cells (Super E-mix) with RT-PCR and conventional cell culture for diagnosing enteroviral meningitis. *Abstracts of the Eighteenth Annual Clinical Virology Symposium*, T13.

Chrystie, I.L. 1996. Electron microscopy. In: Mahy, B.W.J. and Kangro, H.O. (eds), *Virology methods manual*. London: Academic Press, 91–106.

Deeks, S.G., Wrin, T., et al. 2001. Virologic and immunologic consequences of discontinuing combination antiretroviral-drug therapy in HIV-infected patients with detectable viremia. *N Engl J Med*, **344**, 472–80.

Docherty, J.J., Pokabla, C.M. and Gay, H. 2000. Peroxidase-antiperoxidase detection of viral antigens in cells. In: Specter, S., Hodinka, R.L. and Young, S.A. (eds), *Clinical virology manual*, 3rd edn. Washington, DC: ASM Press, 105–11.

Farci, P., Shimoda, A., et al. 2000. The outcome of acute hepatitis C predicted by the evolution of the viral quasispecies. *Science*, **288**, 339–44.

Farci, P., Strazzera, R., et al. 2002. Early changes in hepatitis C viral quasispecies during interferon therapy predict the therapeutic outcome. *Proc Natl Acad Sci U S A*, **99**, 3081–6.

Gerna, G., Baldanti, F., et al. 1999. Clinical significance of expression of human cytomegalovirus pp67 late transcripts in heart, lung, and bone marrow transplant recipients as determined by nucleic acid sequence-based amplification. *J Clin Microbiol*, **37**, 902–11.

Gleaves, C.A., Smith, T.F., et al. 1984. Rapid detection of cytomegalovirus in MRC-5 cells inoculated with low-speed centrifugation and monoclonal antibody to an early antigen. *J Clin Microbiol*, **19**, 917–19.

Gomez, J., Martell, M., et al. 1999. Hepatitis C viral quasispecies. *J Viral Hepatol*, **6**, 3–16.

Heegaard, E.D. and Brown, K.E. 2002. Human parvovirus B19. *Clin Microbiol Rev*, **15**, 485–505.

Hsu, M.M., Hsu, W.C., et al. 2001. Specific IgA antibodies to recombinant early and nuclear antigens to Epstein–Barr virus in nasopharyngeal carcinoma. *Clin Otolaryngol*, **26**, 334–8.

Huang, Y.T., Hite, S., et al. 2000. Application of mixed cell lines for the detection of viruses from clinical specimens. *Clin Microbiol Newsl*, **22**, 89–92.

Huang, Y.T., Yam, P., et al. 2002. Engineered BGMK cells for sensitive and rapid detection of enteroviruses. *J Clin Microbiol*, **40**, 366–71.

Ireland, J.H., O'Donnell, B., et al. 2000. Reactivity of 13 in vitro expressed hepatitis B surface antigen variants in 7 commercial diagnostic assays. *Hepatology*, **34**, 1176–82.

Johanson, J., Abravaya, K., et al. 2001. A new ultrasensitive assay for quantitation of HIV-1 in plasma. *J Virol Methods*, **95**, 81–92.

Johnson, F.B. 1990. Transport of viral specimens. *Clin Microbiol Rev*, **3**, 120–31.

Kalantari, M., Blennow, E., et al. 2001. Physical state of HPV 16, and chromosomal mapping of the integrated form in cervical carcinomas. *Diagn Mol Pathol*, **10**, 46–54.

Lam, K.M., Burg, N., et al. 1998. Significance of reverse transcription polymerase chain reaction in the detection of human cytomegalovirus gene transcripts in thoracic organ transplant recipients. *J Heart Lung Transplant*, **17**, 555–65.

Landry, M.L. and Hsiung, G.D. 2000. Primary isolation of viruses. In: Specter, S., Hodinka, R.L. and Young, S.A. (eds), *Clinical virology manual*, 3rd edn. Washington, DC: ASM Press, 27–42.

Lazzarotto, T., Galli, C., et al. 2001. Evaluation of the Abbott AxSYM cytomegalovirus (CMV) immunoglobulin M (IgM) assay in conjunction with other CMV IgM tests and a CMV IgG avidity assay. *Clin Diagn Lab Immunol*, **8**, 196–8.

Leland, D.S. 2000. Enzyme immunoassay. In: Specter, S., Hodinka, R.L. and Young, S.A. (eds), *Clinical virology manual*, 3rd edn. Washington, DC: ASM Press, 93–104.

Loparev, V.N., McCaustland, K., et al. 2000. Rapid genotyping of varicella zoster virus vaccine and wild-type strains with fluorophore-labeled hybridization probes. *J Clin Microbiol*, **38**, 4315–19.

Mackay, I.M., Arden, E.A. and Nitsche, A. 2002. Real-time PCR in virology. *Nucleic Acids Res*, **30**, 1292–305.

Madeley, C.R. and Peiris, J.S.M. 2002. Methods in virus diagnosis: immunofluorescence revisited. *J Clin Virol*, **25**, 121–34.

Maggi, F., Fornai, C., et al. 1997. Differences in hepatitis C virus quasispecies between liver, peripheral blood mononuclear cells and plasma. *J Gen Virol*, **78**, 1521–5.

Mawle, A.C. 1996. Cell mediated immunity. In: Mahy, B.W.J. and Kangro, H.O. (eds), *Virology methods manual*. London: Academic Press, 143–61.

McSharry, J. 2000. Flow cytometry. In: Specter, S., Hodinka, R.L. and Young, S.A. (eds), *Clinical virology manual*, 3rd edn. Washington, DC: ASM Press, 211–24.

Moodley, D., Coovadia, H.M., et al. 1997. HIV-1 specific immunoglobulin A antibodies as an effective marker of perinatal infection in developing countries. *J Trop Pediatr*, **43**, 80–3.

Mullis, K., Faloona, F., et al. 1986. Specific enzymatic amplification of DANN *in vitro*: the polymerase chain reaction. *Cold Spring Harbor Symp Quant Biol*, **51**, 263–73.

Mushahwar, I.K. and Brawner, T.A. 2000. Radioimmunoassay. In: Specter, S., Hodinka, R.L. and Young, S.A. (eds), *Clinical virology manual*, 3rd edn. Washington, DC: ASM Press, 79–92.

Nolte, F.S. 2001. Hepatitis C virus genotyping: clinical implications and methods. *Mol Diagn*, **6**, 265–77.

Nutting, P.A., Main, D.S., et al. 1996. Problems in laboratory testing in primary care. *JAMA*, **275**, 635–9.

Olivo, P.D. 1996. Transgenic cell lines for the detection of animal viruses. *Clin Microbiol Rev*, **9**, 321–34.

Olsen, M.A., Shuck, K.M., et al. 1993. Isolation of seven respiratory viruses in shell vials: a practical and highly sensitive method. *J Clin Microbiol*, **31**, 422–5.

Petric, M. and Szymanski, M. 2000. Electron microscopy and immunoelectron microscopy. In: Specter, S., Hodinka, R.L. and Young, S.A. (eds), *Clinical virology manual*, 3rd edn. Washington, DC: ASM Press, 54–65.

Ropp, S.L., Esposito, J.J., et al. 1999. Poxviruses infecting humans. In: Murray, P. (ed.), *Manual of clinical microbiology*. Washington, DC: ASM Press, 1131–8.

Schröter, M., Zöllner, B., et al. 2002. Genotyping of hepatitis C virus types 1, 2, 3, and 4 by a one-step LightCycler method using three different pairs of hybridization probes. *J Clin Microbiol*, **40**, 2046–50.

Schüpbach, J. and Gallo, R.C. 2000. Human retroviruses. In: Specter, S., Hodinka, R.L. and Young, S.A. (eds), *Clinical virology manual*, 3rd edn. Washington, DC: ASM Press, 513–16.

Schutzbank, T.A. and McGuire, R. 2000. Immunofluorescence. In: Specter, S., Hodinka, R.L. and Young, S.A. (eds), *Clinical virology manual*, 3rd edn. Washington, DC: ASM Press, 69–78.

Shafer, R.W. 2002. Genotypic testing for human immunodeficiency virus type 1 drug resistance. *Clin Microbiol Rev*, **15**, 247–77.

Smith, R.D. and Yassin, R.S. 2000. The cytopathology of virus infections. In: Specter, S., Hodinka, R.L. and Young, S.A. (eds), *Clinical virology manual*, 3rd edn. Washington, DC: ASM Press, 43–53.

Smith, T.F. 2000. Specimen requirements: selection, collection, transport, and processing. In: Specter, S., Hodinka, R.L. and Young, S.A. (eds), *Clinical virology manual*, 3rd edn. Washington, DC: ASM Press, 11–26.

Solomon, D., Schiffman, M., Tarone, R. and the ALTS Group. 2001. Comparison of 3 management strategies for patients with atypical squamous cells of undetermined significance: baseline results from a randomized trial. *J Natl Cancer Inst*, **93**, 293–9.

St George, K., Patel, N.M., et al. 2002. Rapid and sensitive detection of respiratory virus infections for directed antiviral treatment using R-Mix cultures. *J Clin Virol*, **24**, 107–15.

Talarmin, A., Labeau, B., et al. 1998. Immunoglobulin A-specific capture enzyme-linked immunosorbent assay for diagnosis of dengue fever. *J Clin Microbiol*, **36**, 1189–92.

Thomson, M.M., Pérez-Álvarez, L. and Nájera, R. 2002. Molecular epidemiology of HIV-1 genetic forms and its significance for vaccine development and therapy. *Lancet Infect Dis*, **2**, 461–71.

Van den Bosch, G., Locatelli, G., et al. 2001. Development of reverse transcriptase PCR assays for detection of active human herpesvirus 6 infection. *J Clin Microbiol*, **39**, 2308–10.

Voeten, J.T., Groen, J., et al. 1998. Use of recombinant nucleoproteins in enzyme-linked immunosorbent assays for detection of virus-specific immunoglobulin A (IgA) and IgG antibodies in influenza virus A- or B-infected patients. *J Clin Microbiol*, **36**, 3527–3531.

Warford, A. 2000. Quality assurance in clinical virology. In: Specter, S., Hodinka, R.L. and Young, S.A. (eds), *Clinical virology manual*, 3rd edn. Washington, DC: ASM Press, 3–10.

Whiley, D.M., Mackay, I.M. and Sloots, T.P. 2001. Detection and differentiation of human polyomaviruses JC and BK by LightCycler PCR. *J Clin Microbiol*, **39**, 4357–61.

Zein, N.N. 2000. Clinical significance of hepatitis C virus genotypes. *Clin Microbiol Rev*, **13**, 223–35.

Zmuda, J.F., Wagoneer, B., et al. 2001. Recognition of multiple classes of hepatitis C antibodies increases detection sensitivity in oral fluid. *Clin Diagn Lab Immunol*, **8**, 1267–70.

67

Immunoprophylaxis of viral diseases

STEPHEN C. HADLER AND JANE F. SEWARD

INTRODUCTION

Vaccines are among the most effective and cost-effective means for the prevention of disease. The development of viral vaccines predates the recognition of viral agents as causes of disease by over a century; their use has resulted in marked decreases in the incidence or eradication of diseases that were important causes of human mortality. Vaccines are now available to prevent 13 viral diseases, and new generations of vaccines being developed through molecular techniques hold the promise of providing protection against others.

The modern era of vaccine development began with the demonstration by Jenner that inoculation with cowpox virus provided protection against smallpox and the subsequent wide use of variolation to protect against this disease. The effective use of variola vaccine worldwide culminated, in 1980, in the certification of eradication of smallpox after a decade-long campaign coordinated by the World Health Organization (Fenner et al. 1988). By 1977, viral vaccines to prevent rabies, influenza, yellow fever, poliomyelitis, measles, rubella, and mumps had also been developed and used with striking success to reduce the disease burden due to these viruses. Following the eradication of smallpox, global immunization programs to prevent six childhood diseases, including poliomyelitis and measles, were implemented (Galazka 1994). These programs have achieved 70–75 percent global coverage with these vaccines, and are now being expanded to include hepa-

titis B vaccine (all countries) and yellow fever vaccine where this disease is endemic (World Health Organization and UNICEF, 2002; Vaccines and Biologicals 2002a). A goal for global eradication of poliomyelitis was established for the year 2000; to date, disease incidence has been reduced by 99 percent, with disease endemic in only six countries and eradication certified in the Americas (1994), the Western Pacific (2001), and Europe (2002) (Vaccines and Biologicals 2004). The global strategy, which includes achieving high routine infant vaccination coverage for oral polio vaccine, mass vaccination campaigns with house-to-house vaccination to interrupt remaining chains of transmission, and intensive surveillance for acute flaccid paralysis in children, is being implemented in the remaining countries where polio is endemic (Hull et al. 1994). A regional campaign to eliminate measles has interrupted disease transmission in the Americas; the key elements of this strategy are now being implemented in Africa and elsewhere through a global partnership whose goal is to reduce global measles mortality by 50 percent by 2005 (de Quadros et al. 2003; Strebel et al. 2003).

Viral vaccination has also seen new challenges, including a return to the use of smallpox vaccine in response to the threat of bioterrorism, withdrawal of the use of effective rotavirus vaccines in the USA due to rare adverse events (intussusception), and public concern over safety of viral vaccines including measles, mumps, rubella (MMR), and hepatitis B (Centers for Disease Control and Prevention 2003c; Murphy et al. 2001; Institute of Medicine 2001a, 2002a).

IMMUNOPROPHYLAXIS OF VIRAL INFECTIONS

The primary objectives of viral immunoprophylaxis are to prevent viral infection or to modify viral disease. Active immunoprophylaxis with viral vaccines stimulates the immune system to develop antibodies, cell-mediated immunity, or both, to prevent infection (e.g. measles, polio), and is usually given before exposure to disease. Vaccines (e.g. rabies, hepatitis B, and hepatitis A) may be effective in preventing disease after exposure, because the immune system is stimulated during the long incubation periods of these infections. Vaccines intended to modify the course of previously established infection (e.g. human immunodeficiency virus (HIV) infection, varicella vaccine to prevent or modify herpes zoster) are currently undergoing clinical trials.

Passive immunoprophylaxis, using pooled immunoglobulins prepared from human or animal serum or monoclonal antibodies from cell culture, can provide temporary protection against infection (pre-exposure prophylaxis for hepatitis A, respiratory syncytial virus) or can prevent or modify infection after exposure (disease-specific immunoglobulins to prevent rabies, hepatitis B, varicella).

TYPES OF VIRAL VACCINES

The two classic approaches to active viral immunization include inactivated viruses or their purified components, and live-attenuated vaccines. For some viral diseases, both approaches have been used (poliomyelitis, measles, influenza).

Inactivated viral vaccines

Inactivated vaccines may consist of whole virus particles, purified antigenic surface proteins or smaller peptide epitopes (Table 67.1). Inactivated whole virus vaccines are produced by the multiplication of virus in other animal species (e.g. rabies in mouse brain); in eggs, chick embryos or allantoic fluid (influenza, measles, mumps); or in cell culture (rabies in human diploid cells, polio, rubella), followed by purification and inactivation. Whole virus vaccines have the advantage of producing immune responses not only to surface proteins but also internal components, which may help eliminate viral infection. In the past, purified antigenic protein vaccines have been produced either by disruption of whole virus and purification of component proteins (split virus influenza) or by purification from the blood of virus carriers (plasma-derived hepatitis B vaccine). Newer generations of inactivated vaccines have been developed by genetic engineering, inserting DNA that encodes antigenic viral proteins into other micro-organisms (*Escherichia coli*, yeast, CHO cells, other viruses), which produce recombinant proteins that are subsequently purified (hepatitis B surface antigen, human papilloma virus (HPV) capsid polypeptides, and herpes simplex virus (HSV) glycoproteins in yeast). Most inactivated vaccines are combined with an adjuvant such as aluminum hydroxide (alum) to increase the immunogenicity of the vaccine. However, vaccines

Table 67.1 *Currently available inactivated viral vaccines*

Vaccine	Vaccine type	Uses
Inactivated polio	Killed whole virus	Universal childhood immunization (some developed countries); immunization of immunocompromised people
Hepatitis B	Purified HBsAg produced by recombinant yeast, mammalian cells or from plasma	Routine childhood or adolescent immunization; immunization of high risk adults; postexposure immunization with HBIG
Influenza	Killed whole virus, subvirion or purified surface antigen preparations	Vaccination of high risk individuals, elderly, children 6–23 months
Rabies	Killed whole virus	Postexposure vaccination of individuals, with HRIG; pre-exposure: veterinarians/travelers
Hepatitis A	Killed whole virus	Pre-exposure vaccination: high risk people and travelers
Japanese B encephalitis	Killed whole virus	Pre-exposure vaccination of travelers to endemic areas; routine or mass vaccination in endemic areas
Tick-borne encephalitis	Killed whole virus	Pre-exposure vaccination of travelers to endemic areas; (?) routine or mass vaccination in endemic areas
Under development (late stage)		
Human papillomavirus (prophylactic)	Virus-like particles prepared from surface capsid proteins (L1) produced in yeast	Pre-exposure vaccination of at-risk persons
Herpes simplex	Subunit glycoproteins D and B producd in yeast	Pre-exposure vaccination of at-risk persons

adjuvanted with alum lose potency when the vaccine is frozen.

New approaches to development

Other methods for producing inactivated vaccines include the use of synthetic peptides and idiotypic antibodies. Synthetic peptides, initially produced in 1963, were thought to have great promise as vaccines, especially as DNA sequencing technologies permitted identification of the precise sequences of antigenic sites of viral proteins (Brown 1988). The antigenic sites of viruses may be identified by determining the three-dimensional structure of the virus, comparing sequences of mutant and wild-type viruses or identifying hydrophilic regions of surface proteins and constructing peptides duplicating these sequences. Production of highly purified peptides is feasible, potentially inexpensive and results in a well-defined product without risk of containing adventitious agents. The feasibility of inducing protection in an immunized animal model has been demonstrated by use of an icosapeptide of the surface protein of the foot-and-mouth disease virus (Murphy and Channock 1990). However, other efforts with human disease viruses have met with less success. Peptides are often poorly immunogenic, may stimulate development of binding but not neutralizing antibodies, do not generally induce T-cell responses unless coupled to larger proteins, and cannot mimic conformational epitopes. Efforts to overcome these limitations include coupling the peptide genetically to a fusion protein (e.g. HBsAg), coupling to peptide carriers containing T-cell helper epitopes, and incorporating antigens into aggregates or self-assembling particles (Ellis 2004). Although experimental vaccines have been produced (influenza, foot-and-mouth disease) and found to be protective in animals (canine parvovirus and mink enteritis virus), at present it is uncertain whether viral vaccines for use in humans will follow (Meloen et al. 1995; Ellis 2004).

Anti-idiotype vaccines are based on the principle that neutralizing antibodies to viral antigens contain the mirror image of these epitopes, known as idiotypes. Anti-idiotype antibodies can be generated that mimic the conformation of the original viral epitope, and can then be used to induce neutralizing antibodies in the host. Immunization with anti-idiotype antibody results in the development of neutralizing antibodies to several viruses (poliovirus, hepatitis B surface antigen (HBsAg), rabies) and protection against disease in animal models (Dalgleish and Kennedy 1988). However, the levels of antibodies induced have been less than those induced by the original antigen, and the practicality of this approach for viral vaccines, for which many alternative production methods are available, remains to be demonstrated (Ellis 2004).

Transgenic plants have been engineered to produce viral antigens (e.g. HBsAg), with the potential advantages of producing low cost vaccines which can be administered orally (fed to recipients). Studies to date have demonstrated production of specific mucosal and serum antibodies against antigens in mouse models and reduction in disease in a pig gastroenteritis model, but studies in humans are still at an early stage (Kapusta et al. 2001).

Inactivation of viral vaccines

Inactivated whole virus vaccines produced in culture, animal tissues, or human serum must be subjected to steps that can inactivate the original virus as well as any adventitious agents that may be present in the initial substrate. Formalin has been most commonly used to ensure inactivation of residual viral activity in such vaccines. A balance between the concentration of formalin and the duration of treatment is needed to eliminate residual infectivity of the virus without destroying immunogenicity. Inadequate inactivation of poliovirus by formalin resulted in an outbreak of paralytic poliomyelitis due to inactivated polio vaccine soon after its introduction in the USA (Nathanson and Langmuir 1963). Review of this incident subsequently led to improvement in methods of viral purification and quality control of formalin inactivation procedures. Other inactivating agents that may be used include heat, acetylethyleneimine, and β-propiolactone. These inactivating agents may also provide protection against adventitious agents which can replicate in the cell or animal substrates used to produce vaccines. However, this protection depends on the sensitivity of the agent to the inactivation process. The failure of formalin to inactivate SV40 virus contamination in inactivated polio vaccine originating from monkey kidney cell substrate between 1955 and 1963 raised concern about the safety of this vaccine (Melnick and Stinebaugh 1962). Although some genomic studies suggest SV40 infection may be associated with rare carcinomas, such as mesothelioma and ependymoma, multiple epidemiological studies have not documented increased risk of any cancers in recipients of inactivated poliovirus vaccine (IPV) produced during this period (Institute of Medicine 2002b).

DNA vaccines (plasmid vaccines)

DNA vaccines represent a highly promising strategy for vaccine development. DNA-encoding antigenic portions of viruses – envelope, core, or nucleoprotein – are inserted into a plasmid, which can be injected directly into the host as 'naked' DNA, free of protein or nucleoprotein complexes. Host cells take up the DNA and may express the encoded proteins. Because the proteins are produced intracellularly, they enter the major histocompatibility complex (MHC) class I pathway and stimulate a strong cell-mediated immune (CMI) response, in contrast to inactivated vaccines, which enter the MHC class II pathway and produce, primarily, an antibody response (Fynan et al. 1995; McDonnell and Askari 1996). This predominantly cell-mediated immune response may assist in immune control of both acute and chronic viral infections. The method of vaccine delivery may determine the nature of the T-helper response; saline injections induce primarily Th1 response (CMI), whilst delivery by microprojectiles ('gene-guns') induces Th2 response (antibody). Multivalent vaccines can be constructed that include multiple antigens from a single organism or antigens from several different organisms, or include chimeric proteins (e.g. interleukin-2 immunoglobulin) constructs that enhance immune response. Although prototype naked DNA vaccines have generally elicited weak immune response, facilitation of immune response has been accomplished by incorporation into gene-guns and by coating with cationic lipids, lipospermines, and other molecules that facilitate transfer across membranes (Ellis 2004).

A prototype naked-DNA vaccine using the core nucleoprotein of influenza virus has been developed that protects mice from lethal doses of both homologous and heterologous strains of influenza virus. This vaccine induces both humoral antibody and CMI. Although antibodies to surface glycoproteins protect against infection from the homologous strain, it is likely that CMI provides protection against heterologous strains. DNA vaccines have been demonstrated to stimulate CMI to surface and internal proteins to HIV, hepatitis B virus, influenza virus, and other viruses in animal and primate models and in human trials (Srivastava and Liu 2003). DNA vaccines have also been shown to elicit antibodies against various viral proteins, including influenza, HIV, HBV, rabies virus glycoprotein, herpes simplex glycoproteins, papillomavirus, and hepatitis C virus. Secretory antibodies can be induced through formulation with cationic lipids, encapsulation in microparticles, and other approaches. Candidate vaccines to prevent hepatitis B virus, HIV, and influenza have reached phase 1 or 2 clinical trials in humans. Candidate HIV vaccines induced weak lymphoproliferative responses and interferon chemochines in naive subjects, but these did not persist. Similar trials in HIV-infected persons increased CMI response to rev, nef, and tat, but produced no changes in lymphocyte subsets. However, an HBV DNA vaccine delivered by gene gun has induced protective levels of antibody in naive subjects. Some candidate vaccines induce strong and long-lasting responses in infant experimental animals, indicating their potential use in routine childhood immunizations (Butts et al. 1998).

A promising new approach is to use DNA vaccines in a sequential vaccination strategy, in which the first dose is a DNA vaccine followed by a dose of a live recombinant vectored vaccine (e.g. vaccinia virus, canarypox virus, or adenovirus) carrying similar genes. This strategy is being pursued most actively for HIV vaccines.

The combination of DNA vaccine containing multiple proteins of simian immunodeficiency virus (SIV) and HIV, boosted with modified Ankara vaccinia strain containing similar antigens, has induced strong cellular and weak antibody immune responses and protected against virulent SIV infection (Amara et al. 2001). Key concerns about DNA vaccines include possible mutagenesis if the DNA plasmid becomes inserted into the host genome; the potential for developing tolerance to the antigen because of ongoing production in host cells; and the potential for immune attack on the cells producing the encoded antigen.

Live-attenuated viral vaccines

Currently available live-attenuated virus vaccines have been prepared by two approaches: (1) from related species of virus (Jennerian approach: vaccinia to prevent smallpox; rhesus rotavirus), and (2) by serial passage of virus through live organisms or through one or more cell culture lines (Table 67.2). Examples of the latter include yellow fever vaccine, developed via passage of wild virus in mice and subsequently in chick embryos; and polio (types 1 and 3) and measles vaccines, initially passaged in monkey kidney cells and chick embryo fibroblasts, respectively. Concern about the presence of adventitious viruses in animal-derived cell lines (SV40 virus in monkey kidney cell lines) has led to increased use of human diploid cell lines for producing live virus vaccines (rubella, varicella, polio). Several cell lines (WI-38 and MRC-5) are now commonly used. The World Health Organization has established guidelines for assessing the safety of vaccines produced in human cell lines (World Health Organization 1987).

Live-attenuated vaccines may also be produced via genetic reassortment. Among viruses with multiple-strand genomes, reassortants that combine the genomes encoding antigenic surface proteins from wild virus strains with genomes from attenuated or related strains of virus (cold-adapted influenza; rhesus- or bovine-based rotavirus vaccines) have been developed and shown to be effective (Murphy 1993; Kapikian 1994).

New approaches to development

Other approaches to the development of live virus vaccines include directed mutagenesis, use of strains of viruses from related species, and use of viral vectors such as vaccinia, and canarypox. Methods for direct mutagenesis include growth in low temperatures (25 or 32–34°C) to select temperature-sensitive or cold-adapted strains which do not grow well at human body temperature (Murphy and Channock 1990). Molecular biological techniques, combined with better understanding of molecular aspects of viral replication, can be used to develop specific mutations, such as deletion mutants,

Table 67.2 *Currently available live-attenuated viral vaccines*

Vaccine	Vaccine type	Uses
Oral polio	Attenuated trivalent	Routine childhood immunization; mass campaigns
Measles	Attenuated (Schwarz, Moraten, others)	Routine childhood immunization; mass campaigns
Rubella	Attenuated (RA 27/3)	Routine childhood immunization; adolescent girls; susceptible women of childbearing age
Mumps	Attenuated (Urabe or Jeryl Lynn)	Routine childhood immunization
Measles, mumps, rubella (MMR)	Attenuated	Routine childhood immunization (one or two doses)
Varicella	Attenuated (Oka strain)	Routine childhood immunization; susceptible adolescents and adults
Influenza	Cold adapted/reassortants	Immunization of high risk children/adolescents/adults
Yellow fever	Attenuated (17D)	Routine immunization or mass vaccination in endemic areas; vaccination of travelers to endemic areas
Smallpox (limited availability)	Vaccinia virus	Vaccination of research workers, military, BT response teams
Under development		
Rotavirus	Rhesus reassortants (four serotypes). Bovine reassortants, human neonatal rotavirus strain	Routine childhood immunization
Herpes zoster	Attenuated (Oka strain)	Adults

which are unlikely to revert to wild strains. Vaccines developed from related animal viruses include rhesus and bovine rotavirus as candidate strains to prevent human rotavirus infection, including reassortants that incorporate the surface protein genes for human rotavirus types 1, 2, 3, and 4 (Kapikian 1994; World Health Organization 2003b). Bovine parainfluenza virus 3 induces neutralizing antibodies to human parainfluenza virus type 3, and is a candidate vaccine to prevent this disease.

Large viruses such as vaccinia, other orthopoxviruses, and adenovirus can incorporate DNA that encodes essential proteins from other viruses (e.g. hepatitis B, rabies, measles hemagglutinin, or fusion proteins), attached to viral promoters that ensure adequate production of these antigens (Perkus et al. 1985; Moss et al. 1988). Vaccination results in replication of the parent virus, production of the encoded viral proteins and stimulation of both humoral and cell-mediated immunity. Although there has been some success in inducing immune response to the encoded proteins (HBsAg, influenza A, herpes simplex glycoprotein, rabies) and protection has been induced in experimental animals, concern about the potential for serious adverse events following vaccinia vaccination and limited success in inducing a strong antibody response have hampered development of vaccinia recombinants for humans. The use of canarypox virus, which undergoes only abortive infection in humans, may overcome concerns about the safety of such vaccines, and candidate vaccines have induced high levels of antibody against rabies glycoprotein and the measles hemagglutinin gene in humans. Yellow fever vaccine virus is being used as a foundation for development of Japanese encephalitis virus (JEV) and West Nile virus vaccines, through substituting JEV

and West Nile surface antigens for those of yellow fever virus (Langevin et al. 2003; Monath et al. 2003).

Sequential vaccination, either live vectored vaccines followed by protein or glycoprotein antigens, or with DNA vaccines followed by genetically engineered live vaccines, has produced stronger antibody and cell-mediated immunity than either antigen alone (Ellis 2004). Vaccination with a DNA-based HIV vaccine followed by canarypox HIV vaccine has produced promising results for preventing HIV infection (Amara et al. 2001), while vaccination with a DNA-based vaccine followed by adenovirus vaccine has provided protection against Ebola virus infection in animals (Sullivan et al. 2003).

RISK OF ADVENTITIOUS AGENTS

Possible contamination with adventitious agents is also a concern with live virus vaccines (Waters et al. 1972). A series of tests for potential contaminating agents is undertaken during vaccine development, safety testing, and postlicensing monitoring of vaccines (World Health Organization 1987). However, concerns regarding agents not detectable by current methods continue to arise despite the apparent safety of these vaccines.

Immunological basis of response to active immunization

Development of an immune response generally requires the interaction of T lymphocytes with antigen processing and presenting cells (dendritic or macrophages) (McDevitt 1980; Lanzavecchia 1985; Claman 1992). T-cell response is induced following the uptake of antigen by mononuclear phagocytes or dendritic cells, and can be enhanced by use of an adjuvant; the antigen is processed and presented, in association with MHC antigens, to T-helper cells. T cells recognize polypeptide antigens of 8–20 amino acids in size, presented in association with specific MHC molecules; the type of MHC molecule with which the antigen is presented by antigen-processing cells depends on the source and processing of the polypeptide. These in turn determine the primary type of T-cell response, either cytotoxic or helper. Presentation to T-helper cells results in secretion of immune mediators (cytokines) that can stimulate the maturation of naive T cells and communicate between leukocytes (via interleukins) to regulate the immune response (Baker 1975; Reinherz and Schlossman 1980; Arai et al. 1990).

Antigens from inactivated vaccines are absorbed into vacuoles, and processed and presented with MHC class II antigens; antigens from live-attenuated vaccines or vectored vaccines, produced within the cell, are processed in microtubules and presented with MHC class I antigens. Depending on the antigen and its MHC presentation, T lymphocytes differentiate into either T-helper type 1 cells (Th1, stimulated by MHC I-associated antigen), which mediate CMI, or T-helper 2 (Th2, with MHC II), which assist B cells in developing antibody production. Each of these subsets produces different interleukins and other immune mediators responsible for modulating the immune response.

An antibody response to an initial dose develops 2–6 weeks after immunization with inactivated antigens but may be incomplete even after two doses; after effective priming, booster responses occur within 4–14 days. The initial response is usually IgM antibodies, followed within weeks by IgG antibodies. Response to live vaccines follows a cycle of replication of the vaccine virus, and a period of several weeks or months for full development of the immune response. Response to measles vaccination is usually maximal by 6 weeks, but in younger children antibody titers may continue to rise for several months after vaccination.

Immune response to inactivated and live-attenuated vaccines

INACTIVATED VACCINES

Inactivated or purified viral vaccines induce responses only to the components present in the vaccine. Multiple doses, usually three or more, are necessary to induce a satisfactory response that will persist for long periods; booster doses may be necessary to ensure lasting protection. Most inactivated vaccines are given parenterally, and induce either no mucosal antibody or lower levels than live-attenuated vaccines administered by the oral or nasal routes. Inactivated vaccines may have limited ability to induce T-cell-mediated immunity, which is induced more strongly by antigens produced intracellularly as occurs with replication of live viral vaccines.

Microencapsulation of inactivated viral vaccine antigens in microparticles prepared from polylactide-coglycocide and polylactide polymers can allow delayed release of these antigens over many months, and shows promise for reducing the number of injections required to successfully immunize with inactivated antigens (e.g. hepatitis B) (Singh et al. 1997).

The advantages of inactivated vaccines are the absence of risk of disease due to the vaccine virus, given adequate inactivation; greater thermal stability and ease of handling in routine vaccination programs; and a lower risk of contamination with active adventitious agents than in live-attenuated vaccines. Nevertheless, examples of both inadequate inactivation and presence of active adventitious agents were documented in the past in inactivated polio vaccine (Nathanson and Langmuir 1963; Mortimer et al. 1982), although these problems have not been observed with hepatitis B, hepatitis A, or any other recently developed inactivated vaccines. Inactivated vaccines can be given safely to people with immuno-suppressive conditions.

A disadvantage of inactivated vaccines is the possible potentiation of the disease that the vaccine is intended to prevent. The original killed measles vaccines induced a detectable immune response, but recipients exposed to wild measles virus developed atypical measles with systemic symptoms and giant cell pneumonia (Annunziato et al. 1982). Subsequent analyses indicated that the formalin treatment destroyed the antigenicity of the measles fusion protein, resulting in an unbalanced response (to hemagglutinin only). Similar accentuation of respiratory syncytial virus disease in recipients of a formalin-inactivated vaccine was observed in early trials, and later shown in experimental animals to result from stimulation of formation of binding, but not neutralizing, antibodies to the surface F and G glycoproteins (Murphy and Channock 1990).

LIVE-ATTENUATED VACCINES

Live-attenuated vaccines have the advantage of inducing a complex immunological response simulating natural infection. Replication of the vaccine organism and processing of antigens mimic those of the natural organism, and both humoral and cell-mediated responses are generated to a variety of antigens. Because these antigens are similar or identical to those of the wild organism, responses are usually more effective and cross-reactive than those induced by inactivated vaccines. In addition, mucosal antibody may be stimulated directly by such vaccines when administered through oral or nasal routes (McGhee et al. 1992). Administration of oral or nasal live vaccines is more convenient than injection of inactivated vaccines. Immunity induced by one dose of a live-attenuated vaccine is long lasting, possibly life-long. However, the strength of humoral response is usually less than that of natural infection, and detectable antibodies may wane with time and result in some loss of protection. Induction of immunity by live vaccines can be inhibited by passively acquired antibody, whether from transplacental acquisition from the mother or from receipt of immunoglobulin-containing blood products; thus, achieving optimal response relies on ensuring that passive antibody (e.g. of maternal origin or acquired through administration of blood products) has declined to noninterfering levels. In addition, because the response may be incomplete (90–95 percent) after a single dose, two or more doses may be necessary to induce sufficient immunity to protect both the individual and the community.

The potential disadvantages of live vaccines include residual virulence of the vaccine in both healthy and immunocompromised hosts; possible contamination with adventitious agents; possible interference of response by other viral infections; and greater lability of the vaccine. Potential reversion to virulence has been well demonstrated with oral polio vaccine, paralytic poliomyelitis occurring in either vaccinees or their contacts at a rate of approximately 1 per 2.5 million vaccine doses distributed, with greatest risk after the first vaccine dose (Strebel et al. 1992). Persistent viral infection may occur in immunocompromised people after inadvertent use of measles and oral polio vaccines, and may rarely occur in healthy adults given rubella vaccine (Institute of Medicine 1991, 1993). However, measles vaccine has not been linked to the development of subacute sclerosing panencephalitis. Early lots of oral polio vaccine and yellow fever vaccine were contaminated with SV40 virus and avian leucosis virus, respectively. Although these were not linked with any long-term consequences (Waters et al. 1972), cell substrates used for vaccine production are now tested to ensure that these and other known pathogenic viruses are not present. Nevertheless, it may not be possible to ensure the absence of any adventitious agents in live virus vaccines. The stability of live virus vaccines depends on appropriate handling. Such vaccines require a sound cold chain, with storage at either 0–4°C (measles; measles, mumps, rubella (MMR)) or −15°C (polio, varicella), which can increase the cost of vaccination and impede their use in developing countries.

Determinants of response to viral vaccines

Vaccine and host characteristics are the primary determinants of vaccine response. Response may be affected by vaccine dosage, adjuvant, route and site of administration, number and timing of doses, and vaccine handling. Vaccine doses are determined before licensing to ensure a high level of response; adjuvants such as aluminum salts (hydroxide or phosphate), used only with inactivated antigens, stimulate a better response with a lower dose of antigen. New adjuvants based on improved understanding of immunology of vaccine response are now in clinical trials, and promise further to enhance the immune response in future inactivated viral vaccines (Jennings et al. 1998). An oil–water emulsion MF59 is now used in a split virion influenza vaccine that increases immunogenicity compared with that achieved with alum adjuvant (Ellis 2004). The route of administration – intradermal, subcutaneous, intramuscular, or mucosal – can determine both the strength and the nature of the immune response. Mucosal administration (intranasal or oral) stimulates higher levels of mucosal immunity (IgA antibodies), which may inhibit disease transmission with greater effectiveness than parenteral administration, which induces limited or no mucosal response (McGhee et al. 1992). Intradermal vaccination with low doses may induce antibody responses similar to those induced by intramuscular or subcutaneous administration of recommended doses, but is more difficult to deliver precisely and achieves less predictable responses. Intramuscular injections should be given in the anterior thigh (infants) or deltoid (older children and adults); injection into the buttocks produces a lower response in adults, probably owing to delivery of the vaccine into adipose tissue (Centers for Disease Control and Prevention 1991). The timing of vaccine doses is important: a minimum interval of 1 month between primary doses is usual for inactivated vaccines; delay of a third or reinforcing dose for 6 or more months after the first enhances the response and duration of antibody persistence, and is preferred unless high risk of disease necessitates shorter intervals. Intervals of 4–6 weeks are considered necessary to ensure optimal response to successive doses of live virus vaccines. The recommended routes and sites of administration and the timing of doses are devised to ensure optimal effectiveness in disease prevention and should therefore be used.

Host factors

Host factors that affect immune response include genetic factors (MHC polymorphism), age, nutritional and immune status, gender, pregnancy, and smoking. Although genetic factors, such as MHC polymorphism, are known to affect response at a molecular level, they have a limited effect on population response to available vaccines. Age is an important factor in response to immunization. Newborn infants generally do not develop as strong a response to inactivated vaccines as older infants or children (hepatitis B), and with certain vaccines maternal antibody may inhibit response (IPV, hepatitis A). For live vaccines such as measles, inhibition of the response by maternal antibodies determines the optimal timing for vaccination in early childhood.

The response to vaccines is excellent in young and adolescent children and in young adults, but decreases with increasing age. Male gender in adults and pregnancy have minor negative effects on antibody response of limited clinical significance; smoking decreases response to many antigens, and may increase the risk of nonresponse when other negative factors are present (Hadler and Margolis 1992). Extreme debilitation, acquired or congenital immunodeficiency disorders, diseases or treatments that cause immunosuppression, and some chronic diseases (renal disease, diabetes) can decrease immune response. For people with such conditions, inactivated vaccines are recommended despite lower effectiveness but may require higher or more frequent doses to achieve optimal response; live vaccines are often contraindicated owing to the risk of disseminated disease and possible death due to the vaccine organism (Centers for Disease Control and Prevention 2002a).

Measurement of response

Ideally, reliable laboratory tests should be available to measure the presence and strength of each of the major effectors of protection against the disease. In practice, tests for the presence of antibody are usually available (e.g. radioimmunoassay (RIA), enzyme immunoassay (EIA), complement fixation, immunofluorescent techniques), but these often do not measure the presence of functional (neutralizing or opsonizing) antibody. Tests for CMI are generally available only in research facilities. For some diseases, such as hepatitis B, polio, and measles, there are reliable tests for neutralizing antibodies and the levels needed to confer protection are known; however, only for hepatitis B are inexpensive tests widely available. For other diseases such as rubella and measles, commercial tests are available, often using EIA methods, but specificity is often less well defined, and sensitivity may be lower than that of neutralization assays. Development of better laboratory methods to measure protection and to permit rapid diagnosis of acute disease will remain a priority of disease control programs.

PRELICENSURE VACCINE EVALUATION

Licenses are granted only after extensive review of safety and efficacy data. Before licensing, vaccines are studied first in animals and then in small numbers of humans to determine safety, immunogenicity, and optimal dosages and schedules (phase I and II trials). Phase III trials examine safety and efficacy in larger numbers (1 000–10 000) of subjects. Nevertheless, prelicensing trials are limited in their ability to detect rare adverse reactions (frequency less than one per 1 000–10 000 doses) to vaccination, or adverse events in specific risk groups. Phase IV trials postlicensing may include larger numbers of vaccinees and can better define the frequency of uncommon adverse events. Linking the records of vaccination and of medical outcome in large numbers of children in health maintenance organizations (HMO) or other providers of comprehensive medical care can provide a way to assess causality of temporally related adverse events. In addition, postmarketing surveillance permits detection of new or unanticipated adverse events; reporting of such events observed after vaccination is required in many countries.

PRINCIPLES OF IMMUNIZATION PROGRAMS

The development of successful disease control programs requires safe and effective vaccines and effective public health strategies to prevent disease. Strategies for vaccine use are based on knowledge of epidemiology, consideration of whether eradication or reduction of disease is the primary goal, and the potential for implementing effective programs to deliver vaccines either to the entire population or to target groups (Table 67.3). Among the critical aspects of disease epidemiology are: (1) whether the disease causes infection universally in humans (e.g. poliomyelitis, measles, rubella, varicella, and hepatitis B in some populations) or only in certain geographic areas or in specific groups (hepatitis B in developed countries, rabies, yellow fever); (2) the primary age groups affected; (3) the primary reservoir for infection, including whether an animal reservoir exists (rabies, yellow fever) or infection occurs naturally only in humans (hepatitis B, hepatitis A, measles, mumps, rubella, varicella, poliomyelitis); and (4) whether the virus causes only acute infection or results in chronic or latent infection. Strategies targeted at eradication may be considered for diseases without substantial animal reservoirs or chronic or latent infection in humans, whereas reduction must be the initial goal when animal (rabies) or human reservoirs (hepatitis B, varicella) exist (Centers for Disease Control and Prevention 1993c). Mathematical modeling of the possible impact of vaccines on disease incidence may be helpful for selecting immunization strategies (Fox et al. 1972; Anderson and May 1990; Halloran et al. 1994).

Considerations of cost-effectiveness of vaccination programs have also become increasingly important when developing vaccination strategies. Universal use of vaccines to prevent polio, measles, mumps, and rubella saves money when direct costs of health care are considered (Hatziandreu et al. 1994). Studies showing that universal use of varicella and hepatitis B vaccines resulted in savings in combined direct (health care) and indirect costs influenced the development of policy for universal use of these vaccines in the USA (Lieu et al.

Table 67.3 *Approaches to the control of viral diseases with vaccines*

Disease	Proportion of population infected	Primary age of infection[a]	Chronic carrier	Animal reservoir	Eradicable with vaccine	Type of vaccination program
Polio	High	Child	No[b]	No	Yes	Child; mass campaigns
Smallpox[c]	High	Child	No	No	Yes	Child; containment
Measles	Universal	Child	No	No	Yes	Child; mass campaigns
Rubella	Universal	Child/adult	No	No	Yes	Child; adolescent girls/women
Varicella	Universal	Child	Yes[d]	No	Possible[e]	Child; adolescent; adult (susceptible)
Hepatitis B	Variable	Child/adult	Yes	No	Possible[e]	Infant; adolescent; high risk adult
Influenza	High	All	No	H + A[f]	No	High risk persons (e.g. elderly, chronic medical conditions, infants 6–23 months)
Yellow fever	None to high	All	No	Yes	No	High risk; universal
Rabies	Very low	All	No	Yes	No	High risk; post-exposure

a) Prior to wide use of vaccine.
b) On rare occasions immunodefficient individuals have excreted poliovirus for several years (Kew et al. 1998).
c) Smallpox was certified as eradicated in 1980.
d) Latent infection.
e) Potentially eradicable after several generations of vaccination or if human carriage of virus can be eliminated, or latency-defective vaccine can be developed.
f) Human and animal.

1994; Margolis et al. 1995). More recently, cost-effectiveness studies of varicella vaccine considering both the effect of a vaccination program on varicella and estimated effects on herpes zoster morbidity from modeled data have suggested that a childhood vaccination program may not be cost saving if varicella vaccination leads to an increase in herpes zoster (Brisson and Edmunds 2002).

Programs based on universal vaccination of infants or young children have been implemented successfully (poliomyelitis, measles) in both developed and developing countries (Hinman et al. 1999). Alternative approaches include universal vaccination of adolescents (rubella, hepatitis B), universal vaccination of all or some adults (influenza), and vaccination only of certain target groups or exposed people (rabies, hepatitis B, influenza). Mass immunization campaigns targeted at specific age groups are important in efforts to reduce the incidence of disease rapidly and in eradication and elimination programs for poliomyelitis and measles (Hull et al. 1994; de Quadros et al., 2003).

Vaccine schedules

Childhood immunization programs are now recommended in all countries and have resulted in substantial declines in the occurrence of vaccine-preventable diseases in both developed and developing countries (Galazka 1994; Centers for Disease Control and Prevention 1999b,c; Vaccines and Biologicals 2002a). Childhood immunization schedules are usually established by national governments or advisory bodies. In the USA, policy is established by the Advisory Committee on Immunization Practices (ACIP) of the US Public Health Service and the Committee on Infectious Diseases of the American Academy of Pediatrics (AAP), in consultation with the American Academy of Family Physicians (Centers for Disease Control and Prevention 2002a; Committee on Infectious Diseases 2003; Zimmerman et al 2003; Centers for Disease Control and Prevention 2005a). With effect from July 2004, the unified childhood and adolescent immunization schedule recommends use of vaccines to prevent six viral diseases in all children and adolescents: measles, mumps, rubella, polio, hepatitis B, and varicella (Figure 67.1). In addition, influenza vaccine is recommended for all children 6–23 months of age and their contacts, as well as contacts of infants <6 months of age, because children in this age group are at substantially increased risk for influenza-related hospitalization. Two viral vaccines are also recommended for select groups: hepatitis A vaccine for children and adolescents in areas of the country with high disease incidence and influenza vaccine for children ≥6 months with certain risk factors (including asthma, cardiac disease, sickle-cell disease, diabetes). With recommended universal hepatitis B vaccination of children, immunization can start at birth or any time up to 2 months of age, although the schedule indicates a preference for administering the first HepB dose to all newborns soon after birth and before hospital discharge. Routine doses are scheduled at 2, 4, and 6 months of age (diphtheria and tetanus toxoids and acellular pertussis vaccine (DTaP); *Haemophilus influenzae* type b (Hib); polio vaccine (IPV only); and hepatitis B). MMR is recommended at 12–15 months of age and varicella vaccine at 12 to

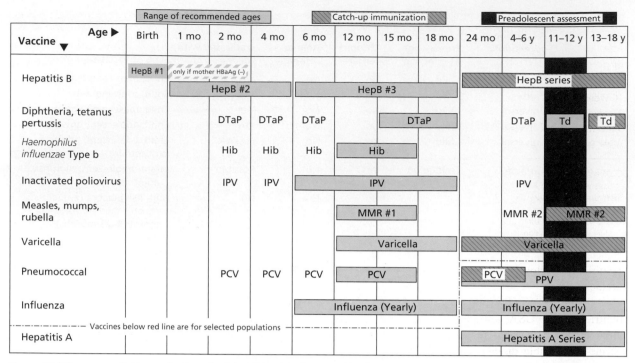

Figure 67.1 *Recommended immunization schedule, USA, 2005 (approved by the Advisory Committee on Immunization Practices, the American Academy of Pediatrics, and the American Academy of Family Physicians). This schedule indicates the recommended ages for routine administration of currently licensed childhood vaccines for children through age 18 years. Any dose not administered at the recommended age should be administered at any subsequent visit when indicated and feasible. Green bar with diagonal lines indicates age groups that warrant special effort to administer those vaccines not previously administered. Licensed combination vaccines may be used whenever any components of the combination are indicated and other components of the vaccine are not contraindicated. Providers should consult the manufacturers' package inserts for detailed recommendations. Readers should consult www.cdc.gov/nip/ acip/recs/child-schedule.htm for footnotes and additional information.*

18 months. Booster doses of DTaP and polio vaccine are recommended at school entry, with the second MMR dose given at primary school entry (Centers for Disease Control and Prevention 1998).

During the early adolescent years (age 11–16 years), immunization status should be assessed to provide a Td booster to ensure that the second dose of MMR has been given, to provide the primary series of hepatitis B vaccine to children who have not already received it and to ensure immunity to varicella. More detail is provided in footnotes to the schedule available at: www.cdc.gov/nip/ recs/child-schedule.htm#julydec. Another version of the schedule is provided for children and adolescents who start immunization late or who are at least 1 month behind.

In the UK, recommendations for immunization are issued and periodically updated by the Departments of Health (Joint Committee on Vaccination and Immunization 1996, update available at www.immunisation.nhs.uk. Differences between the USA and UK schedules include, in the USA, a Hib booster between 12–18 months, a dose of DTaP at 15–18 months, and routine use of hepatitis B, varicella, pneumococcal conjugate, and influenza (for children 6–23 months) vaccines, use of hepatitis A vaccine in high incidence areas and use of influenza vaccine in children >6 months with high risk

conditions, and in the UK use of meningococcal C conjugate vaccine for all children, and bacillus Calmette–Guerin (BCG) vaccine, and an IPV booster dose at age 13–18 years (as Td/IPV).

Routine childhood vaccinations and schedules vary in other countries (Hinman et al. 1999; Salisbury and Olive 2004). Polio and measles vaccination are universal, and rubella, mumps, and hepatitis B vaccination are offered by most developed and some developing countries. The World Health Organization recommends that all countries provide immunization to prevent seven diseases, including polio and measles, vaccinations being given at birth, at 6, 10, and 14 weeks of age, and at 9 months of age, respectively (Table 67.4) (Vaccines and Biologicals 2003). Hepatitis B vaccination, beginning at birth or 6 weeks of age, is now recommended in all countries, with primary goal to prevent perinatal and infant HBV transmission in countries with high or intermediate HBV endemicity. Yellow fever vaccination is recommended at 9 months of age in areas where this disease occurs. The World Health Organization (WHO) recommends that a second opportunity for measles vaccination should be offered either through routine immunization or in a vaccination campaign. The Global Alliance for Vaccines and Immunization (GAVI) provides support for the poorest countries to introduce previously under-utilized

Table 67.4 *Vaccine schedule for Expanded Program on Immunization, World Health Organization*

Age	Vaccine(s)
Birth	TOPV, BCG, Hep B
6 weeks	TOPV, DTP, Hep B, Hib
10 weeks	TOPV, DTP, Hep B, Hib
14 weeks	TOPV, DTP, Hep B, Hib
9 months	Measles, yellow fever (in endemic areas)
After 9 months	Measles second opportunity

BCG, bacillus Calmette–Guérin; DTP, diphtheria and tetanus toxoids and pertussis vaccine; Hep B, hepatitis B; three-dose series beginning at birth; Hib, *Haemophilus influenzae* type b, recommended in high incidence countries; TOPV, trivalent oral polio vaccine dose at birth (optional). Measles second opportunity may be done either as part of the routine schedule or in a campaign.

hepatitis B, yellow fever, and *H. influenzae* type b vaccines.

Vaccination of adults is also recommended in many countries. In the USA, although the childhood immunization program has greatly reduced the burden of vaccine-preventable disease among children, substantial vaccine-preventable morbidity and mortality from diseases such as hepatitis A, hepatitis B, influenza, and pneumococcal infections continue to occur among adults. Each year the ACIP approves the schedule for the routine vaccination of persons aged >19 years (Figure 67.2). The Adult Immunization Schedule is a harmonized schedule accepted by the American Academy of Family Physicians (AAFP) and the American College of Obstetricians and Gynecologists (ACOG) (Centers for Disease Control and Prevention 2003a).

Influenza vaccination is recommended for high-risk groups and in some countries for all older people (>50 years in the USA) (Figure 67.2) (Centers for Disease Control and Prevention 2004; Hinman et al. 1999), and >65 years in many developed countries including UK, France, Canada (National Advisory Committee on Immunization, Canada (NACI) 2002 www.hc-sc.gc/pphb-dgspsp/naci-ccni) and Australia (www1.health.gov.au/immhandbook). In addition, vaccination of adults at risk for hepatitis B, hepatitis A, pneumococcal disease, meningococcal disease, measles, mumps, rubella, and varicella may be recommended on the basis of licensing of vaccines and the burden of disease in a risk group, as well as a lack of history of previous disease or immunization. A Td booster is recommended every 10 years.

Simultaneous administration of vaccines

All childhood vaccines may be given simultaneously if necessary, on the basis of data from many studies showing that most vaccines can be given at the same time without compromising safety or immunogenicity. Simultaneous administration of all vaccines for which a person is eligible increases the probability that a child will be fully immunized at the appropriate age. Use of combination vaccines can reduce the number of injections required at a single visit and is preferred over separate injection of their equivalent components (Centers for Disease Control and Prevention 1999d, 2002a). Thus, DTP, Hib, IPV, hepatitis B, MMR, and varicella vaccines may be given simultaneously (King and Hadler 1994). Interference between live virus vaccines other than OPV (e.g. MMR, varicella) can, theoretically, occur if they are given not simultaneously but within close intervals; therefore, live virus vaccines should either be given simultaneously or at least 28 days apart (Centers for Disease Control and Prevention 2002a). Data are limited concerning interference between live vaccines. Interference has been found between certain vaccines for travelers (cholera and yellow fever) (Centers for Disease Control and Prevention 2002a) and in a study conducted in two US health maintenance organizations, children who received varicella vaccine <28 days after MMR vaccination had a greater risk (2.5-fold higher) of varicella vaccine failure compared with those who received varicella and MMR vaccines simultaneously or ≥28 days apart (Verstraeten et al. 2003). In contrast, one study did not show interference with seroresponse to yellow fever vaccine among persons who received monovalent measles vaccine 1–27 days earlier (Stefano et al. 1999). Immunoglobulins or blood products containing immunoglobulins inhibit the response to certain live virus vaccines (MMR, varicella). The duration of inhibition of response is related to the dose of immunoglobulins, and algorithms have been devised for calculating appropriate delays of MMR, measles, or varicella vaccination after administration of such products (Centers for Disease Control and Prevention 2002a; Siber et al. 1993). In general, MMR and varicella vaccines should be delayed at least 3 months after giving the usual doses of immunoglobulin (to prevent hepatitis A) or blood products, for 5 months after administration of measles immune globulin (IG) or varicella-zoster immune globulin (VZIG) and for longer after higher doses (e.g. ≥11 months after 2 g/kg IGIV for treatment of Kawasaki disease) (Centers for Disease Control and Prevention 2002a).

Vaccination in specific situations

VACCINATION OF PREMATURE INFANTS

Infants born prematurely, regardless of birth weight, should be vaccinated at the same chronological age and with the same schedule as full-term infants. Some studies suggest that response to hepatitis B vaccine may be diminished in infants with birth weights below

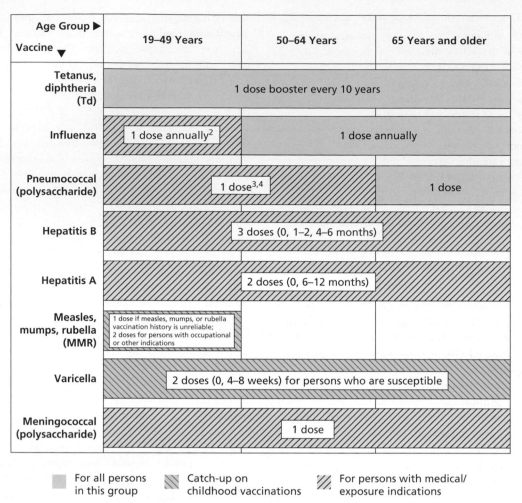

Age Group ▶ Vaccine ▼	19–49 Years	50–64 Years	65 Years and older
Tetanus, diphtheria (Td)	1 dose booster every 10 years		
Influenza	1 dose annually[2]	1 dose annually	
Pneumococcal (polysaccharide)	1 dose[3,4]		1 dose
Hepatitis B	3 doses (0, 1–2, 4–6 months)		
Hepatitis A	2 doses (0, 6–12 months)		
Measles, mumps, rubella (MMR)	1 dose if measles, mumps, or rubella vaccination history is unreliable; 2 doses for persons with occupational or other indications		
Varicella	2 doses (0, 4–8 weeks) for persons who are susceptible		
Meningococcal (polysaccharide)	1 dose		

For all persons in this group   Catch-up on childhood vaccinations   For persons with medical/exposure indications

Figure 67.2 *Recommended Adult Immunization Schedule, 2003–2004 (approved by the Advisory Committee on Immunization Practices, and accepted by the American College of Obstetricians and Gynecologists, and the American Academy of Family Physicians) (Centers for Disease Control and Prevention, 2003a). Readers should consult www.cdc.gov/nip/acip/recs/child-schedule.htm for footnotes and additional information.*

2 000 g; in an infant born to a HBsAg-positive mother and mothers with unknown serostatus, the premature infant should receive hepatitis B vaccine and hepatitis B immune globulin (HBIG) ⩽12 h after birth. If these infants weigh <2 000 g at birth, the initial vaccine dose should not count towards the completion of the hepatitis B vaccine series and three additional doses should be administered, beginning at 1 month of age. In an infant born to an HBsAg-negative mother, vaccination can be initiated either when the infant reaches 2 000 g or at 2 months of age with administration of other childhood vaccines (Centers for Disease Control and Prevention 2002a; Committee on Infectious Diseases 2003).

VACCINATION OF PREGNANT WOMEN

The risk from vaccination during pregnancy is largely theoretical and no evidence exists of risk from vaccinating pregnant women with inactivated virus or bacterial vaccines or toxoids. Hepatitis B and influenza

vaccines may be given to those at high risk of these diseases. Because women in the second and third trimester of pregnancy have an increased risk for hospitalization due to influenza (Neuzil et al. 1998), influenza vaccine is recommended for all women who will be pregnant during the influenza season (Centers for Disease Control and Prevention 2004). Live viral vaccines, in general, should not be administered during pregnancy or to women who may become pregnant in the next 4 weeks. However in some circumstances, the benefit of vaccinating a pregnant woman with a live viral vaccine may outweigh the risk when the probability of exposure is high and when infection might cause harm to the mother or the infant, but the vaccine is unlikely to do so (Centers for Disease Control and Prevention 2002a). Live virus vaccines, such as MMR and varicella, are contraindicated in pregnant women on theoretical grounds; however, as no cases of congenital rubella syndrome or congenital varicella syndrome have been reported after MMR or varicella vaccination among over 200 susceptible women exposed during the first trimester of pregnancy (for rubella vaccine) and >100 susceptible women (for varicella vaccine), inadvertent vaccination is not a reason to interrupt pregnancy (Centers for Disease Control 1989; Shields et al. 2001). Pregnant women may receive OPV (or IPV) and yellow fever vaccines if there is a risk of exposure. Vaccination of family members with MMR live virus vaccine does not pose a risk to pregnant women and because the risk of transmission of varicella vaccine virus is very low, MMR and varicella vaccine should be administered, as indicated, to the children and other household contacts of pregnant women (Centers for Disease Control and Prevention 1996, 1998). Breast-feeding does not adversely affect the responses to live or killed vaccines.

VACCINATION OF PEOPLE WITH ALTERED IMMUNOCOMPETENCE

People with altered immunocompetence require special consideration for vaccination (Centers for Disease Control and Prevention 1993b). Such individuals are often at increased risk of serious adverse consequences of disease; they may also be at increased risk of serious consequences of vaccination or of a poor response. Important groups of immunocompromised people include those with congenital immunodeficiency diseases; acquired immune deficiency syndrome (AIDS); hematopoietic or disseminated malignancy; immunosuppression because of administration of chemotherapy, systemic corticosteroids, radiation or other toxic drugs; and other chronic conditions, including splenectomy and diabetes. All such people can be vaccinated safely with killed, recombinant, subunit, and conjugate vaccines, which are usually recommended in the same doses and schedules as for immunocompetent individuals. Certain vaccines (e.g. influenza) may be specifically indicated for such people. The response to both killed and live vaccines, however, may be suboptimal, and higher doses or an increased number of doses may be needed to ensure protection. Live viral vaccines are generally not recommended for any of these groups, except for people with chronic medical conditions (e.g. diabetes), because of a known or theoretical risk of disseminated infection due to the vaccine. An exception is the recommendation of MMR vaccine for persons with HIV infection without severe immunocompromise, because of the high risk of serious consequences of wild measles infection (Onorato et al. 1988; Centers for Disease Control and Prevention 1998). Similarly, because of the high risk of serious consequences of wild varicella disease, varicella vaccine is licensed for use in immunocompromised people in Europe and in the USA is available under a research protocol for children with acute lymphoblastic leukemia in remission, can be used in persons with impaired humoral immunity, and should be considered for asymptomatic or mildly symptomatic HIV-infected children who should receive two doses of varicella vaccine,

3 months apart (Centers for Disease Control and Prevention, 1999e).

INTERNATIONAL TRAVELERS

International travelers may be at increased risk of exposure to vaccine-preventable diseases, even in developed countries. All children, adolescents, and adults planning international travel should be up to date for all routine childhood immunizations. For certain vaccines, children who travel overseas or live abroad should be vaccinated at an earlier age than recommended for children remaining in the USA. Before their departure, children aged ≥12 months should have received two doses of MMR vaccine separated by at least 28 days. Children aged 6–11 months should receive a dose of monovalent measles vaccine before departure or MMR if monovalent vaccine is not available (Centers for Disease Control and Prevention 1998). Other viral vaccines that should be considered before travel include hepatitis A and B vaccines, yellow fever, Japanese encephalitis, and rabies (if exposure to rabid animals is anticipated). The need for these vaccines should be determined by consulting specific guidelines for travelers (Centers for Disease Control and Prevention 2003b).

Vaccine safety and vaccine injury compensation

Viral vaccines, like other vaccines, usually cause only minor local and systemic adverse reactions, such as induration and pain at the injection site, fever, and malaise. Serious or life-threatening reactions can occur after some viral vaccines, such as paralytic poliomyelitis following oral polio vaccine, disseminated measles vaccine virus infection in immunocompromised children, or encephalitis or viscerotropic disease following yellow fever vaccine. The Institute of Medicine (IOM) in the USA has reviewed available information regarding the possible causality of serious adverse events following each of the licensed childhood vaccines (Institute of Medicine 1991, 1993, 2001a, 2002a), and continues to regularly review evidence regarding potential adverse events caused by vaccination. For many events, information is considered insufficient to determine causality. However, the panels have been able to classify some events definitively, as summarized in Table 67.5. These comprise the most comprehensive compilation of data on vaccine safety, although controversy still persists about some events. The panel has also examined broader issues of vaccine safety, concluding that evidence favors rejection of the hypothesis that multiple immunizations cause immune dysfunction or type 1 diabetes. Most recently, the panel rejected the hypothesis of a causal relationship between MMR vaccine or thimerosal-containing vaccines and autism (Institute of Medicine 2004). Based on a previous IOM report that

Table 67.5 *Summary of Institute of Medicine findings on the relationship of adverse events to individual vaccines*

Vaccine	Establishes causation	Favoring causation	Favoring rejection of causation
Measles (see also MMR)	Death from measles vaccine strain in immunocompromised people	Anaphylaxis	None
MMR (see also measles, mumps, and rubella)	Anaphylaxis/thrombocytopenia	None	Autism spectrum disorders
Mumps (see MMR)	None	None	None
OPV	Poliomyelitis in recipient or contact Death from polio vaccine strain in immunocompromised people	Guillain–Barré syndrome[a]	None
IPV	None	None	None
Hepatitis B	Anaphylaxis	None	Multiple sclerosis
Rubella[b] (see also MMR)	Acute arthritis	Chronic arthritis	None

a) A review of all additional information by the USPHS, which included a re-analysis of the Finnish data, concluded that the available data do not support a causal association.

b) Reviewed by an earlier committee. Initial report categories corresponding to those table headings were 'Evidence indicates a causal relationship,' 'Evidence is consistent with a causal relationship,' and 'Evidence does not indicate a causal relationship.'

found evidence inadequate to reject or accept a relationship between thimerosal preservative in some killed vaccines and neurodevelopmental disorders in children (attention deficit disorder and speech or language delays) (Institute of Medicine 2001b), the USA has removed thimerosal from childhood vaccines, although other countries and WHO have concluded there is insufficient evidence of risk to necessitate its removal from vaccines (see www.who.int/vaccine_safety/topics/thimerosal/statement200308).

Contraindications and precautions for each viral vaccine are usually described in the recommendations for use and in vaccine package inserts. For inactivated vaccines, anaphylactic reaction to a constituent or to a previous dose is usually the only contraindication, whereas, for live virus vaccines, any condition that results in immunocompromise (blood dyscrasias, HIV infection, steroid or chemotherapy, etc.) contraindicates use of the vaccine. Pregnancy is usually a contraindication for live vaccines that might be teratogenic (rubella, varicella), but not for inactivated vaccines. Potential recipients should be questioned regarding the presence of such conditions before any vaccine is administered.

Because viral vaccines may, rarely, cause serious adverse events, some countries have established programs to compensate people who develop permanent injury following vaccination (Centers for Disease Control 1988). A specific table of injuries may describe conditions for which compensation is routinely provided; in addition, anyone who can provide medical evidence of causality may be compensated. In the USA, this program is funded by a special excise tax on each dose of vaccine to which the program applies (DTP, OPV, MMR, Hib, hepatitis B, pneumococcal conjugate, and varicella vaccines). Assuring safe injection is also an essential part of immunization programs. Either single-use disposable or autodisable (AD) syringes should be used for each injection. However, improper reuse of disposable syringes, faulty sterilization of reusable syringes, and needlestick injuries pose a substantial risk of transmission of bloodborne infections (HIV, HBV, hepatitis C virus), and potentially add to the burden of these diseases in many developing countries (Hauri et al. 2004). United Nations International Children's Emergency Fund (UNICEF) and WHO now recommend use of AD syringes in all developing countries, to reduce the risk of transmission of bloodborne pathogens (Vaccines and Biologicals 2002b). GAVI is providing funds for purchase of AD syringes to assist the poorest countries to change from sterilized reusable or single-use syringes. WHO and UNICEF also recommend developing systems for the safe use and destruction of all injection equipment. Jet injectors eliminate the risk of needlestick injuries, but also may pose small risk of transmission of bloodborne diseases (Global Programme for Vaccines and Immunization, 1998).

Surveillance for vaccine-preventable diseases and vaccine supply, coverage, effectiveness, and adverse events

Monitoring the impact of vaccination programs and of the safety of vaccines is critical for refining immunization strategies and for assuring the public and medical community that vaccines are safe. Surveillance has shown the high effectiveness of universal childhood vaccines; compared with the prevaccine era, reductions of over 95 percent in the incidence of disease have been observed in the USA for polio, measles, mumps, and rubella (Centers for Disease Control and Prevention 1999b) and a reduction in varicella cases, hospitalizations and deaths of 70 to 80 percent by 2000 (Seward et al. 2002; Davis et al. 2004; Nguyen et al. 2005).

Surveillance for communicable diseases is maintained in each country, and may include any or all vaccine-preventable diseases (Wharton and Strebel 1995). These data should be monitored to assess the effectiveness of the vaccines and of the vaccination program. Surveillance needs vary according to the stage of the vaccination program. Early in implementation of a new vaccination program or before disease control has been achieved, aggregate reporting of total cases may be adequate. As the program progresses to the disease control stage, surveillance should become case-based; for each reported case of disease, confirmation by laboratory testing (virus isolation or serologic testing) and determination of vaccination status are essential to monitor whether continuing infections are due to failure to deliver vaccine or to low vaccine effectiveness. Information on age of cases is used to describe current epidemiology and to refine vaccine strategies. As the elimination of particular indigenous diseases approaches (achieved in the 1990s for measles in Finland, the UK and the USA), determination of chains of transmission, whether the case is indigenous or imported, and rapid implementation of control measures also become crucial (Peltola et al. 1994; Ramsay et al. 2003; Papania et al. 2004). At the elimination stage of a vaccination program, all healthcare providers are urged to report every suspected case of vaccine-preventable disease promptly to the local or national authorities. Monitoring the effectiveness of vaccines after licensing is essential, particularly during outbreaks in highly vaccinated populations, to reassess effectiveness in wide use and to maintain public confidence in vaccination (Orenstein et al. 1988). Monitoring vaccine coverage is also essential to track national and state vaccine coverage levels to identify pockets of unvaccinated people to target vaccination efforts and to maintain high levels of awareness for disease outbreaks (Vaccines and Biologicals 2002a). Documenting high vaccine coverage is also important; measles cases imported into the USA now have very limited spread due to the high levels of population immunity (Centers for Disease Control and Prevention 2002b).

Monitoring of adverse events after vaccination is also usually required in each country; in the USA it is the joint responsibility of the Food and Drug Administration (FDA) and the Centers for Disease Control and Prevention (CDC). Physicians are required by law to report certain events that occur after vaccination, and should report all suspected adverse reactions after vaccination to the vaccine adverse events reporting system (VAERS) (Centers for Disease Control 1988; Chen et al. 1994). Within a year of licensure of live rotavirus vaccine in the USA in 1999, the VAERS received an unexpectedly high number of reported cases of intussusception clustered 3–7 days after rotavirus vaccine. These reports were the signal that led to the decision to conduct scientific studies to determine whether Rhesus–human reassortant rotavirus (RVV) was associated with intussusception. Based on the results from three studies (case–control, case series, and retrospective cohort) which demonstrated a $\geqslant 20$-fold increase in risk of intussusception with use of RVV, the ACIP voted to withdraw their recommendation of use of this vaccine in the childhood vaccination program in the USA (Centers for Disease Control and Prevention 1999f).

Vaccine handling and storage

Vaccines are perishable products that require specific care in handling and storage. Ensuring that a vaccine maintains potency and safety is a responsibility shared by the manufacturer and everyone handling the vaccine. Live-attenuated vaccines, especially MMR, yellow fever, and varicella vaccines, are more susceptible to rises in temperature than are inactivated vaccines or toxoids. Vaccinia (smallpox) vaccine, the freeze-dried preparation available for the smallpox eradication program, is an exception and is extremely stable at high temperatures. All adjuvanted inactivated vaccines are sensitive to freezing and must be protected from freezing to ensure potency. Vaccines that are exposed to damaging environmental conditions may suffer loss of potency without a change in appearance. Live-attenuated virus vaccines should be administered promptly after reconstitution, $\leqslant 30$ min for varicella vaccine, $\leqslant 1$ h for yellow fever vaccine and $\leqslant 8$ h after reconstitution for measles and MMR vaccine (Centers for Disease Control and Prevention 2002a). A vaccine quality control program should be established in each clinical practice, focusing on education of personnel, maintenance of equipment, and adherence to routine daily monitoring of vaccines (Committee on Infectious Diseases 2003).

PASSIVE IMMUNOPROPHYLAXIS

Passive immunoprophylaxis consists of the use of purified antibodies prepared from human or animal serum to prevent infection or to modify the course of infection, when given either before or after exposure. The use of such antibodies was developed in the late nineteenth century, when sera from hyperimmunized horses and rabbits were used to treat diphtheria and tetanus. Although the use of antibiotics has largely reduced the use of passive immunoprophylaxis for bacterial infections (except tetanus, diphtheria, and replacement prophylaxis for those who are agamma- or hypogammaglobulinemic or immunocompromised), passive prophylaxis has maintained a role in preventing the serious consequences of several viral infections.

Immunoglobulin preparations currently used for viral immunoprophylaxis or treatment are prepared from human serum by cold ethanol precipitation (Cohn et al.

1946; Oncley et al. 1949). This yields three fractions, enriched in cryoprecipitates, globulins, and albumin, respectively, determined by the specific ethanol concentration, temperature, pH, and ion and protein concentrations. Immunoglobulin prepared by Cohn fractionation consists of mainly IgG types 1, 2, and 3, but is relatively depleted in IgG4. Immunoglobulin preparations maintain the properties of complement activation and opsonization associated with Fc receptors, and may also have immunomodulatory functions. In 1998, a new type of immunoglobulin product – humanized monoclonal antibodies against respiratory syncytial virus – became available in the USA. This immunoglobulin is produced in the NSO cell line and purified by ion exchange and other chromatography. This product has no known adverse reactions and is free from potential contamination from bloodborne agents.

Types of immunoglobulin

Four types of immunoglobulin products are used for viral immunoprophylaxis: pooled human immunoglobulin (prophylaxis for hepatitis A, measles) for intramuscular use; specific immunoglobulins (hepatitis B immunoglobulin (HBIG), rabies immunoglobulin (HRIG), varicella-zoster immunoglobulin (VZIG), vaccinia immunoglobulin (VIG) used to prevent the respective diseases); intravenous immunoglobulin, used for immunoprophylaxis for persons with primary or acquired immunodeficiencies; and specific intravenous immunoglobulin (IVIG) (RSV-IVIG, CMV-IVIG) used to prevent specific diseases in persons at risk (Table 67.6) (Finlayson 2003). Pooled human immunoglobulin for both intramuscular and intravenous use is generally prepared from large pools of donors (>1 000) who are not screened for specific antibodies; however, the final immunoglobulin preparation is required to have minimal levels of antibodies to measles and polio (neutralizing), diphtheria (antitoxin), and to hepatitis B surface antigen (anti-HBs). Antibodies to other viral pathogens, including enteroviruses, hepatitis A (HAV) and respiratory syncytial virus (RSV), are also present, although titers may vary widely in different lots. Owing to the relatively high frequency of hepatitis A infection in the general population, anti-HAV titers in immunoglobulin lots produced in the USA have remained relatively constant, although they have decreased in recent years in the UK.

Specific immunoglobulins are produced from a smaller donor pool that has either been screened for high titers of the specific antibody (RSV, cytomegalovirus (CMV)) or been boosted by vaccination of donors (hepatitis B, rabies, varicella-zoster) to ensure high levels of antibody. RSV monoclonal antibody is produced in cell culture, in which the human IgG1 gene has had grafted variable regions of murine monoclonal antibody directed against the F glycoprotein of RSV.

Intravenous immunoglobulin preparations are suitable for administering the larger doses needed by certain groups of immunodeficient patients. To prevent the occurrence of immunoglobulin aggregates, which could activate complement and cause serious reactions if given intravenously, techniques to break them down have been developed, including pepsin or plasmin digestion, reduction and alkylation, β-propiolactone treatment, or ultrafiltration and diafiltration (Waldvogel 1981). These are intended to ensure that >80 percent of IgG is present in monomeric form and that minimal aggregates of dimeric or larger forms exist. Since the mid-1990s, IVIG preparations also undergo steps to inactivate any residual viruses, either the solvent-detergent or heat inactivation or nanofiltration (Finlayson 2003). Manufacturing techniques vary among manufacturers and are continually evolving; package inserts should be consulted for each preparation.

Uses of passive immunoprophylaxis

Immunoglobulin preparations may be used as pre-exposure prophylaxis, given before anticipated exposure to a specific viral agent or as postexposure prophylaxis, either to prevent clinical disease (measles, hepatitis B, rabies) or to modify the course of infection (varicella) (Table 67.6).

PRE-EXPOSURE PROPHYLAXIS

Pre-exposure prophylaxis with immunoglobulin (NHIG) is now limited to hepatitis A prevention. Immunoglobulin is about 80 percent effective when given in a dose of 0.02 ml/kg for short-term protection to travelers to countries where HAV is endemic, or 0.06 ml/kg for protection for up to 6 months. In developed countries, hepatitis A vaccine is now preferred for pre-exposure prevention of hepatitis A.

IVIG is the treatment of choice for preventing bacterial and viral infections in people with primary immunodeficiency disorders associated with low serum IgG levels (Committee on Infectious Diseases 2003). Doses are usually given every 3–4 weeks, but the frequency of treatment may be tailored to the patient's clinical course and trough levels of IgG. Although IVIG treatment is most valuable in preventing bacterial infections, IVIG also reduces the risk of viral infections, including measles, enteroviruses, and RSV. IVIG is recommended to prevent infection in children with HIV infection with hypogammaglobulinemia (AIDS), people with chronic lymphocytic leukemia, and bone marrow transplantation, and is being studied for use in multiple myeloma.

Specific CMV IVIG is indicated for preventing serious outcomes of CMV infection in recipients of solid organ or bone marrow transplants. A 6-week course of therapy beginning within 72 h of transplantation may be used for

Table 67.6 *Immunoglobulins currently available for use in viral diseases*

Preparation	Route of injection	Uses
Human immunoglobulin (NHIG)	Intramuscular	Pre- and postexposure prophylaxis for hepatitis A; postexposure prophylaxis for measles; treatment of hypogammaglobulinemia
Hepatitis B immunoglobulin (HBIG)	Intramuscular	Postexposure prophylaxis for hepatitis B (with hepatitis B vaccine): perinatal, sexual, blood/body fluid exposure
Human rabies immunoglobulin (HRIG)	Intramuscular + intralesion	Postexposure prophylaxis for rabies (with rabies vaccine)
Varicella-zoster immunoglobulin (VZIG)	Intramuscular	Postexposure prophylaxis for susceptible infants, immunocompromised people, adults
Vaccinia immunoglobulin (VIG)	Intramuscular	Treatment of complications of vaccinia (disseminated vaccinia)
Immunoglobulin (IVIG)	Intravenous	Treatment of agamma- and hypogammaglobulinemia; prevention of viral infections in immunocompromised
Respiratory syncytial immunoglobulin (RSV IVIG)	Intravenous	Prevention of respiratory syncytial virus infection in premature infants and children with pulmonary dysplasia
RSV monoclonal antibody	Intramuscular	Uses same as RSV-IG
Cytomegalovirus immunoglobulin (CMV IVIG)	Intravenous	Prevention of serious CMV infection in transplant patients (experimental)

kidney, liver, lung, pancreas, or heart transplants. CMV IVIG may be used in conjunction with drugs (gancyclovir) to reduce risk of illness when an organ from a CMV-positive donor is transplanted into a CMV-negative recipient.

Two products, high titer RSV IVIG and RSV monoclonal antibodies, are now available in the USA to prevent RSV infection in children with bronchopulmonary dysplasia and in premature infants (<32 weeks of gestation) (Committee on Infectious Diseases 1998, 2003). These products are 40–55 percent effective in preventing the most serious complications of RSV disease in these children. RSV monoclonal antibody is given intramuscularly monthly in doses of 15 mg/kg during the RSV season (November–April in USA) to children up to 24 months of age, and is generally preferred because of ease of administration and because it does not interfere with live virus vaccines. RSV IVIG is given intravenously monthly in doses of 750 mg/kg, and may be preferred in infants with severe pulmonary disease in whom respiratory infections other than those caused by RSV may be important.

POSTEXPOSURE PROPHYLAXIS

Immunoglobulin (0.02 ml/kg) is recommended for postexposure prophylaxis to prevent hepatitis A in susceptible people with household or other close exposure if it can be given within 2 weeks of exposure. Immunoglobulin prophylaxis may modify hepatitis A disease without preventing virus excretion, and therefore should

only be given to food handlers with the caution that strict hygienic precautions should be followed for 6 weeks. Some experts prefer not to give immunoglobulin to food handlers. Immunoglobulin may also be given to prevent measles (0.5 ml/kg) in susceptible people at high risk of severe measles (<12 months of age, immunocompromised) if it is given within 1 week of exposure. Postexposure prophylaxis with specific immunoglobulins is recommended to prevent hepatitis B, rabies, and varicella infection. Hepatitis B immunoglobulin (HBIG) is usually given with hepatitis B vaccine to provide passive–active prophylaxis, which may enhance short-term protection and ensure long-lasting immunity: indications for HBIG include perinatal exposure to an HBsAg-positive mother (given as soon as possible after birth); sexual exposure to an HBsAg-positive person; and needlestick, blood, or other percutaneous exposure to HBsAg-positive blood or body secretions (Centers for Disease Control and Prevention 1991). Rabies immunoglobulin is also given as passive–active immunization with rabies vaccine after exposure to a rabies-infected animal; part of the HRIG dose is administered at the wound site and part at a separate site (Centers for Disease Control and Prevention, 1999i). VZIG is indicated for susceptible people at high risk of severe varicella who have household or other sustained contact (at least 1 h direct contact) with an infected individual. Those with highest priority include neonates exposed to maternal varicella (manifest between 2 days before and 5 days after birth), susceptible immunocompromised people, and premature infants born to varicella-susceptible mothers (Centers for Disease Control and Prevention 1996). It may also be used for exposed adults, although pre-exposure use of varicella vaccine should greatly reduce the use of VZIG over all and particularly in this population.

THERAPEUTIC USES

Immunoglobulin products may, rarely, be used to treat diseases. Vaccinia immunoglobulin (VIG) is the recommended treatment for people with serious complications of vaccinia immunization (disseminated disease, vaccinia necrosum). IVIG has also been used to successfully treat parvovirus B19 aplastic crises and RSV infection (Finlayson 2003).

Immune plasma is still used very rarely to treat established infections with highly lethal infections such as those due to hemorrhagic fever viruses (Maiztegui et al. 1979; Peters et al. 1991). Such experimental treatment employs convalescent serum from a previously infected patient, but poses the risk of serious adverse events, including immune complex deposition and serum sickness.

Adverse reactions

Immunoglobulin products for intramuscular use are very safe, with few adverse events and no risk of transmission of bloodborne diseases. Adverse reactions to intramuscular immunoglobulin are uncommon and usually mild, consisting of local pain or low-grade fever (Barundun and Morell 1981; Finlayson 2003). Allergic reactions may, rarely, occur; the risk is greater in people with isolated IgA deficiency. The risk of systemic reactions is greater (5–20 percent) with IVIG, and is highest in those with agamma- or hypogammaglobulinemia who are beginning therapy. The risk of reaction may be reduced by decreasing the rate of administration or by premedication with antihistamines, analgesics (aspirin or paracetamol/acetaminophen), or steroids. Infrequent serious reactions may include aseptic meningitis, acute renal failure, and anaphylaxis.

Immune globulins may interfere with response to live virus vaccines, particularly measles vaccine. Measles, MMR, and varicella vaccination should be delayed for 3 or more months after HNIG or IVIG, depending on dose.

Intramuscular IgG produced in developed countries has never been implicated in the transmission of bloodborne diseases, such as hepatitis B, HIV infection, or hepatitis C, even before the screening of donor blood for these agents. This elimination of infectious agents is probably due to a combination of exposure to high concentrations of ethanol (20–25 percent) and the presence of antiviral antibodies that neutralize activity or enhance the removal of virus during precipitation and centrifugation (Wells et al. 1986; Cuthbertson et al. 1987). All plasma donors in developed countries are now screened for these agents. Several incidents of

transmission of hepatitis C virus (HCV) infection by intravenous immunoglobulin preparations have been reported, including from one US manufacturer after screening of plasma donors for HCV antibodies was initiated (Rousell, 1988; Williams et al. 1988b; Centers for Disease Control and Prevention 1994). Although this step was intended to eliminate most HCV-positive plasma donors, the removal of HCV antibodies may have permitted HCV not complexed with antibodies to remain in the final product. To eliminate this potential hazard, methods of manufacture have been modified using solvent-detergent, heat treatment, or nanofiltration to eliminate the risk. Rarely, immunoglobulin produced in less developed countries has transmitted bloodborne disease, possibly owing to inadequate quality control (Finlayson 2003).

VACCINES RECOMMENDED FOR ROUTINE USE IN CHILDREN

Measles, mumps, and rubella

Live-attenuated measles vaccine is a universally recommended childhood vaccine and is administered most commonly as a single vaccine according to the WHO/EPI schedule at 9 months of age to children in countries following the basic expanded program on immunization (EPI) schedule and as a combined MMR vaccine to children 12–15 months in countries with expanded immunization programs, which include rubella and mumps. The immune response to each component vaccine is similar whether a combined or single product vaccine is administered. Simultaneous administration of MMR vaccine (or individual component vaccines) and other childhood vaccines does not alter the immune responses to any of them. Vaccination with MMR and its component vaccines is contraindicated for pregnant women and for people with moderate or severe febrile illnesses, with a previous anaphylactic reaction to any of the components of the vaccine, or with immunocompromising conditions (Centers for Disease Control and Prevention, 1998). Recent studies suggest that anaphylactic reactions to eggs are not contraindications to vaccination with measles, mumps, or MMR vaccines (James et al. 1995).

In addition to universal immunization of children with a first dose, the World Health Organization recommends that all children should be given a second opportunity for measles vaccination, either through routine vaccination or in a vaccination campaign (Vaccines and Biologicals 2003). Most developed countries have also implemented a schedule calling for a second dose of MMR vaccine The first dose is most commonly administered between 12 and 18 months with some countries administering the second dose before school entry (4–6 years) and others in early adolescence (11–13 years) (Hinman et al. 1999; Salisbury and Olive 2004). The primary aims are to assure that all children receive at least one dose of measles vaccine and to induce protective immunity in children who have not responded to the first dose of the measles component, but there is the added benefit of increasing the proportion of people immune to mumps and rubella (Centers for Disease Control and Prevention 1998).

MEASLES

Within a few years of the initial isolation of the measles virus by Enders and Peebles (1954), an attenuated vaccine was developed by serial passage of the virus in chick embryo fibroblasts. The first measles vaccine was approved for use in 1963. The most common strains of measles vaccine in current use include the Moraten, Schwarz, and Edmonstron–Zagreb strains (Strebel et al. 2004). An inactivated measles vaccine was withdrawn from production following reports of an atypical measles syndrome characterized by high fever, pneumonia, and an unusual rash that occurred after exposure to wild-type measles virus (Annunziato et al. 1982).

In different countries, measles vaccine routinely administered at 8 months (China), 9 months (EPI schedule), 12–15 months of age (USA, Australia, New Zealand, and many countries in Europe), although some countries administer the vaccine at 18 months (Sweden) or even 2 years (Slovenia, Croatia) (Salisbury and Olive 2004). The maternal antibodies to measles transferred to the fetus across the placenta are sufficient to prevent or reduce the immune response to vaccination in young children (Albrecht et al. 1977). Selecting the most appropriate age for vaccination against measles requires balancing the likelihood of a child retaining maternal antibodies against the possibility of being without antibody protection and being exposed to measles. The rates of seroconversion range from 80–85 percent in 9-month-old children to 95 percent and higher in 15-month-old children (Halsey 1983). However, as mothers acquire immunity from vaccination rather than from natural disease, the levels of maternally acquired antibodies in their infants are lower and they decline earlier (Strebel et al. 2004). Measles vaccine is extremely safe, although 5 percent of children who receive it have a raised temperature of $\geqslant 103°F$ ($\geqslant 39.4°C$) 7–12 days after immunization (Peltola and Heinonen 1986; Centers for Disease Control and Prevention 1998). A smaller proportion of children develop a rash, usually about 10 days after immunization. Rarely, the raised temperature provokes a febrile convulsion. Serious adverse events that are even less common include thrombocytopenia (one per 25 000–40 000 doses) and anaphylaxis (Institute of Medicine 1993).

The worldwide administration of measles vaccine has sharply reduced both the number of cases and the number of deaths attributed to measles. However, in 2001, the use of measles vaccine among children aged 12–23 months had remained between 70 and 75 percent

for the last decade. It is estimated that in 2000, there were 40 million cases of measles and 777 000 deaths from measles (Stein et al. 2003) and that measles remained the fifth leading cause of child mortality, accounting for 5 percent of deaths among children <5 years). In the prevaccine era, as many as 130 million cases and 5.8 million deaths may have occurred globally (World Health Organization 1998b). In 2002, the United Nations Special Session for Children endorsed a measles mortality reduction goal of reducing measles deaths by 50 percent by 2005, compared with 1999 estimates. The main strategies for achieving this goal are to achieve high coverage with both the first dose of vaccine and with the second opportunity for measles vaccination. In developing countries, the best strategy for the second opportunity is through supplementary immunization campaigns targeting children 9 months to 14 years, with follow-up campaigns in those aged 9–59 months every 3–5 years. In addition, increased routine coverage to 90 percent or higher will be needed to reduce and maintain absence of measles deaths in these countries (Otten et al. 2003). These strategies were developed in the Americas and are now being implemented in sub-Saharan Africa and many countries in other regions. In the period 2001–2002, 60 million African children in 13 countries received measles vaccine through supplementary immunization activities, and the measles partnership is on target to achieve the 50 percent mortality reduction goal by 2005.

Because measles infection results in lifelong protective immunity, there is no carrier state and humans are the only host, measles is theoretically eradicable (Centers for Disease Control and Prevention 1993c). The availability of an effective vaccine and the successful control of measles in the Americas and some countries in Europe and Asia make measles a potential candidate for eradication after polio (Centers for Disease Control and Prevention 1999g). In 1967, elimination of measles was achieved in the Gambia, and sustained for a 4-year period (Foege 1971). Since that time, strategies for its elimination have evolved that deliver two doses of vaccine using either routine two-dose vaccination, routine vaccination with supplemental mass vaccination campaigns or routine vaccination with a single mass catch-up campaign followed by a routine two-dose schedule. Finland and the USA have achieved elimination based on a routine two-dose program (Peltola et al. 1994; Papania et al. 2004). Most countries in the Americas have used supplemental mass vaccination against measles and by 2003, measles cases had declined 99 percent compared with 1990 and indigenous transmission had been interrupted (de Quadros et al. 2003). The UK, Australia, and some other countries have achieved or are close to achieving elimination using a combination of single mass catch-up campaigns and a routine two-dose schedule (Ramsay et al. 2003; McFarland et al. 2003). Further progress in reducing mortality and morbidity from measles depends on other countries implementing accelerated activities to achieve its elimination. Molecular epidemiological techniques will take on increasing importance in tracking the transmission of the measles virus and identifying importations (Rota et al. 1996). The World Health Organization has developed a standardized nomenclature to characterize the genetic variability in wildtype measles viruses (World Health Organization 1998a).

MUMPS

The mumps virus was first cultured in 1945 in chick embryos, leading to the development of vaccines that were first licensed in the Soviet Union and the USA in the 1960s (Plotkin 2004a). Several strains of mumps virus have been used to produce vaccine; until recently, the most widely used have been the Jeryl Lynn, Rubini, Urabe, Leningrad-3, L-Zagreb, and Hoshino. All produce seroconversion rates of 90–95 percent. Protective efficacy in clinical trials ranged from 92 to 96 percent. Post-licensure, vaccine effectiveness studied in outbreak investigations have been lower, from approximately 65 to 90 percent (Cheek et al. 1995; Wharton et al. 1988; Plotkin 2004a).

Mumps vaccine is well tolerated and, except for aseptic meningitis, few adverse events have been directly associated with vaccination. Aseptic meningitis has been associated mainly with vaccination with the Urabe and Leningrad strains of mumps vaccine (Plotkin 2004a; Ki et al. 2003; Dourado et al. 2000). When MMR vaccine has been used in mass campaigns, clusters of meningitis cases have been reported, highlighting that a specific vaccine strategy may influence the visibility of relatively rare adverse events and undermine public confidence in the vaccine (Dourado et al. 2000). Many developed countries, including Japan, UK, and other European countries, have removed the Urabe mumps vaccine from the market. These adverse events have had a detrimental effect on vaccination programs, in particular reducing acceptance of the combined MMR vaccine in routine vaccination programs, as well as in mass campaigns. The Jeryl Lynn strain has not been associated with aseptic meningitis and remains the mumps vaccine of choice throughout the world.

Widespread vaccination has greatly reduced the reported incidence of mumps in every country that has introduced mumps vaccine. As a disease without a carrier state and without a nonhuman host, the highly efficacious vaccine makes mumps, like measles, potentially eradicable (Centers for Disease Control and Prevention 1993c). It is not yet known whether a single dose can provide adequate population immunity to eradicate mumps, but it is unlikely given experience with single dose vaccine effectiveness under field conditions. Countries that use MMR in their childhood immunization schedule commonly have a two-dose policy for

measles vaccine that also results in two doses of mumps being administered. Russia recommends two doses of mumps-containing vaccine at 12–15 months and 6 years. Using a two-dose schedule of MMR at 14–18 months and 6 years since 1983, Finland has eliminated mumps (Peltola et al. 1994, 2000).

RUBELLA

The mild febrile rash illness due to rubella is important because of the congenital rubella syndrome (CRS). Women infected with rubella during the first trimester of pregnancy frequently give birth to babies with characteristic birth defects. The association between rubella and this congenital syndrome was first recognized as a triad of ocular abnormalities, cardiac defects, and deafness in newborns in Australia in 1941 (Gregg 1941). Subsequent studies have expanded the list of abnormalities in the CRS to include mental retardation, hepato- and splenomegaly, as well as thrombocytopenia, hypothyroidism, and diabetes mellitus. Infection in the first trimester of pregnancy results in the highest frequency of, and most devastating, abnormalities, although infection in the third trimester may cause cataracts (Centers for Disease Control and Prevention 1998).

In the years following the isolation of the virus in 1962, several vaccines were developed. The RA27/3 vaccine strain is now the most commonly used throughout the world (replacing the Cendehill and HPV 77 vaccines in the USA), although the T0-336 and BRD-2 strains are used in Asia and have potency similar to the RA27/3 strain (Plotkin and Reef 2004). Rubella vaccine induces an effective immune response in >95 percent of recipients, which seems to be less affected by maternal antibody than is the response to measles vaccine. Vaccine effectiveness with a single dose, studied during outbreak settings for the RA27/3, as well as some Japanese vaccine strains, has most commonly been >94 percent (Plotkin and Reef 2004).

Rubella vaccination is usually well tolerated, although arthritis or arthropathy may occur. This side-effect is more common in susceptible adult women than in children or adult men (Institute of Medicine 1991; Centers for Disease Control and Prevention 1998). Joint symptoms are usually self-limited, although chronic arthritis associated with rubella vaccine has been reported (Tingle et al. 1986). Symptoms may be less common following vaccination with RA27/3 than after vaccination with other strains. Some workers have found no association with rubella vaccination and the subsequent development of persistent joint symptoms. Inadvertent rubella vaccination during pregnancy has not been associated with congenital defects, but vaccination is contraindicated in pregnancy (Centers for Disease Control, 1989, 1998) and women who receive rubella vaccine should be counseled to avoid pregnancy for 28 days after vaccination (Centers for Disease Control and Prevention, 2001b).

Several strategies have been implemented to control rubella and CRS. Some countries have opted to immunize only women of childbearing age, in practice girls 12–13 years of age, just before their reproductive years. With complete implementation of the program, virus continues to circulate among unvaccinated children and men, providing periodic boosting of immunity in vaccinated women. In theory, the control of CRS is achieved by protecting all women who might become pregnant. In the UK, an immunity level of 97 percent was found to be inadequate to prevent all cases of CRS (Miller 1991). The second strategy is universal vaccination of children. The ultimate aim here is the elimination of rubella transmission and the reduction of CRS by vaccination-induced immunity and herd immunity (Centers for Disease Control and Prevention 1998). Currently, most developed countries combine the two strategies, through universal immunization of children at 12–15 months of age with MMR vaccine or measles, rubella vaccine and immunization of susceptible women with rubella vaccine, and 119 countries have included rubella in routine immunization programs (Salisbury and Olive 2004; Vaccines and Biologicals 2002a). Some countries have conducted mass vaccination campaigns of adults of reproductive age in conjunction with initiating universal child vaccination against rubella (Hinman et al. 1998). Experience with various vaccination strategies in the Pan American Health Organization (PAHO) region in the late 1990s has lead to adoption of one-time mass vaccination of males and females (sometimes ranging from 5–39 years and administered as a combined MR campaign), in addition to introducing MMR in the childhood vaccination program as the most effective way to rapidly reduce virus transmission and more rapidly prevent congenital rubella syndrome. (Castillo-Solórzano et al. 2003). Cuba was the first country to eliminate rubella and CRS through two mass campaigns during 1985 and 1986 that initially targeted women aged 18–30 years followed by children 1–14 years (World Health Organization 2000).

Rubella, like measles, has only a human host and no chronic carrier state, so can theoretically be eradicated. Mathematical modeling suggests that a single dose of vaccine, given universally, should be sufficient to eliminate or even eradicate rubella. To date, Finland and Cuba have declared success in this effort, although the elimination of transmission in the USA is suggested by prolonged periods of no reported disease since the late 1990s, as well as by the epidemiology of CRS between 1997 and 1999, where 41 percent of mothers with CRS births were infected outside the country (Peltola et al. 2000; Reef et al. 2002). Molecular epidemiological methods, similar to those used in measles elimination efforts, in which the genetic information of wildtype viruses is characterized, will aid efforts to track and eliminate rubella virus transmission (Frey et al. 1998; Reef et al. 2002). The major constraints to eradication are a perceived lack of importance because of the mild clinical syndrome and the difficulty in maintaining surveillance for a disease in which half the cases may lack any clinical symptoms. These constraints are changing, however, as experience has been gained with combining rubella with measles surveillance mainly in the Americas (Irons et al. 2003). In developing countries, inadequate surveillance for CRS has meant that its importance is not known. Although rubella is not included in the World Health Organization's Expanded Program on Immunization (Robertson et al. 1997), there has been considerable progress in rubella control and CRS prevention especially in the region of the Americas where almost all countries are now using MMR vaccine in their routine childhood vaccination programs, are integrating measles and rubella surveillance including laboratory testing, and some of which have also initiated mass vaccination campaigns to accelerate rubella control/CRS prevention (Castillo-Solórzano et al. 2003; Irons et al. 2003). The European region has established a target for reducing incidence of CRS to <1 per 100 000 births by 2010. Strategies to achieve the goal of measles elimination by 2007 in this region have included mass campaigns using measles vaccine which have also provided opportunities for countries to launch or accelerate rubella and CRS prevention programs (Spika et al. 2003; Dayan et al. 2003).

Poliomyelitis

Poliomyelitis was a widespread cause of childhood morbidity and mortality in the prevaccine era (Strebel et al. 1992). In 1949, the discovery that poliovirus could be propagated in nonnervous human tissue permitted the large-scale production necessary for vaccine manufacture (Enders et al. 1949). Two standard approaches were pursued: inactivation and attenuation of poliovirus.

Following large-scale field trials of inactivated poliovirus vaccine (IPV) developed by Jonas Salk, IPV became, in 1955, the first poliovirus vaccine to be licensed in the USA (Francis et al. 1957; Salk et al. 1994). IPV contains formalin-inactivated poliovirus types 1, 2, and 3. In 1961, monovalent oral poliovirus vaccines (OPV) developed by Albert Sabin were licensed. Two years later, a balanced formulation of the three monovalent vaccines (trivalent OPV) became available and rapidly replaced IPV as the vaccine of choice for preventing poliomyelitis in the USA and in most other countries. OPV contains live-attenuated polioviruses of the three poliovirus serotypes formulated ratio 10:1:6, with 10^6 median tissue culture infective dose ($TCID_{50}$) of poliovirus type 1, 10^5 $TCID_{50}$ of poliovirus type 2, and $10^{5.8}$ $TCID_{50}$ of poliovirus type 3 (Centers for Disease Control 1982). In the 1980s, enhanced-potency IPVs (eIPV) were developed; eIPV containing 40:8:32

D-antigen units of poliovirus types 1, 2, and 3, respectively, was licensed in the USA in 1987 (Centers for Disease Control 1987).

In most industrialized countries, including the USA before 1997, and virtually all developed countries, the vaccine of choice for the prevention of poliomyelitis is OPV (Centers for Disease Control 1982; Hinman et al. 1999). The primary series of OPV usually consists of three doses in the first 6 months of life, followed by one or more additional doses between 1–2 years of age or at school entry. In the United States prior to 1997, doses were given at 2, 4, and 6–18 months of age, followed by a supplemental dose of OPV at school entry (i.e. 4–6 years). The primary series of IPV consists of between four and seven doses, with two to three doses given in the first year of life and at least one booster dose 6–12 months after the primary series. In the USA, doses are given at 2, 4, and 6–18 months of age, followed by a fourth dose of IPV at school entry. Until 1997, IPV in the USA was indicated primarily for immunologically abnormal infants and their family contacts, and for unvaccinated adults (Centers for Disease Control 1987). Following primary reliance on OPV between 1961 and 1996, the USA revised its poliomyelitis prevention policy with effect from early 1997. Recognizing the absence of indigenous wild poliovirus circulation since 1979, the occurrence of eight to nine cases of vaccine-associated paralytic poliomyelitis (VAPP) annually in the USA and the rapid progress in global polio eradication, the USA revised its policy first to increase the use of IPV, the first two doses of poliovirus vaccine as IPV given at 2 and 4 months of age followed by two doses of OPV at 12–18 months and 4–6 years of age (Centers for Disease Control and Prevention 1997). In 2000, the policy was revised to an IPV-only schedule (Centers for Disease Control and Prevention 2000). OPV is no longer recommended, except in special circumstances such as a child who will be traveling to a polio-endemic area. This schedule ensures development of good humoral immunity, while eliminating the risk of VAPP (McBean and Modlin 1987; Centers for Disease Control and Prevention 2000). IPV has been used exclusively in many northern European countries, including Finland, Sweden, and the Netherlands, and has led to eradication in these countries. Currently, 22 developed countries use exclusive IPV, and an additional eight countries use a sequential schedule of IPV followed by OPV (World Health Organization 2003a).

The Expanded Program on Immunization of the World Health Organization recommends a schedule of four OPV doses administered at birth (zero week), 6, 10, and 14 weeks to ensure earlier protection against poliomyelitis in infants residing in the developing world. Many developing countries also recommend a dose of OPV in the second year of life.

The objective of the routine series of poliovirus vaccine is to induce humoral immunity for individual protection against poliomyelitis and mucosal immunity for community protection against its circulation. In industrialized countries, three doses of OPV or IPV result in seroconversion or seroprevalence levels of >90 percent to all three poliovirus serotypes. In developing countries, the immunogenicity of OPV is substantially lower, with median seroconversion levels of 72, 95, and 65 percent (Patriarca et al. 1991) to poliovirus types 1, 2, and 3, respectively, following the administration of three doses of OPV. The lower immunogenicity of OPV in developing countries may be due to interference by concurrent enterovirus infection, diarrhea, nonspecific inhibition, or other factors. In addition, the immunogenicity of OPV may be lower under program conditions because of suboptimal storage, handling, and administration. When given by the WHO/EPI schedule, the immunogenicity of IPV has varied widely, from 67–99 percent for type 1, 65–99 percent for type 2, and 91–100 percent against type 3 (World Health Organization 2003a). The response to early administration of IPV may be inversely affected by maternally derived type-specific antibody (WHO Collaborative Study Group 1996). Whereas OPV and IPV induce a similarly high-level humoral immune response in infants residing in industrialized countries, the intestinal mucosal immunity induced by OPV is clearly superior to that induced by IPV in limiting the replication and excretion of circulating poliovirus (Sutter and Patriarca 1993).

The widespread use of IPV, starting in 1955, led to a major reduction in the incidence of poliomyelitis in the USA, from 57 879 cases in 1952 to 5 485 cases by 1957. The widespread use of OPV led to the elimination of indigenous circulation of wild poliovirus in the 1960s. The last endemic and epidemic cases of poliomyelitis were reported in 1979. Between 1980 and 1997, aside from a few imported cases of poliomyelitis, approximately eight cases of VAPP were reported each year in the USA (Strebel et al. 1992). Of these eight VAPP cases, three each occurred in OPV recipients and in people in contact with OPV recipients and two cases in immunologically abnormal people. Since the adoption of the IPV schedule, no VAPP cases have been reported in the USA.

The occurrence of VAPP is the most serious adverse event following use of OPV and has been reported from most industrialized countries (Esteves 1988; Joce et al. 1992; Strebel et al. 1992). Among immunocompetent people, the highest risk of VAPP is in recipients of the first dose of OPV (one VAPP case per 1.5 million infants) and in unvaccinated contacts (one VAPP case per 2.2 million contacts) of recently vaccinated infants. However, the risk of VAPP is highest in the presence of immunological abnormality (either congenital or acquired), particularly people with B-cell deficiencies. In Romania, a country that had reported very high rates of VAPP for many years, a case–control study suggested that the apparently increased incidence was primarily due to multiple intramuscular injections of antibiotics following administration of OPV (Strebel et al. 1995). An estimated 250–500 VAPP cases occur annually. An additional risk of OPV use is circulating vaccine-derived polioviruses (cVDPV), in which vaccine-derived polioviruses have reverted to wild-type virulence and developed the ability to circulate widely in the population. Since 1988, four outbreaks of cVDPV have occurred, causing between three and 30 cases of paralytic poliomyelitis (World Health Organization, 2003a). These outbreaks have generally originated in populations with low vaccine coverage, allowing vaccine viruses to circulate for long periods and reattain virulence. IPV is not known to cause serious adverse reactions.

Progress toward poliomyelitis control in industrialized and developing countries prompted the member countries of the WHO region of the Americas to adopt the goal, in 1985, of regional elimination of poliomyelitis from the western hemisphere by the year 1990. Following the implementation of key strategies, the last case of poliomyelitis associated with wild poliovirus isolation was reported from Peru in September 1991, and the region was certified free of indigenous wild poliovirus by an International Certification Commission in September 1994 (Pan American Health Organization 1994). In 1988, the World Health Assembly, the governing body of WHO, adopted the goal of global eradication of poliomyelitis by the year 2000 (World Health Organization 1988). A unique partnership of governmental and private organizations is supporting this initiative; Rotary International, a private service organization, has provided more than US$500 million and immeasurable volunteer time to achieve the goal of eradication.

The poliomyelitis eradication initiative relies on four strategies:

1 high routine coverage with OPV;
2 supplemental immunization, including national immunization days (NID) twice a year to vaccinate all children in order to eliminate the remaining poliovirus reservoirs;
3 enhanced epidemiological and virologic surveillance to detect cases immediately, institute control measures, and eventually assist in eliminating wild poliovirus circulation;
4 house-to-house campaigns to interrupt remaining chains of transmission (Hull et al. 1994). Additional house-to-house campaigns have become the key strategy in the remaining polio-endemic countries.

At present, use of IPV in developing countries is not recommended because of its inferior protection against virus transmission (mucosal immunity), potential lower response to vaccination with the EPI schedule, higher cost, and greater complexity of administration (e.g.

injection, combination vaccines) (World Health Organization 2003a). This recommendation is being reviewed as progress toward eradication continues.

Progress towards eradication can be measured both by outcome evaluation (e.g. the incidence of poliomyelitis) and by process evaluation (e.g. the number of countries conducting NIDs). Worldwide, the number of polio cases has decreased by over 99 percent, from over 200 000 cases in 1980 to 1 250 in 2004. Eradication of polio has been certified in the American (1994), Western Pacific (2001), and European (2002) regions. However, the virus remains endemic in six countries (Nigeria, India, Pakistan, Niger, Afghanistan, Egypt), and in 2004 polio cases caused by wild poliovirus originating from northern Nigeria were reported in ten sub-Saharan countries in Africa and in Saudi Arabia, re-establishing transmission (for more than 6 months) in five countries bordering or near Nigeria (Vaccines and Biologicals 2004; Centers for Disease Control and Prevention 2005b). During this period, NIDs were conducted in up to 96 countries, and supplemental doses were given to 500 million of the world's children < 5 years of age during 266 rounds of NIDs, supplemental immunization days, or mopping up activities in 2002. During 2004, supplemental immunization was conducted in 23 contiguous countries in Africa, and up to 6–8 rounds of vaccination were conducted in the remaining polio-endemic countries.

The progress toward global eradication of poliomyelitis suggests that this objective may be within reach in Asia and Egypt by the end of 2005, and in Africa soon thereafter. However, increased efforts are necessary to ensure that adequate resources are made available to eliminate the remaining poliovirus reservoirs, particularly those in southern Asia and Africa.

Hepatitis B vaccine

Hepatitis B vaccines initially consisted of HBsAg particles purified from the plasma of HBV carriers. Plasma-derived vaccines were highly effective in preventing hepatitis B, were used in developed countries throughout the early 1980s, and continue to be used in a few developing countries (Szmuness et al. 1981; Kane 1993). In 1985, the first recombinant HB vaccines became available. These consist of purified HBsAg produced by recombinant DNA technology in yeast or in mammalian cells. Newer generation vaccines, which may include the pre-S1 or pre-S2 antigens, or both, in addition to HBsAg have also been developed but have not replaced the vaccines based solely on HBsAg (Hadler and Margolis 1992).

Hepatitis B vaccine is usually given as a three-dose series. The licensed schedule in developed countries includes doses at 0, 1, and 6 months, with an alternative schedule of four doses given at 0, 1, 2, and 12 months. However, schedules that vary the timing of the second and third doses to permit integration into the routine childhood immunization schedule have been highly immunogenic (Centers for Disease Control and Prevention 1991). Dosages vary by age, vaccine, and whether the child is born to an HBsAg-positive mother; in the USA, dosages for infants and children are one-half those required for adults.

The response to a three-dose series is excellent in all age groups, with anti-HBs produced in 85–99 percent of vaccinees; response is highest in children aged 2–19 years, and decreases with increasing age (Hadler and Margolis 1992). People with immunocompromising conditions such as renal failure have poorer responses, and higher dosages are recommended. Placebo-controlled trials both in high-risk children in HBV-endemic countries and in high risk adults in the USA and elsewhere have shown short-term efficacy of 80–95 percent (Szmuness et al. 1981; Stevens et al. 1992). Long-term follow up of both children and adults for up to 14 years has demonstrated protection against serious consequences of infection (chronic carriage and chronic liver disease) in virtually all people who respond to the initial series (anti-HBs $\geqslant$10 miu/ml) (Hadler and Margolis 1992; West and Calendra 1996; Mast et al. 2004). Booster doses are not currently recommended for any age group, but the need for them continues to be evaluated.

Hepatitis B vaccine causes few adverse reactions, mainly fever and soreness at the injection site. Rarely, anaphylaxis can occur, and contraindicates additional doses of vaccine. Serious neurological injuries such as Guillain–Barré syndrome and other demyelinating conditions (multiple sclerosis, optic neuritis, and transverse myelitis) have been reported, rarely, following hepatitis B vaccination, but available information favors rejection of a causal link with multiple sclerosis, and is insufficient to accept or reject a relation between other demyelinating conditions and hepatitis B vaccine (Centers for Disease Control and Prevention 1991; Institute of Medicine 1993, 2002a).

In developed countries, including the USA and Europe, hepatitis B vaccine was initially recommended only for infants of HBV-carrier mothers and high risk adults. However, in the USA, the lack of impact on disease incidence led to implementation of a comprehensive strategy for eliminating hepatitis B transmission (Centers for Disease Control and Prevention 1991). This strategy includes: (1) universal screening of pregnant women for HBsAg, and providing hepatitis B immunoglobulin and initiating hepatitis B vaccination within 12 h of birth for infants born to hepatitis B-carrier mothers; (2) universal vaccination of all infants, preferentially beginning at birth, but at least by 2 months of age when other routine childhood vaccines are initiated; (3) vaccination of all previously unvaccinated children at 11–12 years of age; and (4) vaccination of children, adolescents and adults in high risk groups, including people who live in households with HBsAg carriers;

children $\leqslant$11 years old of immigrants from areas of high HBV endemicity; people who abuse drugs parenterally; the sexually active, whether homosexual or heterosexual; and those at occupational risk. The recommendation for universal vaccination of infants was based on several considerations: the low dose of vaccine required for this age group; the feasibility of integration into the routine childhood immunization schedule; the need to prevent chronic infection in high risk children; and data showing that protection persists to the age when high-risk behaviors begin.

Vaccination of all previously unvaccinated adolescents at 11–12 years of age is the primary strategy for hepatitis B control in Canada and some countries in Europe (Committee on Infectious Diseases 2003; Hinman et al. 1999). This approach has the advantage of ensuring that adolescents will be protected before beginning high-risk behaviors, that immunity will be high and that a booster dose of vaccine will not be needed. A key challenge is providing the three-dose vaccine series to this age group in the absence of regular preventive healthcare visits. The vaccination of adolescents has been implemented successfully in British Columbia via school-based programs (Dobson et al. 1995).

The World Health Organization now recommends that all countries should include HB vaccine in their routine immunization schedules, with emphasis on routine infant immunization and prevention of perinatal HBV transmission (Vaccines and Biologicals 2003). In all developing countries, universal vaccination of infants is the recommended strategy for disease control (Kane 1993). The initial dose should be given as soon after birth as possible, particularly in countries in which perinatal disease transmission is predominant (e.g. eastern Asia). Infant immunization has been shown to be highly effective in reducing the frequency of HBV carriers among children in many high risk countries (Mast et al. 2004), and has been associated with reduced risk of liver cancer among children in Taiwan (Chang et al. 2003). Introduction of hepatitis B vaccination in the poorest countries is now supported by funding from the Global Alliance for Vaccines and Immunization, and by 2003, 151 countries had hepatitis B programs, based mainly on universal vaccination of infants (World Health Organization 2003c). A few countries with extremely low HBV endemicity (Scandinavia, UK) continue to rely only on vaccination of high-risk adults.

Varicella vaccine

Live-attenuated varicella-zoster virus vaccine was developed in Japan in the 1970s, has been available in Japan and Korea and some European countries for many years, and is now widely available throughout the world. In 1995, it was licensed for primary prevention of varicella in healthy American children and adults. Clinical efficacy trials conducted with this vaccine, developed from the Oka strain of varicella virus, used varying vaccine potencies and formulations that were not necessarily comparable. For the formulation of vaccine most similar to the currently licensed product, the vaccine is approximately 70–90 percent effective in prevention of varicella disease and over 95 percent effective in providing protection against severe varicella disease (Centers for Disease Control and Prevention 1996; Seward 2001). Moreover, the 1–4 percent of children and adults who experience breakthrough infection annually develop mild disease with an average of ⩽50 lesions, compared with 300 lesions in typical varicella (Bernstein et al. 1993). Post-exposure vaccination, if given within 5 days of exposure, appears effective in preventing or reducing severity of varicella in household contacts of cases (Salzman and Garcia 1998; Centers for Disease Control and Prevention 1999e).

For primary prevention, varicella vaccine is given as a single dose for children age either 9 or 12 months (depending on vaccine manufacturer directions) to 12 years, and two doses separated by at least 1 month for older children and adults (Centers for Disease Control and Prevention 1996; Arvin 2002). Varicella vaccine may be given simultaneously with all other childhood vaccines, but should not be administered within 4 weeks of receipt of another live, viral vaccine. For adolescents and adults, serological screening of people without a history of varicella is likely to be cost-effective, because 70–91 percent of them will be immune to varicella.

Varicella vaccine induces a mild varicelliform rash and fever in 5–10 percent of vaccinees. However, these data are from uncontrolled clinical trials. In the only two placebo-controlled trials conducted among children, one trial reported no difference in rash or fever between vaccine and placebo recipients (Varis and Vesikari 1996). The second trial found no difference in fever and a small difference in rash: 3 percent of vaccine recipients developed noninjection site rashes compared with 2 percent of placebo recipients and 1 percent of vaccine recipients developed a generalized varicella-like rash compared with no placebo recipients (Weibel et al. 1984). Among adults, rash and fever may be more common, but there are no placebo-controlled trial data available. No unanticipated rare, serious adverse effects have occurred postlicensure (Wise et al. 2000). In the USA, varicella vaccine is contraindicated in people who are immunocompromised due to cell-mediated immunodeficiency (any malignant condition, including blood dyscrasias, leukemia, lymphomas of any type, or other malignant neoplasms affecting the bone marrow or lymphatic systems), in pregnant women and in anyone who has an anaphylactic reaction to varicella vaccine or any component, including gelatin. However, vaccine is available to any physician through an investigational drug protocol for use in patients who

have acute lymphoblastic leukemia (ALL) in remission who meet specified criteria) (Centers for Disease Control and Prevention 1996). Vaccination should be delayed for 5 months after the administration of immunoglobulin or blood products, because the response to vaccine administered within this interval is unknown. The risk of herpes zoster after varicella vaccination appears to be lower than after natural varicella infection.

Strategies for the use of varicella vaccine include universal vaccination of children at 12–18 months of age (with or without a catch-up program) and/or targeted vaccination for high-risk groups for severe disease or those in contact with such persons. The latter groups could include children with leukemia, as well as older susceptible children, adolescents and adults, healthcare workers, and family contacts of immunocompromised persons. Targeted programs, although they will provide protection to the individual or their close contacts, will have little impact on varicella epidemiology. Universal vaccination is intended to reduce disease transmission greatly and provide herd immunity to those who remain unvaccinated, and is the strategy adopted by the USA (Centers for Disease Control and Prevention 1996). Varicella vaccine is recommended for all children at 12–18 months of age and for all susceptible older children (with no prior history of varicella). All children who have not had natural varicella infection should be vaccinated at 11–12 years of age. Varicella vaccine is also recommended for susceptible healthcare workers and others in close contact with immunocompromised people who might experience severe varicella if infected, for susceptible adults at high risk for exposure or transmission, such as teachers, childcare center workers, and adults who live in households with children. It should be considered for any adolescents and adults with no prior history of varicella (Centers for Disease Control and Prevention 1999e).

In the USA where experience has been gained with the universal childhood program, varicella cases and hospitalizations and deaths had declined approximately 70 to 80 percent 6 years after implementation of the vaccination program (Seward et al. 2002; Davis et al. 2004; Nguyen et al. 2005). Although the greatest decline in incidence is among children 1–4 years, incidence has declined in all age groups including infants <12 months and adults indicating reduced disease transmission.

OTHER VIRAL VACCINES

Hepatitis A vaccine

Both killed and live-attenuated hepatitis A vaccines have been under development since the 1980s (D'Hondt 1992). Killed vaccines produced in cell culture, purified and inactivated with formalin first became commercially available in 1992. Inactivated hepatitis A vaccines are highly immunogenic (94–100 percent) and over 94 percent effective in preventing hepatitis A infection when given as a two- to three-dose series to children or a two-dose series to adults (Werzberger et al. 1992; Innis et al. 1994). The duration of protection is not known but, on the basis of high antibody levels induced by the vaccine, is expected to exceed 20 years (Van Damme et al. 1994). This vaccine may also provide protection post-exposure, and has been shown to be effective in controlling hepatitis A outbreaks in well-defined populations (Centers for Disease Control and Prevention 1999h). Development of live attenuated vaccines has been impeded by difficulty in achieving an appropriate balance of attenuation and protection, but one Chinese vaccine (H-2 strain) has been reported to be both immunogenic and effective, and has been licensed and used in China since 1992. This vaccine is reported to induce high rates of seroconversion and have high efficacy when given as a single dose subcutaneously to school-age children (Mao et al. 1997).

Licensed inactivated hepatitis A vaccine is given as a two- or three-dose series, with doses at 0 and 6–12 months (or 0, 1, and 6–12 months) to children ≥2 years of age, and as a two-dose series given 6–12 months apart to adults (Centers for Disease Control and Prevention 1999h). The known adverse reactions are limited to pain at the injection site. Rare serious adverse events (e.g. Guillain–Barré syndrome) have been reported following hepatitis A vaccination, but rates of such events have not exceeded those expected in the absence of vaccination. Hepatitis A vaccine may be given simultaneously with other childhood vaccines or vaccines for international travelers. The administration of passive immunoglobulin or maternal antibody interferes with response to the first dose of vaccine, but differences in final antibody response after the multidose series seem unlikely to be of clinical importance.

In developed countries, hepatitis A vaccine is recommended for people at high risk of infection, and is most widely used in those traveling to or working in countries where hepatitis A is highly endemic. In the USA, vaccine is recommended for native Americans and other groups that experience cyclic hepatitis A epidemics, for children age 2–18 years in states that historically had high incidence of hepatitis A, as well as for others at risk such as people with clotting disorders, homosexual men, users of illicit drugs, those at occupational risk, and people who have chronic liver disease (Centers for Disease Control and Prevention 1999h). Universal vaccination of children at age 2 years, with or without catch-up vaccination of susceptible older children, has resulted in marked decline in incidence in Native Americans and in states that previously had high disease incidence. Vaccination also may be considered for the prevention or control of community-wide outbreaks, although the data on effectiveness in this situation are limited. Ultimately, universal vaccination would be the best option to reduce the burden of disease in countries with substantial clinical disease burden such as the USA; however, this will probably require a less costly preparation and its incorporation into combination childhood vaccines.

Influenza virus vaccines

Influenza viruses continue to cause considerable mortality and morbidity throughout the world on an annual basis with the potential for much greater mortality and morbidity during pandemics. The 1918–19 pandemic is estimated to have caused more than 20 million deaths worldwide, more than 500 000 of which occurred in the USA. Recent estimates of influenza-associated deaths in the USA for the seasons 1990–91 through 1998–99 range from 36 000 underlying respiratory and circulatory deaths to 51 000 all-cause deaths (Thompson et al. 2003). The increase in influenza-associated deaths since the 1970s is believed to be partly due to the aging of the US population.

INACTIVATED INFLUENZA VACCINE

Influenza virus was first isolated from humans in 1933 and the first effective vaccine was administered in studies in Pennsylvania soon after that time. Since the 1940s, influenza virus has been grown in chick embryo allantoic sacs; this medium greatly increased yield of virus and promoted vaccine production. Because of the frequent antigenic changes in influenza viruses, the antigenic content of both types of vaccine is changed annually to optimize protection against the influenza type A and B strains expected to circulate during the following winter and spring. Influenza viruses of type A (H1N1 and H3N2) and B are selected according to their immunological match with circulating strains, grown in chicken embryos, inactivated with formalin and combined into vaccine. In the USA, inactivated vaccine is either subvirion vaccine, prepared by disrupting the lipid-containing membrane of the virus, or purified surface-antigen vaccine; whole-cell influenza vaccine is no longer available. The efficacy of vaccine is related to the degree of match between the vaccine and the circulating influenza viruses, as well as age and immunocompetence of the vaccine recipient. In recent years, effectiveness has been estimated to be 70–90 percent in adults <65 years, but lower in older adults (Centers for Disease Control and Prevention 2004; Bridges et al. 2000). Protection against serious complications, including hospitalization and death, is higher than against uncomplicated influenza (Nichol et al. 1994; Gross et al. 1995). Among healthy children, inactivated influenza vaccine efficacy in various studies has ranged from 77 to 91 percent for prevention of influenza respiratory illness and 66 percent for prevention of culture-confirmed influenza. Inactivated influenza vaccine has also been reported to reduce influenza-associated otitis media in children by approximately 30 percent (Centers for Disease Control and Prevention 2004; Neuzil et al. 2001). When major antigenic shifts occur, vaccine effectiveness may be substantially less in all age groups. Annual vaccination is necessary to ensure protection against the current strains.

For previously unvaccinated children 6 months to 8 years of age, two doses of vaccine (0.25 ml), given at 4-week intervals, are recommended (Centers for Disease Control and Prevention 2004). For other groups, only a single dose (0.5 ml) is necessary. About 3–5 percent of vaccinees experience local tenderness or fever after vaccination. The occurrence of Guillain–Barré syndrome within 6 weeks of influenza vaccination was observed in adults after the swine influenza vaccine campaign in 1976, but was not observed subsequently until 1990, when a case–control study suggested a slightly elevated risk in 18–64-year-olds, but not in those over 65 years of age (Schonberger et al. 1979; Chen et al. 1992). A similar small elevated risk was shown in adults age 18 years and older during the 1992–93 and 1993–94 influenza vaccine seasons (Lasky et al. 1998). Given the substantial benefits of influenza vaccination among the target populations, the risk of Guillain–Barré syndrome, if any, is greatly exceeded by the benefits. A previous anaphylactic reaction to egg protein is the only contraindication to influenza vaccination.

Vaccination is intended to reduce the complications and mortality due to influenza infection. Annual immunization is recommended for those at highest risk of these complications (Centers for Disease Control and Prevention 2004). In most developed countries, vaccination is recommended for people with certain chronic medical conditions, including cardiovascular and pulmonary disorders, asthma, other medical disorders such as metabolic disease (including diabetes mellitus), renal disease, hemoglobinopathies (including sickle-cell disease), and for people with immunosuppressive disorders or treatments, and children on long-term aspirin therapy. In many countries, annual vaccination is recommended for all adults aged ⩾65 years. Although immunogenicity and efficacy have not been established in all these high-risk groups, the risk from vaccine virus is extremely low because vaccine is inactivated. Healthcare workers and people caring for or living with those at high risk should also be vaccinated. In the USA, annual vaccination is also recommended for women who will be pregnant during the influenza season, and for adults 50–64 years. Because children aged 6–23 months are at substantially increased risk for influenza-related hospitalizations, vaccine policy setting groups in the USA (ACIP, American Academy of Pediatrics, American Academy of Family Physicians), recommend vaccination of all children in this age group (Centers for

Disease Control and Prevention 2004; Committee on Infectious Diseases 2003). Many countries have developed plans to prepare for pandemic influenza, which occurs every 10–40 years and can have devastating mortality. Such plans include the rapid production and availability of vaccine to ensure the vaccination either of people at highest risk or of the entire population.

LIVE-ATTENUATED INFLUENZA VACCINE

Cold-adapted live-attenuated influenza vaccines (LAIV) have been used in Russia since 1977 (Murphy 1993; Maassab et al. 1994). These vaccines incorporate influenza virus strains attenuated through growth at 25°C, but with reduced growth at 37°C. The genes for relevant circulating influenza strains can be incorporated into these vaccines by reassortment, and the vaccine is administered intranasally. In controled trials, these vaccines have similar efficacy to inactivated influenza vaccines in older children and adults (Belshe et al. 1998; Nichol et al. 1999; Treanor et al. 1999). In children, where the vaccine was studied during two influenza seasons, vaccine efficacy was also high (86 percent) in the season where the vaccine and circulating virus strains were not well matched (Belshe et al. 2000). In 2003, a LAIV was licensed in the USA and is currently approved for use among healthy persons age 5–49 years (Centers for Disease Control and Prevention 2004).

Japanese encephalitis vaccine

Three types of Japanese encephalitis (JE) vaccines have been developed and used to substantially reduce disease incidence in Asia where the disease is endemic. Inactivated Japanese encephalitis vaccine, currently available in Japan, Taiwan, and other developed countries, is a purified preparation of whole virus (Beijing-1 or Nakayama strain) grown in mouse brain and inactivated with formalin. When given as a three-dose series, the vaccine has 91 percent efficacy in adults (Hoke et al. 1988). Antibody persists for at least 2 years; the need for booster doses is uncertain. Primary immunization consists of three doses given at 0, 7, and 30 days; the third dose may be given at 14 days if the schedule does not permit the longer interval (Centers for Disease Control and Prevention 1993a). Vaccination schedules vary in different countries; some countries use a primary series of two doses 4 weeks apart followed by a booster dose after 1 year. The optimal interval for boosting is not defined, but some countries recommend booster doses every 3 years (Vaccines and Biologicals 2003). The dose for young children (1–3 years) is 0.5 ml, and that for older children and adults is 1.0 ml. No data are available on safety and immunogenicity in children <1 year of age. Adverse events include local reactions (20 percent) and minor systemic symptoms (10 percent). Generalized allergic reactions (angioedema, urticaria) may occur in 1–6 per 1 000 vaccinees; more rarely, anaphylaxis, respiratory distress, and hypotension have been reported. Rare neurological events such as fatal acute encephalitis have been reported. China also produces an inactivated vaccine (Beijing P-3 strain) grown in hamster kidney cell cultures, which has 85 percent efficacy for a primary series. This vaccine has been widely used in China, but is being replaced with the live-attenuated vaccine.

A live-attenuated vaccine (SA 14-14-2 strain), produced in primary hamster kidney cells, has been developed and widely distributed in China since 1989. Recent studies have confirmed the safety in 13 000 vaccinated children, and demonstrated 80 percent efficacy of one dose and 98 percent efficacy of two doses in children in China (Chambers et al. 1997). The cost of this vaccine (US$0.06 per dose) is substantially lower than that of the inactivated vaccine, and this vaccine is being investigated as a candidate for inclusion in the Expanded Program on Immunization in JE endemic countries. Developing a vaccine schedule compatible with the EPI childhood schedule, and assuring quality of manufacturing are two challenges for this goal.

JE vaccine is recommended for travelers or residents in areas where the disease is endemic (south and east Asia), who potentially will be exposed during the transmission season particularly in rural areas when traveling for 30 or more days (Centers for Disease Control and Prevention 1993a). JE vaccine is used routinely in many of these countries, but use should be expanded to all endemic countries. Assuring a sufficient supply of effective and inexpensive vaccine will be necessary to meet these disease control objectives (Vaccines and Biologicals 2003).

Rabies vaccine

The first attenuated and inactivated rabies vaccines were developed by Pasteur from desiccated infected rabbit brains. Subsequent vaccines were developed from virus harvested from the brains of rabbits, sheep, or goats, but caused neuroparalytic disease in about one per 2 000 recipients, due to residual myelin derivatives. Nerve tissue-derived vaccines continue to be locally produced and used in many developing countries. Vaccines developed from duck embryos reduced the risk of serious adverse events about tenfold (Hattwick 1974). However, in developed countries these vaccines have now been replaced by those grown in diploid human cell lines (World Health Organization 1992). Rabies virus is harvested from cell culture and inactivated with β-propiolactone. This vaccine (human diploid cell strain (HDCS)) is highly immunogenic when given as a multidose series, either alone (pre-exposure) or with human rabies immunoglobulin (HRIG) (postexposure). The vaccine schedule for pre-exposure prophylaxis is a three-dose series at weekly intervals. For people at high conti-

nuing risk of infection (e.g. veterinarians, travelers to endemic areas), testing for the presence of neutralizing antibody should be done at 2-year intervals and booster doses given if inadequate antibody is present. Alternatively, booster doses may be given at 2-year intervals without testing. Post-exposure prophylaxis includes a five-dose series: the first dose with HRIG, half infiltrated at the site of the bite and half given intramuscularly elsewhere, followed by additional vaccine doses 3, 7, 14, and 28 days later (Centers for Disease Control and Prevention 1999i). Although episodes of rabies have rarely followed the use of HDCS alone, there have been no reports of vaccine failure with HDCS given with HRIG (Devriendt et al. 1982; Centers for Disease Control and Prevention 1999i). The WHO strongly encourages that more potent and safe cell-derived vaccines should replace nerve tissue-derived vaccines (Vaccines and Biologicals 2003).

HDCS causes few adverse events. Local and mild systemic symptoms may occur in 5–40 percent of recipients. Type III hypersensitivity similar to serum sickness can occur with repeated doses. Although cases of neurological disease, such as Guillain–Barré syndrome, have been reported following HDCS, these are not conclusively linked to the vaccine. New vaccines under investigation include recombinant vaccines containing the surface glycoprotein produced in *E. coli*, mammalian or yeast cells, or vectored into vaccinia and canarypox viruses.

Smallpox (vaccinia) vaccine

Variola virus is the causative agent of smallpox. The mortality and morbidity caused by smallpox lead to development of the first vaccine to prevent human disease. In 1796, Edward Jenner demonstrated that material from a human cowpox lesion could be inoculated into the skin of another person to produce a similar infection and this person was later protected from inoculation with smallpox virus. Smallpox vaccine was initially administered by arm-to-arm inoculation. Advances in vaccine development occurred in the 1800s when growth of vaccinia virus on the flank of a calf provided an adequate and safer supply of vaccine material (Fenner et al. 1988; Henderson et al. 2004). However, the vaccine did not remain viable for more than 1 or 2 days at room temperature. Finally, a process for production of a stable freeze-dried vaccine was perfected in the late 1940s. Though Jenner is believed to have used cowpox virus in vaccination, vaccinia virus strains are neither cowpox nor variola and neutralizing antibodies induced by the vaccine are crossprotective for other orthopoxviruses, including monkeypox virus, cowpox virus, and variola virus (Henderson et al. 2004).

Many vaccinia virus strains were used in vaccine production. In the USA, the New York City Board of

Health strain was used exclusively. Other strains used globally included Lister, Temple of Heaven, Tashkent, Copenhagan, and Patwadanger. Attempts to produce less reactogenic vaccines (e.g. Rivers, MVA (modified vaccinia virus Ankara), CVI-78, and LC 16m8) were successful, but some resulted in lowered immunogenicity. The most satisfactory attenuated strain, the LC16m8 from Japan, did produce a satisfactory immune response in humans and had markedly lower rates of adverse reactions compared with other strains. However, the eradication of smallpox precluded testing this vaccine for efficacy (Henderson et al. 2004).

Smallpox vaccine is administered by intradermal inoculation most commonly using a bifurcated needle, though high pressure jet injectors were also used during the smallpox eradication effort. The vaccine is extremely stable even when stored at extremes of temperature. When the vaccine was being used in routine vaccination programs, it was recommended for healthy infants $\geqslant$12 months of age. Adverse reactions varied by vaccine strain and included severe reactions, including generalized vaccinia, eczema vaccinatum, progressive vaccinia, postvaccinial encephalitis, and vaccinial keratitis, and mild to moderate reactions, such as inadvertent inoculation, urticarial rashes, and Steven's Johnson syndrome (Lane et al. 1970; Centers for Disease Control and Prevention 2001a). Reported complications were more common among primary vaccinees and resulted in death in approximately one per million primary vaccinees.

Smallpox was a major cause of mortality worldwide with overall mortality rates of 20–30 percent. Variola major had case-fatality rates of approximately 30 percent and people who survived the infection were commonly left with residual facial pockmarks. Other serious sequelae included blindness and limb deformities. Variola minor produced less severe illness with case-fatality rates of 1 percent or less (Fenner et al. 1988). In the 1950s, when the disease had been eliminated in developed countries, 50 million cases a year were estimated to still occur globally resulting in 6 million deaths. By the 1960s, 15 million cases and 2 million deaths were estimated to occur per year. This stimulated efforts to eradicate the disease globally which were successful; the last naturally occurring case was in Somalia in 1977 and the World Health Assembly certified global eradication in 1980. Smallpox eradication is one of the greatest public health triumphs of the twentieth century.

After smallpox eradication, the vaccine was withdrawn from routine use globally and recommended only for selected persons at high risk for exposure (Centers for Disease Control 1980). In the USA, the vaccine was recommended for laboratory workers who directly handle cultures or animals contaminated or infected with non-highly attenuated vaccinia virus, recombinant vaccinia viruses derived from non-highly attenuated vaccinia strains, or other Orthopox viruses that infect humans (e.g. monkeypox virus, cowpox virus, vaccinia virus, and variola virus) (Centers for Disease Control and Prevention, 2001a). Vaccination could also be offered to healthcare workers who have contact with contaminated materials from non-highly attenuated vaccinia viruses. In 2002–2003, because of heightened concerns over the use of smallpox virus as a bioterrorism agent, the USA and some other countries reinstituted smallpox (vaccinia) vaccination for national and state teams of clinical and public health workers who were designated to respond to and care for smallpox cases if such cases were to occur (Centers for Disease Control and Prevention 2003c) and for military personnel. Through August 2003, approximately 450 000 military personnel and 37 000 clinical and public health workers had been vaccinated. Serious adverse events following vaccination have been very rare with no cases reported of progressive vaccinia, eczema vaccinatum, or transmission of vaccine virus in a healthcare setting. This may be due to the stringent screening procedures that were in place for this vaccination program among both vaccinees and their close contacts. Unexpected serious adverse events, previously described only in occasional case reports with the NYBOH vaccine strain, have included myo/pericarditis seen among both civilian and military vaccinees (Grabenstein and Winkenwerder 2003; Centers for Disease Control and Prevention 2003d; Cassimatis et al. 2004; Eckart et al. 2004).

New generation smallpox vaccines, grown in cell culture, have been developed. Several of these vaccines have produced major cutaneous reactions (takes) and evoked neutralizing antibody and cell-mediated immune responses in the vast majority of subjects with a reactogenicity profile similar to that of Dryvax (Weltzin et al. 2003; Monath et al. 2004; Greenberg et al. 2005). Other smallpox vaccines under development include more attenuated and replication-deficient vaccinia strains including modified vaccinia Ankara and NYVAC vaccinia viruses. These vaccines hold promise as safer vaccines against smallpox or against complications from vaccinia virus and may also have application for immunization of immunocompromised persons (Belyakov et al. 2003).

Yellow fever vaccine

Yellow fever (YF) vaccine, available since the 1930s, is the live-attenuated 17D strain of yellow fever virus. A single dose, given subcutaneously, is highly effective in inducing protection that lasts for 10 or more years; booster doses are recommended only at 10-year intervals (Centers for Disease Control and Prevention 2002c). YF vaccine causes local and limited systemic symptoms in 2–5 percent of recipients 5–10 days after vaccination. Serious reactions including encephalitis are rare; the risk is highest in children <9 months of age, and the vaccine is not recommended for children <9 months of age and contraindicated in those younger than 6 months. During recent years, serious vaccine-associated viscerotropic and neurologic adverse events have been reported globally and have resulted in deaths, primarily in the elderly (Barwick et al. 2003; Kitchener 2004; Yellow Fever Vaccine Safety Working Group 2004). Serious viscerotropic disease has been identified in 23 persons, with >60% case fatality, at an estimated rate of 3 per million vaccines. Serious neurologic disease cases, totaling 19 to present, have included encephalitis, encephalomyelitis, and Guillain Barre syndrome, with an estimated incidence of 4 per million vaccines. Both systemic and neurologic reactions are more likely after the first vaccine dose and do not appear due to mutation of the vaccine virus. Risk appears to be elevated in persons with prior thymectomy (Barwick et al. 2003). YF vaccine should not be administered to pregnant women; however, if a pregnant woman is traveling to an endemic area and cannot avoid potential exposure, YF vaccine may be given. YF vaccine is contraindicated in people with anaphylactic allergy to egg or who are immunocompromised. The response to YF vaccine can be inhibited by cholera vaccine; these vaccines should be given at least 3 weeks apart. Because cholera vaccine is rarely indicated, YF should be given first.

Vaccine is recommended for travelers 9 months of age and older going to areas where YF is endemic, and may be required for entry into such countries. Routine YF vaccination at 9 months of age is recommended in all endemic areas; vaccine may also be given in mass campaigns, which are often initiated by the occurrence of outbreaks. The incorporation of YF vaccine into the routine childhood immunization schedule at 9 months of age was initially recommended by the Expanded Program on Immunization in 1988, and its need reinforced by resurgence of yellow fever outbreaks in West Africa during the 1990s (Monath 2001). Through 2002, 26 of 44 endemic countries have implemented the recommendation, but coverage remains low in many of the highest-risk African countries (Global Programme for Vaccines and Immunization 2003).

VACCINES IN DEVELOPMENT

Rotavirus vaccines

Rotavirus is the most common cause of severe, dehydrating gastroenteritis in children throughout the world. Virtually every child becomes infected with rotavirus at least once in the first 5 years of life. Rotavirus has been estimated to cause 20 percent of all diarrhea deaths in children less than 5 years of age resulting in about 500 000 global deaths annually, most of them in developing countries. Even in developed countries, rotavirus infections cause significant morbidity and some mortality. In the USA, approximately 50 000 children are hospitalized with rotavirus gastroenteritis each year and there are 20–40 deaths due to this infection (Centers

for Disease Control and Prevention 1999a). Studies in developed countries have found incidence per 100 000 children ranging from 250 (Spain) to >1 000 (Ireland) (Cunliffe et al. 2002).

Rotavirus is a double-stranded RNA virus composed of three concentric shells, the outer capsid contains two structural proteins: VP7, the glycoprotein (G protein) and VP4, the protease-cleaved protein (P protein). These two proteins define the serotype of the virus and are considered critical to vaccine development because they are the target of neutralizing antibodies that are considered important for protection. The first natural infection with rotavirus results in a predominantly homotypic response to the virus; however, subsequent infections elicit a broader, heterotypic response. After a single natural infection, 40 percent of children are protected against any subsequent infection with any serotype, 75 percent are protected against severe rotavirus infection and 88 percent are protected against severe diarrhea (Velazquez et al. 1996).

Live-attenuated rotavirus vaccines have been developed from human rotaviruses, as well as from rotaviruses of other species (rhesus, bovine, and lamb). All rotavirus vaccines in development are live, orally administered vaccines that aim to mimic the protection acquired from naturally occurring rotavirus infection (Cunliffe et al. 2002). Vaccines based on animal viral strains are developed using a Jennerian approach enhanced with modern virological techniques. Animal rotaviruses are considered naturally attenuated for humans. Human rotaviruses recovered from children with acute rotavirus infection have been attenuated by passage in tissue culture and rotaviruses isolated from asymptomatic neonates are considered to be less virulent and have also been tested in clinical trials.

Taking advantage of the segmented genome of rotavirus, reassortants have been developed that retain most of the genome of the parent virus, but include one or both of two key surface glycoproteins, VP7 and VP4, of the human viruses. Multivalent vaccines were developed following the recognition that rotavirus disease is caused by four major serotypes (G1, G2, G3, G4, and P1a). Monovalent vaccines also appear to confer protection against other serotypes (Offit 2002).

In 1998, a tetravalent, rhesus-human reassortant rotavirus vaccine (RRV-TV) was licensed and recommended for routine childhood immunization in the United States (Centers for Disease Control and Prevention 1999a). However, within a year of use, the recommendations for vaccine use were withdrawn due to the risk of a rare but serious adverse event, intussusception, that occurred in approximately 1 in 10 000 infants vaccinated (Centers for Disease Control and Prevention 1999f; Kramarz et al. 2001; Murphy et al. 2001). WHO has strongly encouraged the rapid development of new and safe rotavirus vaccines (World Health Organization 2003b) and the Global Alliance for Vaccines and Immunization (GAVI) and The Vaccine Fund have supported a project to accelerate development of rotavirus vaccines for the developing world (McCarthy 2003).

In January 2005, a new vaccine for prevention of rotavirus infections was licensed in Mexico. This monovalent live-attenuated human rotavirus vaccine (G1) produced by GlaxoSmithKline (derived from strain 89–12 which was isolated from a rotavirus-infected child in Cincinnati, Ohio, USA) is administered to infants using a two-dose schedule six to ten weeks apart. The first dose is administered between 6 and 14 weeks of age and the second dose between 14 and 24 weeks of age. Vaccine efficacy data from Finland and Latin America show 70–73 percent protection against rotavirus gastroenteritis, 85–86 percent protection against severe rotavirus gastroenteritis and 93 percent protection against rotavirus illness requiring hospitalization (Bernstein et al. 2002, De Vos et al. 2004, Vesikari et al, 2004). Vaccine efficacy was observed against severe rotavirus gastroenteritis caused by G1 and non-G1 types including the emerging G9 type in Latin America. Safety data available on 5024 immunized infants was reassuring with no increases in any solicited symptoms (including fever, vomiting, diarrhea) compared with placebo, however, the sample size from the combined trials was not intended to draw conclusions about the risk for intussusception which was 0.05 percent in the vaccine group and 0.08 percent in the placebo group (De Vos et al. 2004). The other licensed rotavirus vaccine is a lamb rotavirus vaccine, which is available for use in China, however there are few data available on efficacy and safety of this vaccine.

Several other rotavirus vaccines are currently in development. A pentavalent vaccine based on a bovine rotavirus strain (WC-3) reassorted with the common *VP7* and *VP4* genes of human rotaviruses (G1, G2, G3, G4, and PIa) has been well tolerated in phase I and phase II studies (World Health Organization 2003b). Various bovine reassortant vaccines have been studied as three-dose series in infants; a monovalent WC3 reassortant vaccine was 64–100 percent effective and a quadrivalent WC3 reassortant vaccine was 67 percent protective against all rotavirus disease with essentially complete protection against more serious disease (Clark et al. 1996). This protection is similar to that afforded by RRV-TV, which, when given during infancy in trials in the USA, Finland, and Venezuela, had demonstrated 49–68 percent efficacy against any rotavirus diarrhea and 69–91 percent efficacy against severe diarrhea (Rennels et al. 1996; Joensuu et al. 1997; Perez-Schael et al. 1997). The bovine pentavalent vaccine is currently undergoing large-scale safety trials to examine risks for intussusception, the rare serious adverse event of primary concern. Bovine rotaviruses do not replicate well in the infant small intestine and have lower first dose side-effects than the RRV-TV vaccine. Other vaccine candidates under development include human neonatal RV strains and other human-bovine reassortant vaccines.

Additional approaches to the development of rotavirus vaccines include DNA vaccination and subunit vaccines (Barnes et al. 1997; Cunliffe et al. 2002; World Health Organization 2003b).

Other viral vaccines

Vaccines for prevention or treatment of human papillomavirus (HPV) infections, herpes simplex virus infections (types 1 and 2), and cytomegalovirus (CMV) are in various stages of development and testing. An Institute of Medicine committee to assess vaccine needs for the twenty-first century placed two viral vaccines in its highest priority category (cost savings and QALYs) for vaccine development in the USA: CMV vaccine administration for 12 year olds and influenza virus vaccine administered to the general population and four viral vaccines in the second priority category for vaccine development (costs <$10 000 per QALY saved): hepatitis C virus vaccine for infants, herpes simplex virus vaccine for 12 year olds, HPV vaccine for 12 year olds and RSV vaccine for infants and 12-year-old females (Institute of Medicine 2000). Among these, HPV and HSV are in the late stages of development and with stage III clinical efficacy trials already conducted.

HUMAN PAPILLOMAVIRUS

HPV infection is the most common sexually transmitted disease; the spectrum of disease caused by this virus ranges from benign anogenital warts to cervical and anal cancer. Cancer of the uterine cervix is the third most common cancer in women. Worldwide, approximately 450 000 new cases are diagnosed each year with a 50 percent mortality rate. More than 100 types of HPV have been identified, approximately 30 of these infecting the anogenital region and about 15 of these types causing almost all cervical cancer. HPV-16 accounts for 50 percent of cases of cervical cancer. Thus effective vaccines to prevent and/or treat HPV infection would have enormous global public health impact.

Prophylactic vaccines are designed to prevent infection; the most common type of prophylactic vaccine is made up of viruslike particles (late structural proteins that make up the viral capsid) which are easily synthesized. Animal studies have provided convincing evidence that neutralizing antibodies can block new infection. A number of prophylactic HPV vaccines have been developed and are currently being tested in phase II and phase III trials, including monovalent HPV-16 and HPV-11 vaccines, multivalent HPV-16 and HPV-18 vaccine and a quadrivalent vaccine against types 6, 11, 16, and 18. Titers achieved following vaccination have frequently been 50 times higher than the titers seen in natural infection (Harro et al. 2001; Berry and Palefsky 2003; Schiffman and Castle 2003; Galloway 2003; Kahn and Bernstein 2003). A large placebo-controlled trial of a HPV-16 L1 VLP vaccine with aluminum hydroxyphosphate sulfate adjuvant administered as three doses at 0, 2, and 6 months in >2 000 young adult HPV-16 seronegative women followed for a median duration of 17.5 months demonstrated 100 percent efficacy for prevention of persistent HPV infection (Koutsky et al. 2002). All nine cases of HPV-related cervical intraepithelial neoplasia occurred among the placebo recipients. The authors concluded that immunizing HPV-16-negative women may eventually reduce the incidence of cervical cancer. Large phase III trials of vaccines targeted against multiple oncogenic types are under way.

Therapeutic vaccines are designed to eradicate or reduce infected calls and are therefore aimed at stimulating cytotoxic T lymphocytes and are directed against early proteins (E6 and E7) which are thought to be responsible for the oncogenic potential of HPV. HPV theraupeutic vaccines have been tested in phase I and phase II trials against cervical cancer and anal dysplasia and include subunit, recombinant vaccinia virus, recombinant fusion protein, and plasmid DNA vaccines (Berry and Palefsky 2003; Stanley 2003).

HERPES SIMPLEX VIRUS

The herpes simplex virus has two biologically distinct serotypes, HSV-1 and HSV-2. HSV-2 infection is acquired either by sexual contact causing herpes genitalis (300 000 new infections per year in the USA) or may be vertically transmitted from a maternal genital infection to a newborn resulting in severe neurological sequelae and death (Morrison 2002; Schleiss 2003; Koelle and Corey 2003; Cunningham and Mikloska 2001). Vaccines to protect against or modify established genital herpes infections have been under development for decades. Many types of vaccines have been evaluated in clinical trials of immunogenicity and prophylactic and therapeutic efficacy (Morrison 2002; Koelle and Corey 2003). Two similar subunit vaccines prepared from recombinant glycoproteins with different adjuvants have completed phase III trials using a three-dose schedule at 0, 1, and 6 months. The HSV-2 glycoprotein B and D subunit vaccine combined with MF59 adjuvant was immunogenic, but not effective in preventing HSV-2 infections (Corey et al. 1999). In contrast, a glycoprotein D-subunit vaccine with alum and MPL adjuvant was 73–74 percent effective in prevention of HSV-2 infections among women who were seronegative for both HSV-1 and HSV-2. The vaccine was not efficacious in women who were seropositive for HSV-1 and seronegative for HSV-2 prior to the study or in men (Stanberry et al. 2002). A prophylactic plasmid vaccine using the gene for gD of HSV-2 has completed phase I studies. Other prophylactic and therapeutic HSV-2 vaccines are in various stages of development and preclinical and clinical testing. Several therapeutic vaccines (plasmid, subunit,

and live replication-deficient virus (DISC)) have completed phase I and phase II trials (Koelle and Corey 2003; Morrison 2002).

CYTOMEGALOVIRUS

Cytomegalovirus (CMV) is the most important cause of congenital viral infection, affecting 0.5–1.5 percent of births in the USA. Though most babies with congenital CMV infection have no abnormalities detected at or after birth, 15–25 percent of affected births have abnormalities with sensorineural hearing loss, mental retardation, cerebral palsy, or impaired vision detected at birth or on follow up (Pass and Burke 2002). A vaccine to prevent congenital CMV infection has been designated a top priority for development in the USA by the Institute of Medicine of the National Academy of Sciences (Institute of Medicine 2000). For vaccine development, the major barrier has been the knowledge that naturally acquired infection does not prevent reinfection with a new strain of CMV and that immunity acquired before conception does not always prevent transmission to the infant. These and other issues relevant to development of an effective CMV vaccine have been reviewed (Plotkin 2004b).

An effective vaccine will need to stimulate high levels of neutralizing antibody and cytotoxic lymphocytes and would ideally also stimulate mucosal antibodies (Plotkin 2004b). Vaccines tested to date in phase 1 or phase 2 trials or preclinical studies include various formulations of a live-attenuated vaccine (Towne strain) (phase 1 and phase 2 trials), a recombinant glycoprotein B subunit vaccine (phase 1 and phase 2 trials), chimeric live virus vaccine (Towne and Toledo strains, phase 1 trials), a canarypox vector vaccine with recombinant gB or pp65 (phase 1 trials) and DNA vaccines (preclinical studies) (Pass and Burke 2002; Temperton et al. 2003; Plotkin 2002).

VZV zoster vaccine for prevention of herpes zoster and its complications

Herpes zoster and its complications including postherpetic neuralgia cause a significant public health burden among the aging population in the USA and other developed countries. The incidence of herpes zoster increases with age and it is estimated that about 20 percent of people will develop herpes zoster during their lifetime, resulting in about 600 000 cases of herpes zoster in the USA each year (Hope-Simpson 1965; Schmader 2001). Declines in VZV-specific cell-mediated immunity are associated with increased risk and severity of herpes zoster (Arvin 1996; Oxman 1995). Early studies on administration of a live VZV vaccine (with higher titers than the licensed varicella vaccine) to older adults 55+ have shown that vaccinated persons experience increased VZV-specific cell-mediated immunity responses to levels typical of those observed in younger persons, in whom the incidence and severity of herpes zoster are lower (Levin 2001). A booster dose of VZV vaccine administered ⩾5 years after the first dose resulted in boosting in VZV-specific cell-mediated immunity (Levin et al. 2003). A large (ca. 37 000) placebo-controlled clinical trial has been conducted in the USA to test whether a VZV 'zoster' vaccine in persons ⩾60 years will prevent or reduce the risk or severity of herpes zoster and its complications. Results of this trial are expected in late 2005. This may lead to a future zoster vaccine to reduce the incidence of herpes zoster or reduce/attenuate the severity of post-herpetic neuralgia and other herpes zoster complications.

SOURCES OF INFORMATION ON VACCINES

Important sources for information on vaccines include the following:

World Health Organization. Provides extensive information on vaccines, vaccine preventable diseases, and global and national statistics on immunization programs and vaccine preventable diseases. Additional information about the World Health Organization and international vaccine programs may be found at www.who.int/vaccines/. Training materials may be found at www.who.int/vaccines-diseases/epitraining.

United Nations Children's Fund. Provides information about state of the world's children and women of child-bearing age, including statistics on immunization coverage and progress of initiatives to eliminate neonatal tetanus and measles, and eradicate polio. Websites include www.unicef.org/ and www.childinfo.org.

Global Alliance for Vaccines and Immunization. Information on the Global Alliance for Vaccines and Immunization may be found at the website www.vaccinealliance.org.

National Health Service, UK. Provides information about immunization recommendations for the UK (www.immunisation.nhs.uk or www.immunisation.org.uk).

National Immunization Program, Centers for Disease Control and Prevention, Atlanta, GA 30333, USA. Extensive resources provide specific information on immunization and vaccine preventable diseases (www.cdc.gov/nip/).

The Report of the Committee on Infectious Diseases of the American Academy of Pediatrics (Red Book). The full report containing recommendations on all licensed vaccines is usually updated every 3 years. The most recent *Red Book* was published in 2003. It can be ordered from the American Academy of Pediatrics, 141 Northwest Point Blvd., PO Box 927, Elk Grove Village, IL 60009-0927, USA or from the AAP website (www.aap.org).

Morbidity and Mortality Weekly Report. This report is published weekly by the Centers for Disease Control and Prevention (CDC) and contains vaccine recommendations, reports of specific disease activity, policy statements, and regular and special recommendations of the ACIP. The MMWR is available online at www.cdc.gov/mmwr/ or www.cdc.gov/nip/acip.

Allied Vaccine Group. A partnership of six independent websites providing science-based, reliable information about immunization (www.vaccines.org).

Immunization Action Coalition. The Immunization Action Coalition promotes physician, community, and family awareness of and responsibility for appropriate immunization of all children and adults against all vaccine-preventable diseases. This US-based site has a wealth of education materials (www.immunize.org).

Official Package Circular. Manufacturers provide product-specific information for each vaccine. Some of these are reproduced in their entirety in the *Physicians' Desk Reference* (PDR) and are dated.

Control of Communicable Diseases in Man. The American Public Health Association publishes a manual at approximately 5-year intervals. The 18th edition (2004) is currently available. The manual contains valuable information concerning infectious diseases; their occurrence worldwide; immunization, diagnostic, and therapeutic information; and up-to-date recommendations on isolation and other control measures for each disease presented. It can be ordered from the American Public Health Association, 800 St. NW, Washington, DC 20001, USA.

REFERENCES

Albrecht, P., Ennis, F.A., et al. 1977. Persistence of maternal antibody in infants beyond 12 months: mechanism of measles vaccine failure. *J Pediatr*, **91**, 715–18.

Amara, R.R., Villinger, F., et al. 2001. Control of a mucosal challenge and prevention of AIDS by a multiprotein DNA/mva vaccine. *Science*, **292**, 69–74.

Anderson, R.M. and May, R.M. 1990. Immunization and herd immunity. *Lancet*, **335**, 641–5.

Annunziato, D., Kaplan, M.H., et al. 1982. Atypical measles syndrome: pathologic and serologic findings. *Pediatrics*, **70**, 203–9.

Arai, K., Lee, F., et al. 1990. Cytokines: coordinators of immune and inflammatory responses. *Annu Rev Biochem*, **59**, 783–836.

Arvin, A.M. 1996. Varicella-zoster virus: overview and clinical manifestations. *Semin Dermatol*, **15**, 4–7.

Arvin, A.M. 2002. Varlirix (GlaxoSmithKline). *Curr Opin Investig Drugs*, **3**, 996–9.

Baker, P.J. 1975. Homeostatic control of antibody responses. A model based on the recognition of cell-associated antibody by regulatory T-cells. *Transplant Rev*, **26**, 3–20.

Barnes, G.L., Lund, J.S., et al. 1997. Phase 1 trial of a candidate rotavirus vaccine (RV3) derived from a human neonate. *J Paediatr Child Health*, **33**, 300–4.

Barundun, S. and Morell, A. 1981. Adverse reactions to immunoglobulin preparations. In: Nydegger, U.E. (ed.), *Immunotherapy. A guide to immunoglobulin prophylaxis and therapy*. New York: Academic Press, 223–7.

Barwick, R.S., Marfin, A.A. and Cetron, M.S. 2003. Yellow fever vaccine associated disease. In: Scheld, W.M., Murray, B.E. and Hughes, J.M. (eds), *Emerging infections*, 6th edn. Washington, DC: ASM Press, 25–34.

Belshe, R.B., Mendelman, P.M., et al. 1998. The efficacy of live attenuated, cold adapted, trivalent intranasal influenzavirus vaccine in children. *N Engl J Med*, **338**, 1405–12.

Belshe, R.B., Gruber, W.C., et al. 2000. Efficacy of vaccination with live attenuated, cold-adapted, trivalent, intranasal influenza virus vaccine against a variant (A/Sydney) not contained in the vaccine. *J Pediatr*, **136**, 168–75.

Belyakov, I.M., Earl, P., et al. 2003. Shared modes of protection against poxvirus infection by attenuated and conventional smallpox vaccine viruses. *Proc Natl Acad Sci USA*, **100**, 9458–63.

Bernstein, H.H., Rothstein, E.P., et al. 1993. Clinical survey of natural varicella compared with breakthrough varicella after immunization with live attenuated Oka/Merck varicella vaccine. *Pediatrics*, **92**, 833–7.

Bernstein, D.I., Sack, D.A., et al. 2002. Second year follow-up evaluation of live attenuated human rotavirus vaccine 89-12 in healthy infants. *J Infect Dis* **186**, 1487–9.

Berry, J.M. and Palefsky, J.M. 2003. A review of human papillomavirus vaccines: from basic science to clinical trials. *Front Biosci*, **8**, S333–345.

Bridges, C.B., Thompson, W.W., et al. 2000. Effectiveness and cost–benefit of influenza vaccination of healthy working adults: a randomized controlled trial. *J Am Med Assoc*, **284**, 1655–63.

Brisson, M. and Edmunds, W.J. 2002. The cost-effectiveness of varicella vaccination in Canada. *Vaccine*, **20**, 1113–25.

Brown, F. 1988. Use of peptide vaccines for immunization against foot and mouth disease. *Vaccine*, **6**, 180–2.

Butts, C., Zubkoff, I., et al. 1998. DNA immunization of infants: potential and limitations. *Vaccine*, **16**, 1444–9.

Castillo-Solórzano, C., Carrasco, P., et al. 2003. New horizons in the control of rubella and prevention of congenital rubella syndrome in the Americas. *J Infect Dis*, **187**, Suppl. 1, S146–52.

Centers for Disease Control. 1980. Smallpox vaccine. *Morbid Mortal Wkly Rep* **29**, 417–20.

Centers for Disease Control. 1982, Recommendation of the Immunization Practices Advisory Committee (ACIP). Poliomyelitis prevention. *Morbid Mortal Wkly Rep*, **31**, 22–31.

Centers for Disease Control. 1987. Recommendation of the Immunization Practices Advisory Committee (ACIP). Poliomyelitis prevention: enhanced potency inactivated poliomyelitis vaccine – supplementary statement. *Morbid Mortal Wkly Rep*, **36**, 795–8.

Centers for Disease Control. 1988. National Childhood Vaccine Injury Act: requirements for permanent vaccination records and for reporting of selected events after vaccination. *Morbid Mortal Wkly Rep*, **37**, 197–200.

Centers for Disease Control. 1989. Rubella vaccination during pregnancy: United States, 1971–88. *Morbid Mortal Wkly Rep*, **38**, 289–93.

Centers for Disease Control and Prevention. 1991. Recommendations of the Immunization Practices Advisory Committee. Hepatitis B virus: a comprehensive strategy for eliminating transmission in the United States through universal childhood vaccination. *Morbid Mortal Wkly Rep*, **40** (RR-13), 1–25.

Centers for Disease Control and Prevention. 1993a. Recommendations of the Immunization Practices Advisory Committee (ACIP). Inactivated Japanese encephalitis virus vaccine. *Morbid Mortal Wkly Rep*, **42** (RR-1), 1–15.

Centers for Disease Control and Prevention. 1993b. Recommendations of the Advisory Committee on Immunization Practices (ACIP). Use of vaccines and immune globulins in persons with altered immunocompetence. *Morbid Mortal Wkly Rep*, **42** (RR-4), 1–18.

Centers for Disease Control and Prevention. 1993c. Recommendations of the International Task Force for Disease Eradication. *Morbid Mortal Wkly Rep*, **42** (RR-16), 1–38.

Centers for Disease Control and Prevention. 1994. Outbreak of hepatitis C associated with intravenous immunoglobulin administration: United States, October 1993–June 1994. *Morbid Mortal Wkly Rep*, **43**, 505–9.

Centers for Disease Control and Prevention. 1996. Varicella prevention. Recommendations of the Advisory Committee on Immunization Practices. *Morbid Mortal Wkly Rep*, **45** (RR-11), 1–36.

Centers for Disease Control and Prevention. 1997. Poliomyelitis prevention in the United States: introduction of a sequential schedule of inactivated poliovirus vaccine (IPV) followed by oral poliovirus vaccine (OPV). *Morbid Mortal Wkly Rep*, **46** (RR-2), 1–26.

Centers for Disease Control and Prevention. 1998. Measles, mumps and rubella vaccine use and strategies for elimination of measles, rubella, and congenital rubella syndrome and control of mumps: recommendations of the Advisory Committee on Immunization Practices (ACIP). *Morbid Mortal Wkly Rep*, **47** (RR-8), 1–57.

Centers for Disease Control and Prevention. 1999a. Rotavirus vaccine for prevention of rotavirus gastroenteritis in children. *Morbid Mortal Wkly Rep*, **48** (RR-2), 1–20.

Centers for Disease Control and Prevention. 1999b. Ten great public health achievements – United States, 1990–1998. *Morbid Mortal Wkly Rep*, **48**, 241–3.

Centers for Disease Control and Prevention. 1999c. Impact of vaccines universally recommended for children – United States, 1900–1998. *Morbid Mortal Wkly Rep*, **48**, 243–8.

Centers for Disease Control and Prevention. 1999d. Combination vaccines for childhood immunization: recommendations of the Advisory Committee on Immunization Practices (ACIP), the American Academy of Pediatrics (AAP) and the American Academy of Family Physicians (AAFP). *Morbid Mortal Rec Rep*, **48** (RR-5), 1–15.

Centers for Disease Control and Prevention. 1999e. Prevention and control of varicella: updated recommendations of the Advisory Committee on Immunization Practices (ACIP). *Morbid Mortal Rec Rep*, **48** (RR-6), 1–6.

Centers for Disease Control and Prevention. 1999f. Withdrawal of rotavirus vaccine recommendation. *Morbid Mortal Mortal Wkly Rep*, **48**, 1007.

Centers for Disease Control and Prevention. 1999g. Global disease elimination and eradication as public health strategies. *Morbid Mortal Mortal Wkly Rep*, **48** Suppl., 1–208.

Centers for Disease Control and Prevention. 1999h. Prevention of Hepatitis A through active or passive immunization. Recommendations of the Advisory Committee on Immunization Practices. *Morbid Mortal Wkly Rep*, **48** (RR-12), 1–35.

Centers for Disease Control and Prevention. 1999i. Human rabies prevention: United States, 1999: recommendations of the Advisory Committee on Immunization Practices (ACIP). *Morbid Mortal Wkly Rep*, **48** (RR-1), 1–21.

Centers for Disease Control and Prevention. 2000. Poliomyelitis prevention in the United States: updated recommendations of the Advisory Committee on Immunization Practices (ACIP). *Morbid Mortal Rec Rep*, **49** (RR-5), 1–22.

Centers for Disease Control and Prevention. 2001a. Vaccinia (smallpox) vaccine. Recommendations of the Advisory Committee on Immunization Practices (ACIP), 2001. *Morbid Mortal Rec Rep*, **50** (RR-10), 1–26.

Centers for Disease Control and Prevention. 2001b. Notice to readers: revised ACIP Recommendation for avoiding pregnancy after receiving a rubella-containing vaccine. *Morbid Mortal Wkly Reports* **50**, 1117.

Centers for Disease Control and Prevention. 2002a. General recommendations on immunization. Recommendations of the Advisory Committee on Immunization Practices (ACIP) and the American Academy of Family Physicians (AAFP). *Morbid Mortal Rec Rep*, **51** (RR-2), 1–36.

Centers for Disease Control and Prevention. 2002b. Measles – United States, 2000. *Morbid Mortal Wkly Rep*, **51**, 120–3.

Centers for Disease Control and Prevention. 2002c. Yellow fever vaccine: recommendations of the Advisory Committee on Immunization Practices (ACIP). *Morbid Mortal Wkly Rep*, **51** (RR-17), 1–13.

Centers for Disease Control and Prevention. 2003a. Recommended adult immunization schedule – United States, 2003–2004. *Morbid Mortal Wkly Rep*, **52**, 965–9.

Centers for Disease Control and Prevention. 2003b. *The yellow book. Health information for international travel, 2003–2004.* Washington, DC: US Government Printing Office. Also available online at http://www.cdc.gov/travel/yb/index.htm.

Centers for Disease Control and Prevention. 2003c. Recommendations for using smallpox vaccine in a pre-event vaccination program. Supplemental recommendations of the Advisory Committee on Immunization Practices (ACIP) and the Healthcare Infection Control Practices Advisory Committee (HICPAC). *Morbid Mortal Wkly Rep*, **52** (RR-07), 1–16.

Centers for Disease Control and Prevention. 2003d. Update: adverse events following civilian smallpox vaccination – United States, 2003. *Morbid Mortal Wkly Rep* **52** (34), 819–20.

Centers for Disease Control and Prevention. 2004. Prevention and control of influenza. Recommendations of the Advisory Committee on Immunization Practices (ACIP). *Morbid Mortal Rec Rep*, **53** (RR-06), 1–39.

Centers for Disease Control and Prevention. 2005a. Recommended Childhood and Adolescent Immunization Schedule – United States, 2005. *Morbid Mortal Rec Rep*, **53** (51/52), Q1–3.

Centers for Disease Control and Prevention. 2005b. Progress toward poliomyelitis eradication – Poliomyelitis outbreak in Sudan, 2004. *Morbid Mortal Wkly Rep*, **54**, 97–99.

Chambers, T.J., Tsai, T.F., et al. 1997. Vaccine development against dengue and Japanese encephalitis: report of a World Health Organization meeting. *Vaccine*, **15**, 1494–502.

Chang, M.H., Cen, C.J., et al. 2003. Universal hepatitis B vaccination in Taiwan and the incidence of hepatocellular carcinoma in children. *N Engl J Med*, **336**, 1855–9.

Cheek, J.E., Baron, R., et al. 1995. Mumps outbreak in a highly vaccinated school population. *Arch Pediatr Adolesc Med*, **149**, 774–8.

Chen, R., Kent, J., et al. 1992. Investigation of a possible association between influenza vaccination and Guillain-Barré syndrome in the United States, 1990–1991. *Post Market Surveill*, **6**, 5–6, abstract.

Chen, R.T., Rastogi, S.C., et al. 1994. The vaccine adverse events reporting system (VAERS). *Vaccine*, **12**, 542–50.

Claman, H.N. 1992. The biology of the immune response. *J Am Med Assoc*, **268**, 2790–6.

Clark, H.F., Offit, P.A., et al. 1996. The development of multivalent bovine rotavirus (strain WC3) reassortant vaccine for infants. *J Infect Dis*, **174**, Suppl. 1, S73–80.

Cohn, E.J., Strong, L.E., et al. 1946. Preparation and properties of serum and plasma proteins. IV. A system for the separation into fractions of protein and lipoprotein components of the biological tissues and fluids. *J Am Chem Soc*, **68**, 459–75.

Committee on Infectious Diseases and Committee on Fetus and Newborn, American Academy of Pediatrics. 1998. Prevention of respiratory syncytial virus infections: indications for the use of Palivizumab and update on the use of RSV-IG. *Pediatrics*, **102**, 1211–16.

Committee on Infectious Diseases, American Academy of Pediatrics. 2003. *Report of the Committee on Infectious Diseases*, 26th edn. Elk Grove Village, IL: American Academy of Pediatrics.

Corey, L., Langenberg, A.G., et al. 1999. Two double-blind placebo-controlled trials of a vaccine containing recombinant gD2 and gB2 antigens in MF59 adjuvant for the prevention of genital HSV-2 infection. *J Am Med Assoc*, **282**, 331–40.

Cunliffe, N.A., Bresee, J.S. and Hart, C.A. 2002. Rotavirus vaccines: development, current issues and future prospects. *J Infect*, **45**, 1, 1–9.

Cunningham, A.L. and Mikloska, Z. 2001. The Holy Grail: immune control of human herpes simplex virus infection and disease. *Herpes*, **8**, Suppl. 1, 6A–10A.

Cuthbertson, B., Perry, R.J., et al. 1987. The viral safety of intravenous immunoglobulin. *J Infect*, **15**, 125–33.

Dalgleish, A.C. and Kennedy, R.C. 1988. Anti-idiotype antibodies as immunogens: idiotype-based vaccines. *Vaccine*, **6**, 215–20.

Davis, M.M., Patel, M.S. and Gebremariam, A. 2004. Decline in varicella-related hospitalizations and expenditures for children and adults after introduction of varicella vaccine in the United States. *Pediatrics*, **114**, 786–92.

Dayan, G.H., Zimmerman, L., et al. 2003. Investigation of a rubella outbreak in Kyrgyzstan in 2001: implications for an integrated approach to measles elimination and prevention of congenital rubella syndrome. *J Infect Dis*, **187**, Suppl. 1, S235–40.

de Quadros, C., Olive, J.M., et al. 2003. Progress toward measles elimination in the Americas. *J Infect Dis*, **187**, Suppl. 1, S102–10.

De Vos B., Vesikari, T. et al. 2004. A rotavirus vaccine for prophylaxis of infants against rotavirus gastroenteritis. *Pediatr Infect Dis J*, **158**, 1253–60.

Devriendt, J., Staroukine, M., et al. 1982. Fatal encephalitis apparently due to rabies occurrence after treatment with human diploid cell vaccine but not rabies immune globulin. *J Am Med Assoc*, **248**, 2304–6.

D'Hondt, E. 1992. Possible approaches to develop vaccines against hepatitis A. *Vaccine*, **10**, Suppl. 1, S48–52.

Dobson, S., Schiefle, D. and Bell, A. 1995. Assessment of a universal, school based hepatitis B vaccination program. *J Am Med Assoc*, **274**, 1209–13.

Dourado, I., Cunha, S., et al. 2000. Outbreak of aseptic meningitis associated with mass vaccination with a Urabe-containing measles-mumps-rubella vaccine. *Am J Epidemiol*, **151**, 524–30.

Ellis, R.W. 2004. New technologies for making vaccines. In: Plotkin, S. and Orenstein, W.A. (eds), *Vaccines*, 4th edn. Philadelphia: W.B. Saunders, 1177–98.

Enders, J.F. and Peebles, T.C. 1954. Propagation in tissue cultures of cytopathogenic agents from patients with measles. *Proc Soc Exp Biol Med*, **86**, 277–86.

Enders, J.F., Weller, T.H. and Robbins, F.C. 1949. Cultivation of the Lansing strain of poliomyelitis virus in cultures of various human embryonic tissues. *Science*, **109**, 85–7.

Esteves, K. 1988. Safety of oral poliomyelitis vaccine: results of a WHO enquiry. *Bull WHO*, **66**, 739–46.

Fenner, F., Henderson, D.A., et al. 1988. *Smallpox and its eradication*. Geneva: World Health Organization. Available at www.who.int/emc/diseases/smallpox/Smallpoxeradication.html.

Finlayson, J.S. 2003. Passive immunization. In: Long, S.S. and Pickering, L.K. (eds), *Pediatric infectious diseases*, 2nd edn. Philadelphia, PA: Churchill Livingston, 37–44.

Foege, W.H. 1971. Measles vaccination in Africa. *Proceedings of the International Conference on the Application of Vaccines against Viral, Rickettsial and Bacterial Diseases in Man*. PAHO scientific publication 226. Washington, DC: Pan American Health Organization, 207–12.

Fox, J.P., Elveback, L., et al. 1972. Herd immunity: basic concept and relevance to public health immunization practices. *Am J Epidemiol*, **94**, 179–89.

Francis, T., Napier, J.A., et al. 1957. *Evaluation of the 1954 field trial of poliomyelitis vaccine. Final report.* Ann Arbor, MI: Department of Epidemiology, School of Public Health, University of Michigan.

Frey, T.K., Abernathy, E.S., et al. 1998. Molecular analysis of rubella virus epidemiology across three continents, North America, Europe and Asia, 1961–1997. *J Infect Dis*, **178**, 642–50.

Fynan, E.F., Webster, R.G., et al. 1995. DNA vaccines: a novel approach to immunization. *Int J Immunopharmacol*, **17**, 79–83.

Galazka, A.M. 1994. Achievements, problems and perspectives of the expanded program on immunization. *Int J Med Microbiol*, **281**, 353–64.

Galloway, D.A. 2003. Papillomavirus vaccines in clinical trials. *Lancet Infect Dis*, **3**, 8, 469–75.

Global Programme for Vaccines and Immunization. 1998. *Programme report*, 1997, 98.01. Geneva: World Health Organization.

Global Programme for Vaccines and Immunization. 2003. *Vaccines and biologicals*, WHO/V&B/03.20. Geneva: World Health Organization.

Grabenstein, J.D. and Winkenwerder, W. Jr. 2003. US military smallpox vaccination program experience. *J Am Med Assoc*, **289**, 24, 3278–82.

Greenberg, R.N., Kennedy, J.S., et al. 2005. Safety and immunogenicity of new cell-cultured smallpox vaccine compared with calf-lymph derived vaccine: a blind, single-centre randomised controlled trial. *Lancet*, **365**, 398–409.

Gregg, N.A. 1941. Congenital cataract following german measles in the mother. *Trans Ophthalmol Soc Aust*, **3**, 35–46.

Gross, P.A., Hermogenes, A.W., et al. 1995. The efficacy of influenza vaccine in elderly persons. A meta-analysis and review of the literature. *Ann Intern Med*, **123**, 518–27.

Hadler, S.C. and Margolis, H.S. 1992. Hepatitis B immunization: vaccine types, efficacy, and indications for immunization. In: Remington, J.S. and Swartz, M.N. (eds), *Current topics in clinical infectious diseases*. Boston, MA: Blackwell Scientific, 283–308.

Halloran, M.E., Cochi, S.L., et al. 1994. Epidemiologic effects of routine immunization with varicella vaccine in the United States. *Am J Epidemiol*, **140**, 81–104.

Halsey, N.A. 1983. The optimal age for administering measles vaccine in developing countries. In: Halsey, N.A. and de Quadros, C.A. (eds), *Recent advances in immunization. A bibliographic review*. Washington, DC: Pan American Health Organization, 4–17, PAHO publication 451.

Harro, C.D., Pang, Y.K., et al. 2001. Safety and immunogenicity trial in adult volunteers of a human papillomavirus 16 L1 virus-like particle vaccine. *J Natl Cancer Inst*, **93**, 284–92.

Hattwick, M.A.W. 1974. Human rabies. *Public Health Rev*, **3**, 229–74.

Hatziandreu, E.J., Palmer, C.S., et al. 1994. *A cost benefit analysis of the diphtheria–tetanus–pertussis vaccine*. Arlington VA: Battelle.

Hauri, A., Armstrong, G. and Hutin, Y.F. 2003. Estimation of the global burden of disease attributable to contaminated injections given in health care settings. *Int J STD AIDS*, **15**, 7–16.

Henderson, D.A., Borio, L.L. and Lane, J.M. 2004. Smallpox and vaccinia. In: Plotkin, S.A. and Orenstein, W.A. (eds), *Vaccine*, 4th edn. Philadelphia: W.B. Saunders, 123–54.

Hinman, A.R., Hersch, B.S. and de Quadros, C.A. 1998. Rational use of rubella vaccine for prevention of congenital rubella syndrome in the Americas. *Pan Am J Public Health*, **4**, 156–60.

Hinman, A.R., Orenstein, W.A. and Rodewald, L.E. 1999. Public health considerations. In: Plotkin, S.A. and Orenstein, W.A. (eds), *Vaccines*, 3rd edn. Philadelphia: W.B. Saunders, 1006–32.

Hoke, C.H., Nisalak, A., et al. 1988. Protection against Japanese encephalitis by inactivated vaccines. *N Engl J Med*, **319**, 609–14.

Hope-Simpson, R.E. 1965. The nature of herpes zoster: a long-term study and a new hypothesis. *Proc R Soc Med*, **58**, 2–20.

Hull, H.F., Ward, N.A., et al. 1994. Paralytic poliomyelitis: seasoned strategies, disappearing disease. *Lancet*, **343**, 1331–7.

Innis, B.L., Snitbhan, R., et al. 1994. Protection against hepatitis A by an inactivated vaccine. *J Am Med Assoc*, **271**, 1363–4.

Institute of Medicine. 1991. *Adverse effects of pertussis and rubella vaccines*. In Howson C.P., Howe, C.J. and Fineberg, H.V. (eds), Washington, DC: National Academy Press.

Institute of Medicine. 1993. *Adverse events associated with childhood vaccines. Evidence bearing on causation*. In Stratton, K.R., Howe, C.J. and Johnston, R.B. (eds), Washington, DC: National Academy Press.

Institute of Medicine. 2000. Committee to study priorities for vaccine development. *Vaccines for the 21st century: a tool for decision making*. In Stratton, K.R., Durch, J.S. and Lawrence, R.S. (eds), Washington, DC: National Academy Press.

Institute of Medicine. 2001a. *Immunization safety review: measles, mumps, and rubella vaccine and autism*. Stratton, K.R., Gable, A., et al. (eds), Washington, DC: National Academy Press.

Institute of Medicine. 2001b. *Immunization safety review: thimerosal-containing vaccines and neurodevelopmental disorders*. In Stratton, K.R., Gable, A., McCormick, M.C. (eds), Washington, DC: National Academy Press.

Institute of Medicine. 2002a. *Immunization safety review: hepatitis B and demyelinating neurologic disorders*. In Stratton, K.R., Almario, D.A., McCormick, M.C. (eds), Washington, DC: National Academy Press.

Institute of Medicine. 2002b. *Immunization safety review: SV40 contamination of poliovaccine and cancer*. In Stratton, K.R., Almario, D.A., McCormick, M.C. (eds), Washington, DC: National Academy Press.

Institute of Medicine. 2004. Immunization safety review: Vaccines and Autism. Washington, DC: National Academies Press.

Irons, B., Carrasco, P., et al. 2003. Integrating measles and rubella surveillance: the experience in the Caribbean. *J Infect Dis*, **187**, Suppl. 1, S153–7.

James, J.M., Burks, W., et al. 1995. Safe administration of the measles vaccine to children allergic to eggs. *N Engl J Med*, **332**, 1262–6.

Jennings, R., Simms, J.R. and Heath, A.W. 1998. Adjuvants and delivery systems for viral vaccines – mechanisms and potential. *Dev Biol Stand*, **92**, 19–28.

Joce, R., Wood, D., et al. 1992. Paralytic poliomyelitis in England and Wales, 1985–1991. *Br Med J*, **305**, 79–82.

Joensuu, J., Koskenniemi, E., et al. 1997. Randomized placebo-controlled trial of rhesus-human reassortant rotavirus vaccine for prevention of severe rotavirus gastroenteritis. *Lancet*, **1997**, 1205–9.

Joint Committee on Vaccination and Immunization. 1996. *Immunization against infectious disease 1996: The green book*. United Kingdom: Department of Health (updated at www.doh.gov.uk/greenbook).

Kahn, J.A. and Bernstein, D.I. 2003. Human papillomavirus vaccines. *Pediatr Infect Dis J*, **22**, 5, 443–5.

Kane, M.A. 1993. Progress in control of hepatitis B infection through immunization. *Gut*, **34**, Suppl. 2, S10–12.

Kapikian, A.Z. 1994. Rhesus rotavirus-based human vaccines and observations on selected non-Jennerian approaches to rotavirus vaccination. In: Kapikian, A.Z. (ed.), *Viral Infections of the Gastrointestinal Tract*. New York: Marcel Dekker, 443–69.

Kapusta, J., Modelska, A., et al. 2001. Oral immunization with transgenic lettuce expressing hepatitis B surface antigen. *Adv Exp Med Biol*, **495**, 299–303.

Kew, O.M., Sutter, R.W., et al. 1998. Prolonged replication of a type 1 vaccine-derived poliovirus in an immunodeficient patient. *J Clin Microbiol*, **36**, 2893–9.

Ki, M., Park, T., et al. 2003. Risk analysis of aseptic meningitis after measles–mumps–rubella vaccination in Korean children by using a case-crossover design. *Am J Epidemiol*, **157**, 158–65.

King, G.E. and Hadler, S.C. 1994. Simultaneous administration of childhood vaccines: an important public health policy that is safe and efficacious. *Pediatr Infect Dis J*, **13**, 394–407.

Kitchener, S. 2004. Viscerotropic and neurotropic disease following vaccination with the 17D yellow fever vaccine, ARILVAX. *Vaccine*, **22**, 2103–5.

Koelle, D.M. and Corey, L. 2003. Recent progress in herpes simplex virus immunobiology and vaccine research. *Clin Microbiol Rev*, **16**, 1, 96–113.

Koutsky, L.A., Ault, K.A., et al. 2002. A controlled trial of a human papillomavirus type 16 vaccine. *N Engl J Med*, **347**, 1645–51.

Kramarz, P., France, E.K., et al. 2001. Population-based study of rotavirus vaccination and intussusception. *Pediatr Infect Dis J*, **20**, 410–16.

Lane, J.M., Ruben, F.L., et al. 1970. Complications of smallpox vaccination, 1968: results of ten statewide surveys. *J Infect Dis*, **122**, 303.

Langevin, S.A., Arroyo, J., et al. 2003. Host range restriction of chimeric yellow fever–West Nile vaccine in fish crows. *Am J Trop Med Hyg*, **69**, 78–80.

Lanzavecchia, A. 1985. Antigen-specific interaction between T and B cells. *Nature (Lond)*, **314**, 537–9.

Lasky, T., Terracciano, G., et al. 1998. The Guillain-Barré syndrome and the 1992–1993 and 1993–1994 influenza vaccines. *N Engl J Med*, **339**, 1797–802.

Levin, M.J. 2001. Use of varicella vaccines to prevent herpes zoster in older individuals. *Arch Virol Suppl*, **17**, 151–60.

Levin, M.J., Smith, J.G., et al. 2003. Decline in varicella-zoster virus (VZV)-specific cell-mediated immunity with increasing age and boosting with a high-dose VZV vaccine. *J Infect Dis*, **188**, 1336–44.

Lieu, T.A., Cochi, S.L. et al. 1994. Cost-effectiveness of a routine varicella vaccination program for US children. *J Am Med Assoc*, **271**, 375–81.

Maassab, H.F., Shaw, M.W. and Heilman, C.A. 1994. Live influenza virus vaccine. In: Plotkin, S. and Mortimer, E.A. Jr. (eds), *Vaccines*, 2nd edn. Philadelphia: W.B. Saunders, 781–801.

Maiztegui, J.I., Fernandez, N.J. and DeDamilano, A.J. 1979. Efficacy of immune plasma in treatment of Argentinian heamorrhagic fever and association between treatment and a late neurological syndrome. *Lancet*, **2**, 1216–17.

Mao, J.S., Chai, S.A., et al. 1997. Further evaluation of the safety and protective efficacy of live attenuated hepatitis A vaccine (H2-strain) in humans. *Vaccine*, **15**, 944–7.

Margolis, H.S., Coleman, P.J., et al. 1995. Prevention of hepatitis B virus transmission by immunization. An economic analysis of current recommendations. *J Am Med Assoc*, **274**, 1201–8.

Mast, E., Mahoney, F., et al. 2004. Hepatitis B vaccine. In: Plotkin, S. and Orenstein, W.A. (eds), *Vaccines*, 4th edn. Philadelphia: W.B. Saunders, 299–338.

McBean, A.M. and Modlin, J.F. 1987. Rationale for the sequential use of inactivated poliovirus vaccine and live attenuated poliovirus vaccine for routine poliomyelitis immunization in the United States. *Pediatr Infect Dis J*, **6**, 881–7.

McCarthy, M. 2003. Project seeks to fast track rotavirus vaccine. *Lancet*, **361**, 9357, 582.

McDevitt, H.O. 1980. Regulation of the immune response by the major histocompatibility complex system. *N Engl J Med*, **303**, 1514–17.

McDonnell, W.M. and Askari, F.K. 1996. DNA vaccines. *N Engl J Med*, **334**, 42–5.

McFarland, J.W., Mansoor, O.D., et al. 2003. Accelerated measles control in the Western Pacific region. *J Infect Dis*, **187**, Suppl. 1, S246–51.

McGhee, J.R., Mestecky, J., et al. 1992. The mucosal immune system: from fundamental concepts to vaccine development. *Vaccine*, **10**, 75–88.

Melnick, J.L. and Stinebaugh, S. 1962. Excretion of vacuolating SV40 virus (papovavirus group) after ingestion as contaminant of oral polio vaccine. *Proc Soc Exp Biol Med*, **109**, 965–8.

Meloen, R.H., Casal, J.I., et al. 1995. Synthetic peptides vaccines: success at last. *Vaccine*, **13**, 885–6.

Miller, E. 1991. Rubella in the United Kingdom. *Epidemiol Infect*, **107**, 31–42.

Monath, T.P. 2001. Yellow fever: an update. *Lancet Infect Dis*, **1**, 11–20.

Monath, T.P., Guirakhoo, F., et al. 2003. Chimeric live, attenuated vaccine against Japanese Encephalitis (ChimeriVax-JE): Phase 2 clinical trails for safety and immunogenicity, effect of vaccine dose and schedule, and memory response to challenge with inactivated Japanese Encephalitis antigen. *J Infect Dis*, **188**, 1213–30.

Monath, T.P., Caldwell, J.R., et al. 2004. ACAM2000 clonal Vero cell culture vaccinia virus (New York City Board of Health strain) — a second-generation smallpox vaccine for biological defense. *Int J Infect Dis*, Suppl. 2, S31–44.

Morrison, L.A. 2002. Vaccines against genital herpes: progress and limitations. *Drugs*, **62**, 8, 1119–29.

Mortimer, E.A., Lepow, M.L., et al. 1982. Long-term follow-up of persons inadvertently inoculated with SV40 as neonates. *N Engl J Med*, **305**, 1517–18.

Moss, B., Fuerst, T.R., et al. 1988. Roles of vaccinia virus in the development of new vaccines. *Vaccine*, **6**, 161–3.

Murphy, B.R. 1993. Use of live attenuated cold-adapted influenza A reassortant virus vaccines in infants, children, young adults, and elderly adults. *Infect Dis Clin Pract*, **2**, 174–81.

Murphy, B.R. and Channock, R.M. 1990. Immunization against viruses. In: Fields, B.N., Knipe, D.M., et al. (eds), *Fields' virology*, 2nd edn. New York: Raven Press, 469–502.

Murphy, T.V., Gargiullo, P.M., Rotavirus Intussusception Investigation Team, et al. 2001. Intussusception among infants given an oral rotavirus vaccine. *N Engl J Med*, **344**, 564–72.

Nathanson, N. and Langmuir, A.D. 1963. The Cutter incident. Poliomyelitis following formaldehyde-inactivated poliovirus vaccination in the United States during the spring of 1955. *Am J Hygiene*, **78**, 16–60.

Neuzil, K.M., Reed, G.W., et al. 1998. Impact of influenza on acute cardiopulmonary hospitalizations in pregnant women. *Am J Epidemiol*, **148**, 1094–102.

Neuzil, K.M., Dupont, W.D., et al. 2001. Efficacy of inactivated and cold-adapted vaccines against influenza A infection, 1985 to 1990: the pediatric experience. *Pediatr Infect Dis J*, **20**, 733–40.

Nguyen, H.Q., Jumaan, A.O. and Seward, J.F. 2005. Decline in mortality due to varicella after implementation of varicella vaccination in the United States. *N Engl J Med*, **352**, 450–8.

Nichol, K.L., Margolis, K.L., et al. 1994. The efficacy and cost effectiveness of vaccination against influenza among elderly persons living in the community. *N Engl J Med*, **331**, 778–84.

Nichol, K.L., Mendelman, P.M., et al. 1999. Effectiveness of live, attenuated intranasal influenza vaccine in healthy working adults: a randomized controlled trial. *J Am Med Assoc*, **281**, 137–44.

Offit, P.A. 2002. The future of rotavirus vaccines. *Sem Pediatr Infect Dis*, **13**, 3, 190–5.

Oncley, J.L., Melin, M., et al. 1949. The separation of antibodies, isoagglutinins, prothrombin, plasminogen and B-lipoproteins into sub-fractions of human plasma. *J Am Chem Soc*, **71**, 541–50.

Onorato, I.M., Markowitz, L.E. and Oxtoby, M.J. 1988. Childhood immunization, vaccine-preventable diseases and HIV infection. *Pediatr Infect Dis J*, **7**, 588–95.

Orenstein, W.A., Bernier, R.H. and Hinman, A.R. 1988. Assessing vaccine efficacy in the field. *Epidemiol Rev*, **10**, 212–41.

Otten, M.W. Jr., Okwo-Bele, J.M., et al. 2003. Impact of alternative approaches to accelerated measles control: experience in the African region, 1996–2002. *J Infect Dis*, **187**, Suppl. 1, S36–43.

Oxman, M.N. 1995. Immunization to reduce the frequency and severity of herpes zoster and its complications. *Neurology*, **45**, (Suppl. 8), S41–6.

Pan American Health Organization. 1994. Certification of poliomyelitis eradication – the Americas, 1994. *Morbid Mortal Wkly Rep*, **43**, 720–2.

Papania, M., Seward, J., et al. 2004. The epidemiology of measles in the United States, 1997–2001. *J Infect Dis*, **188**, Suppl. 1, S54–68.

Pass, R.F. and Burke, R.L. 2002. Development of cytomegalovirus vaccines: prospects for prevention of congenital CMV infection. *Semin Pediatr Infect Dis*, **13**, 3, 196–204.

Patriarca, P.A., Wright, P.F. and John, T.J. 1991. Factors affecting the immunogenicity of oral poliovirus vaccine in developing countries: a review. *Rev Infect Dis*, **13**, 926–39.

Peltola, H. and Heinonen, O.P. 1986. Frequency of true adverse reactions to measles–mumps–rubella vaccine; a double blind, placebo-controlled trial in twins. *Lancet*, **1**, 939–42.

Peltola, H., Heinonen, O.P., et al. 1994. The elimination of indigenous measles, mumps, and rubella from Finland by a 12-year, two-dose vaccination program. *N Engl J Med*, **331**, 1397–402.

Peltola, H., Davidkin, I., et al. 2000. Mumps and rubella eliminated from Finland. *J Am Med Assoc*, **284**, 2643–7.

Perez-Schael, I., Guntinas, M.J., et al. 1997. Efficacy of the rhesus rotavirus-based quadrivalent vaccine in infants and young children in Venezuela. *N Engl J Med*, **337**, 1181–7.

Perkus, M.E., Piccini, A., et al. 1985. Recombinant vaccinia virus: immunization against multiple pathogens. *Science*, **229**, 981–4.

Peters, C.J., Johnson, E.D. and McKee, K.T. Jr. 1991. Filoviruses and management of viral hemorrhagic fevers. In: Belshe, R.B. (ed.), *Textbook of human virology*, 2nd edn. St Louis, MO: Mosby Yearbook, 699–712.

Plotkin, S.A. 2002. Is there a formula for an effective CMV vaccine? *J Clin Virol*, **25**, S13–21.

Plotkin, S.A. 2004a. Mumps vaccine. In: Plotkin, S.A. and Orenstein, W.A. (eds), *Vaccines*, 4th edn. Philadelphia: W.B. Saunders, 441–70.

Plotkin, S.A. 2004b. Cytomegalovirus and herpes simplex vaccines. In: Plotkin, S.A. and Orenstein, W.A. (eds), *Vaccines*, 4th edn. Philadelphia: W.B. Saunders, 1199–208.

Plotkin, S.A. and Reef, S. 2004. Rubella vaccine. In: Plotkin, S.A. and Orenstein, W.A. (eds), *Vaccines*, 4th edn. Philadelphia: W.B. Saunders, 707–43.

Ramsay, M.E., Jin, L., et al. 2003. The elimination of indigenous measles transmission in England and Wales. *J Infect Dis*, **187**, Suppl. 1, S198–207.

Reef, S.E., Frey, T.K., et al. 2002. The changing epidemiology of rubella in the 1990s: on the verge of elimination and new challenges for control and prevention. *J Am Med Assoc*, **287**, 464–72.

Reinherz, E.L. and Schlossman, S.F. 1980. Regulation of the immune response – inducer and suppressor T lymphocyte subsets in human beings. *N Engl J Med*, **303**, 370–3.

Rennels, M.B., Glass, R.I., et al. 1996. Safety and efficacy of high-dose rhesus-human rotavirus vaccines – report of the national multicenter trial. *Pediatrics*, **97**, 7–13.

Robertson, S.E., Cutts, F.T., et al. 1997. Control of rubella and congenital rubella syndrome (CRS) in developing countries. Part 2: Vaccination against rubella. *Bull WHO*, **75**, 69–80.

Rota, J.S., Heath, J.L., et al. 1996. Molecular epidemiology of measles virus: identification of pathways of transmission and implications for measles elimination. *J Infect Dis*, **173**, 32–7.

Rousell, R.H. 1988. Clinical safety of intravenous immune globulin and freedom from transmission of viral disease. *J Hosp Infect*, **12**, Suppl. D, 17–27.

Salisbury, D.M. and Olive, J.M. 2004. Immunization in Europe. In: Plotkin, S.A. and Orenstein, W.A. (eds), *Vaccines*, 4th edn. Philadelphia: W.B. Saunders, 1387–406.

Salk, J., Drucker, J.A. and Malvin, D. 2004. Noninfectious poliovirus vaccine. In: Plotkin, S.A. and Orenstein, W.A. (eds), *Vaccines*, 4th edn. Philadelphia: W.B. Saunders, 205–27.

Salzman, M.B. and Garcia, C. 1998. Postexposure varicella vaccination in siblings of children with active varicella. *Pediatr Infect Dis J*, **17**, 250–1.

Schiffman, M. and Castle, P.E. 2003. Human papillomavirus: epidemiology and public health. *Arch Pathol Lab Med*, **127**, 930–4.

Schleiss, M.R. 2003. Vertically transmitted herpesvirus infections. *Herpes*, **10**, 4–11.

Schmader, K. 2001. Herpes zoster in older adults. *Clin Infect Dis*, **32**, 1481–6.

Schonberger, L.B., Bregman, D.J., et al. 1979. Guillain-Barré syndrome following vaccination in the National Influenza Immunization program, United States, 1976–1977. *Am J Epidemiol*, **110**, 105–23.

Seward, J.F. 2001. Update on varicella. *Pediatr Infect Dis J*, **20**, 619–21.

Seward, J.F., Watson, B.M., et al. 2002. Varicella disease after introduction of varicella vaccine in the United States, 1995–2000. *J Am Med Assoc*, **287**, 606–11.

Shields, K.E., Galil, K.G., et al. 2001. Varicella vaccine exposure during pregnancy: data from the first 5 years of the pregnancy registry. *Obstet Gynecol*, **98**, 14–19.

Siber, G.R., Werner, B.C. and Halsey, N.A. 1993. Interference of immune globulins with measles and rubella immunization. *J Pediatr*, **122**, 204–11.

Singh, M., Li, X.-M., et al. 1997. Controlled release microparticles as a single dose hepatitis B vaccine: evaluation of immunogenicity in mice. *Vaccine*, **15**, 4775–81.

Spika, J.S., Wassilak, S., et al. 2003. Measles and rubella in the World Health Organization European region: diversity creates challenges. *J Infect Dis*, **187**, Suppl. 1, S191–7.

Srivastava, I.K. and Liu, M. 2003. Gene vaccines. *Ann Intern Med*, **138**, 550–9.

Stanberry, L.R., Spotswood, L.S., et al. 2002. Glycoprotein-D-adjuvant vaccine to prevent genital herpes. *N Engl J Med*, **347**, 1652–61.

Stanley, M.A. 2003. Progress in prophylactic and therapeutic vaccines for human papillomavirus infection. *Exp Rev Vaccines*, **2**, 381–9.

Stefano, I., Sato, H.K., et al. 1999. Recent immunization against measles does not interfere with the sero-response to yellow fever vaccinations. *Vaccine*, **17**, 1042–6.

Stein, C.E., Birmingham, M., et al. 2003. The global burden of measles in the year 2000: a model that uses country-specific indicators. *J Infect Dis*, **187**, Suppl. 1, S8–S14.

Stevens, C.E., Toy, P.T., et al. 1992. Prospects for control of hepatitis B virus infection: implications of childhood vaccination and long term protection. *Pediatrics*, **90**, 170–3.

Strebel, P.M., Sutter, R.W., et al. 1992. Epidemiology of poliomyelitis in the United States one decade after the last reported case of indigenous wild virus-associated disease. *Clin Infect Dis*, **14**, 568–79.

Strebel, P.M., Ion-Nedelcu, I., et al. 1995. Intramuscular injections within 30 days of immunization with oral poliovirus vaccine – a risk factor for vaccine-associated paralytic poliomyelitis. *N Engl J Med*, **332**, 500–6.

Strebel, P.M., Cochi, S., et al. 2003. The unfinished measles immunization agenda. *J Infect Dis*, **187**, Suppl. 1, S1–7.

Strebel, P.M., Papania, M.J. and Halsey, N.A. 2004. Measles vaccine. In: Plotkin, S.A. and Orenstein, W.A. (eds), *Vaccines*, 4th edn. Philadelphia: W.B. Saunders, 389–440.

Sullivan, N.J., Geisbert, T.W., et al. 2003. Accelerated vaccination for Ebola virus haemorrhagic fever in non-human primates. *Nature*, **424**, 681–4.

Sutter, R.W. and Patriarca, P.A. 1993. Inactivated and live, attenuated poliovirus vaccines: mucosal immunity. In: Kurstak, E. (ed.), *Measles and poliomyelitis. Vaccines, immunization, and control*. Vienna: Springer-Verlag, 279–94.

Szmuness, W., Stevens, C.E., et al. 1981. A controlled clinical trial of the efficacy of hepatitis B vaccine (Heptavax B): a final report. *Hepatology*, **1**, 377–85.

Temperton, N.J., Quenelle, D.C., et al. 2003. Enhancement of humoral immune responses to a human cytomegalovirus DNA vaccine: adjuvant effects of aluminum phosphate and CpG oligodeoxynucleotides. *J Med Virol*, **70**, 1, 86–90.

Thompson, W.W., Shay, D.K., et al. 2003. Mortality associated with influenza and respiratory syncytial virus in the United States. *J Am Med Assoc*, **289**, 179–86.

Tingle, A.J., Allen, M. and Petty, R.E. 1986. Rubella associated arthritis. I. Comparative study of joint manifestations associated with natural rubella infection and RA 27/3 rubella immunization. *Ann Rheum Dis*, **45**, 110–14.

Treanor, J.J., Kotloff, K., et al. 1999. Evaluation of trivalent, live, cold-adapted (CAIV-T) and inactivated (TIV) influenza vaccines in prevention of virus infection and illness following challenge of adults with wild-type influenza A (H1N1), A (H3N2) and B viruses. *Vaccine*, **18**, 899–906.

Vaccines and Biologicals. 2002a. WHO vaccine preventable disease monitoring system, 2002 Global summary. Geneva: World Health Organization, WHO/V & B/02.20.

Vaccines and Biologicals. 2002b. First do no harm. Introducing auto-disable syringes and ensuring injection safety in immunization systems in developing countries. World Health Organization: Geneva, WHO/V & B/02.26.

Vaccines and Biologicals. 2003. Core information for the development of immunization policy. World Health Organization: Geneva, WHO/V & B/02.28.

Vaccines and Biologicals. 2004. Progress toward global eradication of poliomyelitis, January 2003–April 2004. *Morbid Mortal Wkly Rpt* **53**, 532–5.

Van Damme, P., Thoelen, S., et al. 1994. Inactivated hepatitis A vaccine: reactogenicity, immunogenicity, and long-term antibody persistence. *J Med Virol*, **44**, 446–51.

Varis, T. and Vesikari, T. 1996. Efficacy of high titer live attenuated varicella vaccine in healthy young children. *J Infect Dis*, **174**, S330–4.

Velazquez, F.R., Matson, D.O., et al. 1996. Rotavirus infections in infants as protection against subsequent infections. *N Engl J Med*, **335**, 1022–8.

Verstraeten, T., Jumaan, A., et al. 2003. A retrospective cohort study of the association of varicella vaccine failure with asthma, steroid use, age at vaccination, and measles–mumps–rubella vaccination. *Pediatrics*, **112**, 2, 98–103.

Vesikari, T., Karvonen, A et al. 2004. Efficacy of RIX4414 live attenuated human rotavirus vaccine in Finnish infants. *Pediatr Infect Dis J*, **158**, 937–43.

Waldvogel, F.A. 1981. *Immunotherapy: a guide to immunoglobulin prophylaxis and therapy*, Nyedegger, U.E. (ed.), London: Academic Press, 357.

Waters, T.D. and Anderson, P.S. Jr. 1972. Yellow fever vaccination, avian leukosis virus and cancer risk in man. *Science*, **177**, 76–7.

Weibel, R., Neff, B.J., et al. 1984. Live Oka/Merck varicella vaccine in healthy children: efficacy trials in healthy children. *N Engl J Med*, **310**, 1409–15.

Wells, M.A., Wittek, A.E., et al. 1986. Inactivation and partition of human T-cell lymphotropic virus type III during ethanol fractionation of plasma. *Transfusion*, **26**, 210–13.

Weltzin, R., Liu, J., et al. 2003. Clonal vaccinia virus grown in cell culture as a new smallpox vaccine. *Nat Med*, **9**, 1125–30.

Werzberger, A., Mensch, B., et al. 1992. A controlled trial of a formalin inactivated hepatitis A vaccine in healthy children. *N Engl J Med*, **327**, 453–7.

West, D.J. and Calendra, G.B. 1996. Vaccine-induced immunologic memory for hepatitis B surface antigen: implications for policy on booster vaccination. *Vaccine*, **12**, 1019–27.

Wharton, M., Cochi, S.L., et al. 1988. A large outbreak of mumps in the postvaccine era. *J Infect Dis*, **158**, 1253–60.

Wharton, M. and Strebel, P.M. 1995. Vaccine preventable diseases. In: Wilcox, L.S. and Marks, J.S. (eds), *From data to action. CDC's public health surveillance for women, infants and children*. Atlanta GA: US Department of Health and Human Services, 281–90.

WHO Collaborative Study Group on Oral and Inactivated Poliovirus Vaccine. 1996. Combined immunization of infants with oral and inactivated poliovirus vaccines: results of a randomized trial in the Gambia, Oman, and Thailand. *Bull WHO*, **74**, 251–68.

Williams, P.E., Yap, P.L., et al. 1988b. Non-A non-B hepatitis transmission by intravenous immunoglobulin. *Lancet*, **2**, 501.

Wise, R.P., Salive, M.E., et al. 2000. Postlicensure safety surveillance for varicella vaccine. *J Am Med Assoc*, **284**, 1271–9.

World Health Organization. 1987. Acceptability of cell substrates for production of biologicals. *Technical Report Series*, **747**, 1.

World Health Organization. 1988. *Report of the forty-first World Health Assembly*. Geneva: WHO.

World Health Organization. 1992. WHO Expert Committee on Rabies. Eighth Report, *Technical Report Series*, **824.**

World Health Organization. 1998a. Expanded programme on immunization (EPI) – standardization of the nomenclature for describing the genetic characteristics of wild-type measles virus. *Wkly Epidemiol Rec*, **73**, 265–72.

World Health Organization. 1998b. Measles – progress toward global control and regional elimination, 1990–1998. *Wkly Epidemiol Rec* **73**, 389–94.

World Health Organization. 2000. WHO report of a meeting on preventing congenital rubella syndrome: immunization strategies, surveillance needs. Experience with CRS prevention and rubella control in the Americas. Geneva: World Health Organization, WHO/ V & B/00.10:20.

World Health Organization. 2003a. Introduction of inactivated poliovirus vaccine into oral poliovirus vaccine-using countries. *Wkly Epidemiol Rec*, **78**, 241–52.

World Health Organization. 2003b. Rotavirus vaccines, an update. *Wkly Epidemiol Rec* **78**, 2–3.

World Health Organization. 2003c. Global progress towards universal childhood hepatitis B vaccination, 2003. *Wkly Epidemiol Rec* **78**, 366–71.

World Health Organization and United Nations Children's Fund. 2002. *State of the world's vaccines and immunization*. Geneva: World Health Organization.

Yellow Fever Vaccine Safety Working Group. 2004. History of thymoma and yellow fever vaccination. *Lancet* **364**, 936.

Zimmerman, R.K. 2003. Recommended childhood and adolescent immunization schedule, United States, 2003 and update on childhood immunizations. *Am Fam Physician*, **67**, 188, 190, 195–196.

68

Viral vectors for gene therapy

R. MICHAEL LINDEN AND KENNETH I. BERNS

INTRODUCTION

Our increased knowledge of the human genome and the understanding that a large number of human illnesses have a genetic basis have led to a desire to correct the genetic defects underlying these diseases. Human gene therapy has two basic requirements: 1) the wild type gene sequence, and 2) a means of delivering the wild type sequence to the cell so that it may be expressed in an appropriate manner. In the case of a deleterious mutation, which is dominant when heterologous, the therapeutic gene may encode a product which selectively inactivates the deleterious mutant product. While we know and have in hand large numbers of potentially corrective genes, development of successful delivery vehicles or vectors is still at a relatively early stage. To be successful, a vector should be able to introduce the corrective gene (transgene) into the target cell, in most cases transport it to the nucleus, establish a stable state in the nucleus, and express the desired levels of the product encoded by the transgene for extended periods of time. (The latter need not be the case when the intent of the therapy is to engender a protective immune response, i.e. a vaccine or a product intended as a lethal, anticancer agent.) Finally, the vector should not elicit an inflammatory or immune response against the cells that contain the vector.

A variety of delivery systems have been tried including viruses, artificial lipid envelopes, and direct injection of naked DNA (e.g. via the 'gene gun'). Viruses have been the favored instrument since they naturally deliver genes into human cells. The viral genes are expressed in a regulated manner and in many instances persist for extended periods of time. However, there have been only a moderate number of clinical trials and only one has offered good evidence of therapeutic benefit (see below). Several significant problems have been encountered. Either the level of transgene expression has been inadequate or of insufficient duration. The latter is a common problem and is thought to relate to the host immune response to the vector. An immune response to structural proteins in the vector virion leads to inhibition of successful vector delivery on subsequent administration. However, often there is an immune response to expression of the viral genes remaining in the vector. This leads to cell death and frequently is an inflammatory response. It was such a response which led to the only death of a patient in a gene therapy clinical trial after administration of a high dose of an adenovirus vector (see below). Thus, development of vectors which allow sustained expression of the transgene is a common goal; success in this implies the absence of deleterious host response. As an aside, if the patient has a null mutation, it is conceivable that expression of the wild type gene product would elicit an immune response. This is of concern and must be carefully monitored in each case. Another potential concern of gene therapy is the location of the vector within the nucleus. If it remains extrachromosomal and is not able to replicate in synchrony with cell DNA, then it is likely to be diluted out if the cell divides; extrachromosomal vectors are not useful if the goal is introduction of the transgene into progenitor cells. Thus, it would be advantageous to develop vectors that can integrate into the cell genome so that the transgene can be replicated in synchrony. Almost all of the current vectors do integrate to an extent; retroviral-based vectors do so frequently, other current viral vectors integrate at a low frequency. However, of great significance is the possibility of insertional mutagenesis. If the vector integrates into an important cellular gene, it may inactivate the gene or convert its product into one that is deleterious to the cell. As indicated below, in the only clinically successful use of gene therapy a retroviral vector derived from Moloney murine leukemia virus was used to treat patients with severe combined immunodeficiency disease. However, two of the patients developed a leukemia-like disease because of the site of integration of the vector. While these two have been successfully treated for the complication, the risks inherent in vector integration at random sites remain (Hacein-Bey-Abina et al. 2003).

Although human gene therapy is in its infancy, significant progress has been made in the development of viral vectors. In this chapter we will describe such work with the four viruses that are most commonly used as vectors: adenovirus, herpes simplex virus, retrovirus, and adeno-associated virus.

RETROVIRAL VECTORS

Both in vitro and in vivo gene delivery strategies were pioneered using retroviral vector systems. In the early 1970s the concept of gene transfer using retroviruses for a variety of purposes had been put forward. Although nearly 35 years have passed since, the successful application of this system has mainly been limited to a range of laboratory uses. Only recently has clinical investigation resulted in unambiguous evidence that a therapeutically beneficial result can be achieved. Notwithstanding the long development phase, it must be noted that retroviruses have served as a guiding frontrunner in the development of a range of vector systems that are built on many different animal viruses.

Due to the large amount of research involving retroviruses the aim of this section is not to represent a comprehensive review of the virus and all possible applications, but rather to limit the discussion to those characteristics of retroviruses that are essential to understanding the complexities inherent in this promising gene transfer system.

Retrovirus Biology

The *Retroviridae* represent a large group of viruses that are widely distributed throughout the vertebrates (Coffin et al. 1997). The taxonomy of this virus family has recently been adjusted to reflect our understanding of the molecular biology of the different genera. In general, retroviruses can be divided into two groups, the 'simple'

retroviruses among which the alpha-, beta-, and gamma retroviruses are counted and the 'complex' retroviruses with the genera delta-, epsilon-, spuma-, and lenti-retroviruses. Representative members of the retrovirus genera are avian leukosis virus (ALV) for alpha viruses, *Mouse mammary tumor virus* for beta-, and *Murine leukemia virus* (MLV) for the gamma retroviruses. The genera of complex viruses are represented by human T-lymphotropic viruses (HTLV) (delta virus), *Human foamy virus* (spumaviruses) and human immunodeficiency virus (HIV) (lentiviruses). Epsilon viruses are exclusively found in fish and reptiles and will not be further discussed. Based on the observation that the alpha-, beta-, and gamma retroviruses have oncogenic potential these genera have been also collectively called onco-retroviruses. There are several potential mechanisms that can contribute to the transforming potential of these viruses (Suzuki et al. 2002; Mikkers et al. 2002; Lund et al. 2002). First, these viruses are known to undergo recombination at high frequencies resulting in the generation of defective genomes that can be complemented by wild type retroviruses. These contaminating defective genomes have been shown to be able to acquire host cell sequences that, in very rare events can be biologically active. Among those sequences that have been identified to have a significant (detectable) effect on the cell cycle are a number of proto-oncogenes. A second mechanism is inherent to the viral life cycle through the retroviral strategy of integrating a copy of the cDNA into the host genome in a manner that is nonspecific with respect to the chromosomal locus (Stocking et al. 1993). Theoretically the viral cDNA can integrate into or close to a tumor suppressor or a proto-oncogene, respectively. We will discuss the events that have made this theoretical possibility a reality which, in the context of gene therapy, needs consideration.

The members of all retrovirus genera share three coding regions, *gag* (group-specific antigen), *env* (envelope), and *pol* (polymerase) (Goff 2001). The *env* region encodes the envelope protein, the *pol* region the reverse transcriptase, integrase, and a viral protease, and the *gag* region encodes the nucleoproteins as well as the matrix and capsid proteins. The complex retroviruses distinguish themselves from the 'simple' viruses by the presence of additional accessory genes that significantly alter the viral life style.

In general, retroviruses are diploid in that they contain two identical copies of the viral single-stranded RNA. The sizes of positive-strand virus genomes range from seven to 13 kb. As the retrovirus genome is generated by cellular transcription complexes it resembles cellular RNA through the presence of both a 5′ cap and a poly(A) sequence. Additional sequences that are essential to the viral life cycle include the packaging signal (ψ) and the *att*-sites that are required for provirus integration.

Retrovirus life cycle

The life cycle of retroviruses is somewhat complex and in addition to receptor binding, fusion, and uncoating involves reverse transcription (hence *Retro*viruses), nuclear import (either passive through cell division for onco-retroviruses or active in the case of lentiviruses), and integration of the proviral DNA. In order to generate daughter virions, the integrated provirus is transcribed by cellular proteins, followed by splicing and nuclear export. The cytoplasmic RNA is then translated into precursor proteins, and the life cycle is concluded by packaging of full length RNA into the assembled virions. A new round of infection can commence after budding of the virion and proteolytic processing and maturation of the virion. Each of these steps had to be taken into account for the development of retrovirus-based gene transfer strategies. Early problems with this vector system included the contamination by replication competent virus (in this class of viruses a certainly significant concern), low titers of the vectors, only low levels of expression by the transgene, and promoter down-regulation after successful transduction. Overall, the retrovirus gene therapy field has been able to overcome these hurdles to a large extent through many variations of vector design and production. One of the hurdles was the efficiency of receptor binding by retroviruses. All retroviruses that are used for gene therapy purposes are enveloped by a glycolipid membrane. This envelope contains proteins that are responsible for receptor binding and thereby defines the tropism of the viruses and vectors. In general, this receptor-mediated fusion triggers all of the subsequent steps in the viral entry process that are necessary for successful transduction. However, the viral glycoproteins of the envelope also define – and in some cases restrict – the efficiency of gene transfer. A significant development in this regard was the introduction of pseudotyping, a strategy that allowed for the replacement of the native glycoprotein with one of a broader tropism. In the early clinical trials that utilized retroviruses and that were aimed at the transduction of hematopoietic stem cells (HSC), the vectors were pseudotyped with the MLV amphotropic envelope (Chien et al. 1997). A disadvantage of these amphotropic viruses, however, is the relatively low amount of this specific receptor on HSCs. This observation possibly explains the relatively low efficiency transduction of HSCs by amphotropic retroviruses. The protein of choice for the expansion of the tissue tropism was the glycoprotein G from vesicular stomatitis virus (VSV-G) (Yang et al. 1995). While only replacing a single envelope protein, this variation shifts the mode of vector uptake from receptor-mediated fusion to endocytosis that, in addition, requires endosome escape as a result of vesicle acidification. The advantage of this pseudotyping strategy is several-fold. First, the receptor for VSV-G is believed to be a membrane lipid that is ubiquitous in all cells. Second, VSV-G itself mediates pH-dependent endosome escape in addition to its receptor attachment function (Yamada and Ohnishi 1986). As a result, this simple envelope modification conferred a broad tissue tropism and efficient cellular trafficking to many retroviruses, including the increasingly utilized lentiviruses. Conceptually, the introduction of pseudotyping has opened the door to many applications ranging from the broadening of tissue tropism to strategies aimed at the targeting of specific cell types.

Subsequent to membrane fusion, or endocytosis and endosome escape, are several steps that are of importance with respect to retrovirus gene transfer and vector production. Several viral gene products are required for these steps, including reverse transcriptase, integrase, and protease. Although in current vectors the genes encoding these proteins are not present, these, as well as other proteins, are part of the virion and, therefore, do not need to be encoded by the recombinant transfer vector genome.

The reverse transcriptase step during viral replication is of importance with respect to vector design and quality control based on its biochemical properties. The enzyme is characterized by a comparatively slow incorporation rate of <100 nucleotides per second, a poor processivity, a relatively low fidelity with a mis-incorporation rate of approximately one in 104 and the absence of a proof-reading activity (Kerr and Anderson 1997; Oude Essink and Berkhout 1999; Harrison et al. 1998). Although these values have been determined in vitro they do correspond somewhat to the high mutation rate in vivo of ca. one mutation per genome (Burns and Temin 1994). This error rate has been associated to the unique capacity of lentiviruses to evade either host cell responses or the effects of antiviral pharmaceuticals and is therefore biologically significant. With respect to vectors, however, the mis-incorporation rate is somewhat problematic, particularly since it has been documented that the error rate is template-dependent and can therefore not be predicted (Bebenek et al. 1993). An additional characteristic of retroviruses is their diploid genome that, theoretically, could provide a certain genetic stability to the viruses. It has, however, been documented that when genetically different genomes are present the reverse transcription process utilizes both RNA strands resulting in a high degree of recombination.

Nuclear import

In the field of retrovirus gene transfer a frequently discussed 'roadblock' is the transport of the viral cDNA into the nucleus. The onco-retroviruses do not encode for a machinery that would actively facilitate nuclear import. On the level of gene transfer application this reliance on passive import translates into the requirement for cell division prior to transduction (Roe et al. 1993; Lewis and Emerman 1994). Although the majority of applications to date focus on HSC this dependency defines a limitation for the ultimate usefulness of 'simple' retroviruses as it has been demonstrated that even primitive HSC cells are predominantly in a quiescent, nondividing state. This roadblock has been central to the efforts of developing vectors that are based on the complex retroviruses such as the spumavirus human foamy virus (HFV) and, most importantly, lentiviruses. Possibly the most widely explored lentivirus remains HIV-1 (Weinberg et al. 1991; Blomer et al. 1997). Although it might appear counter-intuitive that a virus with such devastating effects on human health would be pursued as an ultimately nonpathogenic gene transfer vector, it has been exactly this phenomenon that resulted in the accumulation of an impressive body of information about the biology of the virus, which has allowed the accelerated development of this class of gene transfer vectors. Among the viruses explored in this class are both HIV-1 and 2, simian immunodeficiency virus (SIV), feline immunodeficiency virus (FIV), bovine immunodeficiency virus (BIV), and equine infectious anemia virus (EIAV) and visna virus. Despite this reorientation of the field towards the complex retroviruses that is mainly based on their nuclear import potential, the underlying mechanisms have not yet been identified and the subject is somewhat plagued by controversy. Similarly, foamy virus nuclear import is not understood, although a pathway that involves different cellular components (and is therefore distinct from lentiviruses) has been proposed (Saib et al. 1997). It must be pointed out that aspects of these unknown mechanisms possibly underlie the observation that in some differentiated tissue in vivo transduction by lentiviruses might require cell division (Park et al. 2000).

Provirus integration

The subsequent step in viral infection, cDNA integration, is one of the clearly attractive features of retroviruses. This step is an essential component of the viral life cycle and it is thus not surprising that the mechanism is quite efficient. Consistent with the life cycle of retroviruses in vivo the integration allows persistence of the viral genome in dividing cells.

Mechanistically, after formation of the double-stranded cDNA and nuclear import, the generation of circular molecules has been observed. To date, it is believed that the presence of certain circular species can be used to detect nuclear import, but it also has become clear that these molecules are poor substrates for the integration process (Lobel et al. 1989). This leaves unanswered the question of function of these circularized retroviral genomes. It is reasonable to assume that these

structures represent a side product of integration rather than an essential part of the mechanism. However, of some concern is the possibility that the circular molecules can – transiently – contribute to transduction efficiency thereby skewing the estimated gene transfer rate (Haas et al. 2000).

A key concern, however, with respect to retroviral gene transfer, has been the potential of insertional mutagenesis. In general, the risk for tumor transformation as a result of a single insertion event could be estimated to be rather low in light of the well-documented notion that the establishment of malignancy in differentiated tissue requires multiple 'hits'. Nevertheless, the application of vectors that integrate in a nonspecific manner into the genome in rapidly dividing cells adds the additional level of selection to the consideration. That is, if virus genomes randomly integrate in cells that are first expanded (either in vivo through growth advantage over nontransduced cells or ex vivo through selective pressure) and then differentiated, it is feasible to hypothesize that cells with integration events into a tumor suppressor gene or close to a proto-oncogene are likely to be enriched. In this 'selection' scenario, a single-hit, vector-induced mutation might be sufficient to contribute to the subsequent establishment of malignancies. In this context it must be emphasized that in nearly 15 years of clinical experimentation with retroviruses, no integration-related cancer has been reported. Recently, however, in what might represent the first clinically successful gene therapy trial to date, two patients developed a T-cell leukemia that was correlated to the insertion of the retroviral vector. The trial was designed to treat X-linked severe combined immunodeficiency (X-SCID) using an MLV-based vector expressing the γ-c chain cytokine receptor. In the affected children the absence of this receptor function results in the inability to respond to cytokine signaling and therefore the absence of functional T- and natural killer (NK) cells (Hacein-Bey-Abina et al. 2002; Fischer 2000; Soudais et al. 2000). Approximately 30 months after the engraftment of retrovirally transduced cells, two of the patients developed a leukemia-like condition that required chemotherapeutic treatment. Since, it has been determined that in both patients the retroviral cDNA had integrated into and close to the LMO2 locus, respectively. Understandably, these adverse side effects have caused considerable anxiety within the gene therapy community, the government regulators, and beyond (Hacein-Bey-Abina et al. 2003; Check 2002a,b). However, this case, that was characterized by the unique willingness of the investigators to share the pertinent information with the scientific community and the public, deserves further analysis. First, among the more than ten treated patients, only two have fallen ill with leukemia. Second, a third patient is said to have insertion into the LMO2 locus but did not develop leukemia within a comparable time frame. Third, within the context of numerous clinical and preclinical experiments employing retroviruses these are the first serious adverse effects documented to result from insertional mutagenesis by a retrovirus. Taken together, these observations indicate that several parameters came together in this case. It is unlikely that random integration (in these cases into the *LMO2* oncogene that has previously been reported to play a role in leukemia development) by the vectors alone caused the development of the malignancies. It is more likely that the cancer in these two patients has resulted from a combination of factors that include the *LMO2* alterations, the unregulated transgene expression (note that the γ-chain of the cytokine receptor for IL2, 4, 7, 9, 15, and 21 naturally confers a selective advantage for the transduced cell) and the nature of this particular treatment strategy that is based on the proliferation of a few cells to repopulate this component of the hematopoietic system. Therefore, the importance of these events to retrovirus-mediated gene therapy in general is unclear and will likely only be assessed through further pre-clinical and clinical trials.

The further steps in the retroviral life cycle, transcription of the provirus, packaging and maturation are mainly important for considerations regarding the vector production and purification. Although most clinical trials to date have been conducted ex vivo, increasingly efforts are underway to develop strategies that employ in vivo delivery. These approaches confront the retrovirus gene therapy with issues related to anti-virus immunity. For example, it has been shown that the glycoprotein G of VSV can serve as an efficient antigen through which the vector can be inactivated (DePolo et al. 2000) by human serum. In order to address this concern, alternative envelopes or PEGylation of these vectors have been proposed (Croyle et al. 2004).

Vector design strategies

Both simple and complex retrovirus vector development have undergone numerous generations, including many variations in the strategy to provide the helper functions necessary to generate infectious virions (for a review of these developments see Brenner and Malech (2003)). Of particular concern in this regard has been, and still are, the attempts to minimize and exclude the risk of generating replication-competent viruses through recombination events. In brief, the approaches can be summarized by two different strategies: first, the use of stable cell lines that contain the genes encoding all necessary helper functions stably integrated within the genome of the producer cell line. A construct containing the transfer vector is then transiently transfected into the producer cell line and the recombinant virus is shed into the medium. Notably, only the essential retrovirus components are retained within the transfer vector, including the packaging signal ψ and the viral LTRs. In

lentiviruses these elements also include the rev responsive element (RRE). The second strategy, transient transfection of both the helper functions and the transfer vector has been more employed during the development of lentivectors. The overall theme during this development process, that has now undergone more than three generations, has been to delete as many of the accessory factors as possible. This was particularly important since some of these factors are toxic to cells and enhanced the likelihood of eliminating the generation of replication competent virus. In exchange, however, both titers and transgene expression levels after gene transfer have been reduced. This problem has then been addressed by the addition of different promoters driving the transgene and the incorporation of post-transcriptional regulatory elements such as the one identified in Woodchuck hepatitis B virus (WHV). An additional safety element has been introduced through the use of self-inactivating (SIN) vectors (Zufferey et al. 1998). In these vectors there is a deletion in the 3′LTR including the TATA box. This deletion is transferred to the 5′ LTR resulting in its inactivation. While this modification does not result in lower titers or reduced transduction efficiency it considerably adds to the safety of these vectors.

Finally, retrovirus based systems have been the front-runners of viral vector development and are likely to contribute significantly to both experimental and therapeutic gene transfer in the future. Several hurdles, however, will need to be overcome. These include the moderate titers achieved with current production schemes as well as regulatory restrictions with regard to the use of a vector that is derived from a serious human pathogen.

ADENOVIRAL VECTORS

The development of gene transfer for the future treatment of a variety of diseases has been accompanied by a number of breakthroughs and prominent setbacks. Due to their early presence in the gene therapy field, adenovirus-based vectors have been at the center of some of the most widely publicized events. In the following section we will outline the basic aspects of adenovirus biology, the early contributions to gene transfer, the culmination of extensive research, and vector-development efforts in the serious adverse effects leading to the death of Jessie Gelsinger and the redefinition of the entire gene therapy field as a direct result.

Adenovirus biology

Adenoviruses were discovered in the 1950s as pathogenic agents found in human adenoid tissue (Rowe et al. 1953) and from military recruits suffering from respiratory illness (Hilleman and Werner 1954). Soon thereafter, these agents were named *adenoviruses*. Since then many viruses with similar characteristics have been isolated from humans and animals resulting in more than a hundred members of this virus group, 47 of which are classified as human adenoviruses. To date the family of *Adenoviridae* is divided into four genera, the *Mastadenoviruses* to which the human viruses belong, those limited to bird infections, the *Aviadenoviruses* (Norrby et al. 1976), the ovine *Atadenoviruses* (Both 2004), and the *Siadenoviruses* that are found in frogs and turkey (Davison 2000). During the early studies on adenovirus biology a key observation was made in 1962 when Trentin found that a human serotype of adenovirus (Ad12) could induce tumors in newborn hamsters (Trentin et al. 1962). Although to date no evidence has been found that adenoviruses are capable of inducing cancer in humans, this first notion of DNA viruses as tumor-inducing agents set precedence for numerous subsequent discoveries in the field of DNA tumor viruses. Furthermore, the use of adenoviruses as model systems to study cellular phenomena led to a number of highly significant findings related to cell cycle regulation, DNA replication, and gene expression. The most prominent discovery was made by Sharp and colleagues and, independently, the laboratory of Roberts who demonstrated the presence of spliced mRNA segments in adenovirus late genes (Berget et al. 1977). This discovery led to the identification of introns and ultimately to our current understanding of splicing and was awarded the Nobel Prize in 1993.

The capsids of adenovirus are not enveloped and form an icosahedral structure of approximately 100 nm in diameter. Each capsomer (one of 252 capsid subunits) contains hexons (at the six-fold axis), pentons (at the five-fold axis), a penton base, and an extending fiber that gives adenoviruses their characteristic appearance (Table 68.1).

The genome of adenoviruses (Shenk 2001) is flanked by inverted terminal repeats (TR) of approximately 160 nucleotides that contain origins of DNA replication. The TRs are covalently attached to terminal protein that is essential to the virus replication cycle. In addition, the left-end DNA contains a number of signals between nucleotides 200 to 400 that are essential for the packaging of the viral genome into preformed empty capsids (Grable and Hearing 1992; Hearing et al. 1987). Together, the packaging elements, the TRs and the 5' covalently attached terminal proteins are sufficient *cis* elements for efficient packaging. This has enabled the development of a new generation of adenoviral vector (gutless vectors) that contain only these minimal *cis* elements flanking the gene cassette of interest (potential therapeutic gene). The viral genome is divided into two regions, the early region (encoding the E1, E2, E3, and E4 transcription units) with two delayed early transcripts (IV and IX) and the late region (L1–L5). In addition, the only RNA polymerase III product, VA, from the adenovirus genome is also expressed in the late phase. In general, the transcription units of adenovirus encode proteins of related functions. E1 units encode proteins involved in transcription (E1A) and the inhibition of apoptosis (E1B), while E2 products are involved in DNA replication. E3 products have functions involved in overcoming host defense mechanisms. It might be noteworthy that a generation of viral vector constructs has omitted the E3 region in order to gain larger capacity for transgene cassettes. The exception to the functional unity within the transcriptional units is provided by the E4 region that encodes proteins that are involved in a range of different functions, including transcription, replication, RNA trafficking, and apoptosis (Leppard 1997). Finally, the family of late genes is responsible for the generation and maturation of the viral capsids.

Vector design strategies

The rich history in adenovirus research has left us with a wealth of tools for the generation of recombinant Ad-based vectors. Strategies have been developed that allowed the generation of mutated and deletion variants

Table 68.1 *Selected characteristics of the most frequently used gene delivery vectors*

Vector	Genome capacity	Tropism	Immune response	Genome persistence	Limitations
Onco-retrovirus	8 kb RNA	Dividing cells	Limited	Integrated, long-term	Require cell division, insertional mutagenesis
Lentiretrovirus	8 kb RNA	Dividing and arrested cells	Limited	Integrated, long-term	Limited titers and some applications, insertional mutagenesis
Herpes virus	40–150 kb dsDNA	Particularly suited for neurons	Strong	Episomal, long-term possible in neurons	Immune rejection of infected tissue (except neurons)
Adenovirus	8–30 kb dsDNA	Broad	Strong	Episomal, transient	Innate and cellular immunity
AAV	5 kb ssDNA	Broad	Limited	Episomal, long-term	Limited packaging capacity, slow onset of transduction

of the adenovirus genome that could still be grown to appreciable titers of recombinant viruses. One of the essential reagents to this end is the human embryonic kidney cell line 293 (HEK293) (Graham et al. 1977). This cell line contains the E1 genes of Ad5 and thus allows the production of high titer stock of E1 deleted adenoviruses. Many of the recently employed recombinants simply replaced the E1 region by the transgene of interest. A corollary of the E1 deletion is, that because of the transcriptional activation functions of E1A, the remaining genes of the Ad-vectors cannot be expressed to appreciable amounts. A second aspect of adenovirus biology that has facilitated the development of viral vectors is the capacity of the virus for genome recombination and thus the possibility for insertion of transgenes into the approximately 36 000 bp genome. Wild type adenovirus undergoes recombination at high efficiency in cells that are co-infected with different serotypes (Williams et al. 1975). The precise mechanism of these recombination events is not entirely dissected to date. However, it has been demonstrated that DNA replication is required for these events to occur (Young et al. 1984). This requirement hints at DNA replication intermediates as likely substrates for the extraordinarily efficient recombination reaction. The proposed model for adenovirus DNA replication predicts that replication initiates at both origins within the TRs and proceeds in a unidirectional manner resulting in the displacement of the strand that is opposite of the replicated strand. This strand displacement mechanism results in generation of a single-stranded genome that can form a panhandle structure through hydrogen bonds between the terminal repeats (Lechner and Kelly 1977). It is this single-strand replication intermediate that is hypothesized to be involved in recombination with other serotypes through either strand-invasion of double-stranded genomes or simple annealing to single-strand intermediates of the other serotype followed by DNA repair (Flint et al. 1976). In order to conclude the DNA replication cycle, both products generated in the first round of replication, the double-stranded genome as well as the single-stranded displaced strand, can serve as templates for further replication.

Adenovirus pathogenesis

Much is known about the pathology and pathogenesis of adenovirus infection in humans and it would exceed the purpose of this chapter to summarize the extensive literature addressing these aspects. However, in view of the application of adenovirus as a gene transfer tool, several observations are noteworthy. With respect to preclinical evaluation of the safety of recombinant adenovirus, a key feature is the species dependent replication cycle of these viruses. Although there is some cross-permissivity in closely related species, no

frequently used animal model is suited, e.g. to evaluate the replication of human adenoviruses. This species specificity is illustrated by the requirement of SV40 co-infection to achieve productive replication of human adenovirus 2 even in monkey cells (Klessig and Anderson 1975). Possibly the only model that was able to faithfully replicate the clinical consequences of wild type adenovirus infection in both the respiratory tract as well as in the eye was the cotton rat (Prince et al. 1993; Tsai et al. 1992). Host range mutants have also been described that allow replication of Ad2 and 5 in simian cells (Klessig and Grodzicker 1979; Klessig and Hassell 1978). Although it appears of limited importance with respect to toxicity evaluation of replication deficient recombinant adenoviruses, the availability of faithful animal models would facilitate the evaluation, e.g. of contaminating wild type particles.

An additional aspect of the infectious cycle of adenovirus is the general absence of toxins. Possibly the only exception to this rule is the capsid component penton. It has been demonstrated that, when added to cells in culture, penton leads to a clear cytopathic effect, even though the mechanism of this phenomenon is not yet fully understood (Pettersson and Hoglund 1969; Seth et al. 1984).

A more complex phenomenon of adenovirus infection is the host immune response to infection. Although a comprehensive description of the immunity to adenoviruses is certainly beyond the scope of this chapter, certain aspects deserve further elaboration in light of the death of Jessie Gelsinger, a patient at the University of Pennsylvania who died of the consequences of adenovirus mediated gene transfer that resulted in an overwhelming immune response and ultimately fatal multiple organ failure. It should be pointed out that this event resulted in profound and lasting changes in the then emerging field of gene therapy research.

Much like many viruses, wild type adenovirus encodes a number of immunomodulatory functions and it must be highlighted that recombinant adenoviruses that are devoid of the expression of viral genes are consequently vulnerable to the effects of capsid-mediated host responses. It has been known for more than a decade now that non-permissive infection by adenovirus results in an activation of cytokine networks (including IL1, IL6, and TNF responses) (Ginsberg et al. 1991; Ginsberg and Prince 1994). Immediately after infection the product of the early gene E1A inhibits interferon-controlled gene regulation while VA-RNA blocks PKR activity. Subsequently, the products of the early region 3 counteract apoptosis and the pro-inflammatory actions of TNF-α. Due to the deletion of E1 (involved in the regulation of both cellular and viral gene expression) in most recombinant adenoviral vectors, there is no controlled expression of the adenovirus 'stealth factors' that in fact make up approximately one third of the wild type genome. It can therefore be of no surprise that the high-dose delivery of recombinant adenovirus (deleted for E1 and E4) could result in severe adverse effects observed in one of the patients enrolled in the study.

In general, a major hurdle in the development of future gene therapy is represented by the multifaceted host responses against viral infections. Adenovirus vectors have demonstrated this problem starting from the observation that transgene expression in all tissues was of transient nature in immune competent animals and culminating in the death of Jessie Gelsinger that is now understood to have resulted from the innate immunity to the viral vector (Marshall 1999, 2002).

Adenovirus vectors

To date, several strategies have been employed to engineer adenovirus vectors. It is noteworthy that most of the more recent strategies were designed to minimize the immune-mediated toxicity of the vectors. While first-generation vectors were deleted for E1 and E3 in order to both prevent late-gene expression and to allow for deficient cloning capacity, subsequent modifications such as the deletion of E2 and E4 were designed to lower the toxicity in animal models (Marshall 1999, 2002). The most recent variation on adenoviral vector design represents a more conceptual development in that all of the adenoviral genes are deleted, leaving only the terminal repeats and a packaging signal. These vectors are termed 'gutless' or helper dependent (HD) adenovirus vectors and clearly resemble the design of first-generation adeno-associated virus vectors (Morsy and Caskey 1999; Cregan et al. 2000; Zhou et al. 2002; Palmer and Ng 2003; Imperiale and Kochanek 2004; Mitani et al. 1995; Parks et al. 1996). Although a number of studies clearly demonstrated that transgene expression as a result of HD-adenovirus delivery, it has become evident that transduction is not persistent for the life span of the animal. It remains to be addressed whether the, albeit delayed, loss of transgene expression is due to vector genome loss, residual immune response to capsid components or to contaminating replication competent helper adenovirus. Although a number of strategies have been designed in order to purify the HD vectors, the biophysical similarity between HD-vectors and their helper virus have made this attempt challenging (Palmer and Ng 2003).

Finally, a different strategy takes advantage of the toxicity of replicating adenoviruses and has been proposed for use in cancer gene therapy. The first strategy proposed involved ONYX015, an adenovirus vector that was deleted in E1B (Bischoff et al. 1996). It was hypothesized that the deletion of the inactivating p53 binding partner would render this virus conditionally permissive in p53 deficient cells. Preclinical studies using this construct were sufficiently promising for clinical studies to be conducted (Nemunaitis et al. 2000; Lamont et al. 2001; Nemunaitis and O'Brien 2002a,b).

This study, however, that is in progress in patients suffering from head and neck cancers, has not yet been able to demonstrate a clinical benefit although tumor-specificity was documented (Lamont et al. 2001). It is not clear what additional, possibly cellular, factors are required in order to convert tumor selectivity into clinical benefit. A number of current preclinical and clinical studies are underway to address this question and to validate this promising approach.

HERPES SIMPLEX VIRUS (HSV) VECTORS

Herpes simplex virus is a large DNA virus that has been well characterized (Roizman and Knipe 2001). It has a predilection for infection of neural tissue; for this reason it has been of special interest as a potential vector for gene therapy of the central nervous system. The genome is a linear, double stranded DNA composed of 152 kb which contains two unique segments, each bounded by an inverted terminal repeat. The two segments can be arranged in either orientation with respect to one another so that there are four possible sequence arrangements. The overall genome is bounded by two short terminal repeats. The capsid is icosahedral and enveloped in a trilaminar lipid membrane into which are embedded ten virally encoded glycoproteins, some of which are involved in cellular attachment. A protein matrix, the tegument, separates the nucleocapsid from the envelope. Functions of proteins in the tegument include regulation of induction of viral gene expression and the shutoff of cellular protein synthesis.

HSV life cycle

HSV gene expression is temporally regulated. Induction of immediate early (IE) gene expression requires VP16, a structural protein in the virion tegument. Only two (ICP 4 and 27) of the five IE proteins are required to turn on later gene expression, the other three (ICP 0, 22, and 47) are not required for productive infection of cell cultures. (One of the non essential genes, ICP 47, is involved in immune evasion in the intact host.) Early (E) gene expression products are required for viral DNA replication, while late (L) genes encode the structural proteins. Overall, the HSV genome encodes 84 proteins (Roizman and Knipe 2001). While deletion of the nonessential early genes helps reduce potential pathogenicity in the intact host, deletion of the required IE genes renders the mutant virus unable to replicate and, therefore, absolutely defective. In this manner it is possible to construct HSV vector viruses which should be nonpathogenic, as long as they do not elicit a toxic immune response in the host. The ability to delete significant regions of the genome and the overall large size of the DNA means that the space available for transgene insertion is large. Vector production can be carried out in cell lines which constitutively express the IE genes which have been deleted from the vector construct. In practice, high titer preparations of recombinant HSV can be made (Advani et al. 2002).

The HSV life cycle is notable for the ability of the virus to establish persistent infections in various ganglia. Primary infection occurs through the skin or mucosal surface where the initial round of viral replication occurs. Progeny virions enter neural axons and are transported in a retrograde manner to the cell body where the virus can establish a latent state in which the viral genome is maintained as an extrachromosomal, duplex circular molecule. Latency can be maintained for periods of months or years until activation, usually induced by some form of stress to the host (e.g. superinfection or exposure to toxic stimuli). Activation leads to production of infectious virus, an event typically manifested in the case of HSV as a cold sore. To the extent that persistent infection can be maintained without the threat of multiplication during the primary infection or during reactivation, HSV represents a good potential vector for human gene therapy.

HSV vectors

An alternative approach to the construction of HSV-based vectors, known as amplicons, is to create plasmids which contain both bacterial and HSV origins of DNA replication, viral genomic packaging, and cleavage signals. All of the HSV functions which are required for DNA replication, structural proteins, etc. can be supplied in trans. If the complementing genes have none of the signals required for replication or packaging and no sequences homologous to the amplicon sequences, only the amplicon should be replicated and packaged into vector virion particles. Thus, amplicons are potentially capable of containing extremely large transgenic sequences. However, despite the lack of homology between amplicon and the HSV helper sequences, in practice it has proven difficult to produce vector preparations devoid of wild type virus.

All of the IE genes, with the exception of ICP 47, are cytotoxic; thus deletion of the other four would be desirable. However, it is difficult to achieve high titer preparations if all of the IE genes are deleted. ICP 0, which is a potent transactivator, appears to greatly facilitate vector production. ICP 0 is metabolized differentially in neurons and glial cells; it appears to be degraded in the former. If so, it is possible that vectors containing ICP 0 could have two potential benefits. They could be used for persistent infection of neurons without toxicity, yet they would retain cytotoxic properties which would make them of value in the treatment of central nervous system tumors of glial cells.

There is extremely limited transcription of the HSV genome during a latent infection. Overlapping transcripts are produced from two promoters, LAP1 and LAP2. One approach to vector construction is to create hybrid promoter enhancers which would incorporate a latency promoter so that expression would occur in the latent state. This has proven possible to do. Transgenes inserted into the latency transcript have been found to be expressed in dorsal root ganglia and motor neurons, as well as in the brainstem motor nuclei of mice.

In a primary HSV infection, virus enters at an epithelial surface and undergoes a round of replication before entering the axon and being transported to the body of the neuron in a ganglion. A consideration was whether replication-defective vectors could be expected to get to the axon and be transported in a retrograde fashion. The potential requirement for an initial round of replication at the site of entry can be overcome by introducing a sufficient amount of the vector. Another way of enhancing vector uptake by axons is to inject the vector intramuscularly in which case it is in proximity to the synapse between the axon and muscle. Of course, it is possible to inject virus directly into the brain in cases where the severity of the disease (i.e. glial cell tumors) would warrant a neurosurgically mediated method of introduction of the vector.

ADENO-ASSOCIATED VIRUS VECTORS

The human parvovirus adeno-associated virus (AAV) has been appreciated to have considerable promise as a vector for human gene therapy (Samulski 2003). AAV is a small, nonencapsidated, icosahedral virus with a linear single-stranded DNA genome (Linden and Berns 2000). The virion has a diameter of ~26 nm. The species type virus AAV2 genome contains 4.68 kb. Although the small size of the genome presumably constrains the size of any transgene, the biological properties of the virus have prompted its development as a gene therapy vector. Additionally, recent experiments have suggested that the constraints on transgene size may be overcome (see below). AAV is widespread in nature throughout vertebrate species. There are at least six human serotypes. The most common are the closely related AAV2/3; about 90 percent of adult humans are seropositive (Blacklow et al. 1971). In spite of this evidence for very common infection by the virus, there has been no evidence of association of the infection with any human disease. Indeed there have been several studies which suggest that infection by AAV may protect women against developing cervical carcinoma (Georg-Fries et al. 1984; Mayor et al. 1976; Sprecher-Goldberger et al. 1971).

AAV life cycle

AAV does not undergo productive infection in healthy cells in culture unless there is concomitant infection with a helper virus, such as an adenovirus or a herpesvirus (Berns and Linden 1995). Several types of the latter have been shown to help AAV multiplication. It is possible to render cells permissive for low levels of AAV replication by treatment of the cells with various genotoxic agents (e.g. UV or gamma irradiation, or various chemical carcinogens) (Yakobson et al. 1987). If AAV infects a healthy cell in the absence of a helper virus coinfection, the viral DNA is uncoated, but undergoes minimal, barely detectable conversion into the double-stranded form and is then integrated into a specific site on the q arm of chromosome 19. As long as the cell remains healthy the viral genome remains relatively quiescent in the integrated form; rescue and replication seems to be inhibited by a very low level of expression of a viral regulatory protein. If the cell is stressed by superinfection with an adenovirus or a herpesvirus or by exposure to certain genotoxic agents, the integrated genome is 'activated,' rescued, replicated, and infectious virus made. As described here, AAV is close to a perfect parasite in that it uses the host to perpetuate the viral genome while doing no harm to the host. If, for unrelated reasons, the host is stressed, the virus activates its genome to form infectious particles to find a new host to infect. The facts that AAV causes no apparent disease, yet can persist for extended periods of time in an integrated state, were significant in alerting investigators to the potential use of AAV as a vector for human gene therapy (Hermonat and Muzyczka 1984).

AAV genetics

The linear, single stranded DNA genome contains two open reading frames bounded by inverted terminal repeats (ITR) of 145 nucleotides (nt). The outer 125 nt constitute an overall palindrome which contains two smaller palindromic sequences, one on either side of the midpoint of the overall palindrome (Lusby et al. 1980). Thus, when the terminal 125 nt sequence is folded on itself to maximize potential base pairing, a T- or Y-shaped structure is formed. The open reading frame in the left half of the genome encodes four regulatory proteins (Rep 78, 68, 52, 40) which have overlapping sequences and which regulate all phases of the AAV life cycle. The four proteins are the consequence of two promoters (P5, P19) and an intron (Lusby and Berns 1982; Mendelson et al. 1986). Both spliced and unspliced forms of the two mRNAs are translated, hence four Rep proteins.

The open reading frame in the right half of the genome encodes three structural proteins (P85, P75, P60), again with overlapping sequences (Srivastava et al. 1983). The three coat proteins are the consequence of alternative splicing and the use of an unusual ACG start codon for translation of the middle protein (Muralidhar et al. 1994).

Site specific integration

AAV integration into the human genome is unique in that it is the only known example of a human virus integrating at a specific site (Kotin et al. 1990, 1992; Samulski et al. 1991). The site (at 19q 13.4) is just upstream from the gene for one of the myosin binding proteins (MBS85) and downstream from the troponin I gene (Dutheil et al. 2000, 2004). The integration site sequence has been dubbed *AAVS1* and is a potential promoter. It is likely that the sequence has a relatively open chromatin structure that would render it susceptible to AAV integration. Within the AAV ITR there is a Rep binding site (RBS) and a terminal resolution sequence (TRS) that is nicked by Rep in a sequence-specific manner. A similar sequence arrangement is present in *AAVS1*. Genetic analyses have shown that both the RBS and the TRS are required for site-specific integration (Linden et al. 1996a,b). Interestingly, the length of the intervening sequence is not absolutely fixed, but the sequence significantly influences the frequency of integration (Meneses et al. 2000). About half of the junctions between viral and cellular DNA occur within the viral ITR; the other half occur just upstream of the viral promoter for Rep at map position 5 (p5 promoter) on the genome (Samulski et al. 1991; Giraud et al. 1995). This is of potential significance because studies of plasmid based integration suggest that the sequence from the end of the ITR to the p5 promoter greatly facilitates the frequency of site specific integration. In model systems where *AAVS1* is on a plasmid, the specific integration site clusters around the *AAVS1* RBS. Integration into the genome does not appear to be as tightly clustered. At the cellular level, integration into the q arm of chromosome 19 has been estimated to occur with a relative frequency of 70–100 percent. More recent studies have trended toward the higher figure. At the cellular level the AAV genome is integrated as a tandem repeat which undoubtedly facilitates rescue. Both head-to-head and head-to-tail repeats have been reported (Cheung et al. 1980; McLaughlin et al. 1988). Whether the tandem arrangement is the consequence of limited viral replication or recombination has not been determined.

AAV vectors

Despite the fact that one of the attractive features of the AAV life cycle, which suggested its use as a vector for human gene therapy, was its ability to persist in a latent form by site-specific integration, all of the AAV vectors which have been tested to date lack the Rep gene. The typical AAV vector consists of the transgene(s) with appropriate regulatory sequences flanked at the ends by the AAV ITR. Omission of Rep has been a consequence of two considerations: 1) the Rep gene occupies half of a small genome, so omission doubles the transgene capacity of the vector; 2) Rep is a potent regulatory protein which might be toxic under certain conditions. Since almost all vectors also lack the p5 promoter sequence which has been found to enhance the frequency of site specific integration (Philpott et al. 2002), the current AAV vectors do not have a propensity for site specific integration and most often persist as extrachromosomal elements. The extrachromosomal elements are quite stable and can persist for a year in the mouse model. It seems likely that structures, which can be assumed by the AAV ITR protect the vectors from exonucleolytic degradation. One year after introduction of AAV vectors into skeletal muscle in the mouse a significant fraction of the vector DNA was found to be integrated at apparently random sites in the SCID mouse genome (Song et al. 2001).

AAV virion vector production requires three elements: 1) the vector construct, a transgene flanked by AAV ITRs within a plasmid vector; 2) the AAV genes for Rep and the structural proteins, either in a plasmid or integrated into the genome of a cell line; 3) required adenovirus helper functions, again either on a plasmid or integrated into the genome of the cell line. The appropriate combination of plasmids are transfected into cells in culture to produce vector virions. The major concern is vector production without contamination with either wild type AAV or adenovirus. Using only the adenovirus helper genes, which constitute a small fraction of the adenovirus genome, means that contamination with adenovirus is not a significant concern. Contamination with wild type AAV, on the other hand, is a major concern. Recombination between the vector construct and the AAV helper construct can occur readily if any homology remains between the two DNAs. Even in the absence of overlap homology illegitimate recombination can occur; hence, it is difficult to produce AAV vectors in which no contamination with wild type virus is detectable. In the past it was difficult to generate high titer preparations of AAV vectors. However, development of new cell lines, better helper plasmids, the use of cell factories, and column-based methods of purification have greatly improved the ability to generate sufficient amounts of clinical grade virus so that human gene therapy trials are feasible.

Several AAV serotypes have been tested with respect to their relative abilities to transduce various tissues. Hybrid vectors have been used in which an AAV2 vector genome is packaged into capsids of various AAV serotypes. Striking differences have been observed with respect to the frequency of transduction observed with the different hybrids. Rabinowitz et al. (2002) observed that in vivo Type 1 was the most efficient in transducing liver and muscle, followed by types 5, 3, 2, and 4, in that order. However, when transduction of the rat retina was attempted, types 4 and 5 were the most efficient, followed by type 1. Although others have found some

relative differences in the ability of specific serotypes to transduce various tissues, the general principle is that there are significant differences and that these differences should be taken into account when it is desirable to transduce a specific tissue. All of the available data are consistent with the notion that the differences in efficiency of transduction reflect the fact that different AAV serotypes use different cell receptors. No evidence has emerged to suggest that the differences reflect regulatory variability within the transfected cells. Additional efforts to modify tissue specificity have involved chemical linkage of cell-specific ligands to vector virions or genetic modification of the coat proteins. Limited success has been achieved so far and, with the ever-increasing number of AAV serotypes which are becoming available, the need for specificity may be able to be met naturally. One likely exception to this conclusion would involve vectors designed to kill tumor cells. In this case, a likely vector would be linked to a monoclonal antibody to a specific tumor surface antigen.

Animal models

There have been numerous reports of successful transductions by AAV vectors in animal models. Most often these have been rodent models, especially genetically defined mice, but other species have been tested, including dogs, rabbits, and nonhuman primates. Among the many genetic lesions reported to have been corrected in mice or rats are a model for asthma, hemophilia B, retinopathy of prematurity, erectile dysfunction, phenylketonuria, diabetes, obesity, a model for acute macular degeneration, and Fabry's disease (Samulski 2003). The hemophilia B model is of particular interest because part of the transgene was in one AAV vector and the other was in a second vector construct. Apparently the two polypeptides were able at either the RNA or protein level to come together to form a functional protein (Duan et al. 2001). In the canine model, AAV has been used to correct Factor IX hemophilia and Leber's disease. The latter is of particular interest. Leber's disease, which also occurs in people, involves a defect in a protein, RPE65, affecting the retinal pigmented epithelium, so that puppies are born blind (as are the human patients). However, the disease is potentially reversible if treatment is instituted early enough. Acland et al. (2001) were able to treat blind puppies with an AAV vector containing a wild type RPE gene by injection into the eye. The treated eye gained visual function, but the contralateral eye did not.

A genetic disease which is relatively common, cystic fibrosis (CF), has been modeled in mice and safety tested in both rabbits and nonhuman primates. The AAV vectors have persisted for a long time and there has been no significant toxicity noted.

There have been several general conclusions noted from these animal studies. The first is regarding the relative safety of the vectors. There has been one report of tumor formation subsequent to AAV-mediated liver transduction (Daly et al. 2001), but analysis of the tumors did not reveal the presence of vector sequences and such tumor formation has not been observed in other experiments (Nakai et al. 2003). The affected animals had a specific genotype. The immune response elicited by the vectors has been limited. There has been at least one report of an immune response to the transgene product, but again this is a rare occurrence. Different strains of mice show variable immune responses to the vector coat proteins, thus the ability to re-administer the original vector is also variable. Recent reports of novel serotypes isolated from nonhuman primates (Gao et al. 2004) opens the possibility of a large increase in the number of vector serotypes, so that immune resistance to readministration may be largely mitigated. Various routes of administration have been used, in part depending on the target tissue. All of the routes, including direct injection, iv injection, and inhalation have been successful in specific cases. Of particular note are the high levels of transgene expression achieved in many instances, of ten at therapeutic levels, and the length of time which expression persists. In many cases the duration of expression has approached the normal life span of the mouse.

Clinical trials

Clinical trials using an AAV vector have been carried out with a limited number of diseases. The first studies concerned patients with CF with moderate symptoms. The first trial involved bronchoscopic administration to 19 patients (Flotte et al. 2003). The major finding was the lack of any detectable toxicity over a wide range of dosages. No significant enhancement in clinical status was noted. A second Phase I trial involving 12 patients was conducted by another group who administered the vector by an aerosolized spray. The experiment was monitored by bronchoscopy to gather experimental samples. Vector transfer was dose related: after nebulization involving 1 013 infectious particles, 0.6 copies per brushed cell were noted after 14 days and 0.1 vector copies were found after 30 days. No vector could be detected by 90 days. Vector was noted to the fourth airway generation after the nebulization administration. Although the conclusion from this experiment was that the protocol had been safe, there were six 'serious' adverse events, three of which might have been related to the vector. In a Phase II trial involving CF patients, vector was administered by spray to the maxillary sinus on one side, the other side serving as the control. No statistically significant differences were noted when relapse of clinically defined sinusitis was measured, or

when sinus transepithelial potential difference, histopathology, or sinus fluid IL-8 measurements were made. Only the level of IL-10 was significantly increased at day 90. However, again the safety of the vector was noted. Trials have been carried out on three patients with Factor IX hemophilia. Since adequate serum levels of Factor IX are the goal, the site of protein synthesis is not critical. In this trial intramuscular injection was used. No evidence for toxicity was noted. Vector sequences were detectable in muscle and there was immunohistochemical evidence for expression of Factor IX, along with evidence for a moderate increase in serum levels (Margaritis et al. 2004). A clinical trial has been announced to test the use of AAV to deliver the aspartoacylase gene to patients with Canavan Disease, a neurodegenerative disease characterized by failure to cleave N-acetyl-aspartate leading to inhibition of normal myelination in the central nervous system. Finally, a clinical trial to see whether an AAV vector can lead to therapeutic levels of alpha-1-antitrypsin in serum is close to initiation. It seems likely that an increasing number of trials involving AAV will take place in the near future.

AAV has demonstrated significant promise as a vector for human gene therapy. To date, in both animal and human studies there has been minimal toxicity observed. The major question has been the extent to which humoral antibody to the virion coat might inhibit subsequent administration of the original vector. Occasional reports of possible AAV vector toxicity in animal models either have not been reproducible or have not been demonstrated to have been caused by the vector. There have been no reports of significant toxicity in several human trials. On the positive side, high levels of transgene expression have been noted in a large number of animal trials. This has not yet been achieved in any of the human trials, although lower levels have been observed. In the animal models, expression occurs rapidly and is sustained at potentially therapeutic levels for more than a year in several instances (essentially the life span of the mice used). This is in distinction to the results observed for either retrovirus or adenovirus vectors. The reason for this difference is not known, but may be a reflection of the fact that there is no expression of AAV genes.

Results to date are highly encouraging for the potential of AAV to be used as a vector for human gene therapy. However, before its utility in this context can be considered established, there are a number of questions that need to be answered. Long-term safety will have to be ascertained. The propensity for the vector to integrate in an apparently random manner after long periods of time raises the question of insertional mutagenesis and its potential consequences. Will the results using a Moloney murine leukemia virus-based vector to treat children with severe combined immunodeficiency (i.e. a leukemoid reaction similar to leukemia which was observed more than a year after therapy) occur? Would it be better to develop AAV vector systems which involve Rep expression like that seen with wild type infection so that site-specific integration would occur? Would such systems have toxicity associated either directly with Rep expression or as a consequence of site-specific integration? If the experience with natural infection is a reasonable model, neither of these concerns would appear to have a high probability, but until there is direct testing of vectors, one cannot be sure. A related question is whether integration into *AAVS1* leads to expression at levels comparable to those observed with the vector as an extrachromosomal element. Another issue to be resolved is whether there is a preferred route of administration or does the optimal route depend upon the specific use of the vector. While the latter would seem to be the more likely answer, the extent to which there may be a preferred general route of administration remains to be determined. Animal models have shown that different AAV serotypes have differing levels of effectiveness depending on the cells to be infected. While this stands to reason, the details of tissue and cell specificity remain to be worked out. Also to be refined is the extent to which vector coat proteins can be selectively modified to both enhance and narrow the specificity of tissue or cellular susceptibility to infection by the vector.

Thus, while the effective application of AAV to human gene therapy has not yet been achieved, AAV remains one of the most promising of the viral vectors.

CONCLUSION

Considerable progress has been achieved in the development of viral vectors. After an early rush to clinical trials with an attendant lack of success, it has become clear that the key to success in human gene therapy is a detailed understanding of the basic biology of the viruses relevant to their use as vectors. Areas of continuing concern include tissue and cell specificity, persistent expression, host response, the possibility of insertional mutagenesis, and maintenance of the vector in dividing cells. Because use of gene transfer for therapeutic purposes is not a major philosophical concern, but altering the germ line is, vectors are monitored for their presence in germ cells. Although most viral vectors cannot replicate and often are delivered locally, systemic spread might be considered to be infrequent; but this is not the case. Much of the time at least some of the vector does reach the circulation and is distributed throughout the body. One way to avoid the possibility of germ line contamination would be to develop viral vectors whose tissue tropism was sufficiently narrow that infection of germ cells would not occur. Another concern stated above is insertional mutagenesis. Potentially, it would be possible to minimize this problem by designing vectors which would integrate at specific sites

in the human genome which would not be deleterious. Wild type AAV is the only human virus which is known to do this. However site-specific integration in this case requires the *rep* gene product and cis-active sites on the vector DNA. Work is proceeding to develop such vectors. Another approach would be to develop a system that can lead to efficient homologous recombination between the resident gene and the transgene to correct the inherent defect. Work is progressing in this direction as well. Each of the viruses discussed in this chapter has inherent drawbacks. Three of the four are significant human pathogens. The challenge is to modify such viruses so that they are no longer virulent but retain the capabilities required of a vector. Although not known to be a pathogen, AAV has a limited transgene capacity and the Rep protein required for site specific integration is a powerful transactivator. Hence it must be demonstrated that AAV-based vectors designed to integrate site-specifically are both safe and effective. A similar issue bedevils retrovirus vectors; we have already seen one instance where the use of what was thought to be a 'disarmed' retroviral vector led to the development of a leukemia-like disease of the type naturally caused in mice by the virus used.

In summary, use of viral vectors for human gene therapy retains its considerable promise. We do have one instance in which a lethal disease has been 'cured,' albeit with some therapeutic complications. However, it is clear that a greater understanding of the biology involved with vector administration and more sophisticated engineering of vectors will be required.

REFERENCES

Acland, G.M., Aguirre, G.D., et al. 2001. Gene therapy restores vision in a canine model of childhood blindness. *Nat Genet*, **28**, 92–5.

Advani, S.J., Weichselbaum, R.R., et al. 2002. Friendly fire: redirecting herpes simplex virus-1 for therapeutic applications. *Clin Microbiol Infect*, **8**, 551–63.

Bebenek, K., Abbotts, J., et al. 1993. Error-prone polymerization by HIV-1 reverse transcriptase. Contribution of template-primer misalignment, miscoding, and termination probability to mutational hot spots. *J Biol Chem*, **268**, 10324–34.

Berget, S.M., Moore, C., et al. 1977. Spliced segments at the 5' terminus of adenovirus 2 late mRNA. *Proc Natl Acad Sci USA*, **74**, 3171–5.

Berns, K.I. and Linden, R.M. 1995. The cryptic life style of adeno-associated virus. *Bioessays*, **17**, 237–45.

Bischoff, J.R., Kirn, D.H., et al. 1996. An adenovirus mutant that replicates selectively in p53-deficient human tumor cells. *Science*, **274**, 373–6.

Blacklow, N.R., Hoggan, M.D., et al. 1971. A seroepidemiologic study of adenovirus-associated virus infection in infants and children. *Am J Epidemiol*, **94**, 359–66.

Blomer, U., Naldini, L., et al. 1997. Highly efficient and sustained gene transfer in adult neurons with a lentivirus vector. *J Virol*, **71**, 6641–9.

Both, G.W. 2004. Ovine atadenovirus: a review of its biology, biosafety profile and application as a gene delivery vector. *Immunol Cell Biol*, **82**, 189–95.

Brenner, S. and Malech, H.L. 2003. Current developments in the design of onco-retrovirus and lentivirus vector systems for hematopoietic cell gene therapy. *Biochim Biophys Acta*, **1640**, 1–24.

Burns, D.P. and Temin, H.M. 1994. High rates of frameshift mutations within homo-oligomeric runs during a single cycle of retroviral replication. *J Virol*, **68**, 4196–203.

Check, E. 2002a. Gene therapy: shining hopes dented – but not dashed. *Nature*, **420**, 735, .

Check, E. 2002b. A tragic setback. *Nature*, **420**, 116–18.

Cheung, A.K., Hoggan, M.D., et al. 1980. Integration of the adeno-associated virus genome into cellular DNA in latently infected human Detroit 6 cells. *J Virol*, **33**, 739–48.

Chien, M.L., Foster, J.L., et al. 1997. The amphotropic murine leukemia virus receptor gene encodes a 71-kilodalton protein that is induced by phosphate depletion. *J Virol*, **71**, 4564–70.

Coffin, J.M., Hughes, S.H., et al. 1997. *Retroviruses*. Cold Spring Harbor, NY: Cold Spring Harbor Press.

Cregan, S.P., MacLaurin, J., et al. 2000. Helper-dependent adenovirus vectors: their use as a gene delivery system to neurons. *Gene Ther*, **7**, 1200–9.

Croyle, M.A., Callahan, S.M., et al. 2004. PEGylation of a vesicular stomatitis virus G pseudotyped lentivirus vector prevents inactivation in serum. *J Virol*, **78**, 912–21.

Daly, T.M., Ohlemiller, K.K., et al. 2001. Prevention of systemic clinical disease in MPS VII mice following AAV-mediated neonatal gene transfer. *Gene Ther*, **8**, 1291–8.

Davison, A.J., Wright, K.M. and Harrach, B. 2000. DNA sequence of frog adenovirus. *J Gen Virol*, **81**, 2431–9.

DePolo, N.J., Reed, J.D., et al. 2000. VSV-G pseudotyped lentiviral vector particles produced in human cells are inactivated by human serum. *Mol Ther*, **2**, 218–22.

Duan, D., Yue, Y., et al. 2001. Expanding AAV packaging capacity with trans-splicing or overlapping vectors: a quantitative comparison. *Mol Ther*, **4**, 383–91.

Dutheil, N., Shi, F., et al. 2000. Adeno-associated virus site-specifically integrates into a muscle-specific DNA region. *Proc Natl Acad Sci USA*, **97**, 4862–6.

Dutheil, N., Yoon-Robarts, M., et al. 2004. Characterization of the mouse AAVS1 ortholog. *J Virol*, **78**, 8917–21.

Fischer, A. 2000. Severe combined immunodeficiencies (SCID). *Clin Exp Immunol*, **122**, 143–9.

Flint, S.J., Berget, S.M., et al. 1976. Characterization of single-stranded viral DNA sequences present during replication of adenovirus types 2 and 5. *Cell*, **9**, 559–71.

Flotte, T.R., Zeitlin, P.L., et al. 2003. Phase I trial of intranasal and endobronchial administration of a recombinant adeno-associated virus serotype 2 (rAAV2)-CFTR vector in adult cystic fibrosis patients: a two-part clinical study. *Hum Gene Ther*, **14**, 1079–88.

Gao, G., Vandenberghe, L.H., et al. 2004. Clades of Adeno-associated viruses are widely disseminated in human tissues. *J Virol*, **78**, 6381–8.

Georg-Fries, B., Biederlack, S., et al. 1984. Analysis of proteins, helper dependence, and seroepidemiology of a new human parvovirus. *Virology*, **134**, 64–71.

Ginsberg, H.S., Moldawer, L.L., et al. 1991. A mouse model for investigating the molecular pathogenesis of adenovirus pneumonia. *Proc Natl Acad Sci USA*, **88**, 1651–5.

Ginsberg, H.S. and Prince, G.A. 1994. The molecular basis of adenovirus pathogenesis. *Infect Agents Dis*, **3**, 1–8.

Giraud, C., Winocour, E., et al. 1995. Recombinant junctions formed by site-specific integration of adeno-associated virus into an episome. *J Virol*, **69**, 6917–24.

Goff, S.P. 2001. *Retroviridae*: The viruses and their replication. In: Knipe, D.M. and Howley, P.M. (eds), *Fields virology*, Vol. 2. Philadelphia: Lippincott-Raven, 1871–939.

Grable, M. and Hearing, P. 1992. cis and trans requirements for the selective packaging of adenovirus type 5 DNA. *J Virol*, **66**, 723–31.

Graham, F.L., Smiley, J., et al. 1977. Characteristics of a human cell line transformed by DNA from human adenovirus type 5. *J Gen Virol*, **36**, 59–74.

Haas, D.L., Case, S.S., et al. 2000. Critical factors influencing stable transduction of human CD34(+) cells with HIV-1-derived lentiviral vectors. *Mol Ther*, **2**, 71–80.

Hacein-Bey-Abina, S., Le Deist, F., et al. 2002. Sustained correction of X-linked severe combined immunodeficiency by ex vivo gene therapy. *N Engl J Med*, **346**, 1185–93.

Hacein-Bey-Abina, S., von Kalle, C., et al. 2003. A serious adverse event after successful gene therapy for X-linked severe combined immunodeficiency. *N Engl J Med*, **348**, 255–6.

Harrison, G.P., Mayo, M.S., et al. 1998. Pausing of reverse transcriptase on retroviral RNA templates is influenced by secondary structures both 5' and 3' of the catalytic site. *Nucleic Acids Res*, **26**, 3433–42.

Hearing, P., Samulski, R.J., et al. 1987. Identification of a repeated sequence element required for efficient encapsidation of the adenovirus type 5 chromosome. *J Virol*, **61**, 2555–8.

Hermonat, P.L. and Muzyczka, N. 1984. Use of adeno-associated virus as a mammalian DNA cloning vector: transduction of neomycin resistance into mammalian tissue culture cells. *Proc Natl Acad Sci USA*, **81**, 6466–70.

Hilleman, M.R. and Werner, J.H. 1954. Recovery of new agent from patients with acute respiratory illness. *Proc Soc Exp Biol Med*, **85**, 183–8.

Imperiale, M.J. and Kochanek, S. 2004. Adenovirus vectors: biology, design, and production. *Curr Top Microbiol Immunol*, **273**, 335–57.

Kerr, S.G. and Anderson, K.S. 1997. RNA dependent DNA replication fidelity of HIV-1 reverse transcriptase: evidence of discrimination between DNA and RNA substrates. *Biochemistry*, **36**, 14056–63.

Klessig, D.F. and Anderson, C.W. 1975. Block to multiplication of adenovirus serotype 2 in monkey cells. *J Virol*, **16**, 1650–68.

Klessig, D.F. and Grodzicker, T. 1979. Mutations that allow human Ad2 and Ad5 to express late genes in monkey cells map in the viral gene encoding the 72K DNA binding protein. *Cell*, **17**, 957–66.

Klessig, D.F. and Hassell, J.A. 1978. Characterization of a variant of human adenovirus type 2 which multiples efficiently in simian cells. *J Virol*, **28**, 945–56.

Kotin, R.M., Siniscalco, M., et al. 1990. Site-specific integration by adeno-associated virus. *Proc Natl Acad Sci USA*, **87**, 2211–15.

Kotin, R.M., Linden, R.M., et al. 1992. Characterization of a preferred site on human chromosome 19q for integration of adeno-associated virus DNA by non-homologous recombination. *EMBO J*, **11**, 5071–8.

Lamont, J.P., Kuhn, J.A., et al. 2001. Gene therapy for head and neck cancers. *Oncology (Huntingt)*, **15**, 303–8, discussion 311–4.

Lechner, R.L. and Kelly, T.J. Jr 1977. The structure of replicating adenovirus 2 DNA molecules. *Cell*, **12**, 1007–20.

Leppard, K.N. 1997. E4 gene function in adenovirus, adenovirus vector and adeno-associated virus infections. *J Gen Virol*, **78**, 2131–8.

Lewis, P.F. and Emerman, M. 1994. Passage through mitosis is required for oncoretroviruses but not for the human immunodeficiency virus. *J Virol*, **68**, 510–16.

Linden, R.M. and Berns, K.I. 2000. Molecular biology of adeno-associated viruses. *Contrib Microbiol*, **4**, 68–84.

Linden, R.M., Ward, P., et al. 1996a. Site-specific integration by adeno-associated virus. *Proc Natl Acad Sci USA*, **93**, 11288–94.

Linden, R.M., Winocour, E., et al. 1996b. The recombination signals for adeno-associated virus site-specific integration. *Proc Natl Acad Sci USA*, **93**, 7966–72.

Lobel, L.I., Murphy, J.E., et al. 1989. The palindromic LTR-LTR junction of Moloney murine leukemia virus is not an efficient substrate for proviral integration. *J Virol*, **63**, 2629–37.

Lund, A.H., Turner, G., et al. 2002. Genome-wide retroviral insertional tagging of genes involved in cancer in Cdkn2a-deficient mice. *Nat Genet*, **32**, 160–5.

Lusby, E., Fife, K.H., et al. 1980. Nucleotide sequence of the inverted terminal repetition in adeno-associated virus DNA. *J Virol*, **34**, 402–9.

Lusby, E.W. and Berns, K.I. 1982. Mapping of the 5' termini of two adeno-associated virus 2 RNAs in the left half of the genome. *J Virol*, **41**, 518–26.

Margaritis, P., Arruda, V.R., et al. 2004. Novel therapeutic approach for hemophilia using gene delivery of an engineered secreted activated Factor VII. *J Clin Invest*, **113**, 1025–31.

Marshall, E. 1999. Gene therapy death prompts review of adenovirus vector. *Science*, **286**, 2244–5.

Marshall, E. 2002. Gene therapy. What to do when clear success comes with an unclear risk? *Science*, **298**, 510–11.

Mayor, H.D., Drake, S., et al. 1976. Antibodies to adeno-associated satellite virus and herpes simplex in sera from cancer patients and normal adults. *Am J Obstet Gynecol*, **126**, 100–4.

McLaughlin, S.K., Collis, P., et al. 1988. Adeno-associated virus general transduction vectors: analysis of proviral structures. *J Virol*, **62**, 1963–73.

Mendelson, E., Trempe, J.P., et al. 1986. Identification of the trans-acting Rep proteins of adeno-associated virus by antibodies to a synthetic oligopeptide. *J Virol*, **60**, 823–32.

Meneses, P., Berns, K.I., et al. 2000. DNA sequence motifs which direct adeno-associated virus site-specific integration in a model system. *J Virol*, **74**, 6213–16.

Mikkers, H., Allen, J., et al. 2002. Proviral activation of the tumor suppressor E2a contributes to T cell lymphomagenesis in EmuMyc transgenic mice. *Oncogene*, **21**, 6559–66.

Mitani, K., Graham, F.L., et al. 1995. Rescue, propagation, and partial purification of a helper virus-dependent adenovirus vector. *Proc Natl Acad Sci USA*, **92**, 3854–8.

Morsy, M.A. and Caskey, C.T. 1999. Expanded-capacity adenoviral vectors--the helper-dependent vectors. *Mol Med Today*, **5**, 18–24.

Muralidhar, S., Becerra, S.P., et al. 1994. Site-directed mutagenesis of adeno-associated virus type 2 structural protein initiation codons: effects on regulation of synthesis and biological activity. *J Virol*, **68**, 170–6.

Nakai, H., Montini, E., et al. 2003. AAV serotype 2 vectors preferentially integrate into active genes in mice. *Nat Genet*, **34**, 297–302.

Nemunaitis, J. and O'Brien, J. 2002a. Head and neck cancer: gene therapy approaches. Part 1: adenoviral vectors. *Expert Opin Biol Ther*, **2**, 177–85.

Nemunaitis, J. and O'Brien, J. 2002b. Head and neck cancer: gene therapy approaches. Part II: genes delivered. *Expert Opin Biol Ther*, **2**, 311–24.

Nemunaitis, J., Swisher, S.G., et al. 2000. Adenovirus-mediated p53 gene transfer in sequence with cisplatin to tumors of patients with non-small-cell lung cancer. *J Clin Oncol*, **18**, 609–22.

Norrby, E., Bartha, A., et al. 1976. Adenoviridae. *Intervirology*, **7**, 117–25.

Oude Essink, B.B. and Berkhout, B. 1999. The fidelity of reverse transcription differs in reactions primed with RNA versus DNA primers. *J Biomed Sci*, **6**, 121–32.

Palmer, D. and Ng, P. 2003. Improved system for helper-dependent adenoviral vector production. *Mol Ther*, **8**, 846–52.

Park, F., Ohashi, K., et al. 2000. Efficient lentiviral transduction of liver requires cell cycling in vivo. *Nat Genet*, **24**, 49–52.

Parks, R.J., Chen, L., et al. 1996. A helper-dependent adenovirus vector system: removal of helper virus by Cre-mediated excision of the viral packaging signal. *Proc Natl Acad Sci USA*, **93**, 13565–70.

Pettersson, U. and Hoglund, S. 1969. Structural aspects of the adenovirus type 2 penton antigen. *J Gen Microbiol*, **57**, xix–xx.

Philpott, N.J., Gomos, J., et al. 2002. A p5 integration efficiency element mediates Rep-dependent integration into AAVS1 at chromosome 19. *Proc Natl Acad Sci USA*, **99**, 12381–5.

Prince, G.A., Porter, D.D., et al. 1993. Pathogenesis of adenovirus type 5 pneumonia in cotton rats (*Sigmodon hispidus*). *J Virol*, **67**, 101–11.

Rabinowitz, J.E., Rolling, F., et al. 2002. Cross-packaging of a single adeno-associated virus (AAV) type 2 vector genome into multiple AAV serotypes enables transduction with broad specificity. *J Virol*, **76**, 791–801.

Roe, T., Reynolds, T.C., et al. 1993. Integration of murine leukemia virus DNA depends on mitosis. *EMBO J*, **12**, 2099–108.

Roizman, B. and Knipe, D.M. 2001. Herpes simplex viruses and their replication. In: Knipe, D.M. and Howley, P.M. (eds), *Fields Virology*, Vol. 2. Philadelphia: Lippincott-Raven, 2399–459.

Rowe, W.P., Huebner, R.J., et al. 1953. Isolation of a cytopathogenic agent from human adenoids undergoing spontaneous degeneration in tissue culture. *Proc Soc Exp Biol Med*, **84**, 570–3.

Saib, A., Puvion-Dutilleul, F., et al. 1997. Nuclear targeting of incoming human foamy virus Gag proteins involves a centriolar step. *J Virol*, **71**, 1155–61.

Samulski, R.J. 2003. AAV vectors, the future workhorse of human gene therapy. *Ernst Schering Res Found Workshop*, **43**, 25–40.

Samulski, R.J., Zhu, X., et al. 1991. Targeted integration of adeno-associated virus (AAV) into human chromosome 19. *EMBO J*, **10**, 3941–50.

Seth, P., Fitzgerald, D., et al. 1984. Evidence that the penton base of adenovirus is involved in potentiation of toxicity of Pseudomonas exotoxin conjugated to epidermal growth factor. *Mol Cell Biol*, **4**, 1528–33.

Shenk, T.E. 2001. *Adenoviridae*: the viruses and their replication. In: Knipe, D.M. and Howley, P.M. (eds), *Fields Virology*, Vol. 2. Philadelphia, PA: Lippincott Williams and Wilkins, 2265–300.

Song, S., Laipis, P.J., et al. 2001. Effect of DNA-dependent protein kinase on the molecular fate of the rAAV2 genome in skeletal muscle. *Proc Natl Acad Sci USA*, **98**, 4084–8.

Soudais, C., Shiho, T., et al. 2000. Stable and functional lymphoid reconstitution of common cytokine receptor gamma chain deficient mice by retroviral-mediated gene transfer. *Blood*, **95**, 3071–7.

Sprecher-Goldberger, S., Thiry, L., et al. 1971. Complement-fixation antibodies to adenovirus-associated viruses, cytomegaloviruses and herpes simplex viruses in patients with tumors and in control individuals. *Am J Epidemiol*, **94**, 351–8.

Srivastava, A., Lusby, E.W., et al. 1983. Nucleotide sequence and organization of the adeno-associated virus 2 genome. *J Virol*, **45**, 555–64.

Stocking, C., Bergholz, U., et al. 1993. Distinct classes of factor-independent mutants can be isolated after retroviral mutagenesis of a human myeloid stem cell line. *Growth Factors*, **8**, 197–209.

Suzuki, T., Shen, H., et al. 2002. New genes involved in cancer identified by retroviral tagging. *Nat Genet*, **32**, 166–74.

Trentin, J.J., Yabe, Y., et al. 1962. The quest for human cancer viruses. *Science*, **137**, 835–41.

Tsai, J.C., Garlinghouse, G., et al. 1992. An experimental animal model of adenovirus-induced ocular disease. The cotton rat. *Arch Ophthalmol*, **110**, 1167–70.

Weinberg, J.B., Matthews, T.J., et al. 1991. Productive human immunodeficiency virus type 1 (HIV-1) infection of nonproliferating human monocytes. *J Exp Med*, **174**, 1477–82.

Williams, J., Grodzicker, T., et al. 1975. Adenovirus recombination: physical mapping of crossover events. *Cell*, **4**, 113–19.

Yakobson, B., Koch, T., et al. 1987. Replication of adeno-associated virus in synchronized cells without the addition of a helper virus. *J Virol*, **61**, 972–81.

Yamada, S. and Ohnishi, S. 1986. Vesicular stomatitis virus binds and fuses with phospholipid domain in target cell membranes. *Biochemistry*, **25**, 3703–8.

Yang, Y., Vanin, E.F., et al. 1995. Inducible, high-level production of infectious murine leukemia retroviral vector particles pseudotyped with vesicular stomatitis virus G envelope protein. *Hum Gene Ther*, **6**, 1203–13.

Young, C.S., Cachianes, G., et al. 1984. Replication and recombination in adenovirus-infected cells are temporally and functionally related. *J Virol*, **51**, 571–7.

Zhou, H., Pastore, L., et al. 2002. Helper-dependent adenoviral vectors. *Methods Enzymol*, **346**, 177–98.

Zufferey, R., Dull, T., et al. 1998. Self-inactivating lentivirus vector for safe and efficient in vivo gene delivery. *J Virol*, **72**, 9873–80.

69

Antiviral chemotherapy

HUGH J. FIELD AND RICHARD J. WHITLEY

INTRODUCTION

The science of antiviral chemotherapy has developed over the last 40 years; in the last two decades the rate of progress has accelerated markedly and more new chemical therapeutics to treat viral diseases have been introduced since 1990 than during the whole of the preceding 30 years. Viruses are obligate intracellular parasites that are completely dependent on an intact host cell to provide the ribosomal machinery for protein synthesis. As such, many scientists claimed that 'selective toxicity' towards viruses was unattainable and that the cost of interfering with virus replication would necessarily be unacceptable damage to the host. Historically, lack of susceptibility to antibiotics was considered to be one of the hallmarks of a virus. This gloomy prospect was transformed by a series of discoveries that has now led to effective and safe systemic chemotherapy for many different virus infections. The mechanisms of action and mode of application of some of the best known are covered in this chapter.

Achieving selective toxicity against human viruses

Although the potential toxicity of antiviral compounds remains important, over the last three decades the prescription of safe, systemic antiviral chemotherapy has gradually come to be taken for granted. This revolution was largely brought about by the development of the nucleoside analogue, acyclovir (also known as aciclovir),

which became one of the world's best known medicines with more than 33 million patients treated by the end of the millennium (Darby 1995). Such is the confidence in its safety that it has been administered prophylactically for over 20 years to individuals, apparently without ill-effects, to suppress recurrences of genital herpes (Whitley and Gnann 1992; Tilson et al. 1993). The confidence generated by this one compound provided a completely new background to our current thinking about the development of antiviral chemotherapy and the encouraging prospects for future therapeutic strategies. The emergence of human immunodeficiency virus (HIV) during the 1980s provided a monumental stimulus to the antiviral field; driving research which led to the many new antiretroviral drugs currently available or in clinical development. Herpesviruses, which were historically the most important targets for chemotherapy are currently attracting less interest (Field and Fitzmaurice 2001), while alternative virus targets such as influenza and hepatitis viruses have come to the fore.

The importance of specific diagnosis and early therapy

Useful inhibitors are generally specific for one family of virus and, in some cases, to individual members of that family (e.g. particular members of the *Herpesviridae*). Initiating the appropriate therapy therefore depends on rapid and accurate diagnosis. In fact, often, significant tissue damage occurs before the etiology of virus infection is determined. For many acute respiratory infections that have both short incubation periods and similar clinical signs early in the infection (e.g. caused by rhinoviruses, myxoviruses, or paramyxoviruses) there is a narrow window of opportunity for intervention by chemotherapy following specific diagnosis and this is an important barrier to the development of new compounds. However, experience with aciclovir demonstrated that therapy can be beneficial, even when the infection has progressed for several days, although, as defined below, early therapy is of paramount importance in determining the outcome when treating herpes zoster, herpes simplex encephalitis, and the complications of cytomegalovirus infection. With several virus infections, however, the slow development of clinical signs over many weeks or months allows ample opportunity, following specific diagnosis, to provide benefit to patients with such diseases as HIV, hepatitis B virus (HBV), hepatitis C virus (HCV) and Papillomavirus (HPV). Furthermore, rapid 'bedside tests' to confirm diagnosis of many different virus infections are becoming available and will be increasingly reliable.

The importance of an intact immune system

Another widely held view at the outset of antiviral chemotherapy was that an intact immune system would be a prerequisite for clearing infection. Experience with several excellent inhibitors of viral replication has shown that this is untrue. Indeed, some of the most spectacular successes with antiviral chemotherapy and prophylaxis have been obtained using aciclovir in severely immunosuppressed patients suffering from herpesvirus infections (Meyers et al. 1982) and subsequently highly active antiretroviral therapy (HAART) administered to HIV-infected patients who have severely compromised immunity (Jain et al. 2003). A particular problem in such patients, however, is their tendency to develop infections resistant to antiviral drugs and the approaches to countering this problem are discussed below.

DISCOVERY AND ASSESSMENT OF NEW ANTIVIRAL COMPOUNDS

Molecular targets for inhibition

The obligate intracellular parasitic mode of viral replication determines that it must pass through a series of stages common to all viruses: adsorption; entry; uncoating of the nucleic acid; expression of the genome; transcription and translation of proteins; replication of nucleic acids; assembly and release of mature progeny (Figure 69.1).

So far, almost all the useful inhibitors of viral replication are targeted to one or other of these steps. The mechanism of action of many compounds in current use

involves interference with nucleic acid metabolism; they include the many nucleoside analogues that inhibit herpesviruses and nucleoside and nonnucleoside analogues that interact with HIV reverse transcriptase (reviewed by De Clercq 1992). Several of the early influenza virus inhibitors affect the disassembly of particles by blocking a virus protein complex that acts as an ion channel (Wang et al. 1993). Most viruses induce one or more proteases involved in processing virus polypeptides into functional components. The HIV protease was the first such enzyme to be targeted, and novel inhibitors of the proteases of other viruses are now being developed (Mills 1993). Finally, a series of inhibitors of picornaviruses act by binding directly to the virion capsid, thus blocking the interaction between the virion and the receptor on the cell surface that facilitates its entry and disassembly (Rossmann 1990).

Now that many compounds have been discovered that possess potent selective toxicity against particular viruses, it is ironic that there is renewed interest in compounds that appear to depend upon a cellular function that has a role in virus replication, e.g. the cyclin-dependent kinases as targets for the inhibition of herpes simplex virus (HSV) (Schang 2001). Furthermore, there is considerable interest in compounds that modify the host response to virus infection such as the induction of cytokines or the accelerated apoptosis of virus-infected cells. Examples of such immune response modifiers are imiquimod, which is reported as a treatment for HSV (Harrison et al. 1988) and HPV (Beutner et al. 1998), and resiquimod, which is also used to treat HSV (Tomai et al. 1995).

Drug discovery

SERENDIPITOUS DISCOVERY

In the early days, most new antiviral compounds were discovered by chance (often referred to as serendipity); indeed, several of the earliest antiviral compounds (e.g. idoxuridine) originated from cancer research where there was an interest in using nucleoside analogues to interfere with DNA synthesis and hence to inhibit the rapid division of tumor cells (Darby 1994).

RATIONAL DRUG DESIGN

With thorough understanding of the molecular basis of the replication of many important viruses, the availability of the entire nucleotide sequences of their genomes and the three-dimensional protein structure derived from X-ray diffraction analysis, compounds can be designed to interact with specific targets involved in the virus replication cycle. Among the first molecular targets were virus-induced enzymes which have properties differing from those of counterpart enzymes induced by the host cell. The best known examples are neuraminidase (NA) induced by orthomyxoviruses;

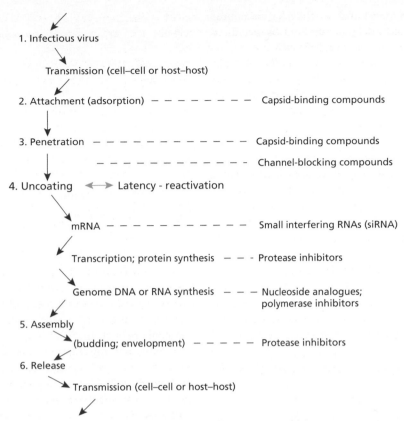

Figure 69.1 *Sites of action for several important classes of virus inhibitors. The classical progression of the virus replication cycle is denoted by the blue arrows. The sites at which the current successful antiviral compounds act are indicated by red dashed lines.*

thymidine kinase (TK) and DNA polymerase (DNApol) induced by some herpesviruses; transcriptase and reverse transcriptases induced by hepadnaviruses and retroviruses; and proteases induced by retroviruses and herpesviruses. Knowledge of such enzymes enables the establishment of biochemical screens to test hundreds of thousands of potential inhibitors and to develop structure–activity relationships. When the enzyme concerned can be crystallized and its three-dimensional structure solved, the synthesis of appropriate molecules to interact with particular sites on that enzyme can be attempted (Laver and Air 1990). For example, the crystal structure of two members of the herpesvirus proteinase family (human cytomegalovirus (CMV) and varicella-zoster virus (VZV)) revealed that they belong to a new class of proteinase with a completely novel protein fold and catalytic site. In some cases, potent inhibitors have been discovered that bind in a region away from the enzyme active site. Such is the case with several useful inhibitors of HIV, the so-called nonnucleoside reverse transcriptase inhibitors (NNRTI) and these will be elaborated on in the HIV section below. This molecular approach to the rational design of new inhibitors is being pursued in relation to HIV reverse transcriptase and protease; influenza neuraminidase and some potential nonenzymatic virus targets, e.g. the picornavirus capsid-binding molecules (Jones 1998).

Although the discovery of future antiviral compounds will rely heavily on these methods, the development of successful drugs still depends on finding molecules with the appropriate pharmacokinetic properties and lack of toxicity, and which can be synthesized inexpensively in large quantities from available precursors; thus, even with the best efforts of the medicinal chemist, relatively few new antiviral agents are likely to become successful antiviral drugs.

Methods for detecting the inhibition of molecular targets directly

STRATEGIES FOR ANTIVIRAL DRUG DISCOVERY

The methods for discovering new antiviral drugs have evolved over the past half century to a high degree of sophistication. The general principles, however, are unchanged. The first or most promising member of a family of related chemical structures that shows antiviral activity is referred to as a 'lead' compound. The overall process of developing an antiviral compound for clinical evaluation can be broken down into the stages of lead generation, lead optimization, and lead development. The virus genome sequence and the study at a molecular level of virus proteins and their functions enables potential molecular targets for attack to be identified.

Methods have been developed in the pharmaceutical industry for screening literally hundreds of thousands of compounds against particular targets. Much use is now made of X-ray crystallographic data obtained from target-inhibitor complexes in drug design and the optimization of lead compounds, in particular the ever-expanding databases of chemical structures such as the Cambridge Structural Database (CSD) for small organic and metallo-organic compounds and the Protein Database (PDB) for polypeptides and polysaccharides. To date, virus-induced enzymes have been particularly useful targets for attack by this means.

VIRUS ENZYME SCREENS

Viruses induce enzyme activities in the infected cells and there are now many examples of the assay of such enzymes in vitro and the screening of potential inhibitors for activity (Öberg 1983b). DNA and RNA polymerases were originally the best-studied systems, particularly in herpes and retroviruses, respectively. The herpesvirus TK was one of the earliest viral enzymes to be studied, because, as well as being a target for inhibition itself (Wright 1994), it is responsible for the phosphorylation of many nucleoside analogues that then become virus DNApol inhibitors. HIV research has largely been responsible for revolutionizing the study of enzyme-inhibitors at the molecular level and the classes of enzyme under investigation has extended beyond the conventional nucleic acid polymerases. In recent years the list of virus-induced enzymes to become targets for effective inhibitors includes retrovirus protease, herpesvirus protease, and helicase primase and orthomyxovirus neuraminidase, and there is no doubt that these will soon be joined by many others.

EFFECTIVE CONCENTRATION (EC$_{50}$) AND TOXIC CONCENTRATION

Antiviral compounds are usually assessed at an early stage for their ability to inhibit viral growth in tissue culture. The virus is generally titrated by means of cytopathic effect, plaque production or some other measure (e.g. infectious center assay). The percentage reduction is usually plotted against the log$_{10}$ of the drug concentration. The concentration of compound that reduces the titer of virus by 50 percent is measured and is usually expressed as the effective dose 50 concentration (ED$_{50}$), inhibitory concentration (IC$_{50}$) or something similar (Figure 69.2). Although the ED$_{50}$ provides the most reproducible value, in some cases the ability to reduce virus yield by 90 percent (ED$_{90}$) is regarded as a more realistic measurement and is sometimes quoted. When expressing results it is important to state the type of cell culture used for the test and the multiplicity of infection because the species of origin, the tissue from which the cells are derived, and whether the cells are resting or dividing can all influence the result. The multiplicity of infection may also be important: plaque reduction tests

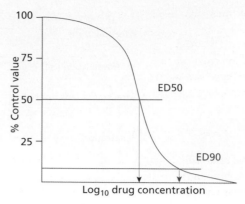

Figure 69.2 *Determination in cell culture of effective dose (ED$_{50}$; ED$_{90}$) for an inhibitor*

are necessarily conducted at low multiplicity but those based on reduction of cytopathic effect or virus yield may be carried out at different multiplicities and this can profoundly affect the result (Harmenberg et al. 1980; Harmenberg et al. 1985b).

A number of important human viruses that are targets for chemotherapy are extremely difficult to grow in convenient tissue culture systems, presenting a major hurdle in the identification and early development of inhibitors. Examples are HPV (Stanley 1993; Stanley et al. 1997; Phelps et al. 1998) and HBV and HCV (Murphy 1993; Main et al. 1998; Walker et al. 2003; Yuen and Lai 2003).

The quantification of compound toxicity is very much more difficult to assess in tissue culture and many methods have been employed (Dayan and Anderson 1988; Newton 1988). They include effects on cell division; cell generation time over several rounds of replication (Field and Reading 1987); cell replication measured by thymidine uptake; cell volume; and various other more subjective measurements of cytopathic effect. Several assays employ vital dyes to assess cell viability, and in these cases colorimetric apparatus can be used to automate the readings (McLaren et al. 1983). Further tests have been devised to assess genetic damage (Evans 1983) and effects on DNA repair systems (Collins et al. 1984) The problems of assessing potential long-term genetic damage by nucleosides is reviewed well by Wutzler and Thust (2001).

An important consideration for both toxicity and antiviral activity in cell culture is that cells from species other than humans are often employed and may give different results (Harmenberg et al. 1985a). Furthermore, cells adapted for tissue culture may provide misleading data in comparison with those actually involved in the natural pathogenesis (Perno and Calio 1994). Experimental work with differentiated cells (e.g. human macrophages or neuroblastomas) or organ fragments (e.g. tracheal rings or ganglion explants) have been used in attempts to circumvent these difficulties. Two important examples of the latter exist. For HPV, raft cultures have been developed Similarly, the trimeric mouse has been utilized to study compounds directed against HCV. Although these methods can provide additional information the results may be difficult to interpret (Bartenschlager 2002a, b; Bartenschlager and Lohmann 2001)

Structure–activity relationships

Having established that a particular chemical inhibitor (lead compound) has a useful selective index against a particular virus or family of viruses, many closely related chemical analogues are synthesized, if possible. These are then screened for antiviral and toxic activity. It often emerges that particular features of the molecule are important and further modifications may be attempted in order to improve or refine the properties of the leading drug for further development. The analysis of such series led to the concept of structure–activity relationship (SAR) and this has been most important in the development of many new drugs. Examples of such series are the 5-substituted 2′-deoxyuridine inhibitors of herpesviruses (De Clercq et al. 1982) and the non-nucleoside reverse transcriptase inhibitors and peptidomimetic protease inhibitors of HIV (Roberts et al. 1990).

ANIMAL MODELS

Animal infection models were essential to the programme of development of most major antiviral compounds in clinical use. This is less true of compounds active against HIV because there is a paucity of suitable models (Koch and Ruprecht 1992).

Infection models for HSV dating back to the 1920s (Goodpasture and Teague 1923) have been developed in mice, rabbits, and guinea-pigs. There is thus a very large amount of published information on the pathogenesis of experimental infections, which aids the interpretation of the different models and the extent to which the results can be extrapolated to human disease (reviewed by Field and Brown 1989). Table 69.1 indicates some of the most important models for studying HSV as a cause of labial, genital, and ocular lesions, and of encephalitis and disease in the immunocompromised host. Such models have been used to provide further evidence of efficacy, to compare different compounds and to study therapeutic regimens. However, their particular strength is the ability to investigate complex features of pathogenesis and their interaction with potential inhibitors. For example, the effects of antiviral compounds on the establishment, maintenance, and reactivation of latency are extremely difficult to study in humans (reviewed by Darby and Field 1984).

Many viruses, including other herpesviruses (e.g. human cytomegalovirus (HCMV) and VZV), have a restricted host range and cannot establish infections in laboratory animals comparable with those in humans. It is, however, sometimes possible to do so using a different member of the same family of viruses, for example murine CMV (Sandford et al. 1985) and feline immunodeficiency virus (North et al. 1993). Clearly, the range of questions that may be asked of such models may be limited, but they can provide powerful systems for studying both the dynamics of drug resistance developing during therapy and counter-measures (e.g. the use of combinations or alternations of drugs).

Table 69.1 *Examples of the many animal models used to study and evaluate inhibitors of herpes simplex virus*

Type of disease	Animal species	Route of inoculation
Orofacial herpes	Guinea-pig	Flank
	Mouse	Ear pinna
		Flank
		Lip
		Foot pad
	Hairless mouse	Flank
	Nude mouse/human skin	Skin
Genital herpes	Guinea-pig (female)	Vagina
Ocular herpes	Rabbit	Cornea
	Mouse	Cornea
Herpes encephalitis	Mouse	Nares
		Vagina
		Cerebrum
		Tail vein
		Peripheral nerve (sciatic)
		Peritoneal cavity
	Rabbit	Olfactory bulb
Disease in immunocompromised host	Mouse (X-irradiated, cyclosporin-treated; nude transgenic knockout, etc.)	Various routes

Animals also play a vital role in the study of toxicity, and a number of statutory tests, both short and long term, are performed in several species in attempts to evaluate the risks of side effects before new compounds enter clinical trials. An important component of evaluation of any drug in animal species, generally two, is the assessment of adsorption, distribution, metabolism and elimination.

Selective index and therapeutic index

The ratio of the 50 percent toxic concentration to the 50 percent virus inhibitory concentration for the compound is often termed the *selective index*. When this is close to unity, the compound is generally taken to be toxic and is very unlikely to become useful. Conversely, a high selective toxicity index suggests a potentially useful compound. It should be stressed, however, that this ratio can be extremely misleading. For example, trifluorothymidine (Kaufman and Heidelberger 1964) has a selective index close to unity yet has been licensed as a topical agent against ocular HSV, for which it has enjoyed some success (Kaufman 1979). There are, of course, many compounds with high selective indices in vitro that demonstrate toxicity only when tested in vivo. Thus, when possible, compounds are tested in animals infected with the target virus itself or a suitable relative for comparison. If inhibition of virus growth and of clinical signs are observed with doses that are tolerated by the host, an estimate of *therapeutic index* (the ratio of the toxic dose to the therapeutic dose) can be made (Field 1988a). This value is generally obtained in suitable animal models; it may remain theoretical for humans.

CLINICAL TRIALS

The evaluation of a potential antiviral drug in humans generally proceeds through several phases, numbered I to IV (Rees and Brigden 1988). Although the boundaries are not always exact, this terminology is widely employed.

Phase I studies

The evaluation begins with the administration of the drug to a limited number of healthy volunteers. It is normally given in small single doses at first, increasing by stages to multiple doses in an attempt to mimic the probable clinical use of the compound. During these studies the pharmacokinetics, pharmacology, and metabolism of the compound are closely monitored. If these results are favorable the investigation may proceed to studies on virus-infected patients.

Phase II studies

The compound is administered to patients with disease, and data similar to those in phase I are collected. This is important because the metabolism of the drug in patients with disease may differ from that in healthy subjects. Phase II studies usually employ controls in order to provide 'proof of principle' data. These data are essential in order to estimate the extent of the drug's effect – information essential for the design of Phase III trials. Limited numbers of patients (<100) are utilized. One should be wary of claims of therapeutic benefit derived from such studies.

Phase III studies

Phase III studies are designed for registration whereby the drug is usually compared against placebo or standard licensed therapies. The main aim is to establish the therapeutic spectrum of the drug and the benefits to be gained from therapy compared with the risks associated with its use (the risk/benefit ratio). These studies require 100–1000 patients.

Phase IV studies

These are generally defined as investigations conducted after obtaining marketing approval. Phase IV studies increase experience of treating patients and provide more information about safety and efficacy. Different formulations, dosages, durations of therapy, drug interactions, and comparisons or combinations with other drugs may be evaluated and special problems such as the selection of drug-resistant mutants detected.

There are many reports of antiviral compounds that demonstrate good selective indices against particular viruses in cell culture and, in some cases, high therapeutic indices in animal models. However, in the absence of appropriate pharmacokinetic properties in humans, only a minority have proved clinically useful.

In practice, most compounds described during the preclinical investigation as active in enzyme screens, cell culture, and animal models, fail to pass through all the phases of clinical studies and many are withdrawn during these evaluations. Nevertheless, for severe and life-threatening diseases, the degree of toxicity allowed to certain compounds may be quite high, including zidovudine for therapy of HIV infections and ganciclovir for treating CMV in immunosuppressed patients.

The remainder of this chapter is confined to the relatively small, but rapidly growing, group of compounds that are currently used for chemotherapy of virus infections or are likely to become clinically useful in the near future.

MECHANISM OF ACTION OF IMPORTANT ANTIVIRAL COMPOUNDS

Of the innumerable compounds known to inhibit one or other of the viruses, only very few have proved useful for treating human infections. The early antiviral compounds that were licensed for use in one or more indications were dominated by those for use against herpesviruses, especially HSV. Subsequently, this emphasis moved to the many new therapies for patients infected with HIV. Currently, the viruses attracting most attention for novel therapies include not only HIV but especially those causing hepatitis. Renewed interest exists for antiviral therapy for influenza. Interest in herpesviruses has, of course, continued in the background and there has been particular progress with the development of treatments for HCMV in immunocompromised patients and newborns.

Inhibitors of herpesviruses

HSV offered one of the most attractive targets for chemotherapy, and thousands of compounds have been discovered that inhibit it selectively. The infections are extremely common and a 1997 survey showed that 62 percent and 16 percent of adolescents in the USA were seropositive for HSV-1 and HSV-2, respectively (Rosenthal et al. 1997). Latent infection is lifelong and is associated with both symptomatic and asymptomatic recurrences with viral shedding on between 15 percent and 25 percent of all days (Wald et al. 1997). With this disease, clinical signs are characteristic, and specific diagnosis (including self-diagnosis) is possible and in many but not all cases can be made when prodromal symptoms occur (Griffiths 1995; Whitley and Roizman 2001). Ocular lesions offer the possibility of topical application. In the normal host, mucocutaneous lesions are almost always

self-limiting; thus, it can be difficult to prove a clinical benefit or, indeed, a lack of benefit from a particular therapy.

ACYCLOVIR; ACICLOVIR; A PARADIGM FOR SELECTIVE TOXICITY

Acyclovir (first published under the name acycloguanosine and now as aciclovir (ACV), Zovirax) is a nucleoside analogue structurally related to the natural nucleoside guanosine (Figure 69.3) (Elion et al. 1977; Schaeffer et al. 1978, reviewed by Elion 1993). To become active, the nucleoside must be converted by three phosphorylation steps to ACV monophosphate (ACV-MP), ACV di- and then ACV triphosphate (ACV-TP) (Figure 69.4) (Fyfe et al. 1978).

ACV is a poor substrate for cellular enzymes, and uninfected human cells convert very little ACV to its triphosphate (ACV-TP). In contrast, the HSV-induced enzyme TK can, albeit with relatively low efficiency, convert ACV to ACV-MP. Thus the HSV TK recognizes ACV as thymidine but the fact that cellular enzymes convert ACV-MP successively to the di- and triphosphate only within virus-infected cells accounts for the extremely high selective index of the compound (Darby 1995). ACV-TP enters the cellular nucleotide pool where it competes with guanosine triphosphate as a substrate for HSV DNApol. ACV-TP is a particularly potent inhibitor of HSV DNApol (the inhibition constant, K_i, versus the natural substrate, deoxyguanosine, is ca. 0.01 μm) and this appears to provide further selectivity, because cellular DNApols are much less sensitive to

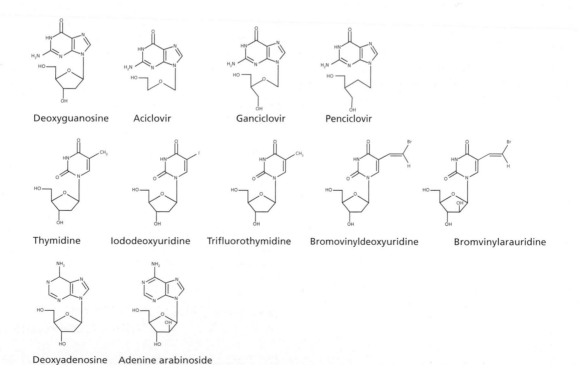

Figure 69.3 *Nucleoside analogues related to the natural nucleosides, deoxyguanosine, thymidine, and deoxyadenosine. The natural molecules are shown in blue. Red denotes those parts of the synthetic compounds that vary from the natural structures.*

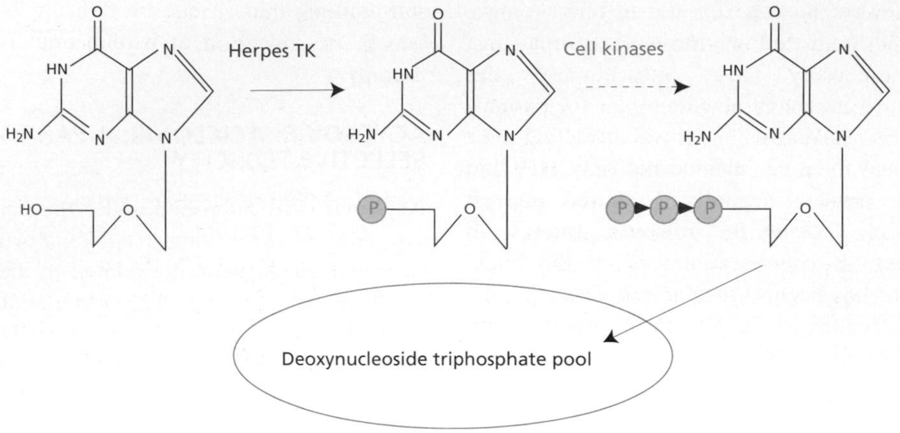

Figure 69.4 *The mechanism of action of aciclovir: activation*

inhibition. As the ACV residue is linked to the growing chain of virus DNA, it forms a chain terminator since there is no 3'-OH group on the ACV sugar moiety to link to the next residue in the growing chain of virus DNA (Figure 69.5) (Furman et al. 1979). ACV may thus be described as an obligate chain terminator.

In summary, ACV is taken up and phosphorylated in significant amounts only by HSV-infected cells and inhibits virus DNA synthesis, thus preventing the production and release of infectious progeny virus.

Clinically, ACV is licensed worldwide in topical, oral, and intravenous formulations. Generally, the drug is effective when given systemically for primary and recurrent genital HSV infections (Bryson et al. 1983; Mertz et al. 1984; Goldberg et al. 1993), mucocutaneous HSV in immunocompromised hosts and life-threatening infections, e.g. encephalitis and neonatal disease (Whitley et al. 1986, 1991). It is also an effective therapy for chickenpox (Balfour et al. 1990; Dunkle et al. 1991; Wallace et al. 1992) and herpes zoster in normal (Crooks et al. 1991) and immunocompromised hosts (Griffiths 1995).

NUCLEOSIDE ANALOGUES RELATED TO ACV

Following the discovery and development of ACV, many other nucleoside analogues with similar modes of

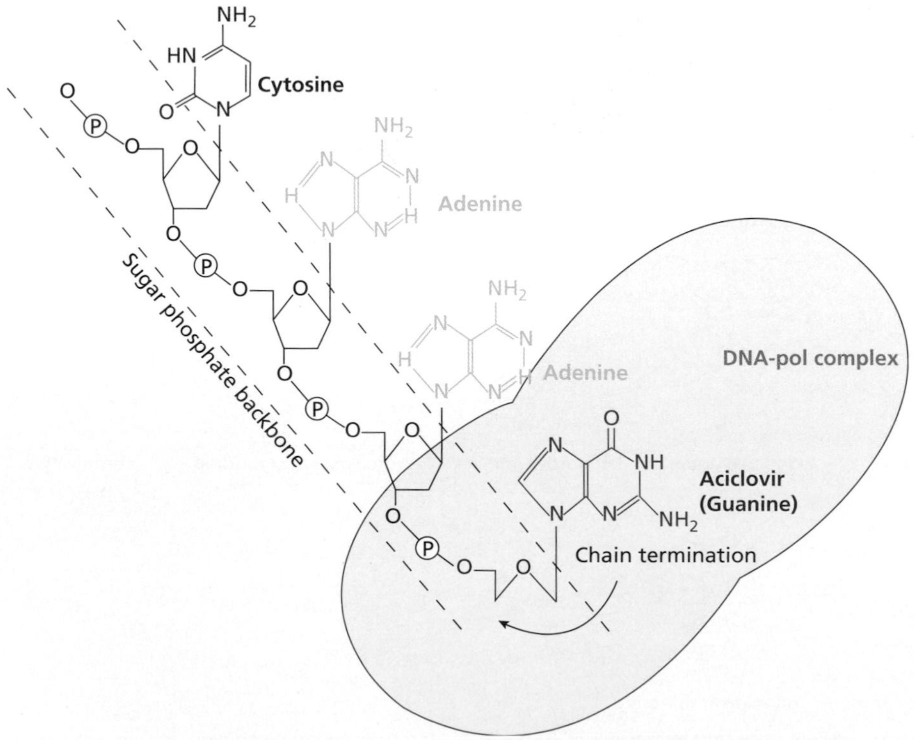

Figure 69.5 *The mechanism of action of aciclovir: inhibition of DNA synthesis and chain termination*

action were described. Some have high selective indices similar to or higher than that of ACV and several have been developed for clinical use. Each new compound, even those with close structural similarities with ACV (e.g. ganciclovir and penciclovir), has individual properties that differ from those of ACV, although the differences may be very subtle (Darby 1995). It is most important that this is kept in mind when comparing the antiviral efficacy and potential toxicity of such compounds with those of ACV (Wutzler and Thust 2001).

Ganciclovir

Figure 69.3 shows that ganciclovir (GCV), Cymevene or Cytovene has a structure similar to ACV, with an additional carbon atom in the sugar moiety and the presence of a 3'-OH group (Smee et al. 1983). The compound therefore differs from ACV in that further extension of the DNA chain is possible after incorporation of GCV triphosphate (GCV-TP). Although the compound shows significant toxicity in humans, its spectrum of action is broader than that of ACV and includes HCMV (Freitas et al. 1985; Matthews and Boehme 1988). Unlike HSV, HCMV does not encode a TK. Studies of viruses with acquired resistance to GCV have, however, revealed that a previously unsuspected virus enzyme is responsible for the metabolic conversion from GCV to GCV monophosphate (GCV-MP) (Littler et al. 1992; Sullivan et al. 1992). The enzyme is a product of CMV gene *UL97*, a discovery that focused attention on this gene which codes for a protein with close homology to several

eukaryotic protein kinases. The precise function of the virus enzyme is thought to concern export of HCMV nucleocapsids from the nucleus (Krosky et al. 2002). Once formed in the CMV-infected cells, GCV-TP inhibits CMV DNApol and virus replication is prevented.

Clinical use of GCV has focused on patients at high risk for CMV disease (Fan-Havard et al. 1989; Levinson and Jacobson 1992; Balfour 1999). Thus, individuals with AIDS benefit from GCV therapy of retinitis and gastrointestinal disease. Oral administration of GCV delays onset of end-organ disease in patients with AIDS who have CD4 counts <200/μl. Similarly, GCV delays the onset of CMV disease in organ transplant recipients. Poor bioavailability and the problem of toxicity limit the value of the compound. The prodrug of GCV, val-ganciclovir (Figure 69.6), has been proven to provide higher oral bioavailability and is now licensed for the treatment of CMV retinitis. However, toxicity remains a problem.

Recently, intravenous GCV has been shown useful for the treatment of symptomatic congenital CMV infection (Kimberlin et al. 2003).

Penciclovir

Penciclovir (PCV), Vectavir or Adenovir, is another nucleoside analogue in which the base, guanine, is normal but the sugar moiety has a structural modification (Boyd et al. 1987). The structural similarity to ACV is apparent (see Figure 69.3); there is, however, no oxygen atom in the acyclic 'sugar' moiety although an OH group exists in the position equivalent to that of the 3'-OH group in the normal nucleoside, guanosine. Like

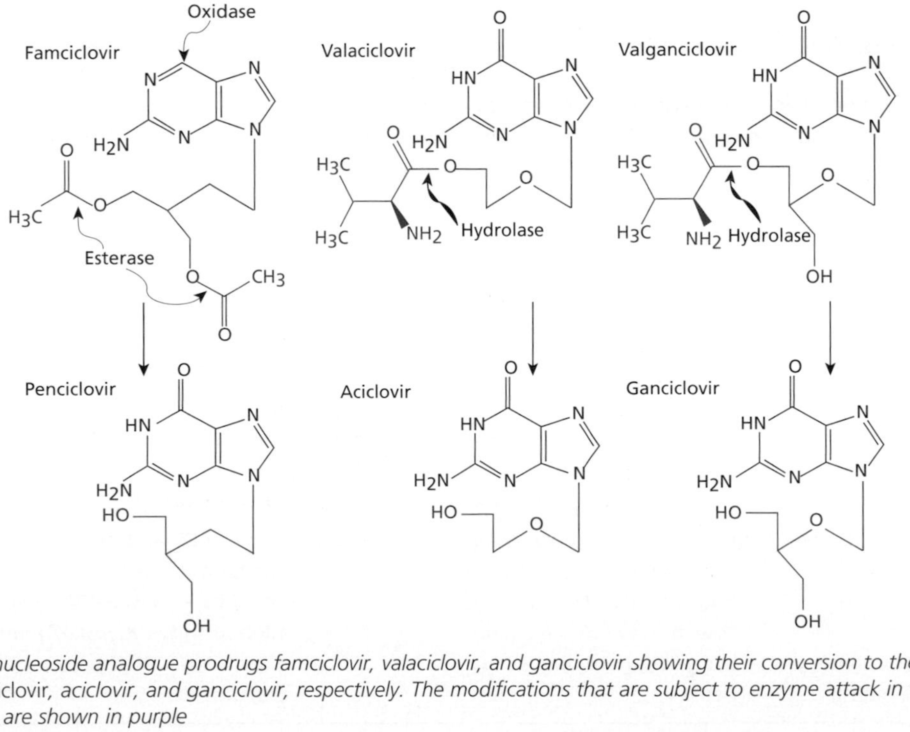

Figure 69.6 The nucleoside analogue prodrugs famciclovir, valaciclovir, and ganciclovir showing their conversion to the active metabolites, penciclovir, aciclovir, and ganciclovir, respectively. The modifications that are subject to enzyme attack in vivo, providing oral bioavailability are shown in purple

ACV, PCV is converted to PCV-monophosphate (PCV-MP) by the HSV or VZV TK (Vere Hodge and Cheng 1993), and PCV-triphosphate (PCV-TP) inhibits the viral DNApol but with the possibility of internal incorporation of PVC residues into viral DNA and further chain extension (Vere Hodge and Perkins 1989). The initial conversion of PVC to PCV-MP is more efficient than the phosphorylation of ACV, but the PCV-TP formed in infected cells is less active than ACV-TP as an inhibitor of HSV DNApol (Table 69.2) (Earnshaw et al. 1992).

PCV-TP has a significantly longer intracellular half-life than ACV-TP (Vere Hodge and Perkins 1989). Although the full implications of this observation have yet to be elucidated, it does seem that the compound may have more long-lasting inhibitory effects in infected tissues; this supposition is supported by tests in animals that compared famciclovir (FCV) and valaciclovir (VACV) (Sutton and Kern 1993; Field et al. 1995). It remains to be seen whether this biochemical feature translates into clinical benefit in humans. Although the compound seems to have a very high selective index, the bioavailability is poor (<5 percent in man) and the drug chosen initially for clinical development is a prodrug of PCV termed FCV, increasing the bioavailability of PCV to >70 percent.

As well as good activity against members of the *Herpesviridae*, PCV has limited activity against HBV (Boker et al. 1994; Locarnini et al. 1994). Thus far, no mechanism of action for this unexpected activity has been reported; it is, however, likely to involve specific inhibition of the HBV-induced DNApol although there is no explanation as yet for the phosphorylation of PCV in the infected hepatocytes.

Brivudin; bromovinyl deoxyuridine

Historically, brivudin, or bromovinyl deoxyuridine (BVDU), Helpin or Zostrex was discovered at about the same time as ACV (De Clercq et al. 1979) and, in vitro, appeared to be even more active than ACV against HSV-1 and VZV (De Clercq et al. 1980). However, the drug proved less useful than was anticipated. It is much more closely related to the natural substrate for TK (i.e. thymidine) with the modification of the bromovinyl group at the five position of the pyrimidine ring (see Figure 69.3).

The mechanism of action resembles that of ACV except that the conversion of BVDU-monophosphate (BVDU-MP) to BVDU-diphosphate (BVDU-DP) seems also to be achieved by the HSV TK (Descamps et al. 1982). The virus (but not cellular) TK thus possesses a thymidylate kinase activity. BVDU is significantly less active against HSV-2, probably because of the lack of conversion of BVDU-MP to BVDU-DP by the HSV-2 TK (De Clercq et al. 1981). A limitation of the compound in vivo is attack by phosphorylases that convert BVDU to bromovinyl ara-uracil, which is inactive. This, and concern about toxicity, has limited the development of the compound for clinical use; even so, the principles discovered during the development of this drug and SAR studies have led to several compounds (e.g. bromovinyl ara-uridine) that seem more promising. For a comprehensive review of brivudin see De Clercq (2004).

Sorivudine; bromovinylarabinosyl-uracil; brovavir

The mechanism of action of sorivudine, or bromovinylarabinosyl-uracil (BVaraU), Usevir (see Figure 69.3), seems similar to that of BVDU (Yokota et al. 1989; Machida 1990); its spectrum of action is, however, different and it seems to be some 2 000-fold more active than ACV or BVDU against VZV replication in cell culture (ED$_{50}$ = 0.001 μm, compared with 14 μM for ACV) (Machida and Nishitani 1990). Like BVDU, however, the compound is poorly active against HSV-2. It is an extremely good substrate for VZV TK and its antiviral activity is attributed to the inhibition by BVaraU-TP of VZV DNApol; the compound is thought not to be incorporated into virus DNA. Unfortunately, one of the metabolites is bromovinylarabinosyl-uracil (BVU), a potent inhibitor of dihydrothymine dehydrogenase which is responsible for degrading drugs such as 5-fluorouracil that are used in cancer chemotherapy. Although this interaction was predicted, a number of deaths have occurred as a result of co-administration of the two drugs (Meeting Report 1995) (see section entitled The problem of toxicity of antiviral compounds). As a consequence, the compound will not be licensed in the USA. However, clinical benefit has been demonstrated against VZV disease in a

Table 69.2 *Comparison of key biochemical properties of the guanosine analogues aciclovir and penciclovir which are produced in vivo by their respective prodrugs, valaciclovir and famciclovir*

	Famciclovir	Valaciclovir
Oral absorption and blood pharmacokinetics parental compounds and production of PCV and ACV are similar		
	Penciclovir	Aciclovir
HSV1 thymidine kinase	High affinity (K_i = 1.5 μ m)	Low affinity (K_i = 173 μ m)
HSV1 DNApol	Low affinity (K_i = 8.5 μ m)	High affinity (K_i = 0.07 μ m)
Stability of triphosphate	Long ($t_{1/2}$ = 10 h)	Short ($t_{1/2}$ = 0.7 h)
DNA chain terminating	Rapid	Obligate

well-controlled clinical trial in comparison with ACV (Gnann et al. 1998).

Vidarabine; adenine arabinoside

Vidarabine, or adenine arabinoside (AraA), was an important landmark in the development of antiviral chemotherapy (Schabel 1968), being among the early compounds that achieved proven clinical benefit with relatively little acute toxicity, particularly in the systemic treatment of severe HSV infections (Whitley et al. 1977). The compound is a close analogue of adenine except that the OH group in the 2′ position on the 'sugar' moiety is in the unnatural 'arabinosyl' configuration (see Figure 69.3). The nucleotides formed from the phosphorylation of AraA have the potential to interfere with many different steps in the metabolism of DNA and its precursors, for example blocking of S-adenosyl homocysteine hydrolase (Hersfield 1979). The relative importance of these effects is unknown but, as with the other nucleoside analogues, the primary target for AraA-triphosphate (AraA-TP) seems to be the HSV-induced DNApol. The compound has low toxicity and may be used systemically, but its poor solubility necessitates the intravenous administration of large quantities of fluids. Secondly, its activity in vivo is limited by rapid deamination of AraA by adenosine deaminase, yielding arabinosyl-hypoxanthine which has no antiviral activity (Whitley et al. 1980a). Attempts to circumvent this problem by the administration of AraA-monophosphate (ARA-MP) have enjoyed little success (Whitley et al. 1980b). Today, vidarabine has largely been replaced in the physician's armamentarium for systemic therapy by more active and less toxic medications.

Idoxuridine

The pyrimidine analogue, idoxuridine (IDU), (e.g. Herpid, Kerecid, Virudox, Idurin, Stoxil) was the first specific antiviral compound to be discovered (Prusoff 1959). and is the best known example of the 5-substituted thymidine series; it is similar to BVDU. However, IDU does not possess the high selectivity associated with the more modern drugs. This 'first generation' nucleoside analogue is readily phosphorylated by cellular enzymes and thus can be converted to the active nucleotide in normal, as well as in virus-infected, cells although the conversion is much more efficient in the latter. The IDU triphosphate (IDU-TP) inhibits viral (and cellular) DNA synthesis, but a major part of the antiviral action may be due to incorporation of the analogue into viral nucleic acids and subsequent perturbation of virus gene expression (De Clercq 1982). The exact mechanism of action is unknown but some selectivity is assumed to result from the comparatively greater accumulation of IDU-TP in infected cells. IDU is, however, severely toxic upon systemic administration

and is useful only as a topical agent, for which it continues to be useful both for herpes zoster and HSV keratitis. Skin penetration is a problem for topical administration. While formulations have been prepared in dimethyl sulfoxide (DMSO) for treating zoster (Dawber 1974; reviewed by Spruance 1994), they have been replaced by oral therapy with ACV, VACV, and FCV. Notwithstanding its traditional use for treating HSV in humans, the potential long-term genetic toxicity of this compound remains a major concern.

Trifluridine; trifluorothymidine

Like IDU, trifluridine (TFT), or trifluorothymidine Viroptic, (see Figure 69.3), synthesized in 1964 (Heidelberger et al. 1964), is also highly toxic and is unsuitable for systemic use. Even to demonstrate its selective antiviral effect in cell culture requires the use of cells lacking TK that are resistant to its toxic effects (Field et al. 1981). However, the compound is very soluble and has found a particular use in the topical treatment of ocular infections (Wellings et al. 1972). The very rapid hydrolysis of TFT to harmless metabolites probably accounts for the lack of toxicity in this application (Dexter et al. 1972). It is the treatment of choice for HSV keratoconjunctivitis (reviewed by Bigar 1979). The compound is reported to be effective against drug-resistant strains and remains in the armoury of anti-herpes drugs despite its toxicity in vitro.

NUCLEOSIDE ANALOGUE PRODRUGS

An important limitation of many nucleoside analogues is their poor bioavailability following oral administration. The development of orally bioavailable compounds that are converted in vivo to yield the relevant nucleoside analogues thus represents a major advance. The first compounds of this type were developed for herpes chemotherapy and the first to be licensed for use in humans were derived from ACV and PCV. Following this paradigm, a similar strategy has now been successfully applied to many different compounds including nucleosides active against alternative virus targets. Note that, technically, ACV itself is a 'prodrug' since the mechanism of action involves conversion of absorbed ACV to the active metabolite (ACV-TP) in vivo. However, in the antiviral field, the term prodrug is usually reserved for compounds where the first chemical conversion in vivo is primarily concerned with significantly improving bioavailability.

Valaciclovir

VACV Valtrex, Zelitrex is the L-valine ester of ACV (Figure 69.6) which, following oral administration, is cleaved in the gastrointestinal tract by an enzyme referred to as VACV hydrolase to yield ACV and the natural amino acid L-valine, little VACV being detected in plasma (Beauchamp et al. 1992). Multiple oral doses of VACV (>1 g four times daily) result in plasma ACV concentrations similar to those achieved with intravenous ACV (5 or 10 mg/kg three times daily) but without the sharp peak concentrations (Carrington 1994; Crooks 1995). Once formed and distributed to the infected tissues, the mode of action is, of course, identical to that of simple ACV. This compound offers a formulation that is more convenient to administer for the treatment of herpes zoster than ACV (Murray 1995).

Famciclovir

The concept that led to VACV also resulted in FCV (Vere Hodge et al. 1989), the diacetyl ester of 6-deoxy-penciclovir (Figure 69.6). In this case two enzymes are involved, first in removing one ester preferentially, then the second, followed by oxidation by aldehyde oxidase to yield PCV (Vere Hodge 1993). The only degradation products from this reaction are harmless carboxylic acid and PCV and, as with VACV, little FCV is detected in plasma. Ease of administration provides a distinct advantage over ACV in the treatment of herpes zoster (Carrington 1994).

Have the nucleoside analogue prodrugs VACV and FCV met the clinical challenge? Following a decade of clinical experience with these nucleoside prodrugs, have the hoped-for improvements in antiviral efficacy been realized? The consensus is that both compounds do offer significant clinical benefits over oral ACV (Field 1996; Baker and Eisen 2003). However, the relative merits of the two new compounds in comparison with one another remain controversial (Carrington 1994, 1997). The disruption to the preclinical and clinical development teams associated with these drugs caused by the merger of the two giant pharmaceutical companies, GlaxoWellcome and SmithKlineBeecham, in the year 2000 may help to explain why there is still a paucity of data from clinical trials on the relative advantages and disadvantages of the two compounds under circumstances where they may be compared directly (Field and Fitzmaurice 2001).

NUCLEOTIDE ANALOGUES

A series of acyclic purine and pyrimidine nucleoside phosphonates was first described in 1986 (De Clercq et al. 1986). Several of these compounds showed a broad spectrum of activity against viruses, including both DNA and RNA viruses. Unlike the natural nucleotides, the acyclic nucleoside phosphonates (ANP) resist phosphorolytic cleavage by cellular esterases. The negative charge on the phosphate moiety impairs their cellular uptake which may occur by an endocytosis-like process. Once inside the cells, the ANP compounds need to be activated by cellular enzymes to catalyse their conversion to di- and tri-phosphorylated forms. The virus inhibitory

effects then result from a selective interaction of their diphosphate metabolites with virus DNA pol (Votruba et al. 1987), thus their ultimate antiviral target is the same as that described above for the regular nucleoside analogues. A general feature of ANPs is the long intracellular half-life of the diphosphate metabolite, which may help to explain their long-lasting antiviral effects allowing infrequent dosing. The mechanisms of action of this series of compounds are thoroughly reviewed by De Clercq (1997)

Cidofovir (Vistide)

Cidofovir, (S)-1-(3-hydroxy-2-phosphonylmethoxypropyl) cytosine (HPMPC, Forvade) (Figure 69.7). As mentioned above, HPMPC viz. has a very long tissue half-life; it has been shown in many animal models that long intervals between doses can be allowed without loss of antiviral effect. Thus, once weekly dosing is employed in humans with apparent success (Snoeck et al. 1993). The compound has significant toxic side effects, particularly nephrotoxicity, although this can be minimized by co-administration of probenecid (which competitively inhibits the transport of drugs through the glomeruli) and intravenous hydration. Intravenous HPMPC is licensed for treatment of HCMV retinitis and topical gel used for the treatment of refractory HSV lesions in AIDS patients. Its spectrum of action extends beyond herpesviruses and includes poxviruses, HPV and HBV (see below). Other important compounds in this series include 9-(2-phosphonylmethoxyethyl) adenine (PMEA) (adefovir), which is active against herpes- retro- and hepadnaviruses, and R-9-(2-phosphonylmethoxypropyl) adenine (PMPA), which is active against retro- and hepadnaviruses. Following the prodrug strategy outlined above for the guanosine nucleosides, the oral prodrug of PMEA, bis(pivaloyloxymethyl) PMEA or adefovir dipivoxil (Naesens et al. 1996) is a very promising compound for the treatment of HBV (see section entitled Inhibitors of hepatitis viruses below)

PYROPHOSPHATE ANALOGUES

A series of compounds has been known for many years whose members interact directly with herpesvirus DNApol at the pyrophosphate binding site. This was first shown with phosphonacetic acid (Purifoy et al. 1977), a compound too toxic for humans. However, the closely related compound phosphonoformate (Figure 69.8) has been developed for use in man in the treatment of CMV disease in immunocompromised hosts. Its administration is associated with toxicity as evidenced by electrolyte imbalances (reviewed by Öberg 1983a).

Phosphonoformic acid

Phosphonoformate (PFA), foscarnet, foscavir (Figure 69.8) seems to have a relatively simple mode of action, being a

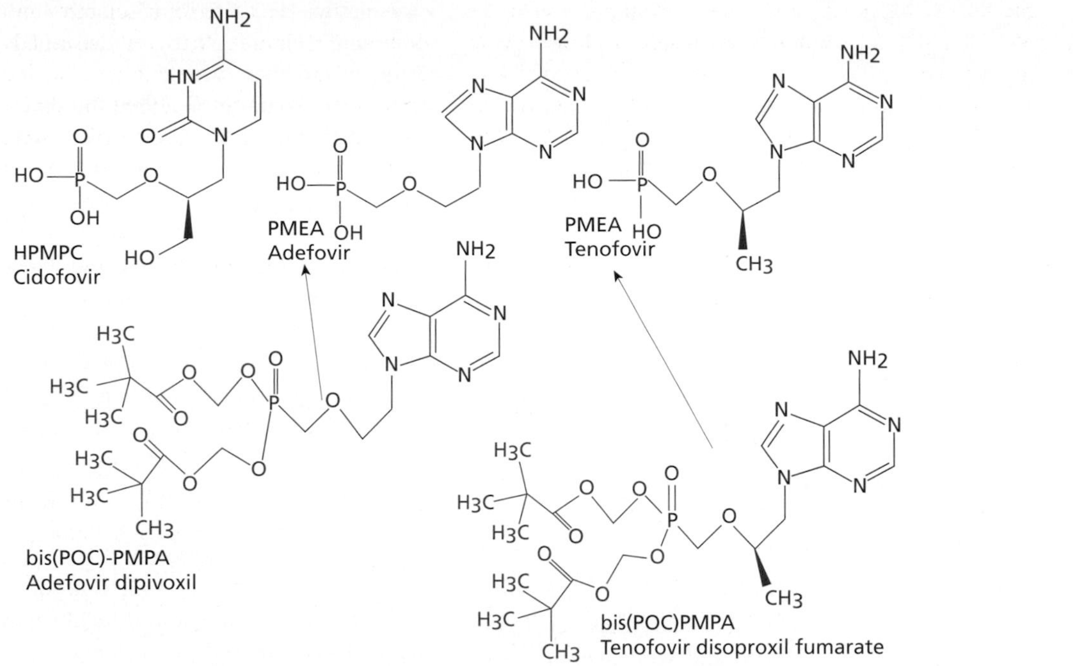

Figure 69.7 *Examples of effective inhibitors of virus polymerase: phosphonyl compounds cidofovir, adefovir, and tenofovir and two prodrugs that yield adefovir and tenofovir, respectively. The modifications to the compounds that provide oral bioavailability are shown in purple.*

direct inhibitor of HSV DNApol (Leinback et al. 1976). The compound suffers from some toxic features, and its tendency to accumulate in bone (Crisp and Clissold 1991) is of particular concern. It does, however, offer an alternative strategy for treating both infections with ACV-resistant strains of HSV and CMV retinitis in AIDS patients (Fanning et al. 1990).

ALTERNATIVE ENZYME TARGETS FOR HERPESVIRUS INHIBITORS

Most of the successful antiherpetic agents, to date, target the virus DNApol. Among the more than 80 distinct genes in the HSV genome, there are several other obvious enzyme targets for inhibition including ribonucleotide reductase (RR), protease, and helicase primase. There has been much effort to target herpes RR including synthetic oligopeptides directed to the enzyme

active site. To date, none of these approaches has resulted in useful therapies. Given the success of compounds directed to the HIV protease (see section entitled Inhibitors of human immunodeficiency virus, below). It is likely that compounds designed to interfere with the herpes proteases will be effective (reviewed by Waxman and Darke 2000), but to date, none have been developed for clinical use. Another function that has been exploited is the HSV helicase primase. This is a virus enzyme that promotes the ATP-dependent unwinding of the DNA duplex during replication and it appears that compounds directed to it can inhibit virus replication at nanomolar concentrations.

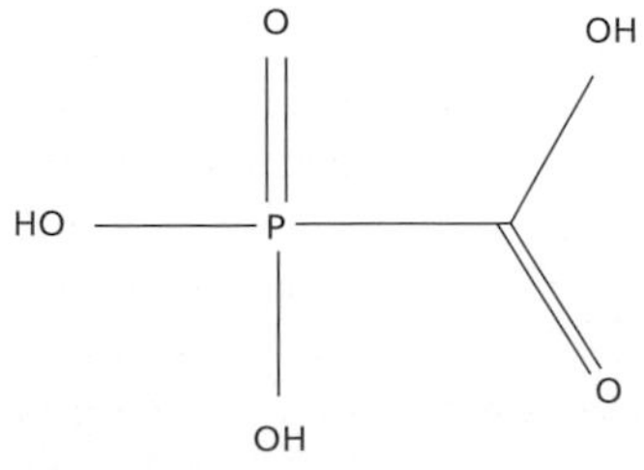

BAY-57-1293

The thiazolylsulfonamide, BAY-57-1293 (N-[5-(aminosulfonyl)-4-methyl-1,3-thiazol-2-yl)-N-methyl-[4-(2pyridinyl)phenyl]acetamide) (Figure 69.9) is an example of an inhibitor of herpes helicase primase (Kleymann et al. 2002, 2004). The compound is highly selective and extremely active in vitro with an IC_{50} concentration of approximately 20 nM (i.e. some 500-fold more active than ACV), furthermore, it is reported to be remarkably effective in several different laboratory animal HSV infection models. Other similarly potent molecules from different chemical series have also been described (Field and Fitzmaurice 2001). Although these particular compounds may not progress to the clinic, the experimental data clearly show that inhibition of this target has considerable potential and it is likely that effective

Figure 69.8 *An inhibitor of herpes DNA polymerase: the pyrophosphate analogue, foscarnet*

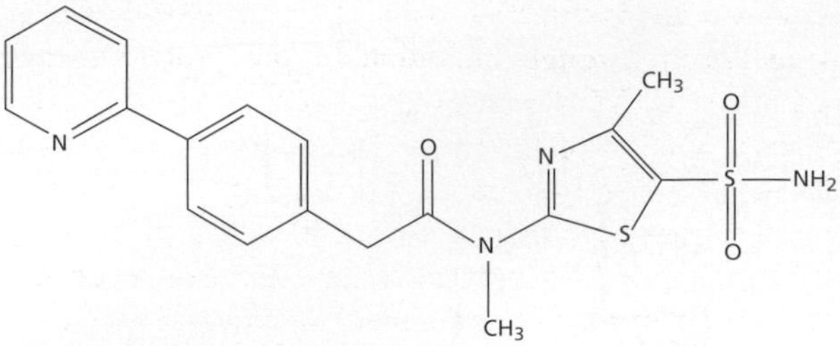

BAY-57-1293

Figure 69.9 *An inhibitor of the herpes simplex virus enzyme, helicase primase: BAY-57-1293*

compounds suitable for clinical development will emerge in the foreseeable future (Kleymann 2003, 2004).

DRUG COMBINATIONS TO MANAGE HERPESVIRUSES

Historically, there has been little enthusiasm for the use of drugs in combination against herpesviruses. Recently, the introduction of combination therapy has revolutionized the management of HIV and viral hepatitis (see sections below). Given the success obtained with different viruses, the possibility of this approach for HSV is currently being assessed – it is the turn for herpes virologists to learn from the younger areas of antiviral research! Actually, there is a long history of anti-inflammatory agents being used in combination with specific antiviral agents to manage severe lesions in recurrent herpes keratitis. One problem with this approach is that some effective anti-inflammatory agents also up-regulate and prolong virus shedding. This can be controlled by using a specific virus inhibitor (Harmenberg et al. 2003), thus a recent trial reported beneficial effects in patients with experimentally induced cutaneous HSV lesions using a combination of topical 5 percent ACV and 1 percent cortisone (Evans et al. 2002). There is no doubt that the further use of combinations of two or more specific antiviral drugs will be the subject of future studies and are likely to become more common in the future.

IMMUNOMODULATORS AS ANTIVIRAL TREATMENTS FOR HERPES

Compounds have been discovered that inhibit HSV replication by interference with a cellular target involved in virus replication (e.g. cyclin-dependent kinases) yet appear to behave as selective inhibitors of virus replication (Schang 2002). It remains to be seen whether such compounds will have a value either alone or in combination with conventional inhibitors of virus functions. Another approach is to stimulate the host to react more effectively to the reactivating virus so as to minimize the clinical signs generally referred to as immunomodulators.

Resiquimod

One compound of this type that is claimed to be effective is known as resiquimod (4-amino-2-ethoxymethyl-

α,α-dimethyl-1H-imidazo[4,5-c]quinoline-1-ethenol). The compound (Figure 69.10) is described as an immune response modifier which induces cytokines including interferons (Tomai et al. 1995), however clinical trials as a topical therapy for genital herpes were recently abandoned.

HCMV INFECTION

HCMV is another member of the *Herpesviridae* that is very widespread among human populations worldwide. Infection is rarely associated with clinical signs in otherwise healthy individuals except when primary infection occurs during pregnancy when congenital disease can result. However, when the immune system is compromised, e.g. associated with allograft transplantation, clinical signs of infection often become apparent and may be extremely damaging. The coming of HIV heightened awareness of the condition and HCMV retinitis became one of the most feared complications of the retrovirus infection. The introduction of highly active antiretroviral therapy has decreased the incidence of this complication substantially, but this and other manifestations of HCMV infection still account for considerable morbidity and there is much interest in developing improved drugs to treat or prevent these conditions (Field 1999). Currently there are five compounds that have been officially licensed for the treatment of HCMV infections. These are ganciclovir and phosphonoformic acid and cidofovir (see above) and two further compounds.

Formivirsen

There have been many unsuccessful attempts to employ antisense oligonucleotides in an effort to block or

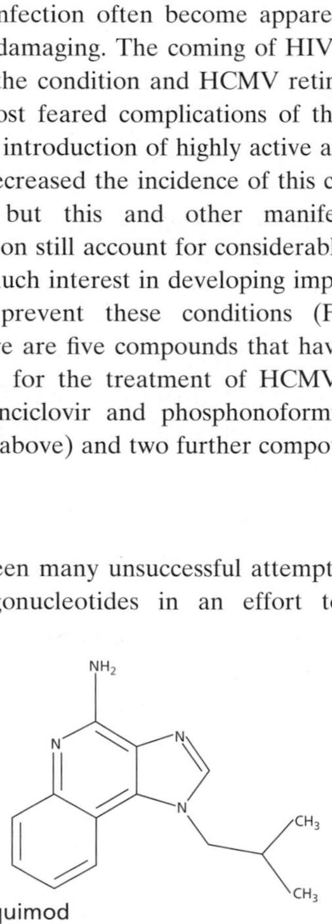

Imiquimod

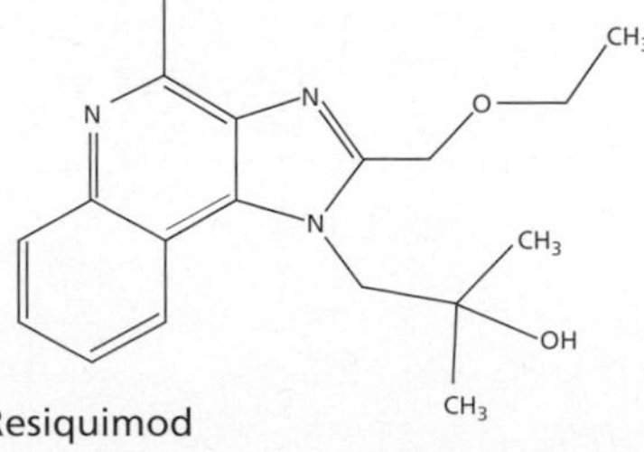

Resiquimod

Figure 69.10 *Examples of antiviral compounds whose primary activity is thought to be as immunomodulators: imiquimod and resiquimod*

5'-d-[G*C*G*T*T*T*G*C*T*C*T*T*C*T*T*C*T*T*G*C*G]3'

sodium salt

*: racemic phosphothorioate antisense oligonucleotide

Formivirsen sodium, Vitravene

Figure 69.11 *Formisvirsen, an antisense oligonucleotide active against human cytomegalovirus*

attenuate virus replication. There have been some more optimistic results, however, and formivirsen (ISIS 2922), vitravene is an antisense oligodeoxynucleotide (Figure 69.11) comprising 21 phosphorothioate-linked nucleosides that is complementary to the RNA of the HCMV major immediate–early region (Azad et al. 1993) and is one of the most promising compounds of this type.

Valganciclovir

Using the same oral prodrug strategy that led to valaciclovir and FCV, the orally bio-available valine ester of ganciclovir was synthesized and found to be effective. Valganciclovir (Valcyte) (Pescovitz et al. 2000; Reusser 2001) (Figure 69.6), when administered orally (two 450 mg tablets twice daily), gives equivalent systemic ganciclovir levels as intravenous ganciclovir at 5 mg/kg twice daily. Oral valganciclovir is expected to replace intravenous ganciclovir in both the therapy and prevention of CMV infections.

1263W94, Maribavir

There are currently many new compounds in development to combat HCMV (briefly reviewed by De Clercq 2003). Currently, one of the most promising of these is 1263W94 or maribavir. This is a novel benzimidazole compound, 5,6-dichloro-2-(isopropylamino)-1,β-L-ribofuranosyl-1-*H*-benzimidazole. (Figure 69.12). The compound has been demonstrated to potently selectively inhibit HCMV in vitro and to have favorable safety profiles in animal species and it is currently undergoing

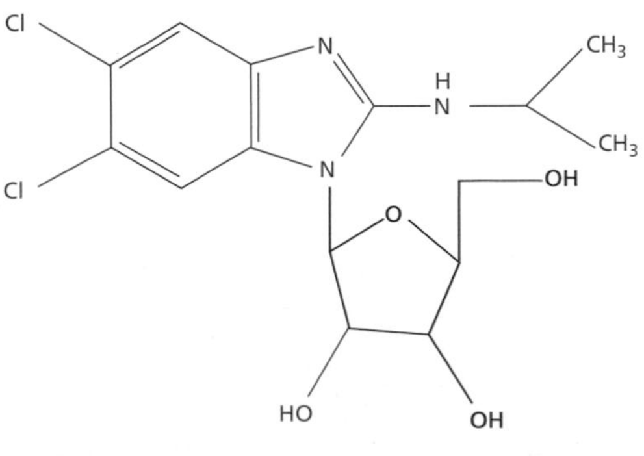

1263W94 Maribavir

Figure 69.12 *A new inhibitor, 1263W94,* maribavir, *which targets the human cytomegalovirus protein kinase*

trials in man (Wang et al. 2003). Its mechanism of action is mediated through inhibition of the protein kinase activity of the *UL97* gene product (Wang et al. 2003). The precise function of this virus product has recently been elucidated, it is thought to concern export of HCMV nucleocapsids from the nucleus (Krosky et al. 2002) and it is the same gene product that is responsible for phosphorylation of ganciclovir to its monophosphate (see above).

Inhibitors of human immunodeficiency virus

NUCLEOSIDE REVERSE TRANSCRIPTASE INHIBITORS (NRTI)

The emergence of HIV as a major pathogen resulted in an unprecedented effort to develop new antiviral agents. The earliest compounds to enjoy limited therapeutic success were all nucleoside analogues; the first to be widely prescribed was 3'-azido-3'-deoxythymidine (azidothymidine).

Zidovudine; azidothymidine

Zidovudine, or azidothymidine (AZT), is an analogue of thymidine (Figure 69.13) (Mitsuya et al. 1985), and is readily phosphorylated in actively dividing cells. The drug is initially phosphorylated by cellular TK, the rate-limiting step being its conversion to AZT diphosphate (AZT-DP) by cellular thymidylate kinase. AZT triphosphate (AZT-TP) competitively inhibits HIV reverse transcriptase with respect to thymidine triphosphate (TTP) and, because the 3'-azido group prevents the formation of 5',3'-phosphodiester linkages, AZT-TP acts as a chain terminator of DNA synthesis (Darby 1995). The compound, via its metabolites, also inhibits a variety of cellular enzymes, including DNA-polymerase-γ, which undoubtedly contributes to the range of toxic effects associated with prolonged clinical use of the drug (Fischl et al. 1987). It was the first drug to be used to treat HIV, and is still accepted as conferring at least transient benefit.

Stavudine; didehydrodideoxyuridine

Stavudine, or 2',3'-didehydro-2'-deoxythymidine (D4T), is similar to AZT in that it is a thymidine nucleoside analogue (Figure 69.13) (Baba et al. 1987). It readily enters cells but, in contrast to AZT, the rate-limiting step is the initial phosphorylation by cellular TK. Once formed, D4T triphosphate (D4T-TP) is rapidly converted to D4T diphosphate (D4T-DP) and triphosphate derivatives. The mechanism of action at the level of reverse transcriptase seems to be similar to that of AZT (reviewed by Hitchcock 1991); toxicity in the form of peripheral neuropathy is, however, more common. The clinical use of D4T is variable worldwide.

AZT azidothymidine, zidovudine   3TC dideoxy3thiacytidine, lamivudine   D4T dideoxydidehydrothymidine, stavudine

DDC dideoxycytidine, zalcitabine, HIVID   DDI dideoxinosine, didanosine

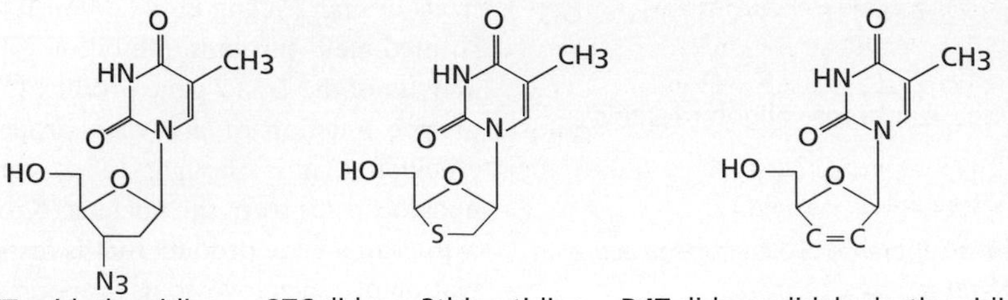

Figure 69.13 *Nucleoside analogue inhibitors of HIV reverse transcriptase (NRTI)*

Didanosine; dideoxyinosine (Videx)

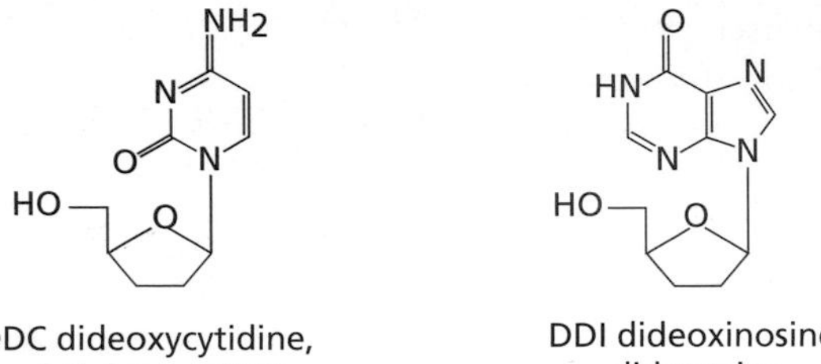

Didanosine, or 2′,3′-dideoxyinosine (DDI), is a purine nucleoside analogue (Figure 69.13) (Mitsuya and Broder 1986) which is taken up intracellularly and converted by 5′ nucleotidase to DDI monophosphate (DDI-MP) and further metabolized by cellular enzymes to DDA triphosphate (DDA-TP), which has a prolonged intracellular half-life (8–24 h). Again, the molecular target for the drug action is the HIV reverse transcriptase (reviewed by McLaren et al. 1991). Clinical trials have been conducted in AIDS patients (Darbyshire and Aboulker 1992; Kahn et al. 1992) but the clinical use of DDI has been limited by its oral formulation which may cause gastrointestinal discomfort.

Zalcitabine; dideoxycytidine (HIVID)

Zalcitabine, or 2′,3′-dideoxycytidine (DDC) (Figure 69.13), is active against HIV-1 and 2 and against some strains that are resistant to AZT (Mitsuya and Broder 1986). The drug seems to be similar in potency to AZT (Bozzette et al. 1995).

Lamivudine; thiacytidine (Epivir)

Next, in this series of nucleoside analogue inhibitors of reverse transcriptase, lamivudine, or 2′-deoxy-3′-thiacytidine (3TC) (Figure 69.13), is synergistic with AZT in vitro and is active against HIV-resistant strains (Soudeyns et al. 1991). It seems to be relatively nontoxic but is less active than AZT in monotherapy. This drug is of particular interest for combination studies with AZT and a protease inhibitor. Lamivudine is also an active inhibitor of HBV DNApol in vitro (Doong et al. 1991) and against HBV infection in vivo (Honkoop and de Man 1995). Lamivudine has been coformulated with AZT and marketed as combivir.

Carbovir, Abacavir (Ziagen)

Abacavir is a carbocyclic synthetic nucleoside analogue (Figure 69.14). Intracellularly, abacavir is phosphorylated by cellular enzymes to its active metabolite, carbovir triphosphate, which is an analogue of deoxyguanosine-5′-TP. Carbovir-TP then inhibits the activity of HIV reverse transcriptase both by competing with the

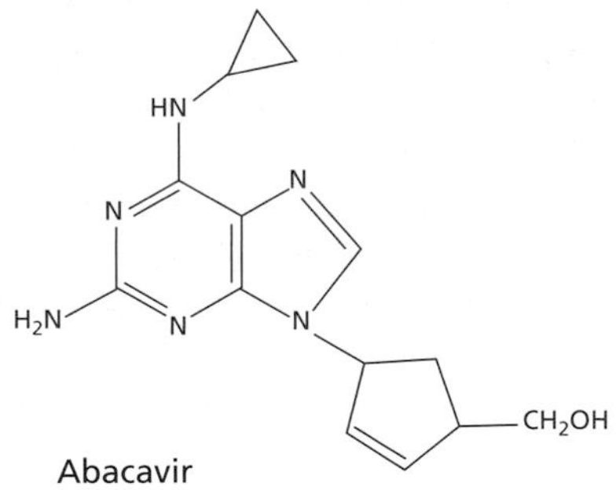

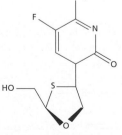

Abacavir

Emtricitabine

Figure 69.14 *Further examples of HIV nucleoside reverse transcriptase inhibitors: NRTI*

natural substrate dGTP and by its incorporation into viral DNA. The lack of a 3'-OH group in the incorporated nucleoside analogue prevents the formation of the 5' to 3' phosphodiester linkage essential for DNA chain elongation, producing chain termination. Abacavir is often used in combination with lamivudine and zidovudine, as well as with either a nonnucleoside reverse transcriptase inhibitor or protease inhibitor.

Adverse reactions associated with abacavir therapy include nausea, headache, stomach pain, diarrhea, insomnia, rash, fever, and dizziness. Importantly, fatal hypersensitivity reactions have been associated with abacavir use.

Abacavir resistance is conferred by mutations in the HIV reverse transcriptase gene that resulted in amino acid substitutions at positions K65R, L74V, Y115F, and M184V. M184V and L74V are the most frequently observed mutations among clinical isolates. Multiple reverse transcriptase mutations conferring abacavir resistance exhibit cross-resistance to lamivudine, didanosine, and zalcitabine in vitro.

Emtricitabine (FTC) (Emtriva)

Emtricitabine is a synthetic nucleoside analogue of cytosine (Figure 69.14) active against the reverse transcriptase of HIV-1. Following triphosphorylation by cellular enzymes, it competes with the natural substrate deoxycytidine 5'-triphosphate and, following incorporation into the nascent viral DNA, results in chain termination.

Other related compounds, e.g. Entecavir, have been found to be more useful against HBV infection and are under investigation for the treatment of chronic HBV infection (see section on Inhibitors of hepatitis viruses, below). Entecavir is a promising new drug that has entered a Phase III clinical trial for efficacy. The compound is a cyclopentile guanosine nucleoside analogue (Figure 69.15) with selective activity against hepatitis B viral DNApol. It is orally bioavailable, and due to a long terminal elimination half life of approximately 110 h, is clearly suitable for once daily therapy. Similarly, a series of L-nucleosides is advancing through Phase II and III clinical trials. Hepatitis viruses are considered in more detail and a description of further inhibitors is dealt with in the section entitled Inhibitors of hepatitis viruses.

NONNUCLEOSIDE REVERSE TRANSCRIPTASE INHIBITORS (NNRTI)

The intensive screening of compounds for anti-HIV activity led to the discovery of several families of inhibitors that, although they differ from one another in structure, share the property of inhibiting reverse transcriptase by binding to sites other than that which normally interacts with the nucleosides. Some act at concentrations in the nanomolar range and are cytotoxic only at 10 000- to 100 000-fold higher concentrations. HIV-1 (but, notably, not HIV-2) reverse transcriptase is

Ribavirin

Entecavir

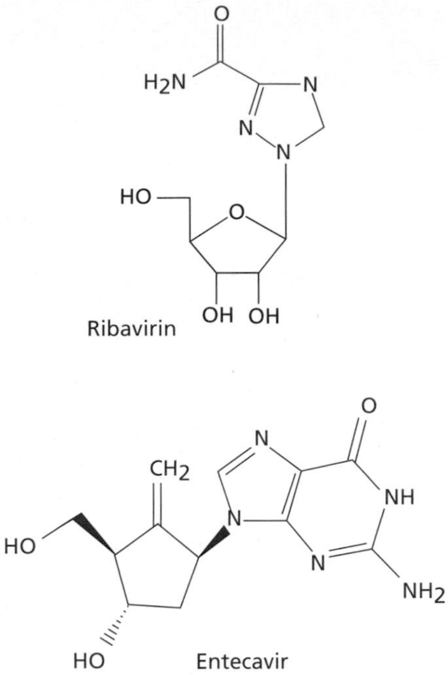

Ac-YTSLIHSLIEESQNQQEKNEQELLELDKWASLWNWF-NH2-

T-20, Enfuvirtide

Figure 69.15 *The broad spectrum nucleoside inhibitor, ribavirin, entecavir, and the synthetic peptide, T-20 which is anti-HIV fusion inhibitor*

the target sensitive to inhibition. Enzyme studies, however, indicated that such compounds inhibit reverse transcriptase in a noncompetitive fashion (De Clercq 1992). The site on the enzyme at which these compounds bind has been termed the TIBO site (Pauwels et al. 1990) and certain other compounds (e.g. HEPT, an acyclic uridine derivative) seem to interact with the same site (Baba et al. 1989) (TIBO and HEPT are discussed below). These compounds have been collectively described as allosteric inhibitors. The rapid selection of drug-resistance seems to be a major limitation of the success of these compounds, which, however, are likely to have an important role when used in combination both with other nonreverse transcriptase inhibitors and with other classes of inhibitor.

TIBO, nevirapine and HEPT

A series of nonnucleoside inhibitors was discovered that are tetrahydro-imidazo[4,5,1-jk][1,4]-benzodiazepin-2H (1H)-thione derivatives (Figure 69.16) (Debyser et al. 1991). This almost unpronounceable name is usually shortened to TIBO. This benzodiazepine-like drug was the first of the NNTRI to be identified (De Clercq 1992). Early trials showed a large but transient reduction in viral

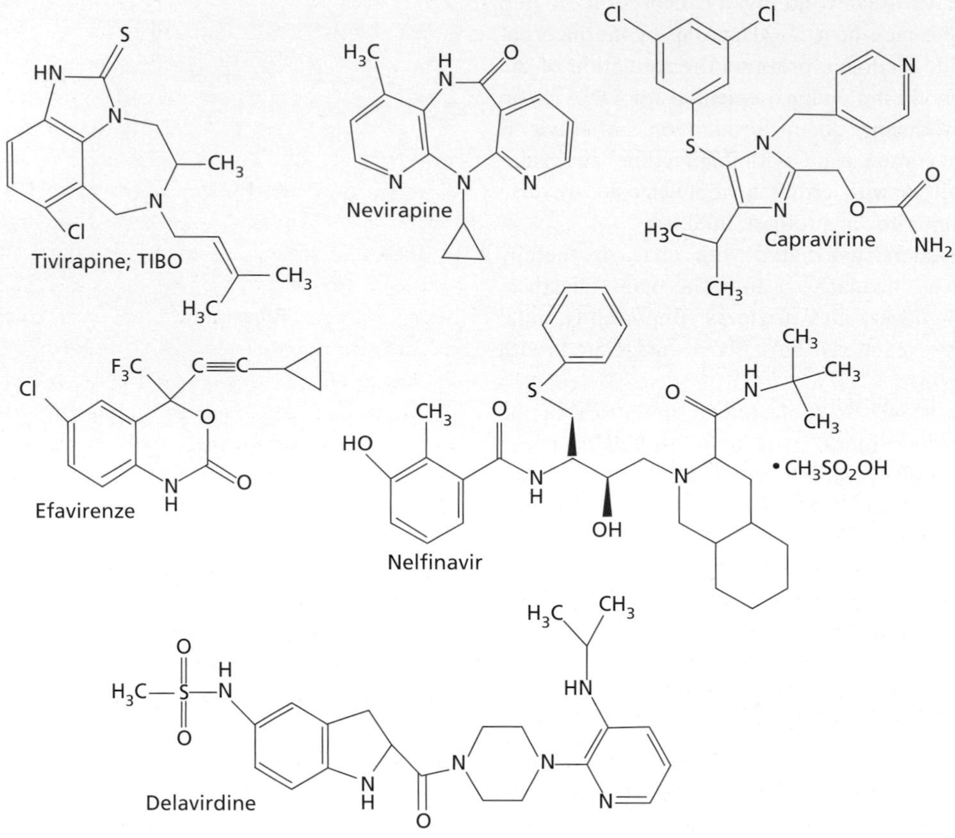

Figure 69.16 *Nonnucleoside analogue inhibitors of HIV reverse transcriptase (NNRTI)*

load. The drug is of relatively low toxicity but its oral bioavailability is poor. Nevirapine (Figure 69.16) is another noncompetitive inhibitor of reverse transcriptase that interacts with tyrosine residues on the enzyme (Merluzzi et al. 1990) and yet another series of compounds of this general type, hydroxyethoxy-methylphenylthiothymine derivatives, has been given the acronym HEPT (Figure 69.16) (Miyasaka et al. 1989).

Nevirapine (Viramune)

Nevirapine is a nonnucleoside (dizyridodiazepinone) reverse transcriptase inhibitor that is structurally similar to benzodiazepines (Figure 69.16) (Merluzzi et al. 1990). Binding of nevirapine to reverse transcriptase is noncompetitive. It selectively inhibits HIV-1, but not HIV-2, reverse transcriptase without significant inhibition of other cellular polymerases. It is currently used in combination with nucleoside reverse transcriptase inhibitors and/or protease inhibitors. Because of the rapid and certain appearance of resistance, it is not used as monotherapy. The major side effect of nevirapine is the development of a cutaneous rash including 'Stevens Johnson syndrome' which is a severe rash, often drug-induced. Other less common side effects include altered liver function tests, fever, and myalgia. Since nevirapine is metabolized by the liver, there is the potential for interaction with other hepatically metabolized medications

metabolized by this organ, including rifabutin, rifampin, ketoconazole, and the protease inhibitors.

Resistance to nevirapine occurs at codons 181, 188, 103, 106, 108, and 190, all of which result in a significant reduction in nevirapine susceptibility to treatment. A nevirapine-associated mutation at codon 181, concurrent with the presence of the most common zidovudine resistant mutation (codon 215), appears to restore susceptibility to zidovudine.

Delavirdine (Rescriptor)

Delavirdine binds directly to reverse transcriptase and blocks RNA-dependent and DNA-dependent DNApol activities (Figure 69.16). HIV-2 reverse transcriptase and human cellular DNApol are not inhibited by delavirdine. In addition, HIV-1 group O, a group of highly divergent strains that are uncommon in North America, may not be inhibited by delavirdine. Delavirdine is frequently used as combination therapy with two nucleoside reverse transcriptase inhibitors, such as zidovudine and didanosine, with or without a protease inhibitor. Adverse reactions associated with delavirdine therapy include rash (which may be maculopapular or pruritic), headache, increased transaminases, nausea, diarrhea, fatigue, and, rarely, Stevens Johnson syndrome. Delavirdine increases concentrations of the protease inhibitors saquinavir, nelfinavir, and indinavir when given in combination.

Mutations conferring resistance to delavirdine occur predominantly at position 103 and less frequently at positions 181 and 236. Combination therapy with delavirdine and zidovudine may result in increased zidovudine sensitivity of patient isolates after 24 weeks on therapy. Mutations at positions 103 and 181 have been associated with resistance to other NNRTI.

Efavirenz (Sustiva)

Efavirenz is mediated predominantly by noncompetitive inhibition of HIV-1 reverse transcriptase (Figure 69.16). HIV-2 reverse transcriptase and human cellular DNApol are not inhibited by efavirenz. Efavirenz is frequently used in combination with two or more nucleoside reverse transcriptase inhibitors, with or without a protease inhibitor. Side effects include headache, dizziness, diarrhea, skin rash, impaired concentration, anxiety, visual disturbances, nausea, vomiting, insomnia, fatigue, and flulike symptoms. Efavirenz has produced numerous birth defects in animal models, and is contraindicated in pregnancy. No clinically significant drug interactions occur between efavirenz and nucleoside reverse transcriptase inhibitors. Efavirenz decreases indinavir concentrations, necessitating an increase in indinavir dosing when given concomitantly with efavirenz. Saquinavir concentrations are diminished to such a degree by efavirenz that the two should not be used in combination.

Mutations at the reverse transcriptase amino acid positions 98, 100, 101, 103, 106, 108, 188, 190, and 225 confer efavirenz resistance. The mutation at position 103 (lysine to asparagine) is the most frequently observed. Efavirenz-resistant isolates are frequently resistant to others in the same class.

Capravirine

Capravirine (Figure 69.16) is the last of this series of NNRTIs currently under investigation. It has potent activity in vitro against HIV variants but RT substitutions are detected including K103N that confer broad cross resistance to the other drugs in this class.

PROTEASE INHIBITORS

HIV encodes an enzyme that specifically cleaves protein precursors in the maturation of gag and pol polyproteins (Pearly and Taylor 1987). Inhibition of this enzyme results in the production of noninfectious virus (Kohl et al. 1988). This virus-induced enzyme has no known cellular function, but a number of highly specific inhibitors of HIV whose action is based on inhibition of the HIV protease have been reported (De Clercq 1995).

Saquinavir (Fortovase, Invirase)

This was the first active virus protease inhibitor to be described. It is a peptide-based transition-state mimetic of an Asn.Phe.{ }Pro. substrate sequence, in which { } indicates the cleavage site (Roberts et al. 1990).

Saquinavir (Figure 69.17) is an extremely active inhibitor of HIV replication in cell culture, with a very high selective index and was the first licensed protease inhibitor worldwide. Its pharmacokinetic properties are, however, not ideal for use in vivo (Roberts 1995). Furthermore, viruses of many other families encode proteases, including pathogens as diverse as polio, HCV, influenza, and HSV, against which a similar approach is being directed. The potential for these compounds to be valuable inhibitors seems to be great but their ultimate success in clinical use cannot yet be predicted. Adverse reactions include diarrhea, abdominal discomfort, and nausea. Photosensitization can occur. Saquinavir is metabolized by the liver enzyme system: cytochrome P-450; thus, ketoconazole and itraconazone increase the plasma levels of saquinavir, as does ritonavir, a fact that has been utilized in the development of combination protease inhibitor therapies.

Saquinavir-resistant HIV occurs most commonly at the HIV protease L90M site. Saquinavir is effective against ritonavir- and indinavir-resistant mutants.

Ritonavir (Norvir)

Ritonavir (Figure 69.17) is a peptide-like inhibitor of HIV proteases and one that renders them incapable of processing the gag–pol polyprotein precursors required for assembly of progeny virions. Ritonavir is used in combination with NRTI and/or NNRTI. Ritonavir is also metabolized by the cytochrome P450 system, as is saquinavir. Ritonavir increases plasma levels of macrolides, particularly clarithromycin and erythromycin, anticonvulsants, tricyclic antidepressants, and the azole antifungals. Ritonavir also increases levels of saquinavir, and, as such, low doses of ritonavir are sometimes used in combination with saquinavir to achieve higher saquinavir concentrations. Adverse reactions include nausea, vomiting, anorexia, abdominal pain, taste perversion, and circumoral and peripheral paresthesia. Furthermore, there are alterations in triglyceride metabolism and elevation of liver function tests have also been described. Clinically, fat redistribution can appear.

Ritonavir resistance occurs with mutations in HIV protease at codons 84, 82, 71, 46, 54, and 36. The development of mutations is stepwise, occurring first at codon 82. Cross-resistance with indinavir but not saquinavir is common.

Indinavir (Crixivan)

Indinavir (Figure 69.17) binds to cleavage sites of HIV protease; thereby, it prevents cleavage of viral polyprotein precursors into individual proteins required for progeny virions assembly. Adverse reactions associated with indinavir therapy include nephrolithiasis, hematuria, and occasionally hyperbilirubinemia.

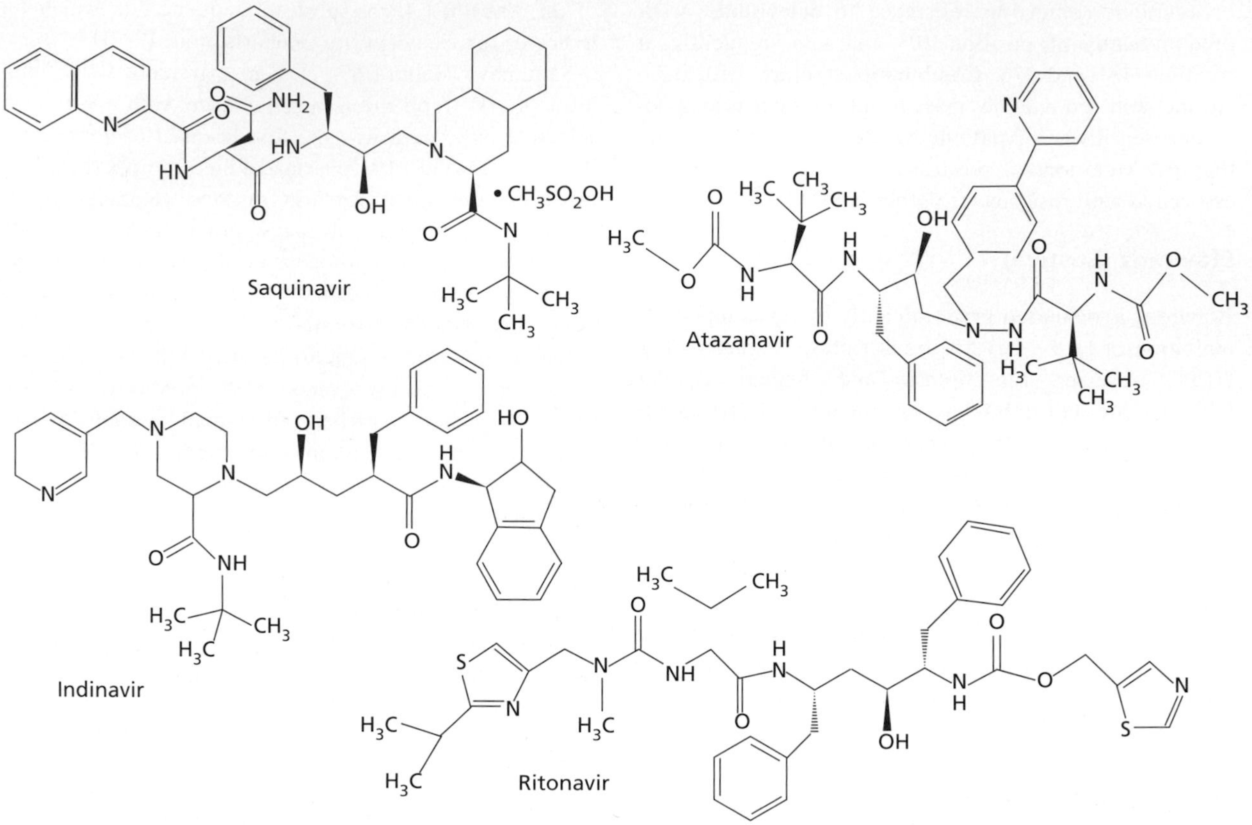

Figure 69.17 *Highly active inhibitors of the HIV protease (PI)*

Administration of indinavir selects for resistant mutants with alterations in HIV protease at a variety of different amino acid sites. Increased resistance is a function of stepwise acquisition of multiple mutations in HIV protease.

Nelfinavir (Viracept)

Nelfinavir (Figure 69.18) is a nonpeptidic inhibitor of HIV protease that inhibits or interferes with processing of viral polyprotein precursors, resulting in non-infectious progeny virions. It is given in combination with NRTI and/or NNRTI. Nelfinavir is metabolized by the cytochrome P450 system. Adverse events associated with nelfinavir administration include diarrhea, rash, leukopenia, and neutropenia.

Resistance to nelfinavir occurs by mutations in HIV protease, particularly at codons 30, 35, 36, 46, 71, 77, and 88. Importantly, these sites are all different from those that confer resistance to other protease inhibitors. However, once resistance to a protease inhibitor develops, it is likely that cross-resistance will occur.

Amprenavir (Agenerase)

Amprenavir (Figure 69.18) acts by binding to the active site of HIV-1 protease, preventing the processing of viral gag and gag–pol polyprotein precursors and results in the formation of immature non-infectious viral parti-

cles. In vitro, amprenavir has synergistic anti-HIV-1 activity in combination with abacavir, zidovudine, dida-nosine, or saquinavir, and additive anti-HIV-1 activity in combination with indinavir, nelfinavir, and ritonavir. Adverse effects associated with amprenavir administration include rash, nausea, vomiting, diarrhea, abdominal pain, and perioral paresthesias. Amprenavir is metabolized by the P450 system.

Resistance to amprenavir is conferred by amino acid substitutions primarily at positions M46I/L, I47V, I50V, I54L/V, and I84V, as well as mutations in the viral protease p1/p6 cleavage site. Cross-resistance between amprenavir and the other protease inhibitors is possible.

Lopinavir/Ritonavir (Kaletra)

Lopinavir/ritonavir combination interferes with processing of viral polyprotein precursors, resulting in non-infectious progeny virions (Figure 69.18). The addition of ritonavir enhances the concentrations of lopinavir that can be achieved following oral administration. It is given in combination with NRTI and/or NNRTI. Side effects of lopinavir/ritonavir include diarrhea, nausea, abdominal pain, and headache.

As lopinavir/ritonavir is a relatively new addition to the protease inhibitors; a complete understanding of resistance profiles will await its widespread utilization.

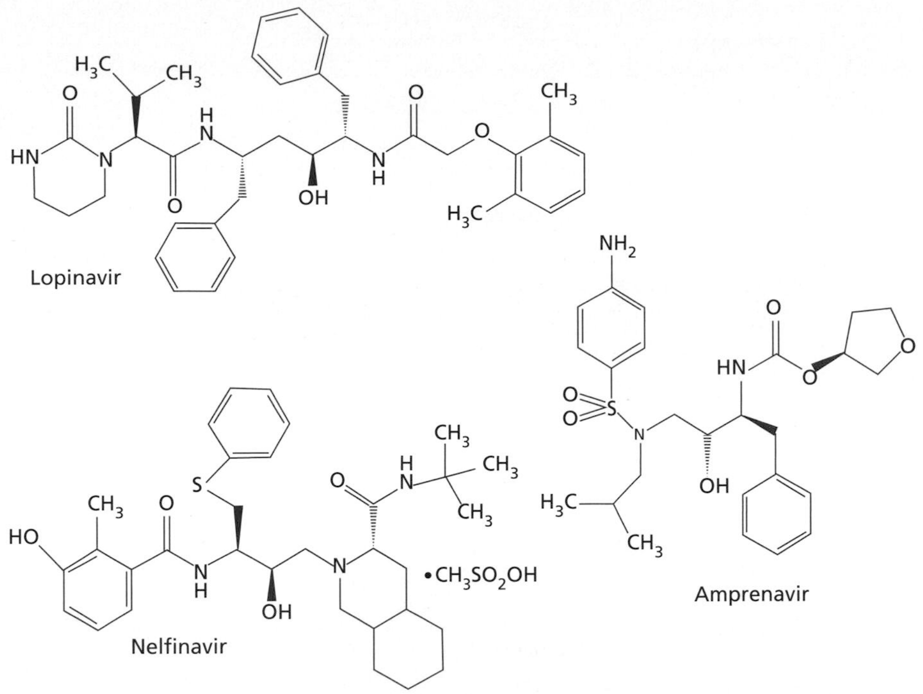

Figure 69.18 *Further examples of PI which are highly active against HIV*

Atazanavir (Reyataz)

Atazanavir (Figure 69.17) is a protease inhibitor. It prevents cells infected by HIV from producing new virus, reducing the amount of virus in the patient. It must be used in combination with at least two other anti-HIV drugs (Prober and Kimberlin 2005).

NUCLEOTIDE ANALOGUES

Tenofovir (tenofovir disoproxil fumarate) (Viread)

Tenofovir or disproxil fumarate salt (Figure 69.7) is an acyclic nucleoside phosphonate diester analogue of adenosine monophosphate. In vitro, the 50 percent inhibitor concentration for HIV is 0.04–8.5 µmol. After diester hydrolysis, tenofovir is phosphorylated to tenofovir-DP that then inhibits HIV reverse transcriptase by competing with the natural substrate deoxyadenosine 5-TP and, after incorporation into DNA, by DNA chain termination. Tenofovir DP is a weak inhibitor of mammalian DNApols α, β, and mitochondrial DNApol γ. Additive or synergic anti-HIV activity with nucleoside analogue, nonnucleoside analogue and protease inhibitors has been demonstrated in vitro. Side effects include lactic acidosis, hepatomegaly with steatosis, and diarrhea, (De Clercq 2002). Resistance is uncommon and occurs at codon 65.

Entecavir

Entecavir (Figure 69.19) is a cyclopentile guanosine nucleoside analogue with selective activity against hepatitis B viral DNApol. It is orally bioavailable, and due to a long terminal elimination half life of approximately 110 h is clearly suitable for once daily therapy.

HIV FUSION INHIBITORS

Enfuvirtide (Fuzeon)

The recent licensing of a fusion inhibitor introduces a new class of antiviral compounds for the treatment of HIV. T-20n (Figure 69.15) (Lalezari et al. 2003) is an inhibitor of fusion of HIV-1 with CD4$^+$ cells that consists of a 36 amino acid synthetic peptide with the N terminus acetylated and the C terminus is a carboxamide. Medication is administered subcutaneously.

Inhibitors of orthomyxo- and paramyxoviruses

EARLY PROGRESS WITH ION CHANNEL BLOCKERS

Amantadine and rimantadine

The compound amantadine (Figure 69.20) has long been known as a specific inhibitor of influenza virus A; influenza B and C are not affected. Clinical experience with amantadine and the chemically related rimantadine, dates from the early 1960s (Davies et al. 1964) and, although these compounds have lately been replaced, they represent major milestones in the history of the development of antiviral chemotherapy. The mechanisms of action of amantadine, and subsequently of rimantadine, which is very similar but with superior

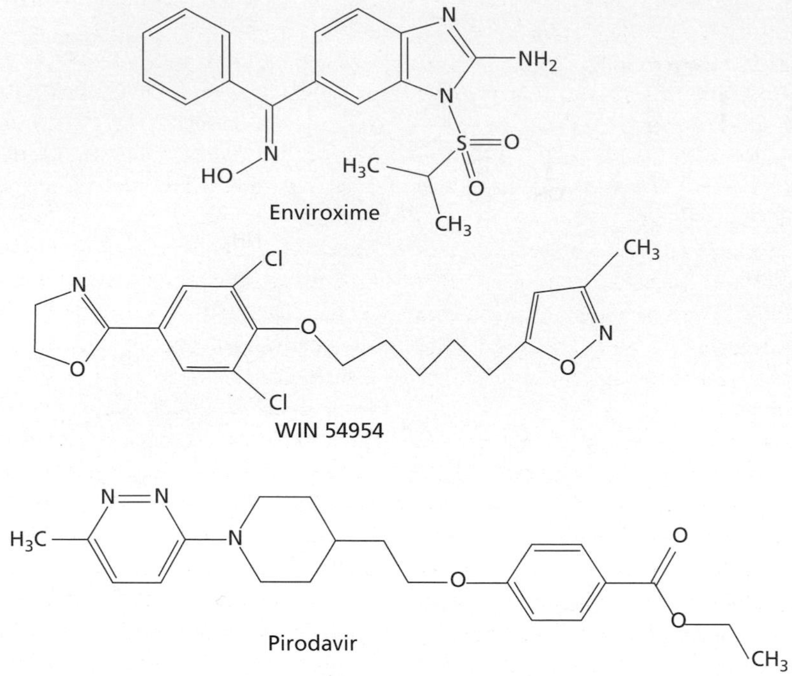

Figure 69.19 *Compounds with activity against the common cold – picornavirus inhibitors*

pharmacological properties (Hayden et al. 1981, 1985), were not elucidated until many years after they had been introduced into the clinic (Hay 1992).

Following attachment to host-cell plasma membrane receptors by means of the influenza envelope glycoprotein spikes, or hemagglutinin (HA), virus is taken up by cells into clathrin-coated pits. The virus, at this early stage of its replication cycle, is contained within lysosomes. Low pH within the lysosome results in conformational changes in the HA which exposes the amino-terminus region of the HA2; this region is hydrophobic and triggers a fusion between the endosomal membrane and the virus envelope, releasing the nucleocapsid into the cytoplasm of the host cell. Originally, amantadine was thought to work simply by raising lysosomal pH, thereby interfering with the conformational change leading to virus fusion with membrane. It now appears

that the process of inhibition is more subtle. The M2 protein in the nucleocapsid seems to form a polymeric tube-like structure which behaves as an ion channel through which protons pass. Amantadine and rimantadine seem to act by binding to M2, possibly being inserted into the channel itself, and thus interfering with the penetration of hydrogen ions into the virion; a process essential for uncoating the single-stranded RNA genome (Wang et al. 1993). Resistant mutations map to the *M2* gene and such variants may ultimately limit the success of chemotherapy (Hayden 1994). Both amantadine and rimantadine have a basketlike hydrocarbon structure and further active compounds of this type are under study. The knowledge of how these compounds interact with the M2 proton channel should enable the rational design of further influenza inhibitors of this type.

The clinical efficacy of the prophylaxis and treatment of influenza virus infections with amantadine and rimantadine has been reviewed by Hayden (1997). The effectiveness of both compounds is limited by the adverse side effects, lack of activity against influenza B viruses, and rapid emergence of transmissible and pathogenic resistant viruses that remain transmissible and pathogenic emerge readily during clinical use (Hayden and Couch 1992; Monto and Arden 1992).

NEURAMINIDASE INHIBITORS

Zanamivir (Relenza) and Oseltamivir (Tamiflu)

While the study of HA dominated the early molecular characterization of influenza, it became apparent that

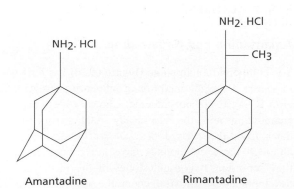

Figure 69.20 *Amantadine and rimantadine, early inhibitors of influenza which target the M2 protein*

the influenza envelope is decorated with a second glyco-protein spike, much less numerous than HA, but with a distinctive long-stalked 'mushroom' shape. Neur-aminidase (NA) was discovered to possess an enzymatic ability to cleave sialic acid from sialylated glycoproteins to yield free sialic acid. Known at first as sialidase, the term neuraminidase is now used universally. Sialic acid (Figure 69.21) is the receptor for the influenza virus on mammalian cells and interference with NA by muta-tions, anti-NA antibody or chemical compounds that bind to NA, all inhibit release of virus from infected cells. NA is also thought to have a role in the passage of virus through mucus to facilitate its colonization of respiratory mucosal cells.

An important molecule in research is Neu5Ac2en (Figure 69.21); this is a dehydrated neuraminidase acid derivative that mimics the geometry of the transition state during the enzymatic reaction. In the early 1990s the high resolution crystal structure of sialic acid and the transition state analogue Neu5Ac2en bound to influenza A and B NAs was solved. The NA active site contains some well-formed, large, and relatively rigid pockets that enable the rational design of molecules to interact with this virus component (reviewed by Kim et al. 1999). Several important inhibitors emerged from such studies. The guanidinyl group was substituted for a hydroxyl carbon atom of Neu5Ac2en to produce the compound 4-Guanidino-Neu5Ac2en (von Itzstein et al. 1993) or zanamivir (Relenza®; Figure 69.21). The polar zwitter-ionic properties of zanamivir give low oral bio-avail-ability and, with rapid excretion, the compound must be

administered intranasally or by inhalation. Another active compound introduced a cyclohexene ring and replaced a polar glycerol with lipophilic side chains (Tai et al. 1998; Sidwell et al. 1998; Mendel et al. 1998) to produce oseltamivir (Tamiflu®; Figure 69.22). This is an ethyl ester that is orally bio-available (30–100 percent) and is readily converted to the active carboxylate by esterases in the liver (Hitchcock 1996; Figure 69.22). Laboratory animal studies using infected mice and ferret models of influenza showed good dose-dependent anti-viral effects and subsequently, both oseltamivir and zanamivir have proved successful when used prophyl-actically or therapeutically in clinical trials (reviewed by Oxford et al. 2002). Relatively few side-effects have been reported although a concern about zanamivir has been exacerbation of reactive airway disease (Cheer and Wagstaff 2002), however, compliance with the inhaler has been good. Oseltamivir causes some gastro-intestinal effects such as nausea. Several studies of prophylaxis among contacts in the workplace and among family members suggest a protective efficacy for zanamivir of 60–70 percent. The therapeutic use of either drug has been encouraging, and they have been shown to signifi-cantly alleviate the clinical signs of influenza (Oxford et al. 2002). Drug resistance mutations are detected following passage in cell culture. The mutations occur in both NA and HA hinting at functional interdependence between the two virus glycoproteins. However, the clin-ical data to date allow optimism. The incidence of resis-tance has been low compared to previous experience with rimantadine and where it does occur, resistance is

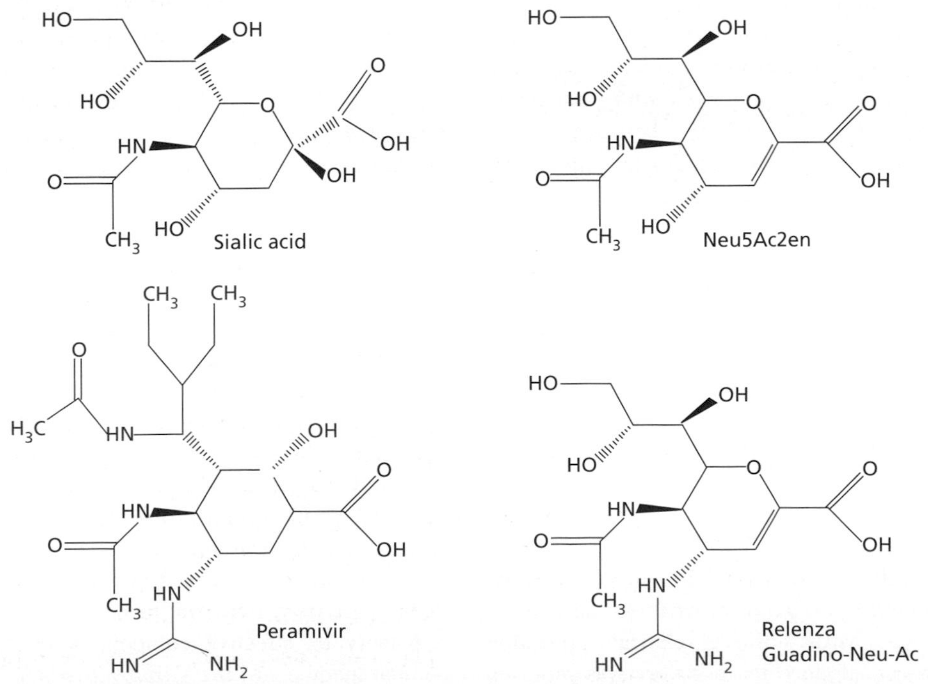

Figure 69.21 *The natural compound sialic acid showing its relationship to Neu5Ac2en and the first effective influenza virus neuraminidase inhibitor, relenza. Chemical modifications that vary from the natural compound are shown in red.*

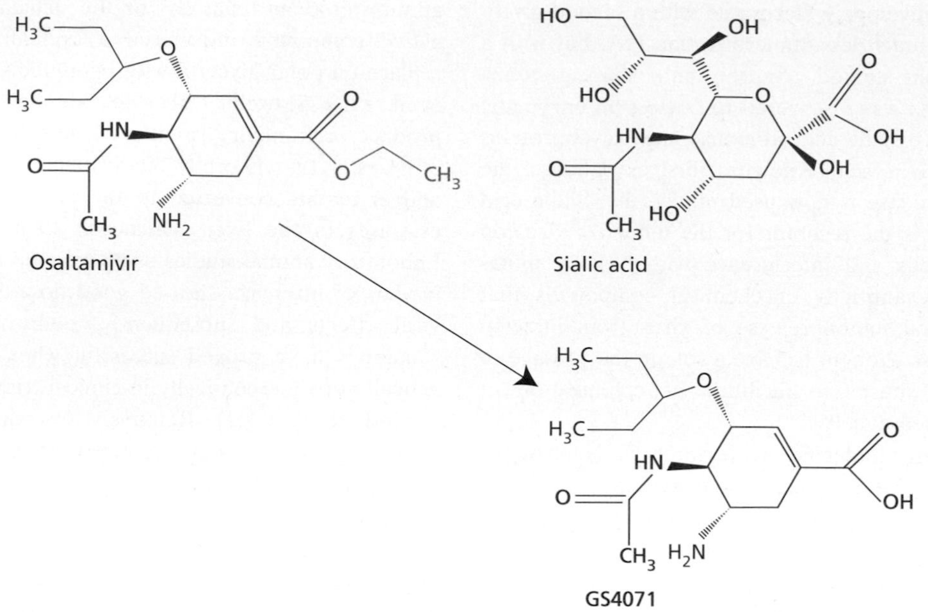

Figure 69.22 *Sialic acid and an orally bioavailable neuraminidase inhibitor, oseltamivir, showing its conversion to the active metabolite. The parts of the molecule shown in purple are removed by host enzyme attack to release the NA inhibitor in vivo.*

detected only transiently, arising late in infection and being cleared normally (Treanor et al. 2000). There is evidence that some of the mutants, at least, are attenuated in mice and ferret models (Herlocher et al. 2002). Thus early clinical data are very encouraging, however, the true potential of zanamivir, oseltamivir, and similar NA inhibitors now awaits the test of the next pandemic influenza outbreak.

Currently, the search for alternative NA inhibitors is active and it is likely that improved drugs will emerge. One novel compound is a dimerised zanamivir molecule that was suggested to be 100-fold more potent than zanamivir in vitro. It was shown to be retained longer in laboratory animal lungs compared with zanamivir, permitting much longer intervals between doses. Another Neu5Ac2en-derived analogue, peramivir (Figure 69.21) was also claimed to be more potent than zanamivir or oseltamivir in cell culture (Boivin and Goyette 2002). Phase II trials were promising, although Phase III less so, and currently development has stopped. Although these particular compounds may not be progressed, the preliminary results strongly suggest that the NA inhibitors presently in use have not achieved maximum efficacy and that more potent drugs in this class will become available in due course.

Ribavirin

Ribavirin 1-β-D-ribofuranosyl-1H-1,2,4-tiazole-3-carboxamide is an inhibitor of paramyxoviruses, particularly respiratory syncytial virus; however, clinical application has been controversial since its discovery was reported in 1972 (Sidwell et al. 1972). The compound is a guanosine analogue (Figure 69.15); evidence has been

obtained for at least three distinct modes of action but the important molecular targets have yet to be confirmed (reviewed by Sidwell et al. 1985). It is a structural analogue of guanosine and is converted successively to ribavirin-MP, -DP, and -TP by cellular enzymes. The inhibition of virus is not, however, reversed by adding guanosine, suggesting a more complicated mode of action (Gilbert and Knight 1986). The enzyme inosine-MP dehydrogenase is effectively inhibited in vitro by ribavirin-MP, with a resulting decrease in pool size of GTP. However, this is not thought to be the single inhibitory factor. Ribavirin-resistant mutants have been very difficult, if not impossible, to isolate in the laboratory. This may be because the compound interferes with multiple virus targets; alternatively, there may be one or more important cellular effects that are not virus-specific. Clinically, aerosolized ribavirin has been reported to be efficacious for treating respiratory syncytial virus infection of infants (Sidwell et al. 1985); however, the results of more recent clinical trials cast doubt on the value of this agent (Wald et al. 1988). Ribavirin has proved to be a useful antiviral drug against several disparate virus families, e.g. hepatitis (see below). Paramyxoviruses cause a wide variety of human and animal diseases and there is a constant threat from new and dangerous viruses to emerge with pandemic potential. In molecular terms, the family has many similarities to the *Orthomyxoviridae* which includes influenza with similar potential targets for inhibition yet, to date, apart from ribavirin, to be screened there remains a paucity of effective compounds in development to combat members of the *Paramyxoviridae*.

As noted below, ribavirin is used in combination with interferon to treat HCV.

Inhibitors of hepatitis viruses

Several distinct viruses infect the liver and cause hepatitis. Furthermore, virus infections of this organ are prone to become persistent leading to chronic hepatitis and pathological sequelae including cirrhosis and liver cancer. Of the many hepatitis viruses discovered, to date, the most important are HBV and HCV. The former is a member of the *Hepadnoviridae*, a family of enveloped icosahedral viruses that contain a double-stranded, circular DNA genome and reverse transcriptase step in the replication cycle analogous to that in HIV. By contrast, HCV particles are nonenveloped and contain a small, positive single-stranded RNA genome. HCV is classified in the genus *Hepacivirus* within the family *Flaviviridae*. HCV does not replicate in conventional tissue culture systems and this has severely hampered research on potential inhibitors.

Both these viruses are major causes of human disease; there are estimated to be 300–400 million carriers of HBV worldwide (reviewed by Main et al. 1998) and some 170 million chronic HCV carriers (Walker et al. 2003), causing an estimated 10–12 000 deaths per annum in the USA alone. In both cases, chronic infection can lead to progressive liver disease, especially cirrhosis, with the increased risk of hepatocellular carcinoma. There is an effective subunit vaccine for HBV but this has no benefit for those already infected. The aim of antiviral chemotherapy is to clear the virus from the liver and thus prevent the life-threatening complications of chronic virus hepatitis and reduce the risk of transmission to others.

INTERFERONS

Since the early 1970s, interferon-α (IFN-α) has been used to treat chronic HBV and success rates of up to 40 percent have been reported for those who acquired infection as adults although treatment of carriers who acquired infection perinatally is less successful. Leucocyte and lymphoblastoid interferon (IFN), of both human and recombinant origin, have been reported as effective in decreasing viral replication in patients (Hoofnagle 1994). The mechanism of action is uncertain but may include the effects of increasing natural killer cell activity and enhancing MHC class-1 activity bearing in mind that hepatocytes naturally have little MHC -1 display. A typical regimen is 5–10 MU/m^2 three times weekly for 3–4 months. IFN-α treatment of Asian patients does not prevent the occurrence of cirrhosis-related complications and hepatocellular carcinoma (Yuen et al. 2001). For the treatment of HCV, like HBV, IFN-α monotherapy has enjoyed some success. Recently, PEG–IFN is now the preferred IFN molecule which is chemically modified form using mono-methoxy polyethylene glycol (PEG) or a branched PEG molecule. This modification has the effect of slowing IFN absorption, decreasing the rate of systemic clearance and produces an approximately 5–10-fold increase in serum half-life. For the treatment of HCV infection, PEG-IFN is used only in combination with ribavirin.

NUCLEOSIDE AND NUCLEOTIDE ANALOGUES

Apart from IFN-γ, there are currently several antiviral compounds in clinical use for the treatment of HBV. While treatment with several nucleoside analogues (e.g. fialuridine, ribavirin, and lamivudine) have been investigated (Honkoop and de Man 1995) only two are licensed: lamivudine and adefovir dipivoxil (Figures 69.7 and 69.13). The L-isomer of 3TC is more active against HBV replication and less cytotoxic than the D-isomer and is assumed to act on the HBV reverse transcriptase step and it may also inhibit the completion of double-stranded DNA. The drug is remarkably free of side effects but there is a high relapse rate, thus, after 6–9 months therapy, drug resistance develops due to mutations in the catalytic domain of the HBV polymerase gene. There is some evidence that the resistant viruses may be less replication-competent compared with the parental virus, however, resistant virus is thought to be responsible for the flare-up of hepatitis. Trials showed a rapid decrease in levels of HBV DNA in treated patients but a return to baseline at the end of therapy.

The nucleotide analogue adefovir dipivoxil (9-2-phosphonylmethoxyethyl) adenine (bis(POM)PMEA) (Figure 69.7) appears to be less susceptible to the development of resistance. The dose of adefovir is significantly lower than that used in studies of HIV infection where renal toxicity was observed. Whether this poses a problem on long-term administration remains to be determined.

COMBINATION THERAPY

Treatment of chronic HBV infection is associated with relapse on cessation of therapy and the emergence of drug-resistance. Following the success of combination therapy for HIV, the use of combinations of drugs to treat HBV and HCV have become common. IFN-α plus lamivudine or adefovir or the use of lamivudine and adefovir combinations are currently under investigation (Yuen and Lai 2003).

The combination of ribavirin with PEG–IFN-α-2a (rebetron) or PEG–IFN-α-2b, typically for 12–24 weeks, results in sustained virologic responses in the range of 40 to 50 percent, however, outcome is phenotype dependent.

Animal models for studying hepatitis virus chemotherapy

HBV and HCV are extremely difficult viruses to manipulate in tissue culture. Stably transfected lines of HepG2 cells can be used to study the replication of HBV; it is tetracyclin regulated. These cells can be used to screen and study inhibitors. However, much development work for antiviral therapy has depended on the use of laboratory animal infection models. Chimpanzees provide reliable HBV and HCV models for evaluation of vaccines and therapeutic agents (Farci and Purcell 1993; Caselmann 1994; Purcell 1994) but severe restrictions are imposed on the use of nonhuman primates including ethical concerns, welfare considerations, and simply the very high cost of maintaining primates. Tree shrews (*Tupaia belangeri*) can be infected by inoculation with human serum positive with HBV and duck hepatitis has been studied in Pekin ducks. A virus related to HBV was discovered in woodchucks (WHV) that mimics human disease, including the progression of chronic liver infection to hepatocellular carcinoma. HBV is also studied in specially prepared mice: the HBV-Trimera mouse in which mice irradiated lethal total whole body irradiation reconstituted with severe combined immunodeficiency (SCID) mouse bone marrow cells. Human HCV- or HBV-infected liver tissue can be engrafted under the murine kidney capsule which then models the chronically infected tissue in vivo and is available for the study of therapeutic regimens (Ilan et al. 1999). Finally, the pestivirus bovine diarrhea virus (BVDV) is genetically related to HCV and has been used as a surrogate in cell culture system for evaluating anti-HCV compounds. This is currently an extremely active area of research among many academic institutions and pharmaceutical research laboratories. Likely progress will occur with the production of improved tissue culture systems and more convenient and reliable in vivo models to study the prevention and therapy of virus hepatitis; one of the most exciting major growth areas in antiviral therapy today.

Inhibitors of picornaviruses

PIRODAVIR AND PLECONARIL

The *Picornaviridae* are among the smallest of the RNA viruses and cause a broad spectrum of human and animal diseases. Among the *Picornaviridae* are the rhinoviruses. Scientists seeking to develop antiviral chemotherapy are often reproached with failure to 'cure the common cold.' An increasing number of compounds has been reported as potent inhibitors of rhinoviruses; they comprise an assorted collection that fall into two classes, with different antiviral targets. The first class (noncapsid binding) includes compounds such as enviroxime (Figure 69.19) (De Long 1984). Compounds of this type seem to act shortly after uncoating, inhibiting the formation of the virus RNA-dependent RNA polymerase complex. These compounds are no longer under investigation.

The second class of compounds (capsid binding) has a quite different target of inhibition. Picornaviruses possess a capsid comprising three types of protein subunit (VP1, VP2, and VP3) assembled into an icosa-

hedral shell. The virions are not enveloped and therefore rely on receptor sites on their protein shell to engage and dock on to protein receptor molecules in the plasma membrane of the host cell. X-ray crystallographic studies revealed that attachment of the virus is mediated by a canyon-shaped receptor site which encircles each of the 12 pentameric vertices of the icosahedral capsid. Selective inhibitory compounds, e.g. pirodavir and WIN-54954, work by binding into a hydrophobic pocket (the 'win pocket') situated in VP1 beneath the canyon floor (Figure 69.23) (Rossmann 1990). Likely, this pocket forms a natural molecular hinge in the protein which may give flexibility to the molecule during disassembly and assembly of the icosahedral structure required when uncoating, and again during production of new virus particles. When the inhibitor is bound into the pocket it may have two effects. First it can interfere with virus attachment to the cell receptor. Secondly, and more important, it may interfere with uncoating (Woods et al. 1989; Andries et al. 1992).

The most promising antipicornavirus compound to progress into clinical development is known as pleconaril. It is a capsid-binding agent, structurally related to WIN 54954 (Pleconaril) (Figure 69.19) In vitro, pleconaril inhibits the replication of most rhinoviruses (responsible for >50 percent of all common colds) and enteroviruses. Oral treatment has been studied in randomized double-blind, placebo-controlled trials and was found to produce significant benefits (Hayden et al.

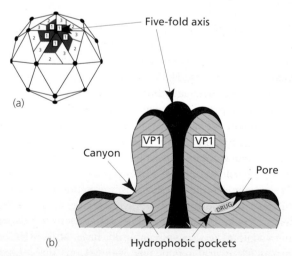

Figure 69.23 *The proposed mechanism of action for capsid-binding inhibitors of picornaviruses, including rhinoviruses.* **(a)** *Icosahedral capsid of a rhinovirus, depicting the arrangement of the three capsid proteins about a five-fold axis.* **(b)** *Three of the five VP1 proteins at the five-fold axis. A typical rhinovirus inhibitor is binding into the hydrophobic pocket at the base of the canyon, probably reducing the flexibility of the VP1 protein and affecting receptor binding and uncoating. An amino acid substitution in the region forming the pocket may lead to resistance because of the lost ability to bind drug. (Field and Goldthorpe (1985), with permission.)*

2003). Phase III clinical trials involving over 2 000 patients who took the drug showed early and substantial reduction in symptom severity and a 1 day reduction in disease duration. However, an unexpected problem was encountered; namely an interaction with oral contraceptives. Breakthrough bleeding was evident in 3 percent of women taking oral contraceptives during a 5 day course of pleconaril.

During 2002, the US Food and Drug Administration (FDA) rejected pleconaril (Picovir) as an antiviral drug being developed to treat the common cold on the grounds that this may encourage the development of resistant strains and may reduce the effectiveness of oral contraceptives (Senior 2002). Furthermore, a more recent 6 week prophylaxis study found that pleconaril induces cytochrome P-450 3A enzymes which metabolize a variety of drugs (Hayden et al. 2003).

Despite the encouraging early clinical data on the antiviral effects, the compound is unlikely to be widely used for the less severe upper respiratory virus infections at least until the pharmacological phenomena have been elucidated. It was hoped that the drug may be beneficial for the treatment of more serious picornavirus infections, however early data are less encouraging and a double-blind, placebo-controlled trial of pleconaril in infants suffering from enterovirus meningitis was inconclusive (Abzug et al. 2003).

Inhibitors of other DNA viruses

POXVIRUSES

Smallpox was officially declared to have been eradicated from the world in 1980 after a 10-year campaign of intensive surveillance and vaccination. Although smallpox has not afflicted humans for more than 20 years now, large quantities of the virus are thought to remain in storage and there is concern that this virus might be employed as a weapon of terrorism or biowarfare (Baker et al. 2003). The *Poxviridae* comprise several genera including *Orthopoxvirus* which contains variola (smallpox), vaccinia and monkeypox; *Capripoxvirus* which contains lumpy skin disease; and *Parapoxvirus* which contains orf of sheep and pseudocowpox of cattle. All these infections can infect humans and produce severe disease, especially when the subject is immunocompromised. For all these reasons there is a perceived need for effective antiviral chemotherapy. Historically, 1-methyl-isatin-β-thiosemicarbazones methisazone, Marboran (Bauer et al. 1969) (Figure 69.24) was among the first selective antiviral agents to be used in humans. It was used with some success during the 1960s to treat smallpox and the severe complication of vaccinia, namely *excema vaccinatum*. The mechanism of action was thought to involve interference with late virus protein synthesis (Hovi 1988). The further development of

Methisazone

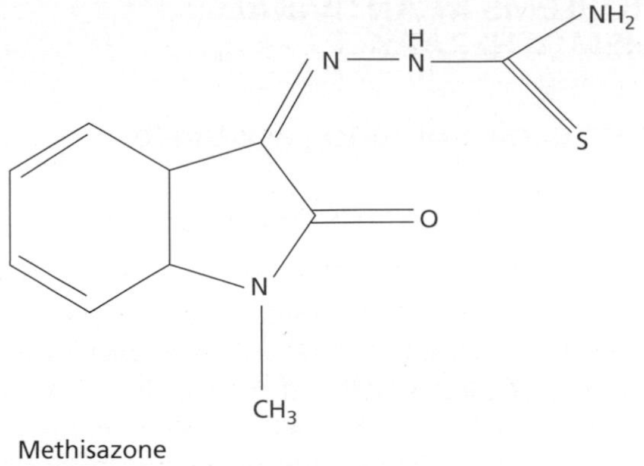

Figure 69.24 *An very early inhibitor of poxviruses – methisazone*

thiosemicarbazones was overtaken by the eradication of smallpox. Furthermore, modern criteria for laboratory assessment of compounds suggests that the potency of marboran is, at best, modest. Members of the acyclic nucleoside phosphonate family of compounds (see Herpesvirus section above) are found to be much more promising; in particular cidofovir and adefovir derivatives (Whitley 2003; Kern 2003). Beneficial clinical responses in severe orf infections in immunocompromised patients have been claimed in single patient studies (Geerinck et al. 2001). The potential for these compounds as inhibitors of poxviruses and a comprehensive catalogue of alternative antiviral strategies for prophylaxis and therapy of poxviruses is documented by Baker et al. (2003).

PAPILLOMAVIRUSES AND ADENOVIRUSES

Human papillomavirus infections most often cause genital warts or juvenile laryngeal papillomatosis. Interferons have been extensively evaluated for treating such infections (see Chapter 16, Viral evasion of the host immune response) The local (intralesional) therapy of genital warts refractory to cytodestructive therapy is sometimes effective. The association between genital warts and cervical carcinomas provides further impetus for the development of antiviral agents to treat diseases associated with these viruses. The broad spectrum of action of the acyclic nucleoside phosphonates includes both HPV and adenoviruses. Success has been claimed in small studies (Stragier et al. 2002) providing some optimism for the clinical utility of this family of compounds in such severe cases that are relatively rare, but clinically very difficult to manage. The potential molecular targets offered by HPV for potential antiviral attack are reviewed by Phelps et al. (1998). There has also been much interest in the compound, 1-(2-methyl-propyl)-1H-imidazo[4,5-C]quinolin-4-amine), given the generic name imiquimod (Figure 69.10) (Miller et al. 1995). Similar to resiquimod, the antiviral activity seems to result from interferon-α induction and, if so, would place this compound among the immunomodulators.

PROBLEMS IN ANTIVIRAL CHEMOTHERAPY

Virus evolution and resistance

A DEFINITION OF VIRUS DRUG RESISTANCE

As for all forms of microorganism, including eukaryotic cells, viruses can readily become resistant to inhibitors. This may be defined as: 'An acquired genetic change such that the virus is relieved from inhibition at drug concentrations that are normally inhibitory in the therapeutic range'. For viruses, this is always the result of one or more mutations in the virus genome.

Thus, drug resistance in viruses implies the emergence of strains for which the ED_{50} significantly exceeds the inhibitory concentration normally achieved in vivo (Field 1988b). When possible, a drug-resistant variant is compared directly with its drug-sensitive parent (Figure 69.25), but in clinical practice the latter may not be available. Criteria have been established to define acquired drug resistance which are particular to each family of virus and are related to the appropriate laboratory tests. Assays which detect mutations known to be associated with resistance are called 'genotypic tests' whereas 'phenotypic tests' are applied to infectious virus (Table 69.3). There are advantages and disadvantages associated with each type of test (Blaise et al. 2002). Virus families that are naturally insensitive to a compound should not properly be included within the definition of drug resistance.

REASONS FOR STUDYING DRUG RESISTANCE IN VIRUSES

Clearly, drug resistance is an important medical problem which may subvert otherwise successful therapy. However, the phenomenon also has some uses. The detection of resistant mutants is a very important criterion for demonstrating that a particular drug is

selective for the target virus. Once drug-resistant mutants have been obtained, the location and nature of drug resistance mutations enables the identification of the target gene(s) in the virus and functional domains in target proteins to be defined at a molecular level. In turn, this enables patterns of cross resistance to be predicted and is often important in the development of further compounds with improved antiviral characteristics. Thus, the selection and study of drug-resistant variants plays a vital part in the development process of all new compounds

VIRUS EVOLUTION

Point mutations, or small groups of mutations, can readily lead to substantial increases in resistance to various specific antiviral drugs (Coen 1986; Field and Owen 1988; Mellors et al. 1995). Viruses are susceptible to natural mutations which may occur as a result of

- damage due to chemical mutagens, ionizing radiation cosmic rays etc
- enzymatic modification after replication
- errors by the polymerase during replication.

Of the three possibilities, the last is the most important. Some antiviral drugs are potential chemical mutagens, notwithstanding, most mutants appear to arise naturally and have a selective advantage in the presence of the inhibitor. Several types of mutation are possible: transition ($A \leftrightarrow G$, $C \leftrightarrow T$); transversion ($A \leftrightarrow C \leftrightarrow G$, $A \leftrightarrow T \leftrightarrow G$), insertion; and deletion. Insertions and deletions are particularly common when there are runs of identical nucleotides such as several consecutive guanosine residues, sometimes referred to as a 'G-string'. Insertions or deletions into such a sequence may introduce a frame-shift and disruption of the normal polypeptide.

VIRUS POLYMERASES ARE ERROR-PRONE

DNA viruses have a relatively low intrinsic error rate (1×10^{-7} to 1×10^{-8} errors per nucleotide). In double-stranded DNA viruses, a $3'-5'$ exonuclease proofreading function can edit out errors giving an overall rate of $<1 \times 10^{-9}$. However, given the large number of viruses in an infected host, this is still sufficiently high for DNA viruses to evolve very rapidly relative to higher life forms.

RNA viruses have very high intrinsic mutation rates and there are no proofreading or repair mechanisms available. This high rate of mutation ($\geqslant 1 \times 10^{-4}$), coupled with a large population size, can quickly lead to enormous genetic diversity within a single infected host. For example, HIV has a single-stranded RNA genome of approximately 9 000 nucleotides. The replication rate in an infected individual has been estimated to be approximately 10^9 daily, thus, $10^{-4} \times 9\ 000 \times 10^9 = 9 \times 10^8$ mutants occur each day. This means that, in theory, every point mutation occurs 10^5 times per day in an HIV-infected individual and every double mutant ten

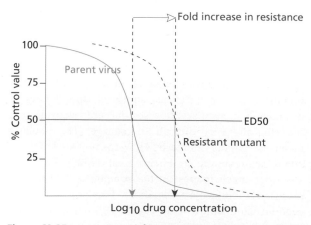

Figure 69.25 *Measurement of increase in resistance, e.g. when the ED_{50} of the mutant is 10 μg/ml and the parental strain is 0.1. This would represent an increased resistance of 100-fold.*

Table 69.3 *Methods for detecting resistance in clinical specimens*

Advantages and disadvantages	
Phenotypic[a]	**Genotypic**[b]
Slow	More rapid
Cumbersome	Less cumbersome
Expensive	Less expensive
Clinically relevant	May not correlate with phenotype
May underestimate reResistance in vivo	May exaggerate resistance in vivo
May not detect mixtures	Insensitive to minor species

a) Usually tissue-culture based
b) Usually PCR-based

times per day! As a result, HIV actually exists as a 'quasi species' or 'swarm' around a particular consensus sequence.

PRIMARY, SECONDARY, AND COMPENSATING DRUG RESISTANCE MUTATIONS

Mutations that give rise to amino acid substitutions in, or close to, the site that interacts with the inhibitor and that are clearly associated with a biochemical change in the interaction leading to resistance, are termed 'primary mutations.' Such mutations characterize variants that arise early upon exposure to the inhibitor. Further mutations may accumulate – and these are termed 'secondary mutations' and these may contribute to the overall level of resistance. However, yet further mutations may appear which are apparently unrelated to the sites on proteins that interact with the drug. Such mutations may have no direct effect on biochemical drug sensitivity but may increase enzyme efficiency so as to compensate for the deleterious effects of the primary and secondary mutations. Another example has been observed in HIV where a mutation may change the protease cleavage site in the target protein that compensates for a change in the substrate specificity of the HIV protease itself due to a primary resistance mutations. Many compensating mutations are suspected but, in most cases, their precise role has yet to be elucidated (Swanstrom and Erona 2000).

BIOCHEMICAL VS CLINICAL DRUG RESISTANCE

From the earliest attempts at therapy of ocular herpesvirus, it was realized that treatment failure did not necessarily correlate with biochemical resistance in virus isolates. Conversely, patients carrying HIV with multiple drug resistance mutations may still respond to therapy; virus replication remains suppressed and immune function near normal despite the presence of highly resistant variants. There are likely to be several different explanations for these observations. First, the assay methods to measure resistance may not accurately reflect the conditions in the host, e.g. cell type (including the species/ tissue of origin), the growth rate of cells (resting or multiplying), the complexity of media components (that

may interfere with specific drugs), the multiplicity of infection, heterogeneous virus populations, and the existence of latently infected cells. Other possible host factors include noncompliance or changes in the patient that effect metabolism of the drug. Furthermore, the fact that many mutations may result in attenuation is probably a factor in resistance development by all types of virus (see below).

MATHEMATICAL MODELS TO PREDICT FUTURE RESISTANCE TRENDS

Based upon virus mutation rates (see above) alone, it would follow that virus infections would evolve to resist any specific inhibitor within a few days, rendering any drug useless. However, experience shows that this is rarely the case because the possession of drug resistance mutations usually has a biological price. For example, many mutations in the reverse transcriptase nucleotide binding site or protease active site in HIV or neuramidase of influenza are thought to reduce the catalytic activity of these enzymes and negatively affect replication and/or transmission efficiency. Similarly, HSV TK^{-ve} mutants are highly resistant to aciclovir; while such mutants replicate efficiently in tissue culture, normal TK activity is required for virus replication in neurons and to enable HSV to reactivate from latency. In some cases the attenuation may be reduced by compensating mutations although such effects are likely to be difficult to define.

VIRUS FITNESS

Some drug-resistant mutant viruses are clearly attenuated or 'less fit.' The biochemical changes resulting from mutations in the virus genome may, of course, be extremely subtle and the biological effects very difficult to measure. Much effort has been directed to the establishment of relevant laboratory tests to estimate attenuation (e.g. Weber et al. 2003). Certain constellations of changes may give rise to more successful drug-resistant viruses that will then dominate the population. These effects have been quantified by mathematical modelers. With increased understanding of virus pathogenesis and the mechanism of action of virus inhibitors, the theoretical models have become increasingly sophisti-cated. Some predictions are optimistic, e.g. the likely future development of aciclovir resistance in genital herpes (Gershengorn et al. 2003), and influenza virus resistance to neuraminidase inhibitors (Ferguson et al. 2003) are both expected to remain low. However, for HIV, the predictions are more pessimistic and the expectation from the models is that, despite combination therapy, HIV drug resistance will eventually overtake the therapeutic effort. (Blower and Volberding 2002). However, this is a dynamic situation and viruses will continue to evolve. Resistance thus remains a threat for all types of antiviral therapy. The key general features of virus drug resistance are summarized in Table 69.4 and the methods for isolating and study of resistance in Tables 69.5 and 69.6.

DRUG RESISTANCE IN HERPES SIMPLEX AND VARICELLA-ZOSTER VIRUS

In the immunologically normal host

Historically, HSV was among the first viruses where the phenomenon of drug resistance was studied. A single

Table 69.4 *Acquired drug resistance*

Summary of general features
Results from one or more mutations in genes coding for target proteins
Develops spontaneously due to high mutation rates in viruses
Found in all viruses, for almost all classes[a] of specific inhibitor
Resistance is the hall-mark of selectivity for antiviral compound
Useful for elucidation of mechanism of drug action
Many resistance mutations alter virus pathogenicity (fitness)
Variants may be present among heterogeneous populations
Clinical importance varies among virus families
Incidence predicted from mathematical models
Especially important in immunocompromised host

a) Exceptions are immunomodulators and compounds with a cellular target for virus inhibition. It is arguable whether such compounds are true 'antiviral' compounds.

Table 69.5 *Methods for obtaining laboratory drug-resistant strains*

Methods
Passage of virus in presence of subinhibitory concentrations
Selection by using alternative drug with same target e.g. TK
Genetic recombination with resistant virus
Obtain molecular clone with induced mutation; recombine with wild-type
Obtain virus strains from clinical isolates following therapy

Table 69.6 *Sequence for the study of drug resistance to a new compound*

Sequence
Virus selected for resistance
Resistance demonstrated in tissue culture and, if possible, in animal model
Mutations mapped to specific gene
DNA sequence reveals: deletion, insertion, point mutation (homopolymers in TK)
Protein is analyzed and single amino acid substitutions/ truncations predicted
Enzyme shown to have lower affinity for substrate or be insensitive in vitro
Site-directed mutagenesis generate new mutants; then shown to be resistant
Patterns of cross-resistance to alternative drugs explored
Clinical isolates from treated patients shown with identical mutations

passage of virus in the presence of a subinhibitory concentration of the compound (e.g. aciclovir, penci-clovir or brivudin) results in significant decrease in sensi-tivity to the respective compound (Larder and Darby 1984). Clinical isolates, including those obtained from normal patients who have never received chemotherapy, contain a small proportion (perhaps 0.1 percent) of pre-existing drug-resistant mutants (Paris and Harrington 1982) that can continue to multiply when selective pres-sure is applied.

Selection for resistance in the laboratory

Aciclovir and similar nucleoside analogues were found to select for resistance mutations in two loci: DNApol and TK (Larder and Darby 1984; Coen 1986) (Table 69.7). Several laboratory mutants of each type shown in this table have been fully characterized (Larder and Darby 1984; Coen 1986). The mutant proteins (TK or DNApol) undergo changes in their enzymatic properties and DNA sequencing has identi-fied the specific base substitutions of other changes that give rise to the drug-resistant phenotype; thus, the origin of resistance is fully explained (Collins and Darby 1991). The most common mutations are probably single G insertions into the G-string motif (Sasadeusz et al. 1997; Harris et al. 2003). Furthermore, several drug-resistant strains obtained from clinical isolates (almost all from immunocompromised patients following drug failure) proved to have genotypes identical to the previously characterized laboratory-selected strains (Larder and Darby 1984).

Herpesvirus DNApol is essential for virus replication and resistance mutations are generally single base substi-tutions that alter the affinity of the enzyme for nucleo-side analogue triphosphates. Pyrophosphate analogues (e.g. foscarnet) also select for resistance mutations in DNApol. In contrast to DNApol, HSV TK is not essen-

Table 69.7 *Nature of herpes virus drug-resistant mutants so far isolated*

Genetic locus	Genetic change	Resistance	Frequency in clinical isolates
TK (TK⁻)	Base: substitution, insertion or deletion	Little or no TK enzyme to phosphorylate thymidine or thymidine analogue	Relatively common (in mixtures) but usually attenuated
Mutations in promoter site TK (TKʳ)	Base substitution	Altered TK substrate specificity; reduced phosphorylation of inhibitor but whole or partial phosphorylation of thymidine analogue	Quite rare
DNApolʳ (DNApolʳ)	Base substitution	Low affinity for nucleoside analogue triphosphate	Very rare

tial for replication and TK^{-ve} viruses grow with normal kinetics in actively dividing cell cultures. In resting cells, however, TK^{-ve} viruses are less efficient and have restricted ability to replicate in neurons. Mutants with drug-resistance mutations in the TK gene may produce full-length polypeptides with base substitutions leading to altered enzyme substrate specificity (TK-altered) or the enzyme activity may be absent (TK-defective or TK^{-ve}). In laboratory animal infection models both DNApol and TK mutants of both types have been shown to be attenuated and, TK^{-ve} mutants show particularly marked reductions in neuropathogenicity.

In clinical practice, the incidence of resistant viruses is very low (<1 percent) in virus isolates obtained from immunocompetent patients. Large surveys measuring the sensitivity of virus isolates to aciclovir have been carried out regularly from 1979 to the present day and these show no significant changes in the mean sensitivity of isolates (ED$_{50}$ approximately 1 μM). There is no evidence of increased incidence of resistance after more than 20 years use including oral prescription and widespread availability of topical formulations over the counter. Furthermore, daily administration to individual patients for more than 10 years for suppression of their recurrent disease has not been associated with resistance development. Recent surveys for penciclovir sensitivity among clinical isolates also show no evidence for increase in resistance (Bacon et al. 2002; Shin et al. 2003)

The explanation for the lack of resistance to HSV antiviral drugs in clinical practice appears to be that the majority of resistance mutations are of reduced pathogenicity. In cell culture, the kinetics and yields of such mutants are similar to those of their parental strains, but they are usually more or less attenuated when tested in animal models (Field et al. 1980, reviewed by Field 1989). It may be that the early establishment of neuronal latency with sensitive virus is another important factor (Field 2001).

Occasionally, TK^{-ve} viruses have been isolated that appear to be highly pathogenic in animal models. One such virus was recently elucidated. Sequencing showed that the TK^{-ve} phenotype resulted from a double G

insertion into a G-string giving rise to a truncated polypeptide. However, this virus underwent a high frequency mutation event inserting a further G into the G-string thus restoring the open reading frame. Passage of this virus through the nervous system of mice resulted in rapid selection of the TK^{+ve} variant (Grey et al. 2003). Such viruses are likely to remain rare in nature, but this work reminds us of the potential for new and unexpected possibilities in the future.

Varicella-zoster virus resistance appears to follow the same pattern as HSV although there are no convenient rodent laboratory infection models to explore the pathogenicity of resistant strains as has been the case for HSV (Kimberlin et al. 1995). Currently, drug resistance is not regarded as a problem for either of these viruses except in immunocompetent patients.

Resistance to herpes simplex in the immunocompromised patient

Drug resistance to ACV has been encountered among immunocompromised patients, of whom several large surveys suggest that about 5 percent shed resistant virus (Wade et al. 1982; Englund et al. 1990). All three mechanisms of drug resistance have been observed (Table 69.3) and, in some cases, clinical isolates comprise mixtures of sensitive and resistant viruses, perhaps with more than one type of resistant virus present (Martin et al. 1985; Christophers and Sutton 1987; Sacks et al. 1989). Viruses that are resistant through lack of TK are, naturally, cross-resistant to other drugs that depend on virus TK for activation, whereas viruses of the TKʳ phenotype show varying patterns of cross-resistance. Foscarnet selects for resistance only at the DNApol locus and is a possible alternative for therapeutic use when resistance develops to the nucleoside analogues. However, multiple drug resistance has occurred in some patients (Crumpacker et al. 1982). In summary, although drug resistance in the immunocompetent patient does not seem to be a problem at present, it may prove to be a very serious matter in the individual patient with defective immunity.

DRUG RESISTANCE IN HCMV

HCMV infection is one of the major virological problems in the immunocompromised patient and, unfortunately, drug resistance has emerged as a significant additional problem in these cases (Drew et al. 1991). Viruses that have acquired resistance to GCV have been encountered, and analysis of these strains led to the discovery of a hitherto unsuspected site of action of the drug (Drew et al. 1991; Drew et al. 1993). The drug-resistance mutations were traced to gene *UL97*, which, as mentioned under 'Ganciclovir', encodes a protein kinase function (Littler et al. 1992; Sullivan et al. 1992). Although this finding confirms a serious problem in these patients that renders the therapy ineffective, at a biochemical level it was an exciting discovery because it revealed a novel potential target for the design of inhibitors against this and other viruses (Birch and Mills 1994; Biron 1994). Relevantly, documentation of GCV resistance in transplant recipients may occur as frequently as 20 percent of the time.

Drug resistance in HIV

In contrast to the earlier experience with herpesviruses, antiviral drug resistance has emerged as one of the major problems in the management of HIV. Indeed, the study of resistance has had a central role in HIV drug development; it is the subject of numerous research communications and thus the subject has necessarily been covered in the consideration of HIV as a target for chemotherapy (see section on Inhibitors of human immunodeficiency virus above). HIV drug resistance is considered to be the most important factor limiting the continued effectiveness of all three classes of anti-HIV drug currently in use (RT inhibitors, nonnucleoside RT inhibitors, and protease inhibitors (Bean et al. 1987; Ljungman et al. 1990; Safrin et al. 1994) in patients undergoing monotherapy. This problem led to the introduction of the successful strategy of drug combinations in HAART.

At first it was difficult to show the development of resistance to the early drugs directed against HIV such as AZT. Unfortunately, this turned out to be due to a technical problem and, once the methods for detection were improved, virus drug resistance was revealed as a universal feature of all chemotherapeutic strategies so far employed against this infection.

Drug resistance in HIV results from point mutations leading to alterations in the affinity of reverse transcriptase for the inhibitor (the most important mutations are documented for individual HIV drugs in the section on Inhibitors of human immunodeficiency virus above) although this has, in many cases, been very difficult to prove by testing the enzyme functions for reduced sensitivity to inhibition in vitro. Development of resistance was first shown for zidovudine (Larder et al. 1989; Larder and Kemp 1989), and subsequently for all other nucleoside inhibitors. Resistance to the NNRTI apparently occurs even more readily and the resistant strains are cross-resistant (Richman et al. 1991; Condra et al. 1992). Resistance to the various proteinase inhibitors has also been clearly demonstrated (Otto et al. 1993; Kaplan et al. 1994; Mellors et al. 1995). Several hundred resistance mutations have now been documented and the sequential patterns of mutations are well understood (D'Aquila et al. 2003; Swanstrom and Erona 2000).

Particular mutations (and in some cases sequences of mutations) lead to progressively more resistant virus populations in the patient. Knowledge of resistance patterns to individual drugs enables rational strategies for combinations of drugs. The monitoring for resistance in individual patients has led to the possibility of tailoring therapeutic regimens to the patient. However, the success of triple or quadruple drug regimens has produced long-term suppression of virus growth in the patient and sustained normality of T-cell populations. Furthermore, it has come to light that among the heterogeneous population of virions in the patient, highly drug-resistant variants are present. The fact that the patient appears to be able to tolerate their presence may be explained by the fact that the resistant variants are of lower pathogenicity, i.e. less fit (discussed above).

A North American study (Little et al. 2000) showed that between 1–11 percent HIV infections were already resistant to one or more compounds when acquired and the proportion of new HIV infections involving resistance is increasing. Even taking into account the reduced fitness of some drug-resistant variants, mathematical models remain pessimistic, predicting that the long term future for the continued success of current antiviral agents is fairly bleak

DRUG RESISTANCE IN ORTHOMYXOVIRUSES

Influenza A virus has long been known to develop resistance to amantadine (Cochran et al. 1965; Oxford et al. 1970). Resistance was mapped first to the hemagglutinin and subsequently to the *M2* gene (Lamb et al. 1985; Hay et al. 1986) which codes for a component of the nucleocapsid. Of the two sites, changes in the M2 protein are the more important (Hay et al. 1985). Analyses of such drug-resistant mutants were of paramount importance in defining the mechanism of action of amantadine and similar compounds (Field and Owen 1988) (see section on Inhibitors of orthomyxo- and paramyxoviruses).

The rapid development of resistance following transmission to susceptible birds was reported following the experimental infection and therapy of chickens with highly virulent avian influenza virus causing fowl plague (Webster et al. 1986), and more recently a similar rapid development of drug resistance has been observed in humans infected with influenza A (Belshe et al. 1989;

Hayden et al. 1989, 1991; Hayden 1994). Although drug resistance is readily selected for in cell culture, there has been much debate on the significance of published surveys to assess the impact of resistance in humans to amantadine (Stilianakis et al. 1998).

The neuraminidase inhibitors zanamivir and oseltamivir select for resistance mutations in the neuraminidase gene and polymorphisms in the hemagglutinin may be important in determining the sensitivity of isolates (Gubareva et al. 2001a, 2001b). The new inhibitors were introduced into clinical practice in various parts of the world between 1999 and 2002. In order to monitor the potential development of resistance, the 'Neuraminidase Inhibitor Susceptibility Network' was established to coordinate testing of clinical isolates (McKimm-Breschkin et al. 2003). This has established a base line susceptibility of over 1 000 clinical isolates. It will enable accurate monitoring of resistance emerging in the future, particularly in the inevitable widespread use of anti-influenza virus therapy during an influenza pandemic. To date, resistance to the neuraminidase inhibitors appears to be limited in clinical practice and taken with the predictions from mathematical models (Ferguson et al. 2003), this allows cautious optimisms regarding the future impact of resistance in the treatment and prevention of influenza.

DRUG RESISTANCE IN HEPATITIS VIRUSES

Although there are relatively few data on clinical resistance compared to that for HIV, the development of resistance during HBV therapy appears to parallel that observed among retroviruses. Lamivudine treatment is associated with the rapid development of drug-resistance variants with specific polymerase mutations. Similarly, adefovir dipivoxil therapy is associated with the selection of mutations in the HBV polymerase, however, at a very low rate of occurrence (Angus et al. 2003). Compared with the monotherapy of HIV, resistance development is slower to emerge during HBV treatment, possible reflecting the slow rate of infected hepatocyte turnover which is significantly slower than infected lymphocyte turnover during HIV (Mutimer 1998). Similar to HIV, the most important approach is thought to be the introduction of combination therapy using two or more different drugs simultaneously. Treatment failures are also observed in HCV therapy by means of combinations of an antiviral drug with pegylated interferon. These failures are suspected to involve drug resistance although the mechanisms are, to date, unknown.

DRUG RESISTANCE IN PICORNAVIRUSES

The action of capsid-binding molecules that interact with rhinoviruses is readily reversed by the growth of mutants with point mutations in the genes coding for the capsid proteins concerned (Ninomiya et al. 1985). The patterns of cross-resistance have been widely studied (Yasin et al. 1990a) and in some cases, cross-resistance to the effects of neutralizing antibodies occurs (Dutko and Diana 1990; Rossmann 1990). Such antibodies also depend on capsid-binding at a nearby site in order to achieve neutralization. Although the study of such resistance is very useful in elucidating precise virus-inhibitor mechanisms, its implication for the future use of anti-picornavirus compounds of this type is far from clear. Resistance has the potential to arise very rapidly in vitro, and the unresolved question is whether such resistant variants will have impaired pathogenicity or reduced ability to spread. One trial suggested that this may indeed be the case (Dearden et al. 1989; Yasin et al. 1990b); however, there is as yet far too little information to predict the possible impact of drug resistance in the clinic of such compounds becoming widely used (Al-Nakib 1993). Pleconaril readily selects for drug resistant variants in tissue culture. There has been too little experience with the compound to determine whether or not this will be important in clinical practice. However, concern about resistance development has been cited among the reasons for the 2002 US Food and Drug Administration ruling that pleconaril should be rejected as an antiviral drug being developed to treat the common cold.

VIRUS DRUG RESISTANCE – CODA

Although drug resistance may be seen as a setback after many years of otherwise successful development of new drugs, it does have useful aspects: the isolation of resistant variants defines the compound as having a virus-specific mode of action; it enables the molecular targets for drug action to be identified with certainty; and, particularly when such targets are unsuspected, it may reveal hitherto unknown targets for the design of further inhibitors. Finally, when the precise mechanisms of drug resistance are elucidated, this information may provide a rationale for alternative therapeutic strategies to minimize or circumvent the impact of drug resistance in the patient.

The problem of toxicity of antiviral compounds

As stated at the outset of this chapter, the principal obstacle to the development of antiviral compounds has been to obtain selective toxicity. Having established both in in vitro and animal models that a compound has a high selective index, problems may be encountered when the compounds are administered to humans. In some cases the toxic effects may be caused by minor metabolites of the original compound.

Nucleoside analogues often cause a variety of acute effects, including malaise, weight loss, tremors, mutism, peripheral neuropathy, acute liver and kidney damage as well as the more common complaints of nausea and vomiting. In some cases these effects have been related to the inhibition of cellular enzymes, particularly mitochondrial enzymes, by the antiviral compounds. (The problems encountered when treating patients with particular HIV drugs are considered in the section entitled Inhibitors of human immunodeficiency virus, above). Amantadine administration is associated with reversible neurological change (rimantadine is used successfully in the control of Parkinson's disease) and these effects are thought to relate to the release and uptake of dopamine in the central nervous system (Mizoguchi et al. 1994). To these problems must be added the long-term concern regarding possible teratogenicity and genetic damage caused by agents that interact with DNA (Griffiths 1995). The latter can theoretically occur when nucleoside analogues are incorporated into host-cell DNA or, indirectly, as a result of inhibition of DNA repair systems (Darby 1995).

'Familiarity breeds contempt' and there have been two incidences of toxicity in patients that resulted in deaths, reminding us of the need for constant attention to the potential that antiviral agents have for producing serious side-effects.

TWO EXAMPLES OF SEVERE TOXICITY PROBLEMS IN HUMANS

Fialuridine toxicity

Fialuridine (1-2′-deoxy-2′-fluoro-1-β-D-arabinofuranosyl-5-iodouracil; FIAU) is an orally bioavailable compound active against HBV (Fried et al. 1992). Pilot studies with a four-week course were encouraging and showed that significant reduction in virus replication could be achieved. However, further trials with a longer treatment period were stopped after 12 weeks when patients developed myopathy, lactic acidosis, peripheral neuropathy, pancreatitis and liver failure; there were several deaths (Meeting Report 1995). The mechanism for this unexpected delayed toxicity seems to be a consequence of FIAU incorporation into mitochondrial DNA.

Sorivudine, BVaraU: toxic interactions with 5-fluoruracil

Sorivudine, or BVaraU, is a potent inhibitor of VZV (see section on Inhibitors of herpesviruses) and the drug is currently undergoing clinical trials. It was licensed in Japan in 1993 but the license was withdrawn when several deaths occurred in patients also receiving 5-fluorouracil. The toxicity resulted from the formation of the metabolite bromovinyluracil (Ashida et al. 1993) which inhibits dihydrothymine dehydrogenase, normally responsible for degrading 5-fluorouracil. This drug interaction led to the accumulation of 5-uracil in cancer patients receiving both drugs, and thus to fatal bone marrow suppression.

The problem of virus latency

HERPESVIRUS LATENCY

Several viruses are capable of establishing latency in infected cells. This is a particular feature of all the herpesviruses, and both HSV and VZV can remain latent in neurons for the lifetime of the infected individual (Wildy et al. 1982). Periodic reactivations may cause clinical recurrences. In some cases they are subclinical but, whether or not disease is apparent, the infection may be transmitted during the episode to a susceptible contact. Because, during the latent phase, the virus does not express the genes coding for virus proteins, including TK and DNApol, it is unaffected by any of the conventional nucleoside analogues or drugs that rely on viral protein targets. Experimental infection in animal models suggests that latency is established early, and foci of latently infected neurons are detected a few hours after the first round of virus replication at the mucosal site of infection (Thackray and Field 2000). In man, the process of establishing latency may take a little longer, but the implication is that chemotherapy is unlikely to be started early enough to prevent the establishment of latency during a primary infection. Even if chemotherapy is successful in limiting the clinical signs of disease, the virus will persist, to reactivate later (Darby and Field 1984). However, both famiclovir and aciclovir do suppress recurrent infections and patients have taken suppressive therapy for this purpose over periods up to 10 years (Douglas et al. 1984; Straus et al. 1984; Goldberg et al. 1993; Mertz et al. 1997). Furthermore, prophylaxis can prevent episodes of herpes resulting from reactivation in immunosuppressed patients. The problem of eradicating herpesvirus DNA harbored in latently infected cells is one for which there remains no obvious solution however, the early establishment of latency and the subsequent role of the nervous system in the reactivation and recurrence of infection may underlie the very low incidence (discussed above in section entitled The problem of toxicity of antiviral compounds), of HSV drug resistance (Field 2001).

RETROVIRUS LATENCY

HIV can establish a different kind of latency in which the viral DNA, always formed as an intermediate during replication, may become stably integrated into the chromosome of the host cell. In some cases the cells survive infection and continue to harbor the viral genes, which are not expressed, or are expressed at a very low level, with the potential to become active later. Furthermore, the stimulation of resting lymphocytes is associated with the activation of latent HIV (Hermankova et al. 2003). HAART has been effective in reducing the plasma levels of HIV-1 RNA below the limits of detection of most clinical assays. However, the infection has not been eradicated by HAART and this is likely due to latent HIV-1 replication-competent provirus in resting CD4$^+$ T-lymphocytes (Pomerantz 2003).

COMBINATION CHEMOTHERAPY FOR VIRAL INFECTIONS

As with the treatment of some bacterial diseases, especially mycobacterial infections, combinations of drugs have proven exceedingly valuable. The recognition that monotherapy of HIV infections has not resulted in a cure has led to numerous clinical trials evaluating various combinations of antiretroviral therapy (e.g. nucleoside analogues combined with nonnucleoside analogues and/or protease inhibitors) (Schinazi 1991, 1995). This has led to the concept of HAART. This strategy has proved extremely successful with suppression of virus to below the level of detection and a marked and sustained benefit (De Clercq 1998). However, the toxic effects of the chronic use of the current compounds remains a limiting factor in the medium to long term. Similarly, for life-threatening herpesvirus infections (e.g. encephalitis or neonatal herpes), combination therapies will be tested, including the combined use of drugs and immunoglobulins or cytokines, including interferons.

CONCLUSIONS AND FUTURE PROSPECTS

The rapid application of molecular biology to the study of viruses most assuredly will lead to the development of novel antiviral drugs. Already, the identification of protease in a variety of viruses other than HIV has led to a great increase in research directed toward the synthesis of peptidomimetics that inhibit these enzymes. Hepatitis C, HSV, CMV etc. are prime targets. For HSV alone, many genes provide targets for debilitation of viral replication; they include both those essential for viral replication and others that are not. The application of antisense RNA, triplex-forming oligonucleotides, ribozymes and direct DNA targeting, although intellectually appealing, poses drug delivery problems that have yet to be overcome in clinical practice.

REFERENCES

Abzug, M.J., Cloud, G., et al. 2003. Double blind placebo-controlled trial of pleconaril in infants with enterovirus meningitis. *Pediatr Infect Dis J*, **4**, 335–41.

Al-Nakib, W. 1993. Drug resistance in rhinoviruses. *Int Antiviral News*, **1**, 100.

Andries, K., Dewindt, B., et al. 1992. In vitro activity of pirodavir (R 77975), a substituted phenoxy-pyridazinamine with broad-spectrum antipicornaviral activity. *Antimicrob Agents Chemother*, **36**, 100–7.

Angus, P., Vaughan, R., et al. 2003. Resistance to adefovir dipivoxil therapy associated with the selection of a novel mutation in the HBV polymerase. *Gastroenterology*, **125**, 292–7.

Ashida, N., Ljichi, K., et al. 1993. Metabolism of 5′-ether prodrugs of 1-beta-d-arabinofuranosyl-E-5-(2-bromovinyl)uracil in rats. *Biochem Pharmacol*, **46**, 2201–7.

Azad, R.F., Driver, V.B., et al. 1993. Antiviral activity of a phosphorothioate oligonucleotide complementary to RNA of the human cytomegalovirus major immediate-early region. *Antimicrob Agents Chemother*, **37**, 1945–54.

Baba, M., Pauwels, R., et al. 1987. Both 2′,3′-dideoxythymidine and its 2′,3′-unsaturated derivative (2′,3′-dideoxythymidinene) are potent and selective inhibitors of human immunodeficiency virus replication in vitro. *Biochem Biophys Res Commun*, **142**, 128–34.

Baba, M., Tanaka, H., et al. 1989. Highly specific inhibition of human immunodeficiency virus type 1 by a novel 6-substituted acyclouridine derivative. *Biochem Biophys Res Commun*, **165**, 1375–81.

Bacon, T.H., Boon, R.J., et al. 2002. Surveillance for antiviral-agent-resistant herpes simplex virus in the general population with recurrent herpes labialis. *Antimicrob Agents Chemother*, **46**, 3042–4.

Baker, D. and Eisen, D. 2003. Valacyclovir for prevention of recurrent herpes labialis: 2 double-blind, placebo-controlled studies. *Cutis*, **71**, 239–42.

Baker, R.O., Bray, M. and Huggins, J.W. 2003. Potential antiviral therapeutics for smallpox, monkeypox and other orthopoxvirus infections. *Antiviral Res*, **57**, 13–23.

Balfour, H.H. Jr. 1999. Antiviral drugs. *N Engl J Med*, **340**, 1255–68.

Balfour, H.H. Jr, Kelly, J.M., et al. 1990. Acyclovir treatment of varicella in otherwise healthy children. *J Pediatr*, **116**, 633–9.

Bartenschlager, R. 2002a. Hepatitis C virus replicons: potential role for drug development. *Nature Reviews, Drug Discovery*, **1**, 911–16.

Bartenschlager, R. 2002b. In vitro models for hepatitis C. *Virus Res*, **8**, 25–32.

Bartenschlager, R. and Lohmann, V. 2001. Novel cell culture systems for the hepatitis C virus. *Antiviral Res*, **52**, 1–17.

Bauer, J.J., St Vincent, L., et al. 1969. Prophylaxis of smallpox with methisazone. *Am J Epidemiol*, **90**, 130–45.

Bean, B., Fletcher, C., et al. 1987. Progressive mucocutaneous herpes simplex infection due to acyclovir-resistant virus in an immunocompromised patient: correlation of viral susceptibilities and plasma levels with response to therapy. *Diagn Microbiol Infect Dis*, **7**, 199–204.

Beauchamp, L.M., Orr, G.F., et al. 1992. Amino acid ester prodrugs of acyclovir. *Antiviral Chem Chemother*, **3**, 157–64.

Belshe, R.B., Burk, B., et al. 1989. Resistance of influenza A virus to amantadine and rimantadine: results of one decade of surveillance. *J Infect Dis*, **159**, 430–5.

Beutner, K.R., Douglas, J.M., et al. 1998. Treatment of genital warts with an immune response modifier (imiquimod). *J Am Acad Dermatol*, **38**, 230–9.

Bigar, F. 1979. Clinical experiences with trifluorothymidine in herpes simplex keratitis. *Adv Ophthalmol*, **38**, 110–15.

Birch, C. and Mills, J. 1994. Cytomegalovirus and drug resistance. *Int Antiviral News*, **2**, 119–20.

Biron, K. 1994. Ganciclovir resistance of cytomegalovirus: mechanisms and prospects for rapid detection. *Int Antiviral News*, **2**, 117–18.

Blaise, P., Clevenbergh, P., et al. 2002. HIV resistance to antiretroviral drugs: mechanisms, genotypic and phenotypic resistance testing in clinical practice. *Acta Clin Belg*, **57**, 191–201.

Blower, S. and Volberding, P. 2002. What can modeling tell us about the threat of antiviral drug resistance? *Opin Infect Dis*, **6**, 609–14.

Boivin, G. and Goyette, N. 2002. Susceptibility of recent Canadian influenza A and B virus isolates to different neuraminidase inhibitors. *Antiviral Res*, **54**, 143–7.

Boker, K.H., Ringe, B., et al. 1994. Prostaglandin E plus famciclovir – a new concept for the treatment of severe hepatitis B after liver transplantation. *Transplantation*, **57**, 1706–8.

Boyd, M.R., Bacon, T.H., et al. 1987. Antiherpesvirus activity of 9-(4-hydroxy-3-hydroxymethylbut-1-yl)guanine (BRL39123) in cell culture. *Antimicrob Agents Chemother*, **31**, 1238–42.

Bozzette, S.A., Kanouse, D.E., et al. 1995. Health status and function with zidovudine or zalcitabine as initial therapy for AIDS: a randomized controlled trial. Roche 3300/ACTG Study Group. *JAMA*, **273**, 295–301.

Bryson, Y.J., Dillon, M., et al. 1983. Treatment of first episodes of genital herpes simplex virus infection with oral acyclovir. A randomized double-blind controlled trial in normal subjects. *N Engl J Med*, **308**, 916–21.

Carrington, D. 1994. Prospects for improved efficacy with antiviral prodrugs: will valaciclovir and famciclovir meet the clinical challenge? *Int Antiviral News*, **2**, 50–3.

Carrington, D. 1997. Valaciclovir and famciclovir under the clinical microscope – have improvements in antiviral efficacy been realized? *Internat Antiviral News*, **5**, 53–7.

Caselmann, W.H. 1994. HBV and HDV replication in experimental models: effect of interferon. *Antiviral Res*, **24**, 124–9.

Cheer, S.M. and Wagstaff, A.J. 2002. Zanamivir: an update of its use in influenza. *Drug*, **62**, 71–106.

Christophers, J. and Sutton, R.N.P. 1987. Characterization of acyclovir-resistant and sensitive clinical isolates of herpes simplex virus from an immunocompromised patient. *J Antimicrob Chemother*, **20**, 389–98.

Cochran, K.W., Massab, H.R., et al. 1965. Studies on the antiviral activity of amantadine hydrochloride. *Ann NY Acad Sci*, **130**, 432–9.

Coen, D.M. 1986. General aspects of virus drug resistance with special reference to herpes simplex virus. *J Antimicrob Chemother*, **18**, suppl B, 1–10.

Collins, A., Downes, C.S. and Johnson, R.T. 1984. *DNA repair and its inhibition*. Oxford: IRL Press.

Collins, P. and Darby, G. 1991. Laboratory studies of herpes simplex virus strains resistant to acyclovir. *Rev Med Virol*, **1**, 19–28.

Condra, J.H., Emini, E.A., et al. 1992. Identification of the human immunodeficiency virus reverse transcriptase residues that contribute to the activity of diverse nonnucleoside inhibitors. *Antimicrob Agents Chemother*, **36**, 1441–6.

Crisp, P.L. and Clissold, S.P. 1991. Foscarnet. *Drugs*, **41**, 104–29.

Crooks, R.J. 1995. Valaciclovir – a review of its potential in the management of genital herpes. *Antiviral Chem Chemother*, **6**, suppl 1, 39–44.

Crooks, R.J., Jones, D.A. and Fiddian, A.P. 1991. Zoster-associated chronic pain: an overview of clinical trials with acyclovir. *Scand J Infect Dis*, **80**, suppl 1, 62–8.

Crumpacker, C.S., Schnipper, L.E., et al. 1982. Resistance to antiviral drugs of herpes simplex virus isolated from a patient treated with acyclovir. *N Engl J Med*, **306**, 343–6.

D'Aquila, R.T., Schapiro, J.M., et al. 2003. Drug resistance mutations in HIV-1. *Top HIV Med*, **11**, 92–6.

Darby, G. 1994. A history of antiherpes research. *Antivir Chem Chemother*, **5**, suppl 1, 3–9.

Darby, G. 1995. In search of the perfect antiviral. *Antivir Chem Chemother*, **6**, suppl 1, 54–63.

Darby, G. and Field, H.J. 1984. Latency and acquired resistance – problems in chemotherapy of herpes infections. *Pharmacol Ther*, **23**, 217–51.

Darbyshire, J.H. and Aboulker, J.-P. 1992. Didanosine for zidovudine-intolerant patients with HIV disease. *Lancet*, **340**, 1346–7.

Dawber, R. 1974. Idoxuridine in herpes zoster: further evaluation of intermittent topical therapy. *Br Med J*, **2**, 526–7.

Davies, W.L., Grunert, R.R., et al. 1964. Antiviral activity of 1-adamantanamine (amantadine). *Science*, **144**, 862–3.

Dayan, A.D. and Anderson, D. 1988. Toxicity of antiviral compounds. In: Field, H.J. (ed.), *Antiviral agents: the development and assessment of antiviral chemotherapy*, Vol. 1. . Boca Raton, FL: CRC Press, 111–25.

De Clercq, E. 1982. Specific targets for antiviral drugs. *Biochem J*, **205**, 1–13.

De Clercq, E. 1992. HIV inhibitors targeted at the reverse transcriptase. *AIDS Res Hum Retroviruses*, **8**, 119–34.

De Clercq, E. 1995. Antiviral chemotherapy: where do we stand and what can we expect? *Int Antiviral News*, **3**, 52–4.

De Clercq, E. 1997. Acyclic nucleoside phosphonates in the chemotherapy of DNA virus and retrovirus infections. *Intervirology*, **40**, 295–303.

De Clercq, E. 1998. Current progress in antiviral therapy. *Int Antiviral News*, **6**, 75.

De Clercq, E. 2002. New anti-HIV agents and targets (Review). *Med Res Rev*, **22**, 531–65.

De Clercq, E. 2003. New Inhibitors of HCMV (human cytomegalovirus) on the horizon. *J Antimicrob Chemother*, **51**, 1079–83.

De Clercq, E. 2004. Discovery and development of BVDU (brivudin) as a therapeutic for the treatment of herpes zoster. *Biochem Pharmacol*, **68**, 2301–15.

De Clercq, E., Descamps, J., et al. 1979. (E)-5-(2-bromovinyl)-2'-deoxyuridine: a potent and selective antiherpes agent. *Proc Natl Acad Sci USA*, **76**, 2947–51.

De Clercq, E., Descamps, J., et al. 1980. Comparative efficacy of antiherpes drugs against different strains of herpes simplex virus. *J Infect Dis*, **141**, 563–74.

De Clercq, E., Verhelst, G., et al. 1981. Differential inhibition of herpes simplex viruses type 1 (HSV-1) and type 2 (HSV-2), by (E)-5-(2-X-vinyl)-2'-deoxyuridines. *Acta Microbiol Acad Sci Hung*, **28**, 307–12.

De Clercq, E., Balzarini, J., et al. 1982. Antiviral, antimetabolic, and cytotoxic activities of 5-substituted 2'-deoxycytidines. *Mol Pharmacol*, **21**, 217–23.

De Clercq, E., Holy, A., et al. 1986. A novel selective broad-spectrum anti-DNA virus agent. *Nature (London)*, **323**, 464–7.

De Long, D.C. 1984. Effect of enviroxime on rhinovirus infections in humans. In: Leive, L. and Schlessinger, D. (eds), *Microbiology*. Washington DC: American Society of Microbiology, 431–4.

Dearden, C., Al-Nakib, W., et al. 1989. Drug-resistant rhinoviruses from the nose of experimentally treated volunteers. *Arch Virol*, **109**, 71–81.

Debyser, Z., Pauwels, R., et al. 1991. An antiviral target on reverse transcriptase of human immmunodeficiency virus type 1 revealed by tetrahydroimidazo-[4,5,1-jk][1,4]benzodiazepin-2(1H)-one and thione derivatives. *Proc Natl Acad Sci USA*, **88**, 1451–5.

Descamps, J., Sehgal, R.K., et al. 1982. Inhibitory effect of E-5-(2-bromovinyl)-1-beta-d-arabinofuranosyluracil on herpes simplex virus replication and DNA synthesis. *J Virol*, **43**, 332–6.

Dexter, D.L., Wolberg, W.H., et al. 1972. The clinical pharmacology of 5-trifluoromethyl-2'-deoxyuridine. *Cancer Res*, **32**, 47.

Doong, S.L., Tsai, C.H., et al. 1991. Inhibition of the replication of hepatitis B virus in vitro by 2',3'-dideoxy-3'-thiacytidine and related analogues. *Proc Natl Acad Sci USA*, **88**, 8495–9.

Douglas, J.M., Critchlow, C., et al. 1984. A double-blind study of oral acyclovir for suppression of recurrences of genital herpes simplex virus infection. *N Engl J Med*, **310**, 1551–6.

Drew, W.L., Miner, R.C., et al. 1991. Prevalence of resistance in patients receiving ganciclovir for serious cytomegalovirus infection. *J Infect Dis*, **163**, 716–19.

Drew, W.L., Miner, R.C. and Saleh, E. 1993. Antiviral susceptibility testing of cytomegalovirus: criteria for detecting resistance to antivirals. *Clin Diagn Virol*, **1**, 179–85.

Dunkle, L.M., Arvin, A.M., et al. 1991. A controlled trial of acyclovir for chickenpox in normal children. *N Engl J Med*, **325**, 1539–44.

Dutko, F.J. and Diana, G.D. 1990. Quantitative structure-activity relationships and biological consequence of picornavirus capsid-binding compounds. In: Laver, W.G. and Air, G.M. (eds), *Use of X-ray crystallography in the design of antiviral agents*. San Diego CA: Academic Press, 187–98.

Earnshaw, D.L., Bacon, T.H. and Darlison, S.J. 1992. Penciclovir: mode of action of penciclovir in MRC-5 cells infected with herpes simplex virus (HSV-1), HSV-2 and varicella-zoster virus. *Antimicrob Agents Chemother*, **36**, 2747–57.

Elion, G.B. 1993. Acyclovir: discovery, mechanism of action and selectivity. *J Med Virol*, suppl 1. S2–6.

Elion, G.B., Furman, P.A., et al. 1977. Selectivity of action of an antiherpetic agent 9-(2-hydroxyethoxymethyl)guanine. *Proc Natl Acad Sci USA*, **74**, 5716–20.

Englund, J.A., Zimmerman, M.E., et al. 1990. Herpes simplex virus resistant to acyclovir: a study in a tertiary care center. *Ann Intern Med*, **112**, 416–22.

Evans, H.J. 1983. Cytogenetic methods for detecting effects of chemical mutagens. *Ann NY Acad Sci*, **407**, 131.

Evans, T.G., Bernstein, D.I., et al. 2002. Double-blind, randomized, placebo-controlled study of topical 5 percent acyclovir-1 percent hydorcortisone cream (ME-609) for treatment of UV radiation-induced herpes labialis. *Antimicrob Agents Chemother*, **46**, 1870–4.

Fan-Havard, P., Nahata, M.C. and Brady, M.T. 1989. Ganciclovir: a review of pharmacology, therapeutic efficacy and potential use for treatment of congenital cytomegalovirus infections. *J Clin Pharm Ther*, **14**, 329–40.

Fanning, M.M., Read, S.E., et al. 1990. Foscarnet therapy of cytomegalovirus retinitis in AIDS. *J Acquired Immune Defic Syndr*, **3**, 472–9.

Farci, P.F. and Purcell, R.H. 1993. Natural history deduced from experimental infections in primates. In: Zuckerman, A.J. and Thomas, H.C. (eds), *Viral hepatitis: scientific basis and clinical management*. Edinburgh: Livingstone, 241–67.

Ferguson, N.M., Mallett, S., et al. 2003. A population-dynamic model for evaluating the potential spread of drug-resistant influenza virus infections during community-based use of antivirals. *J Antimicrob Agents Chemother*, **4**, 977–90.

Field, A.K. 1999. Human cytomegalovirus: challenges, opportunities and new drug developement. *Antivir Chem Chemother*, **10**, 219–32.

Field, H.J. 1988. Animal models in the evaluation of antiviral chemotherapy, *Antiviral Agents: the development and assessment of antiviral chemotherapy*, Vol I. Boca Raton FL: CRC Press, 67–84.

Field, H.J. 1988. The development of antiviral drug resistance, *Antiviral Agents: the development and assessment of antiviral chemotherapy*, Vol. I. Boca Raton FL: CRC Press, 127–49.

Field, H.J. 1989. Persistent herpes simplex virus infection and mechanisms of virus drug resistance. *Eur J Clin Microbiol Infect Dis*, **8**, 671–80.

Field, H.J. 1996. Famciclovir origins, progress and prospects. *Expert Opin Investig Drugs*, **5**, 925–38.

Field, H.J. 2001. Herpes simplex virus antiviral drug resistance – current trends and future prospects. *J Clin Virol*, **3**, 261–9.

Field, H.J. and Brown, G.A. 1989. Animal models for antiviral chemotherapy. *Antiviral Res*, **12**, 165–80.

Field, H.J. and Fitzmaurice, T.J. 2001. Reflections on herpesvirus chemotherapy 1992-2002. *Int Antivir News*, **9**, 189–93.

Field, H.J. and Goldthorpe, S.E. 1989. Antiviral drug resistance. *Trends Pharmacol Sci*, **10**, 333–7.

Field, H.J. and Owen, L.J. 1988. Virus drug resistance. In: De Clerq, E. and Walker, R.T. (eds), *Antiviral drug development. Life Sciences Series A 143*. New York: Plenum Press 203–36.

Field, H.J. and Reading, M.J. 1987. The inhibition of bovine herpesvirus-1 by methyl 2-pyridyl ketone thiosemicarbazone and its effects on bovine cells. *Antiviral Res*, **7**, 245–56.

Field, H.J., Darby, G. and Wildy, P. 1980. Isolation and characterization of acyclovir-resistant mutants of herpes simplex virus. *J Gen Virol*, **49**, 115–24.

Field, H., McMillan, A. and Darby, G. 1981. The sensitivity of acyclovir-resistant mutants of herpes simplex virus to other antiviral drugs. *J Infect Dis*, **143**, 281–5.

Field, H.J., Tewari, D., et al. 1995. Comparison of efficacies of famciclovir and valaciclovir against herpes simplex virus type 1 in a murine immunosuppression model. *Antimicrob Agents Chemother*, **39**, 1114–19.

Fischl, M.A., Richman, D.D., et al. 1987. The efficacy of azidothymidine (AZT) in the treatment of patients with AIDS and AIDS-related complex: a double blind, placebo-controlled trial. *N Engl J Med*, **317**, 185–91.

Freitas, V.R., Smee, D.F., et al. 1985. Activity of 9-(1,3-dihydroxy-2-propoxymethyl)guanine compared with that of acyclovir against human, monkey and rodent cytomegaloviruses. *Antimicrob Agents Chemother*, **28**, 240–5.

Fried, M.W., Dibisceglie, A.M., et al. 1992. FIAU, a new oral antiviral agent, profoundly inhibits HBV DNA in patients with chronic hepatitis B. *Hepatology*, **16**, 127A.

Furman, P.A., St Clair, M.H., et al. 1979. Inhibition of herpes simplex virus induced DNA polymerase activity and viral DNA replication by 9-(2-hydroxyethoxymethyl)guanine. *J Virol*, **32**, 72–7.

Fyfe, J.A., Keller, P.M., et al. 1978. Thymidine kinase from herpes simplex virus phosphorylates the new antiviral compound 9-(2-hydroxyethoxymethyl)guanine. *J Biol Chem*, **253**, 8721–7.

Geerinck, K., Lukito, G., et al. 2001. A case of human orf in an immunocompromised patient treated successfully with cidofovir cream. *J Med Virol*, **4**, 543–9.

Gershengorn, H.B., Darby, G. and Blower, S.M. 2003. Predicting the emergence of drug-resistant HSV-2; new predictions. *Infect Dis*, **3**, 1.

Gilbert, B.E. and Knight, V. 1986. Biochemistry and clinical applications of ribavirin. *Antimicrob Agents Chemother*, **30**, 201–5.

Gnann, G.W., Crumpacker, C.S., et al. 1998. Sorivudine versus acyclovir for treatment of dermatomal herpes zoster in human immunodeficiency virus-infected patients: results from a randomized, controlled clinical trial. Collaborative Antiviral Study Group/AIDS Clinical Trials Group, Herpes Zoster Study Group. *Antimicrob Agents Chemother*, **42**, 1139–45.

Goldberg, L.H., Kaufman, R., et al. 1993. Long-term suppression of recurrent genital herpes with acyclovir: a 5-year bench mark. Acyclovir study group. *Arch Dermatol*, **129**, 582–7.

Goodpasture, E.W. and Teague, O. 1923. Transmission of the virus herpes febrilis along nerves in experimentally infected rabbits. *J Med Res*, **44**, 139–84.

Grey, F., Sowa, M., et al. 2003. Characterization of a neurovirulent aciclovir resistant variant of herpes simplex virus. *J Gen Virol*, **84**, 1403–10.

Griffiths, P.D. 1995. Progress in the clinical management of herpesvirus infections. *Antivir Chem Chemother*, **6**, 191–209.

Gubareva, L.V., Kaiser, L., et al. 2001a. Selection of influenza virus mutants in experimentally infected volunteers treated with oseltamivir. *J Infect Dis*, **183**, 523–31.

Gubareva, L.V., Webster, R.G. and Hayden, F.G. 2001b. Comparison of the activities of zanamivir, oseltamivir and RWJ-270201 against clinical isolates of influenza virus and neuraminidase inhibitor-resistant variants. *Antimicrob Agents Chemother*, **45**, 3403–8.

Harmenberg, J., Wahren, B. and Öberg, B. 1980. Influence of cells and virus multiplicity on the inhibition of herpesvirus with acycloguanosine. *Intervirology*, **14**, 239–44.

Harmenberg, J., Abele, G. and Malm, M. 1985a. Deoxythymidine pools in animal and human skin with reference to antiviral drugs. *Arch Dermatol Res*, **277**, 402–3.

Harmenberg, J., Wahren, B., et al. 1985b. Multiplicity dependence and sensitivity of herpes simplex virus isolates to antiviral compounds. *J Antimicrob Chemother*, **15**, 567–73.

Harmenberg, J.G., Awan, A.R., et al. 2003. ME-609, a treatment for recurrent herpes simplex virus infections. *Antivir Chem Chemother*, **14**, 205–15.

Harris, W., Collins, P., et al. 2003. Phenotypic and genotypic characterisation of isolates of herpes simplex virus resistant to aciclovir. *J Gen Virol*, **84**, 1393–401.

Harrison, C.J., Jenski, L., et al. 1988. Modification of immunological responses and clinical disease during topical R-837 treatment of genital HSV02 infection. *Antiviral Res*, **10**, 209–23.

Hay, A.J. 1992. The action of adamantanamines against influenza A viruses: inhibition of the M2 ion channel protein. *Semin Virol*, **3**, 21–30.

Hay, A.J., Wolstenholme, A.J., et al. 1985. The molecular basis of the specific anti-influenza action of amantadine. *EMBO J*, **4**, 3621–4.

Hay, A.J., Zambon, M.C., et al. 1986. Molecular basis of resistance of influenza A viruses to amantadine. *J Antimicrob Chemother*, **18**, suppl B, 19–29.

Hayden, F.G. 1994. Amantadine and rimantadine resistance in influenza A viruses. *Curr Opinion Infect Dis*, **7**, 674–7.

Hayden, F.G. 1997. Antivirals for pandemic influenza. *J Inf Dis*, **176**, 556–61.

Hayden, F.G. and Couch, R.B. 1992. Clinical and epidemiological importance of influenza A viruses resistant to amantadine and rimantadine. *Rev Med Virol*, **2**, 89–96.

Hayden, F.G., Gwaltney, J.M., et al. 1981. Comparative toxicity of amantadine hydrochloride and rimantadine hydrochloride in healthy adults. *Antimicrob Agents Chemother*, **19**, 226–33.

Hayden, F.G., Minocha, A., et al. 1985. Comparative single dose pharmacokinetics of amantadine hydrochloride and rimantadine hydrochloride in young and elderly adults. *Antimicrob Agents Chemother*, **28**, 216–21.

Hayden, F.G., Belshe, R.B., et al. 1989. Emergence and apparent transmission of rimantadine-resistant influenza A virus in families. *N Engl J Med*, **321**, 1696–702.

Hayden, F.G., Sperber, S.J., et al. 1991. Recovery of drug-resistant influenza A virus during therapeutic use of rimantadine. *Antimicrob Agents Chemother*, **35**, 1741–7.

Hayden, F.G., Herrington, D.T., et al. 2003. Efficacy and safety of oral pleconaril for treatment of colds due to picornaviruses in adults: results of 2 double-blind, randomized, placebo-controlled trials. *Clin Infect Dis*, **36**, 1523–32.

Heidelberger, C., Parsons, D.G. and Remy, D. 1964. Synthesis of 5-trifluoromethyluracil and 5-trifluoromethyl-2′-deoxyuridine. *J Med Chem*, **7**, 1.

Herlocher, M.L., Carr, J., et al. 2002. Influenza virus carrying an R292K mutation in the neuraminidase gene is not transmitted in ferrets. *Antiviral Res*, **54**, 99–111.

Hermankova, M., Siliciano, J.D., et al. 2003. Analysis of human immunodeficiency virus type 1 gene expression in latently infected resting CD4+ T lymphocytes in vivo. *J Virol*, **77**, 7383–92.

Hersfield, M.S. 1979. Apparent suicide inactivation of human lymphoblast S-adenosyl homocysteine hydrolase by 2′-deoxyadenosine and adenine arabinoside. *J Biol Chem*, **254**, 223.

Hitchcock, M.J. 1991. 2′,3′-Didehydro-2′,3′-dideoxythymidine (D4T), an anti-HIV agent. *Antivir Chem Chemother*, **2**, 125–32.

Hitchcock, M.J. 1996. GS4104: a new orally administered anti-influenza drug candidate. *Int Antiviral News*, **4**, 175.

Honkoop, P. and de Man, R.A. 1995. Clinical aspects of nucleoside analogues for chronic hepatitis B. *Int Antiviral News*, **3**, 78–80.

Hoofnagle, J.H. 1994. Therapy of acute and chronic viral-hepatitis. *Adv Intern Med*, **39**, 241–75.

Hovi, T. 1988. Successful selective inhibitors of herpesviruses. In: Field, H.J. (ed.), *Antiviral agents: the development and assessment of antiviral chemotherapy*. Boca Raton, RL: CRC Press, 1–22.

Ilan, E., Burakova, T., et al. 1999. The hepatitis B virus-Trimera mouse: a model for human HBV infection and evaluation of anti-HBV therapeutic agents. *Hepatology*, **29**, 553–62.

Jain, M.K., Skiest, D.J., et al. 2003. Changes in mortality related to human immunodeficiency virus infection: comparative analysis of inpatient deaths in 1995 and in 1999–2000. *Clin Infect Dis*, **36**, 1030–8.

Jones, P.S. 1998. Strategies for antiviral drug discovery. *Antivir Chem Chemother*, **9**, 283–302.

Kahn, J.O., Lagakos, S.W., et al. 1992. A controlled trial comparing continued zidovudine with didanosine in human immunodeficiency virus infection. *N Engl J Med*, **327**, 581–7.

Kaplan, A.H., Michael, S.F., et al. 1994. Selection of multiple human immunodeficiency virus type 1 variants that encode viral proteases with decreased sensitivity to an inhibitor of the viral protease. *Proc Natl Acad Sci USA*, **91**, 5597–601.

Kaufman, H.E. 1979. Antiviral update. *Ophthalmology*, **86**, 131–6.

Kaufman, H.E. and Heidelberger, C. 1964. Therapeutic antiviral action of 5-trifluormethyl-2′-deoxyuridine in herpes simplex keratitis. *Science*, **145**, 585–6.

Kern, E.R. 2003. In vitro activity of potential anti-poxvirus agents. *Antiviral Res*, **57**, 35–40.

Kim, C.U., Chen, X. and Mendel, D.B. 1999. Neuraminidase inhibitors as anti-influenza virus agents. *Antivir Chem Chemother*, **10**, 141–54.

Kimberlin, D.W., Kern, E.R., et al. 1995. Models of antiviral resistance. *Antiviral Res*, **26**, 415–22.

Kimberlin, D.W., Lin, C.Y., et al. 2003. Effect of ganciclovir therapy on hearing in symptomatic congenital cytomegalovirus disease involving the central nervous system: a randomized, controlled trial, 2003. *J Pediatr*, **143**, 16–25.

Kleymann, G. 2003. Novel agents and strategies to treat herpes simplex virus infections. *Expert Opin Invest Drugs*, **12**, 165–83.

Kleymann, G. 2004. Helicase primase: targeting the Achilles heel of herpes simplex virus. *Antivir Chem Chemother*, **15**, 135–40.

Kleymann, G., Fischer, R., et al. 2002. New helicase-primase inhibitors as drug candidates for the treatment of herpes simplex disease. *Nat Med*, **8**, 392–8.

Koch, J.A. and Ruprecht, R.M. 1992. Animal models for anti-AIDS therapy. *Antiviral Res*, **19**, 81–109.

Kohl, N.E., Emini, E.A., et al. 1988. Active human immunodeficiency virus protease is required for viral infectivity. *Proc Natl Acad Sci USA*, **85**, 4686–90.

Krosky, P.M., Baek, M.-C. and Coen, D.M. 2002. The human cytomegalovirus UL97 protein kinase, an antiviral drug target, is required at the stage of nuclear egress. *J Virol*, **77**, 905–14.

Lalezari, J.P., Henry, K., et al. 2003. Enfuvirtide, an HIV-1 fusion inhibitor for drug resistant HIV infection in North and South America. *N Engl J Med*, **348**, 2175–85.

Lamb, R.A., Zebedee, S.L. and Richardson, C.D. 1985. Influenza virus M2 protein is an integral membrane protein expressed on the infected cell surface. *Cell*, **40**, 627–33.

Larder, B.A. and Darby, G. 1984. Virus drug-resistance: mechanisms and consequences. *Antiviral Res*, **4**, 1–42.

Larder, B.A. and Kemp, S.D. 1989. Multiple mutations in HIV-1 reverse transcriptase confer high-level resistance to zidovudine (AZT). *Science*, **246**, 1155–8.

Larder, B.A., Darby, G. and Richman, D.D. 1989. HIV with reduced sensitivity to zidovudine (AZT) isolated during prolonged therapy. *Science*, **243**, 1731–4.

Laver, G.W. and Air, G.M. 1990. *Use of X-ray crystallography in the design of antiviral agents*. London: Academic Press.

Leinback, S.S., Reno, G.M., et al. 1976. Mechanisms of phosphonoacetate inhibitions on herpes virus-induced DNA polymerase. *Biochemistry*, **15**, 426–30.

Levinson, M.L. and Jacobson, P.A. 1992. Treatment and prophylaxis of cytomegalovirus disease. *Pharmacotherapy*, **12**, 300–18.

Little, S.J., Holte, S., et al. 2002. Antiretroviral-drug resistance among patients recently infected with HIV. *N Engl J Med*, **347**, 385–94.

Littler, E., Stuart, A.D. and Chee, M.S. 1992. Human cytomegalovirus open reading frame encodes a protein that phosphorylates the antiviral nucleoside analogue ganciclovir. *Nature (London)*, **358**, 160–2.

Ljungman, P., Ellis, M.N., et al. 1990. Acyclovir-resistant herpes simplex virus causing pneumonia after marrow transplantation. *J Infect Dis*, **162**, 711–15.

Locarnini, S.A., Shaw, T., et al. 1994. Antiviral activity of penciclovir, a novel antiherpesvirus compound, against duck hepatitis B in vitro. *Antiviral Res*, **23**, suppl 1, S79.

Machida, H. 1990. In vitro anti-herpes virus action of a novel antiviral agent, brovavir (BV-araU). *Chemotherapy (Tokyo)*, **38**, 256–61.

Machida, H. and Nishitani, M. 1990. Drug susceptibilities of isolates of varicella-zoster virus in a clinical study of oral brovavir. *Microbiol Immunol*, **34**, 407–11.

Main, J., McCarron, B. and Thomas, H.C. 1998. Treatment of chronic viral hepatitis. *Antivir Chem Chemother*, **9**, 449–460.

Martin, J.L., Ellis, M.N., et al. 1985. Plaque autoradiographic assay for the detection and quantitation of thymidine kinase-deficient and thymidine kinase-altered mutants of herpes simplex in clincial isolates. *Antimicrob Agents Chemother*, **28**, 181–7.

Matthews, T. and Boehme, R. 1988. Antiviral activity and mechanism of action of ganciclovir. *Rev Infect Dis*, **10**, suppl 3, S490–4.

McKimm-Breschkin, J., Trivedi, T., et al. 2003. Neuraminidase sequence analysis and susceptibilities of influenza virus clinical isolates to zanamivir and oseltamivir. *Antimicrob Agents Chemother*, **47**, 2264–72.

McLaren, C., Ellis, M.N. and Hunter, G.A. 1983. A colorimetric assay for the measurement of the sensitivity of herpes simplex virus to antiviral agents. *Antiviral Res*, **3**, 223–34.

McLaren, C., Datema, R., et al. 1991. Didanosine. *Antivir Chem Chemother*, **2**, 321–8.

Meeting Report, 1995. 8th International Conference on Antiviral Research. *Int Antiviral News*, **3**, 101.

Mellors, J.W., Larder, B.A. and Schinazi, R.F. 1995. Mutations in HIV-reverse transcriptase and protease associated with drug resistance. *Int Antiviral News*, **3**, 8–13.

Mendel, D.B., Tai, C.Y., et al. 1998. Oral administration of a prodrug of the influenza virus neuraminidase inhibitor GS 4071 protects mice and ferrets against influenza infection. *Antimicro Agents Chemother*, **42**, 640–6.

Merluzzi, V.J., Hargrave, K.D., et al. 1990. Inhibition of HIV-1 replication by a non-nucleoside reverse transcriptase inhibitor. *Science*, **250**, 1411–33.

Mertz, G.J., Critchlow, C.W., et al. 1984. Double-blind placebo-controlled trial of oral acyclovir in first-episode genital herpes simplex virus infection. *JAMA*, **252**, 1147–51.

Mertz, G.J., Loveless, M.O., et al. 1997. Oral famciclovir for suppression of recurrent genital herpes simplex virus infection in women. A multicenter, double-blind, placebo-controlled trial. *Arch Intern Med*, **157**, 343–9.

Meyers, J.D., Wade, J.C., et al. 1982. Multicenter collaborative trial of intravenous acyclovir for treatment of herpes simplex virus infection in the immunocompromised host. *Am J Med*, **73**, 229–35.

Miller, R., Birmachu, W., et al. 1995. Imiquimod: cytokine induction and antiviral activity. *Int Antiviral News*, **3**, 111–13.

Mills, J.S. 1993. Discovery of the HIV proteinase inhibitor Ro 31-8959: a paradigm for drug discovery. *Int Antiviral News*, **1**, 18–19.

Mitsuya, H. and Broder, S. 1986. Inhibition of the in vitro infectivity and cytopathic effect of human T-lymphotrophic virus type III/lymphadenopathy-associated virus (HTLV-III/LAV) by 2′,3′-dideoxynucleosides. *Proc Natl Acad Sci USA*, **83**, 1911–15.

Mitsuya, H., Weinhold, K.J., et al. 1985. 3′-Azido-3′-deoxythymidine (BWA 509U): an antiviral agent that inhibits infectivity and cytopathic effects of human T-lymphotropic virus type III lymphadenopathy associated virus in vitro. *Proc Natl Acad Sci USA*, **82**, 7096–100.

Miyasaka, T., Tanaka, H., et al. 1989. A novel lead for specific anti-HIV-1 agents: 1-[(2-hydroxyethoxy)methyl]-6-(phenylthio)thymine. *J Med Chem*, **32**, 2507–9.

Mizoguchi, K., Yokoo, H., et al. 1994. Amantadine increases the extracellular dopamine levels in the striatum by re-uptake inhibition and by N-methyl-d-aspartate antagonism. *Brain Res*, **662**, 255–8.

Monto, A.S. and Arden, N.H. 1992. Implications of viral resistance to amantadine in control of influenza A. *Clin Infect Dis*, **15**, 362–7.

Murphy, V.F. 1993. Molecular targets for novel antiviral agents in the treatment of hepatitis C virus infection. *Int Antiviral News*, **1**, 115–17.

Murray, A.B. 1995. Valaciclovir – an improvement over aciclovir for the treatment of zoster. *Antivir Chem Chemother*, **6**, suppl 1, 34–8.

Mutimer, D. 1998. Hepatitis B virus antiviral drug resistance: from the laboratory to the patient. *Antivir Ther*, **3**, 243–6.

Naesens, L., Balzarini, J., et al. 1996. Antiretroviral activity and pharmacokinetics in mice of oral bis-(pivaloyloxymethyl)-9-(2-phosponylmethoxyethyl) andenine, the bis(pivaloyloxymethyl)-ester

prodrug of 9-(2-phosponylmethoxyethyl) andenine. *Antimicrob Agents Chemother*, **40**, 22–8.

Newton, A.A. 1988. Tissue culture methods for assessing antivirals and their harmful effects. In: Field, H. (ed.), *Antiviral agents: the development and assessment of antiviral chemotherapy*. Boca Raton, FL: CRC Press, 2–66.

Ninomiya, Y., Aoyama, M., et al. 1985. Comparative studies on the modes of action of the antirhinovirus agents Ro 09-0410, Ro 09-0179, RMI-15,731, 6-dichloroflavan, and enviroxime. *Antimicrob Agents Chemother*, **27**, 595–9.

North, T.W., Remington, K.M., et al. 1993. Feline immunodeficiency virus: a unique model for studies of viral resistance to AIDS chemotherapy. *Int Antiviral News*, **1**, 71–2.

Öberg, B. 1983a. Antiviral effects of phosphonoformate (PFA, foscarnet sodium). *Pharmacol Ther*, **19**, 387–415.

Öberg, B. 1983b. Inhibitors of virus-specific enzymes. In: Stuart-Harris, C.H. and Oxford, J. (eds), *Problems of antiviral therapy*. London: Academic Press, 35–69.

Otto, M.J., Garber, S., et al. 1993. In vitro isolation and identification of human immunodeficiency virus (HIV) variants with reduced sensivity to C-2 symmetrical inhibitors of HIV type 1 protease. *Proc Natl Acad Sci USA*, **90**, 7543–7.

Oxford, J.S., Logan, I.S. and Potter, C.W. 1970. The in vivo selection of an influenza A2 strain resistant to amantadine. *Nature (London)*, **226**, 82–3.

Oxford, J.S., Novelli, P., et al. 2002. New millennium antivirals against pandemic and epidemic influenza: the neuraminidase inhibitors. *Antivir Chem Chemother*, **13**, 205–17.

Paris, D.S. and Harrington, J.E. 1982. Herpes simplex virus variants resistant to high concentrations of acyclovir exist in clinical isolates. *Antimicrob Agents Chemother*, **22**, 71–7.

Pauwels, R., Andries, K., et al. 1990. Potent and selective inhibition of HIV-1 replication in vitro by a novel series of tetrahydro-imidazo[4,5,1-jk][1,4]-benzodiazepin-2(1H)-one and -thione (TIBO) derivatives. In: De Clercq, E. (ed.), *Design of anti-aids drugs*. *Pharmacochemistry Library*, **14**. Amsterdam: Elsevier, 103–22.

Pearly, L.H. and Taylor, W.R. 1987. A structural model for the retroviral protease. *Nature (London)*, **329**, 351–4.

Perno, C.-F. and Calio, R. 1994. Evaluation of anti-HIV compounds in monoctye/macrophages: importance and clinical implications. *Int Antiviral News*, **2**, 88–9.

Pescovitz, M.D., Rabkin, J., et al. 2000. Valganciclovir results in improved oral absorption of ganciclovir in liver transplant recipients. *Antimicrob Agents Chemother*, **10**, 2811–15.

Phelps, W.C., Barnes, J.A. and Lobe, D.C. 1998. Molecular targets for human papillomaviruses: prospects for antiviral therapy. *Antivir Chem Chemother*, **9**, 359–77.

Pomerantz, R.J. 2003. Reservoirs, sanctuaries, and residual disease: the hiding spots of HIV-1. *HIV Clin Trials*, **4**, 137–43.

Purcell, R.H. 1994. Hepatitis C virus: historical perspective and current concepts. *FEMS Microb Rev*, **14**, 181–92.

Prober, C.G. and Kimberlin, A.W. 2005. Antiviral drugs. In: Yaffe, S.J. and Avanda, J.V. (eds), *Neonatal and pediatric pharmacology*, 3rd edn. Philadelphia: Lippincott, Williams & Wilkins, 475–503.

Prusoff, W.H. 1959. Synthesis and biological actiivities of iodo-deoxyuridine, an analogue of thymidine. *Biochim Biophys Acta*, **39**, 295–6.

Purifoy, D.J., Lewis, R.B. and Powell, K.L. 1977. Identification of the herpes simplex virus DNA polymerase gene. *Nature (London)*, **269**, 621–3.

Rees, P.J. and Brigden, W.D. 1988. Problems of assessing antiviral agents in man. In: Field, H.J. (ed.), *Antiviral agents: the development and assessment of antiviral chemotherapy*. Boca Raton, FL: CRC Press, 85–109.

Reusser, P. 2001. Oral valganciclovir: a new option for treatment of cytomegalovirus infection and disease in immunocompromised host. *Expert Opin Investig Drugs*, **10**, 1745–53.

Richman, D., Shih, C.K., et al. 1991. Human immunodeficiency virus type 1 mutants resistant to nonnucleoside inhibitors of reverse transcriptase arise in tissue culture. *Proc Natl Acad Sci USA*, **88**, 11241–5.

Roberts, N.A. 1995. Progress of saquinavir (Ro 31-8959) in clinical trials. *Int Antiviral News*, **3**, 2–3.

Roberts, N.A., Martin, J.A., et al. 1990. Rational design of peptide-based HIV proteinase inhibitors. *Science*, **248**, 358–61.

Rosenthal, S.L., Stanberry, L.R., et al. 1997. Seroprevalence of herpes simplex virus types 1 and 2 and cytomegalovirus in adolescents. *Clin Infect Dis*, **24**, 135–9.

Rossmann, M.G. 1990. Neutralizing rhinoviruses with antiviral agents that inhibit attachment and uncoating. In: Laver, W.G. and Air, G.M. (eds), *Use of X-ray crystallography in the design of antiviral agents*. San Diego CA: Academic Press, 115–37.

Sacks, S.L., Wanklin, R.J., et al. 1989. Progressive esophagitis from acyclovir-resistant herpes simplex. Clinical roles for DNA polymerase mutants and viral heterogeneity. *Ann Intern Med*, **111**, 893–9.

Safrin, S., Elbeik, T., et al. 1994. Correlation between response to acyclovir and foscarnet therapy and in vitro susceptibility result for isolates of herpes simplex virus from human immunodeficiency virus-infected patients. *Antimicrob Agents Chemother*, **38**, 1246–50.

Sandford, G.P., Wingard, J.R., et al. 1985. Genetic analysis of the susceptibility of mouse cytomegalovirus to acyclovir. *J Virol*, **53**, 104–13.

Sasadeusz, J.J., Tufaro, F., et al. 1997. Homopolymer mutational hot spots mediate herpes simplex virus resistance to acyclovir. *J Virol*, **71**, 3872–8.

Schabel, G.M. Jr 1968. The antiviral activity of 9-beta-D-arabinofuranosyladenine (araA). *Chemotherapy (Basel)*, **13**, 321–38.

Schaeffer, H.J., Beauchamp, L., et al. 1978. 9-(2-hydroxyethoxymethyl)guanine activity against viruses of the herpes group. *Nature (London)*, **272**, 583–5.

Schang, L.M. 2001. Cellular proteins (cyclin-dependent kinases) as potential targets for antiviral drugs. *Antiviral Chem Chemother*, **12**, suppl 1, 157–78.

Schang, L.M. 2002. Cyclin-dependent kinases as cellular targets for antiviral drugs. *J Antimicrob Chemother*, **50**, 779–92.

Schinazi, R.F. 1991. Combined chemotherapeutic modalities for viral infections: rationale and clinical potential. In: Chou, T.-C. and Rideout, D.C. (eds), *Synergism and antagonism in chemotherapy*. Orlando FL: Academic Press, 109–82.

Schinazi, R.F. 1995. A brighter future for nucleoside antiviral agents. *Int Antiviral News*, **3**, 45–6.

Senior, K. 2002. FDA panel rejects common cold treatment. *Lancet Infect Dis*, **2**, 264.

Shin, Y.K., Weinberg, A., et al. 2003. Susceptibility of herpes simplex virus isolates to nucleoside analogues and the proportion of nucleoside-resistant variants after repeated topical application of penciclovir to recurrent herpes labialis. *J Infect Dis*, **187**, 1241–5.

Sidwell, R.W., Huffman, J.H., et al. 1972. Broad-spectrum antiviral activity of virazole: 1-beta-D-ribofuranosyl-1,2,4-triazole-3-carboxamide. *Science*, **177**, 705.

Sidwell, R., Revankar, G. and Robins, R. 1985. Ribavirin: review of a broad-spectrum antiviral agent. In: Shugar, D. (ed.), *International encyclopedia of pharmacology and therapeutics*, Vol. 2, section 116. Oxford: Pergamon Press, 49–108.

Sidwell, R.W., Huffman, J.H., et al. 1998. Inhibition of influenza virus infections in mice by GS 4104, an orally effective influenza virus neuraminidase inhibitor. *Antiviral Res*, **37**, 107–20.

Smee, D.F., Martin, J.C., et al. 1983. Antiherpes activity of the acyclic nucleoside 9-(1,3-dihydroxy-2-propoxymethyl)guanine. *Antimicrob Agents Chemother*, **23**, 676–82.

Snoeck, R., Neyts, J. and De Clercq, E. 1993. Strategies for the treatment of cytomegalovirus infections. In: Michelson, S. and Plotkin, S.A. (eds), *Multidisciplinary approach to understanding cytomegalovirus disease*. Amsterdam: Elsevier, 269–78.

Soudeyns, H., Yao, X.-J., et al. 1991. Anti-human immunodeficiency virus type 1 activity and in vitro toxicity of 2′,3′-dideoxy-3′-thiacytidine

(BCH-189) a novel heterocyclic nucleoside analog. *Antimicrob Agents Chemother*, **35**, 1386–90.

Spruance, S.L. 1994. Topical therapy of mucocutaneous herpesvirus infections. *Int Antiviral News*, **2**, 86–7.

Stanley, M. 1993. In vitro culture systems for papillomaviruses. *Int Antiviral News*, **1**, 85–6.

Stanley, M.A., Masterton, P.J. and Nichols, P.K. 1997. In vitro and animal models for antiviral therapy in papillomavirus infections. *Antivir Chem Chemother*, **8**, 381–400.

Stilianakis, N.I., Perelson, A.S. and Hayden, F.G. 1998. Emergence of drug resistance during an influenza epidemic: insights from a mathematical model. *J Infect Dis*, **177**, 863–73.

Stragier, I., Snoeck, R., et al. 2002. Local treatment of HPV-induced skin lesions by Cidofovir. *J Med Virol*, **67**, 241–5.

Straus, S.E., Takiff, H.E., et al. 1984. Suppression of frequently recurring genital herpes. A placebo-controlled double-blind trial of oral acyclovir. *N Engl J Med*, **310**, 1545–50.

Sullivan, V., Talarico, C.L., et al. 1992. A protein kinase homologue controls phosphorylation of ganciclovir in human cytomegalovirus-infected cells. *Nature (London)*, **358**, 162–4.

Sutton, D. and Kern, E.R. 1993. Activity of famciclovir and penciclovir in HSV-infected animals: a review. *Antivir Chem Chemother*, **4**, suppl 1, 37–46.

Swanstrom, R. and Erona, J. 2000. Human immunodeficiency virus type-1 protease inhibitors: therapeutic successes and failures, suppression and resistance. *Pharm Therapeut*, **86**, 145–70.

Tai, C.Y., Escarpe, P.A., et al. 1998. Characterization of human influenza virus variants selected in vitro in the presence of neuraminidase inhibitor GS 4071. *Antimicrob Agents Chemother*, **42**, 3234–41.

Thackray, A.M. and Field, H.J. 2000. The effects of antiviral therapy on the distribution of herpes simplex virus type 1 to ganglionic neurons and its consequences during, immediately following and several months after treatment. *J Gen Virol*, **81**, 2385–96.

Tilson, H.H., Engle, C.R. and Andrews, E.B. 1993. Safety of acyclovir: a summary of the first 10 years' experience. *J Med Virol*, suppl 1, S67–3.

Tomai, M.A., Gibson, S.J., et al. 1995. Immunomodulating and antiviral activitities of the imidazoquinoline S-28463. *Antiviral Res*, **28**, 285–64.

Treanor, J.J., Hayden, F.G., et al. 2000. Efficacy and safety of the oral neuraminidase inhibitor Oseltamivir in treating acute influenza. *JAMA*, **283**, 1016–24.

Vere Hodge, R.A. 1993. Famciclovir and penciclovir. The mode of action of famciclovir including its conversion to penciclovir. *Antivir Chem Chemother*, **4**, 67–84.

Vere Hodge, R.A. and Cheng, Y.C. 1993. The mode of action of penciclovir. *Antivir Chem Chemother*, **4**, 13–24.

Vere Hodge, R.A. and Perkins, R.M. 1989. Mode of action of 9-(4-hydroxy-3-hydroxymethylbut-1-yl)guanine (BRL 39123) against herpes simplex virus in MRC-5 cells. *Antimicrob Agents Chemother*, **33**, 223–9.

Vere Hodge, R.A., Sutton, D., et al. 1989. Selection of an oral prodrug (BRL 42810; famciclovir) for the antiherpesvirus agent BRL 39123 [9-(4-hydroxy-3-hydroxymethylbut-1-yl)guanine; penciclovir]. *Antimicrob Agents Chemother*, **33**, 1765–73.

von Itzstein, M., Wu, W.-Y., et al. 1993. Rational design of potent sialidase-based inhibitors of influenza virus replication. *Nature (London)*, **363**, 418–23.

Votruba, I., Bernaerts, R., et al. 1987. Intracellular phosphorylation of broad-spectrum anti-DNA virus agent (S)-9-(3-hydroxy-2-phosphonylmethoxypropyl)adenine and inhibition of viral DNA synthesis. *Mol Pharmacol*, **32**, 524–9.

Wade, J.C., Newton, B., et al. 1982. Intravenous acyclovir to treat mucocutaneous herpes simplex virus infection after marrow transplantation: a double blind trial. *N Engl J Med*, **96**, 265–9.

Wald, E.R., Dashefsky, B. and Green, M. 1988. Ribavirin: case of premature adjudication. *J Pediatr*, **112**, 154–8.

Wald, A., Corey, L., et al. 1997. Frequent genital herpes simplex virus 2 shedding in immunocompetent women: effect of acyclovir treatment. *J Clin Invest*, **99**, 1092–7.

Walker, M.P., Appleby, T.C., et al. 2003. Hepatitis C virus therapies: current treatments, targets and future perspectives. *Antivir Chem Chemother*, **14**, 325–44.

Wallace, M.R., Bowler, W.A., et al. 1992. Treatment of adult varicella with oral acyclovir. A randomized placebo-controlled trial. *Ann Intern Med*, **117**, 358–63.

Wang, C., Takeuchi, K., et al. 1993. Ion channel activity of influenza A virus M2 protein: characterization of the amantadine block. *J Virol*, **67**, 5585–94.

Wang, L.H., Peck, R.W., et al. 2003. Phase I safety and pharmacokinetic trials of 1263W94, a novel oral anti-human cytomegalovirus agent, in healthy and human immunodeficiencey virus-infected subjects. *Antimicrob Agents Chemother*, **47**, 1334–42.

Waxman, L. and Darke, P.L. 2000. The herpesvirus proteases as targets for antiviral chemotherapy. *Antivir Chem Chemother*, **11**, 1–22.

Weber, J., Rangel, H.R., et al. 2003. Role of baseline pol genotype in HIV-1 fitness evolution. *J Acquir Immune Defic Syndr*, **33**, 448–60.

Webster, R.G., Kawoaka, Y. and Bean, W.J. 1986. Vaccination as a strategy to reduce the emergence of amantadine and rimantadine resistant strains of A/chick/Pennsylvania/83 (H5N2) influenza virus. *J Antimicrob Chemother*, **18**, suppl B, 157–64.

Wellings, P.C., Awdry, P.N., et al. 1972. Clinical evaluation of trifluorothymidine in the treatment of herpes simplex corneal ulcers. *Am J Ophthalmol*, **73**, 932.

Whitley, R.J. 2003. Smallpox: A potential agent of bioterrorism. *Antiviral Res*, **57**, 7–12.

Whitley, R. and Gnann, J.W. 1992. Acyclovir: a decade later. *N Engl J Med*, **327**, 782–9.

Whitley, R.J. and Roizman, B. 2001. Herpes simplex viruses: from structure to function. *Lancet*, **357**, 1513–18.

Whitley, R.J., Soong, S.J., et al. 1977. Adenine arabinoside therapy of biopsy-proved herpes simplex encephalitis. *N Engl J Med*, **297**, 289–94.

Whitley, R., Alford, C., et al. 1980a. Vidarabine: a preliminary review of its pharmacological properties and therapeutic use. *Drugs*, **20**, 267–82.

Whitley, R.J., Tucker, B.C., et al. 1980b. Pharmacology, tolerance, and antiviral activity of vidarabine monophosphate in humans. *Antimicrob Agents Chemother*, **18**, 709–15.

Whitley, R.J., Alford, C.A., et al. 1986. Vidarabin vs acyclovir therapy in herpes simplex encephalitis. *N Engl J Med*, **314**, 144–9.

Whitley, R., Arvin, A., et al. 1991. A controlled trial comparing vidarabine with acyclovir in neonatal herpes simplex virus infection. Infectious Diseases Antiviral Collaborative Study Group. *N Engl J Med*, **324**, 444–9.

Wildy, P., Field, H.J. and Nash, A.A. 1982. Classical herpes latency revisited. In: Mahy, B.W.J., Minson, A.C. and Darby, G.K. (eds), *Virus persistence. SGM Symposium*, **33**. 133–67, Cambridge: Cambridge University Press, 133–67.

Woods, M.G., Diana, G.D., et al. 1989. In vitro and in vivo activities of WIN 54954, a new broad-spectrum antipicornavirus drug. *Antimicrob Agents Chemother*, **33**, 2069–74.

Wright, G.E. 1994. Herpesvirus thymidine kinase inhibitors. *Int Antiviral News*, **2**, 84–6.

Wutzler, P. and Thust, R. 2001. Genetic risks of antiviral nucleosides – a survey. *Antiviral Res*, **49**, 55–74.

Yasin, S.R., Al-Nakib, W. and Tyrrell, D.A. 1990a. Pathogenicity for humans of human rhinovirus type 2 mutants resistant to or dependent on chalcone Ro 09-0410. *Antimicrob Agents Chemother*, **34**, 936–66.

Yasin, S.R., Al-Nakib, W. and Tyrrell, D.A. 1990b. Isolation and preliminary characterization of chalcone Ro 09-0410-T resistant human rhinovirus type 2. *Antivir Chem Chemother*, **1**, 149–54.

Yokota, T., Konno, K., et al. 1989. Mechanism of selective inhibition of varicella-zoster virus replication by 1-beta-D-arabinofuranosyl-E-5-(2-bromovinyl)uracil. *Mol Pharmacol*, **36**, 312–16.

Yuen, M.-F. and Lai, C.-L. 2003. Current and future antiviral agents for chronic hepatitis B. *J Antimicrob Chemother*, **51**, 481–5.

Yuen, M.F., Hui, C.K., et al. 2001. Long term follow up of interferon-alpha treatment in Chinese patients with chronic hepatitis B infection: the effect on HBeAg seroconversion and the development of cirrhosis-related complications. *Hepatology*, **34**, 139–45.

70

The emergence and re-emergence of viral diseases

BRIAN W. J. MAHY AND FREDERICK A. MURPHY

INTRODUCTION

The emergence of new diseases

New or previously unrecognized viral diseases are constantly being identified. In most cases, there is no way to predict when or where the next important new viral pathogen will emerge. Neither is there any way to predict the ultimate importance of a virus as it first emerges: it may be the cause of a geographically limited curiosity, of intermittent outbreaks of disease or of a new epidemic. New viral diseases seem to be emerging globally with increasing frequency, as suggested by published reports of cases, outbreaks, and epidemics and by the rate of identification of new pathogenic viruses (Mahy 2000). The list of newly emergent viruses of humans and animals is impressive (Figure 70.1; Tables 70.1 and 70.2).

DETERMINANTS CONTRIBUTING TO THE EMERGENCE OF NEW DISEASES

Many different factors can contribute to the emergence of a new viral disease. These include: (1) virological determinants such as mutation, recombination, reassortment, natural selection, fitness adaptation, and evolutionary progression; (2) individual host determinants such as specific risk behaviors, innate resistance, acquired immunity, and physiological factors such as age, nutritional status, and pregnancy; (3) host population determinants such as community, behavioral, societal, transport, commercial, and iatrogenic factors; (4) environmental determinants such as ecological and zoonotic influences; (5) viruses intentionally used for harm – the threat of bioterrorism. These determinants need to be understood if we are to develop control measures to prevent the occurrence and spread of specific diseases within human and/or animal populations. In this chapter we consider the underlying causes for emergence and re-emergence and illustrate them with selected examples.

Initial recognition of new, emerging diseases

Since 1986, following upon the development of the polymerase chain reaction (PCR) and other very sensitive, very specific, high-throughput detection and diagnostic

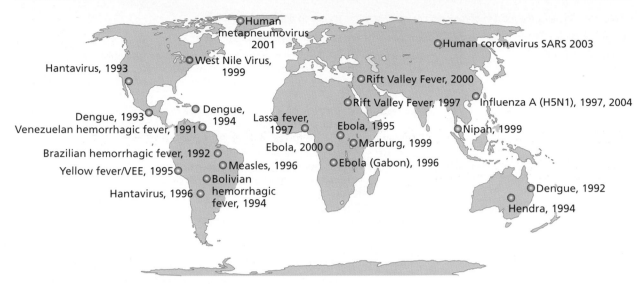

Figure 70.1 *Recent emergence and reemergence of human viral diseases, examples.*

methods, we have seen a dramatic increase in the direct detection of viruses, whether in diseased tissues, in cultured cells inoculated with clinical materials or in appropriate environmental samples. As a consequence, an impressive number of new, important viruses have been recognized (Table 70.3). In fact, some new viruses have been detected, described, and named solely on the basis of genomic sequences amplified by reverse transcription and polymerase chain reaction from postmortem tissues. For example, Bayou virus (a hantavirus distantly related to Sin Nombre virus, and an etiologic agent of hantavirus pulmonary syndrome in North America) is a case in point (Khan et al. 1995) – its significance as a human pathogen was determined entirely by indirect molecular methods.

As another example, the diversity of human papillomaviruses has been recognized solely by genomic nucleotide sequencing. The 100 or more human papillomaviruses have never been cultivated in cell culture or animals, and serotyping has not proven useful, so their pathogenic significance was not appreciated for many years. Since the advent of genomic sequence analysis, our appreciation of the importance of papillomaviruses has changed dramatically.

Human papillomaviruses can now be differentiated by sequence analysis, and exist in more than 100 recognized types in the human population (De Villiers et al. 2004) There is a clear causal relationship between certain papillomavirus types and genital cancers, especially cervical cancer (see Chapter 23, Papillomaviruses). Papillomavirus genome DNA is a small circular molecule that is easily cloned from biopsy specimens of infected tissues. Originally these viruses were classified by DNA hybridization, and considered to be different types if they shared less than 50 percent homology. It was soon realized that certain types were frequently associated with cervical and other forms of genital

cancer (for example types 16, 18, and 31), and other types were found in malignant respiratory papillomas (for example, types 6 and 11) so it was important to determine the human papillomavirus type as an aid in diagnosis. With the advent of simpler methods for DNA sequencing, some of the original hybridization data proved to be inconsistent, and a human papillomavirus type is now defined as new when the genome DNA is more than 10 percent dissimilar in the combined nucleotide sequences of 3 genes, E6, E7, and L1. This requires determination of 2.4 kbp of sequence (one-third of the genome) for each new isolate. More than 100 human papillomaviruses have now been recognized as types by this method, and divided into supergroups. For example, 54 papillomavirus types of genital origin form one supergroup (A) by sequence analysis, and another includes 24 types associated with epidermodysplasia verruciformis and other cutaneous lesions (Chan et al. 1995). Those human papillomavirus types that are presently known to be associated with a high risk of genital cancer are types 16, 18, 31–35, 51–52, 56, 58, 61, 66, 68, 70, and 73.

Another major advance in public health which stemmed directly from the application of molecular methods was the identification of hepatitis C virus. In 1989, as a result of a collaboration between CDC and Chiron Corporation to search for the cause of non-A non-B hepatitis, a new hepatitis virus, hepatitis C virus, was cloned from the blood of a chimpanzee that had been experimentally infected with blood factor VIII that was known to transmit non-A non-B hepatitis (Choo et al. 1989; Matsuura and Miyamura 1993). RNA extracted from the chimpanzee blood was reverse-transcribed to make cDNAs using random primers. The DNA was cloned in the bacteriophage gt 11 expression vector, and the resultant bacterial colonies were screened using sera from patients with non-A non-B hepatitis. After screening thousands of clones in this

Table 70.1 *Some of the most important new, emerging and re-emerging human viral pathogens*

Virus	Association of the virus(es) with human disease
Alkhurma virus[a]	Newly recognized member virus of the family *Flaviviridae*; the etiologic agent of severe hemorrhagic fever with a 25 percent mortality rate; tick-borne; first recognized in 1995 in Saudi Arabia where it has caused substantial morbidity and mortality
Australian bat lyssavirus	Newly recognized member virus of the genus *Lyssavirus*, family *Rhabdoviridae*; the etiologic agent of fatal rabies-like disease in humans and domestic animals; reservoir host fruit bats; found throughout eastern Australia
B-virus	Member virus of the family *Herpesviridae*; the common herpesvirus of macaques, especially rhesus macaques; the etiologic agent of severe, often lethal, encephalitis in humans; increasing as a threat because of increasing use of these animals in medical research
Crimean–Congo hemorrhagic fever virus[a]	Member virus of the genus *Nairovirus*, family *Bunyaviridae*; etiologic agent of severe hemorrhagic fever in humans with 10 percent mortality; tick-borne; reservoir in wildlife, sheep, and goats; widespread across Africa, the Middle East and Asia
Dengue viruses[a]	Member viruses of the family *Flaviviridae*; the etiologic agent of febrile disease with rash; mosquito-borne; the cause of millions of cases of febrile disease in the tropics and subtropics, and of dengue hemorrhagic fever (dengue shock syndrome), a life-threatening disease, especially in children
Ebola virus and Marburg virus[a]	Member viruses of the family *Filoviridae*; the etiologic agents of the most lethal hemorrhagic fevers known; zoonotic, but natural reservoir(s) unknown; there have been several recent substantial epidemics of Ebola hemorrhagic fever in central Africa
GB virus-C/hepatitis G virus	Newly recognized member viruses of the family *Flaviviridae*; disease association unproven, but there is a lifelong infection in humans and non-human primates world-wide
Guanarito virus[a]	Member virus of the family *Arenaviridae*; etiologic agent of Venezuelan hemorrhagic fever; rodent-borne
Hantaan virus and other Old World hantaviruses[a]	Member viruses of the genus *Hantavirus*, family *Bunyaviridae*; etiologic agents of hemorrhagic fever with renal syndrome; rodent-borne; an important cause of severe disease and death in Asia and Europe
Hendra virus	Newly recognized member virus of the genus *Henipavirus*, family *Paramyxoviridae*; etiologic agent of acute, often fatal, respiratory distress syndrome in humans and horses; zoonotic, reservoir host fruit bats (flying foxes); found in eastern Australia
Hepatitis C virus	Member virus of the family *Flaviviridae*; etiologic agent of hepatitis; associated with severe, chronic liver disease leading to hepatocellular carcinoma
Hepatitis delta virus	Member virus of the genus *Deltavirus*; etiologic agent is an unusual 'helper' virus; its presence makes hepatitis B more lethal
Hepatitis E virus	Member virus of the family *Picornaviridae*; etiologic agent of epidemic hepatitis, especially in Asia; recently recognized as widespread along the US–Mexico border; infection is associated with a high mortality rate in pregnant women
Human herpesvirus 8 (Kaposi sarcoma-associated herpesvirus)	Member virus of the family *Herpesviridae*; etiologically associated with Kaposi sarcoma; serologic studies show that HHV8 infection is tightly linked to KS risk; infection also associated with several uncommon lymphoproliferative syndromes in AIDS patients, including multicentric Castleman's disease and primary effusion lymphoma
Human herpesviruses 6 A and B and 7	Member viruses of the family *Herpesviridae*; etiologic agents of febrile illnesses in infants; HHV6B is the etiologic agent of roseola infantum (exanthem subitum); lifelong persistent/latent infections which may reactivate to cause disease in immunosuppressed people, typically AIDS patients and transplant recipients, sometimes culminating in rejection of transplanted organs and death
Human immunodeficiency viruses (HIV-1 and HIV-2)	Member viruses of the family *Retroviridae*; the etiologic agents of AIDS; the most important emerging infectious disease globally; still expanding in many parts of the world
Human metapneumovirus	Newly recognized member virus of the family *Paramyxoviridae*; the etiologic agent of respiratory disease in young children; first recognized in the Netherlands in 2001, now known to be distributed worldwide
Human papillomaviruses	Member viruses of the family *Papillomaviridae*; over 100 viruses, some etiologically associated with cervical, esophageal and rectal carcinomas

(Continued over)

Table 70.1 *Some of the most important new, emerging and re-emerging human viral pathogens (Continued)*

Virus	Association of the virus(es) with human disease
Human parvovirus B19	Member virus of the family *Parvoviridae*; etiologic agent of erythema infectiosum in children and a possible cause of fetal damage when pregnant women become infected
Human T-lymphotropic viruses (HTLV-I and HTLV-II)	Member viruses of the family *Retroviridae*; the etiologic agents of adult leukemia and neurological disease, especially in the tropics
Influenza viruses	Member viruses of the family *Orthomyxoviridae*; etiologic agents of influenza, causing thousands of deaths every winter in the elderly; the cause of the single most deadly epidemic ever recorded – the worldwide epidemic of 1918, in which 20–40 million people died; since 1997, highly pathogenic strains of avian influenza virus (H5N1, H7N1, and H9N2) have caused severe influenza in humans, with many fatalities, mainly in Asia, in persons in close contact with poultry
Japanese encephalitis virus	Member virus of the family *Flavivirus*; the etiologic agent of severe, often lethal, encephalitis; mosquito-borne; now spreading across southern Asia; potential for great epidemic and geographic expansion
Junin virus[a]	Member virus of the family *Arenaviridae*; etiologic agent of Argentine hemorrhagic fever; rodent-borne
Lassa virus[a]	Member virus of the family *Arenaviridae*; etiologic agent of Lassa fever; rodent-borne; a very important disease in West Africa; imported into a Chicago hospital in 1990
Machupo virus[a]	Member virus of the family *Arenaviridae*; etiologic agent of Bolivian hemorrhagic fever; rodent-borne
Measles virus	Member virus of the family *Paramyxoviridae*; the etiologic agent of the systemic disease measles; re-emerging in adolescents and young adults in many countries due to waning immunity; re-emerging in children in some countries due to poor vaccine coverage and infection in infancy before vaccination
Monkeypox virus	Member virus of the family *Poxviridae*; etiologic agent of vesiculo-pustular disease resembling a mild form of smallpox; repeated outbreaks in west Africa; reservoir in African squirrels; in 2003 mammals imported from Ghana into the USA transmitted the virus to prairie dogs from which an outbreak of monkeypox occurred in humans who had contact with infected prairie dogs
Nipah virus	Newly recognized member virus of the genus *Henipavirus*, family *Paramyxoviridae*; etiologic agent of severe, often fatal, encephalitis; zoonotic, reservoir in fruit bats; epidemic in Malaysian peninsula in 1999 with more than 100 human fatalities; since 2003 has caused outbreaks with high fatality rates in India and Bangladesh
Noroviruses	Member viruses of the family *Caliciviridae*; etiologic agents of explosive outbreaks of diarrhea and enteric disease throughout the world; increasingly associated with contaminated drinking water in institutional settings (schools, child care facilities, nursing homes) or other group settings (banquet halls, cruise ships, campgrounds)
Polioviruses	Member viruses of the family *Picornaviridae*; etiologic agents of poliomyelitis; still an important problem in developing countries of Africa and Asia; targeted by WHO for worldwide eradication by the year 2006
Rabies virus	Member virus of the genus *Lyssavirus*, family *Rhabdoviridae*; the etiologic agent of fatal encephalitis in humans and many animals; zoonotic, transmitted by the bite of rabid animals; raccoon epidemic still spreading across eastern USA; still an important human disease with ~30 000 human deaths per year globally
Rift Valley fever virus[a]	Member virus of the genus *Phlebovirus*, family *Bunyaviridae*; etiologic agent of febrile disease with hepatitis and hemorrhagic fever; mosquito-borne; the cause of one of the most explosive epidemics ever seen in Africa; recently spread from Africa to the middle East
Ross River virus	Member virus of the family *Togaviridae*; etiologic agent of febrile disease and epidemic polyarthritis; mosquito-borne; has moved from Australia across the Pacific region several times
Rotaviruses (Group A, B, and C rotaviruses)	Many member viruses of the genus *Rotavirus*, family *Reoviridae*; etiologic agents of diarrhea / enteric disease; the second leading cause of death among infants in the world; emergent when sanitary conditions deteriorate
Sabía virus[a]	Member virus of the family *Arenaviridae*; etiologic agent of Brazilian hemorrhagic fever; rodent-borne; high mortality rate, including two laboratory-acquired cases

(Continued over)

Table 70.1 *Some of the most important new, emerging and re-emerging human viral pathogens (Continued)*

Virus	Association of the virus(es) with human disease
SARS coronavirus	Newly recognized member virus of the family *Coronaviridae*; etiologic agent of severe acute respiratory distress syndrome; worldwide epidemic originating in China in 2002
Sin Nombre virus and other New World hantaviruses	Member viruses of the genus *Hantavirus*, family *Bunyaviridae*; Sin Nombre virus is the etiologic agents of hantavirus pulmonary syndrome; rodent-borne
Variant Creutzfeldt-Jakob disease prion	BSE prion; etiologic agent of invariably fatal spongiform encephalopathy; zoonotic, originating as the BSE prion; more than 150 cases in the United Kingdom in recent years
Venezuelan encephalitis virus	Member virus of the family *Togaviridae*; etiologic agent of febrile disease and encephalitis; mosquito-borne; the cause of recent major epidemics in Central and South America
West Nile virus	Member virus of the family *Flaviviridae*; etiologic agent of febrile disease and encephalitis; mosquito-borne, introduced into New York in 1999, now spread throughout the USA, north to Canada and south to Mexico and beyond
Yellow fever virus[a]	Member virus of the family *Flaviviridae*; etiologic agent of hepatitis and hemorrhagic fever; mosquito-borne; one of the most deadly diseases in history

a) The viruses that cause hemorrhagic fever in humans.

way, one was found that reacted with antibodies in the sera of infected patients but not controls. DNA from the positive clone was then used to screen other clones by DNA hybridization, and eventually the full length sequence of hepatitis C virus was determined. This enabled the development of specific diagnostic tests, including enzyme immunoassays that could be used to screen the blood supply, largely eliminating transfusion-associated transmission of hepatitis. We now recognize multiple genotypic variants of the original hepatitis C virus (see Chapter 54, Hepatitis C virus).

Since the discovery of hepatitis C virus, additional viruses with similar characteristics (member viruses of the family *Flaviviridae*), have been found using molecular techniques (Muerhoff et al. 1995; Linnen et al. 1996). These viruses, known as GB virus A, GB virus B, and GB virus C/hepatitis G virus, appear to be widespread in human and nonhuman primate populations (Robertson 2001) but so far no human disease has been definitively ascribed to their presence (Mushahwar 2000). The search for possible new viruses causing hepatitis has revealed yet another new class of viruses, currently termed anelloviruses and typified by TT virus (Nishizawa et al. 1997). These viruses are ubiquitous in human and nonhuman primate populations, and consist of a single-stranded DNA genome of negative sense, about 3 800 nucleotides in length (Mushahwar et al. 1999; Hino 2002). So far, no specific disease association has been found for these viruses, but infection may alter the severity of other infectious diseases, such as gastritis caused by *Helicobacter pylori* (Maggi et al. 2003) (see Chapter 57, TT virus and other Anelloviruses).

It should be emphasized that although molecular techniques may be crucial to the initial discovery of a new, emerging virus, classical techniques still have their place. For example, virus isolation in cell culture or even in experimental animals followed by characterization by histopathology, electron microscopy, immunofluorescence, and other specialized microscopy technologies still find their place in the discovery and initial characterization of new viruses. A case in point is the epidemic of severe acute respiratory syndrome, known as SARS (see Chapter 39, Coronaviruses, toroviruses, and arteriviruses), which first appeared in China in November 2002 and then spread via Hong Kong to many countries in 2003. The importance of this epidemic and the interactive methods used to identify its cause provides lessons worthy of more detail.

An outbreak of severe pneumonia was first recognized in Guangdong Province, China, in November 2002, initially with 300 cases of unknown etiology and five deaths. This was reported to the World Health Organization (WHO) in February 2003, and initially it was thought that these pneumonia cases might be due to a novel influenza virus.

Within the next two weeks, a WHO official working in Hanoi, Vietnam reported an unusual case of severe acute respiratory disease to WHO, and this disease was soon recognized in a large number of sick health care workers in Hong Kong and Vietnam. WHO issued a global alert about these cases, and on March 14th cases of a similar disease syndrome were reported from Canada.

Over the next few weeks it became clear that all these cases of severe respiratory disease could be linked to a single hotel in Hong Kong where the index case, a 65-year old doctor from Guangdong province in China, had stayed one might before his admittance to a hospital. Eventually the disease spread from this hotel to eight countries worldwide. These countries included Vietnam, Singapore, Canada, Hong Kong, USA, Ireland, Germany, and Thailand. Cases were also exported to France from Vietnam. Virus isolated from patients was grown in Vero (African Green monkey kidney) cells, and when examined by electron microscopy was found

Table 70.2 *Some of the most important new, emerging and re-emerging viral pathogens of animals*

Virus	Association of the virus(es) with animal disease
African horse sickness viruses	Member viruses of the genus *Orbivirus*, family *Reoviridae*; etiologic agents of acute respiratory distress syndrome, myocarditis and massive edema in horses with a 95 percent mortality rate; zoonotic with some human cases of febrile disease; mosquito-borne; an historic problem in southern Africa; a major threat to horses world-wide
African swine fever virus	Member virus of the family *Asfarviridae*; etiologic agent of systemic febrile disease with very high mortality rate in swine; tick-borne and also spread by contact; endemic in Africa and recently has been present in Europe and South America; a major threat to commercial swine industries globally
Avian influenza viruses	Member viruses of the family *Orthomyxoviridae*; etiologic agents of avian influenza; very high mortality rate associated with some virus strains; spread by wild birds; a major threat to commercial poultry industries globally
Bluetongue viruses	Member viruses of the genus *Orbivirus*, family *Reoviridae*; etiologic agents of systemic febrile disease; culicoides-borne; the isolation of several strains in Australia became an important non-tariff trade barrier issue in the 1980s
Bovine spongiform encephalopathy prion	BSE prion; etiologic agent of invariably fatal spongiform encephalopathy; first recognized in 1986; the cause of a major epidemic in cattle in the UK, resulting in major economic loss and trade embargo; zoonotic, causing fatal variant Creutzfeld-Jakob disease (vCJD) in humans
Canine parvovirus	Member viruses of the family *Parvoviridae*; etiologic agent of systemic disease, with diarrhea and enteric disease, cardiomyopathy; a new virus in the late 1970s, originating by mutation from feline panleucopenia virus; the virus rapidly swept round the world in the 1980s causing a pandemic of severe disease in dogs; now has become endemic globally
Chronic wasting disease of deer and elk prion	CWD prion; etiologic agent of invariably fatal spongiform encephalopathy; discovered in captive animals in the USA and now spreading in captive and wild deer and elk in the USA and Canada; the question of whether this disease might be zoonotic is raising concern and prompting appropriate research
Dolphin, porpoise, and phocine (seal) morbilliviruses	Member viruses of the family *Paramyxoviridae*; the etiologic agents of epidemic respiratory disease in several species of marine mammals; first identified in 1988 in European seals; emerging pathogens endangering several marine species
Feline immunodeficiency virus and Simian immunodeficiency viruses	Member viruses of the family *Retroviridae*; etiologic agent of AIDS-like syndrome; important new viruses, the one affecting cats in nature and all serving as important models in AIDS research
Foot-and-mouth disease viruses	Member viruses of the family *Picornaviridae*; systemic vesicular disease; still considered the most dangerous disease of livestock in the world because of the great capacity for rapid transmission and great economic loss; still entrenched in Africa, the Middle East, and Asia; caused a devastating epidemic in the United Kingdom in 2001
Hendra virus	Newly recognized member virus of the genus *Henipavirus*, family *Paramyxoviridae*; etiologic agent of acute, often fatal, respiratory distress syndrome in horses and humans; reservoir host fruit bats (flying foxes); found in eastern Australia
Malignant catarrhal fever virus (Alcelaphine herpesvirus 1)	Member virus of family *Herpesviridae*; etiologic agent of systemic disease with fever and acute inflammation of nasal and oral membranes and involvement of pharynx and lungs; usually fatal; etiologic agent is silently carried by certain African wildlife species such as gnu, wildebeest, and hartebeest; it can occur in zoos, and its presence is an important non-tariff trade barrier issue throughout the world
Monkeypox virus	Member virus of the family *Poxviridae*; etiologic agent of vesiculo-pustular disease resembling a mild form of smallpox in wild and captive monkeys in contact with squirrels and other small rodents in Central and West Africa; reservoir in African squirrels; in 2003 mammals imported from Ghana into the USA transmitted the virus to prairie dogs from which an outbreak of monkeypox occurred in humans who had contact with infected prairie dogs

(Continued over)

Table 70.2 *Some of the most important new, emerging and re-emerging viral pathogens of animals (Continued)*

Virus	Association of the virus(es) with animal disease
Myxoma virus	Member virus of the family *Poxviridae*; etiologic agent of systemic exanthematous disease in rabbits; had been used to control rabbits in Australia, but with diminishing success; a damaging virus in commercial rabbit industries in some countries
Nipah virus	Newly recognized member virus of the genus *Henipavirus*, family *Paramyxoviridae*; etiologic agent of encephalitis and respiratory disease in swine; reservoir in fruit bats; massive epidemic in swine in southern Asia in 1999; zoonotic, with often fatal encephalitis in humans in contact with infected swine
Porcine reproductive and respiratory syndrome virus (PRRS virus)	Member virus of family *Arteriviridae*; etiologic agent of respiratory disease and reproductive tract disease; an important disease in commercial swine industries of several countries, with major economic impact
Rabbit hemorrhagic disease virus	Member virus of family *Caliciviridae*; etiologic agent of universally fatal hemorrhagic disease in rabbits; being used to control rabbits in Australia
Rinderpest virus	Member virus of the family *Paramyxoviridae*; etiologic agent of systemic disease with very high mortality rate in cattle and many other species of cloven footed animals; still considered very dangerous, with potential for causing great economic loss; still entrenched in limited areas in Africa and Asia; target of ongoing global eradication campaign
West Nile virus	Member virus of the family *Flaviviridae*; etiologic agent of febrile disease and encephalitis in birds and mammals, especially horses; mosquito-borne; in 1999 a particularly virulent strain from Israel moved to the USA, where it has caused thousands of deaths in crows and other passerine birds as well as horses; zoonotic, has become very important human pathogen

to resemble a coronavirus. Cultures of the virus showed immunofluorescence when reacted with serum from recovered patients (Ksiazek et al. 2003; Drosten et al. 2003). Subsequently, knowing that it was a coronavirus by electron microscopy, consensus primers were used in PCR amplification, and the complete genetic sequence of the virus was determined by several groups (Rota et al. 2003; Marra et al. 2003; Ruan et al. 2003; Thiel et al. 2003). Despite the availability of this sequence information, numerous studies have so far not determined the precise origin of the SARS coronavirus, although it is speculated that it arose from an animal reservoir, perhaps in palm civets (Guan et al. 2003).

THE VIRUS: VARIATION AND THE EMERGENCE OF NEW VIRAL PHENOTYPES

The variety and diversity of viruses

As knowledge of the molecular structure and replication of viruses has increased, we have learned that the viruses that we know to be responsible for human and animal diseases represent only a small fraction of a large, diverse global virus population. Currently, some 3 600 virus species are recognized taxonomically, but international reference centers and culture collections keep track of more than 30 000 viral strains (Murphy et al. 1995). This number continues to increase because each time a potential host species or a new disease is studied in detail, new viruses are found. In addition,

clues to the existence of new viruses may sometimes be found in other species (ecological niches). For example, the picobirnaviruses, with a genome of two segments of double-stranded RNA, 2.6 and 1.5 kb in length, were first found in rat feces (Pereira et al. 1988), and only later in humans, where they may be a cause of diarrhea (Grohmann et al. 1993; Gallimore et al. 1995).

Polygenic basis for viral variation

There are several genetic mechanisms that drive virus evolution: discussed below are mutation, recombination, and reassortment of genes. However, many of the most important variances among viruses are polygenic, and of ancient derivation, the result of the natural selection of the most fit variants (Nathanson et al. 1993). A classic example of such variation was the definition many years ago of smallpox virus variants, variola major (Indian subcontinent and Europe, mortality up to 30 percent), and variola minor (South America, mortality about 1 percent) (Fenner et al. 1988). Another example was naturally occurring attenuated poliovirus variants, some of which inspired the development of Sabin live-attenuated polio vaccines (Sabin 1981). Only recently has it been possible to begin to explain such phenotypic differences from a molecular genetic perspective

Mutation

The replication of viruses involves copying the genome nucleic acid millions of times; mistakes in the copying process introduce mutations (see Chapter 2, The origin

Table 70.3 *Emerging human viral diseases: recognition by molecular techniques*

Virus	Disease	Method
Human papillomaviruses (more than 100 types)	Warts, anogenital carcinomas, laryngeal papillomas, and carcinomas	Cloning and restriction fragment analysis or sequencing of viral genomic DNA from infected tissues
Hepatitis C virus	Hepatitis, often chronic, leading to hepatocellular carcinoma	Cloning, sequencing, expression, and immunoselection with specific sera
Hepatitis E virus	Acute epidemic hepatitis	Cloning, sequencing, expression, and immunoselection with specific sera
Human herpesvirus 8	Kaposi sarcoma	Representational DNA difference analysis (RDA) of normal vs. sarcoma tissue
Hepatitis G virus/GB virus-C	Unknown	Cloning, sequencing, expression, and immunoselection with specific sera
Human metapneumovirus	Respiratory disease in children	Random primer polymerase chain reaction
GBV-A, GBV-B	Unknown	Representational difference analysis
GBV-C – Hepatitis G virus	Unknown	Cloning, sequencing, expression, and immunoselection with specific sera
Sin Nombre virus	Hantavirus pulmonary syndrome	Reverse transcription and consensus sequence polymerase chain reaction amplification from infected human and rodent tissues
Bayou virus	Hantavirus pulmonary syndrome	Reverse transcription and polymerase chain reaction amplification from infected human tissues and sequence analysis
TT virus	Not known	Representational DNA difference analysis of human sera

and evolution of viruses). When such mutations lead to new phenotypic characters that enable the virus to replicate in a new host or cell type, to replicate to a higher titer or at a faster rate, or to better escape host defenses, the potential exists for emergence of a new viral disease. Genetically, mutational changes affecting phenotype may be minimal, involving one or a few nucleotides, or they may be large and complex, involving the addition of new genes into viral genomes by recombination or reassortment (see below). In any case, it is the expression of genotypic change as a new phenotype that is important in nature, and usually it is phenotypic change affecting transmission that is at the heart of the emergence of a new disease. Mutations that affect antigenic determinants on the viral surface proteins may be selected for, especially when viruses replicate in the presence of antibody. This has been clearly documented in the case of influenza. New antigenic variants of influenza viruses occur so pervasively that reformulation of vaccine is required on an annual basis.

The emergence of influenza virus variants by the accumulation of point mutations is termed genetic drift (see Chapter 32, Orthomyxoviruses: influenza). Such mutations may dramatically alter viral pathogenicity, but more importantly they may result in new viral surface epitopes that the population does not recognize, when it is termed antigenic drift. An example of genetic drift occurred in 1983, when an outbreak of avian influenza A virus (H5N3) in Pennsylvania spread through the poultry industry of the region, leading to the destruction of 17 million fowl and a loss of about US$60 million. When the virus was sequenced, it was found to have acquired a single point mutation that altered the cleavability of its hemagglutinin, thereby greatly increasing its pathogenicity.

A dramatic example of the emergence of a new virus by mutation is afforded by canine parvovirus (Parrish 1990, 1994). Serological evidence suggests that this virus made its first appearance as a new pathogen of dogs in 1976. The virus was isolated in 1978 as the cause of severe enteritis, sometimes fatal, that occurred in dogs in North America, Europe, and Australia. Outbreaks of sudden death in puppies due to myocarditis were also linked to the new virus. Soon after its isolation, it became clear from antigenic analysis and restriction endonuclease mapping that the canine virus was closely related to feline panleukopenia virus, a pathogen that had been recognized since the 1920s. Sequence analysis of isolates of the canine virus revealed that it differed from feline panleucopenia virus in only six nucleotides, and probably originated as a result of two amino-acid changes in the viral capsid, which for the first time allowed the feline virus to replicate in dog cells. The rapidity with which canine parvovirus disease spread round the world has not been explained, but the extreme physical stability of the virus probably made fomite carriage by humans very efficient.

The special case of high frequency mutation and quasispecies formation in RNA viruses

Given their great potential for generating new genotypes, the RNA viruses seem to represent an enormous and continuous risk with regard to the emergence of new epidemic diseases, but in fact the frequency of emergence of such new diseases is lower than might be expected (see Chapter 2, The origin and evolution of viruses). New genotypes are tested severely by natural selection and few represent a better fit than current wild types. Better fit and better adaptation to an econiche require that a new genotype or a new virus has certain improved traits, such as improved transmissibility, and perhaps improved capacity for surviving 'lean times' such as those presented by a highly immune population or even a harsh physical environment. There is no doubt that the mode of transmission is the critically important element in this regard; viruses transmitted by the respiratory route fit their econiches very well indeed, and represent the threats to our civilization of major epidemic or pandemic disease (Mims 1991). However, as we are learning from the insidious spread of human immunodeficiency virus (HIV) in Africa and Asia, other transmission patterns can be equally deadly.

Recombination

Genetic recombination involves an interaction between two or more viral genomes during mixed infection of a cell, giving rise to progeny having a genome with characteristics derived from two or more parental genotypes. Recombination is observed with both DNA and RNA viruses, but surprisingly few examples have been documented of emergence of new viruses through this mechanism. For example, although experimental evidence exists for recombination in vivo among herpesviruses, and many individuals are dually infected by more than one herpesvirus, no herpesvirus disease manifestation in humans has ever been attributed to recombinational events (Javier et al. 1986).

There is one major exception to the dearth of evidence that recombination is important in the emergence of viral diseases: Western equine encephalitis virus (WEE) is a recombinant, its two glycoprotein genes being derived from a Sindbis-like virus progenitor and the remainder of its genome derived from Eastern equine encephalitis virus (Hahn et al. 1988). It is estimated that two cross-over events were required to produce WEEV from its progenitors, and that this probably occurred during persistent infection in a mosquito host more than 1 000 years ago (Strauss and Strauss 1994). Recombination is also well documented between serotypes of polioviruses, for example after administration of trivalent Sabin vaccine to infants, recombinant variant viruses are shed in the stool of some individuals (Liu et al. 2003). This confirms the potential for generation of recombinant viruses with altered pathogenicity or altered host range, yet it is surprising that so few examples have been found.

Reassortment

Closely related viruses that have segmented genomes often undergo genetic recombination during dual infections. This special case of recombination in which whole genome segments are recombined is termed reassortment. Different influenza A viruses can reassort their genome segments, forming viable progeny; when this results in replacement of the hemagglutinin or neuraminidase genes it is termed 'antigenic shift'. No reassortment occurs between influenza A and influenza B viruses; the basis for this restriction is not known. Each of the major human influenza pandemics of this century (1918, 1957, and 1968) was caused by reassortment of genome segments between an existing human virus and an avian virus (Webster and Kawaoka 1994). Several new strains of human influenza arose by reassortment between the prevailing human influenza virus and genes from the avian influenza virus gene pool that exists in wild ducks. For example, in 1957 the virus causing a worldwide pandemic of influenza (the Asian influenza pandemic) acquired three genes (PB1, HA, and NA) by reassortment with the influenza gene pool in ducks, and kept five other genes from the circulating human strain (Kawaoka et al. 1989). Swine may provide an important intermediate host in the stabilization of reassortants between avian and human influenza viruses. In 1997, reassortment between avian influenza virus genomes resulted in an avian influenza virus with a highly cleavable hemagglutinin. The hemagglutinin gene was apparently acquired from influenza A/ Goose/Guandong/1/96 virus (Xu et al. 1999). This change allowed the variant virus to infect 18 humans, six of whom died. Fortunately this emergent virus did not readily transmit from human to human, but the virus has remained in poultry in Eastern Asia, causing many outbreaks of disease in birds and a significant number of influenza cases and deaths in humans. Clearly the danger is that the viruses now established in poultry will continue to mutate and could acquire the necessary phenotype for efficient human to human transmission through mutation, or through reassortment with a prevailing human influenza virus. Such an event would undoubtedly result in an influenza pandemic, as the H5 hemagglutinin molecule has not previously circulated widely in the human population (Li et al. 2004; Stephenson et al. 2004).

Reassortment between animal and human viruses also seems to be important in generating new pathogenic strains of rotaviruses (Gentsch et al. 1993; Iturriza-Gómara et al. 2001). Such novel viruses have been isolated as predominant outbreak strains in the USA (Ramachandran et al. 1998) and in the UK (Iturriza-Gomara et al. 2002).

Epidemic potential of newly evolved viruses

The epidemic potential of newly emergent viruses varies, depending upon the mode of transmission, the immunological and genetic susceptibility of the host population, the size of the population at risk, and other epidemiological and pathogenetic factors. Epidemic potential is greatest for an agent that is readily transmitted from host to host, particularly via the respiratory route. Conversely, zoonotic agents and arthropod-borne agents are usually limited in their geographic range, although the latter are certainly not limited in their capacity for causing very large epidemics.

Certain kinds of phenotypic change are most notable as the bases for the epidemic potential of particular viruses. An extension in host range can permit a virus to spread into a new species with devastating consequences. An increase in virulence (based on any of several mechanisms) can convert a nonpathogenic or trivially pathogenic virus into one with devastating pathogenic qualities. A change in antigenic signature can permit a virus to infect a population already immune to parental strains of the same virus.

THE INDIVIDUAL HOST: SUSCEPTIBILITY/RESISTANCE FACTORS FAVORING THE EMERGENCE OF VIRAL DISEASES

In many ways, the influence of the host on the emergence of viral diseases is more important than influences attributed to the virus per se. The host brings a much more complex genome to the battle between virus and host that involves the qualities of the virus that are crucial for its transmission and survival, and the resistance of the host. These host factors are usually categorized under (1) innate resistance, mostly dependent on poorly understood nonspecific resistance factors, (2) acquired resistance (e.g. macrophages and the cellular and humoral immune responses), and (3) physiological factors affecting resistance (e.g. age, nutritional status, hormonal effects especially in pregnancy, fever). When host resistance is optimal, infection may be subclinical or abortive, but when host response is inadequate qualitatively or quantitatively, disease is the usual outcome. Furthermore, when an overly exuberant immune response occurs there can be immunopathological disease.

The host immune response

Studies with inbred mice have identified a large repertoire of genes that confer survival potential on the host. Most of these genes are specific for a single family of viruses, although a few map to the major histocompatibility locus and encode proteins that influence host immune responses to multiple agents. Polygenic resistance characteristics are less well understood, but seemingly are even more important. For example, line-breeding and inbreeding experiments led to the development of the classic strains of mice that are exquisitely sensitive to certain viruses: these mice have been used for many years to isolate arboviruses, rabies virus, and picornaviruses. The genes selected for in these mice may be unknown, but the implication is that many genes may affect host resistance to viral infections.

The age of the host

The age of the host may also affect viral pathogenesis. This is true of poliomyelitis, a disease which emerged concurrently with improved sanitation and hygiene. It is likely that poliomyelitis occurred as a sporadic disease since ancient times. During the eighteenth and first half of the nineteenth centuries a few clusters of cases were reported, but from about 1905 onwards epidemics were reported annually in the USA. The same pattern of emergence of poliomyelitis as an epidemic disease has been repeated many times since, first in developed and then in developing countries. What accounts for this emergence of epidemic poliomyelitis? There is no evidence that it was due to the appearance of virus strains of increased virulence. Epidemiological data suggest that there is a correlation between age at the time of infection and risk of paralytic disease. Before vaccines were used to control the disease, it was apparent that in virgin soil epidemics in isolated communities without prior experience of the virus, most severe cases and deaths occurred in adults. It was proposed by Nathanson and Martin (1979) that the appearance of epidemic poliomyelitis was due, paradoxically, to improvements in public sanitation and personal hygiene, which led to a reduction in virus transmission. A delay in the age of initial infection, beyond the age when infants are protected by passively acquired maternal antibody, is postulated to have increased the risk of clinical disease. However, at the present time the phenomenon of increased disease severity of poliovirus infection in adults is still not completely understood.

Persistent infection and chronic shedding

The dynamics of emergence of a new viral disease can vary greatly, depending on the incubation period, whether the infection is rapidly self-limiting or persistent and whether the resulting disease (and shedding pattern) is acute or chronic. When associated with a short incubation period and acute disease, emergence can be a dramatic event. However, when the emerging agent is associated with a long incubation period, the resulting epidemic may rise over a period of years before it reaches a peak. Furthermore, a long interval between infection and disease occurrence may obscure the identification of the causal agent and its mode of transmission and may thereby delay intervention actions. Finally, if the disease is chronic, the impact on the healthcare system may spread over decades rather than weeks, with major economic consequences beyond those ordinarily associated with an acute epidemic.

HIV AND ACQUIRED IMMUNODEFICIENCY SYNDROME (AIDS)

The premier example of the importance of a long incubation period disease in the emergence of a new disease is AIDS. In fact, the length of the incubation period, which averages 8–10 years, repeatedly led to underestimates of the true extent of spread and penetration of the epidemic (Figure 70.2). Associated with this was uncertainty regarding the proportion of infections that would lead to death. The long incubation period led to the initial assumption that only a small proportion of infections, perhaps no more than 10 percent, would be fatal; projections of total AIDS incidence were correspondingly low. Also important was a failure to appreciate the epidemiological impact of life-long persistence of infection and virus shedding. It proved difficult to devise a model of the number of potentially infectious individuals in the population at any given time, and their impact on transmission dynamics. Finally, it was not appreciated that the chronic nature of AIDS would produce a vast new burden upon the healthcare system.

Coincident change in viral virulence and host resistance

The best documented example of coincident change in host and virus leading to the emergence of a variant disease involves the rabbit and myxoma virus. The disease, myxomatosis of rabbits, is caused by the poxvirus, myxoma virus; it occurs naturally as a mild infection of rabbits in South America and California (*Sylvilagus* spp.) where it produces a skin tumor from which virus is transmitted mechanically by biting insects. However, in the European rabbit (*Oryctolagus cuniculus*), myxoma virus causes a lethal infection, a finding that led to its use for biological control of wild rabbits in Australia. The European rabbit was introduced into Australia in 1859 for sporting purposes and rapidly spread to become the major animal pest of agricultural and pastoral industries. Myxoma virus was successfully introduced into this rabbit population in 1950; when originally introduced the virus produced case-fatality rates of over 99 percent. This highly virulent virus was readily transmitted by mosquitoes. Farmers operated 'inoculation campaigns' to introduce the virus into wild rabbit populations.

It might have been predicted that the disease, and with it the virus, would disappear at the end of each summer, owing to the greatly diminished numbers of susceptible rabbits and mosquitoes during the winter. This must have occurred often in localized areas, but it did not happen over the continent as a whole. The capacity of virus to survive the winter conferred a great selective advantage on viral mutants of reduced lethality: during this period,

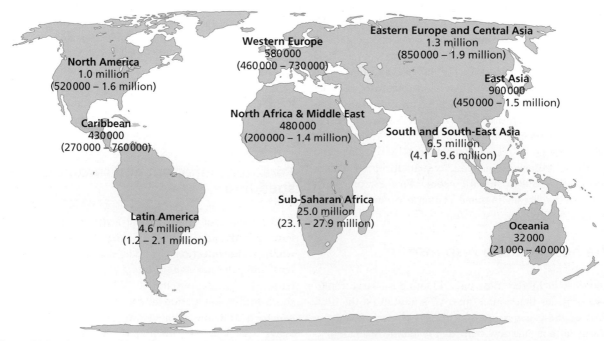

Figure 70.2 *Adults and children estimated to be living with HIV as of the end of 2003. Source WHO UNAIDS Programme.*

Table 70.4 *Emerging viral diseases: examples of probable crossings of the species barrier*

Year	Virus	Disease	Species Involved	Cause
1931	HIV-1	AIDS	Chimpanzees to humans	? Mutation
1940	HIV-2	AIDS	Sooty Mangabies to humans	? Mutation
1978	Canine parvovirus	Pandemic enteritis, myocarditis	Cat to dog	Mutation of feline panleucopenia virus
1988	Phocid distemper virus 1	Fatal respiratory disease (distemper)	Harp seals to harbor seals	Migration of harp seals due to climatic conditions
1989	Phocid distemper virus 2	Fatal respiratory disease (distemper)	Dogs to Siberian seals	Contact between different marine species or contact with terrestial animals (dogs)
1994	Hendra virus	Acute respiratory distress syndrome (ARDS), and encephalitis	Fruit bats to horses and humans	Unknown
1999	Nipah virus	Severe respiratory disease and encephalitis	Fruit bats to pigs and humans	Unknown

when mosquito numbers were low, rabbits infected by such mutants survived in an infectious condition for weeks instead of a few days and thereby contributed disproportionately to the progeny pool. Within 3 years such 'attenuated' mutants became the dominant strains throughout Australia. Thus, the original highly lethal virus was progressively replaced by a heterogeneous collection of strains of lower virulence, but most of them were still virulent enough to kill 70–90 percent of genetically unselected rabbits.

Rabbits that recover from myxomatosis are immune to reinfection. However, because most wild rabbits have a life-span of less than a year, herd immunity is not an important factor in the epidemiology of myxomatosis. Selection for more genetically resistant animals operated from the outset of the 'inoculation campaigns'. In areas where repeated outbreaks occurred, the genetic resistance of surviving rabbits increased progressively. The early appearance of viral strains of lower virulence, which allowed 10 percent of genetically unselected rabbits to recover, was an important factor in allowing the number of genetically resistant rabbits to increase. In areas where annual outbreaks occurred, the case-fatality rate fell from 90 percent to 25 percent within 7 years. Subsequently, in areas where there were frequent outbreaks, somewhat more virulent strains of virus became dominant, because they produced the kind of disease that was best transmitted in populations of genetically resistant rabbits. Thus, the ultimate balance struck between myxoma virus and Australian rabbits involved adaptations of virus and host populations, reaching a dynamic equilibrium that finds rabbits still greatly reduced compared with their pre-myxomatosis numbers, but too numerous for the wishes of farmers and conservationists.

'Species-jumping' – crossing the species barrier

The ability of animal viruses to cross the species barrier as a result of mutations has been documented in several

cases (Mahy and Brown, 2000; Table 70.4) but in many cases involving humans, further transmission does not occur, and humans are a 'dead-end ' host (e.g. hantavirus pulmonary syndrome) (Mims 1991). Among important human viral pathogens, HIV-1 and HIV-2 provide the best examples of crossing the species barrier (Korber et al. 2000).

HIV-1 AND HIV-2

Perhaps the most significant example of species-jumping occurred when HIV entered the human population from a simian reservoir. Although the disease went unrecognized in the human population until 1977, careful molecular dating analysis suggests that HIV-1 entered the human population around 1931 (Korber et al. 2000) and HIV-2 around 1940 (Lemey et al. 2003).

Both HIV-1 and HIV-2 viruses have a narrow host range, seemingly limited to humans. The viruses can experimentally infect certain nonhuman primates, in which replication usually occurs without apparent disease. However, simian lentiviruses (simian immunodeficiency viruses (SIV)) can be recovered from a range of African monkey species, and phylogenetic analysis has confirmed the simian origins of both HIV-1 and HIV-2 (Myers et al. 1992; Korber et al. 2000). HIV-1 seems to have arisen as a cause of immunodeficiency in humans by species-jumping from the chimpanzee, and HIV-2 came from sooty-mangabeys in West Africa (Hahn et al. 2000); there is clear overlap between the areas in Africa where HIV-2 was first detected and the range of known SIV-infected monkey species (Smallman-Raynor and Cliff 1991). Humans in close contact with nonhuman primates are susceptible to infection with SIVs (Gao et al. 1992; Khabbaz et al. 1994), but these infections are usually asymptomatic and the precise mutational changes that led to the emergence of HIV as an epidemic disease spreading in the human population are unknown.

HENDRA VIRUS AND NIPAH VIRUS

The emergence of Hendra virus provides yet another lesson-filled example of the importance of species-jumping. In 1994 a horse trainer and a stablehand in Hendra, Queensland, Australia, became ill with interstitial pneumonia (acute respiratory distress syndrome (ARDS)) while nursing a sick horse that had recently been brought onto the property. The disease spread to other horses in the stables, and 14 of 21 infected horses died from a pulmonary disease with hemorrhagic manifestations that was caused by a previously unknown virus. Although the stablehand survived the infection, the trainer died. A virus was isolated from both equine lung tissue and human kidney tissue taken at autopsy, and from structural and antigenic studies was named an 'equine morbillivirus' (Murray et al. 1995), though subsequently it was renamed 'Hendra virus'. One year later a horse farmer 600 miles away, in Mackay, Queensland died of encephalitis from the same virus. He had assisted at the necropsy of two of his horses that had died (one with acute respiratory disease, and the other with neurological symptoms). Although he became ill initially with mild meningitis, one year elapsed before the farmer became severely ill and died, when at autopsy Hendra virus was found in his brain (O'Sullivan et al. 1997).

In an investigation as to the origin of Hendra virus, an extensive serological survey involving over 5 000 animals was carried out. Of all species tested, only fruit-eating bats (flying foxes) of the genus *Pteropus* were found seropositive (Young et al. 1996). Subsequently, Hendra virus was directly isolated from pteropid bats, and a sampling over a wide geographic range found that almost 50 percent of pteropid bats had serological evidence of infection (Field et al. 2001).

Hendra virus clearly belongs to the *Paramyxoviridae,* but has a longer genome (19 kb in length) than any previously studied members of the family, and genome sequence analysis clearly showed many unique features (Gould 1996; Wang et al. 2000). In 1999, a related virus was discovered in Malaysia following a major outbreak of respiratory disease in pigs and severe neurological disease in humans in close contact with diseased pigs. More than 100 humans died, and in a successful effort to control the disease 1.1 million pigs were slaughtered. A virus was isolated from brain tissue from a fatal human case – the patient had lived in Nipah River Village, and so the virus was named Nipah virus (Chua et al. 2000). Hendra virus and Nipah virus cross-react antigenically, and once the two viruses were compared by sequence analysis it was obvious that they belong to the same genus, which has been named '*Henipavirus*'. Although all human cases from the original Nipah virus outbreak had close contact with pigs, a 'mystery disease' recognized in India in 2003, and seen subsequently in Bangladesh in 2004 (Hsu et al. 2004), seems to involve direct infection of humans by Nipah virus without an intermediate domestic animal host. These new outbreaks seem to be due to direct transmission between Nipah virus-infected pteropid bats or their excreta and humans, most of whom have been young boys who climb trees in which infected bats can be found.

Spread in the human population

Many viruses can cross the species barrier and infect humans, but transmission to humans represents a 'dead end' for the virus and no further transmission occurs (Mims 1991). On the other hand, some are regularly or irregularly transmitted from human-to-human, but without establishing an independent long-term exclusively human reservoir. All of these variations define the terms 'zoonosis' and 'zoonoses'. Many of these zoonotic viruses are arthropod-borne, including alphaviruses such as Eastern equine encephalitis virus and Western equine encephalitis virus, flaviviruses such as West Nile virus and Japanese encephalitis virus and St. Louis encephalitis virus, and bunyaviruses such as La Crosse virus and Rift Valley fever virus. Other viruses are transmitted directly to humans from zoonotic animal reservoirs, most commonly from rodent reservoirs. Examples include bunyaviruses such as Hantaan virus (the etiologic agent of hemorrhagic fever with renal syndrome), Seoul virus, Puumala virus (the etiologic agent of nephropathia epidemica), and Sin Nombre virus (the etiologic agent of hantavirus pulmonary syndrome), and arenaviruses such as Machupo virus (the etiologic agent of Bolivian hemorrhagic fever), Junin virus (the etiologic agent of Argentine hemorrhagic fever) and Lassa virus (the etiologic agent of Lassa fever). Historically, each of these viruses has been responsible for the emergence of a 'new' human disease.

THE HOST POPULATION: INDIVIDUAL AND SOCIETAL BEHAVIORAL FACTORS FAVORING THE EMERGENCE OF VIRAL DISEASES

Several influences pertaining to human behavior (individual and societal behavior) have favored the emergence of new virus diseases; all of these influences seem to have accelerated over the last century. The global human population has continued to grow inexorably, bringing increasingly larger numbers of people into close contact. There have been successive revolutions in the speed of transportation, making it possible to circumnavigate the globe in less than the incubation period of most viral infections (Murphy and Nathanson 1994). For this reason, viral diseases occurring anywhere in the world can no longer be presumed to stay confined to their country or continent of origin. The death of a patient from Lassa fever in a hospital in Chicago in 1989 provided sobering testimony to the distance and speed that exotic viruses can move around the world (Holmes et al. 1990). The patient, an American citizen who had visited Nigeria to attend his mother's funeral, became ill 2 days after his return to Chicago. A total of 102 people had contact with him in the hospital. Fortunately, none of these contacts became infected. However, the incident illustrates the potential vulnerability of populations remote from the normal locale of geographically limited diseases. More recently, at least four cases of Lassa fever virus infection in European persons who had visited West Africa have been recorded, raising concern regarding the clinical management of such cases in diverse European settings (Crowcroft 2002).

The influence of individual behavioral factors

There are diverse influences pertaining to the behavior of individuals that can lead to the emergence of new diseases or new patterns of disease transmission. Many diseases that depend upon such factors are emergent or re-emergent. Behavioral influences include: (1) risk factors leading to sexually transmitted diseases (e.g. multiple sex partners, homosexual risk behaviors); (2) behavioral risk factors associated with day care and school; (3) behavioral risk factors favoring the transmission of childhood diseases in the community; (4) risk factors pertaining to food preparation and storage in the home; (5) risk factors associated with keeping pet animals in the home; and (6) viruses intentionally used for harm by bioterrorists.

SEXUALLY TRANSMITTED DISEASES

After declining over many years in developed countries, sexually transmitted diseases are now increasing at epidemic rates in urban populations in Europe, the USA, and many developing countries. Changes in sexual attitudes and behavior, combined with injectable drug use, have led to rapid amplification of certain viral diseases that are spread sexually. This is especially disturbing because many of the sexually transmitted diseases enhance the risk of transmission of each other (via new bacteria and viruses entering through established lesions). Thus, the risk of transmission is increased beyond expected rates and 'curable' diseases, such as gonorrhea and syphilis, support the spread of 'incurable' diseases, such as genital herpes and HIV infection/AIDS. The major societal failing in this regard stems from declining support for public health programmes, but in some instances emergence reflects advances in our ability to detect new viruses. One example is the emergence of human papillomavirus infection, genital papillomatosis, and cervical cancer. Multiple risk factors contribute to cervical cancer; these include behavioral (sexual behavior), dietary, hormonal, and viral risk factors (zur Hausen 2002). There are several theories but no real proof as to how these risk factors, in concert, lead to cervical neoplasia. Now that one risk factor for cervical cancer is known to be infection with certain types of human papillomaviruses, DNA probes for these viruses are being added to cytological screening programmes.

DAY CARE AND VIRAL INFECTIONS

Shifts in the structure of the family in all developed countries have resulted in a dramatic increase in the proportion of children in day care; currently in the USA, 35 million children under 14 years with working mothers spend 22–40 hours per week in day care. This trend is likely to continue, and in the year 2001 it was estimated that more than nine million families included working mothers with children under 5 years of age. Viral diseases represent the most important problems in day care, respiratory and diarrheal illnesses being most common. Children attending day care facilities may also become silent reservoir hosts for some agents of disease, such as hepatitis A virus and several enteroviruses. Depending on the disease, children attending day care have a 2- to 18-fold increased risk of becoming ill compared with children at home. The most common viral diarrheal pathogens acquired in day-care centers are rotaviruses. Rotaviruses, first discovered in 1973, infect every child in its first 3–4 years of life; this leads, in the USA, to an estimated 3 million cases of diarrhea, 500 000 doctor visits, 70 000 hospitalizations for 300 000 inpatient days and 75–125 deaths, and the costs for hospital care total US$200–400 million per year. Worldwide, some 600 000 children die each year of rotavirus diarrhea (Bern et al. 1992).

KEEPING PET ANIMALS

There have been many episodes of the introduction of new pathogens, such as exotic *Salmonella* types, via reptiles and amphibians kept as pets, but until recently viruses received little attention in this regard. The introduction in 2003 of monkeypox virus into the USA from Africa changed all this (CDC 2003b). A pet supplier in Texas, USA imported a shipment of rodents from Accra, Ghana which included giant Gambian rats, tree squirrels, rope squirrels, dormice, and several other African rodent species. One or more of these species were infected with monkeypox virus, which is endemic in Africa. These animals were housed by the importer together with prairie dogs, an American ground squirrel (*Cynomys* sp.) that is very popular as a family pet. The prairie dogs readily became infected with monkeypox virus, and when sold as pets human cases of monkeypox began to emerge in the mid-western United States (Guarner et al. 2004b). As a result, more than eighty human cases of monkeypox occurred in the USA, and there was a real danger that monkeypox virus could become endemic in wild rodent populations. Following this episode, regulation of imports and interstate movement of exotic mammals have been upgraded, but it seems likely that we will see more of this kind of threat from imported pathogens in the future.

VIRUSES INTENTIONALLY USED FOR HARM

Since the terrorist attacks of September 11th 2001 in the USA, and the subsequent anthrax attacks through the US mail system, the possible use of viruses as weapons of bioterrorism must be considered (Smolinski et al. 2003). Although smallpox was eradicated in 1980, the possibility that the virus could be deliberately reintroduced into the world population remains the subject of considerable concern (Henderson 1999; Mahy 2003) and several countries are taking steps to prepare for such an event. Many other viral pathogens are also considered to be possible agents of biological warfare, including viruses causing severe hemorrhagic fever such as filoviruses (e.g. Ebola virus and Marburg virus), arenaviruses (e.g. Lassa fever, Machupo virus), and viruses causing severe encephalitis (e.g. Venezuelan equine encephalitis virus, Eastern equine encephalitis virus, Western equine encephalitis virus). The possible use of a virus to cause harm to the agricultural economy must also be considered, and in this context foot-and-mouth disease virus must be a prime candidate.

These threats also include the potential which now exists for deliberate genetic engineering of an existing virus so as to alter properties like pathogenicity or susceptibility to control by vaccination. The future emergence of a harmful virus disease by deliberate human action remains uncertain, but only by recognizing the possibilities can we prepare for, and minimize, the impact of such an event.

The influence of societal, commercial, and iatrogenic factors

There are diverse societal, commercial, and medical care factors that lead to the emergence of new diseases or new disease patterns. Again, many diseases that depend on such factors are emergent or re-emergent. Such risk factors include: (1) those associated with the commercial food industries, from sources on the farm to processing, transportation, wholesaling, and retailing; (2) those associated with water supply, (3) those associated with pharmaceuticals and biologicals; (4) those causing iatrogenic diseases.

DISEASES ASSOCIATED WITH ADVANCED MEDICAL CARE

Diseases such as those associated with immunosuppressive drug therapy, organ transplantation (including xenotransplantation), blood banking, and kidney dialysis are all increasing substantially in all developed countries.

Since the early 1980s there has been an unprecedented rise in opportunistic infections associated with these medical care practices. In particular, the increase in organ transplantation and cancer chemotherapy, with their associated immunosuppressive drug therapies, has combined with the emerging AIDS epidemic to create a large, highly susceptible population at risk for a variety of viral diseases (see Chapter 43, Reoviruses, orbiviruses and coltiviruses). In many cases viruses cause diseases of greatly increased severity in such individuals. These include diseases caused by DNA viruses, such as cytomegalovirus, Epstein-Barr virus, varicella-zoster virus, human herpesvirus 6, human papillomaviruses, human parvovirus B19, human polyomaviruses JC and BK, adenoviruses, hepatitis B virus, and molluscum contagiosum virus, and RNA viruses such as measles virus, hepatitis C virus, influenza, respiratory syncytial virus and parainfluenza virus.

Human herpesvirus 8, which is strongly associated with and may be the cause of Kaposi's sarcoma, is an example of an emerging virus that might not have been recognized except for its association with HIV and its immunosuppressive effects (Chang et al. 1994). As the number of naturally and therapeutically immunosuppressed people continues to expand throughout the world, it is likely that more and more new viral diseases, or new manifestations of old viral diseases, will continue to be seen.

MODERN AGRICULTURAL AND FOOD INDUSTRY PRACTICES AND VIRAL INFECTIONS

Changes in every aspect of the food industry, from on-the-farm technologies to processing technologies, favor the emergence of new viral disease problems. Animal husbandry has changed in ways that increase stress and promote viral transmission and endemic infection cycles in livestock and poultry. Large numbers of animals are being confined in limited space and at very high density, cared for by a few, inadequately trained workers. Elaborate housing systems are used, with good evaluation of cost:benefit, but with inadequate evaluation of health effects of systems for ventilation, feeding, waste disposal, and cleaning. In addition, some diseases are favored by the global expansion of agricultural markets, involving the global transport of animals, animal products, and animal semen and embryos. Yet, other diseases can emerge as a consequence of changes in processing systems and distribution systems for finished foods.

In 1997 there was an outbreak of hepatitis A which was first noticed in Michigan schoolchildren and later in Maine. Investigation of these two outbreaks linked them to the consumption of frozen strawberries commercially prepared by the same processor. By genetic sequence analysis, the virus causing illness in 126 patients from Michigan and Maine was identical. Later investigation found virus of the same sequence in patients with hepatitis A in Arizona, Louisiana, and Wisconsin, all of whom had eaten strawberries supplied by the same food processor

(Hutin et al. 1999). In 2003, an outbreak of hepatitis A in Pennsylvania was linked to the consumption of green onions in a Mexican restaurant where they were served in salsa. As a result of this food-borne outbreak immune globulin was provided to approximately 9 000 persons. Traceback investigations showed that the green onions consumed in Pennsylvania came from one or more farms in Mexico. By genetic sequence analysis, this outbreak was linked to similar hepatitis A outbreaks in Tennessee, Georgia, and North Carolina that also were associated with eating green onions (CDC 2003c).

Hepatitis A virus outbreaks provide good examples of the ease with which a pathogen can be widely dispersed in the population due to current food processing and distribution systems (Tauxe 1997).

Nipah virus, which emerged in Malaysia in an intense pig farming area, and then spread with movement of infected animals to several other parts of Malaysia and even to Singapore, may have stemmed in part from certain newly-introduced farming practices. The disease caused severe respiratory distress and some encephalitis in the pigs, but when a large number of workers on the pig farms developed encephalitis, and more than 100 died, it was decided to slaughter more than a million pigs, and this stopped the disease spread to humans. Fortunately, as noted above, humans were a dead-end host for Nipah virus infection, and no secondary spread was noted in the human community. The virus was identified because of its close relationship to Hendra virus. Using antiserum against Hendra virus, cell cultures growing the Nipah virus fluoresced, and this soon led to complete characterization and sequencing of the Nipah virus (Chua et al. 2000).

LIVESTOCK DISEASES

We usually think of the importance of livestock diseases in terms of financial losses, because the capacity of the commercial livestock food and fiber industries of developed countries are such that surpluses are a greater problem than are shortages. However, in developing countries this is not the case: livestock diseases, especially new, emerging or re-emerging diseases, cause immediate human suffering by substantially compromising scarce human food resources, especially the supply of high-quality protein.

Epidemiological considerations

Perpetuation of a virus in nature depends on the maintenance of serial infections, i.e. a chain of transmission; the occurrence of disease is neither required nor necessarily advantageous. Although clinical cases may be somewhat more productive sources of virus than inapparent or mild infections, the latter are generally more numerous and do not restrict the movement of infectious individuals, and thus provide a major mechanism of viral dissemination and emergence.

Epidemics are classically divided according to their means of spread into two major categories, propagated and common source (Nathanson 1996).

PROPAGATED EPIDEMICS AND CRITICAL COMMUNITY SIZE

In propagated epidemics, spread from host to host continues to expand as long as each infection gives rise to more than one new infection. The rate of transmission depends on a number of variables, such as the density of the population, the proportion of the population that is susceptible, the degree and duration of contagiousness, and the frequency of contacts leading to transmission. The classic large epidemics of viral diseases have all been propagated epidemics.

In most instances, for viruses that produce acute self-limiting infections to survive, the susceptible host population must be both large and relatively dense. Such viruses may disappear from a population because they exhaust the supply of susceptible hosts as they acquire immunity to reinfection. Persistent viruses, on the other hand, may survive in very small populations, sometimes by spanning generations. Depending on the duration of immunity and the pattern of virus shedding, the critical community size varies considerably with different viruses.

MEASLES

Much was learned about the dynamics of the viral transmission chain by Panum, who studied the devastating measles epidemic of 1846 in the Faroe Islands; this was at a time when even the concept of a virus was unknown (Panum 1939). Nevertheless, Panum described the incubation period of measles and the lifelong immunity that follows infection. With an incubation period of about 12 days, maximum viral excretion for the next 6 days and solid immunity to reinfection, between 20 and 30 susceptibles would need to be infected in series to maintain measles transmission for a year. Since nothing like such precise one-to-one transmission occurs, many more than 30 susceptibles are needed to maintain endemicity. Analyses of the incidence of measles in different size communities have shown that a population of about half a million people is needed to ensure a large enough annual input of new susceptibles, provided by the annual birth cohort, to maintain measles indefinitely as an endemic disease. Because infection depends on close contact, the duration of epidemics of measles is correlated inversely with population density. If a population is dispersed over a large area, the rate of spread is reduced and the epidemic will last longer, so the number of susceptible persons needed to maintain endemicity is reduced. On the other hand, in such a situation, a break in the transmission cycle is much more likely. If a large proportion of the population is initially susceptible, the intensity of the epidemic builds up very quickly, often reaching almost 100 percent. Virgin-soil epidemics in isolated communities have had devastating consequences owing to lack of medical care and the disruption of work capacity. In large urban communities, before the era of vaccination, measles epidemics occurred every 2–3 years, each time exhausting available susceptibles; this epidemic cycle occurred on a continental scale. Before the introduction of vaccine, the cyclic occurrence of measles epidemics was influenced by several variables besides the build-up of susceptibles; these included the dynamics of reintroduction of the virus and seasonal influences.

COMMON SOURCE EPIDEMICS

Common source epidemics occur when a virus is disseminated from a single focus; they usually result from contamination of air, food, water, drugs, biomedical devices or the like. If a virus is introduced from a common source into a large population, disease can emerge on an epidemic scale. An excellent example is provided by the unwitting introduction of hepatitis B virus during immunization against yellow fever.

In the early stages of World War II, it was decided to immunize large numbers of American troops with 17D yellow fever vaccine. In order to stabilize the infectivity of the live attenuated 17D virus, protein was added to the final vaccine formulation. To prevent serum sickness, human serum was selected as the protein source. Almost 1 000 donors were used; unfortunately, at least one donor was a carrier of hepatitis B virus. Consequently, in the spring of 1942 over 400 000 troops received contaminated vaccine, causing about 20 000 cases of hepatitis (Sawyer et al. 1944). Although the onset of disease was spread over a considerable time, when plotted according to the interval from administration of the vaccine the timeline formed a classic log-normal curve, thereby providing statistical proof of the association of the epidemic with the administration of the vaccine. This epidemic clearly established hepatitis B as a distinct entity, separable from hepatitis A (e.g. different mean incubation periods: 3 months for hepatitis B, one month for hepatitis A).

THE ENVIRONMENT: ECOLOGICAL AND ZOONOTIC FACTORS FAVORING THE EMERGENCE OF VIRAL DISEASES

Ecological factors pertaining to unique environments and geographic isolation often underpin the emergence of new viruses and thereby new viral diseases. Such factors favor the adaptation of viruses to new econiches. When ecosystems are altered, viral infections of humans and animals follow. Population movements and the intrusion of humans and domestic animals into new arthropod habitats have resulted in many new emergent disease episodes. The classic example of this was the emergence of yellow fever when susceptible humans entered the Central American jungle to build the Panama Canal; there are many contemporary examples suggesting that similar events will continue to happen, in most cases in unanticipated circumstances. Deforestation has been the key to the exposure of farmers and domestic animals to new arthropods and the viruses they carry. The occurrence of Mayaro virus disease in Brazilian wood-cutters as they cleared the Amazonian forest in recent years is a case in point. Increased long-distance transportation facilitates the carriage of exotic arthropod vectors around the world. The carriage of the Asian mosquito, *Aedes albopictus*, a vector for dengue viruses and California encephalitis virus, into the USA in the water contained in imported used tyres, represents an unsolved problem of this kind. Increased long-distance transportation of livestock facilitates the carriage of viral agents and arthropods (especially ticks) around the world. The introduction of the tick-borne agent, African swine fever virus, from Africa into Portugal (1957), Spain (1960), and South America (1960s and 1970s) is thought to have occurred in this way; it is just a matter of time until this virus makes further international forays.

A recent dramatic example is provided by West Nile virus (WNV), a flavivirus which appeared for the first time in the Western hemisphere in 1999 (Briese et al. 1999; Lanciotti et al. 1999). Although originally isolated in Uganda in 1937, from where it spread to Egypt, Israel, India, and other parts of Africa, the virus caused occasional outbreaks of human disease in the 50 years following its discovery, but was not considered a serious public health problem. However in the mid-1990s, the virulence of WNV apparently changed (Hubalek and Halouzka 1999; Murgue et al. 2001a,b) and epidemics associated with severe neurological disease in humans and high mortality in birds began to occur in the Mediterranean basin and surrounding countries before WNV appeared in New York in 1999 (Ostlund et al. 2001). Following its isolation and characterization, the New York virus was found to be virtually identical in nucleotide sequence to an isolate of WNV made in Israel (Lanciotti et al. 1999). The mode by which the virus moved across the Atlantic ocean is unknown, but transport of an infected mosquito or bird in the hold of a jetliner are reasonable possibilities. An infected human or other mammal seems unlikely to have seeded the virus in the US, because the level of viremia would be rather low compared to that in a bird or carried in a mosquito. From its origin in New York, the virus has spread at an alarming rate throughout the continent, and reached California by August 2003, also spreading north into Canada and south into Mexico and the Caribbean. (Petersen et al. 2003). Many of the human cases have involved severe encephalomyelitis (Guarner et al. 2004a), but this represents the tip of the iceberg, and many asymptomatic infections also occur. Direct human-to-human transmission through blood has been documented with WNV; this is the first time that the US blood supply has had to be checked for a mosquito-borne virus (Armstrong et al. 2003; CDC 2003a).

Changing routes of long-distance bird migrations, brought about by new water impoundments, represent an important yet still untested additional risk of introduction of arboviruses into new areas. This may be a key to some of the movement of Japanese encephalitis virus into new areas of Asia. Ecological factors pertaining to environmental pollution and uncontrolled urbanization are contributing to many new, emergent disease episodes. Arthropod vectors breeding in accumulations of water (tin cans, old tyres, etc.) is a problem world-wide. Environmental chemical toxicants (herbicides, pesticides, residues) can also affect vector–virus relationships directly or indirectly. For example, mosquito resistance to all licensed insecticides in parts of California is a known direct effect of unsound mosquito abatement programmes, augmented indirectly by poorly regulated pesticide usage against crop pests. Ecological factors relating to water use (i.e. increasing irrigation and the expanding reuse of water) are becoming important factors in the emergence of viral diseases. The problem with primitive water and irrigation systems that are developed without attention to arthropod control is exemplified in the emergence of Japanese encephalitis in new areas of southeast Asia and the Indian subcontinent. Global warming, affecting sea level, estuarine wetlands, swamps, and human habitation patterns, may be affecting arthropod vector relationships throughout the tropics; however, data are scarce and too many programmes to study the effect of global warming have not included the participation of viral disease experts.

Dengue

Dengue is one of the most rapidly emerging diseases in the tropical parts of the world, millions of cases occurring each year. For example, Puerto Rico had five dengue epidemics in the first 75 years of the 20th century, but more recently has had epidemics nearly every year, at an estimated cost of over US$150 million. At the same time, a record number of cases have occurred elsewhere in the Americas; Brazil, Bolivia, Colombia, Paraguay, Ecuador, Venezuela, Nicaragua, Cuba, and Mexico have experienced major dengue epidemics. These epidemics have involved multiple virus types: all four dengue virus types are now circulating in the Caribbean region. These are the circumstances that lead to dengue hemorrhagic fever (dengue shock syndrome): the lethal end of the dengue disease spectrum. Dengue hemorrhagic fever first occurred in the Americas in 1981; since then, most countries have reported cases, and in 1998 more than a million cases of dengue/dengue hemorrhagic fever were reported to WHO. By the beginning of the 21st century it was estimated that, globally, between 50 million and 100 million cases of dengue fever and several hundred thousands of cases of dengue hemorrhagic fever occur each year, the latter accompanied by case fatality rates of 1–10 percent, depending on the country (Gubler 2002).

Why is dengue emerging, especially in the Americas? The answer is simple: urban mosquito habitats are expanding (the vector mosquito, *Aedes aegypti*, is extremely well adapted to human proximity), mosquito density is increasing, and mosquito control is failing. This is occurring not just in the least developed countries but also in many developed countries. Financial resources for public health are severely limited and, too often, mosquito control, which is very expensive, falls off the bottom of the priority list. Meanwhile, mosquito control is becoming more expensive as older, cheaper chemicals lose effectiveness or are banned as damaging to the environment. As mosquito control fails, dengue follows quickly.

Yellow fever

An even more frightening situation associated with failing mosquito control is that yellow fever virus, which is transmitted by the same mosquito vector as dengue, *Aedes aegypti*, might also re-emerge. Where dengue occurs, the conditions are also appropriate for yellow fever (initiated by importation via an infected person or an infected mosquito). It is one of the mysteries of tropical medicine that yellow fever has not occurred more often where vector density and a susceptible human population coexist (Monath 2001). However, since the 1980s there has been a resurgence of yellow fever both across Africa and in South America: this is a potential risk to the USA, since *Aedes aegypti* is present in urban areas in the South (Robertson et al. 1996).

In fact, no one knows where, when or even if yellow fever virus will re-emerge in the kinds of epidemics that were the scourge of tropical and subtropical cities of the western hemisphere and Africa throughout the seventeenth, eighteenth, and nineteenth centuries; however, because this virus is so dangerous, the possibility is constantly on the mind of national and international health officials.

Hantaviruses and hemorrhagic fever with renal syndrome

Hantaviruses provide an example of a virus species that no doubt has existed for a long time in the same habitats, but was only recognized relatively recently. The first well characterized hantavirus disease was Korean hemorrhagic fever, which emerged during the Korean war of 1950–52. Thousands of United Nations troops developed a mysterious disease marked by fever, headache, hemorrhage, and acute renal failure; the mortality rate was 5–10 percent. Despite much research, the agent of this disease remained unknown for 26 years; then, in

1976, a new virus, named Hantaan virus, was isolated in Korea from fieldmice. The discovery of this virus was, however, just 'the tip of an iceberg.' In subsequent years, related viruses have been found in many parts of the world in association with different rodents and as the cause of human diseases with more than 150 different local names (Schmaljohn and Hjelle 1997). It has been found in recent years that, from an ecological perspective, there are seven or eight different subgroups of viruses and three different transmission patterns: rural, urban, and laboratory acquired. From a clinical perspective, two disease patterns are described, one marked by severe disease (hemorrhagic fever with renal syndrome, with significant mortality) and the other by mild disease (febrile disease, without mortality). The rural, severe disease is widespread in the Far East (e.g. Korean hemorrhagic fever in Korea; 'epidemic hemorrhagic fever' in China, causing more than 100 000 cases per year). A similar rural, severe disease is emerging in the Balkans (mortality rate c. 20 percent).

Hantaviruses and acute respiratory distress syndrome

In May 1993, a new hantavirus disease was recognized in the southwestern region of the USA. The disease appeared as an acute respiratory distress syndrome. Clinical signs include fever, headache, and cough, followed by acute pulmonary congestion and edema leading to hypoxia, shock, and, in many cases, death. Within a short time, cases were found in 23 states and eventually throughout the USA. By July 2004, 366 cases of hantavirus pulmonary syndrome have been confirmed in the United States, with an overall case fatality rate of 38 per cent.

The causative virus was shown to be a previously unknown hantavirus (Nichol et al. 1993), now named Sin Nombre virus, that has a reservoir in the deer mouse (*Peromyscus maniculatus*). Horizontal transmission, via biting, is believed to be an important route of transmission between rodents. Human infection occurs following inhalation of virus particles from rodent urine, feces, and saliva, from contact of broken skin or mucous membranes with infectious virus, or by rodent bite. Viral RNA amplified from patients' specimens by PCR, when sequenced and compared to sequences obtained from specimens from different areas, indicates that several different variant viruses, all new and previously unknown, are active in different rodent species and subspecies in the USA, some causing human disease and others merely present in rodent populations without any human disease association. Hantavirus sequences have been used in expression systems to produce homologous antigens for further studies and diagnostic services. The same serological and molecular biological methods were applied to large numbers of rodents collected in the areas where patients lived; this proved that at least eight

species of rodents were involved, the primary reservoir host in the southwest being *Peromyscus maniculatus*, the deer mouse (c. 30 percent of this species were found to harbor the viruses in several areas of southwestern USA) (Morzunov et al. 1998). The viruses have very likely always been present in the large area of the western region of the USA inhabited by *Peromyscus* species; they were recognized in 1993 only because of the number and clustering of human cases, which in turn were probably caused by a great increase in rodent numbers consequent on an increase in piñon seeds and other rodent food. As a result of this kind of rapid field and laboratory investigation, the public is being advised about reducing the risk of infection, mostly by reducing rodent habitats and food supplies in and near homes and taking precautions when cleaning rodent-contaminated areas. Fortunately, human-to-human transmission has not been observed with hantaviruses in North America. Humans become infected by contact with or inhalation of rodent excreta, but are then dead-end hosts.

In 1996 it was recognized that hantaviruses are also present in rodent populations in South America, and here there has been some evidence for human-human transmission of Andes virus, which occurs mainly in Argentina and Chile (Wells et al. 1997). As in North America, there are both pathogenic and nonpathogenic hantaviruses in South America, and since the first report several hundred cases of human hantavirus pulmonary syndrome have been recorded. Fortunately, the rodents which transmit hantavirus pulmonary syndrome are confined to the S*igmodontinae*, a subfamily of the *Muridae*, members of which are only found in the Western hemisphere (Figure 70.3). The other murid subfamilies that transmit hantaviruses are the *Murinae*, (e.g. Hantaan virus, Dobrava-Belgrade virus, and Seoul virus) and the *Arvicolinae* (e.g. Puumala virus) both associated with hemorrhagic fever with renal syndrome in Europe and Asia. Interestingly, although several hantavirus species are associated with arvicoline rodent species in North America, none has been associated with human disease (Table 70.5).

Rabies

Rabies can serve as an example of ecological factors relating to the adaptation and emergence of viruses in new econiches. The most dramatic illustration of this in recent years has been the appearance of epidemic raccoon rabies in eastern USA. The epizootic has been traced to the importation of raccoons from Florida to West Virginia in 1977. This epidemic demonstrates dramatically how human disturbance of the environment, in this instance involving the transportation of wild animals, can lead to emergence of a disease in a previously unaffected area. A key to our understanding of this episode was the discovery that rabies virus is not one virus; rather, it is a set of

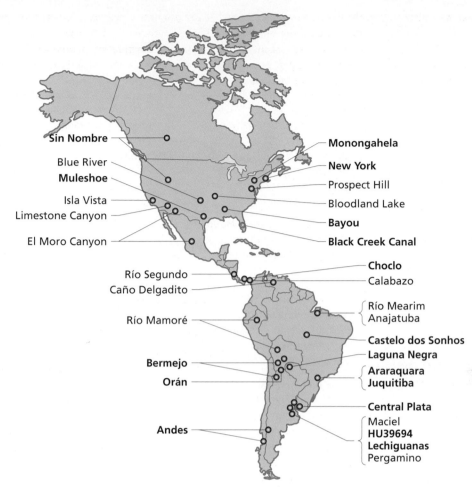

Figure 70.3 *Geographical distribution of New World hantaviruses recognized as of 2004. Viruses named in Roman face have not been associated with human disease – those named in bold face are known to cause hantavirus pulmonary syndrome. (Courtesy of James Mills, CDC).*

different genotypes, each transmitted within a separate reservoir host niche. In North America, there are about six terrestrial animal genotypes, one involving the skunk in the north-central states, one the skunk in the south-central states, one the Arctic fox and red fox in Alaska and Canada, one the grey fox in Arizona, one the coyote and feral dog in southern Texas and northern Mexico, and one the raccoon in eastern states. 'Raccoons-bite-raccoons-bite-raccoons' and after some time their virus becomes a distinct genotype, highly adapted to the host cycle and inefficient if introduced into another host cycle. When this discovery was made (first using monoclonal antibody panels and more recently partial viral genomic sequencing), many mysteries of rabies ecology were clarified.

THE PREVENTION AND CONTROL OF NEW, EMERGING, AND RE-EMERGING VIRAL DISEASES

Since 1991 we have witnessed the emergence or re-emergence of a large number of new human viruses (Figure 70.4). When a new virus disease is suspected, a complex continuum of prevention and control activities may be called into action, but, given financial and resource constraints, decisions must be made and priorities must be set. The full continuum comprises the following activities and resources, which may be divided into investigative and interventional phases.

The investigative phase

- The disease must be characterized (usually the work of clinicians and pathologists).
- There is nearly always need for epidemiological field investigation to assess the risk to the population (usually the work of medical epidemiologists).
- The agent must always be sought. When a new virus is suspected, it must be isolated, identified, characterized.
- There is usually need for diagnostics development, to provide and authenticate primary, reference, and confirmatory tests.
- An integrated research programme is usually needed (but not always implemented), covering sciences as diverse as molecular virology, pathogenesis, pathophysiology, immunology, ecology, epidemiology, sociology and behavior, vector biology, etc.

Table 70.5 *Recognized hantaviruses in the world, their hosts, the recognized geographic occurrence of the virus, and the diseases caused*

Virus	Host species (subspecies)[a]	Distribution of virus	Disease
Order *Rodentia*, Family *Muridae*, Subfamily *Murinae*			
Hantaan virus (HTNV)[b]	*Apodemus agrarius (mantchuricus)*	Eastern Russia, Northern Asia, Balkans	Severe HFRS
Seoul virus (SEOV)[b]	*Rattus norvegicus*	Nearly Worldwide	Mild/Moderate HFRS
Dobrava-Belgrade virus (DOBV)[b]	*Apodemus flavicollis*	Balkans	Severe HFRS
Thailand virus (THAIV)[b]	*Bandicota indica*	India	NR
Saarema virus (SAAV)[b]	*Apodemus agrarius (agrarius)*	Europe	Mild HFRS
Amur virus (AMRV)	*Apodemus peninsulae*	Far Eastern Russia	HFRS
Order *Rodentia*, Family *Muridae*, Subfamily *Arvicolinae*			
Puumala virus (PUUV)[b]	*Clethrionomys glareolus*	Europe, Scandinavia, Russia, Balkans	Mild HFRS
Prospect Hill virus (PHV)[b]	*Microtus pennsylvanicus*	North America	NR
Bloodland Lake virus (BLLV)	*Microtus ochrogaster*	North America	NR
Isla Vista virus (ISLAV)	*Microtus californicus*	North America	NR
Tula virus (TULV)	*Microtus arvalis/ M. rossiaemeridionalis*	Russia, Slovakia	NR
Khabarovsk virus (KBRV)	*Microtus fortis*	Eastern Russia	NR
Topografov virus (TOPV)	*Lemmus sibericus*	Siberia	NR
Order *Rodentia*, Family *Muridae*, Subfamily *Sigmontinae*			
Sin Nombre virus (SNV)[b]	*Peromyscus maniculatus*	North America	HPS
New York virus (NYV) [b]	*Peromyscus leucopus*	Eastern USA and Central USA	HPS
Black Creek Canal virus (BCCV)[b]	*Sigmodon hispidus*	Southeastern USA	HPS
Bayou virus (BAYV)[b]	*Oryzomys palustris*	Southeastern USA	HPS
Muleshoe virus (MULEV)	*Sigmodon hispidus (texianus)*	Southern USA	HPS
Monongahela virus (MONV)	*Peromyscus maniculatus (nubiterrae)*	Eastern USA and Canada	HPS
Limestone Canyon virus (LSCV)	*Peromyscus boylii*	Southwestern USA	NR
Blue River virus (BRV)	*Peromyscus leucopus*	Central USA	NR
El Moro Canyon virus (ELMCV)[b]	*Reithrodontomys megalotis*	Western USA and Mexico	NR
Río Segundo virus (RIOSV)	*Reithrodontomys mexicanus*	Costa Rica	NR
Caño Delgadito virus (CDGV)[b]	*Sigmodon alstoni*	Venezuela	NR
Juquitiba virus (JUQV)	Unknown	Southeastern Brazil	HPS
Araraquara virus (ARAV)	Unknown	Southeastern Brazil	HPS
Castelo dos Sonhos virus (CASV)	Unknown	Central Brazil	HPS
Anajatuba virus (AJV)	*Oligoryzomys fornesi*	Northern Brazil	NR
Río Mearim virus (RMV)	*Holochilus sciureus*	Northen Brazil	NR
Río Mamoré virus (RIOMV)	*Oligoryzomys microtus*	Bolivia, Peru	NR
Laguna Negra virus (LNV)[b]	*Calomys laucha*	Western Paraguay and Bolivia	HPS
Andes virus (ANDV)[b]	*Oligoryzomys longicaudatus*	Southern Argentina and Chile	HPS
Lechiguanas virus (LECV)[b]	*Oligoryzomys flavescens*	Central Argentina	HPS
Bermejo virus (BMJV)	*Oligoryzomys chacoensis*	Northwestern Argentina, Southern Bolivia	HPS
Orán virus (ORNV)	*Oligoryzomys longicaudatus*[c]	Northwestern Argentina, Southern Bolivia	HPS
Maciel virus (MACV)	*Bolomys obscurus*	Central Argentina	NR
Hu39694	Unknown	Central Argentina	HPS
Pergamino virus	*Akodon azarae*	Central Argentina	NR

(Continued over)

Table 70.5 *Recognized hantaviruses in the world, their hosts, the recognized geographic occurrence of the virus, and the diseases caused (Continued)*

Virus	Host species (subspecies)[a]	Distribution of virus	Disease
Choclo virus	*Oligoryzomys fulvescens (costaricensis)*	Southwestern Panama	HPS
Calabazo virus	*Zygodontomys brevicauda (cherriei)*	Southwestern Panama	NR
Maporal virus	*Oecomys bicolor*	Central Venezuela	NR
	Order *Insectivora*, Family *Soricidae*		
Thottapalayam[b]	*Suncus murinus*	India	NR

HFRS = hemorrhagic fever with renal syndrome; HPS = hantavirus pulmonary syndrome; NR = None Recognized.
a) Taxonomy follows Wilson and Reeder (1992).
b) Virus isolated in cell culture; others identified from genetic sequence.

The interventional phase

- There is always a need for comprehensive communications systems.
- There is often need for technology transfer (transfer of diagnostics technology to local agencies and transfer of information pertinent to vaccine and drug development to the commercial sector).
- There is usually need for training and clinical continuing education.
- Comprehensive public health systems may need to be adapted to the disease at hand. This may involve new public education programmes, new vital record and disease register systems, rapid case reporting, new surveillance systems, expanded laboratory diagnostics services, new staffing and staff support, new logistical systems (facilities, equipment, supplies, transport), and the like.
- There may be a need for new policy decisions, new risk management decisions. These may involve new legislation and regulations, new law enforcement action, and even new administrative and management systems.
- There may be need for new clinical medical systems (isolation of cases by quarantine, barrier nursing, physical biocontainment, and extra disinfection and sterilization). There may be need for new patient management systems and even need for improving the general health of the population at risk (better nutrition, housing, primary medical care).
- There may be need for specialist systems, such as vector control, reservoir host control, environmental control (water, animal, and arthropod habitats, etc.) and sanitary engineering (to provide safe food and water, sewage treatment, etc.).
- In the largest epidemics there are also global issues to be dealt with, such as control of international movement of people and animals, establishment of international disease control task forces, and the like. Finally, there is the global issue of adequate funding for such programmes.

All these activities must be integrated to construct a comprehensive view of the immediate problem at hand and strategy and programmes for its control. Today, this kind of integrated investigative, problem-solving activity is usually thought to be the sole responsibility of government agencies, but, in fact, many professionals from throughout the health sector have played central roles in recent episodes. As it turns out, assessing risk and guiding intervention involve quite diverse activities; for example, in some cases complex field studies of the incidence of infection in the general population or in a selected subpopulation are necessary to determine risk factors for infection, mode of transmission, targets for intervention, etc., whereas in other cases, studies of the pathogenetic mechanisms underpinning the clinical presentation in the individual patient might hold the key. Today, in nearly every instance, important clues lie in characterizing the molecular structure and replication strategy of the virus and the cellular pathobiology of the infection.

REFERENCES

Armstrong, W.S., Bashour, C.A., et al. 2003. A case of fatal West Nile virus meningoencephalitis associated with receipt of blood transfusions after open heart surgery. *Ann Thorac Surg*, **76**, 605–707.

Bern, C., Martines, J., et al. 1992. The magnitude of the global problem of diarrhoeal disease: a ten year update. *Bull WHO*, **70**, 705–14.

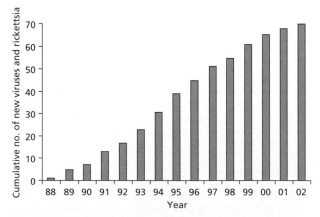

Figure 70.4 *Emergence of newly recognized viruses affecting humans over the period 1988–2002. Cumulative plot showing the annual increase in numbers of new viruses. (Courtesy of CDC)*

Briese, T., Jia, X.Y., et al. 1999. Identification of a Kunjin/West Nile-like flavivirus in brains of patients with New York encephalitis. *Lancet*, **354**, 1261–2.

CDC, 2003a. Detection of West Nile virus in blood donations – United States 2003. *MMWR*, **52**, 769.

CDC, 2003b. Update: multistate outbreak of monkeypox – Illinois, Indiana, Kansas, Missouri, Ohio, and Wisconsin, 2003. *MMWR*, **52**, 642.

CDC, 2003c. Hepatitis A outbreak associated with green onions at a restaurant - Monaca, Pennsylvania, 2003. *MMWR*, **52**, 1155–7.

Chan, S.-Y., Delius, H., et al. 1995. Analysis of genomic sequences of 95 papillomavirus types: uniting typing, phylogeny and taxonomy. *J Virol*, **69**, 3074–83.

Chang, Y., Cesarman, E., et al. 1994. Identification of herpes-like DNA sequences in AIDS-associated Kaposi's sarcoma. *Science*, **266**, 1865–9.

Choo, Q.L., Kuo, G., et al. 1989. Isolation of a cDNA clone derived from a blood-borne non-A, non-B viral hepatitis genome. *Science*, **244**, 359–62.

Chua, K.B., Bellini, W.J., et al. 2000. Nipah virus: a recently emergent deadly Paramyxovirus. *Science*, **288**, 1432–5.

Crowcroft, N.S. 2002. Management of Lassa fever in European countries. *Euro Surveill*, **7**, 50–2.

De Villiers, E.M., Fauquet, C., et al. 2004. Classification of papillomaviruses. *Virology*, **324**, 17–27.

Drosten, C., Guenther, S., et al. 2003. Identification of a novel coronavirus in patients with severe acute respiratory syndrome. *N Engl J Med*, **348**, 1967–76.

Fenner, F., Henderson, D.A., et al. 1988. *Smallpox and its eradication*. Geneva: World Health Organization.

Field, H., Young, P., et al. 2001. The natural history of Hendra and Nipah viruses. *Microbes Infect*, **3**, 307–14.

Gallimore, C.I., Appleton, H., et al. 1995. Detection and characterization of bisegmented double-stranded RNA viruses (picobirnaviruses) in human faecal specimens. *J Med Virol*, **45**, 135–40.

Gao, F., Yue, L., et al. 1992. Human infection by genetically diverse SIVsm-related HIV-2 in West Africa. *Nature (London)*, **358**, 495–9.

Gentsch, J.R., Das, B.K., et al. 1993. Similarity of the VP4 protein of human rotavirus strain 116E to that of the bovine B223 strain. *Virology*, **194**, 424–30.

Gould, A.R. 1996. Comparison of the deduced matrix and fusion protein sequences of equine morbillivirus with cognate genes of the *Paramyxoviridae*. *Virus Res*, **43**, 17–31.

Grohmann, G.S., Glass, R.I., et al. 1993. Enteric viruses and diarrhea in HIV-infected patients. *N Engl J Med*, **329**, 14–20.

Guan, Y., Zheng, B.J., et al. 2003. Isolation and characterization of viruses related to the SARS coronavirus from animals in southern China. *Science*, **302**, 276–8.

Guarner, J., Shieh, W.J., et al. 2004a. Clinicopathological study and laboratory diagnosis of 23 cases with West Nile virus encephalomyelitis. *Hum Pathol*, **35**, 983–90.

Guarner, J., Johnson, B.J., et al. 2004b. Monkeypox transmission and pathogenesis in prairie dogs. *Emerg Inf Dis*, **10**, 426–31.

Gubler, D.J. 2002. Epidemic dengue/dengue hemorrhagic fever as a public health, social and economic problem in the 21st century. *Trends Microbiol*, **10**, 100–3.

Hahn, B.H., Shaw, G.M., et al. 2000. AIDS as a zoonosis: scientific and public health implications. *Science*, **287**, 607–14.

Hahn, C.S., Lustig, S., et al. 1988. Western equine encephalitis virus is a recombinant virus. *Proc Natl Acad Sci USA*, **85**, 5997–6001.

Henderson, D.A. 1999. The looming threat of bioterrorism. *Science*, **283**, 1279–82.

Hino, S. 2002. TTV, a new human virus with single stranded circular DNA genome. *Rev Med Virol*, **12**, 151–8.

Holmes, G.P., McCormick, J.B., et al. 1990. Lassa fever in the United States. Investigation of a case and new guidelines for management. *N Engl J Med*, **323**, 1120–3.

Hsu, V.P., Hossain, J., et al. 2004. Reemergence of Nipah virus in two outbreaks in Bangladesh. *Emerg Inf Dis*, **10**, 2082–7.

Hubalek, Z. and Halouzka, J. 1999. West Nile Fever – a reemerging mosquito-borne viral disease in Europe. *Emerg Inf Dis*, **5**, 643–50.

Hutin, Y.J., Pool, V., et al. 1999. A multistate, foodborne outbreak of hepatitis A. *N Engl J Med*, **340**, 644–5.

Iturriza-Gómara, M., Isherwood, B., et al. 2001. Reassortment *in vivo*: driving force for diversity of human rotavirus strains isolated in the United Kingdom between 1995 and 1999. *J Virol*, **75**, 3696–705.

Iturriza-Gomara, M., Cubitt, D., et al. 2002. Characterization of rotavirus G9 strains isolated in the UK between 1995 and 1998. *J Med Virol*, **61**, 510–17.

Javier, R.T., Sedarati, F. and Stevens, J. 1986. Two avirulent herpes simplex viruses generate lethal recombinants in vivo. *Science*, **234**, 746–8.

Kawaoka, Y., Krauss, S. and Webster, R.G. 1989. Avian-to-human transmission of the PB1 gene of influenza A virus in the 1957 and 1968 pandemics. *J Virol*, **63**, 4603–8.

Ksiazek, T.G., Erdman, D., et al. 2003. A novel coronavirus associated with severe acute respiratory syndrome. *New Engl J Med*, **348**, 1947–58.

Lanciotti, R.S., Roehrig, J.T., et al. 1999. Origin of the West Nile virus responsible for an outbreak of encephalitis in the northeastern United States. *Science*, **286**, 2333–7.

Li, K.S., Guan, Y., et al. 2004. Genesis of a highly pathogenic and potentially pandemic H5N1 influenza virus in eastern Asia. *Nature*, **430**, 209–13.

Liu, H.M., Zheng, D.P., et al. 2003. Serial recombination during circulation of type 1 wild-vaccine recombinant polioviruses in China. *J Virol*, **77**, 10994–1005.

Khabbaz, R.F., Heneine, W., et al. 1994. Brief report: infection of a laboratory worker with simian immunodeficiency virus. *N Engl J Med*, **330**, 172–7.

Khan, A.S., Spiropoulou, C.F., et al. 1995. Fatal illness associated with a new hantavirus in Louisiana. *J Med Virol*, **46**, 281–6.

Korber, B., Muldoon, M., et al. 2000. Timing the ancestor of the HIV-1 pandemic strains. *Science*, **288**, 1789–96.

Lemey, P., Pybus, O.G., et al. 2003. Tracing the origin and history of the HIV-2 epidemic. *Proc Nat Acad Sci*, **100**, 6588–92.

Linnen, J., Wages, J., et al. 1996. Molecular cloning and disease association of hepatitis G virus: a transfusion transmissible agent. *Science*, **271**, 505–8.

Maggi, F., Marchi, S., et al. 2003. Relationship of TT virus and *Helicobacter pylori* infections in gastric tissues of patients with gastritis. *J Med Virol*, **71**, 160–5.

Mahy, B.W.J. 2000. The global threat of emerging infectious diseases. In: Andrew, P.W., Oyston, P., et al. (eds), *Fighting infection in the 21st century*. Oxford: Blackwell Science, 1–16.

Mahy, B.W.J. 2003. An overview on the use of a viral pathogen as a bioterrorist agent: why smallpox? *Antiviral Res*, **57**, 1–5.

Mahy, B.W.J. and Brown, C.C. 2000. Emerging zoonoses: crossing the species barrier. *Rev Sci Tech Off Int Epiz*, **19**, 33–40.

Marra, M.A., Jones, S.J., et al. 2003. The genome sequence of the SARS-associated coronavirus. *Science*, **300**, 1399–404.

Matsuura, Y. and Miyamura, T. 1993. The molecular biology of hepatitis C virus. *Semin Virol*, **4**, 297–304.

Mims, C.A. 1991. The origin of major human infections and the crucial role of person-to-person spread. *Epidemiol Infect*, **106**, 423–33.

Monath, T.P. 2001. Yellow fever: an update. *Lancet Inf Dis*, **1**, 11–20.

Morzunov, S.P., Rowe, J.E., et al. 1998. Genetic analysis of the diversity and origin of hantaviruses in *Peromyscus leucopus* mice in North America. *J Virol*, **72**, 57–64.

Muerhoff, A.S., Leary, T.P., et al. 1995. Genomic organization of GB viruses A and B: two new members of the flaviviruses associated with GB agent hepatitis. *J Virol*, **69**, 5621–30.

Murgue, B., Murri, S., et al. 2001a. West Nile outbreak in horses in southern France; the return after 35 years. *Emerg Inf Dis*, **7**, 692–6.

Murgue, B., Murri, S., et al. 2001b. West Nile in the Mediterranean basin: 1950–2000. *Ann NY Acad Sci*, **951**, 117–26.

Murphy, F.A. and Nathanson, N. 1994. The emergence of new viral diseases: an overview. *Semin Virol*, **5**, 87–102.

Murphy, F.A., Fauquet, C.M., et al. 1995. *Virus taxonomy, Sixth Report of the International Committee on Taxonomy of Viruses*. New York: Springer-Verlag.

Murray, K., Selleck, P., et al. 1995. A morbillivirus that caused fatal disease in horses and humans. *Science*, **268**, 94–7.

Mushahwar, I.K. 2000. Recently discovered blood-borne viruses: are they hepatitis viruses or merely endosymbionts? *J Med Virol*, **62**, 399–404.

Mushahwar, I.K., Erker, J.C., et al. 1999. Molecular and biophysical characterization of TT virus: evidence for a new virus infecting humans. *Proc Nat Acad Sci*, **96**, 1177–82.

Myers, G., MacInnes, K. and Korber, B. 1992. The emergence of simian/human immunodeficiency viruses. *AIDS Res Hum Retroviruses*, **8**, 373–86.

Nathanson, N. 1996. Epidemiology. In: Fields, B.N. and Knipe, D. (eds), *Fields' virology*, 3rd edn. New York: Raven Press, 251–71.

Nathanson, N. and Martin, J.R. 1979. The epidemiology of poliomyelitis: enigmas surrounding its appearance, epidemicity, and disappearance. *Am J Epidemiol*, **110**, 672–92.

Nathanson, N., McGann, K.A., et al. 1993. The evolution of viral diseases: their emergence, epidemicity, and control. *Virus Res*, **29**, 3–20.

Nichol, S.T., Spiropolou, C.F., et al. 1993. Genetic identification of a hantavirus associated with an outbreak of acute respiratory illness. *Science*, **262**, 914–17.

Nishizawa, T., Okamoto, H., et al. 1997. A novel DNA virus (TTV) associated with elevated transaminase levels in posttransfusion hepatitis of unknown etiology. *Biochem Biophys Res Comms*, **241**, 92–7.

Ostlund, E.N., Crom, D.D., et al. 2001. Equine West Nile encephalitis, United States. *Emerg Inf Dis*, **7**, 665–9.

O'Sullivan, J.D., Allworth, A.M., et al. 1997. Fatal encephalitis due to novel paramyxovirus transmitted from horses. *Lancet*, **349**, 93–5.

Panum, P.L. 1939. Observations made during the epidemic of measles in the Faroe Islands in the year 1846. *Med Classics*, **3**, 839–86.

Parrish, C.R. 1990. Emergence, natural history and variation of canine, mink and feline parvoviruses. *Adv Virus Res*, **38**, 403–50.

Parrish, C.R. 1994. The emergence and evolution of canine parvovirus – an example of recent host range mutation. *Semin Virol*, **5**, 121–32.

Pereira, H.G., Flewett, T.H., et al. 1988. A virus with bisegmented double-stranded RNA genome in rat (*Oryzomys nigripes*) intestines. *J Gen Virol*, **69**, 2749–54.

Petersen, L.R., Marfin, A.A. and Gubler, D.J. 2003. West Nile virus. *JAMA*, **290**, 524–8.

Ramachandran, M., Gentsch, J.R., et al. 1998. Detection and characterization of novel rotavirus strains in the United States. *J Clin Microbiol*, **36**, 3223–9.

Robertson, B.H. 2001. Viral hepatitis and primates: historical and molecular analysis of human and nonhuman primate hepatitis A, B and the GB-related viruses. *J Viral Hepatitis*, **8**, 233–42.

Robertson, S.E., Hull, B.P., et al. 1996. Yellow fever: a decade of reemergence. *J Am Med Assoc*, **276**, 1157–62.

Rota, P.A., Oberste, S., et al. 2003. Characterization of a novel coronavirus associated with severe acute respiratory syndrome. *Science*, **300**, 1394–9.

Ruan, Y., Wel, C.L., et al. 2003. Comparative full-length genome sequence analysis of 14 SARS coronavirus isolates and common mutations associated with putative origins of infection. *Lancet*, **361**, 1779–85.

Sabin, A.E. 1981. Paralytic poliomyelitis: old dogma and new perspectives. *Rev Infect Dis*, **3**, 543–64.

Sawyer, W.A., Meyer, K.F., et al. 1944. Jaundice in army personnel in the western region of the United States and its relation to vaccination against yellow fever. *Am J Hyg*, **39**, 337–87.

Schmaljohn, C. and Hjelle, B. 1997. Hantaviruses: a global disease problem. *Emerg Inf Dis*, **3**, 95–104.

Smallman-Raynor, M. and Cliff, A. 1991. The spread of human immunodeficiency virus type 2 into Europe: a geographic analysis. *Int J Epidemiol*, **20**, 480–9.

Smolinski, M.S., Hamburg, M.A. and Lederberg, J. (eds) 2003. *Microbial threats to health: emergence, detection, and response*. Washington: The National Academies Press, 367 pp.

Stephenson, I., Nicholson, K., et al. 2004. Confronting the avian influenza threat: vaccine development for a potential pandemic. *Lancet Inf Dis*, **4**, 499–509.

Strauss, J.H. and Strauss, E.G. 1994. The alphaviruses: gene expression, replication and evolution. *Microbiol Rev*, **58**, 491–562.

Tauxe, R.V. 1997. Emerging foodborne diseases: an evolving public health challenge. *Emerg Infect Dis*, **3**, 425–34.

Thiel, V., Ivanov, K.A., et al. 2003. Mechanisms and enzymes involved in SARS coronavirus genome expression. *J Gen Virol*, **84**, 2305–15.

Wang, L.F., Yu, M., et al. 2000. The exceptionally large genome of Hendra virus: support for creation of a new genus within the family *Paramyxoviridae*. *J Virol*, **74**, 9972–9.

Webster, R.G. and Kawaoka, Y. 1994. Influenza – an emerging and re-emerging disease. *Semin Virol*, **5**, 103–11.

Wells, R.M., Estani, S.S., et al. 1997. An unusual hantavirus outbreak in Southern Argentina: person-to-person transmission? *Emerg Inf Dis*, **3**, 171–4.

Wilson, D.E. and Reeder, D.M. (eds) 1992. *Mammal species of the world: A taxonomic and geographic reference*, 2nd edn. Washington: Smithsonian Institution Press.

Xu, X., Subbarao, K., et al. 1999. Genetic characterization of the pathogenic influenza A Goose/Guangdong/1/96 (H5N1) virus: similarity of its hemagglutinin gene to those of H5N1 viruses from the 1997 outbreaks in Hong Kong. *Virology*, **261**, 15–19.

Young, P.L., Halpin, K., et al. 1996. Serologic evidence for the presence in *Pteropus* bats of a paramyxovirus related to equine morbillivirus. *Emerg Inf Dis*, **2**, 239–40.

zur Hausen, H. 2002. Papillomaviruses and cancer: from basic studies to clinical application. *Nat Rev Cancer*, **2**, 342–50.

Index

Notes

(Fig.) and (Tab.) refer to figures and tables respectively. *vs.* indicates a comparison or differential diagnosis.

To save space in the index, the following abbreviations have been used:

EBV - Epstein–Barr virus
HCMV - Human cytomegalovirus
HHV - human herpesvirus
HIV - human immunodeficiency virus
HPV - human papillomavirus
HSV - herpes simplex virus
HTLV - Human T-cell leukemia (lymphotrophic) virus
IL- interleukin
LCMV - Lymphocytic choriomeningitis virus
MHC - major histocompatibility complex
SV40 - Simian virus 40
VZV - varicella-zoster virus

Complete table of contents for *Topley & Wilson's Microbiology and Microbial Infections*

VIROLOGY, VOLUMES 1 AND 2

BACTERIOLOGY, VOLUMES 1 AND 2

MEDICAL MYCOLOGY

PARASITOLOGY

IMMUNOLOGY